North American Nursing Diagnosis Association (NANDA) Accepted Nursing Diagnoses

- Activity Intolerance
- Activity Intolerance, Risk for
- Adaptive Capacity: Intracranial, Decreased
- Adjustment, Impaired
- Airway Clearance, Ineffective
- Anxiety
- Aspiration, Risk for
- Body Image Disturbance
- Body Temperature, Risk for Altered
- Breastfeeding, Effective
- Breastfeeding, Ineffective
- Breastfeeding, Interrupted
- Breathing Pattern, Ineffective
- Caregiver Role Strain
- Caregiver Role Strain, Risk for
- Communication, Impaired Verbal
- Community Coping, Ineffective
- Community Coping, Potential for Enhanced
- Confusion, Acute
- Confusion, Chronic
- Constipation
- Constipation, Colonic
- Constipation, Perceived
- Decisional Conflict (Specify)
- Decreased Cardiac Output
- Defensive Coping
- Denial, Ineffective
- Diarrhea
- Disorganized Infant Behavior
- Disorganized Infant Behavior, Risk for
- Disuse Syndrome, Risk for
- Diversional Activity Deficit
- Dysfunctional Grieving
- Dysfunctional Ventilatory Weaning Response
- Dysreflexia
- Energy Field Disturbance
- Environmental Interpretation Syndrome, Impaired
- Family Coping: Compromised, Ineffective
- Family Coping: Disabling, Ineffective
- Family Coping: Potential for Growth
- Family Process: Alcoholism, Altered
- Family Processes, Altered
- Fatigue
- Fear
- Fluid Volume Deficit
- Fluid Volume Deficit, Risk for
- Fluid Volume Excess
- Functional Incontinence
- Gas Exchange, Impaired
- Grieving, Anticipatory
- Grieving, Dysfunctional
- Growth and Development, Altered
- Health Maintenance, Altered
- Health Seeking Behaviors (Specify)
- Home Maintenance Management, Impaired
- Hopelessness
- Hyperthermia
- Hypothermia
- Incontinence, Bowel
- Incontinence, Functional
- Incontinence, Reflex
- Incontinence, Stress
- Incontinence, Total
- Incontinence, Urge
- Individual Coping, Ineffective
- Infant Feeding Pattern, Ineffective
- Infection, Risk for
- Injury, Risk for
- Knowledge Deficit (Specify)
- Loneliness, Risk for
- Management of Therapeutic Regimen: Community, Ineffective
- Management of Therapeutic Regimen: Families; Ineffective
- Management of Therapeutic Regimen: Individual, Effective
- Management of Therapeutic Regimen: (Individuals), Ineffective
- Memory, Impaired
- Noncompliance (Specify)
- Nutrition: Less than Body Requirements, Altered
- Nutrition: More than Body Requirements, Altered
- Nutrition: Potential for more than Body Requirements, Altered
- Oral Mucous Membrane, Altered
- Organized Infant Behavior, Potential for Enhanced
- Pain
- Pain, Chronic
- Parent/Infant/Child Attachment, Risk for Altered
- Parental Role Conflict
- Parenting, Altered
- Parenting, Risk for Altered
- Perceived Constipation
- Perioperative Positioning Injury, Risk for
- Peripheral Neurovascular Dysfunction, Risk for
- Personal Identity Disturbance
- Physical Mobility, Impaired
- Poisoning, Risk for
- Post-Trauma Response
- Powerlessness
- Protection, Altered
- Rape-Trauma Syndrome
- Rape-Trauma Syndrome: Compound Reaction
- Rape-Trauma Syndrome: Silent Reaction
- Reflex Incontinence
- Relocation Stress Syndrome
- Role Performance, Altered
- Self Care Deficit
  - Bathing/Hygiene
  - Feeding
  - Dressing/Grooming
  - Toileting
- Self Esteem, Chronic Low
- Self Esteem, Situational Low
- Self Esteem Disturbance
- Self-Mutilation, Risk for
- Sensory/Perceptual Alterations (Specify) (visual, auditory, kinesthetic, gustatory, tactile, olfactory)
- Sexual Dysfunction
- Sexuality Patterns, Altered
- Skin Integrity, Impaired
- Skin Integrity, Risk for Impaired
- Sleep Pattern Disturbance
- Social Interaction, Impaired
- Social Isolation
- Spiritual Distress
- Spiritual Well-Being, Potential for Enhanced
- Suffocation, Risk for
- Sustain Spontaneous Ventilation, Inability to
- Swallowing, Impaired
- Thermoregulation, Ineffective
- Thought Processes, Altered
- Tissue Integrity, Impaired
- Tissue Perfusion, Altered (Specify Type) (Renal, cerebral, cardiopulmonary, gastrointestinal, peripheral)
- Trauma, Risk for
- Unilateral Neglect
- Urinary Elimination, Altered
- Urinary Retention
- Violence, Risk for: Self-directed or directed at others

NANDA Nursing Diagnoses: Definitions & Classification 1995–1996. North American Nursing Diagnosis Association. Philadelphia, 1994

Ruth F. Craven, EdD, RN

Associate Professor
Department of Biobehavioral Nursing and Health Systems

Assistant Dean
Continuing Nursing Education
University of Washington School of Nursing
Seattle WA

Constance J. Hirnle, MN, RN

Assistant Professor
Seattle University School of Nursing
Seattle WA

Lippincott
Philadelphia • New York

Fundamental

Fundamentals of Nursing

HUMAN HEALTH AND FUNCTION

Second Edition

To Bob, Scott, John, and Sarah Hirnle
Bill, Brent, Judy, and Kyle Craven

for their love, support, sacrifice, and encouragement that allowed us to make this book a reality.

Sponsoring Editors: Donna L. Hilton, BSN, RN and Mary Gyetvan, MSN, RN
Developmental Editor: Eleanor Faven
Project Editor: Susan Deitch
Production Manager: Helen Ewan
Production Coordinator: Nannette Winski
Senior Design Coordinator: Kathy Kelley-Luedtke

Second Edition

Printed in the United States of America. For information write Lippincott-Raven Publishers, 227 East Washington Square, Philadelphia, PA 19106.

Library of Congress Cataloging in Publications Data

Craven, Ruth F.
Fundamentals of nursing : human health and function / Ruth F. Craven, Constance J. Hirnle. — 2nd ed.
p. cm.
Includes bibliographical references and index.
ISBN 0-397-55169-X
1. Nursing I. Hirnle, Constance J. II. Title
[DNLM: 1. Nursing. 2. Nursing Process. 3. Nursing Diagnosis.
WY 100 C898f 1996]
RT41. C86 1996
610.73—dc20
DNLM/DLC
for Library of Congress 95-32206
CIP

9 8 7 6 5 4 3 2 1

Contributors

Catherine Broom, ARNP, CS
Psychosocial Clinical Nurse Specialist/
Psychiatric Nurse Practitioner
University of Washington Medical Center
Seattle, WA

*3: Ethical and Legal Concerns**

Margaret Bruya, DNSc, RN, CS
Professor
Intercollegiate Center for Nursing Education
Spokane, WA

5: Nursing Research

Dona Marie Carpenter, EdD, RN, CS
Associate Professor of Nursing
Department of Nursing
University of Scranton
Scranton, PA

1: The Profession of Nursing
2: Conceptual Frameworks and Nursing Theories

B. Jane Cornman, PhD, RN
Assistant Professor
School of Nursing
University of Southern Maine
Portland, ME

15: Health and Wellness

Susanna Cunningham, PhD, RN, FAAN
Associate Professor
Department of Biobehavioral Nursing and Health Systems
University of Washington
Seattle, WA

36: Fluid, Electrolyte, and Acid-Base Balance

Alice S. Demi, DNS, FAAN
Professor
Georgia State University
Atlanta, GA

50: Loss and Grieving

Laina M. Gerace, PhD, RN
Associate Professor
University of Illinois at Chicago-
Rockford Regional Program
Rockford, IL

20: Communication: The Nurse-Client Relationship

Kathryn Van Dyke Hayes, PhD, RN, C
Division of Nursing
Holy Family College
Philadelphia, PA

*9: Nursing Process: Foundation for Practice**
*10: Nursing Assessment**
*11: Nursing Diagnosis**
*12: Outcome Identification and Planning**
*13: Implementation and Evaluation**

Robert W. Hirnle, MS, RRT
Program Director, Respiratory Care
Highline Community College
Des Moines, WA

34: Oxygenation: Respiratory Function

Emily Wurster Hitchens, EdD, RN
Professor and Associate Dean
Seattle Pacific University
Seattle, WA

19: Values
53: Spiritual Health

Sharon Jensen, MN, RN
Lecturer
Seattle University
Seattle, WA

21: Health Assessment of Human Function

Ann E. Kelly, MSN, RN, CS
Clinical Nurse Specialist
San Diego Veterans Affairs Medical Center
San Diego, CA

47: Self-Concept

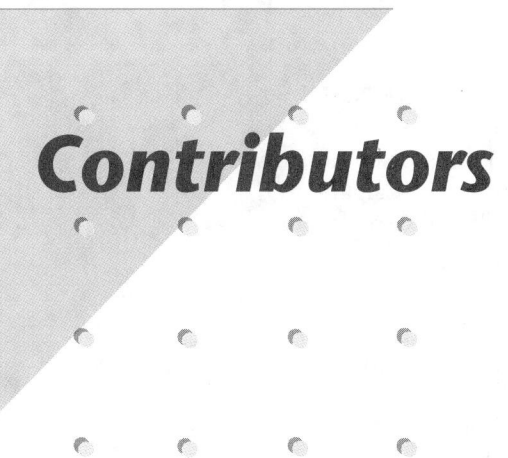

Barbara S. Levine, PhD, ARNP, CS
Assistant Professor
Department of Biobehavioral Nursing and Health Systems
University of Washington
Seattle, WA
46: Cognitive Processes

Katherine E. Matas, PhD, RN
Assistant Professor
College of Nursing
Arizona State University
Tempe, AZ
*7: Community-Based Nursing and Continuity of Care**

Donna Moniz, MN, RN, JD
Attorney
Seattle, WA
*3: Ethical and Legal Concerns**

Marjorie A. Muecke, PhD, RN, FAAN
Program Officer, Reproductive Health
The Ford Foundation
New York, NY
18: Culture and Ethnicity

Connie Nakao, PhD, RN
Associate Professor
School of Nursing
Seattle University
Seattle, WA
16: Lifespan Development

Georgia L. Roberts Narsavage, PhD, RN
Associate Professor of Nursing
Department of Nursing
University of Scranton
Scranton, PA
49: Families and Their Relationships

Ellen F. Olshansky, DNSc, RNC
Associate Professor
Coordinator, Women's Primary Care Nurse Practitioner Program
Department of Family and Child Nursing
University of Washington
Seattle, WA
52: Human Sexuality

Jane W. Peterson, PhD, RN
Professor
School of Nursing
Seattle University
Seattle, WA
17: Individual, Family, and Community

Marlene Reimer, MN, RN
PhD Candidate
Associate Professor of Nursing
The University of Calgary
Calgary, Alberta, Canada
43: Sleep and Rest

Bonnie Reinert, PhD, RN
Senior Research Fellow
School of Nursing
University of Washington
Seattle, WA
6: The Healthcare Delivery System

Gaie Rubenfeld, MS, RN
Assistant Professor, Nursing
Eastern Michigan University
Ypsilanti, MI
*8: Critical Thinking**

Jill Salisbury, MSN, RN, CS
Clinical Director, Eating Disorders Program
Swedish Medical Center/Ballard
Seattle, WA
37: Nutrition

Ginger Salvadalena, MN, RN, CS, CETN
Surgical Clinical Nurse Specialist
Enterostomal Therapy Nurse
Northwest Hospital
Seattle, WA
38: Skin Integrity and Wound Healing

Jennifer M. Schaller-Ayers, PhD, RN, C
Assistant Professor and Director of
Community Health Nursing Family Nurse
Practitioner Programs
University of Texas
El Paso, TX
30: Health Maintenance

Anita Shoup, MN, RN
Clinical Nurse Specialist, Regent Hospital Products, Ltd.
Clinical Faculty, School of Nursing
University of Washington
Seattle, WA
28: Perioperative Nursing

Barbara Scheffer, MS, RN
Assistant Professor, Nursing
Eastern Michigan University
Ypsilanti, MI
*8: Critical Thinking**

Sheila M. Sparks, DNSc, RN, CS
Assistant Professor
Georgetown University
School of Nursing
Washington, DC
*9: Nursing Process: Foundation for Practice**
*10: Nursing Assessment**
*11: Nursing Diagnosis**
*12: Outcome Identification and Planning**
*13: Implementation and Evaluation**

Marchelle Thobaben, MS, PHN, RN, FNP
Professor
Humboldt State University
Arcata, CA
*7: Community-Based Nursing and Continuity of Care**

Sharon Weinstein, MS, RN, CRNI
Director, Office of International Affairs
Premier Hospitals Alliance, Inc.
Westchester, IL
26: Intravenous Therapy

Diana Wilkie, PhD, RN, FAAN
Associate Professor and
American Cancer Society Professor of Oncology Nursing
Department of Biobehavioral Nursing and Health Systems
University of Washington
Seattle, WA
44: Pain Perception and Comfort

Karen S. Wulff, MN, EdD, RN
Assistant Administrator, Patient Care Services
Fred Hutchinson Cancer Research Center
Seattle, WA
4: Nursing Leadership and Management

Terry Cicero, MN, RN, CCRN
Lecturer
School of Nursing
Seattle University
Seattle, WA
Procedures

Elaine A. Furst, MA, RN
Lecturer
School of Nursing
Seattle University
Seattle, WA
Therapeutic Dialogues

*Chapter cowritten with another contributor

Mary Kay Flynn, MA, RN, CCRN
Associate Professor
Grand Canyon University
Phoenix, AZ
Collaborative Care Plan: Critical Pathway

Contributors to First Edition

Joan M. Baker, MS, RN, CS
Sensory Perception

Debra A. Beauchaine, MN, RN
Urinary Elimination*
Bowel Elimination

Diane Britt, MN, RN
Cognitive Processes

Karen K. Carlson, MN, RN, CCRN
Vital Sign Assessment*

Ann Tyler Chadwick, MN, RN, CRRN
Safety

Teresa A. Delarose, EdD, RN, CNOR
Perioperative Nursing
Nutrition

Mary P. Farley, MN, RN, CCRN
Asepsis
The Body's Defenses Against Infection

Polly E. Gardner, MN, RN
Medication Administration

Mikell Goe, MN, RN, CCRN
Diagnostic Tests and Procedures*
Oxygenation: Cardiac Function and Perfusion

Joanne Woodhull Goepfert, MN, PHC, RN
Self-Care and Hygiene

Mary Sue Gorski, MN, RNC
Communication of the Nursing Process: Recording and Reporting

Celia L. Hartley, MN, RN
The Health-Care Delivery System

Judy A. Hartmann, MSN, RN
Communication: Social Interaction

L. Michele Issel, PhD, RN
Home Maintenance Management

Don Johnson, PhD, RN
Fluid, Electrolyte, and Acid-Base Balance

Joan M. Jenks, MSN, RN
Consultant

Joy Miller Knopp, MN, RN, OCN
Pain Perception and Comfort*

Kathleen Kovarik, MN, RN
Skin Integrity and Wound Healing*

Claudia Kroll, MSEd, MSN, ARNP
Skin Integrity and Wound Healing*

Valerie G. Larson, MN, ARNP, CS
Diagnostic Tests and Procedures

Alice Lind, BSN, RN
Ethical and Legal Concerns

Mary McGregor, MN, RN, CDE
Medication Administration*

Beverly S. McKenna, MN, RN
Pain Perception and Comfort*

Kristine Iwersen Moore, MN, RN, CDE
Patient Teaching

Cheryl M. Prandoni, MSN, RNC
Human Needs

Barbara J. Ruff, MN, RN
Stress, Coping, and Adaptation

Margaret L. Snyder, MN, RN, CCRN
Vital Sign Assessment*

Karen A. Thomas, PhD, RN
Lifespan Development

Wendy L. Walker, MN, RN
Urinary Elimination*

Lorraine A. Watson, PhD, RN
Thermoregulation

Reviewers

Judy Davy, FNP, MHS, RN
Professor of Nursing
Homboldt State University
Arcata, CA

Kathy Dougherty, MS, MSN, RN
Assistant Professor and Program Coordinator
University of Texas at Brownsville
Brownsville, TX

Susan Dudek, BS, RD
Consultant Dietician
Bertrand Chaffee Hospital
Jennie B. Richmond Nursing Home
Springville, NY

Janet R. Ericksen, MA, RN
Senior Instructor
University of British Columbia, School of Nursing
Vancouver, BC

Jayne KauzLoric, MN, RN
Seattle—King County Department of Public Health
Seattle, WA

Mary DeMarino Lavin, MS, RN
Lecturer
University of Rhode Island, College of Nursing
Kingston, RI

Margaret M. Lockwood, BSN, MSN, EdD, RNC
Assistant Professor
University of Cincinatti, College of Nursing and Health
Cincinatti, OH

Anita Mobrak, BSN, MSN, RN
Curriculum Chair
Baptist Memorial Hospital School of Nursing
Memphis, TN

Joan C. Murphy, MS, NP, RN
Associate Professor of Nursing
Utica College of Syracuse University
Utica, NY

Dicey Ann O'Malley, BSW, MSN, EdD, RN
Chairperson, Nursing Department
Hudson Valley Community College
Troy, NY

Barbara Rideout, MSN, CETN, RN
Assistant Professor of Nursing
Temple University
Philadelphia, PA

Rosalie Stevenson, MSN, RN
Coordinator for Associate Nursing Program
Piedmont Technical College
Greenwood, SC

Toni Vezeau, PhD, RN
Assistant Professor of Nursing
Seattle University
Seattle, WA

Janet Weber, EdD, RN
Department of Nursing
Southeast Missouri State University
Cape Girardeau, MO

Stephanie Yewcic, MSN, RN
Course Coordinator for Basic Concepts
Conemaugh School of Nursing
Johnstown, PA

Reviewers for First Edition

Donna Adams, DNSc, RN

Janet S. Anderson, MSN, RN

Mary Ann Anglim, ME, BSN, RN

Shirley Bell, EdD, MSN, BSN, RN

Barbara Boland, MSN, RN

Penny S. Brooke, JD, MSN, RN

Bonita M. Cavanaugh, PhD, RN

Mary F. Crowley, MSN, BA, RN

Marjorie L. Garrity, MS, RN

Judith A. Halstead, RNC, MSN

Phyllis G. Hummel, MSN, RN

Mary Sue Jack, PhD, RN

Judy Johnson, PhD, MSN, RN

Margaret Ann Kerr, MSN, BS, RN, ANP

Mary L. Killeen, PhD, RN

Kathryn Lackey, MSN, BSN, RN

Peggy Tracy Leapley, PhD, RN

Ruth Lindquist, PhD, RN

Judith Maroni, DNSc, RN, CS

Edwina A. McConnell, PhD, RN

Faye Medley, MSN, RN

Sandra Millon-Underwood, PhD, RN

Suzanne M. Philip, MA, BEd, BScNEd, RN

Mildred M. Russin, MSN, RN

Mariah Snyder, PhD, RN, FAAN

Barbara Thomas, EdD, RN

Darla Ura, MN, RN

Judith A. Vessey, PhD, RN, C

Nancy Wells, DNSc, RN

Ann Windsor, DNS, RN

Preface

As nursing approaches the turn of the century, its focus has not changed. Promotion and maintenance of individual, family, and community health function; management of a healthy environment; and care of the ill are at the center of nursing. Two basic premises of *Fundamentals of Nursing: Human Health and Function* relate to these foci.

The first premise is that the art and science of professional nursing practice focus on the health, function, and wellness of the person, with the goals of maintaining, supporting, and restoring health and function in a variety of contemporary settings. Achieving these goals requires that the nurse promptly identify potential altered function and recognize manifestations of altered function and their impact on the clients' activities of daily living.

The second premise is that contemporary nursing practice is based on the appropriate selection and use of nursing interventions. In nursing practice, these activities involve the "diagnosis and treatment of human responses to potential or actual health problems" (ANA. (1980). *Nursing: A Social Policy Statement.* Kansas City, MO, ANA).

Through the incorporation of both of these premises, we have attempted to create an innovative text that helps nursing faculty prepare beginning students for the challenging and dynamic nursing practice of the twenty-first century. The intent is to provide the student with the knowledge base to assess a client's ability to function independently, evaluate the client's ability to cope with altered function, help the client identify realistic outcomes and intervene to maximize function. These nursing responsibilities are critical as healthcare delivery moves away from the hospital-based setting to care in a variety of community settings and focuses on promoting the client's self-responsibility. Both nurses and clients find themselves in a rapidly changing healthcare environment with evolving healthcare delivery patterns.

Organization of the Text

The text is organized in two main sections: **Section I, Conceptual Foundations of Nursing,** and **Section II, Human Function and Clinical Nursing Therapeutics.**

Section I presents the professional and clinical concepts essential to nursing today. This section contains six units.

Unit I, Concepts Essential for Professional Nursing, introduces the student to the profession of nursing. *Chapter 1, The Profession of Nursing,* provides the foundation. Frameworks and theories basic to nursing are summarized in Chapter 2. The remaining chapters discuss topics that underscore nursing's vital role: ethical and legal concerns, leadership and management, and nursing research.

Unit II, The Delivery of Nursing Care, is a new unit and discusses the current healthcare delivery system and its future in Chapter 6. Chapter 7 develops the subject further as it shows how healthcare and nursing are moving out into the community. Continuity of care, important in seeing that the client doesn't get lost in the system, is included in Chapter 7.

Unit III, The Nursing Process: Framework for Clinical Nursing Therapeutics, explains the nursing process to the beginning student and explores each component in detail. The student is introduced first to critical thinking and its importance to nursing. Following an overview of nursing process, the unit continues as it discusses the skills and activities needed to assess a client's health status, analyze and cluster data to formulate a nursing diagnosis, identify realistic outcomes, formulate a plan of care, select nursing interventions, and evaluate the effectiveness of those interventions using outcome criteria. The final chapter discusses forms of recording and reporting, the communication aspect of the nursing process. This unit provides the framework for the application of the nursing process throughout the text.

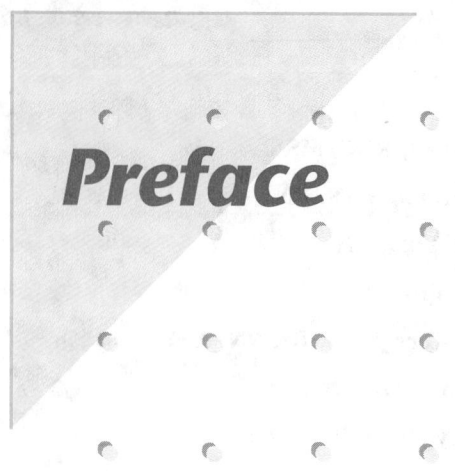

Unit IV, Concepts Essential for Human Function and Nursing Management, provides foundational concepts and knowledge about clients essential for providing safe, effective nursing care. This unit begins with a discussion of the concepts of health, wellness, and illness. *Chapter 16, Lifespan Development,* presents the concepts of human growth and development. The information in this chapter sets the stage for the "Lifespan Considerations" section in each nursing care chapter in Section II. Other chapters explore the individual as part of a family and a community; culture and ethnicity; and values. *Chapter 20, Communication: The Nurse–Client Relationship,* focuses on the skills needed to establish a therapeutic nurse–client relationship. This chapter has been coordinated with *Chapter 48, Communication: Social Interaction,* to focus strongly on communication and its importance in all human relationships.

Unit V, Essential Assessment Components, explores the fundamental skills in each component of health assessment. *Chapter 21, Health Assessment of Human Function,* details an overall health assessment. Additional chapters provide information on vital signs and laboratory and diagnostic tests.

Unit VI, Selected Clinical Nursing Therapeutics, focuses on nursing responsibilities associated with common clinical situations that provide the basis for many aspects of nursing care, including client teaching, asepsis, intravenous therapy, medication administration, and caring for the client before and after surgery.

Section II, Human Function and Clinical Nursing Therapeutics, is organized by areas of human function and uses a consistent nursing process format to present the concepts and nursing responsibilities for helping clients with healthcare needs in each area of function. Each clinical nursing care chapter in the 11 units in this section focuses on assessment and diagnosis of altered function and human responses, identification of outcome criteria, followed by implementation of appropriate nursing care strategies and evaluation of those interventions.

Normal function is discussed first in each chapter, to allow the student to fully understand normal or expected function before proceeding to altered function. Both normal and altered function set the framework for assessment of subjective and objective data and for the nursing interventions. Each chapter in this section emphasizes North American Nursing Diagnosis Association (NANDA) nursing diagnoses, outcome identification, and possible outcome criteria. Additionally, each clinical chapter in Section II includes step-by-step, illustrated procedures that cover purpose, assessment, equipment, and procedure steps with rationale. "Lifespan Considerations" and "Home Care Modifications" assist the student in modifying a procedure or making adjustments while caring for all types of clients regardless of the environment in which they live.

Special chapters in Section II focus on timely nursing care topics. These chapters provide the student with an expanded knowledge base and give a contemporary focus to information presented in traditional fundamentals texts. *Chapter 30, Health Maintenance,* discusses how people perceive their own health, what they do to improve or maintain it, and how a nurse can assist in this endeavor. *Chapter 31, Home Management,* explores how clients can maintain their own environment and types of support needed to manage altered health in the home setting. Essential information for appropriate discharge planning is provided.

In *Chapter 35,* the clinical topic of *Oxygenation: Cardiac Function and Tissue Perfusion* explores the essential role of circulation in fulfilling the body's need for oxygenation, which are particularly relevant topics as cardiovascular disease continues to be the leading cause of death in the United States. *Chapter 40, Thermoregulation,* and *Chapter 46, Cognitive Processes,* focus on two areas of particular concern in the elderly population. Finally, *Chapter 48, Communication: Social Interaction,* and *Chapter 49, Families and Their Relationships,* emphasize the impact these areas of psychosocial function have on human health and wellness.

Chapters New to This Edition

New chapters help the student keep pace with scientific changes and the ever-evolving profession of nursing. The following chapters are new to the second edition:

2, Conceptual Frameworks and Nursing Theories. This new chapter with some new information expanded from the first edition helps the student understand how a variety of theorists look at nursing and nursing care.

7, Community-Based Nursing and Continuity of Care. This completely new chapter defines and describes community-based care and discusses the relationship of consumerism, continuity of care, and discharge planning.

8, Critical Thinking. This chapter explores the importance of critical thinking specific to nursing. The student is led through various strategies and characteristics, a sample model, and development of critical thinking skills.

12, Outcome Identification and Planning. This text is the first to separately discuss the 1991 addition to ANA *Standards of Clinical Nursing Process:* outcome identification. Planning is included in this chapter because of its close relationship to outcome identification.

26, Intravenous Therapy. The importance and common use of IV therapy prompted the addition of a separate chapter on the subject.

Learning About Nursing Process

Fundamentals of Nursing: Human Health and Function provides students with a solid grounding in the nursing process and nursing diagnosis. Each clinical nursing care chapter in Section II employs a nursing process format in which each component is examined in relation to an area of human function. The assessment portion of each chapter presents both subjective and objective data collection. Each chapter then explores the definition, defining characteristics, and related factors of appropriate nursing diagnoses as defined by NANDA. This provides the beginning student with a firm foundation in the knowledge and application of nursing diagnoses. A section on related diagnoses demonstrates the interrelationship among diagnoses in the spectrum of human responses.

Outcome identification, with possible outcome goals, is presented consistently throughout the clinical chapters to help the student understand the relationship between outcome identification and planning of care.

Each chapter presents implementation in three categories to illustrate the scope of nursing care for client needs in each area of function. The first category, "Nursing Interventions to Promote Health and Function," focuses on nursing activities that promote wellness, maximize client strengths, and maintain health and function. "Nursing Interventions for Altered Function," the second section, covers those basic nursing interventions that address the nursing care needs for common problems associated with dysfunction. The last category, "Community-Based Nursing," emphasizes those nursing activities that promote continuity of care and help the client move from one level of care to another within the various settings in the community.

The final section, "Evaluation," uses the Client Goals identified in the "Outcome Identification" section and adds "Possible Outcome Criteria," thus showing the relationship between outcome identification and planning and evaluation of care. Finally, Nursing Plans of Care in each chapter teach students how to use nursing diagnoses and provide examples of appropriate nursing interventions along with scientific rationale.

Key Features

Fundamentals of Nursing: Human Health and Function presents the essential concepts, processes, and skills that help students build a solid foundation for professional nursing practice. To achieve this goal, the text includes key features from the first edition and incorporates new features.

- **Emphasizes human health, function, and wellness.** Building on the foundational sciences helps students fully understand normal function, which provides a solid foundation for understanding the scientific rationale for basic nursing care.
- **Emphasizes how normal function and dysfunction vary throughout the life cycle.** This emphasis encourages students to view people and their differing needs within the context of their developmental stage.
- **Discusses the impact of dysfunction on activities of daily living.** Understanding how a person's daily life is affected by dysfunction enables students to better assist clients to maintain optimal function.
- **Reinforces nursing responsibility for promoting optimal function in wellness and illness.** This thread runs throughout the text and helps students to understand the impact of health and illness on human response and to implement nursing care strategies for people throughout the health–illness continuum.
- **Emphasizes holistic care across the life cycle.** This emphasis helps students to see people as having equally important physiologic, psychosocial, and spiritual needs.
- **Provides a strong nursing process and nursing diagnosis framework.** The nursing process is fundamental to nursing care. This organizing structure creates a strong theoretical underpinning and assists student understanding of how to use nursing process and nursing diagnosis in clinical practice.
- **Emphasizes client goals and outcome criteria.** Nursing interventions relate to outcome, and measurable client behaviors help students evaluate the effectiveness of the interventions carried out.
- **Explores community-based nursing.** Discharge planning and home care were a key feature of the first edition. This feature has been expanded in this edition to meet the changing environments for care in the healthcare system and to help the student understand the importance of continuity of care.
- **Emphasizes collaborative care.** An integral part of community-based care is collaboration among a variety of healthcare professionals. The nurse is part of this team and, in fact, often manages the care. To help the student understand collaborative care, several displays called "Collaborative Care Plan: Critical Pathways" appear in the text.
- **Features a family focus.** This perspective encourages students to view clients in light of their family relationships and roles and to view families as critical members of the team that helps the client meet his or her needs.
- **Emphasizes communication.** Communication is an essential component of all human relationships. This text helps students become effective listeners and reliable communicators in the healthcare team. New to this edition are boxed displays called "Therapeutic Dialogues" that compare effective and less effective means of com-

munication between the nurse and colleagues or clients. These dialogues provide an excellent learning tool.

- **Emphasizes nursing research.** By introducing research early, beginning students learn to be discriminating consumers of nursing research, understand its relevance to clinical practice, and value the importance of research in the advancement of professional nursing.
- **Introduces critical thinking.** The student learns to apply critical thinking to a growing knowledge base of nursing care. Each chapter begins with a vignette to enhance thinking in relation to the chapter subject. At the end of the chapter, the student is challenged to apply critical thinking to the clinical situation at the beginning of the chapter.
- **Considers the client as an individual.** The student learns that at the center of all the applied knowledge and care is an individual with human needs. The text avoids gender bias and emphasizes ethnic and cultural needs without stereotyping individuals.

Features for Student Learning

To reinforce and enhance learning and involve the student in the learning process, numerous features summarize or highlight text information.

- **Learning Objectives, Key Terms, and Chapter Outlines** alert students as to what to expect in the chapter, provide important terms, and help them focus on the flow of chapter content.
- **Critical Thinking** clinical vignettes at the beginning of each chapter show and emphasize the real-world of nursing practice. Critical Thinking Challenges at the end of each chapter that relate to these vignettes prepare the student for developing critical thinking and decision-making skills.
- **References and Bibliographies** provide students with classic references, current nursing research, and a broad base of authoritative resources.
- **Boxed displays and tables** throughout the text emphasize essential material. Recurring displays include "Therapeutic Dialogue," "Nursing Research," "Safety Alert," "Client Teaching," "Planning: Examples of Nursing Interventions," "Nursing Assessment," "Nursing Care Guidelines," and "Nursing Plan of Care."
- **Abundant color photos and art** clarify the text, illustrate procedures, and enhance understanding.

Summary of New Features

All of the following elements to guide student learning are new to this edition:

- Five new chapters
- "Therapeutic Dialogue" displays
- Clinical vignettes and Critical Thinking Challenges
- "Collaborative Care Plans: Critical Pathways"
- Many new full-color photos and art
- Vivid four-color design
- Latest NANDA Nursing Diagnoses
- Latest CDC information on isolation and precautions
- New procedures

Teaching–Learning Package

Fundamentals of Nursing: Human Health and Function has an extensive ancillary package, designed with both the student and instructor in mind. A student *Study Guide* augments the text and provides a means of student self-evaluation. An *Interactive Self-Study Computer Disk* in the back of the book is new to this edition. It has multiple choice NCLEX-style questions, with feedback to enhance the student's learning.

Procedure Checklists provide guidelines for student practice and evaluation tools for faculty. The *Instructor's Manual* includes teaching–learning plans. Four-color transparency acetates allow the instructor to visually augment teaching. A printed and computerized testing program, ParTEST, facilitates instructor-designed queries and examinations. For the first time, *Lippincott's Clinical Skills Series* ($18\frac{1}{2}''$ VHS video cassettes) and *Lippincott's Clinical Interactive Skills Series* (laser discs) are available.

Ruth F. Craven, EdD, RN
Constance J. Hirnle, MN, RN

Acknowledgments

Sincere appreciation and warmest thanks are extended to the many people who contributed to the production of this book

- The contributors, who worked diligently to provide content in their areas of expertise and were patient with revision.
- Our students, for their contributions and opinions regarding organization and level of content and their ideas regarding what would facilitate learning.
- Donna Hilton, Vice President and Publisher, Eleanor Faven, Senior Developmental Editor, and Mary Gyetvan, Editor, for encouragement, patience, competence, and faith that "it would work!"
- Susan Deitch, Project Editor, for her patience, reliability, and good-natured support while completing the book.
- Kathy Kelley-Luedtke, Senior Design Coordinator, and Nannette Winski, Production Coordinator, for seeing the production process through with patience and professionalism.
- Barbara Sullivan, RN, MN, Director of Learning Resource Center at Seattle University, Debbie McDaniel, BSN, RN, Bessie Burton Sullivan Skilled Nursing Residence, Terry Cicero, MN, CCRN, Lecturer, Seattle University, and Daniel Hallett, photographer, Swedish Hospital Medical Center for their assistance with photographs used in this text.
- Seattle University, Bessie Burton Sullivan Skilled Nursing Residence, University of Washington School of Nursing, University of Washington Medical Center, Seattle Pacific University, Overlake Hospital Medical Center, friends, colleagues, and all others who contributed photos for use in this text.

Finally, but most importantly, we acknowledge with love and gratitude the constant support and encouragement of family, friends, and colleagues throughout this revision.

Contents

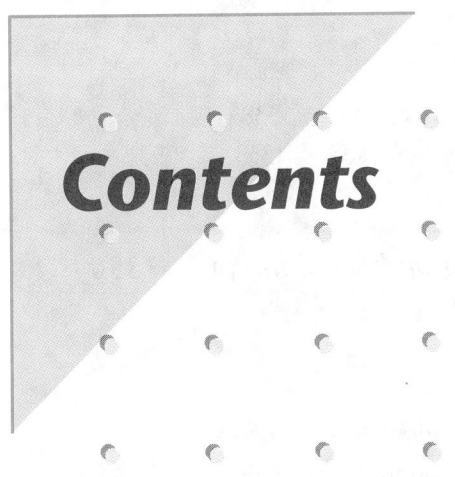

Expanded Contents

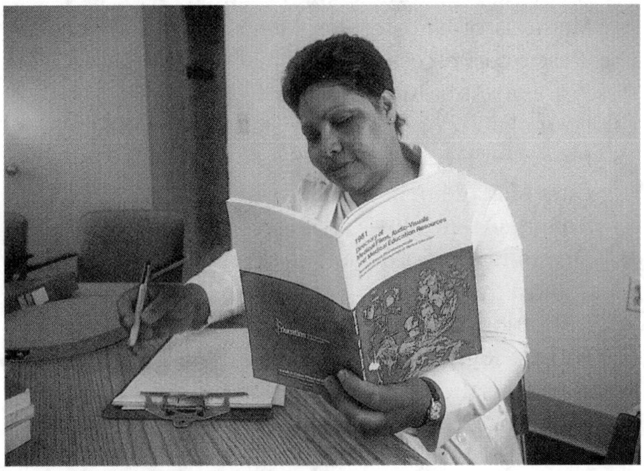

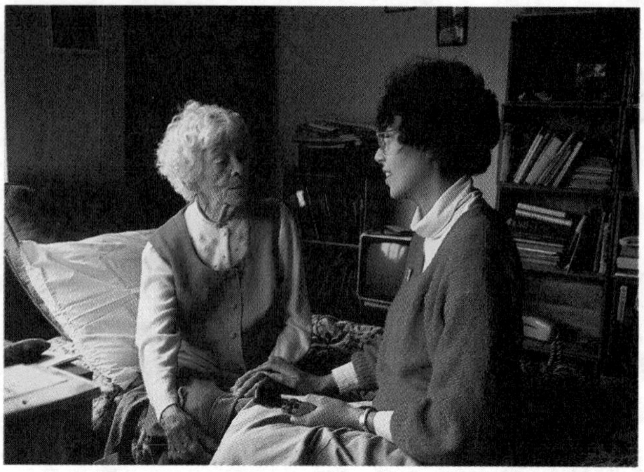

Chapter 18
Culture and Ethnicity 302

Chapter 19
Values 320

Chapter 20
Communication: The Nurse–Client Relationship 340

Unit V
Essential Assessment Components 362

Chapter 21
Health Assessment of Human Function 364

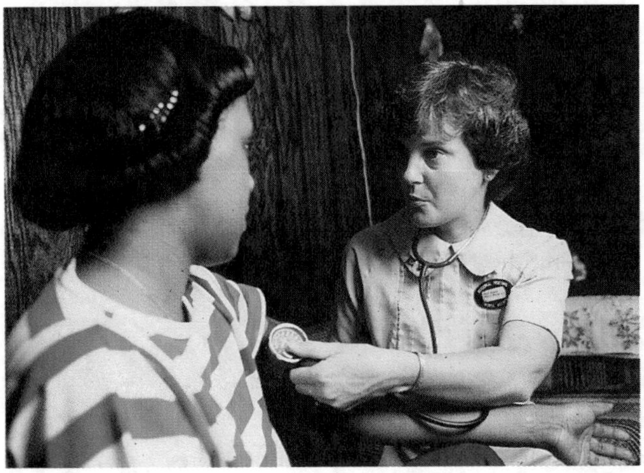

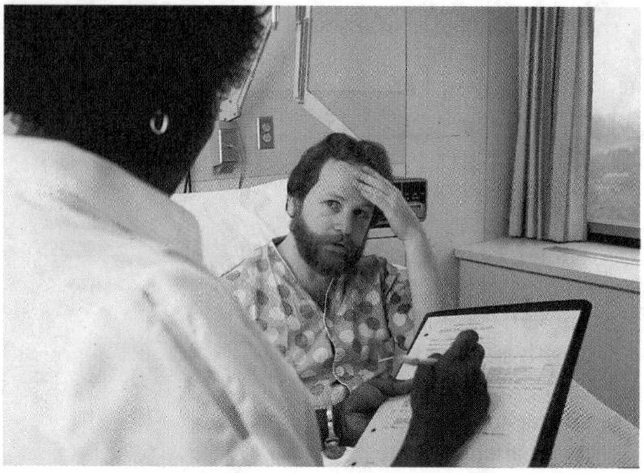

Unit VI
Selected Clinical Nursing Therapeutics 486

Chapter 24
Client Teaching 488

Chapter 25
Asepsis 510

Chapter 26
Intravenous Therapy 546

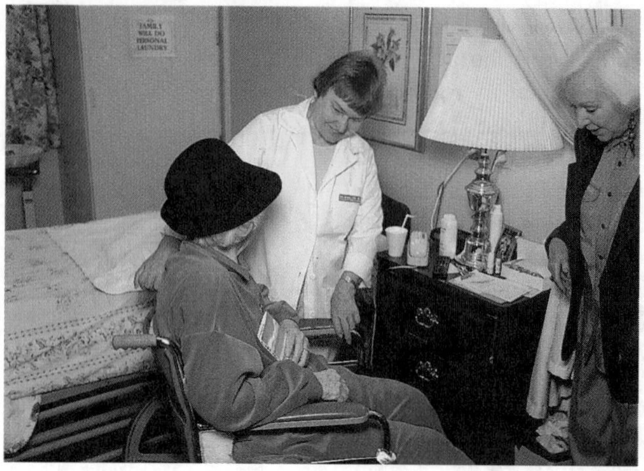

Unit VIII
Activity and Exercise 768

Chapter 32
Self-Care and Hygiene 770

Chapter 33
Body Mechanics and Mobility 822

Chapter 34
Oxygenation: Respiratory Function 882

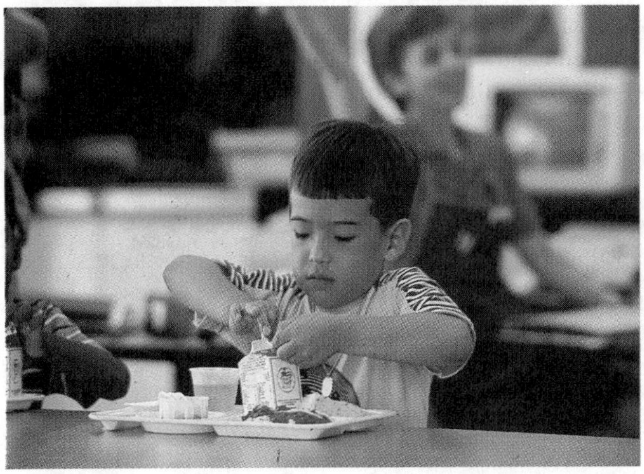

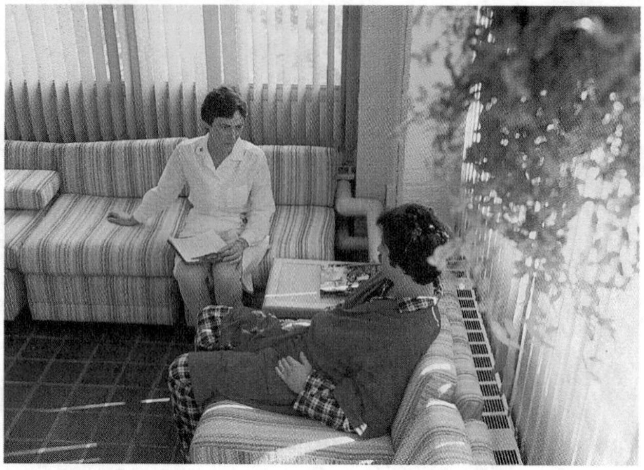

Chapter 37
Nutrition 1018

Chapter 38
Skin Integrity and Wound Healing 1062

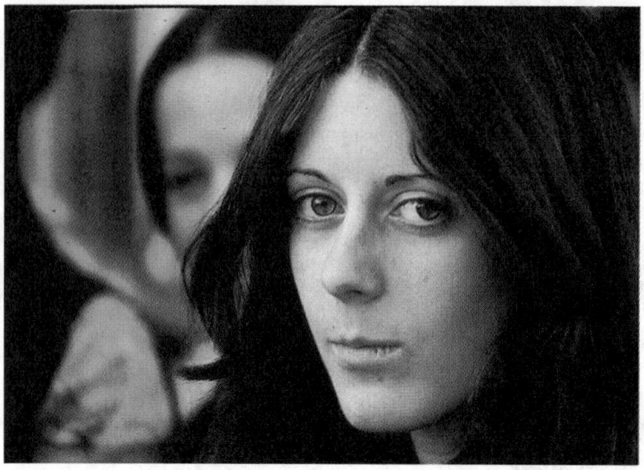

Unit XIII
Self-Perception and Self-Concept 1390

Chapter 47
Self-Concept 1392

Unit XIV
Roles and Relationships 1416

Chapter 48
Communication: Social Interaction 1418

Chapter 49
Families and Their Relationships 1440

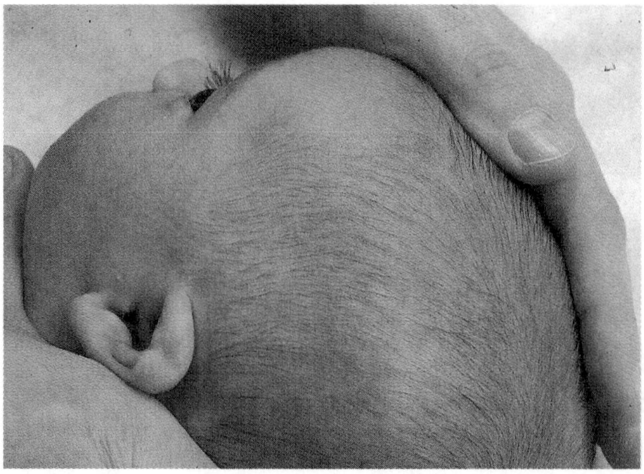

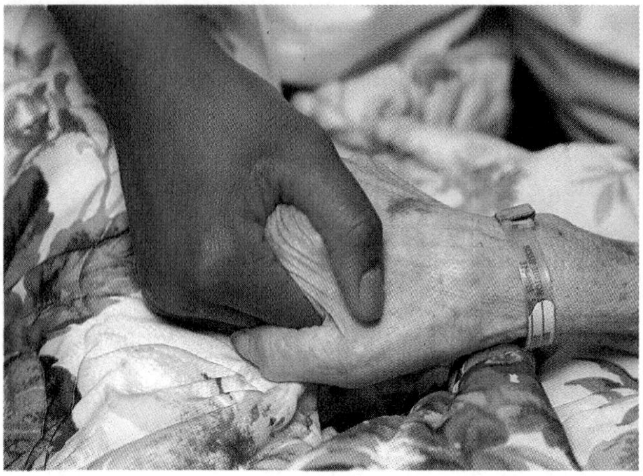

Nursing Procedures and Skills

Nursing Diagnoses Used in This Textbook

Nursing Plans of Care

Summary of Recurring Displays

SECTION I

Conceptual Foundations of Nursing

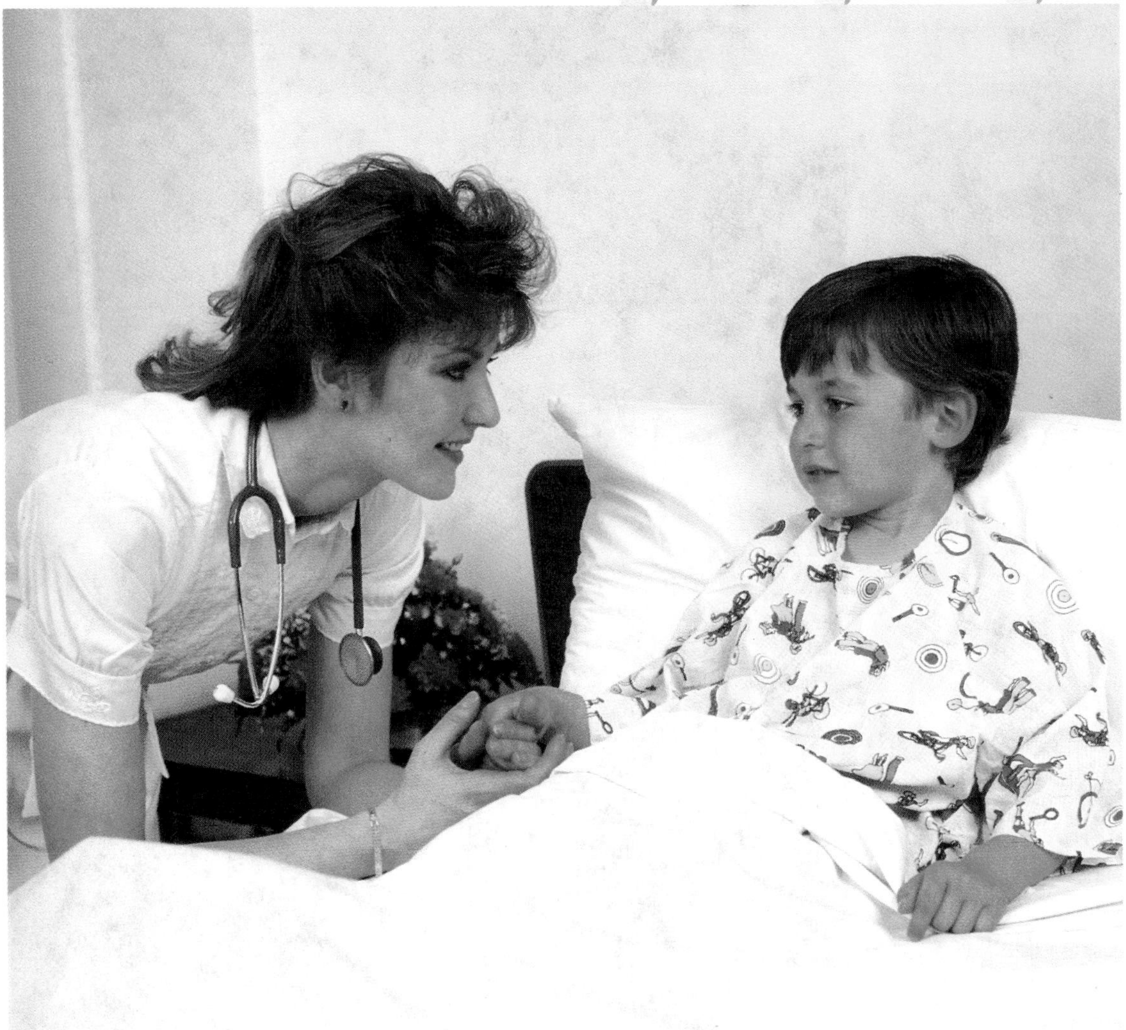

Concepts Essential for Professional Nursing

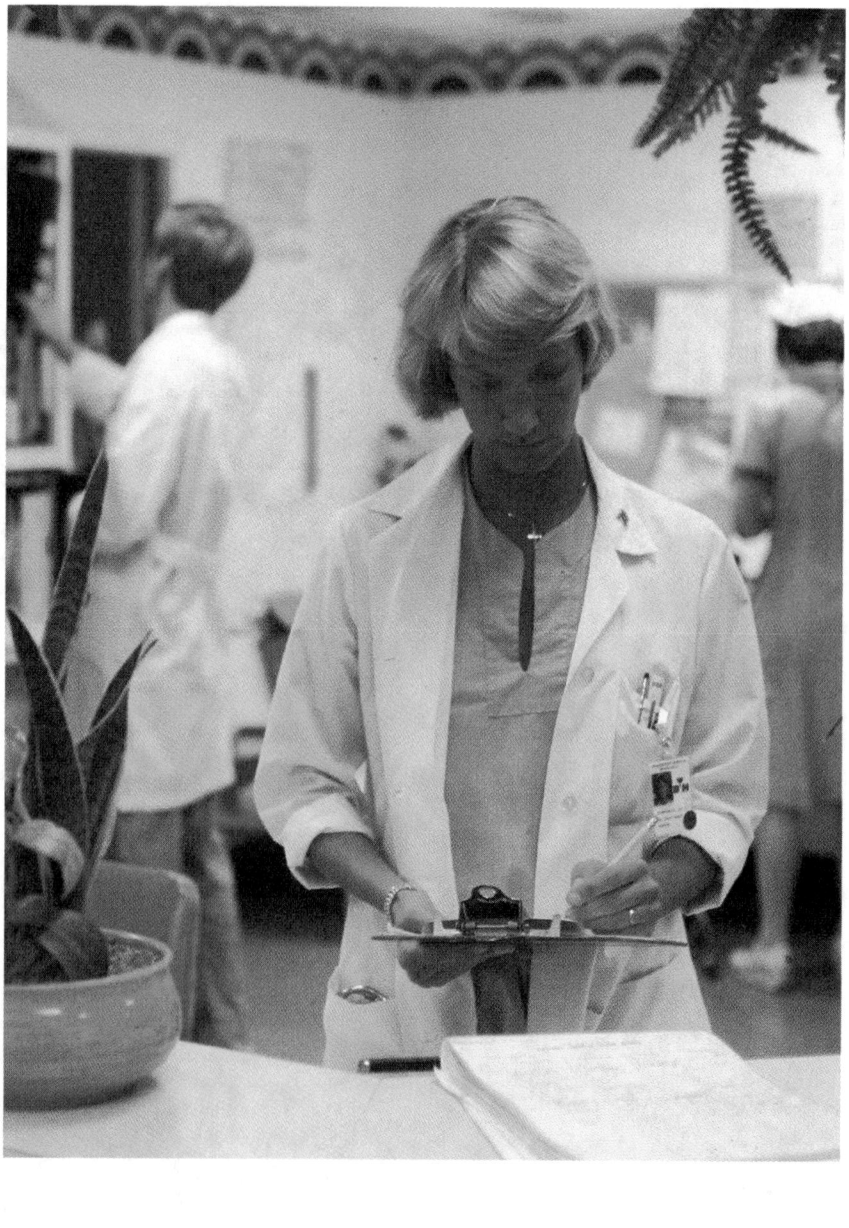

UNIT I

Professional nursing has an impressive history and a solid foundation in theory and education. Today's nursing practice is built on historical and theoretical foundations, which make it dynamic and challenging. Unit I introduces the profession of nursing and explores the principles and concepts that underlie its theory, education, and practice.

The first chapter provides the knowledge base for understanding professional nursing and explores its history, practice guidelines, education, and organizations. The next chapter presents the work of various nursing theorists to promote a beginning understanding and appreciation of this important framework for professional nursing. Chapter 3 considers the ethical and legal principles and concepts that underlie professional nursing practice and relationships. Chapter 4 provides a beginning discussion of leadership and management, skills and knowledge essential for practicing roles in today's demanding and diverse healthcare environment. The final chapter in this unit introduces the research process, emphasizing nursing research. Such an introduction allows beginning practitioners to appreciate the relevance of research to clinical practice, to learn to be discriminating consumers of nursing research, and to value the importance of research in the advancement of professional nursing.

Unit I provides a strong foundation for understanding the many facets of the profession of nursing. The concepts learned in this unit will help the student develop a knowledge base for skills learned later in the book.

The Profession of Nursing

Key Terms	Learning Objectives

Key Terms

American Nurses Association
Clinical Nurse Specialist
International Council of Nurses
Licensed Practical Nurse
National League for Nursing
Nurse Administrator
Nurse Anesthetist
Nurse Educator
Nurse Midwife
Nurse Practice Acts
Nurse Practitioner
Nurse Researcher
Staff Development

Learning Objectives

Upon completion of this chapter, the student will be able to do the following:

- *Describe the evolution of professional nursing.*
- *Discuss the influence of nursing's historic development on contemporary views of professional nursing.*
- *Identify three distinct pathways for entrance into professional nursing practice.*
- *Explain types of graduate educational programs in nursing.*
- *Identify roles and responsibilities of professional nursing within the healthcare delivery system.*
- *Describe career development opportunities and expanded nursing roles.*
- *Describe the purpose and function of professional nursing organizations.*
- *Discuss the impact of current and future social trends on professional nursing practice.*

1

You are a nursing student beginning your first clinical rotation on a medical-surgical unit. This is your first experience caring for clients in the hospital setting. When you arrive on the unit to review your client assignment, a member of the nursing staff pulls you aside and asks: "Why are you entering the nursing profession? You should change your major while you have the chance. Get out now before it's too late!"

Why are you entering the nursing profession? You must have reasons for making the decision, although you may not have been asked to put them into words. When you have completed this chapter, you will have an initial knowledge about nursing history, education needed, career opportunities, and nursing practice. Much is happening in the field of healthcare and within nursing. Although the focus of nursing remains the same, settings for healthcare are changing. You will be part of the revolutionary changes. The Critical Thinking Challenges at the end of the chapter will help you think through your reasons for wanting to become a nurse.

The word *nursing* brings to mind a multitude of ideas and images. For some these images include white uniforms, nursing caps, needles, and bedpans; for others they include kindness, skill, compassion, and intelligence. Many factors influence the way nursing is perceived by the public, by nursing professionals and their colleagues, and by those beginning their nursing careers. Socialization of women, the portrayal of nursing in the media, and our history have had a considerable impact on the image of nursing today.

Nursing is caring, commitment, and dedication to meeting functional health needs (physiologic, psychological, and sociologic) of all people. Nurses are individuals committed to identifying and meeting the healthcare needs of other individuals, families, communities, and groups. As technology increases and society's healthcare changes, the need for well-educated nurses who are committed to maintaining expertise in the theory and practice of professional nursing will continue to grow.

Providing nursing care in settings outside the hospital, such as in a client's home or in ambulatory clinics, is becoming more common. The assumption that the majority of clients will be cared for in the hospital environment is no longer valid. Changes in reimbursement for healthcare services and cost-containment measures have moved nursing practice to areas beyond the hospital setting. Nursing means caring for communities and groups of people, such as the homeless, and addressing issues, such as human rights and acquired immunodeficiency syndrome. Nursing means being socially responsible, involved, and committed to the health of all people.

As society's healthcare needs continue to change, nursing will continue to grow and change in response to those needs. Nursing offers a multitude of challenging, exciting career opportunities. As a profession, nursing continues to promote excellence in healthcare by attracting the brightest and most dedicated people. Students embarking on a professional nursing career accept responsibility for society's healthcare needs and for the advancement of nursing as a profession. This chapter provides a starting point for your understanding where nursing has been, where it is now, and where it is headed as we move into the 21st century.

The Profession of Nursing

The practice of professional nursing has evolved over many years, but issues affecting the profession today are connected to its history. Developing an understanding of nursing's evolution provides the background necessary to understand current nursing practice (Fig. 1-1). Table 1-1 highlights events in nursing's history and shows how the past affects current nursing issues.

Historic Evolution of Modern Nursing

Although nursing in some form has probably existed throughout human history, documentation of the history of nursing goes back only 150 years. Nursing probably began as women intuitively identified and provided for their families' healthcare needs. As certain individuals emerged with the desire and ability to nurture and provide care, the profession of nursing began.

Pre-Christian Era

Pre-Christian history makes few references to nursing; any discussions of nursing or medical roles were blurred. Brief accounts of men and women engaging in practices that may be associated with nursing have been found. For example, in ancient Egypt, maternal-child nursing was the responsibility of nurse midwives, and wet nurses were hired to breast-feed infants. Priests were primarily responsible for healing practices, and the security of the people was directly related to keeping the gods appeased. Israelites practiced principles of sanitation by using boiled or filtered water and carefully inspecting meat for spoilage. Purification rites, such as bathing and isolation, practiced in ancient times continue to be practiced today by Orthodox Jews (Mitchell & Grippando, 1993).

In ancient Babylonia, Egypt, and Sumeria, wealthy families were the primary recipients of nursing care. If and when nursing care was available outside wealthy homes, the nurse was primarily a servant. Subservient

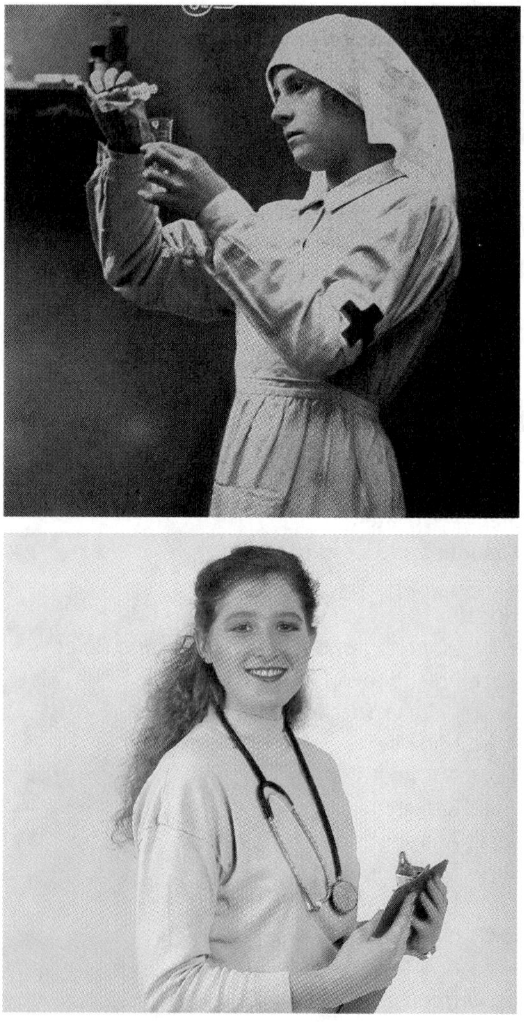

Figure 1-1 • *Comparison of the nurse at the beginning of the 20th century and a professional nurse at the end of the 20th century.*

Table 1-1 • Then and Now—A Selection of Significant Events in the History of Nursing

Date	Then	Now
1–500 (approximately)	Nursing care primarily involves meeting the hygiene and comfort needs of individuals and families. Care is provided by Christians working in close association with an organized church.	Nursing care today involves a high degree of technical skill and includes responsibilities above and beyond hygiene and comfort measures, although these components of care continue to be important. Today's nurse must be highly skilled and up to date with technologic advances, computer literate, and have a strong foundation in the sciences and humanities. Responsibilities are complex and require critical thinking skills. Nursing is no longer tied to the church, and nurses are educated in colleges and universities.
1836	Theodor Fliedner opens a small hospital and training school in Kaiserworth, Germany, where Florence Nightingale, "the founder of modern nursing," receives her nursing education.	Hospital-based schools of nursing continue to exist, but these programs have been declining in number as the profession moves forward and requires education in academic settings.
1854–1860	Florence Nightingale makes major contributions to modern nursing, is named Super-intendent of Nursing, cares for soldiers in the Crimean War, opens a training school at St. Thomas Hospital in London, and publishes "Notes on Nursing, What it is, What it is not."	Nightingale's many contributions to nursing continue to impact on the profession. The components of her theory apply even today, and nurses around the world recognize the courage, dedication, and work of this early professional leader.
1861–1865	Dorothea Dix establishes the Nurse Corps of the United States Army. Dix was not a nurse but an advocate for the mentally ill.	Nurses continue to choose careers in the armed services where opportunities for exciting and rewarding careers are offered.
1872	America's first trained nurse, Linda Richards, graduates from the New England Hospital for Women in Boston.	Nursing continues to prepare educated, competent individuals to provide nursing care in institutions of higher education.
1873	Three nursing schools patterned after the Nightingale plan develop in the United States: Bellevue Training School, Connecticut Training School, and Boston Training School. In 1874, the first "Nightingale model" school of Nursing in Canada is set up in St. Catherines, Ontario.	New nursing programs continue to develop. The profession now offers several routes to a career in nursing, including diploma, associate degree, baccalaureate degree, the generic master's, and doctoral degree.
1882	American National Red Cross is organized by Clara Barton	The Red Cross continues to exist today, offering care to victims of disasters, maintaining the nation's blood supply, and educating the nation about AIDS.
1893	Lillian Wald and Mary Brewster found the Henry Street Settlement, the first home visiting nurse organization in the United States. The Henry Street Settlement can still be visited in New York City.	Visiting nurse associations have grown and become essential healthcare components in society. Today, nursing care is provided in this setting to a large extent. Cost containment and healthcare reform concerns have moved nursing from the hospital setting to the community once again.
1897	The American Society of Superintendents of Training Schools of the United States and Canada is organized. Renamed the American Nurses Association in 1911 and the Canadian Nurses Association in 1907.	The American Nurses Association and the Canadian Nurses Association continue to function as nursing's professional organizations.
1899	International Council of Nurses (ICN) is established.	ICN continues to represent and speak to international nursing concerns.
1900	American Journal of Nursing—first nursing journal to be owned, operated, and published by nurses—is developed.	American Journal of Nursing and The Canadian Nurse continue to be major references for clinical nursing practice.

(continued)

Table 1-1 *(Continued)*

Date	Then	Now
1923	Goldmark report of the Rockefeller foundation is published, advocating financial support of University-based schools of nursing. A similar report, The Weir Report, is published in Canada in 1932.	There is a decline in available financial support to incoming students of nursing. However, nursing organizations and leaders are working to improve financial assistance to students.
1940	World War II results in another nursing shortage. Esther Lucille Brown completes the Brown report on nursing education, advocating that education for nursing belongs in colleges and universities, not in hospitals.	Although hospital-based schools of nursing continue to exist, they are declining in number, and students are more frequently choosing college and university educations.
1953	National Student Nurses' Association (NSNA) is established.	NSNA continues today to encourage students of nursing to become involved in professional issues. Students are given opportunities to hold leadership positions at state and national levels. The equivalent organization in Canada is known as the Canadian University Nursing Students Association.
1965	ANA issues its first "position paper on nursing education," calling for all nursing education to take place in institutions of higher education and stipulating the baccalaureate as minimum preparation for professional nursing and the associate degree for technical nursing practice.	The entry level debate has not been completely resolved. Preparation of nurses for the future continues to be one of professional nursing's concerns.
1985	National Center for Nursing Research is established at the National Institutes of Health in Bethesda, Maryland.	1993—The National Center for Nursing Research is upgraded by President Clinton to Institute status.
1994	Healthcare reform is a discussion that permeates professional circles. Cost-containment measures, access to health care, and the need for health promotion are integral components of the issues.	Healthcare reform will continue to be an integral issue to the nursing profession. Nurses will continue to explore options for advanced practice nurses to maintain nursing's role and move it forward in this environment of change.

roles for women and nurses were rooted in the sexual discrimination and overall devaluation of human life reflective of this era. Cultural attitudes toward the sick combined with the low status of women provided major obstacles to nursing (Dolan, Fitzpatrick, & Herrmann, 1983).

Early Christian Era

Evidence of nursing roles became more apparent in the early Christian era. Women performed roles that reflected components of today's nursing practice: dietitian, physical therapist, pharmacist, and counselor. Providing hygiene and comfort measures was the central focus of nursing (Dolan, et al., 1983). Men and women committed to the church spread the philosophy of Christianity while providing nursing care to the ill.

The influence of Christianity raised nursing's social position by placing more value on human life and individuality. Compassion, charity, and willingness to serve were qualities associated with nurses. Deacons and deaconesses (individuals working for the church ministry) were designated to perform services for the sick because women's roles primarily involved marriage and childbearing (Kelly, 1985).

Deaconesses functioned as visiting nurses and dedicated their lives to charity work. This role allowed widowed or unmarried women to hold a respectable place in society. Phoebe (55 A.D.) is the most noted deaconess identified in nursing's history. A need for hospitals to care for the sick was identified by the early deaconesses and resulted in the emergence of several Christian hospitals. Fabiola established the first general hospital in Rome around 380 A.D. and dedicated her life to the care of the sick (Mitchell & Grippando, 1993).

Contributions of the Greeks

The Greeks made significant contributions to the care of the sick and to a certain extent, to the profession of nursing. Hippocrates, known as "the father of medicine," made a major advance in medicine by rejecting the belief that diseases had supernatural causes. He also is credited with developing assessment standards for clients, establishing overall medical standards, and recognizing a need for nurses (Kelly, 1985).

The Middle Ages

Poverty was a critical problem during the Middle Ages, but nursing continued to shape the purpose and direction of healthcare and provide leadership in the field. These advancements were enhanced by the continuing spread of Christianity, which had positive effects on cultural values and institutions. The influence of Christianity also improved the status of nursing by attracting intelligent individuals from respected families (Dolan, et al., 1983). The Crusades resulted in the establishment of military nursing orders and the recruitment of men into nursing. Nursing was well organized at this time and had many similarities to traditional nursing practice (Mitchell & Grippando, 1993). The Church dictated the scope of nursing practice, and the spiritual needs of the client were viewed as the priority for care. Obedience and devotion were maintained with rigid discipline and remained central to organized nursing for centuries (Mitchell & Grippando, 1993).

The Renaissance

During the Renaissance (1400–1600) recognition of the need for sound educational preparation in nursing contributed to further advancement of the profession. Unfortunately, the continuing lack of effective sanitation and increasing poverty resulted in serious healthcare problems. The immediate need for healthcare providers, due to a significant increase in medical problems, further delayed the move toward improving nursing education (Dolan, et al., 1983).

The Reformation

Nursing encountered a severe setback during the Reformation. The dispersion of religious orders, which had been the primary source of healthcare, resulted in a serious deterioration in hospital conditions and nursing care. Attempts to improve nursing education and the image of nurses were destroyed (Dolan, et al., 1983). The role of women changed dramatically during the Reformation. Women were viewed as subordinate to men and were expected to remain at home caring for children, thus decreasing the number of qualified women practicing nursing (Mitchell & Grippando, 1993).

Nursing in the 18th Century

Revolutions and epidemics resulted in further expansion of nursing roles. The prevention of illness became a primary objective of the nursing profession. Continuing problems of poor sanitation and low standards of living increased the need for what we know today as public-health nursing (Dolan, et al., 1983). By the end of the 18th century, nursing was present in hospitals, but nurses' working conditions were poor, resulting in a loss of social status for the profession. As nursing's social status deteriorated, fewer qualified individuals chose to enter the profession. Nursing was considered a last-resort occupation.

Society's attitudes about nursing during this time were reflected in Charles Dickens' *Martin Chuzzlewit* (1884), in which nursing care was provided by criminals and women of low moral standards. One of the book's characters, Sarah Gamp, was a nurse who abused alcohol and was cruel to her clients. This negative portrayal of nursing seriously damaged the profession's image, and fragments of such images can still be found in media portrayals of nursing today (Dolan, et al., 1983).

Nursing in the 19th Century

Nursing in the 19th century brought new problems and social changes that affected the profession and the nurse's role. The 19th century brought the industrial revolution and was characterized by political, economic, and social expansion. Poverty, long work days for women and children, and the prevalence of disease increased the need for community health nurses. Continued emphasis was placed on the need for proper preparation of nurses. Nursing was once again influenced by religion; the caring image of the nurse was believed to be based on a spiritual calling to the profession. Poverty, innocence, and submissiveness were qualities associated with potential nursing candidates (Dolan, et al., 1983).

Florence Nightingale. Florence Nightingale has been called the founder of modern nursing. Stubborn and unyielding, Nightingale improved health laws, reformed hospitals, reorganized military medical services, and established nursing as a profession with two missions: sick nursing and health nursing. Nightingale saw "sick nursing" as helping clients use their own reparative processes to get well and "health nursing" as the prevention of illness (Dolan, et al., 1983; Kelly, 1985).

Nightingale was born May 12, 1820, in Florence, Italy, to a wealthy English family and was educated in languages, philosophy, and the liberal arts. Much to her family's dismay, she entered nurses' training when she was 31 years old in the hope of replacing the "Sarah Gamp" image with that of education, intelligence, and kindness (Dolan, et al., 1983).

Nightingale's contributions to nursing were many. She was the superintendent of nurses at King's College Hospital until she left to care for soldiers during the Crimean War. Her efforts during this war were credited with halving the mortality rate, and she soon became known as "the lady with the lamp," because she made midnight rounds to the soldiers. In 1859, Nightingale published *Notes on Nursing* and in 1860 started the

Nightingale Training School for Nurses. Nightingale was gracious and hard working, and her contributions continue to influence the profession today (Dolan, et al., 1983).

Nursing During the American Civil War. During the Civil War (1861–1865), more hospitals and more and better prepared nurses were needed. Although she was not a nurse, Dorothea Dix established the Nurse Corps of the U.S. Army, further expanding nursing's role. Another early nursing leader, Clara Barton, practiced nursing on Civil War battlefields. Barton founded the American Red Cross, an organization that continues to make significant contributions to society and healthcare today (Dolan, et al., 1983).

Nursing Education in the 19th Century. In 1869, the American Medical Association developed the Committee on the Training of Nurses, and as a result of this committee's recommendations, hospital-based schools of nursing under medical supervision emerged. In 1874, Linda Richards, America's first trained nurse, graduated from the Bellevue Hospital Training School in New York City.

The central focus of nursing during this time was caring for the sick. Despite improvements in nursing education, major problems remained. Nursing students were expected to perform such non-nursing duties as scrubbing floors and doing laundry. They also were used as free labor in hospitals as they gained clinical experience (Dolan, et al., 1983).

The end of the 19th century brought with it the emergence of public-health nursing. Two early nursing leaders, Lillian Wald and Mary Brewster, established the first public-health nursing service for the sick and poor, the Henry Street Settlement on New York City's Lower East Side. The Henry Street Settlement is now a famous center of public-health nursing (Dolan, et al., 1983).

Nursing in the 20th Century

The First Half of the Century. In the early 20th century, professional organizations such as the American Nurses Association (ANA), the Canadian Nurses Association (CNA), the International Council of Nurses, and the National League for Nursing (NLN) emerged. Nursing journals were developed and research was conducted into the need for higher education in nursing. The American Journal of Nursing (AJN), first published in 1900, was the first nursing journal to be owned, operated, and published by nurses. AJN continues to be a significant nursing publication (Dolan, et al., 1983).

A noteworthy milestone in the history of nursing education occurred in 1923 with the publication of the Goldmark Report, which advocated financial support for university-based schools of nursing. This report's findings eased the transition from hospital-based schools of nursing to university settings, marking a major advance in nursing education (Dolan, et al., 1983).

Military Influences. Military influences on nursing education in the 20th century have been numerous. During the Spanish American War, the Volunteer Nurse Corps (1898) was established, and in 1901, become the Army Nurse Corps. In 1908, the Navy Nurse Corps was also authorized by Congress (Mitchell & Grippando, 1993). World War I saw nurses being transported to war areas in Europe and the Far East to care for the sick and wounded.

The casualties of World War II brought a critical nursing shortage, prompting quick solutions to increase the number of nurses and providing a setback for the move toward university-based nursing education. Nonetheless, Esther Lucille Brown, in her report on nursing education published at that time, wrote that nursing education belonged in colleges and universities, not in hospitals. This report provided further documentation of the need for university-based nursing education programs (Dolan, et al., 1983).

During the Korean War, Congress authorized the creation of the Air Force Nurse Corps (1949), and by 1950, Air Force Nurses were evacuating wounded soldiers from Korea. In 1956, the Army Student Nurse Program was established (Mitchell & Grippando, 1993).

The Vietnam War saw many nurses involved in the Army and Navy Nurse Corps caring for the wounded. In addition, Air Force Nurses were assigned to Vietnam. In 1970, Anna Mae Hayes, Chief of the Army Nurse Corps, was promoted to Brigadier General.

Operation Desert Shield/Desert Storm once again saw the mobilization of nurses to Saudi Arabia (1991). Similar to other war situations, the nursing shortage in the United States placed pressure on the military to provide nursing and medical care.

The Second Half of the Century. In 1965, a report by the National Commission on Nursing and Nursing Education addressed several nursing issues, including supply and demand for nurses, clarification of nursing roles and functions, nursing education, and available career opportunities for nurses. The report, called the Lysaught Report in honor of the study's director, helped clarify the role of professional nursing practice (Dolan, et al., 1983).

The latter part of the 20th century has been marked by rapid scientific advances and increasingly complex technology. Longer lifespans, increased incidence of chronic illness, and new family structures have had a dramatic impact on where and how nurses practice. Despite these changes, nursing continues to focus on the delivery of care that is safe, comprehensive, and effective. Nursing's historic antecedents affect the profession today. Education, practice settings, and roles have been influenced by the profession's history. Likewise, when, how, and why the profession evolves will be directly related to the contributions made by present and future nursing professionals. Social forces can be expected to influence future definitions of nursing, just as these forces have affected nursing practice to date.

Socialization to Professional Nursing

Socialization is a process that involves learning theory and skills and internalizing an identity appropriate to a specific role. Internalizing a specific role allows one to participate as a member of a group.

Students often enter nursing with the perception that their professional identity will center on providing service to individuals who are ill or who require care in regaining health. Although this initial perception may be true, it is only a small part of the professional identity that students must internalize when they join the profession. Socialization to nursing involves changes that ultimately affect a student's knowledge base, attitudes, and values regarding professional nursing practice. This socialization is a lifelong process that occurs as the individual grows personally and professionally. As the student becomes socialized to nursing, an understanding of the nursing profession develops and is internalized.

Professions generally have a specific body of knowledge, a specific set of values, and specific skills that differentiate them from one another. Professional nursing curriculums teach foundations of the discipline of nursing. Theoretical and clinical instruction facilitates the development of a professional identity and prepares students to function as beginning professional nurses. Beyond this initial socialization to nursing, continuing socialization occurs as the nurse gains experience in the workplace and perhaps pursues advanced education.

Patricia Benner, in *From Novice to Expert* (1984), discusses socialization and skill acquisition in nursing using the Dreyfuss model (Table 1-2). According to this model, a student passes through five levels of profi-

Table 1-2 • Dreyfuss Model of Skill Acquisition Applied to Nursing

Level of Proficiency	*Summary Description*
Novice	A beginning nursing student or any nurse entering a situation in which he or she has had no previous experience. Behavior is governed by established rules and is limited and inflexible.
Advanced beginner	The advanced beginner can demonstrate marginally acceptable performance. He or she has had enough experience in actual situations to identify meaningful aspects or global characteristics that can be identified only through prior experience.
Competent	Competence is reflected by the nurse who has been on the same job for 2 or 3 years and who consciously and deliberately plans nursing care in terms of long-range goals.
Proficient	The proficient nurse perceives situations as whole rather than in terms of aspects and manages nursing care rather than performing tasks.
Expert	The expert nurse no longer relies on rules or guidelines to connect understanding of a situation to an appropriate action. The expert nurse, with an enormous background of experience, has an intuitive grasp of the situation and zeroes in on the problem.

The five levels of proficiency listed in the left column were developed by Stuart Dreyfuss and Hubert Dreyfuss. The second column reflects the author's summary of a discussion by Patricia Benner in *From novice to expert: Excellence and power in clinical nursing practice*. San Francisco: Addison-Wesley, 1984.

ciency when acquiring and developing a skill: novice, advanced beginner, competent, proficient, and expert. Differences in each level reflect changes in three areas of skill performance. In the first level, the student moves from relying on abstract principles to using concrete experiences. The second level involves a change from seeing situations in parts to seeing them more conceptually, or as a whole. Finally, in the third level, the student is no longer outside the situation observing, but is directly involved in the situation.

Nursing and Professionalism Defined

Because definitions of nursing reflect the values and influences of society, the profession is subject to misinterpretation. One common misconception is that nurses are handmaidens to physicians; other misconceptions can readily be seen on television and in films and novels. Beginning nursing professionals must form a clear, accurate understanding of professional nursing practice if precise interpretations of the role of the nurse are to be shared by other members of the healthcare team and the public.

Nursing is a multifaceted profession and as such, has been defined in a variety of ways. Florence Nightingale defined nursing as "the act of utilizing the environment of the client to assist him in his recovery" (Nightingale, 1859/1992). The ANA defined nursing as "the diagnosis and treatment of human responses to actual or potential health problems" (ANA Social Policy Statement, 1980, pg. 1). The CNA published the following definition (CNA, 1987).

The nursing profession exists in response to a need of society and holds ideals related to human health throughout the lifespan. Nurses direct their energies toward the promotion, maintenance, and restoration of health; the prevention of illness; the alleviation of suffering and the ensurance of a peaceful death when life can no longer be sustained. Nurses value a holistic view and regard an individual as a biopsychosocial being who has the capacity to set goals and make decisions and who has the right and responsibility to make informed choices congruent with personal beliefs and values. Nursing, a dynamic and supportive profession guided by its code of ethics, is rooted in caring, a concept evident throughout its four fields of activity: practice, education, administration, and research.

Despite the multitude of definitions of nursing, common themes are evident. Holism, caring, teaching, advocacy, supporting, promoting, maintaining, and restoring health are all components of nursing practice. Nursing care involves creativity, sensitivity, and care based on scientific rationale. All of these components are part of the practice, but nurses should not limit themselves to these themes.

The question of whether nursing is a profession has been a topic of ongoing debate. To answer this question, it is first helpful to examine the established criteria for a profession. Several criteria to evaluate nursing's professional status have been proposed, including the need for higher education, a specific body of knowledge, public interest and responsibility, and internal organization. Table 1-3 compares the patterns identified in developing professions with characteristics specific to nursing. Table 1-3 shows that nursing is an evolving profession. The growth of professionalism in nursing has been influenced by higher and more specialized education and by increased autonomy in practice. Increased levels of research activity, accountability, and responsibility have contributed to enhance nursing's status as a profession. As more nurses obtain master's and doctoral degrees and research contributions grow, the profession's specific body of knowledge becomes clearer and more accurately defined.

Educational Preparation and Career Opportunities

Educational preparation in nursing has long been a topic of debate among members of the profession.

Table 1-3 • *Professional Development Patterns Compared With Nursing*

Patterns of Developing Professions	*Nursing Profession*
Professions require critical thinking ability and higher education.	Nurses are educated in institutions of higher learning and function in a responsible and accountable manner. Critical thinking is now being emphasized to great extent in all levels of nursing education.
Professions are based on specific body of knowledge.	Nursing has identified and continues to develop its own specific body of knowledge from which nursing practice emerges. Application of theory derived from research provides rationale for action.
Professions characteristically are accompanied by acceptance of responsibility and are fueled by public interest.	Nursing professionals accept a great deal of responsibility for providing for healthcare needs of people. The profession evolved in response to needs identified by society and is guided by an ethical code.

Three distinct pathways exist for entrance into professional nursing practice, and new approaches emerge continually. Basic preparation and selected examples of newer approaches are presented in this section.

Directly related to the issue of educational preparation is the topic of career opportunities in nursing. Depending on the individual's educational preparation and area of clinical expertise, many career opportunities exist in professional nursing.

Accelerated changes in healthcare with an emphasis on primary care have intensified interest in **advanced practice nurses**. "Regulation of advanced practice nursing is done by statute or by certification. Regulation by statute involves modification of the state nurse practice act to regulate advanced nursing practice and involves issuance of a second license. Regulation by certification involves a process whereby professional boards validate an individual nurse's advanced qualifications in a particular area of nursing" (Ziemer, 1994, p. 7). An example of advanced practice nursing would be the role of the nurse practitioner.

Nursing Education

The issue of educational preparation for entry into practice has been debated since the 1930s and 1940s, when the Brown and Goldmark reports recommended two levels of nursing preparation. In 1965, the ANA adopted a resolution proposing that minimum preparation for beginning professional practice should be a baccalaureate degree in nursing, and the minimum preparation for technical practice should be an associate degree in nursing. The ANA's 1965 resolution also prompted the 1985 ANA statement adopting the titles of **associate nurse**, a nurse prepared in an associate degree program, and **professional nurse**, a nurse possessing the baccalaureate degree in nursing, for these two levels of educational preparation.

In Canada there is one level of nursing practice: the professional level. Although nurses are educated at the diploma and university levels, all are considered to be professional nurses. The CNA endorsed the baccalaureate standard for entry to practice in 1982, although several provinces had adopted this standard earlier. The goal is to prepare all "entering" students at the baccalaureate level by 2000.

Many critical issues in professional nursing practice continue to be affected by the debate over entry-level preparation. Included in this debate are the competencies of new nursing graduates, the public view of nursing roles, the need for professional status within the healthcare community, the organization of nursing education, and the supply and demand for nursing professionals. Finally, the variety of programs available for entry into nursing practice is confusing to students, employers, and the public. Professional nursing must resolve the problems of entry-level requirements.

Nursing in the United States continues to have three major routes leading to the *registered nurse* licensure. Educational preparation may be the diploma, associate, or baccalaureate degree. Now emerging are programs that have the master's degree and nursing doctorate degree as entry-level preparation.

All nursing programs require a minimum of state or provincial approval. In addition to state approval, the NLN provides accreditation standards for all types of nursing programs in the United States. Accreditation from the NLN signifies excellence in nursing education. Accreditation from the Canadian Association of University Schools of Nursing signifies excellence in Canada.

Types of Educational Programs

Would-be nurses may enter licensed practical nursing programs or may pursue diploma, associate, baccalaureate, master's, or doctoral degrees. Students may choose the educational route that best suits their needs and goals.

Practical Nursing Program. People interested in a practical nursing career attend 1-year programs that prepare them to perform technical skills under the supervision of a registered nurse. In the United States, students successfully completing the program requirements may sit for the licensure examination given by the state board of nursing to become a **licensed practical nurse** (LPN) or licensed vocational nurse. A similar process controlled by the provincial association is in place in Canada. LPNs are employed in hospitals, long-term care facilities, and rehabilitation centers and by healthcare providers, such as physicians. LPNs differ from registered nurses in two areas: educational preparation and scope of practice. Practical nursing was established to prepare healthcare providers for client care and to assist the professional nurse with routine technical procedures.

Diploma Nursing Program. Diploma nursing schools were the first type of educational preparation available for registered nurses. In the United States, diploma programs usually require 3 years of study. Students earn some college credit, but college credit is not awarded for nursing courses. Clinical experience is extensive, which is an advantage of this route. In Canada, diploma programs can be at the hospital (3-year) level or at the college (2-year) level. College credit is awarded for all courses at the college level.

Students successfully completing diploma programs take the state or provincial board of nursing examination for registered nurse licensure. Graduates of diploma programs work as beginning practitioners in acute, intermediate, long-term, and ambulatory healthcare facilities. Graduates must demonstrate competency in the assessment, planning, implementation, and evaluation phases of the nursing process (National League for Nursing, 1978b).

The number of diploma programs is declining as nursing education moves into institutions of higher learning. This decline is related to nursing's efforts to achieve professional status and control over practice.

Associate Degree Nursing Program. Associate degree nursing began in 1952 in the Division of Nursing Education of Teachers College, Columbia University, under the direction of Mildred Montag. Developed in response to a nursing shortage, associate degree nursing education continues to exist successfully today. The student pursuing this degree attends a junior college for 2 years, receiving college credit for all courses and clinical experience in nursing. The goal of this program is to prepare a technical nurse, who is capable of functioning as a quality practitioner under the supervision of a professional nurse. The student successfully completing the requirements of an associate degree program also takes the state board of nursing examination for registered nurse licensure. (Canada does not have an associate degree nursing program.)

As a provider of nursing care, the associate degree nurse uses the nursing process to formulate and maintain individualized nursing plans of care. The associate degree nurse also teaches clients who need information or support to maintain health. As a manager, the associate degree nurse provides care for a group of clients with common, well-defined health problems in structured settings (National League for Nursing, 1978c).

Baccalaureate Degree Nursing Program. The baccalaureate degree in nursing offers the student a full college or university education with a background in liberal arts. The programs are rigorous and provide the student with credits for nursing courses and clinical experience in all areas of nursing practice. There is an added emphasis in baccalaureate degree programs on community health nursing, research, leadership, and management. Baccalaureate programs in nursing are offered in college or university settings.

Students successfully completing the baccalaureate degree in nursing take the state board of nursing examination for registered nurse licensure. In Canada, students take a provincial board examination for registration; there is no licensure. Nurses are prepared as generalists at the baccalaureate level and provide comprehensive service that assesses, promotes, and maintains the health of individuals, families, communities, and groups (National League for Nursing, 1978a).

Advanced Nursing Education Opportunities

Master's Degree Nursing Program. Master's level education in nursing began in the last quarter of the 19th century in response to a need for better educated faculty and supervisory staff (Mitchell & Grippando, 1993). Nurses interested in attaining advanced education in a specialty area may complete graduate programs in their area of interest. Graduate education prepares the nurse for advanced, independent practice with continued emphasis on research. Graduate education requires independent critical thinking, and nurses pursuing graduate education must have a high degree of scholastic ability.

In an innovative movement, several colleges in the United States offer a generic master of science degree in nursing in preparation for professional nursing practice. Usually students begin the programs with a baccalaureate degree in a field of study other than nursing. Students completing generic master's programs have advanced research capabilities and some opportunity for clinical concentration in a nursing specialty.

Doctoral Degree Program. The first four doctoral degree programs in the United States were offered at Boston University, New York University, Teachers College at Columbia University, and the University of Pittsburgh. In Canada, the first doctoral degree programs were at McGill University, the University of Alberta, the University of British Columbia, and the University of Toronto. Students may earn a Doctor of Philosophy (PhD), a Doctor of Education (EdD), or a Doctor of Nursing Science (DNS). Individuals interested in careers as nurse researchers or nurse educators usually must obtain doctoral degrees. Doctoral education has become more available to nurses, and the number of nurses earning doctoral degrees continues to increase. Doctoral education in nursing is usually obtained after completing a master's program. Many PhD programs incorporate the master's degree for students who enter from BSN programs.

An innovative program combines entrance into professional nursing practice with a professional nurse doctorate program. Case Western Reserve University began the first program in 1985, and the University of Colorado has recently begun a program. Advanced preparation in clinical research is a major component of the program.

Graduate Degree Programs. Master's level education in nursing began in the last quarter of the 19th century in response to a need for better educated faculty and supervisory staff (Mitchell & Grippando, 1993). Nurses interested in attaining advanced education in a specialty area may complete graduate programs in their area of interest. Graduate education prepares the nurse for advanced, independent practice with continued emphasis on research. Graduate education requires independent critical thinking, and nurses pursuing graduate education must have a high degree of scholastic ability.

Doctoral Degree Programs. The first four doctoral degree programs in the United States were offered at Boston University, New York University, Teachers College at Columbia University, and the University of Pittsburgh. In Canada, the first doctoral degree programs

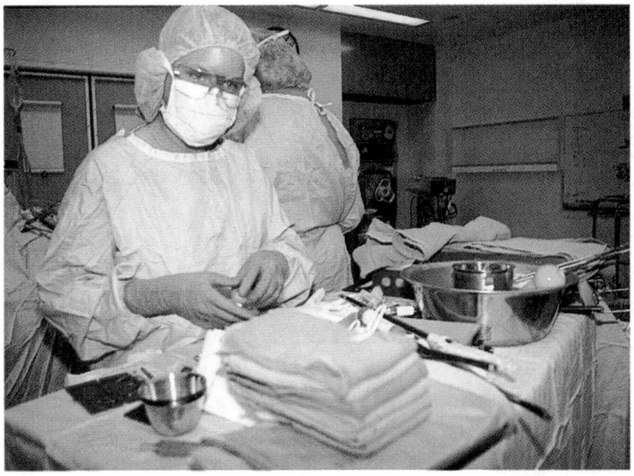

Figure 1-2 • *Hospital nursing may involve a specialty area, such as the operating room.*

were at McGill University, the University of Alberta, the University of British Columbia, and the University of Toronto. Students may earn a Doctor of Philosophy (PhD), a Doctor of Education (EdD), or a Doctor of Nursing Science (DNS). Individuals interested in careers as nurse researchers or nurse educators usually must obtain doctoral degrees. Doctoral education has become more available to nurses, and the number of nurses earning doctoral degrees continues to increase. Doctoral education in nursing may be obtained after completing a generic program, or students may enter doctoral nursing programs directly from high school as their generic program (N.D.—Nurse Doctorate).

Staff Development

Staff development is provided by hospital employees to newly hired nurses or other healthcare providers to ensure quality care. Staff development helps nurses provide the most accurate and up-to-date care to clients. For example, staff development educators may provide information on a new piece of equipment or on fire safety. A primary goal of in-service educators is to upgrade employees' knowledge and skills.

Nursing Practice Settings

Settings for nursing practice change as healthcare needs of society change and the cost of healthcare rises. These changes will continue through the beginning of the new century. This section gives a sample of the variety of settings in which a nurse may practice. These settings are discussed further in Chapter 6.

Hospital

Nurses have always been and probably always will be at the bedside caring for clients and helping to meet their healthcare needs. Hospital nursing involves caring for acutely ill clients with medical and surgical needs. It may include specialty areas, such as orthopedics, obstetrics and gynecology, ambulatory chemotherapy, emergency room nursing, operating room nursing, cardiac rehabilitation, and pediatrics (Fig. 1-2). Opportunities are diversified and challenging in the hospital as nurses continually meet their clients' complex healthcare needs. Changes in healthcare and reimbursement programs move clients away from the hospital setting more quickly. As a consequence, more service is being provided outside the traditional hospital setting.

Community

The number of nurses employed in community-based practice has increased substantially because of the increased cost of hospital care and the focus on health promotion and disease prevention. Community health nurses are responsible for teaching about health and for providing care to clients as they recover or live with chronic conditions in their home. With the increasing cost of hospitalization, the need for community health nurses will grow.

Private Duty

Private-duty nursing, which involves caring for one client for the duration of his or her illness, may take place in the hospital or at home. The request for a private-duty nurse is usually made by the client or family. Private-duty nurses help meet the healthcare needs of clients with complex problems that require individualized, continuous attention.

Health Promotion Centers

Prevention and health promotion provide the major focus of healthcare today, and nursing plays a significant role in this setting. Nurses' involvement in health promotion activities is increasing. Nurses serve in a teaching and supportive role, helping clients achieve goals, such as losing weight, quitting smoking, and establishing exercise programs. Nurses working in health promotion centers may be employed by a hospital, or they may work independently.

Long-Term Care Facilities

Long-term care facilities provide nursing care to those who require long-term assistance in meeting healthcare needs. Clients in a long-term care facility have complex needs and require intensive nursing care. As the population of older adults increases and technology helps individuals live longer lives, special healthcare needs of the community will continue to grow.

Rehabilitation Centers. Nurses care for clients who need help regaining their abilities to perform activities

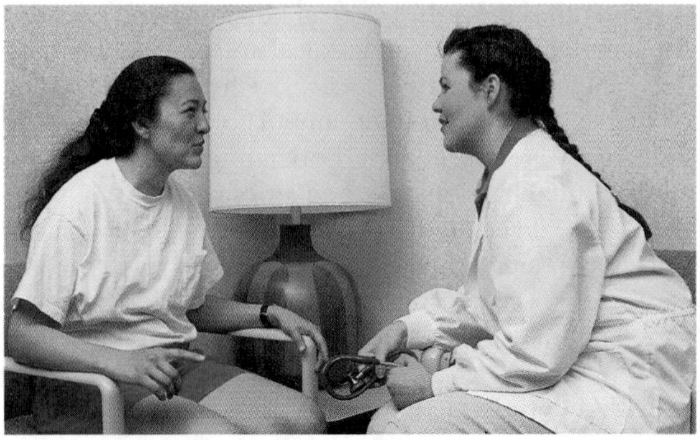

Figure 1-3 • *Nursing centers are healthcare facilities that address basic needs of both individuals and their communities.*

of daily living in rehabilitation centers. Nurses in these centers work with clients who may have experienced traumatic injury and need long-term assistance and therapy to regain maximum independence.

Nursing Centers. Nursing centers are one of the newest arenas for the practice of nursing (Fig. 1-3). Colleges and universities have been among the first to develop nursing centers to meet their students' healthcare needs and to provide settings for nursing practice. Nursing centers help meet the community's healthcare needs by providing such services as physical examinations, basic diagnostic studies, and physician referrals when indicated.

Nursing Roles and Responsibilities

Historically, the sole duty of a nurse was to provide care and comfort to the sick. The expansion of technology, knowledge, health promotion, and prevention has expanded the roles and functions of the nurse. Nursing functions include activities that the nurse performs independently or collaboratively. For instance, the nurse may initiate activities, such as turning or positioning a bed client every 2 hours, which is a nurse-prescribed intervention (Carpenito, 1995). On the other hand, when a physician delegates an action (a physician-prescribed intervention) that requires the nurse to use his or her own judgment, he or she is addressing a collaborative problem. For example, although the physician must prescribe the medication, he or she relies on the nurse's judgment. The nurse must have a thorough understanding of the medication, observe for side effects, and teach the client about the medication. Nurse- and physician-prescribed interventions are discussed further in Unit III.

In addition to these roles, the profession has many other requirements, including assertiveness; a sound knowledge base in the sciences, humanities, and arts; the ability to make safe judgments; the ability to communicate the healthcare needs of clients in written and oral form; and a spirit of collegiality with other members of the healthcare team. The professional nurse is autonomous and assumes the responsibilities of caregiver, decision-maker, client advocate, manager and coordinator of healthcare needs, educator, and communicator.

Caregiver

As a provider of care, the nurse assumes responsibility for helping the client promote, restore, and maintain health and wellness (Fig. 1-4). The client is seen as unique, and the "whole" person is considered in the caring process. Not only physiologic concerns are addressed, but also spiritual, emotional, and social needs. Nurses must set priorities for care and assist clients in meeting all their needs in the most timely and cost-effective manner possible, while ensuring excellence in client care.

Decision-Maker

Nurses are continually identifying obstacles or difficulties in the promotion, restoration, and maintenance of health. Problem resolution requires the ability to make sound judgments and decisions. Nurses must make choices about the best approach to client care, help clients participate in this decision-making process, and use safe and effective judgments when providing client care. The nurse also is responsible for involving other members of the healthcare team and the client's family in the decision-making process to ensure that sound choices are made (Fig. 1-5).

Client Advocate

One of the nurse's most important functions is to protect the client. Nurses act as client advocates in many

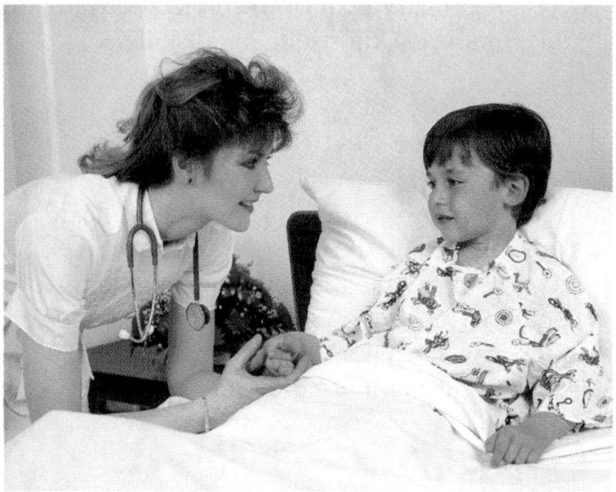

Figure 1-4 • *The nurse provides care across the lifespan.*

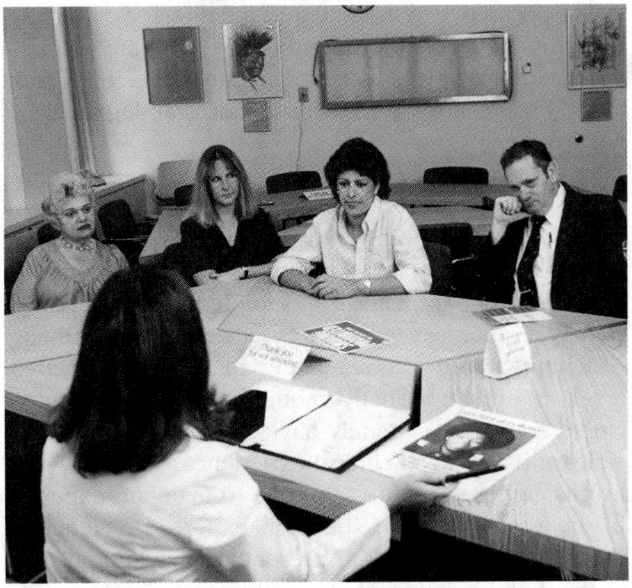

Figure 1-5 • *The nurse is responsible for involving other members of the healthcare team in decision making.*

situations; examples include communicating the client's needs and concerns and ensuring that clients understand their treatment. Nurses must promote a safe environment that facilitates the restoration of health. Nurses are responsible for having a thorough understanding of their clients' health problems, history, and potential problems. Nurses consistently take responsibility for protecting their clients' legal rights and helping clients assert these rights.

Manager and Coordinator

Promoting, restoring, and maintaining health involves coordinating the services offered by a variety of healthcare professionals. In addition to managing his or her own time, the nurse also must coordinate all activities or treatments that involve the client. The goal of the manager/coordinator role is to have client care completed effectively and efficiently and in a manner that benefits the client.

Communicator

Central to all other roles is the role of communicator. Because the nurse spends the most time with the client, he or she has the greatest opportunity for observing, communicating, and identifying problems or improvements in the plan of care. The nurse is responsible for communicating findings to the healthcare team in oral and written form. The quality of communication is a critical factor in meeting clients' healthcare needs; the nurse must be knowledgeable, articulate, and capable of effective written and verbal expression.

Educator

Health promotion and illness prevention have become a growing concern and focus of the healthcare delivery system. Educating clients about the disease process, disease prevention, nutritional factors, and healthy behaviors is essential. The nurse must explain treatments and procedures for which he or she is responsible, answer any questions the client has, and evaluate the client's progress toward health. Education is involved in all nursing activities.

Career Development and Expanded Nursing Roles

There are many additional opportunities for career development and advancement in nursing. These opportunities, some requiring advanced education, lead to new and varied roles and exciting challenges. Some of these expanded nursing roles include nurse practitioner, clinical nurse specialist, nurse midwife, nurse anesthetist, nurse researcher, nurse administrator, and nurse educator.

Nurse Practitioner

Nurse practitioners have advanced education, often a master's degree in nursing, and are graduates of a nurse practitioner program. Nurse practitioners function with more independence and autonomy and are highly skilled at making nursing assessments, performing physical examinations, counseling, teaching, and treating minor health problems. Nurse practitioners may be generalists or may have a specialty, such as obstetrics or pediatrics.

Clinical Nurse Specialist

Clinical nurse specialists have a master's degree in nursing and may have advanced experience and expertise in a specialized area of practice (eg, gerontology, pediatrics, critical care, oncology, endocrinology, or cardiovascular or pulmonary disease). They work in a variety of settings, depending on their specialty (Fig. 1-6). Their roles include clinician, educator, manager, consultant, and researcher.

Nurse Midwife

A **nurse midwife** is educated in nursing and midwifery and in the United States, is certified by the American College of Nurse Midwives. The nurse midwife provides independent care for women during normal pregnancy, labor, and delivery. The nurse midwife practices in conjunction with a specific healthcare agency in which medical services are available if the client develops complications. The nurse midwife also may do routine

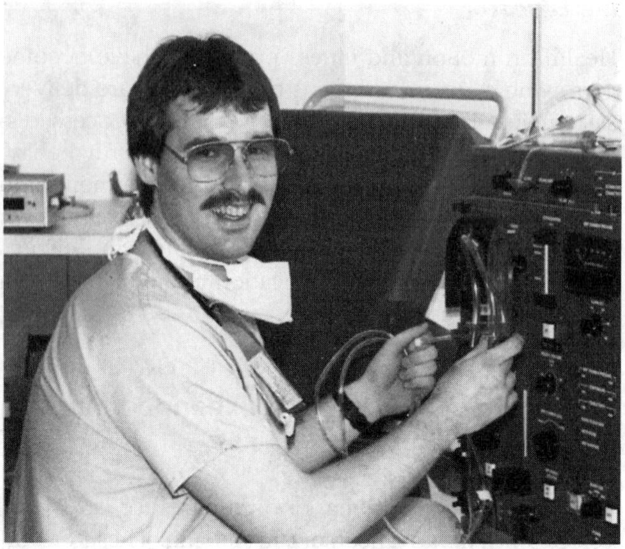

Figure 1-6 • Nurses in the renal dialysis unit specialize in helping clients with specific health problems.

Pap smears, breast examinations, and family planning. In Canada, midwives are trained as autonomous professionals and may or may not be nurses. Provincial Colleges of Midwives (similar to State Board of Nursing) are being established to set and enforce standards of education.

Nurse Anesthetist

Nurse anesthetists provide general anesthesia for clients undergoing surgery under the supervision of a physician prepared in anesthesiology. The nurse anesthetist is a registered nurse with advanced education in anesthesiology. He or she works in a hospital. There are no nurse anesthetists in Canada.

Nurse Researcher

Nurse researchers are responsible for the continued development and refinement of nursing knowledge and practice through the investigation of nursing problems. Nurse researchers have advanced education, usually at the doctoral level. They work in large teaching hospitals and research centers, such as the National Institute for Nursing Research in Bethesda, Maryland. Many nurse researchers also are employed in academic settings. All nurses have a responsibility to do research to improve nursing care. Even nurses without advanced preparation in research can work with individuals who have such training.

Nurse Administrator

Nurse administrators manage and control client care. They are responsible for specific nursing units and serve as liaisons between the staff and the director of nursing. Educational preparation for the role of nurse administrator requires at least a baccalaureate degree in nursing and, in some cases, a master's or doctoral degree.

Nurse Educator

The **nurse educator** role can be developed in a variety of settings, in schools of nursing or hospital staff development departments, for example. Advanced education is required, usually a master's degree in nursing. Teaching at the baccalaureate, master's, or doctoral level in nursing usually requires a doctoral degree. Nurse educators generally have a specific clinical specialty and advanced clinical experience. The individual in this career role must continue to maintain expertise in the practice setting, develop expert knowledge of theory, perfect classroom presentation style, and have in-depth knowledge of curriculum development and higher education.

Professional Nursing Practice

Standards of Practice

As nursing became an independent profession, it began to develop its own standards of practice. Standards of practice are essential because they serve as guidelines for providing and evaluating nursing care. Standards of practice ensure high-quality care and serve as criteria in legal questions of whether adequate care was provided. Standards of practice for the United States and Canada appear in the accompanying display.

ANA's standards include two lists: standards of care and standards of professional performance. Measurement criteria are printed in ANA's booklet: "Standards of Clinical Nursing Practice" (1991). The standards of care list designates professional nursing responsibilities as assessment, diagnosis, outcome identification, planning, implementation, and evaluation. These responsibilities are inherent in the nursing process and are discussed throughout the text. Standards of professional performance include quality of care, performance appraisal, education, collegiality, ethics, collaboration, research, and use of resources. All of these performance standards are integrated into the text under related discussions.

Similar standards of practice have been set by the CNA. The CNA's four central standards of nursing practice are the use of a conceptual model for nursing, effective use of the nursing process, initiation of helping relationships between the client and nurse, and the fulfillment of professional responsibilities. In addition, each province has written standards of nursing practice for which nurses are accountable.

Standards of Practice

American Nurses Association Standards of Clinical Nursing Practice Standards of Care

Standard I. Assessment
The nurse collects client health data.

Standard II. Diagnosis
The nurse analyzes the assessment date when determining diagnoses.

Standard III. Outcome identification
The nurse identifies expected outcomes individualized to the client

Standard IV. Planning
The nurse develops a plan of care that prescribes interventions to attain expected outcomes.

Standard V. Implementation
The nurse implements the interventions identified in the plan of care.

Standard VI. Evaluation
The nurse evaluates the client's progress toward attainment of outcomes.

Standards of Professional Performance.

Standard I. Quality of care
The nurse systematically evaluates the quality and effectiveness of nursing practice.

Standard II. Performance appraisal
The nurse evaluates his or her own nursing practice in relation to professional practice standards and relevant statutes and regulations.

Standard III. Education
The nurse acquires and maintains knowledge in nursing practice.

Standard IV. Collegiality
The nurse contributes to the professional development of peers, colleagues, and others.

Standard V. Ethics
The nurse's decisions and actions on behalf of clients are determined in an ethical manner.

Standard VI. Collaboration
The nurse collaborates with the client, significant others, and healthcare providers in providing client care.

Standard VII. Research
The nurse uses research findings in practice.

Standard VIII. Resource utilization
The nurse considers factors related to safety, effectiveness, and cost when planning and delivering client care.

Canadian Nurses Association Standards for Nursing Practice

Standard I.
Nursing practice requires that a conceptual model(s) for nursing be the basis for that practice.

Standard II.
Nursing practice requires the effective use of the nursing process.

Standard III.
Nursing practice requires that the helping relationship be the nature of client–nurse interaction.

Standard IV.
Nursing practice requires nurses to fulfill professional responsibilities.

From American Nurses Association (1991). *Standards of clinical nursing practice.* Kansas City, MO: Author. (Measurement Criteria for these standards are listed in their publication.)
From Canadian Nurses Association (1987). *A definition of nursing practice: Standards for nursing practice.* Ottawa: Author. (Sets of related behaviors are included with their standards.)

Nurse Practice Acts

Each state or province's **nurse practice act** defines the practice of nursing within that state or province. Requirements for licensure in the United States are set by the state licensing board in conjunction with the board of nursing. Requirements for registration in Canada are set by the provincial nursing association. New graduates must take and pass the nursing licensure examination to qualify for a nursing license or registration. With the emergence of more autonomous and expanded roles for nurses, many states have begun to revise their nurse practice acts to reflect those changes.

Nursing Organizations

As the nursing profession has developed and advanced, the organizations that have become an integral part of the profession also have increased. The number of associations continues to grow at local, state, and national levels. Nursing organizations may be related to a specialty or they may encompass all areas of nursing.

The organizations that involve most nurses or student nurses are the ANA, the CNA, the NLN, the National Student Nurses' Association (NSNA), and the Canadian University Nursing Students Association. The International Council of Nurses includes nurses throughout the world and addresses international healthcare concerns in nursing. See the display for a sample list of nursing specialty organizations.

American Nurses Association

The **ANA** is American nursing's professional organization. Membership in state constituents of the ANA is open only to registered professional nurses. The ANA is important because it makes decisions about the functions, activities, and goals of the nursing profession. The ANA is a voice for nurses because it acts on issues and wishes expressed by the membership (Kelly, 1985).

The ANA's functions and activities have been adapted or expanded in accordance with the changing needs of the profession and the public. Its goals, as stated in the current bylaws, are to work for the improvement of health standards and the availability of healthcare services for all, to foster high standards of nursing, and to stimulate and promote the professional development of nurses and advance their economic and general welfare (Kelly, 1985).

Canadian Nurses Association

The CNA, Canada's professional nursing organization, promotes high standards of practice and professional development for Canadian nursing. It functions in a similar fashion to the ANA.

National League for Nursing

The main purpose of the **NLN** is to ensure that the public need for nursing will be met. The NLN's members include nurses and other members of the health team, lay people, and agencies concerned with nursing education and service. The NLN works within the community and in association with individuals and groups outside of nursing. Nursing education programs seek accreditation through the NLN, signifying excellence in nursing education (Kelly, 1985).

National Student Nurses' Association

The NSNA, established in 1953, is the national organization for nursing students in the United States. Its goals are to contribute to nursing education to provide for the highest quality healthcare; to provide programs representative of fundamental and current professional interests and concerns; and to aid in the development of the whole person, his or her professional role, and his or her responsibility for the healthcare of people in all walks of life. The NSNA is autonomous, student-financed, and student-run. It serves as the voice of nursing students, speaking out on issues of concern to nursing students and the nursing profession (Kelly, 1985).

International Council of Nurses

The oldest international association of professional women is the **International Council of Nurses**. This nonpolitical group brings together people from many countries who have a common interest in nursing and the common purpose of developing nursing throughout the world (Kelly, 1985).

Current and Future Trends in Nursing Practice

Professional nursing is changing to reflect society's values. Examples of issues and trends that affect the profession include healthcare cost containment, scientific and technologic advances, and the women's movement.

Selected Nursing Specialty Organizations

Academy of Medical Surgical Nursing
American Association of Critical Care Nurses
American Association of Occupational Health Nurses
American Nephrology Nurses' Association
American Association of Neurosurgical Nurses
American Association of Nurse Anesthetists
American College of Nurse Midwives
Association of Operating Room Nurses
Nurses' Association of the American College of Obstetricians and Gynecologists
American Organization of Nurse Executives
American Society of Post Anesthesia Nurses
Association of Rehabilitation Nurses
International Association for Enterostomal Therapy
National Association of Pediatric Nurse Practitioners
National Intravenous Therapy Association
Oncology Nursing Society
American Assembly for Men in Nursing
American Association of Colleges of Nursing
American Association for the History of Nursing
American Association of Neuroscience Nurses
American Association of Nurse Attorneys
National Black Nurses Association
Canadian Association of Neuroscience Nurses
National Emergency Nurses Association
Canadian Association of Nurses in Oncology
Canadian Nursing Research Group
Canadian Clinical Nurses Specialty Group

Given the limits on resources, cost containment has become imperative. Clients enter the healthcare system acutely ill and leave much sooner than they did in the past, increasing the demand on nurses to ensure high quality, comprehensive care before discharge. The healthcare system must shift its focus: emphasis is increasingly placed on such areas as illness prevention, nutrition, and healthy lifestyles.

Nursing practice must change in response to current social transitions and directions. Current trends in nursing practice include the development of nursing centers, wellness promotion programs, care of the elderly, birthing centers, and home and community healthcare. As nursing practice changes, so too must the preparation of its practitioners.

Science and technology continue to affect the nursing profession. In the past, nurses relied on their experience, observation, and intuition. Today nursing has defined a body of knowledge specific to the profession and continues to develop this knowledge through research and practice. Contemporary nurses work in a more technical and more controversial healthcare delivery system that demands a high degree of skill. New ethical dilemmas and questions continue to arise in the process of providing healthcare.

The women's movement has affected nursing practice. The movement has brought attention to the need for equality and the recognition of universal human rights; as a result, nurses have become more assertive as professionals and are demanding more autonomy in client care. Some believe, however, that the movement has hurt nursing by encouraging women to enter nontraditional careers, thus diminishing the pool of capable women from which nursing has traditionally drawn.

Social issues and concerns are intimately linked to the provision of healthcare. Just as social issues of the past have affected today's nursing practice, the issues of today will influence what happens in the future. The profession must remain dynamic in its attempts to meet the healthcare needs of society.

Key Concepts

- The nursing profession has evolved over hundreds of years and continues to grow in response to the needs of society.
- The history of nursing has affected the modern profession's educational requirements, roles, and practice settings.
- Educational preparation and career opportunities in nursing are numerous. Diploma, associate, baccalaureate, master's, and doctoral degrees are available to those seeking a career in nursing.
- Nursing roles have expanded as nursing has developed more autonomy and gained status as a profession.
- Nurses function as caregivers, decision-makers, client advocates, managers, communicators, and educators.
- The practice of nursing is governed by individual state nurse practice acts that define the scope of nursing practice within each state.
- The ANA's standards of practice guide and direct the practice of nursing, designating nursing responsibilities to include collecting data, making nursing diagnoses, planning and implementing care, and evaluating outcomes of client care.
- Nursing organizations have emerged to represent nurses in general and nurses involved in specialties.
- The ANA is the professional organization for American nurses.
- Trends in nursing practice develop in response to changes in society. Trends affecting modern nursing practice include advances in technology, shorter hospital stays for clients, and the women's movement.

Critical Thinking Challenges

Now that you have studied this chapter, turn back to the situation at the beginning of the chapter, and consider the following questions.

1. *Describe your immediate reaction to this situation, and reflect on your choice of nursing as a career.*
2. *Examine the rationale or conclusions that led you to your decision to become a nurse.*
3. *Analyze what you think the nurse may be experiencing that resulted in the question asked in the situation.*
4. *List all the "pros" and "cons" of a career in nursing. Prioritize the list, and discuss your rationale for choosing or not choosing nursing as a career.*

References

American Nurses Association. (1991). *Standards of clinical practice.* Kansas City, MO: Author.

American Nurses Association. (1980). *Nursing: A social policy statement.* Kansas City, MO: Author.

Benner, P. (1984). *From novice to expert: Excellence and power in clinical nursing practice.* Menlo Park, CA: Addison-Wesley.

Canadian Nurses Association. (1987). *A definition of nursing practice: Standards for nursing practice.* Ottawa: Author.

Carpenito, L. (1995). *Nursing diagnosis: Application to clinical practice* (5th ed.). Philadelphia: J.B. Lippincott.

Dolan, A. J., Fitzpatrick, M. L., & Herrmann, E. K. (1983). *Nursing in society: A historical perspective* (15th ed.). Philadelphia: W.B. Saunders.

Kelly, L. Y. (1985). *Dimensions of professional nursing* (5th ed.). New York: Macmillan.

Mitchell, P. R., & Grippando, G. M. (1993). *Nursing perspectives and issues* (5th ed.). New York: Delmar Publishers.

National League for Nursing. (1978a). *Characteristics of baccalaureate education in nursing,* Pub. No. 15-1758. New York: Author.

National League for Nursing. (1978b). *Roles and competencies of graduate of diploma programs in nursing,* Pub. No. 16-1735. New York: Author.

National League for Nursing. (1978c). *Roles and competencies of the associate degree nurse on entry into practice,* Pub. No. 23-17211. New York: Author.

Nightingale, F. N. (1992). *Notes on nursing: What it is and what it is not.* Philadelphia: J.B. Lippincott (originial publication, 1859).

Ziemer, M. (1994). Advanced practice nursing. *The Pennsylvania Nurse, August,* 7.

Bibliography

Ashley, J. (1976). *Hospitals, paternalism, and the role of the nurse.* New York: Teachers College Press.

Buhler-Wilkerson, K., et al. (1987). Missing data: Nurses with their patients. *Nursing Research, 36*(1), 38–41.

Fairman, J. (1992). Watchful vigilance: Nursing care, technology, and the development of intensive care units. *Nursing Research, 41*(1), 56–60.

O'Brian, P. A. (1987). All a woman's life can bring: The domestic roots of nursing in Philadelphia, 1830–1885. *Nursing Research, 36*(1), 12–17.

Pokorney, M. E. (1992). An historical perspective of Confederate nursing during the Civil War, 1861–1865. *Nursing Research, 41*(1), 28–32.

Reverby, S. (1987). A caring dilemma: Womanhood and nursing in historical perspective. *Nursing Research, 36*(10), 5–11.

Thibodeau, J. A., & Hawkins, J. W. (1994). Moving Toward a Nursing Model in Advanced Practice. *Western Journal of Nursing Research, 16*(2), 205–218.

Widerquist, J. G. (1992). The spirituality of Florence Nightingale. *Nursing Research, 41*(1), 49–55.

Conceptual Frameworks and Nursing Theories

Key Terms	Learning Objectives

Key Terms

Change theory
Conceptual framework
Environments
Freezing
Functional health patterns
General Systems Theory
Health
Human needs
Maslow's hierarchy of human needs
Movement
Nursing theory
Person
Refreezing
Self-actualization
Theory
Unfreezing

Learning Objectives

Upon completion of this chapter, the student will be able to do the following:

- *Define nursing theory and conceptual framework.*
- *Recognize major nursing theories and their relevance to nursing practice.*
- *Discuss the relationship of nursing theories to non-nursing theories.*
- *Summarize non-nursing theories and their use in nursing.*
- *Discuss the relationship of functional health pattern typology to nursing.*

2

You are a nursing major completing your clinical laboratory in a local hospital. You are assigned to a unit that cares primarily for clients with diabetes mellitus and clients with cancer. The unit is quite large. Usually there are 40 clients on the unit. Each client room is private. Nurses care for five to six clients as part of their regular assignment. A nursing theory is being chosen for this unit.

In the first chapter you were introduced to the nursing profession. In this chapter you will add to your knowledge base by studying about theories and frameworks. You will learn why nurses do what they do in the way they do it. You will see how the approach to nursing may vary from facility to facility or agency to agency. The Critical Thinking Challenges at the end of the chapter will help you think through the previous situation and apply your knowledge about theories.

Although many people view nursing as a practice discipline, the *art* of practice is grounded in scientific principles. The science and practice of nursing are recognized as nursing's two major dimensions. Without nursing science, nursing practice could not exist (Rogers, 1970). Developing the science and practice of nursing is an essential component of the discipline that should generate knowledge that supports and advances professional nursing practice and healthcare. The contemporary move to use, refine, and or develop theoretical models for nursing practice and education reinforces the nursing profession's emphasis on theory-based practice.

The science of nursing incorporates the study of relationships among nurses, clients, and their environments within the context of health. Conceptual and theoretical nursing models generate knowledge that will improve nursing practice, guide nursing research, and facilitate the organization of curricula for all levels of nursing education (Marriner-Tomey, 1993; Fawcett, 1994). From nursing science, conceptual models and nursing theories evolve. As the nursing profession continues to develop its own body of knowledge, concepts and theories will continue to develop to support the practice component of nursing.

Through the years, nursing has incorporated ideas from non-nursing theories, such as systems, human needs, change, problem-solving, and decision-making theories. More recently, a functional health approach to nursing has become popular. The development and clarification of theoretical frameworks applied to the practice of professional nursing describes what nurses do and how they do it. This chapter provides an introduction to theory with definitions of conceptual frameworks, an overview of the major nursing theories and theorists, and a discussion of non-nursing theories and functional health patterns as methods of organizing and explaining nursing.

Nursing Theory

A **conceptual framework** or model is defined as a set of concepts and the propositions that integrate them into a meaningful configuration (Nye & Berardo, 1981). Conceptual frameworks are composed of concepts that describe ideas about individuals, groups, situations, and events of particular interest to a discipline, in this instance, nursing. The concepts and propositions of a conceptual model are highly abstract and general. Conceptual models have the "basic purpose of focusing, ruling some things in as relevant, and ruling others out due to their lesser importance" (Williams, 1979, p. 96). Barnum (1994) defines **theory** as "a construct that accounts for or organizes some phenomenon. A nursing theory, then describes or explains nursing" (p. 1). Theories are made up of concepts and propositions, similar to conceptual frameworks. A theory, however, goes one step beyond a conceptual framework: A theory is a way to relate concepts by using definitions that state significant relationships between concepts. The concepts and propositions of a theory are much more specific than those of a conceptual framework.

Nursing theory provides the foundation for nursing knowledge and gives direction to nursing practice. The development and future direction of nursing research should be guided by nursing theory. Barnum (1994) offers this vivid analogy to describe nursing theory:

> A theory is like a map of a territory as opposed to an aerial photograph. The map does not display the full terrain (buildings, moving vehicles, or grazing livestock); instead, it picks out those parts that are important for its purpose. If its aim is to guide travelers, the map will highlight roads; if its purpose is to describe the physical terrain, it shows mountains, plains, and rivers. But no map (or theory) reflects all that is contained within a phenomenon. Such a map would defeat its purpose: giving one a handle on the phenomenon. The handle is created by making the essential parts stand out in relief (p. 1).

Development of Nursing Theory

Conceptual frameworks and nursing theories are important to the nursing profession. The development of nursing theory has provided direction for the structure of professional nursing practice, education, and research. Chinn and Jacobs (1987) emphasize the importance of nursing theory to nursing students and practicing professionals, emphasizing that "Nursing theory ought to guide research and practice, generate new ideas, and differentiate the focus of nursing from other professions" (p. 145).

The introduction of nursing theory historically begins with Florence Nightingale (1860). She was the first nurse to write about a framework for nursing in her book *Notes on Nursing*. Nightingale conceptualized the nurse's role as manipulating the environment to facilitate and encourage the reparative process by attending to ventilation, warmth, light, diet, cleanliness, and noise. Her framework for nursing can be seen in the practice of professional nursing today in terms of clients' nutritional status and the importance of universal precautions.

Throughout history, nursing theories have become increasingly sophisticated. Some theories and frameworks are easily adapted to the practice setting, while others are better suited as a framework for research. Nurse theorists continue to contribute to the development of nursing's body of knowledge.

Four Major Concepts

Nurses have developed a variety of conceptual models and theoretical frameworks that provide explanations of the nursing discipline according to the nurse theorist's view. Nursing theories, as varied as they may be, have in common four central concepts: person, environment, health, and nursing. Each theory defines, relates, and emphasizes these concepts in different ways.

The concept of **person** in a broad sense refers to all human beings. People are the recipients of nursing care and include individuals, families, communities, and groups. **Environment** includes factors that affect the individual internally and externally. The environment includes not only the everyday surroundings of the person but also the settings where nursing care is provided. **Health** generally addresses the person's state of well-being. The concept of **Nursing** is central to all nursing theories. Definitions of nursing describe what nursing is, what nurses do, and what the role of the nurse is in his or her interaction with clients. Most nursing theories address each of the four central concepts implicitly of explicitly. Table 2-1 lists each major nursing theorist, the central purpose of each theory, and each theorist's definitions of the four major concepts.

text continues on page 31

Table 2-1 • Overview of Major Nursing Theorists

Nurse Theorist	Purpose	Person	Environment	Health	Nursing
Florence Nightingale (1860) "Notes on Nursing, What it is and what it is not"	To help individuals responsible for caring for the sick to "think how to nurse." The theory addresses fundamental needs of the sick and basic principles of good healthcare.	An individual with vital reparative processes to deal with disease	External conditions that affect life and the development of the individual. Focus is on ventilation, warmth, odors, and light.	The focus is on the reparative process of getting well.	The goal of nursing is to place the individual in the best condition for nature to act by manipulating the environment
Hildegard E. Peplau (1952) "Interpersonal Relations in Nursing"	To develop an interpersonal interaction between the client and the nurse	An organism striving to reduce tension generated by needs	Environment is implicitly defined. The interpersonal process is always included, and the psychodynamic milieu is given attention with emphasis on the client's culture and mores.	Ongoing human process that implies forward movement of personality and other ongoing human processes in the direction of creative, constructive, productive, personal, and community living.	Interpersonal therapeutic process. "It functions cooperatively with other human processes that make health possible for individuals in communities. Nursing is an educative instrument, a maturing force that aims to promote forward movement of personality.
Virginia Henderson (1955) "The Nature of Nursing"	To assist the client in gaining independence as rapidly as possible	Individual requiring assistance to achieve health and independence or a peaceful death. Mind and body are inseparable.	All external conditions and influences that affect life and development	Health is equated with independence. Health is viewed in terms of the client's ability to perform the 14 components of nursing care unaided. These include breathing, eating, drinking, maintaining comfort, sleeping, resting, clothing, maintaining body temperature, ensuring safety, communicating, worshiping, working, recreation, and continuing development.	Assists and supports the individual in life activities and the attainment of independence

(continued)

Table 2-1 *(continued)*

Nurse Theorist	Purpose	Person	Environment	Health	Nursing
Faye Glenn Abdellah (1960) "Patient-Centered Approaches to Nursing"	To deliver nursing care for the whole individual	The recipient of nursing care having physical, emotional, and sociologic needs that may be overt or covert	Not clearly defined or discussed in-depth. Some discussion indicates that clients interact with their environment, of which the nurse is a part.	Implicitly defined as a state when the individual has no unmet needs and no anticipated or actual impairments	Broadly grouped in "21 nursing problems," which center around needs for hygiene, comfort, activity, rest, safety, oxygen, nutrition, elimination, hydration, physical and emotional health promotion, interpersonal relationships, and development of self-awareness. Nursing care is doing something for an individual.
Ida Jean Orlando (1961) "The Dynamic Nurse–Patient Relationship"	To interact with clients to meet immediate needs by identifying client behaviors, reactions of the nurse, and nursing actions to be taken	Unique individual behaving verbally and nonverbally. Assumption is made that individuals may at times be able to meet their own needs for help and at other times be unable to do so.	Environment is not defined.	Does not define health. Assumption is made that if one is without emotional or physical discomfort and has a sense of well-being, these contribute to a healthy state.	Professional nursing is conceptualized as finding out and meeting the client's immediate need for help. Medicine and nursing are viewed as distinctly different.
Lydia E. Hall (1964) "Nursing—What is it?"	To provide professional nursing care to people past the acute stage of illness	Client is composed of body, pathology, and person. People set their own goals and are capable of learning and growing.	The environment should facilitate the achievement of the client's personal goals.	Development of a mature, self-identity that assists in the conscious selection of actions that facilitate growth.	Caring is the primary function of the nurse. Professional nursing is most important during the client's period of recuperation.
Ernestine Weidenbach (1964) "Clinical Nursing—A Helping Art"	To assist individuals in overcoming obstacles that prevent meeting healthcare needs	Any individual who is receiving help (care, instruction, or advice) from a member of the health profession or from a worker in the field of health.	Not specifically addressed	Not defined. Concepts of nursing, client, and need for help and the relationships among these concepts imply health-related concerns in the nurse–client relationship (Marriner-Tomey, p. 245).	A functioning human being who acts, thinks, and feels. All actions, thoughts, and feelings underlie what the nurse does.

(continued)

Table 2-1 *(continued)*

Nurse Theorist	Purpose	Person	Environment	Health	Nursing
Myra Estrin Levin (1973) "Conservation Model"	To use conservation activities aimed at optimal use of client's resources	A holistic being	Viewed broadly and includes all experiences of the individual	The maintenance of unity and integrity of the client	A discipline rooted in the organic dependency of the individual human being on his or her relationships with other human beings.
Dorothy E. Johnson (1980) "The Behavioral System Model for Nursing"	To reduce stress so the client can recover as quickly as possible	A system of interdependent parts with patterned, repetitive, and purposeful ways of behaving.	All forces that impact on the person and that influence the behavioral system	Focus on person, not illness. Health is a dynamic state influence by biologic, psychological, and social factors.	Promotion of behavioral system, balance, and stability. An art and a science providing external assistance before and during system balance disturbances.
Martha E. Rogers (1970) "The Science of Unitary Man"	To assist the client in achieving a maximum level of wellness	Unitary man, a four-dimensional energy field	Encompasses all that is outside any given human field. Person exchanging matter and energy.	Not specifically addressed, but emerges out of interaction with the human and the environment, is forward moving, and maximizes human potential	A learned profession that is both science and art. The professional practice of nursing is creative and imaginative and exists to serve people.
Dorothea E. Orem (1971) "Nursing: Concepts of Practice"	To provide care and to assist the client to attain self-care	Biopsychosocial being capable of self-care. Includes physical, psychological, interpersonal, and social aspects of human functioning.	Internal and external stimuli. Requisites for self-care have their origins in human beings and the environment.	State of wholeness or integrity of human beings, including physical, mental, and social well-being	A creative effort of one human being to help another human being. consists of three nursing systems, wholly compensatory, partially compensatory, and supportive/educative.
Imogene M. King (1971) "Open Systems Model"	To use communication to help the client reestablish a positive adaptation to his or her environment	Biopsychosocial being	Internal and external environment continually interacting to assist in the adjustment to change.	A dynamic life experience with continued goal attainment and adjustment to stressors.	Perceiving, thinking, relating, judging, and acting with an individual who comes to a nursing situation

(continued)

Table 2-1 *(continued)*

Nurse Theorist	Purpose	Person	Environment	Health	Nursing
Joyce Travelbee (1966, 1971) "Interpersonal Aspects of Nursing"	To assist individuals, families, communities, and groups to prevent or cope with illness and regain health	A unique, irreplaceable individual who is in a continuous process of becoming, evolving, and changing.	Health includes the individual's perceptions of health and the absence of disease.	Not explicitly defined	An interpersonal process where-by the professional nurse practitioner assists an individual, family, or community to prevent or cope with the experience of illness and suffering and, if necessary, to find meaning in these experiences
Betty Neuman, (1972) "The Neuman Systems Model"	To address the effects of stress and reactions to stress on the development and maintenance of health	A client system that is composed of physiologic, psychological, sociocultural, and environmental variables	The internal and external forces surrounding humans at any time	Health or wellness exists if all parts and subparts are in harmony with the whole person.	A unique profession concerned with all the variables affecting an individual's response to stressors.
Sister Callista Roy (1979)	To identify the types of demands placed on a client and the client's adaptation to the demands	A biopsychosocial being and the recipient of nursing care.	All conditions, circumstances, and influences surrounding and affecting the development of an organism or groups of organisms	The person encounters adaptation problems in changing environments.	A theoretical system of knowledge that prescribes a process of analysis and action related to the care of the ill or potentially ill person.
Jean Watson (1979) "Nursing: Human Science and Human Care"	To focus on curative factors derived from a humanistic perspective and from scientific knowledge	A valued person to be care for, respected, nurtured, understood, and assisted; a fully functional, integrated self	Social environment, caring, and the culture of caring impact on health.	Physical, mental, and social well-being	A human science of people and human health; illness experiences that are mediated by profession, personal, scientific, aesthetic, and ethical human care transactions
Rosemarie Rizzo Parse (1981) "Man—Living—Health: A Theory of Nursing"	To focus on humans as living unity and humans' qualitative participation with health experience	A major reason for nursing's existence, evidenced by a "pattern of patterns of relating" (p. 26)	"Man and environment interchange energy to create what is in the world, and man chooses the meaning given to the situations he creates" (p. 27).	A lived experience that is a process of being and becoming	"Nursing practice is directed toward illuminating and mobilizing family interrelationships in light of the meaning assigned to health and its possibilities as language in the cocreated patterns of relating" (p. 82).

Concerns About Nursing Theory

Questions have been raised about the applicability and need for nursing theory. One of the most critical arguments related to theory development is that there is not enough evidence that nursing theories are grounded in practice. Those arguing this view believe that theories look good on paper but cannot be applied in the practice setting. Others have demonstrated by numerous examples how nursing theories and models have been used as guides or organizing frameworks for nursing practice (Firlit, 1990). Research in the application of nursing theory to practice settings would provide valuable data to resolve this argument.

Because nursing is a multifaceted profession, some have questioned whether only one theory is needed, when probably theories from basic science and social sciences are needed. Cohesive arguments can be made in support of one theory or multidisciplinary theories (Stevens, 1985). Differences in opinions and beliefs regarding single- or multiple-theory approaches stem from differing philosophies about what constitutes nursing science and practice.

Studies and discussions on theory development in nursing have proliferated since the publication of *Theory Development: What? Why? How?* by the National League for Nursing in 1975 and will continue as the nursing profession continues to develop a scientific base for practice. No definitive answer to the questions asked about nursing theory exists, but all nursing theories challenge the reader to approach the world of nursing in different and increasingly complex ways (Moccia, 1986).

Non-Nursing Theories Used in Nursing

The nursing profession also has used non-nursing theories to guide practice. The non-nursing theories reviewed in this chapter include general systems theory, human needs theory, and change theory. Relationships among nursing and non-nursing theories are included. Other non-nursing theories in relation to the nursing process are presented in Chapter 9.

General Systems Theory

The general systems theory, or a systems framework, provides another approach for studying individuals in their environments. Many disciplines have used general systems theory. **General systems theory** includes purpose, content, and process. It explains breaking down the "whole" and analyzing the parts. The relationships between the parts of the whole are examined to learn how they work together.

General systems theory was developed by von Bertalanffy (1969; 1976) and assumes the following:

- All systems must be goal directed.
- A system is more than the sum of its parts.
- A system is ever changing, and any change in one part affects the whole.
- Boundaries are implicit and in human systems are open and dynamic (von Bertalanffy, 1969; 1976)

Nursing Theorists' Use of General Systems Theory

Examples of nursing theories that have used the systems approach to client care include Roy's adaptation model (1980), Hall's philosophy of nursing (1964), Neuman's healthcare systems model (1972), Johnson's behavioral model (1968), and Parse's theory for nursing (1981). These theories are summarized in Table 2-1.

Human Needs Theory: Maslow's Hierarchy of Human Needs

Human needs are any physiologic or psychological factors necessary for a healthy existence. The most prominent theorist to focus on human needs has been Abraham Maslow (1970). Maslow's hierarchy of human needs states that all humans are born with instinctive needs, which he grouped into five categories. These needs are arranged in order of importance from those essential for physical survival to those necessary to develop to the fullest human potential. Maslow's hierarchy of human needs provides a framework for recognizing and prioritizing basic human needs.

Maslow's hierarchy is constructed as a pyramid, as shown in Figure 2-1. Just as a pyramid must be constructed from its base to its apex, people must meet lower-level needs to some degree before they can address higher-level needs. A person is not motivated by all five categories of human needs at the same time. The category most relevant to the person's circumstances at a particular time is the primary motivator. Meeting needs is a dynamic process and involves the continual resolution of, progression beyond, and return to any given category of needs.

Human needs are motivational forces (Yura & Walsh, 1988). The motivational strength and manner of expression of these needs are influenced by culture, socioecomonic factors, personal values, and health state. All people develop behaviors that help them meet their needs. They can learn to delay meeting needs and modify the specific behaviors that satisfy a need, depending on the need's motivational strength. If a need goes unmet, physical illness, psychological disequilibrium, or death can occur.

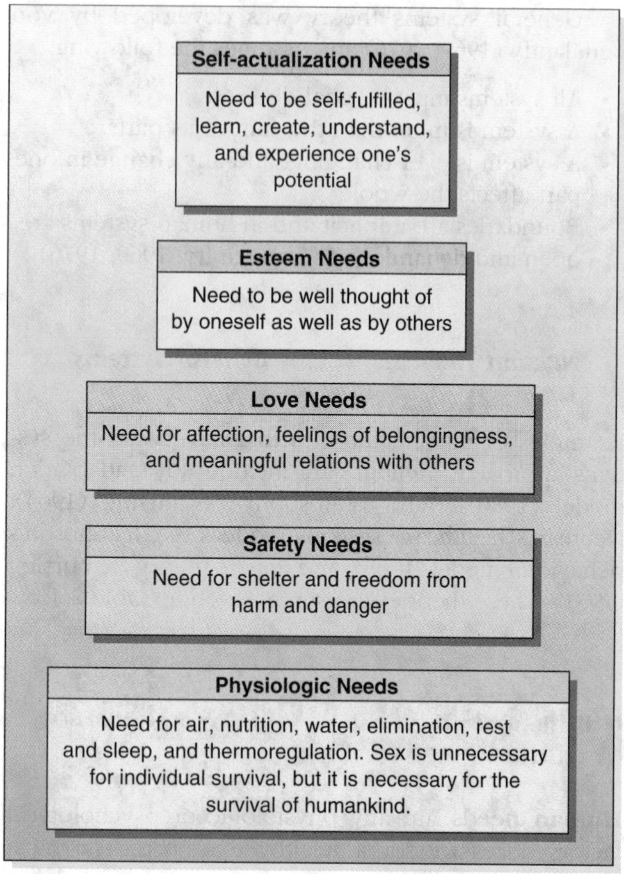
Self-actualization Needs
Need to be self-fulfilled, learn, create, understand, and experience one's potential
Esteem Needs
Need to be well thought of by oneself as well as by others
Love Needs
Need for affection, feelings of belongingness, and meaningful relations with others
Safety Needs
Need for shelter and freedom from harm and danger
Physiologic Needs
Need for air, nutrition, water, elimination, rest and sleep, and thermoregulation. Sex is unnecessary for individual survival, but it is necessary for the survival of humankind.

Figure 2-1 • *A pyramid represents Maslow's heirarchy of human needs. According to Maslow, basic physiologic needs, such as nutrition and water, must be met before the person can move on to higher-level needs. Nursing helps people to meet needs they cannot meet by themselves.*

Physiologic Needs

Physiologic needs are the fundamental motivating force in human existence and provide the base for Maslow's pyramid. Existence requires oxygen, food, water, elimination, activity, rest, temperature maintenance, and sexuality. Nurses assess the client's ability to meet his or her physiologic needs and identify the nature and degree of nursing interventions necessary to enable the person to satisfy these needs.

Air. Oxygen is essential for the body's metabolic processes. Satisfying this need requires a properly functioning respiratory and cardiovascular system.

Nutrition. Proper nutrition is essential for energy production and the body's metabolic processes. Satisfying this need requires adequate food and a properly functioning gastrointestinal tract.

Water. Fluids are necessary for metabolic processes of the body, and proper fluid balance is critical for life.

Elimination. Elimination, a crucial part of the metabolic process, enables the body to dispose of waste products and maintain fluid and electrolyte balance.

Sleep and Rest. Sleep and rest are necessary for the body to revitalize itself. People vary considerably in the total amount, frequency, and duration of sleep and rest periods required. Requirements for sleep and rest also vary throughout the lifespan. Failure to meet this need leads to fatigue, irritability, behavioral changes, difficulty concentrating, and eventual exhaustion.

Thermoregulation. Temperature maintenance is necessary for life. Extremes in either direction can lead to death. The body monitors and maintains its temperature through sensors in the skin, hypothalamus, and the effector system. Any alteration in these structures can affect temperature regulation. The body can adapt to environmental temperatures within broad limits, but age and health status greatly affect this capacity.

Sex. Sexual relations are not essential for an individual's survival but are necessary for the continuation of the human race. The importance of this need varies widely among people. Meeting this need can affect how the person deals with higher-order needs, such as love, belonging, and self-esteem.

Safety Needs

After basic physiologic needs are met, the person must address safety needs. Humans need to be physically safe and free from the fear and anxiety that can result from a lack of security and protection. Safety often can be a dominant motivating need. For example, in a country at war, safety becomes a primary motivating force as long as physiologic needs are met at a minimal level. The same is true during natural disasters, such as floods or tornadoes. Such events cause major disruptions in personal, family, and societal routines and can lead to chaos. According to Maslow (1970), an essential aspect of safety is the need for predictability and routine.

Love Needs

The need for love and belonging is the next tier on the pyramid. After a sense of safety is achieved, people need to feel that they belong and are loved to avoid loneliness and isolation. To meet this need, a person must give and receive love.

Esteem Needs

According to Maslow (1970), there are two types of esteem needs: esteem derived from others and self-esteem. People need to know that others think well of them and admire and respect them. Self-esteem is a person's sense of his or her own adequacy and worth. To be genuine, it must be firmly grounded in a realistic appraisal of strengths and weaknesses. If esteem needs go unmet, the person faces a life characterized by self-doubt and feelings of helplessness and worthlessness. What others value in a person and what that person values in himself or herself vary greatly and are influenced by cultural, social, and psychological variables.

Self-Actualization Needs

According to Maslow (1970), the need for **self-actualization** is the innate need to realize fully all of one's abilities and qualities, to develop one's maximum potential. Maslow sees this as a never-ending process. Although it is affected by early life experiences, individuals have the capacity to change and reach a stage of optimal psychological health as they strive for self-actualization.

Nursing Theorists' Perceptions of Human Needs

Through the years, nursing theories have incorporated ideas from human needs theory. Typically, nurses identify a client's needs and base the care they deliver on this information. Human needs theory led to the development of nursing models and frameworks for holistic nursing discussed earlier in this chapter. Examples nurse theorists who have used human needs theory in their work are given in Table 2-2.

Table 2-2 • Nurse Theorists and Human Needs

Nurse Theorist	Integration of Human Needs
Florence Nightingale	In *Notes on Nursing* (1860/1946), Nightingale wrote that nurses should create an environment in which healing could take place; the need for a positive environment, free from filth and vermin, is as paramount to the client's recovery.
Virginia Henderson	Henderson (1966) described 14 principles of nursing that focus on physiologic, social, psychological, and spiritual needs.
Ida Jean Orlando	The concept of need is central to Orlando's theory, which focuses on clients and their unmet needs. Orlando believed that the purpose of nursing is to provide the assistance that a client requires to meet his or her needs.
Dorothea Orem	Orem placed human needs into three categories: universal self-care requisites, developmental self-care requisites, and health deviations. Universal healthcare requisites include the need for air, food, water, elimination, and safety. Developmental requisites address human needs throughout the lifespan. Finally, health deviations addressed needs that developed as a result of an illness.
Imogene M. King	King viewed nursing as a process that involves action, reaction, interaction, and transaction. The nurse operates on the belief that each person is an open system who interacts with interpersonal and societal systems. The client and nurse establish a relationship to cope with or improve a health state.
Sister Callista Roy	Roy's adaptation model identifies five essential elements: person, goal of nursing, nursing activities, health, and environment. Each person constantly interacts with the environment. She includes four modes of adaption: physiologic needs (adaptation to satisfy basic needs), self-concept (adaptation to maintain psychological integrity), role function (adaptation to society's roles and duties), and interdependence (adaptation to enable need fulfillment; support systems).
Martha E. Rogers	Rogers (1970) described nursing as a humanistic science dedicated to compassionate concern for maintaining and promoting health. Preventing illness and rehabilitating the sick and disabled are primary goals.
Lydia E. Hall	Hall saw nursing as having different functions in three interlocking circles: care circle (client's body), cure circle (disease), and core circle (client's inner feelings and motivations). The nurse helps the client become aware of his or her needs, feelings, and motivations. It then becomes the client's task to set goals and priorities. This learning process encourages maximum growth. The client freely expresses ideas regarding the disease process and his or her own needs, and through this expression the client gains self-identity.
Jean Watson	Watson believed that caring is central to nursing. Watson's hierarchy of 10 carative factors is similar to Maslow's: Clients must satisfy lower-order needs before attaining higher ones.
Faye Glenn Abdellah	Abdellah described nursing as a service to people, families, and society. The nurse helps people, sick or well, to cope with their health needs. In Abdellah's model, nursing care means providing information to the client or doing something to the client with the goal of meeting needs or alleviating an impairment.

Change Theory

People grow and change throughout their lives. This growth and change is evident in the dynamic nature of basic human needs and how they are met. Change happens daily. It is subtle, continuous, and manifested in everyday life events and in more disruptive life events. Reactions to change are grounded in our basic human needs for self-esteem, safety, and security.

Change involves modification or alteration in something and may be planned or unplanned. Although a variety of change theories exist, Kurt Lewin developed the classic theory of change. Lewin's (1962) change theory identifies six components of change:

1. Recognition of the area where change is needed
2. Analysis of a situation to determine what forces exist to maintain the situation as it is and what forces are working to change it
3. Identification of methods by which change can occur
4. Recognition of the influence of group mores or customs on change
5. Identification of the methods that the reference group uses to bring about change
6. The actual process of change

Lewin (1962) identified three states of change: unfreezing, movement, and refreezing. **Unfreezing** is the recognition of the need for change and the dissolution of previously held patterns of behavior. **Movement** is the shift of behavior toward a new and more healthful pattern. Movement marks the initiation of change. **Refreezing** is the long-term solidification of the new pattern of behavior.

The healthcare delivery system and the practice of professional nursing are continually changing and evolving. Nurses must continually recognize the dynamic nature of change and assist individuals and groups to adapt to change (Tiffany, 1994; Lutjens & Tiffany, 1994). The impact of change on basic human needs is constant and should be recognized to best use this framework to organize nursing care.

Nursing Theorists' Use of Change Theory

Change theory offers insight into the expected behaviors that evolve when significant change occurs within an environment. Nurse theorists have incorporated various aspects of change theory in their nursing theories. For example, Peplau's (1952) use of the nursing process applies aspects of change theory as client needs are assessed and needed changes in specific patterns of behavior are determined.

Functional Health Patterns As a Framework for Nursing

The nurse deals with the "whole" person: the physical, psychological, interpersonal, and spiritual aspects of his or her life. The whole person concept emphasizes a holistic approach to professional nursing. The client's family and community are considered in holistic practice, which has become important because the community has become a common location for the delivery of healthcare.

Nursing faculty and clinicians have struggled with a way of organizing information that is more nursing focused. In addition to specific nursing theories, another way to organize nursing information in a holistic way is by using Marjory Gordon's **functional health patterns**. These patterns delineate the human needs of the person, family, community, and group. The patterns, which focus on behaviors that occur with time, present a total picture of the client, rather than just a small part of his or her life. Functional health patterns represent basic health needs, and they develop as people strive to meet their needs. These patterns are unique because they are interrelated: One pattern often provides answers to another. No pattern can be studied as a separate category.

Gordon's patterns are consistent with the human needs philosophy and general systems theory and can provide a framework for holistic nursing assessment (Fig. 2-2). Gordon provides a comprehensive discussion of client needs; Maslow's hierarchy offers a rationale for determining the order in which needs should be addressed; and systems theory requires an analysis of relationships, purposes, reasons, and tasks.

The *Health perception–health management* pattern is the first in a series of 11 patterns addressed by Gordon (1994). This pattern focuses on health values and beliefs and the resources in the community available to meet health needs. It is based on the awareness that although nursing promotes health as one of its primary functions, the client actually manages his or her own health. Success in meeting human needs by the person, family, and community in this pattern relies heavily on culture, societal beliefs, personal expectations, and one's own health. The client's family may play an important part in this function because a family member may make major health decisions for other family members.

The *nutritional/metabolic* health pattern is the second function identified by Gordon. Life cannot be sustained without meeting human needs in this category. People establish patterns for meeting these needs early in life, and many of these behaviors are learned in the family setting. It is not simply a matter of eating; it is a complex pattern of food knowledge, food preparation,

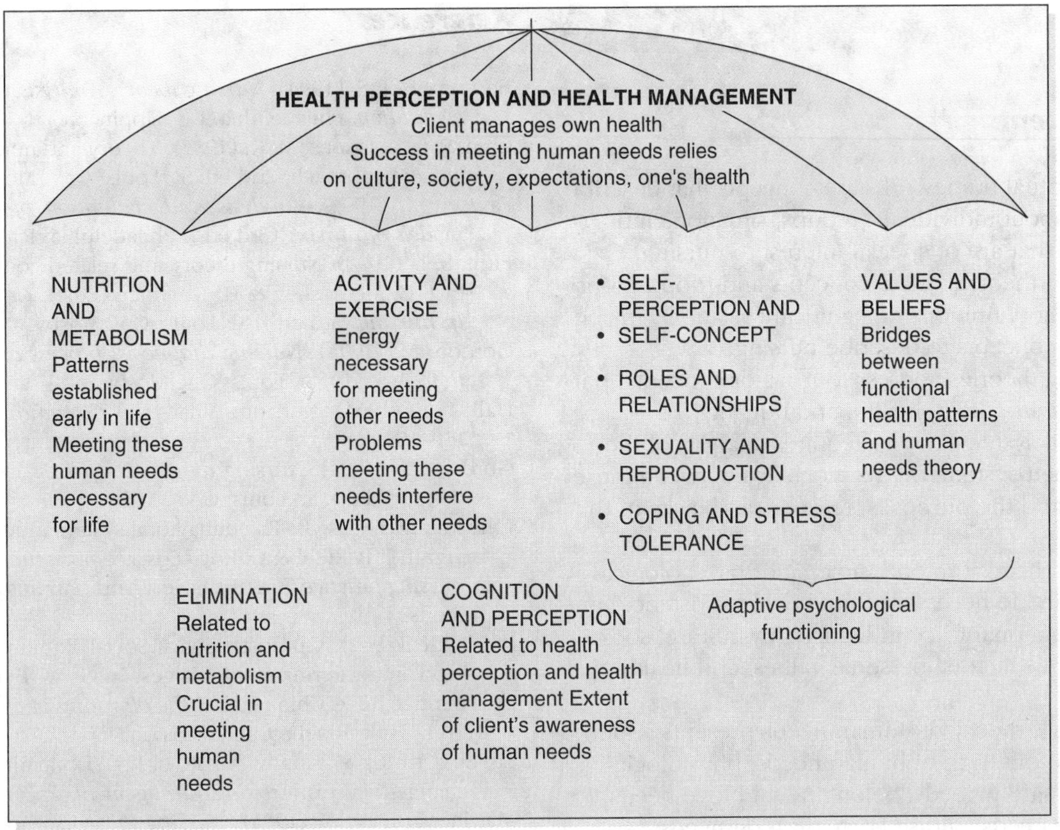
HEALTH PERCEPTION AND HEALTH MANAGEMENT
Client manages own health
Success in meeting human needs relies
on culture, society, expectations, one's health
NUTRITION AND METABOLISM
Patterns established early in life
Meeting these human needs necessary for life
ACTIVITY AND EXERCISE
Energy necessary for meeting other needs
Problems meeting these needs interfere with other needs
• SELF-PERCEPTION AND
• SELF-CONCEPT
• ROLES AND RELATIONSHIPS
• SEXUALITY AND REPRODUCTION
• COPING AND STRESS TOLERANCE
VALUES AND BELIEFS
Bridges between functional health patterns and human needs theory
ELIMINATION
Related to nutrition and metabolism
Crucial in meeting human needs
COGNITION AND PERCEPTION
Related to health perception and health management Extent of client's awareness of human needs
Adaptive psychological functioning

Figure 2-2 • *Relationship of functional health patterns, human needs theory, and delivery of nursing care. The first function, health perception and health management, forms an umbrella for the remaining ten.*

financial limits, and cultural ideas. The community is important because of the resources it can offer.

The third function, *elimination*, is closely related to nutrition and metabolism, and often these areas can be assessed simultaneously. Both are crucial to understanding the client's needs.

Energy must be expended to meet human needs; this is examined in *activity and exercise*. Clients must be evaluated for their ability to engage in self-care activities to meet basic physiologic needs. Another aspect involves determining how much energy they have to ensure the safety of their environment. For example, the requirements for an elderly person living alone are vastly different from those of a young adult living in an intact family. The relationship to health perception –health management is evident because the nurse must learn the importance the client places on the person, family, or community. The community may not have adequate transportation for its members to engage in such activities. Problems meeting needs in this category may affect other needs, such as human companionship and food.

Sleep and rest are primary human needs. Patterns begin to develop at birth and change throughout life. Newborns, for example, spend a great deal of time sleeping. Parents can reveal the amount of time and how the infant sleeps, thus showing a pattern. The person's environment may help or hinder this category of needs. The *cognitive–perceptual* pattern examines the extent of the client's awareness of human needs, which ties in with the first pattern. Lifespan considerations are important when evaluating this pattern.

The last functions, *self-perception–self-concept, role–relationship, sexuality–reproductive, coping–stress tolerance*, and *value–belief*, involve a complex group of needs that are intimately related to the person's level of adaptive psychological functioning. Adequate examination of these patterns requires assessment of the client's intrapsychic and interpersonal functioning, which means looking at the client in relation to himself or herself, the family, significant others, and the community.

Values and beliefs provide the bridge between functional health patterns and human needs and other theories. Understanding the client's value and belief system is crucial: this information tells the nurse the importance of each human need as a motivating factor in the client's life, his or her life as a community member, and the life of his or her family.

Key Concepts

- Conceptual frameworks are concepts that describe ideas about individuals, groups, situation, and events that are of special interest to nursing.
- Nursing theories relate concepts and propositions by using definitions of significant relationships between concepts to describe nursing.
- Nursing theories address four major concepts: person, environment, health, and nursing.
- General systems theory requires analysis of the parts of a system, the relationships between these parts, and the purposes, reasons, and tasks of the system.
- Human needs (any physiologic or psychological factor in life necessary for a healthy existence) are a motivational force influenced by culture, socioeconomic factors, personal values, and health status.
- Maslow's theory of human needs presents a hierarchical ordering of human needs: physiologic needs, safety needs, belonging and love needs, esteem needs, and self-actualization needs.
- Change theory recognizes the dynamic nature of growth and the need for constant reevaluation of nursing practice.
- Using functional health patterns is a holistic approach to nursing. Patterns delineate the human needs of the client, family, and community.
- Functional health patterns provide a comprehensive discussion of client needs by incorporating other nursing and non-nursing theories.

Critical Thinking Challenges

Now that you have learned about conceptual frameworks and nursing theories, turn to the situation about the nursing unit in the beginning of the chapter and consider these questions.

1. *Select a nursing theory you believe would best apply to this type of unit, and state your rationale.*
2. *Illustrate how the four concepts of the theory selected might be addressed on this unit.*
3. *Compare arguments for and against using your chosen theory in this practice setting.*
4. *Formulate a plan for how you might convince your colleagues that this theory applies to the practice setting.*

References

Barnum, B. J. S. (1994). *Nursing theory: Analysis, application, evaluation.* Philadelphia: J.B. Lippincott.

Chin, P. L., & Jacobs, M. K. (1987). Theory and nursing. A systematic approach, 2nd ed. St. Louis: C. V. Mosby.

Fawcett, J. (1994). *Analysis and evaluation of conceptual models of nursing* (3rd ed.). Philadelphia: F.A. Davis.

Firlit, S. L. (1990). Nursing theory and related considerations. In J. C. McCloskey & H. K. Grace (Eds.), *Current issues in nursing* (3rd ed.). St. Louis: C.V. Mosby.

Gordon, M. (1994). *Nursing diagnosis, process and application* (3rd ed.). St. Louis: C.V. Mosby.

Hall, L. E. (1964). Nursing: What is it? *Canadian Nurse, 60,* 150–154.

Gordon, M. (1994). *Nursing diagnosis: Process and application* (3rd ed.). St. Louis: C.V. Mosby.

Johnson, D. E. (1968). The behavioral system model for nursing. In J. P. Riehl & C. Roy (Eds.), *Conceptual models for nursing practice* (3rd. ed.). New York: Appleton-Century-Crofts.

Lewin, K. (1962). Quasi-stationary Social Equilibria and the Problem of Permanent Changes. In G. W. Bennis, K. D. Bennee, & R. Chin (Eds.), *The planning of change.* New York: Holt, Rinehart and Winston.

Lutjens, L. R., & Tiffany, C. R. (1994) Evaluating planned change theories. *Nursing Management, 25*(3), 54–57.

Marriner-Tomey, A. (1993). *Nursing theorists and their work* (3rd ed.). St. Louis: C.V. Mosby.

Maslow, A. H. (1970). *Motivation and personality* (2nd ed.). New York: Harper & Row.

Moccia, P. (Ed) (1986). *New approach to theory development.* New York: National League for Nursing.

Neuman, B. (1972). *The Neuman systems model: Application to nursing education and practice.* New York: Appleton-Century-Crofts.

Nightingale, F. (1860). *Notes on nursing: What it is and what it is not.* London: Harrison & Sons.

Nye, F. I., & Berardo, F. N. (1981). *Emerging conceptual frameworks in family analysis.* New York: Macmillan.

Parse, R. R. (1981). *Man-living-health: Theory of nursing.* New York: John Wiley and Sons.

Peplau, H. E.(1952). *Interpersonal relations in nursing.* New York: Putnam.

Rogers, M. E. (1970). *An introduction to the theoretical basis of nursing.* Philadelphia: F.A. Davis.

Roy, C. (1980). *The Roy adaptation model.* In J. P. Riehl & C. Roy (Eds.), *Conceptual models for nursing practice.* New York: Appleton-Century Crofts.

Stevens, B. J. (1985). Nursing theories: One or many? In J. C. McCloskey & H. K. Grace (Eds.), *Current issues in nursing* (2nd ed.). St. Louis: Blackwell Mosby Book Distributors.

Tiffany, C. R. (1994) Analysis of planned change theories. *Nursing Management, 25*(2), 60–62.

von Bertalanffy, L. (1969). *General system theory.* New York: George Braziller.

von Bertalanffy, L. (1976). *Perspectives on general system theory: Scientific-philosophical studies.* New York: George Braziller.

Williams, C. A. (1979). *The nature and development of conceptual frameworks.* In Downs, F. S., & Fleming, J. W., *Issues in nursing research.* New York: Appleton-Century-Crofts.

Yura, H., & Walsh, M. (1988). *The nursing process: Assessing, planning, implementing, and evaluating* (5th ed.). Norwalk, CT: Appleton & Lange.

Bibliography

Abdellah, F. G. (1960). *Patient centered approaches to nursing.* New York: Macmillan.

Barrett, E. A. (1994) *Rogerian scientists, artists, revolutionaries.* NLN Publication (15-2610): 61-87. New York: National League for Nursing.

Bunting, S. (1993). *Rosemarie Parse: Theory of human becoming.* Newburg Park: Sage.

Conway, J. (1994) Reflection, the art and science of nursing and the theory-practice gap. *British Journal of Nursing, 3*(3), 114–118.

Elkan, R., & Robinson, J. (1993). Project 2000: The gap between theory and practice. *Nurse Education Today, 13*(4), 295–298.

Evans, C. L. S. (1993). *Imogene King: A conceptual framework for nursing.* Newbury Park: Sage.

Forchuk, C. (1993). *Hildegard E. Peplau: Interpersonal nursing theory.* Newbury Park: Sage.

Hagerman, Z. J., & Tiffany, C. R. (1994). Evaluation of two planned change theories. *Nursing Management, 25*(4), 57–60, 62.

Hartweg, D. L. (1993). *Dorothea Orem: Self-care deficit theory.* Newbury Park: Sage.

Henderson, V. (1966). *The nature of nursing.* New York: Macmillan.

King, I. M. (1971). *Toward a theory of nursing.* New York: Wiley.

Levine, M. C. (1973). *An introduction to clinical nursing* (2nd. ed.). Philadelphia: F.A. Davis.

Lutjens, L. R. J. (1993). *Martha Rogers: The science of unitary human beings.* Newbury Park: Sage.

Lutjens, L. R. J. (1993). *Callista Roy: An adaptation model.* Newbury Park: Sage.

Marchione, J. (1993). *Margaret Newman: Health as expanding consciousness.* Newburg Park: Sage.

Montague, A. (1970). *The direction of human development.* New York: Hawthorne.

Nursing Theories Conference Group. (1980). *Nursing theories: The base for professional nursing practice.* Englewood Cliffs, NJ: Prentice Hall.

O'Connor, N. (1993). *Paterson and Zderad: Humanistic nursing theory.* Newbury Park: Sage.

Orem, D. E. (1971). *Nursing: Concepts of practice* (3rd. ed.). New York: McGraw-Hill.

Orem, D. E. (1990). *Nursing: Concepts of practice* (3rd. ed.). St. Louis: Mosby–Year Book.

Orlando, I. J. (1961). *The dynamic nurse-patient relationship: Function, process, and principles.* New York: Putnam.

Reed, S. (1993). *Betty Neuman: The systems model.* Newbury Park: Sage.

Reynolds, C. L., & Leininger, M. M. (1993). *Madeleine Leininger: Cultural care diversity and universality theory.* Newbury Park: Sage.

Rogers, M. E. (1994) *Nursing science evolves.* NLN Publication (15-2610): 3–9, New York: National League for Nursing.

Schmieding, N. J. (1993). *Ida Jean Orlando: A nursing process theory.* Newbury Park: Sage.

Selanders, L. C. (1993). *Florence Nightingale: An environmental adaptation theory.* Newbury Park: Sage.

Travelbee, J. (1971). *Interpersonal aspects of nursing.* Philadelphia: F.A. Davis.

Vander, A. J., Sherman, J. H., & Luciano, D. S. (1993). *Human physiology: The mechanisms of body function* (6th ed.). San Francisco: McGraw Hill.

Watson, J. (1985). *Nursing:The philosophy and science of caring.* Boulder, CO: University Press.

Wright, P. S., Piazza, D., Holcombe, J., & Foote, A. (1994) A comparison of three theories of nursing used as a guide for the nursing care of an 8-year-old child with leukemia. *Journal of Pediatric Oncology Nursing, 11*(1), 14–19.

Ethical and Legal Concerns

Key Terms	Learning Objectives
Advance directives *Assault* *Autonomy* *Battery* *Beneficence* *Crime* *Double effect* *Ethics* *Justice* *Laws* *Liability* *Malpractice* *Negligence* *Nonmaleficence* *Respondeat superior* *Tort* *Veracity*	*Upon completion of this chapter, the student will be able to do the following:* • *Define key terms in the chapter.* • *Differentiate morals from values.* • *Explain ethical philosophy.* • *Describe the principles and rules of healthcare ethics.* • *Describe a systematic approach to resolve ethical dilemmas.* • *Analyze an ethical dilemma, citing ethical principles.* • *Explain licensure.* • *Describe standard of care.* • *Explain and give examples of crimes and torts.* • *Define four elements of negligence.* • *Describe legal protections for nurses, and cite measures to be taken.*

3

As a home health nurse, you regularly see a client who is 69 years old, lives alone, and has chronic restrictive pulmonary disease. At each visit, your client is weaker and more fatigued. He struggles with shortness of breath and has lost approximately 10 lb during the last month. His two adult children live nearby. They take turns transporting their father to clinic appointments. The daughter is concerned about her father's worsening respiratory condition and the increasing amount of care he requires. She mentions this to you. You know that clients with this disease deteriorate with time, and they often require ventilator support when they no longer have the strength to breathe on their own.

In previous chapters, you learned about the professionalism of nursing. In this chapter, you extend your knowledge base of professional nursing to include ethical and legal practice. When you have completed this chapter, you should be familiar with laws that concern you now as a student nurse and later as a registered nurse. You should be able to apply critical thinking to your ethical decisions. Critical Thinking Challenges at the end of the chapter will help you work your way through the ethical dilemmas presented in the previous situation.

Healthcare delivery has undergone notable changes during the last decade. Client participation in decision-making has become more prominent. Hospital stays are shorter than ever. Services have been restructured to provide care in alternative settings, such as ambulatory clinics, short-stay units, long-term, and in-home care. Multidisciplinary collaboration and care coordination are emphasized to ensure that clients' needs are met throughout the health and illness continuum. For nurses, these changes have contributed to the development of new clinical environments and expanded practice. In the course of their work, nurses encounter situations in which it is difficult to discern the best course of action.

Nurses are obligated to provide ethical and legal client care that demonstrates respect. Fundamental principles and rules of healthcare ethics and laws governing the scope of nursing guide nurses in all situations. Ethical nursing practice is promoted by applying ethical thinking and moral reasoning to the decisions and actions inherent in client care. Legal nursing practice is based on standards of care and the applicable nurse practice act.

Addressing ethical problems in clinical practice is empowering for nurses. It increases their satisfaction about what they are able to achieve for their clients. Nurses achieve personal and professional success when they are able to identify ethical problems and legal responsibilities in clinical practice and then use their knowledge and skills to bring about resolution.

Ethics in Nursing

The branch of philosophy dealing with standards of conduct and moral judgment is called **ethics**. Healthcare ethics pertain to how professionals fulfill their responsibilities and how care is provided to clients. There is no set of absolute guidelines that provides answers for all problems, but the fundamental principles of ethics are a basis for interpreting and analyzing clinical situations to make decisions.

Ethics are based on moral reasoning and reflect sets of values. Morals are standards of right and wrong that help individuals judge what is the correct or permissible action to take in a situation. Values are ideas or beliefs an individual considers important and feels strongly about. Values are rooted in each person's unique experience. They develop through family relationships, religious affiliations, education, and associations with friends and other professionals. Together, morals and values are the basis for establishing priorities and making choices (Munson, 1992).

Morals and values are not always consistent within a society or a culture. In a pluralistic society, there are numerous, diverse ways of thinking about what is important and right. Life choices and healthcare decisions vary according to each person's values and beliefs. When opposing values arise in a situation, decision-making can be very challenging. For example, Jehovah's Witnesses often refuse blood products in their treatment. This affects how surgery will be conducted and whether it is done. Though there are conflicting values in such a situation, the client must receive respectful treatment.

Value judgments influence how we respond to the needs of clients. When human immunodeficiency virus (HIV) and acquired immunodeficiency syndrome (AIDS) were first brought into the public eye, they were highly associated with homosexual men and injection drug users. This heightened society's judgmental response and may have slowed constructive action to pursue information about the causes, prevention, and treatment of the disease (Shilts, 1988). The American Nurses Association (ANA) has formulated a National Action Agenda for the comprehensive, holistic, and humane care of clients and their families, including the need to respect the dignity and value of all clients, regardless of sexual preference or ethnicity (ANA, 1993). Particular attention has been paid to ethical and legal concerns, such as protecting confidentiality and planning for guardianship for people in the late stages of the disease.

Nurses must distinguish between personal values and professional ethics. Personal values are what each individual holds as significant and true for himself or herself. These personal convictions apply only to the situations and decisions pertaining to that individual. Professional ethics involve principles that have universal application and standards of conduct that must be upheld in all situations. In ethical practice, a nurse avoids allowing personal judgments from biasing treatment of clients. Healthcare ethics is the application of moral reasoning to all aspects of healthcare. Decisions about client care, research endeavors, public policy, and service delivery must reflect ethical practice. Every provider must show respect for people, act in the best interest of clients, and be honest and fair with clients.

The ANA has published a Code for Nurses (ANA, 1985), which delineates the conduct and responsibilities nurses are expected to maintain in their practice. Nurses' ethical obligations include acting in the best interest of their clients, not only as individual practitioners, but also as members of the nursing profession, the healthcare team, and the community. A nurse is responsible to know and comply with the standards of ethical practice and to ensure that all nurses also comply. Interpretive statements have been developed that explain how each item in the code is manifested in nursing practice. The complete document can be obtained from the ANA. The Canadian Nurses Association and the International Council of Nurses also have published codes of ethics that reflect the basic tenets of nursing practice. These codes are summarized in the accompanying display.

Foundations for Ethical Practice

Healthcare professionals must be able to use ethical thinking in their decision-making and clinical practice. The foundations for ethical practice include knowledge of basic ethical concepts and the ability to understand their significance for professional responsibilities and everyday client care.

Theoretical Frameworks in Ethics

Frameworks in ethics provide a systematic way of organizing reasons that are a basis for choosing the best

Professional Codes of Ethics for Nurses

American Nurses Association Code for Nurses*

1. The nurse provides services with respect for human dignity and the uniqueness of the client unrestricted by considerations of social or economic status, personal attributes, or the nature of health problems.
2. The nurse safeguards the client's right to privacy by judiciously protecting information of a confidential nature.
3. The nurse acts to safeguard the client and the public when healthcare and safety are affected by the incompetent, unethical, or illegal practice of any person.
4. The nurse assumes responsibility and accountability for individual nursing judgments and actions.
5. The nurse maintains competence in nursing.
6. The nurse exercises informed judgment and uses individual competence and qualifications as criteria in seeking consultation, accepting responsibilities, and delegating nursing activities to others.
7. The nurse participates in activities that contribute to the ongoing development of the profession's body of knowledge.
8. The nurse participates in the profession's efforts to implement and improve standards of nursing.
9. The nurse participates in the profession's efforts to establish and maintain conditions of employment conducive to high-quality nursing care.
10. The nurse participates in the profession's effort to protect the public from misinformation and misrepresentation and to maintain the integrity of nursing.
11. The nurse collaborates with members of the health professions and other citizens in promoting community and national efforts to meet the health needs of the public.

Canadian Nurses Association Code of Ethics for Nursing†

I. A nurse treats clients with respect for their individual needs and values.
II. Based on respect for clients and regard for their right to control their own care, nursing care reflects respect for the right of choice held by clients.
III. The nurse holds confidential all information about a client learned in the healthcare setting.
IV. The nurse is guided by consideration for the dignity of clients.
V. The nurse provides competent care to clients.
VI. The nurse maintains trust in nurses and nursing.
VII. The nurse recognizes the contribution and expertise of colleagues from nursing and other disciplines as essential to excellent healthcare.
VIII. The nurse takes steps to ensure that the client receives competent and ethical care.
IX. Conditions of employment should contribute in a positive way to client care and the professional satisfaction of nurses.
X. Job action by nurses is directed toward securing conditions of employment that enable safe and appropriate care for clients and contribute to the professional satisfaction of nurses.
XI. The nurse advocates the interests of clients.
XII. The nurse represents the values and ethics of nursing before colleagues and others.
XIII. Professional nurses' organizations are responsible for clarifying, securing, and sustaining ethical nursing conduct. The fulfillment of these tasks requires that professional nurses' organizations remain responsive to the rights, needs, and legitimate interests of clients and nurses.

International Council of Nurses Code for Nurses‡

The fundamental responsibility of the nurse is fourfold: to promote health, to prevent illness, to restore health, and to alleviate suffering.

The need for nursing is universal. Inherent in nursing is respect for life, dignity, and rights of humans. It is unrestricted by considerations of nation ality, race, creed, color, age, sex, politics, or social status.

Nurses render health services to the individual, the family, and the community and coordinate their services with those of related groups.

Nurses and People

The nurse's primary responsibility is to people who require nursing care.

The nurse, in providing care, promotes an environment in which the values, customs, and spiritual beliefs of the individual are respected.

The nurse holds in confidence personal information and uses judgments in sharing this information.

Nurses and Practice

The nurse carries personal responsibility for nursing practice and for maintaining competence by continual learning. The nurse maintains the highest standards of nursing care possible within the reality of a specific situation.

The nurse uses judgment in relation to individual competence when accepting and delegating responsibilities.

(continued)

Professional Codes of Ethics for Nurses (continued)

The nurse when acting in a professional capacity should at all times maintain standards of personal conduct that reflect credit on the profession.

Nurses and Society
The nurse shares with other citizens the responsibility for initiating and supporting action to meet the health and social needs of the public.

Nurses and Coworkers
The nurse sustains a cooperative relationship with coworkers in nursing and other fields. The nurse takes appropriate action to safeguard the individual whose care is endangered by a coworker or any other person.

Nurses and the Profession
The nurse plays a major role in determining and implementing desirable standards of nursing practice and nursing education.

The nurse is active in developing a core of professional knowledge.

The nurse, acting through the professional organization, participates in establishing and maintaining equitable social and economic working conditions in nursing.

*From American Nurses Association (1985). *Code for nurses.* Kansas City, MO: Author.
†From Canadian Nurses Association (1991). *Code of ethics for nursing.* Ottawa, Ontario: Author.
‡*Adapted from* International Council of Nurses (1973). *ICN Code for nurses: Ethical concepts applied to nursing.* Geneva: Imprimeries Populaires.
This represents only one element of the code—values. Obligations and limitations are provided with each value in the publication.

actions. Major theoretical frameworks in ethics are differentiated according to which values are emphasized as most important. Goals, duties, and rights are central considerations to all ethics theories, but they vary in how they are assigned priority within each of the frameworks (Benjamin & Curtis, 1986). Conceptualization of a particular situation within each framework yields different conclusions.

In frameworks that emphasize goals, actions are judged to be right based on whether they contribute to the achievement of identified outcomes. In the utilitarian framework, actions are right when they contribute to the greatest good and wrong when they detract from the greatest good (Gorovitz, 1971). The greatest good may refer to the greatest happiness for an individual. For cancer clients, alternatives such as radical surgery, chemotherapy, or radiation are evaluated according to which one will give the client the greatest comfort and chance of survival.

Some utilitarian theories define "good consequences" according to whether an action results in the greatest good for the greatest number. A decision might be made not to fund very expensive or experimental treatments needed by only a few to reserve dollars for wellness and prevention services that benefit more people.

The emphasis within deontologic frameworks is on the set of roles or responsibilities one is morally obligated to fulfill. One is expected to remain faithful to a certain set of duties, which takes precedence over other considerations (Munson, 1992). Decisions about the right action are based on which action is in keeping with these duties, not with regard to consequences. An example of a duty is a nurse's obligation to protect a client's confidentiality.

When *rights* are identified as the primary consideration, focus is on the claims or entitlements of each individual (Benjamin & Curtis, 1986). Actions are judged according to whether they uphold each individual's rights. The "right to life" campaign is an example of an ethical position based on rights. The central element is an unborn child's entitlement to life. Judgments about actions are based on whether or not they support this right.

Principles and Rules of Healthcare Ethics

Principles

Principles are basic ideas that are a starting point for understanding and working through a problem (Jonsen, 1994). The principles are tenets that are important to uphold in all situations. The major principles of healthcare ethics are beneficence and nonmaleficence, autonomy, and justice. These principles are the basis for rules that govern the relationships between healthcare providers and clients.

Beneficence and Nonmaleficence. **Beneficence** means doing or promoting good. This principle is the basis for all healthcare. Nurses, physicians, and all other healthcare practitioners work to accomplish good for clients by promoting their best interest and striving to achieve optimal client outcomes. Nurses take beneficent actions when they administer pain medication, perform a dressing change to promote wound healing, or provide emotional support to a client who is anxious or depressed. Overall, healthcare reform is a beneficent effort to provide accessible, affordable care to those who need it.

Nonmaleficence is the converse of beneficence. The principle of nonmaleficence means to avoid doing harm. When working with clients, healthcare workers must not cause injury or suffering. Nurses uphold the principle of nonmaleficence by providing medication to prevent a client from further suffering, protecting clients from a chemically impaired practitioner, or reporting suspected child abuse for investigation to prevent further victimization.

Doing good and avoiding harm seem fairly simple, but in many cases, this is complex and difficult to discern. Bone marrow transplantation often saves lives; however, the client experiences a great deal of pain and suffering to benefit from the intervention. Saving the life of an expectant mother with a cardiac problem who is not likely to survive childbirth may require harm to the unborn child in the form an abortion. Confronting a colleague's substance abuse may help that person obtain therapy. However, it also may mean a temporary suspension from employment for that individual and can elicit embarrassment or hostility.

Autonomy. **Autonomy** essentially means independence and the ability to be self-directed. In healthcare, respect for autonomy is the basis for the client's right to self-determination, which means the client is entitled to make decisions about what will happen to him or her and his or her body. Competent adult clients have the right to consent or refuse treatment. Even if healthcare providers do not agree with clients' decisions, their wishes must be respected (Beauchamp & Childress, 1989).

Infants, young children, mentally handicapped or incapacitated people, and people in a persistent vegetative state or coma do not have the capacity to participate in decision-making about their healthcare. For these individuals, a surrogate decision-maker must be identified to act on behalf of the client. Through nursing assessment and therapeutic relationships, nurses gain an in-depth understanding of what clients need and want from their healthcare. Nurses promote client autonomy by integrating clients' wishes into the treatment plan.

Clients communicate their wishes to healthcare providers through documents called **advance directives** to physicians. These documents specify what interventions the client would or would not want if he or she became terminally ill or sustained an injury or illness that impeded the ability to make or communicate decisions (Fig. 3-1). Through the use of a Durable Power of Attorney for Healthcare Decisions, an individual designates another person to make decisions. If the client becomes incapacitated and unable to make decisions for himself or herself, this "surrogate decision-maker" would act on the client's behalf. The legal aspects of these documents are discussed later in this chapter.

Clients are entitled to rescind or change their directives at any time. Nurses are often the first to learn about changes a client is contemplating. The nurse must then document the client's wishes and notify the client's physician and other involved professionals so that the plan of care is altered to reflect the client's wishes.

The Patient Bill of Rights (see display), published by the American Hospital Association (1992), identifies key elements of clients' rights and responsibilities in their relationship with healthcare providers. A client is entitled to considerate and respectful care. This includes assurances of confidentiality, complete information, continuity of care, and access to treatment providers. The bill also identifies the client's right to information about costs and financial liabilities and whether or not there are rules and regulations in the organization by which he or she must abide.

Cultural diversity has implications for upholding client autonomy. Care must be modified to reflect respect for values and beliefs of different ethnic or social groups. Some cultures prefer that information about severe or terminal illness be withheld from a client. Religious beliefs and allegiance to tradition affect how much information a client will share and how receptive he or she is to the recommendations of a healthcare provider.

Justice. **Justice**, the principle of fairness, is the basis for the obligation to treat all clients in an equal and fair way. It is the foundation for decisions about resource allocation throughout a society or a group. Unfortunately, resource limitations constrain our ability to do everything for every person in our society (Stopes-Roe, 1994).

Nurses face issues of justice when organizing care for a group of clients and deciding how much time will be spent with each client. A *just* decision is based on client need and a fair distribution resources. It would be *unjust* to make such a decision based on how much he or she likes each client. Nurses may identify ethical conflicts when a client is disruptive and therefore receives more attention than more cooperative clients. Another example is when a terminally ill client receives life-sustaining treatment in an intensive care unit, while another client with a greater chance for recovery cannot be admitted due to lack of beds. In such situations, nurses promote justice by requesting that realistic outcomes and a clear treatment plan be identified.

Issues of justice, such as whether all individuals have access to healthcare and how such care is funded, have implications for the community. With healthcare reform, insurance companies have been required to

text continues on p. 46

DECLARATION

I, *Mildred Jones*, being of sound mind, willfully and voluntarily make this declaration to be followed if I become incompetent. This declaration reflects my firm and settled commitment to refuse life-sustaining treatment under the circumstances indicated below.

I direct my attending physician to withhold or withdraw life-sustaining treatment that serves only to prolong the process of my dying, if I should be in a terminal condition or in a state of permanent unconsciousness.

I direct that treatment be limited to measures to keep me comfortable and to relieve pain, including any pain that might occur by withholding or withdrawing life-sustaining treatment.

In addition, if I am in the condition described above, I feel especially strongly about the following forms of treatment. **I realize that if I do not specifically indicate my preference regarding any of the forms of treatment listed below, I may receive that form of treatment.**

• Cardiac resuscitation:	I do want (x)	I do not want( )
• Mechanical respiration:	I do want ( )	I do not want (x)
• Tube feeding or any other artificial or invasive form of nutrition (food):	I do want ( )	I do not want (x)
• Any artificial or invasive form of hydration (water):	I do want ( )	I do not want (x)
• Blood or blood products:	I do want ( )	I do not want (x)
• Any invasive diagnostic tests:	I do want ( )	I do not want (x)
• Any form of surgery:	I do want ( )	I do not want (x)
• Kidney dialysis:	I do want ( )	I do not want (x)
• Antibiotics:	I do want (x)	I do not want ( )

Other instructions:

I(x) do ( ) do not want to designate another person as my surrogate to make medical treatment decisions for me if I should be incompetent and in a terminal condition or in a state of permanent unconsciousness.

Name and address of surrogate (if applicable):

Jonathan Jones
423 Main Street
Crossroads SC

Name and address of substitute surrogate (if surrogate designated above is unable to serve):

Trudy Conover
619 Wyoming Drive
Crossroads SC

I made this declaration on the *21* day of *10/95* (month, year).

Declarant's signature: *Mildred Jones*

Declarant's address: *423 Main Street*
Crossroads SC

The declarant or the person on behalf of and at the direction of the declarant knowingly and voluntarily signed this writing by signature or mark in my presence.

1. Witness's signature: *Mary Martin*
   Witness's address: *818 Hill Drive*
   Bayside GA

2. Witness's signature: *Rosa Diaz*
   Witness's address: *1043 River Road*
   Summit SC

Figure 3-1 • *Sample of an advance directive.*

A Patient's Bill of Rights

Introduction

Effective healthcare requires collaboration between patients and physicians and other healthcare professionals. Open and honest communication, respect for personal and professional values, and sensitivity to differences are integral to optimal patient care. As the setting for the provision of health services, hospitals must provide a foundation for understanding and respecting the rights and responsibilities of patients, their families, physicians, and other caregivers. Hospitals must ensure a health care ethic that respects the role of patients in decision making about treatment choices and other aspects of their care. Hospitals must be sensitive to cultural, racial, linguistic, religious, age, gender, and other differences as well as the needs of persons with disabilities.

The American Hospital Association presents *A Patient's Bill of Rights* with the expectation that it will contribute to more effective patient care and be supported by the hospital on behalf of the institution, its medical staff, employees, and patients. The American Hospital Association encourages health care institutions to tailor this bill of rights to their patient community by translating and/or simplifying the language of this bill of rights as may be necessary to ensure that patients and their families understand their rights and responsibilities.

Bill of Rights*

1. The patient has the right to considerate and respectful care.
2. The patient has the right to and is encouraged to obtain from physicians and other direct caregivers relevant, current, and understandable information concerning diagnosis, treatment, and prognosis.

   Except in emergencies when the patient lacks decision-making capacity and the need for treatment is urgent, the patient is entitled to the opportunity to discuss and request information related to the specific procedures and/or treatments, the risks involved, the possible length of recuperation, and the medically reasonable alternatives and their accompanying risks and benefits.

   Patients have the right to know the identity of physicians, nurses, and others involved in their care, as well as when those involved are students, residents, or other trainees. The patient also has the right to know the immediate and long-term financial implications of treatment choices, insofar as they are known.
3. The patient has the right to make decisions about the plan of care prior to and during the course of treatment and to refuse a recommended treatment or plan of care to the extent permitted by law and hospital policy and to be informed of the medical consequences of this action. In case of such refusal, the patient is entitled to other appropriate care and services that the hospital provides or transfer to another hospital. The hospital should notify patients of any policy that might affect patient choice within the institution.
4. The patient has the right to have an advance directive (such as living will, health care proxy, or durable power of attorney for health care) concerning treatment or designating a surrogate decision maker with the expectation that the hospital will honor the intent of that directive to the extent permitted by law and hospital policy.

   Health care institutions must advise patients of their rights under state law and hospital policy to make informed medical choices, ask if the patient has an advance directive, and include that information in patient records. The patient has the right to timely information about hospital policy that may limit its ability to implement fully a legally valid advance directive.
5. The patient has the right to every consideration of privacy. Case discussion, consultation, examination, and treatment should be conducted so as to protect each patient's privacy.
6. The patient has the right to expect that all communications and records pertaining to his/her care will be treated as confidential by the hospital, except in cases such as suspected abuse and public health hazards when reporting is permitted or required by law. The patient has the right to expect that the hospital will emphasize the confidentiality of this information when it releases it to any other parties entitled to review information in these records.
7. The patient has the right to review the records pertaining to his/her medical care and to have the information explained or interpreted as necessary, except when restricted by law.
8. The patient has the right to expect that, within its capacity and policies, a hospital will make reasonable response to the request of a patient for appropriate and medically indicated care and services. The hospital must provide evaluation, service, and/or referral as indicated by the urgency of the case. When medically appropri-

(continued)

A Patient's Bill of Rights *(continued)*

ate and legally permissible, or when a patient has so requested, a patient may be transferred to another facility. The institution to which the patient is to be transferred must first have accepted the patient for transfer. The patient must also have the benefit of complete information and explanation concerning the need for, risks, benefits, and alternatives to such a transfer.

9. The patient has the right to ask for and be informed of the existence of business relationships among the hospital, educational institutions, other health care providers, or payers that may influence the patient's treatment and care.
10. The patient has the right to consent to or decline to participate in proposed research studies or human experimentation affecting care and treatment or requiring direct patient involvement, and to have those studies fully explained prior to consent. A patient who declines to participate in research or experimentation is entitled to the most effective care that the hospital can otherwise provide.
11. The patient has the right to expect reasonable continuity of care when appropriate and to be informed by physicians and other caregivers of available and realistic patient care options when hospital care is no longer appropriate.
12. The patient has the right to be informed of hospital policies and practices that relate to patient care, treatment, and responsibilities. The patient has the right to be informed of available resources for resolving disputes, grievances, and conflicts, such as ethics committees, patient representatives, or other mechanisms available in the institution. The patient has the right to be informed of the hospital's charges for services and available payment methods.

The collaborative nature of health care requires that patients, or their families/surrogates, participate in their care. The effectiveness of care and patient satisfaction with the course of treatment depend, in part, on the patient fulfilling certain responsibilities. Patients are responsible for providing information about past illnesses, hospitalizations, medications, and other matters related to health status. To participate effectively in decision making, patients must be encouraged to take responsibility for requesting additional information or clarification about their health status or treatment when they do not fully understand information and instructions. Patients are also responsible for ensuring that the health care institution has a copy of their written advance directive if they have one. Patients are responsible for informing their physicians and other caregivers if they anticipate problems in following prescribed treatment.

Patients should also be aware of the hospital's obligation to be reasonably efficient and equitable in providing care to other patients and the community. The hospital's rules and regulations are designed to help the hospital meet this obligation. Patients and their families are responsible for making reasonable accommodations to the needs of the hospital, other patients, medical staff, and hospital employees. Patients are responsible for providing necessary information for insurance claims and for working with the hospital to make payment arrangements, when necessary.

Conclusion

Hospitals have many functions to perform, including the enhancement of health status, health promotion, and the prevention and treatment of injury and disease; the immediate and ongoing care and rehabilitation of patients; the education of health professionals, patients, and the community; and research. All these activities must be conducted with an overriding concern for the values and dignity of patients.

*These rights can be exercised on the patient's behalf by a legally designated surrogate or proxy decision maker if the patient lacks decision-making capacity, is legally incompetent, or is a minor. Reprinted with permission of the American Hospital Association. © 1992.

make changes so that all individuals have access to coverage. Public policy must reflect just distribution of services. Nurses contribute their knowledge about client needs and healthcare systems to public debate and decisions.

Rules

The principles of healthcare ethics must be upheld in all situations. They are the foundation for the ethical rules, veracity, fidelity, and confidentiality. These rules are guidelines for the relationship between clients and healthcare providers. Some circumstances may create exceptions to the rules, but for the most part, nurses are required to adhere to these obligations.

Veracity. **Veracity** means telling the truth, which is essential to the integrity of the client–provider relationship. Healthcare professionals are obliged to be honest with clients. The right to self-determination becomes meaningless if the client does not receive accurate, unbiased, and understandable information (President's Commission for the Study of Ethical Problems in Medicine and Biomedical and Behavioral Research, 1982).

Clients and families frequently disclose their questions and concerns to nurses. Nurses help them obtain information and understand how it applies to their situation by arranging discussions between the client, family, and physician and providing emotional support to those adjusting to illness. Telling a client about serious health problems can be distressing for the client and the healthcare professional. Several studies reveal that clients prefer to be given accurate information about their condition and prognosis even when the outlook is bleak (Woodard & Parmies, 1992; Sardell & Trierweiler, 1993). Candid discussions about their condition and treatment is reassuring to some clients (Sell, et al., 1993). A study of cancer clients shows a large percentage of clients want more information than their physicians are inclined to reveal and that informed clients are less anxious and more cooperative (Espinosa, Gonzales-Baron, Poveda, Ordonez, & Zamora, 1993).

Fidelity. Fidelity means being faithful to one's commitments and promises. Nurses' commitments to clients include providing safe care and maintaining competence in nursing practice. In some instances, a promise is made to a client in an overt way. In psychiatric day treatment programs, detailed client care contracts are made between the client and the team. If a nurse agrees to be the resource to the client when he or she is in crisis, the nurse must fulfill this commitment. If the nurse cannot be available, the ethical action is to discuss this with the client and arrange a substitute when needed.

Nurses must use good judgment when making promises to clients. Being responsive to a client's request is important, but the nurse must evaluate whether agreements can be upheld.

Dave Meyers, RN, admitted a client with a history of alcohol abuse. The client asked for assurance that leather restraints would not be used under any circumstances. In an attempt to calm the client, Dave agreed to this request. Following surgery, the client grew agitated, delirious, and combative. Though restraints were indicated to preserve the client's safety, Dave opposed using them because of the promise he made. This promise was not safe. Ethical practice in this case would have incorporated the client's concerns and an explanation of circumstances in which restraints would be applied.

Confidentiality. The rule of confidentiality requires that information about a client be kept private. What is documented in client's record is accessible only to those providing care to that client. No one else is entitled to the information unless that client has signed a *consent for release of information* identifying with whom information may be shared and for what purpose. Discussing clients outside the clinical setting, telling friends or family about clients, or discussing clients in an elevator or public area violate client confidentiality and must be avoided.

In some situations, it may be troubling not to share information.

Joseph Adams, a 32-year-old diagnosed with HIV 4 years ago, has developed several AIDS symptoms and is now hospitalized. He is not expected to live much longer. Joseph's parents and sister live in another state and have not seen him for a few years. Joe does not want his family to know he is homosexual. His parents are now at the hospital and have asked for information about Joe's illness.

The nurse is obligated in this situation to protect the client's confidentiality and not to give the family information about the diagnosis. One approach the nurse can take is to talk with Joe and his partner about information that Joe would permit the family to have and how best to share this information with them. Nursing has provided significant leadership in the care and treatment of AIDS clients.

Breaking confidentiality may be ethically justified if there is a well-defined reason to share the information. Information can be shared only if this would substantially benefit someone else and if the benefit outweighs or overrides the harm that would come from a breach of confidentiality (Walters, 1988).

Model for Case Analysis

When any client enters treatment, a decision must be made regarding what is best to do. Ethical issues are relevant in all cases and affect how this decision is made. The ability to analyze clinical situations to integrate ethical considerations with relevant clinical data and surrounding issues is an essential skill for ethical clinical practice. There are various models for clinical decision-making, such as the GUIDE model (Levenson & Pettery, 1994) and case analysis (Silva, 1990). For this text, we have chosen the case analysis model developed by Jonsen, Siegler, and Winslade (1992), which aids in organizing the salient features of a clinical situation to promote problem-solving and decision-making. In this model, information about the case is divided into four categories: Indications for Medical Intervention, Patient Preference, Quality of Life, and Contextual Features. The accompanying display presents the model.

Model for Case Analysis

Indications for Medical Intervention

- Client's condition and prognosis
- Risks and benefits of intervention

What "good" can be done for the client?

Patient Preference

- Consent or refusal of treatment
- Informed and competent

What are the client's wishes?

Quality of Life

- Satisfaction with current situation
- Evaluation of future possibilities

Is it satisfying? Can it be improved?

Contextual Features

- Benefits and burdens for others
- Costs, policies, values of others

Is this use of resources justifiable?

Adapted from Jonsen, A. R., Siegler, M., & Winslade, W. (1992). Clinical ethics (3rd ed.). New York: McGraw-Hill.

The ethical considerations pertinent in each category are discussed in the following section.

Indications for Medical Intervention

For each person entering the healthcare system as a client, there are questions to be answered about the client's need for treatment and what interventions will be used. Indications for medical treatment include consideration of the client's diagnosis and condition. Treatment alternatives are then evaluated according to whether they are indicated and what they can accomplish for that client.

Beneficence and nonmaleficence are relevant in this category. A clinical judgment must be made about whether a treatment alternative will produce a benefit and what will achieve the greatest good for the client. The distinction between available treatment and that which is truly indicated is important. The criterion on which this distinction rests is whether the intervention can achieve a therapeutic or desired benefit for the client. Nurses participate in determining whether interventions are indicated by continually assessing the client's condition and response to treatment and then integrating this information into the plan of care.

Available interventions are not always beneficial for every client. Liver transplantation is a treatment alternative for many clients with cirrhotic liver disease. However, pneumonia and bleeding problems diminish a client's chance of surviving a transplant. The client would be at high risk for being ventilator dependent following surgery, for acquiring generalized infection from the pneumonia, and experiencing intraoperative and postoperative bleeding. Although liver transplantation might be life saving for some clients, it would not produce a positive outcome or therapeutic benefit for clients with these serious complications.

Double Effect

The concept of **double effect** means that an action can produce two outcomes. It may be helpful and harmful at the same time. Usually, one of the outcomes is desired; the other is not intended. The reason for taking an action must be important enough to justify the negative consequences. An infant in intensive care may require painful interventions to save his or her life. Administering large doses of morphine to someone who is dying relieves pain but also may diminish respirations and hasten death.

Futility

When interventions are not likely to preserve life, restore health, or relieve suffering, they are considered futile (Schneiderman, Jecker, & Jonsen, 1990). Determinations of futility are defined in reference to the goals; therefore, a treatment course is best designed around outcomes that are mutually agreed on by the client and the healthcare provider.

Paula Hastings, a 30-year-old woman, has had cancer for several years. After surgical tumor resections, chemotherapy, and radiation, she is found to have several tumors, including lung metastases, and is considered terminal. The physician discusses with Paula that no further aggressive interventions will be used, and care will be directed toward making her as comfortable as possible. Weeks later, Paula presents in the emergency room with bleeding through an enterocutaneous fistula near her colostomy. The resident on call admits Paula and orders blood products to be given. The assistant head nurse on the unit where Paula is admitted is familiar with her case. He recalls the do-not-resuscitate order for this client. He is concerned that resuscitating this terminally ill client would be providing futile treatment. The nurse identifies that the goals of treatment need to be reviewed and that interventions should be discussed in light of these goals.

Client Preference

A client's choice about what is done is essential to healthcare decision-making. Each individual is uniquely qualified to make decisions about his or her own best interest (Munson, 1992). After a clinical judgment has been made about the client's condition and indicated interventions have been determined, this information is discussed with the client who may then accept or refuse the treatment alternatives. The wishes of an informed, competent client must always be respected and incorporated into the plan of care because it is the ultimate expression of autonomy.

Grace Hall, 73, was diagnosed with cancer 10 years ago. Over the years, she has undergone several forms of treatment. She has suffered most of the negative side effects of these treatments, such as nausea and vomiting, hair loss, fatigue, and pain. When another mass is discovered, her physician presents the treatment options to her and informs her that without treatment, chances of surviving for more than 6 months are very poor. The physician indicates that he will be scheduling her for radiation treatment. Mrs. Hall tells the nurse that she does not want treatment. She is worried that if she tells the doctor this, he will not want her as a client any more. Because she is in a great deal of pain and needs medication, this concern of abandonment is frightening to her.

One of the primary ethical responsibilities of the nurse in this case is to advocate for the client's wishes by informing the physician of the client's statement and assisting the client to talk with the physician. Even though the physician believes treatment would provide a substantial therapeutic gain, he must respect the client's preference to forego further intervention. Ethical care in this case also would include preserving the client's function and preventing suffering to whatever degree possible.

Informed Consent

Clients' right to self-determination means they are entitled to make decisions about the care they will receive. To derive a preference, the client must have information about his or her condition, the proposed treatment, the risks and benefits of the specified treatment, and the alternatives, including not having the proposed interventions (Appelbaum, Lidz, & Meisel, 1987). Ethically valid consent is meant to be a process of shared decision-making with mutual respect and participation.

Clients frequently disclose their concerns and fears to nurses. When this happens, the nurse must listen carefully to identify whether the client needs further information, clarification, or reassurance. Ethical nursing action is to advocate for the client by answering questions, arranging more information to be given, or accommodating the client's need for time to adjust to the implications of the information. All of these actions help to ensure that the client's preferences will be known, respected, and incorporated into decisions about care.

> **Client Teaching**
> *Ethical and Legal Concerns*
>
> *Instruct the client as follows:*
> - *Ask questions about all procedures and treatments so that you can be fully informed.*
> - *Prepare a living will, or make your wishes known to your family and healthcare providers.*
> - *If you do noy feel you are supported by your healthcare providers (nurse, physician, others), seek other healthcare providers.*

Quality of Life

Quality of life refers to how satisfying a person's life is according to the client's point of view and the evaluation by others. The client makes a subjective assessment of his or her experience and situation. For example, a male client evaluates how satisfied he is with his level of functioning following a severe back injury. He may not be able to walk, he may be able to walk but not participate in sports that he previously enjoyed, or he may have persistent leg pain. Some clients feel life is not worth living if they are not able to return to favorite activities. Some feel some states of being are worse than death (Pearlman, et al., 1993). Others make adjustments and feel satisfied to be alive even if they are disabled.

Onlookers, such as professionals working with the client, family members, or friends, also assess the client's quality of life and judge it according to their own subjective assessment about what is satisfying. Nurses assess a client's quality of life when they observe how a client is managing or adapting to constraints resulting from illness or injury. In a rehabilitation center, a nurse assesses whether a woman who now requires a wheelchair is able to get around or will require constant assistance. The nurse makes a judgment about the quality of the woman's life in light of the required adjustment. If the woman has always preferred to be independent, she may experience a greater sense of loss and may be less satisfied with her quality of life than someone who accepts assistance readily and has family available to help.

Contextual Features

Contextual features are benefits and burdens that affect individuals or groups other than the client but have compelling influence on the situation. Factors considered in this category include matters of finance, family situations, availability and use of resources, pressures from family or friends, and organizational or public policy.

The significance of these issues can be illustrated by comparing the perspectives that these features lend to a case. A baby boy born with several congenital malformations may require numerous surgeries to survive. Intensive care would be necessary for several months, and after a prolonged hospitalization, he would require extensive care, including a ventilator. He would never be able to eat normally.

Consider this same infant in two different contexts. In one scenario, the baby is born into a stable family environment. Family income is secure, and the family has generous healthcare insurance. The mother is willing to stay at the hospital and learn the care required for her son. A large extended family has been lending assistance and support. In contrast, the baby might be born to a single mother who leaves the hospital indicating that it is too painful to look at the baby. She says she cannot be a good mother to him and relinquishes parental rights to a state welfare agency. The young mother is estranged from her family, and no one has come forward to be involved in the care of the infant.

This situation involves a dilemma about whether to provide life-sustaining treatment for an infant with severe problems. When a case such as this is presented, it is not unusual to first conclude that the baby would have whatever treatment is needed to preserve life. However, the decision becomes more complex because of the problems that will remain even after extensive intervention. At this point, the contextual considerations would weigh heavily on the decision.

Resolving Ethical Dilemmas

Nurses' responsibilities for ethical practice encompass managing oneself as a moral being, functioning as a member of the healthcare team, being an accountable employee in an organization, and participating in the community. Nurses can take action in any of these spheres to promote ethical client care (Broom, 1990). In each of these areas, nurses must be able to recognize an ethical dilemma and then take steps to resolve the situation.

A dilemma is a situation in which the following exist:

- Two or more choices are available.
- It is difficult to determine which choice is best.
- The needs of all those involved cannot be solved by the available alternatives.

The alternatives in a dilemma may each have favorable and unfavorable features. Ethical dilemmas in healthcare involve issues surrounding professional actions and client care decisions. They can lead to discomfort and conflict among the members of the healthcare team or between the providers and the client and family. Nurses can use several strategies to prevent and resolve ethical dilemmas.

Validate Feelings and Values. Emotions affect how individuals think and act in any situation. Doctors and nurses have strong feelings and values about their work with clients. When a client is dying despite extensive treatment efforts, it is normal for professionals to grieve. When a client does not adhere to treatment, thereby compromising his or her own safety, physicians and nurses may share frustration and anger. Sometimes team members blame each other when things go wrong. This can cause conflict.

Validation is a way of acknowledging and identifying feelings as credible. When an individual is validated, he or she feels accepted. This promotes communication necessary for well-coordinated healthcare. Because conflict may erupt in situations involving ethical dilemmas, conflict resolution strategies, such as clarifying misunderstanding, validating, consensus building, and collaborating, also contribute to resolution of the ethical dilemmas.

Conduct a Case Analysis. Analyzing the case according to the model presented in the preceding section organizes the facts of the case and elucidates the ethical issues that must be considered. Using the model also prompts consideration of areas that otherwise may be overlooked. A case analysis can be done by those directly involved in the case, or assistance may be requested from a member of the organizational ethics committee. Gathering the team together to conduct the analysis in a team conference format promotes information sharing.

Various individuals involved in a case fulfill different roles and have different data to contribute to the case analysis and management. The physician contributes facts about the medical condition and prognosis. Nurses describe the client's adaptation to illness and response to treatment. A physical therapist describes how physical capabilities will affect quality of life. Social workers provide information about community resources.

Compiling all the information about the case helps clarify problems and issues. Ethical conflicts become more evident. The significance of various factors becomes more apparent. Alternatives are weighed in light of the ethical considerations and the specifics of that case.

Identify Outcomes. Planning care according to outcomes gives focus and consistency to a treatment plan.

Often ethical conflicts arise in a case because the parties involved hold different ideas about the goals of intervention. Once information in all the categories has been considered, realistic outcomes can be formulated.

Identify Short- and Long-Term Goals. Outcomes for the care and treatment of a terminally ill client may include such goals as planning for pain relief, setting up hospice care, identifying a surrogate decision-maker, and determining whether or not the client will be resuscitated if he or she experiences cardiac arrest. Clarifying what will be done in relation to each of these concerns promotes a sense of well-being for the client. For the healthcare team members, answers to such questions prevent confusion about what care is meant to achieve. Crisis management is avoided. Cost savings result from working toward realistic and desirable goals rather than allowing a situation to linger or to grow more complex without a clear plan.

Clarify Accountabilities. Different individuals may be accountable for actions that have been identified as part of the plan. For instance, if the team has received information that the client has a living will, a nurse or social worker can take responsibility for contacting the family and requesting a copy of this document for re-

Therapeutic Dialogue
Ethical Issues

Scenes for Thought

Mrs. Miller's 23-year-old daughter, Melanie, is in a meeting with the physician, and you are the primary nurse. Mrs. Miller, who has been unconscious since major abdominal surgery for metastatic cancer, has been in the intensive care unit for 3 weeks. The purpose of this meeting is to re-explain the plan for Mrs. Miller and its rationale because Melanie seems to be confused about the prognosis.

Effective

Physician: *We need to talk with you again about why we're decreasing your mom's IVs and oxygen.*
Melanie: *I thought the reason you were taking them away was because she was getting well! I don't understand!* She looks angry and begins to cry.
Physician: *I really thought you understood, Melanie. I'm sorry you're upset about this.*
Nurse: *Could you tell us what you see when you go in to visit your mother, Melanie? (Assessing her point of view before making any assumptions.)*
Melanie: *I see that she's lying there, resting quietly, looking like she's asleep.* Still crying quietly, face is set in a stiff frown.
Nurse: *We've all noticed some changes in her over the last few weeks. Have you? (Assessing her perceptions.)*
Melanie: *Well . . . um, I have noticed that her color is getting paler and that she doesn't move around at all anymore, even when you do something to her. I suppose you think that means something!* She looks frightened and angry at the same time.
Nurse: *Yes, we think it means that your mom is going deeper into her coma and that there is very little chance that she'll ever come out. (Further explanation of coma and its relationship to the cancer by both nurse and physician.)*
Melanie: Puts her head in her hands and cries quietly. The room is quiet. She looks up. *I knew this. The doctor said that before. I didn't want to believe it.*
Nurse: *We know it's difficult to say "give up" on someone you love. It might be helpful to you to talk some more about what to expect over the next few days and how you can help us with your mother's care. Would that be good for you? (Help her participate in the decision.)*
Melanie: *Yes, that would be helpful. I hope you don't mind if I cry, though. I thought she would get better.* Cries.
Nurse: *That's a very reasonable thing to do. We won't mind. (Discussion with Melanie continues. Support from clergy, father, and sibling suggested. Family meeting arranged the next day to include all.)*

Less Effective

Melanie: *I thought you were taking her oxygen and IVs away because she's getting better! I don't understand what you're doing to her.* Crying and looking angry.
Nurse: *I thought you understood, Miss Miller, that your mother isn't getting any better and that, in fact, she probably won't come out of her coma at all. (Said softly but firmly.)*
Melanie: *No, I didn't get that! My mother is still a young woman, and she's never been sick like this. How can she be dying? How can you take away the things she needs to live?*
Nurse: *I know it's hard for you to understand. I think it would be a good thing if you called your minister and the rest of your family so you can talk it over and decide what to do.*
Melanie: *I think I'll call our family lawyer, too. There's something funny going on here!* Crying as she strides purposefully away to the phone.

Critical Thinking Challenge

• Determine which of the 11 items of the ANA Code of Ethics the first nurse reflected in her care of the Miller family. • After studying the Patient's Bill of Rights, propose those rights that are particularly relevant to the Miller family's situation • Explain who is the client: Mrs. Miller, Melanie, or the family. • Critique the second nurse's failure to meet Melanie's needs. • Construct some emotional reasons that you think cause clients and their families to sue healthcare professionals and agencies.

view. If questions remain about whether a medical condition would be responsive to treatment, the physicians may need to pursue further tests or request consultation. If client preference is unclear, a psychosocial clinical nurse specialist may be designated to work with the client to assess what he or she wants or hopes from treatment. When a decision is made to withhold medically futile care, the physician is accountable to communicate this to the family.

Follow Through. Once a plan has been established, participants are ethically bound to uphold their accountabilities and professional responsibilities by following through with their part of the plan. Failing to do so is an infraction against the integrity of their profession and the healthcare system. Such failure also undermines the public's confidence and trust in healthcare professionals.

Resolving Reactions. Healthcare decisions are complex and often have dramatic consequences. The existence of an ethical dilemma can make the situation more vexing and add to the emotional reactions of those involved. By working through reactions to an event, healthcare members learn from the experience and prevent the residual feelings from hampering their ability to work through similar situations in the future. Discussing feelings and reactions among the team, with peers, or with a supervisor is an important step for promoting resolution. This type of discussion can lead to planning care for future clients to avoid repeating the same problems.

Ethics Committees. Organizational ethics committees help to work through ethical issues in practice. The American Hospital Association encourages the development of these committees as interdisciplinary vehicles for identifying and addressing ethical issues. These committees have three primary functions: policy development, education, and consultation (American Hospital Association, 1984b). As part of the educational and consultative functions, regular case reviews can promote ethical practice by assisting staff to recognize the ethical implications in practice and to develop strategies for resolution (Walker, 1993).

Additional Actions. Beyond case-by-case intervention, nurses help identify and resolve ethical problems by participating in their organization and community. Nurses also can contribute to the development of a healthcare system that reflects respect for all individuals and upholds the fundamentals of ethical practice. Nurses should be educated voters and participate in public forums in which decisions are made about healthcare. They should inform public officials about how the decisions they make affect healthcare.

Nursing Research
Ethical and Legal Issues

Selected Nursing Research Studies

Cassidy, V. R., (1991). Ethical responsibilities in nursing: Research findings and issues. *Journal of Professional Nursing, 7*(2), 112–118.

Duncan, S. M., (1992). Ethical challenges in community health nursing. *Journal of Advanced Nursing, 17*(9), 1035–1034.

Millette, B. E. (1993). Client advocacy and the moral orientation of nurses. *Western Journal of Nursing Research, 15*(5), 607–618.

Warren, J. J. (1992). Ethical concerns about noncompliance in the chronically ill patient. *Progress in Cardiovascular Nursing, 9*(4), 10–15.

Possible Topics for Nursing Inquiry

- What are the ethical dilemmas encountered by nurses in long-term care who work with ill and frail elderly clients?
- How do nurses in critical care balance ethics and the life-sustaining need of critically ill clients?
- What are the most useful methods for teaching ethics to nursing students?
- What are the most common documentation errors by nurses in cases that are brought to litigation?

Legal Issues In Nursing

Laws are rules or standards of human conduct established by government. They are established through legislative bodies and interpreted by courts to protect the rights of citizens. As a society changes its moral standards, the laws generally evolve to correspond with current thinking about morality and ethics. At any time, different views about morality or ethics may not conform to law.

In healthcare and other areas of society where technology has a major impact, moral and legal standards lag behind technologic advances. As a result, the law alone may not provide specific answers to difficult healthcare dilemmas. Nurses have a responsibility to understand the current legal and ethical guidelines that govern client care.

Sources of Laws

Three kinds of law have potential for affecting nursing practice:

- Civil law generally governs actions by one individual or corporation against another.

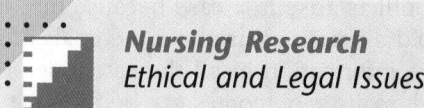

- Criminal law involves actions by the state against an individual for violations of criminal statutes.
- Administrative law involves actions by state administrative agencies against individuals or organizations.

The kinds of cases commonly affecting nursing practice are set forth in the chart. Malpractice cases are civil cases that most often involve nursing. A client or family member sues the nurse or the nurse's employer for malpractice because of a claim of client injury caused by the nursing care. Fortunately, criminal prosecution of nurses is rare. Examples of criminal law violations are drug diversion, client assault, or mercy killing. Administrative agencies govern the practice of nursing through boards or commissions of nursing in each state.

Laws come from three major sources. Statutes are passed by state and federal legislatures. Specific details of statutory implementation are governed by regulations adopted by state or federal agencies. Courts decide individual cases, which develop a precedent for how civil statutes will be interpreted. In addition, courts will interpret federal and state constitutions.

Licensure

The major type of administrative law that governs nursing is licensing law. Each state has a nurse practice act, although the language of each state act is different. Generally nurse practice acts define nursing, address the scope and expectations of practice, describe how the profession will be governed, and provide criteria for nursing education. Licensure is mandatory (that is, to practice nursing, one must be licensed as a nurse). In all states, there are exceptions for those who provide nursing care to ill friends or family members (Creighton, 1986).

Two of the current challenges to state boards of nursing are increasing the scope of practice to include the nurse's expanding role in entrepreneurial positions and establishing the baccalaureate degree as the educational requirement for registered nursing. The North Dakota Board of Nursing in 1986 was the first to tackle the latter challenge and was supported in this change by the North Dakota Supreme Court in 1987 (McCarty, 1987). Liability for licensing arises in several areas. Care given below nursing standards can result in liability to the Board of Nursing for malpractice. In addition, the Board of Nursing is concerned with nurses practicing beyond the scope of their license, even when the practice meets quality standards. For example, a nurse without an advanced practice license who decides to suture wounds or prescribe medicine may be liable for practice beyond their scope in accordance with the Nurse Practice Act. Drug diversion or abuse gives rise to a number of licensing actions, although some states now provide an alternative program that promotes treatment and rehabilitation rather than discipline. Unfortunately, client abuse and sexual contact with clients is an increasing area of liability in licensing cases. Although more significant in psychiatric nursing, sexual contact with clients *or former* clients may be a violation of standards. In addition, violation of other statutes or regulations may give rise to licensing action.

Standards of Care

Standards of care are important in malpractice and licensing cases. Each state's nurse practice act provides one set of guidelines for the standard that nursing care should meet. These guidelines vary as to how specifically they govern practice. The standards of care also are defined on the national level by the ANA and other specialty organizations. The Joint Commission on Accreditation of Healthcare Organizations (JCAHO) accredits hospitals and sets nursing standards for some aspects of care, such as documentation.

Institutions or agencies may have their own policies and procedures that define the agency standards for nursing care. Standardized nursing plans of care or protocols also may reflect the care expected for a specific client group. Healthcare reform efforts are likely to raise new issues for nursing boards or commissions (Moniz, 1992). The care provided by each nurse also is measured against the expected behavior of a nurse with a similar level of expertise and experience. Nurses involved in setting standards should be certain that the standards are realistic in light of the resources available. Standards set by an agency should by updated frequently to reflect changes in technology. Nurses *must* familiarize themselves with the standards. Standards of practice are discussed in Chapter 1. When circumstances prevent compliance with standards, nurses should document the reasons for deviation.

Informed Consent

Nurses have a moral obligation to ensure that clients give informed consent for their care. Healthcare providers are *legally* required to involve clients in healthcare decisions. The law has evolved from first demanding that physicians simply obtain permission for experimental treatment and surgery to the modern concept of giving clients full information regarding all therapeutic and diagnostic procedures. These elements must be covered for consent to be "informed:"

- The client's current medical status and the general course of the illness
- The proposed treatment and its rationale
- Risks and benefits of the proposed treatment
- Risks of not consenting to the treatment

- Alternatives to the proposed treatment, including nontreatment, and their associated risks and benefits

The healthcare provider who performs a procedure is charged with obtaining informed consent; however, it is generally the nurse's responsibility to obtain the client's signature verifying that he or she was informed about a proposed treatment. The JCAHO stipulates that agencies specify in their policies which procedures require signed consent. Once a consent form is signed, the burden of proof falls to the plaintiff in a legal action against the hospital or employee. A sample informed consent form is shown in Chapter 28.

As of 1991, 18 of the 50 states had informed consent statutes. In the other states, case law governed ("Informed Consent," 24 Creighton L. Rev. 888, 914, 1991). These statutes may define the criteria for informed consent, address the need for legal competency of the client, and stipulate who is authorized to give consent for an incompetent client. Statutory and case law grant permission to administer emergency treatment without consent if it is impossible to obtain.

Torts and Crimes

Torts and crimes are legal wrongs committed against a person or property. A **tort** is subject to action in a civil court; a crime is a violation punishable by the state. Types of torts and crimes are listed in the accompanying display.

Tort actions compensate for damages. Successful tort actions result in money damages paid to the victim. Torts may be intentional (assault and battery, invasion of privacy, false imprisonment, defamation of character) or unintentional (negligence, malpractice).

A **crime** is any wrong punishable by the state. Two elements are necessary: evil intent and a criminal act. However, crimes may exist in which intent is not absolutely clear (eg, reckless driving). Crimes are prosecuted in the criminal justice system and classified as felonies (eg, rape, murder) or misdemeanors (lesser offenses generally punishable by a fine of less than $1,000 or imprisonment of less than 1 year).

Differences Between Crimes and Torts

Crime

Results in prison term or fine or short jail sentence to punish offender.

Felony

Intentional (first-degree murder)
Unintentional (second-degree murder; manslaughter)

Misdemeanor

An offense punishable by imprisonment of less than 1 year or a fine of less than $1,000. Does not amount to a felony.

Tort

Results in civil trial to assess compensation for plaintiff.

Intentional

Assault and battery
Defamation of character
Fraud
Invasion of privacy
False imprisonment

Unintentional

Negligence (eg, error in sponge counts, causing a burn, failure to use aseptic technique, falls, medical errors, misadministration of blood)
Malpractice

Intentional Torts

Assault and Battery. **Assault** is the threat of touching another person without his or her consent. **Battery** is the actual carrying out of such a threat (ie, the unlawful touching of a person's body). A nurse can be sued for battery any time he or she fails to get consent for a procedure. For example, if an alert, competent client refuses an injection, it is unlawful for a nurse to apply restraints to carry out the procedure.

Defamation of Character. Defamation of character includes false communication resulting in injury to a person's reputation by means of print (libel) or spoken word (slander). The nurse is permitted to make statements about clients *only* as part of his or her nursing practice and *only* within the limits provided by law.

Fraud. *Fraud* is the willful, purposeful misrepresentation of self or an act that may cause harm to a person or property. A nurse who misrepresents his or her qualifications or bills for care not given may be committing a fraud.

Invasion of Privacy. The nurse is bound to limit discussion of the client to appropriate parties. Disclosing confidential information to an inappropriate third party subjects the nurse to liability for invasion of privacy, even if the information is true. The nurse should discuss the client with others only when the discussion is necessary for treatment and care or when the client consents to disclosure.

The AIDS epidemic has highlighted issues regarding defamation and invasion of privacy. A nurse who discloses that a client is HIV positive may be liable for invasion of privacy. Disclosure of a false AIDS diagnosis may constitute defamation of character.

False Imprisonment. Prevention of movement or unjustified retention of a person without consent may be *false imprisonment.* Nurses must use restraints only in accordance with agency policies and usually with the order of a physician. A client cannot be forced to remain in the hospital against his or her will (assuming that the client is mentally alert, oriented, and capable of participating in care decisions). If the client refuses to remain in the hospital, the agency will have him or her sign a release stating that he or she left without medical approval. Those with mental impairments may be committed involuntarily in accordance with court proceedings if they are dangerous to themselves or others.

Unintentional Torts

Negligence. **Negligence** may be an act of omission or commission (neglecting to do something that a reasonably prudent person would do or doing something that a reasonably prudent person would not do). **Malpractice** is negligence on the part of a professional. Intent to harm is not an element of a malpractice suit.

To prove nursing malpractice, a lawyer must prove that there has been a deviation from the standard of care that has caused damage to a client. In a malpractice case, violations of the standard of care are generally proven or disproven by expert testimony. A nurse expert in a given field of nursing will be called to testify about the standard of practice as it relates to the particular case.

To prove malpractice, four elements are necessary:

- A duty to the plaintiff
- A failure to meet the standard of care, or a breach of duty, which may be an act of omission
- Causation (that is, that the breach of duty produced the injury in a natural and continuous sequence)
- Damages, which require an actual injury to the client

Duty. *Duty* describes the relationship between the plaintiff (the person bringing suit) and the defendant (the person being sued). Nurses have a duty to care for their clients. The existence of a duty is rarely an issue in a malpractice suit.

Breach of Duty. *Breach of duty* is the failure to conform to the standard of practice, thus creating a risk for a person that a reasonable person would have foreseen. Breach of duty may be charged when a client falls in a hospital; falls used to be common causes for malpractice suits against nurses. Although the use of restraints is controversial, the courts have held that the appropriate use of siderails and restraints is a nursing judgment (O'Reilly-Yob, 1988). Nurses can best assess their clients' needs for safety measures, while following their facility's policies and procedures regarding restraints. In addition, recent nursing home regulations restrict the circumstances in which restraints legally may be used (42 CFR 483.13[a]).

Although some nursing malpractice cases involve use of highly technical equipment, many cases involve assessment of routine indicators of client well-being, such as vital signs. For example, a client underwent surgery for correction of incontinence. During her 11-day hospitalization, she suffered a fluctuating temperature. On the morning of discharge, her temperature was 102°F. Despite her elevated temperature, she was sent home in accordance with the doctor's orders. The client was readmitted with sepsis after 3 days and died 2 months later of multiple organ failure. An appellate court held that the standard of care for nurses requires them to evaluate independently a client's condition prior to hospital discharge and to discuss any concerns with physicians (*Koeniguer v. Eckrich*, 422 N.W.2d 600 [S.D. 1988]).

Proximate Cause. Causation must be proven for the courts to find negligence. A nurse's carelessness might not result in injury, or injury may occur without the nurse's carelessness as its proximate cause. This was true in the case of one client who suffered a cardiovascular accident. The court found that the nurse failed to meet the standard of care because she failed to take vital signs as frequently as ordered. The client's paralysis was not directly caused by the nurse's failure to take the client's blood pressure, however (Fiesta, 1988).

Courts frequently use foreseeability as a criterion for determining whether a cause is considered proximate (Prosser, 1984). The question becomes whether a reasonable person should have foreseen that injury would result from a failure to conform to the standard of care.

A nurse or hospital may not be liable for damage to a client even if the nurse is negligent when the negligence does not cause the plaintiff's injury. In one case, a plaintiff alleged that the discharge nurse's failure to relate the plaintiff's complaint of chest pain to an attending physician was negligent. However, an expert testified that if the nurse had reported to the physician, the result would not have been different because there was no evidence the doctor would have reexamined the plaintiff. The doctor already knew of the pain and had misdiagnosed it (*Gill v. Foster* [1992, 4th Dist.] 232 Ill. App.3d 768, 173 Ill.Dec. 802, 597 N.E.2d 776).

It is difficult to prove proximate cause with hospital-acquired infections; however, in one case, a hospital was found liable for a client's infection after he testified that the nurses did not wash their hands after caring for his roommate, who had a staphylococcal infection

(Fiesta, 1988). The nurse should have foreseen that failure to wash her hands after caring for the roommate could spread infection to the plaintiff.

Res Ipsa Loquitur. When it is obvious that the client's injury was the result of someone's negligence, but it is impossible to prove who was at fault, the doctrine of *res ipsa loquitur* ("the thing speaks for itself") may be invoked. Three elements must be proven (Fiesta, 1988):

- The injury could not have occurred if negligence were not present.
- The defendant or defendants (eg, nurse, doctor, or hospital) were in complete control of the instrument causing the injury.
- The plaintiff (client) did not voluntarily create the injury.

Damages. For a plaintiff to prevail in a malpractice suit, the plaintiff must have suffered damages. The purpose of the suit is to compensate for these damages. *General* damages include pain and suffering, disfigurement, and disability. *Special* damages are for the losses and expenses related to the injury, such as medical expenses and lost wages. *Punitive* damages are for especially malicious behavior on the part of the defendant and generally result in a larger judgment (Fiesta, 1988).

Manning v. Twin Falls Clinic and Hospital (830 P.2d 1185 [Id. 1992]) involves a lawsuit by the family of a deceased client against a nurse and hospital. The client was 67 years old when he was admitted to the hospital with a lengthy history of respiratory problems, including chronic obstructive pulmonary disease and carbon dioxide retention. He had been on oxygen for several years. He was on no code status and on oxygen in the hospital. However, the client was to be moved to a private room because he was already near death. The nurse elected to move him without using portable oxygen for transport. The client's family protested, claiming he could not survive without his oxygen and requested a portable oxygen unit. The nurse refused. The court affirmed punitive damages against the nurse personally because the care given was found to be a deviation from the community standard of nursing care (830 P.2d 1191).

Trends in Nursing Malpractice. In the past, nurses generally were not named in malpractice suits because it was considered better to sue the person or institution with the most money or insurance. Nurses are increasingly named in malpractice litigation, however, because of higher income or insurance and because of their increasing autonomy.

During the past few decades, medical care has seen dramatic advances in knowledge about disease processes and technology for diagnosis and treatment of illnesses. The number of malpractice suits has increased as a result of these highly complex and advanced methods of delivering healthcare (Benninger, 1988). The result has been higher standards of care for nurses, with a corresponding increase in liability (Salatka, 1992). The public's change in perception of the healthcare community's roles and responsibilities when caring for critically ill clients has caused an additional area of increased exposure to liability (Salatka, 1992). Increasingly, institutions are sued successfully for nurses' failure to follow the standard of care in recognizing abnormal client conditions and initiating appropriate nursing intervention, including timely notification of the attending physician (*Fairfax Hospital System, Inc. v. McCarty*, 419 S.E.2d 621 [Va. 1992]). Awards for the damages resulting from such a breach in the standard of care may be in the millions. As the pressures of healthcare reform mount, problems of chronic substandard staffing are likely to lead to more lawsuits against nurses and their institutional employers (Pruett, 1993).

Liability

Liability denotes legal responsibility to pay damages. When the four elements of negligence are proven (ie, when the nurse's breach of a duty owed to the client was the proximate cause of injury to the client), the nurse can be found liable. The hospital, clinic, or visiting nurse service may be held responsible for a nurse's negligence under the doctrine of **respondeat superior** ("let the master answer"). This notion of vicarious liability can be applied whenever the nurse is acting within the scope of employment. The employer may attempt to prove that the nurse was not acting within the scope of employment when the negligent act occurred; this is one reason why all nurses should have liability insurance. Defining scope of employment has been a difficult legal question, but nurses are generally covered by vicarious liability when they are acting under the control of their employer. General areas of liability are summarized in Table 3-1.

Hospitals have a legal duty to treat clients who come to their emergency rooms; nurses as hospital employees have a duty to treat clients admitted by the hospital (42 USC 1395 dd). In a few recent cases, clients were denied emergency treatment because they could not pay hospital fees. A nurse who refuses care to a client can be held liable for injuries resulting from such refusal.

Crimes

Criminal proceedings may be distinguished from civil tort proceedings in that the state brings charges against a defendant who has violated a criminal statute (eg, robbery, rape, or manslaughter). The state seeks punishment for that wrongdoing. Negligence that leads to the death of a client is tried as a civil tort, a lawsuit filed by the client's family. Only rarely will the state file a criminal action. In a criminal procedure, the prosecution must prove guilt beyond a reasonable doubt; in a

Table 3-1 • General Areas of Liability

	To Whom Is Healthcare Provider Responsible?	Client Injury Necessary?	Result if Successful
Malpractice or negligence	Client	Yes	Money paid to client by healthcare provider
Administrative/ Licensing	Board of nursing	No	Loss of license or keeping license on certain conditions; fine
Criminal	State represented by prosecutors	No	Jail or fine

civil case, the plaintiff need only prove a preponderance of evidence in his or her favor.

Assault and battery (described previously) also may be criminally tried. Other examples of crimes for which nurses have been tried include robbery, narcotics laws violations, and murder. In one notorious case, a nurse who wanted to prove the need for a pediatric intensive care unit administered succinylcholine to several children in a pediatrician's office. The first five children experienced respiratory arrest and survived. When the sixth child died, she was tried and convicted for murder (Tammelleo, 1986a).

Another case resulted in criminal charges when a nurse forcefully searched a client whom she suspected of stealing money from another client. When the client objected to being searched, a guard held the client's arms so the nurse could search the pockets. Finding no money, they left the client, who subsequently suffered a cardiac arrest and died. Criminal intent was shown because the nurse should have been aware that her search was illegal (Tammelleo, 1985).

Controlled Substances

In 1970, the Comprehensive Drug Abuse Prevention and Control Act was passed in the United States. In most states, nurses may administer controlled substances (narcotics, depressants, stimulants, and hallucinogens) only under the direction of a licensed physician. Misuse can lead to criminal penalties unless the substances are authorized under advanced practice licenses. In institutions, most controlled substances must be kept secure and monitored closely in accordance with institutional policies and state regulations.

Death and Dying

Death occurs when there is an absence of brain function, despite the function of other body organs. It is the nurse's duty to recognize legal death. In some states, the nurse may pronounce death at the bedside; however, in most states the physician has the legal responsibility of pronouncing the person dead.

Euthansia. Physician- or nurse-assisted death (active euthanasia) is a controversial issue. Many healthcare providers believe that actively causing a client's death would violate professional ethics. Active euthanasia is considered murder in all states and almost all other countries. Despite most practitioners' reluctance to participate in active euthanasia, there is growing support for its legalization.

Advance Directives. In 1990, the federal legislature passed the Patient Self-Determination Act. This requires that each hospital, nursing home, or visiting nurse agency admitting clients to their services inform clients about their rights regarding end-of-life decisions. The agency is required to inform clients of state law and local policy and agency policies, if any, regarding end-of-life decisions. Nurses should become familiar with statutes in their own states regarding the execution of living wills or directives to physicians, a person's signed request to be allowed to die when life can be supported only by mechanical or artificial measures. These statutes list specific procedures to follow while granting civil and criminal immunity to those following the guidelines. The living will should be prepared before people become incapacitated. Nurses should be aware of the requirements for witnessing a living will. Usually, the state's Natural Death Act prohibits an employee of the healthcare provider caring for the client to be a witness.

Resuscitation. The nurse must know the code status of his or her clients. The nurse verifies the code status on the client's order sheet and follows agency policy. When nurses are unaware and encounter a client in cardiac arrest, the client should be resuscitated pending confirmation that there is a no code order. If there is a no code order, resuscitation may be stopped once initiated.

Death Certificate. Laws are specific in the United States and Canada regarding death certificates. It is the physician's responsibility to sign a death certificate.

Care of the Body. After the death pronouncement by the physician, the nurse is responsible for preparing the body for the morgue or mortuary. The nurse must be familiar with the hospital's instructions for care and the wishes of the deceased and family. The body should be treated with dignity.

Organ Donation. The nurse must check to see if the deceased wished to donate organs to a transplant program. If the death was accidental and no donor card is available, the nurse may discuss with the family the possibility of donating the organs of the deceased. Figure 3-2 shows a sample organ donor card. A section of the living will, discussed previously in this chapter, also may provide this information. If functional organs are to be donated, the hospital should have specific care instructions for the body. The Uniform Anatomical Gift Act was promulgated in 1968 and adopted in all 50 states and the District of Columbia. The act was revised in 1987 and is in the process of adoption by the states with some variation. The new act facilitates the procurement process while safeguarding donor intentions and improves procedures for use and distribution (Uniform Anatomical Gift Act, 1987).

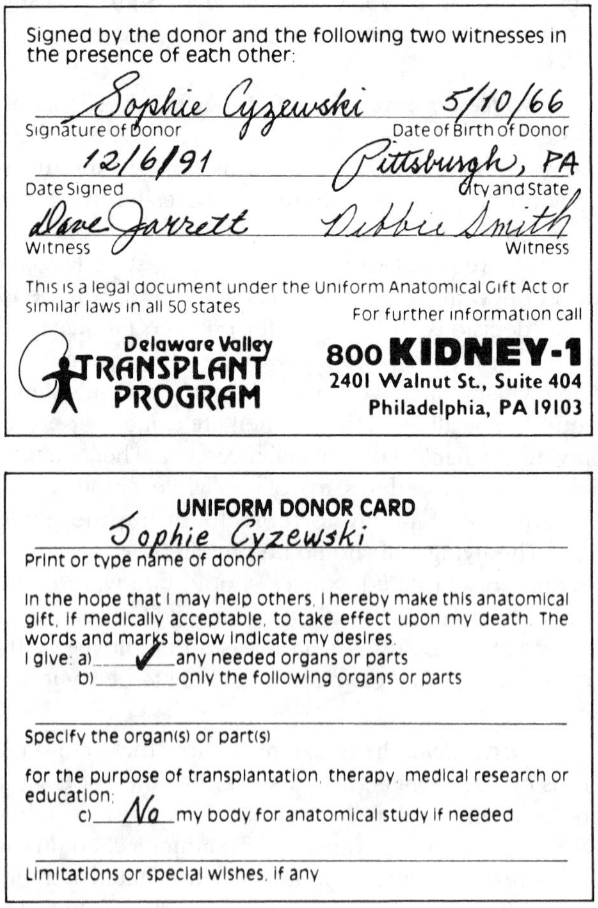

Signed by the donor and the following two witnesses in the presence of each other:

Sophie Cyzewski — 5/10/66
Signature of Donor — Date of Birth of Donor

12/6/91 — Pittsburgh, PA
Date Signed — City and State

Dave Jarrett — Debbie Smith
Witness — Witness

This is a legal document under the Uniform Anatomical Gift Act or similar laws in all 50 states

For further information call

Delaware Valley TRANSPLANT PROGRAM

800 KIDNEY-1
2401 Walnut St., Suite 404
Philadelphia, PA 19103

UNIFORM DONOR CARD

Sophie Cyzewski
Print or type name of donor

In the hope that I may help others, I hereby make this anatomical gift, if medically acceptable, to take effect upon my death. The words and marks below indicate my desires.
I give: a) ✓ any needed organs or parts
b) ______ only the following organs or parts

Specify the organ(s) or part(s)

for the purpose of transplantation, therapy, medical research or education;
c) No my body for anatomical study if needed

Limitations or special wishes, if any

Figure 3-2 • *Sample organ donor card.*

Autopsy. An *autopsy* is a postmortem examination of the organs and tissues of the body to determine the cause of death or pathologic conditions contributing to the death. Consent for an autopsy is a legal requirement. It is the physician's responsibility to request an autopsy, but family members may ask the nurse for clarification. Consent may be given by the deceased before death or by a close family member. Because of religious beliefs, some families may not consent to an autopsy, but the consent law is overruled if the death was by murder, suicide, or suspicious.

Wills. The nurse may be asked to witness a *will,* a person's declaration regarding how his or her property is to be handled after death. Many institutions have policies about nurses witnessing legal documents. If a nurse does witness a will, the nurse makes a note on the client's chart about the client's mental and physical condition at the time of the signing and of the nurse's role in the procedures. A nurse cannot be a beneficiary to any will he or she witnesses.

Good Samaritan Law

The Good Samaritan Law offers legal immunity for healthcare professionals who assist in an emergency and render reasonable care under such circumstances. Because most states do not require nurses or citizens to aid the distressed, such assistance becomes an ethical, rather than a legal, duty. Although this law limits liability for the nurse, he or she may be liable for *gross* negligence. A nurse who stops to help is obligated to remain until additional assistance is obtained. The nurse should then relinquish care to official rescue personnel unless asked to remain. Because emergency assistance is generally outside the scope of the nurse's employment, the employer's malpractice insurance will not provide coverage. This is another reason for nurses to carry their own insurance.

Protecting Yourself

Nurses may minimize the risk of legal problems, including malpractice, in a number of ways. First, nurses must keep current with advances in practice. Continuing education is absolutely essential to stay knowledgeable regarding general and particular expectations of nurses. Likewise, nurses should be familiar with state regulations governing nursing and with standards of professional organizations.

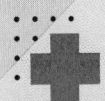

Safety Alert
Ethical and Legal Issues

- Use responsible professional judgment in performing all procedures; you are legally accountable for your actions.
- Carry out physicians' orders. Question orders you feel are detrimental or in error; you are accountable independent of the physician.
- Take responsibility only for assignments for which you have been prepared; ask for supervision for tasks in which you have less skill.
- Know the limits of the nurse practice act in your state; you are accountable for practice within the limits of that act.

Nurses involved in the development of policies, procedures, protocols, or standardized nursing plans of care should be sure to make them realistic, whether for home or an agency. Such measures of the standard of care should not be made unless they can be applied with the resources available. Staffing and equipment to conform to these guidelines must be available on nights, weekends, holidays, and weekdays. Those who develop standards to apply to various practice settings should keep in mind the differences in resources and facilities of different sizes, acuity, and geographic area. Those involved in policy making need to continue to update the policies to be timely and sensible in accordance with the demands of nursing. New knowledge must be applied. Policies, procedures, and protocols must be followed. Propounding unrealistic policies and procedures and then not following them is an invitation to malpractice suits.

The condition of the client must be monitored and the observations documented. Whether the client is in a hospital recovering from surgery, in home care coping with a chronic illness, or dealing with long-term, multiple drug administration, assessment of the client must be recorded. Significant changes in the client's condition need to be reported to the physician in a timely manner. The report to the physician also must be documented. When physicians do not follow up with assessment intervention, their care needs to be challenged by the nurse. Hospitals may be liable when nurses do not challenge physicians in the face of obvious negligence (*Schoening v. Grays Harbor Hospital*, 40 Wn. App. 331, 698 P.2d 593 [1985]).

Documentation

Documentation should be accurate, complete, and contemporaneous with the care given (Fig. 3-3). Documentation should include normal findings in the form of a flow sheet, checklist, or narrative. When critical events occur, the precise time should be noted in the records. Vital signs need to be assessed in accordance with agency policy and recorded. Documentation should be objective. Criticism of other providers does not belong in the medical record. Negative comments about the client or family also should not be included in the medical record, unless they constitute objective documentation of behavior or accurate quotations of statements made. Errors should be corrected by marking a line through the error and recording the nurse's initials. An entry should never be obliterated. The presumption will be that the matter erased is more damaging than whatever was actually written. If a specific incident, such as a fall or medication error, occurs, follow these principles:

- Maintain rapport with the client. Do not avoid communication with the client who is experiencing stress and uncertainty. Offer simple explanations if you can do so honestly, calmly, and without blaming anyone.
- Document the incident in the progress notes and the appropriate forms used by your institution. Incident reports are useful to remind you of the events surrounding the incident (Doll, 1980), and they are useful to bring about needed changes in the institution (Communique, 1988).

Nursing students must perform *only* duties that are in the scope of their professional training to date. These acts are performed with the same degree of competence an RN would exhibit. Under the auspices of a clinical supervisor, they may carry out assignments. Nursing students assume liability for their negligent or wrong acts. The clinical supervisor or school may be held liable as well.

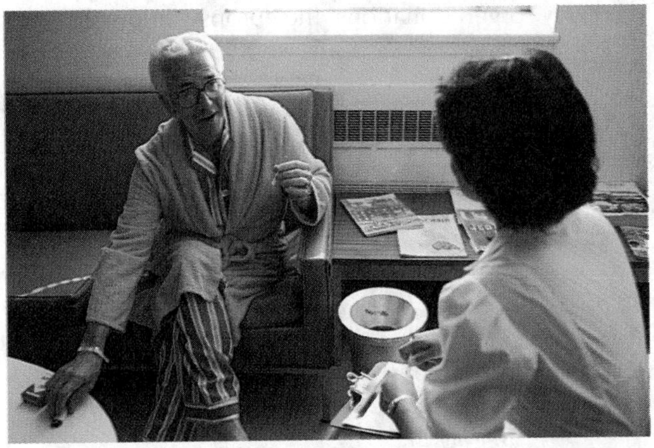

Figure 3-3 • *The nurse is responsible for documenting what assessments he or she makes; what planning is done with the client; what actions he or she takes, including teaching; and the results of those actions.*

Key Concepts

- Morals are standards of right and wrong. Values are ideas and beliefs that and individual holds to be important.
- Nurses must be able to use ethical and legal reasoning in their clinical practice.
- The ANA code of ethics is the nurse's value statement to the public.
- Universal moral principles include beneficence, nonmaleficence, autonomy, and justice. Rules include confidentiality, veracity, and fidelity.
- An ethical dilemma involves choosing between conflicting values. Resolution of a dilemma involves the application of structured analysis based on moral principles.
- Nurses are potentially subject to discipline by the licensing authority when malpractice occurs, which involves care below the standard of care or when care rendered is beyond the scope of nursing practice.
- Individual state nurse practice acts provide some guidance for standards of nursing care.
- The four elements of negligence are duty, breach of duty, proximate cause, and damage.
- Although the Good Samaritan Law provides immunity for professionals under specific circumstances, nurses should carry personal liability insurance.
- One way to avoid malpractice litigation is to follow the current standard of nursing care as evidenced in state statutes and regulations, standards of professional organizations, and current literature.
- The nurse has legal responsibilities regarding the dying client and the deceased (eg, euthanasia, living wills, resuscitation, the death certificate, care of the body, organ donations, the autopsy, and wills).

Critical Thinking Challenges

Legal and ethical information is an important addition to your developing knowledge base of the nursing profession. Now you should be able to turn to the situation at the beginning of the chapter, and apply your new information to the following.

1. *Design assessments of the client's and family's comprehension and expectations of the client's deteriorating health.*
2. *Based on those data, identify planning and interventions that you believe are needed.*
3. *Propose additional information you need to supply the family, so you can assist them in planning realistic possibilities for the future.*
4. *Detect the ethical dilemmas that may be part of the planning decisions.*
5. *Determine the legal concerns you see as inherent in this situation.*

References

24 Creighton L.Rev. 888, 914 (1991). Informed Consent.

American Hospital Association (1984a). *A patient's bill of rights.* Chicago: Author.

American Hospital Association (1984b). *Hospital Committees on biomedical ethics. American Hospital Association Guidelines.* Catalog #025001.15M-2/84-0387. Chicago: Author.

American Nurses' Association (1985). *Code for nurses with interpretive statements.* Kansas City, MO: Author.

American Nurses Association (1993). *Nursing and HIV/AIDS national action agenda, 1993 update.* Kansas City, MO: Author.

Appelbaum, P. S., Lidz, C. W., & Meisel, A. (1987). *Informed consent. Legal theory and clinical practice.* New York: Oxford University Press.

Beauchamp, T. L., & Childress, J. F. (1989). *Principles of biomedical ethics* (3rd ed.). New York: Oxford University Press.

Benjamin, M., & Curtis, J. (1986). *Ethics in nursing.* New York: Oxford University Press.

Broom, C. (1990). Conflict resolutions strategies for ethical dilemmas: When ethical dilemmas evolve to conflict. *Dimensions of Critical Care Nursing, 10*(6): 354–363.

Communique, Q. A. (1988). Development of an incident reporting system. *Quarterly Review Bulletin, 14,* 245–250.

Creighton, H. (1986). *Law every nurse should know* (5th ed.) (pp. 2, 148, 227, 233). Philadelphia: W.B. Saunders.

Doll, A. (1980). What to do after an incident. *Nursing '80, 10,* 73–79.

Espinosa, E., Gonzales-Baron, M., Poveda, J., Ordonez, A., & Zamora, P. (1993). The information given to the terminal patient with cancer. *European Journal of Cancer, 29(12),* 1795–1796.

Fiesta, J. (1988). *The law and liability: A guide for nurses* (2nd ed.). St. Paul, MN: John Wiley & Sons.

Gorovitz, S. (Ed.) (1971). *Utilitarianism with critical essays* (pp. 18, 21). New York: Bobbs-Merrill.

Jonsen, A. R. (1994). Clinical ethics and the four principles. In R. Gillon & A. Lloyd (Eds.), *Principles of health care ethics* (pp. 13–22). Chichester: John Wiley & Sons.

Jonsen, A. R., Siegler, M., & Winslade, W. (1992). Clinical ethics (3rd ed.). New York: McGraw-Hill.

Levinson, J. L., & Pettrey, L. (1994). Controversial decisions regarding treatment and DNR: An algorithmic guide for the uncertain in decision-making ethics (GUIDE). *American Journal of Critical Care,* 3(2), 87–91.

McCarty, M. (Ed.) (1987). Legislature upholds North Dakota Board of Nursing's power. *The American Nurse, 19,* 3.

Moniz, D. M. (1992). The legal danger of written protocols and standards of practice. *The Nurse Practitioner, The American Journal of Primary Health Care, 17*(9).

Munson, R. (1992). *Intervention and reflection: Basic issues in medical ethics* (4th ed.). Belmont, CA: Wadsworth.

O'Reilly-Yob, M. (1988). Use of restraints: Too much or not enough? *Focus of Critical Care, 15,* 32–33.

Patient Self-Determination Act. 42 USC 1396a(a); 42 USC 1396m(1)(a); 42 USC 1396n(c)(2).

Pearlman, R. A., Cain, K. C., Patrick, D. L., Appelbaum-Maizel, M., Starks, H. E., Jecker, N. S., & Uhlmann, R. F. (1993). Insights pertaining to patient assessment of states worse than death. *Journal of Clinical Ethics, 4*(1), 33–41.

President's Commission for the Study of Ethical Problems in Medicine and Biomedical and Behavioral Research (1982). *Making health care decisions* (Vol. 1) (pp. 2, 32, 44, 46). Washington, DC: U.S. Government Printing Office.

Prosser, W. L. (1984). *Handbook of the law of torts* (4th ed.) (p. 267). St. Paul, MN: West.

Pruett (1993). Chronic substandard staffing and the nurses' liability. *Critical Care Nurse,* 88.

Salatka (1992). Professional liability in critical care nursing. *Ohio Northern University Law Review, 19,* 85.

Sardell, A. N., & Trierweiler, S. J. (1993). Disclosing the cancer diagnosis. *Cancer, 72*(11), *3355–3365.*

Schneiderman, L. J., Jecker, N. S., & Jonsen, A. R. (1990). Medical Futility: Its meaning and ethical implications. *Annals of Internal Medicine, 112*(12), *949–954.*

Sell, L., Devlin, B., Bourke, S. J., Munro, N. C., Corris, P. A., & Gibson, G. J. (1993). Communicating the diagnosis of lung cancer. *Respiratory Medicine, 87,* 61–63.

Shilts, R. (1988). *And the band played on: Politics, people and the AIDS epidemic.* New York: Penguin Books.

Silva, M. C. (1990). Preparation of nurse executives for ethical decision making. *Nursing Connections, 3*(2), 28–31.

Stopes-Roe, H. (1994). Principles and life stances: A humanist view. In R. Gillon & A. Lloyd (Eds.), *Principles of health care ethics* (pp. 117–133). Chichester: John Wiley & Sons.

Tammelleo, A. D. (Ed.). (1985). Chaos in the O.R. *The Regan Report on Nursing Law, 26,* 4.

Tammelleo, A. D. (Ed.) (1986a). Nurse murders pediatric patient. *The Regan Report on Nursing Law, 27,* 6.

Tammelleo, A. D. (Ed.) (1986b). R.N. searches patient—Death results. *The Regan Report on Nursing Law, 27,* 2.

Walker, M. U. (1993). Keeping moral space open: New images of ethics consulting. *Hastings Center Report, 23*(2), 33–40.

Walters, L. (1988). Ethical issues in the prevention and treatment of HIV infection and AIDS. *Science, 239,* 597–603.

Woodard, L. J., & Parmies, R. J. (1992). The disclosure of the diagnosis of cancer. *Primary Care, V19*(4), 657–663.

Bibliography

American Nurses' Association Congress for Nursing Practice (1973). *Standards for nursing practice.* Kansas City, MO: Author.

American Nurses' Association (1980). *Nursing: A social policy statement.* Kansas City, MO: Author.

Annas, G. J. (1985). Adam Smith in the emergency room. *Hastings Center Report, 15,* 4.

Astrom, G., Jansson, L., Norberg, A., & Hallberg, I. R. (1993). Experienced nurses' narratives of their being in ethically difficult care situations. The problem to act in accordance with one's ethical reasoning and feelings. *Cancer Nursing, 16*(3), *179–187.*

Broom, C. (1994). Patient-family conflicting issues: Part 2: Case analysis. *Dimensions of Critcal Care Nursing, 13*(1), *44–50.*

Callahan, D. (1990). *What Kind of Life?* New York: Simon and Schuster.

Canadian Nurses Association (1985). *Code of ethics for nursing.* Ottawa: Author.

Cameron, M. E., Crisham, P., & Lewis, D. E. (1993). The basic nature of ethical problems experienced by persons with acquired immunodeficiency syndrome: Implications for nursing ethics education and practice. *Journal of Professional Nursing, 9*(6), *327–335.*

Curtin, L. L., & Flaherty, M. J (1982). *Nursing ethics: Theories and pragmatics.* Bowie, MD: Robert J. Brady.

Cushing, M. (1982). Gaps in documentation. *American Journal of Nursing, 82,* 1899–1900.

Davis, A. J., & Aroskar, M. A. (1983). *Ethical dilemmas and nursing practice* (2nd ed.). Norwalk, CN: Appleton-Century-Crofts.

Davis, A. J. (1991). Dilemmas in alternative care settings. *Western Journal of Nursing Research, 13*(5), 650–652.

Francoeur, R. T. (1983). *Biomedical ethics.* New York: John Wiley & Sons.

Gilligan, C. (1982). *In a different voice* (p. 74). Cambridge, MA: Harvard University Press.

Greenlaw, J. (1982). When leaving siderails down can bring you up on charges. *RN, 45,* 75–78.

Guarrielo, D. L. (1984). Legal booby-traps in nursing standards. *RN, 47,* 19–21.

International Council of Nurses (1973). *ICN code for nurses: Ethical concepts applied to nursing.* Geneva: Imprimeries Polpularies.

Jameton, A. (1984). *Nursing practice: The ethical issues* (p. 5). Englewood Cliffs, NJ: Prentice-Hall.

Kadish, S., Schulhofer, S., & Paulsen, M. (1983). *Criminal law and its processes* (4th ed.) (p. 274). Boston: Little, Brown.

Kant, I. (1785). *Groundwork of the metaphysics of morals* (pp. 22, 63). New York: Bobbs-Merrill.

Kaufmann, W. (1970). Prologue. In M. Buber (Ed.), *I and Thou* (p. 20). New York: Charles Scribner's Sons.

Killian, W. H. (1990). Nurses face increasing liability. *American Nurse, 22,* 43.

Mancini, M. (1984). What you should know about malpractice insurance. *American Journal of Nursing, 84,* 985–986.

Murphy, E. K. (1990). Legal concerns of the next decade. *Association of Operating Room Nurses, 51,* 258, 260–261.

Penticuff, J. H. (1990). Ethical issues in redefining death. *Journal of Neuroscience Nurses, 22,* 48–49.

Putsch, R. W. (1985). Cross-cultural communication: The special case of interpreters in health care. *JAMA, 254*(23), *3344–3348.*

Reinert, B. R., & Buck, E. A. (1989). Issues in liability insurance and the nursing consultant. *Clinical Nurse Specialist, 3,* 42–45.

Rozovsky, F. A. (1993 Supplement). *Consent to treatment* (pp. 16–17). Little, Brown and Company.

Singer, P. A., Pellegrino, E. D., & Siegler, M. (1990). Ethics committees and consultants. *Journal of Clinical Ethics, 1*(4), *263–267.*

Trandel-Korenchuk, D. M., & Trandel-Korenchuk, K. M. (1980). Current legal issues facing nursing practice. *Nursing Administration Quarterly, 5,* 37–45.

Turner, J. S., & Helms, D. B. (1987). *Lifespan development.* New York: Holt, Rinehart & Winston.

Watson, C. (1993). The role of the nurse in ethical decision making in intensive care units. *Intensive Critical Care Nursing, 9*(3), *191–194.*

Nursing Leadership and Management

Key Terms	Learning Objectives

Key Terms

Charge nurse
Clinical nurse specialist
Controlling
Directing
Directive leadership
Leadership
Managed care
Management
Nurse anesthetist
Nurse executive
Nurse midwife
Nurse practitioner
Organizing
Participative leadership
Planning
Primary nursing
Problem-solving
Team leader
Team nursing

Learning Objectives

Upon completion of this chapter, the student will be able to do the following:

- *Define the differences between leadership and management.*
- *Describe the four components of the management process.*
- *Identify three skills required for effective management.*
- *List interventions that can control perceptions and reactions to change.*
- *Describe common clinical practice, management, and education roles in nursing.*
- *Characterize leadership and management functions of common nursing roles.*
- *Identify and describe the three most popular models of nursing care delivery.*
- *Explain why problem-solving, management, and nursing processes are similar.*

4

Your charge nurse wants to change the practice model on your unit from team nursing to primary nursing. You have been working on the unit for 3 years. You are pleased with the present system and wonder how the change will affect you. Will you be happy with a new model?

In previous chapters, you learned about many concepts related to professional nursing: education, standards, theory, and ethical and legal concerns. In this chapter, you will learn about two more features of nursing: leadership and management. As you develop new skills, you will expand your knowledge base about the profession you are entering. Critical Thinking Challenges at the end of the chapter will help you apply your body of knowledge to the previous situation.

As professionals, nurses have a responsibility to provide a defined service that meets the needs of society. The American Nurses Association's (1980) social policy statement defines that service as "the diagnosis and treatment of human responses to actual or potential health problems." The American Organization of Nurse Executives (1993) further defines three essential role components of nursing as: "1) a contingent component which requires medical authorization for treatment, 2) an independent component of practice, and 3) a role as integrator and coordinator of care, across the lifespan of individuals, as well as across settings and among disciplines" (AONE 1993). For the professionals in nursing to meet the service responsibilities to society and fulfill the accountabilities of the three component roles of nursing, the profession needs internal organization and leadership. At the institutional level, leadership abilities and management skills are required to provide the circumstances in which nurses can practice. At the individual nurse–client level, leadership and good management skills are required to determine the plan of nursing care, integrate that plan of care effectively with other healthcare professionals, and coordinate the interdisciplinary treatment plan for the client.

Because of the diverse specialties, the variety of work settings in which nurses practice, and the vast number of roles, each nursing leadership role cannot be addressed. Nurses may decide to specialize in medical, surgical, parent–child, psychiatric, or home health fields or any subcomponent of these specialties, such as cardiac, oncology, or gerontology nursing. Nurses also may choose to care for clients with either acute or chronic illnesses. Although most nurses work in hospitals, others work in home health nursing, clinics, physicians' offices, nursing homes, schools, industry, the military, or missionary work. Nurses may choose among clinical practice roles, teaching roles, or management roles. Although most nurses are clinicians, education and management roles exist in most organizations where nurses practice to provide the education, management, communication, and representation required for nurses to practice nursing.

Many options are available to new nursing graduates. Throughout their nursing careers, they may choose different work settings and roles in nursing. This chapter discusses leadership, the management process, management skills, and leadership and management aspects of some common roles in nursing.

Leadership

Leadership is the ability to influence others to strive for a vision or goal or to change. Leadership results from the effective practice of behaviors that are selected to meet the needs of the situation. These behaviors can be learned.

There is no one best way (or one best set of behaviors) for effective leadership. Research on leaders and leadership has shown that different leaders have different inherent traits and abilities (Bass, 1990; Yukl, 1989). Although certain personality traits are more common in leaders than in followers, no single set of traits is always found in leaders. Although many leaders are assertive, decisive, logical, thorough, and innovative, some followers also have these traits. According to more recent leadership research, a leader's effectiveness depends not only on his or her traits, skills, and behaviors, but also on characteristics of the followers, the relationship between the leader and followers, and factors in the situation, such as their shared purpose and desire for change (Bass, 1990; Rost, 1993; Yukl, 1989).

Styles of Leadership

Effective leadership occurs when a person with the right combination of personality traits and abilities uses behaviors appropriate for the circumstance. A leader who is effective in one situation may not be effective in another. Leaders are often described by the style of leadership they predominantly use. Leadership style describes how the leader interacts with followers, which reflects his or her traits, values, abilities, and behaviors.

In a classic article that has been the basis for many subsequent leadership theories, Tannenbaum and Schmidt (1973) describe leadership styles along a continuum from directive to participative (Fig. 4-1).

Directive leadership describes a leader who makes all the decisions and tells followers what to do. The leader is in complete control. The directive leader does not involve followers in problem-solving, discus-

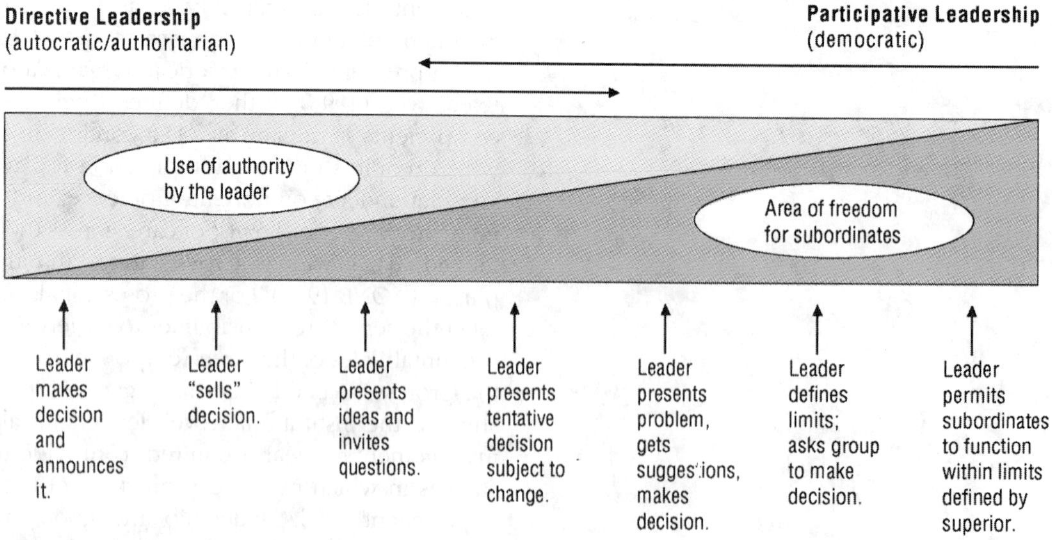

Figure 4-1 • *Leadership style is often described along a continuum from directive to participative. Directive leadership is sometimes called* autocratic, authoritative, *or* boss-centered. *The opposite end of the continuum is participative leadership, also called* democratic *or* subordinate-centered *leadership. (Adapted by permission of* Harvard Business Review. *An exhibit from "how to choose a leadership pattern" by Tannenbaum, R. & Schmidt, W.H. (May/June, 1973). Copyright © 1973 by the Presidents and Fellows of Harvard College; all rights reserved.)*

sion, or decision-making. This type of leadership is also called authoritarian or autocratic. It was formerly used in hospitals: Physicians told nurses what to do, and nurses told clients what to do. As the roles of nurses and clients have changed, leadership style also has changed. A participative or democratic leadership usually is preferred. In an emergency, however, leadership may require one person to make decisions and instruct others what to do.

Participative leadership, also referred to as democratic, is at the opposite end of the continuum. The participative leader involves followers in goal-setting, problem-solving, and decision-making. This involvement acknowledges the importance of followers in goal achievement and effective organization and promotes a sense of control over individual situations. Participative leadership also tends to involve those most familiar with the details of the situation in the decision. To be effective, a participative leader also must provide overall direction to the group process.

Under most circumstances, some degree of participation is appropriate to promote job satisfaction and commitment, but in a crisis or emergency, there is no time for group discussion and decision, so directive leadership is most appropriate. A more directive style also may be appropriate when the leader is sharing new skills or knowledge with immature, insecure, or unskilled followers. The effective leader learns how to vary his or her style to match the circumstances.

Today's postindustrial, information age has seen rapid change and major transitions; for example, much of healthcare has moved from the hospital to the home, and the focus of nursing has changed from tasks and treatments to coordination of the interdisciplinary treatment plan for clients. Therefore, certain leadership competencies and actions are more effective today. Effective leaders are driven by their own values and sense of purpose. They communicate a vision and coach, facilitate, and empower others to master change and work toward that vision (Bass & Avolio, 1994; Covey, 1991; Noer, 1993; Senge, 1990).

Management

Management is a systematic process similar to the problem-solving and nursing processes (see Chap. 9). All are similar because they are based on the scientific or research process.

Functions of Managers

Management is getting a job done or accomplishing a goal by planning, organizing, directing, and controlling (Fig. 4-2). In any setting, these four management functions provide a way to organize people, things, and ac-

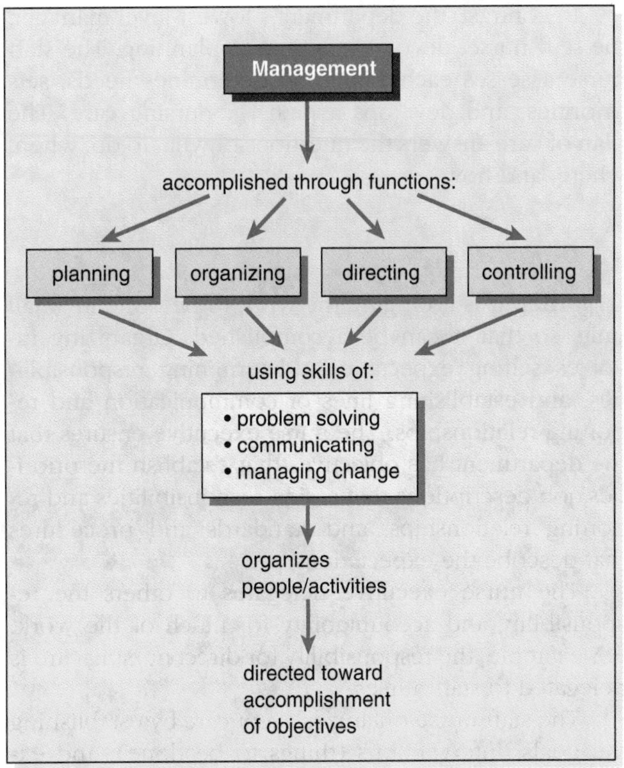

Figure 4-2 • *The management process includes the functions of planning, organizing, directing, and controlling. To perform each of these functions effectively, managers must be skilled in problem-solving, communicating, and managing change.*

tivities and to direct them toward overall objectives. These management functions provide the glue that holds the organization together. In healthcare organizations, managers must organize the healthcare professionals and support staff; the building space, supplies, and equipment; and the client care and support activities. The four management functions help to accomplish the overall objective of providing quality client care.

Planning

Planning is deciding what to do, when, where, how, by whom, and with what resources. Planning is an ongoing process that involves assessing, setting goals, establishing priorities, developing action plans, and evaluating whether the actions are meeting the objectives. Planning provides direction for the people involved, meaning for the work activities, and a scheme for efficient use of the people, space, and equipment.

In a nursing department, the top-level manager, the **nurse executive,** devotes a great deal of time to planning. The nurse executive plans the department's goals and services and determines the numbers and types of nurses and other personnel required to provide those services.

In contrast, the department's lowest-level manager, the staff nurse, devotes less time to planning. The staff nurse assesses each client and determines needs, sets priorities, and develops a plan for nursing care. The plan of care answers the questions of what to do, when, where, and how.

Organizing

Organizing is arranging the work to be done in small units so that it can be accomplished. Organizing involves setting expectations, determining responsibilities, and establishing lines of communication and reporting relationships. The nurse executive ensures that the department has objectives that establish the priorities, job descriptions that assign responsibilities and reporting relationships, and standards and procedures that describe the expectations.

The nurse executive delegates to others the responsibility and accountability for much of the work. For example, the responsibility for direct nursing care is delegated to staff nurses.

The staff nurse organizes client care by establishing the goals, interventions (things to be done), and expected outcomes of the care. The plan of care, nursing documentation, and nursing shift report communicate priorities to other nurses who are delegated responsibility for delivering some of the nursing care.

Directing

Directing involves supervision and ongoing decision-making to carry out the plans. Directing includes assigning responsibilities for the work to be done, providing instructions, communicating expectations, and guiding others as needed to reach the overall objectives. The nurse executive directs much of the change for the department of nursing by supervising the next level managers; he or she devotes much less time to directing than to planning and controlling.

The **charge nurse** directs the work of the shift by assigning clients, scheduling meal and break times, and determining who will admit and care for clients admitted during the shift. The staff nurse directs the care for clients by ordering nursing care, communicating the care on the written plan of care and in shift reports, and supervising the care delivered by others.

Controlling

Controlling is checking that plans are being carried out as planned and evaluating the outcomes of the actions. Controlling also includes evaluating staff. Some steps in the control process are measuring results against pre-established standards or expectations and taking action to reinforce effective actions and to change ineffective ones.

The nurse executive monitors the results of recruitment, staff turnover, and budget performance against expectations. He or she uses the performance appraisal process to acknowledge positive performance and to promote further growth in staff.

The staff nurse reassesses the client to determine whether the prescribed nursing interventions and interdisciplinary treatments are resulting in client improvement, whether interventions need to be changed, and whether other interventions should be added.

Skills for Effective Management

Because managers deal with people, ideas, and things, the effective manager must be skilled in problem-solving, communicating, and managing change.

Problem-Solving

Problem-solving is a systematic process (see Chap. 9) that involves the following steps:

1. Identifying and analyzing the problem
2. Determining possible solutions

Skills for Effective Management

Abilities to Problem Solve

- Identify and analyze the problem.
- Determine possible solutions.
- Consider consequences, and choose solution.
- Implement the solution.
- Evaluate results.

Abilities to Communicate

- Send a clear message.
- Receive and objectively interpret the message.
- Have verbal skills: writing and speaking.
- Be able to listen.
    - Pay full attention to speaker.
    - Listen to facts and feelings.
    - Avoid prematurely judging meaning.
    - Avoid prematurely formulating a response.
    - Use questions to clarify.
- Use nonverbal skills: body language.

Abilities to Manage Change

- Compare current to anticipated future.
- Determine if change is needed.
- Involve appropriate people.
- Communicate goals or vision.
- Provide required information, skills, knowledge, and resources.
- Reinforce progress, and overcome resistance.

3. Considering the consequences of each possible solution and choosing a solution
4. Implementing the solution
5. Evaluating the results

Identifying and analyzing the problem involves collecting information about the issue to clarify the problem and its circumstances. Gathering information helps to clarify the problem and also offers clues to possible solutions and their consequences. After speculating on the possible consequences of each proposed solution, the manager chooses the solution that is expected to result in the most positive outcome. After the solution is implemented, another assessment will determine whether the desired results were obtained.

Managers use problem-solving in each step of the management process (planning, organizing, directing, and controlling). Staff nurses use problem-solving in each step of the nursing process to manage client care.

Communication

Communication is a prerequisite to problem-solving and one of the fundamental skills of management. Research shows that managers spend 75% to 90% of their time communicating in one form or another with others (Glueck, 1980). Staff nurses spend a large amount of their time communicating with clients, families, other nurses, physicians, and other healthcare professionals and support staff.

To implement the management process successfully, managers must have effective writing, speaking, and listening skills. For effective communication, the sender must be able to translate what they mean into what they say, and the receiver must be able to receive and objectively interpret that message. The interpretation of the message can be influenced by factors such as differences in the sender's and receiver's skills, background experiences, education, trust, values, semantics, and emotional states. The status difference between the leader and followers also may affect communication effectiveness.

The nonverbal cues accompanying the message are essential aspects of verbal communication. If the sender's tone, speed, inflection of voice, facial expression, or other nonverbal behaviors are consistent with the verbal message, communication will be enhanced; however, if any of these are inconsistent with the verbal message, the receiver will believe the nonverbal message instead of the verbal one.

Listening is an important part of effective verbal communication. Listening can be hampered by the listener's lack of interest in the topic, premature interpretation of the message, or preoccupation with preparing a response. Good listening is a choice of actions that can be improved with practice. To be more effective, the listener should do the following:

- Give full attention to what the speaker is saying.
- Listen to the facts and feelings.
- Avoid formulating a response or judging the meaning until the speaker has finished.
- Use questions to clarify meanings.

Communication skills are necessary for successful implementation of the management process. Managers depend on communication to stay informed, to assist with planning and decision-making, and to convey decisions to others. Effective leaders inspire followers by successfully communicating a shared meaning of goals, direction, and vision. Staff nurses rely on communication to care for clients and families, to relate to coworkers, and to function as an effective interdisciplinary team member.

Managing Change

Charles Handy defines change as growth or learning (Handy, 1990). To be effective, managers must be masters of the change process. They need to be able to assess a situation and anticipate future needs, to determine when change is needed, and to implement the needed change. Managers also must be able to manage change that is imposed by others.

Managers need to know how to overcome resistance to change in themselves, their followers, and the overall organization (Fig. 4-3). Lack of knowledge, inaccurate information, fear of the unknown, threats to status or position, and threats to economic benefits can cause resistance to change. Education and enhanced communication are the best ways to reduce resistance caused by a lack of information or inaccurate information. Participation and involvement are effective approaches when the initiators of the change do not have all the information they need to design the change and when others have the power to resist the change. When people are resisting the change because of emotional adjustment problems, the best interventions are facilitation and support. Negotiation and agreement may be appropriate when the change adversely affects the person's position or economic status.

People can control their perceptions and reactions to change by being aware of emotional reactions associated with change and by actively seeking information, increasing communication, and getting involved in the change process. Those who perceive change as an opportunity for learning and personal growth see it as positive and offer less resistance to the change.

To implement change effectively, managers must assess the implications of any change for themselves and their followers and must intervene by providing needed communication, information, support, and involvement. For instance, illness represents a change for clients and their family members. The nurse increases communication, teaches, involves the client and family

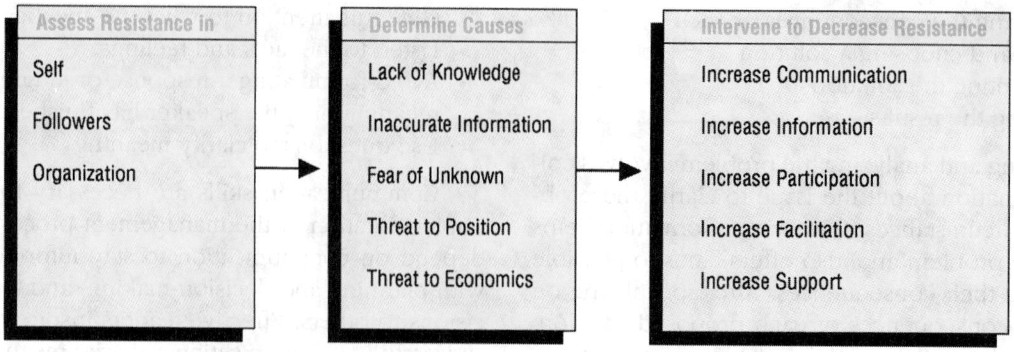

Figure 4-3 • *To be effective, managers must be masters of the change process. They need to know how to intervene in order to overcome resistance to change in themselves, their followers, and the overall organization.*

in care, and offers support to ease client and family adjustment to illness.

Applying Leadership and Management to Nursing Roles

There is a subtle difference between leadership and management. Leadership focuses on people and inspiring them to perform or change. Management focuses on getting the job done by planning, organizing, directing, and controlling people and activities. To be effective, managers must also have leadership abilities. To be effective, nurses also use both management and leadership skills in the various professional nursing roles as discussed in the following section (Marquis & Huston, 1994).

Clinical Practice Roles

Nursing delivers its service to society through clinical practice roles. The teaching and administrative roles within the profession exist to support and represent the clinical practice roles. Circumstances, such as the availability of nurses, changing client populations, changes in technology, hospital system variations, and altered financial conditions, lead to the development of new models of care delivery or variations in current models. Nurses use their knowledge of systems, the current circumstances, and the priorities of care to adjust the current model of care delivery or to create a new one.

> ***Difference Between Leadership and Management***
>
> - **Leadership** is focused on personnel and inspiring them to perform or change.
> - **Management** is focused on getting the job done by planning, organizing, directing, and controlling people and activities.

Staff Nurse

The core role of nursing is the staff nurse role. Most nurses are staff nurses, and they deliver most of the nursing care directly to clients, whether in the hospital, long-term care, or home. The staff nurse fulfills many functions in the delivery of client care: provider of care, decision-maker, client advocate, team member, communicator, and educator. Whether working in a hospital, clinic or office setting, or in the community, the staff nurse initiates the nursing process. He or she assesses the client and family, determines nursing diagnoses, establishes a plan of care (nursing orders), and evaluates the outcome of the care. In addition, the staff nurse consults with other healthcare professionals, reports the most current client status, and coordinates the care by those professionals. The staff nurse uses management skills to integrate the nursing plan of care with the therapy plans of the other healthcare professionals and leadership skills to coordinate the interdisciplinary care for the client.

The most popular models of care delivery are team nursing, primary nursing, and managed care.

Team Nursing. In **team nursing**, a team cares for a group of clients, with team members assigned specific care functions or procedures to perform for all the clients. Members of the team usually include at least nurses, licensed practical nurses, and nursing assistants. The **team leader** is the nurse who manages the team by using the management process (planning, organizing, directing, and controlling).

Some of the advantages of team nursing include the natural group discussion and decision-making about the plan of care for each client. Team nursing in an inpatient setting also provides an easy mechanism for more experienced nurses to supervise and teach less experienced nurses.

Applying Roles of Leadership and Management to Nursing in Clinical Practice

Staff Nurse

- Functions as provider of care, decision-maker, client advocate, team member, communicator, coordinator, educator
- Initiates the nursing process
- Consults with other health professionals
- Reports current client status
- Integrates the plan of nursing with therapy plans of other professionals
- Coordinates client care

Team Nurse

Cares for a group of clients; different team members are assigned specific care functions for all clients. The team leader, a nurse, manages the team.

- Organizes group discussion and decision-making on the plan of care for each client
- Provides a mechanism for more experienced nurses to supervise and teach less experienced nurses

Primary Nurse

- Assumes responsibility for developing a 24-hour plan for nursing care
- Integrates that plan with the therapy plan of the other healthcare professionals
- Accepts total responsibility for quality of care
- Has autonomy and professional accountability
- Delegates appropriate tasks and procedures to assistive personnel

Managed Care

- Primary nurse works jointly with a physician to develop and individualize a standard plan of care, which includes a time frame
- Evaluates daily the client's progress with the physician and plans corrections and changes

Advanced Clinical Practice Roles

Clinical Nurse Specialist

(Registered nurse with a master's degree and advanced preparation in a specialty area)

- Gives direct client care
- Consults with staff nurses
- Provides advanced education for nurses in specialty areas
- Evaluates nursing care outcomes
- Develops new nursing practice to support new therapy or new technology

Nurse Practitioner

(Registered nurse with advanced degree in a specialty area and either certification or advanced licensing)

- Practices independently in a specialty area (usually practices in community clinics or offices as independent practitioner or as member of a group practice)
- Uses good management techniques in planning and implementing client care, consultation efforts, and educational programs
- Delivers advanced care
- Consults on complex care issues
- Develops new nursing practice
- Participates in nursing research and publication

One disadvantage is that more staff members deliver care to each client. This fragmentation may result in decreased accountability for the overall plan and delivery of care and can result in decreased quality of client outcome. The client and family also are less likely to develop rapport with the nursing staff and are less likely to receive consistent care.

Primary Nursing. In **primary nursing** within a hospital, a professional nurse assumes responsibility for developing a 24-hour nursing plan of care and for integrating that plan with the therapy plan of the other healthcare professionals. The primary nurse accepts total responsibility for the quality of the nursing care for a client. He or she uses good management skills in planning and coordinating client care. The primary nurse also uses leadership abilities to ensure that the prescribed plan is implemented and that the nursing care is integrated with the care delivered by others.

Primary nursing results in increased continuity of care, improved interdisciplinary communication, and enhanced coordination of the total therapy plan. Primary nursing provides improved quality and consistency of nursing care for clients. The primary nursing model can result in increased job satisfaction for nurses because it provides increased autonomy in practice, a close working relationship with clients and families, enhanced collaboration with other healthcare professionals, and increased focus of the nurse's role on planning and delivering client care.

Primary nursing requires enough registered nurses so that all clients have a nurse responsible for their plan of care, while allowing a reasonable caseload for each registered nurse. A staff of all registered nurses may be impossible because of availability and cost. The professional nurse must have enough direct contact with the client to make critical judgments about the client's diagnoses, required care, response to therapy, and ongoing disease process.

Potential disadvantages of the primary nursing model are the lack of a built-in system for experienced nurses to supervise and teach less experienced nurses and the lack of a natural nurse-to-nurse consultation. The busy routine in the work setting detracts from nurse-to-nurse consultation and joint decision-making. With economic changes in healthcare delivery, primary nursing may be viewed as economically inefficient.

Managed Care. In some healthcare agencies, primary nursing has evolved into a **managed care** delivery model. In the managed care model, the primary nurse uses a predetermined critical pathway to establish and monitor the extent and timing of care within an anticipated length of hospital stay. (Critical pathways are discussed and an example is given in Chap. 12.) For commonly treated conditions, a team of nurses and physicians jointly develops a standard plan of care that includes a time frame. Some of the key elements that are slotted at specific times in the plan include diagnostic tests, consultations, treatments, activities, procedures, and discharge planning and teaching.

Within the first day after admission, the primary nurse reviews the standard critical pathway with the client's physician. They jointly individualize the plan to reflect unique client circumstances that are expected to alter the timing or type of care required. They evaluate the client's progress daily against the critical pathway and deal with variances. If the variance is due to a hospital system or the actions or inaction of caregivers, corrections are made. If the variance is due to an unanticipated client reaction, changes in care are considered and added to the plan as needed. The primary nurse manages and closely controls client care, using the critical pathways to evaluate client progress and to determine the need for corrective action (Zander, 1989).

Confronted with nursing shortages and cost-reduction efforts, the nursing profession is currently going through another transition in using *assistive personnel* to do tasks and procedures delegated by the professional nurse. This allows the nurse to focus on the nursing process and on coordination of interdisciplinary care. In some cases, the primary nurse has available *nursing assistants* to help as needed. Others have formalized this process and have a *care partner*, who is hired by the professional nurse and who works the same schedule with that nurse. In other settings, unit-based *multiskilled technical roles* have been developed, not only to assist the professional nurse with client care but also to decentralize to the unit many of the activities previously done in other departments by many different staff (ie, client registration, venipuncture, electrocardiography). This *client-focused model* is intended not only to allow the nurse to focus on professional practice but also to provide increased responsiveness and consistency for client care.

Advanced Clinical Practice Roles

Advanced nurses provide direct client care and consultation to staff nurses. Some provide direct nursing care through group or independent practice. To be effective, these advanced practitioners must use good management techniques when planning and implementing client care, consultations, and educational programs. Others in the nursing profession also expect these advanced practitioners to be leaders in the profession through delivery of advanced care, consultation on

Nursing Research
Leadership and Management

Selected Nursing Research Studies

Chase, L. (1994). Nurse manager competencies. *Journal of Nursing Administration, 24,* 56–64.

Irurita, V. F. (1994). Optimism, values, and commitment as forces in nursing leadership. *Journal of Nursing Administration, 24,* 61–71.

McDaniel, C. & Patrick, T. (1992). Leadership, nurses, and patient satisfaction: A pilot study. *Nursing Administration Quarterly, 16,* 72–74.

Nugent, K. E., & Lambert, V. A. (1994). Empowering faculty through intrapreneurship: A change model. *Journal of Nursing Education, 33,* 226–229.

Pedersen, A. (1993). Qualities of the excellent head nurse. *Nursing Administration Quarterly, 18,* 40–50.

Young, S. W. (1992). Educational experiences of transformational nurse leaders. *Nursing Administration Quarterly, 17,* 25–33.

Possible Topics for Nursing Inquiry

- What are the leadership behaviors of staff nurses who are identified as experts by their peers?
- What are the relative priorities of various management skills of staff nurses at different career stages?
- What is the impact of varying leadership styles of head nurses on staff nurse job satisfaction and retention?
- What effects do various staff nurse roles and the use of assistive personnel have on client care outcomes?

complex care issues, development of new nursing practices, and participation in nursing research and publication. Often through their pioneering efforts, nursing is clarified, refined, and in some instances, redefined.

Clinical Nurse Specialists. **Clinical nurse specialists** are registered nurses who have a master's degree and advanced preparation in a specialty area of nursing (eg, cardiovascular, neuroscience, critical care, psychosocial, or rehabilitation). Clinical nurse specialists usually practice in hospitals, hospital clinics, community home health agencies, or private practice. They provide direct client care, consult with staff nurses, offer advanced education for nurses in specialty areas, evaluate nursing care outcomes, and develop new nursing practices to support new therapies or new technology.

Nurse Practitioners. **Nurse practitioners** are registered nurses with advanced degrees and preparation in health assessment in a specialty area, such as pediatrics, geriatrics, women's health, or adult health. These nurses also hold either certification or advanced licensing to allow them to practice independently in a specialty area. They usually work in community clinics or offices as independent practitioners or as a member of a group practice.

Other advanced specialty roles within the nursing profession include nurse midwives and nurse anesthetists. A **nurse midwife** is a registered nurse with advanced education and certification in the care of women during uncomplicated pregnancy and delivery. The **nurse anesthetist** is a registered nurse with additional education in anesthesiology. The nurse anesthetist administers anesthesia to surgical clients under the supervision of an anesthesiologist.

Nursing Management Roles

Some of the many management positions are summarized in Figure 4-4.

Beginning Managers. Through experience, staff nurses gain increasing abilities to manage care for a group of clients, assist team members, and serve as a resource for new nurses. These enhanced abilities are an indication to supervisors that staff nurses are ready to assume beginning management functions. Two such beginning management roles are team leader and charge nurse.

In hospitals or community nursing, in which team leading is the model of nursing care delivery, the team leader manages a team of nurses, licensed practical nurses, and nursing assistants to provide nursing care for a group of clients. The team leader is responsible for the performance of team members and the quality of nursing care delivered.

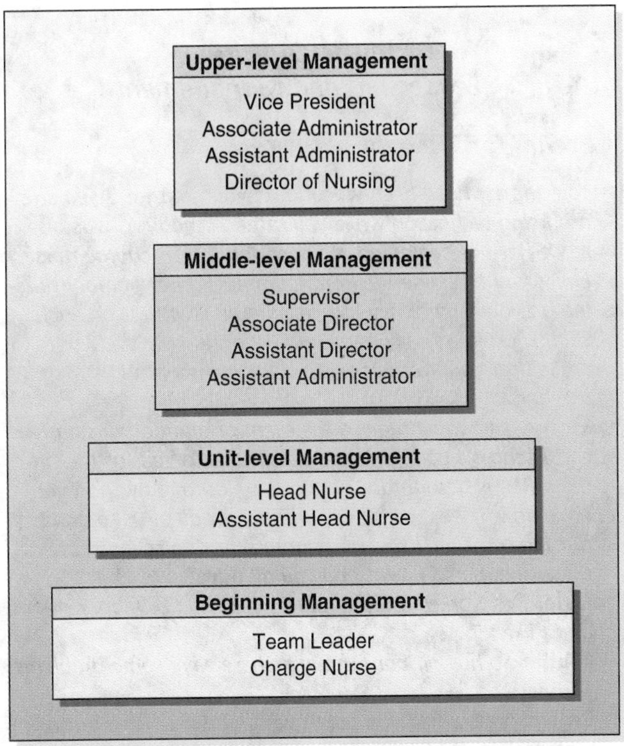

Figure 4-4 • *Depending on the size and complexity of the hospital or agency, there may be several levels and roles in management. These management roles exist to support and represent the clinical practice roles in nursing.*

The charge nurse is responsible for the functioning of a nursing unit for a particular work shift. The charge nurse makes management decisions and supervises the unit's staff as needed to provide quality client care on that shift. The charge nurse is a resource person for other staff members and may be pulled into issues that require interdepartmental or interdisciplinary problem-solving. During the shift, the charge nurse determines staff work assignments and evaluates whether the numbers and skills of the staff on the next shift are adequate to meet current client needs safely.

Although the staff supervision and decision-making functions of the team leader and the charge nurse are similar, the scope of responsibility is different. The charge nurse has responsibility for the entire unit, which may have more than one team. The charge nurse supervises the team leaders (or if primary, managed, or other model of care delivery is used, supervises the total unit staff) and facilitates communication and work between the teams (or staff).

Unit Managers. Permanent management roles at the hospital unit level are *head nurse* and *assistant head nurse*. The head nurse role is a pivotal role within the hospital. In many hospitals, the head nurse is recognized as a department head and is held accountable for 24-hour operations of the nursing unit. Operations in-

Therapeutic Dialogue
Leadership and Management

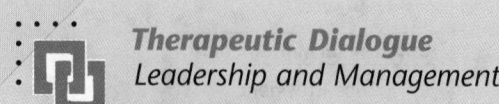

Scenes for Thought

You, James, have been working on your unit for 3 years as a nursing technician while you attend school. As was discussed at the beginning of the chapter, your charge nurse, Emily, wants to change from team nursing to primary nursing on your unit. Emily has called staff meetings on each shift to explain the change and why and how she wants to make that change. Below is a short transcript of your shift meeting.

Emily: *The advantage to the client of primary nursing is consistency of care, and the advantage to you, as the primary RN, is accountability and more autonomy than you have now. I see it as an opportunity for all of us to practice nursing the way we were taught in nursing school: care of the whole person. What do you all think?*

Jane: *I've worked in other places that had primary care, and I liked it.*

Millie: *So have I, but I thought there were some problems with it.*

Emily: *Jane, could you tell us what you liked about the system? Then, Millie, could you tell us what some of the problems were?*

Jane: *Well, I liked being responsible for total care of my clients. I was the "expert" on them and their care, and the families and doctors came to me for information about them. I felt as though we were all on the client's team.*

Millie: *I saw some problems with nurses sharing clients. After all, we can't work 24 hours a day, 7 days a week. Someone has to take over on my day off, and some of the nurses I worked with were terrible about passing on vital information. My head nurse at the time wasn't good at training people to communicate, so we all ended up feeling angry. I left because of that.*

James: *What is the place of the nursing tech in this primary care system? Who will I take care of? Who will be my supervisor? I feel a little left out here!*

Emily: *I know it sounds a little confusing right now. You'll be assigned to a primary nurse to work with clients, and we can work out the details together. One vision I have about this system is that we can tailor it to who we are and how well we already work together. This is only the first meeting to define the new system. I want to take more questions and comments now so everyone is on the same track. Connie, what do you think? (Discussion continues)*

Critical Thinking Challenges

- *Based on the descriptions of leadership style in this chapter, select the style Emily uses, and explain your choice.*
- *Analyze which one (or all) of the four management functions she demonstrates.*
- *Give examples of how she goes about problem-solving, communicating, and managing change.*

clude such functions as staff scheduling and supervision, budget management, staff education, and quality client care. The head nurse provides a vital communication link between clients, direct caregivers, and the administration. The head nurse alerts the administration to changing client needs and care preferences and changing staff characteristics. The head nurse also represents the administration to the staff and clients by communicating changes in the organization that may affect them.

The assistant head nurse helps the head nurse with overall management of the nursing unit by performing functions delegated by the head nurse (eg, hiring, evaluating, and counseling staff; preparing work schedules; and preparing and monitoring the unit budget). In addition to performing delegated management functions, the assistant head nurse often serves as a unit-based clinical resource and educator.

In community home health agencies, staff nurses are similarly organized into teams by geographic or specialty areas. A supervisor, coordinator, or director manages each team and is the pivotal person and communication link between the clients, staff, and agency administration.

Middle Managers. Depending on the size and complexity of the hospital or agency, there may be several levels of middle management. Between the head nurse or coordinator and the nurse executive may be managers with titles of supervisor, assistant director, associate director, or assistant administrator. These middle managers are usually responsible for the activities of several departments and programs. They spend more of their time in strategic planning and interdepartmental or interdisciplinary problem-solving than the head nurse but spend less of their time dealing with day-to-day client care management than the head nurse does.

Nurse Executives. The nurse executive has a variety of titles and duties, depending on the type and complexity of the institution or healthcare agency (Fig. 4-5). Some of the titles are vice president, associate administrator, assistant administrator, or director of nursing. The nurse executive is an administrator and a leader of professionals. Because he or she is involved in strategic planning and decision-making for the institution, the nurse executive must effectively negotiate with nonclinical administrators and the medical director (the other top-level clinical administrator). The nurse executive also must be able to lead, influence, and represent nursing professionals.

To be effective in all of these management roles, people must be skilled in the techniques of planning, organizing, directing, and controlling. The proportion of time spent doing each of these activities varies with each role. The beginning managers, head nurse, and assistant head nurses primarily focus on current operations and client care management. The nurse executive primarily focuses on strategic planning and issues within the agency that affect nursing practice or issues with the community or other agencies.

A manager's success depends on strong management techniques and effective leadership practices. The higher the level of the manager, the more essential it is for him or her to be an effective leader. Nurse executives are expected to be leaders within their agency and in the nursing profession itself. Effective nurse executives establish circumstances that allow nurses to function as professionals when providing quality client care.

Teaching Roles

Formal or informal teaching is an inherent part of all roles in nursing. The staff nurse teaches the client and family about health, disease, and self-care. The experienced nurse teaches the less experienced nurse. The head nurse coaches staff nurses, team leaders, and charge nurses. The nurse executive coaches middle managers. In addition, most agencies have an educator who is responsible for orientation and continuing education programs. Effective teachers influence others through leadership skills and role-modeling (Fig. 4-6).

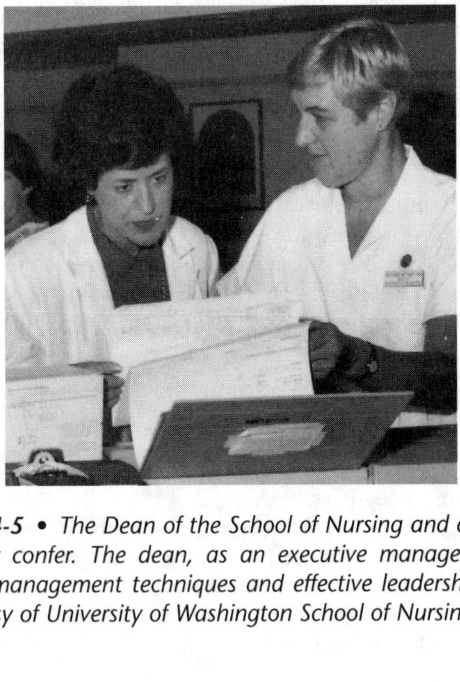

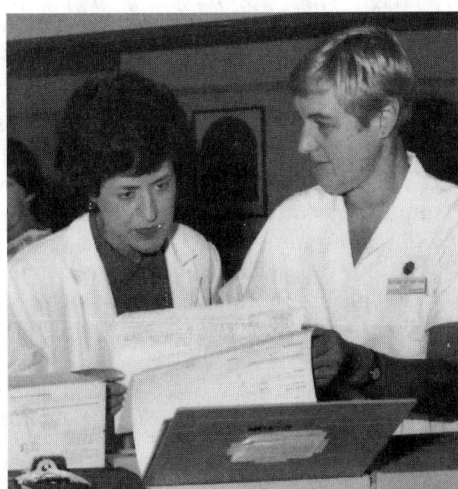

Figure 4-5 • *The Dean of the School of Nursing and a faculty member confer. The dean, as an executive manager, needs strong management techniques and effective leadership skills. (Courtesy of University of Washington School of Nursing)*

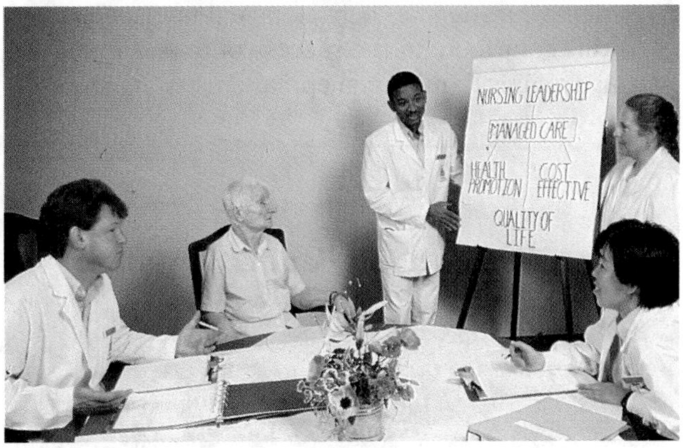

Figure 4-6 • *Leaders strengthen each other in their management skills as they meet to discuss their roles in programs.*

Key Concepts

- Nurses are professionals responsible for providing a service to society through effective leadership behaviors and management skills.
- Leadership is the ability to influence others to strive for a goal or vision or to change. Management is getting the job done or the goal accomplished through planning, organizing, directing, and controlling.
- The management process is similar to the problem-solving and the nursing processes because all are based on the scientific or research process.
- As managers, nurses need to be skilled in problem-solving, communicating, and managing change.
- The five steps of the problem-solving process are identifying and analyzing the problem, determining possible solutions, considering the consequences of each possible solution and choosing a solution, implementing the solution, and evaluating the results.
- Effective communication involves transferring the meaning of information between people, using good verbal communication and effective listening.
- Change is inevitable. People can influence their own perceptions and reactions to change by being aware of the emotions associated with it and by actively seeking information, increasing communication, and getting involved in the change process.
- New nursing graduates have many options available in work settings and roles within nursing.

- Effective leadership behaviors and management skills contribute to the success of nurses in the many clinical, management, and teaching roles.

Critical Thinking Challenges

Now that you have added leadership and management to your knowledge base of the nursing profession, turn to the situation at the beginning of the chapter. You should be able to apply what you have learned to the following challenges.

1. *Compare and contrast client advantages of team nursing with primary nursing. Do the same for nurses in the two situations.*
2. *Determine reasons why the hospital or the charge nurse might want to change the current model.*
3. *Considering your skill and knowledge, select the model in which you would like to participate. List your reasons.*
4. *If you were practicing under case management, analyze how you would collaborate with other nurses and with other staff members.*

References

American Nurses Association. (1980). *Nursing: A social policy statement.* Kansas City, MO: Author.

American Organization of Nurse Executives (1993). *Nursing's contibution to the health of the American people.* Chicago, IL: Author.

Bass, B. M. (1990). *Bass and Stogdill's handbook of leadership: Theory, research, and managerial applications* (pp. 76, 87, 361). New York: Free Press.

Bass, B. M., & Avolio, B. J. (1994). *Improving organizational effectiveness through transformational leadership* (p. 80, 132, 154–155). Thousand Oaks, CA: Sage.

Covey, S. R. (1991). *Principle-centered leadership* (pp. 40–47, 138). New York: Summit.

Glueck, W. G. (1980). *Management* (pp. 564–565). Hinsdale, IL: Dryden Press.

Handy, C. (1990). *The age of unreason* (p. 5). Boston: Harvard Business School Press.

Marquis, B. L., & Huston, C. J. (1994). *Management decision making for nurses* (pp. 35, 38) (2nd ed.). Philadelphia: J.B. Lippincott.

Noer, D. M. (1993). *Healing the wounds: Overcoming the trauma of layoffs and revitalizing downsized organizations* (pp. 197–202). San Francisco: Jossey-Bass.

Rost, J. C. (1993). *Leadership for the twenty-first century* (p. 102). Westport, CT: Praeger.

Senge, P. M. (1990). *The fifth discipline: The art and practice of the learning organization* (pp. 340, 343, 345, 356). New York: Doubleday Currenc.

Tannenbaum, R., & Schmidt, W. H. (1973). How to choose a leadership pattern. *Harvard Business Review, 51,* 164–173.

Yukl, G. A. (1989). *Leadership in organizations* (pp. 9, 174, 273, 274) (2nd ed.). Englewood Cliffs, NJ: Prentice-Hall.

Zander, K. (1994). Nurses and case management: To control or to collaborate (p. 257). In J. C. McCloskey & H. K. Grace (Eds.), *Current issues in nursing* (4th ed.). St. Louis: CV Mosby.

Bibliography

Arnold, W. W., & Plas, J. M. (1993). *The human touch.* New York: John Wiley & Sons.

Barnum, B. S. (1994). Realities in nursing practice: A strategic view. *Nursing & Health Care, 15*(8), 400–405.

Bellman, G. M. (1992). *Getting things done when you are not in charge.* New York: Fireside.

Conger, J. A. (1992). *Learning to lead: The art of transforming managers into leaders.* San Francisco: Jossey-Bass.

DePree, M. (1992). *Leadership jazz.* New York: Dell.

Douglass, L. M. (1992). *The effective nurse leader and manager* (4th ed.). St. Louis: C.V. Mosby.

Dunham-Taylor, J., Fisher, E., & Kinion, E. (1993). Experiences, events, people: Do they influence the leadership style of nurse executives? *Journal of Nursing Administration, 23*(7/8), 30–34.

Gillies, D. A. (1994). *Nursing management: A systems approach* (3rd ed.). Philadelphia: W.B. Saunders.

Forbes, B. A. (1993). *Profile of the leader of the future: Origin, premises, values, and characteristics of the Theory F Transformational Leadership Model.* Unpublished monograph, Seattle, WA.

Gunden, E., & Crissman, S. (1992). Leadership skills for empowerment. *Nursing Administration Quarterly, 16*(3), 6–10.

Hitt, W. D. (1990). *Ethics and leadership: Putting theory into practice.* Columbus: Battelle.

Jaco, P. R., Price, S. A., & Davidson, A. M. (1994). The nurse executive in the public sector: Responsibilities, activities, and characteristics. *Journal of Nursing Administration, 24*(3), 55–62.

Johnson, L. M. (1992). Structures, strategies, and synthesis: The nurse executive as social architect. *Nursing Administration Quarterly, 17*(1), 10–16.

Kerfoot, K. M. (1994). Leaders: Yesterday, today, and tomorrow. In R. Spitzer-Lehmann (Ed.), *Nursing management desk reference: Concepts, skills, & strategies.* Philadelphia: W.B. Saunders.

Koerner, J. G., & Bunkers, S. S. (1992). Transformational leadership: The power of symbol. *Nursing Administration Quarterly, 17*(1), 1–9.

Kouzes, J. M., & Posner, B. Z. (1993). *Credibility.* San Francisco: Jossey-Bass.

Mark, B. A. (1994). The emerging role of the nurse manager: Implications for educational preparation. *Journal of Nursing Administration, 24*(1), 48–55.

Marriner-Torrey, A. (1992). *Guide to nursing management* (8th ed.). St. Louis: C.V. Mosby.

Porter-O'Grady, T. (1992). Transformational leadership in an age of chaos. *Nursing Administation Quarterly, 17*(1), 17–24.

Sergiovanni, T. J. (1992). *Moral leadership.* San Francisco: Jossey-Bass.

Simmons, G. F., Vasquez, C., & Harris, P. R. (1993). *Transcultural leadership: Empowering the diverse workforce.* Houston: Gulf.

Sullivan, E. J., & Decker, P. J. (1992). *Effective management in nursing* (3rd ed.). Menlo Park: Addison-Wesley.

Wall, B., Solum, R. S., & Sabol, M. R. (1992). *The visionary leader.* Rocklin, CA: Prima.

Wheatley, M. J. (1994). *Leadership and the new science.* San Francisco: Bennett-Koehler.

Wilson, C. K. (1992). *Building new organizations: Visions and realities.* Gaithersburg, MD: Aspen.

Zaleznik, A. (1992). Managers and leaders: Are they different? *Harvard Business Review, 70*(2), 126–135.

Nursing Research

Key Terms	Learning Objectives

Key Terms

Anonymity
Confidentiality
Dependent variable
Hypothesis
Independent variable
Literature review
Method
Nursing research
Problem statement
Qualitative research
Quantitative research
Research design
Theory

Learning Objectives

Upon completion of this chapter, the student will be able to do the following:

- *Explain the contributions that research has made to nursing.*
- *Discuss the role of research in nursing.*
- *Review the research process for the beginning professional student in nursing.*
- *Summarize legal and ethical issues related to nursing research.*

5

You are a nurse working in a rehabilitation center. You enter a client's room to conduct a follow-up assessment and find the client engrossed in a conversation with a woman in a lab coat. She introduces herself, and you learn that this woman is a graduate student from a nearby university who is conducting research for her master's thesis. You know that no arrangements have been made for this student to collect data in this setting. You also know that no consent form has been signed by the client as a participant in the study. The student states that she was only interviewing the client, not providing any treatment, and was not putting the client at any risk. Therefore, she did not think she needed to obtain a consent.

In previous chapters, you learned about the profession of nursing and the application of theory and ethical and legal issues to the practice of nursing. This chapter expands your knowledge base with information about the application of research to nursing care. When you finish the chapter, you will be able to apply this information to the previous situation. Critical Thinking Challenges at the end of the chapter will help you apply your body of knowledge to the situation.

Biomedical and sociologic research have resulted in monumental advances in modern healthcare. Research into the human immune system has led to the ability to transplant body organs and has provided essential information about the care and treatment of individuals with acquired immunodeficiency syndrome. A major reason for conducting research is to expand a profession's knowledge base.

Nursing practice is enhanced when the nurse decides to use a method of treatment with a research base instead of an untested treatment. Research-based nursing practice leads to improved care. The science of nursing draws heavily on other sciences. In particular, nursing draws on the biopsychosocial fields, such as physiology, pharmacology, psychology, and sociology. A nurse must be able to discriminate "good" research from "poor" research to know what to use in clinical nursing.

Therefore, the nurse must have a beginning working knowledge of research methods and a beginning ability to read for application and to critique research. This chapter helps the nursing student understand the research process and, in particular, the application of research to the practice of nursing.

Research and Nursing

For the purposes of this chapter, research is defined as a formalized process of systematic investigation designed to test a research question or **hypothesis** and draw conclusions from the data collected. Many similarities exist between the formalized research process and the nursing process format that is an integral part of nursing education.

Nursing research is defined as a "systematic inquiry into the problems encountered in nursing practice and into the modalities of client care, such as support and comfort, prevention of trauma, promotion of recovery, health education, health appraisal and coordination of health care" (Gortner, 1975). Waltz and Bausell (1981) include the precision of the research process to "gain solutions to problems and/or discover and interpret new facts and relationships" (p. 1). "Nursing research concerns nursing and things nurses do that are different from the actions of other disciplines" (Nieswiadomy, 1993, p. 4).

Nursing research is similar to that of any other discipline in which practitioners are interested in seeking the truth. Nurses interested in discovering the truth about nursing practice attempt to describe events and phenomena, define and describe the relationships among the phenomena, and eventually control and predict the phenomena studied (Munhall & Boyd, 1993).

Nurse researchers hope to affect the clinical practice of nurses in their speciality, particularly in relation to the goals of nursing (Fig. 5-1). Nursing research "develops knowledge about health and the promotion of health over the full lifespan, care of persons with health problems and disabilities, and nursing actions to enhance the ability of individuals to respond to actual or potential health problems" (American Nurses Association [ANA], 1981). Nurses interested in critical care might be interested in a study on oral temperature accuracy (Fallis, Gupton, & Kassum, 1994), whereas nurses working in geriatrics (older people) might be more interested in Bader's (1993) work on physical health impairment and depression. Each specialist becomes familiar with research related to his or her speciality.

Although many problems nurses encounter in their clinical practice affect people of all ages, some problems are age- or person-specific. One nurse may be interested in the health benefits of aerobic exercise in a healthy geriatric population; another nurse may be interested in the effect of positioning on the oxygen saturation of postoperative coronary artery bypass surgery clients. Every nurse needs to be interested in prevention in the cost-conscious healthcare arena (Griffith, 1993). Each researcher contributes to the body of nursing knowledge in a specific way, and all nurses should contribute in some fashion to the expansion of nursing knowledge.

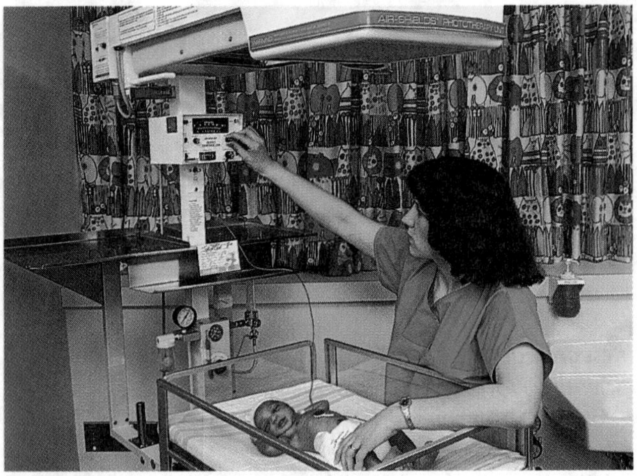

Figure 5-1 • Clinical research defines nursing practice and raises the standards of nursing care.

The focus of nursing research must be on generating fundamental knowledge to guide nursing practice (Barnard, 1980; LoBiondo-Wood & Haber, 1994). Making progress in nursing service, nursing practice, or the administration of nursing requires systematic analyses of research applicable to a nurse's area of expertise (Mason & Leavitt, 1993).

Scientific Process and Nursing Research

In general, research means the search for a valid answer to a question. How the question is raised and by whom often is the key to solving the problem. The scientific method, the problem-solving method, and the nursing process all use a method of research. The problem-solving method and nursing process are compared in Chapter 9. In this section, scientific process is compared with nursing practice.

Ways of seeking and finding answers and acquiring knowledge in any field include classes, clinical experience, discussions with classmates, scientific problem-solving, continuing education, and research studies relevant to the area of interest. These methods of seeking knowledge have the following in common:

- Identifying what one needs to know
- Deciding how to approach the goal of answering the problem
- Devising a plan to do so
- Implementing the plan
- Assessing the results

The first step for the practicing nurse is to assess a problem, and for the researcher, the first step is to recognize the general problem area. The next step for the practicing nurse is to make a nursing diagnosis, whereas defining the specific problem is the second step in the research process. The clinical nurse then proceeds with planning and intervention, whereas the nurse researcher proposes hypotheses and manages data. In the final step, the clinician evaluates outcomes, whereas the researcher analyzes results and disseminates his or her findings.

Beginning nurses can use the nursing process framework to begin to formulate and answer questions. The outcome will be improved client care and services and the advancement of nursing as a profession. Another way to become involved in research is to be a research subject or a data collecter for another person's research project (Glass, 1991).

Evolution of Nursing Research

Appreciation of the place of research in nursing has grown significantly in the last 30 years, but nursing research has been an integral part of the profession since Florence Nightingale documented the care of soldiers in the Crimean War (Sarkis & Conners, 1986). Nightingale's carefully kept statistical records are a model for nurses and social scientists (Cohen, 1984).

According to multiple authors (LoBiondo-Wood & Haber, 1994; Nieswaidomy, 1993; Polit & Hungler, 1995), several historic events led to recent developments in nursing research. From 1900 to 1940, research centered around nursing education, methods of teaching, and methods of evaluating how nurses learned. During World War II, research interest turned to the supply and demand of nurses because of the increased need for nurses to serve military and civilian needs.

During the 1950s, more master's programs specific to nursing were developed, and most of these programs included courses on research methods. Increased federal funding enabled more nurses to continue their studies at the master's level, and publications of nursing research became more common. The journal *Nursing Research* began publishing the results of studies by individuals and schools of nursing. At about the same time, a 5-year research project sponsored by the ANA focused on nurses' activities and functions.

Federal funding for graduate study and research continued in the 1960s. The profession of nursing was strengthened with the development of conceptual frameworks (an early stage of theory development wherein interrelated concepts help shape the proposed research) and the use of scientific method in nursing practice. Nursing organizations established priorities for research investigations. Such research endeavors led to improvements in the quality and specificity of nursing care.

Rapid growth in nursing research continued during the 1970s and 1980s. Three more journals of nursing research were born in the 1970s: *Advances in Nursing Science*, *Research in Nursing and Health*, and *Western Journal of Nursing Research*. The ANA Commission on Nursing Research in 1980 recommended further research in areas of health promotion, illness prevention, cost-effective healthcare, and nursing care for high-risk clients. Researchers examined the conceptual frameworks that arose in the 1960s and 1970s.

The Institute of Medicine, in a 1983 study, urged the federal government to increase the level of funding for nursing. As a result, the National Center for Nursing Research was established under the National Institutes of Health. The purpose of the center was to place nursing securely in the sphere of scientific investigation and to support research and training into client care, health promotion, disease prevention, and the mitigation of effects of acute and chronic disabilities (Merritt, 1986). This center has continued to fund and support nursing research.

Groups began to establish priorities in nursing research during the 1980s (Polit & Hungler, 1993). In 1985, the ANA Cabinet on Nursing Research identified 11 priorities for nursing research (Polit & Hungler, 1995), as listed in the accompanying display. In the late 1980s, *Applied Nursing Research*, a journal with studies related to the practice of nursing, began.

Polit and Hungler (1995) state, "the question areas that interest nurse researchers are as diverse as the types of positions held by nurses, the multiplicity of settings in which nurses practice, the complexity of human nature, and the personality of each nurse." They list the following as the current topics of interest:

- Promotion of positive health practices
- The nursing process of clinical judgments
- Groups at risk for specific health problems
- Description of holistic nursing situations
- Minority groups
- Compliance with prescribed programs of treatment

Characteristics of Nursing Research

Traditionally, nursing has been concerned with the whole person, not the individual parts. Likewise, nursing research differs from biomedical research in that it has a *holistic* perspective. When nurses do research, they focus on the physiologic, psychological, sociologic, cultural, and economic factors that affect that person. They view events from different perspectives and ask questions about what they see (Mateo & Kirchhoff, 1991). Diers (1979) listed four properties of nursing research that maintain the holistic perspective:

- The focus of nursing research must be on a variance that makes a difference in improving client care.

The 11 Priorities for Nursing Research

1. Promote the health, well-being, and ability to care for oneself among all age, social, and cultural groups.
2. Minimize or prevent behaviorally and environmentally induced health problems that compromise the quality of life and reduce productivity.
3. Minimize the negative effects of new health technologies on the adaptive abilities of individuals and families experiencing acute or chronic health problems.
4. Ensure that the care needs of particularly vulnerable groups, such as the elderly, children with congenital health problems, individuals from diverse cultures, mentally ill people, and the poor, are met in effective and acceptable ways.
5. Classify nursing practice phenomena.
6. Ensure that principles of ethics guide nursing research.
7. Develop instruments to measure nursing outcomes.
8. Develop integrative methodologies for the holistic study of human beings as they relate to their families and lifestyles.
9. Design and evaluate alternative models for delivering healthcare and for administering healthcare systems so that nurses will be able to balance high quality and cost-effectiveness when meeting the nursing needs of identified populations.
10. Evaluate the effectiveness of alternative approaches to nursing education for the kind of practice that requires broad knowledge and a wide repertoire of skills and for the kind of practice that requires specialized knowledge and a focused set of skills.
11. Identify and analyze historical and contemporary factors that influence the shaping of nursing professionals' involvement in national health policy development.

From American Nurses' Association Cabinet on Nursing Research (1985). *Directions for nursing research: Toward the twenty-first century.* Kansas City, MO: ANA, with permission.

- Nursing research has the potential for contributing to theory development and the body of scientific nursing knowledge.
- A research problem is a nursing research problem when nurses have access to and control over phenomena being studied.
- A nurse interested in research must have an inquisitive, curious, and questioning mind.

Methods of Nursing Research

Just as subjects of studies are diverse, so are the methods of study. Two broad approaches to research are quantitative and qualitative research. Polit and Hungler (1995) define the two: "**Quantitative research** involves the systematic collection of numeric information, usually under conditions of considerable control, and the analysis of that information using statistical procedures. **Qualitative research** involves the systematic collection and analysis of more subjective narrative materials, using procedures in which there tends to be a minimum of researcher-imposed control." Furthermore, quantitative researchers tend to use deductive reasoning, logic, and measurable attributes of human experience. Qualitative researchers tend to use dynamic, individual aspects of the human experience in a holistic approach (Polit & Hungler, 1995). The two are compared in Table 5-1. Both methods have strengths and weaknesses and specific applications.

The Research Process

An understanding of the step-by-step process used by nurse researchers is essential for the beginning practitioner and user of nursing research. Understanding the process helps the nurse judge the appropriateness of the research presented and allows him or her to apply the findings to the clinical situation. The following sections summarize steps in the research process.

Problem Area Identification

Practical experience, scientific literature, and untested theories influence the development of a research idea. For the practicing nurse, clinical practice can provide daily opportunities to piece together observations that may lead to a researchable problem. For example, nurses working in the recovery room observe that temperatures taken with an aural (in the ear) device appear more quickly determined and just as accurate as the more traditional oral or rectal methods. The nurses note the differences in methods and speculate about other factors that might contribute to the ultimate adoption of

Table 5-1 • Comparison of Quantitative and Qualitative Research

	Quantitative Research	Qualitative Research
Focus	Focuses on a relatively small number of specific concepts	Attempts to understand entirety of some phenomenon rather than focusing on specific concepts
Initial concept	Begins with preconceived ideas about how concepts are interrelated	Has few preconceived ideas: stresses importance of people's interpretations of events and circumstances rather than researcher's interpretation
Method	Uses structured procedures and formal instruments to collect information	Collects information without formal, structured instruments
Controls	Collects information under conditions of control	Does not attempt to control the context of the research, but attempts to capture that context in its entirety
Objectivity versus Subjectivity	Emphasizes objectivity in collection and analysis of information	Attempts to capitalize on subjective data as a means for understanding and interpreting human experiences
Analysis	Analyzes numeric information through statistical procedures	Analyzes narrative information in an organized, but intuitive, fashion

Information adapted from Polit, D. F., & Hungler, B. P. (1993). *Essentials of nursing research: Methods, appraisal, and utilization* (3rd ed.) (pp. 19–20). Philadelphia: J.B. Lippincott.

the aural method rather than the traditional methods. Nurses can work together to design and implement different methods for researchable problems (Dilorio, Hockenberry-Eaton, Maibach, & Rivero, 1994).

Review of Scientific Literature

Literature review is the process of selecting published materials (both research based and anecdotal) that contribute to and substantiate a summary of the concepts to be studied.

Scientific literature may be a valuable source for research ideas. For example, articles on how a family adapts to a child's head injury (Baker, 1990) or how prepared childbirth classes affect obstetric outcome (Hetherington, 1990) may be valuable for your clinical practice area.

Untested theories are good starts for nursing research. For example, Haase (1987) studied critically ill adolescents using a "courage" theory. The study gave insight into this special population and served to further develop a knowledge base surrounding adolescent care. Research interviews can help a researcher understand people's responses to illness or a particular situation (Hutchinson, Wilson, & Wilson, 1994).

Critical appraisal of the scientific literature may lead a nurse to speculate about a problem area, particularly if the literature is in conflict or inconsistent with his or her practice. For example, a nurse working in coronary care may read two articles on pain management in percutaneous transluminal coronary angioplasty clients that suggest two different protocols. The nurse may wonder which protocol is the most valid. Because of the conflict in the literature, an evaluation of the area may give the answer.

The literature review must be systematic and exhaustive. The researcher must take a critical, almost dubious, approach to the material. Because the critical appraisal of the literature is the basis for the current study, such review is essential. All research builds on previous work; hence, an extensive literature review, properly executed, allows the researcher to place current ideas in the context of previous work. A complete review also helps develop the conceptual frame of reference for the study. It gives clues on how to study the problem (the **methods**) and suggests instruments that might help.

The search for nursing literature can seem overwhelming to a beginner. An indispensable skill is the ability to identify and locate pertinent documentation on a particular topic. To do so, the student must know which library sources to use. Books and indexes of journals, reports, and abstracts are a few places to start. Books provide an overview of a topic or deal with a specific detailed topic. Bibliographies in books are valuable resources because they provide information about past references. Indexes are the gateway to the enormous volume of literature in the health sciences. Indexes, such as the *International Nursing Index, Index Medicus, Nursing Studies Index, Grateful Med,* and *Nursing Research Index,* are invaluable to the nursing researcher. They are available in print and on computer databases; consult a librarian for details.

To help you understand the use of nursing research, displays on nursing research are provided throughout this textbook. An example of the displays is given here. The displays are divided into two sections: "Selected Nursing Research Studies" and "Possible Topics for Nursing Inquiry." The first section lists recent research articles; the second section may lead to class discussion or future study.

Nursing Research
Examples of Nursing Research

Selected Nursing Research Studies

- Badger, T. A. (1993). Physical health impairment and depression among older adults. *Image 25*(4), 326–330.
- Hetherington, S. L. (1990). A controlled study of the effects of prepared childbirth classes on obstetric outcome. *Birth, 17*(2), 64–80.

Possible Topics for Nursing Inquiry

- How does age affect the understanding of consent forms?
- What cultural indicators are at play in active participation in flu and pneumonia shots?

Theoretical Framework

Nursing science and theory development are in the early stages of refinement. A **theory** is a set of interrelated constructs or propositions that attempt to present or explain systematically some phenomenon. Several nursing theorists have developed models and theories that remain incompletely tested. This incomplete testing and the evolving nature of models and theories give the researcher an opportunity to use the work of a nursing theorist to test concepts from that theory for practice application. An example might be a nurse who wants to study Orem's self-care model for clients undergoing ambulatory surgical procedures. The nurse might design a study to investigate factors influencing self-care abilities of the adult surgical client before and after surgery.

The nursing model or theory should be a guide to identify and study systematically the logical relationships between variables. Each nursing model depends on the individual researcher's philosophy of human behavior and how that philosophical behavior meshes with other ways of looking at science (Fawcett & Downs, 1992).

Often a theoretical framework is likened to an architectural blueprint. These renderings, although not exact models of the real item, help the user move from one place to another. They help the nurse construct theories that deal with the phenomena of concern to nursing and help distinguish nursing from other disciplines.

Formulation of a Problem Statement

One of the key steps in the research process is the ability to formulate the problem statement. The **problem statement** identifies the direction that a research project will take. As a beginning consumer of research literature, the nursing student is in a position to evaluate whether the study is a logical extension of that problem. Sometimes the problem area is not clearly stated, and the reader is unsure of the direction of the study. The problem statement should be clear and unambiguous, express a relationship between two or more variables, identify the population to be studied, and encourage empirical testing. The problem statement is introduced early in the research and should reflect a well-defined, specific focus.

Stating the problem requires specifying the population to be studied. In the problem statement, the researcher states who will be the focus. For instance, the problem statement "Is there a relationship between fathers who have been abused as children and their school-aged sons' emergency room records for suspicious injury?" suggests that the populations to be studied are fathers and sons.

The researcher must consider the problem's significance for nursing. Research should be applicable to nursing practice, education, or administration. It should have the potential for altering nursing practice or protocol and benefiting clients, other nurses, or students. It should be theoretically relevant.

Questions about judgments, ethics, morals, or values are not amenable to the scientific research process. For example, the question "Is it better to tell clients about their diagnosis of terminal cancer or let them discover it themselves?" is impossible to answer. What is meant by "better?" Whose value system is being considered? The study of values has no right answer. If the question were framed differently, it would be researchable through clinical inquiry. For instance, a nurse interested in determining how often each method was used could investigate attitudes toward each method.

Proposed Hypotheses

In the problem statement, the relationship is expressed between two or more variables, or operationalized concepts. Variables, or properties that vary from each other, are the focus of the study. For example, a researcher studying postoperative clients might be interested in preoperative preparation in relation to the outcome of respiratory function.

Variables can be dependent or independent, depending on their role in a particular study. An **independent variable** has the presumed effect on the dependent variable. It may be manipulated if the researcher is doing an experimental study; in a nonexperimental study, it is assumed to have occurred naturally before or during the study. The **dependent variable** is the consequence or presumed effect that varies as changes occur in the independent variable. The dependent variable is the one that the researcher is interested in understanding and explaining.

For example, a nurse may study the problem that cardiac output measurement (the dependent variable) will vary with the temperature of the injectate solution (the independent variable). In this case, the researcher would try to explain the effects of temperature on the measurements.

Data Management

Research Design

Research design is the overall plan for the collection and analysis of the data. The design of a study is crucial. If the design can limit the number of research problems before the study, the outcome may be more useful. If an instrument is to be used in a study or a new instrument needs to be developed, a consultant in methods (methodologist) can alleviate some reliability and validity problems by helping the novice researcher select or develop an instrument.

Because most nursing research occurs outside a laboratory setting, the policies, parameters, and constraints of the institution must be taken into account. The researcher must consider the costs of the facilities, equipment, and personnel time (Fig. 5-2). Sometimes a study cannot be conducted because the costs outweigh the benefits.

Testability

The final consideration when evaluating a research problem is testability. The problem must be measurable by qualitative or quantitative methods. If the question is posed in such a way that there is a relationship between an independent and a dependent variable and that relationship can be measured, it is probably a researchable question.

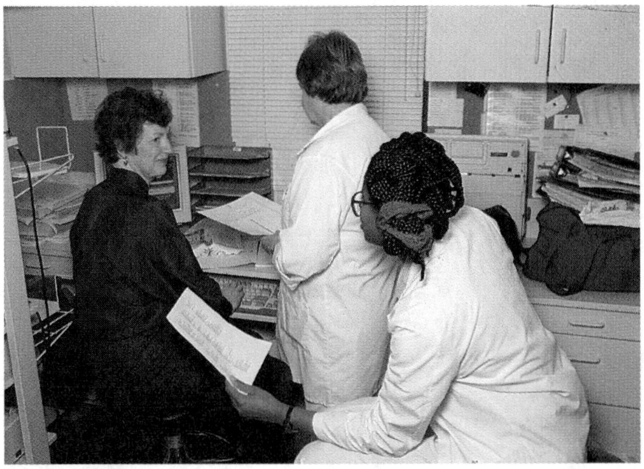

Figure 5-2 • *Nursing research can be time consuming for personnel, and the value of research must be weighed against the cost.*

Analysis of Results

Data are not the final result. They are a raw form of the answer. The reviewer puts the data through various types of analysis and interpretation. These are managed in an orderly, preplanned method. The researcher looks for patterns of information. The information may be analyzed objectively or subjectively (see Table 5-1) by quantitative or qualitative analysis.

The results must make sense, and this is part of the researcher's responsibility in interpretation. The implications are examined. The following question is asked: "How do these implications apply in the broader context?" The researcher returns to his or her original question or problem statement. It should be answered with the analysis and interpretation of the results.

Dissemination of Results

Once the results of a study are determined, the findings must be disseminated so that clinical application or research replication by other nurses can occur. Conclusions are strengthened and validated by similar findings in more than one research study.

Communication of Findings

Findings can be disseminated by oral and poster presentations at research meetings or in print through research and clinical journals. Presenting and publishing study results allows other nurses interested in improving nursing practice to act on the findings. Nurses may adopt the finding for clinical practice. Another nurse may choose to do the same study but with a different group of study subjects or subjects in another clinical area. Others may extend the same study or stop using a clinical procedure or therapy that has shown little or no merit. A bonus of presenting at meetings or publishing the results of studies may be that the researcher will meet other nurses with similar interests. This is called "networking" and is a good way to disseminate and expand one's knowledge.

Adoption of Findings

When a research report is being considered for use in the clinical practice area, preparation for change is made. It is essential to bring together all those professionals who are affected if the change is to be made smoothly. For example, nurses in one unit may read a study concluding that selective decontamination of the digestive tract of mechanically ventilated clients may reduce the incidence of nosocomial infections (Meijer, Van Saene, & Hill, 1990) and decide they want to implement the findings. To make such a change, nurses would collaborate with physicians, hospital microbiologists, pharmacists, and respiratory therapists to consider how this change would influence client care. During the evaluation, everyone involved in client care must be aware that each client in the study should be treated according to the existing standards of care in the unit. Research subjects need to be given the same treatment as nonresearch subjects to be compared with each other on outcome variables, if this is the design of the study.

Legal and Ethical Issues

Legal and ethical issues related to the review process arise. The primary issue is that of human rights or subject rights. In the past, research has been conducted without proper consent or without any consent from the participants.

Institutional Review Boards

In 1974, the National Research Act was passed, requiring any agency applying for funding for any project involving biomedical or behavioral research on humans to submit assurances that it had an institutional review board to review the research and protect the rights of human subjects. At agencies where no federal money has been awarded, there is usually a review mechanism similar to the institutional review board.

Why are institutional review boards necessary? After World War II, the Nuremberg military tribunal was charged with prosecuting Nazis who had done biomedical research on concentration camp prisoners. Because the tribunal had no measures against which to test the defendants, a set of basic principles of ethical, moral, and legal concepts for the conduct of acceptable experiments had to be written. The Articles of the Nuremberg Tribunal are listed in the display.

Subject Rights

The first tenet of the Nuremberg code, developed in 1949, addressed the rights of research subjects. Paramount are voluntary consent; the right to withdraw from investigations; protection from physical and mental suffering, injury, disability, and death; and a balance between benefits and risks (Levine, 1981). Nursing researchers must provide the following information to human subjects (Commission on Nursing Research, 1981):

- Explanation of the study
- Procedures to be followed and their purposes

Articles of the Nuremberg Tribunal Related to Ethical, Moral, and Legal Concepts for the Conduct of Experiments

- The voluntary consent of the human subject is absolutely essential.
- The experiment should be such as to yield fruitful results for the good of society, unprocurable by other means of study, and not random and unnecessary in nature.
- The experiment should be so designed and based on the results of animal experimentation and knowledge of the natural history of the disease or other problems under study that the anticipated results will justify the performance of the experiment.
- The experiment should be conducted to avoid all unnecessary physical and mental suffering and injury.
- No experiment should be conducted where there is a prior reason to believe that death or disabling injury will occur.
- The degree of risk to be taken should never exceed that determined by the humanitarian importance of the problem to be solved by the experiment.
- Proper preparations should be made and adequate facilities provided to protect the subject against...injury, disability, or death.
- The experiment should be conducted only by scientifically qualified persons.
- The human subject should be at liberty to bring the experiment to an end.
- During the experiment the scientist...if he has probable cause to believe that a continuation of the experiment is likely to result in injury, disability, or death due to the experiment subject...will bring it to a close.

(Reprinted from Katz, J. et al. [1972]. *Experimentation with human beings* [pp. 289–290]. Copyright © 1972 Russell Sage Foundation.)

- Clear description of physical and mental discomforts, any invasion of privacy, and any threat to dignity
- Methods used to protect the anonymity and ensure confidentiality

These may seem obvious, but before 1974, several human research studies were conducted in the United States that probably would not be allowed today. Subjects in these studies underwent unethical experimental procedures, including sterilization, euthanasia, injection with live cancer cells, and the withholding of treatment for syphilis (Diers, 1979; Faulder, 1985; LoBiondo-Wood & Haber, 1994; Tetting, 1990).

Clients involved in research assume that their privacy is being protected. **Anonymity** is the protection of the subject so that not even the researcher can link the subject with the information provided. **Confidentiality** ensures that the subjects' identities will not be linked with the information they provide and will not be publicly divulged.

Although a student may have few opportunities to seek or obtain informed consent from individuals selected as potential subjects for research, a student may have a role in data collection or may provide medications or treatments in a research study. The role that a nurse or student is to play in a research study must be clarified with the involved faculty member.

Research and the Professional Nurse

Different Levels of Nursing Participation

Some nurses may think they have little to contribute to research, but this is not so. Nurses actually have a great deal to contribute by observing client responses to treatments and techniques. A nurse with several years of clinical experience in a particular unit may generate many unanswered questions. He or she would be in a position to initiate research with a skilled researcher or would value assisting with client management or data collection in someone else's research project.

The education of nurses who are clinical specialists often emphasizes clinically relevant research. In the practice arena, they can do their own research, act as consultants to novice researchers, and collaborate with other healthcare professionals on more complex client situations. For example, a clinical specialist in oncology may collaborate with a clinical psychologist to study stressors of pain or side effects related to therapy.

The ANA's Commission on Nursing Education has developed guidelines for the investigative function of nurses. They are listed in the accompanying display. These standards give information about how different educational levels may enhance the research contributions that nurses can make.

Clinical Nursing Practice

Clinical Research

The problem-solving methods used by nurses can help practicing nurses translate clinical problems into research projects. Nurses in clinical areas regularly raise questions that could be considered researchable. Because of daily interactions with clients, nurses have the opportunity to solve problems, but in the strict sense, do not research nursing questions.

A nurse interested in research, especially in the clinical area, uses the resources at hand: clients. Client care allows the nurse to define and seek solutions to a variety of problems. Using observation skills, discussions with colleagues, and personal clinical experience, the nurse can learn to organize priorities and offer the client the most efficient and timely care.

Nurse researchers use techniques similar to those they developed first as a student and then refined as a skilled clinician. The nurse researcher broadens the area of study and tries to discover the variety of conditions (variables) that affect the situation. For example, a nurse in the neonatal unit might be concerned with the temperature balance of neonates receiving phototherapy for physiologic jaundice. The researcher recognizes that to study this problem, the related fields of physical thermodynamics and developmental physiology have to be investigated. The researcher also needs to investigate the placement of temperature probes, site selection, nurse technique, and the soundness of previous research.

The nurse researcher recognizes that other experts need to be consulted and other organizational patterns must be considered. Recruitment of those skilled in particular areas ensures that the results will be more useful and gives the design and statistical analysis more merit. Often the skills of a statistician, for example, are needed.

Applying Research to Practice

The student nurse and the beginning practicing nurse are not usually involved in direct research, except in the role of data collection or administering medications and treatments as a protocol in a research project. Even with limited direct participation in research, the beginning nurse should be a consumer of research. He or she can read research literature applicable to the practice setting and attempt to evaluate it or use it in clinical practice after collaboration with more expert practitioners. For the beginning nurse, the ability to read articles carefully and critically is important. Critiquing does not necessarily mean finding flaws and faults. It is the conscious decision to undertake an objective and careful evaluation of the research project in light of how the practicing nurse, working directly with a client or client population, would be able to use this knowledge.

Guidelines for Investigative Function of Nurses

Associate Degree in Nursing

- Demonstrates awareness of the value or relevance of research in nursing
- Assists in identifying problem areas in nursing practice
- Assists in collection of data within an established, structured format

Baccalaureate in Nursing

- Reads, interprets, and evaluates research for applicability to nursing practice
- Identifies nursing problems that need to be investigated, and participates in implementation of scientific studies
- Uses nursing practice as a means of gathering data for refining and extending practice
- Applies established findings of nursing and other health-related research to nursing practice
- Shares research finding with colleagues

Master's Degree in Nursing

- Analyzes and reformulates nursing practice problems so that scientific knowledge and scientific methods can be used to find solutions
- Enhances the quality and clinical relevance of nursing research by providing expertise in clinical problems and by providing knowledge about the way in which these clinical services are delivered
- Facilitates investigation of problems in clinical settings through such activities as contributing to a climate supportive of investigative activities, collaborating with others in investigations, and enhancing nursing's access to clients and data
- Conducts investigations for the purpose of monitoring the quality of the practice of nursing in a clinical setting
- Assists others to apply scientific knowledge in nursing practice

Doctoral Degree in Nursing or Related Discipline

Graduate of a practice-oriented doctoral program

- Provides leadership for the integration of scientific knowledge with other sources of knowledge for the advancement of practice
- Conducts investigations to evaluate the contribution of nursing activities to the well-being of clients
- Develops methods to monitor the quality of the practice of nursing in a clinical setting and to evaluate contributions of nursing activities to the well-being of clients

Graduate of a research-oriented doctoral program

- Develops theoretical explanations of phenomena relevant to nursing by empirical research and analytical processes
- Uses analytic and empirical methods to discover ways to modify or extend existing scientific knowledge so that it is relevant to nursing
- Develops methods for scientific inquiry of phenomena relevant to nursing

This language was developed as a part of the work of the ANA Commission on Nursing Education and was included in the report of that commission to the 1980 ANA House of Delegates. From Commission on Nursing Research (1981). *Guidelines for the investigative function of nurses.* Kansas City, MO: Author.

After a study or research project has been evaluated, the findings might be used in clinical practice. However, the nurse should not assume that just because something has been published, it is appropriate for clinical practice. On the contrary, because something is published, the contents should be viewed with some degree of skepticism before adopting for the reader's clinical setting.

Applying research findings to clinical practice has utility. Nurses need to narrow the gap between research and application by selecting useful studies to put into place. The expanding use of community-based nursing and family-centered care offers a whole new area of research.

In the meantime, while research continues, a planned program of evaluation and implementation will help nurses find appropriate approaches to client care situations. For example, the journal *Focus on Critical Care* has a column, "Research Review," which helps critical care nurses apply relevant research to their practice. Other journals provide similar information.

Key Concepts

- Expanding the knowledge base of nursing is an important goal of nursing research.
- Nursing research is the systematic inquiry into clinical practice problems and modes of client care.

- The scientific method of research and the nursing process are similar.
- Research is a step-by-step process of defining ideas, reviewing the literature, developing a theoretical framework, formulating a problem statement, proceeding with the study, and disseminating findings.
- Nursing research must be disseminated so that the profession can evaluate and apply the findings.
- Ethical consideration of the rights of human subjects, anonymity, and confidentiality are central to any research study.
- Practicing nurses encounter many questions that may be a basis for a research study.

Critical Thinking Challenges

Now that you have studied about research, the process of research, and the relationship of research to nursing, turn back to the situation at the beginning of the chapter. Read again about the nurse who is doing research in your clinical area, and complete the following challenges.

1. *Critique the actions of the graduate student in your client's room in light of how you understand the protection of client rights in research.*
2. *Based on your understanding of client rights, describe your reaction to the graduate student's response.*
3. *Now that you have clarified your understanding and considered the graduate student's response, identify how you will proceed.*

References

American Nurses Association. (1981). *Research priorities for the 1980s: Generating a scientific base for nursing practice.* Publication #D-68. Kansas City, MO: Author.

American Nurses Association Cabinet on Nursing Research (1985). *Directions for nursing research: Toward the twenty-first century.* Kansas City, MO: American Nurses Association.

Bader, A. (1993). Physical health impairment and depression among older adults. *Image, 25*(4), 326–330.

Baker, J. L. (1990). Family adaptation when one member has a head injury. *Journal of Neuroscience Nursing,* 22, 232–237.

Barnard, K. E. (1980). Knowledge for practice: Directions for the future. *Nursing Research,* 29, 208 212.

Cohen, I. B. (1984). Florence Nightingale. *Scientific American,* 250(3), 128–137.

Commission on Nursing Research. (1981). *Guidelines for the investigative function of nurses.* Kansas City, MO: Author.

Diers, D. (1979). *Research in nursing practice.* Philadelphia: J.B. Lippincott.

Dilorio, C., Hockenberry-Eaton, M., Maibach, E., & Rivero, T. (1994). Focus groups: An interview method for nursing research. *Journal of Neuroscience Nursing, 26*(3), 175–180.

Fallis, W. M., Gupton, A., & Kassum, D. (1994). Determination of oral temperature accuracy in adult critical care patients who are orally intubated. *Heart & Lung,* 23(4), 300–307.

Faulder, C. (1985). *Whose body is it?* London: Virago.

Fawcett, J., & Downs, F. S. (1992). *The relationship of theory and research* (2nd ed.). Philadelphia: F.A. Davis.

Glass, E. C. (1991). Importance of research to practice. In M. A. Mateo & K. T. Kirchhoff (Eds.), *Conducting and using nursing research in the clinical setting.* Baltimore: Williams & Wilkins.

Gortner, S. (1975). Research for a practice profession. *Nursing Research, 24*(6), 193–197.

Griffith, H. M. (1993). Needed—a strong nursing position on preventive service. *Image, 25*(4), 272.

Haase, J. E. (1987). Components of courage in critically ill adolescents: A phenomenological study. *Advances in Nursing Science, 19*(2), 64–80.

Hetherington, S. L. (1990). A controlled study of the effects of prepared childbirth classes on obstetric outcome. *Birth,*17(2), 86–89.

Hutchinson, S. A., Wilson, M. E., & Wilson, H. S. (1994). Benefits of participating in research interviews. *Image,26*(2), 161–164.

Levine, R. J. (1981). *Ethics and regulation of clinical research.* Baltimore: Urban & Schwarzenberg.

LoBiondo-Wood, G., & Haber, J. (1994) *Nursing research: Critical appraisal and utilization* (3rd ed.). St. Louis: C.V. Mosby.

Mason, D. J., & Leavitt, J. K. (1993). Policy and politics: A framework for action. In D. J. Mason, S. W. Talbott, & J. K. Leavitt (Eds.), *Policy and politics for nurses* (2nd ed.). Philadelphia: W.B. Saunders.

Mateo, M. A., & Kirchhoff, K. T. (1991). *Conducting and using nursing research in the clinical setting.* Baltimore: Williams & Wilkins.

Meijer, K., Van Saene, R., & Hill, J. (1990). Infection control in patients undergoing mechanical ventilation: Traditional approach versus a new development—Selective decontamination of the digestive tract. *Heart & Lung, 19*(10), 11–20.

Merritt, D. H. (1986). The National Center for Nursing Research. *Image: Journal of Nursing Scholarship, 18*(2), 84.

Munhall, P. L., & Boyd, C. O. (1993). *Nursing research: A qualitative perspective,* Publication #19-2535. New York: National League for Nursing Press.

Neiswaidomy, R. M. (1993). *Foundations of nursing research* (2nd ed.). Norwalk, CT: Appleton & Lange.

Polit, D. F., & Hungler, B. P. (1995). *Nursing research: Principles and methods* (3rd ed.). Philadelphia: J.B. Lippincott.

Sarkis, J. M., & Conners, V. L. (1986). Nursing research: Historical background and teaching information strategies. *Nursing Research, 4*(2), 121–125.

Tetting, D. W. (1990). Preparing for human subjects review. *Critical Care Nursing Quarterly, 12*(4), 10–16.

Waltz, C., & Bausell, R. P. (1991). Nursing research: Design, statistics and computer analysis. Philadelphia: F.A. Davis.

Bibliography

American Nurses Association (1976). *Research in nursing: Toward a science of health care.* Publication #D-525M. Kansas City, MO: Author.

Bostrom, A. C., et al. (1989). Staff nurses' attitudes toward nursing research: A descriptive survey. *Journal of Advanced Nursing, 14,* 915–923.

Brent, N. J. (1990). Legal issues in research: Informed consent. *Journal of Neuroscience Nursing, 22*(3), 189–191.

Briones, T., & Bruya, M. A. (1990). The professional imperative: Research utilization in the search for scientifically based nursing practice. *Focus on Critical Care, 17*(1), 78–81.

Burns, N. (1989). The research process and the nursing process: Distinctly different. *Nursing Science Quarterly, 2*(4), 162–171.

Chicuye, P. S. (1989). Nursing in action: Nurses' influence in research and health policy development. *Journal of Professional Nursing, 5,* 326–329.

Clayton, G. M. (1989). Instruments for use in nursing education research, New York: Publication #15–2248, 1–70. *NLN Council on Social Research in Nursing Education.*

Craig, H. M. (1985). Accuracy of indirect measures of medication compliance in hypertension. *Research in Nursing and Health, 8,* 61–66.

Fonteyn, M. E. (1990). The need for nurse involvement in critical care research. *Critical Care Quarterly,* 12(4), 1–4.

Heaney, R. P., & Barger-Lux, M. J. (1986). Priming students to read research critically. *Nursing and Health Care, 7,* 421–424.

Hinshaw, A. S. (1989). Nursing science: The challenge to develop knowledge. *Nursing Science Quarterly, 2*(4), 162–171.

Jackre, M. (1989). Presenting research to nurses in clinical practice. *Applied Nursing Research, 2*(4), 191–193.

Jones, J. A. (1989). The verbal protocol: A research technique for nursing. *Journal of Advanced Nursing, 14,* 1062–1070.

Kingry, M. J., Tiedje, L. B., & Friedman, L. L. (1990). Focus groups: A research technique for nursing. *Nursing Research, 39*(2), 124–125.

Leininger, M. (1990). Ethnomethods: The philosophic and epistemic bases to explicate transcultural nursing knowledge. *Journal of Transcultural Nursing, 1*(2), 40–51.

Lindeman, C. A. (1989). Using nursing research. Research in nursing practice. NLN Publication #15–2232, 1–17.

LoBiondo-Wood, G., & Haber, J. (1994). *Nursing research: Methods, critical appraisal and utilization.* St. Louis: C.V. Mosby.

Maerker, M., Lisper, H., & Rickberg, S. (1990). Role-playing as a method in nursing research. *Journal of Advanced Nursing, 15*(2), 180–186.

Marchette, L. (1986). Professional survival tips: Basing your practice decisions on research. *Perioperative Nursing Quarterly, 2*(2), 68–70.

Moody, L. E. (1986). Generating researchable problems. *Nurse Educator, 11*(5), 8–9.

Neidich, B. (1990). A method to facilitate student interest in research: Chart review. *Nurse Educator, 29*(3), 139–140.

O'Brien, D., & Heyman, B. (1989). Changes in nurse education and the facilitation of nursing research: An exploratory study. *Nurse Education Today, 9*(6), 392–396.

Oddi, L. F., & Cassidy, V. R. (1989). Nursing research in the United States: The protection of human subjects. *International Journal of Nursing Studies, 27*(1), 21–33.

Rempusheski, V. F. (1990). Ask an expert: Formulating research questions. *Applied Nursing Research, 3*(1), 44–46.

Selby, M. L., Tornquist, E. M., & Finerty, E. J. (1989). How to present your research: The ABCs of creating and using visual aids to enhance your research presentation, part 2. *Nursing Outlook, 37,* 236–238.

Stark, J. L. (1989). A multiple-strategy leased research program for staff nurse involvement. *Journal of Nursing Administration, 19*(9), 7–8.

Thiele, J. E. (1989). Guidelines for collaborative research. *Applied Nursing Research, 2*(4), 150–153.

The Delivery of Nursing Care

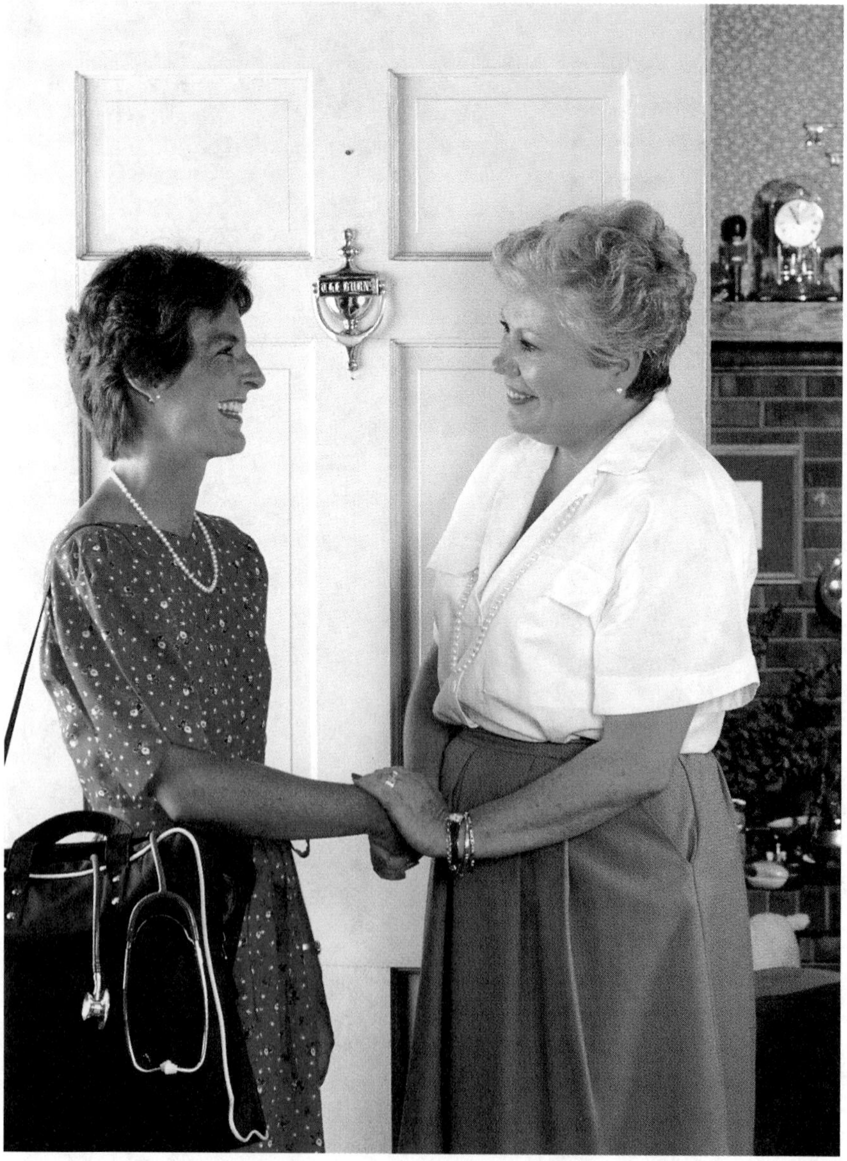

UNIT II

The delivery of healthcare and nursing care constantly changes to meet the needs of citizens of a community, whether it is worldwide, national, state (or provincial), or a small group. Related to this care, however, is the individual's ability or the community's ability to finance care. Ethical and legal concerns come into play, so healthcare will be on a continuum, be family oriented, and address the needs of all people equally. Unit II examines the rapidly changing delivery of care in the United States.

Chapter 6 discusses factors affecting the delivery of care, types of services, and the variety of healthcare settings. Colleagues providing services are defined, and the economics of healthcare services are further explained. The chapter ends with issues of healthcare delivery that are a constant challenge to providing safe, quality care. After a discussion of healthcare delivery in general, Chapter 7 looks at how nurses provide care through these outlets. A vital responsibility of the professional nurse is to see that a client's care is continued from one setting to another through careful, documented discharge planning.

Despite changes in types of healthcare or the actual setting in which nursing care is provided, there is one constant to healthcare: quality care. While Unit II provides a setting for these services, Unit I and the remainder of the units in this book provide a foundation for the student nurse to use in performing quality care as a professional nurse.

The Healthcare Delivery System

Key Terms

Alternative healthcare
Ambulatory care center
Consumerism
Healthcare delivery system
Healthcare reform
Health insurance
Health maintenance organization
Hospices
Long-term care
Medicaid
Medicare
Preferred provider organization
Prospective payment
Quality assurance

Learning Objectives

Upon completion of this chapter, the student will be able to do the following:

- *Discuss current factors affecting delivery of healthcare services.*
- *Explain the four types of healthcare services.*
- *Identify the various healthcare settings.*
- *Outline the role and educational preparation of at least 10 colleagues in the healthcare delivery system.*
- *Identify several methods of healthcare funding.*
- *Explain how quality assurance (improvement) can be evaluated and why it is important.*
- *Discuss current issues and the future in healthcare delivery and healthcare reform.*

6

You work at a day-care center as a nurse. One day a young mother confides to you that she has some recurring health problems. As you listen to her, you recognize that her problems could be effectively treated if she sought medical help. When you inquire about her reluctance to seek care, she tells you that she does not have healthcare benefits at her place of employment. When she goes to an emergency room, she is told that her problems are not life-threatening and she should see her primary healthcare provider. However, because she does not have health benefits, primary care providers are reluctant to see her or to add her to their practice panel. She asks how she should obtain healthcare for herself and her toddler.

In previous chapters, you studied about concepts essential to professional nursing. In this chapter, you will learn about the healthcare delivery system: its problems, its variety, and its future. When you have completed the chapter, you will have expanded your knowledge base so that you can address the questions asked by the young mother in the day-care center. The Critical Thinking Challenges at the end of the chapter will guide you further in your thinking.

The healthcare delivery system is one of the largest industries in the United States. It employs an estimated 8.5 million people (U.S. Department of Commerce, 1993). A tremendous variety of products are consumed by the system in the form of supplies, equipment, and medication. However, despite all of the resources that have been invested in the system, it remains a rather poorly repaired, fragile net of services full of holes and clumsy patches.

The term **healthcare delivery system** refers to a complex industry that transforms a variety of resources into services designed to meet the healthcare needs of society. These services are preventive, therapeutic, supportive, and rehabilitative. They are provided in traditional settings, such as hospitals, nursing homes, physicians' offices, and clinics. Increasingly, they also are provided in less traditional settings, such as shelters, shopping malls, schools, and mobile clinics. Healthcare is provided by a long list of health professionals; it is paid for by clients, private insurance companies, charitable organizations, and government agencies. Finally, the industry is guided by rules and regulations developed by federal, state, and local government agencies.

As the healthcare delivery system grows in size and complexity, it also becomes more expensive. According to the U.S. Department of Commerce, healthcare expenditures have been growing in excess of 10% per year for the last several years (1993). In 1987, $500 billion was spent on healthcare, which doubles the expenditures of 1977. By 1994, that figure had grown to more than $800 billion. By 2000, if costs are allowed to continue without controls, healthcare is expected to exceed $1.7 trillion (Lee & Estes, 1994). This annual spending on healthcare is higher than that of any other nation.

The healthcare delivery system is undergoing dramatic changes. In response to a need to control healthcare costs, ensure quality care, and meet consumer demands, a number of new and innovative organizations are emerging, and many traditional components of the system are changing (Harrington, Estes, & Davis, 1994).

Commonly Used Abbreviations in Healthcare Delivery

AHA	American Hospital Association
AMA	American Medical Association
ANA	American Nurses Association
APHA	American Public Health Association
APhA	American Pharmaceutical Association
CAHEA	Committee on Allied Health Education and Accreditation
CDC	Centers for Disease Control and Prevention
CHAMPUS	Civilian Health and Medical Program of the Uniformed Services
CNA	Canadian Nurses Association
DHHS	Department of Health and Human Services (formerly the Department of Health, Education and Welfare)
DRG(s)	Diagnosis-Related Group(s)
EPA	Environmental Protection Agency
FDA	Food and Drug Administration
GNP	Gross National Product
HCFA	Health-Care Financing Administration
HMO	Health Maintenance Organization
HSA	Health Service Administration
ICF	Intermediate-Care Facility
ICN	International Council of Nurses
JCAHO	Joint Commission on Accreditation of Healthcare Organizations
MCH	Maternal–Child Health
NCHS	National Center for Health Statistics
NINR	National Institute for Nursing Research
NIH	National Institutes of Health
NHI	National Health Insurance
NIA	National Institute on Aging
NFSNO	National Federation for Specialty Nursing Organizations
NLN	National League for Nursing
OSHA	Occupational Safety and Health Administration
PHS	Public Health Service
PPO	Preferred provider organization
RFP	Request for Proposal
SMI	Supplementary Medical Insurance
SNF	Skilled Nursing Facility
UR	Utilization Review
VA	Veterans Affairs (or Administration)
VNA	Visiting Nurses Association
WHO	World Health Organization

Factors Affecting Healthcare Delivery

Several factors have contributed to the growth, complexity, and expense of our healthcare delivery system: increasing longevity of Americans, technologic advances, rising consumerism, changing health services, and the politics of healthcare.

Increasing Longevity of Americans

Americans born in 1995 can expect to live an average of 76 years (men 73, women 80), compared with 47.3 years for those born in 1900 (U.S. Department of Commerce, 1993). The fastest growing age group is that of people 85 years and older (Fig. 6-1). Because the heaviest users of health services are the elderly, more emphasis is being placed on their needs; the need for services has increased, and gerontology has become a significant branch of medicine and nursing. New legal and ethical dilemmas arise as the public becomes concerned about the ability to maintain life and the quality of that life.

Technologic Advances

Advances made in technology have drastically changed healthcare and significantly altered the profile of the hospitalized client. For example, after insulin was developed in the 1920s, people with diabetes could manage their disease at home instead of in the hospital. The polio vaccine eliminated the need for clients to undergo long hospital stays in an iron lung. Antibiotics have

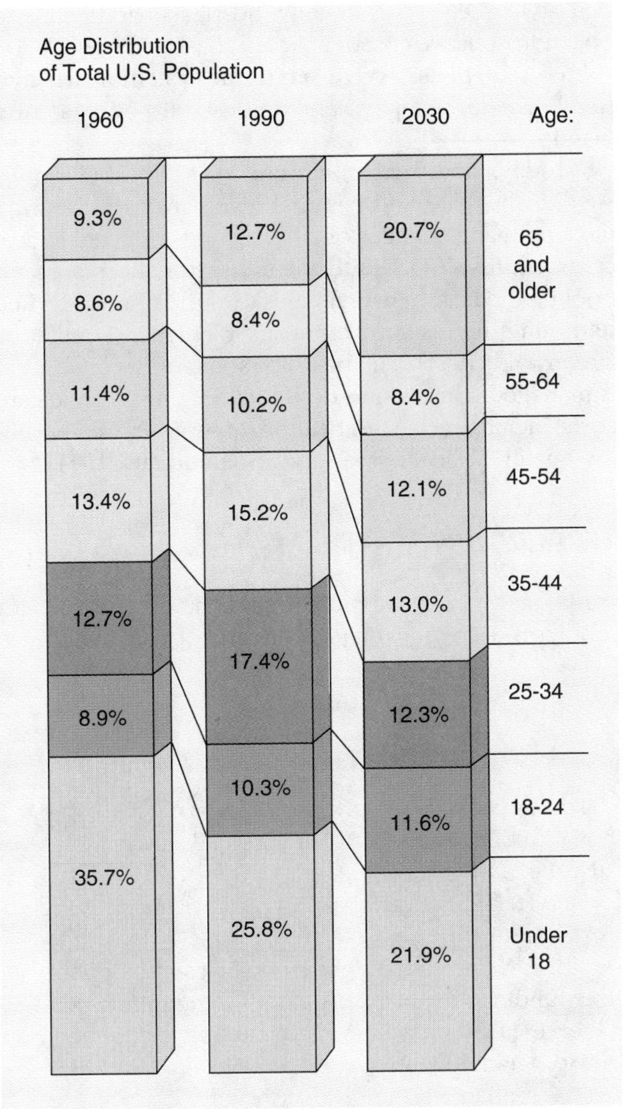

Figure 6-1 • *The U.S. Census Bureau data indicate the population of the United States is aging. A comparison of 1960, 1990, and projections for 2030 shows where growth and decline are taking place. (From U.S. Census Bureau.)*

been discovered that can ward off previously deadly diseases. Less invasive diagnostic tools can assist in identifying conditions at an early stage while they are still treatable. All these advances have reduced hospital stays and allowed people to live longer.

Many previously incurable diseases can now be treated. Life can now be maintained mechanically long after biologic systems have stopped functioning. Heart, lung, and liver transplants, unheard of 2 decades ago, are becoming common. However, new technology is expensive, and some advances raise formidable questions. For example, should insurance plans cover expensive transplants? How do we decide when to remove an individual from life-support equipment? Who decides to whom the organs should be given?

Rising Consumerism

Consumerism is the public's expectation that it will have a voice in determining the type, quality, and cost of healthcare. Consumers are better informed today than ever before and are asserting their rights in the area of healthcare delivery. The consumer movement was fostered by the advent of health maintenance organizations (HMOs), which promote the prevention and treatment of illness.

The movement was further encouraged by legislation that required facilities to obtain informed consents from clients before beginning certain treatments. Previously, the healthcare system operated on the assumption that physicians knew what was best for clients and should make decisions for them. Now clients expect—and demand—to be involved in healthcare decisions.

The right to healthcare also has became a consumer issue. Historically, the poor either had to be satisfied with a decreased quality of care or do without care. Today, many Americans view equal access to healthcare as everyone's right. An ongoing debate centers around who pays for these additional healthcare needs.

Changing Health Services

Health services in the 1980s and 1990s have been marked by a move to a more holistic approach. Health promotion and disease prevention are beginning to receive as much emphasis as the diagnosis and treatment of disease (Fig. 6-2). When people began to realize the importance of exercise, specialties such as sports medicine emerged. Gerontology developed as a specialty interested in the needs of the older adult. As people with diseases like diabetes, acquired immun-

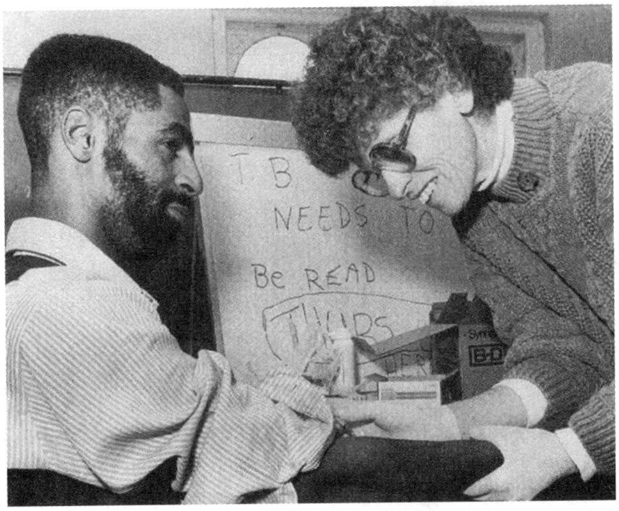

Figure 6-2 • *Outreach programs are designed to help prevent the spread of communicable diseases. A public health nurse is performing tuberculin testing in a local soup kitchen. (Photo courtesy of MCOSS, Inc., Red Bank, NJ, Home News Photo.)*

odeficiency syndrome (AIDS), and cancer began to live longer, treatment of chronic disease became more important.

Politics of Healthcare

Nothing has affected the healthcare delivery system more than federal legislation. For example, the Hill-Burton Act of 1946 provided funds for the construction of many small rural hospitals. In 1965, the Social Security Act was amended to incorporate Medicare and Medicaid; until that time, no branch of the government had been responsible for providing aid to nonindigent people when they were ill. **Medicare** provides health insurance to people who are either older than 65 years or disabled. **Medicaid** provides health benefits to the poor. These two programs are discussed later in this chapter.

In 1984, hospital funding based on diagnosis-related groups (DRGs) was established; it was determined that most hospital clients could be classified into one of 467 DRGs. Historically, hospitals had been paid on a retrospective cost or near-cost basis. This legislation shifted to a **prospective payment** system in which a fixed schedule of payment was established based on diagnosis.

Today, **healthcare reform** legislation being pursued at the state and national levels may result in the most dramatic changes of all. Reform is directed at cost control, providing health insurance for the poor, and pooling the health insurance risks of the nonpoor while reforming the insurance industry (Schieber, Poullier, & Greenwald, 1994). The basis for some of the legislation is managed competition designed to control healthcare costs, increase access to healthcare services, and ensure the quality of healthcare services (Buerhaus, 1994).

Types of Healthcare Services

Traditionally diagnosis and treatment of acute health problems were the major concern of the healthcare

Healthcare Delivery in Canada

Similar forces have affected healthcare delivery in Canada, but they have been handled in a substantially different manner because of intrinsic differences in the healthcare delivery systems. Healthcare in Canada is based on five fundamental principles (Canada Health Act, 1984):

- *Universality*—the entitlement of all citizens to insured health services
- *Accessibility*—the availability of health services on uniform terms and conditions without extra charges and user fees
- *Comprehensiveness*—the insurance of all essential health services provided by hospitals and physicians and, where legislated in the provinces, similar or additional services provided by other healthcare practitioners
- *Portability*—the continuation of health insurance coverage when residents are temporarily absent or move between provinces
- *Public administration*—the administration and operation of provincial healthcare insurance plans on a nonprofit basis by an appointed or designated public authority.

In other words, comprehensive healthcare insurance is provided to all Canadians through government sources. Constitutionally, healthcare is a provincial responsibility, but it is financed largely through transfer payments from the federal government.

The early 1960s saw increasing erosion of the previously mentioned principles. Hospital costs were escalating. Many physicians were augmenting the fees for service set by various provincial plans by direct extra billing to clients. Through the 1984 Canada Health Act, the federal government used its control over funding to reverse the extra billing trend and to increase health promotion, community, and home care program incentives (Canada Health Act, 1984).

The Canadian Nurses Association (CNA) has played a major role in the lobbying for healthcare reform. It was a major breakthrough to have included in the Canada Health Act the provisions for access to the healthcare system through physicians *and* other practitioners. Unlike the United States, where other healthcare providers such as nurse practitioners have been an access point for healthcare, physicians have been essentially the sole entry point for insured services in Canada. The CNA continues to press for reallocation of resources to further emphasize health promotion, illness prevention, and community involvement in decision-making. This position is in keeping with the move toward primary healthcare. As defined by the World Health Organization (1978), primary healthcare is "essential health care made universally accessible to individuals and families in the community by means acceptable to them, through their full participation and at a cost that the community and country can afford."

The section on healthcare delivery in Canada was written by Marlene Reimer, RN, MN, Associate Professor, University of Calgary, Calgary, Alberta, Canada.

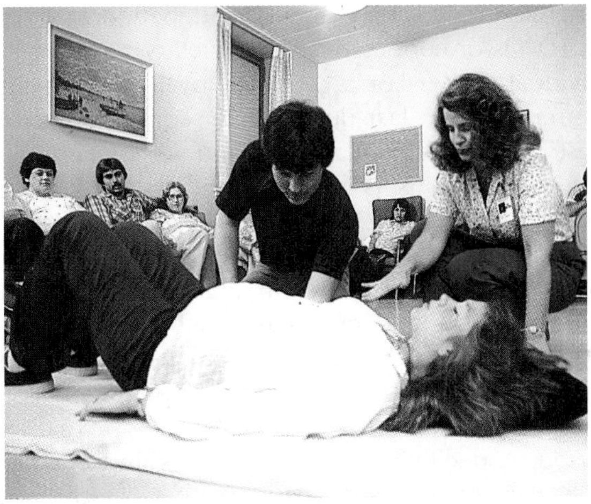

Figure 6-3 • *Nurse practitioners actively participate in health promotion activities at all levels.*

delivery system. Other types of care were used only to augment medical treatment regimens. As the healthcare market changed, health promotion and illness prevention, nurturing and support, and rehabilitative services have become more important.

Health Promotion and Illness Prevention

Health promotion and illness prevention services have grown in popularity in the last decade as Americans have taken more responsibility for their own health (Fig. 6-3). Many types of healthcare providers offer health information classes and counseling on topics such as nutrition, weight control, stress reduction, smoking cessation, and moderation in the use of alcohol. Nurses can provide individualized information or assist clients in selecting the appropriate classes or counseling based on their individual needs and history.

Nurture and Support

Nurturing and supportive nursing care includes services designed to assist individuals with the self-care activities they are unable to accomplish for themselves. These services are especially important for clients in hospitals, long-term care facilities, hospices, and home care. Nurturing and supportive services that include things such as comfort measures, activities of daily living, nutrition, mobility, or safety are usually provided by a registered nurse or by practical nurses and aides under the direction of a registered nurse. This type of nursing care has become more important as we have learned how to extend the lives of people who are dying or have debilitating and chronic diseases.

Diagnosis and Treatment

The therapeutic treatment of illness may take many forms and may occur in a variety of settings depending on the seriousness of the diagnosis and the equipment and facilities required to correct the condition. In the past, this care was generally provided in a physician's office; if needed, the client was admitted to a hospital for treatment and nursing care. Now diagnostic services, such as mammograms, blood tests, and chest x-rays, have moved to clinics, walk-in emergent care facilities, and even temporary mobile settings in parking lots. Surgical procedures that used to require overnight hospitalization are now carried out in ambulatory care settings with conscious sedation. Hospital stays have been shortened or eliminated, and high-tech treatments often occur in the client's own home. The nurse's role in these settings becomes even more essential because of the limited time the client is available for assessment and education. Coordination of the multiple resources needed by the client, or case management, also becomes critical.

Rehabilitation

The goal of rehabilitation is to help the client with an injury or disabling illness to achieve maximum function and independence. Rehabilitative services may be offered at a large medical complex or a free-standing agency. Often the rehabilitation program involves a team of health professionals, including physicians, nurses, physical therapists, and social workers.

Healthcare Settings

A person seeking healthcare today faces a tremendous array of settings in which care is provided. Some suggest that this maze is so complex that the average person needs an advocate to help him or her move through it. Services may vary: Some concentrate on health promotion and illness prevention, while others focus on diagnosis and treatment, rehabilitation, or supportive care. Because of the recent increases in the number and variety of agencies that provide healthcare, any attempt to categorize them in this chapter would be incomplete.

Until recently, hospitals and medical centers were the largest and most organized of healthcare agencies. Because of rising hospital costs, more procedures and treatments are being performed on an ambulatory basis. Clients come to an ambulatory care facility and usually do not stay overnight. A hallmark of good ambulatory care is thorough family and client education. The role of nurses in an ambulatory center may vary considerably, depending on their education and the management of the center.

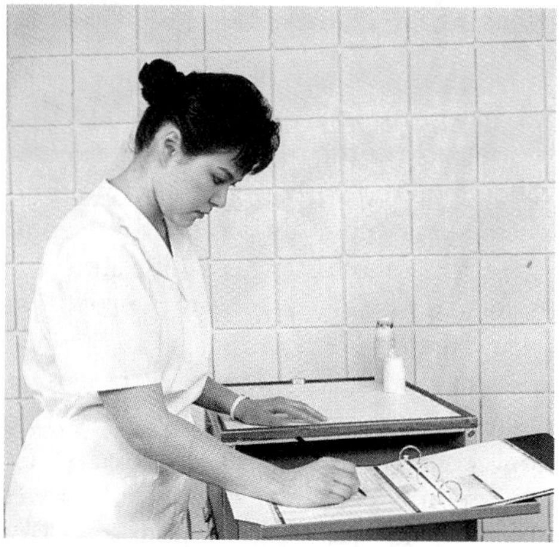

Figure 6-4 • Hospital care involves careful documentation and coordination of services. (© B. Proud)

Community healthcare agencies offer care to a neighborhood or community. Many of the care facilities, such as day-care centers or ambulatory care centers, also may be community based. Many have come into existence as a result of federal legislation.

Acute-Care Hospitals

Hospitals provide a wide range of services, including surgical treatment, diagnostic procedures, care of mothers and babies, rehabilitation, emergency services, and more recently ambulatory care. They are seen as acute-care facilities; that is, they provide care during the acute phase of an illness, surgery, or trauma. Many hospitals have added substance-abuse treatment units, oncology units, health-promotion programs, and home health services. The size of a hospital is generally reported as the number of available beds; the average size in the United States is about 200 beds (American Hospital Association, 1993).

Hospitals can be classified as those owned by the federal, state, or local government or by a private organization. The federal government owns the hospitals that are run by the Department of Veterans Affairs; the Department of Defense; the Department of Health and Human Services (DHHS); the Alcohol, Drug Abuse and Mental Health Administration, which functions under DHHS; and the Department of Transportation. Also included in this category are hospitals in federal prisons.

States own the hospitals at state-run medical schools and prisons. They also often own hospitals that offer long-term care, such as psychiatric facilities.

On the local government level are hospitals organized by a district, county, or city. These hospitals are usually funded by local bonds and often have an elected board of directors or commissioners.

Privately owned hospitals are further classified as being voluntary (not for profit) and proprietary (for profit). Voluntary hospitals are operated by religious or charitable groups; they may be independent or represent HMOs or cooperatives. Proprietary hospitals have individual owners or are owned by a partnership or corporation. The last decade has seen an increase in investor-owned hospital corporations; the stock of these corporations is traded on the stock exchange (Harrington, et al., 1994).

Today hospitals are the largest component of the U.S. healthcare delivery system (Fig. 6-4) and accounted for 40% of the total personal health expenditures in 1991 (U.S. Department of Commerce, 1993). However, as hospital expenditures have increased, the number of operating hospitals in this country has actually decreased. A decline in admission rates and client care days has resulted in a dramatic number of closures, especially among small, nonaccredited, financially struggling hospitals.

Long-Term Care Facilities

Long-term care is social, personal, and supportive services, in addition to medical care, needed by individuals who have lost some or all capacity for self-care because of chronic disease or disabling physical or mental conditions (Lee & Estes, 1994). Long-term care is most often provided to the elderly, but some people need long-term care from birth; others need long-term care after an injury or because of a debilitating disease, such as multiple sclerosis. Long-term care focuses on maintaining as much function as possible and emphasizes activities of daily living (basic needs, such as eating, dressing, toileting, bathing, and ambulating).

The term long-term care is used because clients spend much longer in one of these facilities than in an acute-care facility; often clients spend their last days at a long-term care center. Because of this, clients may see the facility as their home. Greater accommodation must be made for visits from family and friends and for outings (Fig. 6-5). Because clients have varying degrees of functional ability, the staff must be flexible and tailor their care to each client's needs.

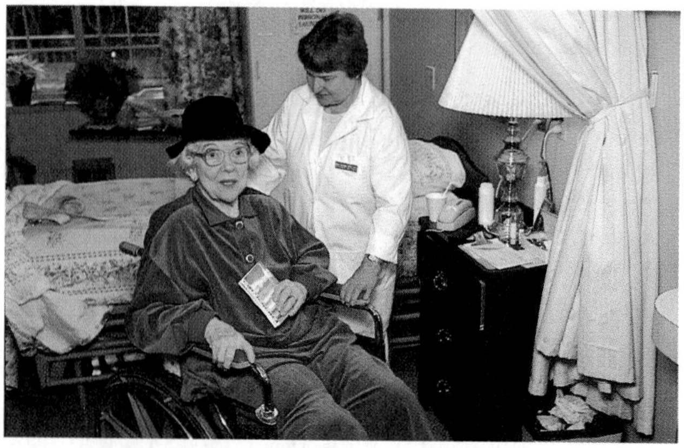

Figure 6-5 • Nurses in a long-term care facility try to make the environment as homelike as possible. Clients are encouraged to dress and go on outings.

Most long-term care is provided by nursing homes. An estimated 5% of the population older than 65 years lives in nursing homes, and one in every four Americans will spend some time in a nursing home (U.S. Senate Special Committee Report on Aging, 1991). Nursing homes also may be certified as skilled nursing facilities, intermediate-care facilities, or both. As with acute-care facilities, the ownership of nursing homes may be voluntary, proprietary, or governmental; in 1985, almost 75% of the homes were proprietary, with an average bed capacity of 85 (Kane & Kane, 1987).

Specialized Facilities

Some facilities offer only specialized services, such as psychiatric hospitals and alcohol and drug rehabilitation centers. Another example would be respite care facilities, which provide short-term inpatient services to individuals who usually are cared for at home. The purpose of respite care is to offer relief to the primary caregiver, usually a family member.

Rehabilitation centers also might be considered specialized inpatient facilities, although ambulatory services may be available. Rehabilitation centers focus on helping clients return to normal functioning or achieve the highest possible level of functioning after an illness or injury.

Physicians' Offices

In the physician's office, the traditional center for ambulatory care, clients are treated for minor injuries and illnesses and may have diagnostic workups, such as electrocardiograms, radiographs, and ultrasonograms. Laboratory diagnostic services, such as analysis of blood and urine specimens, may be available. Other services also may be offered, depending on the physician's specialty. Many physicians are extending their office hours to accommodate the work schedules of their clients and are hiring nurse practitioners (NPs) and physician assistants to increase access and control expenses.

Ambulatory Care Centers and Clinics

Clients can receive care for conditions not requiring hospitalization at **ambulatory care centers.** Many ambulatory care centers and clinics are affiliated with a hospital, but others operate independently, often in poorer areas. Traditional "walk-in" clinics have existed for many years and are often supported by government funding or charitable organizations. They frequently are designed to be used by people of lower economic status in lieu of a family physician. Centers may operate on an appointment or drop-in basis. Some clinics are specialized, such as family-planning clinics or those offering women's healthcare only. Much of the care in ambulatory care centers and clinics is provided by NPs or physician assistants.

Urgent care centers, which operate in a manner similar to walk-in clinics, are often owned by larger corporations that specialize in ambulatory healthcare. They are frequently located in major shopping areas or malls and may only be open during regular business hours. Clients who need services at other hours of the day must seek care elsewhere, such as emergency departments. Urgent care centers offer a variety of primary care services.

Day-Care Centers

Day-care centers target a particular client population; for instance, many day-care centers serve older adults who cannot be left alone for long periods of time but who can carry out activities of daily living. Other day-care centers serve clients who are physically or mentally challenged, such as those with cerebral palsy or Down syndrome, or people with chemical dependencies. These centers care for clients when family members are working and offer such services as meals, rehabilitation, and occupational therapy.

Mental Health Centers

Mental health centers offer a wide range of mental health services within a given "catchment" area. They may be part of a network of coordinated services rather than a single entity. They may be staffed with a variety of healthcare providers, including physicians, nurses, and social workers, and they usually provide short-term and crisis intervention approaches to treatment (Fig. 6-6). Centers may be associated with a hospital or may operate as independent nonprofit entities.

Rural Health Centers

Developed as a result of federal financing, rural health centers were established to provide care in rural, impoverished areas that have few physicians (Fig. 6-7). Much of the care in rural health centers is provided by residents and physicians who work on a rotating basis and from NPs and physician assistants.

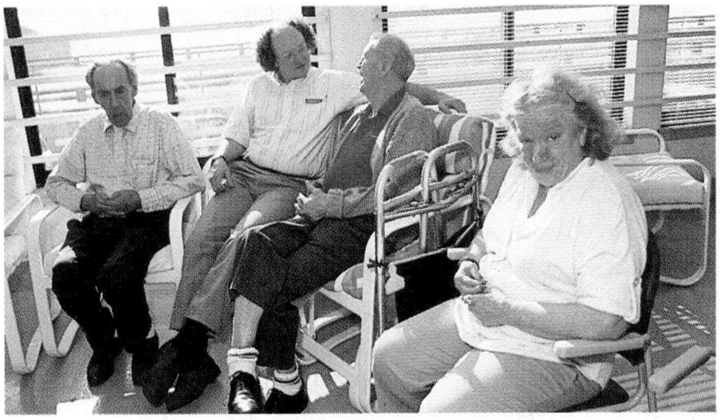

Figure 6-6 • *A nurse may provide mental health counseling within a community group.*

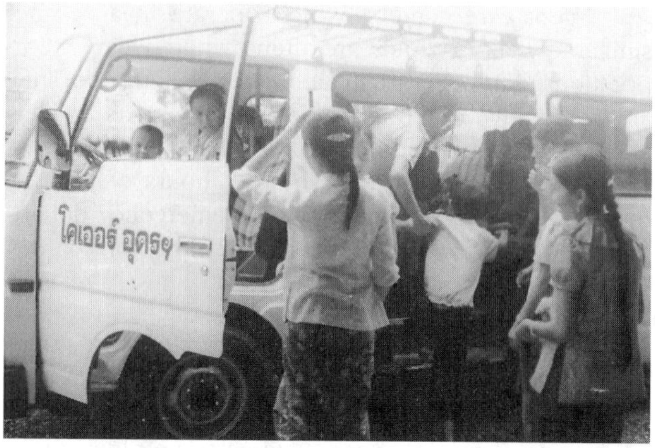

Figure 6-7 • Transportation is often necessary to help people in rural areas gain access to healthcare. This is especially true when immigrants do not speak the language or do not have their own transportation facilities. (Photo courtesy of Marjorie A. Muecke.)

Home Care Agencies

As the impact of prospective payment has forced clients to be discharged from the hospital earlier, home healthcare has become an essential part of the healthcare delivery system. Much of the care is given by registered nurses skilled in assessment, but practical nurses and aides also are employed.

Agencies receiving reimbursement under the Medicare program must be certified and must meet conditions and standards established by federal legislation. These services may be provided by a visiting nurse association, the local health department, or proprietary or voluntary agencies established for this purpose.

Technology previously found only in hospitals is now provided by home care agencies. Treatments may include intravenous feedings and medications, ventilators, portable dialysis machines, and cardiac monitoring.

In addition to skilled nursing care, home healthcare may include therapeutic services, such as physical, occupational, or speech therapy. Home care in a broader sense also may include homemaker services, in-home services to the elderly, and home-delivered meals.

Hospice

Hospices, run by public or private agencies, are designed to care for terminally ill clients and their families by providing supportive, palliative services (Castro, 1994). Many clients receiving these services are suffering from cancer, although conditions such as AIDS, multiple sclerosis, congestive heart failure, or end-stage renal disease also may require hospice care. The first hospice in the United States was established in 1974 in New Haven, Connecticut, and was modeled after St. Christopher's Hospice in London (Baker, 1992).

Nurses play a major role in hospice care; a team approach involving physicians, therapists, trained volunteers, and members of the clergy is often used. Nurses focus on managing pain, treating symptoms, and helping the client and family live life to the fullest until the death of the client (Fig. 6-8); they then work with family members to assist in bereavement and reorganizing their lives. Hospice care was initially provided in the home and still is; however, more recently, hospital- and community-based units have developed as well.

Retirement Communities

In the last 20 years, the number of retirement communities has increased significantly. These communities take many forms. They may occupy entire small towns, retirement subdivisions, apartments or condominiums, and continuing-care communities. Although the services vary, retirement communities usually provide a number of levels of care. In an arrangement known as assisted living, older people can live independently and have care nearby when they need it. A convalescent center may be associated with the facility, and services such as physical and occupational therapy may be provided. Other healthcare services, such as dental care, also may be available.

Residents are guaranteed access to various healthcare services, and the financial responsibilities are spread over the entire community. Some of the fees, such as entry fees, must be prepaid and may be very expensive. Monthly maintenance fees also are high; thus, access to these facilities is limited to more affluent retirees.

Colleagues in the Healthcare System

As healthcare has become more complex, the number and variety of providers involved in the healthcare field have increased proportionately. Raffel and Raffel (1989) identify 24 allied health training occupations accredited

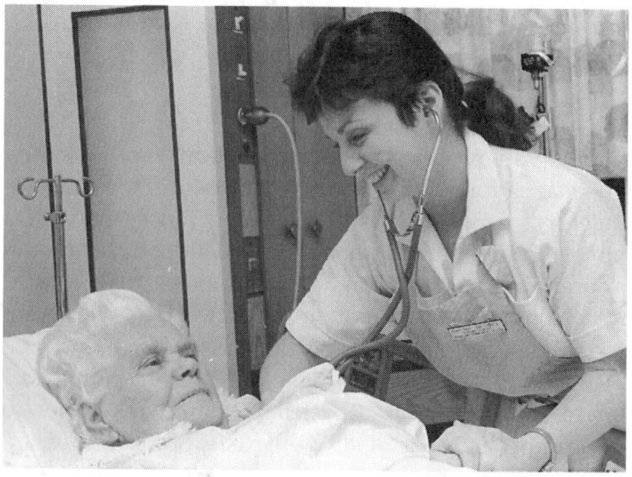

Figure 6-8 • Hospice nursing provides care to both the client and the family. The nurse helps the client with comfort measures. (Photo courtesy of Shoreline Community College.)

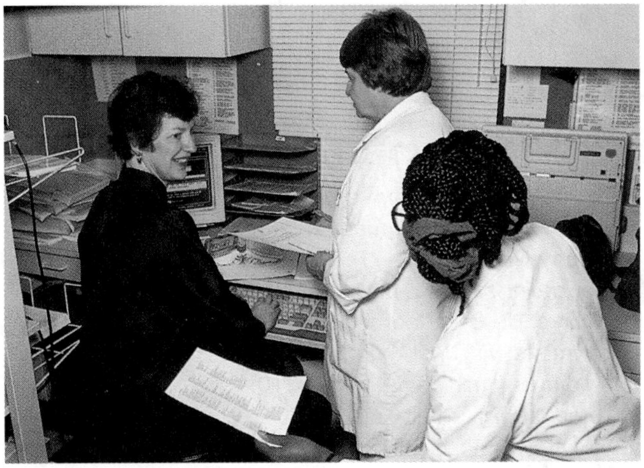

Figure 6-9 • *Quality healthcare delivery requires planning and coordination among colleagues.*

through the Committee on Allied Health Education and Accreditation, and many other jobs are accredited by other groups. Collaboration among professionals is critical to providing quality care (Fig. 6-9).

Registered Nurses and Nurse Practitioners

Registered nurses are the single largest group of healthcare professionals. Nurses address clients' self-care deficits, assist them in their adjustment to healthcare changes, and control their environments as a means of promoting health. In the past, most nurses worked in hospitals. In response to the changes occurring with healthcare reform, more nurses are moving to community-based practices.

NPs assume many of the responsibilities of physicians, and they can substitute for physicians when a shortage exists. NPs are skillful in diagnosing and managing acute and chronic health problems with health promotion as a central focus.

The first formal NP programs started in the 1960s and were designed to prepare nurses to provide primary medical care services and advanced nursing care to ambulatory clients. NP programs started as continuing education classes, but today most programs are offered through master's coursework in schools of nursing. NP coursework builds on the educational and practice experience of registered nurses and focuses on medical and nursing science, along with clinical skill. NPs work under their own nursing license and are responsible for their own performance. They work collaboratively with physicians to provide primary healthcare services.

Physicians and Physician Assistants

Physicians make up the second-largest group of healthcare professionals. They diagnose and treat clients in an attempt to cure or improve the condition. Nurses collaborate with physicians and assist them by carrying out the day-to-day treatments and care. Because they generally are responsible for the client's entry into the healthcare system, physicians are considered primary healthcare providers; however, nurses working in extended roles also may serve in this capacity.

Physicians attend 4 years of college, 4 years of medical school, and then train as residents. The practice of medicine has become highly specialized, either around a body part (eg, cardiology, gynecology) or around conditions and their treatment (eg, oncology, rheumatology).

In the past, most physicians were in solo practice. Today, many physicians are joining group practices or contracting with healthcare corporations. Many physicians employ physician extenders or assistants.

The physician assistant is a relative newcomer to the healthcare delivery system; the first training program for physician assistants was started at Duke University in 1966 (Raffel & Raffel, 1989). The training program is typically 2 years long, is part of an undergraduate program, and focuses on medical science and clinical skills. Physician assistants work directly under the supervision of physicians, who are responsible for their performance.

Focused Care Providers

Within the healthcare delivery system, certain groups of professionals provide focused care services (those limited to or concentrated on a particular aspect of healthy living). Examples are clinical psychologists, dentists, podiatrists, and optometrists. (Optometrists are often confused with ophthalmologists. Ophthalmologists are medical specialists; optometrists are trained and licensed to examine eyes for vision problems and to prescribe and fit eyeglasses but do not diagnose or treat eye diseases or injuries.) These professionals are licensed, although standards vary from state to state. They are usually addressed as "doctor." Their prescriptive authority also varies from state to state. In some areas, they may have hospital privileges (that is, they can admit and treat clients in a hospital setting).

Technicians and Technologists

Many people who provide ancillary healthcare services are called technicians or technologists. Examples include the medical laboratory technician or medical technologist, the medical record technician, the radiologic technician, and the dietary technician. At one time, the term technologist was used for people with a bachelor's degree and the term technician for those with a 2-year degree. In recent years, the terms have been applied indiscriminately; therefore, no conclusions can be drawn from the titles. Technicians or technologists provide a service that contributes to client care. For example, the medical laboratory technician works in the hospital's clinical laboratory, testing body fluids and tissues to help diagnose a client's condition.

Therapists

Other professionals are called therapists; examples are respiratory, occupational, physical, mental health, and speech therapists. Each is educated and licensed to provide a specific service. For example, the respiratory therapist helps clients with pulmonary function and oxygenation, and the speech therapist helps the client speak more clearly or correct speech disturbances.

Others Providing Necessary Services

Pharmacists make up the third largest group of healthcare providers. They are specialists in the science of drugs and can make recommendations about drug therapy. Most programs preparing pharmacists are 5 years long and include an internship.

The role of social workers is becoming increasingly important in today's healthcare delivery system. These professionals counsel clients and families and are involved in planning for discharge from the hospital. They are knowledgable in various healthcare resources. Social workers have bachelor's degrees, although many have a master's degree, which is preferred for healthcare employment.

Chaplains try to meet the spiritual and emotional needs of clients and families. Usually they are nondenominational in their approach. If the client prefers, the chaplain may contact a member of the clergy or a spiritual leader from the client's faith.

Nursing Research
Healthcare Delivery

Selected Nursing Research Studies

Mahoney, D. (1994). Appropriateness of geriatric prescribing decisions made by nurse practitioners and physicians. *Image—The Journal of Nursing Scholarship, 26*(1), 41–46.

Clarke, H., & Beddome, G. (1993). Public health nurses' vision of their future reflects changing paradigms. *Image, 25*(4), 305–310.

Cloonan, P., & Belyea, M. (1993). Limits of using patient characteristics in predicting home health care coordination. *Western Journal of Nursing Research, 15*(6), 742–751.

Gennaro, S., Klein, A., & Miranda, L. (1992). Health policy dilemmas: Related to high technology infertility services. *Image, 24*(3), 191–194.

McCullock, C., & Mclnyk, K. (1990). Barriers to care: Operationalizing the variable. *Nursing Research, 39*(2), 108–112.

Saver, B., & Peterfreund, N. (1993). Insurance, income, and access to ambulatory care in King County, Washington, *American Journal of Public Health, 83*(11), 1583–1588.

Possible Topics for Nursing Inquiry

- When nurses are added to hospital ethics committees, are decisions more client centered?
- Is there a relationship between the amount of time nurse practitioners spend providing client education information and client care outcomes?
- Is there a relationship between the hospital staff ratio of registered nurses to other healthcare providers and client care outcomes?
- Do clients receiving care through an HMO exhibit more health promotion behaviors than those receiving care from physicians in private or group practice?

Economics of Healthcare Services

How did the U.S. healthcare delivery system become so expensive? Who should pay for the ever-increasing costs of healthcare and hospitalization? These questions have become the impetus for untold numbers of reports, articles, studies, and documentaries. The astronomical cost of some forms of treatment has made it impossible for the average client to pay personally for all medical and nursing services. Bills exceeding $10,000 are no longer the exception. **Health insurance** provides protection against the cost of medical care and hospitalization arising from illness or injury.

There has been much debate about whether the United States should adopt a national health insurance plan. Under a national plan, taxpayers would pay for the coverage, much as insurance companies collect funds from subscribers. No health insurance plan, national or private, is free.

Private Health Insurance

Many people have private health insurance plans, which are offered as a benefit by employers or purchased by individuals. Because the insurance company pays the medical bill, this system is known as third-party reimbursement. One of the earliest health insurance programs in the United States was started at Baylor University Hospital in Texas in 1929. Teachers prepaid a monthly payment to insure up to 21 days of semiprivate hospitalization annually (Rothman, 1993). From this evolved the Blue Cross program.

Many organizations provide private health insurance programs. Health insurance benefits have become a major negotiable item in labor contracts. The available programs vary tremendously: Some cover all medical costs; others have sizable deductibles and force subscribers to shoulder some of the cost. Whether policies should cover extremely expensive procedures, such as transplants, is a subject of debate.

The term *catastrophic health insurance* generally refers to plans that protect the insured (particularly the older adult) and their families from bankruptcy due to major or long-term illness. A workable plan for catastrophic health coverage has yet to be developed.

Private and group insurance policies can provide significant assistance to people struggling to meet rising healthcare costs but provide no assistance to people who are unemployed or those who do not receive health insurance benefits. Who pays for healthcare services for the growing segment of the population who are ineligible for health insurance?

Government Involvement in Healthcare Funding

The federal government helps to cover healthcare costs for some citizens. The DHHS is the second-largest department of the federal government; only the Department of Defense is larger. Some of the services offered by the federal government are mentioned earlier in this chapter, such as services provided in government hospitals. Care also is provided under the Medicare and Medicaid programs, started in 1965.

Medicare and Medicaid

Medicare provides medical and hospital insurance to people 65 years or older and to disabled people. Hospital insurance, provided under Part A of the plan, covers inpatient care, care in a skilled nursing facility, and home healthcare. It is financed by social security taxes. Part B of Medicare, which provides supplemental medical insurance, is optional. People choosing to enroll in this plan in addition to Part A must pay for the services, and the cost is deducted from their social security check. Part B covers physicians' charges, ambulatory or emergency room services, unlimited home health visits, and other services, such as speech and physical therapy, x-rays, and wheelchairs and similar supplies. The Healthcare Financing Administration oversees the Medicare program. Medicare expenditures are increasing each year, raising concerns for the program and the public it serves.

Medicaid is a federally funded program administered through the states to provide services to two groups of people:

- The *categorically needy* are blind, disabled, or aged people and those receiving public assistance from Aid to Families with Dependent Children.
- The *medically needy* are those who meet other low-income standards as defined by the state in which they live.

Medicaid's benefit structure varies from state to state. Some states pay for dental care, eyeglasses, or prescription drugs, but other states do not. Like Medicare, the cost of this program has grown and is a matter of public concern.

Prospective Payment

Two acts passed by Congress have significantly affected the methods by which hospitals are reimbursed for care. The Tax Equity and Fiscal Responsibility Act of 1982 established a cost-per-case basis for hospital payment. Of even greater significance were the 1983 amendments to the Social Security Act, which established a method of paying for inpatient care for Medicare clients based on DRGs. In an attempt to control rising costs, a predetermined (prospective) and fixed rate was established to reimburse for the care for each of 467 diagnoses or procedures. Hospitals receive no more than this figure, regardless of the cost they may have incurred delivering the care. Costs above the established amount must be absorbed by the hospital, but if the care is delivered for less than the established amount, the hospital keeps the difference and makes a profit. Different rates were set for urban and rural hospitals, and rates are adjusted each year to reflect the increasing costs of goods and services. DRGs have been adopted as the basis for reimbursement of care provided to clients other than those covered by Medicare.

Integrated Healthcare Systems

Historically, the healthcare delivery system in the United States has been composed of informally connected providers working together to produce healthcare services. The result was often fragmented and costly care. The healthcare delivery system of the future is likely to be very different. HMOs and preferred provider organizations (PPOs) are examples of formal healthcare networks that are already operating in the United States.

Health Maintenance Organizations

HMOs are prepaid health management plans that offer complete healthcare services to their members for an established fee and minimal copayments; thus, they combine traditional insurance and healthcare delivery in one organization. HMOs are expected to be leaders in the healthcare field of the future.

HMOs provide a wide range of services, including inpatient and ambulatory hospital care, infertility and mental health services, therapeutic radiologic treatment, alcohol and drug addiction treatment, and physical therapy.

HMOs were first established in 1973 under a federal program. The number of HMOs in existence grew from 175 in 1976 to 556 in 1992 (U.S. Department of Commerce, 1993). Enrollment is voluntary; members have the option to select another plan. Because the fee paid by members is fixed, the organization tries to minimize its costs. To do this, HMOs place greater emphasis on health promotion and disease prevention. Physicians who work for HMOs may receive a monthly salary regardless of the number of clients they see, and costs such as malpractice insurance are paid by the organization.

Preferred Provider Organizations

A PPO is a group of physicians, and possibly one or more hospitals, that offers a prepaid healthcare plan to employers. In a preferred provider arrangement, clients select their healthcare providers from the list of people, groups, or institutions that have contracted to offer services at a certain price. Generally, the cost of care is somewhat lower because these arrangements place a greater emphasis on health maintenance and limit expensive procedures. If a consumer seeks services from a provider who has not contracted with the plan, a substantial deductible fee is assessed, or the service is not covered at all. In the future, PPOs are likely to grow larger and include a broader range of providers.

Charitable Funding of Healthcare

The largest percentage of charitable care is offered by hospitals to the uninsured. Some charitable funding is directed toward special populations, such as children suffering from muscular dystrophy or cancer.

Issues of Healthcare Delivery

As the delivery of healthcare services has become more complex and sophisticated, many ethical and bioethical issues have resulted. Six major issues are addressed here.

Limited Medical and Financial Resources

As discussed previously, healthcare costs in the United States are increasing steadily. Some of the reasons are the growing population of older adults, increasing technology, increasing specialization in services, and changing values. In an effort to offset some of the rising costs, several measures have been adopted. For example, healthcare delivery through organizations like HMOs has been encouraged, and the government has established prospective payment for Medicare. However, as the availability of resources has decreased, a number of issues have emerged. With limited resources, the question of healthcare rationing must be addressed. The change to lower cost providers by hospitals and clinics has created job security concerns for many nurses. All healthcare providers are being asked to put a dollar value on their services, inside and outside of hospitals, and relate these costs to client outcomes. Finally, quality versus quantity of life questions are being debated at all levels.

Access to Healthcare

Access to healthcare services is an individual's ability to find a healthcare provider. Access has been a public health issue for many years. Although more people are involved in the healthcare system than ever before, some areas of the United States still lack adequate healthcare resources. Research has suggested that access varies depending on the individual's income, race, and geographic location (Saver & Peterfreund, 1993). Numerous plans have been tried to solve the access issue. The healthcare reform movement is the latest attempt to provide a solution through universal coverage.

Fragmentation of Service

The explosive growth in medical information has led to specialization throughout the healthcare system. The traditional family physician who treats cuts and fractures, delivers babies, performs minor surgery, and treats medical emergencies with equal poise and confidence is seldom found today. Likewise, the nurse who can work on any hospital unit has become a rarity. The sophisticated technology throughout today's hospital requires more than a generalist's knowledge and skill.

The price for these technologic advances is fragmented care. For example, a surgical client who suffers from diabetes receives care from a surgeon and an endocrinologist or internist. If that same client has heart problems during surgery, a cardiologist is called in. The client may spend time in surgery, the recovery room, the intensive or coronary care unit, a step-down unit, or a medical or surgical unit; the same client may spend some time in all these areas. After discharge, this fragmentation may continue as different specialists prescribe different medications and require follow-up visits. This can confuse and upset the client and family.

The nurse can help ensure that the healthcare delivery system always puts the client's needs first and can help minimize fragmented care. As a coordinator of care and a client advocate, the nurse can advise clients and reduce confusion (Fig. 6-10).

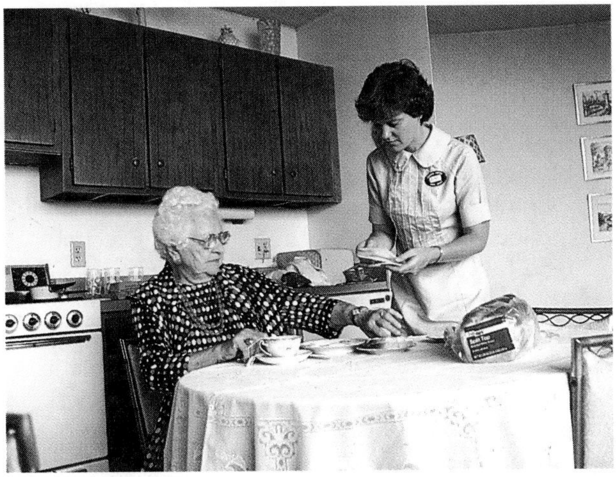

Figure 6-10 • Nursing is one step in eliminating fragmentation of service. The nurse is responsible for teaching and coordinating healthcare and works with the client and family to plan for discharge. The nurse is a facilitator in providing nursing care in the home.

Quality of Care

Quality assurance, one of the most discussed topics in healthcare today, is the methods used to measure the quality of care provided by people or institutions. Licensing, accreditation, and certification are examples of attempts to guarantee that people and places are prepared to do what the public expects. Some of the titles given to this process of ensuring quality care are quality assurance, quality improvement, or continuous quality improvement. The goal remains the same: measuring and ensuring the quality of care being provided.

Both people and institutions may be licensed. Mechanisms, often tests, are established to recognize minimal competence in a profession. Practicing without a license is a criminal offense. Institutions are licensed based on their ability to meet established criteria. Typical factors considered are physical structure, administration, qualification of personnel, and standards for provision of services. Hospitals, nursing homes, and pharmacies are licensed in all states; licensing of other facilities and nonhospital services varies from state to state.

Accreditation, a popular approach to quality measurement, is a voluntary system used in institutions. Groups with mutual interests establish standards of quality and inspect themselves according to these standards. Although not a legal requirement, strong incentives exist to attain and maintain accreditation. In many instances, accreditation is required for securing federal funding. For hospitals, an important accrediting organization is the Joint Commission on Accreditation of Healthcare Organizations. Nursing programs can seek accreditation from the National League for Nursing.

Certification, the third approach to quality control, combines features of licensing and accreditation. Standards for education, experience, and performance on examinations are used to determine a person's competence. Although certification is usually voluntary, there are incentives for people to become certified. Certification is often used to designate a person's professional specialty.

More recently, quality assurance methods have been used to evaluate the care of clients or groups of clients. Often these methods of evaluating care compare the care given to clients with an established standard. This type of assessment requires that peer review, either retrospective or concurrent, be built into the system.

A popular method of evaluating care is to review client care outcomes. In this system, medical charts are reviewed, and clients are reexamined and interviewed; this information is then compared with established standards that are usually based on indicators of health status. Quality assurance checks or audits are done by third-party payers, who review a hospital's charts and records to determine the quality and appropriateness of the care provided.

Quality assurance is a critical element of the healthcare delivery system, but it is time consuming and therefore costly. Standards for assessment must be developed and refined, which requires time and constant updates.

Ethical and Bioethical Decisions

Should terminally ill clients be placed on respirators? Should a person be required to donate bone marrow if that person is the only acceptable match? Should major health insurance plans cover expensive transplants? Should tissue from a fetus be used to treat illnesses? As technology makes available more options of care, ethical and bioethical decision-making becomes critical. Many hospitals have formed ethics committees that make decisions and establish policies on such controversial issues as allocation of scarce medical and financial resources and development of appropriate treatment protocols. Nurses play a critical role in making decisions on bioethical issues and often serve on these ethics committees. Because they have the most contact with the client, nurses are in a unique position to know the client's and family's wishes and to be advocates on the client's behalf. See Chapter 3 for more discussion on ethical concerns in nursing.

Alternative Healthcare Services

Alternative healthcare is care composed of nontraditional treatments. These treatments may include acupressure, acupuncture, therapeutic touch, herbal treatments, hypnosis, imagery, or homeopathy. Alternative healthcare treatments are being studied to see how they can be used to support more traditional plans of care. Congress established the Office of Alternative Medicine in 1992 to sponsor research in this field to determine the value of nontraditional treatments on client outcomes. The value of even testing the efficacy of alternative healthcare, however, has been the center of much controversy.

Future for Healthcare Delivery

Several factors are forcing the healthcare delivery system to change. Consumers and payers of healthcare services are demanding more cost-efficient and effective care. Consumers are demanding that providers offer them a continuum of different types of services and that those services be available in a broad geographic area (Riley, 1994).

Experts believe that future integrated models of healthcare will be able to supply a broad range of services, from in-house care to ambulatory, within their own system (vertically integrated) or arrange for the services to be provided by other systems (horizontally integrated) through corporate agreements (Riley, 1994). Primary care providers, hospitals, retirement communities, pharmacies, rehabilitation centers, and other types of providers from a large geographic area will be connected in a formal way.

Formal integration of services is expected to restructure the economic activity of the healthcare delivery system (Buerhaus, 1994). Networks are expected to compete for clients by becoming more efficient, charging lower prices, and providing quality services. They will guarantee quality care for a fixed cost for the life of the individual and maintain a central database to ensure comprehensive care as the client moves from provider to provider within the system. Whether it is government mandated or initiated by consumers and corporations, the future of healthcare will continue to change.

Key Concepts

- The U.S. healthcare delivery system has experienced phenomenal growth, and this pattern will continue.
- Nurses are assuming increasingly significant roles in the delivery of care. They are primary caregivers, develop collaborative roles, and respond to the increasing specialization in healthcare.
- Americans have come to view healthcare as a right rather than a privilege and are demanding a greater voice in determining the type and quality of care.
- Two other factors affecting the healthcare system are increasing longevity and increasing technology.
- The federal government continues to assume a large role in the healthcare system.
- Several types of health services are available in the United States: health promotion and illness prevention, diagnosis and treatment, support, and rehabilitation.
- Healthcare settings include acute care hospitals, long-term care facilities, physicians' offices, ambulatory care centers and clinics, day-care centers, mental health centers, rural health centers, home care agencies, hospice, and retirement communities.
- Healthcare benefits are available to consumers through private health insurance, programs initiated by the federal government (such as Medicare and Medicaid), and charitable funding.
- To provide quality care, a collaborative approach is needed between nurses and other healthcare professionals.
- Among current issues of healthcare delivery are limited medical and financial resources, access to healthcare, fragmentation of services, quality of care, ethical and bioethical decisions, and alternative healthcare services.

Critical Thinking Challenges

You have added the vastness of the healthcare delivery system to your knowledge base of the nursing profession. Now turn to the situation at the beginning of the chapter, and consider these challenges.

1. *Describe how you think this mother might feel right now. Associate that with how you would feel if you were in her position.*
2. *Define the kind of response you believe this mother is seeking from you.*
3. *Outline possible responses you could make to this mother.*
4. *Based on your analysis of your previous responses, identify the match between the healthcare delivery system and the needs of this mother.*
5. *Present some options for how you and she might proceed.*

References

American Hospital Association (1993). *Hospital statistics.* Chicago: Author.

Baker, M. (1992). Cost effective management of the hospital-based hospice program. *Journal of Nursing Administration, 22*(1), 40–45.

Buerhaus, P. (1994). Economics of managed competition and consequences to nurses. *Nursing Economics, 12*(2), 75–80, 106.

Castro, J. (1994). *The American way of health.* Boston: Little, Brown.

Harrington, C., Estes, C., & Davis, S. (1994). The medical-industrial complex. In C. Harrington & C. Estes (Eds.), *Health policy and nursing.* Boston: Jones & Bartlett.

Kane, R. A., & Kane, R. L. (1987). *Long-term care: Principles, programs and policies.* New York: Springer.

Lee, P., & Estes, C. (1994). *The Nation's Health* (4th ed.). Boston: Jones & Bartlett.

Raffel, M. W., & Raffel, N. K. (1989). *The U.S. health system: Origins and functions* (3rd ed.). New York: John Wiley & Sons.

Riley, D. (1994). Integrated health care systems: Emerging models. *Nursing Economics, 12*(4), 201–206.

Rothman, D. (1993). A century of failure: Health care reform in America. *Journal of Health, Politics, and Law, 18*(2).

Saver, B., & Peterfreund, N. (1993). Insurance, income, and access to ambulatory care in King County, Washington. *American Journal of Public Health, 83*(100), 1583–1588.

Schieber, G., Poullier, J., & Greenwald, L. (1994). U.S. health expenditure performance: An international comparison and data update. In C. Harrington & C. Estes (Eds.), *Health policy and nursing.* Boston: Jones & Bartlett.

U.S. Department of Health and Human Services (1990). *Vital statistics for the United States: 1987 life tables* (Vol. 2, Sec. 6). Publication #PHS 90-1104. Hyattsville, MD: U.S. Government Printing Office.

U.S. Senate Special Committee Report on Aging. (1991). *Aging America: Trends and projections* (1991 ed.). Washington, DC: Public Health Service, Department of Health and Human Services.

U.S. Department of Commerce (1993). *Statistical abstract of the United States 1993.* (113th ed.). Washington, DC: Government Printing Office.

Bibliography

Aiken, L., & Fagin, C. (1992). *Charting nursing's future.* New York: J.B. Lippincott.

Buerhaus, P. (1994). Managed competition and critical issues facing nurses. *Nursing and Health Care, 15*(1), 22–26.

Buerhaus, P. (1994). Economics of managed competition and consequences to nurses: Part I. *Nursing Economics, 12*(1), 10–17.

Callahan, D. (1990). *What kind of life: The limits of medical progress.* New York: Simon & Schuster.

Clawson, D., & Osterweis, M. (1993). *Roles of physician assistants and nurse practitioners in primary care.* Kansas City: Academic Health Centers.

Cranford, R. E. (1990). A hostage to technology. *Hastings Center Report, 20*(5), 9–10.

Donley, Sr. R. (1993). Ethics in the age of health care reform. *Nursing Economics, 11*(1), 18–24.

Kassirer, J. P. (1994). Access to specialty care. *New England Journal of Medicine, 331*(17), 1151–1153.

Lynn, J., & Glover, J. (1990). Cruzan and caring for others. *Hastings Center Report, 20*(5), 10–11.

McKenzie, N. (1994). *Beyond crisis: Confronting health care in the United States.* New York: Meridian Publishing.

Schroeder, C. (1993). Nursing's response to the crisis of access, costs, and quality in health care. *Advances in Nursing Science, 16*(1), 1–20.

Sherman, V. (1994). *Creating the new American hospital.* San Francisco: Jossey-Bass.

Star, P. (1994). *The logic of health care reform.* New York: Whittle Books.

Stevens, N. (1993). Marginalized women's access to health care: A feminist narrative analysis. *Advances in Nursing Science, 16*(2), 39–56.

Weil, T., & Stack, M. (1993). Health reform: Its potential impact on hospital nursing service. *Nursing Economics, 11*(4), 200–207.

Community-Based Nursing and Continuity of Care

Key Terms	Learning Objectives
Community-based healthcare *Community-based nursing care* *Continuity of care* *Discharge planning* *Managed care* *Seamless care*	*Upon completion of this chapter, the student will be able to do the following:* • *Discuss consumerism and the part it plays in healthcare services.* • *Identify three levels of healthcare and the services under each.* • *Trace hospitals through their traditional services, the current transition, and into the future.* • *Using goals of various planning groups for the future, state visions of community-based care.* • *Discuss the holistic focus of nursing care in various settings and situations.* • *List and define community healthcare delivery settings and community-based nursing settings.* • *Relate home healthcare nursing to other aspects of professional nursing.* • *Create a list of discharge planning guidelines for continuity of care.*

7

You are employed as a nurse case manager working in an integrated healthcare organization. A new client on your caseload was just readmitted to the hospital with a history of recurrent exacerbations of chronic obstructive lung disease with two hospitalizations in the last 6 months. You visit the client in her hospital room after reading her chart and talking with her primary nurse. At this time, you take a more detailed history, including information about her family and support system, home environment, and healthcare insurance coverage. You begin the discharge planning process by discussing with the client the kind of support services she might need to help her chronic condition to stabilize within the context of the healthcare resources available to her. Later you visit one of your clients who was recently transferred to a long-term care facility after hospitalization. You assess the client and discuss with the nursing staff the client's progress. Next you make several home visits to clients in need of health monitoring, support, and teaching. You finish your day with several telephone calls to clients who are more independent but still in need of support, and you make additional consultative calls to several physicians and a social worker.

In previous chapters, you learned about concepts essential for professional nursing. You were introduced to the healthcare delivery system and issues affecting it. With this chapter, you will add community-based nursing to your growing knowledge base. The opening scenario describes a form of nursing practice that is community based and "without walls." That is, your practice setting is wherever your clients are, which may be anywhere along a continuum of healthcare services. The Critical Thinking Challenges at the end of the chapter will strengthen your understanding of nursing in the community.

The American healthcare system at the end of the 20th century is in the midst of a major transition. As a citizen and a consumer, you have read about, probably discussed with your family and friends, and perhaps participated in the national healthcare reform town hall meetings, congressional hearings, and debates. The American healthcare system is in a state of crisis (American Nurses Association [ANA], 1991). A crisis, however, presents opportunity. Healthcare policy and decision makers are eager to find solutions that will work. The pivotal problem is how to deliver *cost-effective* and *quality* healthcare that will be *accessible* to everyone and will result in *positive health outcomes.*

Most legislative discussions for national healthcare have several key strategies in common: primary healthcare and health promotion or disease prevention services. In addition, the World Health Organization (WHO, 1978), an agency of the United Nations that promotes health for people worldwide, includes the components of universality, essentiality, community empowerment, community participation, and community development in its definition of primary healthcare.

Because hospital stays are getting shorter, care provided in the community must expand (Laffrey, 1994). As the emphasis on primary healthcare and prevention increases, community-based care will become more significant than institution-based healthcare. It is predicted that more nurses will work in community-based settings than in institution-based (hospital) settings in the future.

To provide a better understanding of current and future trends in healthcare delivery and in nursing care, this chapter presents background information related to traditional care and changes, focusing on continuity of care and describing emerging models of community-based nursing practice. Although everything in this textbook is related to community-based nursing (because the hospital is part of community-based nursing), the clinical chapters in Section II use community-based nursing as an integral part of their "Implementation" section.

Consumerism and Its Effect on Current Healthcare Trends

"Americans are moving away from a narrow concept of health as the absence of disease to a broader definition that encompasses quality of life issues" (Healthcare Forum, 1994, p. 3). In a random survey of 1,000 households conducted to determine what the public considers vital to individual health and the health of their communities, results revealed that Americans are moving away from a passive approach to health and toward an approach that emphasizes actively "creating" health. Values commonly held among survey participants include the following:

- Individuals can influence their own health through behavior and lifestyle changes.
- Prevention strategies are important.
- Health and well-being include quality of life issues.

A significant finding is that quality of life is believed to be synonymous with what people think makes a healthy community. The public's current perspective sees lowering crime rates, strengthening families and their lifestyles, improving environmental quality, and providing behavioral or mental healthcare as critical elements to creating healthy communities. The Healthcare Forum (1993) further states the following:

> These results show the emergence of public recognition that one's own health is somehow related to the health of one's neighbors; suggesting that perhaps, the most practical approach to pursuing a healthier life is the *pursuit of a healthier community* (italics added; p. 5).

In relation to healthcare within the community, the Healthcare Forum (1994) found that desire for high quality healthcare, affordable healthcare, and good access to healthcare were almost equal (Fig. 7-1).

Findings of this survey support predictions made in 1992 by the National League for Nursing (Executive Wire, 1992). The predicted trends for healthcare included the following:

- Nurses will emerge as community leaders.
- Community nursing centers and community health programs to assist in preventing disease and promoting health will expand and become more available to the consumer.
- Home care will become the center of healthcare.
- Health will become a value with moral force for the American public, creating a demand for consumer-driven services (Executive Wire, 1992).

The use of nontraditional healthcare must be considered in any discussion of consumerism and healthcare choices. Eisenberg et al. (1993) report the following. A random sample of American adults (N = 1539) responded to a telephone survey. One in three of the respondents (34%) reported using at least one unconventional therapy in the last year. Most respondents (72%) did not inform their physicians of these actions.

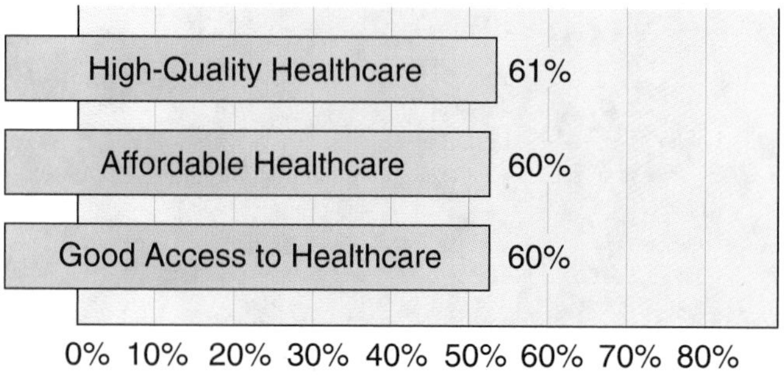

Figure 7-1 • *Critical determinants of healthcare in a healthy community. (Data from Healthcare Forum (1994). What creates health? San Francisco.)*

When these results are extrapolated to the U.S. population, in 1990, an estimated 425 million visits were made to providers of unconventional therapy; this exceeds the number of visits to all U.S. primary healthcare physicians (388 million). The researchers conclude that the use of unconventional therapy is far higher than previously reported.

Studies from reliable sources (Eisenberg, et al., 1993; Healthcare Forum, 1994; Gruman, 1995) predict that in the future, healthcare delivery will be community based, will include a much broader array of traditional and nontraditional services, and will include programs formerly not considered related to health, all of which have the potential to be provided by or managed by nurses.

Levels of Healthcare

The Division of Nursing of the Department of Health and Human Services has analyzed current nursing practice and education in relation to population healthcare needs. Levels of healthcare are categorized as primary, secondary, and tertiary healthcare. The majority of current resources, services, nursing practice, and nursing education exist within the category of secondary healthcare (emergency care, acute and critical care, diagnosis and treatment), as illustrated in Figure 7-2. The needs of the population, however, lie mainly within the categories of primary healthcare (health promotion, education, protection, screening) and tertiary healthcare (rehabilitation, long-term care and support services, hospice care), also illustrated in Figure 7-2. The majority of primary and tertiary healthcare services are most appropriately delivered from community-based settings, and historically, they have been. Healthcare at the end of this century and the beginning of the next century must address how to bring these levels of need and provisions of care into better alignment.

Community-Based Healthcare Delivery

One of the major criticisms of the current system in national healthcare reform discussions is that there really is no system. That is, care is fragmented, with little or no coordination across settings or among providers. With few formal linkages between acute care, long-term care, and home healthcare, complete information is difficult to transmit between systems and multiple providers.

The trend in current healthcare delivery is in the direction of community-based care. **Community-based healthcare** is healthcare directed toward a specific group within the community. This group may be formed by an employer, a school district attendance area, a managed care insurance provider, geographic boundaries, and categoric or medical need. To understand community-based healthcare, it is wise to study the traditional care provided by the hospital and the transition it is undergoing.

Traditional Hospital-Based Delivery System

During the latter half of the 20th century, the hospital was an institution in which physicians admitted clients

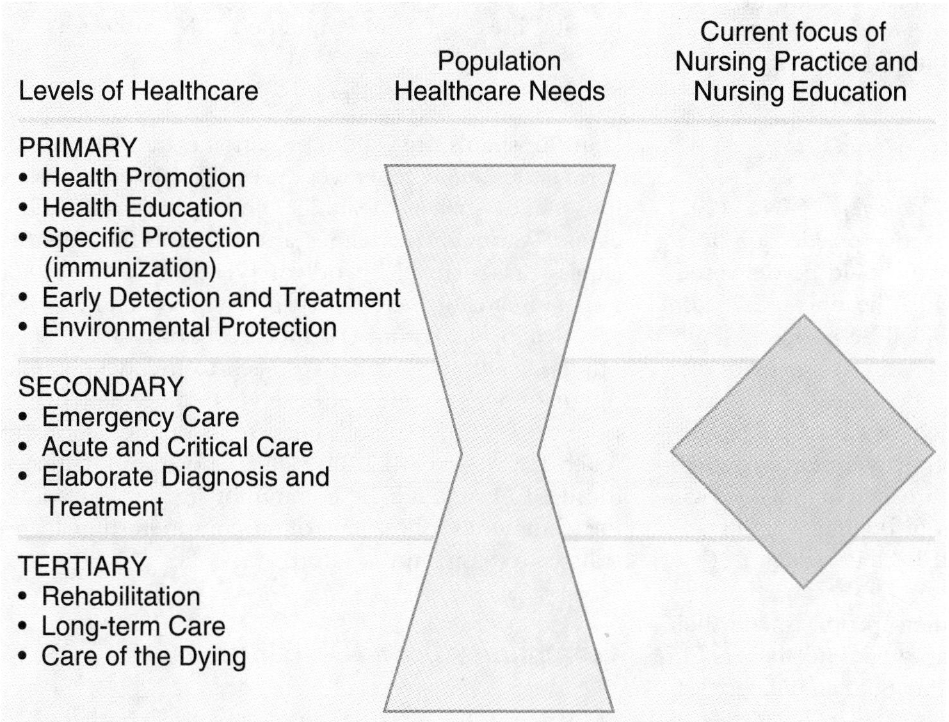

Figure 7-2 • *Levels of healthcare, with a comparison of population healthcare needs and the current focus of nursing practice and nursing education. (Developed by the Nursing Practice Branch, Division of Nursing of the Department of Health and Human Services.)*

in need of intense medical and nursing care or surgery and other highly technical procedures. It was not uncommon for a person to stay in the hospital for 7 to 10 days for uncomplicated conditions or surgery in the 1960s and 1970s. With the implementation of diagnostic related groupings, as explained in Chapter 6, hospital stays began to shorten.

Hospital Care in Transition

Because hospitals no longer receive payment for all services rendered and instead receive a set payment, it is financially advantageous for the hospital if clients have shorter stays. With additional efforts to contain rising medical costs, more care is being delivered outside of the "traditional" hospital. Care once considered safe only within the hospital is now routinely delivered in settings such as ambulatory surgical centers, dialysis centers, rehabilitation centers, and the home.

The healthcare approach is broadening from treatment of the acutely ill or injured individual to the general health of the community served by the hospital. Such concerns are reflected in changes of names. For instance, the national organization responsible for hospital accreditation has changed its name from the Joint Commission for the Accreditation of Hospitals to the Joint Commission for the Accreditation of Hospital Organizations. Other organizations are following suit. In such a move, the Arizona Hospital Association changed its name in 1995 to the Arizona Hospital and Healthcare Organization Association. These examples reflect a deeper philosophical and operational change in the nature of the way hospitals conduct business. The hospital of the future will be known as a healthcare organization or an integrated healthcare system, which already exists in many parts of the country.

Newer Community-Based Structures

Nursing's Agenda for Health Care Reform (ANA, 1991) is the nursing community's proactive position on how, where, and by whom healthcare should be delivered. It promotes an approach in which healthcare is taken to the consumer who, in turn, will be an increasingly informed participant in decisions affecting his or her care. Healthcare services will be delivered in such places as the place of employment or school-based clinics. Hospitals and other institutions will remain significant components of the healthcare system, but they will no longer be the central focus or dominant influence. That position will be assumed by the consumer (National League for Nursing, 1994).

Healthcare will increase where people spend their time—at home, in schools, at work, in shelters, in churches, in senior citizen gatherings, in ambulatory settings, in long-term care facilities, and in hospitals—in other words, in the community. Common to all programs will be the need for greater individual authority, accountability, and responsibility with a lesser reliability on institutional authority and policies (National League for Nursing, 1994). This type of care is emerging in various forms. Several are mentioned here; more are discussed in the section, "Community-Based Nursing."

Managed Care

Ellis and Hartley (1995, p. 301) define **managed care** as "any system in which the care of an individual from the time of contact with the healthcare system to discharge is carefully planned and monitored to ensure that standards are followed and costs are minimized." Managed care has been a favored model in the restructuring of healthcare delivery. In a managed care model, healthcare providers join to meet health needs across the continuum of care from health promotion and disease prevention to hospice care. The managed care model can include hospitals, physicians, nurse practitioners, physician assistants, and insurance carriers in a joint venture; it also can include the more traditional health maintenance organization. (Chapter 6 discussed the economics of healthcare services.) It is predicted that 90% of Americans will be in some type of managed care plan by the end of the century (Smith, 1993).

Seamless Care

Healthcare organizations (integrated healthcare systems) are developing systems of **seamless care**, in which all levels of care are available in an integrated form. Continuity of care facilitates recovery and positive health outcomes. Health promotion and disease prevention programs have long-term benefits when potentially harmful lifestyles can be modified (ANA, 1994).

Community Initiatives

Many hospitals are joining a national trend by sponsoring community initiatives. These initiatives have various names, such as "healthier communities" or "healthy cities." Although the names are different, the intent is similar. Based on the work of WHO (Tsouros, 1990), nurse-researcher Beverly Flynn (Flynn & Rains, 1993), the Healthcare Forum (Healthcare Forum, 1994), and others, healthy city initiatives seek to involve community members at a grass roots level to determine health priorities, set measurable goals, and define actions to reach these goals. If a hospital is not the initiator of these efforts and a local community agency is leading, the community's hospitals often contribute human resources to assist in the effort.

Community-Based Nursing

A change in healthcare delivery results in a change in delivery of nursing care. Nursing education is in the midst of making these changes and redirecting its emphasis. In the past, nurses were trained in caring for clients in hospitals; now their energies and knowledge must be redirected to providing care within the community. Nurses have a critical role to play in the evolving models of community-based care.

Community-based nursing can be defined as nursing care directed toward a specific group or population within the community and may be provided to individuals and groups. The level of care can be primary, secondary, or tertiary. In community-based nursing, the nurse has more authority, is accountable for his or her actions, and is responsible to the consumer rather than an institution. The emphasis is on a "flowing" kind of care that does not necessarily take place in one setting. Community-based nursing is the wave of future practice. It presents a special opportunity for nurses to practice their discipline, perhaps more fully than ever before.

Focus of Nursing Care

The site for nursing care and the type of intervention may change, but the focus is always the same. Wherever nursing is practiced, the nurse's concern is for the whole person (not only physiologic needs but psychosocial and spiritual needs as well) in relation to that person's environment.

In nursing practice in the hospital, physiologic stabilization is a primary goal for most clients. Needs may include physiologic monitoring, complete or partial personal care (from bowel and bladder care to bathing), exercise (from assistance with positioning to range of motion exercises, ambulating, and strengthening exercises), nutritional support (from feeding to administering total parenteral nutrition), pain management, treatment and medication administration, anticipatory guidance, counseling, and teaching. Care needs are complex, and because of the trend toward shorter lengths of stay, the client may be discharged before counseling and teaching can be completed.

In nursing practice in community-based settings following discharge from a hospital, activities change. If nursing care is directed toward an individual, as, for example, home healthcare, the physiologic crisis is past, although care needs may still be intense. Assessment of the home environment and involvement of family in direct care are essential. Planning and intervention center on restoring health to the maximum functioning possible, while continuing to monitor for possible side effects to treatment or complications of the person's condition.

If community-based nursing is directed toward a population, the needs of that population, as determined by epidemiologic and demographic data and input from the population itself, help to set priorities. For example, worksite healthcare services are individualized to the industry involved (factory versus white collar workers).

Nursing Research
Community-Based Nursing

Selected Nursing Research Studies

Burkhart, P. V. (1993). Health-perceptions of mothers of children with chronic conditions. *Maternal-Child Nursing Journal, 21*(4), 122–129.

Lamb, G. S., & Stempel, J. E. (1994). Nurse case management from the client's view: Growing as insider-expert. *Nursing Outlook, 42*(1), 7–13.

Neary, M. A. (1993). Community services in the 1990s: Are they meeting the needs of caregivers? *Journal of Community Health Nursing, 10*(2), 105–111.

Possible Topics for Nursing Inquiry

- What effect does the caregiver's perception of a family member's chronic disability have on their ability to cope with their family situation?
- How does understanding the client's point of view enhance the case management process?
- How can nurses help older clients and family caregivers access the community services they need?

Traditional Community-Based Nursing Practice in Transition

Traditional community-based settings for nursing practice include county and state health departments. The Institute of Medicine's report *The Future of Public Health* (1988) concludes that public health in the United States is in a state of disarray. Health departments attempting to carry out the traditional functions of public health (assessing community health status, ensuring health, and health policy development) have experienced funding reductions in recent years. National, state, and county departments of health continue to attempt to carry out their mission with limited resources. While public health nurses still conduct some home visits, nursing practice in health departments in many states focuses on contact with clients during clinic visits for maternity and child care, infectious diseases, and primary healthcare.

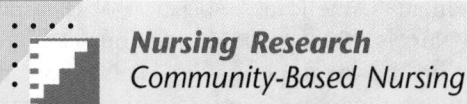

Other traditional community-based settings for nursing practice include schools (school nursing), the workplace (occupational health nursing), and homes (hospice and home healthcare nursing). School nurses focus their practice on the population of children attending their school. Health screening, health education, and first aid or acute care are some of the functions within school nursing practice. Occupational health nurses focus their practice on worker populations. "The practice focuses on promotion, protection and restoration of workers' health within the context of a safe and healthy work environment" (American Association of Occupational Health Nurses, 1994, p. 2). Hospice nurses focus their practice on the dying population. Palliative care within a multidisciplinary team and family support are included in hospice nursing practice. Home healthcare nurses focus their practice on populations in need of restorative care and health maintenance. Geographic boundaries often define the group with which they work. Practice is primarily with "individuals, in collaboration with the family and designated caregivers" (ANA, 1992, p. 3). Healthcare services provided in the home can range from dressing changes or insulin injections to intravenous antibiotics, dialysis, and teaching related to self-care and health promotion.

Newer Community-Based Nursing Settings

Community Nursing Centers

Newer forms of community-based nursing practice include community nursing centers, which may be located in schools, workplaces, or other sites within the community. Nurse-managed centers deliver primary healthcare to specific populations. Nurse practitioners and community health nurses staff these centers with physician backup and consultation as needed. The NLN defines a community nursing center as the following:

- A nurse occupies the chief management position.
- Accountability and responsibility for client care and professional practice remain with nursing staff.
- Nurses are the primary providers seen by clients visiting the center (Murphy, 1995, p. 3).

Nursing centers, however, are not only a site where clients visit. They also are a concept that shapes broader services offered by nurses in practice arrangements within the community (Sharp, 1992). "It must allow for an actual site for care but also support nurse-managed services to clients in their home, community, hospital, nursing home, or a site across the healthcare continuum" (Murphy, 1995, p. 3). A further description of types of centers is given in the accompanying display.

Categories of Community Nursing Centers

Community outreach: free-standing clinics similar to traditional community public health clinics

Institution based: derive their mission from a large parent organization, such as a hospital, university, or corporation

Wellness/health-promotion models: provide triage, screening, education, counseling, and health maintenance services

Independent practice nurses: faculty, nurse entrepreneurs

The first three categories are described in Riesch, S. K. (1992). Nursing centers: an analysis of the anecdotal literature. Journal of Professional Nursing, 8(1), 16–25. The fourth category is described in Aydelotte, M. K., Hardy, M. A., & Hope K.P. (1988). Nurses in private practice. Kansas City MO: American Nurses Association.

Employee Assistance Programs and Wellness Programs

Employee assistance programs (EAPs; Masi, 1992) and wellness programs represent additional settings for community-based nursing practice. EAPs historically have focused on assistance with behavioral health and substance abuse problems. Currently, EAPs are incorporating wellness programs into their services (Erfurt, Foote, & Heirich, 1992). Future EAP programs will likely integrate wellness strategies and programs with more traditional human services (Mermis & Matas, 1995). One example is the Arizona State University (ASU) EAP and Wellness Program. Community health graduate nursing students were involved in the program planning and development of a campus-wide coalition for 2 years (Fig. 7-3). The resulting program model and evaluation plan (Matas & Mermis, 1993; 1994) have strong support from the ASU community, that is administration, faculty, and staff. Nursing theory and practice form the core of the model (Fig. 7-4). The new program was implemented in September 1995.

Wellness programs can be found in a variety of settings and are often managed and staffed by nurses. These programs exist in integrated healthcare systems, such as the nursing network of the Carondelet system in Tucson (Lamb & Huggins, 1990), and as a component of healthy cities projects (Matas, 1994). In the Carondelet Healthcare System, the professional nursing network model extends beyond institutional boundaries to include community-based services. One of the important components of the nursing network has been the development of community health centers, which were established as an outreach program for the assessment and evaluation of health needs of older adults. An example of a nursing network model is illustrated in Figure 7-5.

Other wellness programs have been established in the workplace and schools. Nursing theory and current research literature on wellness programs (Pelletier, 1991; 1992) suggest that to be effective, a wellness program must be comprehensive and oriented to the whole person within the context of community and family needs.

Other Forms of Practice

Other emerging forms of community-based nursing practice include parish nursing, developing lay health

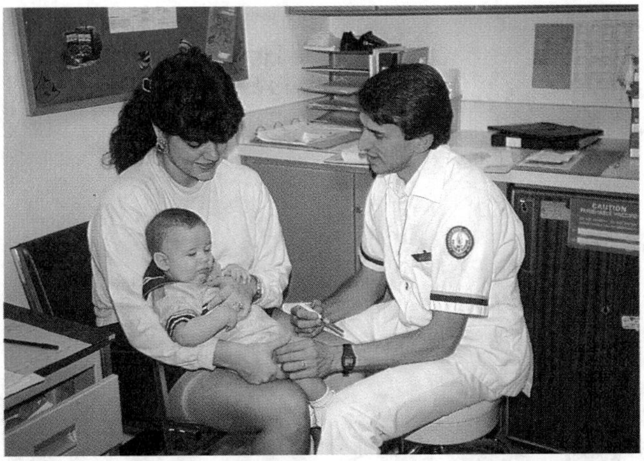

Figure 7-3 • A student nurse interviewing a woman with her infant at Community Health Services of Arizona State University, College of Nursing, Tempe, AZ.

worker networks (McFarlane, Kelly, Rodriguez, & Fehir, 1994), case management, independent nursing practice, and work with community coalitions, such as the healthy cities projects (Butterfoss, Goodman, & Wandersman, 1993). Nurses have been active in parish nursing in the Midwest for some time. Prior to that, they were common as public health nurses in rural and mountainous regions. Many churches have full-time nurses on their staff. Others work part time in consultation. Others plan health fairs for the parish. As the population ages, churches may find the addition of a nurse to the staff a help in meeting the needs of their senior citizens.

In some communities, lay health workers are the critical link between under served or high-risk populations and the formal healthcare system. Nurses have partnered with community members to identify, support, and provide training and consultation to lay health workers, who are members of the community and committed to assisting themselves and their neighbors through outreach networks. In this way, nurses can significantly impact eliminating barriers to healthcare, increase accessibility of needed services, and thus improve the health status of the community.

Case management involves healthcare provided through the direction of a case manager, usually a nurse. The case manager plans, coordinates, and tracks client care through a variety of settings, thus providing continuity of care. This type of care is useful when the client is high risk, and care is more complex. Nurses involved in case management are primary care nurses or skilled clinicians.

Some nurse practitioners work independently, setting up their own offices for consultation. Some state laws require that the independent nurse practitioner have some link with a medical backup. "Success depends on the possession of specific resources, such as adequate skills, finances, emotional support, and the desire to be one's own boss" (Calmelat, 1993).

"Community coalitions unite individuals and groups in a shared purpose" (Butterfoss, Goodman & Wandersman, 1994, p. 316). In recent years, many efforts have been focused on building community coalitions for the purpose of improving communities' health. These efforts usually take multifaceted approaches, such as developing gang prevention programs or substance abuse programs along with the more traditional public health approaches of health status assessment or assurance of health. Nurses are key participants and contributors in community coalitions and are well prepared to assume leadership positions.

One example of such an effort is the Building a Healthy Mesa project under the sponsorship of the Mesa United Way in Mesa, Arizona. Several faculty members, undergraduate community health nursing students, and graduate community health students contributed significantly to the work of the coalition. The undergraduate students conducted community assessments in several neighborhoods over the last 2 years. In a two-semester project, the graduate students worked in a neighborhood assessing, planning, implementing, and evaluating an immunization program for an ethnically diverse

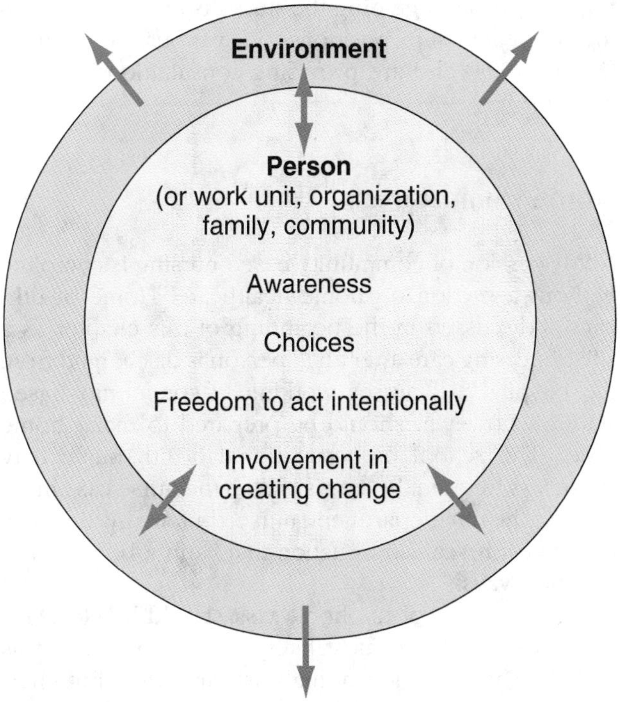

Figure 7-4 • The Arizona State University Well-Being Model is a model for the dynamic process of knowing participation in change. Well-being is defined as actualizing choices based on awareness of intentional action and involvement in a changing environment. Power is defined as the capacity to knowingly participate in change. Well-being enhances power of the individual, the organization, and the community within a continuous mutual process. It is based on Barrett's Power Theory (1983). (© K. Matas, 1994.)

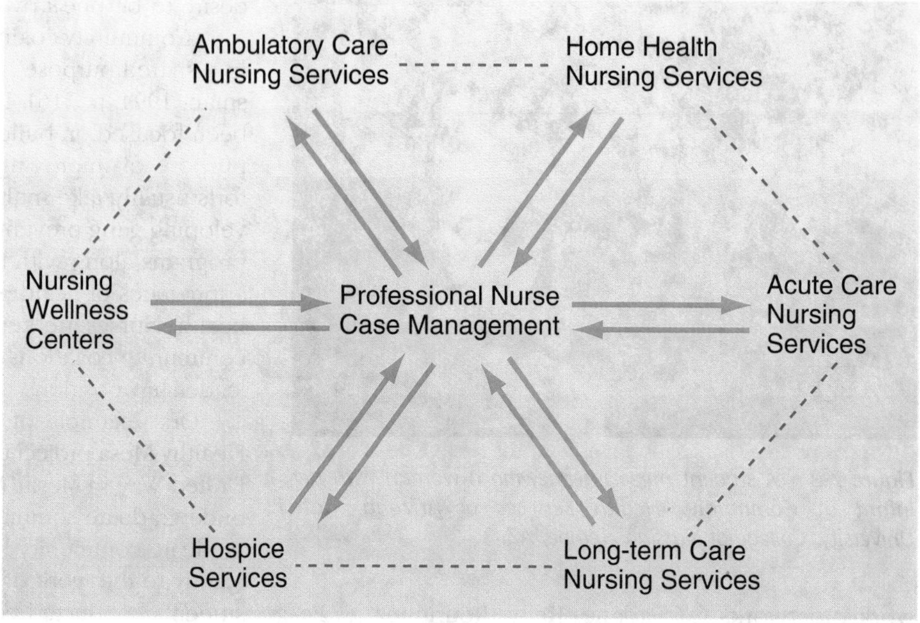

Figure 7-5 • *Carondelet St. Mary's professional nursing network model. (Lamb and Huggins, 1990.)*

and economically vulnerable high-risk group, which included developing a lay health worker outreach program. Funding has now been received from the City of Mesa to develop a community resource center in one of the neighborhood schools. Faculty have contributed, not only through guiding the students but also by serving in leadership positions on various committees (Matas, 1994) and are providing consultation for grant writing.

Home Healthcare

No discussion of community-based nursing is complete without a section on home healthcare. Home healthcare is discussed in the beginning of this chapter as a site of nursing care after an ill person is discharged from the hospital. All nurses working in community-based settings, however, should be prepared to make home visits. The school or occupational health nurse may make less frequent home visits than the nurse case manager or health department nurse, but many times, a home visit reveals information that cannot be gathered in other ways.

The *purpose* of the home visit should be clear. Individuals at risk are most likely to be in need of this service. The definition of high risk may vary, but characteristics such as no health insurance, single parent, chronic health problems, and low socioeconomic status are indicators. Focusing on the whole person within his or her environment, the home visit may help the nurse determine optimal interventions. For example, a single parent may have a high absenteeism rate because of inadequate child care for sick children. The home healthcare nurse may be able to make referrals for child care or find medical help for chronically ill children and support groups for the single parent.

The nurse in the home can observe family interaction patterns and nonverbal behaviors (Fig. 7-6). Cues may become apparent in family photos or heirlooms. The nurse observes the general state of the home and yard or neighborhood (ie, state of repair, clutter, cleanliness).

The home healthcare nurse evaluates the need for additional home visits and jointly plans with the client or family the form that follow-up may take. If it is agreed that additional home visits are needed, a date and time are set, and a plan of care is drawn up for what is to be accomplished. Following through will help to build a therapeutic relationship. Home visits are discussed further in Chapter 31.

Competencies Needed for Community-Based Nursing Care

Nurses play a critical role in the evolving models of community-based care. As mentioned previously in this section, educational programs are restructuring to prepare nurses for professional practice in the community.

The Pew Health Professions Commission (1991) issued a report entitled *Healthy America: Practitioners for 2005.* The Commission's "agenda for action" identifies 17 competencies that future health professionals must possess. These competencies, which are listed in the accompanying display, emphasize community and public health principles and call for nurses to have highly developed skills in the areas of accessible, cost-effective healthcare; integrated healthcare systems; information management; interdisciplinary team work; promoting consumer self-responsibility and cultural diversity; and others.

Nursing practice in community-based integrated healthcare systems will require basic competencies in

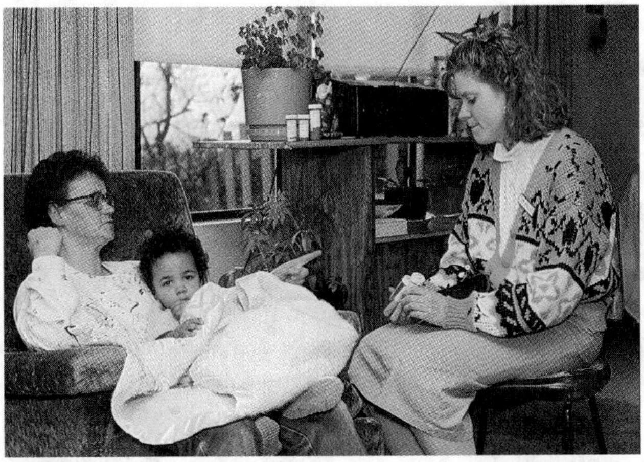

Figure 7-6 • *The nurse who visits in the home can observe family interactions and verbal and nonverbal behaviors. (Courtesy of Yesler Terrace.)*

community health nursing, including primary, secondary, and tertiary prevention; community health assessment; knowledge and use of epidemiologic principles; community planning and coalition building; population health interventions (such as screening and educational programs); case management; and evaluating outcomes of community- or population-focused care (Association of Community Health Nurse Educators, 1990).

Familiarity with current major national and state documents concerning health is critical to community-based nursing practice. An example of a national document is *Healthy People 2000: National Health Promotion and Disease Prevention Objectives* (U.S. Department of Health and Human Services, 1990). An example of a state document is *Arizona 2000: Plan for a Healthy Tomorrow* (Arizona Department of Health Services, 1993). At the national and state level, both of these documents identify health priorities for communities and at-risk groups. Goals for *Healthy People 2000* are:

- Increase the span of healthy life for Americans
- Reduce health disparities among Americans
- Achieve access to preventive services for all Americans

Other important recent documents providing direction for the future of community-based healthcare include the Pew Health Professions Commission report (1991), the Institute of Medicine's report on *The Future of Public Health* (1988), and *Nursing's Agenda for Healthcare Reform* (ANA, 1991).

Continuity of Care and Entrance and Exit Within the System

Continuity of care is the provision of health services without disruption, regardless of the client's movement between settings. Continuity of care has been highlighted in provision of healthcare across the continuum. All models of community-based nursing address it. There has to be an organizational structure in place to ensure continuity of care from one healthcare setting to another and between and among professionals.

Admission to the Healthcare System

The client's admission into the healthcare system generally is filled with some apprehension. Clients may fear the unknown, or they may be afraid of becoming dependent and losing control over themselves or their decisions by placing themselves in the care of healthcare professionals. Because the admission process is so significant to the client's well-being, the nurse's confidence and competence can exert a lasting influence on the course of care. To lessen fear or anxiety over loss of personal control, the nurse can assist the client by:

- Establishing rapport and a willingness to listen
- Clearly defining the purpose and expectations of this admission
- Aiding the client in understanding how to participate as fully as possible in care-related decisions
- Clarifying the nursing role in relation to the client's healthcare needs
- Documenting the procedure

Chapter 20 discusses how to communicate effectively with the client.

Whether it is a short visit in an emergency room or a longer stay in another type of healthcare facility, the client receives an identification bracelet. The bracelet is provided at the admissions desk at the same time required paperwork (admissions questions, insurance coverage, consents, and other forms) is completed. The identification bracelet contains the client's name, healthcare provider's name, unit and room number, and, possibly, allergies. For the client's safety, the identification bracelet must be checked before any diagnostic test, medication, or other treatment is carried out.

When the client is escorted to the unit or room, the nurse welcomes the client and addresses the client by name, introduces herself or himself, and gives full attention to the client. While this may be a routine admission to the nurse, no admission into a healthcare setting is routine for a client. Conveying empathy and concern will help put the client at ease. Cultural and spiritual needs among clients must be considered at the time of admission, eg, the need for an interpreter, awareness of what this admission means culturally, or respect for spiritual beliefs. Chapters 18 and 53 provide more in-depth discussion on these subjects.

Whether the client is admitted to a unit within an emergency or outpatient setting, a hospital, or a long-term care room, the client and family need to know the following:

- How to access assistance (call bell signal, tele-

*Pew Commission Competencies for Practitioners**

1. *Care for the community health.* Practitioners should have a broad understanding of the determinants of health, such as the environment, socioeconomic conditions, behavior, medical care, and genetics, and be able to work with others in the community to integrate a range of services and activities that promote, protect and improve health.
2. *Expand access to effective care.* Practitioners should participate in efforts to ensure access to healthcare for individuals, families, and communities and to improve the public's health
3. *Provide contemporary clinical care.* Practitioners should possess up-to-date clinical skills to meet the public's healthcare needs.
4. *Emphasize primary care.* Practitioners should be willing and able to function in new healthcare settings and interdisciplinary team arrangements designed to meet the primary healthcare needs of the public.
5. *Participate in coordinated care.* Practitioners should be able to work effectively as team members in organized settings and emphasize high-quality, cost-effective integrated services.
6. *Ensure cost-effective and appropriate care.* Practitioners should incorporate and balance cost and quality in the decision-making process.
7. *Practice prevention.* Practitioners should emphasize primary and secondary preventive strategies for all people.
8. *Involve clients and families in the decision-making process.* Practitioners should expect patients and their families to participate actively in decisions regarding their personal healthcare and in evaluating its quality and acceptability.
9. *Promote healthy lifestyles.* Practitioners should help individuals, families, and communities maintain and promote health behavior.
10. *Assess and use technology appropriately.* Practitioners should understand and use appropriately increasingly complex an often costly technology.
11. *Improve the healthcare system.* Practitioners should understand the determinates and operations of the healthcare system from a broad political, economic, social, and legal perspective to improve continuously the operations and accountability of that system.
12. *Manage information.* Practitioners should manage and use large volumes of scientific, technologic, and client information.
13. *Understand the role of the physical environment.* Practitioners should assess, prevent, and mitigate the impact of environmental hazards on the health of the population.
14. *Provide counseling on ethical issues.* Practitioners should provide counseling for clients when ethical issues arise and should participate in discussion of ethical issues in healthcare as they affect communities, society, and the health professions.
15. *Accommodate expanded accountability.* Practitioners should be responsive to increasing levels of public, governmental, and third-party participation in, and scrutiny of, the shape and direction of the healthcare system.
16. *Participate in a racially and culturally diverse society.* Practitioners should appreciate the growing diversity of the population and the need to understand health status and healthcare needs through differing cultural values.
17. *Continue to learn.* Practitioners should anticipate changes in healthcare and respond to redefining and maintaining professional competency throughout practice life.

Adapted from deTornyay, R. (1992). Reconsidering nursing education: The report of the Pew Health Profession Commission. *Journal of Nursing Education, 31*(7), 296-301.
*Although these competencies apply to all healthcare professionals, the term "nurse" can be substituted in place of the term "practitioners" in the above statements.

phone number, or other electronic alerting)
- What the physical environment and healthcare arrangements are (unit or room arrangement)
- Basic care equipment
- Frequency of contact with care provider

Table 7-1 lists possible admission procedures performed by the nurse at admission.

When clients are admitted to a setting other than their own home, the nurse needs to orient them to the organization of the facility, the caregiving supplies in the unit, and safety equipment in the unit and facility. Orientation to the client unit for maximizing safety is discussed in Chapter 29. Teaching the client and family about the safe operation of the bed, use of side rails, the overbed table, and the lighting system and controls gives them control of some aspects of their care and makes the client unit less intimidating.

The nurse supports the family by familiarizing them with the location of waiting rooms, restrooms, public telephones, the nurses' station or desk, and other areas. This information helps to ease the sense of anxiety. It gives them an opportunity to call other family members or a spiritual leader.

Client units also have other equipment for use in caregiving, such as the sphygmomanometer, outlets for oxygen and suction, and the personal care materials in the bedside stand, such as bath basin, bedpan or urinal, emesis basin, and personal articles like soap, tooth paste and toothbrush, and extra linen. Explaining the location and purpose of equipment increases the comfort level of the client and family. If the client is expected to stay overnight in a unit, generally there is a telephone and television or radio.

The nurse takes complete admission information. The slant will depend on the setting. In the emergency department a focused admission is done, ie, focusing on the purpose of this current visit, symptoms, and information pertaining to the current problem. For hospital admission a more in-depth admission form is completed. In some hospitals this form runs to 12 pages. Again it focuses on the current problem but contains other aspects of the client and his or her lifestyle. In a community-related facility, or if the client's condition is not life-threatening, an even more-detailed admission assessment may be made. This would include multi problems and information about the family or the client's environment. A sample admission form based on functional health is given in Figure 21-1, where focused and comprehensive health assessments are discussed.

During the assessment phase, the nurse can help the client understand how the client can participate in decisions and planning. For instance, the nurse may say, "After the physical examination your physician will talk to you in his office."

Leaving the client alone in the room without any information increases anxiety level. The nurse gives as much information as he or she knows or is permitted to give. For example, the nurse may say, "Your physician expects to come in before lunch," "Some techicians will be here shortly to take an x-ray and take some blood for tests," or "I will bring you a pill for the pain as soon as I get permission from your physician."

Discharge Within the System

Discharge planning is the process of coordinating, planning, and arranging for the transition from one healthcare setting to another. The discharge planner is the healthcare professional who coordinates these services. Discharge planning has long been associated with discharge from the hospital, but in the current healthcare scene, discharge planning can occur from any healthcare system, including home healthcare. (Continuity of care and discharge planning are discussed in more detail in Chapter 31.) The discharge planner must

Table 7-1 • Overview of Admission to Various Healthcare Facilities

Facility	*Possible Admission Procedures*
Hospital	Introduction; orientation to room and equipment; complete nursing history, vital signs, and other physical assessment
Emergency room	Introduction; ABCs (airway, breathing, and circulation); vital signs; focused assessment for acute problems; orientation to surroundings
Clinic or physician's office	Introduction; explore reason for seeking medical care and focused assessment of that problem; vital signs
Nursing home	Introduction; review of written or verbal report from transferring agency; nursing history and assessment focusing on functional abilities, orientation to new surroundings
Hospice	Introduction; review of referral; nursing history and assessment focusing on pain control, functional abilities, coping, and support; wishes concerning terminal care and death (eg, living will); orientation to procedures and care
Psychiatric facility	Introduction; mental health evaluation, including history, mood state, suicide risk, use of drugs, support system
Home visit	Introduction; review of referral and client's medical and nursing problems, home environment, caretaker and family support, community resources

be familiar with physiologic processes, the illness and its treatment, and community resources and support groups. Communication and skills in documentation also are necessary for competent discharge planning.

The discharge planning role of the hospital nurse has become more important than ever in the reality of the rapidly changing healthcare system. Some clients are discharged to their homes directly from intensive care units. Most are discharged at a higher acuity level than was found several years ago.

Working in an integrated healthcare system will require attention to continuity of care and discharge planning across multiple settings: from hospital to extended nursing care or rehabilitation facility to home to possibly hospice or self-care or family care.

Discharge from a community-based healthcare setting needs the same, or possibly greater, level of attention than from acute care facilities. Discharge from home healthcare, for example, requires that the nurse be familiar with community resources that families can access for continuing needs. This includes home-delivered meals, transportation, and personal care. For an occupational health nurse, continuity of care may mean referring a worker to appropriate community mental health systems and evaluating treatment effectiveness in follow-up. For a school nurse, continuity of care may mean child advocacy and family referral to child protective services.

Key Concepts

- At the root of healthcare reform is how to deliver cost-effective and quality healthcare that will be accessible to everyone and will result in positive health outcomes.
- Levels of healthcare are categorized as primary, secondary, and tertiary. The majority of current resources and services are in secondary healthcare, while the needs of the population lie within the categories of primary and tertiary healthcare.
- Care once considered safe only within the hospital is now routinely delivered in community-based settings.
- Common to all community-based programs will be the need for greater individual authority, accountability, responsibility, and allegiance to the client, with less reliability on institutional authority and policies.
- Although the site and circumstances of nursing care may change, the focus remains the same: the nurse's concern for the whole person in relation to that person's environment.
- Community nursing centers deliver primary healthcare to a specific population, are managed and staffed by nurses, and have physician backup and consultation as needed.
- An organizational structure must be in place to ensure continuity of care from one healthcare setting to another and between and among professionals. This occurs through discharge planning.

Critical Thinking Challenges

Now that you have added the concepts of continuity of care and community-based nursing to your knowledge base of the healthcare delivery system and professional nursing, review the description of the nurse case manager's day at the beginning of the chapter. Consider the following, and be creative in your thinking.

1. *Describe what it would be like to work in an integrated healthcare system.*
2. *Explain the importance of continuity of care and discharge planning in the emerging healthcare system.*
3. *Propose how various healthcare professionals will work with nurses in the community.*
4. *Predict the opportunities for the nursing profession within the changing healthcare system.*
5. *Calculate what will happen to hospitals in the future.*

References

American Association of Occupational Health Nurses (1994). *Standards of occupational health nursing practice.* Atlanta: Author.

American Nurses Association (1991). *Nursing's agenda for health care reform.* Kansas City, MO: Author.

American Nurses Association (1992). *Nursing case management.* Kansas City, MO: Author.

American Nurses Association (1992). *A statement on the scope of home health nursing practice.* Washington, DC: Author.

American Nurses Association (1994). *Clinician's handbook of preventive services.* Waldorf, MD: American Nurses Publishing.

Arizona Department of Health Services (1993). *Arizona 2000: Plan for a healthy tomorrow.* Phoenix: Author.

Association of Community Health Nurse Educators (1990). *Essentials of baccalaureate nursing education for entry level practice in community health nursing.* Louisville, KY: Author.

Butterfoss, F. D., Goodman, R. M., & Wandersman, A. (1993). Community coalitions for prevention and health promotion. *Health Education Research, 8*(3), 315–330.

Calmelat, A. (1993). Tips for starting your own nurse practitioner practice. *Nurse Practitioner, 18*(4), 58.

Eisenberg, D. N., Kessler, R. C., Foster, C., Norlock, F. E., Calkins, D. R., & Delbono, T. L. (1993). Unconventional medicine in the United States. *New England Journal of Medicine, 328*(4), 246–252.

Ellis, J. R., & Hartley, C. L. (1995). *Nursing in today's world: Challenges, issues, and trends* (5th ed.). Philadelphia: J. B. Lippincott.

Erfurt, F. C., Foote, A., & Heinrich, M. A. (1992). Integrating employee assistance and wellness: Current and future core technologies of a megabrush program. *Journal of Employee Assistance Research, 1*(1), 1–31.

Executive Wire. (1992). *Trends to watch for in '92: Health highest on American agenda*. New York: National League for Nursing.

Flynn B. C., & Rains, J. W. (1993). Establishing community coalitions for prevention: Healthy cities Indiana. In R. N. Knollmueller (Ed.), *Prevention across the lifespan*. Washington, DC: American Nurses Publishing.

Gruman, F. (1995). An expanded view of health: implications for how healthcare works. *Healing, 3*(2), 23–26.

Healthcare Forum (1994). *What creates health?* San Francisco: Author.

Institute of Medicine. (1988). *The future of public health*. Washington, DC: National Academy Press.

Laffrey, S. (1994). Guest editorial: Primary care or primary health care: Which model will we choose for community health nursing? *Association of Community Health Nurse Educators Newsletter, 12*(11), 6.

Lamb, G., & Huggins, D. (1990). The professional nursing network. In G. M. Mayer, M. J. Madden, & E. Lowrenz (Eds.), *Patient care delivery models*. Rockville, MD: Aspen.

Masi, D. (Ed.) (1992). *Handbook for developing employee assistance and counseling programs*. New York: American Management Association.

Matas, K. E. (1994). *Health theme team framework: Building a healthy mesa*. (Unpublished manuscript.) Mesa, AZ: United Way.

Matas, K. E., & Mermis, W. L. (1993). *Campus wellness project*. Report submitted to the Department of Human Resources, Tempe, AZ: Arizona State University.

Matas, K. E., & Mermis, W. L. (1994). *Campus wellness project: Year 2*. Report submitted to the Department of Human Resources, Tempe, AZ: Arizona State University.

McFarlane, J., Kelly, E., Rodriguez, R., & Fehir, J. (1994). De madres a madres: Women building community coalitions for health. *Health Care for Women International, 15*(5), 465–476.

Mermis, W. L., & Matas, K. E. (1995). EAPs and wellness: A partnership for health (Unpublished Manuscript). Tempe, AZ: Arizona State University.

Murphy, B. (Ed.) (1995). *Nursing centers: The time is now*. New York: National League for Nursing Press.

National League for Nursing. (1994). *A vision for nursing education*. New York: Author.

Pelletier, K. R. (1991). A review and analysis of the health and cost-effective outcome studies of comprehensive health promotion and disease prevention programs. *American Journal of Health Promotion, 5*(4), 311–315.

Pelletier, K. R. (1993). A review and analysis of the health and cost-effective outcome studies of comprehensive health promotion and disease prevention programs at the worksite: 1991–1993. *American Journal of Health Promotion, 8*(1), 50–62.

Pew Health Professions Commission (1991). *Healthy America: Practitioners for 2005*. Durham, NC: Author.

Sharp, N. (1992). Community nursing centers: Coming of age. *Nursing Management, 23*(8), 18–20.

Smith, L. (1993). The coming health care shakeout. *Fortune, 127*(10), 70–75.

Tsouros, A. O. (1990). *World Health organization healthy cities project: A project becomes a movement*. Copenhagen: FADL Publishers.

U.S. Department of Health and Human Services (1990). *Healthy people 2000: National health promotion and disease prevention objectives*. Washington, DC: U.S. Government Printing Office. DHHS Pub. #(PHS)91–50212.

World Health Organization (1978). *Primary health care: Report of the international conference on primary health care*. Geneva, Switzerland: Author.

Bibliography

Allen, S. A. (1994). Medicare case management. *Home Healthcare Nurse, 12*(3), 21–27.

Burge, B. J. (1994). Occupational health: Nursing in the workplace. *Nursing Clinics of North America, 29*(3), 431–441.

Burgel, C. J. (1993). *Innovation at the work site*. Washington DC: American Nurses Publishing.

deTornyay, R. (1992). Reconsidering nursing education: The report of the Pew Health Profession Commission. *Journal of Nursing Education, 31*(7), 296–301.

Elliott, B. (1993). *Vision 2010: Families and health care*. Minneapolis: National Council on Family Relations.

Flarey, D. L. (1995). Redesigning nursing care delivery: Transforming our future. Philadelphia: J.B. Lippincott.

Pollock, A. J., & Biester, D. J. (1994) Community nursing center: An approach to caring for the underserved. *Journal of Pediatric Nursing, 9*(5), 333–334.

Rogers, B. (1994). *Occupational health nursing: Concepts and practice*. Philadelphia: W.B. Saunders.

Swanson, J. M., & Albrecht, M. (1993). *Community health nursing: Promoting the health of aggregates*. Philadelphia: W.B. Saunders.

The Nursing Process: Framework for Clinical Nursing Therapeutics

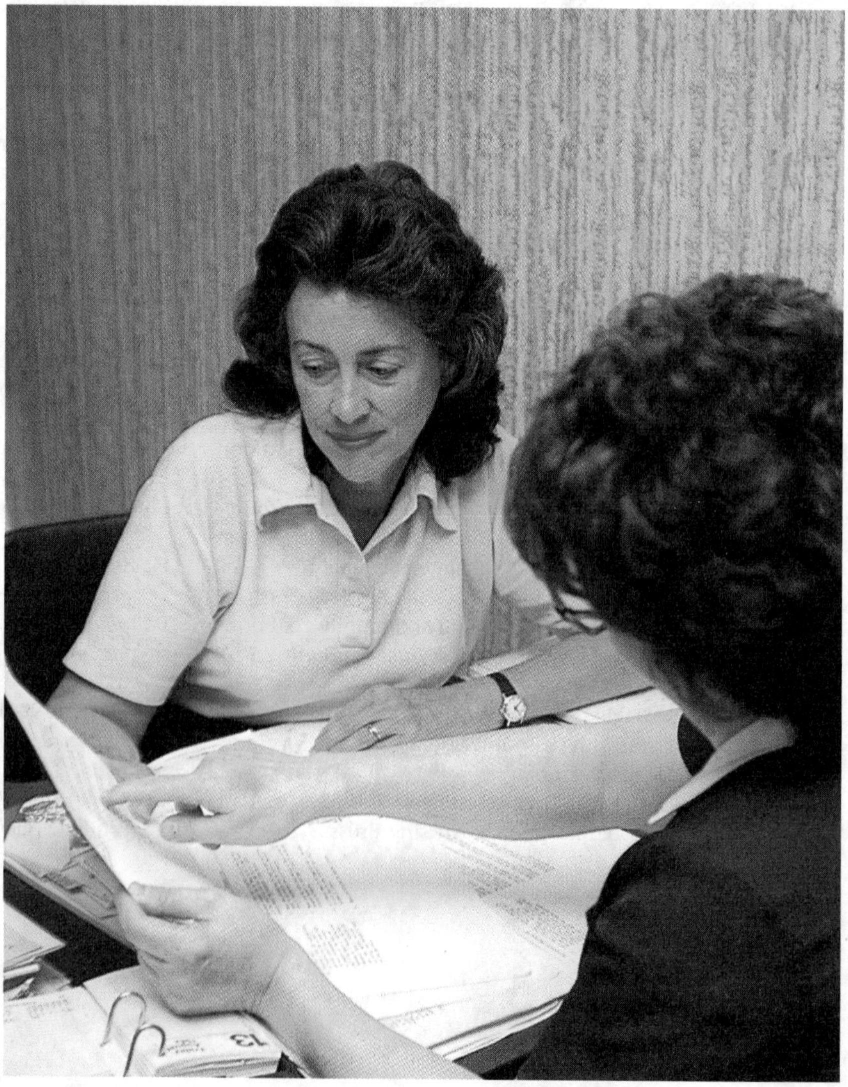

UNIT III

The nursing process is a systematic method of providing holistic, individualized nursing care that is goal directed and client centered. Unit III discusses the five phases of the nursing process in detail. This discussion provides a solid grounding in the essential concepts.

Critical thinking, integral in using the nursing process, is launched in Chapter 8. The relevance of critical thinking to nursing and the nursing process is introduced, along with strategies and skills. The reader is led through means of developing critical thinking skills. Chapter 9 provides an overview of the nursing process, describing historical development of the nursing process, components and their relationships, theoretical foundations, and skill requirements. The nursing process takes a cyclical rather than linear approach, allowing the nurse to use knowledge, experience, and skills to help clients maintain, support, and restore health and function. The next four chapters in the unit explore the skills and activities needed to assess a client's health status, to analyze and cluster data to formulate a nursing diagnosis, to identify desired outcomes and their criteria, to prepare a plan of care and select nursing interventions based on mutually decided client goals, and to evaluate the effectiveness of those interventions using outcome criteria. A final chapter discusses the variety of methods for recording and reporting—communicating the nursing process.

The nursing process underlies nursing actions. This unit provides the framework for the application of the nursing process throughout the clinical nursing care chapters of the text.

Critical Thinking

Key Terms	Learning Objectives
Acronym *Critical thinking* *Dualism* *Inquiry* *Metacognition* *Mnemonic* *Relativism* *Self-Efficacy* *Thinking*	*Upon completion of this chapter, the student will be able to do the following:* • *Recognize the importance of critical thinking in nursing.* • *Discuss definitions, characteristics of, and skills in critical thinking.* • *Identify various physical and emotional factors that affect thinking.* • *Appreciate existing personal thinking skills.* • *Explore ways to enhance and develop critical thinking skills, especially as applied to nursing.* • *Set personal goals for thinking skill development.*

8

You are a nursing student beginning your first quarter of clinical nursing. You carry a heavy load this semester: you are taking five courses, including the dreaded Pathophysiology. You have three children younger than 12 years of age, and a spouse who is beginning to feel less positive about your return to school. This week will be your first week at the hospital taking care of a real client. You get your assignment and find you will be caring for an older gentleman who fractured his hip yesterday. Your client has 5 other medical problems and takes 10 medications. At this point, you feel overwhelmed and unsure that you are ready for this experience.

Most students can identify with this scenario. Although some details may be different, the average beginning student worries about being capable of handling clinical situations with a limited knowledge base and no experience. Every chapter you have studied in this text so far has built your knowledge base in nursing. The other courses you are taking and your life experiences are also components of your knowledge base. Other chapters later in this text will help you build a solid base of knowledge about therapeutics and clinical practice. In this chapter, you will learn how critical thinking will help you in your personal life and in your nursing career. The Critical Thinking Challenges at the end of the chapter will assist you in evaluating your thinking as well as practicing further critical thinking.

Thinking is a skill each human being practices in his or her own way (Fig. 8-1). Each person, for instance, thinks about what to wear in the morning and how to organize the day's activities. Thinking is so automatic that we do not pay much attention to how we think. On the other hand, thinking is a complex process. Because thinking is so abstract and individualized, it is a challenging subject for beginning nursing students.

Beginning students may believe that "nurse-thinking" is a totally new skill to learn. Approached as a new skill, critical thinking would appear overwhelming, but this would ignore the students' *existing* thinking

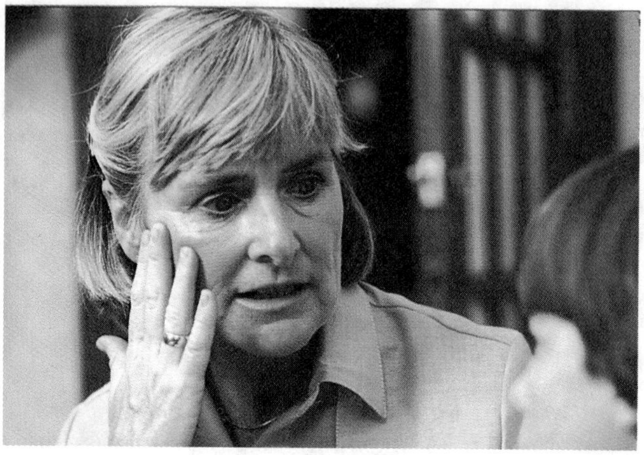

Figure 8-1 • Thinking is a human skill. Nursing is a complex human skill. Student nurses build on their previous ability to think in order to complement the other nursing skills they learn.

skills. Indeed, it would be a waste of time and energy if the student did not build on existing skills. Many experts in education believe the best way to learn is through the "assimilative approach," linking new knowledge to existing knowledge. This chapter builds on that premise.

Reading one chapter or even one book on thinking will not make the reader a great thinker, but it should provide a stimulus for thinking about thinking. This chapter focuses on what thinking is. An overview provides definitions, discusses the conceptual development and characteristics of critical thinking, and uses one model of critical thinking as an example of the application of critical thinking to nursing. The student is given an opportunity to evaluate his or her own personal thinking strategies, to select a framework for thinking, and to develop further critical thinking skills.

Importance of Critical Thinking in Nursing

As you will learn in this chapter, critical thinking helps the nurse find options for solving client care problems. Both the nurse and the client need to be effective thinkers so together they can identify problems accurately and set realistic outcomes. Using critical thinking, they plan, implement, and evaluate high-quality care. In some cases the nurse will be required to help the client or family develop thinking skills for their own use in the home.

There is an enormous amount of information in healthcare, and it changes continually. Simple memorization-style thinking cannot keep up with the nurse's task of sorting, organizing, and identifying relevant information so that it can be used in the most effective and efficient ways. Critical thinking helps the nurse choose solutions in client care situations or identify options from which to choose. The growing complexity of healthcare demands the use of critical thinking for effective, creative, and efficient nursing care.

Nurses are required to think critically in all client interactions, for example in the home, in ambulatory

Table 8-1 • *Thinking Strategies*

Strategy	Advantages	Disadvantages
Problem-solving process 1. Recognize existence of problem 2. Collect data 3. Analyze data; specify problem 4. Determine ways to achieve solution of problem 5. Execute the planned actions 6. Judge the effectiveness of selected actions	Logical, methodical, Socratic approach	Very linear; does not consider affective domain, creativity, or context of situation
Decision making 1. Define the goal 2. Identify alternatives 3. Analyze alternatives 4. Rank alternatives 5. Judge highest-ranked alternatives	Logical, methodical, Socratic approach	Very linear; does not consider affective domain, creativity, or context of situation
Critical thinking • Metacognition • Contextual description of problem issue • Divergent/convergent focus • Take action and assess outcomes	Reflective condition and culturally focused; creativity required	Requires flexibility and tolerance for ambiguity

Selected Definitions of Critical Thinking

Matthews and Gaul (1979)
Critical thinking is "an attitude of inquiry which involves the use of facts, principles, theories, abstractions, deductions, interpretations and evaluation of arguments."

Ennis (1985)
Critical thinking is "reflective and reasonable thinking that is focused on deciding what to believe or do."

Bandman and Bandman (1988)
Critical thinking is "the rational explanation of ideas, inferences, assumptions, principles, arguments, conclusions, issues, statements, beliefs, and actions."

Facione (1990)
"We understand critical thinking to be purposeful, self-regulatory judgement which results in interpretation, analysis, evaluation, and inference as well as explanation . . . upon which judgement is based. Critical thinking is essential as a tool of inquiry. . . . Critical thinking is a pervasive and self-rectifying human phenomenon. . . ."

Paul (1992)
Critical thinking is "the art of thinking about your thinking while you are thinking in order to make your thinking better: more clear, more accurate, or more defensible."

Rubenfeld and Scheffer (1995)
Critical thinking is a "blend of five modes of thinking: Total Recall, Habits, Inquiry, New Ideas and Creativity, and Knowing How You Think."

care, in the critical care unit, or in some form of disaster relief. The focus of nursing care as it enters the 21st century will be on individuals, families, communities, and the world. The nurse's ability to think critically will be one of his or her most important skills.

Thinking About Thinking

Dictionaries describe **thinking** as a mental activity in which one forms thoughts in the mind, forms intentions, determines by reflection, or attains clear ideas. "Inference," "facts," "beliefs," "opinions," "judgment," "logical," "rational," and other terms are used when people discuss thinking. Descriptions of these are beyond the scope of this chapter; some of these terms, however, are discussed further in Chapter 46.

Critical is defined as a turning point or especially important juncture. It is the point at which a definite change is made. *Critical thinking*, then, assumes a turning point because of a thought process. Definitions of critical thinking are given later in this chapter in the section on Conceptual Development of Critical Thinking.

Thinking Strategies

"Problem-solving," "decision-making," and "critical thinking," common terms used in the nursing profession, are major thinking strategies or processes. Table 8-1 compares these processes. Similarities among them become evident when they are studied, and each has advantages and disadvantages.

In the next chapter, the nursing process is presented. It is a means of practicing nursing care through problem-solving and critical thinking. Critical thinking is essential in each of the phases of the nursing process. A new approach, critical thinking (Scheffer & Rubenfeld), looks at thinking as not just a series of linear steps but as a contextual creative process.

Conceptual Development of Critical Thinking

The term "critical thinking" is not new. It has been prominent in the general educational literature since the early 1980s. Originally it was called "higher-order thinking skills." The initial emphasis was on students in elementary school, middle school, and high school. Costa (1985) compiled a book of several papers describing the key role of critical thinking in education as well as how to teach critical thinking. Costa and contributors (1985) proposed a system of critical thinking using the six Rs: remembering, repeating, reasoning, reorganizing, relating, and reflecting.

There is no one definition of critical thinking. Definitions vary, as do the systems or models for critical thinking. Ennis (1985) described critical thinking as "reflective and reasonable thinking that is focused on deciding what to believe or do" (p. 45). He continued by emphasizing that critical thinking requires the ability to see clearly, make inferences, support inferences, and achieve orderly and effective decision-making.

Paul, the founder of the Foundation for Critical Thinking, offered several definitions for critical thinking, one of which is, "critical thinking is the art of thinking about your thinking while you are thinking in order to make your thinking better: more clear, more accurate, or more defensible" (1992, p. 643). Part of what he described was **metacognition**, or thinking about thinking. In another definition, Paul (1993) states, "Critical thinking is the intellectually disciplined process of actively and skillfully conceptualizing, applying, analyzing, synthesizing, or evaluating information gathered from, or generated by, observation, experience, reflection, reasoning, or communication, as a guide to belief and action" (p. 110).

The most comprehensive attempt to define critical thinking in general was made by Facione (1990). Using the Delphi method, he surveyed 46 experts from all over the United States, from the disciplines of philosophy, education, social science, and physical science. The consensus statement from this survey addressed both critical thinking and the ideal critical thinker.

> We understand critical thinking to be purposeful, self-regulatory judgment which results in interpretation, analysis, evaluation, and inference as well as explanation . . . upon which judgement is based. Critical thinking is essential as a tool of inquiry. . . . Critical thinking is a pervasive and self-rectifying human phenomenon (p. 2).

Nursing and Critical Thinking

Critical thinking has always been an integral part of nursing, even if it was not always labeled as such. Yura and Walsh (1973) were two of the first nursing authors to emphasize "intellectual skills" as an essential component of nursing through the use of the nursing process.

Matthews and Gaul (1979) wrote of the relationship between critical thinking and diagnostic reasoning. They defined critical thinking as "an attitude of inquiry which involves the use of facts, principles, theories, abstractions, deductions, interpretations and evaluation of arguments" (p. 19).

In 1988, Bandman and Bandman wrote a book to help nurses examine the role of scientific reasoning, logic, and philosophy in improving thinking in nursing. They defined critical thinking in nursing as "the rational explanation of ideas, inferences, assumptions, principles, arguments, conclusions, issues, statements, beliefs and actions" (p. 5).

Miller and Malcolm's (1990) article, "Critical Thinking in the Nursing Curriculum," helped set the stage for the 1990s, focusing nursing education on critical thinking. They did not define critical thinking beyond their literature review, but posed several questions to the profession to begin a serious examination of the concept, how it relates to clinical judgment, and how to evaluate it.

In 1991, Kintgen-Andrews conducted a literature review of critical thinking in nursing and education after she found that students did not show growth of critical thinking skills. She questioned the connections between critical thinking and clinical judgment. Kintgen-Andrews found that although student-subjects performed well on standard critical thinking tests, often measured by the Watson-Glaser Critical Thinking Appraisal, those same subjects did not make sound nursing clinical judgments. She concluded that critical thinking is more complex than what was usually measured and that metacognition, linking thinking to action, intuition, creativity, reasoning, and flexibility, was important. Furthermore, she developed recommendations for better understanding of the process of thinking, allowing time for thinking and linking content knowledge to thinking. She concluded that critical thinking needed to be better defined in nursing and that better measuring instruments were needed.

Jones and Brown (1991) described how critical thinking is misunderstood in the nursing community. Their survey of nursing schools indicated that critical thinking usually is closely equated with the scientific method, and that it is used in a linear problem-solving format.

Rubenfeld and Scheffer (1995) define critical thinking as a blend of five modes (types) of thinking, all working together as a whole. The best critical thinking demands synergy among all the modes, resulting in sound clinical judgment. The modes include Total Recall, Habits, Inquiry, New Ideas and Creativity, and Knowing How You Think.

Characteristics of Critical Thinking

The definitions of critical thinking are summarized in the accompanying display. From this review, it is easy to see that a critical thinker has many characteristics. Facione (1990) surveyed a large group of experts from around the country and found consensus for seven characteristics of an ideal critical thinker. According to those experts, an ideal thinker is inquisitive, open-minded, analytical, systematic, confident, truth-seeking, and mature.

At the beginning of this chapter, thinking was described as individual, automatic, and complex. Critical thinking is all of that and more, as one can see from the preceding descriptions. What is most important for beginning nursing students is to understand that they already have the basic thinking skills necessary to become good critical thinking nurses. Their responsibility is to increase their awareness of those skills, nurture and develop them, and allow them to grow in depth and breadth. The next section of this chapter will help increase the reader's awareness of thinking by exploring one model of critical thinking specifically designed for beginning-level nursing students.

The THINK Model of Critical Thinking

There are several models for studying and developing critical thinking; one model is given here as an example. Because it is easy to use, Rubenfeld and Scheffer's THINK model (1995) is useful for beginning-level stu-

Characteristics of Critical Thinking

In defining critical thinking, proponents have outlined characteristics. A summary of definitions reveals the following characteristics:

- Reflective and reasonable thinking (Ennis, 1985)
- Focus on deciding what to believe or do (Ennis, 1985)
- Intellectually disciplined process of actively and skillfully conceptualizing, applying, analyzing, synthesizing, or evaluating information (Paul, 1993)
- Collection of data gathered from or generated by observation, experience, reflection, reasoning, or communication (Ennis, 1993)
- Purposeful, self-regulatory judgment (Facione, 1990)
- Results in interpretation, analysis, evaluation, and inference (Facione, 1990)
- Essential as a tool of inquiry (Facione, 1990)
- Pervasive and self-rectifying human phenomenon (Facione, 1990)
- Involvement of facts, principles, theories, abstractions, deductions, interpretations, and evaluation (Matthews & Gaul, 1979)
- Rational explanation of ideas, inferences, assumptions, principles, arguments, conclusions, issues, statements, beliefs, and actions (Bandman & Bandman, 1988)

Although authors have used different terms, the above characteristics of critical thinking can be narrowed down to the following:

- It is purposeful: it clarifies and improves one's understanding
- It is disciplined
- It is pervasive
- It is active and skillful
- It uses a variety of methods to obtain information
- It is reflective, reasonable, and rational
- It is essential to gathering useful information

dents. The model uses a **mnemonic** (a memory tool) to describe the five modes (types) of thinking. The modes are

Total recall
Habits
Inquiry
New ideas and creativity
Knowing how you think

The first letter of each mode creates the word **THINK**. The model can be remembered by its association with "think." Table 8-2 briefly defines each mode and gives examples. Although experts use all five THINK modes simultaneously when they think, it is important for beginners in nursing to examine each mode for its special qualities.

Total Recall

Total recall thinking involves the brain's memory storage and retrieval system. The information learned in nursing and supporting courses and in life experiences can be stored in memory. If information itself is not stored, then knowing where to look for the information can be recalled. In everyday life, people need to remember phone numbers, the highways and streets used to drive to school, and where to find a recipe for pineapple upside-down cake. Nurses need to remember normal vital sign measurements, how to maintain a sterile field when changing a dressing, and where to go to find normal laboratory values for red blood cells. This is part of recall and retrieval.

Habit

Habits are behavior patterns that, because of repetition, have become nearly or completely involuntary. *Habit* thinking is both a help and a hindrance. Helpful habits save time, money, and energy. They allow a driver to stop a car safely when a truck cuts off the car. Helpful habits allow nurses to administer cardiopulmonary resuscitation efficiently without having to look up information in a book as the client becomes cyanotic. Other helpful nursing thinking habits include always collecting complete information, consistently validating information, and automatically using the nursing process as a dynamic whole instead of like steps in a recipe book.

Habits become a hindrance when they are used to replace other modes of thinking. It is easy to get into the habit of eating potato chips to relieve stress while ignoring the content of what is being eaten and its effect on the body's nutrition.

Habit thinking in nursing can become "ruts." These thinking ruts are illustrated by statements like, "We have always done dressing changes like this." They are used when nurses assume that all clients who are overweight need to be on weight reduction diets, or that all clients who have suffered heart attacks can be provided high-quality care with the same standardized plan of care.

Inquiry

Inquiry thinking is most simply described as thoughtful questioning, not accepting everything at face value, asking why and why not, and then making conclusions.

Table 8-2 • Rubenfeld and Scheffer's Five Modes of Thinking

Situation: The clinic nurse, Joan, reads the chart of the next client. Joan notes the client has a headache.

Initial and Mode	Description	Example
T Total Recall	Remembering facts or remembering where to look for them	Joan recalls all she can about headaches from personal and professional experience; she also remembers a specific reference book to confirm information or to identify signs and symptoms of headaches.
H Habits	Accepted ways of doing things that work, save time, or are necessary; thinking approaches that are repeated so often they become second nature	Joan systematically and automatically collects relevant data: questions are asked about the pain—where it is, how it started, how it progressed, how long it has existed; what makes it better or worse; what the client thinks is causing it.
I Inquiry	Examining issues in depth and questioning what may seem immediately obvious	Joan questions the relationships among data (Are headaches connected to nursing examinations?); looks for patterns) Do headaches occur with all examinations?); identifies missing data; interprets the data; questions things that do not seem to fit together; and makes conclusions about what is going on before and after care is provided to determine changes.
N New Ideas and Creativity	Individualized thinking that goes beyond the usual to reconfigure the norm	Joan designs a customized plan of care with the client. This might include teaching the client some relaxation exercises, massaging the client's neck, or referring the problem to a physician.
K Knowing How You Think	Thinking about one's thinking; metacognition	Before, during, and after the interaction, Joan reflects on *how* she thinks: Did my personal biases influence the interpretation of data? Did I collect enough data to make accurate conclusions? Did I consider all possible conclusions? How well did the solution fit this particular client's needs?

(Adapted from Rubenfeld, M. G., & Scheffer, B. K. (1995). *Critical thinking in nursing: An interactive approach.* Philadelphia: J. B. Lippincott.)

Anyone who has been around a 3-year-old who is constantly asking "why?" is familiar with the early stages of inquiry thinking. Although the 3-year-old's ability to process the answers and draw accurate conclusions is limited, his or her ability to ask the questions is unlimited.

In adult life, inquiry thinking helps us formulate questions and arrive at the most accurate conclusions. For example, you get in the car to leave for school and the car will not start. You must figure out why the car will not start. You might suspect the battery, so you collect information on the sound when you turn the key and check to see if the lights work. If everything indicates that the battery is working, you might then think, "Am I out of gas?" This process of inquiry thinking continues until you come up with a conclusion, or decide you need more expert assistance.

Inquiry thinking requires the nurse to be a health detective, to delve deeper for better information, and to ask questions that lead to answers for developing the most accurate conclusions. For example, consider a client with hypertension who periodically fails to take his medications. The nurse could consider the client to be noncompliant, forgetful, lazy, or uninterested in his health. If the nurse has an inquiring mind, however, he or she wonders if there are still other possibilities. The nurse has to ask more questions of the client. For instance, what are the client's priorities in life? This client's priority is to get to work, which requires driving. Because the client experienced dizziness while taking the medication, he decided it was dangerous to drive. Rather than stop driving, his choice was to stop the medication on days that he worked. In this situation, a conclusion of "priority conflicts" versus "noncompliance" will better focus care to meet this client's individual needs.

Making accurate conclusions requires that nurses ask useful questions and not jump to the most obvious conclusions, but keep an open mind and maintain an inquiring attitude. Much of the thinking in nursing is focused on "ruling in" and "ruling out" hunches. Nurses need continually to expand their thinking to consider all possibilities, and then narrow their thinking to select the hunch or conclusion with the highest probability of accuracy.

New Ideas and Creativity

New ideas and creativity is the thinking mode that is most closely linked to individualization of nursing care. This mode is unique to each thinker. It involves combining information and ideas to create something that did not exist before, and permits the nurse to customize care to fit each client's needs and situations.

Many people consider themselves very creative, whereas others consider their creativity limited, but everyone has some creative ability that can be nurtured. Examples of creativity include such varied efforts as creating a study space with two old nightstands and a door that was sitting in the basement, making an elegant and delicious meal out of ordinary leftovers, painting a picture, or writing an interesting letter to a friend.

Creativity and new ideas in nursing are demonstrated daily. One rural community health nurse discovered during her first home visit that the client had been taught in the hospital to do his colostomy care using a bathroom sink and toilet. The client had no indoor plumbing. (The nurse doing discharge planning and teaching in the hospital had neglected to discover this.) Creativity and new ideas were necessary to help the client find a safe and efficient way to do his irrigations and dressing changes without indoor plumbing. In this case, the nurse worked with the client to design a plan together. The client was able to heat pump water for his irrigations and dressing changes, to use available materials to set up an irrigation system, and to identify a safe way to dispose of the soiled water and fecal material in his outhouse.

Knowing How You Think

Knowing how you think is the key to putting all the modes together successfully. Thinking about thinking is referred to as "metacognition." Studies of how experts think reveal that the best thinkers are able to articulate *how* as well as *what* they think. Each person's thinking style is unique. Some people think quickly on their feet; others take a more deliberate, slower approach. Some people have very good memories; others need additional memory aids. How we think is also affected by our values and beliefs, physical and emotional states, experience, and self-perceptions. Rubenfeld and Scheffer (1995) believe a healthy balance in critical thinking comes when nurses use all five modes simultaneously.

Factors Affecting Thinking

Many factors influence thinking. A great many have to do with cognitive function (see Chapter 46); among these are the person's physical state, the amount of sleep or rest a person gets, nutrition, fluid and electrolyte balance, and cognitive processes. The individ-

Nursing Research
Critical Thinking

Selected Nursing Research Studies

Bechtel, G., Smith, J., Printz, V., & Gronseth, D. (1993). Critical thinking and clinical judgement of professional nurses in a career mobility program. *Journal of Nursing Staff Development, 9*(5) 218–222.

Brooks, K., & Sheppard, J. (1992). Professionalism versus general critical thinking abilities of senior nursing students in four types of nursing curricula. *Journal of Professional Nursing, 8*(2), 87–95.

Miller, M. (1992). Outcome evaluation: Measuring critical thinking. *Journal of Advanced Nursing, 17*(12), 1401–1407.

Plunkett, E. (1994). The development of cognitive diagnostic reasoning skills in undergraduate nursing students across a four-semester time period. In M. Carroll-Johnson & M. Paquette (Eds.), *Classification of nursing diagnosis: Proceedings of the Tenth Conference.* Philadelphia: J. B. Lippincott.

Saarmann, L., Freitas, L., Rapps, J., & Riegel, B. (1992). The relationship of education to critical thinking ability and values among nurses: Socialization into professional nursing. *Journal of Professional Nursing, 8*(1), 26–34.

Possible Topics for Nursing Inquiry

- What factors contribute to the development of relativistic thinking?
- How frequently are students asked to reflect on their own thinking process during their nursing education?
- Will the new NLN accreditation criterion for critical thinking foster increased critical thinking in nursing students?
- What clinical and classroom teaching strategies foster critical thinking in nursing students?
- How does the ability to think critically develop further during the first 5 years after graduation?

ual's age and developmental level also affect thinking. The amount and complexity of the information to be thought about is important.

This section of the chapter focuses on three very important factors that affect thinking: self-efficacy, anxiety, and intellectual development. Although these are not the only factors, they are particularly important for beginning-level students to address to increase their awareness of their own thinking skills.

Self-Efficacy

Self-efficacy refers to the person's belief that he or she is capable of doing something. The theory of self-efficacy, developed in the late 1980s, is important in the sense that it views intelligence as fluid and ever-changing (ie, not constant). This theory encourages learners to achieve beyond what someone else says they are capable of doing (Angelo & Cross, 1993). Self-efficacy is particularly appropriate in the area of critical thinking in nursing because beginning-level students need to believe they can be good critical thinkers.

It is important for beginning-level students to know they already have the basics and, with increased awareness and nurturing, they can become experts in critical thinking. Students who feel good about their thinking skills and their ability to learn are more likely to take thinking risks, to ask questions, to challenge the status quo, and to use mistakes as opportunities to learn and grow.

Anxiety

Life is full of anxiety-producing situations. The nursing profession certainly has more than its share of life-and-death, health-and-illness situations that are anxiety producing. Too little anxiety limits thinking; some anxiety can stimulate thinking. Too much anxiety can paralyze higher-order thinking skills (Angelo & Cross, 1993). A proper balance of anxiety is the key to high-level thinking. Determining ways to reduce excessive anxiety is essential to maintaining an effective balance. For example, one nursing student who was overanxious about how to survive his very busy schedule of family, work, school expectations, and the long drive to campus, came up with a creative way to study. He would read aloud his class notes onto an audiotape, and then listen to the tapes as he drove to and from classes each day. This significantly reduced his anxiety about his limited study time and freed up more time for other life responsibilities.

Intellectual Development

Intellectual development, as described by Perry (1970), explains how people perceive and function in their world. Perry examined intellectual development on a continuum from dualism to relativism. People who practice **dualism** in their thinking assume there is one right answer for every question, that authorities have all the answers, and the best way to learn is to memorize *all* the information. People who think in this way see things only as good or bad, right or wrong. A study by Valiga (1983) found that beginning-level nursing students are predominantly dualistic in their thinking.

Dualistic approaches assume perfection is possible. Perfection, however, is an ideal, not an actuality. Most judgments, in nursing for instance, are probabilities not absolutes. Effective nurses acknowledge these level of gray and aim for the "best" not the "perfect."

Dualistic approaches also prevent nurses from being creative and adapting learned nursing care to different settings or circumstances. Expecting a right/wrong answer (one answer is right; all others are wrong) is a dualistic way of thinking. Many traditional learning approaches have promoted dualistic thinking habits, so learners often expect there to be one correct answer to a given problem. For example, a nurse is planning care for a homebound client who must have the head of his bed elevated 30 degrees. The nurse has learned that the right way to elevate a hospital bed is to adjust the levers to the required elevation. But this client cannot afford a hospital bed, and insurance will not pay for it. Because she cannot do it the "right" way, the nurse is at a loss for planning care for this client. A bit of "New Ideas and Creativity" would be useful here.

On the other hand, **relativism** defines knowledge as relative to individuals, groups, and conditions. Perceiving life as relativistic means that one recognizes there are a variety of effective approaches to any situation. There is not just one "right" way, with all others being wrong. The nurse who is able to perceive the world as relativistic is better able to apply the principles of nursing to a variety of situations in a variety of settings. In the above situation, a nurse who thinks relativistically knows she cannot use a hospital bed, so she thinks about options. The nurse asks herself how she can elevate the client's head in another way, and realizes she can use more pillows to raise the client's head, or she can place blocks under the head of the bed to raise it. She knows there is more than one solution.

Nursing, because of its focus on human function and responses, is full of relativistic situations. What is best for one person is not necessarily best for another. Often, standardized, "fixed" approaches cannot be used but have to be adapted to individual situations.

Development of Critical Thinking Skills

Optimal nurse-thinking does not occur automatically. It takes self-reflection and practice (Fig. 8-2).

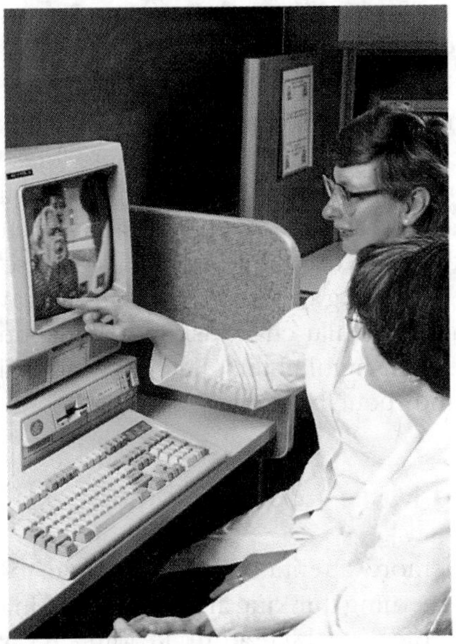

Figure 8-2 • Interactive video is a technology that allows the nursing student to make clinical decisions in a safe laboratory environment as he or she develops critical thinking skills.

Self-Reflection on Thinking Skills

The nursing student asks himself or herself, "How do I think? Where did I acquire my thinking modes? How will my thinking styles help me in providing nursing care as a student? As a nurse in the future?" Identifying your unique style of thinking will help you think about thinking. The accompanying self-reflection inventory will help you think about your thinking. There are no "right" or "wrong" answers to these questions; if you took this same inventory later in the day, you might find that you answered the questions very differently. The purpose of this exercise is simply to increase your awareness. As you become more aware of your unique thinking style, you may find that some things work well in nursing situations, whereas others may need some adjusting. As you consciously focus on your thinking in client care situations, you will see your thinking develop.

Building on Existing Thinking Skills

The basic types of thinking used in nursing are the same as those used in everyday life. There are differences, however, in the content focus of that thinking and the relative amounts of one type of thinking or another used in given situations. For example, the decision about what to wear today was based on thinking that may have included collecting information about the weather, what clothes were clean, the person's mood, the occasion, and who the person might be with during the day. Based on thinking about those issues, the person made a decision about what to wear. A similar kind of thought process is used when the nurse thinks about a client's problem and discusses with the client how to solve the problem. The difference between a wardrobe selection situation and a nursing situation lies in the kind of information that needs to be processed and the importance of the outcome; the thinking process itself is the same. Because the issues in nursing are usually more significant than selecting one's attire, the term "critical thinking" is commonly used for

Self-Reflection Inventory: Knowing How You Think

Do you remember isolated facts easily, or do you search for patterns so you can store information in your brain more easily?

Do you tend to accept what you are told by authorities, or do you question most things you hear or read?

Are you comfortable with ambiguity, or do you prefer situations to have one "right" answer?

Is it easier to think about information after you hear it or after you see it, or both?

What happens to your thinking when you are anxious, and what makes you anxious?

What are your biases (about cultures, health, illness, eating, exercise, economic status, education, and so forth), and how do they affect your thinking?

How creative are you? What does creativity mean to you?

Are you comfortable thinking aloud, or do you wait to say something until you have your ideas firmly in place?

How do you deal with ideas that conflict with yours?

Do you like to examine the reasons behind answers, or do you like to be told the "correct" answer?

Do you like to think about things for a long time before coming to a conclusion, or do you like to come to conclusions quickly and save time?

Are you comfortable with debate on issues, or do you prefer that everyone be in agreement?

Can you describe your thinking, or do you just "think?"

How intuitive are you?

Nurturing Your Thinking Skills

1. Make a list of your current thinking skills.
2. Keep a log (diary) of how you use thinking skills on a regular basis.
3. Share your log with a classmate. Learn from and applaud each other.
4. Read an article or book on thinking in nursing and discuss it with a classmate.
5. Draw a picture or write a paragraph that describes how you would like to enhance your thinking and the factors that hinder your thinking. Share it with a classmate.
6. Promise yourself always to consider at least three possible answers (hunches/conclusions) for every question.
7. Remind yourself that the path to responsible nursing care is along the path of critical thinking.
8. Give yourself a reward for your development of thinking skills.
9. Set goals for further development of your thinking skills.

the thinking expected of nurses. Learning how to think critically in nursing is best accomplished when the student or nurse actively thinks about existing thinking skills and styles and builds on them. The accompanying display on nurturing thinking skills will help the student use existing skills, strengthening and building on them.

Optimizing Thinking

The nursing student can learn to identify optimum conditions for cognitive functioning. A person who has difficulty remembering isolated facts may want to devise a way of patterning information so facts can be related to something else. One way of making patterns is the use of mnemonics; mnemonics were discussed earlier as memory tools. Mnemonics are easier to remember because they trigger connections. The THINK model was an example. Learning acronyms is one memory enhancer. An **acronym**, a type of mnemonic, is a word formed from the initial letter or letters of each of the successive parts or major parts of a compound term. An example is MASH for Mobile Army Surgical Hospital. THINK is another example.

Another system is to make logical linkages of information. For example, associating the **l** in **l**eft hemisphere cerebral strokes with the initial **l** in **l**anguage difficulties can help one remember which clients are likely to have communication difficulties associated with their strokes.

If a person realizes he or she thinks better at certain times of the day, that person may be able to schedule studying or work for those times. Some people think and learn better when they write notes while listening to lectures. Others find note-taking interferes with their information processing. The former should take notes, but the latter would be better off taping lectures.

Some people use thinking aids as diverse as eating chocolate, listening to music, wearing certain clothing, sitting on a particular chair, using a special desk, or using fluorescent highlighters. Such aids are valuable for comfort and reducing anxiety.

Learning More About Thinking

More and more attention is being given to thinking. Topics concerning thinking are showing up in both popular and professional literature. Reading about and discussing thinking improves one's understanding.

Finding role models is another method for learning more about thinking. Nurses who appear to be skilled thinkers, for example, can be asked to describe how they think. Students can describe their thinking to fellow students or family members and ask them for feedback. Working with peers allows one to hear others' descriptions of their thinking, and different styles of thinking can be compared and contrasted. Sharing best approaches helps each student strengthen his or her repertoire.

Both oral and written descriptions of thinking are helpful. Sometimes one is forced to find more specific words when one writes a description, whereas more circuitous descriptions may be made verbally. However, both of these approaches are valuable to expanding knowledge about thinking.

Setting Goals in Thinking Skill Development

When students know what thinking skills they have and what skills they want or need to develop, they can better set goals for themselves. The following are examples of goals to improve thinking skills:

- Distinguish between facts and assumptions regarding client information, and give rationale
- Describe relevant information in a client situation, and explain why it is relevant
- List several biases you have about health, nursing, and clients, and analyze how these biases developed
- Describe the process you use to problem-solve, why you have been using it, and how well it works
- Explain how your anxiety affects your unique thinking
- Appreciate and value your unique thinking skills

The nursing student may be surprised to find that he or she already has some of the thinking skills needed to achieve these goals. Periodic evaluations help the student set additional goals for developing further skills, thus improving critical thinking.

Opportunities for Critical Thinking in This Text

Because critical thinking is such an important element in nursing, activities to help the student think critically are given in every chapter of this text. A situation for contemplation is given at the beginning of the chapter, and then a Critical Thinking Challenge related to that situation appears at the end of the chapter to strengthen and focus the knowledge gained from the chapter. The student may opt to take the challenge before reading the chapter, and then again for evaluation after studying the material. Critical Thinking Challenges are also provided at the end of Therapeutic Dialogue displays.

Key Concepts

- Critical thinking is important in all nursing–client interactions.
- There are different ways of thinking, and each has a specific purpose.
- Critical thinking is essential for using the nursing process, an important element in effective nursing practice.
- Many authors have defined critical thinking. Each definition may differ slightly, but all view critical thinking as a positive, reflective process that helps people make decisions and take action.
- Many factors affect thinking. Important emotional factors are self-efficacy, anxiety, and intellectual development.
- The student can develop critical thinking skills through self-reflection, building on existing skills, optimizing thinking, observing role models, expressing thinking both verbally and in writing, reading about and discussing critical thinking, setting goals, and practicing critical thinking.

Critical Thinking Challenges

Now you have added information on critical thinking to your knowledge base of professional nursing. In the remaining chapters in this unit, you will learn to apply critical thinking to the nursing process. But you still have your situation to solve from the beginning of the chapter. Turn back to that situation and consider these questions.

1. *Identify factors that could affect your ability to think during your first clinical experience.*
2. *Reflect on at least five of your qualities that will be helpful in having a successful first clinical experience. Write them down and share them with one other person.*
3. *Reflect on two other "first-time" experiences in your life. Determine what methods of coping and thinking helped make these new experiences positive and growth-producing.*
4. *Determine what your choices are in the situation, and give rationales for each. Evaluate which of your choices are helpful to you, your client, or your spouse.*

References

Angelo, T. A., & Cross, K. P. (1993). *Classroom assessment techniques: A handbook for college teachers* (2nd ed.). San Francisco: Jossey-Bass.

Bandman, E. L., & Bandman, B. (1988). *Critical thinking in nursing*. East Norwalk, CT: Appleton & Lange.

Costa, A. L. (Ed). (1985). *Developing minds: A resource book for teaching thinking*. Alexandria, VA: Association for Supervision and Curriculum Development.

Ennis, R. H. (1985). A logical basis for measuring critical thinking skills. *Educational Leadership, 10*, 44–48.

Facione, P. A. (1990). *"The Delphi Report" executive summary critical thinking: A statement of expert consensus for purposes of educational assessment and instruction.* Millbrae, CA: The California Academic Press.

Jones, S. A., & Brown, L. N. (1991). Critical thinking: Impact on nursing education. *J Adv Nurs, 16*, 529–533.

Kintgen-Andrews, J. (1991). Critical thinking and nursing education: Perplexities and insights. *Journal of Nursing Education, 30* (4), 152–157.

Matthews, C. A., & Gaul, A. L. (1979). Nursing diagnosis from the perspective of concept attainment and critical thinking. *Advanced Nursing Science, 2* (1), 17–26.

Miller, M. A., & Malcolm, N. S. (1990). Critical thinking in the nursing curriculum. *Nursing and Health Care, 11*(2), 67–73.

Paul, R. (1992). *Critical thinking: What every person needs to survive in a rapidly changing world* (2nd ed.). Santa Rosa, CA: The Foundation for Critical Thinking.

Perry, W. G. (1970). *Forms of intellectual and ethical development in the college years: A scheme.* New York: Holt, Reinhart & Winston.

Rubenfeld, M. G., & Scheffer, B. K. (1995). *Critical thinking in nursing: An interactive approach*. Philadelphia: J. B. Lippincott.

Scheffer, B. K., & Rubenfeld, M. G. (1994). *Strategies to improve critical thinking.* Unpublished manuscript.

Valiga, T. M. (1983). Cognitive development: A critical component of baccalaureate nursing education. *Image, 15* (4), 115–117.

Yura, H., & Walsh, M. B. (1973). *The nursing process: Assessing, planning, implementing, evaluating* (2nd ed.). New York: Appleton-Century-Crofts.

Bibliography

Bevis, E. O. (1993). All in all, it was a pretty good funeral. *Journal of Nursing Education, 32,* 101–105.

Brookfield, S. (1993). On impostorship, cultural suicide, and other dangers: How nurses learn critical thinking. *Journal of Continuing Education in Nursing, 24* (5), 197–205.

Carnevali, D. L., & Thomas, M. D. (1993). *Diagnostic reasoning and treatment decision making in nursing.* Philadelphia: J. B. Lippincott.

Dewey, J. (1910). *How we think.* Boston: D. C. Heath & Co.

Eyres, S. J., Loustau, A., & Ersek, M. (1992). Ways of knowing among beginning students in nursing. *Journal of Nursing Education, 31*(4), 75–180.

Gehrke, P. (1994). Finding voices through writing. *Nurse Educator, 19* (2), 28–30.

Heinrich, K. T. (1992). The intimate dialogue: Journal writing by students. *Nurse Educator, 17* (6), 17–21.

Jones, E. A., & Ratcliff, G. (1993). *Critical thinking skills for college students.* University Park, PA: National Center on Postsecondary Teaching, Learning, and Assessment.

Klaassens, E. (1992). Strategies to enhance problem solving. *Nurse Educator, 17* (3), 28–30.

McKeachie, W. J., Pintrich, P. R., Lin, Y., et al. (1986). *Teaching and learning in the college classroom: A review of the research literature.* Ann Arbor, MI: National Center for Research to Improve Post Secondary Teaching and Learning, University of Michigan.

Polin, L. (1993). Three ways writing is thinking. *Writing-Notebook: Visions for Learning, 10* (4), 31–33.

Reinsmith, W. A. (1993). Ten fundamental truths about learning. *The National Teaching and Learning Forum, 2* (4), 7–8.

Schank, M. J. (1990) Wanted: Nurses with critical thinking skills. *Journal of Continuing Education in Nursing, 21* (2), 86–89.

Villas, P. (1993). Thinking and writing. *Journal of Health Education, 24* (1), 57.

Nursing Process: Foundation for Practice

Key Terms	Learning Objectives
Decision making Diagnostic reasoning process Functional health pattern Information-processing theory Nursing process Primary source Problem-solving process Secondary source Systems theory	Upon completion of this chapter, the student will be able to do the following: • Identify the components of the nursing process. • Recognize significant historic developments in the evolution of the nursing process. • Discuss the requirements for effective use of the nursing process. • Explain the major theoretical foundations on which the nursing process is based. • Describe the functional health approach to the nursing process. • Appraise future trends that influence the nursing process.

9

You are assigned to care for a client who had a total hip replacement 3 days ago. As you enter the room, the client is awake and greets you cheerfully. You introduce yourself and ask the client how she is feeling. The client replies, "I'm doing as well as can be expected." Your morning assessment reveals the following:

- *Vital signs: blood pressure 148/84, pulse 86, respirations 18, temperature 36.5°C*
- *Pain controlled adequately while in bed but complains of pain when ambulating with PT*
- *Eating soft diet; no BM since surgery; bowel sounds present*
- *Incision dry with no signs of inflammation*
- *Ambulated twice yesterday with PT; complained of dizziness and pain; states she does not know how she will manage walking at home because she lives alone, and her house is large with steps*

In previous chapters, you learned about concepts essential to your nursing career and how nursing care is delivered in the 1990s. This chapter introduces you to the nursing process and further expands your knowledge base. As you proceed through this chapter, you will learn how the nursing process provides a foundation for care of your clients. The Critical Thinking Challenges at the end of the chapter will help you apply your knowledge to this client's care.

The foundation of the nursing profession is nursing process. Skill in using nursing process is necessary for the clinical application of knowledge and theory in nursing practice. Concepts related to nursing process continue to evolve. For instance, what was previously a five-phase process has now become a six-phase process. This textbook uses the six-step process, so it can be on the cutting edge in nursing education and in the nursing profession. The six phases of the nursing process are assessment, diagnosis, outcome identification, planning, implementation, and evaluation.

This chapter discusses the historic development of nursing process, summarizes each phase, and gives a brief review of the theoretical foundations of the nursing process. This chapter also describes the requirements for the effective use and professional relevance of the nursing process. The chapter concludes with a discussion of a functional health approach to the nursing process and future nursing process trends.

Historic Development of the Nursing Process

The term **nursing process** is synonymous with the problem-solving approach for discovering the healthcare and nursing care needs of clients and their families. Before the widespread use of the term nursing process in the late 1960s, nurses cared for clients using a loosely structured framework based on the medical model. Since then, several nursing leaders have been instrumental in developing today's nursing process, and many models of the nursing process have been developed.

Lydia Hall is credited with originally introducing the term "nursing process" in 1955 (George, 1990), but it was not used extensively in nursing publications until the 1960s. A few years later, a three-step nursing process was described by Dorothy Johnson (1959), Ida Jean Orlando (1961), and Ernestine Wiedenbach (1963). In 1967 Lois Knowles published a five-step nursing process using "the five Ds:" discover, delve, decide, do, and discriminate. The *discover* and *delve* steps are synonymous with the assessment phase; *decide* is the planning stage; *do* is the implementation phase; and *discriminate* is the evaluation of client responses to nursing interventions.

In 1967, several publications defined the nursing process and delineated the steps. The Western Interstate Commission on Higher Education (WICHE) and the faculty at The Catholic University of America were instrumental in moving the nursing process forward. WICHE published this definition: "The nursing process is that which goes on between a client and a nurse in a given setting; it records the behaviors of client and nurse and the resulting interaction. The steps of the process are perception, communication, interpretation, and evaluation" (Western Interstate Commission on Higher Education, 1967, p. 6). Although this definition was never widely accepted, it was an impetus to the development of the nursing process.

Helen Yura and Mary Walsh, along with the nursing faculty at The Catholic University of America, identified the steps of the nursing process as assessing, planning, implementing, and evaluating. Since 1967, Yura and Walsh have continued to develop and refine the nursing process concept.

In 1973, the American Nurses Association (ANA) distinguished diagnosis as a separate step of the nursing process in their *Standards of Nursing Practice*. The

Table 9-1 • Contributions of Selected Individuals and Organizations to the Development and Evolution of the Nursing Process

Decade	Individual/Organization	Contribution
1950s	L. Hall (1955)	Originally used the term "nursing process." Identified three aspects of nursing care as care, cure, and core. Three steps of nursing process: note observations, ministration of care, validation.
	D. Johnson (1959)	Nursing seen as fostering the behavioral functioning of the client. Three steps of nursing process: assessment, decision, nursing action.
1960s	I. J. Orlando (1961)	Nursing process set into motion by client behavior. Three steps of nursing process: client behavior, nurse reaction, nurse's actions.
	Western Interstate Commission of Higher Education (1967)	Nursing defined as an interactive process between client and nurse. Four steps of nursing process: perception, communication, interpretation, evaluation.
	H. Yura & M. Walsh (1967)	Four components of nursing process: assessing, planning, implementing, evaluating.
	Knowles (1967)	Described nursing practice as discover, delve, decide, do, discriminate.
1970s	American Nurses Association (1973)	Published *Standards of Nursing Practice.* Diagnosis distinguished as separate step of nursing process.
1980s	American Nurses Association (1980)	Published *Nursing: A Social Policy Statement.* Diagnosis of actual and potential health problems delineated as integral part of nursing practice.
1990s	American Nurses Association (1991)	Published *Standards of Clinical Nursing Practice.* Outcome identification differentiated as a distinct step of the nursing process. Six steps of nursing process: assessment, diagnosis, outcome identification, planning, implementation, evaluation.

standards were arranged according to the five steps of the nursing process (see Chap. 1). Thus, the use of the five-step nursing process model by nursing educators and practitioners began around this time.

In the 1980s, further support was gained for making diagnosis a distinct nursing function and a separate step of the nursing process. In *Nursing: A Social Policy Statement,* the ANA (1980) again identified diagnosis of actual and potential health problems as an integral part of nursing practice.

The newest development in nursing process is the six-step nursing process model, which was introduced by ANA (1991) in its *Standards of Clinical Nursing Practice.* In this six-step model, outcome identification was distinguished as the third step of the nursing process. These six steps are used thoughout this text. Table 9-1 summarizes selected contributions of people and organizations to the development and evolution of the nursing process.

Components of the Nursing Process

Definition

The **nursing process** generally is defined as a systematic problem-solving approach of giving individualized nursing care. It has been defined in various ways by a number of authors. A few definitions are included in the display for your consideration. Note the similarities among the definitions. Whatever definition is used, the nursing process is used by nurses as a problem-solving method in all settings with clients of all ages to identify and treat human responses to potential or actual health problems. By incorporating the unique aspects of each client, the nursing process facilitates the development of individualized care.

The nursing process complements the current role of consumers in healthcare; that is, clients play an active role in decisions affecting their health. Clients no longer passively accept the decisions made by healthcare professionals.

The nursing process serves as a guide for professional nursing practice. It has the following characteristics:

- It is a framework for providing nursing care to clients, families, and communities.
- It is orderly and systematic.
- It is interdependent.
- It provides individual care.
- It is client centered and uses the client's strengths.
- It is appropriate for use throughout the lifespan.
- It can be used in all settings.

Figure 9-1 illustrates the six phases (assessment, diagnosis, outcome identification, planning, implementation, and evaluation) of the nursing process.

Definitions of Nursing Process by Several Authors

"The nursing process is an organized, systematic method of giving goal-oriented, humanistic care that's both *effective* and *efficient.* It's *organized* and *systematic* in that it consists of five sequential and interrelated steps—Assessment, Diagnosis, Planning, Implementation, and Evaluation—during which you perform deliberate activities designed to maximize long-term results. It is *humanistic* in that the plan of care is developed and implemented in such a way that the unique interests and ideals of consumers and their significant others are given great consideration" (Alfaro-LeFever, 1994, p. 3).

"Nursing process is a method of problem identification and problem solving. Although derived from the supposedly objective scientific method, nursing process is not applied in an objective, value-free way. *Human values influence both problem identification and problem solving.* The components of nursing process discussed in textbooks vary but generally include assessment and diagnosis. These are the problem-identification components. Outcome projection, intervention, and outcome evaluation are the problem-solving components" (Gordon, 1994, pp. 9–10).

"The nursing process is an orderly, systematic manner of determining the client's health status, specifying problems defined as alterations in human need fulfillment, making plans to solve them, initiating and implementing the plan, and evaluating the extent to which the plan was effective in promoting optimum wellness and resolving the problems identified" (Yura & Walsh, 1988, p. 1).

"After a client has sought healthcare in his or her home, office, clinic, or hospital, the nurse uses systematic assessment and problem-solving techniques to evaluate his functional status: Is it positive or altered, or is he at risk for altered functioning? Does he identify a problem with his health status? The nurse and client collaborate on planning and implementing appropriate interventions and on evaluating the effectiveness of these interventions. The nursing process describes this method, for through its five components—assessment, diagnosis, planning, intervention, and evaluation—it sets the practice of nursing in motion" (Carpenito, 1993, p. 46).

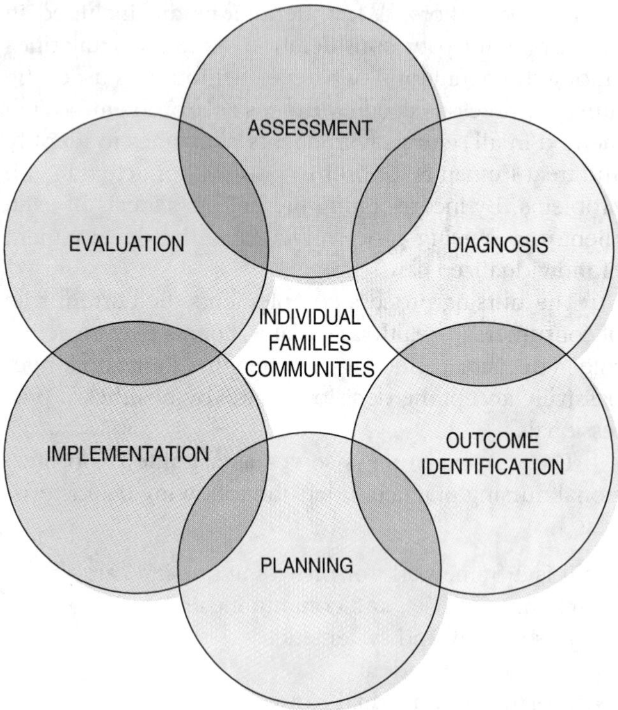

Figure 9-1 • *Six phases of the nursing process.*

Phases

Assessment

Assessment commonly refers to evaluation or appraisal. In nursing, assessment is the systematic collection of subjective and objective data with the goal of making a clinical nursing judgment about a client, family, or community. During assessment, the nurse appraises the client's total situation by considering the physical, psychological, emotional, sociocultural, and spiritual factors that may affect his or her health status.

All relevant information about the client's present, past, or potential problems must be gathered to develop a complete database. Data collection takes place during every nurse–client interaction and from many other available sources (Gordon, 1987; 1994). The client is the **primary source** of information for assessment. **Secondary sources** include family members, significant others, other healthcare professionals, health records, and literature review.

Assessment data are gathered by observing, interviewing, and examining the client and interpreting laboratory data. Observation begins with the first encounter with the client and is an ongoing process. The nursing interview allows for the systematic assessment of functional health, including the client's perception and interpretation of problems (Gordon, 1982; 1987; 1994). During the physical examination, the nurse uses the techniques of inspection, percussion, palpation, and auscultation to obtain data. Objective information from health records, including laboratory and diagnostic data, completes the database.

An in-depth nursing history and physical assessment are usually required at admission. This initial database becomes the reference point for all further nursing assessments. Thorough assessment data provide the foundation for nursing diagnoses (Yura & Walsh, 1988).

Diagnosis

Diagnosing human responses to actual or potential health problems is the second phase of the nursing process. Diagnosis is the clinical act of identifing problems and also the term given to the client's problem. To diagnose means to analyze assessment information and derive meaning from this analysis.

Registered nurses are educated and licensed to make nursing diagnoses. They are responsible for identifying nursing diagnoses for their clients and for identifying and planning client management based on nursing diagnoses. The North American Nursing Diagnosis Association (1992) defines nursing diagnosis as "a clinical judgment about individual, family, or community responses to actual or potential health problems/life processes. Nursing diagnoses provide the basis for selection of nursing interventions to achieve outcomes for which the nurse is accountable" (p. 5). The registered nurse is responsible for identifying nursing diagnoses for clients under his or her care.

The clinical skills used to make nursing diagnoses are the nursing diagnostic process and the formulation of a nursing diagnostic statement. The nursing diagnostic process uses cue clustering, cluster interpretation, and diagnostic validation to ensure accuracy in the selection of the correct diagnoses. Formulating the diagnostic statement requires knowledge of the differences among actual, risk, possible, and wellness nursing diagnoses.

Outcome Identification

According to the ANA's new (1991) *Standards of Clinical Nursing Practice*, outcome identification refers to the formulation and documentation of measurable, realistic, client-focused goals. Outcome identification is an integral phase that carries the consideration of problems and use of strengths into the planning of interventions.

Planning

Once nursing diagnoses have been determined, priorities established, and expected outcomes written, the planning phase begins. The nurse and the client work together to identify client goals and intervention strate-

Nursing Research
Nursing Process

Selected Nursing Research Studies

Chase, S. (1994). Clinical judgement by critical care nurses: An ethnographic study. In R. M. Carroll-Johnson & Pacquette (Eds.), *Classification of nursing diagnosis: Proceedings of the ninth conference, North American Nursing Diagnosis Association* (pp. 367–368). Philadelphia: J.B. Lippincott.

Lunney, M. (1992). Divergent productive thinking factors and accuracy of nursing diagnoses. *Research in Nursing and Health*, 15(4), 303–312.

Miller, V. G. (1993). Measurement of self-perception of intuitiveness. *Western Journal of Nursing Research*, 15, 595–606.

Staggers, N., & Mills, M. E. (1994). Nurse-computer interaction: Staff performance outcomes. *Nursing Research*, 43(3), 144–150.

Possible Topics for Nursing Inquiry

- What is the relationship between intuitive nursing knowledge and the diagnostic process in nurses with 10 years of experience?
- Do nursing students use more intuitive skill in the first clinical course or the last clinical course of a nursing program?
- How widely is outcome identification incorporated in the nursing process by practicing nurses?
- What teaching styles help promote the development of critical thinking in the nursing student?
- How have practicing nurses changed their view of the nursing process during the past 10 years?

gies that will reduce identified client problems. The planning phase involves preparing a nursing plan of care, which directs the activities of the nursing staff in the provision of client care.

The nursing plan of care is a written summary of the care to be given a client. The Joint Commission on Accreditation of Healthcare Organizations (1993) requires a written plan of care for each client. Although many institutions have developed standardized plans of care, all plans must be individualized. Nursing plans of care are further discussed in Chapter 12. The skills involved in planning include establishing client goals and outcome criteria and determining nursing interventions.

Writing the plan of care on the client record formally recognizes what the nurse planned and accomplished to assist the client. Because the plan of care remains a permanent part of the record, the beginning practitioner is sometimes intimidated to write information that may be criticized or changed by another nurse. As nurses develop their skill in writing plans and begin to recognize their responsibility to carry out other nurses' plans of care, this fear should be reduced. Once the plan of care is written, it must be implemented on behalf of the client.

Implementation

Implementation is the action phase of the nursing process. It is the actual initiation of the plan, evaluation of response to the plan, and recording of nursing actions and client response to these actions. To implement means to carry out, to perform, to intervene, or to do something. Implementation may include the delegating or coordinating of interventions within the plan of care (ANA, 1991). This phase also may include the designation of the client, significant others, or health-care providers to implement the pre-established plan of care (ANA, 1991). Nursing actions are goal directed and should assist the client to reach maximum functional health. Because nursing care is provided to assist in meeting client goals, it is imperative that nurses focus on their actions. The nurse should make sure that each action undertaken is necessary and required.

The components of implementation are reassessment, initiation of the plan, evaluation of the response, and recording of actions taken. Nursing actions focus on resolving or diminishing a client's functional health status problems.

Implementation requires the use of intellectual, interpersonal, and technical skills. Developing expertise in each of these skills is required for professional nursing practice. Once the care has been provided, it is evaluated.

Evaluation

Evaluation commonly refers to rating, grading, and judging. In the evaluation phase, the nurse discovers why the nursing plan of care was a success or failure (Alfaro-LeFevre, 1994). The nurse determines the client's reaction to nursing interventions and judges whether the goals of the plan of care have been achieved. The plan of care provides the basis for evaluation. Reassessing the client provides new information for changing or eliminating nursing diagnoses, goals, or interventions. Determining goal achievement is a joint decision between the client and the nurse (Yura & Walsh, 1988).

Evaluation focuses on individual clients and groups of clients. Quality assurance monitors provide input for development and refinement of standards of care for groups of similar clients.

Although evaluation is a separate and distinct phase, it also is an ongoing and continuous process performed throughout all phases of the nursing

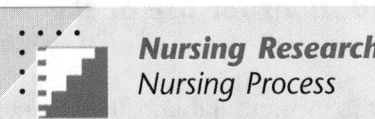

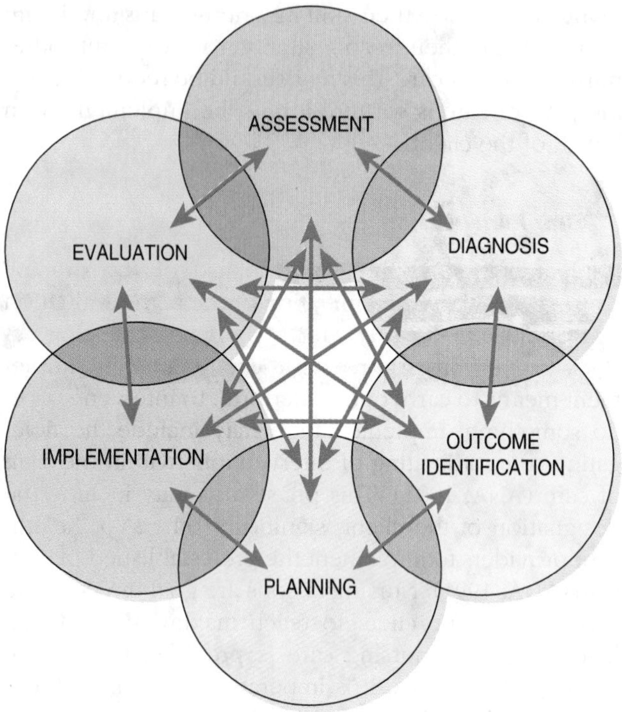

Figure 9-2 • Interactive nature of the nursing process.

process. Judgments in previous phases of the nursing process result in prompt reassessment, rediagnosing, and replanning. The evaluation phase involves a detailed reassessment of the entire plan of care. An in-depth, comprehensive judgment about client goal attainment and fulfillment of outcome criteria takes place in this phase (Yura & Walsh, 1988).

The process of evaluation requires a variety of skills for judging the nursing plan of care. These include knowledge of standards of care, knowledge of normal client responses, knowledge of conceptual models of nursing, ability to monitor the effectiveness of nursing interventions, and awareness of clinical research.

Interactive Nature of Each Phase

Each phase of the nursing process interacts with and is influenced by the other phases (Fig. 9-2). For example, a nurse collecting assessment information may implement some aspects of care at the same time. In a similar manner, as the nurse evaluates nursing care, new plans are made and implemented. During an emergency, all phases of the nursing process may be carried out with no apparent division among them.

As the client's condition changes, new data are gathered and incorporated into the plan of care. When care is provided, evaluation of the client's response may indicate a need for immediate revision of the plan or for the identification of new nursing diagnoses.

Theoretical Foundations for Use of the Nursing Process

An understanding of the theoretical foundations of the nursing process is necessary to apply it effectively. Systems theory, problem-solving process, decision-making process, information processing theory, and diagnostic reasoning process are the basic structural units of the nursing process.

Systems Theory

Systems theory is one conceptual foundation on which nursing process is built. Systems theory illustrates how the steps of the nursing process interact with each other, forming a unique blend that is greater than the sum of its parts (Fig. 9-3). Systems terminology provides a common language for the members of the healthcare team (Fawcett, 1995; George, 1990).

All systems have cyclical patterns, and the nursing process is no exception. The steps of the nursing process overlap and influence subsequent steps. A system is composed of a set of subsystems, and each higher level is made up of systems of the lower levels. The nursing process has six subsystems: assessment, diagnosis, outcome identification, planning, implementation, and evaluation.

Input, the information that enters a system, is the data collected during the assessment step (the nursing

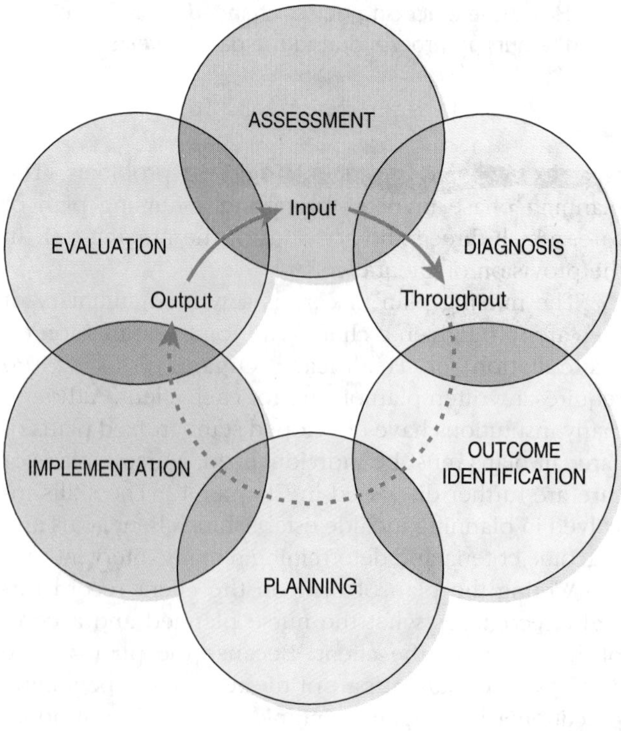

Figure 9-3 • Systems theory in comparison to the nursing process.

interview and physical examination). Input includes assessment data about the client and his or her immediate environment. *Throughput* is the process by which a system transforms, creates, and organizes input, resulting in a reorganization of the input. After the nurse identifies nursing diagnoses and outcomes and plans and implements nursing care, throughput takes place. *Output,* the end-product of a system, is the client's health status (that is, whether the client's health has been maintained or improved). Evaluation of the attainment of goals and the need for modification provide feedback for revising the plan, thereby completing the cycle. See Figure 9-3 for a comparison of systems theory to the nursing process.

Problem-Solving Process

Nurses encounter problems that require solutions, ranging from a simple question to a complex clinical situation. Nurses confront problems with clients, family members, other healthcare team members, or equipment. Approaches to problem solving vary depending on the nature of the problem (eg, complex or simple); the problem solver's experience, knowledge, and mental ability; and the alternative or option chosen to solve the problem.

Problem solving is the basis for the nursing process. The **problem-solving process** is a modified version of the scientific problem-solving method, which focuses on one problem, is carried out in a laboratory, has an extended time element, and controls as many variables or factors as possible. In contrast, the problem-solving process takes place in a clinical setting and involves clients with multiple problems. It occurs under shorter time constraints, and unforeseeable factors and events frequently intervene. The problem-solving process allows for the flexibility needed in the "real world" of clinical nursing practice.

Problem solving does not occur in isolation. The nurse solves problems by interacting and working with clients, family members, and other healthcare team members. It is an interpersonal approach that may involve two or more people (Sinnott, 1989). The client, whenever possible, is involved in solving problems.

The problem-solving process is composed of six steps. The phases of the nursing process are similar to the steps of the problem-solving process. Table 9-2 illustrates the similarities of the scientific problem-solving method, the problem-solving process, and the nursing process.

Decision-Making Process

Making decisions about client care is the essence of nursing practice. Decision-making is integral to every step of the nursing process. In its simplest form, **decision-making** consists of three phases: identifying the problem, determining the alternatives, and selecting the most appropriate alternative. People make decisions constantly, such as what to wear, what to eat, and when to study. All of the decisions we make are influenced by past experiences and exposure to different life events.

In a clinical situation, the nurse must decide which client should receive care first, when care may be delegated to other healthcare team members, and which client-care activity is needed. Each decision is carried out or changed depending on the immediate circumstances. Some days, decisions made early in the day present no problems, but usually, priorities change to meet emergent needs. The nurse must deal with uncertainty and must be adept at making astute clinical decisions.

The steps used in this process can be compared with the phases of the nursing process. Gathering information is analogous to assessment; identifying the

Table 9-2 • *Similarities and Differences Among the Scientific Problem-Solving Method, the Problem-Solving Process, and the Nursing Process*

Scientific Problem-Solving Method	*Problem-Solving Process*	*Nursing Process*
Define problem	Recognize existence of problem	Assessment
Collect data	Collect data	Assessment
Formulate a hypothesis	Analyze data; specify problem	Diagnosis
Select method to test hypothesis	Determine ways to achieve solution to problem	Outcome identification, planning
Test hypothesis	Execute the planned actions	Implementation
Formulate conclusion; evaluate hypothesis	Judge the effectiveness of selected actions	Evaluation

problem area is similar to diagnosing; considering alternative courses of action and selecting a course may be likened to the planning phase. Evaluating information and the course of action is implied in this process.

Information-Processing Theory

After the interview is completed, the chart reviewed, and the client examined, the nurse must synthesize the data. This is a complex task (Benner & Tanner, 1987): the processing of information requires the cognitive skills of logical and inductive–deductive thinking and the decision-making and diagnostic processes.

Information-processing theory (Fig. 9-4) can be used to help cluster data to arrive at a diagnosis (Newell & Simon, 1972; Simon, 1979). Because the brain can process only five to seven pieces of information at once, data need to be organized in a framework or outline. The model used in this textbook is functional health. In this way, the nurse can see how each piece fits into the whole. Studies have shown that experienced nurses need fewer cues to make accurate diagnoses (Benner, 1984).

Gathering and processing information can proceed inductively or deductively. Nurses use both approaches to identify and resolve problems. *Induction* is a reasoning process that proceeds from the specific to the general:

A rose has petals.
A daisy has petals.
A petunia has petals.
Therefore, all flowers have petals.

Deduction proceeds from the general to the specific:

All flowers have petals.
A rose has petals.
Therefore, a rose is a flower.

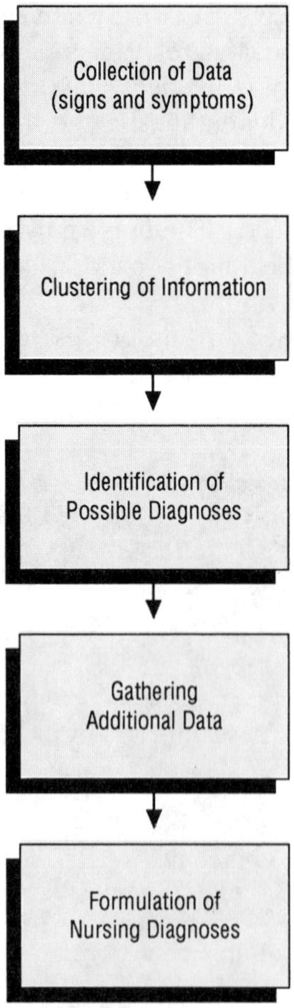

Figure 9-4 • *Information processing model.*

Diagnostic Reasoning Process

The **diagnostic reasoning process** is used to make accurate clinical diagnoses about client problems. It is a complex process composed of several interrelated steps and affected by variables, such as the background of the diagnostician and the client. Although the steps are discussed sequentially, in practice, there is much overlap until the diagnosis is made and confirmed (Woods, 1984). The steps include the following:

- Consideration of background of the diagnostician and client
- Initiation of the process
- Gathering individual cues
- Development of cue clusters
- Identification of possible diagnoses
- Collection of specific data
- Confirmation or refutation of the diagnosis.

Skill Requirements

Sound Knowledge Base

To use the nursing process successfully, the nurse must have a general understanding of the basic sciences and humanities. Nursing uses this scientific knowledge during assessment, planning, implementing, and evaluating client care. For example, in a client with chronic obstructive pulmonary disease, several factors may produce changes in the physiology of his or her lungs. He or she must adapt based on culture and ethnic background. Also, the course of the disease may have been influenced by exposure to pollutants acquired at work. Drawing all the pieces together to plan care requires a broad knowledge base.

Nurses add to their basic knowledge formally and informally by attending continuing education programs, reading professional journals, learning about related fields, and having discussions with peers and others. Incorporating new research findings into practice is necessary to achieve better client outcomes, develop

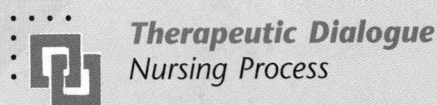

Therapeutic Dialogue
Nursing Process

Scenes for Thought

Linda Castro, a 34-year-old mother of two, was admitted yesterday for a course of chemotherapy for leukemia. She has been in the hospital for this treatment twice before and is known to the staff on this floor. She is lying in bed.

Nurse: *Hi, Ms. Castro. I'm Lesley Jory; do you remember me from last time?*
Client: *Yes. Hi, Lesley. I'm glad you're still here.* Client looks tired and pale.
Nurse: *Is it good to see a familiar face? (Checking out the client's perception.)*
Client: *Yes. I was worried that there would be a lot of changes since I was here last.*
Nurse: *We're all still here. How have you been since we last saw each other? (Assessment of coping outside the hospital.)*
Client: *Not too bad. The kids are a handful, but my husband helps most of the time, and I manage. And then I get so tired I can't do anything. The bruising is back again, too; look.* Shows several large bruises on her arms and legs.
Nurse: *I see. They look painful. You look kind of tired now. Is there something I can help you with or get for you? (Assessment of immediate needs.)*
Client: *I'd love it if you could fix these pillows for me. I can't seem to move today.*
Nurse: *Sure. Is that okay? (Evaluation of intervention.)*
Client: *Ah, that's good. When do the treatments start, Lesley?*
Nurse: *This afternoon, I think. The lab results have to come up yet. Then we can get started. Is there something you're concerned about? (Assessment.)*
Client: *Well, I'm wondering if I'll have the same problem with my veins as the last time.* Looks worried.
Nurse: *Let me check your old chart. I think we did some magic with warm compresses that seemed to work last time; remember? (Evaluation of prior intervention.)*
Client: *Oh yeah. That worked great. I'm glad you remembered.*
Nurse: *Is there anything else you need before I see to those labs?*
Client: *Yes. Could you get me a laxative order? I have been too tired to eat or drink much, so I guess it's all out of whack right now.* Laughs, a little embarrassed.
Nurse: *Not a problem. Perhaps you could also order a salad along with dinner and some fruit. I'll bring in some ice water. We'll work on it together. (Planning with the client.)*

Critical Thinking Challenge

• *Identify all the phases of the nursing process you could see Lesley using* • *Analyze whether it was an orderly progression or whether she skipped phases and then returned to them* • *Using Activity Intolerance, Fatigue, and Anxiety (mild) as nursing diagnoses for Ms. Castro, describe some of your plans for caring for her* • *Determine what other information you would need to assess Ms. Castro's functional health and make further diagnoses.*

new standards for practice, and provide cost-effective care.

Ability to Communicate in Writing

Writing skills are needed to communicate information on the client's health record and other agency forms. Writing enables others to develop a picture of the client at the time of the assessment. Records are often the only way to discover historic information about the progression of a disease and the client's response to it. Skillful writing requires the ability to summarize information while remaining comprehensive and accurate. Succinct descriptive terms are useful for providing an accurate, detailed written report.

Ability to Listen

One way to obtain information for written reports is by listening. Active listening implies that the nurse is responsive to the cues the client is sending. If clients are anxious or preoccupied, they may respond to questions with short or inappropriate answers. The astute nurse listens to what the client says to follow up on misconceptions and misunderstandings or to correct misinformation.

Being an active listener is hard work. It involves paying attention to nonverbal cues and the spoken response. Clients may hesitate to give certain information. Although it is important to respect the client and not to pry, the nurse needs to gather data essential for good client care. As interviewing skills develop, the nurse learns how to phrase certain questions and how to approach personal matters. Often the way a question is asked can make the difference between a complete or a superficial response.

Professional Relevance

The nursing process is a systematic, organized way of providing nursing care for any client in any situation. Its adaptability and practicality contribute to high-quality nursing care. Because a concise nursing plan of care is written, continuity of care is facilitated, and communication among nurses is enhanced.

The nursing process focuses on the client's unique problems. The client or family members are involved in setting priorities, developing goals and outcome criteria, and selecting nursing interventions. Because of this involvement, they play an important role in decisions that directly affect client care. The client's responses to nursing interventions are continually assessed and evaluated, which fosters individualized nursing care.

Legally, the nursing process is recognized as the standard for nursing practice. The nurse is held accountable to practice according to legal statutes and the nurse practice act of the state. Most states use the term nursing process when describing the act of nursing.

Professionally, the nursing process is recognized as the method of practicing nursing. It is the model on which professional nursing standards are based. Although sometimes criticized for not being adaptable to the changing healthcare environment, the nursing process remains the almost universally accepted method for providing nursing care.

Functional Health Approach

Gordon (1982; 1987; 1994) developed a method for organizing nursing assessment data that involves the appraisal of 11 **functional health patterns.** These functional health patterns provide a framework for the collection of assessment data.

Gordon originally developed the functional health pattern typology (a systematic classification) in 1974 while teaching nursing assessment and diagnosis to nursing students at Boston College. The incorporation of comments from nurse scholars, nurse educators, clinical nurse specialists, and students who used the categories in their practice resulted in some modification of the original health pattern categories.

Functional health patterns help the nurse ascertain the client's strengths and any dysfunctional or potentially dysfunctional pattern that exists. All 11 patterns are considered a composite of the client–environment situation and are examined collectively. The typology of the 11 patterns is given in the display. The patterns are built on the data collected during the interview and physical examination and are relevant for the individual, family, or community (Gordon, 1982; 1987; 1994).

Functional health patterns are the blueprint for the rest of the nursing process. In this way, the functional health approach permeates every phase of the nursing process. Although functional health patterns guide the collection of assessment data, they also serve as a guide for the identification of nursing diagnoses, development of the plan of care, implementation of the plan, and the organization of evaluative data for revision of the plan. Figure 9-5 diagrams the relationships between functional health and the nursing process.

Typology of 11 Functional Health Patterns

Health perception–health management: Describes client's perceived pattern of health and well-being and how health is managed

Nutritional–metabolic: Describes pattern of food and fluid consumption relative to metabolic need and pattern indicators of local nutrient supply

Elimination: Describes patterns of excretory function (bowel, bladder, skin)

Activity–exercise: Describes pattern of exercise, activity, leisure, and recreation

Cognitive–perceptual: Describes sensory-perceptual and cognitive pattern

Sleep–rest: Describes patterns of sleep, rest, and relaxation

Self-perception–self-concept: Describes self-concept pattern and perceptions of self (eg, body comfort, body image, feeling state)

Role–relationship: Describes pattern of role-engagements and relationships

Sexuality–reproductive: Describes client's patterns of satisfaction and dissatisfaction with sexuality pattern; describes reproductive patterns

Coping–stress tolerance: Describes general coping pattern and effectiveness of the pattern in terms of stress tolerance

Value–belief: Describes patterns of values, beliefs (including spiritual), or goals that guide choices or decisions.

(From Gordon, M. [1994]. *Nursing diagnosis: Process and application* [3rd ed]. St. Louis: C.V. Mosby.

Future Nursing Process Trends

Although the steps of the nursing process are likely to remain the same, the way the nursing process is used will change. Many institutions have computerized their data-collection methods and nursing plans of care. Written documentation is often minimal; instead, the nurse systematically enters data into a computer terminal, often at the client's bedside, providing easy access to all types of information necessary for quality client care. For example, a client's laboratory test results may be available for rapid interpretation and possible changes in the nursing plan of care.

Computerization should not be equated with a lack of personalized care. Computerization aims to provide a larger, more comprehensive database to provide improved client care and outcomes. Frequently clients require complex medical treatment and nursing care.

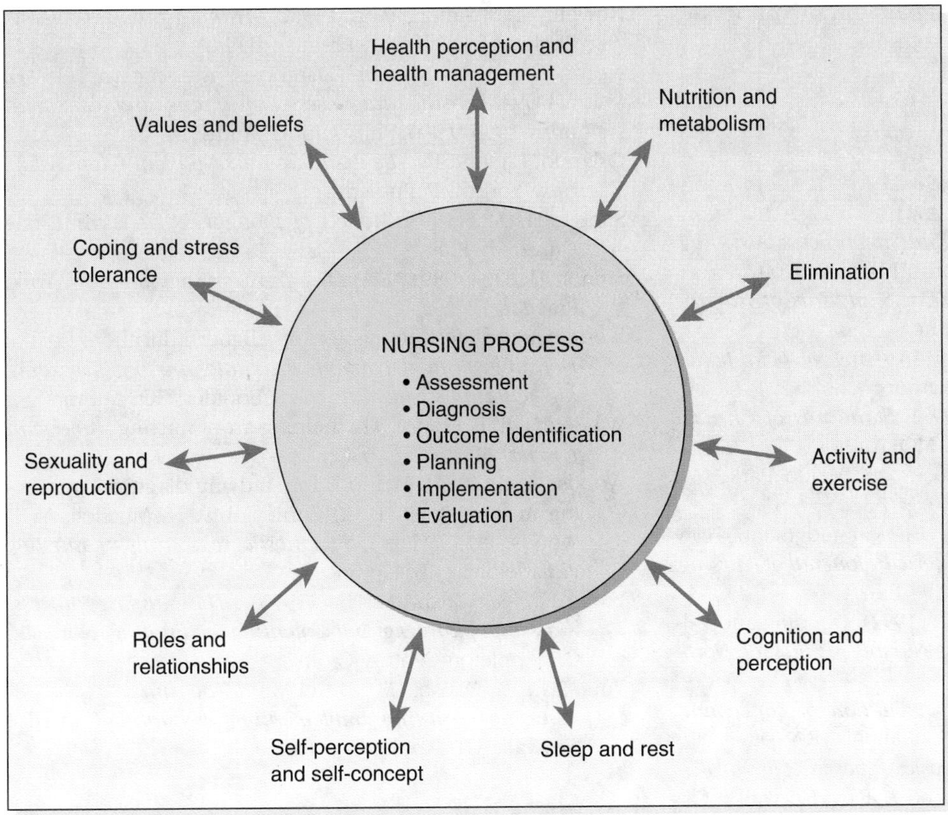

Figure 9-5 *• Functional health permeates every phase of the nursing process.*

Often the treatment involves the use of sophisticated technologic devices. In this technologic environment, it is important not to lose sight of the client's need for human touch.

As nursing diagnoses are researched and the taxonomy is scientifically validated, approaches to nursing care delivery can be standardized. Use of national health data bases will assist in evaluating and modifying nursing care. Nursing efforts are focusing on the development of a nursing intervention taxonomy and a client outcome taxonomy (Bulechek & McCloskey, 1992; Lang & Marek, 1990; McCloskey & Bulechek, 1994). There may be a need to develop a nursing assessment taxonomy as well.

Key Concepts

- The nursing process is the systematic, problem-solving approach to providing nursing care to clients, families, and communities.
- The nursing process has evolved over the last 40 years to consist of six phases: assessment, diagnosis, outcome identification, planning, implementation, and evaluation.
- The nursing process is used in all settings with clients of all ages to identify actual and potential health problems and design strategies to resolve them.
- Systems theory, the problem-solving process, decision-making process, information processing theory, and diagnostic reasoning process are the theoretical foundations for the nursing process.

Critical Thinking Challenges

Now turn back to the situation at the beginning of the chapter. You should be able to apply your basic information about nursing process to the care of the client when you consider the following critical thinking.

1. *Reflect on the assessment data of the client with the total hip replacement, and consider what you think are the client's problems. State whether they are actual problems or potential problems.*
2. *Determine the information processing methods (inductive and deductive) that you used to arrive at these problems, and validate your conclusions.*
3. *Explain how a sound knowledge base, ability to listen, and ability to communicate in writing are important in developing and implementing an*

individualized and effective plan of care for this client.

References

Alfaro-LeFevre, R. (1994). *Applying nursing process: A step-by-step guide* (3rd ed.). Philadelphia: J.B. Lippincott.

American Nurses Association. (1973). *Standards of nursing practice.* Kansas City, MO: Author.

American Nurses Association (1980). *Nursing: A social policy statement.* Kansas City, MO: Author.

American Nurses Association. (1991). *Standards of Clinical Nursing Practice.* Kansas City, MO: Author.

Benner, P. (1984). *From novice to expert.* Menlo Park, CA: Addison-Wesley.

Benner, P., & Tanner, C. (1987). Clinical judgment: How expert nurses use intuition. *American Journal of Nursing, 87,* 23–31.

Bulechek, G. M., & McCloskey, J. C. (1992). Defining and validating nursing interventions. *Nursing Clinics of North America, 27,* 289–297.

Fawcett, J. (1995). *Analysis and evaluation of conceptual models of nursing* (3rd ed.). Philadelphia: F.A. Davis.

George, J. B. (1990). *Nursing theories: The base for professional nursing practice* (3rd ed.). East Norwalk, CT: Appleton & Lange.

Gordon, M. (1982). *Nursing diagnosis: Process and application.* New York: McGraw-Hill.

Gordon, M. (1987). *Nursing diagnosis: Process and application* (2nd ed.). New York: McGraw-Hill.

Gordon, M. (1994). *Nursing diagnosis: Process and application* (3rd ed.). St. Louis: CV Mosby.

Johnson, D. (1959). A philosophy of nursing. *Nursing Outlook, 7,* 198–200.

Joint Commission on Accreditation of Healthcare Organizations. (1993). *1994 Accreditation manual for hospitals. Vol. 1. Standards.* Chicago: Author.

Knowles, L. (1967). *Decision-making in nursing: A necessity for doing.* New York: Appleton-Century-Crofts.

Lang, N. M., & Marek, K. D. (1990). The classification of patient outcomes. *Journal of Professional Nursing, 6*(3), 158–163.

McCloskey, J. C., & Bulechek, G. M. (1994). Standardizing the language for nursing treatments: An overview of the issues. *Nursing Outlook, 42,* 56–63.

Newell, A., & Simon, H. A. (1972). *Human problem-solving.* Englewood Cliffs, NJ: Prentice-Hall.

North American Nursing Diagnosis Association. (1994). *NANDA nursing diagnoses: Definitions and classifications 1995–1996.* Philadelphia: Author.

Orlando, I. J. (1961). *The dynamic nurse–patient relationship.* New York: G.P. Putnam.

Simon, H. A. (1979). *Models of thought.* New Haven: Yale University Press.

Sinnott, J. D. (1989). *Everyday problem-solving.* New York: Praeger.

Western Interstate Commission on Higher Education. (1967). *Defining clinical content, graduate nursing programs, medical and surgical nursing.* Boulder, CO: Author.

Wiedenbach, E. (1963). The helping art of nursing. *American Journal of Nursing, 63*(11), 54–57.

Woods, N. F. (1984). Methods for studying diagnostic reasoning in nursing. In D. L. Carnevali, P. H. Mitchell, N. F. Woods, et al. (Eds.), *Diagnostic reasoning in nursing.* Philadelphia: J.B. Lippincott.

Yura, H., & Walsh, M. B. (1973). *The nursing process: Assessing, planning, implementing, evaluating.* Norwalk, CT: Appleton-Century-Crofts.

Yura, H., & Walsh, M. B. (1988). *The nursing process: Assessing, planning, implementing, evaluating* (5th ed.). Norwalk, CT: Appleton & Lange.

Bibliography

Carpenito, L. J. (1995). *Nursing diagnosis: Application to clinical practice* (6th ed.). Philadelphia: J. B. Lippincott.

Coyle, L. A., & Sokop, A. G. (1990). Innovation adoption behavior among nurses. *Nursing Research, 39,* 176–180.

Hamers, J. P. H., Abu-Saad, H. H., & Halfens, R. J. G. (1994). Diagnostic process and decision making in nursing: A literature review. *Journal of Professional Nursing 10* (3), 154–163.

Harvey, R. M. (1991). Nursing diagnosis by neural networks: A new aid for nursing practice. In R. M. Carroll-Johnson (Ed.), *Classification of nursing diagnoses: Proceedings of the ninth conference.* Philadelphia: J.B. Lippincott.

Roberts, J. D., While, A. E., & Fitzpatrick, J. M. (1993). Problem solving in nursing practice: Application, process, skill acquisition and measurement. *Journal of Advanced Nursing, 18,* 886–891.

Solomon, J. (1990). Physical assessment skills in undergraduate curricula. *Nursing Outlook, 38,* 194–195.

Nursing Assessment

Key Terms	Learning Objectives

Key Terms

Assessment
Auscultation
Cue
Inspection
Interviewing
Intuition
Objective data
Observation
Palpation
Percussion
Physical examination
Subjective data
Validation

Learning Objectives

Upon completion of this chapter, the student will be able to do the following:

- *Define the assessment phase of the nursing process.*
- *Discuss the purpose of assessment in nursing practice.*
- *Identify the skills required for nursing assessment.*
- *Differentiate the three major activities involved in nursing assessment.*
- *Describe the process of data collection.*
- *Explain the rationale for data validation.*
- *Discuss the frameworks used to organize assessment data.*
- *Perform a nursing assessment using a functional health approach.*

10

You are a nurse working in a busy medical clinic attached to a large medical center. An older man comes alone to the health clinic. You are asked to make an initial health assessment. His major complaint is generalized abdominal pain and decreased appetite. His wife of 51 years died 2 months ago. He moves slowly but appears steady on his feet. He is able to answer questions, but he does not look directly at you and mumbles his responses. You have 15 minutes to complete your health assessment.

In the previous chapter you were introduced to the nursing process. Now, as you study this chapter, you will begin to focus more closely on the aspect of nursing assessment. When you have completed the chapter you will have expanded your knowledge base about nursing process and be better able to address the older man's complaints and problems. Critical Thinking Challenges at the end of the chapter will help you consider your assessment skills.

The first phase of the nursing process is called **assessment**. Assessment is the collection of data for nursing purposes. The nurse uses many skills to collect information, including observation, interviewing, physical examination, and intuition. Data or information are collected from many sources, including clients, their family members or significant others, health records, other health team members, and literature review. Figure 10-1 shows the assessment phase in relation to the other phases in the nursing process. Interpretation or analysis of the data takes place in the diagnosis phase of the nursing process. Many frameworks have been developed to organize assessment data; they are discussed at the end of this chapter.

Assessment is the phase of the nursing process during which data are gathered for the purpose of identifying actual or potential health problems. Accurate assessment information is essential for the provision of high-quality nursing care.

Although there may be overlap in the collection of some data by other members of the healthcare team, the specific way in which the data are used differs from

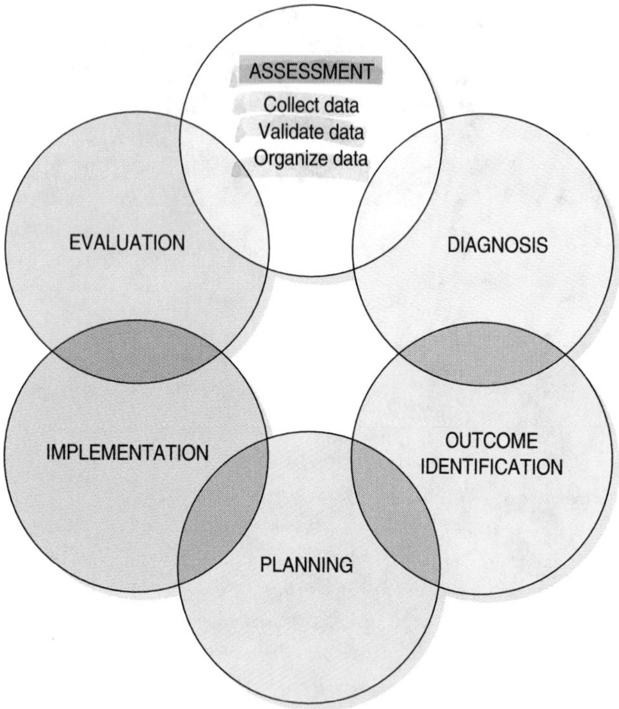

Figure 10-1 • *ANA Standard I states: The nurse collects client health data. This illustration shows activities used in the Assessment phase and also the relationship of Assessment to the other phases of the nursing process.*

one profession to another. Nursing assessment focuses on the gathering of data about a client's state of wellness, functional ability, physical status, strengths, and responses to actual and potential health problems (Gordon, 1987; 1994).

The purpose of nursing assessment is to gather data about the client that can be used in diagnosing, identifying outcomes, planning, and implementing care. Assessment is done to

- Establish baseline information on the client
- Determine the client's normal function
- Determine the presence or absence of dysfunction
- Determine the client's strengths
- Provide data for the diagnosis phase.

The activities that make up the assessment phase are

- Collect data
- Validate data
- Organize data.

These activities and various frameworks to organize assessment data are discussed later in this chapter.

Preparing for Assessment

Types of Assessment

Assessment takes many forms depending on the clinical situation, client status, time available, and purpose of data collection. The types of assessment are the initial assessment, focus assessment, time-lapsed reassessment, and emergency assessment (Table 10-1).

Initial Assessment

An initial assessment, also called an admission assessment, is performed at the time the client enters the healthcare facility. The purposes are to evaluate the client's health status, to identify functional health patterns that are problematic, and to provide an in-depth, comprehensive database, which is critical for evaluating changes in the client's health status in subsequent assessments (Gordon, 1982; 1987; 1994).

This type of assessment is usually performed by a professional registered nurse. If a thorough assessment cannot be completed because of the client's health status or urgency of specific health problems, it is finished at a later time. Frequently, parts of the admission assessment are delegated to nonprofessional staff members. Even if parts of the assessment are delegated to others, however, the professional registered nurse is ultimately responsible for the completeness and accuracy of the information. The Joint Commission on the Accreditation of Healthcare Organizations (1993) mandates that each client have a documented nursing admission assessment that follows institutional policies.

Focus Assessment

The goal of the focus assessment is to collect data about a problem already identified. This type of assessment has a narrower scope and a shorter time frame than the initial assessment. The nurse determines if the problem still exists and whether the status of the problem has changed (eg, improved, worsened, or resolved). This assessment also includes the appraisal of any new, overlooked, or misdiagnosed problems. In the intensive care unit, the nurse may perform focus assessments every few minutes for a critically ill client.

Often, the nurse assesses the client for a specific problem and provides nursing care at the same time. For example, while bathing a client with weakness in the lower extremities, the nurse can assess the client's muscular strength and ability to perform self-care activities (Gordon, 1982; 1987; 1994).

Time-Lapsed Reassessment

Time-lapsed reassessment is another type of assessment that takes place after the initial assessment is performed. The aim of the time-lapsed reassessment is to evaluate any changes in the client's functional health. It is performed when substantial periods of time have elapsed between assessments. Like the focus assessment, it determines the status of problems already identified. Because of the varying time interval between reassessments (eg, 3 to 12 months), a complete review of all functional health patterns is carried out. For exam-

Table 10-1 • Types, Aims, and Time Frame for Assessment

Type	Aim	Time Frame
Initial assessment	Initial identification of normal function, functional status, and collection of data concerning actual or potential dysfunction Provide baseline for reference and future comparison	Within the specified time frame after admission to a hospital, nursing home, ambulatory healthcare center, or home healthcare setting
Focus assessment	Determine status of a specific problem identified during previous assessment	Ongoing process; integrated with nursing care; a few minutes to a few hours between assessments
Time-lapsed reassessment	Comparison of client's current status to baseline obtained previously; detection of changes in all functional health patterns after an extended period of time has passed	Several months (3, 6, or 9 months or more) between assessments
Emergency assessment	Identification of life-threatening situation	Anytime a physiologic, psychological, or emotional crisis occurs

ple, several weeks or months may lapse between reassessments of a client in an ambulatory setting. Time-lapsed reassessment is usually less comprehensive than the initial assessment (Gordon, 1987; 1994).

Emergency Assessment

Emergency assessment takes place in life-threatening situations in which the preservation of life is the top priority. Time is of the essence for rapid identification of and intervention for the client's health problems. Often the client's difficulties involve airway, breathing, and circulatory problems (the ABCs). Abrupt changes in self-concept (suicidal thoughts) or roles or relationships (social conflict leading to violent acts) can also initiate an emergency (Gordon, 1987; 1994). Emergency assessment focuses on a few essential health patterns, and is not comprehensive.

Setting and Environment

Assessment can take place in any setting where nurses care for clients and their family members: in the client's home, at a clinic, in a hospital room, at a health fair, or at the client's workplace. The client's physical comfort helps facilitate data collection, so the assessment should be scheduled at an appropriate time of day so that the client is not tired, hungry, or in pain.

The nurse must be aware of environmental factors conducive to the collection of accurate and complete assessment data. An assessment is best performed in a quiet, private setting that lends itself to the discussion of sensitive, personal, and confidential information. The setting must be restricted or secluded to prevent the client's undue embarrassment during the interview and physical examination. The nurse may ask visitors and family members to leave the room temporarily (Smeltzer & Bare, 1992). Distractions should be minimized (eg, television or radio, announcements over the intercom, a too-hot or too-cold room). The nurse may need to close the door, pull the curtains, turn down the heat, or move the client to another place if the environment cannot be modified.

Assessment Skills

Nurses use a variety of skills as they assess clients and their family members. Assessment skills are important in obtaining comprehensive data. One can read about various skills, but it is through actual clinical experience and use of these skills that proficiency in nursing assessment is developed. Assessment involves recognizing and collecting **cues**, pieces of information about a client's health status. Cues may be overt (objective) or covert (subjective). Examples of overt cues are a description of an incision site ("reddened, swollen") or a blood pressure measurement (180/110); an example of a covert clue is the client's statement, "I have a sharp pain in my shoulder." In the diagnosis phase, these cues are interpreted, clustered, and analyzed. Subjective and objective data are further defined in the section on Assessment Activities in this chapter.

The clinical skills of observation, interviewing, physical examination, and intuition are used to assess

Table 10-2 • *Clinical Skills Used in Assessment*

Type	Definition
Observation	The act of noticing client cues
Interviewing	Interaction and communication process for gathering data by questioning and information exchange
Physical examination	Analysis of bodily functioning using the techniques of inspection, palpation, percussion, and auscultation
Intuition	Use of insights, instincts, or clinical experience to make judgments about client care

clients across the lifespan in a variety of settings. The nurse uses these skills simultaneously when assessing clients. For example, during the client interview, the nurse asks questions, observes the client, listens to the client's answers, and mentally stores information for further exploration during the physical examination. The clinical skills used in assessment are summarized in Table 10-2.

Nurses come in contact with clients of all ages. Assessment techniques are modified according to the age and developmental stage of the client. Assessing a child often involves parental assistance; the parent may hold the child on his or her lap to facilitate examination. Distraction techniques, such as flashing a light or moving an object, are helpful to divert an infant's attention during assessment (eg, when examining the ear) (Bates, 1995). When assessing an obese client, a larger blood pressure cuff may be needed. The nurse may need to speak more slowly and distinctly when examining an elderly client with degenerative hearing loss. An elderly client with joint problems or muscular weakness may require additional time to change positions during the physical examination.

Observation

Observation lays the groundwork for collecting other kinds of assessment data. As assessment proceeds, the nurse anticipates the type of information that will be necessary or appropriate to obtain for a particular client. **Observation** comprises more than the nurse's ability to "see" the client; the nurse uses the senses of vision, smell, hearing, and touch (the sense of taste is rarely used) (Gordon, 1987, 1994; Yura & Walsh, 1988).

Observation begins the moment the nurse meets the client. As the client walks into the room, gets out of the wheelchair, or is assisted into bed, the nurse is constantly observing, using all the appropriate sensory modalities. Observation includes looking, watching, examining, scrutinizing, surveying, scanning, or appraising. Using his or her knowledge of nursing care, physical assessment, basic sciences, social sciences, and pathophysiology, the nurse observes clients in a sophisticated manner. Intellectual skills also come into play as the nurse makes decisions about what data are needed to complete the assessment.

Vision

The sense of vision is used in a specialized manner. The nurse's ability to survey how the client "looks" is key. Does the client show signs of distress or discomfort, such as grimacing, scowling, or frowning, and guarding or holding a body part? Is the client sitting upright in a chair with arms resting comfortably at the sides, or curled up in bed? What is the client's body size and nutritional status: overweight, obese, normal weight, or undernourished and emaciated? What is the client's preferred posture? Can he or she walk? Are there abnormal movements?

How is the client groomed and dressed? Is the client's clothing clean, excessively worn, or inappropriate for the season or weather? If a client's appearance and clothing are disheveled, further information is needed to determine if the client is homeless or has a physical or mental condition contributing to self-neglect. The nurse must compare the client's appearance to the probable norm for the client, taking into account the client's lifestyle, occupation, age, and socioeconomic group (Bates, 1995; Yura & Walsh, 1988).

Nonverbal behavior is noted during every interaction with the client. The client's nonverbal demeanor yields information about feelings toward the nurse, staff, and family (Sundeen, et al., 1994). Does the client show any signs of anger, suspicion, anxiety, or hostility? For example, the client may deny any anxiety or apprehension about health problems, but may have an anxious facial expression or tear-filled eyes. The client may be argumentative and hostile with family members, but cooperative and friendly with staff.

Smell

A keen sense of smell is used when observing the client. The nurse notes any body or breath odors that may indicate an underlying physical condition. For example, foul-smelling breath may signify an oral or pulmonary infection. A fruity breath odor may indicate a metabolic disorder such as ketosis in diabetes mellitus. Alcohol on the client's breath can mean that alcohol intake is one explanation for mental and physical findings (Bates, 1995). Body odors indicate sweat and sebaceous gland function and the client's overall cleanliness. A homeless person may have body odors related to lifestyle circumstances and the inability to bathe.

Hearing

Observation includes the nurse's ability to listen to and hear what the client says. The client's level of consciousness and awareness of the surroundings are noted. The client's ability to state his or her name, location, and date accurately is determined as the nurse asks questions and observes how the client answers. The ability to initiate conversation or to respond only when spoken to gives clues about the client's mental and physical condition. If the client is confused, the nurse should question the validity of the information obtained; family members or significant others, if available, can provide information for the confused or incapacitated client.

Touch

General observations continue through the use of touch. Touch is used to greet the client (a handshake), to provide nonverbal communication and reassurance, and to perform a preliminary appraisal of skin temperature and moisture. The nurse observes the presence of perspiration, warmth or coldness, and strength of the client's handshake. A gentle touch on the arm or hand may reassure the client and at the same time reveal dry, scaly skin indicative of dehydration or thyroid problems. A specialized kind of touching called palpation is performed during the physical examination.

The nurse must consider the client's sociocultural background when using touch. In some cultures, the use of touch must be modified to minimize the client's sense that privacy has been invaded. Clients of some cultures may interpret touching as a hostile action.

Interviewing

The nurse must be an effective communicator to conduct a successful interview. Among the factors affecting the quality and comprehensiveness of the interview are the nurse's skill and experience and the client's willingness to share information.

There are several techniques that facilitate communication between the nurse and the client. These techniques establish rapport, help the nurse elicit the client's thoughts and feelings, encourage conversation, and ensure mutual understanding (Stuart & Cash, 1985; Sundeen, et al., 1994). Barriers that hinder interaction have the opposite effect on communication (Carpenito, 1995; Sundeen, et al., 1994). Table 10-3 summarizes the facilitators and barriers to effective communication. Communication techniques are further discussed in Chapter 20.

Interviewing is an essential skill for obtaining information for the nursing history, which consists of questions designed to elicit subjective data from the client or family members. The nursing history focuses on the client's account of the impact of actual or potential health problems on his or her functional health status. The nursing history helps to

- Clarify and verify the client's perception of his or her functional health status
- Compare the client's present and past functional health status, lifestyle behaviors, and coping abilities
- Identify actual and potential nursing diagnoses
- Develop the nursing management plan
- Implement nursing interventions supportive of the client's adaptive responses.

Healthcare institutions usually have a form for the systematic collection and documentation of the nursing history. Such documentation improves communication between nursing staff and other health team members.

A nursing history can take 30 to 60 minutes to perform. Although usually completed in one session, it may be obtained over several sessions. If the client's condition (eg, severe pain, breathing difficulties) or the setting (eg, excessive noise, lack of privacy) makes data collection difficult, the nurse can collect information

Table 10-3 • Techniques that Facilitate and Block Communication During an Interview

Facilitators of Communication	Barriers to Communication
Use broad opening statements	Make stereotyped comments
Give general leads	Give advice or state your opinion
Listen	Agree with the client
Acknowledge the client's feelings	Defend
Use silence	Give approval
Give information	Use reassuring clichés
Reflect or repeat the client's words	Request an explanation
Share observations	Express disapproval
Clarify	Belittle the patient's feelings
Summarize	Change the subject
Validate	Disagree with the client
Verbalize implied thoughts or feelings	

about urgent problems and defer other questions until a more suitable time.

An interview can be divided into four phases: preparatory, introductory, maintenance, and concluding.

Preparatory Phase

The preparatory or preinteraction phase occurs before the nurse meets the client. Actions taken in this phase help ensure that the interview will be as productive as possible. The nurse's attention is directed toward preparing for the first nurse–client interaction. During this phase, the nurse does the following (Sundeen, et al., 1994):

- Reviews as much information as possible about the client
- Decides what data are needed and what type of data collection form will be used
- Reviews the literature pertinent to the client's developmental age, psychosocial aspects, and pathophysiologic considerations, if needed
- Assesses his or her feelings or reactions to previous clients that may interfere with the nurse–client relationship
- Seeks assistance from more experienced nurses, mentors, or supervisors if concerned about how to carry out the interview
- Plans for a private, quiet setting for the interview, schedules a mutually convenient time of day, and determines the length of time needed for data collection
- Modifies the environment to facilitate the interview.

Introductory Phase

The second phase of an interview is called the introductory phase. Also known as the orientation phase, the introductory phase begins when the nurse and client meet. The nurse's actions in this phase assist in establishing rapport, clarifying roles, and alleviating anxiety. The nurse and client are actively involved in asking questions, getting acquainted, and exchanging their expectations for the interview and health assessment. During this phase, the nurse does the following (Sundeen, et al., 1994):

- Introduces self by name and position and explains the purpose and content of the interview
- Begins to establish rapport with the client by conveying a caring, interested attitude; rapport is essential for a trusting, helpful nurse–client relationship
- Observes the client's behavior and listens attentively to determine the client's self-perceptions and the way the client sees his or her health problems; validates the client's perceptions as the interview progresses
- Lets the client know how long the nurse–client relationship is expected to last
- Informs the client how the information collected will be used
- Starts with nonthreatening, specific questions and proceeds to open-ended questions
- Establishes a verbal contract with the client, incorporating the goals of the interview.

Maintenance Phase

The maintenance phase is the third phase of an interview. In the maintenance or working phase, the nurse and client work toward achieving the specific task or goal agreed on in the introductory phase. Both participants maintain the interaction for the purpose of getting the "work" done, but it is the nurse's responsibility to ensure that the goals are met. The goals may be mutually revised by the client and nurse. In this phase, the nurse does the following (Sundeen, et al., 1994):

- Keeps focused on the tasks or goals to ensure that needed data are obtained and goals are achieved
- Encourages the client to express his or her feelings, concerns, and questions
- Uses techniques that facilitate communication between the nurse and client (eg, silence, using general leads, validating)
- Observes the nonverbal behavior that accompanies verbal responses (eg, a client may say she is not nervous, worried, or anxious, but she bites her fingernails, moves constantly, and smokes throughout the interview)
- Assesses the client's ability to continue the interview (eg, grimace of pain, shortness of breath, fatigue)
- Facilitates goal attainment by moving to the next topic of discussion after needed data are collected.

Concluding Phase

In the concluding or termination phase, the nurse–client relationship is completed. Actions taken in this phase can help ensure that the termination will be a positive experience for both participants. The nurse focuses on reviewing goals or tasks attained and expressing concerns related to this phase. In this phase, the nurse does the following (Sundeen, et al., 1994):

- Reviews goal or task attainment; such a review can foster a sense of achievement in the client and nurse
- Summarizes the highlights of the interview and its meaning to the nurse and the client
- Encourages the client to express and share his or her feelings regarding the termination of the nurse–client relationship

- Uses language congruent with the client's cultural background and local custom (eg, "good-bye" may mean a final farewell in some cultures; promises to contact the client in the future may be taken literally).

Physical Examination Techniques

The **physical examination** is a systematic data collection method that uses the senses of sight, hearing, smell, and touch to detect health problems. It is divided into four techniques: inspection, palpation, percussion, and auscultation. Usually, the nursing interview is completed before the physical examination is performed. The physical examination is used to verify and expand the data gathered during the nursing interview (Gordon, 1982; 1987; 1994). More details on physical examination techniques can be found in Chapter 21.

Inspection

Inspection is a visual examination of the client done in a methodical and deliberate manner. It begins with the nurse's first contact with the client and is conducted intentionally and continuously so that important data are not omitted. Inspection is not haphazard or passive. It is an important first step in the physical examination process. As the nurse inspects the client, the underlying anatomic structures are considered and any abnormalities that may be present are identified. Factors such as color, shape, symmetry, movement, pulsations, and texture of the involved body part are noted (Bates, 1995; Fuller & Schaller-Ayers, 1994).

Inspection is carried out during the interview and subsequent physical examination. For example, an enlarged thyroid or growth in the neck may be visible while interviewing a client. Detailed inspection of the neck would take place after the interview.

Palpation

Palpation is the specialized use of touch for the collection of data that augment the inspection process. By using the fingertips and palms of the hand, the nurse can determine the size, shape, and configuration of underlying body structures. The pulsations of blood vessels; the outline of organs such as the thyroid, spleen, or liver; the size, shape, and mobility of masses; the temperature of the skin; vibration or movement of blood in a blood vessel; and tenderness or sensitivity of a body part are detected.

Percussion

Percussion is a technique in which one or both hands are used to strike the body surface to produce a sound called a percussion note. Underlying body structures have characteristic percussion notes that indicate their denseness or hollowness. Percussion is used to discover the location and level of organs (liver, heart, diaphragm), the consistency of body structures (fluid-filled, air-filled, or solid), the presence of tenderness (over the kidneys or near the spine), and the identification of masses or tumors.

Nursing Research
Nursing Assessment

Selected Nursing Research Studies

Cronin-Stubbs, D., Swanson, B., Dean-Baar, S., et al. (1992). The effects of a training program on nurses' functional performance assessments. *Applied Nursing Research, 5*(1), 38–43.

Henning, M. (1991). Comparison of nursing diagnostic statements using a functional health pattern and health history/body systems format. In R. M. Carroll-Johnson (Ed.), *Classification of nursing diagnoses: Proceedings of the ninth conference, North American Nursing Diagnosis Association* (pp. 278–279). Philadelphia: J. B. Lippincott.

Miller, V. G. (1993). Measurement of self-perception of intuitiveness. *Western Journal of Nursing Research, 15,* 595–606.

Minton, J. A., & Creason, N. S. (1991). Evaluation of admission nursing diagnoses. *Nursing Diagnosis, 2,* 119–125.

Monninger, E., Padgett, D., & Fleeger, M. E. (1994). Functional health pattern nursing assessment for BSN students. In R. M. Carroll-Johnson & M. Pacquette (Eds.), *Classification of nursing diagnoses: Proceedings of the tenth conference, North American Nursing Diagnosis Association* (p. 341). Philadelphia: J. B. Lippincott.

Possible Topics for Nursing Inquiry

- Do graduate nurses and experienced nurses differ in the way they view functional health pattern assessment?
- What is the effect of the documentation of functional health pattern assessment on nurses' participation in client-care decisions?
- Does functional health pattern assessment facilitate the development of new nursing diagnoses?

Auscultation

Auscultation is the technique of listening to body sounds with a stethoscope. It yields information about the movement of air or fluid in the body. The stethoscope is placed on the body surface to amplify normal and abnormal sounds. Mastery of auscultation lies in the interpretation of the findings. Consulting nurses who are more experienced and proficient in identification of auscultation sounds can be helpful in developing proficiency. Various body systems, including the respiratory, cardiovascular, and gastrointestinal systems are auscultated for characteristic sounds. Bowel sounds, breath sounds, heart sounds, and the sound of blood moving through a narrowed or twisted blood vessel (known as a bruit) are heard through auscultation.

Intuition

Intuition has only recently been acknowledged as a legitimate part of nursing practice. It is defined as the use of insight, instinct, and clinical experience to make clinical judgments about the client. "Although not validated or valued in traditional ways, intuitive knowledge appears to be used by nurses, particularly expert nurses, in many aspects of clinical practice" (Beckett, 1990).

Intuition plays a role in the nurse's ability to analyze cues rapidly, make clinical decisions, and implement nursing actions even though assessment data may be incomplete or ambiguous (Rew, 1988). In the past, the concept of intuition appeared infrequently in nursing literature, but nurse researchers and scholars are beginning to examine its role in the various phases of the nursing process. Research results imply that the nursing process addresses only part of the problem-solving process used by nurses (Rew & Barrow, 1989). Rew (1988) found that most experienced nurses used intuition in the assessment and implementation phases of the nursing process.

Intuition comes into play when assessment data are incomplete, sketchy, or vague, or when the client looks all right on the surface but the nurse senses that something is not quite right. For example, before obtaining complete assessment data, a nurse may enter a client's room and get a strong "feel" about the client's condition without performing a physical examination or reading the chart. Or a nurse may sense that a client with normal vital signs, skin color, and neurologic status is going to have a cardiac or respiratory arrest (Rew, 1988). In the two situations described, the nurse uses intuitive knowledge to analyze cues, make clinical decisions, and implement nursing interventions on behalf of the client. Intuition results in decisions that might not have been made had the nurse used the nursing process alone.

Assessment Activities

During the assessment phase, the nurse collects, validates, and organizes data. Because these activities are so closely related, the nurse often shifts from one to another, perhaps collecting and organizing data at the same time. The nurse may choose to validate information as it is collected rather than at the completion of data collection. As data are organized, the nurse may discover an ambiguous cue that requires further clarification and validation with the client.

Collect Data

The process of compiling information about the client is called data collection. Data collection begins with the first contact with the client and is done by observation, interviewing, and physical examination. Usually, data are collected using a systematic format that ensures comprehensive, accurate information.

Types of Data

Objective and subjective data, both integral parts of assessment, are obtained during data collection. Table 10-4 shows the differences in the methods of obtaining subjective and objective data, and provides examples of each type.

Subjective data, also known as symptoms or covert cues, include the client's feelings and statements about his or her health problems. Subjective data are supplied by the client, and it is not always feasible to validate, confirm, or substantiate them through other sources. Often the nurse tries to validate subjective data through objective data collection. Subjective data are obtained through the interview, and are best recorded as a direct quote from the client:

"I haven't felt good for the last couple of months."
"I get a sharp pain in my stomach after I eat."
"Every time I move, I feel nauseated."

Objective data, also known as signs or overt cues, are observable, perceptible, and measurable. They can be validated or verified by others. Examples include bowel sounds, temperature reading, peripheral pulses, distended neck vessels, and skin rashes. Objective data may be obtained by the senses (eg, vision, touch, smell) or by measuring devices or equipment (eg, thermometer, sphygmomanometer), laboratory studies (eg, complete blood count), or diagnostic procedures (eg, colonoscopy).

Sources of Data

Two major sources of data exist for the collection of information about the client. The client is considered the

Table 10-4 • Comparison of Subjective and Objective Data

	Subjective Data (Covert Cues)	Objective Data (Overt Cues)
Method of Obtaining Data	Interview	Techniques of inspection, palpation, percussion, and auscultation Measurement devices Health record Laboratory studies, radiologic tests, diagnostic procedures
Examples	Symptoms Values Perceptions Feelings Attitudes Sensations Beliefs	Physical examination findings: heart sounds, palpable tumor, discolored skin Blood pressure, temperature, intracranial pressure Written reports of other health-team members on health record Complete blood count results, chest radiography results

primary source of data because only he or she can give a first-hand description of the health problem and its effects on his or her lifestyle. All other sources, such as family members, significant others, other members of the healthcare team, laboratory tests, and literature review are considered secondary sources.

Primary Sources. The client is the primary source of data. Information collected from the client is considered to be the most reliable. Skills used for obtaining information from the client include observation, interview, and physical examination. Assessment data are elicited from the client unless circumstances such as altered level of consciousness, severe pain, impending surgery, acute illness, or age make data collection impossible. The client is deemed unreliable if he or she is confused or suffering from physical or mental conditions that alter thinking, judgment, or memory. In situations in which the client is unreliable, secondary sources help provide the necessary assessment information.

Secondary Sources. There are several secondary sources of data. Secondary sources provide data that supplement, clarify, and validate information obtained from the client. These include family members or significant others, the health record, laboratory tests and diagnostic procedures, health team members, and literature review.

Family members or significant others supplement and verify information obtained from the client. They can provide information that the client forgets to mention or is unwilling to reveal. They may be the only source of data for children or for confused, unresponsive, or severely ill clients. Data provided by family members and significant others include a description of how the client reacts to illness, the client's perceptions of changes in functional health, the client's ability to cope with life stressors, and information about the client's home situation.

Usually the client's permission is obtained *before* seeking information from family members or significant others. All people involved must understand the confidential nature of the information they provide. The client's permission must also be obtained to divulge any information (eg, diagnosis of cancer, AIDS, pregnancy) to family members or significant others.

Past and current health records—items such as consultation reports, medical and nursing histories, and physical examination findings—contain a wealth of information about the client and are helpful in completing assessment data. Facts about the client's previous illnesses, hospitalizations, function, and dysfunction are obtained. The health record may also reveal data not expressed by the client or picked up by the nurse. Reviewing health records can also reduce the number of times a client is asked the same questions by various health team members.

Laboratory tests and diagnostic procedures are another secondary source of data for the completion of the data base. They clarify, supplement, and verify findings from the interview and physical examination. Laboratory tests are always interpreted in relation to the client's underlying health problems and treatment modalities. These results can also identify actual or potential health problems not disclosed by the client or explored by the nurse. Sometimes laboratory tests and diagnostic procedures are used to judge the effectiveness of nursing interventions.

Written and verbal reports from other health team members are another source of assessment data. The nurse can take advantage of the expertise of other colleagues caring for the client: all of them are valuable sources of information about the client's current and past health status. By consulting other health team members, the nurse verifies and supplements the assessment data. Health team members include professional staff such as nurses, social workers, physical therapists, physicians, clergy, and respiratory therapists, and nonprofessional personnel such as nursing assistants.

Reviewing the literature helps complete the client's database. Pertinent literature includes textbooks, journals, dissertation abstracts, and unpublished monographs presented at professional meetings. The client's health patterns must be viewed in relation to current knowledge and theory. A thorough review of the literature provides information on recent developments in nursing and medical practice.

Recording Data

Using a framework or outline, assessment data are systematically recorded and become a permanent part of the medical record. Institutions usually have a specific form for recording data and facilitating its use by other nurses caring for the client. Baseline assessment data are referred to periodically to reaffirm assessment findings and to compare the client's current status to his or her initial condition. Two methods can be used: the traditional written assessment record and the computerized assessment record. Chapter 14 discusses documentation of client assessment in detail.

Traditional Written Assessment Record. Traditionally, while assessment data are collected, the nurse takes notes throughout the nursing interview and physical examination. After the health assessment, an in-depth recording of findings is made. The nurse follows institutional policy and records the data by hand on the appropriate forms. Depending on the examiner's skill and the number of health problems the client has, recording assessment data can be time consuming. The more experienced nurse can take notes on the appropriate forms as the interview proceeds and summarize comments quickly and efficiently.

Computerized Assessment Record. Computerization of health records has led to a new format for recording assessment data: the computerized nursing assessment record. In many institutions, assessment data can be entered into a computer at the client's bedside using a computer screen format (Meyer, 1992). Instead of writing the data on client record forms, data are entered into the computer by typing on the keyboard. The time required to enter the data depends on the nurse's familiarity with computers and typing proficiency. Some computerized systems incorporate other types of data,

Examples of Cues and Inferences

Example 1

Group of Cues

Client has

- Blurry vision or visual defect
- Headache
- Tingling and numbness in extremities
- Dizziness

Possible Inferences

- Client has a brain tumor.
- Client is having warning signals of a stroke
- Client may be diabetic
- Client is anxious

Example 2

Cue

Mr. Spencer has dry, flaky skin

Possible Inferences

1. Mr. Spencer may be dehydrated.
2. Mr. Spencer has hypothyroidism.
3. Mr. Spencer has some type of dermatitis.

Example 3

Cue

Client has frequency and burning on urination.

Inference

Client has a urinary tract infection.

Example 4

Cue

Mrs. Smith's blood sugar is 55 mg/dL.

Inference

Mrs. Smith is suffering from a hypoglycemic reaction.

Example 5

Cue

Client states, "I just can't seem to shake this pain in my joints."

Inference

Client has inadequate pain management.

such as laboratory test data and diagnostic study results. This facilitates the retrieval of these data for nursing purposes. For example, a laboratory blood test result can be obtained by computer, rather than waiting for the report to arrive on the client care unit or calling the laboratory personnel for a verbal report. The nurse can immediately incorporate these data into the client's functional health assessment.

Validate Data

Validation is the process of confirming the accuracy of assessment data collected. It is commonly referred to as double-checking the information at hand. As the nurse collects data, multiple cues are identified. Inferences are made about the cues; that is, a meaning or interpretation is attached to the cue. One or more inferences can be made about a particular cue or group of cues (Alfaro-LeFevre, 1994), as seen in the examples provided in the display.

The nurse must make sure that the cues and inferences are correct. Validation assists in the verification and clarification of cues and inferences and increases the likelihood that cues and inferences are accurate, free from bias, and interpreted correctly (Alfaro-LeFevre, 1994). Incorrect cues and inferences lead to the development of inappropriate nursing diagnoses and nursing management plans. Figure 10-2 illustrates the connection between cues and inferences and methods for the validation of data.

Identification of relevant cues and correct inferences depends on the nurse's clinical nursing knowledge, assessment skills, personal values, and past experience (Alfaro-LeFevre, 1994). Inferences must be validated before the clustering and analysis of cues and identification of nursing diagnoses.

Methods of validating data include (Alfaro-LeFevre, 1994)

- Comparing cues to normal function. For example, Mr. Jones is a professional athlete and has a resting pulse of 50 beats per minute; the nurse knows that physiologic heart changes in physically fit people can result in a slower pulse rate (bradycardia).
- Referring to textbooks, journals, and research reports. For example, the nurse may consider brown macules or "liver spots" on the hands and forearms of an elderly client as abnormal. After checking a textbook on physical changes that occur with aging, the nurse learns that they are common in the elderly.
- Checking consistency of cues. Data can be checked, for example, by retaking the client's temperature or blood pressure or by using another piece of equipment. Subjective and objective data can be compared. For example, the client may state, "I feel hot," but his or her temperature is 98.6°F, or the client may state, "I can't get my breath," but respirations are 20 and lung sounds are clear.

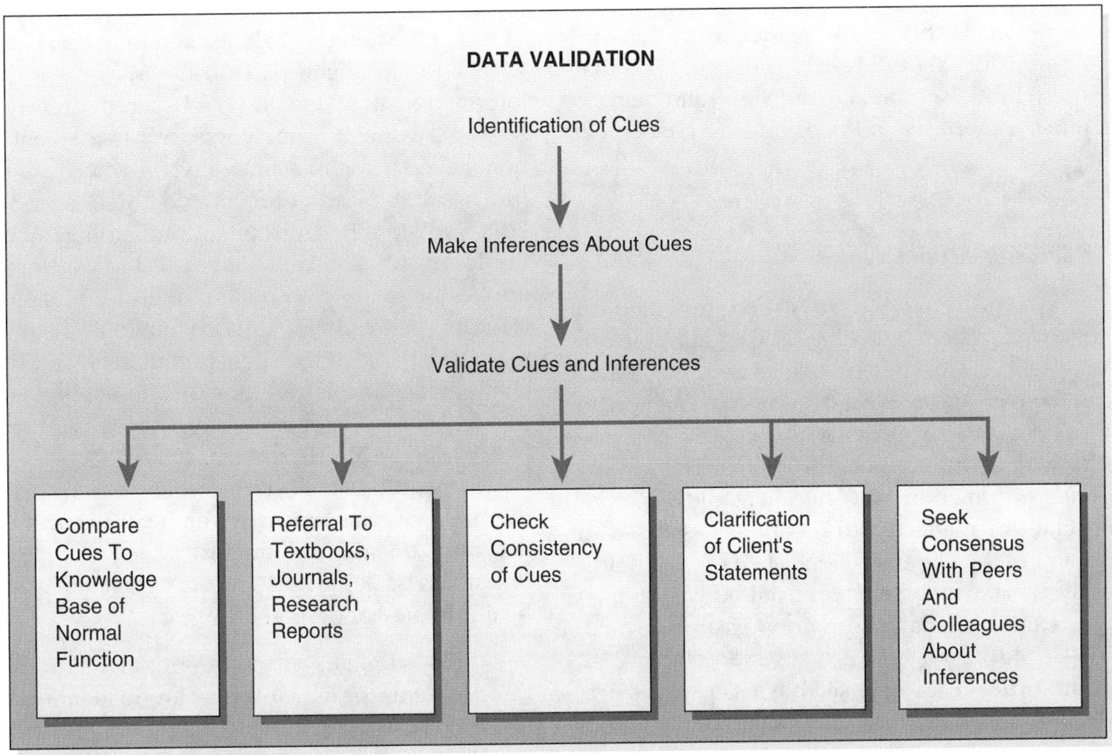

Figure 10-2 • *Methods for the validation of cues and inferences.*

- Clarifying the client's statements. Ask specific, closed-ended questions, share observations with the client and family members, clarify ambiguous or vague statements, and verify inferences.
- Seeking consensus with colleagues about inferences. This is usually done after the data have been validated using the above methods. If peers or colleagues independently reach the same conclusion as you, and that conclusion is based on valid data, your inferences are supported. If colleagues present an alternative view, it assists the nurse in questioning the validity of his or her own inferences.

Organize Data

There are a variety of frameworks for the orderly collection and recording of assessment data. The framework serves as a guide during the nursing interview and physical examination, helps prevent the omission of pertinent information, and fosters data analysis in the diagnosis phase. The framework may be modified based on the client's physical status and on the nurse's personal preference (Fuller & Schaller-Ayers, 1994).

Nursing conceptual models provide one such framework. Institutions, nursing schools, and individual nurses use one or more of these frameworks to guide their nursing practice. Each conceptual framework has a frame of reference for carrying out nursing care. Some examples are Orem's self-care model, Roy's adaptation model, Neuman's systems model, and Johnson's behavioral model (Fawcett, 1995). The reader who uses one of these frameworks should refer to specific texts that describe these models in detail. Table 10-5 summarizes selected nursing theorists and their nursing conceptual models.

Body Systems Model

The body systems model (also called the medical model, review of systems) focuses on the client's major anatomic systems. This framework is used to collect data about the past and present condition of each organ or body system and to examine thoroughly all body systems for actual and potential problems. This review often reveals information that the client did not consider important or neglected to mention. It starts with an assessment of the client's general state of health, followed by systematic assessment of each body system—neurologic, cardiovascular, respiratory, gastrointestinal, and so on—until all systems are assessed. Table 21-2 indicates the order of the physical assessment as performed by the staff nurse using a body systems framework.

Table 10-5 • Selected Nursing Theorists and Their Nursing Conceptual Models

Theorist	Conceptual Model
Orem	Self-care model
Roy	Adaptation model
Neuman	Systems model
Johnson	Behavioral system model
Rogers	Life process model
King	Open systems model
Levine	Conservation model
Parse	Man-living-health model
Paterson & Zderad	Humanistic nursing model
Yura & Walsh	Human needs model

Head-to-Toe Model

Using the head-to-toe framework for assessment, the nurse systematically examines every part of the body starting from the head and progressing down to the toes. Similar to the body systems model, the head-to-toe method first assesses the client's general state of health. Vital signs may be taken before the physical examination is begun. Table 21-1 indicates the order of physical assessment when the head-to-toe assessment framework is used. Modifications of the head-to-toe framework can be used for young children to ensure that invasive techniques, such as examining the ears with an otoscope, are done last.

Functional Health Patterns

The client's strengths, talents, and functional health patterns are an integral part of the assessment data. This information occasionally is obscured or forgotten in some assessment frameworks. An assessment of functional health focuses not only on the client's normal function but on his or her altered function or risk for altered function. Because the information gathered using the 11 functional health patterns is basic to nursing, it is applicable to all conceptual models of nursing practice (Gordon, 1982; 1987; 1994). Functional health assessment can be used for clients of all ages and in all specialty areas, and is relevant for the assessment of the person, family, or community (Beyea & Matzo, 1989; Nettle et al., 1993; Tompkins, 1989).

Some nurses collect physical assessment data using the body systems model or the head-to-toe model, but use a functional health framework to organize and document assessment data. The advantages of a functional health framework are

- Client strengths or assets—not merely deficits, problems, or limitations—can be identified.
- The focus is on nursing diagnoses, not medical diagnoses.

- Clustering is easier to do because of the simple categories and concise typology.
- It may contribute to the delineation of basic assessment areas relevant for all clients.

Components of Functional Health Assessment. There are several components of functional health assessment: the pattern label, assessment parameters for each pattern, and recording of assessment data.

The *pattern label* is the name given to a category of assessment data. Eleven categories of assessment data, called functional health patterns, have been identified by Gordon (1982; 1987; 1994). Pattern labels indicate if the client has a functional (asset, strength) or dysfunctional (nursing diagnosis) health pattern.

Assessment parameters help the nurse gather specific information about each functional health pattern. Assessment parameters have been identified for each functional health pattern. Specific interview questions, physical examination techniques, and other information such as laboratory data or health records help the nurse identify health problems in each pattern.

There are various forms for *recording assessment parameters* and identifying the client's functional or dysfunctional health patterns (Beyea & Matzo, 1989; Gordon, 1987; 1994). The nurse uses the approved institutional form at the place of employment or school of nursing. Data may be recorded by hand on a form, or by entering the information into a computer.

Description of Functional Health Patterns. The 11 functional health patterns identified by Gordon (1982; 1987; 1994) are described here. For in-depth information about the assessment parameters for each functional health pattern, see Chapter 21.

Health perception and health management focuses on the client's perception of his or her state of health and well-being and general management of health. Assessment parameters include a general survey of the client's health status and usual health behaviors.

Nutrition and metabolism focuses on the client's dietary pattern and food and fluid consumption in relation to metabolic need. The client's skin integrity and wound-healing status are also considered. Assessment parameters include eating habits, appraisal of appetite, weight loss or gain, and changes in skin, hair, or nails.

Elimination centers on excretory function (bowel, bladder, and skin). Routines, laxatives, or devices used to control excretion are examined. Assessment parameters include the client's usual bowel and bladder elimination habits as well as the excretory function of the skin (eg, excessive perspiration).

Activity and exercise focuses on the client's pattern of energy expenditure in exercise, activity, leisure, and recreation. Assessment parameters include the client's mobility status, exercise routine, and leisure activities.

Cognition and perception focuses on cognitive functions such as memory, language, reasoning, and problem solving, and sensory/perceptual abilities such as vision, hearing, and sensory overload and deprivation. Assessment parameters include changes in cognitive function; ability to hear, see, and speak; and the presence of pain, numbness, or other sensations.

Sleep and rest focuses on the client's perception of sleep, rest, and relaxation patterns. Assessment parameters include the client's regular sleep habits and routine.

Self-perception and self-concept focuses on the client's feelings of self-worth and body image. Assessment parameters include the client's descriptions of himself or herself, physical appearance, effects of illness, and major life accomplishments.

Role and relationships focuses on the client's satisfaction and dissatisfaction with family and social roles and relationships. Assessment parameters include the client's perceptions of key relationships and observations of interactions with others.

Sexuality and reproduction focuses on the client's sexual expression in relationship to his or her developmental stage, perceptions of satisfaction and dissatisfaction, and reproductive patterns. Assessment parameters include the client's appraisal of his or her sexual role and sexual health.

Coping and stress tolerance focuses on the client's perception of stressors and coping patterns and their effectiveness in terms of stress tolerance. Assessment parameters concentrate on the client's evaluation of current stress level, coping ability, and ability to endure life stressors. Physiologic responses to stress are also assessed (eg, blood pressure, heart rate).

Values and beliefs focuses on the client's beliefs or goals that guide decision making and preferences in life, including spiritual beliefs. Assessment parameters include the client's identification of valued people and possessions, sources of support, and religious practices.

Key Concepts

- Assessment is the collection of subjective and objective data from the client and other sources for the purpose of describing health problems.
- Types of assessment vary depending on the clinical situation, the client's health status, the time available, and the purpose of data collection.
- An in-depth, comprehensive appraisal of a client's functional health patterns at the time of entry into a healthcare facility is called an admission assessment.

- Environmental factors can facilitate or hinder collection of assessment data.
- Observation helps the nurse anticipate appropriate data to be collected during the nursing interview and physical examination.
- Proficient interviewing skills are necessary for obtaining comprehensive assessment data.
- The physical examination is a systematic analysis using inspection, palpation, percussion, and auscultation.
- Intuition, a legitimate aspect of nursing practice, involves the nurse's use of insight, instinct, and clinical experience.
- The client, family and significant others, health team members, and health records are sources of assessment data.
- Assessment data are recorded and become a permanent part of the health record.
- The functional health pattern assessment provides a framework for the collection and organization of client data and provides a foundation for the development of nursing diagnoses.

Critical Thinking Challenges

Now turn back to the situation at the beginning of the chapter. Consider the following questions concerning your assessment of the older man in the clinic.

1. *Measure the importance of rapport in this assessment, and propose methods you would use to establish rapport.*
2. *From the limited information provided, detect possibilities of what might be wrong with this client, supporting these informed guesses with data from the situation.*
3. *Summarize subjective and objective data collection and plan techniques or questions you will use to obtain data.*
4. *Given your limited time for assessment, determine how you will prioritize collection of essential information.*

References

Alfaro-LeFevre, R. (1994). *Applying nursing diagnosis and nursing process: A step-by-step guide* (3rd ed.). Philadelphia: J. B. Lippincott.

Bates, B. (1995). *A guide to physical examination and history taking* (5th ed.). Philadelphia: J. B. Lippincott.

Beckett, J. E. (1990). Intuition in clinical nursing. *Research Review: Studies in Nursing Practice, 6*(3), 2.

Beyea, S., & Matzo, M. (1989). Assessing elders using the functional health pattern assessment model. *Nurse Educator, 14*(5), 32–37.

Carpenito, L. J. (1995). *Nursing diagnosis: Application to clinical practice* (6th ed.). Philadelphia: J. B. Lippincott.

Fawcett, J. (1995). *Analysis and evaluation of conceptual models of nursing* (2nd ed.) Philadelphia: F. A. Davis.

Fuller, J., & Schaller-Ayers, J. (1994). *Health assessment: A nursing approach* (2nd ed.). Philadelphia: J. B. Lippincott.

Gordon, M. (1982). *Nursing diagnosis: Process and application.* New York: McGraw-Hill.

Gordon, M. (1987). *Nursing diagnosis: Process and application* (2nd ed.). New York: McGraw-Hill.

Gordon, M. (1994). *Nursing diagnosis: Process and application* (3rd ed.). St. Louis: C. V. Mosby.

Joint Commission on Accreditation of Healthcare Organizations. (1993). *1994 Accreditation manual for hospitals. Vol. 1. Standards.* Chicago: Author.

Meyer, C. (1992). Bedside computer charting: Inching toward tomorrow. *Am J Nurs, 92*(4), 38–44.

Nettle, C., Pavelich, J., Jones, N., et al. (1993). Family as client: Using Gordon's health pattern typology. *Journal of Community Health Nursing, 10*(1), 53–61.

Phipps, W. J., Long, B. C., & Woods, N. F. (1983). *Medical-Surgical nursing: Concepts and clinical practice* (2nd ed.). St. Louis: Mosby-Yearbook.

Rew, L. (1988). Intuition in decision-making. *Image, 20,* 150–154.

Rew, L., & Barrow, E. M. (1987). Intuition: A neglected hallmark of nursing knowledge. *Advances in Nursing Science, 10*(1), 49–62.

Smeltzer, S. C., & Bare, B. G. (1996). *Brunner and Suddarth's textbook of medical–surgical nursing* (8th ed.). Philadelphia: J. B. Lippincott.

Stuart, C. J., & Cash, W. B. (1985). *Interviewing principles and practices* (4th ed.). Dubuque, IA: William C. Brown.

Sundeen, S. J., Stuart, G. W., Rankin, E. D., et al. (1994). *Nurse–client interaction: Implementing the nursing process* (5th ed.). St. Louis: C. V. Mosby.

Tompkins, E. S. (1989). In support of the discipline of nursing: A nursing assessment. *Nursing connections, 2*(3), 21–29.

Yura, H., & Walsh, M. B. (1988). *The nursing process: Assessing, planning, implementing, evaluating* (5th ed.). Norwalk, CT: Appleton and Lange.

Bibliography

Correnti, D. (1992). Intuition and nursing practice implications for nurse educators: A review of the literature. *The Journal of Continuing Education in Nursing, 23,* 91–94.

Cronin-Stubbs, D., Swanson, B., Dean-Baar, S., et al. (1992). The effects of a training program on nurse's functional performance assessments. *Applied Nursing Research, 5*(1), 38–43.

Davis, M. J., & Nomura, L. A. (1990). Vital signs of class I surgical patients. *Western Journal of Nursing Research, 12*(1), 28–41.

Jones, D. A. (1994). Alternative conceptualizations of assessment. In R. M. Carroll-Johnson & M. Paquette (Eds.), *Classification of nursing diagnoses: Proceedings of the tenth conference, North American Nursing Diagnosis Association* (pp. 105–112). Philadelphia: J. B. Lippincott.

Latz, P. A. (1992). Computerized nursing documentation systems: Development, implementation. *AORN J, 56,* 300–301, 304–309.

Ruth-Sahd, L. A. (1993). A modification of Benner's hierarchy of clinical practice: The development of clinical intuition in the novice trauma nurse. *Holistic Nursing Practice, 7*(3), 8–14.

Staggers, N., & Mills, M. E. (1994). Nurse–computer interaction: Staff performance outcomes. *Nurs Res, 43,* 144–150.

Woodtli, M., & Van Ort, S. (1991). Nursing diagnosis and functional health patterns in patients receiving external radiation therapy: Cancer of the head and neck. *Nursing Diagnosis, 2,* 171–180.

Vincenz, M. C., & Siskind, M. M. (1994). Functional health patterns: A curricular course model for adult acute care. *Nursing Diagnosis, 5,* 82–87.

Nursing Diagnosis

Key Terms

Actual nursing diagnosis
Cluster
Collaborative health problem
Cue
Medical diagnosis
Nursing diagnosis
Possible nursing diagnosis
Premature closure
Risk nursing diagnosis
Taxonomy
Validation
Wellness nursing diagnosis

Learning Objectives

Upon completion of this chapter, the student will be able to do the following:

- *Define diagnosis in relation to the nursing process.*
- *State the meaning of nursing diagnosis.*
- *Describe the components of a nursing diagnosis.*
- *Discuss the significance of nursing diagnosis for nursing practice.*
- *Differentiate between a nursing diagnosis and other healthcare problems.*
- *Identify the clinical skills needed to make nursing diagnoses.*
- *Formulate nursing diagnoses for a client situation.*
- *Discuss the categorization of nursing diagnoses by functional health patterns.*

11

A middle-aged former carpenter, J.M., comes to the health clinic with a temperature of 101°F. He has been a wheelchair-dependent quadriplegic for 6 months following a construction accident. He is not working but considers himself to be the provider for his family, which is composed of a wife and two children. He displays anger that his wife has to work to pay the bills and that she has the responsibility of disciplining the children. You are the nurse caring for him.

In previous chapters you learned about holistic healthcare and the beginning phase of the nursing process. This chapter expands your knowledge base about nursing process and the next phase, nursing diagnosis. As you study this chapter, you will see how holism is applied when using proper assessment data to determine strengths and problems in the functioning of the quadriplegic client mentioned in this clinical situation. Critical Thinking Challenges at the end of the chapter will help you apply your knowledge to his care.

Diagnosing human responses to actual or potential health problems is the second phase of the nursing process. After the nurse collects relevant client information, the data need to be analyzed and interpreted. The result of this interpretation is the nursing diagnosis. Registered nurses are educated and licensed to make nursing diagnoses. As such, they have a duty to identify and plan care for clients, such as J.M., based on the nursing diagnoses.

The North American Nursing Diagnosis Association (NANDA, 1992) defines **nursing diagnosis** as the following:

> a clinical judgment about individual, family, or community responses to actual and potential health/life processes. Nursing diagnoses provide the basis for selection of nursing interventions to achieve outcomes for which the nurse is accountable (p.5).

The term *nursing diagnosis* serves as the label and the action of describing a client's functional problems.

The purpose of a nursing diagnosis is to identify problems and synthesize the information gathered during the nursing assessment. The following are reasons for doing this:

- Analyze collected data.
- Identify the client's strengths.
- Identify the client's normal functional level and indicators of actual or potential dysfunction.
- Formulate a diagnostic statement in relation to this synthesis.

In the diagnosis phase, the nurse does the following:

- Identifies patterns
- Validates the diagnosis
- Formulates the nursing diagnosis statement

Figure 11-1 shows the diagnosis phase in relation to the other phases of the nursing process.

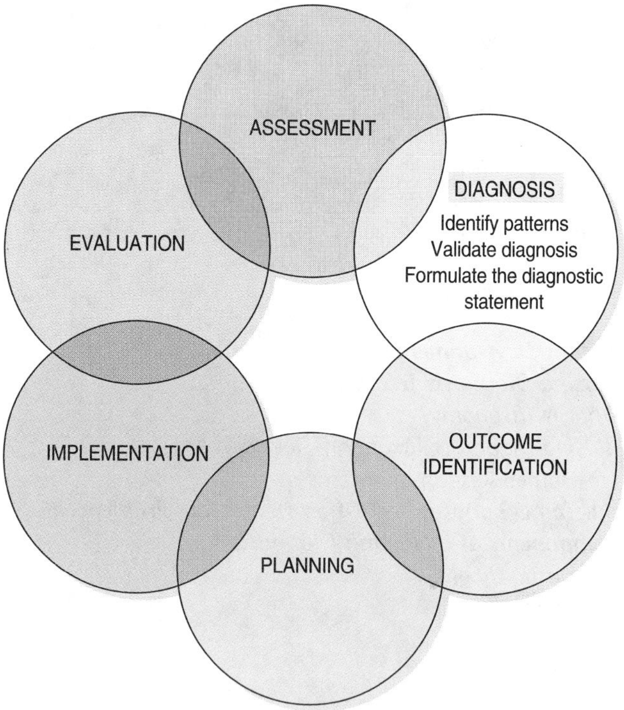

Figure 11-1 • *ANA Standard II states: The nurse analyzes the assessment data in determining diagnoses. This illustration shows activities used in the Nursing Diagnoses phase and also the relationship of Nursing Diagnoses to the other phases of the nursing process.*

Historic Development *

As early as 1926, Harmer suggested that nurses should include problem statements when documenting client care. In 1947, Lesnich and Anderson argued that diagnosis was within the scope of nursing practice. Fry (1953) is generally credited with the first use of the term nursing diagnosis in the nursing literature. During the 1960s, a series of research studies focused on the nurse's ability to make clinical judgments using client cues (Hammond, 1966). These studies revealed that knowledge and interpretation varied widely and that the terms used to describe client problems were not standardized.

In 1972, Gordon completed her dissertation on diagnostic reasoning in nursing. The formal development of the identification and classification of nursing diagnoses began with the first National Conference on the Classification of Nursing Diagnoses convened by Gebbie and Lavin in 1973.

Although implied in the assessment phase of the nursing process (Yura & Walsh, 1973; 1988), nursing diagnosis emerged as a separate phase in the early 1970s. The act of diagnosing was recognized by the American Nurses Association (ANA) in *Standards of Nursing Practice* (1973) and reaffirmed by the publication of revised standards in 1991 (American Nurses Association, 1991). It gained further support when the ANA included diagnosis as a separate activity in *Nursing: A Social Policy Statement* (1980). Since that time, most state nurse practice acts have included diagnosis as part of the domain of nursing practice for which the nurse is held accountable. Standards developed by the Joint Commission on the Accreditation of Healthcare Organizations mandate that each client's nursing care be based on identified nursing diagnoses or client care needs (Joint Commission on the Accreditation of Healthcare Organizations, 1993).

Nurses continue to develop new nursing diagnoses, refine existing diagnoses, and organize them into a classification system useful to practicing nurses. NANDA has been the leader in nursing diagnosis classification and has been endorsed by the ANA as having the responsibility to do so. To date, 11 conferences have been held to refine the classification system for nursing diagnoses.

* Acknowledgment is made to Margaret Lunney (1990) for the outline for this section.

Nursing Diagnosis Taxonomy

Professions require a sound scientific base; the nursing process is nursing's scientific base. To achieve this scientific foundation, nursing requires a **taxonomy**, or classification system, to provide a structure for nursing practice. "The purposes of a taxonomy are to provide vocabulary for classifying phenomena in a discipline, provide new ways of looking at the discipline, and play a part in concept derivation" (NANDA, 1992, p. 2). Developing a classification system for nursing diagnoses involves a knowledge of nursing practice, theoretical frameworks, and the characteristics of taxonomies. NANDA has been acknowledged by the nursing profession as the leader in nursing diagnosis classification. To understand the complexity of this task, a discussion of types of taxonomies and the selection of a nursing taxonomy is presented.

What is Taxonomy?

A taxonomy is a method for ordering complex information. Each classification system is based on a single principle or set of principles (criteria). These principles establish the ground rules for the selection and placement of individual elements in the system. A simple example of an ordering system is an outline:

I.
  A.
  B.
    1.
    2.
      a.
      b.

The set (in this case, I, II, III) is a well-defined collection. The subset is a smaller unit or category of the set (A, B, C). These elements, or subsets, can be further subdivided into smaller units (1 or 2, a or b). The further down the classification, the more concrete the unit becomes. It may name a real thing or may be observable and measurable. An example of a simple classification system is the dictionary: Words are grouped under each letter of the alphabet, which simplifies finding them. (Searching for a word in the dictionary arranged with no organizing principle would be mind-boggling.)

The goal of a taxonomy is to produce a workable classification system. If the system is too complex, it confuses its users. If the system is too simple, the categories may be vague and duplicated. "In every system the component classes must have something different. Without the sameness there is no identifiable class; without the differences there are no discrete entities to group" (Gebbie & Lavin, 1975, p. 34).

The classification of diseases has been evolving since the 1770s. Today, the most widely accepted classification system of diseases is the International Classification of Diseases-10-CM (ICD-10-CM). It is constantly undergoing revision, and NANDA and the ANA are working to incorporate nursing diagnoses into this system (Fitzpatrick et al., 1989). The ICD-10-CM codes diseases by cause or manifestation. Other classification systems include the Systemized Nomenclature of Medicine (SNO MED), published by the College of American Pathologists; Current Procedural Terminology, published by the College of American Pathologists; and Current Procedural Terminology, published by the American Medical Association. In psychiatry, the Diagnostic and Statistical Manual of Mental Disorders (American Psychiatric Association, 1994) is used to classify mental health disorders. All of these systems respond to changes in epidemiology and practice to maintain accuracy.

Nursing Diagnosis Taxonomy Development

NANDA's goal has been to develop a nursing diagnosis taxonomy. At the first conference in 1973, 86 nursing diagnoses were listed alphabetically and published for use and development by all registered nurses (Gebbie & Lavin, 1975). There was no claim as to the validity of the diagnoses, nor was the list considered final. No classification system was selected.

Through the first six conferences, the listing of nursing diagnoses remained alphabetical, but attention was being given to the selection of a classification system. Nursing theorists were involved with the classification from the outset, and in 1977 were formally asked to participate in the development of the classification system.

As of 1994, 109 nursing diagnoses had been accepted by NANDA for clinical use and testing. An additional 18 have been placed on a "to be developed" list (NANDA, 1994). Psychiatric nurses requested inclusion of their nursing diagnoses at the 11th Biennial conference in 1994, and a decision is pending as to the outcome.

A summary of the activities of each conference is presented in Table 11-1. To illustrate the development of taxonomy, one nursing diagnosis, *Grieving*, has been selected to highlight changes made throughout the 11 conferences. The numbers indicate its placement in the classification system.

NANDA Process for Review and Staging Nursing Diagnoses. New or revised nursing diagnoses may be submitted to NANDA for review and staging. To obtain new guidelines for submission and an abstract form, contact them at NANDA, 1211 Locust Street, Philadelphia, PA, 19107 (1-800-647-9002).

After a diagnosis is submitted, the diagnostic review committee completes a review and places the diagnosis into one of four categories.

Level 1: A diagnosis from the time it is recommended with a label through placement on the taxonomy
Level 2: A diagnosis after it is accepted for clinical development; now to be studied clinically
Level 3: A diagnosis after it has been clinically validated and tested
Level 4: Revision or refinement of an existing diagnosis

In 1994, NANDA approved 19 new nursing diagnoses and placed them on the taxonomy for clinical use and testing. They also modified labels for many diag-

Table 11-1 • Summary of the Classification of Nursing Diagnosis Conferences

Year/#	Accomplishments	Chronological Development of the Nursing Diagnosis: Grieving
1973 1st National Conference	86 nursing diagnoses identified, listed alphabetically Established clearing house for nursing nursing diagnoses	11.73 Grieving 11.74 Normal Grieving 11.75 Normal Grieving, Potential 11.76 11.77 Arrested Grieving 11.78 Arrested Grieving, Potential 11.79 Delayed Onset of Grieving 11.80 Delayed Onset of Grieving, Potential
1975 2nd National Conference	Further identification of nursing diagnoses, listed alphabetically	11.73 Grieving, Acute 11.76 Grieving, Anticipatory 11.77 Grieving, Delayed
1978 3rd National Conference	Diagnoses listed alphabetically "Unitary man" schema introduced as classification	11.73 Grieving
1980 4th National Conference	Patterns of nursing diagnoses discussed; no definite recommendations Diagnoses listed alphabetically	11.73 Grieving, Dysfunctional 11.74 Delete 11.75 Delete 11.76 Grieving, Anticipatory 11.77 Delete 11.78 Delete 11.79 Delete 11.80 Delete
1982 5th National Conference	Patterns of unitary man described Diagnoses listed alphabetically Vote to become NANDA	Grieving, Anticipatory Grieving, Dysfunctional
1984 6th Conference	First conference open to nursing public Further refinement to patterns of unitary man Diagnoses listed alphabetically	Grieving, Anticipatory Grieving, Dysfunctional
1986 7th Conference	Endorsement of NANDA taxonomy I Human response patterns replaced patterns of unitary man Development of rules for submission of new diagnoses	9.2.2 Grieving 9.2.2.1 Dysfunctional 9.2.2.2 Anticipatory 9.2.2.3
1988 8th Conference	Endorsement of NANDA taxonomy I (rev.)	9.2.1.1 Dysfunctional Grieving 9.2.1.2 Anticipatory Grieving
1990 9th conference	NANDA taxonomy II proposed Definition of nursing diagnosis approved	Same as 1988
1992 10th Conference	New nursing diagnoses added	Same as 1988
1994 11th Conference	18 "to be developed" nursing diagnoses Psychiatric nursing diagnoses proposed Revised submission guidelines for nursing diagnoses	Same as 1988

noses. One of the most significant changes was substituting the word "Risk" for the previous term "High Risk."

Human Response Patterns

The complete NANDA Taxonomy I (1994) is presented in the accompanying display. The nursing diagnoses are organized according to human response patterns: exchanging, communicating, relating, valuing, choosing, moving, perceiving, knowing, and feeling. Human response patterns characterize the essence of nursing practice. Each pattern describes an abstract concept; together the patterns describe the alterations of human responses that nurses are prepared and educated to treat.

As abstract labels, the title of each pattern is intended to be inclusive of all the nursing diagnoses that fit that particular pattern. The more detailed the taxonomy, the more concrete (real) and clinically useful the entity becomes. This specificity enables the nurse to plan and deliver care that is tailored to resolve specific client problems. The ability and knowledge to assist clients inresolving clearly identified problems enables the nurse to demonstrate what *nursing* does in providing healthcare services. Not all nursing diagnoses are at the same level. Some are broadly stated concepts that must be individualized before they can become clinically useful. In practice, nurses continue to identify new nursing diagnoses and refine existing ones.

Each human response pattern is presented, with a definition and description of the nursing diagnoses included in each. This overview illustrates where there are gaps in nursing knowledge, suggests directions for nursing research, and provides guidance for implementing specific interventions and evaluating client outcomes.

Pattern 1—Exchanging. This pattern involves mutual giving and receiving; to give, relinquish, or lose means giving up something while receiving something in return. The nursing diagnoses are mostly physiologic. The major concepts are nutrition, physical regulation, elimination, circulation, oxygenation, and physical integrity.

Pattern 2—Communicating. This pattern involves sending messages to convey, impart, confer, or transmit thoughts, feelings, or information, either verbally or nonverbally. The only nursing diagnosis in this pattern is Impaired Verbal Communication, but alterations in nonverbal communication probably exist. Other communication problems may be described in the future.

Pattern 3—Relating. This pattern involves establishing bonds: to connect, to establish a link between, to stand in some association to another thing, person, or place. The major concepts in this pattern are socialization, parenting, and sexuality. The individual and the family unit are recognized.

Pattern 4—Valuing. This pattern involves the assigning of relative worth: to be concerned about, to care, to equate in importance. The only nursing diagnosis in this pattern is Spiritual Distress, but again there is a presumed lack of completeness and need for further development in this area.

Pattern 5—Choosing. This pattern involves the selection of alternatives: to determine in favor of a course, to decide in accordance with inclinations. The nursing diagnoses range from Coping to Noncompliance. Two distinct concepts, coping and participation, are evident. The individual and family are recognized by accepted diagnoses; the community is a discrete entity yet to be described.

Pattern 6—Moving. This pattern involves activity; to change the place or position; to put or keep in motion. There are several nursing diagnoses in this category. The main concepts are activity, rest, recreation, and activities of daily living.

Pattern 7—Perceiving. This pattern involves the reception of information; to apprehend what is not open or present to observation. The nursing diagnoses include Disturbance in Body Image, Self-Esteem, or Personal Identity; Sensory-Perceptual Alterations; Hopelessness; and Powerlessness. The major concepts are self-concept, sensory responses, and meaningfulness.

Pattern 8—Knowing. This pattern involves the meaning associated with information: to be cognizant of something through observation, inquiry, or information. The nursing diagnoses include Knowledge Deficit and Altered Thought Processes. The main concepts are knowledge, learning, and thinking. This pattern clearly indicates a need to be able to describe more clearly the subsets of knowing.

Pattern 9—Feeling. This pattern involves the subjective awareness of information; to be consciously or emotionally affected by a fact, event, or state. The nursing diagnoses in this pattern include Pain, Grieving, Post-Trauma Response, Rape-Trauma Syndrome, Violence, Anxiety, and Fear. The major concepts are loss, aggression, and mental or physical distress.

Nursing Diagnoses and Other Healthcare Problems

Nursing diagnoses must be distinguished from medical diagnoses. A **medical diagnosis** describes a disease or pathology of specific organs or body systems that

NANDA-Approved Nursing Diagnoses for Clinical Use and Testing (1994)

Pattern 1: Exchanging

Altered nutrition: More than body requirements
Altered nutrition: Less than body requirements
Altered nutrition: Potential for more than body requirements
Risk for Infection
Risk for Altered Body Temperature
Hypothermia
Hyperthermia
Ineffective Thermoregulation
Dysreflexia
Constipation
Perceived Constipation
Colonic Constipation
Diarrhea
Bowel Incontinence
Altered Urinary Elimination
Stress Incontinence
Reflex Incontinence
Urge Incontinence
Functional Incontinence
Total Incontinence
Urinary Retention
Altered (Specify Type) Tissue Perfusion (Renal, cerebral, cardiopulmonary, gastrointestinal, peripheral)
Fluid Volume Excess
Fluid Volume Deficit
Risk for Fluid Volume Deficit
Decreased Cardiac Output
Impaired Gas Exchange
Ineffective Airway Clearance
Ineffective Breathing Pattern
Inability to Sustain Spontaneous Ventilation
Dysfunctional Ventilatory Weaning Response (DVWR)
Risk for Injury
Risk for Suffocation
Risk for Poisoning
Risk for Trauma
Risk for Aspiration
Risk for Disuse Syndrome
Altered Protection
Impaired Tissue Integrity
Altered Oral Mucous Membrane
Impaired Skin Integrity
Risk for Impaired Skin Integrity
*Decreased Adaptive Capacity: Intracranial
*Energy Field Disturbance

Pattern 2: Communicating

Impaired Verbal Communication

Pattern 3: Relating

Impaired Social Interaction
Social Isolation
*Risk for Loneliness
Altered Role Performance
*Altered Parenting
*Risk for Altered Parent/Infant/Child Attachment
Sexual Dysfunction
Altered Family Processes
Caregiver Role Strain
Risk for Caregiver Role Strain
*Altered Family Process: Alcoholism
Parental Role Conflict
Altered Sexuality Patterns

Pattern 4: Valuing

Spiritual Distress (distress of the human spirit)
*Potential for Enhanced Spiritual Well Being
Distress of the Human Spirit

Pattern 5: Choosing

Ineffective Individual Coping
Impaired Adjustment
Defensive Coping
Ineffective Denial

treatment focuses on correcting or preventing. Medical diagnoses convey information about the signs and symptoms of disease processes and provide a convenient means of communicating treatment requirements. The physician focuses on treating the underlying pathology.

In contrast, a nursing diagnosis describes an actual or high-risk human response to a health problem that nurses are responsible for treating independently. Nursing diagnoses describe the client's response to the disease process, developmental stage, or life process and provide a convenient way to communicate nursing therapies or interventions.

Nursing diagnoses carry legal ramifications. Only healthcare problems within the scope of nursing practice can be identified as nursing diagnoses. The nurse cannot diagnose a medical disease and is not licensed to treat such problems. Care must be taken to identify client problems within the scope, practice abilities, and education of the registered nurse.

When identifying problems from assessment data, the nurse determines if the problem can be addressed legally and independently by nurses, if so, it is a nursing diagnosis. If the problem requires physician-prescribed and nurse-prescribed actions, however, it is

NANDA-Approved Nursing Diagnoses for Clinical Use and Testing (1994) *(Continued)*

Ineffective Family Coping: Disabling
Ineffective Family Coping: Compromised
*Potential for Enhanced Community Coping
*Ineffective Community Coping
Family Coping: Potential for Growth
Ineffective Management of Therapeutic Regimen (Individuals)
Noncompliance (Specify)
*Ineffective Management of Therapeutic Regimen: Families
*Ineffective Management of Therapeutic Regimen: Community
*Ineffective Management of Therapeutic Regimen: Individual
Decisional Conflict (Specify)
Health Seeking Behaviors (Specify)

Pattern 6: Moving

Impaired Physical Mobility
Risk for Peripheral Neurovascular Dysfunction
*Risk for Perioperative Positioning Injury
Activity Intolerance
Fatigue
Risk for Activity Intolerance
Sleep Pattern Disturbance
Diversional Activity Deficit
Impaired Home Maintenance Management
Altered Health Maintenance
Feeding Self Care Deficit
Impaired Swallowing
Ineffective Breastfeeding
Interrupted Breastfeeding
Effective Breastfeeding
Ineffective Infant Feeding Pattern
Bathing/Hygiene Self Care Deficit
Dressing/Grooming Self Care Deficit
Toileting Self Care Deficit
Altered Growth and Development
Relocation Stress Syndrome
*Risk for Disorganized Infant Behavior
*Disorganized Infant Behavior
*Potential for Enhanced Organized Infant Behavior

Pattern 7: Perceiving

Body Image Disturbance
Self Esteem Disturbance
Chronic Low Self Esteem
Situational Low Self Esteem
Personal Identity Disturbance
Sensory/Perceptual Alterations (Specify) (Visual, auditory, kinesthetic, gustatory, tactile, olfactory)
Unilateral Neglect
Hopelessness
Powerlessness

Pattern 8: Knowing

Knowledge Deficit (Specify)
*Impaired Environmental Interpretation Syndrome
*Acute Confusion
*Chronic Confusion
Altered Thought Processes
*Impaired Memory

Pattern 9: Feeling

Pain
Chronic Pain
Dysfunctional Grieving
Anticipatory Grieving
Risk for Violence: Self-directed or directed at others
Risk for Self-Mutilation
Post-Trauma Response
Rape-Trauma Syndrome
Rape-Trauma Syndrome: Compound Reaction
Rape-Trauma Syndrome: Silent Reaction
Anxiety
Fear

*New diagnoses added in 1994.

a **collaborative health problem**. A collaborative problem refers to actual or potential physiologic complications that can result from disease, trauma, treatment, or diagnostic studies for which nurses intervene in collaboration with other disciplines (Carpenito, 1995). Table 11-2 compares nursing diagnoses with collaborative and medical diagnoses, and Figure 11-2 shows how a nurse makes these determinations. Procedures, medical terminology, symptoms, client needs, and treatments are often confused with nursing diagnoses. For example, if the nurse writes "Foley catheter," this is a treatment, not the response the client may have to the treatment. Other examples include "need for oxygen" or "dyspnea," terms that describe symptoms and do not provide enough information to validate the presence of a nursing diagnosis. Another common mistake is to write "lack of adequate nutrition" as the nursing diagnosis. This phrase describes a client need but it is not a nursing diagnosis. The nursing diagnosis, in this case, would be Altered Nutrition: Less Than Body Requirements.

The following list shows the proper use of a variety of terms for a client with a specific breathing problem. These terms are often confused.

Table 11-2 • Comparison of Nursing Diagnoses with Collaborative Problems and Medical Diagnoses

	Nursing Diagnoses	Collaborative Problems and Medical Diagnoses
Focus of assessment activities	Main focus is on monitoring human responses to actual and potential health problems.	Main focus is on monitoring for pathophysiologic response of body organs or systems
Problem identification	Nurse identifies and validates independently that problem exists and can be treated legally by nursing staff.	Nurse may identify problem but is required to refer to physician for validation that problem exists (may require additional diagnostic studies to label the problem). Nurse may not be qualified to diagnose exact nature of problem but refers abnormal data to physician.
Treatment	Nurse legally initiates actions for treatment.	Nurse collaborates with physician to initiate interventions for treatment. Nurse may have standing orders from physician or institution (delegated authority) to initiate diagnostic studies or treatment interventions for the problem without physician's orders.

From Alfaro-LeFevre, R. (1994). *Applying nursing diagnosis and nursing process: A step-by-step guide* (3rd ed.). Philadelphia: J. B. Lippincott, p. 67.

- Medical diagnosis: pneumonia
- Nursing diagnosis: Ineffective Airway Clearance related to tracheobronchial secretions
- Client need: oxygenation
- Procedure: bronchoscopy
- Treatment: oxygen therapy

Formulating an accurate nursing diagnosis is a clinical judgment, but nursing diagnoses should not be written in judgmental terms. For example, it is incorrect to write "failure to carry out medical regimen related to drug use." The reasons for the client's noncompliance with the regimen should be explored and analyzed to avoid labeling or stereotyping a client's behavior based on insufficient evidence.

Components of a Nursing Diagnosis

The parts of a nursing diagnosis are the diagnostic label, definition, defining characteristics (major and minor), risk factors, related factors, and qualifiers. All of the diagnoses discussed in Section II describe each of these points.

Diagnostic Label

The diagnostic label is the name of the nursing diagnosis as listed in the taxonomy. It describes the essence of the problem using as few words as possible. Some examples are Stress Incontinence, Anxiety, and Feeding Self-Care Deficit. Each nursing diagnosis represents a pattern of related client cues.

Qualifiers

Qualifiers are words used to give additional meaning to the nursing diagnosis. They describe changes in condition, state of the client, or some qualification of the specific nursing diagnosis. They accompany the label in the Taxonomy display. Examples used by NANDA (1994) include the following:

- Altered: a change from baseline
- Impaired: made worse, weakened, damaged, reduced, deteriorated
- Depleted: emptied wholly or partially exhausted
- Deficient: inadequate in amount, quality, or degree; defective, not sufficient, incomplete
- Excessive: greater than necessary, desirable, or useful
- Dysfunctional: abnormal or incomplete functioning
- Disturbed: agitated, interrupted, or interfered with
- Ineffective: not producing the desired effect
- Decreased: lessened in size, amount, or degree
- Increased: greater in size, amount, or degree
- Acute: severe but of short duration
- Chronic: lasting a long time, recurring, habitual, or constant

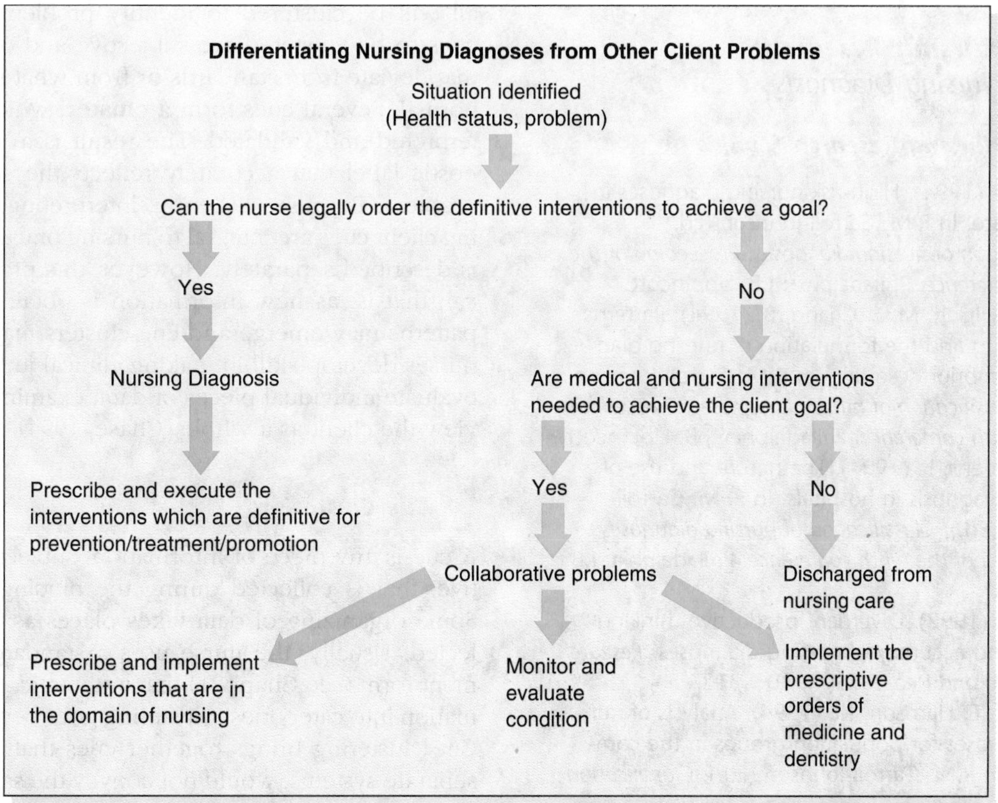
Differentiating Nursing Diagnoses from Other Client Problems
Situation identified
(Health status, problem)
Can the nurse legally order the definitive interventions to achieve a goal?
Yes
No
Nursing Diagnosis
Are medical and nursing interventions needed to achieve the client goal?
Prescribe and execute the interventions which are definitive for prevention/treatment/promotion
Yes
No
Collaborative problems
Discharged from nursing care
Prescribe and implement interventions that are in the domain of nursing
Monitor and evaluate condition
Implement the prescriptive orders of medicine and dentistry

Figure 11-2 • *Differentiating a nursing diagnosis from other client problems. (From Carpenito, L. [1995].* Nursing Diagnosis: Application to Clinical Practice, *[6th ed.]. Philadelphia: J.B. Lippincott.)*

- Intermittent: stopping and starting again at intervals, cyclic, periodic

Definition

Each nursing diagnosis approved by NANDA for clinical use and testing has a definition that describes the characteristics of the human response under consideration. For example, the definition of the diagnostic label hypothermia is "the state in which an individual's body temperature is reduced below normal range" (NANDA, 1992).

Defining Characteristics

Defining characteristics are the major and minor clinical cues that validate the presence of an actual nursing diagnosis. Each piece of client information is considered a clinical cue; a set of clinical cues forms a cluster that is present if the diagnosis is accurate. Major defining characteristics are present 80% to 100% of the time in researched nursing diagnoses. Minor defining characteristics are present 50% to 79% of the time in researched nursing diagnoses. (NANDA, 1994).

Risk Factors

The term *risk factors* is used to describe clinical cues in *risk nursing diagnoses.* They are identifiable intrinsic (inside, somatic) and extrinsic (outside, environmental) characteristics of the client. The presence of specific risk factors indicates that the individual, family, or community is vulnerable to or at risk for a particular problem. Examples of risk factors for the nursing diagnosis Risk for Fluid Volume Deficit include extremes of age, physical immobility, and excessive fluid losses. If the risk factors are not addressed, a potential problem may become an actual problem.

Related Factors

Related factors describe the etiology or likely cause of the problem. Although there is usually not a direct causal relationship between the nursing diagnosis and the cause, some relationships can be described. Terms that can be used are "associated with," "related to," or "contributing to." Identifying related factors helps the nurse to develop specific interventions to resolve the health problem. For example, different nursing interventions would be used when caring for a client with

Nursing Research
Nursing Diagnosis

Selected Nursing Research Studies

Gordon, M. (1994). High-risk nursing diagnoses in critical care. In R.M. Carroll-Johnson (Ed.), *Classification of nursing diagnoses: Proceeding of the tenth conference.* Philadelphia: J.B. Lippincott.

Jensen, K., Hirsch, M. & Chang, B. (1994). Patterns of knowing and the formulation of nursing diagnoses and priority setting. In R.M. Carroll-Johnson (Ed.), *Classification of nursing diagnoses: Proceeding of the tenth conference.* Philadelphia: J.B. Lippincott.

Johnson Lutjens, L. (1994). The nature and use of nursing diagnosis in hospitals. In R. M. Carroll-Johnson (Ed.), *Classification of nursing diagnoses: Proceeding of the tenth conference.* Philadelphia: J.B. Lippincott.

Lunney, M. (1992). Divergent productive thinking factors and accuracy of nursing diagnoses. *Research in Nursing and Health 15*(4), 303–312.

Neufeld, A., & Harrison, M. (1994). Analysis of nursing diagnoses for population groups in the community. In R.M. Carroll-Johnson (Ed.), *Classification of nursing diagnoses: Proceeding of the tenth conference.* Philadelphia: J.B. Lippincott.

Possible Topics for Nursing Inquiry

- What is the relationship between years of nursing practice and the ability to recognize a cue cluster for a selected nursing diagnosis?
- Are there nursing diagnoses that occur together in specific patient situations?
- Is the classification system used to organize nursing diagnoses valid and reliable?
- What is the cost-effectiveness of a reimbursement system using nursing diagnoses as the organizing framework?
- What is the minimum number of cues necessary to make a specific nursing diagnosis?

Stress Incontinence related to high intra-abdominal pressure than for a client with Stress Incontinence related to overdistention between voidings.

Diagnosis Activities

Identify Pattern

After the nurse completes the client assessment, the data obtained are analyzed to identify specific client problems. The data, both subjective symptoms and objective signs, form **cues.** All data are examined, but not all will be clustered to identify problems. Significant cues to be clustered are subjective and objective data that deviate from standards or from what is considered normal. Several cues form a **cluster**, which is then interpreted and validated. The result is a nursing diagnostic label that accurately reflects the specific client problem. Because clustering, interpreting, and validating client cues are integral to nursing practice, each step is described separately. However, this process is cyclical; that is, as new information is obtained, new cue patterns may emerge and cue clusters may change. As nurses develop skill in making clinical judgments, they evaluate individual pieces of data, examine trends, and view the client as a whole (Chase, 1994).

Cue Clustering

A cue is any piece of information, subjective or objective, that is collected during the nursing assessment. Some organizing of data takes places as cues are collected. Usually, the nurse uses a standardized assessment form (see Chap. 21) that automatically puts information into categories. Clustering goes beyond systems. Cue clustering brings together cues that, if viewed in separate systems, would not convey the same meaning. The purpose of cue clustering is to take individual cues and group them to derive meaning.

Cue clustering can be compared with piecing together a puzzle. All the puzzle pieces form one picture (the client problem); each piece is a cue. Figure 11-3 illustrates the puzzle concept. The puzzle shows a circle and two triangles. All the pieces of the puzzle with the circle form a cluster, as do all the pieces for the triangles. Placing the circle pieces into a cluster helps identify the pattern of the puzzle (the diagnosis). A separate and distinct cue cluster forms each nursing diagnosis.

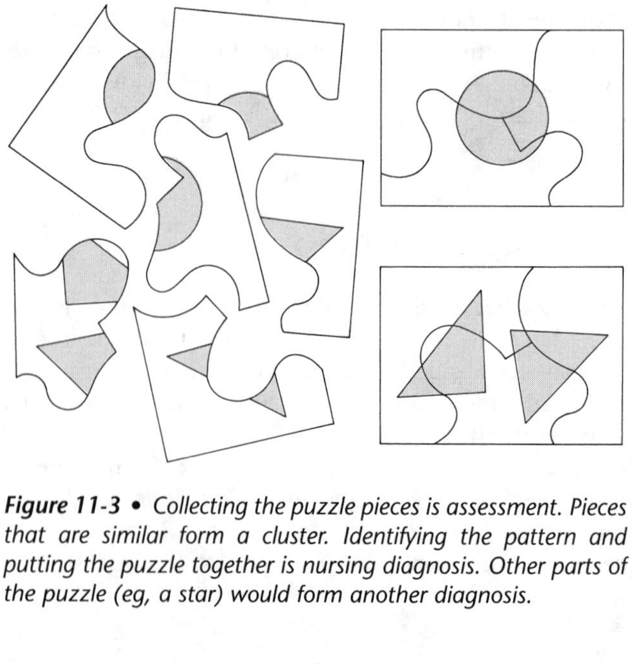

Figure 11-3 • *Collecting the puzzle pieces is assessment. Pieces that are similar form a cluster. Identifying the pattern and putting the puzzle together is nursing diagnosis. Other parts of the puzzle (eg, a star) would form another diagnosis.*

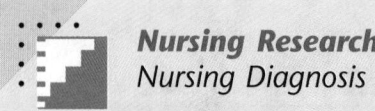

During cue clustering, the nurse uses critical thinking to analyze and synthesize the cues. Each cue is analyzed for its fit into a particular problem. The cues are then put together to form meaningful clusters that describe specific client problems.

To see how this process works, refer to the client in the situation at the beginning of the chapter. Review the situation of the former carpenter (J.M.) and then see which cues belong together when describing a particular problem.

Although the first tendency is to identify Hyperthermia as a nursing diagnosis—and it is present—the nurse also should look at other cues the client has given. For the purpose of illustration, one nursing diagnosis has been selected here, but the reader is encouraged to select other cues and describe additional nursing diagnoses that may be present. The relevant cues follow:

- Not currently working
- Recent change from active, mobile individual to wheelchair-dependent quadriplegic person
- Considers self to be provider
- Angry at wife for carrying out role of breadwinner

Taken together, these cues fit the defining characteristics of a specific nursing diagnosis. The knowledgeable nurse will recognize this cue cluster and proceed with the next step, cluster interpretation. Before doing that, some of the problems that can occur in cue clustering must be described.

Problems in Cue Clustering. The major problems in cue clustering are insufficient, inaccurate, and inconsistent cues. Skill in cue clustering comes with experience and practice. The beginning practitioner should expect to use a variety of reference materials to develop these skills.

Having insufficient cues is a problem: the nurse cannot plan effective care because the problem cannot be determined with confidence. Using the example from the beginning of the chapter, the nurse might select the cue temperature of 101°F and write this nursing diagnosis: Hyperthermia. However, not enough information has been gathered to lead to this conclusion. This lack of adequate cues also can be called **premature closure**, selecting a diagnosis before analyzing pertinent information. Additional cues that would be needed to identify Hyperthermia are flushed skin, warm to touch, increased respiratory rate, tachycardia, or seizures/convulsions (NANDA, 1992).

Inaccurate clustering of cues is a problem because the nurse may be clustering unrelated information and may make judgments based on incorrect clusters. Inaccuracy in clustering occurs when the nurse is unfamiliar with the diagnosis or when the cues for different diagnoses overlap. If, for example, the cues (wheelchair-dependent quadriplegic, not working, and anger) are clustered and the nursing diagnosis of Impaired Mobility related to dependency is made, nursing interventions will be geared toward resolving the dependency, not the problem of impaired mobility.

Inconsistent cues are a problem because the meaning attached to one cue may be altered based on another cue. For example, one client may say that she cannot eat a regular diet, but later she is seen eating a steak and potatoes. Because the cues do not match, further information is needed to validate the problem and the cues.

Cluster Interpretation

Cluster interpretation means synthesizing the cue clusters. It is an intellectual activity that requires the nurse to see the whole picture and to attach meaning to the cluster, looking at the pattern the cluster suggests. It is the ability to derive the meaning and implications of the human response for a client.

A specific cue cluster was presented in the clinical example. Review it now, and think of possible nursing diagnoses. The following nursing diagnoses are listed as possible choices for the client:

- Ineffective Individual Coping related to dependency. Cues: anger, wheelchair-dependent quadriplegic.
- Impaired Adjustment related to disability requiring change in lifestyle. Cues: wheelchair-dependent quadriplegic for 6 months, not working.
- Altered Role Performance related to recent change. Cues: not working, angry at wife for carrying out breadwinner role, perceives self as provider, recent change from active, mobile person to wheelchair-dependent quadriplegic.

Analyzing these suggested nursing diagnostic statements would involve reviewing each definition and associated defining characteristics.

The first two cannot be supported by clinical cues. Ineffective Individual Coping relies on two cues that are not defining characteristics of this diagnosis. This diagnosis requires evidence of a client's verbalization of the inability to cope or ask for help or the inability to solve problems. More information is needed to support the use of this diagnosis. The diagnosis of Impaired Adjustment may or may not describe this client. The nurse has assumed that by becoming a wheelchair-dependent quadriplegic, this client has not made a satisfactory adjustment to his new lifestyle. Additional defining characteristics are needed to evaluate the presence of this problem.

In the third diagnosis, Altered Role Performance, all the cues supporting the defining characteristics for this diagnosis are present. The client had a change in the perception of his role, in his physical capacity to resume a previous role, and in his usual patterns of responsibility. There is evidence of conflict, as shown by his anger toward his wife. The nurse can make this diagnosis with confidence and plan nursing interventions to assist the client in resolving this problem.

Problems in Cluster Interpretation. The analysis of cue clusters can be impeded by incorrect clustering of data and misinterpretation of cue clusters. "Clinical inference is the process of arriving at clinical conclusions. Conscious, logical deliberation is one mode of decision making" (Pinkley, 1994, p. 131).

If the cues are not clustered correctly, the nurse cannot make accurate clinical judgments. For example, if the cues (malnourished, feeds self, and dependent in mobility) are clustered, the nurse may arrive at the erroneous diagnosis of Self-Care Deficit related to inadequate intake. There is no information here about the daily intake of food. The fact that the client feeds himself does not explain the cue of dependent in mobility. Does the client use assistive devices? What is the state of malnourishment? Are supplemental feedings being given? By forming this particular cue cluster, the nurse has neglected other important areas for analysis. In this example, these include defining characteristics for the nursing diagnoses of Altered Nutrition: Less Than Body Requirements and Impaired Physical Mobility.

Misinterpretation of cue clusters occurs when the nurse fails to recognize the correct pattern. This can happen if the nurse is unfamiliar with the nursing diagnosis or is inexperienced in relating how these particular cues fit together. If the defining characteristics for the diagnosis under consideration are complex and require extensive analysis for correct interpretation, it would be prudent to ask the experienced clinician to assist with interpreting the cues.

Validate Diagnosis

After a nursing diagnosis is selected (Altered Role Performance, in the clinical example), it should be validated with the client. **Validation** legitimizes the diagnosis and helps to discover its significance for the client. The client may deny that there is a problem and may not want to deal with it, or he or she may acknowledge it but want to deal with it later. These are acceptable reasons for not dealing with an identified diagnosis, but the presence of the problem and its status should be documented. For most problems, the client will agree that there is a dysfunctional health pattern that can be resolved with nursing assistance.

Diagnostic validation occurs in two stages. In the first stage, the cue clusters that have been interpreted are compared with norms for the client and for clients in general. In the second stage, the specific nursing diagnosis is evaluated for its nursing research base. This research base is different for each diagnosis.

In the clinical example, these diagnoses may be made if additional collection identifies cues to support them:

- Ineffective Individual Coping
- Impaired Adjustment
- Hyperthermia

For each of these diagnoses, the nurse should talk with J.M. about the significance of the problem, determine J.M.'s perception of the reason for the problem, and ask J.M. if help is desired to resolve or diminish the problem. Some clients are not ready or motivated to seek help even when a problem clearly exists.

Problems in Diagnostic Validation

Problems can occur in diagnostic validation because of a nurse's limited experience, lack of a knowledge base about the nursing diagnosis, or insufficient characteristics of a diagnosis.

If the nurse has limited clinical experience, exposure to a variety of clients under the guidance of an instructor, mentor, or expert practitioner can provide an opportunity to practice these skills. Each nursing diagnosis and defining characteristic should be discussed and errors corrected. This requires a nonthreatening environment and patience and understanding for both parties. It is helpful to trace the steps taken to arrive at a particular problem; errors in logic or missing steps in the process can sometimes be identified and suggestions made for avoiding them.

The nurse who is not knowledgeable about specific nursing diagnoses should refer to articles, books, and other material that discuss the identification of the problem and its management. For example, the proceedings of the NANDA conferences on the classification of nursing diagnosis and *Nursing Diagnosis: Application to Clinical Practice* (Carpenito, 1995) can be used to learn about individual nursing diagnoses.

The problem of insufficient research about specific nursing diagnoses can be corrected by participating in clinical research studies sponsored by institutions, organizations, and individual researchers. The registered nurse has an obligation to contribute to the scientific development of the profession. Current research on nursing diagnoses can be found in nursing journals and the previously mentioned proceedings of the NANDA conferences. The term nursing diagnosis is listed as a subject heading in the *Cumulative Index for Nursing and Allied Health*, enabling the nurse to find nursing diagnosis information quickly.

Formulate the Diagnostic Statement

Formulating the nursing diagnostic statement involves writing the label of the actual, risk, wellness, or possible nursing diagnoses that have been made through the

Table 11-3* • *Types of Diagnostic Statements

Type	*Construction*	*Example*
Actual nursing diagnosis	Three-part statement includes diagnostic label, related factors, defining characteristics	Pain related to surgical trauma and inflammation, as evidenced by grimacing and verbal reports of pain
Risk nursing diagnosis	Two-part statement includes diagnostic label, risk factors	Risk for Infection related to surgery and immunosuppression
Possible nursing diagnosis	Two-part statement includes diagnostic label, related factors (unknown)	Possible Self-Esteem Disturbance related to unknown etiology
Wellness diagnosis	One-part statement includes diagnostic label	Potential for Effective Breastfeeding

nursing diagnostic process. The correct way of stating these diagnoses is described in the following section and illustrated in Table 11-3 and Figure 11-4. Accurate and inaccurate examples also are given in the text and in Table 11-4.

Actual Nursing Diagnoses

Actual nursing diagnoses describe a human response to a health problem that is being manifested. They are written as three-part statements: the diagnostic label, related factors, and defining characteristics. Client cues supporting the existence of the problem can be found in the documentation of assessment data. In the nursing diagnosis statement, cues are identified by "as manifested by" or "as evidenced by." Problems sometimes occur when the nurse inverts the label and the "related to" phrase. This problem can be avoided by determining the main focus of the problem (the diagnostic label) and the factor that is contributing to the client's inability to resolve it (related factor).

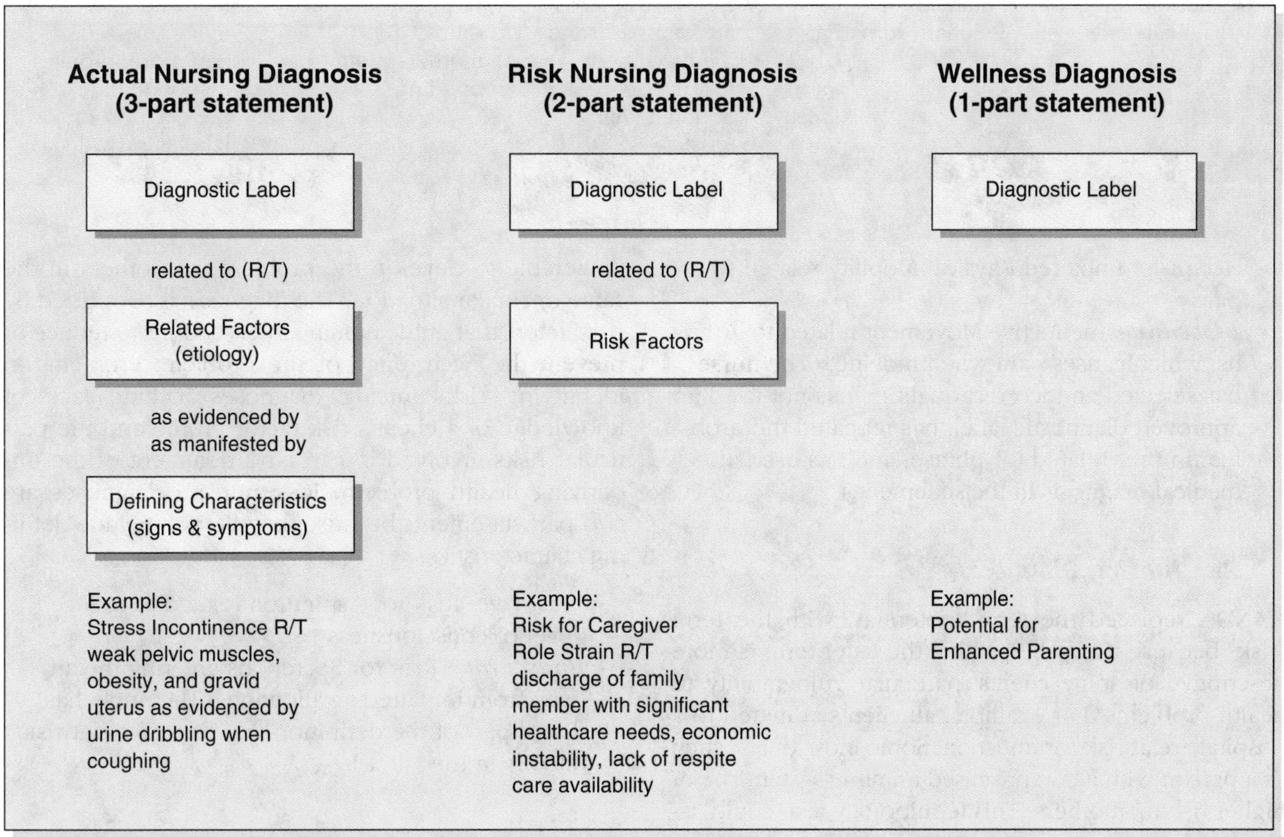

Figure 11-4 • *Examples of a three-part actual nursing diagnostic statement; a two-part risk nursing diagnostic statement; and a one-part wellness nursing diagnostic statement.*

Table 11-4 • Examples of Accurate Versus Inaccurate Statement of Nursing Diagnoses

Type	Accurate Statement	Rationale	Inaccurate Statement	Rationale
Actual nursing diagnosis	Constipation related to decreased activity and fluids as manifested by small, hard, formed stool every 4 days	Properly stated using three-part statement, including diagnostic label (constipation), related factors (decreased activity), and defining characteristics (small, hard, formed stool every 4 days)	Altered Bowel Function related to production of hard stool	Incorrect diagnostic label; altered bowel function is nonspecific and not accepted by NANDA. Only a two-part statement; related factors are omitted, and defining characteristics (hard stool) are substituted.
Risk nursing diagnosis	Risk for Activity Intolerance related to prolonged bedrest	Risk is used rather than "potential." Risk diagnoses use risk factors. Defining characteristics should not be included.	Activity Intolerance, Potential	"Potential" rather than "risk" used; diagnostic label is reversed, and no risk factors are provided.
Possible nursing diagnosis	Possible Impaired Adjustment related to unknown etiology	Unknown etiology used until more data can be collected to validate diagnosis.	Adjustment impaired, possibly due to recent car accident that resulted in quadriplegia	Diagnostic label is reversed, and cues are included in "related to" without validation.
Wellness nursing diagnosis	Potential for enhanced parenting	Wellness diagnoses are one-part statements without risk factors or defining characteristics.	Parenting potential due to good mother–infant bonding	Diagnostic statement reversed, and more information than just the diagnostic label is provided.

- *Accurate*: Impaired Physical Mobility related to pain
- *Inaccurate*: Ineffective Movement related to arthritis, which causes pain when moving. (The nurse has selected an incorrect qualifier, has not used an approved diagnostic label, has repeated the problem in the "related to" phrase, and has used a medical diagnosis in the statement.)

Risk Nursing Diagnoses

NANDA replaced the term "potential" with the term "risk" because it is believed that the latter term is more descriptive of some clients' particular vulnerability to health problems. For example, all clients admitted to a hospital are at risk for infection. Some individuals, such as a person with a compromised immune system, are at higher risk than others. This terminology also could assist in third-party reimbursement for nursing care and is the term in the ICD-10 list of nursing diagnoses. A **risk nursing diagnosis**, as defined by NANDA, is a clinical judgment that a person, family, or community is more vulnerable to develop the problem than others in the same or similar situation. The diagnosis is supported by risk factors that guide nursing interventions to reduce or prevent the occurrence of the problem. Problems in identifying risk nursing diagnoses include lack of knowledge of a client's risk factor profile and the particular risks involved in care and treatment of the underlying health problem. Risk nursing diagnoses are two-part statements because they do not include defining characteristics.

- *Accurate*: Risk for Aspiration related to reduced level of consciousness
- *Inaccurate*: Risk for Secretions entering the airway from impaired swallowing. (The nurse has listed part of the definition and one of the at risk factors in the label.)

Wellness Nursing Diagnoses

A **wellness nursing diagnosis** is a diagnostic statement that describes the human response to levels of wellness in an individual, family, or community that have a potential for enhancement to a higher state (NANDA, 1992). Potential for Enhanced Breastfeeding is an example of wellness nursing diagnosis.

Possible Nursing Diagnoses

A **possible nursing diagnosis** is made when there is not enough evidence to support the presence of the problem, but the nurse thinks it is highly probable and wants to collect more information. The statement is phrased in the same way as an actual problem, except the "related to" phrase is "unknown cause." An example of a possible nursing diagnosis statement follows:

- *Accurate*: Possible Impaired Adjustment related to unknown etiology. (One of the first interventions will be to collect additional assessment data.)
- *Inaccurate*: Adjustment Impaired, Possible due to recent car accident that resulted in quadriplegia. (The nurse has reversed the diagnostic label and included cues in the "related to" phrase.)

Significance of Nursing Diagnosis

Nursing diagnoses provide a means of communicating nursing requirements for client care to other nurses, the healthcare team, and the public. "Nursing diagnoses facilitate the development of nursing autonomy and accountability by focusing the attention of nurses on the phenomena that are uniquely nursing and by providing a common language for communication of the phenomena" (Maas, 1986, p. 39). Nursing diagnostic labels can serve as shorthand for specific client problems.

Although many nursing diagnoses need further research to be clinically useful, all have suggested lists of defining characteristics or risk factors that validate the existence of the problem. Making accurate nursing diagnoses helps to ensure that clients receive quality nursing care.

By focusing attention on the actual or potential health needs of clients, nursing diagnoses increase the specificity of nursing interventions for each client. This specificity can be measured and monitored to make sure that effective interventions are acknowledged for their contribution to resolving the healthcare problem. Coding of nursing diagnoses in computerized systems allows direct reimbursement of nurses. This acknowledgment of nursing's specific contribution in resolving health problems advances professional nursing practice.

Studies of specific nursing diagnoses improve our understanding of the nursing diagnostic process and contribute to examination of the nurse's role in healthcare. As nursing diagnoses become supported by research, a clear description of the scope of nursing practice will emerge. The development and publication of a taxonomy of nursing diagnoses should have a significant impact on practice, education, research, legislation, and nursing as a profession. A nursing diagnosis taxonomy will help to bridge the gap between knowledge and practice and will articulate the scope of nursing practice. This is essential to developing nursing's professional role in healthcare.

Each nurse will decide the usefulness of the nursing diagnosis taxonomy. As the profession develops, the taxonomy will be critically reviewed, revised, and tested. For today's practitioner, the taxonomy meets the need for organization of nursing diagnoses.

The limitations of NANDA Taxonomy I (Rev.) do not mean that it cannot or should not be used in clinical practice. All nurses have the opportunity and responsibility to use the taxonomy in practice. The challenge for each practitioner is to learn the concepts and skills required to assist clients by accurately diagnosing, planning, and implementing nursing care.

Functional Approach to Nursing Diagnosis

Nursing process and nursing diagnosis taxonomy continue to evolve. New nursing diagnoses are added, and existing diagnoses are reworded. The human response pattern evolved from the concept and classification of the Unitary Man. Gordon (1994) has suggested a framework for the organization of nursing diagnoses based on functional health. Functional health offers a convenient way to cluster similar diagnoses. Because this book focuses on function and data collected during the assessment phase is discussed and organized in this fashion, it is useful to organize nursing diagnoses in the same manner. See the complete list of nursing diagnoses organized by function in the display.

Reviewing function and nursing diagnoses for each pattern of function ensures that the nurse has given consideration to all actual, possible, or risk nursing diagnoses. In this manner, the nurse can ensure that physiologic problems do not overshadow the client's emotional, social, or spiritual needs.

Key Concepts

- Collection of assessment data provides the basis for identification of nursing diagnoses.
- Registered nurses are educated and licensed to make nursing diagnoses.
- A nursing diagnosis is a clinical judgment about individual, family, or community responses to actual or potential health problems and life processes.

Nursing Diagnoses Organized by Functional Health Patterns

Health Perception–Health Management

*Energy Field Disturbance
Growth and Development, Altered
Health Maintenance, Altered
Health Seeking Behaviors
Injury, Risk for
  Risk for Suffocation
  Risk for Poisoning
  Risk for Trauma
*Injury, Risk for Perioperative Positioning
*Management of Therapeutic Regimen, Effective
Management of Therapeutic Regimen, Ineffective
*Management of Therapeutic Regimen, Ineffective: Family
*Management of Therapeutic Regimen, Ineffective: Community
Noncompliance

Nutritional–Metabolic

*Adaptive Capacity, Intracranial: Decreased
Body Temperature, Risk for Altered
  Hypothermia
  Hyperthermia
  Thermoregulation, Ineffective
Fluid Volume Deficit
Fluid Volume Excess
Infection, Risk for
Nutrition, Altered: Less Than Body Requirements
Nutrition, Altered: More Than Body Requirements
Nutrition, Altered: Potential for More Than Body Requirements
  Breastfeeding, Effective
  Breastfeeding, Ineffective
  †Breastfeeding, Interrupted
*Feeding Pattern, Ineffective Infant
  Swallowing, Impaired
Protection, Altered
Tissue Integrity, Impaired
  Oral Mucous Membrane, Altered
  Skin Integrity, Impaired
  Skin Integrity, Risk for Impaired

Elimination

Bowel Incontinence
Constipation
Constipation, Colonic
Constipation, Perceived
Diarrhea
Urinary Elimination, Altered
  Urinary Retention
  Total Incontinence
  Functional Incontinence
  Reflex Incontinence
  Urge Incontinence
  Stress Incontinence

Activity–Exercise

Activity Intolerance
Decreased Cardiac Output
Disuse Syndrome, Risk for
Diversional Activity Deficit
Home Maintenance Management, Impaired
*Infant Behavior, Disorganized
*Infant Behavior, Risk for Disorganized
*Infant Behavior, Potential for Enhanced Organized
Mobility, Impaired Physical
*Peripheral Neurovascular Dysfunction, Risk for
†Respiratory Function, Risk for Altered
  Dysfunctional Ventilatory Weaning Response
  Ineffective Airway Clearance
  Ineffective Breathing Patterns
  Impaired Gas Exchange
  Inability to Sustain Spontaneous Ventilation
†Self-Care Deficit (Specify): (Feeding, Bathing/Hygiene, Dressing/Grooming, Toileting)
Tissue Perfusion, Altered: (Specify) (Cerebral, Cardiopulmonary, Renal, Gastrointestinal, Peripheral)

- Activities of nursing diagnoses are pattern identification, diagnostic validation, and formulation of the nursing diagnosis statement.
- NANDA-accepted nursing diagnoses are organized according to human response patterns.
- A nursing diagnosis must address a problem within the scope and education of the registered nurse, and the nurse must be able to intervene legally and independent of physician-prescribed actions.
- The nurse is responsible and accountable to identify and treat collaborative problems, which focus on pathophysiologic responses, in cooperation with the physician.
- The parts of a nursing diagnosis are the diagnostic label, definition, defining characteristics (major and minor), risk factors, related factors, and qualifiers.
- A cue is a piece of information (subjective or objective) collected during the nursing assessment.

Nursing Diagnoses Organized by Functional Health Patterns (Continued)

Sleep–Rest

Sleep Pattern Disturbance

Cognitive–Perceptual

Aspiration, Risk for
Pain
Pain, Chronic
*Confusion, Acute
*Confusion, Chronic
Decisional Conflict
Dysreflexia
*Environmental Interpretation Syndrome, Impaired
Knowledge Deficit: (Specify)
Sensory–Perceptual Alteration: (Specify) (Visual, Auditory, Kinesthetic, Gustatory, Tactile, Olfactory)
Thought Processes, Altered
Unilateral Neglect

Self-Perception

Anxiety
Body Image Disturbance
Fatigue
Fear
Hopelessness
  Personal Identity Disturbance
  Powerlessness
  Self-Esteem Disturbance
    Chronic Low Self-Esteem
    Situational Low Self-Esteem

Role–Relationship

†Communication, Impaired Verbal
*Family Processes, Altered
*Family Process: Alcoholism, Altered
Grieving, Anticipatory
Grieving, Dysfunctional
*Loneliness, Risk for
*Parent/Infant/Child Attachment, Risk for Altered
Parental Role Conflict
Parenting, Altered
Role Performance, Altered
Social Interaction, Impaired
Social Isolation

Sexuality–Reproductive

Sexual Dysfunction
Sexuality Patterns, Altered

Coping–Stress Tolerance

Adjustment, Impaired
*Caregiver Role Strain
Caregiver Role Strain, Risk for
Coping, Ineffective Individual
  Defensive Coping
  Ineffective Denial
Coping, Ineffective Family: Disabling
Coping, Ineffective Family: Compromised
Coping, Family: Potential for Growth
*Coping, Ineffective Community
*Coping, Potential for Enhanced Community
Post-Trauma Response
  Rape-Trauma Syndrome
Relocation Stress Syndrome
Self-Mutilation, Risk for
Violence, Risk for: Self-directed or directed at others

Value–Belief

Spiritual Distress
*Spiritual Well Being, Potential for Enhanced

Source: Carpenito, L. J. (1995). *Handbook of nursing diagnosis (5th ed.).* Philadelphia: J.B. Lippincott; used with permission.

*These diagnoses are staged as Level 1.

- Cluster interpretation is synthesis of the cue clusters. it is an intellectual activity requiring the ability to see the whole picture, attach meaning to the cluster, and discern the pattern the cluster suggests.
- Diagnostic validation occurs in two stages: comparing the clusters with norms and evaluating the specific nursing diagnosis for its particular nursing research base.
- Formulating the nursing diagnostic statement involves writing the actual, risk, wellness, or possible nursing diagnoses.

Critical Thinking Challenges

Now that you have learned about nursing diagnosis, turn back to the situation at the beginning of the chapter, and answer the following questions.

1. *Cluster data provided in this situation under various nursing diagnoses, and provide justification for your decisions regarding data placement. (Note: Some data may fit under several diagnoses.)*
2. *Evaluate patterns in data clustering that indicate adequate support for identifying a nursing diagnosis.*
3. *Construct a list of additional data you need to validate each diagnostic statement, and propose a plan for obtaining this iformation.*
4. *Reflect on factors that could bias your interpretation of this data.*
5. *Create a three-part nursing diagnostic statement.*

References

American Nurses Association. (1973). *Standards of nursing practice.* Kansas City, MO: Author.

American Nurses Association. (1980). *Nursing: A social policy statement.* Kansas City, MO: Author.

American Nurses Association. (1991). *Standards of clinical nursing practice.* Kansas City, MO: Author.

American Psychiatric Association. (1994). *Diagnostic and statistical manual of mental disorders* (4th ed.). Washington, DC: Author.

Carpenito, L. J. (1995). *Nursing diagnosis: Application to clinical practice* (6th ed.). Philadelphia: J.B. Lippincott.

Chase, S. K. (1994). Clinical judgment by critical care nurses: An ethnographic study. In R. M. Carrol-Johnson & M. Paquette (Eds.), *Classification of nursing diagnoses: Proceedings of the tenth conference.* Philadelphia: J.B. Lippincott.

Fitzpatrick, J. J., Kerr, M. E., Saba, V. K., Hoskins, L. M., Hurley, M. E., Mills, W. C., Rottkamp, B. C., Warren, J. J., & Carpenito, L. J. (1989) Translating nursing diagnosis into ICD code. *American Journal of Nursing, 89*(4), 493–495.

Fry, V. (1953). The creative approach to nursing. *American Journal of Nursing, 3,* 301–302.

Gebbie, K., & Lavin, M. (1975). *Classification of nursing diagnoses: Proceedings from the first national conference.* St. Louis: C.V. Mosby.

Gordon, M. (1994). *Manual of nursing diagnosis, 1995-1996.* St. Louis: Mosby-Year Book.

Hammond, K. R. (1966). Clinical inference in nursing: A psychologist's viewpoint. *Nursing Research, 15,* 27–38.

Joint Commission on Accreditation of Healthcare Organizations. (1993). *1994 Accreditation manual for hospitals Vol. 1. Standards.* Chicago: Author.

Maas, M. L. (1986). Nursing diagnoses in a professional model of nursing: Keystones for effective nursing administration. *Journal of Nursing Administration, 16*(12), 39–42.

NANDA. (1994). NANDA News. *Nursing Diagnosis, 5*(2), 52–55.

North American Nursing Diagnosis Association. (1990). *NANDA taxonomy I* (rev.) St. Louis: Author.

North American Nursing Diagnosis Association. (1994). *NANDA nursing diagnoses: Definitions and classification.* Philadelphia: Author.

Pinkley, C. L. (1994). Linking diagnostic judgment with outcomes and interventions. In R. M. Carroll-Johnson & M. Paquette (Eds.), *Classification of nursing diagnoses: Proceedings of the tenth conference.* Philadelphia: J. B. Lippincott.

Yura, H., & Walsh, M. B. (1973). *The nursing process.* Norwalk, CT: Appleton-Century-Crofts.

Yura, H., & Walsh, M. B. (1988). *The nursing process* (5th ed.). Norwalk, CT: Appleton & Lange.

Bibliography

Alfaro-LeFevre, R. (1994). *Applying nursing process: A step-by-step guide* (3rd ed.). Philadelphia: J. B. Lippincott.

Avant, K. C. (1990). The art and science in nursing diagnosis development. *Nursing Diagnosis, 1*(2), 51–55.

Benner, P., & Tanner, C. (1987). Clinical judgment: How expert nurses use intuition. *American Journal of Nursing, 87,* 23–31.

Dickel, C. A., & Mehmert, P. A., (1994). Self-care deficit: Bathing/hygiene replication study: Defining characteristics and related factors documented in acute care. In R. M. Carrol-Johnson & M. Parquette (Eds.), *Classification of nursing diagnoses: Proceedings of the tenth conference* (pp. 325–326). Philadelphia: J. B. Lippincott

Hamers, J. P. H., Huijer Abu-Saad, H., & Halfens, R. M. G. (1994). Diagnostic process and decision making in nursing: A literature review. *Journal of Professional Nursing, 10*(3), 154–163.

Heafey, M. L., Golden-Baker, S. B., & Mahoney, D. W. (1994). Using nursing diagnoses and interventions in an inpatient amputee program. *Rehabilitation Nursing, 19*(93), 163–168.

LeMone, P. (1993). Validation of the defining characteristics of altered sexuality patterns. *Nursing Diagnosis, 4* (2), 56–62.

Lunney, M. (1990). *Concept of nursing diagnosis: History.* Prepared for NANDA. New York.

Radwin, L. E. (1990). Research on diagnostic reasoning in nursing. *Nursing Diagnosis, 1* (2), 70–77.

Outcome Identification and Planning

Key Terms	Learning Objectives
Goal Outcome criteria Outcome identification Planning phase Priority Qualifier Scientific rationale	Upon completion of this chapter, the student will be able to do the following: • Define outcome identification and planning. • Discuss the purposes of outcome identification and planning. • Describe the components of the nursing plan of care. • Formulate a nursing plan of care for a client given a nursing assessment database. • Use a functional health approach to plan client care.

12

You are working as a nurse in an extended care facility. You admit a client from the community hospital who had a total hip replacement 1 week ago. Your admission assessment reveals the following:

Client states, "They sent me here until I could walk better because my daughter isn't willing to take me like this!" Medical history includes arthritis controlled with nonsteroidal anti-inflammatory drugs and irregular heart rhythm controlled with digoxin; vital signs stable (VSS), incision healing well; fair appetite, no swallowing difficulties; BM every 2 or 3 days (often needs laxative); physical therapy twice a day to work on ambulating with a walker and increasing endurance.

From this data, you identify the following nursing diagnoses:

Impaired Physical Mobility related to inability to ambulate or transfer independently, decreased muscle strength, therapeutic restricted adduction of hip

Constipation related to decreased physical mobility and inability to perform toileting tasks

In previous chapters of this unit, you learned about nursing assessment and nursing diagnoses. In this chapter, you will learn how to work with the client to identify outcomes and plan nursing care. When you complete this chapter, you should be able to apply all the information you have learned so far about the nursing process to make plans for caring for this client who underwent total hip replacement. Reflecting on the Critical Thinking Challenges at the end of this chapter will further strengthen your ability to take care of your clients.

After assessment data have been collected and analyzed and nursing diagnoses have been identified and validated, the nurse is ready to begin planning care with the client. Nursing is a practice discipline, which involves application of theoretical knowledge to actual client situations. The nurse and client set realistic goals in what the nursing process calls outcome identification. Plans are then made concerning interventions to be used to meet those goals.

Outcome Identification

Outcome identification is the formulation of goals and measurable outcomes that provide the basis for evaluation for nursing diagnoses. Outcome identification is the most recent addition to the nursing process as described in the current American Nurses Association (ANA) *Standards of Clinical Nursing Practice* (1991). The ANA describes seven measurement criteria for outcome identification. Outcome identification, including client goals and outcome criteria, are an integral part of the format of Chapters 29–53 in Section II of this text. A section discussing outcome identification and planning appears in each chapter after nursing diagnoses. Client goals applicable to each diagnosis are listed. The same client goals with examples of outcome criteria appear in the evaluation section and are included in the plan of care at the end of the chapter.

The purpose of outcome identification includes the following:

- Provide individualized care.
- Promote client participation.
- Plan care that is realistic and measurable.
- Allow for involvement of support people.

Activities performed in this phase of the nursing process are the following:

- Establish priorities.
- Establish client goals and outcome criteria.

Outcome identification in relation to other phases of the nursing process is shown in Figure 12-1.

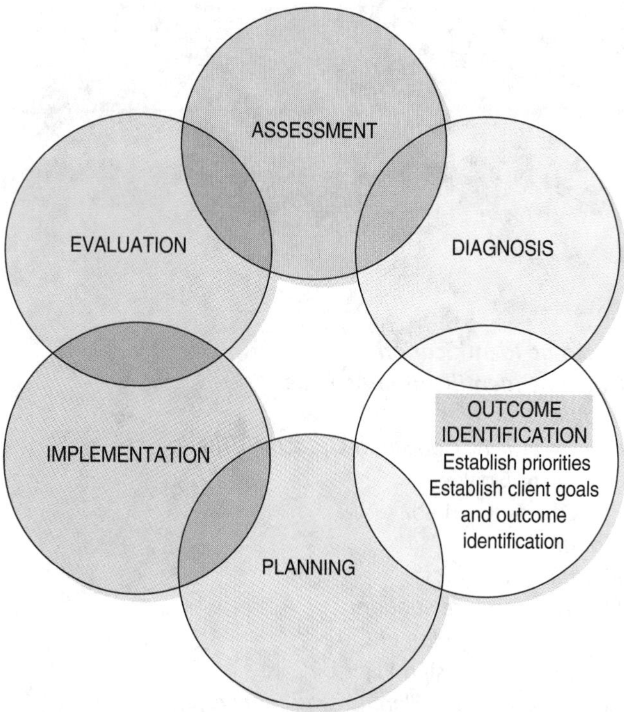

Figure 12-1* • *ANA Standard III states: The nurse identifies expected outcomes individualized to the client. This illustration shows activities used in the Outcome Identification phase and also the relationship of Outcome Identification to the other phases of the nursing process.

Outcome Identification Activities

Establish Priorities

A **priority** is something that takes precedence in position; it is deemed the most important among several items. Priority setting is a decision-making process that ranks the order of nursing diagnoses in terms of importance to the client. Priorities are constantly changing as the client's situation and condition change. Clinical expertise and practice are involved in establishing priorities. The nurse uses experience, knowledge, and assessment data collected from the client to determine priorities. High priorities for the client involve the following:

- Life-threatening situation (eg, difficulty breathing, hemorrhage)
- Something that needs immediate attention (eg, preparation for a test, discharge from the facility that will occur shortly)
- Something that is very important to the client (eg, pain or anxiety)

Life-threatening problems always take precedence over routine care. For instance, maintaining an airway when a client is having respiratory difficulties always takes precedence over client teaching. Often the client's physical condition is more stable, and determining priorities is more subtle. If the client is receiving care in the home, establishing priorities might include determining what should be taught to a newly diagnosed diabetic client during a 60-minute home visit.

High-priority nursing diagnoses are those that are potentially life-threatening and require immediate action. Examples are Impaired Gas Exchange, Dysreflexia (a condition in which a spinal cord–injured client experiences life-threatening inhibited sympathetic responses due to noxious stimuli), or Self-Directed Risk for Violence. In each of these situations, the individual could die if appropriate intervention is not initiated.

Medium-priority nursing diagnoses involve problems that could result in unhealthy consequences, such as physical or emotional impairment, but are not likely to threaten life. Examples include Fatigue, Stress Incontinence, or Dysfunctional Grieving. Assessment data from the client determine how significant and what priority each nursing diagnosis is assigned.

Low-priority nursing diagnoses involve problems that often can be resolved easily with minimal interventions and have little potential to cause significant dysfunction. Often the low-priority status is based on the significance for the client and the high likelihood that the problem will be easily resolved. For example, Pain might be a nursing diagnosis for a client following minor surgery, but because the pain is moderate and probably will last only a short time, the problem is low priority.

Sometimes clients and nurses disagree on the priority that problems are given. For example, a postoperative client may view pain as the most important problem and try to avoid moving or ambulating so that pain will decrease. The nurse might view ineffective breathing pattern as much more significant for this client. Through dialogue, the nurse and client are able to share their opinions, experiences, and values with each other so that an agreeable plan can be determined. After listening to the client, the nurse may say, "I see you are in pain, but it is important to ambulate so that you do not develop respiratory complications. How about planning to get you up 30 minutes after you get your pain medication so that your pain is well controlled by then?" During shift change, client goals and progress can be shared with other staff to promote continuity of care (Fig. 12-2).

Nurses use priorities to plan care and determine the order in which interventions will be carried out. Sometimes availability limits whether all desirable interventions can actually be carried out. For example, a nurse may want to wash a client's hair to promote self-esteem, but time may not allow this if two other clients are scheduled for surgery.

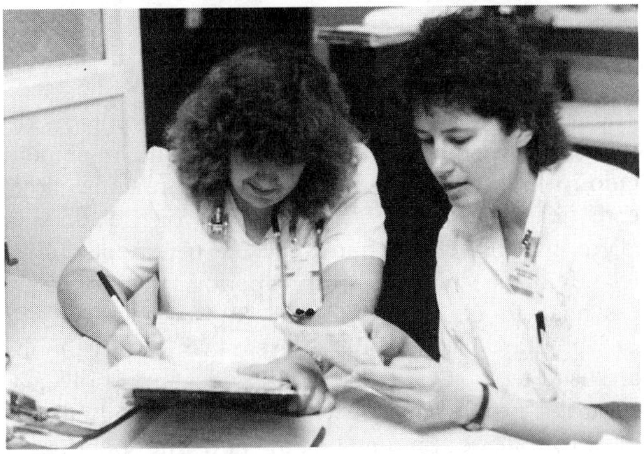

Figure 12-2 • *Outcome criteria clarify what is expected of the client as a result of nursing care. Such criteria, as part of care, are useful when shifts change and for evaluation of the client and care provided.*

Establish Client Goals and Outcome Criteria

Often the terms goals, objectives, and outcomes are used interchangeably because they are statements of expectations. Because of this, nurses should be familiar with the specific use of terms in the clinical setting in which they work. A distinction is made in this textbook: client goals and outcomes are not used interchangeably. Their definitions and use are described in the following sections.

Client Goals

A client **goal** is an educated guess, made as a broad statement, about what the client's state will be after the nursing intervention is carried out. It directly addresses the problem stated in the nursing diagnosis. Using clinical knowledge and experience, the nurse, in collaboration with the client, determines appropriate goals.

Behavioral goals are written to indicate a desired state. They contain an action verb and a qualifier that indicate the level of performance needed to be achieved. Some commonly used behavioral verbs are presented in the accompanying display. The **qualifier** is a description of the parameter for achieving the goal. For instance, "walks" would not be a specific client goal. Restating this client goal as "ambulates safely with one-person assistance" clarifies this goal statement.

Goals may be short-term or long-term. A short-term goal can be met in a relatively short period of time (within days or less than 1 week). A long-term goal requires more time, perhaps several weeks or months. A long-term goal also may indicate ongoing activity. Long-term goals are usually stated by using "every day" or "will maintain" (Alfaro-LeFevre, 1994).

Goals need to be revised if the client's situation or medical condition changes. For example, you are working in the home with a client who has mobility deficits from multiple sclerosis. During the home visit, you and

Behavioral Verbs Used in Care Plans

Calculate	Distinguish	Practice
Classify	Draw	Recall
Communicate	Explain	Recite
Compare	Express	Record
Construct	Identify	Stand
Contrast	List	State
Define	Maintain	Use
Demonstrate	Name	Verbalize
Describe	Participate	Walk
Discuss	Perform	

the client decide that a goal is to be "ambulates safely with a quad cane." Two weeks later during another home visit, you notice increased mobility problems due to an exacerbation of multiple sclerosis. This change in the client's medical condition was unexpected and not within your control. An appropriate revision of a goal might be "transfers safely to a chair, with one-person assistance." As this client's mobility status improves or deteriorates, mobility goals will need to be revised.

Outcome Criteria

Outcome criteria are specific, measurable, realistic statements of goal attainment. They may restate the goal, but they also present information that will guide the evaluation phase of the nursing process. To be specific and measurable, certain requirements must be met when writing outcome criteria. Outcome criteria answer the questions who, what actions, under what circumstances, how well, and when (Alfaro-LeFevre, 1994). According to Alfaro-LeFevre (1994), requirements include the following:

- Subject: *Who* is the person expected to achieve the goal?
- Verb: *What actions* must the person do to achieve the goal?
- Condition: *Under what circumstances* is the person to perform the action?
- Criteria: *How well* is the person to perform the action?
- Specific time: *When* is the person expected to perform the action?

For example, the client (*who*) verbalizes (*what action*) three dietary modifications of a low-salt diet to his wife (*under what circumstances*) accurately (*how well*) following the teaching session (*when*).

Planning

Planning, the fourth phase of the nursing process, refers to the development of nursing strategies designed to ameliorate client problems. A plan of care is developed to direct nursing care activities related to the individual for whom the goals and outcomes were set. The written plan of care directs the activities of the nursing staff in the provision of client care.

Purposes of planning are the following:

- Direct client care activities.
- Promote continuity of care.
- Focus charting requirements.
- Allow for delegation of specific activities.

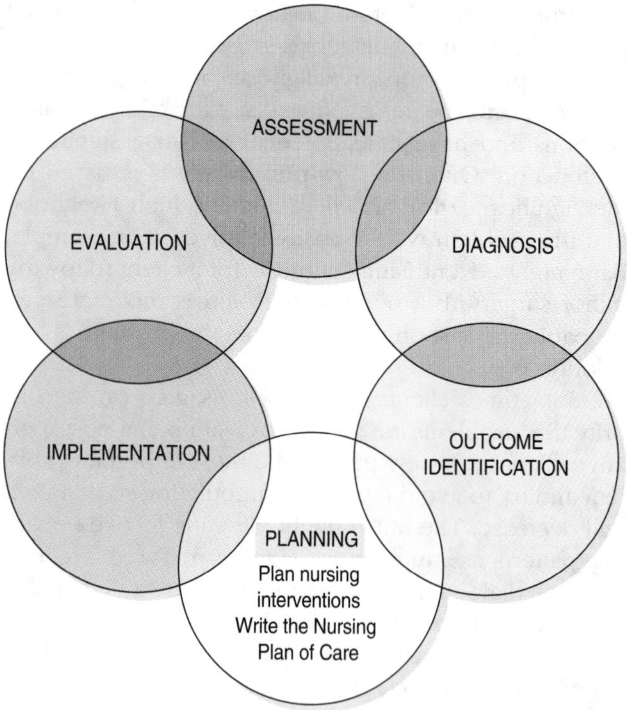

Figure 12-3 • *ANA Standard IV states: The nurse develops a plan of care that prescribes interventions to attain expected outcomes. This illustration shows activities used in the Planning Phase and also the relationship of Planning to the other phases of the nursing process.*

Activities of the planning phase follow:

- Plan nursing interventions.
- Write the nursing plan of care.

Planning in relation to other phases of the nursing process is illustrated in Figure 12-3.

Planning Activities

Plan Nursing Interventions

The selection of appropriate nursing interventions directs activities that will be carried out in the implementation phase. **Nursing interventions** are "any direct care treatment that a nurse performs on behalf of a client, which includes nurse-initiated treatments, physician-initiated treatments, and performance of daily essential functions" (Bulechek & McCloskey, 1992, p. 26). Alfaro-LeFevre (1994) says nursing interventions are used to monitor health status; prevent, resolve, or control a problem; assist with activities of daily living; or promote optimum health and independence. Interventions are written as specific activities on the plan of care.

Determination of appropriate nursing interventions for a specific client requires clinical knowledge and practice. In general, interventions can be grouped to describe the activity being suggested. Work in the area of classification of interventions is just beginning (Bulechek & McCloskey, 1992). At this point, types of interventions include the following:

- Psychomotor (positioning, inserting, applying)
- Psychosocial (supporting, exploring, encouraging)
- Educational (demonstrating, teaching, observing return demonstrations)
- Maintenance (skin care, hygiene)
- Surveillance (detecting changes)
- Supervisory (other healthcare providers)
- Sociocultural (spending time, incorporating cultural differences into care regimen)

Write a Nursing Plan of Care

The problem-solving process is documented in the nursing plan of care. The ability to create the nursing plan of care has become a standard expected of every nurse. The plan is a critical element in focusing nursing activity. To serve as evaluation criteria and meet the standards of the Joint Commission for Accreditation of Healthcare Organizations (JCAHO, 1993), the plan must be developed by a registered nurse, must be documented in the client's health record, and must reflect the standards of care established by the institution and the profession. Medicare and Medicaid standards require nursing plans of care for each client.

The following are two important guidelines when developing a nursing plan of care:

- The plan of care is *nursing* centered.
- The plan of care is a step-by-step process.

Keeping the plan of care *nursing* centered is essential to identify the scope and depth of nursing practice. By focusing on the treatment of human responses to actual or potential health problems, the nurse remains in the nursing practice domain.The following apply to the second guideline:

- Sufficient data are collected to substantiate nursing diagnoses.
- At least one goal must be stated for each nursing diagnosis.
- Outcome criteria must be identified for each goal.
- Nursing interventions must be specifically designed to meet the identified goal.
- Each intervention should be supported by scientific rationale.
- Evaluation must address whether each goal was completely met, partially met, or completely unmet.

Types of Nursing Plans of Care

The nursing plan of care can be written in various ways. Institutions may use a portable metal card file format, a notebook, or a computerized care plan design. Despite these design differences, the plan of care usually contains three key elements: the nursing diagnosis (client problem), client goals, and nursing interventions (nursing orders, nursing actions). The plan of care can be written for the individual client, standardized for a client population, generic for a specific problem, or computer-generated from assessment data. Students learning to write plans use the instructional nursing plan of care format. In practice settings, nurses use the clinical nursing plan of care format. Each of these plans is discussed in the remainder of the chapter.

Instructional Nursing Plans of Care. Instructional nursing plans of care allow the student to learn about a variety of client problems and the processes nurses use to solve them. Scientific rationales from nursing literature are given as references for the information and to illustrate the nurse's decision-making process. Specific recommendations for completing this type of plan of care are given using each step of the nursing process. These guidelines also apply to writing a clinical nursing plan of care as a practicing nurse and are refined further in Section II of this text.

Preparing the Instructional Nursing Plan of Care. Usually student nurses are required to complete some form of an instructional nursing plan of care. The purpose is to demonstrate in a written format an understanding of the problem-solving process used in assisting clients to maintain or regain a higher level of function. Once assessment data have been collected, organized, and synthesized, one or more nursing diagnoses are identified (see Chaps. 10 and 11). Each nursing diagnosis is used in the development of the plan of care.

Components of instructional nursing plans of care usually include nursing diagnoses, client goals or client outcome criteria, nursing interventions, scientific rationale, and evaluation.

The format used in Section II of this text illustrates this format and includes one nursing diagnosis, one or more client goals, several client outcome criteria, nursing interventions, and scientific rationale. The goals and outcome criteria reflect those discussed in that specific chapter. The nursing plans of care are designed in the sample format given in the accompanying display; they appear at the end of Chapters 29 through 53. To help the student understand what to include in each section of the plan, a second copy of the format with instructions for completion is included here.

To assist in learning how to state nursing diagnoses, client goals, outcome criteria, nursing interventions, scientific rationale, and evaluation correctly, refer to Table 12-1.

Nursing Diagnosis. The nursing diagnostic statement is recorded in the space labeled "nursing diagnosis,"

Nursing Plan of Care Format Used in This Text

*Nursing Diagnosis:*______________________________
*Client Goal:*______________________________
Client Outcome Criteria

- ______________________________
- ______________________________
- ______________________________

Nursing Intervention	*Scientific Rationale*
1. ____________________	1. ____________________
2. ____________________	2. ____________________

using NANDA terminology if possible. A three-part statement composed of the diagnostic label, the related factor (*related to*), and the defining characteristics that support the label (*manifested by*) is used. For risk diagnoses, risk factors are provided with the diagnostic label, creating a two-part statement. Wellness nursing diagnoses are one-part statements containing only the diagnostic label. Refer to Chapter 11, Figure 11-4, and Table 11-4 for more examples. All of the identified nursing diagnoses for a client should be listed in order of priority for client care. Using a functional approach helps the nurse focus on real or potential functional problems rather than on disease pathology.

Client Goals. One or more client goals are established for each nursing diagnosis. The goal is a broadly stated objective that indicates an overall picture of the state of the client if the problem is ameliorated or resolved. Each goal must be measurable, realistic, or observable. Some examples of goal statements include maintains present weight, demonstrates no evidence of infection, and administers insulin correctly. The goal describes a client outcome in broad terms. The client goal reflects resolution or correction of the identified problem.

Client Outcome Criteria. Client outcome criteria are specific, measurable, realistic statements that can be

Information to be Placed in Nursing Plan of Care

Nursing Diagnosis (Use the NANDA-accepted list of nursing diagnoses. List in priority order. Use the diagnostic label and "related to" [related factor], followed by "manifested by" [supporting defining characteristics].)

Client Goal (One or more client goals established from nursing diagnosis. A broadly stated objective that indicates an overall picture of the state of the client if the problem is resolved.)

Client Outcome Criteria (Specific, measurable, realistic statements that can be evaluated to judge goal attainment. Stated as behavioral objectives, they include a verb, a short phrase describing the specific measure to be accomplished, and a time reference.)

Nursing Intervention	*Scientific Rationale*
(Write interventions [nursing orders] that are specific and relate to the goal. The "related to" phrase of the nursing diagnostic statement directs choice of nursing interventions. Interventions include who, what, when, and how the order is to be carried out.)	(Gives justification for carrying out the intervention. Demonstrates synthesis of physiologic, psychological, and pathophysiological concepts.)

Table 12-1 • Correct and Incorrect Plan of Care Entries

Entry	Rationale
Nursing Diagnoses	
Correct Feeding self-care deficit (Level 3) related to right-sided weakness manifested by inability to pick up spoon, lack of attention to food on tray, and inability to open containers	Correct statement of actual nursing diagnosis using three-part statement, including diagnostic label, related factors, and defining characteristics.
Incorrect Self-care deficit, Feeding: due to left cerebrovascular accident, manifested by not eating	Incorrect statement of actual diagnosis. Diagnostic label is inverted, a medical diagnosis is used for the causative agent, and defining characteristics are not provided for validation of the diagnosis.
Client Goal	
Correct Client demonstrates correct skin care regimen	Correctly stated client goal: general statement of overall picture of client if problem is resolved; measurable, realistic, and observable.
Incorrect Client's skin is free of eczema	Incorrect statement of client goal. The goal is not achievable through nursing interventions and may be unrealistic even with medical treatment.
Client Outcome Criteria	
Correct Ambulates 30 feet with walker before discharge	Correctly stated client outcome: specific, measurable, and realistic.
Incorrect Walks in the hall	Incorrectly stated outcome criterion because it is not specific and does not include qualifiers for the outcome.
Nursing Interventions	
Correct Staff will perform passive range of motion exercises to all extremities during morning care and evening care	Correctly stated nursing intervention, including who, what, when, and how nursing order will be carried out.
Incorrect Encourage joint mobility	Incorrectly stated nursing intervention because time frame, type of exercise, and who will perform the exercise are not specified.
Scientific Rationale	
Correct Small shifts in body weight promote circulation and help to prevent skin breakdown (Craven & Hirnle, 1995)	Correctly stated rationale: tells scientific basis for nursing action and correctly cites source.
Incorrect Changes position every 2 hours	Incorrectly stated scientific rationale: restates a nursing intervention without documenting why it is an appropriate nursing intervention, and no source is cited.
Evaluation	
Correct Unable to complete passive range of motion to right upper extremity after morning care because of reported pain when arm is elevated above shoulder level. Physician notified, and patient instructed to rest arm.	Correctly stated evaluation because it indicates that goal was not met, with specific documentation providing the data for revision.
Incorrect Range of motion discontinued due to pain	Incorrect evaluation statement: statement does not contain client's response or follow up on the problem.

evaluated to judge goal attainment. They should include a time reference. Outcome criteria are stated in terms of behavioral objectives. They include a verb that denotes the action and a short phrase that describes the specific measure to be accomplished:

- Draws up correct dosage of insulin at next teaching session.
- Demonstrates deep-breathing and coughing exercises at next teaching session.
- Verbalizes to the nurse during evening shift a basic understanding of the relationship between excessive stimuli and feelings of loss of control.

Nursing Interventions. Sometimes called nursing orders, nursing interventions are written in specific terms that relate to the goals. The "related to" phrase of the nursing diagnostic statement directs the choice of nursing interventions. Each nursing intervention must specify who, what, when, and how the order is to be carried out. "Interventions are designed to resolve a problem or to minimize adverse sequalae, traumatic impact, and severity of the problem. In the case of potential problems or high-risk states, interventions reduce risk factors and prevent the problem" (Gordon et al., 1994, p. 66). The statements should be comprehensive but brief; the nurse may refer to procedures, protocols, or standing policies for further information. In some cases, nursing interventions include specific measures needed to carry out the medical regimen and are not directed at a nursing diagnosis. Examples are shown in Table 12-2.

Scientific Rationale. **Scientific rationale** is the justification or reason for carrying out the intervention. It often synthesizes psychological and pathophysiologic concepts. The rationale—the "why" of the intervention—describes a research-based reason for why intervention should be performed. Usually student nurses are required to supply scientific rationale to show they understand the basic reasons for carrying out specific nursing interventions. In clinical practice settings, the nurse may use rationales to illustrate new research findings or support a controversial approach to a problem. A reference for each scientific rationale must be given, citing the author, year, title, and page of the article or book used. Sometimes nurses think that interventions are based on common sense, but this is not so: many nursing interventions previously thought to be sensible have turned out to be unsafe, impractical, or unnecessary. Asking why certain nursing interventions are performed aids in the scientific development of nursing practice.

Evaluation. The evaluation of a nursing intervention is a written statement that determines the client's status in relation to the outcome criteria at a particular time. The evaluation stage answers the question, was the goal achieved? It provides the necessary feedback to guide revision of the plan of care or resolution of the problem. Changes may be needed in the time frame for goal achievement or to facilitate new skill development in the client. In some cases, the student will state what *would* have been evaluated if nursing care had been provided during additional clinical experiences.

Evaluation of care usually is recorded in the narrative nursing note and includes the client's response to the intervention and the objective clinical findings. Each intervention is evaluated for effectiveness, modified if needed, and deleted if not necessary.

Clinical Nursing Plans of Care. The clinical plan of care used in practice is different from the required instructional plan of care done by students. The nursing process is used, but the plan is organized in a practical, concise format for daily use. There is less specific detail, and rationales are not documented. The focus is to individualize the plan of care for each client using findings from the nursing assessment and identified nursing diagnoses.

Individual Plan of Care. Individual plans of care are written for each client by a registered nurse. The nursing diagnoses are listed, along with specific goals and interventions to resolve the problem. This method is ideal, but it is time consuming.

Standardized Plan of Care. Standardized plans of care are written by a group of nurses who are experts in a

Table 12-2 • Examples of Nursing Interventions to Include the Medical Regimen

Medical Order	Nursing Intervention
Weight qd, report loss > 5#	Bedscale weight every day at 6 AM; report weight > (specify #) to team leader and physician.
Increase caloric intake	Provide between-meal snack at 10 AM, 2 PM, and 10 PM. Request consultation with dietitian (done 10/19). Transfer client to chair for each meal and snack.

given area of practice (eg, obstetrics, rehabilitation, or orthopedics). The plan is written for a client population with a specific medical diagnosis (ie, total hip replacement, pressure ulcer, vaginal delivery, or coronary artery bypass surgery). These experts identify the most common nursing diagnoses for this client population and write the goals and interventions usually necessary to resolve the problem. Each time a standardized plan of care is used, it must be individualized for a specific client. This method assures the nurse that the plan is correct for the client. The danger of a standardized plan of care lies in the fact that it may not fit a specific client. Nurses must make judgments as to the degree standardized plans should be modified or if they should not be used in individual cases.

Generic Plan of Care. Generalized plans of care usually are written for a specific nursing diagnosis. They contain the goals and interventions most commonly seen when that particular nursing diagnosis is identified. Again, the generic plan of care must be individualized for a specific client. Because generic plans are written by experts in a particular diagnostic area, they may serve as a learning tool for the inexperienced nurse who is unfamiliar with the content.

Computerized Plan of Care. Computerized plans of care are generated from assessment data entered into a computer about a specific client. The plan is written by experts in the area, and the content is similar to that of the standardized or generic plan of care. Once the plan is on the computer screen, the nurse has an opportunity to customize it for the client. Because these plans are linked to assessment data, it is critical that all pertinent information be collected and entered into the system. The generated plan of care is only as good as the data on which it is based.

Preparing the Clinical Nursing Plan of Care. As the nurse becomes more experienced, he or she continues to refine the process of writing plans of care and actively uses them in implementing daily care. In the clinical nursing plan of care, the nursing process is used, but the plan is organized in a practical, concise format. There is less specific detail, and rationales are not documented. The goal is to individualize the plan for each client using findings from the nursing assessment and identified nursing diagnoses. A well-written, continually updated nursing plan of care is an invaluable tool. The steps of a clinical plan of care follow.

Assessment and Data Collection. The nurse continues data collection and client assessment. The history and physical assessment are guidelines for the initial plan. Data are gathered in each subsequent meeting with the client to revise the plan.

Nursing Diagnosis. The nursing diagnosis in a working plan of care is written using the guidelines in Chapter 11. The instructional plan of care includes all possible client problems; the clinical plan of care focuses on individual client needs and priority nursing problems.

Outcome Identification. Client goals and outcome criteria are often seen in the same statement. The goals are specific to meeting the client problems identified in the nursing diagnoses.

Interventions. Nursing actions specific to each client's needs are documented. The healthcare person responsible for performing the nursing action is identified. The action may be most appropriately completed by the nurse, but in some instances, it is delegated to auxiliary nursing personnel. This leads to better communication and use of plans for daily assignments and is particularly important in practice.

Rationale. Although scientific rationale is not documented in the clinical plan, it is no less important than in the instructional plan. The nurse must know the rationale behind the nursing actions or must question and review the rationale before performing the action. This is a professional responsibility and is expected of every practicing nurse.

Evaluation. Evaluation is ongoing from initial care through resolution of the problem. Evaluation in the

Nursing Research
Outcome Identification

Selected Nursing Research Studies

Buchanan, L.M. (1994). Therapeutic nursing intervention knowledge development and outcome measures for advanced practice. *Nursing & Health Care, 15,* 190–195.

de la Cruz, F.A. (1994). Clinical decision-making styles of home healthcare nurses. *Image: Journal of Nursing Scholarship, 26,* 222–226.

Wanich, C.K., Sullivan-Marx, E.M., Gottlieb, G.L., & Johnson, J.C. (1992). Functional status outcomes of nursing intervention in hospitalized elderly. *Image: Journal of Nursing Scholarship, 24,* 201–207.

Possible Topics for Nursing Inquiry

- What is the effect of the establishment of outcome criteria on the quality of life of clients with chronic illness?
- Does instituting a nursing plan of care collaboratively with the client, family, and healthcare team maximize the client's level of functioning?
- In what ways does the process of developing a nursing plan of care differ in novice nurses and experienced nurses?
- How do the cultural and belief systems of a client influence the formation of the nursing plan of care?
- What is the relationship between healthcare reform and outcome criteria development?

clinical plan is based on the specific observations made of client progress toward the outcome criteria as outlined in the plan. The plan is updated and changed—minute by minute in critical and acute care, weekly or monthly in long-term or home healthcare.

Collaborative Care Plan: Critical Pathways

Critical pathways (paths) are becoming the current standard guideline for nursing care in many hospitals. The focus on outcome management, controlling costs, and continuous quality improvement has been the driving force for most organizations as they convert to critical paths and case management as a system for care delivery (Zander, 1993a). Various terms for critical paths are used: clinical paths, collaborative care plans, CareMaps, multidisciplinary care plan, and case management plans.

The critical path is a cause-and-effect grid that describes a client's problems with intermediate outcomes and multidisciplinary staff actions along a timeline. The critical path tool can be designed for clients with a particular illness, diagnostic-related grouping (DRG), procedure, or condition. Timelines can be developed for a continuum of care in the hospital in terms of hours, days, and months; across geographic care units (emergency room, CCU, telemetry); or for a continuum of care in the community.

To help you understand the use of critical pathways, a generic form is included. In this case, blanks are filled in with generic information. Three more examples of critical pathways are included in Chapters 28, 33, and 35. They follow the format shown here. The format may differ in some agencies.

Information on the critical path is based on the most cost-efficient practice patterns for a particular diagnosis or procedure. This method addresses key events in the treatment process that must be accomplished to achieve predetermined outcomes at a minimal cost. The staff nurse is responsible for initiating, maintaining, and completing the critical path, including documentation of variances. Many hospitals are developing a version of the critical path for clients and families to help increase their understanding of and participation in the plan of care.

Most critical paths incorporate quality indicators and discharge criteria to measure the quality of care provided. The client's progress at the time of discharge is measured against established criteria. The paths reflect the criteria of the Health Care Financing Administration. Clients who do not meet the discharge criteria and are discharged must be monitored for readmissions and premature discharges.

The impetus for critical paths was the Federal government's prospective payment system (DRGs) aimed at controlling costs for Medicare and Medicaid clients in the early 1980s. The reduction in healthcare costs was believed to result from shortening the length of stay (LOS) for hospitalized clients. However, hospitals needed to increase the quality and efficiency in healthcare delivery to achieve the predetermined LOS specified by the DRGs. Consequently, critical paths were specifically written to incorporate the DRG-determined LOS into the timeline. If critical paths were followed and clients were discharged within the predetermined LOS, hospitals were reimbursed the predicted cost.

Critical paths became an ideal tool to help clients achieve the predicted LOS, improve quality, and control costs.

A key to the success of critical paths is that they are collaboratively developed by the multidisciplinary team involved in care of that client population. The collaboration helps ensure that the tool is relevant and will be followed by all members of the health team.

The New England Medical Center Hospital in Boston is credited as being the first hospital to develop critical paths, now called CareMaps™. Their case management and critical path/CareMap system has evolved during the past decade to include a comprehensive tool. Although the critical path was developed primarily as a case management tool, it is being used alone or with case management to guide client care activities in healthcare institutions. In some hospitals, critical paths are used as a guideline for client care in as much as 80% of the hospital's population. The remainder of clients require case management because of complex health problems, complications, or need for follow-up or referral (Zander, 1993b).

A criterion for success of the critical path is consistency in healthcare delivery. Lack of consistency in care delivery usually results in a variance from the critical path. Variances occur when a deviation occurs in the path that alters an expected outcome or the date of discharge. Client, staff, and system variances can occur. Some hospitals also include variances in the community. Variances are monitored concurrently and retrospectively for continuous quality improvement. Variance measurement has the potential for identifying client problems and complications early in hospitalization, variations in practice patterns, and system problems.

A recent development in the critical path movement has been to include documentation as a permanent part of the client's health record. Incorporating documentation in the design of the critical path eliminates much of the redundancy in charting. Critical path documentation consists of writing the provider's initials next to the outcome and intervention or indicating whether a variance occurred. Some hospitals place a "V" next to the outcome or intervention if a variance occurs. Documentation of client variance is written in the progress or nurse's notes. Staff and system variances are documented on a separate variance sheet so that data can be monitored for continuous quality improvement.

Nurses must have a thorough understanding of the nursing process not only because it is the basis for

Generic Collaborative Care Plan: Critical Pathway (and types of information included in such a plan)

Collaborative Care Plan: Critical Pathway

Client Name: ______			
Case Type: ______	Admit Date: ______	Expected LOS: ______	
DRG: ______	Date Path	Actual LOS: ______	Physician: ______
ICD-9: ______	Initiated: ______	Discharge Date: ______	Case Manager: ______

Outcome Criteria

(Timeline)	*(Date) Day 1 (may be expressed in hours, days, or events)*				*Day 2*				*Day 3 (may extend for more days or expected length of stay)*			
CLIENT PROBLEMS	*(Site of Care)*	*D*	*E*	*N*		*D*	*E*	*N*		*D*	*E*	*N*
(May be stated as nursing diagnoses or client problems for individualized care. Usually includes 3–5 problems)	(Intermediate or expected outcome for each problem.)				(Rather than Day, Evening, Night, may be 12-hour shifts with two columns)							
(May include more than one space)												
INTERVENTIONS	(May be stated as nurse, physician, or client actions or actions of any health-care members)											
Consult/Referral (List appropriate referrals to specific health-care providers)												
Diagnostic Tests (Diagnostic or laboratory tests needed for this particular client)												
Assessment (Routine or specific assessments required)												
Treatments (Multidisciplinary procedures such as antiembolic stockings, oxygen administration, dressing changes, Foley catheter)												

(continued)

nursing care, but also because it is the underlying framework for the critical path. The nursing process, however, is a problem-solving process and a mental function, while the critical path is a tool that operationalizes that process. Hospitals that are developing critical paths without listing the client problems (or nursing diagnoses) and intermediate outcomes or discharge outcomes have fragmented the nursing process. When outcome is separated from process, outcomes based on that process cannot be evaluated. The nurse

Generic Collaborative Care Plan: Critical Pathway (and types of information included in such a plan) *(continued)*

	Day 1				Day 2				Day 3			
Patient Problems		D	E	N		D	E	N		D	E	N
Activity (Includes mobility prescriptions or limitations)												
Diet (Prescribed diet, supplement, or restrictions)												
Meds (Regularly scheduled & PRN meds. IV may be included)												
Teaching (Routine teaching expected for client/family—when and by whom)												
Discharge/Transfer Planning (Coordination of services & referrals for transition to home or other healthcare facility. May indicate follow-up services or appointment)												

Initials/Signatures:

____

____

____

____

____

Write "V" for variance in box if expected outcome not met or intervention not performed as stated. Client variances need to be explained in progress notes.

or health team member cannot determine whether a particular outcome was a result of a specific intervention if they are not linked accordingly. Critical paths that function as comprehensive multidisciplinary care plans allow for the evaluation of the nursing process, documentation of that process, and monitoring for continuous quality improvement. Integration of the nursing process within the critical path framework is essential to ensure an outcome-based, accountability-driven system. By including a documentation section next to each outcome and intervention, evaluation of the nursing process is possible, ensuring accountability for the critical path.

Nurses in hospital and community settings will be expected to function as case managers and to develop and use critical paths in their case management role.

Functional Approach to Planning

The nurse must meet high standards to satisfy professional mandates; these include legal, social, and institutional expectations of professional practice. Using a functional approach facilitates professional nursing practice. Because function is useful for organizing assessment data and identifying nursing diagnoses, it also is useful for focusing the plan of care.

Some clients have good function in many areas but may require nursing care for dysfunction in other areas. Understanding the concepts of function and dysfunction allows the nurse to see the client's strengths and limitations. Functional health provides a forceful focus for outcome identification and planning nursing interventions.

Key Concepts

- The nursing plan of care is designed to direct client care activities, promote continuity of care, focus charting requirements, and specify who is to carry out the nursing actions.
- The key elements of the nursing plan of care are the nursing diagnosis, client goals and outcome criteria, and nursing interventions.
- Client goals are stated as behavioral objectives and indicate the desired state of the client if the problem has been resolved.
- Outcome criteria are specific, measurable, realistic statements of goal attainment.
- Nursing interventions are independent, dependent, and interdependent activities that nurses carry out to provide client care.
- The use of critical pathways (paths) is on the rise in many areas. They provide a collaborative plan of care.

Critical Thinking Challenges

Now turn back to the situation at the beginning of the chapter, and apply what you have learned about the nursing process to these questions.

1. *Analyze how you would prioritize the nursing diagnoses for this client, and suggest additional information you may need to collect.*
2. *State possible outcomes for each diagnosis that should be met prior to the client's discharge to the home.*
3. *Construct possible methods to work with the client to individualize the plan of care and develop realistic outcomes.*
4. *Develop a hypothetical written plan of care for one of the above nursing diagnoses, indicating what additional information is needed.*

References

Alfaro-LeFevre, R. (1994). *Applying nursing process: A step-by-step guide* (3rd ed.). Philadelphia: J.B. Lippincott.

American Nurses Association (1991). *Standards of clinical nursing practice.* Kansas City, MO: Author.

Bulechek, G. M., & McCloskey, J. C. (1992). *Nursing interventions: Essential treatments* (2nd ed.). Philadelphia: W.B. Saunders.

Gordon, M., Murphy, C. P., Candee, D., & Hiltunen, E. (1994). Clinical judgment: An integrated model. *Advances in Nursing Science, 16* (4), 55–70.

Joint Commission on the Accreditation of Healthcare Organizations (1993). *1994 Accreditation manual for hospitals. Vol. 1. Standards.* Chicago: Author.

Zander, K. (1993a). Responsive restructuring: Part II: Decision support for coordinated care - Financial and clinical integration. *The New Definition, 8* (4), 1–3.

Zander, K. (1993b). The New England Medical Center (Center for Case Management), at a conference in Scottsdale, AZ.

Bibliography

Avant, K. C. (1994). The link of theory to practice. In R. M. Carroll-Johnson & M. Paquette (Ed.), *Classification of nursing diagnoses: Proceedings of the tenth conference* (pp. 11–16). Philadelphia: J.B. Lippincott.

Bulechek, G. M., & McCloskey, J. C. (1992). Defining and validating nursing interventions. *Nursing Clinics of North America, 27,* 289–297.

McCloskey, J. C., & Bulechek, G. M. (1994). Standardizing the language for nursing treatments: An overview of the issues. *Nursing Outlook, 42,* 56–63.

McCloskey, J. C., Bulechek, G. M., Cohen, M. Z., et al. (1990). Classification of nursing interventions. *Journal of Professional Nursing, 6* (3), 151—157.

Neufeld, K. R., Degner, L. F., & Dick, J. A. M. (1993). A nursing intervention strategy to foster patient involvement in treatment decisions. *Oncology Nursing Forum, 20,* 631–635.

Zander, K. (1994). Case Management series: Part I: Rationale for care-provider organizations. *The New Definition, 9*(3), 1–3.

Implementation and Evaluation

Key Terms	Learning Objectives
Implementation *Nursing monitors* *Peer review* *Quality improvement programs* *Standards*	*Upon completion of this chapter, the student will be able to do the following:* • *Define implementation and evaluation.* • *Discuss the purposes of implementation and evaluation.* • *Describe clinical skills needed to implement the nursing plan of care.* • *Describe methods for revising or modifying the nursing plan of care.* • *Describe activities the nurse carries out during the evaluation phase of the nursing process.* • *Discuss quality assurance monitors used in nursing settings.* • *Use a functional approach to implement and evaluate client care.*

13

You are a nurse recently hired by a nursing home to implement a new total quality improvement (TQI) program. The facility is up for reaccreditation by the Joint Commission on Accreditation of Healthcare Organizations (JCAHO) within the next year. On your first day in the nursing home, you are in the cafeteria and overhear three of the staff members talking about "the new nurse that doesn't really know much but probably will want to change around things that are already working." You are embarrassed by their conversation and decide to leave the cafeteria before they know you overheard them.

In previous chapters, you learned about ethics, legal issues, leadership, and management. This unit has added the first four steps of the nursing process to your knowledge base. In this chapter, you will learn about the remaining two steps of the nursing process: implementation and evaluation. You will see how evaluation is client centered and quality assurance centered. When you have completed the chapter, you should be able to apply your knowledge to the situation given at the beginning of the chapter. Critical Thinking Challenges at the end of the chapter will help you continue to apply your skills.

After the nurse and client identify problems and strengths, they plan together methods of helping the client maintain or return to healthy function. Outcome criteria are set for their goals, and a plan of care is developed. Now they are ready for the implementation phase of the nursing process, the activity that provides planned care, and the evaluation phase, in which the client's status is measured in response to the nursing care provided.

Implementation

Implementation refers to the action phase of the nursing process in which nursing care is provided. It is the actual initiation of the plan and recording of nursing actions. The purpose of implementation is to provide technical and therapeutic nursing care required to help the client achieve an optimal level of health.

Competence in intellectual, interpersonal, and technical skills is required to carry out the implementation phase of the nursing process. Parts of the plan of care can be delegated to other members of the healthcare team, but the registered nurse maintains accountability for the supervision and evaluation of these individuals. The activities of implementation are illustrated in Figure 13-1 and include the following:

- Reassess.
- Set priorities.
- Perform nursing interventions.
- Record actions.

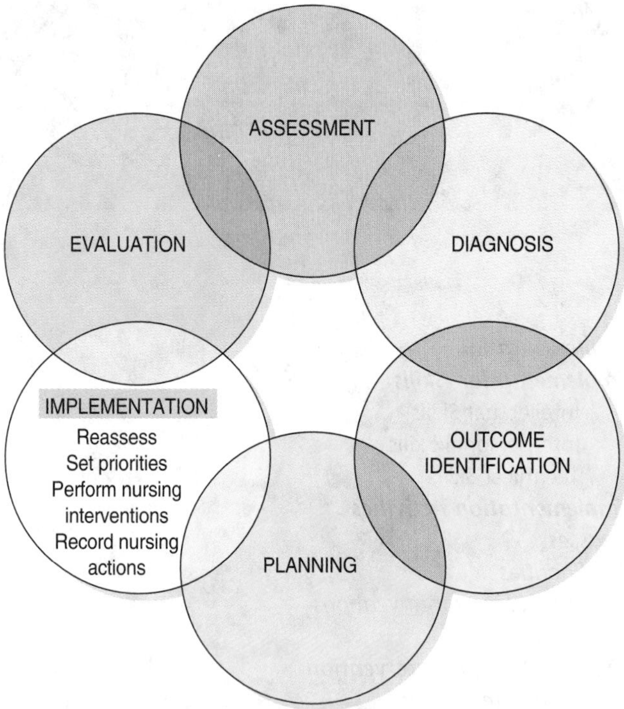

Figure 13-1 • ANA Standard V states: The nurse implements the interventions identified in the plan of care. This illustration shows activities used in the Implementation phase and also the relationship of Implementation to the other phases of the nursing process.

Implementation Skills

Intellectual Skills

The intellectual skills used in implementation include problem solving, decision-making, and teaching. To solve problems, the nurse asks the client pertinent questions, discusses alternatives, and is open to new ideas. To enrich the client's decision-making ability, the nurse gives him or her opportunities to help choose which treatments are performed, when, and in what sequence. Teaching requires a knowledge base of teaching–learning principles and the information to be conveyed.

Interpersonal Skills

The ability to work with others to accomplish a goal is critical to nursing. The nurse uses communication skills to carry out planned nursing interventions. Skill at verbal and nonverbal communication is refined through practice. More details on communication are given in Chapter 20.

Technical Skills

Technical skills are used to carry out treatments and procedures. The specific skills are learned through clinical practice. Technical competence means being able to use equipment, machines, and supplies in a particular specialty. For example, the nurse working in the delivery room must be familiar with fetal monitoring, positioning on the delivery-room table, and neonatal resuscitation devices. On the other hand, the nurse working on a medical unit may need technical competence in using the hypothermia blanket, therapeutic beds, or feeding pumps. A home health nurse must be familiar with adaptive equipment, client-controlled analgesia pumps, and wound dressing supplies.

Implementation Activities

The activities of the implementation phase include reassessment, setting priorities, performing nursing interventions, and recording action.

Reassess

During each client encounter, the nurse assesses the client's function. This ensures that prompt attention is paid to emerging problems. Because the condition of the client can change quickly and dramatically, the astute nurse remains alert to subtle cues and inferences. For example, the client experiencing pain may become quiet and withdraw from external stimuli. Recognizing this change, the nurse can intervene, validate, and assist the client to become more comfortable. A client who is demanding and irritable may be masking anxiety about a surgical procedure or fear about the results of a diagnostic test. As the nursing plan of care is initiated, care must be taken to make sure that the planned interventions are still relevant.

Set Priorities

Priority was discussed in Chapter 12 under outcome identification. Because a person's condition changes, priorities also may change. Priorities are based on information collected during reassessment. When setting priorities, the nurse ranks nursing problems in order of importance based on several factors (Fig. 13-2):

- The client's condition
- New information from reassessment
- Time and resources available for nursing interventions
- Feedback from the client, family, and healthcare staff
- The nurse's experience in assessing situations and setting priorities

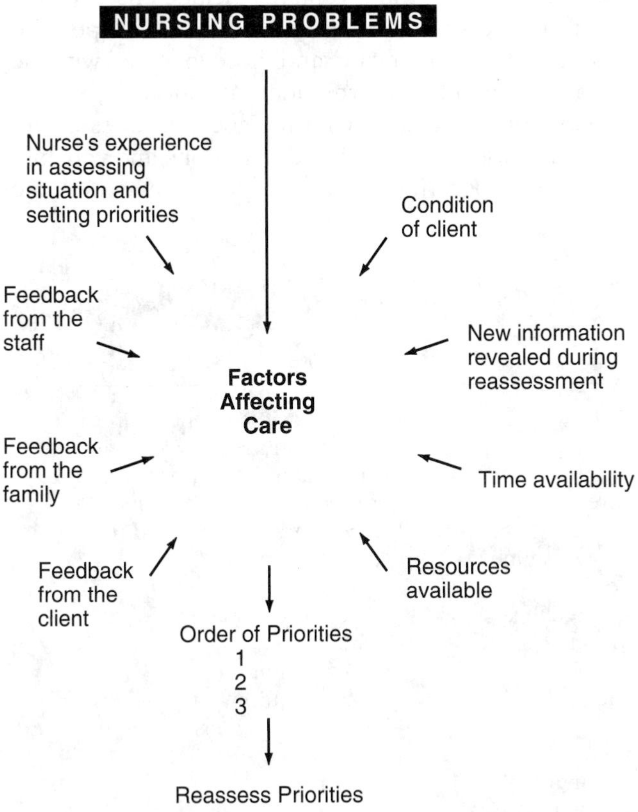

Figure 13-2 • *Priorities (position of prominence) are set by considering factors affecting care.*

A priority problem requires a nursing intervention before another problem is addressed, but setting priorities does not entail skipping any interventions. Setting priorities affects only the order in which nursing interventions are carried out.

Priorities can be set every few minutes, hourly, daily, weekly, or for longer periods. For example, in the critical care unit, priorities may need to be set every few minutes for an unstable multiple trauma client. Usually maintaining a patent airway, breathing, and circulation (the ABCs) are top priorities for these clients. Priorities for home care clients may be set for much longer periods of time. For example, a priority over time may be fostering independent transferring from bed to chair or independent ambulation to the bathroom.

Perform Nursing Intervention

The nurse (or designee) carries out the nursing interventions listed on the nursing plan of care. If the nurse is caring for several clients, a schedule is developed so that all clients may be cared for in a timely fashion.

Intervention for Collaborative Problems. Nurses manage collaborative problems (see Chap. 10) using "physician-prescribed and nursing-prescribed interventions to minimize the complications" (Carpenito, 1995, p. 29). Nursing diagnoses are determined, in part, when the nurse asks, "Is this a problem that a nurse can legally treat without an order from a physician?" Interventions based on such diagnoses are *nurse-prescribed* actions. When the nurse cannot legally make a treatment decision but has to follow the physician's orders, the action is *physician prescribed.* Both types of interventions involve nursing judgment because both require legal mandates. The problem is a *collaborative problem* (Alfaro-LeFevre, 1994) when the nurse uses both nurse-prescribed and physician-prescribed interventions to give nursing care. For instance, the physician prescribes pain medication, but the nurse sometimes makes the decisions when it is given. The nurse also may use alternative methods for pain relief.

Record Actions

After nursing interventions have been carried out, they are recorded in the client's health record. Each institution determines the specific requirements for documentation and should prepare written guidelines for the use of all forms. With today's emphasis on efficiency, new charting methods are being developed. It was anticipated that by 1992, focus charting would be the method of choice in 35% of hospitals, and charting by exception would be used in 27% of hospitals (Wake, 1990). The recording of information is discussed in Chapter 14.

Types of Nursing Intervention

Joanne McCloskey and Gloria Bulechek spearheaded the Iowa Intervention Project, which focuses on the development of a classification system for nursing interventions.

The Nursing Interventions Classification (NIC) assists in defining the role of the professional nurse by listing direct care treatments performed within the nursing role. Similar to NANDA's nursing diagnoses taxonomy, the NIC provides a label or name for each intervention, a definition of the intervention, and a set of defining activities or actions that a nurse performs to implement the intervention (McCloskey & Bulechek, 1992). The NIC is in its early stages and will continue to be refined.

Possible advances from the NIC include the following (McCloskey & Bulechek, 1992):

- Creation of a standardized language that promotes better understanding and communication of nursing interventions
- Expansion of knowledge about similarities and differences across nursing diagnoses
- Exploration of nursing care information systems
- Assistance in determining cost of services provided by nurses
- Demonstration of the impact nurses have within the healthcare system

Nursing interventions fall within three major categories: those using cognitive skills, those using interpersonal skills, and those using technical skills (Table 13-1). Selection of the type of nursing intervention to be used in client situations depends on the client's dysfunction and functional requirements.

Cognitive Interventions

Teaching and supervising others are important cognitive nursing interventions.

Educational Intervention

Educational nursing interventions are carried out by applying general principles about the teaching and learning process. Teaching plans are developed, and instruction is provided about health promotion or specific healthcare problems and their management. The ability to teach clients requires knowledge of normal anatomy and physiology, usual patterns of client response to health changes, and pathophysiology of the disease process. A careful assessment of the client yields information about his or her level of motivation, level of knowledge, willingness to follow the health regimen, and physical and psychological ability to carry out the plan. See Chapter 24 for more information on client teaching.

Once the nurse is aware of the client's readiness for learning, the teaching plan can be implemented. Goals specific to the individual situation are established, and instruction methods that optimize a successful outcome are used.

Supervisory Intervention

Supervisory nursing interventions include ensuring that other members of the nursing team carry out specified aspects of the plan of care, and those involved with the client or family return demonstration of skills. Supervision of nursing team members requires an in-depth knowledge of the job descriptions and capabilities of each person on the team. Nurses may delegate

Table 13-1 • Types of Nursing Interventions

Cognitive	Interpersonal	Technical
Teach/educate	Coordinate activities	Provide basic hygiene, skin care
Relate knowledge to activities of daily living (ADLs)	Provide caregiving	Perform routine nursing activities
Provide feedback	Use therapeutic communication	Detect change from baseline data
Create strategies for clients with dysfunctional communication	Provide a personal presence	Reorganize abnormal responses
Supervise nursing team	Set limits	Provide independent and dependent treatment
Supervise client in performance	Provide opportunity to examine values and attitudes	Assist with ADLs
Supervise family in performance	Explore and legitimize feelings	Provide appropriate sensory stimulation
Alter the environment as needed	Provide spiritual support	Mobilize equipment
	Use humor	Maintain equipment
	Provide individual therapy	Use special abilities or talents
	Provide group therapy	
	Become client's advocate	
	Support client and family plans	
	Make referrals for follow-up	
	Serve as a role model	

specific aspects of care to nonprofessional staff, but the registered nurse is held accountable for the selection of appropriate nursing care measures that can be performed by these personnel. The nurse also maintains the responsibility to ensure that these nursing care measures have been carried out correctly and that important information about the client's response to the care is communicated verbally and in written form to the nurse responsible for the client.

Supervising the client or family in skill performance is essential to provide encouragement, provide feedback about correct and incorrect performance, or facilitate introduction of new skills to be learned. Clients and their families often are unfamiliar with nursing care regimens, equipment, and supplies. They should be given ample opportunity to carry out the intervention under supervision. This requires inclusion of the client and family in planning and implementing initial care. The nurse can help the client or family begin to assume responsibility for self-management. Each nurse taking care of the client subsequently should be informed about the capabilities of the client and family to carry out the intervention. Skills are built with practice; doing an activity once usually is not sufficient for proficiency.

Interpersonal Interventions

Interpersonal nursing interventions involve coordinating care, providing support, and using specific psychosocial skills.

Coordinating Intervention

Coordinating client activities serves many purposes. The nurse carries out the coordination function by acting as a client advocate, making referrals for follow-up care, collaborating with other healthcare team members, and ensuring that the client's schedule is therapeutic.

For some clients, the nurse fulfills the advocate role by speaking for the client or encouraging the client to ask questions. For example, a client may need help in refusing a suggested treatment or requesting a second opinion about surgery. In the advocacy role, the nurse presents the client's point of view and suggests ways in which the client's requests can be met.

The nurse is in a position to know what type of nursing follow-up the client needs. Referrals should be made to home health agencies, visiting nurse associations, or other healthcare providers to facilitate return of optimal function. Many self-help groups and community services are available to provide assistance to clients with health-related problems; creativity in matching clients with these services can help ensure that the client's health status will be monitored and that relapses may be minimized.

Supportive Intervention

Supportive nursing interventions emphasize use of communication skills, relief of spiritual distress, and caring behaviors. A combination of good communication and caring provides comfort and promotes a healthy response to dysfunctional health problems. Being supportive means recognizing the need for encouragement, unconditional acceptance of behaviors, and the positive effects of "being there" for a client during stress or crisis. The nurse may sit with a client who is anxious, listen to a client's experience grieving for the loss of a loved one, or touch the forehead of a client with a spinal-cord injury. This is called "therapeutic use of self."

Spiritual support can be provided by giving the client time to carry out religious practices, meditation, or reading. Respecting the client's privacy during these times conveys acceptance and understanding. If the client wants to talk, the nurse should listen to assess spiritual distress without being judgmental. If the client asks for a spiritual support person, the client's minister, rabbi, priest, or the hospital chaplain can be contacted.

Psychosocial Intervention

Psychosocial nursing interventions focus on resolving emotional, psychological, or social problems. Humor, individual or group therapy, role-modeling social skills, and exploring feelings are all ways of carrying out psychosocial nursing interventions.

Some clients and families respond to stress by joking, teasing, or laughing about it. The nurse can use humor as a way to relieve stress and give the client examples of difficult situations and ways to resolve them. Humor must always be used judiciously, however. The nurse must recognize underlying themes or deeper problems and respond appropriately. A client may jokingly say to the nurse, "Gee, my arm must be target practice for everyone learning how to draw blood." The nurse should pick up on this cue and find out how many times the client has been "stuck," determine why there was such a problem, and instruct the client to speak up and request special consideration for future blood-drawing attempts.

Providing individual and group therapy is the responsibility of nurses in various settings. Individual therapy, used as a means of resolving psychological problems, usually requires additional training or certification. Group therapy is often used to provide support and guidance for clients and their support people with similar needs or problems. Recognizing the need for individual or group therapy, the nurse makes referrals to healthcare providers with the required expertise. In some settings, nurses hold group meetings with families of Alzheimer's clients or families of children with cancer. Most group therapy sessions have a stated purpose

Nursing Research *Implementation and Evaluation*

Selected Nursing Research Studies

Cullen, L., McCloskey, J., & Bulechek, G. (1994). Development and validation of circulatory nursing interventions. In R. M. Carroll-Johnson (Ed.), *Classification of nursing diagnoses: Proceedings of the tenth conference.* Philadelphia: J.B. Lippincott.

Stewart, B., & Archbold, P. (1993). Nursing intervention studies require outcome measures that are sensitive to change (Part II). *Research in Nursing and Health* 1(16) 77–82.

Wesorick, B. (1994). Consensual validation of goals/outcomes and interventions for nursing diagnostic categories. In R. M. Carroll-Johnson (Ed.), *Classification of nursing diagnoses: Proceedings of the tenth conference.* Philadelphia: J.B. Lippincott.

Possible Topics for Nursing Inquiry

- Do certain conceptual nursing models facilitate comprehensive evaluation more than others?
- What is the effect of functional health assessment on the evaluation phase of the nursing process?
- What is the relationship between a nursing conceptual model, personal practice ethics, and the evaluation process in new graduate nurses?

and schedule of activities. Group members rely on their own experiences and gain new ways of dealing with problems from others who have experienced the same problems. The nurse therapist serves as the group facilitator and assists group members to share feelings, advice, and helpful hints with one another.

Sometimes a group member can offer a suggestion that would not be acceptable to the person if made by a healthcare professional. For example, in a group for spouses of Alzheimer's clients, one wife reported that her husband continued to drive even though he admitted that he often got lost and could not remember the way home. Another group member simply said, "Take the keys away! I don't want to be on the street with him." The wife accepted this blunt advice and followed it. She had previously refused this advice from the therapist because she said driving was his only pleasure; she did not want to rob him of this last piece of independence.

Role-modeling social skills is used for clients who have not acquired them because of lack of exposure or lengthy illness. In some long-term care settings, clients have grown to depend on the staff to make all their decisions. In other cases, clients have never practiced acceptable social behaviors. By treating the client with respect and using appropriate language and social behaviors (saying "please" and "thank you" and not interrupting, for instance), the nurse can help the client to become socially adept.

Exploring feelings is another provision of psychosocial nursing. Many clients with chronic or life-threatening illnesses need an opportunity to explore their feelings in a nonjudgmental setting. The nurse is in a prime position to help these clients ventilate their feelings and relieve fears and anxiety.

Technical Interventions

The nurse uses technical interventions to help the client maintain psychological and physiologic well-being, to monitor client status, and to perform psychomotor skills.

Maintenance Intervention

The goal of maintenance nursing interventions is to help the client retain a certain state of health. Maintenance activities prevent deterioration of physical or psychological functioning and preserve independence. Maintenance interventions include basic hygiene, skin care, and other routine nursing activities.

Maintenance nursing interventions are sometimes undervalued or considered insignificant, but they allow the client to preserve function and reduce the chance of developing complications. Nurses should take proper credit for maintaining healthy states and should receive acknowledgment for these activities in their job evaluations and recognition awards for excellence in practice.

Surveillance Intervention

Surveillance nursing interventions include detecting changes from baseline data and recognizing abnormal responses. This activity also can be categorized as observation, inspection, or vigilance. The nurse relies on the senses to detect changes. Hearing, vision, touch, and smell are routinely used. Nurses observe the appearance and characteristics of the client. They hear by auscultation, pitch, and tone. Odors are detected and compared with past experience and knowledge of specific problems. Using touch, the nurse assesses body temperature, skin condition, clamminess, or diaphoresis. All of these surveillance activities are used to determine the client's current status and changes from previous states. Subtle changes in a client's condition are often detected by the nurse and communicated to the physician to minimize problems. Expert nurse clinicians develop skill in detecting and preventing complications and usually receive positive feedback for their accurate and timely interventions based on this "sense" of something being wrong.

Psychomotor Intervention

Psychomotor nursing interventions—those requiring technical expertise—include inserting, removing, changing, applying, administering, cleansing, or any other activity that requires a psychomotor action. The management and care of equipment, supplies, treatments, and procedures also falls into this category of nursing interventions. The nurse gains technical competence by practice.

Functional Approach to Implementation

When thinking about implementation, the nurse should consider the overall perspective of nursing. With a functional approach, nursing tries to maximize a client's functional status and resolve dysfunction. With each client encounter, the nurse reassesses function, revises care when needed, and evaluates the client's response. By focusing on areas of strength or healthy functioning (as discussed in the planning phase of Chapter 12), the nurse can optimize interventions to help the client reach his or her healthiest state.

Evaluation

Evaluation, as the sixth phase of the nursing process, follows implementation of the nursing plan of care. **Evaluation** is defined as the judgment of the effectiveness of nursing care to meet client goals; it is the phase in which the nurse compares the client's behavioral responses with predetermined client goals and outcome criteria. This phase involves a thorough, systematic review of the effectiveness of nursing interventions and a determination of whether client goals have been met and outcome criteria achieved. The nurse uses a variety of skills to judge the effectiveness of nursing care. These skills include knowledge of standards of care, knowledge of normal client responses, knowledge of conceptual models of nursing, ability to monitor the effectiveness of nursing interventions, and awareness of clinical research. Critical appraisal of goal attainment is determined jointly by the nurse and client.

Although evaluation is a separate and distinct phase, it also is ongoing throughout the nursing process (Alfaro-LeFevre, 1994). Judgments made in previous phases usually result in prompt reassessment, rediagnosis, and replanning (Yura & Walsh, 1988). The nurse continually assesses the client's response to a particular nursing intervention, establishes different priorities for nursing diagnoses, and alters the nursing plan of care. An in-depth, comprehensive judgment about goal attainment and fulfillment of outcome criteria is performed only during the evaluation phase of the nursing process (Yura & Walsh, 1988).

The nursing plan of care is the foundation for evaluation. The identified nursing diagnoses, client goals, outcome criteria, and nursing interventions are the guide for evaluation. Through the evaluation process, the appropriateness, accuracy, and relevance of these nursing care components can be determined. Evaluation also helps the nurse discover any errors that may have occurred in previous steps of the nursing process. The nurse always considers evaluation in light of how the client responded or reacted to the planned course of action (Yura & Walsh, 1988). Figure 13-3 illustrates the relationship of the activities of the evaluation phase to the other phases of the nursing process.

There are several purposes for carrying out evaluation:

- Collect subjective and objective data to make judgments about nursing care delivered.
- Examine the client's behavioral responses to nursing interventions.
- Compare the client's behavioral responses with predetermined outcome criteria.
- Appraise the extent to which client goals were attained or problems resolved.
- Appraise involvement and collaboration of the client, family members, nurses, and healthcare team members in healthcare decisions.

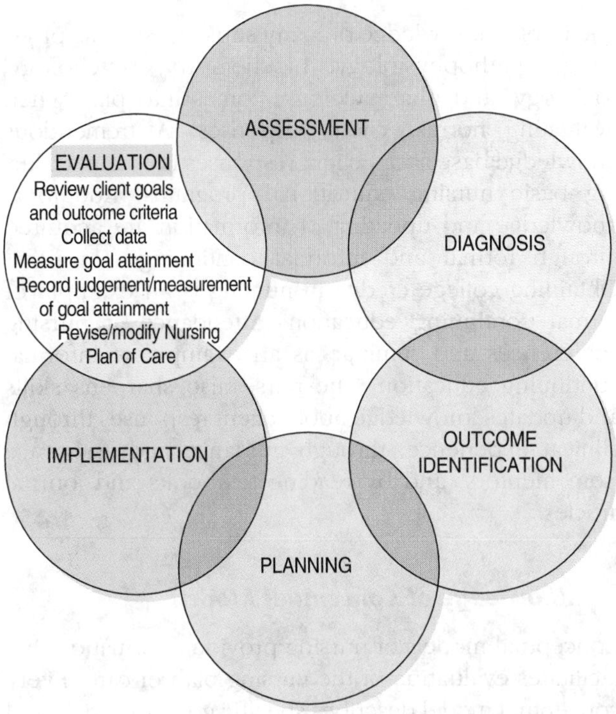

***Figure 13-3** • ANA Standard VI states: The nurse evaluates the client's progress toward attainment of outcomes. This illustration shows activities used in the Evaluation phase and also the relationship of Evaluation to the other phases of the nursing process.*

- Provide a basis for the revision of the nursing plan of care evaluation.
- Monitor the quality of nursing care and its effect on the client's health status (Alfaro-LeFevre, 1994; Carpenito, 1995; Yura & Walsh, 1988).

The evaluation phase consists of a number of specific activities:

- Review client goals and outcome criteria.
- Collect data.
- Measure goal attainment.
- Record judgment or measurement of goal attainment.
- Revise or modify the nursing plan of care.

Evaluation Skills

Knowledge of Standards of Care

The nurse must know about the current standards of care proposed by nursing organizations (eg, the American Nurses Association [ANA, 1991]), external review boards (eg, JCAHO [1993]), and his or her own institution (eg, policies and procedures) to evaluate nursing care. See the section on quality improvement programs for a discussion of these standards.

Knowledge of Normal Client Response

The nurse's knowledge of many subjects, such as physiology, pathophysiology, biochemistry, psychology, sociology, and pharmacology, comes into play when evaluating normal client responses. A tremendous knowledge base about client responses is obtained during basic nursing educational programs. Additional knowledge and updating of information are acquired through formal and informal continuing education. Obtaining college credits in nursing is an example of formal continuing education. Attendance at nursing conferences and seminars is an example of informal continuing education. The nurse also sharpens skills and updates knowledge about client responses through clinical experience, through guidance and assistance from mentors, and by reading textbooks and journal articles.

Knowledge of Conceptual Models

Conceptual models of nursing provide information that facilitates evaluation of the nursing plan of care. Every conceptual model describes specific goals of action and consequences of those actions that assist in the evaluation of care. Because the conceptual model guides development of client goals and outcome criteria, the goal of action or desired result of a particular conceptual model is revealed in these components of the plan (Ziegler, Vaughan-Wrobel, & Erlen, 1986). If a client's behavioral responses match the client goal statements and client outcome criteria, the conceptual model's goal has been reached. For example, the goal of the Roy (Roy & Roberts, 1981) Adaptation Model of Nursing is the adaptation of the client in four adaptive modes. The consequences of nursing actions lead to effective coping mechanisms, maximal level of functioning, and adaptive responses.

Ability to Monitor the Effectiveness of Nursing Interventions

Many intellectual and technical skills are required to monitor the effectiveness of nursing interventions. Interviewing techniques and physical assessment skills are needed to obtain subjective and objective data from the client and family members. Knowledge of interviewing techniques, such as types of questions, interview phases, and the appropriate environment for interviewing, facilitates the collection of subjective data for evaluation of the nursing plan of care. For further information about interviewing, see Chapter 10. Physical and functional assessment skills are necessary to monitor the effectiveness of nursing interventions. The ability to inspect, palpate, percuss, and auscultate proficiently provides objective data about the effectiveness of nursing interventions. For example, if a client has impaired gas exchange related to altered oxygen supply, auscultation of breath sounds yields information about the effectiveness of nursing interventions.

Knowledge and skill in the use of measurement devices yield further information about the effectiveness of nursing interventions. Many technologic advances in medicine and nursing make it mandatory for nurses to have knowledge and skill in the use of multiple measurement devices. Nurses use devices such as blood pressure cuffs, thermometers, arterial lines, intracranial pressure monitors, and central venous pressure lines frequently, depending on the practice setting. Measurement devices provide information for the evaluation of nursing strategies.

Nursing also requires knowledge and skill in interpreting laboratory data. Laboratory studies, such as complete blood counts, arterial blood gases, and routine urinalysis tests, produce data for evaluation of nursing interventions. For example, in the same client with Impaired Gas Exchange related to altered oxygen supply, arterial blood gas measurements help the nurse determine oxygenation, ventilation, metabolic status, and the necessity for suctioning.

Awareness of Clinical Research

Current research findings are used to develop innovative methods to sharpen assessment and diagnostic skills; establish future standards for developing client goals, client outcomes, and nursing interventions in the planning stage; and provide the latest knowledge to enhance nursing practice. Journal clubs are a way to integrate current research findings into clinical practice; including nurse scientists in these meetings facilitates interaction between clinicians and researchers (Avant, 1994).

Types of Evaluation

Evaluation can center on one of three areas: structure, process, or outcome.

Structure Evaluation

Structure evaluation focuses on the attributes of the setting or surroundings where the healthcare is provided. It deals with the environmental aspects that directly or indirectly influence the quality of care provided. Availability of equipment, layout of physical facilities, nurse-client ratios, administrative support, and maintenance of nursing staff competence are some areas of concern for structure evaluation (Miller, 1989; Ziegler, et al., 1986).

Process Evaluation

Process evaluation focuses on the performance of the nurse and whether the nursing care provided was appropriate and competent (Ziegler, et al., 1986). The phases of the nursing process are used as the framework for the evaluation of nursing care. Areas of concern for this type of evaluation include the type of information obtained by interview and physical assessment, the validity of the nursing diagnostic statements, and the technical competence of the nurse.

Outcome Evaluation

Outcome evaluation, which focuses on the client and the client's function, is receiving a great deal of emphasis. Outcome evaluation determines the extent to which the client's behavioral response to nursing intervention reflects the desired client goal and outcome criteria (Ziegler, et al., 1986). Outcome evaluation can take place only after standards have been developed. An example of an outcome evaluation is to establish standards of care for a specific diagnosis and then compare actual client outcomes with that standard.

Evaluation Activities

The evaluation phase of the nursing process includes reviewing client goals and outcome criteria, collecting data, measuring goal attainment, recording judgment of goal attainment, revising the nursing plan of care, and recording judgments made about goal attainment.

Review Client Goals and Outcome Criteria

The nurse begins measuring goal attainment by reviewing the client goals and outcome criteria developed for each nursing diagnosis. Outcome criteria, written in measurable terms in the planning phase, are used to judge goal attainment. Review of the expected client behaviors includes examining the time frames and methods for measurement of goal fulfillment. This review helps the nurse focus on data needed to assess the accuracy and realistic nature of the goals and outcome criteria (Alfaro-LeFevre, 1994).

Collect Data

Systematic data collection is required to determine if goals have been attained and if client outcome criteria have been fulfilled. Subjective and objective data are collected to judge the client's behavioral responses to nursing interventions. Subjective data are collected from many sources, including the client, family members or significant others, nursing staff, and other healthcare team members. Information from observation (eg, posture, skin color, behavior), health records (eg, laboratory results, reports from other healthcare team members), physical assessment (eg, breath sounds, strength of extremities), and measurement devices (eg, blood pressure, temperature) are examples of objective data.

Subjective data also are used to evaluate the effectiveness of nursing care provided. For example, a client with a nursing diagnosis of Pain related to a recent surgical procedure may have as a goal, "Client will state that pain is relieved within 10 minutes after repositioning." The client's subjective statement would be needed to judge whether this goal has been achieved. More information on subjective and objective data can be found in Chapter 21.

Measure Goal Attainment

After collecting data, the nurse forms a comprehensive picture of the client's behavioral responses to nursing interventions. The next activity is to make a judgment about goal attainment. The evaluative data are used to compare the client's actual behavioral responses to the predicted responses or predetermined outcome criteria developed in the planning phase. When possible, the client is involved in the judgment of goal attainment.

The four possible judgments that may be made follow (Alfaro-LeFevre, 1994):

- The goal was completely met.
- The goal was partially met.
- The goal was completely unmet.
- New problems or nursing diagnoses have developed.

The fourth judgment can exist simultaneously with any of the first three. Table 13-2 provides some examples of a completely met goal, a partially met goal, and a completely unmet goal. Once the judgment about the attainment or lack of attainment of the outcome criteria is made, the plan of care is revised. See the section on revision and modification of the nursing plan of care.

Assess Facilitators of Goal Attainment

Clients, family members, significant others, and other healthcare team members are invaluable in facilitating or helping with goal attainment. Occasionally, only those closest to the client can identify the subtle or elusive factors that helped (or hindered) goal achievement. Examples of facilitators include audiovisual materials, written handouts, repetition of material, and easily accessible and interested nursing staff.

Assess Barriers of Goal Attainment

Several barriers to goal attainment have been identified. Barriers may involve the client, family members, significant others, and the nurse or other healthcare team members. Examples of how goal attainment may be blocked include providing incorrect information, withholding information, having an unexpected reaction to treatment (eg, allergic response to therapy), possessing inadequate coping ability, and experiencing worsened underlying pathologic condition (Yura & Walsh, 1988).

Family members also may act as barriers to goal achievement in multiple ways. For example, their lack of understanding of the plan of care, their lack of interest in the client, or their failure to realize the client actu-

Table 13-2 • Clinical Examples of Evaluation of Goal Attainment

Nursing Diagnosis	Client Goal	Subjective Data Collected	Objective Collected	Goal Judgment
Impaired Swallowing related to neuromuscular impairment	Client will demonstrate correct eating techniques to maximize swallowing.	Client states, "I sit up in a chair for a half hour after I eat."	Client wears dentures when eating; performs return demonstration of facial exercises; bends head forward when eating; checks mouth for any remaining food particles; remains in Fowler's position for at least 30 minutes after eating; lies on side while lying in bed.	Goal completely met
Chronic Low Self-Esteem	Client interacts verbally in group therapy session.	Client states, "I feel uncomfortable when speaking in front of others."	Client observed sitting in group session, looking at floor, and not participating in discussion.	Goal partially met
Impaired Mobility related to neuromuscular impair ment	Client will carry out prescribed mobility regimen.	Client states, "I can't do anything by myself. I need a lot of help with everything."	Client unable to perform active range of motion exercises independently; unable to transfer from bed to wheelchair; unable to dress and groom independently.	Goal completely unmet

ally has a problem can impede movement toward goal achievement. The cultural heritage, moral values, and religious influences of a family can be barriers to goal attainment (Yura & Walsh, 1988).

The nurse may unwittingly block goal achievement, for instance, by neglecting to collect pertinent assessment data, assigning an inappropriate priority rating to nursing diagnoses, and delegating nursing care to inappropriate nursing staff members. The nurse may fail to include the client in the planning step, fail to incorporate facets of the medical regimen when developing the nursing plan of care, or neglect to share critical information with other members of the health team (Yura & Walsh, 1988).

Other healthcare team members may be barriers to goal attainment. They may have a lack of communication among themselves, inability to work together as a team, and failure to coordinate the activities of all healthcare team members (Yura & Walsh, 1988). When healthcare team members do not share information among themselves, continuity in the planning and implementation of care is hampered. The evaluation phase identifies the barriers that interfere with the client's advancement toward goal achievement.

Record Judgment or Measurement of Goal Attainment

Written documentation of the subjective and objective data gathered and the judgment made about goal attainment is required on the client's health record. Judgments about goal attainment are written clearly and concisely. Avoid ambiguous terms, such as "inadequate," "good," or "extremely well," which can be interpreted differently by different people (Ziegler, et al., 1986).

Revise or Modify the Nursing Plan of Care

Revision and modification of the nursing plan of care are part of the evaluation phase. This provides a feedback mechanism that starts the entire chain of events again. Figure 13-4 illustrates the feedback mechanism, which starts with a complete reassessment of the client and illustrates the cyclic nature of the nursing process.

Nursing diagnoses that were resolved require no further nursing intervention and may be removed from the nursing plan of care. To maintain the client's "problem-free status," a nursing plan of care is developed that incorporates potential for wellness and other health-promoting nursing diagnoses and focuses nursing actions toward maximal functioning. The nurse periodically reassesses the level of functioning and health status changes to determine if new problems or nursing diagnoses have developed.

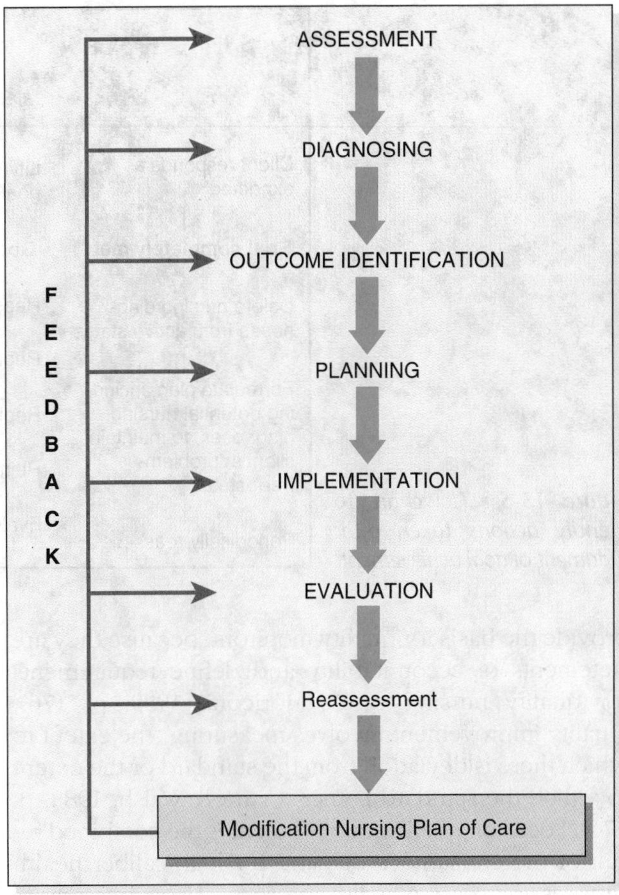

Figure 13-4 • Feedback mechanism and cyclic nature of the nursing process.

Some client goals will be partially met or completely unmet. Modification begins with a complete reassessment of the client. Changes in client goals, client outcome criteria, and nursing interventions are required. If new problems have arisen, new nursing diagnoses must be identified and a nursing plan of care written. Figure 13-5 illustrates the steps taken after judgment of goal attainment and needed revisions of the nursing plan of care.

Quality Improvement Programs

Up to this point, the discussion has centered on evaluation of the individual. The client's nursing plan of care, with unique nursing diagnoses, client goals, outcome criteria, and nursing interventions, has been the center of attention. Another focus is evaluation of the quality of nursing care provided to groups of clients with similar problems or nursing diagnoses. Formerly called quality assurance monitors, total quality management or TQI programs are mechanisms that ensure that quality client care is provided and standards are upheld. They provide input for the development and refinement of standards of care for groups of similar clients. Standards

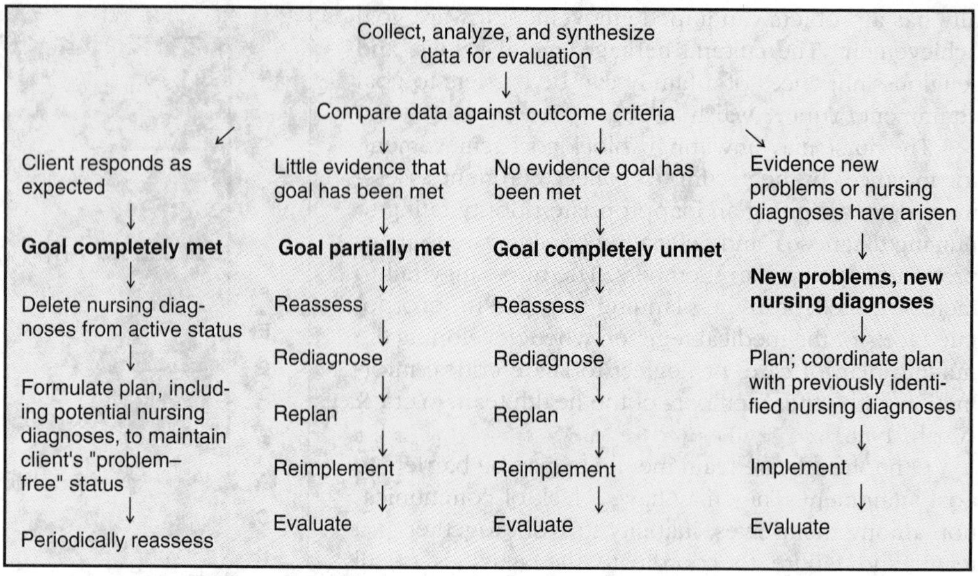

Figure 13-5 • *Flowchart to identify actions taken after judgment of goal achievement.*

provide the basis for quality monitors "because they are statements of accountability and define requirements for quality nursing care" (Moriconi, 1989, p. 176). Quality improvement involves measuring "the extent to which there is deviation from the standard or the extent to which the standard is met" (Yura & Walsh, 1988, p. 174). Focus on quality improvement is the combined result of the consumer's demand for high-caliber health services and soaring healthcare costs. Also, governmental agencies, accreditation groups, and regulatory bodies have pressured the nursing profession to respond to quality improvement issues. Standards of care have been proposed by the ANA, the JCAHO, specialty nursing organizations (eg, the American Association of Neuroscience Nurses, American Association of Spinal Cord Injury Nurses), and by individual healthcare institutions.

American Nurses Association

The ANA established the *Standards of Nursing Practice* in 1973 (see Chap. 1). ANA updated these standards in 1991 with *Standards of Clinical Nursing Practice*, which includes "standards of care" and "standards of professional performance." Based on a nursing process framework, "standards of care" are composed of seven nursing standards for providing nursing care to all clients. The behaviors and roles of professional nurses are described in the eight "standards of professional performance." Both standards include measurement criteria for the evaluation of nursing care and performance.

Some specialty nursing groups, in conjunction with the ANA, have developed processes and outcome criteria for a number of nursing diagnoses. For example, the Association of Rehabilitation Nurses and the American Association of Neuroscience Nurses have set standards based on nursing diagnoses applied to their specialty.

Joint Commission on Accreditation of Healthcare Organizations

The JCAHO is an external review board that establishes standards for institutions. These standards help to ensure that the institution functions within specified guidelines (Miller, 1989). The hospital standards for nursing care are applicable to all clients in every setting where nursing care is provided. Recent changes in the JCAHO guidelines require the continuous monitoring and evaluation of the quality of nursing care provided by the department of nursing. The guidelines are general, and each institution develops a specific quality improvement program suited to its organizational structure (Miller, 1989).

Peer Review

Peer review is the evaluation and judgment of a nurse's performance by other nurses. It is another mechanism for evaluating and monitoring nursing care provided. There are two types of peer review—nursing monitors and individual peer review.

Nursing Monitors. **Nursing monitors**, previously called nursing audits, are "a review, by a nurse, of the client's care or records to determine the extent to which that care or records meet established standards" (Yura & Walsh, 1988, p. 177). Nursing monitoring committees usually establish the "standards against which their observations will be measured" (Yura & Walsh, 1988, p. 178). Although nursing departments develop their own standards for particular nursing care settings, the ANA's (1991) *Standards of Clinical Nursing Practice* is often used as a source of generating unique standards for a particular setting or institution. Members of the monitoring committee may review a nurse's documentation of care in the health record or may determine the client's health status through observation.

Individual Peer Review. The second type of peer review is individual peer review, which focuses on the nurse. An individual nurse's performance is evaluated and judged by other nurses with similar education and experience. This type of review also is based on preestablished standards (Yura & Walsh, 1988). Individual peer review adds to nurse monitoring data.

Functional Approach to Evaluation

Evaluation using the functional health approach requires a specific perspective. In addition to measuring attainment of client goals and client outcomes, the client's functional status for each health pattern is established. The client's functional status is ascertained after the nursing plan of care is implemented and is based on data from the evaluation phase. Subjective and objective data are used to determine the client's movement toward improved function. Evaluation using the functional health approach provides a framework for organization and evaluation of data for revision or modification of the nursing plan of care.

Key Concepts

- Nurse-prescribed actions are based on client interventions that the nurse can legally perform without a physician's order.
- Collaborative problems are those in which the nurse uses both physician-prescribed and nurse-prescribed interventions to give care.
- Implementing the nursing plan of care requires intellectual, interpersonal, and technical skills.
- Evaluation is a judgmental process for determining the effectiveness of nursing interventions to meet client goals.
- Evaluation occurs throughout all steps of the nursing process but also is a distinct, separate step.
- An in-depth, comprehensive judgment about client goal attainment and fulfillment of client outcome criteria is performed during the evaluation step of the nursing process.
- The nursing plan of care forms the foundation for evaluation.
- The nurse and client determine goal attainment.
- The nurse, client, family members, significant others, and other healthcare team members may help or hinder goal attainment.
- Quality improvement involves the monitoring and evaluating of nursing care against standards of nursing practice.
- Revising the nursing plan of care involves reassessment, rediagnosis, and replanning.
- Evaluation determines the reasons why the nursing plan of care was a success or failure.

Critical Thinking Challenges

Now you have studied each step of the nursing process and have added the use of the nursing process to your knowledge base. When you review the situation given at the beginning of this chapter, you should be able to apply your learning to the following questions.

1. *Reflect on factors that may have contributed to the nurses' negative feelings about your being hired to implement the new evaluation program.*
2. *Analyze the impact such feelings could have on the success of any quality improvement program.*
3. *Infer how the nurses' perception of the value of quality improvement might be altered or modified in a positive way.*
4. *Propose possible sources of support that you might use, and give reasons for your answers.*

References

Alfaro-LeFevre, R. (1994). *Applying nursing process: A step-by-step guide* (3rd ed.). Philadelphia: J.B. Lippincott.

American Nurses Association (1973). *Standards of nursing practice.* Kansas City, MO: Author.

American Nurses Association (1991). *Standards of clinical nursing practice* Kansas City MO: Author.

Avant, K. C. (1994). The link of theory to practice. In R. M. Carroll-Johnson & M. Paquette (Eds.), *Classification of nursing diagnoses: Proceedings of the tenth conference* (pp. 11–16). Philadelphia: J.B. Lippincott.

Carpenito, L. J. (1995). *Nursing diagnosis: Application to clinical practice* (6th ed.). Philadelphia: J.B. Lippincott.

Joint Commission on the Accreditation of Healthcare Organizations (1993). *1994 Accreditation manual for hospitals. Vol. 1. Standards.* Chicago: Author.

McCloskey, J., & Bulechek, G. (1992). *Iowa Interventions Project Nursing Interventions Classification (NIC).* St. Louis: C.V. Mosby.

Miller, E. (1989). *How to make nursing diagnosis work: Administrative and clinical strategies.* Norwalk, CT: Appleton & Lange.

Moriconi, D. (1989). Quality assurance in diagnosis-based

nursing practice. In E. Miller (Ed.), *How to make nursing diagnosis work: Administrative and clinical strategies.* Norwalk, CT: Appleton & Lange.

Roy, C., & Roberts, S. L. (1981). *Theory construction in nursing: An adaptation model.* Englewood Cliffs, NJ: Prentice-Hall.

Wake, M. M. (1990). Nursing care delivery systems: Status and vision. *Journal of Nursing Administration, 20*(5), 47–51.

Yura, H., & Walsh, M. B. (1988). *The nursing process: Assessing, planning, implementing, evaluating* (5th ed.). Norwalk, CT: Appleton & Lange.

Ziegler, S. M., Vaughan-Wrobel, B. C., & Erlen, J. A. (1986). *Nursing process, nursing diagnosis, nursing knowledge: Avenues to autonomy.* Norwalk, CT: Appleton-Century-Crofts.

Bibliography

Bulechek, G. M., & McCloskey, J. C. (1992). Defining and validating nursing interventions. *Nursing Clinics of North America, 27,* 289–297.

Gordon, M., Murphy, C. P., Candee, D., & Hiltunen, E. (1994). Clinical judgment: An integrated model. *Advances in Nursing Science, 16*(4), 55–70.

McCloskey, J. C., & Bulechek, G. M. (1994). Standardizing the language for nursing treatments: An overview of the issues. *Nursing Outlook, 42,* 56–63.

Neufeld, K. R., Degner, L. F., & Dick, J. A. M. (1993). A nursing intervention strategy to foster patient involvement in treatment decisions. *Oncology Nursing Forum, 20,* 631–635.

Communication of the Nursing Process: Recording and Reporting

Key Terms	Learning Objectives

Key Terms

Audit
Care plan conferences
Change-of-shift report
Charting by exception
Flowsheets
FOCUS charting
Incident
Kardex
Nursing plan of care
PIE charting
Problem-oriented medical record
Recording
Reporting
SOAP note
Source-oriented record

Learning Objectives

Upon completion of this chapter, the student will be able to do the following:

- *Describe the purposes of the client record.*
- *List principles of charting.*
- *Differentiate formats of source-oriented recording, problem-oriented recording, and charting by exception.*
- *Understand how to use a nursing Kardex.*
- *Properly record nursing progress notes by SOAP, PIE, FOCUS, or narrative format.*
- *Identify flowsheets used in the client record.*
- *Fill out a nursing history admission sheet and a nursing discharge summary.*
- *Identify important data for the change-of-shift report.*
- *Describe the procedure for telephone reporting.*
- *Discuss the importance of confidentiality.*

14

When you come on duty for the morning shift, you check your clients' charts. You examine the following documentation found on one of your client's charts from the previous shift:

"Client had a terrible night. She was bloated and very nauseated. Bowel sounds present in all quadrants. She complained her doctor never came in to see her, and when he did, he didn't seem very interested in how she felt.

Vital signs: BP 176/74, P 92, R 18

Complaining of incisional pain; Demerol given. She was also upset about her family."

In previous chapters in this unit, you learned each step of the nursing process. In this chapter, you will increase your knowledge base with information on how to communicate that process with your coworkers. Recording and reporting client information is important to quality client care. Critical Thinking Challenges at the end of the chapter will help you synthesize the information you have learned.

The nursing process is communicated verbally and in writing. Effective communication enhances client care by ensuring comprehensive, coordinated care by a variety of providers. All members of the healthcare team share information through recording and reporting.

Written communication, or **recording**, serves as a permanent document of client information and care. The client record or chart provides information during the present visit or admission and may be consulted in the future to review the client's history and for educational, research, and legal purposes. **Reporting** takes place when two or more people share information about client care, either face to face (as in a nursing report from one shift to the next), by audiotape, or by telephone (as in laboratory reports given to the nursing unit).

Nurses are responsible for accurate, complete, and timely recording and reporting. As an instrument of continuous client care and as a legal document, the client record should contain all pertinent assessments, planning, interventions, and evaluations for that client.

Written Communication: The Client Record

The client record is essential for the communication of goals, overall plan of care, and progress for each client. It is prepared in written or computerized form and is accessible to members of the healthcare team caring for the client. If a client record is misplaced on a nursing unit, a vital line of communication is blocked.

Nurses must be familiar with the type of recording done in their agency. Nurses' entries on the client record are important because they show medical and nursing orders carried out, independent assessments and interventions performed, the exact dates and times of care delivered, and evaluation.

Purpose

The client record is kept for the following reasons: communication, assessment, care planning, education, reimbursement, research, auditing, and legal documentation.

Communication

Clearly documented information on the client record communicates the plan of care and the client's progress to all members of the healthcare team. Team members who interact with the client at different times and in different ways get a clear picture of what took place in their absence. This communication ensures continuity of care and provides essential data for revision or continuation of care.

Assessment

Nurses and other team members gather assessment data from the client record. By reading about the client's history and initial assessment and comparing additional subjective and objective information that has been documented, the nurse can assess current health status and progress toward goals. Progressive assessments of a wound, for example, might alert the nurse to a developing infection or indicate that the wound is healing properly.

Care Planning

Formulation of a plan of care flows from assessment data recorded on the client record. All data on the client record should be considered when developing nursing diagnoses, goals, outcome criteria, interventions, and evaluation criteria for that client. An individualized nursing plan of care is essential for each client and becomes part of the permanent client record.

Education

Members of the healthcare team, including students of nursing, medicine, and other disciplines, use the client record as an educational tool. It contains valuable information about signs and symptoms of disease, diagnostic tests, treatment modalities, and client responses to the disease and treatment. A nursing student, for example, may read the record of a stroke client to learn what signs and symptoms the client initially experienced, what computerized axial tomography scan results show, what effect medications given to minimize brain injury had, and whether physical therapy is helping the client reach rehabilitation goals.

Research

Nursing and healthcare research are often carried out by studying client records. Data may be gathered from groups of records to determine significant similarities in disease presentation, to identify contributing factors, or to determine the effectiveness of therapies. For example, a nurse researcher may review the records of clients who have had appendectomies to determine how long they needed pain medication postoperatively. This information might be used in preoperative teaching or to plan more effective pain intervention strategies.

Reimbursement

Documentation often provides the basis for decisions regarding payment, either by supporting diagnosis-related group classification or by stating interventions

Nursing Research
Recording and Reporting

Selected Nursing Research Studies

Aaronson, L., & Burman, M. (1994). Use of health records in research: reliability and validity issues. *Research in Nursing and Health, 17*(1), 67–74.

Howse, E., et al. (1992). Resistance to documentation—a nursing research issue. *International Journal of Nursing Studies, 29*(4), 271–281.

Rodgers, B., et al. (1993). The qualitative research audit trail: a complex collection of documentation. *Research in Nursing and Health, 16*(3), 219–226.

Possible Topics for Nursing Inquiry

- What are barriers to documenting nursing care?
- What nursing activities can be documented on flowsheets compared with progress notes?
- What is the relationship between daily nursing documentation and effective discharge planning?

that were actually performed for the client. Documentation provides evidence for decisions made by Medicare, Medicaid, worker's compensation, and third-party insurance companies to cover health-related expenses. For example, to obtain reimbursement when a wound culture is done, documentation would indicate that the test was ordered by a physician and actually carried out by the laboratory. Administration of medication or the use of equipment also may be verified with documentation.

Documentation is essential when determining Medicare eligibility for home care. To qualify, the client must be home bound, so nursing documentation, such as "extremely short of breath after ambulating 30 feet," would provide supporting evidence (Magliozzi, 1990).

Auditing

An **audit** is a review of records. Audits of client records serve a dual purpose: quality assurance and reimbursement. Auditing is done for quality assurance by randomly selecting records to see if certain standards of care have been met and documented. The Joint Commission on Accreditation of Healthcare Organizations (JCAHO) audits client records yearly and encourages hospitals to set up ongoing quality assurance programs. If deficiencies are detected, educational programs can be designed to improve outcomes in these areas.

Legal Documentation

The client record serves as a legal document of the client's health status and the care given. It may be used in court to prove or disprove injuries a client incurred in an accident or to implicate or absolve a healthcare professional for improper care. Because nurses and other healthcare team members cannot remember specific assessments or interventions about a client years after the fact, accurate and complete documentation is essential. The care may have been excellent, but documentation must prove it.

Principles of Charting

Principles of good charting are easier to accept and adopt if the purposes of the record are kept in mind. Remember that any entry made in the nursing notes can serve not only as communication, but also may be scrutinized carefully by students, lawyers, and researchers. Principles of good charting include conciseness, accuracy, completeness, organization, legibility, timeliness, and confidentiality.

Conciseness

Good charting is concise and brief. Use partial sentences and phrases; drop the client's name and terms referring to the client. Use abbreviations but only those that are commonly accepted and approved by your facility. Table 14-1 lists common abbreviations. Unnecessary elaboration confuses important issues. Being concise also is helpful in time management; the nurse will spend less time charting and more time with clients.

Accuracy

Entries must be accurate. The nurse must write only observations that he or she has seen, heard, smelled, or felt; an observation made by another health professional must be clearly identified. Charting that a client "states he is upset that surgery has been postponed" is more accurate than charting "client mad at doctor." Precise measurements and times should be used when possible. For example, a wound should be described as "3 cm by 0.5 cm" rather than "small." To avoid confusion, make sure that the names of physicians or other professionals are correct. Correct spelling and correct use of medical terms are important.

When an error occurs, erasure is not permissible, so a notation about the error must be made (Fig. 14-1). A single line should be drawn through the error, and the word "error" and the nurse's initials should be written above it. Some hospitals require an explanation of the error, such as "charted for wrong client."

Completeness

Obviously, not every observation and intervention is recorded, but information about the nursing process must be complete. Other team members may consider that an action not recorded may not have been done. For example, if a client's temperature of 100.8°F at 2 PM was not recorded, the nurse coming on at 4 PM might not take the client's temperature. It may be significantly higher; the client will be uncomfortable, and infection may be flourishing. Complete, pertinent assessment data, such as other vital signs, wound drainage, client complaints, who was notified, and what interventions were carried out, give the night-shift nurse a complete

text continues on p. 224

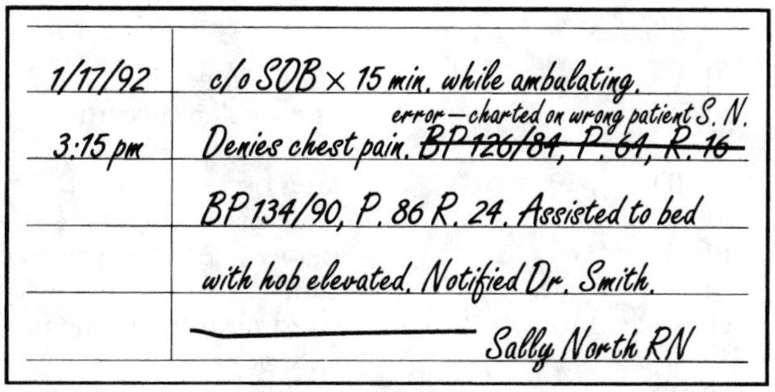

Figure 14-1 • *Sample correction of an error in client charting.*

Table 14-1 • *Abbreviations Commonly Used in Documentation*

Abbreviation	Meaning	Abbreviation	Meaning
ā	before	NG	nasogastric
abd	abdomen	noc	night
ac	before meals	NPO	nothing by mouth
ADLs	activities of daily living	os	mouth
ad lib	as needed	OOB	out of bed
adm.	admitted, admission	oz	ounce
amp.	ampule	p̄	after
ant.	anterior	p.c.	after meals
AP	anterior–posterior	post	posterior
ax.	axillary	prep	preparation
b.i.d.	twice a day	prn	when necessary
BP	blood pressure	q̄, q	every
BR	bed rest	q̄, 2 (3, 4, etc.) hours	every 2 (3, 4, etc.) hours
BRP	bathroom privileges	qd	every day
C	Centigrade	qh	every hour
c̄	with	q.i.d.	four times a day
caps	capsule	q.o.d.	every other day
C.C.	chief complaint	q.s.	quantity sufficient
cc	cubic centimeter (1 cc = 1 mL)	R/O	rule out
CVP	central venous pressure	ROM	range of motion
c/o	complains of	s̄	without
D/C	discontinue	SBA	stand by assistance
disch; DC	discharge	SC	subcutaneous
drsg	dressing	SL	sublingual
dr	dram	SOB	shortness of breath
elix	elixir	sol, soln	solution
ext	extract or external	spec	specimen
F	Fahrenheit	S/P	status post
fx.	fracture, fractional	sp. gr.	specific gravity
gm	gram	S.S.E.	soapsuds edema
gr	grain	ss	one-half
gtt	drop	stat	immediately
"H," SC, or sub q	hypodermic or subcutaneous	tab	tablet
		t.i.d.	three times a day
h	hour	tinct or tr.	tincture
HOB	head of bed	TKO	to keep open
h.s.	bedtime (hour of sleep)	TPN	total parenteral nutrition hyperalimentation,
hx	history		
I & O	intake & output	TPR	temperature, pulse, respiration
IM	intramuscular		
		tsp	teaspoon
IV	intravenous	TO	telephone order
kg	kilogram	TWE	tap water enema
KVO	keep vein open	VO	verbal order
L	left; liter	VS	vital signs
lat	lateral	VSS	vital signs stable
MAE	moves all extremities	W/C	wheelchair
mg	milligram	WNL	within normal limits
ml, mL	milliliter (1 mL = 1 cc)		
NAD	no apparent distress		
Selected Abbreviations Used for Specific Descriptions			
AKA	above-knee amputation	Nsy.	nursery
ASCVD	arteriosclerotic cardiovascular disease	NWB	non–weight-bearing
		O.D.	right eye
ASHD	arteriosclerotic heart disease	O.S.	left eye
BKA	below-knee amputation	O.U.	each eye
ca	cancer	OPD	outpatient department
chest clear to A & P	chest clear to auscultation & percussion	ORIF	open reduction internal fixation
CMS	circulation movement sensation	Ortho	orthopedics
		OT	occupational therapy

Table 14-1 • *(continued)*

Abbreviation	Meaning	Abbreviation	Meaning
CNS	central nervous system	PE	physical examination
DJD	degenerative joint disease	PERRLA	pupils equal, round, & react to light and accommodation
DOE	dyspnea on exertion	PID	pelvic inflammatory disease
DT's	delirium tremens	PI	present illness
D_5W	5% dextrose in water	PM & R	physical medicine & rehabilitation
FUO	fever of unknown origin	Psych	psychology; psychiatric
GB	gall bladder	PT	physical therapy
GI	gastrointestinal	RL (or LR)	Ringer's lactate; lactated Ringer's
GYN	gynecology	RLE	right lower extremity
H_2O_2	hydrogen peroxide	RLQ	right lower quadrant
HA	hyperalimentation; headache	RR, PAR	recovery room, post-anesthesia room
HCVD	hypertensive cardiovascular disease	RUE	right upper extremity
HEENT	head, ear, eye, nose, throat	RUQ	right upper quadrant
HVD	hypertensive vascular disease	Rx	prescription
ICU	intensive care unit	STSG	split-thickness skin graft
I & D	incision and drainage	Surg	surgery, surgical
LLE	left lower extremity	T & A	tonsillectomy & adenoidectomy
LLQ	left lower quadrant	THR, TJR	total hip replacement; total joint replacement
LOC	level of consciousness; laxatives of choice	URI	upper respiratory infection
LMP	last menstrual period	UTI	urinary tract infection
LUE	left upper extremity	vag	vaginal
LUQ	left upper quadrant	VD	venereal disease
MI	myocardial infarction	WNWD	well-nourished, well-developed
Neuro	neurology; neurosurgery		
NS	normal saline		

Selected Abbreviations Related to Common Diagnostic Tests

BE	barium enema	hct	hematocrit
B.M.R.	basal metabolism rate	Hgb	hemoglobin
Ca^{++}	calcium	IVP	intravenous pyelogram
CAT	computed axial tomography	K^+	potassium
CBC	complete blood count	LP	lumbar puncture
Cl^-	chloride	MRI	magnetic resonance imaging
C & S	culture & sensitivity	Na^+	sodium
Dx	diagnosis	RBC	red blood cell
ECG, EKG	electrocardiogram	UGI	upper gastrointestinal x-ray
EEG	electroencephalogram	UA	urinalysis
FBS	fasting blood sugar	WBC	white blood cell

Commonly Used Symbols

$>$	greater than	@	at
$<$	less than	+	positive
=	equal to	−	negative
≈	approximately equal to	±	positive or negative
≤	equal to or less than	F_1	first filial generation
≥	equal to or greater than	F_2	second filial generation
↑	increased	PO_2	partial pressure of oxygen
↓	decreased	PCO_2	partial pressure of carbon dioxide
♀	female	:	ratio
♂	male	∴	therefore
°	degree	%	percent
#	number or pound	2°	secondary to
×	times	Δ	change

picture so that he or she can make objective evaluations and revise the plan as needed.

The following information is essential when charting:

- Any new or changed information
- Signs and symptoms
- Client behavior
- Nursing interventions
- Medications given
- Physician's orders carried out
- Client teaching
- Client responses

Organization

Each entry must clearly show a logical and systematic grouping of important information. Information is grouped by problem or occurrence and flows in a logical format. For example, assessment is recorded with subjective and objective data, the identification of nursing diagnoses, goals, nursing interventions, and the client's response. Information about a routine laboratory test is recorded elsewhere if it does not pertain to this problem.

There must be a chronologic flow of information about client care according to time and procedures completed, with client reaction documented. Recording as the events of the day unfold can prevent out-of-sequence or fragmented entries that can cause confusion.

Legibility

The nurse's writing must be clear and easily read by others. Legibility is especially important when recording numbers and medical terms. For example, a pulse rate of 164 may look similar to 104, but has more serious implications. The term *dysphasia* (difficulty speaking) may be mistaken for *dysphagia* (difficulty swallowing).

Legibility is required on computer documentation as well. Checking the spelling of words will reduce errors, as will proofreading notes to ensure readability.

Timeliness

Time should be indicated for documentation. If litigation occurs, lawyers use charted documentation to reconstruct time sequences (Martin, 1994). Many agencies use military time to avoid possible errors. Some information can be entered for the shift, but when the client's status changes rapidly or frequent assessments are made, specific times should be recorded.

Documentation should occur in a timely manner to avoid errors. For example, suppose a nurse gives a postoperative client an injection of 75 mg of meperidine (Demerol) but does not record the injection. He or she then enters an isolation room to care for another client. Another nurse discovers that the postoperative client's blood pressure has dropped. She notifies the surgeon, who takes steps to determine if the client has internal bleeding. The client was having an adverse reaction to meperidine, but because the injection was not charted, other team members were unaware of it. Nurses should not leave the unit for breaks or other long periods until important information is recorded.

Timeliness also helps avoid forgetting important information. Waiting until the end of the shift to record the day's events on several clients may cause the nurse to omit important data or enter inaccurate information. Recording events in sequence will provide support if needed to demonstrate that appropriate responses were identified and reported. This can be essential for protecting a nurse from negligence or malpractice claims.

Confidentiality

All client care should be confidential. This is a basic nursing responsibility. Nurses treat the client record as a confidential document entrusted to the healthcare team. It should never be left in public areas or where it could be read by unauthorized individuals. Its contents are not to be discussed or shared with anyone not directly involved in the client's care. This includes the client's minister, family members, and physicians or nurses who are friends of the family. The client's right to privacy must be actively guarded. Strangers, such as new students on a unit, should be asked for identification before they are allowed access to the client's record.

The client record is the property of the healthcare facility, agency, or physician's office. The Federal Privacy Act and other federal laws ensure the right for selected individuals (federal government employees, clients receiving care in a Veterans Administration Hospital, Public Health Service facility, or a long-term care facility receiving Medicare or Medicaid payment) to review their health records. In other instances, state law applies, with 18 states providing access to health records within some limits. Agency policy may require that the client reviews his or her record in the presence of a nurse or physician to assist understanding of medical terminology and limit misinterpretation.

Clients should be discussed only in a manner that ensures confidentiality. Specific clients should not be discussed in the cafeteria or elevators, where family or friends could possibly overhear and misinterpret information discussed. When making a telephone report or engaging in other verbal communication, nurses must make sure they are speaking in a private place and that they are speaking to authorized people.

When using computers in documentation, access codes must be issued and kept secret. The computer screen should not be left unattended when client information is displayed. Computer programs used for documentation should not permit deletion of entries once they are logged into a client's record.

Types of Documentation

Documentation may vary depending on the agency. Systems of documentation used include the following:

- Source-oriented record
- Problem-oriented medical record (POMR)
- Charting by exception (CBE)
- Computerized client record

Nurses should become familiar with the type of documentation used in their facility. All health team members should use the same type of documentation system.

Source-oriented record

In the **source-oriented record**, documentation is organized according to who is making the entry. Each type of healthcare provider documents separately. For example, nurses record only in the area designated for nursing; the physician writes in the progress notes, and physical therapists document separately in a section designated for physical therapy. This may cause fragmentation and replication of documentation and may hinder coordination between team members. Table 14-2 explains components of the source-oriented record.

Source-oriented documentation makes recording easier, but it makes it more difficult to review a particular event or to follow the overall progress of a client. For example, if an elderly client falls getting out of bed, the nurse records the event in the nurses' notes. The physician charts his or her assessment on the physician's progress notes and makes orders on the physician's order sheet. A physical therapist who teaches the client how to use a cane records in physical therapy notes. The x-ray report appears in the radiology section. Reviewing the entire incident would require flipping back and forth and scanning information from multiple sources.

Some nurses think that source-oriented recording makes it easier to evaluate nursing care because they can simply review the nurses' notes. In the source-oriented record, traditional narrative nurses' notes are preferred to newer formats for recording nursing care.

Problem-Oriented Medical Record

Weed (1971) introduced a new method of organizing the medical record by using a client problem approach or POMR. The POMR includes a database, problem list, plan of care, and progress notes; the focus is the client's problem list. Because the same problem list and progress notes are used by all team members, the plan of care is coordinated. An example of a POMR-based plan of care is given in Figure 14-2.

The *database* consists of all information known about the client, including physician and nursing histories, physical assessment data, and diagnostic test results. Any team member may provide information for the database. The database provides the basis from

Table 14-2 • The Source-Oriented Record and Its Components

Component	Information Included
Admission sheet	Client's name, address, age, sex, Social Security number, occupation, employer, religion, attending physician, admitting diagnosis, health insurance
Physician's order sheet	Specific orders for medications, treatment, diagnostic tests
Graph/flowsheets	Temperature, pulse, respirations, blood pressure, daily weights, intake and output measurements, urine sugar and acetone, daily activity, routine treatments performed
Nursing admission assessment	Nursing history and functional assessment on admission
Nurses' notes	Chronologic documentation of the nursing process (ongoing assessment, nursing diagnosis, outcome criteria, planning, intervention, and evaluation of care)
Medication sheet	Name, dosage, route, and time of medication given with initials and signature of nurse who gave it
Physician's history and physical examination	Medical history, physical examination, diagnosis, and tentative plan of care
Physician's progress notes	Chronologic assessment and interpretation of client's progress with revisions in plan of care
Discharge summary	Physician's summary of client's course of illness, response to treatment, prognosis, status at discharge, and plan for rehabilitation or follow up
Nurse's discharge sheet	Client's vital signs and health status at discharge, follow up and other instructions
Miscellaneous forms	Laboratory reports, x-ray reports, consultations, respiratory therapy notes, physical therapy notes, dietary notes, social service notes.

LONG TERM GOAL

The patient will maintain optimal gas exchange and a patent airway.

DATE AND HOUR	PROB. NO.	PROBLEMS/NEEDS/ CONCERNS	PATIENT OUTCOMES	INTERVENTIONS/TEACHING AND DISCHARGE PLANS	INITIAL & DATE RESOLVED
1-4	1	Impaired gas exchange related to inflammatory process in lungs.	no dyspnea on exertion; decreased restlessness; arterial blood gases within normal limits	Assess and document respiratory rate, depth, and sounds q 4 hours Administer O_2 2L per nasal cannula Elevate head of bed or have patient up in a chair to maximize air exchange	
1-4	2	Ineffective airway clearance related to pulmonary inflammation.	experiences effective coughing; has adequate fluid intake	Encourage deep breathing and coughing q 2 hours while awake Offer fluids frequently (1000cc /shift) Change position q 2 hours	

PT. NO.

James, John
Age 52

NAME

K. Subramanian, M.D.

D.O.B.

PRIMARY NURSE J. Sidney, RN

UNIVERSITY OF WASHINGTON HOSPITALS
HARBORVIEW MEDICAL CENTER
UNIVERSITY HOSPITAL
SEATTLE, WASHINGTON

PATIENT CARE PLAN

UH 0570 REV SEP 78 1-78-2059

Figure 14-2 • Combined problem list and plan of care.

which client problems can be identified and the plan of care individualized.

The *problem list* is made up of problems identified by different team members as they occur or are discovered. Problems include medical diagnoses, nursing diagnoses, signs and symptoms, abnormal diagnostic test results, behavioral problems, or risk factors. These problems are numbered but not necessarily in order of importance. Problems are dated as to when they happened and when they were resolved.

Following the database and problem list is the *initial plan of care.* Initial medical and nursing plans of care may be listed after each problem. Physician's orders also appear in this section. The nursing plan of care may be located here, rather than in a separate file (or Kardex).

Progress notes document client status in areas indicated in the problem list. Traditionally the POMR system uses a SOAP format of progress recording (S, subjective; O, objective; A, assessment; P, plan) or a variation of the SOAP format. SOAP charting is discussed later in this chapter.

Charting by Exception

First developed in 1985 at St. Luke's Hospital in Milwaukee, Wisconsin, CBE permits the nurse to document only those findings that fall outside the standard of care and norms that have been developed by the institution (Barthel, Reichert, Streff, Twite, 1993). This is a shift away from the concept previously held that "if it hasn't been documented, it hasn't been done."

Agencies develop written norms and standards against which client assessments or client care activities can be compared. These standards are available on each nursing unit and often are included in the back of the client's chart for easy reference. Flowsheets provide a form on which the nurse can indicate, usually by making a checkmark, that assessment findings and care fall within the agency's standards. Standards require periodic assessments and notations, usually once per shift, so that it is easy to note changes in client status. Documentation is required any time the client's status changes significantly. Additional documentation is required when any deviation from standards is detected. Often this documentation is a narrative note on the same form to explain the variance, but it can be a SOAP note, PIE note, or DAR note in the progress notes. (These forms of charting are described in detail later in this chapter.)

CBE has many advantages: it requires less nursing time, guidelines are clear as to expected outcomes and normal assessment parameters, changes in client status can be readily detected, and information is more readily accessible. The most significant disadvantage of the system is the time it takes for each agency to develop standards, flowsheets, and train personnel to chart effectively using this new method. Also CBE seems to work best in agencies where routine care can be anticipated. Settings like home care, where greater differences exist, make this more difficult.

Critical Pathways

The physician may order care according to a critical pathway or CareMap™ for a specific client. He or she can write additional orders as needed for each client to individualize care. The pathway is then placed in the client's chart, providing orders for care. Documentation occurs on the pathway form, usually requiring the nurse to initial when specific interventions have occurred or outcomes have been met. A variance occurs when the client does not proceed along the pathway as planned. Any variances are documented in detail, usually using narrative notes.

Computer Documentation

Computer documentation use is increasing. The computer can save time in storage and retrieval of information. The use of the Hospital Information System for improving documentation of nursing practice started as early as the 1960s (Saba & McCormick, 1986). The functions of the computer in a hospital include ordering supplies and services for a client; storing admission assessment data; developing and revising nursing plans of care; documenting progress notes; listing treatments, procedures, and medications; and storing diagnostic test results. JCAHO requires a plan to safeguard security and confidentiality whenever hospitals use computers.

Computer programs used on nursing units are client centered. Data for a particular client can be entered or retrieved easily (Fig. 14-3). This eliminates

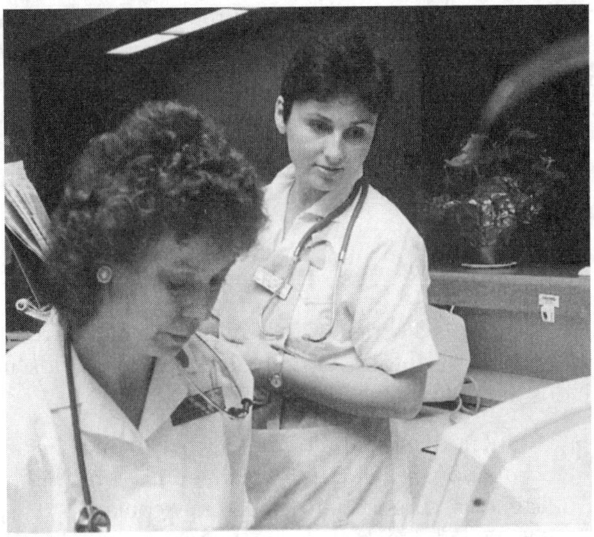

Figure 14-3 • *The computer in the nursing unit is a time-saver for both storage and retrieval of information in the client record.*

phone calls to other departments to order supplies, reading through a whole client record to evaluate progress, or sorting through stacks of reports to determine a client's test result. Client information is permanently recorded, and caregivers in various departments can communicate with one another.

In large agencies, basic computer skills are usually taught through in-service education. Each nursing unit or each bed has a computer screen, a keyboard, and possibly a printer. Appropriate personnel are given an access code, which allows them to retrieve and enter data into the client's record. To maintain confidentiality and avoid unauthorized individuals from entering client records, this access code should not be shared. The entire client record or just parts of it (such as the medication record or laboratory tests) may be computerized.

Computerized documentation systems have many advantages, including legibility, accuracy, rapid communication, definite documentation accountability, enhanced client education, and reduced medication errors (Eggland & Heinemann, 1994). Possible malfunction, impersonal effect, concern for privacy, dissemination of inaccurate information, and cost are some possible disadvantages.

Nursing Entries on the Client Record

Nurses make entries on a variety of components in the client record, including the nursing plan of care, the Kardex, nursing progress notes, flowsheets, admission record, discharge instruction sheet, and medication record.

Nursing Plan of Care

A **nursing plan of care** should be generated at admission and revised to reflect changes in the client's condition. The nursing plan of care must contain nursing diagnoses, goals, outcome criteria, nursing interventions, and evaluation. Standardized plans of care designed for clients with specific medical diagnoses may be used, but they must be individualized. Nursing plans of care are often part of the permanent client record. See Chapter 12 for information on nursing plans of care.

Kardex

The **Kardex** is a series of flip cards kept in a portable file (Fig. 14-4). Information entered on the Kardex includes the following:

- Pertinent demographic data, such as name, age, occupation, religion, physician, admission date, diagnosis, surgery, and emergency contact
- Basic needs, such as diet, activity, hygiene, how bowel and urinary elimination is accomplished, assistive devices, and safety precautions
- Allergies
- Diagnostic tests
- Intravenous therapy
- Daily nursing procedures, such as dressing changes, vital signs, and irrigations
- Medications
- Respiratory therapy, such as use of oxygen, mechanical ventilation, or suctioning

The Kardex is a way to ensure continuity of care from one shift to another and from one day to the next. The Kardex is commonly used for the change-of-shift report and is discussed later in this chapter. This most current record of a client's healthcare is updated at least once every 8 hours or more frequently as the client's condition changes or new physician orders are obtained.

Kardex entries are often in pencil so that they can be changed as the client's condition changes. This means that the Kardex is for planning and communication purposes *only*; nursing care and client progress must be documented in the progress notes and appropriate flowsheets. If the Kardex is to become part of the permanent client record, it is written in ink. In either case, nurses are responsible for initiating and updating the Kardex and ensuring that data have been transcribed correctly from the client record.

Nursing Progress Notes

Nursing progress notes are recorded for all clients but vary in format. Narrative notes are often used in the source-oriented system, SOAP notes, DAR notes, or PIE notes in the POMR system. Table 14-3 compares different formats for writing nursing progress notes.

Narrative Notes. This type of documentation is a method for recording all the client's relevant behavior and activities throughout a shift. The note includes the date and time of the entry and specific activities accomplished (Figure 14-5). Typical notes include the type of morning care given (for example, bath or shower) and the client's response. The meals given are included with the time and how much the client ate. Nursing procedures, such as dressing changes and intravenous care, are documented as they are completed throughout the day. Nursing assessment data are recorded as they are gathered.

Because recording in this method describes nursing actions and procedures, specific nursing identification of client problems is not required. These activities should support information recorded on the nursing plan of care and the nursing Kardex.

A disadvantage of narrative notes is that much reading is required to learn about a specific problem. The use of abbreviations and concise language decreases space and time used in recording. Many hospitals com-

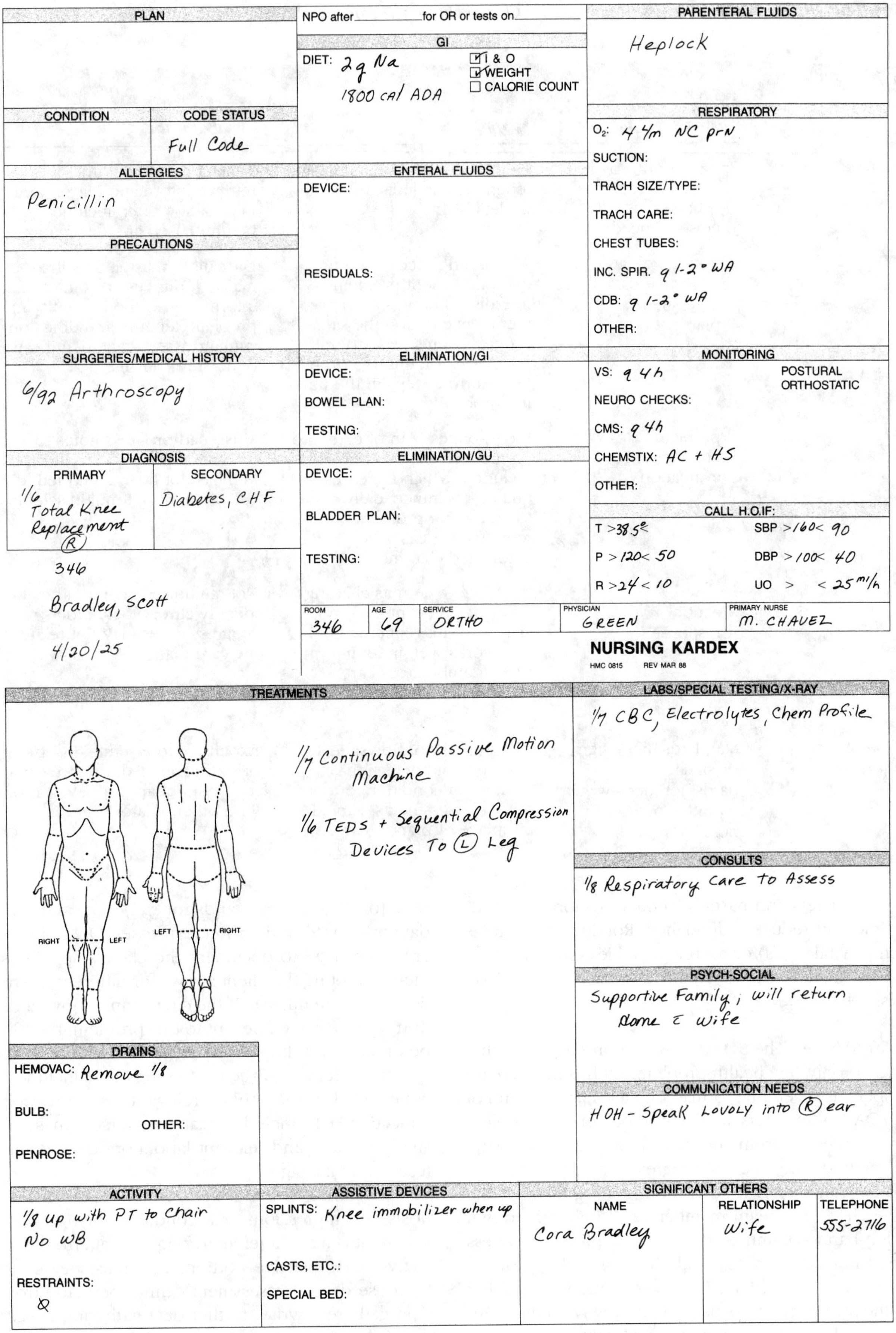

PLAN

NPO after ________ for OR or tests on ________

GI

DIET: 2g Na 1800 cal ADA

☑ I & O
☑ WEIGHT
☐ CALORIE COUNT

PARENTERAL FLUIDS: Heplock

CONDITION:

CODE STATUS: Full Code

ALLERGIES: Penicillin

PRECAUTIONS:

ENTERAL FLUIDS
DEVICE:
RESIDUALS:

RESPIRATORY
O2: 4 l/m NC prn
SUCTION:
TRACH SIZE/TYPE:
TRACH CARE:
CHEST TUBES:
INC. SPIR. q 1-2° WA
CDB: q 1-2° WA
OTHER:

SURGERIES/MEDICAL HISTORY: 6/92 Arthroscopy

ELIMINATION/GI
DEVICE:
BOWEL PLAN:
TESTING:

MONITORING
VS: q 4h
POSTURAL ORTHOSTATIC
NEURO CHECKS:
CMS: q 4h
CHEMSTIX: AC + HS
OTHER:

DIAGNOSIS
PRIMARY: 1/6 Total Knee Replacement Ⓡ
SECONDARY: Diabetes, CHF

ELIMINATION/GU
DEVICE:
BLADDER PLAN:
TESTING:

CALL H.O.IF:
T >38.5°
SBP >160< 90
P >120< 50
DBP >100< 40
R >24 < 10
UO > < 25 ml/h

346
Bradley, Scott
4/20/25

ROOM	AGE	SERVICE	PHYSICIAN	PRIMARY NURSE
346	69	ORTHO	GREEN	M. CHAVEZ

NURSING KARDEX
HMC 0815 REV MAR 88

TREATMENTS
1/7 Continuous Passive Motion Machine
1/6 TEDS + Sequential Compression Devices To Ⓛ Leg

RIGHT LEFT LEFT RIGHT

LABS/SPECIAL TESTING/X-RAY
1/7 CBC, Electrolytes, Chem Profile

CONSULTS
1/8 Respiratory Care to Assess

PSYCH-SOCIAL
Supportive Family; will return Home c̄ wife

DRAINS
HEMOVAC: Remove 1/8
BULB:
OTHER:
PENROSE:

COMMUNICATION NEEDS
HOH - Speak LOUDLY into Ⓡ ear

ACTIVITY
1/8 up with PT to Chair
No WB
RESTRAINTS: Ø

ASSISTIVE DEVICES
SPLINTS: Knee immobilizer when up
CASTS, ETC.:
SPECIAL BED:

SIGNIFICANT OTHERS

NAME	RELATIONSHIP	TELEPHONE
Cora Bradley	Wife	555-2716

Figure 14-4 • Example of a nursing Kardex.

Table 14-3 • Comparing Documentation Notes

	Format	Advantages	Disadvantages
Narrative	Information provided in written sentences or phrases; usually time sequenced.	Easy to learn; easy to adjust length as needed; can explain in detail.	Time consuming; difficult to retrieve information; irrelevant information often included; can be unfocused and disorganized.
SOAP	S subjective data O objective data A assessment P plan	All charting focused around identified client problems; interdisciplinary—all team members chart on the same progress notes; easy to track progress for identified problem; mirrors steps in the nursing process.	Difficult to master. Specific focus makes it difficult to chart general information without identifying a problem; lengthy and time consuming; assessment identification difficult for nurses.
PIE	P problem I interventions E evaluations	Incorporates plan of care into progress notes; outcomes included, which increases quality assurance; daily review to determine progress; less redundancy; easily adapted to automated charting.	Must read progress notes to determine plan of care; if problem has not been identified, difficult to chart; not multidisciplinary
FOCUS	D data A action R response	Broad view permits charting on any significant area, not just problems; concise, flexible; works well in long-term care or ambulatory care.	Not multidisciplinary; difficult to identify chronologic order; progress notes may not relate to the care plan
Charting By Exception (CBE)	Standards met—sign or check off; standards not met—write narrative or SOAP note	Efficient; use of flowsheets permits rapid detection of changes in condition; outline normal assessments; can take the place of plan of care.	Expensive to institute; inservicing of staff is needed; not prevention focused; not appropriate for long-term or ambulatory care.

bine flowsheets and narrative notes to shorten recording time and reduce redundancy. Routine assessments (such as vital signs) or routine activities (such as intravenous care and bowel elimination) are recorded on flowsheets.

SOAP Notes. The **SOAP note** is a progress note that relates to only one health problem. All healthcare team members use the same format. The left-hand column of the SOAP note refers to the number of the problem being addressed from the master problem list. Using this method, the client's progress on that particular problem can be assessed without sorting through the whole chart. The team member need only read down the left-hand column of the interdisciplinary progress notes and read the notes of all disciplines that relate to that numbered problem. However, some nurses think that the SOAP format focuses too narrowly on the identified problem list and does not highlight routine nursing care as well as traditional narrative notes do.

After documenting the problem to be addressed, the next step is organizing the information in the SOAP note format. The "S" stands for *subjective* and refers to data or symptoms the client expresses. Quotation marks are often used to document the client's specific statements; quoting the client allows for different interpretations than the nurse's. If the client cannot give information or gave none relevant to this problem, the "S" may be omitted or followed by "none."

"O" refers to *objective* findings and includes data collected by the nurse relevant to the problem. Objective data include what the nurse can see, feel, smell, or hear and relevant laboratory data, diagnostic tests, and vital signs.

"A" stands for *assessment,* which represents a diagnosis, an impression, or a condition change. This assessment is made after analyzing the data from the subjective and objective portions and must be supported by those data. If assessment cannot be made from the data gathered, write "further data gathering necessary" or "abdominal pain, unknown etiology" under the "A" portion of the SOAP note.

"P" stands for *plan.* This portion deals with nursing interventions specifically related to the identified prob-

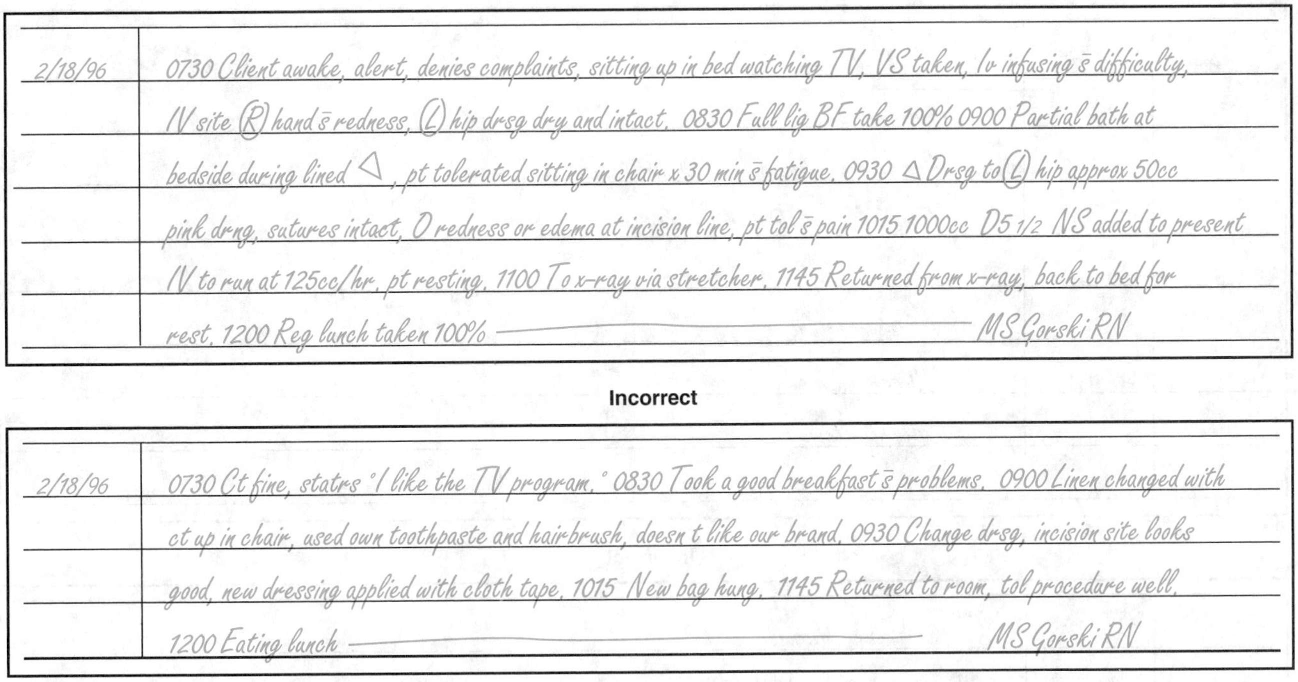
Correct

2/18/96	0730 Client awake, alert, denies complaints, sitting up in bed watching TV, VS taken, Iv infusing s̄ difficulty,
	IV site (R) hand s̄ redness, (L) hip drsg dry and intact, 0830 Full liq BF take 100% 0900 Partial bath at
	bedside during lined △ , pt tolerated sitting in chair x 30 min s̄ fatigue, 0930 △ Drsg to (L) hip approx 50cc
	pink drng, sutures intact, 0 redness or edema at incision line, pt tol s̄ pain 1015 1000cc D5 1/2 NS added to present
	IV to run at 125cc/hr, pt resting, 1100 To x-ray via stretcher, 1145 Returned from x-ray, back to bed for
	rest, 1200 Reg lunch taken 100% ——— MS Gorski RN

Incorrect

2/18/96	0730 Ct fine, statrs "I like the TV program," 0830 Took a good breakfast s̄ problems, 0900 Linen changed with
	ct up in chair, used own toothpaste and hairbrush, doesn t like our brand, 0930 Change drsg, incision site looks
	good, new dressing applied with cloth tape, 1015 New bag hung, 1145 Returned to room, tol procedure well,
	1200 Eating lunch ——— MS Gorski RN

Figure 14-5 • *Example of narrative nursing progress notes. Reflect on why the correct nursing note is better.*

lem. The plan section may simply state "continue present regimen" when the assessment is made that the client is progressing adequately using the plan already outlined. The plan also can specify revisions of the present nursing interventions as the need is assessed. Figure 14-6 provides an example of SOAP nursing progress notes.

Some hospitals use the SOAPIER format of recording (I, intervention; E, evaluation; R, revision). This allows the team member to record interventions, the client's response to the plan, and any revisions needed to the plan. The nurse must remember that all information recorded under the SOAP or SOAPIER headings must pertain to the same problem.

In some circumstances, a full SOAP note may be unnecessary. Routine care may be documented on a flowsheet. Routine nursing assessments need not be written as a SOAP note if they are not specifically related to a problem (for example, routine temperature and blood pressure on a client who has had no problem with fever and has stable blood pressure).

PIE Notes. The **PIE charting system**, first instituted in 1984 at Craven Regional Medical Center, simplifies documentation by incorporating the plan of care into the progress notes. Documentation is entered for each nursing diagnosis every shift using the acronym PIE to structure information according to problem (P), intervention (I), and evaluation (E). Client assessments are not part of the PIE note because this information is recorded on flowsheets for each shift. Figure 14-7 provides an example of a PIE nursing note. At the end of a 24-hour period the nurse reviews client documentation to ascertain client response to therapeutic intervention and progress. In this way, outdated problems can be dropped and new problems added to the documentation record. This daily review of client progress helps promote continuity of care.

Variations for the PIE system can be used when appropriate. To designate new problems or abnormal assessments, "A" can be added to the numbered problem (eg, API), thus allowing the nurse to also provide pertinent assessment data in the documentation. When appropriate, an intervention or an evaluation can be documented without writing the entire PIE statement.

Advantages of the PIE system of documentation include increased efficiency and flexibility, care planning focus, better tracking of client problems, nursing interventions and client outcomes, and less redundancy. This system easily adapts to automated charting, and client care can be easily audited. A disadvantage of the PIE system is that it is not multidisciplinary, providing a documentation system only for nursing. Although the PIE system uses a nursing plan of care format, there is no written plan of care. This necessitates reviewing previous documentation to become knowledgeable about current nursing diagnoses.

Focus DAR Notes. The FOCUS system of documentation organizes data entry around data (D), action (A),

Correct

Problem	8/18/96	"S" My head hurts right in the back of my eyes. Client desribes pain worse bending over, like
#3	0900	sinus headaches in past.
		"O" Eyes closed, lights dim, hesitant to move head when questioned.
		HR80 R20 BP140/90 T98.6
		"A" HA probable 2° sinus pressure.
		"P" 1. Decongestant prn as ordered
		2. Warm wash cloth to eyes
		3. Monitor temp q 4°
		4. Assess pain after med and contact physician as indicated —— MS Gorski RN

Incorrect

	8/18/96	"S" Ct states "My head hurts."
#3	0900	"O" History of constipation, ate well at breakfast, took shower without assist, lungs clear,
		"I hurt all over now."
		"A" Headache
		"P" Contact physician for further orders. —— MS Gorski RN

Figure 14-6 • *Example of SOAP nursing progress notes. Reflect on why the correct SOAP nursing note is better.*

and response (R). This system is broader in its view because a FOCUS can be a problem area (eg, nursing diagnosis) but does not need to be. An entry can be made on a significant event, positive growth, or learning that occurs during a teaching session. In this way, client documentation can focus on the client's strengths and important problem areas.

The data portion of the statement describes subjective and objective data that support the FOCUS of the note. Interventions and treatments are included in the action section of the note, whereas the client's response to therapy is discussed in the response section. Some notes may include all three sections, but flexibility permits the nurse to chart data, action, or response singularly or in combination. An example of a FOCUS nursing note appears in Figure 14-8.

Flowsheets

Flowsheets are designed to document routine nursing procedures and to free the nurse from writing out procedures done repeatedly. One example is a sheet for vital signs that gives a graphic representation of pulse, blood pressure, respirations, and temperature so that trends can be evaluated. (See Figure 22-11 for an example of a vital signs record.) The intake and output sheet is used to maintain an ongoing record of all fluid intake and output. A sample form is given in Chapter 36. On another common flowsheet, shown in Figure 14-9, the nurse documents all routine care, such as activity, dressing changes, meals taken, and breath sounds. Assessments also can be documented in this manner. Critical care flowsheets are used in the intensive care unit to document frequently changing data, specific nursing interventions, client responses, and multiple medications and intravenous fluids administered. In the last decade, flowsheets have evolved in some agencies into CBE, discussed earlier in this chapter.

Admission Entries

When a client enters the system, a nursing history is completed. The data gathered include most or all of the functional health patterns as described by Gordon

9/10 0400	Problem #1	Caregiver role strain related to chronically ill spouse, lack of immediate family support, and financial stress.
	Intervention for P(#1)	IP(#1): Acknowledge and talk with caregiver about stress involved with 24-hour care for loved one.
		IP(#1): Allow caregiver to express feelings.
		IP(#1): Help caregiver identify possible supports within the family and community.
	Evaluation for P(#1)	EP(#1): Caregiver discussed the strain of caring for her husband; crying and demonstrating signs of anxiety
		eg. "I just don't think I will be able to do this for long and then what is going to happen to us all? Sometimes it
		seems so hopeless." Stated she felt her children were supportive but they lived in another state and could not
		help with the day-to-day problems. -R. Wolfe, RN
		Note: as additional data is charted for the problem of caregiver role strain, Problem #1 is used to identify the problem.

Figure 14-7 • *Example of a PIE nursing note arranging information by P (problem), I (intervention), and E (evaluation).*

(1987). The nutrition, activity, sleep, and coping patterns are assessed and documented, as are pertinent medical history and history relating to the reason for current care. A complete physical assessment is performed and fully documented. See Chapter 21 for a full description of nursing history and physical assessment. A sample admission assessment form is shown in Figure 21-1.

In addition to recording a nursing history and physical assessment on admission, the nurse must document the admission procedure. This information may be entered on the nursing admission history and physical assessment sheet, on another standardized form, or in nursing progress notes.

Nursing Discharge Summary

A nursing discharge summary should be started at initiation of care (Fig. 14-10). It should list the discharge planning and client teaching that took place. (Discharge planning in relationship to community-based nursing care is discussed in each chapter in Section II of this text.) The discharge summary notes the client's condition at discharge and provides specific information about care after discharge. A copy of the discharge summary may be given to the client or sent to a home health nurse or extended-care facility.

text continues on page 236

Date / Time	FOCUS	NOTE
10/2	Injection Instruction	Data: Referred to injection room for teaching re injection technique as wife will be discharged and need IM injections of Compazine for
0900		nausea control. Husband states willingness to learn, yet states anxiety re "sticking wife and causing her pain."
		Action: Demonstrate injection technique including drawing up medication in syringe, locationg site, injecting medication, keeping record of
		medication administered. Have husband verbalize steps and then demonstrate technique.
		Response: Husband able to draw up medication correctly in syringe and verbalize step to injection technique without cuing. Husband injected
		model, hands shook, and needed verbal cuing to aspirate. -J. Morales RN
10/3	Injection Instruction	Response: Husband demonstrated good technique giving wife injection, without cuing. Wife will be discharge in AM with Visiting nurse
		follow-up. -J. Morales RN

Figure 14-8 • *Example of a FOCUS nursing note arranging information by D (data), A (action), and R (response).*

EVERGREEN HOSPITAL MEDICAL CENTER
KIRKLAND, WASHINGTON
DAILY NURSING SUMMARY

NUR-010 (REV. 1/90)		DATE: 2-14											
		0700	0800	0900	1000	1100	1200	1300	1400	1500	1600	1700	1800
VITAL SIGNS	TEMPERATURE	36^{2}				36^{6}				37^{2}			
	PULSE	92				88				86			
	RESPIRATIONS	20				22				22			
	BLOOD PRESSURE	110/82				116/92				120/88			
CNS	MENTATION	alert oriented			A/O					A/O			
	RESPONSE / MOTOR VERBAL	appropriate											
SAFETY	SIDERAILS / CALL LIGHT FALL PRECAUTIONS	2↑				2↑				2↑			
	RESTRAINTS												
ACTIVITIES OF DAILY LIVING	REST/ACTIVITY / TYPE TOL	up in room		up walking				up chair					
	PERSONAL HYGIENE			Bath/linen change									
	NUTRITION / TYPE % TAKEN	ice chips			ice chips			ice chips		ice chips			
	FLUID INTAKE												
PHYSICAL CHANGES	FLUID OUTPUT / FOLEY CARE	500				250							
	EMESIS/NG / AMT APPEARANCE												
	BOWEL / GUAIAC APPEARANCE	passing flatus				+ Bowel sounds				flatus			
	LUNGS BS, TCDB / O_2 AMOUNT												
	SKIN	warm dry					warm dry						
	IV CHECK / SOLUTION RATE IV SITE	patent no redness			1cc per hour			1cc per hour		patent			
	DRAINS / CHEST TUBES	J-P = 20 cc recompressed					J-P = 30cc recompressed						
PAIN	TYPE, LOCATION	Abd.											
	INTERVENTION/RESPONSE												
WOUND	HEALING/APPEARANCE	incision intact											
	DRESSING ✓/CHANGE	minimal drainage											
OTHER	PHYSICIAN			Dr. Stuart in									
	NURSES INITIALS	JS	JS	JS	JS	JS	JS	JS	JS	JS			

Identify Initials with Signature on Back

INTAKE

TYPE	DAYS	EVES.	NOCS	24 HR. TOTAL
oral	150	150	100	400
IV	1000	950	1000	2950
TOTAL	1150	1100	1100	3350

TODAY'S MEASURED WEIGHT 146

YESTERDAY'S MEASURED WEIGHT 145

OUTPUT

TYPE	DAYS	EVES.	NOCS	24 HR. TOTAL
urine	750	1250	800	2800
J-P	50	40	20	110
TOTAL	800	1290	820	2910

▼ STAMP HERE ▼

Harvey, Judith
Age 54
K. Stuart, MD

Figure 14-9 • *Example of a nursing assessment flowsheet.*

Diagnosis
Congestive Heart Failure

Procedures/Surguries: (include dates)

How Patient Discharged
☐ Ambulatory ☑ Wheelchair ☐ Ambulance ☐ Cabulance

Who Patient Discharged With:
☐ Alone ☑ M. Hazelet (daughter)
Name and Relationship to Patient

Discharged to:
☐ Nursing Home (name)
☐ Own Home or Apt. ☑ Other (name) Daughter's home

Family/Support System (Name, Relationship, Phone)
May Hazelet (daughter) 698-8650

Sensory Needs
Hearing ☐ within Normal Limits — ☑ Hard of Hearing ☐ Aids ∅
Vision ☐ within Normal Limits — ☑ Aids glasses
Speech ☐ within Normal Limits — ☐ Aphasic ☐ Aids

Languages Spoken:
English

Allergies: ☒ None
☐ Specify

SELF CARE STATUS LEVEL
(Check √ either I - Independent, A - Assistance, U - Unable)

	I	A	U
DRESSES SELF		√	
SHAVES SELF		√	
TRANSFERS SELF		√	
AMBULATES		√	
FEEDS SELF	√		
BATHES SELF ☐ TUB ☑ SHOWER		√	
ORAL HYGENE		√	

• BLADDER

• BOWEL

• WOUNDS/DRESSINGS/TUBES
(Type and Location) none

(Supplies/Amt. Provided)

• SPECIAL EQUIPMENT/APPLIANCES SENT HOME WITH PATIENT

(If Rental, Obtained from:

YOUR MEDICATIONS

NAME	DOSAGE	WHEN TO TAKE	SPECIAL INSTRUCTIONS	LAST DOSE GIVEN AT
Digoxin	0.125 mg	1 tablet q other day in morning		0900 3-21
Lasix	40 mg	1 tablet every morning		0900 3-21
Potassium	40 mEq	every morning		0900 3-21

PATIENT TEACHING	RETURN DEMONSTRATION	NEEDS PRACTICE	NEEDS MORE INSTRUCTION	SATISFACTORY
Skills/Topics				

FOLLOWUP CARE

SPECIAL INSTRUCTIONS	CLINIC NAME / PHYSICIAN	DATE	TIME
Diet 2 Gm Na	Lake Beach Clinic	3-29-96	9:00 am
Activity Up ad lib	Dr. B. Kyle		
Lab Work			
Other			

PHONE NUMBER WHERE YOU CAN BE REACHED
AT UWMC CALL (206) 548-4333 TO MAKE APPOINTMENT(S)
AT HMC CALL ________ TO MAKE APPOINTMENT(S)

REFERRAL AT DISCHARGE
Agency Name
Address
Phone # — Date Phoned
Referral For:
☐ NURSING CARE
☐ P.T. ☐ O.T.
☐ MEAL SERVICE
☐ CHORE WORKER
☐ COMPANION
☐ OTHER

Discharge Date/Time
3-21-96 11:30

I have been informed and I understand my home discharge instructions.

Patient Signature or Care Giver
X Scott Bradley

Primary Nurse Signature
X J. Sidney RN R.N.

Discharge Unit/Phone Number
689-5342

PT.NO. 029345

NAME Bradley, Scott

D.O.B.

UNIVERSITY OF WASHINGTON MEDICAL CENTERS
HARBORVIEW MEDICAL CENTER - UW MEDICAL CENTER
SEATTLE, WASHINGTON
PATIENT DISCHARGE STATUS REPORT
DIVISION OF NURSING

* U 0 0 2 1 *

UH 0021 REV FEB 94

WHITE - MEDICAL RECORD
CANARY - PATIENT (BELOW PERFORATION)
PINK - REFERRAL COPY
GOLDEN ROD - CLINIC

Figure 14-10 • *Example of a patient discharge summary.*

Nursing discharge summary forms are usually standardized and contain space to write specific instructions. Information includes medications, diet, activity, follow-up care, and special instructions, such as heat applications and circumstances requiring notification of the physician (eg, signs of wound infection). Often these forms are carbonized so that a copy can easily be given immediately to the client. Nursing discharge summary forms also contain space for vital signs, condition at discharge, method of discharge, time, and to whom and where the client was discharged.

Any pertinent discharge information should be documented on the nursing progress notes if it is not on the nursing discharge summary, such as assessment of the client's home environment, support system, and self-care abilities. Educational assessment, educational goals, and knowledge or skill criteria to be met by discharge should be documented (Cordell & Smith-Blair, 1994). The client's response to client teaching should be recorded throughout the hospital stay. Any written information or teaching plans given to the client should be documented. A note to the home health provider should mention any further health-education needs.

Home Care Documentation

Documentation should follow each home visit and include such information as the reason for the visit, the client's health status, nursing interventions used, and evaluations of interventions or outcomes. Future plans and recommendations for future home visits are included. Documentation is especially important in the area of home care, because appropriate documentation is essential for reimbursement from Medicare and other forms of third-party payment. Nurses working in home care must be knowledgeable concerning requirement for reimbursement (eg, homebound status or the need for skilled nursing care) and make sure that such information is provided clealy in documentation.

Medication Records

The medication record and intravenous flowsheets are important parts of documentation. Nurses should record administration of medications promptly to avoid confusion about missed doses and to prevent inadvertent double dosing.

The medication record distinguishes between routine medications and as needed (prn) medications (Fig. 14-11). On the form are routine times for medication administration, such as 0800, 1200, 1600, with a space for the initials of the nurse giving the drug. When giving a prn drug, the nurse records the time given and the effectiveness of the drug. When a client refuses or does not receive a drug for any reason, the dose must be circled, and the reason the client did not receive the drug is noted. Intravenous flow records ensure continuity by recording the type of solution, total intake over 8 hours, the volume remaining at the end of shift, and the condition of the infusion site.

Incident Report

An **incident** is any unusual happening, such as a fall, a medication error, a malfunction in equipment, or injury to a visitor or employee, in a healthcare facility. Each agency has a standardized form on which the witnessing nurse can record client or visitor incidents. The form includes the date and time of the incident, the events leading up to it, the client's response, and a full nursing assessment. The nurse is not judgmental or accusatory in documenting the incident. There should be a place on the form for physician notification, which is usually advisable, and an area for additional medical orders and assessment.

Some hospitals use incident reports related to nursing procedures as a way to evaluate the quality of care; these are called quality assurance memos. These reports are used to assess patterns of errors and the need to change the procedures involved. For example, a monthly review of incident reports reveals three identical errors by three different nurses. The same medication was involved in each instance. Discussion with each nurse may reveal that a simple change in the medication's packaging may prevent further incidents. It is difficult to admit that a mistake was made, but it is important to document the error for the client's sake and to prevent future errors. For legal reasons, incident reports do not become attached to the client's chart, nor should reference be made in the chart to any incident reports that have been filed. When an error occurs, it is important to document accurately what occurred but not highlight any mistakes that could result in litigation (Eggland & Heinemann, 1994). For example, if a medication is given at the wrong time, the time that the medication was actually given should be indicated in the chart, but explanation that this was a medication error should not be documented.

Oral Communication: Reporting

Oral communication is used to communicate the nursing process to other healthcare personnel. Reporting is done face to face, on the telephone, by taped messages, or on the computer. Reporting enhances client care and educates caregivers. It should be organized, concise, complete, and professional.

Change-of-Shift Reports

In the **change-of-shift report**, one nurse reports to another about client status and plans of care. This report is a way of ensuring continuity in client care from one

ROUTINE MEDICATIONS

DATE			MEDICATION STRENGTH—DOSAGE—ROUTE		DATE	DATE	DATE	DATE
US	RN	RPh			TIME & INITIAL	TIME & INITIAL	TIME & INITIAL	TIME & INITIAL
3-6			Digoxin 0.125 mg p.o.	2400-0800				
	JJ		qd	0800-1600	0800/JS	0800/JS		
			TIME 0800	1600-2400				
3-6			Procardia 10 mg p.o.	2400-0800				
	JJ		bid	0800-1600	0800/JS	0800/JS		
			TIME 0800 2000	1600-2400	2000/JS	2000/JS		
3-6			Atarax 50 mg p.o.	2400-0800	0600/JS	0600/JS		
	JJ		qid	0800-1600	1200/JS	1200/JS		
			TIME 0600 1200 1800 2400	1600-2400	1800/JS 2400/JS	1800/JS 2400/JS		
3-6			Amitriptyline 50 mg	2400-0800				
	JJ		qhs	0800-1600				
			TIME 2200	1600-2400	2200/JS	2200/JS		
				2400-0800				
				0800-1600				
			TIME	1600-2400				
				2400-0800				
				0800-1600				
			TIME	1600-2400				
				2400-0800				
				0800-1600				
			TIME	1600-2400				
				2400-0800				
				0800-1600				
			TIME	1600-2400				
				2400-0800				
				0800-1600				
			TIME	1600-2400				

I.V. DRIP MEDICATION	DATE	I.V. DRIP MEDICATION	US	RN	RPh	DATE	I.V. DRIP MEDICATION	US	RN	RPh

INITIAL	SIGNATURE	INITIAL	SIGNATURE
1.	J.S. J. Sidney RN	6.	
2.	J.J.A. James RN	7.	
3.		8.	
4.		9.	
5.		10.	

ALLERGY: NKA

DIAGNOSIS: CHF

▼ PATIENT STAMP ▼

Herbert, Howard
Age 58
N. Dean, MD

EVERGREEN HOSPITAL MEDICAL CENTER
KIRKLAND, WASHINGTON
MEDICATION RECORD

A - RIGHT ARM
B - LEFT ARM
C - RIGHT BUTTOCK
D - LEFT BUTTOCK
E - RIGHT THIGH
F - LEFT THIGH
G - RIGHT VENTROGLUTEAL
H - LEFT VENTROGLUTEAL
I - RIGHT ABDOMEN
J - LEFT ABDOMEN

RX-229A

Figure 14-11 • *Example of a medication record.*

Safety Alert
Recording and Reporting

- Familiarize yourself with the type of recording done in your institution.
- Use only commonly accepted abbreviations and symbols on the client record.
- Draw a line through any errors on the record. Do not erase or use wite out.
- Be complete in your notes.
- Write legibly so others can read your notes.
- Record information immediately or as soon as possible for proper care. This is vital in medication administration.
- Keep all client care confidential. Do not leave client information in public areas or where the client or family can read it.
- Document all incidents according to agency protocol. Include everything leading up to the occurrence, response, and a full nursing assessment. Do not be judgmental or accusatory.
- Be accurate when giving and taking telephone reports. Clarify anything not understood.

shift to the next. It may be taped or given face to face (Fig. 14-12); audiotaping saves time but does not allow for clarification of details. A study conducted by Richard (1988) found that taped reports were more likely to have omissions than face to face reports. A change-of-shift report in an acute-care hospital includes the following information:

- Name, age, and room number
- Medical diagnosis(es), surgery (date)
- Physician name or group
- Significant nursing diagnoses and progress toward goals
- Significant assessment findings, including vital signs
- diagnostic and laboratory test results
- Specific treatments (ie, dressing changes, respiratory therapy)
- Intravenous rate and amount remaining

Information about changes in status should be reported comprehensively and should include assessment data, nursing diagnoses pertaining to the change, planning, interventions, and evaluation. The client's emotional response and behavior should be reported as well. Exact times, dosages, and measurements should be given.

Oral and taped reports use the nursing Kardex and nursing plan of care as a basis for the information to be included. The listener also uses the Kardex as a guide to clarify information given by the previous nurse and to fill in the details of routine care.

Variations in shift reports occur according to the specialty nursing area. For example, the report in a critical-care setting may include an in-depth evaluation of each client's body system (ie, respiratory status by assessment and ventilator readings, cardiovascular status by rhythm strips, and blood pressure measurements). The report in a long-term care setting might include only those clients with significant status changes and might not mention those with no change in condition.

Nursing Rounds

Another method of reporting is nursing rounds (also called walking rounds). Rounds may be used for change-of-shift reports or for care planning. Two or more nurses visit a group of clients, and the nurse assigned to each client summarizes the client's current status and plan of care.

The advantage of nursing rounds is that there is optimal communication between nurses, and client status is confirmed by direct observation. For instance, it may be easier to describe various intravenous lines and dressing changes when the oncoming nurse is at the client's bedside. Two disadvantages are that rounds are time consuming because other topics may be discussed and that the client may feel excluded or alienated by the medical terms being used. Using understandable language and encouraging the client to participate can facilitate client's involvement.

Telephone Reports

Telephone reports can be used when transferring a client to another facility or to another unit within the hospital. Telephone reports also are used extensively to update physicians about client status and to communicate between hospital departments. Because telephone

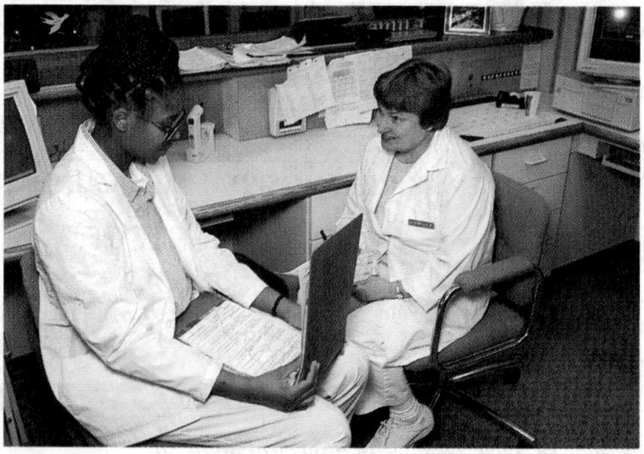

Figure 14-12 • *By reporting to one another, nurses ensure that their clients have continuity of care from one shift to another.*

reports do not rely on written verification or direct observation, accuracy is vital. Clarification should be made if any question exists. The sender should state the message clearly and concisely, and the receiver should repeat pertinent data for verification. Verbal orders need to be cosigned by the ordering physician, usually within a 24-hour period. It is important for the nurse to make sure this occurs to validate the order and avoid possible litigation if problems arise (Martin, 1994).

Client Transfers

When transferring a client to a different facility (such as from the hospital to an extended-care facility), a form must be completed to provide necessary information for the client's continued care. Forms vary, but the basic information includes physician orders, nursing orders, specific client needs, client limitations, and other pertinent data for planning care. The telephone report includes the client's status at the time of transfer and a verbal reiteration of information included on the form. The receiving nurse needs to know what to expect, and the telephone report enables the nurse to prepare for the client before his or her arrival. It also allows the receiving nurse to clarify any information.

When transferring a client to a different unit, the client record is transferred with the client, but the receiving nurse needs to have the most current information on client status and a summary of the client's progress and general care. Information to be included in the transfer report follows:

- Client name and age
- Current diagnosis and medical history
- Reason for transfer
- Most current assessment, particularly abnormalities
- Equipment to be transferred with client (ie, oxygen, intravenous infusion, wheelchair)
- Time and method of expected transport

Report to Physician

A telephone report to a physician usually involves a change in the client's condition. The most important preparation for this type of communication is completion of a focused nursing assessment. The assessment may be focused on the system involved, but all pertinent data should be gathered and communicated as appropriate. It may help to outline on paper the information that needs to be communicated to the physician. Have the client's record handy for reference. Important information to give a physician for status reports or possible medical intervention follows:

- Client name and diagnosis
- Stated symptoms

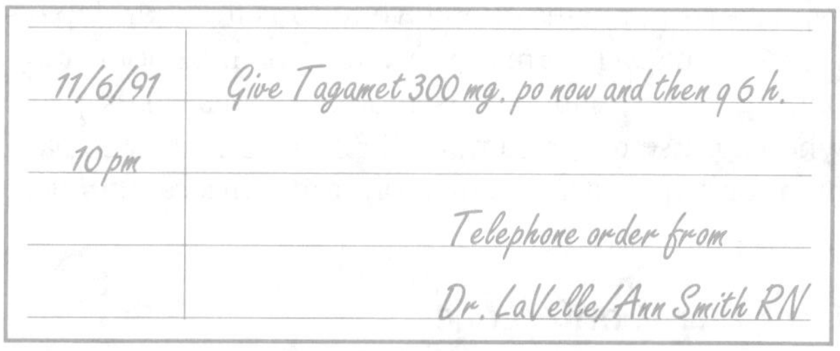

11/6/91	Give Tagamet 300 mg. po now and then q 6 h.
10 pm	
	Telephone order from
	Dr. LaVelle/Ann Smith RN

Figure 14-13 • Example of a documentation of a telephone order from a physician by a nurse.

- Changes in nursing assessment
- Vital signs (compared with baseline)
- Laboratory tests (compared with baseline)
- Nursing treatment initiated and client response

The following is an example of a nurse–physician telephone call:

> Mr. Jones, who is here for knee surgery, has a history of unstable angina. He now complains of epigastric pain; he states it's like "gas pain." The pain does not get worse with ambulation. His vital signs remain normal, and he has no abdominal tenderness or distention. Mylanta 30 mL prn as ordered relieves pain within 15 minutes. I wanted to let you know of this change because of his cardiac history.

A telephone report to a physician is often followed by telephone orders that must be documented in the client record and carried out by the nurse. For example, the physician may order a medication for Mr. Jones that should be started before the physician can visit the client. The nurse writes the order in the client record on the physician's order sheet and labels it as a telephone or verbal order. The nurse is responsible for correctly identifying the medication, dose, time, route, and the physician who ordered it. To ensure accuracy, the nurse should repeat the information and ask the physician to spell the medication or his or her name as necessary. Figure 14-13 is an example of a correctly transcribed telephone order.

Reports from Other Departments

Nurses often receive telephone reports from other departments, such as radiology or the laboratory. Information is exchanged that is crucial to client care, and numbers for laboratory values and complex terminology for diagnostic procedures may easily be misunderstood. When requesting information from another department, the nurse should be courteous. The nurse should identify herself or himself and identify the client, room number, and identification number, if necessary. When a report is given, the nurse should repeat the information and speak clearly to verify numbers.

Likewise, nurses often give reports to other departments. Usually information such as name, room number, age, and diagnosis is reported. This takes place when a nurse reports a new client to the dietary department or requests a consultation from physical therapy.

Care Plan Conferences

Care plan conferences are discussions about client care, involving either several departments or just the nursing staff on the unit.

Interdisciplinary conferences help to coordinate services so that the client's plan of care can be developed and implemented in the most efficient way. Nurses may initiate these conferences and invite members of the healthcare team from other departments, such as physical therapy, social services, and dietary. Clients who most benefit from such conferences are those with multiple, complex problems.

A conference with other nurses may be held to "brainstorm" ideas about a particular client's care. These conferences are initiated by the nurses caring for the client in hopes of enhancing the quality and continuity of care.

Key Concepts

- The purposes of the client record are communication, assessment, care planning, education, research, auditing, and legal documentation.
- Principles of recording are conciseness, accuracy, completeness, organization, legibility, timeliness, and confidentiality.
- A source-oriented record is divided into sections according to the type of caregiver (ie, nurses, physicians, respiratory therapists).
- A problem-oriented medical record is divided into sections by problem. All caregivers record on the same set of progress notes.
- The use of computers is increasing in documentation. Either the entire client record or just parts of it, such as the nursing plan of care, can be computerized.
- The nursing Kardex is a series of cards containing background information, routine care information, and specific treatments for each client. It is used when giving care and for change-of-shift reporting.
- The SOAP format organizes information into subjective, objective, assessment, and plan categories. Chronologic narrative nursing progress notes may be difficult to follow when checking the progress of the client on a specific problem.
- The PIE format incorporates the plan of care into the progress notes. Information is organized according to problem (P), intervention (I), and evaluation (E).
- FOCUS charting permits documentation on any significant topic, not just client problems. Information is organized around data (D), action (A), and response (R).
- Flowsheets for vital signs, intake and output, and routine nursing assessment and care make recording quicker and less redundant.
- CBE enables the nurse to check off normal assessments or treatment administered, writing narrative notes only when deviations from standards or norms are found.
- A nursing discharge summary reports the client's status at discharge and gives instructions for diet, activity, home care, and follow-up.
- Change-of-shift reports should be comprehensive but brief. They should highlight changes in the past 24 hours.
- In telephone reporting, the sender of the message should speak clearly, and the receiver should repeat the message to avoid errors.

Critical Thinking Challenges

In this chapter, you have learned how to share client information with your coworkers. You have studied the importance of complete and accurate documenting. Now turn back to the situation at the beginning of the chapter, and consider the following questions.

1. *Formulate information you would like to have that was not charted about your client.*
2. *Rate positive qualities in the charting. Identify at least five weaknesses in this charting and why you see them as problematic.*
3. *Construct charting for this client using narrative, PIE, and FOCUS formats. Add hypothetical information as necessary to reflect information that would be important to chart. Compare and contrast charting using these different methods.*
4. *Reflect on possible legal or ethical problems with the charting given at the beginning of the chapter.*

References

Barthel, M., Reichert, B., Streff, M., & Twite, K. (1993) Charting by exception eases documentation. *Oncology Nursing Forum, 20*(5), 826.

Cordell, B., & Smith-Blair, N. (1994) Streamlined charting for client education. *Nursing94, 24*(1), 57–59.

Eggland, E., & Heinemann, D. (1994) *Nursing documentation charting, recording, and reporting*. Philadelphia: J.B. Lippincott Company.

Gordon, M. (1987). *Nursing diagnosis: Process and application* (2nd ed.). New York: McGraw-Hill.

Magliozzi, H. (1990). Home care: Charting makes it through the medicare maze. *RN, 53*(6), 75–79.

Martin, F. (1994). Documentation Tips. *Nursing94, 24*(6), 63–64.

Richard, J. A. (1988). Congruence between intershift report and patients' actual condition. *Image, 20*, 4–6.

Saba, V. K., & McCormick, K. A. (1986). *Essentials of computers for nurses.* Philadelphia: J. B. Lippincott.

Weed, L. L. (1971). *Medical records, medical education, and patient care.* Chicago: Year Book.

Bibliography

Campbell, J. M., & Dowd, T., (1993) Capturing scarce resources: Documentation and communication. *Nursing Economics, 11*(2), 103–106.

Gruber, M., & Gruber, J. M. (1990). Nursing malpractice: The importance of documentation, or saved by the pen! *Gastroenterological Nursing, 12*, 255–259.

Kerr, S. (1992) A comparison of four nursing documentation systems. *Journal of Nursing Staff Development, 8*(1), 27–31.

Lucatorto, M., Petras, D. M., Drew, L. A., et al. (1991). Documentation: A focus of cost saving. *Journal of Nursing Administration, 21*(3), 32–36.

Moniz, D., & Belden, L., (1992) Ask the attorney. Co-signing others' charting. *Washington Nurse, 22*(3), 6–7.

Murphy, J., & Burke, L. J. (1990). Charting by exception: A more efficient way to document. *Nursing '90, 20*(5), 65–69.

Rauen, K. K. (1990). Documentation of the nursing process in the outpatient clinic. *Journal of Nursing Quality Assurance, 4*(4), 55–62.

Schmidt, D., Gathers, B., Stewart, M., et al. (1990). Charting for accountability. *Nursing Management, 21*(11), 50–55.

Wakefield, B., Miller, P., Farzad, R., et al. (1990). Documentation of the nursing process in the operating room. *Journal of Nursing Quality Assurance, 4*(4), 45–54.

Woolery, L. K. (1990). Professional standards and ethical dilemmas in nursing information systems. *Journal of Nursing Administration, 20*(10), 50–53.

Concepts Essential for Human Function and Nursing Management

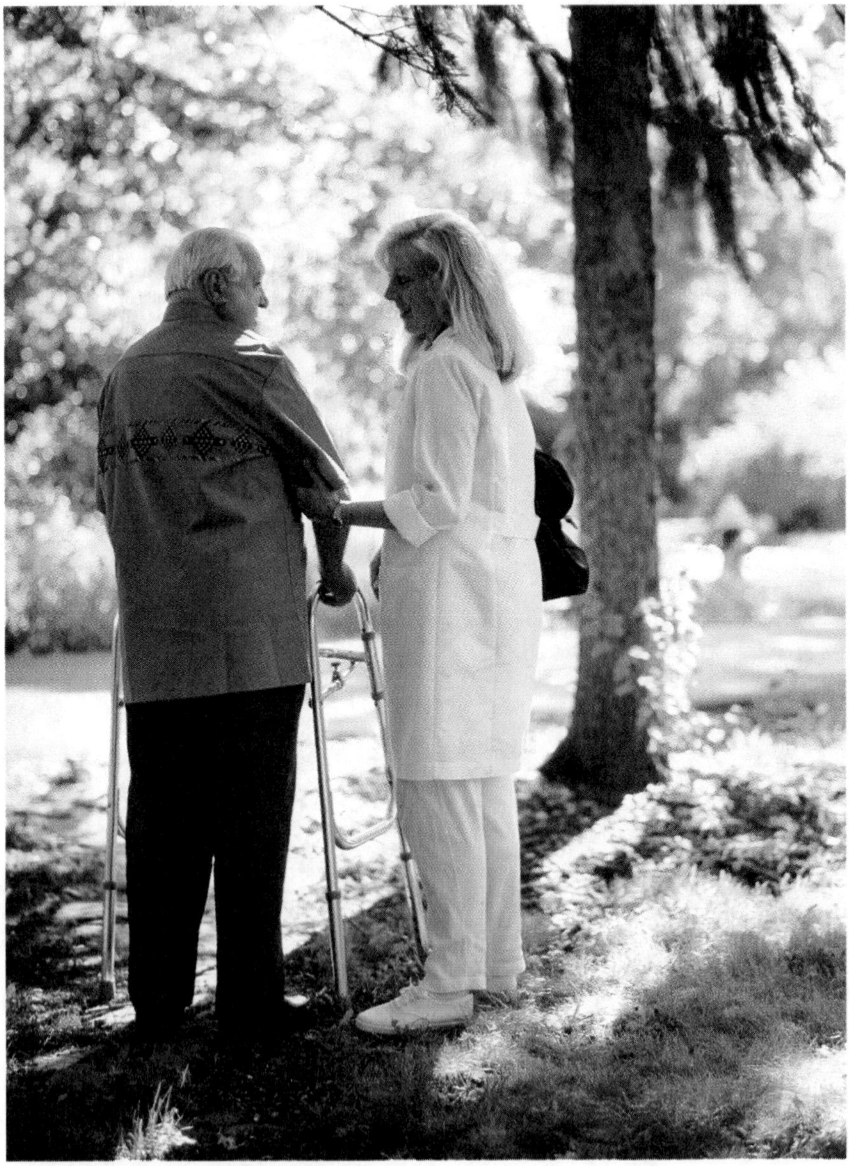

UNIT IV

Unit IV explores the foundational concepts essential for the nurse to provide safe, effective, holistic nursing care across the lifespan and to various cultural and ethnic groups.

Chapter 15 considers the concepts of health and wellness and defines their use with an emphasis on maintaining health and wellness. Chapter 16 discusses human growth and development throughout the lifespan. This chapter sets the stage for the "Lifespan Considerations" in each clinical chapter—an integrated approach that enables the nurse to see how these concepts are applied clinically. The next chapter considers the client as an individual, part of a family, and part of a larger community. This chapter begins a family focus that is evident throughout the text. Culture, ethnicity, and values are considered in Chapters 18 and 19. These issues affect a client's attitudes and feelings about health practices and underlie his or her decisions about health-care. The final chapter in this unit focuses on the knowledge and skills needed to establish an effective nurse–client relationship. This chapter is coordinated with Chapter 48 to focus on communication and its importance in all human relationships.

The chapters in this Unit provide a strong foundation for understanding less tangible client needs and for planning individualized, holistic nursing care. This foundation is basic to nursing care of all people.

Health and Wellness

Key Terms	Learning Objectives

Key Terms

Disease
Dysfunction
Health
High-level wellness
Holism
Homeostasis
Illness
Imagery
Meditation
Self-awareness
Therapeutic Touch
Wellness

Learning Objectives

Upon completion of this chapter, the student will be able to do the following:

- *Define wellness, holism, and holistic care.*
- *Compare and contrast the different methods of healthcare.*
- *Identify the connection between mind, body, and spirit and symptoms.*
- *Explain the role of the holistic nurse as a colleague with the client.*
- *Give examples of holistic healthcare modalities.*

15

Emma Rose lays in her bed, considering her situation. She is 25 years old, independent, and had unexpected surgery and a cast for a broken leg yesterday. She has never been in a hospital before. This morning she overheard the physician on rounds refer to her as "the broken leg in Room 304." Being in a hospital bed and overhearing this comment makes her feel like a piece of furniture one minute and a child the next. No one seems interested in how this relatively simple operation has affected her. She had always taken her health for granted. Now she feels sick and disabled. When you stop by as you begin your morning shift, you tell her you practice holistic nursing. Now Emma Rose wonders what is different about holistic nursing.

In previous chapters, you learned about professional nursing and the delivery of nursing care. This chapter expands your knowledge base with further information about health and wellness and holistic healthcare. As Emma Rose is led through her understanding of holistic care, you will learn how to provide holistic care to your clients. The Critical Thinking Challenges at the end of the chapter will help you apply your knowledge to Emma Rose's care.

During the last half of this century, healthcare professionals have been changing the way they think about health. The concept of holism is in the forefront of current thinking. As Emma Rose's nurse, you have indicated that you practice holistic nursing. This chapter will help you understand current healthcare practices related to health and wellness rather than the outdated theme of illness.

The chapter discusses definitions of health along with concepts related to health and wellness. A summary of the practice of holistic healthcare using Emma Rose and her nurse for illustration is followed with examples of a few holistic healthcare modalities.

Health and Wellness

The World Health Organization (WHO) defines **health** as "a state of complete physical, mental, and social well-being, not merely the absence of disease or infirmity" (WHO, 1947, p. 1–2). This is a dramatic departure from the traditional Western view, which considered a person healthy if he or she were merely symptom-free.

This definition of health is a useful starting point. It considers the total person (functioning physically, psychologically, and socially) as essential to the state of health and wellness. According to Allen (1986), the WHO's definition was designed to prevent health from being defined in a Western "disease" orientation. He suggested that when trying to define health, we should consider historic meanings and implications and understand whose interests were served; this enables us to recognize what is necessary for present and future social change.

Each person has a personal definition of health. Some people describe their state of health as "good," even though they may actually have one or more diagnosed illnesses. That is because each person defines health in relation to personal expectations and values.

The concept of health must allow for this individual variability. Health is a dynamic state in which the person is constantly adapting to changes in the internal and external environments. For example, a person may see himself or herself as healthy while experiencing a respiratory infection. Someone who has a temporary disability related to mobility may consider himself or herself "not healthy," but a person with a permanent disability may consider that a "normal" state and will define health differently.

The concept of wellness also allows for individual variability. **Wellness** can be thought of as a balance of the physical, psychological, social, and spiritual aspects of a person's life. This is a dynamic state. As with health, each person would also define wellness in relation to personal expectations. Wellness behaviors promote healthy functioning and help prevent illness. These include, for example, stress management, nutritional awareness, and physical fitness.

Various models of the concept of health exist. Some models are based narrowly on the presence or absence of definable illness. Others are based more conceptually on health beliefs, wellness, and holism.

Clinical Model

In the clinical model, health is interpreted narrowly as the absence of signs and symptoms of disease or injury; thus, the opposite of health is disease. Dunn (1961, p. 2) defines health in this model as "a relatively passive state of freedom from illness . . . a condition of relative homeostasis." Illness, therefore, is something that happens to a person. Many healthcare providers focus on the relief of signs and symptoms of disease and conclude that when these are no longer present, the person is healthy.

This model may not take into consideration the person's health beliefs or the lifestyle factors that may continue to place him or her at high risk for disease. Relieving obvious signs and symptoms may not address larger issues in the person's life that may affect his or her health. For example, the person who persists in smoking cigarettes and living a sedentary life will eventually develop signs and symptoms that relate to these lifestyle patterns.

Host–Agent–Environment Model

The host–agent–environment model, as illustrated in Figure 15-1, was developed to help identify the cause of an illness (Leavell, 1965). In this model, the following definitions apply:

Host: the person (or group) who may be at risk for or susceptible to an illness
Agent: any factor (internal or external) that can lead to illness by its presence or absence
Environment: factors (physical, social, economic, emotional, spiritual) that may create the likelihood or the predisposition for the person to develop disease

In this model, health and illness depend on the interaction of these three factors (Fig. 15-1). For example, a person (host) may be exposed to the virus for the common cold (agent), but whether or not a cold develops depends on a variety of conditions (environment). Poor nutrition, inadequate sleep, and unusual stress before the exposure predispose the host to develop a cold. Conversely, a person who is well nourished and physically fit and who is in control of the stresses of life is less likely to develop symptoms.

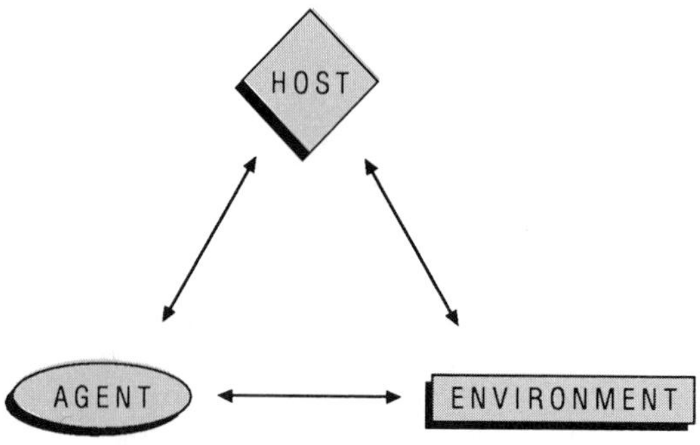

Figure 15-1 • Host–agent–environment model.

Health Belief Model

In the health belief model (Rosenstock, 1974), there is a relation between a person's beliefs and actions (Fig. 15-2). Factors that influence those beliefs include the following:

- Personal expectations in relation to health and illness
- Earlier experiences with illness and health
- Sociocultural context
- Age and developmental state

Someone who expects to have a cold at the same time every year may find that those expectations come true. Conversely, positive, health-oriented expectations might keep the person from developing an illness. Previous experience with an illness has a major influence on how the person reacts to subsequent challenges; previous pain experiences, for example, shape future experiences with pain.

Peer influence, personality characteristics, ethnicity, and socioeconomic factors may affect a person's response to illness. Someone who gets sick but whose experience is similar to that of his or her peers or socioeconomic group may not consider that he or she is in "poor health." Group values influence the health beliefs of each person.

Age and developmental stage are important considerations in the health belief model. For example, an elderly person may be more tolerant of a particular illness or disability than a younger person, because of perceived greater susceptibility to "poor health." Infants and very young children do not differentiate illness from health because they have not developed a conscious memory of one state compared with another.

The health belief model provides insight into the connection between the way a person sees his or her state of health and his or her response to health, illness, and treatment.

High-Level Wellness Model

Dunn (1961) introduced the term **high-level wellness** and recognizes health as an ongoing process toward the person's highest potential of functioning. This

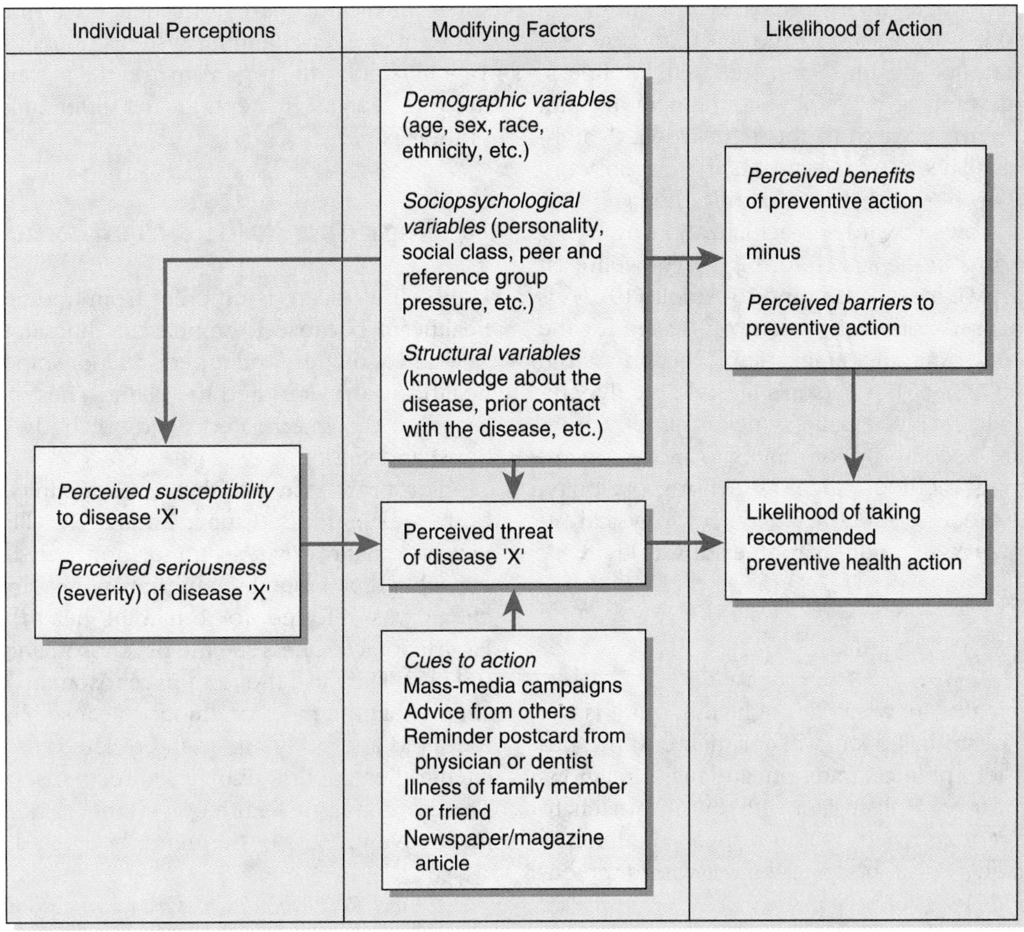

Figure 15-2 • *Health belief model.*

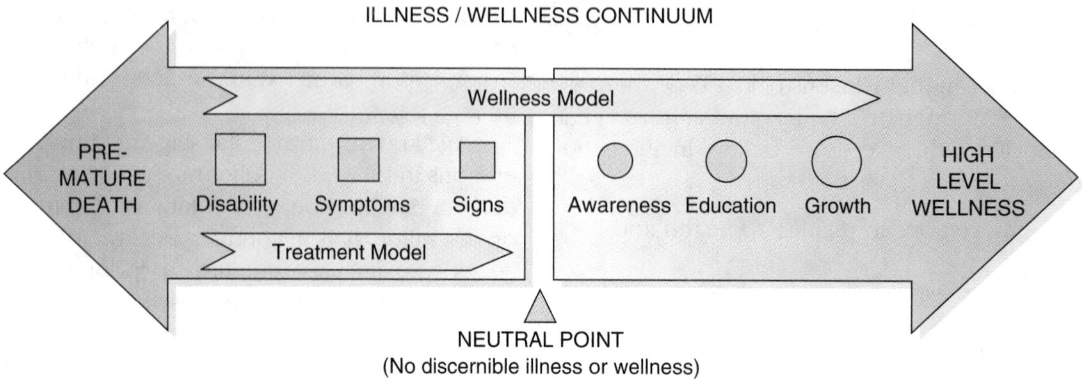

Figure 15-3 • *Illness/wellness continuum. (From Travis, J. W., & Ryan, R.S. (1988). Wellness workbook. Berkeley, CA: Ten-Speed Press.)*

process involves the person, the family, and the community. Dunn describes high-level wellness as "the experience of a person alive with the glow of good health, alive to the tips of their fingers with energy to burn, tingling with vitality—at times like this the world is a glorious place."

The wellness-illness continuum (Travis & Ryan, 1988) is a visual comparison of high-level wellness and traditional medicine's view of wellness (Fig. 15-3). At the neutral point, there are no signs or symptoms of disease. A person moving toward the left experiences a worsening state of health. Someone with wellness-oriented goals wants to move beyond the neutral point (mere absence of disease) to the right (toward high-level wellness). This person evaluates the current conduct of his or her life, learns about the available options, and grows toward self-actualization by trying out these options in the search for high-level wellness.

High-level wellness, according to Ardell (1977), is "a lifestyle-focused approach which you design for the purpose of pursuing the highest-level health within your capability" (p. 65). A person's lifestyle is a dynamic process that involves beliefs, needs, and values. Choices in life become opportunities to move toward wellness, using methods such as self-responsibility, nutritional awareness, stress management, physical fitness, spiritual growth, and environmental sensitivity.

Holistic Health Model

Holism is seen as a "new" model of health, but it is not new at all. Holism has been a major theme in the humanities, Western political tradition, and major religions throughout history. Holism is a different approach to healthcare that acknowledges and respects the interaction of a person's mind, body, and spirit within the environment (Fig. 15-4).

Holism, derived from the Greek *holos* ("whole"), was first used by South African philosopher Jan Christian Smuts (1926) in *Holism and Evolution*. Smuts saw holism as an antidote to the atomistic approach of contemporary science. An atomistic approach takes things apart, examining the person piece by piece in an attempt to understand the larger picture by examining the smallest molecule or atom. In Emma Rose's case, this atomistic approach concentrated on her broken leg and ignored the rest of her life.

Holism is based on the belief that people (or even their parts) cannot be fully understood if examined solely in pieces apart from their environment. People are seen as ever-changing systems of energy. As Figure 15-4 illustrates, the organism and the system in which it lives are seen as greater than and different from the sum of their parts.

Wellness and Holistic Healthcare

Holistic healthcare is different from traditional Western healthcare because it emphasizes humanism, choices, self-care activities, and a peer relationship between the healthcare provider and the client. These interventions focus on the interrelated needs of body, mind, emotions, and spirit.

For years, the healthcare community thought of body and mind as distinct entities. An illness labeled psychosomatic (*psyche,* mind, and *soma,* body) was considered a mental health problem, and often the client was referred to a mental health practitioner. Holistic practitioners see the psychosomatic process differently. They use the term psychosomatic to mean not simply that the mind or emotions cause illness, but that the mind and body are so interrelated that they act on each other in an intimate, direct, inseparable way. Therefore, holistic health practitioners acknowledge the interactive process of the mind, body, and spirit.

Emma Rose decides to talk to you about ideas related to holistic care. You give her some questionnaires to fill out to gather information about her lifestyle, including

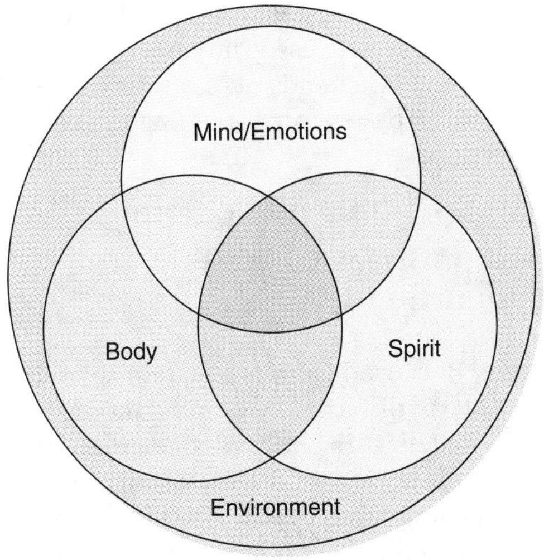

Figure 15-4 • *Schematic representation of holism. The system is greater than and different from the sum of the parts.*

questions on nutrition, exercise, stress reduction, spirituality, expression of feelings, even environmental awareness. Just answering the questions makes Emma Rose think about lifestyle choices and their role in her desire for wellness. For instance, the questionnaire about nutrition made her realize that she usually had a doughnut for breakfast but was hungry by midmorning. Her morning coffee really seemed to increase her jitters.

Holistic Practice

Holistic health practitioners do not want to abandon the established successes of traditional healthcare. Instead, they try to combine the best of both worlds: the proven success of Western modern medicine and a wide range of alternatives. This balance is illustrated by the Tai-chi T'u symbol (Fig. 15-5). This symbol shows the symmetry of *yin* and *yang,* or the feminine and masculine principles of Chinese thought. The diagram depicts the equality of power and mutual interdependence of two major forces. This is the intent of holistic care: to acknowledge and use the best elements of both systems of healthcare.

Holistic practitioners recognize the incredible strides that traditional medicine has made toward wellness (eg, antibiotics and surgery). They are especially mindful of the risk of *iatrogenic* illness, illness that results from treatment and may be traced to the overuse and abuse of prescription medications.

Consumers also are recognizing the need for "alternative therapies." In January 1993, the *New England Journal of Medicine* published a study (Eisenberg, et al.) citing that in 1990, Americans spent 13.7 billion dollars on "unconventional healthcare." One in three of the study's respondents reported using at least one unconventional therapy, including chiropractic, massage, lifestyle diets (eg, macrobiotics), acupuncture, naturopathic medicine, and homeopathy. Partly in recognition of the public's demand for healthcare choices and the need for funding of research and resulting publications on alternative modalities of healing, the National Institutes of Health in 1993 established an Office of Alternative Medicine.

The cost of the traditional Western model of healthcare is staggering. In 1930, Americans spent $2.8 billion on healthcare. In 1990, the country spent 235 times as much on medical care (Gordon, 1992). Holistic practitioners strive to reduce unnecessary, invasive care. For example, stress reduction or relaxation techniques for a hypertensive client can reduce or eliminate the need for medication and its accompanying risk of side effects.

Emma Rose has asked someone for pain medication and was told it was not time and she would have to wait another 30 minutes. When you stop by her room a few minutes later, she is in pain and anxious. You suggest that using imagery might help her relax and feel more comfortable. You lead her into imagery by suggesting she picture herself on a warm, soft stretch of sand, looking out over a calm, blue-green body of water under a clear blue sky. Before long, Emma Rose realizes she is no longer counting the minutes until her pain medication, and she feels calmer.

She realizes that working with a holistic health practitioner means she will be a partner, an active participant in her own care. Later in the day, she again uses the imagery by herself to feel calmer, and she likes feeling that she is in charge.

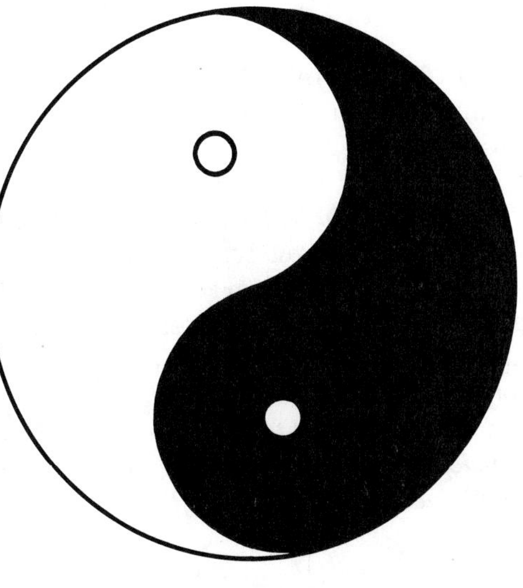

Figure 15-5 • *Tai-chi T'u (yin-yang) symbol.*

Self-Responsibility

The first dimension of a wellness lifestyle is *self-responsibility,* a personal sense of accountability for one's own well-being. As stated in Healthy People 2000, the many roles that each of us fulfills in our daily lives afford us numerous opportunities for promoting health and preventing disease. With these opportunities comes responsibility for our own personal health habits. To make informed choices, the client must first be aware of himself or herself. **Self-awareness** means knowing and caring for oneself, recognizing one's strengths and limitations. Holistic health practices add to self-knowledge. This knowledge of self on all levels (physical, psychological, social, and spiritual) enables the person to identify his or her status of being and decide the priorities of knowledge and service required. Self-knowing may be the first step toward self-caring.

Informed Choices

Making informed choices, being an active participant rather than a passive pawn, can benefit one's self-concept. This altered self-concept may facilitate a fundamental change in the person's belief system. The holistic health practitioner can use this decision to change by encouraging the person to examine his or her lifestyle and consider moving toward high-level wellness.

For example, people learning to use biofeedback to reduce tension headaches must first gather data on their own tension signals and triggers. To initiate relaxation techniques at an early stage, they become aware of the body symptoms or signals that warn of a tension build-up. By becoming aware of the situations that trigger a stress response, they can learn ways to change those situations or change their view of the situation to prevent the stress response before it occurs.

Self-Worth

Psychologist Yetta Bernhard (1975) proposes that self-respect and self-worth are developed in the process of caring for oneself.

After being taught by the holistic nurse what to watch for, Emma Rose begins to monitor her own leg and foot. When she examines her toes, she recognizes that the fact the toes are pink and warm and without swelling indicates her leg and foot have healthy circulation. She feels a sense of control that was not present when her other care provider simply pinched the toenail of her great toe, nodded her head, and left without saying anything.

Participating in self-care gives the client a greater feeling of independence and control. The altered concept of self as an active agent can help the person move toward high-level wellness. The concept of self as an active health agent extends across the wellness-illness continuum and applies to people at all developmental levels.

Meaning of Disease, Illness, and Dysfunction

Disease. Because health is a state of harmony, **disease** is a state of disharmony of mind, body, emotions, and spirit. Pelletier, in *Holistic Medicine* (1979), discusses the holistic view of disease as an opportunity to discover meaning. Traditional medicine often equates disease with failure, either of medicine or of the person. Even language, such as "chief complaint," conveys a negative message. When going to see the school nurse, a child is often asked, "What's wrong?"

According to the holistic view, the manifestation and course of a disease depend on how the client integrates the experience into his or her life. The school nurse can ask the child, "How are things going for you today?" Disease can be transformed into a positive experience of personal value and growth.

Illness. **Illness** is a product of the disharmonious interaction (disease) between mind, body, emotions, and

Nursing Research
Health and Wellness

Selected Nursing Research Studies

Allred, R.H., & Parrish, R.S. (1994). Preventive measures applied by RNs in occupational health settings: A descriptive study. *AAOHN Journal, 42*(1), 23–29.

Bechtel, G. A., & Franklin, R. (1993). Health risk appraisal differences between well elderly and university students. *Journal of Community Health Nursing, 10*(4), 241–247.

Stuifbergen, A. K., Becker, H.A. (1994). Predictors of health-promoting lifestyles in persons with disabilities. *Research in Nursing and Health, 17*(1), 3–13.

Possible Topics for Nursing Inquiry

- How does a person's value of health affect his or her health-promoting behaviors and resulting wellness?
- What are effective noninvasive holistic treatments to reduce unnecessary usage of medications and surgery in treating disease?
- How can nurses support the clients healthcare choices while evaluating the efficacy of these choices objectively?

spirit. Claude Bernard, a 17th-century French physiologist, developed the concept of **homeostasis,** the organism's attempt to restore balance. With self-regulatory mechanisms, our bodies respond to constant challenges from the external environment in an effort to maintain equilibrium or health. Illness is our body's way of signaling that we have exceeded our natural ability to mediate between our internal and external environment. Illness can be an opportunity to discover meaning in life and to heal ourselves. We can identify areas of disharmony or "disease" and determine how to best move toward a natural state of harmony.

Illness is a product of a complementary interaction between mind and body. Meek (1977) observes that if the client's mind is fed a daily diet of anger, remorse, revenge, hate, jealousy, suspicion, and envy, the cells of the client's body reflect this environment. Increased vulnerability to specific diseases seems to correlate with problems expressing certain emotions. For instance, people who deny anxiety seem more prone to cardiac disease. Psychologist Lawrence LeShan (1961) found that cancer clients had a higher-than-normal incidence of feelings of helplessness and hopelessness before their diagnosis. Cancer also seems to correlate with difficulty expressing feelings, such as anger and depression (Eysenck, 1988).

Feelings do not cause disease, but they do interfere with the immune system and may create an atmosphere in which disease can develop. One study of cancer clients and their families found a powerful relationship between negative images surrounding cancer and treatment outcomes (Simonton, Matthews-Simonton, & Creighton, 1978). The authors counseled clients and their support systems about psychological awareness and self-care to achieve the best treatment outcome.

Illness can be a signal that important needs are not being met. It can be an invitation from within to look at the balance between activity and rest or self- and other-oriented care. Do we really prefer to ignore this balance until we become ill (and are forced to curtail our activities)? Should we openly acknowledge or even anticipate these signals and provide ourselves with an opportunity to prevent illness and enjoy ourselves in the process?

Getting Well Again (Simonton, et al., 1978) suggests a simple exercise to identify the needs being met through illness and ways to find other avenues:

> List the five most important benefits you received from an illness in your life. Consider the needs that were met by your illness: relief from stress, love and attention, opportunity to renew energy, and so forth. Identify the rules or beliefs that limit you from meeting each of these needs when you are well.

> *Emma Rose uses this exercise to analyze her situation. Up to this point she has focused only on the negative aspects of her accident. She realizes this event allowed her to take a break from a project at work she didn't enjoy. She decides to ask her supervisor to assign her to a project she would enjoy more. Also the cards and telephone calls from her friends show her that they care for her and miss her. She decides to reorganize her calendar so she can have more contact with caring friends.*

Dysfunction. **Dysfunction** is an action (abnormal, inadequate, or impaired) that does not meet expected norms. The action "generates therapeutic concern on the part of the client, family, or friends, and the nurse" (Gordon, 1991).

> *Emma Rose wonders if she will regain her muscle strength and physical activity. She voices her concerns to you. You tell her she will have altered mobility and reduced strength while she is on crutches and for awhile after she returns to her usual activities. In the meantime, you teach her how to strengthen her quadriceps muscles and wiggle her toes to stimulate the lower leg muscles. You tell Emma Rose to take short walks and then rest and that it is normal to feel tired after exertion. You advise her not to push herself beyond endurance but to move within the limitations of discomfort. "Normal function will return in a few weeks," you say.*

Therapeutic interventions for dysfunctional problems are directed at contributing factors. Interventions for potential dysfunction are directed at prevention by reducing risk factors (Gordon, 1991). "An outgrowth of the disease orientation is a disability orientation; an outgrowth of the health orientation is an ability orientation" (Hopkins & Smith, 1993, p. 435). Therefore, the person with altered function is not necessarily disabled but should be able to adapt strengths toward being abled. This transformation is evident in the lives of famous role models, such as Helen Keller and President Franklin D. Roosevelt.

Effect of Stress

Holistic practitioners recognize that life stresses affect how and when an illness will be manifested. Any change, even a positive one, results in a certain amount of stress. Psychosocial stress, such as the death of a spouse or being diagnosed with a progressively deteriorating illness, can lead to depression, anger, and despair, all of which harm the immune system. A cluster of events that requires life adjustment is associated with illness onset. Underlying cardiovascular disease and cancer, the two leading causes of disability and death, is a prolonged state of sympathetic nervous system activity mediated through the hormonal pathways. This is the body's response to prolonged stress reactivity.

Holistic practitioners recognize the impact of stress on health and teach skills to notice and decrease it when possible. See Chapter 51 for more information on stress.

Nursing in Wellness and Holistic Healthcare

Holistic professionals are committed to participating and cooperating with clients. The holistic nurse acts as a "caring colleague" of the client (Blattner, 1981). Holistic nurses help their clients toward high-level wellness while acknowledging that each has the right to choose his or her own path. Holistic nurses also recognize a duty to provide the healthiest environment for themselves and generations to come. An indication of the shared purpose and mutual support among nurses active in holistic healthcare is the formation in 1980 of the American Holistic Nurses Association.

According to Martha Rogers (1990), the primary purpose of nursing is to help people achieve their maximum health potential. The first line of defense is promotion of health and prevention of illness. By promoting high-level wellness and preventing illness whenever possible, the holistic nurse uses an approach that minimizes risk and empowers the client.

Promoting Health and Preventing Illness

"The goal of holistic nursing is to use preventive, nurturative, and generative activities to assist clients towards achieving their own high-level wellness" (Blattner, 1981, p. 23). A major goal is to prevent unnecessary disruptions in the clients' lives.

Preventive Activities

The prevention aspect of holistic nursing has three levels:

Primary prevention, preventing disease before it occurs, might involve enforcing environmental controls (eg, prohibiting excessive noise in the workplace to prevent hearing loss).

Secondary prevention involves screening or education to promote early diagnosis and treatment (eg, a program identifying hypertensive clients to teach stress-reduction techniques).

Tertiary prevention applies to rehabilitation situations, where the goal is to minimize residual dysfunction. A good example is a program for a myocardial infarction client that includes lifestyle changes, such as dietary and exercise habits, and attitude changes or modified responses to stress.

Prevention is discussed further in Chapter 30.

Nurturative Activities

The nurturative activities of the holistic nurse involve caring, supporting, and sustaining clients. These activities may range from giving antibiotics to giving a massage.

Emma Rose tells you she feels uprooted by being surrounded by unfamiliar objects and wearing a gown. You suggest she ask a friend to bring her own pajamas from home and a few things, such as cassette tapes, that would make the environment more comfortable. "If you can't be home, you can bring some of your home here," you tell her.

Generative Activities

Generative activities encourage self-care. Examples are teaching relaxation techniques to children with cancer to help them cope during traumatic procedures or researching alternate healing methods to provide an objective database for future decision-making.

Nursing as a Therapeutic Partnership

The holistic practitioner sees the nurse-client relationship as a therapeutic partnership rather than a dependent relationship. Some nurses believe the word *patient* connotes a passive, helpless person rather than a person seeking wellness, which at times includes the support of a healthcare provider; as an alternative, many nurses use the term *client.* The nurse is no longer the "pill fairy" in a culture that has become accustomed to a quick fix. Instead, the nurse is an agent for change, helping clients to take responsibility and to take charge of their lives and health.

True helping can occur only when the client wants and needs it. Some helpers become rescuers by entering into what Steiner (1971) calls the victim, rescuer, and persecutor triangle (Fig. 15-6). In the triangle, the client can be seen as a victim, acting as if he or she wants help. The healthcare provider, as a rescuer, decides to help, but the rescuer neglects to determine if the help being offered is needed or wanted. The rescuer usually ends up as a victim of the same person he or she was trying to rescue, because the help is ineffective and the efforts wasted. The rescuer may feel persecuted by the client and experience resentment ("after all I've done for you!").

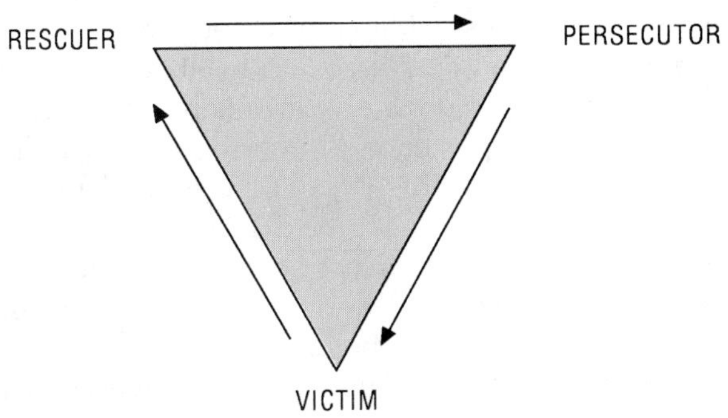

Figure 15-6 • *Victim–rescuer–persecutor triangle.*

People in these roles go around and around the triangle. Rescuing leads to burnout on the part of the healthcare provider, because the energy expended does not result in the desired outcome. Table 15-1 lists characteristics of helpers and rescuers (Travis & Ryan, 1988).

A healthcare provider cannot change or help others unless they want to be changed or helped. Clients cannot be made well unless they want to be well more than they want to be ill (Meek, 1977). Once healed, they will not stay well unless they want to stay well. Clients may be unaware that they want to be well or ill. In these cases, practitioners may help clients clarify and explore their desires in terms of wellness. Is the payoff for becoming well greater than the gains of remaining ill?

Nursing Diagnoses for Wellness

Nursing diagnoses are used to provide organization and clarity when communicating with the healthcare team. Nursing diagnoses for wellness serve several purposes. They encourage the nurse and client to examine positive, life-affirming behaviors that contribute to healthy functioning. When written as part of the client's healthcare record, the diagnoses can be used to reinforce continued health promotion. "Assessment of strengths and health-promoting behaviors, shared and supported in collaboration with the recipient of nursing care, encourages the continued use of positive strategies in similar circumstances" (Houldin, Saltstein, & Ganley, 1987, p. 20). There are four wellness diagnoses on the North American Nursing Diagnostic Association accepted list. These are Effective Breastfeeding; Health Seeking Behaviors; Family Coping, Potential for Growth; and Anticipatory Grieving.

Nurses in all settings can use these and other wellness diagnoses to focus on promoting health. Each person should be seen as a whole person with the physical, psychological, and spiritual potential for optimal functioning across the lifespan.

Examples of Holistic Healthcare Modalities

Lifestyle Modification

Holistic practitioners advocate the use of lifestyle modification skills, such as meditation, exercise, or relaxation, that alleviate stress and promote a state less susceptible to disease. These skills increase energy flow rather than reduce awareness of tension.

Norman Cousins (1976), in his courageous fight against a serious connective tissue disorder, called the placebo effect "the doctor who resides within." He recognized the importance of how he thought about his illness, how much control he perceived himself as having in his life, and how much he was enjoying his life.

Cousins took the bold step of accepting responsibility for his disorder. He decided to check out of the hospital where his condition was termed hopeless and made his relationship with his physician into a partnership. He started a self-care regimen that included

Table 15-1 • *Differences Between Helpers and Rescuers*

Helper	***Rescuer***
Listens for request	Gives when not asked
Presents offer	Neglects to discover if offer is welcome
Gives only what is needed	Gives more help and for longer time than needed
Checks periodically with client	Omit feedback
Checks results that client Functions better Meets goals Solves problems independently Uses suggestions successfully	Does not check results and feels good when accepted, bad when turned down by client

From Travis, J., & Ryan R.S. (1988). *Wellness workbook.* Berkeley, CA: Ten-Speed Press.

watching comedies by the Three Stooges and the Marx Brothers because he had noticed that laughter eased his symptoms. Rather than focusing on the negative connotations of his disease, he became an active agent to change his outlook in a more positive direction. After months of recuperation, he resumed his work, and his mobility improved.

Meditation

Meditation, deep personal thought and reflection, may be one of the most basic and powerful self-care activities that we can incorporate into our lives. It stills the chattering mind and sharpens our understanding of internal and external worlds. Meditation is a way to tune and train the mind that leads to greater efficiency in everyday life. It helps to decrease anxiety and helps us handle stress with less negative impact. Meditators withstand more life changes with less illness.

Although meditation seems like simple tool, it can have powerful results. It is not a strange and complicated technique requiring great effort and skill: it is merely a way of switching our concentration from the external world to the internal world. Many types of meditation are clearly described in Joel Levey's *The Fine Arts of Relaxation, Concentration and Meditation* (1994).

Imagery

Imagery is the "internal experience of a perceptual event in the absence of the actual external stimuli" (Achterberg & Lawlis, 1980, p. 27). In the Simontons' (1978) work with cancer clients, they teach their clients to use daily relaxation and mental imagery to enhance their immune system response. The clients are taught to picture cancer cells being destroyed by the current treatment and by their body's white blood cells. The imagery process includes seeing themselves as whole, well, and full of energy. Using these methods, the Simontons report encouraging results; surviving clients in one study lived on the average twice as long as clients who received medical treatment alone, and even clients who died lived 1.5 times longer than the control group.

Therapeutic Touch

Therapeutic Touch, a technique derived from the ancient "laying on of hands," incorporates many aspects of holism and holistic healthcare. Dora Kunz and Dolores Krieger developed this approach, which has been taught to nurses worldwide. According to their philosophy, the client's state of health is reflected in the vital energy field that surrounds him or her. The Therapeutic Touch practitioner learns to attune to this energy field by first centering, or achieving a sense of peace and wholeness within himself or herself. Krieger described **Therapeutic Touch** as a healing meditation, be-cause the centered state is maintained throughout the process. The practitioner assesses and treats the client's energy field with the goal of restoring harmony. If the flow of energy is perceived as obstructed, disordered, or depleted, the practitioner attempts to direct energy to the client to release congestion and balance the areas where flow may be disordered.

Therapeutic Touch relaxes the client, who experiences slower, deeper breathing; decreased muscle tension; and warmer hands and feet. This method has been reported to alleviate discomfort and to speed healing (MacCrae, 1988; Wirth, 1990). Therapeutic Touch is a noninvasive process that may decrease clients' need for medication and may enable them to tap into their natural healing potential. It is said to be a healing experience for practitioner and client.

Therapeutic Touch is only one healing method in the expanding field of holistic nursing. It represents a powerful shift in medicine that has influenced healthcare practitioners and clients alike.

Key Concepts

- Health, as defined by WHO, is a state of complete physical, mental, and social well-being.
- Wellness is a dynamic state that allows for different personal beliefs about health.
- In the clinical model, health is seen as the absence of indications of illness.
- The host–agent–environment model of health seeks a source or cause of illness.
- The health belief model is characterized by the relationship between a person's beliefs and actions.
- In the high-level wellness model, health is an ongoing process toward the person's highest potential.
- The holistic health model recognizes the unique interaction of a person's mind, body, and spirit within the environment.
- Holistic healthcare combines the proven success of modern medicine, participation of the client, and additional activities to complement medical protocol.
- The nursing diagnoses related to health and wellness are important for initiating and reinforcing health promotion.
- Holistic healthcare interventions include lifestyle modification, exercise, meditation, imagery, and Therapeutic Touch.

Critical Thinking Challenges

Now that you have studied this chapter, you should be able to apply what you have learned about health, wellness, and holistic nursing to the care of Emma Rose.

1. *Examine Emma Rose's dual feelings of being merely a piece of furniture and being a child, explaining why this made her feel disabled and sick.*
2. *Analyze how Emma Rose and you participated in relieving Emma Rose's pain.*
3. *Infer how the connection of mind, body, and spirit accentuated Emma Rose's symptoms and how your nursing care addressed Emma Rose's concerns.*

References

Achterberg, J. A., & Lawlis, G. F. (1980). *Bridges of the bodymind.* Champaign, IL: Institute for Personality and Ability Testing.

Allen, D. G. (1986). Using philosophical and historical methodologies to understand the concept of health. In P. Chinn (Ed.), *Nursing research methodology* (pp. 157–168). Rockville, MD: Aspen.

Ardell, D. B. (1977). *High-level wellness.* Emmaus, PA: Rodale.

Bernhard, Y. (1975). *Self-care.* Millbrae, CA: Celestial Arts.

Blattner, B. (1981). *Holistic nursing.* Englewood Cliffs, NJ: Prentice-Hall.

Cousins, N. (1976). Anatomy of an illness. *New England Journal of Medicine, 12,* 4–51.

Dunn, H. L. (1961). *High-level wellness.* Arlington, VA: R. W. Beatty.

Eisenberg, D. M., Kessler, R. C., Foster, C. F., Norlock, F. E., Calkins, D. R., & Delbanco, T. L. (1993). Unconventional medicine in the United States. *New England Journal of Medicine, 4,* 246–252.

Eysenck, H. J. (1988). Personality, stress and cancer prediction and prophylaxis. *British Journal of Medical Psychology, 61,* 57–75.

Gordon, J. S. (1992). How America's health care fell ill. *American Heritage, May/June,* 49–65.

Gordon, M. G. (1991). *Nursing diagnosis: Process and application* (3rd ed.). St. Louis: Mosby Yearbook.

Hopkins, H. L., & Smith, H. D. (1993). *Willard and Spackman's occupational therapy* (8th ed.). Philadelphia: J. B. Lippincott.

Houldin, A., Saltstein, S., & Ganley, K. (1987). *Nursing diagnosis for wellness.* Philadelphia: J.B. Lippincott.

Leavell, H. R., et al. (1965). *Preventive medicine for the doctor in his community* (3rd ed.). New York: McGraw-Hill.

LeShan, L. (1961). A basic psychological orientation apparently associated with malignant disease. *Psychiatric Quarterly, 35,* 314.

Levey, J. (1994). *The fine arts of relaxation, concentration and meditation: Ancient skills for modern minds.* London: Wisdom Publications.

MacCrae, J. (1988). *Therapeutic Touch: A practical guide.* New York: Alfred A. Knopf.

Meek, G. W. (1977). *Healers and the healing process.* Wheaton, IL: Theosophical Publishing House.

Pelletier, K. (1979). *Holistic medicine.* New York: Delacorte.

Rosenstock, I. (1974). Historical origin of the health belief model. *Health Education Monographs, 2,* 334.

Rogers, M. (1990). *An introduction to the theoretical basis of nursing.* Philadelphia: F. A. Davis.

Simonton, O. C., Matthews-Simonton, S., & Creighton, J. L. (1978). *Getting well again.* New York: Bantam.

Smuts, J. C. (1926). *Holism and evolution.* New York: Macmillan.

Steiner, C. (1971). *Transactional analysis made simple.* San Francisco: Transactional Publications.

Travis, J. W., & Ryan, R. S. (1988). *Wellness workbook.* Berkeley, CA: Ten-Speed Press.

U.S. Department of Health and Human Services, Public Health Service (1992). *Healthy People 2000 Summary Report.* Boston: Jones and Bartlett Publishers.

Wirth, D. P. (1992). The effect of non-contact Therapeutic Touch on the healing rate of full thickness dermal wounds. *Cooperative Connection, Vol III,* (3), International Society for the Study of Subtle Energies and Energy Medicine.

World Health Organization (1947). Constitution of the World Health Organization. *Chronicles of WHO, 1,* 1–2.

Bibliography

Dossey, B. M., Keegan, L., Guzzetta, C. E., & Kilkmeier, L. G., (1993). *Holistic Nursing: A Handbook for Practice* (2nd ed.). Rockville, MD: Aspen.

Dunham-Taylor, J., Oldaker, J., DeCapua, T., Manley, N. K., Oprian, B., & Wrestler, J. (1993) Nurses cut health care costs. *Journal of Holistic Nursing, 11*(4), 398–411.

Gillanders, W. R., Buss, T. F., Gemmel, G., Pomidor, W. (1992). Worried wellness: How meaningful is the concept in managing elderly patients? *Family Practice Research Journal, 12*(1), 27–42.

Jensen, L., Allen, M. (1993). Wellness: the dialectic of illness. *Image The Journal of Nursing Scholarship, 25*(3), 220–224.

Loreno, P., & Drick, C. (1990). Self-care identity formation: A nursing education perspective. *Holistic Nurs Practice, 4*(2), 79–86.

Petit, J. M. (1994) Continuing care retirement communities and the role of the wellness nurse. *Geriatric Nursing, 15*(1), 28–31.

Redland, A. R., & Stuifbergen, A. K. (1993). Strategies for maintenance of health-promoting behaviors. *Nursing Clinics of North America, 28*(2), 427–442.

Rudman, W. J., & Hagiwara, A. F. (1992). Sexual exploitation in advertising health and wellness products. *Women and Health, 18*(4), 77–89.

Volden, C., et al. (1990). The relationship of age, gender, and exercise practices to measures of health, life-style, and self-esteem. *Applied Nursing Research, 3*(1), 20–26.

Lifespan Development

Key Terms	Learning Objectives
Development Developmental tasks Embryo Environment Fetus Genetics Growth Maturation Moral reasoning Neonatal period Perception Puberty	Upon completion of this chapter, the student will be able to do the following: • Relate genetics and environment to human development. • State and discuss the principles of development. • Identify theorists and their theories of development. • Describe the influence of development on health. • Describe the influence of health status on development. • Identify the major health needs of specific developmental age groups.

16

You are doing a well-child assessment on a 13-month-old boy. You ask the mother if there is anything that concerns her. She seems reluctant to answer, but finally says that she is concerned that her son is not yet "potty trained." When you question her further about why she is concerned, she tells you that her mother-in-law said that her son (this 13-month-old's father) was completely potty trained by 12 months, and that either there is something wrong with the child or the mother is not working hard enough to accomplish potty training.

Through your study of previous chapters you have developed a foundation in nursing concepts and practice. In this chapter, you will study about human development across the life continuum and functional health at various stages of development. This will increase your knowledge base so that you can work with individual clients and their families in situations such as the one in the well-child clinic. At the end of the chapter there are Critical Thinking Challenges to help you develop your thinking skills further.

Development is the process of ongoing change, reorganization, and integration occurring throughout life. This process includes changes in body structure and physiologic function as well as changes in psychosocial behaviors, emotional responses, and cognition. As a result of development, a person's competence and capabilities change both quantitatively and qualitatively so he or she can participate more fully in life.

Traditionally, development was seen as a characteristic of infancy and childhood, with little attention given to development beyond adolescence, yet there is mounting evidence that predictable patterns of change occur throughout life. Researchers (Gilligan, 1982; Lynch & Lynch, 1991; Peterson, 1994; Sasser-Coen, 1993) have delineated phases of adult development. Lifespan development is a central and critical issue in attempting to understand human behavior as it relates to health. Beliefs about how individuals grow and mature across the lifespan influence perceptions of the client, nurse–client relationships, and definition of the nurses' roles. When the word "development" is used in this chapter, "lifespan" is always an assumed qualifier.

Genetics and Environment

Two primary factors drive development—genetics and environment. **Genetics** involves the potential for human function determined by the inheritance of 46 single chromosomes carrying genetic information from each birth parent. The code contained in the chromosomes provides complete information governing the growth, differentiation, and function of all body cells. Our knowledge of the inheritance of physical characteristics, such as eye color, is substantial; less well understood is behavioral genetics, or the extent to which behavior is also inherited. Because of the enormous numbers of possible combinations of inherited characteristics, each person possesses a unique genetic make up, contributing to the wide variety of observed individual differences.

Environment defines the context in which the person exists, including both animate and inanimate surroundings (Bronfenbrenner, 1979). The animate environment comprises specific people (parents, siblings, spouses, partners, extended family, friends, classmates, workmates, and colleagues) and, more broadly, social and cultural groups. The inanimate environment includes all aspects of the physical surroundings. Sensory components of the physical environment include sound and light as well as motion. The inanimate environment at a broader level includes housing, transportation, resources, economics, and other ecologic factors. Although genetic make up is stable over generations, surroundings change. Two important factors influencing individual development are history and cohort; that is, environment is decidedly different based on the year of birth and the experiences of the cohort, or generational counterparts, of people born at that time. In 1961, school children across the United States gathered in classrooms and gymnasiums to watch television coverage of Alan Shepherd, the first American astronaut to fly in space—quite a different experience from children in 1927 who learned from the newspaper or radio of Charles Lindbergh's flight to Europe.

Although the environment can be arbitrarily divided into components, the environment is experienced as a whole. **Perception**, a highly individual process, is the neurosensory process that allows the environment to be experienced by each person. Even when environments may appear to be similar, individual perceptions are different. Thus, two siblings who share the same family, home, school, and community have differing perceptions of their environments.

Development is the expression of both genetic inheritance and environmental influences. The question of whether genetics or environment has greater impact on developmental outcomes cannot be easily answered because the individual and environment are, in reality, one indivisible system. Currently, four frameworks are offered to explain the relative contributions of nature (genes) and nurture (environment) (Cole & Cole, 1993). Gesell is a proponent of the *biological maturation* framework, which proposes that the developmental process is governed primarily by internal biologic heritage. Environment plays a secondary role in modifying innate drives. Researchers such as Watson put forth the *environmental learning* theory. This approach states that biologic factors are the foundations of development, but the major causes of change are environmental, in particular changes that occur as a result of learning through social interactions. Piaget's theory is an example of the *universal constructivist* framework, which explains that environment and biology have equal importance as sources of development. Exogeneous and endogenous elements act reciprocally and in concert over time to create the individual person. The *cultural context* framework emphasizes the importance of the environment but focuses on the history of the social group within which the child lives as the major external force. The impact of the social group may, in fact, change the structure of the child.

Although people are different, changes in body structure and function, psychosocial behaviors, and cognition show similar characteristics when described in similar age groups. Development occurs as a pattern, that is, certain predictable processes follow a time course (eg, puberty occurs in early adolescence). Patterns provide a way of describing the commonalities of development while preserving the consideration of individual differences. By understanding patterns of development with change, reorganization, and integration, we can better understand individual behavior at a point in the lifespan.

Change. Development starts with conception and continues through death. Development, although ongoing, is not consistent across time, nor is it a simple linear process. The school-age child's ability to determine that a set volume of liquid is the same, regardless of the shape of the container, does not demonstrate a gradual change. Neither does development peak at 18 years of age and plateau until old age. Development includes periods of both relative stability and change. Infancy and adolescence are short in duration but are known for rapid changes in a multitude of functions, including physical maturation and coordination, and cognitive and social skills.

Although all aspects of human function change with development, not all changes occur on the same time schedule. Body development and social development are not entirely synchronized. The social behaviors of the adolescent may indicate an increasing interest in sexuality, although there may be little change in endocrine activity or physical evidence of puberty. A 3-month-old infant may focus intently on a toy and attempt to reach the toy using a batting motion of the arms. The desire to handle the toy is spurred by cognitive development; however, the infant's motor development has not progressed to the level of obtaining the toy.

Reorganization and Integration. Development is not only a process of continuous, gradual, additive changes in function and abilities, such as an increase in vocabulary, but a process of abrupt, dramatic changes in entire patterns of behavior, such as the ability to use tools to solve problems. That is, developmental changes seem to occur in spirals, with periods of relative quiescence, periods of disorganization and seeming regression, and periods of organization in which new abilities are demonstrated. These newly acquired skills allow the person to view and interact with the environment in entirely different ways. Despite the discontinuities in development, continuities remain whereby experiences during childhood seem to lay the foundations for adulthood.

The question of critical periods in development is another issue related to continuity. Critical periods are times in which specific environmental or biologic events must occur for development to occur normally. Animal studies indicate that such periods exist; however, studies of human development are not so clear. The development of genitalia and language in children does suggest that there are critical periods in the development of the human child (Newport, 1991).

Concepts of Development

Principles of Growth and Development

Knowledge about growth and development is drawn from biologic and psychosocial sciences and involves certain principles that generally affect all people. These principles, as listed in the accompanying display, express commonalities of the process of growth and development.

> **Principles of Growth and Development**
>
> Principle 1: The process of growth and development is continuous and systematic, following a purposeful sequence.
> Principle 2: The process of growth and development is ongoing and complex.
> Principle 3: The process of growth and development is distinctive and predetermined and occurs at a discrete rate for each person.
> Principle 4: The process of growth and development has both quantitative and qualitative aspects.
> Principle 5: The process of growth and development requires experience and practice as well as energy.
> Principle 6: The process of growth and development occurs through adaptation to the conflict of equilibrium versus disequilibrium.
> Principle 7: The process of growth and development produces individuality from interaction of genetic heredity and environment.
> Principle 8: The outcome of growth and development is the attainment of personal potential.

Growth and Development Theory

Theories of development describe why development occurs as it does and what factors shape developmental outcomes. Developmental theories can be categorized under six broad headings, depending on the perspective the theorist takes. Most theories propose that people progress through universal stages of maturation and that each stage must be mastered before entering subsequent ones. However, not all researchers agree.

Psychodynamic theories are based on the perspective that humans are essentially emotional, responding to instinctive drives without rationality. By studying childhood events, psychodynamic theorists attempt to explain human behavior throughout the lifespan. Freud and Erikson are two well known psychodynamic theorists, although Freud's perspectives are currently controversial.

Piaget has conducted considerable research on *cognitive development theory*, which deals with perception and thinking, focusing on intellectual processes at each stage of development. Intellectual growth involves changes in the mental operations of the person at var-

Table 16-1 • Overview of Selected Developmental Theories

Theorist	Stages/Tasks	Characteristics
Sigmund Freud	Oral—birth to 1 year	Seeking pleasure through oral gratification
	Anal—2 to 3 years	Delayed gratification through controlling anal sphincter
	Phallic—4 to 5 years	Curiosity regarding genitals and gender differences
	Latent—6 to 12 years	Transition; peer relationships and identification with parent of same sex
	Genital—13 to death	Sexual interest and maturation
Erik Erikson	Trust vs. mistrust—Birth to 1 year	Development of trust (or mistrust) in parents
	Autonomy vs. shame—2 to 4 years	Gaining independence through parents' encouragement
	Initiative vs. guilt—4 to 6 years	Developing confidence in abilities
	Industry vs. inferiority—8 to 12 years	Pleasure from accomplishments
	Identity vs. role confusion—13 to 20 years	Achieving stable sense of identity
	Intimacy vs. isolation—20 to 30 years	Developing close personal relationships
	Generativity vs. stagnation—30 to 60 years	Creativity, productivity in work
	Integrity vs. despair— > 60 years	Attainment of purpose, fulfillment
Jean Piaget	Sensorimotor—Birth to 2 years, 6 substages	Development of senses, motor activity
	Preoperational—2 to 7 years. 2 substages	Beginning intellectual ability
	Concrete operations—7 to 11 years	Reasoning, organizing, relationships
	Formal operations—11 to death	Abstract thinking, deductive reasoning
Robert Havighurst	Infancy, early childhood	Learning neuromuscular control
	Middle childhood	Developing physical, intellectual, emotional skills
	Adolescence	Achieving gender roles, independence
	Early adulthood	Marriage, family, career
	Middle age	Assisting grown children, parents; social, civic responsibility
	Later maturity	Retirement, declining physical ability, loss of relationships
Abraham Maslow	Physiologic Safety Love and belongingness Esteem Self-actualization	Hierarchic human needs: lower-order needs must be fulfilled to achieve higher-order needs
Lawrence Kohlberg	Premoral (preconventional) Obedience, punishment Hedonistic	Development of moral reasoning: governed by egocentricity
	Conventional morality Approval seeking Respect for authority	Concrete thinking: follows orders and requests for approval
	Postconventional morality Democratic contractual morality Principles of conscience morality	Autonomous decision-making regarding moral issues

ious ages. Children at various ages respond to cognitive tasks in comparable ways, according to this theory.

Other theories include the *developmental task theory* (Havighurst), *human needs theory* (Maslow), and *moral development theory* (Kohlberg). Selected developmental theories are summarized in Table 16-1.

Psychodynamic Theories

Freud. The work of Freud characterizes psychosexual development across the lifespan, encompassing the oral, anal, phallic, latency, and genital phases. In Freud's view, the mind consisted of the *id* (concerned with self-gratification), the *ego* (the mediator between the id and reality), and the *superego* (the conscience). Freud theorized that all people pass through the five phases, confronting and resolving conflicts of the id–ego–superego in the process. If the person does not resolve these conflicts, movement through succeeding stages may not be successful.

Erikson. Although based on Freud's theory, Erikson's theory of development encompassed social and cultural influences as well. He was the first theorist to recognize that development is a lifelong process. The eight stages of his theory progress from birth to death, and are presented as developmental crises (eg, trust versus mistrust) that must be mastered before proceeding to the next stage.

Cognitive Development Theory

Piaget. Piaget's theory of cognitive development is based on the assumption that human nature is essentially rational and that the person's basic goal is to learn to master the environment. The resulting satisfaction received from learning prompts the person's curiosity, problem-solving, imitation, practice, and play activities (Piaget, 1952). Two functions that assist the person in learning and intellectual growth are organization and adaptation. *Organization* involves the rearranging and structuring of one's knowledge and thoughts. *Adaptation* relates to the process of assimilating and accommodating new information. To integrate new learning with old and adapt it to expanding environments, the infant uses the complementary processes of assimilation and accommodation. *Assimilation* is the ongoing process of organizing new information into existing knowledge. *Accommodation* is the process of resolving the disequilibrium resulting from the modifications needed in thought processes to incorporate new data. The four cognitive development stages identified by Piaget are the sensorimotor, preoperational, concrete operations, and formal operations.

Developmental Task Theory

Havighurst. Havighurst's theory of development is based on learning and learned behaviors, called **developmental tasks**, that emanate from biologic, psychological, and social origins during the lifespan. Specific developmental tasks are assigned to the various stages of life. Failure to complete the tasks assigned to each stage may lead to failure in tasks in subsequent stages. According to this theory, success in achieving the developmental tasks leads to success with tasks in later stages of life (Havighurst, 1972).

Human Needs Theory

Maslow. Abraham Maslow is one of the better known humanistic theorists. Humanistic theories (also called phenomenologic theories) propose that people are basically good when born and attempt to become all they are capable of becoming throughout their lives. People vary in their experiences, and have free will and the ability to grow and become what they self-determine.

Maslow organized human needs into a hierarchic framework (discussed in Chapter 2), with a base of physiologic needs and an apex of self-actualization (see Table 16-1). To reach the apex of the hierarchy, a person must have met each of the preceding levels of needs, beginning with physiologic needs and moving up toward self-actualization. Maslow's theory is often used as a guide for holistic health, focusing on promoting high levels of wellness, preventing illness, and encouraging individual responsibility for health (Murray & Zentner, 1993).

Moral Development Theory

Kohlberg. Lawrence Kohlberg (1976, 1984) extended Piaget's work on moral reasoning to develop a theory of moral development. **Moral reasoning** can be defined as judgments individuals make about what is right and wrong behavior within a social context. How do principles such as justice, concern for the welfare of others, or altruism affect behavior? As children's cognitive abilities mature and social experiences increase, appropriate behaviors in relation to others within a given culture and society begin to emerge. Through a series of short vignettes describing concrete moral dilemmas, Kohlberg assessed children's beliefs about what action should be taken and why. Three major levels of moral development corresponding to Piaget's three later stages of cognitive development were identified. Each level has two stages.

The first level of moral development is called preconventional and corresponds with preoperational thinking. In this level, young children make moral judgments based on external rules established by powerful adults and on the consequences of their actions. Stage 1 begins at the end of the preschool period. Responses to moral dilemmas are very egocentric and focus on the outcomes of actions. When the child is about 7 to 8 years of age, the second stage emerges because, although still egocentric, the child can recognize that others may have a different perspective. Major growth in self-reliance occurs during this period. Children no longer rely solely on adults for the regulation of their behaviors. Instead, with increasing exposure to other social groups, children are able to negotiate with one another to decide on a course of action.

Children's moral reasoning during the second level takes into consideration the thoughts and feelings of other people and standards for social conduct. This period corresponds with the period of cognitive development called concrete operations. In Stage 3, children primarily use the "Golden Rule" to judge moral behavior. Stage 4 marks a shift in moral reasoning because children are now guided by rules and laws of society. This stage appears during early adolescence, and is often referred to as the "law-and-order" stage (Cole & Cole, 1993)

Moral reasoning during the third level is characterized by the ability to think about abstract principles of right and wrong. When adolescents and young adults reach the cognitive stage of formal operations, they are able to recognize that social laws may be in conflict with broader moral principles and to look for ways to improve the current social order. Stage 5 is not attained before early adulthood. Adults in Stage 6—a stage rarely encountered—use universal ethical principles to make moral judgments. These ethical principles apply to all of humanity and are upheld without regard to the cost to the individual.

A number of criticisms have been raised in relation to the validity of Kohlberg's theory (Kurtines & Gewirtz, 1991). First, not all studies support the premise that the stages of moral development correspond with Piaget's stages of cognitive development. In addition, some researchers refute the assumption that people progress through each stage in a linear fashion and question whether all individuals progress through each stage. Second, controversy exists as to sex differences in moral reasoning (Gilligan, 1982). Third, the issue of cultural differences and cultural bias in Kohlberg's theory has been raised. Opponents of Kolhberg's theory argue that because his theory depends on Piaget's stages of cognitive development, one can reason that higher levels of moral reasoning imply "superior morality."

Growth and Development Through the Lifespan

Normal growth and development are orderly, predictable processes in the human experience (Table 16-2), yet each person progresses and develops at an individual pace. For example, in the child, there is a time range during which developmental phases are expected to occur (eg, walking, talking). If a child progresses through a stage outside of the usual time range, there may be no significant effect on overall development, or it may affect the ability to move on to or complete subsequent phases of development.

Intrauterine Development

Growth and development are initiated at the moment of conception. During the 9 months of the intrauterine stage, development moves from the single cell of the fertilized ovum to a complete human being at the time of birth. Cognitive and psychosocial development begins during intrauterine development, setting the stage for further development after birth.

Physical Development

The period of intrauterine gestation is divided into three phases or trimesters. The first trimester begins with the fertilization of the ovum by the sperm that unites the two sets of chromosomes, creating the genetic program of the new organism. From this program, genetically produced characteristics, such as eye and hair color, are passed on to the child. The third trimester ends with all organs formed, with their physiologic functioning able to support life outside the womb, and the settling of the fetus into the birth canal.

First Trimester. The first trimester, the developmental period, produces all the organ systems, and the **embryo** (the stage of development between the 2nd and 8th weeks) continues to develop rapidly. By the 8th week, the embryo possesses a face, legs, arms, brain, heartbeat, and a productive digestive system and liver (red blood cell production). The critical development of organ systems during this trimester renders the embryo susceptible to developmental or environmental influences that may cause malformations. When the first bone cells appear in the upper arms, the embryo becomes a **fetus** (child in utero from 3rd month of gestation to birth). The fetus is approximately 3 inches long and weighs 1 oz.

Second Trimester. Fetal movement is felt by the mother during the second trimester. This is a major milestone for the mother. However, fetal activity is believed to be essential for the proper development of the central nervous system (Hamburger, 1975). During this growth period lanugo (downy hair) develops on the fetus' arms, legs, and back. Head hair, eyelashes, eyebrows, fingernails, and toenails appear. Skeletal ossification continues. The skin is red and wrinkled. The fetus is nonviable at this point and cannot survive out of the uterine environment. Toward the 20th week, fetal growth slows and the lower limbs are fully formed. The fetus is 11 to 14 inches long and weighs 1 lb, 4 oz.

Third Trimester. During the last trimester, fetal features are refined. The hair on the head grows, fingernails grow, and lanugo almost disappears. Teeth buds for permanent teeth appear behind milk teeth buds. The fetus responds to bright lights and internal and external sounds. As the fetus increases in growth, his or her activity may diminish because space becomes less available. Arms and legs increase in flexion during the third trimester; early in the third trimester, the fetus is extended. The head remains large in comparison to the body. The lungs mature. The fetus receives short-term immunity from the mother as some antibodies pass through the placenta. Chances for survival improve with the advent of the delivery date.

Cognitive Development

Fetal activity represents a form of mother–baby communication that fosters bonding. During the last trimester, the fetus responds to internal and external sounds by changes in heart rate or movement. Researchers believe that stimulation in utero may influence later development. For example, at birth, neonates

Table 16-2 • *Physical and Psychosocial Development Through the Lifespan*

Stage	Physical	Psychosocial
Neonate (birth to 1 month)	Reflexive physical functioning Major organ systems are stabilizing Heart rate decreases from 130–160 to 120–140 Systole and diastole shorten in length Respiratory movements are primarily abdominal (30–50/min) Fontanelle is palpable between unfused skull bones. Behavior—crying, sucking, sleeping, and activity Sporadic, symmetric movements in all four extremities Smiles reflexively Responds to sensory stimuli (particularly caregiver's voice, face and touch) Reflex—blinks in response to light, and startles to loud sudden noise, Babinski's, Landau, Moro, palmar grasp, placing, rooting, neck righting	Parents and infants develop deep attachment normally. Interactions during routine care enhance or detract from attachment process. Infant's waking hours include feedings and short play periods. Attachment may be altered if either parent or child experiences health problems after birth.
Infant (1 month to 1 year)	Doubles birthweight by 6 months and triples it at 12 months Grows 10 to 12 in Walks on hands and feet like a bear Walks—one hand held Reaches for objects Sucks/mouths objects Progresses from holding head up to sitting alone, crawling, pulling to stand, cruising Throws objects to floor Patterns of body function stabilize—predictable sleep, elimination, and feeding routines Fine motor prehension (cortically controlled individual movements of fingers and thumbs); also uses both hands simultaneously	Differentiates self from others (external world) Smiles responsively Deals with environment through emergence of trust Sensory and cognitive abilities improve; recognizes differences in people Establishes close attachment with caregiver Plays simple social games (peek-a-boo) More meaningful interaction with environment
Toddler (1–3 years)	Rate of increase in height and weight slows (smaller food intake) Heart rate slows to 110 beats, respiration to 24 beats/min Cardiopulmonary system stabilizes—110/60 blood pressure Walks upright with broad gait Gross motor skills advance—walks up and down stairs, kicks a ball, jumps and stands on one foot, rides a tricycle, runs Fine motor—scribbles spontaneously; draws circles, crosses, stick people; stacks a tower of small blocks	Child develops autonomy. Explores immediate environment Needs emotional support and encouragement from parents Parent is most significant person in toddler's life Parallel-plays with others Learns to control possessions and self Extremely active and unable to set limits on own behavior. Parents must set limits

(continued)

Table 16-2 *(Continued)*

Stage	Physical	Psychosocial
	Handedness appears around 19 months Toilet training—develops sphincter control Able to undress	Parents must create safe environment for exploratory behavior (automobile safety, poisoning).
Preschool (3–6 years)	Heart (90 beats/min) and respiratory rates (24 beats/min) continue to stabilize	Relies heavily on parents/primary caregivers for security
	Weight increases 5 lb/year. Average (by age 5) is 45 lb.	Ventures out to seek contact with children and adults
	Height increases 2 in/year. Average (by age 5) is 42 in.	Asks questions
	Large and fine muscle coordination improves.	Is less afraid of strangers
	Runs well, climbs stairs with ease, hops, skips, jumps, throws and catches a ball Fine motor—copies circles, squares, and triangles; begins printing letters and numbers	
School age (6–11 years)	Height increases 1–2 in/year	Develops a sense of achievement
	Variable weight increases (averages 3–6 lb/year)	Psychosocial development is influenced by physical and cognitive skill development.
	Cardiovascular functioning refines: heart rate = 65–90 beats/min, blood pressure = 110/70 mm Hg, and respiratory rate = 16–18 beats/min.	Is independent in activities of daily living
	Until age 9, boys are 1–2 in taller and 2 lb heavier than girls.	Possesses need to maintain control
	Girls begin rapid growth period (9–12 years). At age 12, girls are 2 lb heavier and 1 in taller than boys.	Develops strong preferences (food, clothes)
	Prepubertal physical changes and growth spurts can occur between the ages of 9 and 14 for girls, 12 and 16 for boys. Steady skeletal growth in trunk and extremities	Engages in group-oriented play
	Minimal secondary sex characteristics are present	Prefers same-sex peers
	Strength doubles	Regards rules as necessary
	Most permanent teeth have erupted	Considers motivation and behavior when making judgments
	Refined neuromuscular functioning—good body balance, rides bicycle, engages in team sports, climbs trees; eye–hand coordination improves (punts, writes in script, paints, detailed drawing, plays computer games)	
Adolescence (11–21 years)	Sexual maturation with development of primary and secondary characteristics	Establishes independence from family; close peer relationships
	Increased growth rate of skeleton, muscle, and viscera	Makes major decisions about life and vocation Refines adult cognitive skills Establishes moral code Establishes own identity Adjusts to own sexuality Establishes unique identity (personal and group) Develops moral judgment
Young and middle adulthood (21–65 years)	Physical structure stabilizes and few changes are noted (except for pregnancy).	Emotional health is related to one's ability to resolve personal and social tasks (family, job stresses).
	Young adults—quite active, experience less severe illnesses and tend to ignore physical symptoms when ill	23 to 28 years—refines self-perception and intimacy

(continued)

Table 16-2 *(Continued)*

Stage	Physical	Psychosocial
	Health concerns and risk factors center around lifestyle, family history, and community.	29 to 34 years—energy is put toward achievement in world
	Middle adults—the aging process varies for all individuals; decreases appear in hormone levels, basal metabolic rate, respiratory, cardiovascular and circulatory functioning.	35 to 43 years—examines life goals and relationships Decides between singlehood and marriage Decides on family, parenthood Develops sense of generativity Makes lasting contributions through involvement with others
Late adult (65–77 years)	All systems are affected by the aging process: reproductive, urinary, neurologic, musculoskeletal, respiratory, head and neck, breasts, skin, and nails. Effects vary with the person's lifestyle, genetic predisposition, and freedom from disease.	Puts life in order Recognizes sense of integrity and wisdom Learns to accept life accomplishments, retirement, death

are noted, among other things, to respond differentially to the voice of the mother. Furthermore, researchers (De Casper & Fifer, 1980) found that infants changed their rate of sucking on hearing the story their mothers read while the infants were in utero. Extreme maternal stress and neonatal stressors are thought to affect development adversely (Thompson, 1990). Research tends to show that periods of diminished oxygen and severe, long-term prenatal malnutrition adversely affect later developmental functioning (Worthington-Roberts & Klerman, 1990).

Psychosocial Development

It has not yet been determined if events occurring during intrauterine life affect the psychosocial development of the fetus. The current research methodologies rule out objective study of psychological interactions between fetus and mother. However, it appears that prebirth events do help to mold cognitive, language, and affective development (Schuster & Ashburn, 1992). Because the mother's emotional state influences the fetus' biochemical environment, any stressor may play a significant, although indirect, role in the psychosocial development in utero.

Neonate (Birth to 1 Month)

Physical Development

During the **neonatal period** (from birth to 4 weeks), the neonate depends on others to have all physiologic and emotional needs met. Neonates must learn new ways of taking in food and oxygen and eliminating waste products, while at the same learning to adjust to their families' lifestyle. Although all organs are developed, not all are fully mature. This process occurs throughout the neonatal period and on through adolescence. At birth, the average newborn weighs 3,200 g (7 lb, 1 oz), is 49 cm (19.3 in) in length, and has a head circumference of 34 cm (13.5 in). Arm, leg, and hand movements of the newborn are reflexive. The newborn's movements continue to remain an important means of communicating with others. Although neonates cannot support their head while lying on their abdomen, they are able to lift their head briefly. When pulled to a sitting position, neonates may hold their head in line with the back. The neonate is capable of rolling part way to side from back. One-month-old newborns usually keep their hands fisted or slightly open. If fingers are pried, the neonate is able to grasp the handle of a spoon or rattle briefly. Neonates stare at objects, coordinating their eyes; however, they do not reach for objects.

Cognitive Development

Piaget's first period of cognitive development, the sensorimotor stage, begins with the coordination of such activities as grasping objects and basic reflexes. Although historically neonates were thought to exhibit reflexive behavior only, current knowledge reveals that, even at birth, neonates are capable of a wide range of behaviors, particularly the ability to provide cues to parents and caregivers regarding interactional needs.

Psychosocial Development

The neonate responds positively to comfort and satisfaction and negatively to pain. The neonate smiles back at a face. The primary caregiver is often able to comfort the newborn when making direct eye contact or talking to him or her. Attachment or bonding develops at this time (Karen, 1994).

Infant (1 Month to 1 Year)

Physical Development

The infant progresses physically in a sequential pattern. Weight and height increase at rates faster than during any other period. By 5 months of age, infants double their birth weight and triple it by the end of the first year of life. At 1 year of age, length has increased by 50% over the birth length. Voluntary motor skills begin to replace reflexive behavior (Schuster & Ashburn, 1992). Visual acuity reaches 20/100, facilitating eye–hand coordination. The infant begins by holding his or her head up for brief periods of time and advances to supported sitting, independent sitting, creeping, standing with support, and walking while holding on to objects (Fig. 16-1). The infant gains increasing efficiency in energy expenditure while increasing the speed and accuracy of movement. A pincer grasp (picking up objects) replaces the whole-hand carry. Separation of tongue movement from the jaw indicates maturing oral motor development. With refinement of gross, fine, and oral motor skills coupled with the eruption of deciduous teeth, the infant is able to "munch" on foods and begin self-feeding.

Cognitive Development

Infants engage in systematic imitative behavior. They attach meanings to words and, after a period of babbling, utter a few words. Infants are able to solve simple problems by using previously mastered activities or actions. When an infant discovers a pleasurable activity, he or she repeats this behavior. Through manipulation of objects and motor activities, the infant differentiates self and environment. Infants are fascinated with their own extremities. The infant achieves personal satisfaction from the ability to direct or control objects. Play remains an important component in self-concept development. Sensory impressions and motor activities provide the groundwork for infants' knowledge of the world. They are capable of coordinating one action with another. The "power of association" (Turner & Helms, 1987) assists the infant in understanding a cause–effect relationship. The concept of object permanence develops.

Psychosocial Development

The infant's primary gratification is in sucking and having needs met by the caregiver. Social responsiveness is evident later on as he or she smiles in response to a familiar face. Laughing indicates pleasure as the infant shows preferential treatment or response to caregiver. The infant shows fear of strangers or separation from his or her parent. Many theorists consider attachment to be a lifelong process; nonetheless, the ability to trust and to form attachments during this period of development is critical to the ability to form meaningful relationships as adults (Karen, 1994). The infant begins to explore the environment while separating briefly from parents. He or she is capable of making simple needs known by gestures. The infant enjoys simple games, toys, water and sand play, books, and nursery rhymes.

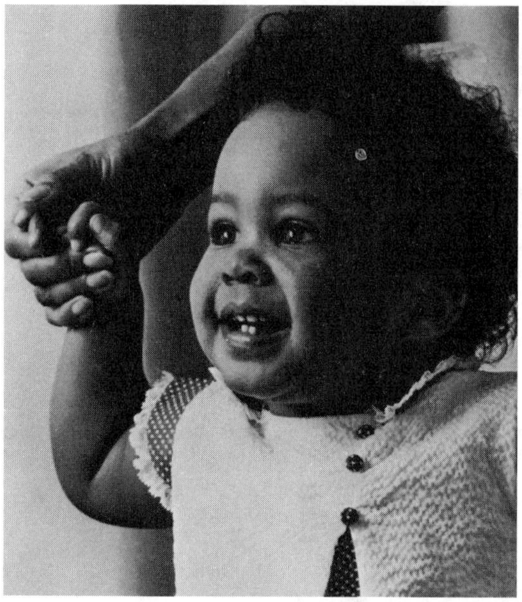

Figure 16-1 • *The 1-year-old takes her first shaky steps with assistance. Note the normal tooth development for the 1-year-old child. (Courtesy of Gerber Products Company.)*

Toddler (1 to 3 Years)

Physical Development

The toddler possesses a large head relative to a long trunk, and short, stubby legs. Weak abdominal muscles account for a "pot-bellied" look. At birth, head size is slightly greater than chest size. They are equal in size until about 2 years of age, after which growth in chest size slowly exceeds head size. During the second year, the growth of legs and arms increases. In comparison to the first 12 months of life, the toddler's growth in height and weight is less accelerated. The toddler gains 5 lb per year until the age of 9 or 10 years, and grows 3 to 5 inches. At the end of this period, all deciduous teeth have erupted and the mature rotary pattern of chewing allows the toddler to meet nutritional needs by the intake of solid foods. The development of the central nervous, musculoskeletal, cardiopulmonary, gastrointestinal, and urinary systems is almost complete. Gross motor skills rapidly develop. Toddlers learn to use upper muscles of the arms and legs before finger or toe muscles. They kick a ball, jump, walk stairs, ride a tricycle, and run. Fine motor abilities progress from stacking a tower of blocks to drawing stick people. The toddler's visual system reaches a more adult level. From 18 to 24 months, visual acuity is 20/40; and by 2 to 3 years, it is 20/30. Accommodation is well developed.

Cognitive Development

Toddlers have definite ideas about how their world should operate, often expressing individual preferences. At the age of 18 months, the toddler responds negatively to requests. "No" is a favorite reply. Self-identity and competency are reflected in common phrases such as "mine" and "I do it." The egocentric characteristic of this age contributes to sense of self. The young child sees the world from his or her perspective and attempts to impose order on the environment. Thus, everything has its place, and rituals develop. Piaget's sensorimotor period extends from birth to approximately 2 years. Concepts mastered include object permanence, causality, spatial relationships, and the use of instruments (Mussen, 1990). Between the ages of 2 and 6 years, young children advance to the preoperational stage, in which children assign meaning or identity to an object governed by their own perceptions. Internal and external reality are one. At approximately 18 months of age, the toddler's use of words seems to increase dramatically. By the time they are 3 years old, they understand well over 2,000 words, and are able to make short sentences and follow simple commands.

Psychosocial Development

The world of the toddler expands to include peers or playmates and other adults. In becoming increasingly autonomous, toddlers see themselves as separate, although emotionally attached to parents. Separation anxiety is at its peak. Toddlers become aware of the approval or disapproval of others. Fear, an emotional response to threat against the self, is expressed (DuPont, 1994). At 2 years, the toddler seems impulsive, inflexible, domineering, defiant, and demanding, and is always on the go. A major transition occurs in imitation and play behavior. Toddlers are able to imitate behaviors not currently present and to engage in symbolic play. Interest in peers is often exhibited in parallel play (side by side). Toddlers begin to acquire basic social skills and, by the end of this period, respond with more socially responsible behavior and cooperation.

Preschooler (3 to 6 Years)

Physical Development

Physical changes occur at a slow, even, continuous pace. The 5-year-old child's head circumference is 50 cm (90% of adult size), whereas leg circumference is 22.5 cm (only 45% of adult size). By 5 years of age, the child weighs 39 lb and is 40 inches tall. Arms and legs grow faster; trunk growth follows later. By 5 years of age, the pot-bellied appearance of the toddler has changed to that of a miniature adult. By the end of this period, permanent teeth may appear. Neuromuscular skills refine. He dresses himself, washes his face and hands, brushes his teeth, and takes care of his own toilet needs. Preschoolers are able to copy figures and draw pictures. By 6 years of age, preschoolers should have a visual acuity of 20/20.

Cognitive Development

In Piaget's preoperational stage, the preschooler can use mental symbols; thinking can include past or future events or events happening elsewhere in the present. Preconceptual thinking (based on concrete perceptions) progresses to intuitive (internally representing events) thinking. Magical thinking occurs in which preschoolers believe their thinking influences the outside world. Questions from the preschooler begin with "why," progressing to "where" and "how." Preschoolers ask meanings of words, talk constantly, count, identify coins, know the day of the week, follow three-step directions in order, and memorize their address. During early childhood, the development of receptive language is critical to the development of later expressive abilities. Between 3 and 5 years, children practice adult speech, and dysfluency or stuttering may result. Sentences are grammatically correct and increasingly complex. Preschoolers may attempt to read simple print.

Psychosocial Development

Play is critical for early development (Johnsen, 1991). The play style of preschoolers is termed associative. Children play together, demonstrating preferences for friends, and sharing materials or objects. There is little organization or goal-oriented behavior. The securely attached preschool child easily tolerates limited separation from parents while enjoying the company of other children. This is a period of rapid fluctuations between dependence and independence, competence and ineptitude, maturity and infantilism, and growing affection and antisocial destructiveness. As the preschool children strive for individuality, they question and explore their own abilities (Turner & Helms, 1987). They learn to express emotions acceptably along with developing a conscience for moral growth and internalizing control of their actions.

School-Age Child (6 to 11 Years)

Physical Development

The school-age child is taller and thinner than the preschooler. Steady growth occurs; height increases 2 to 3 inches per year, and weight increases 6.5 lb per

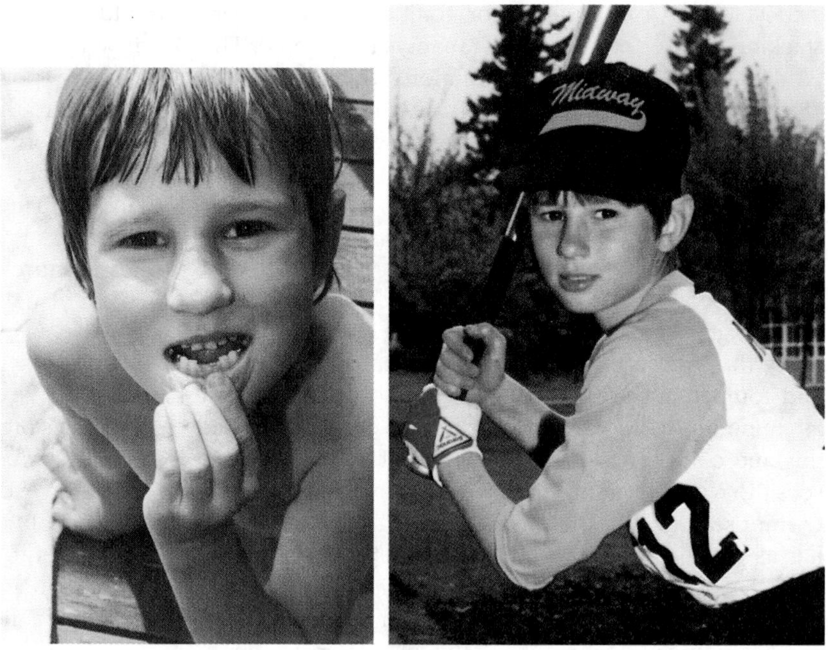

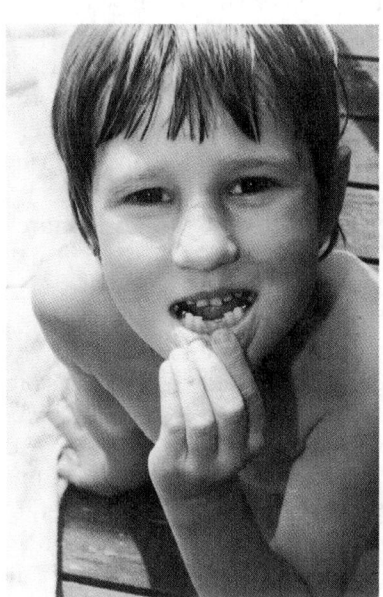

Figure 16-2 • Normal development in a school-age child. Loss of baby teeth occurs in the early school years. The child becomes interested in sports as motor skills develop.

year. Baby fat decreases, followed by a reaccumulation of fat from about 7 to 10 years. The child's body is forming new bony tissue constantly as bones lengthen and harden and muscle mass increases. Proportions continue to be more adult-like. Lordosis of early childhood has disappeared. Facial proportions change (forehead broadens, nose grows larger, lips get fuller, jaw juts out). Head size continues to increase at a slower rate of about one-half inch per 5 years until puberty. During this period, a child loses and gains about four teeth per year (Fig. 16-2). Lymphoid tissues grow rapidly until adult size is reached shortly before adolescence. Advanced motor activities indicate completion of central nervous system myelination. School-age children engage in large muscle activities—walking, running, skating, swimming, riding skateboards and horses, and team sports (see Fig. 16-2). Small muscle activities include sewing, printing and script writing, painting, clay modeling, and model building. Visual function has reached maximum function, and hearing ability is almost complete but does not reach full maturity until adolescence.

Cognitive Development

During middle childhood, tremendous growth in the ability to use words occurs. Vocabulary increases, and the school-age child uses rules of grammar and syntax. The cognitive operation of concrete thinking is mastered. These children use more logic in their thinking (Piaget, 1952); they are able to classify and order objects and to conserve their physical properties despite the shape these objects may take. However, logic is limited to the here and now. Comprehension of cause–effect relationships increases, and the concept of time is better understood. Becoming less egocentric, the school-age child begins to appreciate another's perspective. The school-age child demonstrates a public and private self.

Psychosocial Development

The family and the school are major socializers affecting the school-age child's developing personality and self-image. They enjoy brief separation from family (overnight). Play is cooperative; they play in groups with fixed rules and goals. Friendships are an important part of social contacts, usually with children of the same sex. Rivalry for friends is often evident. Friends are chosen largely by similarity. Although relationships are quickly formed and dissolved, they may be intense. The school-age child observes and imitates the attitudes, values, and behaviors of those significant people in his or her environment. In this age of industry (Erikson, 1963), the child is determined to master tasks, becoming a competent member of his or her culture.

Adolescent (11 to 21 Years)

Physical Development

The early years of adolescence are ones of rapid growth. This period begins with **puberty**, a maturation of the sex organs and reproductive functions along with the appearance of secondary sex characteristics. Girls begin adolescence at approximately 10 to 11 years of age, whereas boys enter at 11 to 12 years (Murray & Zentner, 1993). The end of adolescence varies. Skeletal growth, dependent on the secretion of growth hormones regulated by the pituitary and thyroid glands, occurs through a combination of lengthening of the bones and changes in the ossification centers. Girls (11–13 years of age) achieve a growth spurt 2 years earlier than boys and plateau in height by 17 years of age. Although girls are initially taller than boys, boys grow rapidly between the ages of 14 to 21 years. They then surpass girls in height. Weight gain follows a similar pattern for both sexes. Chronologic age does not always coincide with these changes. One may see a 4-year spread in sexual development among adolescents. These variations become a developmental crisis for some young people. Concern over body normality, sports competition, and social and peer relationships can create major hurdles. Late adolescence (18–22 or 25 years) is often categorized as a period of transition to adulthood.

Cognitive Development

Formal thinking begins to emerge around 12 years of age (Piaget, 1952). This level is characterized by the ability to think abstractly; ideas can be expressed conceptually. The thinking of this age group reflects formal logic. Formal thinking allows a situation to be seen from multiple perspectives. It is not entirely related to chronologic age, and its acquisition may vary with the person. Adolescents engage in introspection, self-examination, and personal critique.

Psychosocial Development

The psychosocial development of the adolescent is characterized by a search for identity and self-discovery. A changing body challenges the sense of identity as physical maturation and sexuality are integrated into the self-image. This process occurs within the context of peers. Piaget refers to this stage as adolescent egocentrism, in which adolescents do not distinguish between their own conceptualizations and those of the rest of society (Freiberg, 1987). Instability and emotional upheaval characterize early adolescence (11–13 years). Increasing independence from parents and family is coupled with increasing time spent with members of peer group, creating changes that may cause tension between the adolescent and family. Drug abuse, alcoholism, and cigarette smoking present challenges to the adolescent as he or she develops a personal value system. Peer contacts and being a part of a group are important. Roles and relationships take on abstract meaning. Initial experience with dating and early intimate relationships occur in adolescence. First forays into the working world are often attempted. The adolescent develop a more mature morality based on his or her own judgment. Late adolescents (17–20 years) develop a smoother relationship with their parents. Physical growth slows, allowing the person to adapt to a new body image. Older adolescents refine interpersonal skills and gain mastery over drives and emotions as they prepare to enter the world of adults.

Young Adult (21 to 40 years)

Physical Development

The young adult's physical structure stabilizes. Maturational development is complete at this time, with most systems operating at peak efficiency. However, weight and muscle mass may change as the result of the environmental influences of diet and exercise. Dental maturity is evident in the mid-20s. Sexuality is fully mature, and function is at a peak.

Cognitive Development

Having reached Piaget's last stage of cognitive development, abstract thinking comes readily. In some groups, the need to achieve intellectually is strong. The young adult is creative, has effective problem-solving abilities, is realistic, and is less egocentric. Formal educational opportunities along with apprenticeship-type education are common.

Psychosocial Development

Young adulthood (18–22 or 25 years) is a period of transition from adolescence to adulthood. The tasks of adulthood emerge: work, intimacy, and parenting. An adult assumes a multitude of roles: citizen, taxpayer, homeowner. Social support is important because role conflict often arises. One must juggle the many roles of parent, grandparent, husband, wife, brother, sister, daughter, friend, and worker while prioritizing to achieve success and happiness.

Middle Adult (40 to 60 years)

Physical Development

The middle adult years are a time of transition between the active, building years of young adulthood and the later years of older adulthood. Physiologically, adults in their middle years begin to slow down. Body tissue tends to redistribute, with increased thickening around the middle portion of the trunk. The earliest signs of aging begin to show. Hair starts to gray, wrinkles begin to show, men may begin to lose hair, and visual acuity for near vision begins to diminish (presbyopia). Decreased function in other body systems is evidenced as beginning loss of muscle strength and agility, decreased cardiac output, decreasing hormone production, and increased fatigue.

The physical changes of the middle years occur gradually and insidiously and do not interfere with the person's vitality or function in life. In the absence of disease or disabilities, the ability to function physically is unaffected. A lifestyle emphasizing adequate diet, regular exercise, control of stress, and limiting or eliminating unhealthful habits (eg, no smoking, moderate alcohol intake) contributes to successful life in the middle years.

Cognitive Development

Adults in their middle years continue to be interested in learning and show no decrease in ability to learn. Education is particularly motivated if the knowledge is relevant and personally applicable. Although the ability to perform may remain unchanged, a reduction in speed of problem-solving or motor skills may interfere with some aspects of functioning (eg, eye–hand coordination is not as keen as before, leading to a slower reaction time).

Psychosocial Development

During the middle years, changes in roles occur. Children may be grown and have left home, although in recent years many parents have delayed having children until they are well into their fourth or fifth decade. If married, the marriage may be stressed or strengthened by these changes. At this time of life, people may be faced with providing support for children who may not be totally independent and at the same time have elderly parents who may require care. Women in particular may feel the burden of both responsibilities. Illness or death of parents often brings grief and lifestyle disruption.

The middle-aged person often views himself or herself more favorably, with more time for social and leisure activities. A greater commitment to enjoying relationships may exist. Interpersonal impoverishment or stagnation may develop if the mature adult does not develop generativity (Erikson, 1963). One accomplishes this by possessing a genuine concern for oneself, one's children, community, peers, and society. Inability to accept the physical changes and psychosocial challenges of this time may foster depression and low self-esteem.

Older Adult (60 Years and Older)

Physical Development

Growth and maturation occur during late life, with the physical changes accompanying old age appearing at different times and manifesting themselves in different ways. All physiologic systems decline in overall function and efficiency. Chronologic age alone is not a predictor of physical decline, however. Genetic influence, lifestyle factors, and self-concept combine in determining aging.

Stamina and strength may decrease. Basal metabolic rate decreases, and the gastrointestinal system has decreased digestive juices, less tone, and slower peristalsis. The older person often finds it difficult to adapt to changing temperatures because there is a decrease in subcutaneous fat, diminished circulation to the skin, and a decrease in core body temperature. Age-related changes in the function of the heart, circulatory, and respiratory systems contribute to diminished output of the left ventricle, less anaerobic support to muscles, less efficient ventilatory ability, and increased time for recuperation and healing.

Neurologic changes in aging include increased time required for impulses to travel over multisynaptic pathways, less efficient sleep, and decline in sense of balance. Special senses that began to decline in middle age continue to show decreased function. Vision and hearing changes (presbyopia and presbycusis) become more prominent in the older adult. Urinary function diminishes with age because the plasma flow to the kidneys may decrease by as much as 50% from 30 to 80 years of age, leading to a comparable decrease in glomerular filtration rate. Decreased urinary bladder tone can contribute to incomplete emptying of the bladder, urinary frequency, and bladder infections in the older adult. Degenerative changes in connective tissue and cartilage, along with demineralization of the bone, can lead to age-related problems with posture, mobility, and injury as a result of accidents (eg, falls).

Although the older adult experiences many physical changes with aging, these changes occur gradually and to varying extents. As a result, the older person has been adapting and accommodating to these changes over a period of years and, in the absence of illness or specific debilities, can function adequately in the later years of life.

Cognitive Development

Although the stereotype of the aging person is one of memory loss and reduced cognitive skills, the actual cognitive changes seen in the latter part of the lifespan do not fit the description (Nemeroff & Colarusso, 1990; Schulz, 1993). With aging, there is a reduction in visual and auditory acuity, potentially affecting function. Changes in cognition are more often a difference in speed rather than ability (ie, learning a new task takes longer and performance time is longer). An older adult is more concerned about accuracy and less concerned about speed of performance than younger adults. Along with age comes increasing experiential knowledge.

Intellectual loss in later life may reflect interrelated physiologic decrements caused by disease (eg, atherosclerosis causes blood vessels to narrow). Perfusion to the brain is diminished. Malignancies may metastasize to the brain and other body parts. Cardiovascular disease, emphysema, high blood pressure, poor nutrition, or effects of surgery may temporarily reduce blood supply to the brain, limiting or altering performance. Cognitive dysfunctions that may result from dementia, delirium, chronic brain disorders, or Alzheimer's disease are not synonymous with old age. Most older adults do not experience cognitive impairments. Physical fitness and intellectual stimulation help maintain intellectual functioning in old age.

Psychosocial Development

Older adults must make the transition from working to retirement. Retirement entails the loss of the work role and relationships at work and substantial changes in one's lifestyle. Some people welcome retirement, with the increased opportunities it brings for activities such as church, community, and leisure projects. Other people find that retirement makes them feel useless and as though they are waiting to die. Losses are common for elderly people, who experience the death of spouses, friends, and possibly children. Women outlive men by an average of 7 years. Social contacts and role performance may be limited by physical changes associated with aging. Preretirement planning and a prior devotion to hobbies make the transition easier (Fig. 16-3).

If an older adult successfully accomplishes "ego" integrity (Erikson, 1963), he or she still participates in life and does not fear death. Family support, friends, and coworkers influence the retiree. Although marriage and divorce occur in later life, marital satisfaction before retirement greatly affects marital satisfaction in retirement. Although many older people maintain their own houses or apartments, a minority live in retirement homes for the aged or nursing homes.

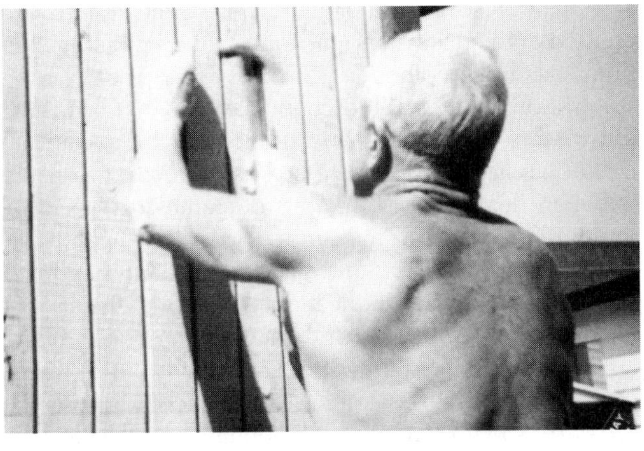

Figure 16-3 • *Developing hobbies and leisure activities promotes successful retirement. (Photo courtesy of the University of Washington School of Nursing.)*

Functional Health and Anticipatory Guidance Across the Lifespan

Knowledge of lifespan development and an understanding of how humans operate physiologically as well as behaviorally are basic components of nursing. A key to appreciating human function is knowledge of how development produces qualitative and quantitative differences in function across the lifespan and how these differences relate to health. The focus of discussion in this section is how functional health varies with age, the way in which health needs are modified by age, and the way in which the nurse uses anticipatory guidance, an educational intervention, to assist with promoting health, maximizing function, and minimizing health problems.

Health Perception and Health Management

Fetus, Newborn, and Infant. The earliest effects of health behaviors are seen during the period of fetal development. The intrauterine environment and its effects on the growing fetus produce a lifelong impact on health and shape how individuals function throughout the remainder of their lifespan. Maternal factors, including general health and health history, drug and alcohol use, smoking, exposure to toxins, diet, and stress are important determinants of fetal outcome. The fetus and the newborn infant may experience dysfunction (eg, problems affecting the cardiac, musculoskeletal, or nervous systems) related to the intrauterine environment.

Getting neonates off to the best possible start is an important means of influencing lifelong health. For this reason, women's health management during the prenatal period is of paramount importance in anticipatory guidance. Pregnant women need to be encouraged to seek prenatal care early in pregnancy and to maintain a lifestyle conducive to creating the optimal environment for the fetus.

An infant continues to depend on the parents' health behaviors. Parents should be encouraged to seek well-child care with regular health monitoring, immunizations, and preventive teaching. Facilitating the transition to the parent role may help prevent future health and relationship problems (Fig. 16-4).

Neonates and young infants are particularly prone to infection because of immaturity of the immune system. Certain behaviors of infants and toddlers, such as mouthing objects, increase the occurrence of infection. Because day-care situations provide more opportunity for exposure, it is not surprising that infants in day care have more infections, especially upper respiratory infections. The effects of economics and living conditions on infant health are evidenced by a greater incidence

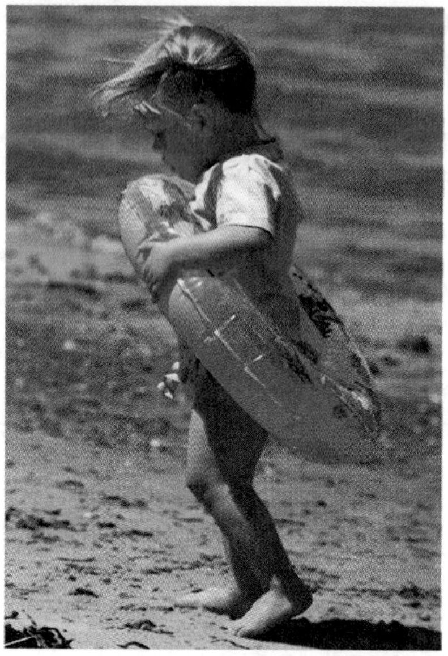

Figure 16-4 • *Young children are active and curious. They place a lot of enthusiasm on their activities, and safety is a factor of concern.*

of infections in infants from families of lower socioeconomic status.

The chief health concern for infants is safety. This includes safe sleeping conditions and prevention of falls, aspiration, and poisoning. The increasing mobility involved in rolling over, creeping, crawling, and walking requires modifications in the home to prevent falls and other hazards. In older infants, hand-to-mouth behavior could cause choking or ingestion of harmful substances. Chapter 29 continues a discussion of safety in the home.

Toddler and Preschooler. The toddler and preschooler continue to be prone to infections and minor illnesses. Although rubella, mumps, and rubeola can be prevented through immunization, chickenpox remains a common communicable disease, often experienced in early childhood. Immunization (discussed in Chapter 39) is a means of reducing the incidence of certain infections and is a component of normal well-child healthcare.

The toddler's advancing motor and cognitive skills promote exploration, and high levels of energy and activity are often the basis for injury. Injuries can range from falls and minor injuries that occur as a part of play, to life-threatening accidents such as drownings, burns, poisonings, or motor vehicle accidents.

Anticipatory guidance for parents of toddlers and preschoolers includes providing a safe environment for exploration, such as storing chemicals, household cleaning products, and medications in safe and protected places. Use of seatbelts in motor vehicles and life vests when around water, as well as providing close supervision wherever there is a potentially dangerous situation (eg, in bathtubs, by swimming pools, at playgrounds), are essential.

The toddler's and preschooler's normal level of curiosity makes them prone to participate in dangerous activities. Parents need to view the world from the level of their child and protect the child from danger at that level (eg, wall outlets, stove burners and knobs, stairs, space heaters).

School-Age and Adolescent. Accidents and minor illnesses continue to be the most common health problems of the school-age child. Exposure to larger numbers of children in school and play environments adds to the kinds and types of infections to which the child may be susceptible. Advances in motor skills throughout childhood are associated with the use of bicycles, tricycles, skateboards, and other riding toys, and, consequently, their related safety concerns become factors. Independent excursions away from home make traffic accidents a concern, and school-age children need to be taught precautions with regard to strangers. Daring exploits, imagination, and industriousness of school-age children determine safety needs.

Adolescence is a time of trying out different identities and testing limits, coupled with the perception of invulnerability. Some of these actions involve health risks, such as smoking, drug use, alcohol consumption, fast driving, drinking and driving, and involvement in sexual activity. In adolescence, the risk of sexually transmitted disease (STD) is increased with sexual activity and is added to the usual infectious possibilities concurrent with youth. AIDS becomes an additional risk, particularly if experimentation with intravenous drugs or unprotected sex occurs. Increasing rates of teenage pregnancy continue to be of concern to healthcare providers, families, and communities (Spitz et al., 1993). Gang activity is on the rise among adolescents, and creates significant concern. Violence within the home and community affects children of all ages; however, it is among adolescents that suicide and homicide have increased dramatically, and the term "children killing children" has been coined.

Although the adolescent may have a working knowledge of how the body functions, there may be limited ability to appreciate a cause–effect relationship between health behaviors and outcomes. In addition, intense privacy needs may impede adequate healthcare.

The nurse teaches and gives counseling regarding safety concerns, sex education, appropriate nutrition, and hygiene. Supporting and encouraging positive family relationships is particularly important during these transitional years. Assisting the adolescent as he or she seeks personal identity and belonging is crucial.

Adult and Older Adult. Young adulthood is characterized by separation from family of origin, career development, and family establishment. Occupation may determine specialized safety concerns. Unhealthy behaviors begun in adolescence, such as smoking, drinking, and promiscuity, may continue into adulthood. During adulthood, the physical effects of health behaviors may become apparent. For example, cigarette smoking results in progressively declining pulmonary function. Health problems common to the middle adulthood group include hypertension, adult-onset diabetes, elevated cholesterol, or serious illness (eg, cancer or cardiac disease).

The older adult may find the ability to manage health independently impaired by changes associated with aging. Alterations in hearing, vision, and mobility affect health management practices such as hygiene, diet, and exercise. Changes in sensory and motor abilities intensify safety needs and make falls a major source of injury. Because the immune response is decreased, older people are at increased risk for infection at a time when poor nutrition and other factors may further impede natural defenses.

Acute and chronic illnesses related to lifestyle patterns are manifested late in life. The cumulative effects of smoking, poor nutrition, inadequate exercise, and other health risks are demonstrated in aging. The common health problems include chronic pulmonary conditions, cardiovascular problems, and joint degeneration.

Anticipatory guidance includes health teaching for behavior modifications, such as a regular program of exercise, lifestyle management, stress reduction, and appropriate diet. Adults need to be encouraged to have regular physical examinations and to seek referrals as may be warranted for physical or mental health as well as for relational challenges. For more information, see Chapter 30.

Nutrition and Metabolism

Newborn and Infant. Infancy is a period of high metabolic rate and nutritional need. Nutrient intake is particularly important because brain growth occupies a large share of the body's metabolic rate. The infant's complex nutritional needs can be met by breast milk or formula during the first 6 months of life. Health problems related to nutrition focus mainly on the infant's receiving adequate amounts of milk and properly prepared formula. With the eruption of teeth and the introduction of solid foods, nutrient intake is expanded to many types of foods, and breast milk or formula becomes less essential in the diet.

Increased metabolic rate and immature renal function lead to high fluid requirements in infancy. Resulting inherent health problems include reduced ability to remove drugs or other substances from the body, greater potential for fluid loss or overload, and difficulty concentrating or diluting urine.

Nursing Research
Growth and Development

Selected Nursing Research Studies

DeSantis, L., & Thomas, J. T. (1994). Childhood independence: Views of Cuban and Haitian immigrant mothers. *Journal of Pediatric Nursing, 9,* 258–267.

Edwards-Beckett, J. (1994). Caregivers' expectations of future learning of dependents with a developmental disability. *Journal of Pediatric Nursing, 9,* 27–32.

Feingold, C. (1994). Correlates of cognitive development in low-birth-weight infants from low-income families. *Journal of Pediatric Nursing, 9,* 91–97.

Gullicks, J. N., & Crase, S. J. (1993). Sibling behavior with a newborn: Parents' expectations and observations. *Journal of Obstetric, Gynecologic and Neonatal Nursing, 22,* 438–444.

Youngblut, J. M., Loveland-Cherry, C. J., & Horan, M. (1994). Maternal employment effects on families and preterm infants at 18 months. *Nursing Research, 43,* 331–337.

Possible Topics for Nursing Inquiry

- What are cultural indicators affecting cognitive development among school-age children?
- What specific stressors affect the accomplishment of developmental tasks of older adults?
- What cultural factors affect parents of infants seeking access to well-child care?

Temperature regulation is less well developed during this period because of less fat storage, increased metabolic rate, and an immature central thermoregulating mechanism.

The nurse teaches parents regarding infant nutrition, proper preparation of formula, and monitoring of the infant's physical growth. Helping parents understand when and how to introduce new foods is supportive. Parents should also be taught how to use a thermometer and when to call a healthcare provider.

Toddler and Preschooler. Appetite during toddlerhood and preschool years is extremely variable, and changes are usually a normal consequence of slowing of growth and change in body composition. The primary health problem relates to parental concerns regarding the adequacy of intake of nutrients because the parent is beginning to have less control over what the child eats. At this age, there is also a potential for children to chew food incompletely and possibly choke on pieces of food.

Parents are encouraged to provide adequate quantity and variety of food. From this, the child generally selects enough for sufficient nutrition. Children should be encouraged to develop good hygiene practices such as washing hands and brushing and flossing their teeth. At this age, parents should clean their children's teeth and, at the same time, model appropriate hygiene behaviors and make learning fun. Sometime around the second birthday, the child should make his or her first visit to the dentist.

School-Age and Adolescent. In general, the school-age period is a time of few health problems. As the child moves beyond the home environment, social influences on food consumption become increasingly important. The food choices of school-age children and adolescents are highly related to peer influences and media advertisements. This is an excellent time to involve children in preparing family meals. Adolescence is a period of rapid growth and high nutritional requirements. It is not uncommon for adolescents to be unable to eat sufficient amounts of food to meet the requirements for physical growth and physiologic change. Adolescents, in particular, are at risk for less than adequate amounts of iron, calcium, and zinc. For some adolescents, the conflict between eating and the desire to be thin is expressed in the health problems of fad dieting, bulimia, or anorexia. For others, the response to stress may be overeating, leading to obesity. These types of health problems may set lifelong patterns. Skin problems are a source of concern during puberty and adolescence.

Anticipatory guidance depends on teaching and attempting to influence peer groups in a positive way to encourage good nutrition. Working with adolescents in groups tends to be more effective in changing behavior. Meeting the nutritional needs of adolescents from poorer families is a challenge and requires the use of community resources to feed adequately all members of the family. Good hygiene practices are paramount. It is not until children reach 9 years of age that they can physically manipulate a toothbrush and dental floss to clean their teeth adequately without adult supervision. Some adolescents may use over-the-counter products to treat skin problems, but most should be encouraged to keep the skin clean and free of harsh chemical, and to avoid direct exposure to the sun.

Adult and Older Adult. Metabolic activity decreases in adults, but not the need for adequate nutrients. Bone growth, which is accelerated during adolescence, continues in young adulthood. During childbearing years, nutrition is particularly important to women and to the outcome of the pregnancy. Health problems can be avoided by an optimal nutritional intake during the active young adult years. Obesity, bulimia, or anorexia may begin or continue to be problems in young adults. Metabolic disorders, such as diabetes, may be manifested in childhood, adolescence, or young adult years.

Through the middle and older adult years, there is increased concern about health problems related to nutrition. Cardiovascular changes make blood cholesterol levels and fat in the diet a concern. The sodium content of food is important for people with disorders of the kidney or with high blood pressure. People with diabetes need to regulate total dietary intake. Meeting nutritional needs using fewer calories is a challenge, and many people must be concerned about excess weight.

Aging changes in the kidney may limit adaptability to fluid changes. Decreased glomerular filtration rate can lead to fluid retention and inability to remove drugs or their metabolites.

Anticipatory guidance in the adult years includes providing the client with access to reliable information about nutrition so that fact and myth can be identified. Referral to dietitians, nutrition classes, and support groups may be beneficial. For more information, see Chapter 37.

Elimination

Newborn and Infant. The infant is too immature to have control over either bowel or bladder elimination. Health problems relate primarily to skin disorders resulting from the need to wear diapers. Monilial infections and diaper rash are common problems. Anticipatory guidance by the nurse is directed toward teaching proper diapering, disposal of stool and diapers, and care of the skin. Parents will want to learn about skin hygiene, frequency of diaper changes, and differences in skin rashes and their treatment.

Toddler and Preschooler. Between 2 and 3 years of age, toddlers have begun to develop control over elimination. Health problems relate to skin care and delay in progressing toward continence. Continence, once achieved, is not guaranteed, and "accidents" are not uncommon during the preschool years.

Anticipatory guidance can help parents understand that the attitudes conveyed during this time of achieving continence and reactions to incidences of incontinence influence not only feelings about body function but also about personal mastery and competency. Neurologic maturation necessary for control over defecation and urination is not achieved until the child is able to walk independently. Patience and allowing the child to progress at his or her own pace are the hallmarks of this stage of development.

School-Age and Adolescent. Older children occasionally have difficulty with nocturnal enuresis or "bed-wetting" after preschool and young school-age years. This problem is often related to maturation of both urinary control mechanisms and sleep but may have emotional or structural causes. Nocturnal enuresis after the age of 6 years is a matter of concern. It is not uncommon to identify a familial pattern of enuresis. The main health problem is related to embarrassment and self-consciousness on the part of the child, who may limit social activities as a result of the enuresis.

Anticipatory guidance is directed toward helping parents and child understand nocturnal enuresis, encouraging a thorough evaluation, and realizing that the child usually matures and becomes continent. Although a physical assessment is essential, psychosocial support also is imperative.

Adult and Older Adult. Continence may be disrupted by "normal" life events, such as pregnancy or childbirth, which result in changes in the pelvic musculature. Decreasing estrogen levels that occur during menopause affect sphincter control, resulting in an increased occurrence of stress incontinence (Lobo, 1994). Illnesses, such as a cerebral vascular accident, or procedures, such as prostatic surgery, ureterostomy placement, or a colostomy, alter normal elimination patterns and threaten the sense of mastery and personal control at any age. In older adults, alterations in innervation and changes in muscle tone may produce incontinence or nocturia.

The nurse shapes client teaching to the specific problem related to elimination, teaching either how to manage the alterations or therapies the client can use to regain continence. For more information, see Chapters 41 and 42.

Activity and Exercise

Newborn and Infant. Newborns and infants are prone to respiratory difficulties as a result of the relative immaturity of the airway and lung structures. Premature infants can be at risk for respiratory distress syndrome, and newborns born by cesarean delivery may have excessive mucus in their lungs. These situations lead to potential health problems related to adequate ventilation.

Developing motor activities can lead to problems related to safety. As infants learn to reach and grasp objects and to roll over, they are placing themselves at risk for injury.

The nurse works with parents to help them understand what factors constitute danger. Close supervision of motor activities and, if needed, of respiratory function are central elements in teaching. At the same time, parents should be given information about ways to provide a stimulating environment.

Toddler and Preschooler. Energy production by the heart and lungs in the toddler and preschooler is adequate. The occurrence of respiratory infections and the management of congenital problems with the heart or lungs are the leading health problems of this age group.

As their motor control increases, the desire to explore and the curiosity of toddlers and preschoolers cause them to be adventurous and to take risks (see Fig. 16-4). Safety and accident prevention are the focus of healthcare.

Anticipatory guidance centers on prevention of respiratory infections, when possible, and early treatment when they occur. Parents of children with congenital problems need support and individual teaching to manage their child's difficulty. Awareness of safety needs remains paramount. (See the section on Health Perception and Health Management, earlier.)

School-Age and Adolescent. The school-age child without congenital abnormalities or chronic problems has few health problems. Respiratory infections continue to occur as a result of contact with classmates. As motor control develops, children become more active, but their bones are not mature and are susceptible to some types of fracture, but because they are not completely ossified, they are somewhat more resistant to fractures. Because the rib cage is not yet rigid, the school-age child is vulnerable to injury to the heart and lungs from blows to the chest. School-age children are constantly "on the go." They must be provided with and encouraged to wear appropriate protective clothing when riding bicycles, skateboards, or rollerblades, and to adhere to safe behaviors. Sports injuries of all kinds are a major cause of morbidity.

The adolescent's health problems are related to lifestyle factors and risk-taking behaviors. Smoking and the use of smokeless tobacco predispose the adolescent to changes in the mucosa of the mouth and the respiratory tract, with the potential for malignant changes in the tissues and in vital capacity changes in ventilation. Increased physical activity in sports, motor vehicle driving, and, possibly, gang activity place the adolescent at risk for serious injuries.

The nurse needs to be a teacher, counselor, and confidant when working with and advising school-age children and adolescents. Helping parents and their children understand ways they can minimize health problems and prevent injury is the nursing focus.

Adult and Older Adult. The effects of smoking or other pollution sources become apparent with aging. When combined with the decline in function that normally occurs with age, the resulting health concerns include decreased vital capacity of the lungs, reduced stroke volume and force of contraction of the heart, and ischemia of tissues that are not adequately perfused. In addition, the vascular system shows accumulation of atherosclerotic plaque and reduced resilience of vessel walls with age.

Changes in motor abilities are noticeable in adulthood. Throughout life the motor system operates under the "use it or lose it" principle. Exercise is increasingly important in maintenance of muscle function. Mobility is affected not only by muscular changes, but also by skeletal changes such as arthritis or loss of bone mineral. Visual and motor changes impair use of means of transportation.

Anticipatory guidance includes encouragement to participate in a regular program of exercise, maintain a low-fat, high-fiber diet, and develop pleasurable leisure activities. The adult is capable of modifying lifestyle to extend wellness late into life (see Chapter 30).

Cognition and Perception

Newborn and Infant. Special senses are important components of cognitive–perceptual development in infancy. Sensory stimulation is a basic human need. Studies of sensory deprivation indicate that sensory stimulation is an important requirement for central nervous system function. Sensory stimulation is critical during the early years of life and essential for normal development.

Although sensory stimulation during early development is extremely important, the central nervous system of the neonate and infant is easily overwhelmed by excess stimulation. Infants provide caregivers with behavioral cues indicating the appropriateness of stimulation for the particular infant's neurobehavioral development (Barratt, et al., 1992).

Health problems that interfere with the accuracy of sensory input (eg, hearing) affect cognitive–perceptual development. In connection with immature anatomy and immune response, the infant is prone to the development of middle ear infections, which, if they become chronic and recurring, may interfere with hearing perception. Infants express pain through pulling on or rubbing the ear, disturbances in sleep or eating, or crying or fussiness.

Observation of the infant's responses to sounds and expressions of pain is an important form of anticipatory guidance for parents. Helping parents understand the need for physical contact and sensory stimulation for adequate cognitive–perceptual development is an important nursing function. Holding and cuddling provide physical sensory stimulation, whereas colorful mobiles, pictures, sounds, and toys in the environment stimulate the special senses.

Toddler and Preschooler. Hearing and vision problems can impede progress in development and may relate to misperceptions by the child. It takes careful and informed observation to identify the subtle pain behaviors in children of this age. Although one might expect to see reduction in activity, children often continue to participate in play despite being in pain. At this age, children are developing cognitive skills, such as language, and are more verbal about indicating the presence of pain. Children as young as 3 years of age can use an objective tool to indicate the level of pain experienced (Beyer, et al., 1992).

Parents are encouraged to have regular hearing and vision examinations as part of well-child care and to follow up with additional assessment if the child's hearing or vision seems to be questionable. Assisting parents in becoming observant of subtle behaviors that may be linked to pain and an underlying health problem is part of client teaching.

School-Age and Adolescent. Health problems for school-age children and adolescents may be related to previous problems of sensory input. On the other hand, difficulty with school work may be the first indication of a sensory impairment. Physiologic, emotional, and environmental factors may also influence cognitive–perceptual function (see Chapter 46). Use of drugs and alcohol alters cognition. Mental health problems become more prominent at these ages than at earlier ages, and suicide is a major health concern.

The nurse provides anticipatory guidance at regular well-child examinations at which vision and hearing are examined. The nurse encourages parents to be aware of indications of substance use or mental health problems, such as poor academic performance, withdrawal, or change in personality, and to seek appropriate care.

Adult and Older Adult. In the absence of chronic conditions, the young and middle adult years are associated with few health problems related to cognition and perception. With aging, the decline in sensory function can contribute to cognitive misperceptions. Pain perception in the older adult may vary from the typical pattern seen in younger people and needs careful evaluation. Chapter 46 presents a complete discussion of the various factors that affect the older adult's cognition. Reversible confusion and dementia are two major health problems for older adults.

The nurse prompts older adults to seek evaluation of pain, sensory deficits, and cognitive changes. Abnormalities should not be accepted as a "normal" part of aging.

Sleep and Rest

Newborn and Infant. Infants are in the process of organizing sleep and rest. As the infant matures, sleep periods consolidate and become longer. Sleep moves from being free-running to becoming linked to nighttime (Murray & Zentner, 1993), such that, at about 3 to 4 months of age, most infants sleep through the night. Health problems of sleep in the infant are usually related to problems in the maturation of neurologic integration. Parents should be advised that infants normally organize their own sleep patterns. Deviations from orderly progression, however, should be assessed by a healthcare provider.

Toddler and Preschooler. Toddlers and preschoolers have organized sleep patterns; most sleep occurs at night, with one or two naps during the day. During the second year of life, nightmares often emerge as cognitive development leads to increased memory and the ability to represent experiences mentally, including fearful situations (Betz, et al., 1994). The nurse advises parents to reassure the anxious child in an unhurried manner and to talk in a quiet voice.

School-Age and Adolescent. Nightmares continue to occur in early school-age children, producing nighttime awakenings. Nighttime bedwetting, a common problem in young children, may disrupt sleep (Nino-Murcia & Keenan, 1987). Parents are encouraged to reassure their children regarding nightmares. As a rule, children outgrow bedwetting, and parents should understand that scolding and punishment are ineffective.

The adolescent actually has increased sleep needs as a result of rapid growth and endocrine changes. Sleep deprivation may, in reality, be a health problem for adolescents who are pressured by school, jobs, and multiple activities (Betz, et al., 1994). Using anticipatory guidance, the nurse counsels the adolescent regarding time management and balance of activities, so that the adolescent can be active and yet get enough sleep.

Adult and Older Adult. Adult sleep problems are often related to stress and schedules that lead to sleep deprivation. Sleep patterns in older adults often are within the range of normal. Environmental situations, such as nighttime problems of children in the family, pregnancy, or late-night exercising or eating, may interfere with sleep as well. Anticipatory guidance includes counseling the adult about activities that foster sleep before bedtime. Insomnia and sleep apnea are frequent sleep disorders for adults. Insomnia, a disorder of initiating or maintaining sleep, may become a health problem for which the adult may choose to seek evaluation. Sleep apnea is the absence of breathing for 10 seconds or longer five times during an hour and may require thorough assessment and intervention. For more information, see Chapter 43.

Self-Perception and Self-Concept

Newborn and Infant. The infant's perception of self begins with the parent–child relationship, in which the infant learns a sense of worthiness. The infant's successful use of cues in conveying and satisfying needs is early evidence of competency. Health problems arise when the infant is unable to respond to the usual parent–child interactions. The nurse provides anticipatory guidance by supporting parents in interactions that engender trust.

Toddler and Preschooler. Toddlers and preschoolers are egocentric in their relationships with peers. Expressions of anger, jealousy, and even regression are not uncommon. Health problems exist for the child who is at either extreme: lack of egocentric response or exaggerated responses. Excessive fears of injury or altered body image may indicate problems with self-concept. The nurse can help parents understand the range of normal behaviors and provide anticipatory guidance about behaviors outside of that range that require further evaluation.

School-Age and Adolescent. At these ages, children's self-concept is tied closely to peers and peer relationships. One's self-concept may be challenged by the response and acceptance given by peers. Use of drugs and exposure to STDs and AIDS may be indications of the need for peer acceptance to have a positive self-concept. The nurse focuses on open communication, interactions with groups that promote development of positive self-concept (church, Scouts, sports), and health education regarding the consequences of drug use and sexual activity.

Adult and Older Adult. Throughout the lifespan, self-concept and self-perception are reinforced or altered as a consequence of life events and interpersonal relationships. In adulthood, this pattern is extremely individual and less predictable, although certain commonalities exist. The older adult may be depressed over life events, or for no definable reason. Evidences of disturbed self-concept that interfere with the ability to carry out activities of daily living require referral for evaluation and treatment. The nurse needs to be supportive of the client and family during periods when self-concept may be altered. Referral to support groups, counselors, or psychiatrists may be the appropriate guidance.

Roles and Relationships

Newborn and Infant. The newborn's primary relationship is with the parents, and attachment is the foundation of its development (Ainsworth, et al., 1978). Attachment is a process in which the ongoing interaction between the infant and parent produces a special bond, offering the infant a safe base from which to launch into the world. The sensitive parent learns to "read" the infant's cues and provides for the infant's needs. The infant in turn responds by cessation of crying, by smiling, or by sleeping. Problems in either party can alter the interaction and interfere with attachment. The

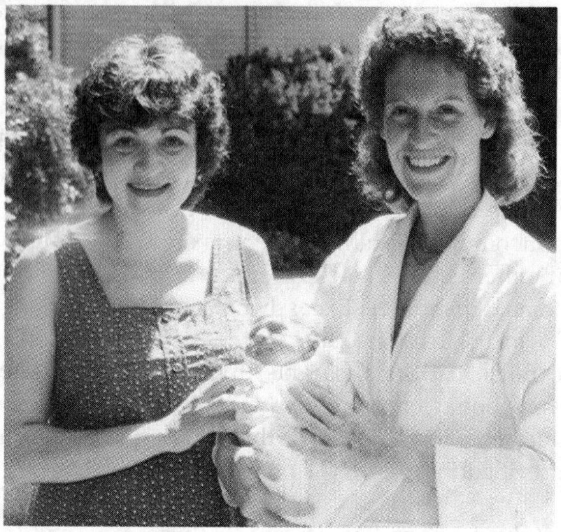

Figure 16-5 • Attachment formation between mother and newborn is an important task of the neonatal and infant period. The nurse encourages attachment and supports the mother in her care of the newborn. (Photo courtesy of former Booth Maternity Center, Philadelphia, PA.)

change in the relationship produces a sense of loss, which leads to an altered ability to form relationships. Problems in roles and relationship during this time are also thought to contribute abuse and neglect. The nurse encourages parent–infant bonding through providing opportunities for positive interaction and by teaching the parent the importance of reciprocal interactions (Fig. 16-5).

Toddler and Preschooler. In late infancy and toddlerhood, the child expresses the sense of loss inherent in changes in relationships through separation anxiety and protest. The degree of anxiety and protest, however, is not necessarily direct evidence of attachment. The nurse can provide anticipatory guidance by assisting the parents in understanding the response of the child and recognizing when it exceeds normal bounds.

School-Age and Adolescent. Peer relationships are increasingly important in the school-age years. The two key influences during adolescence are sexual development and the peer group. Time spent with friends is increased, whereas time spent with parents and family is decreased. The child who has difficulty relating to peers, leaving home and family, or managing sexuality appropriately may be exhibiting problems in roles and relationships. The nurse can be a safe confidant and counselor for the child, a support and encouragement for parents, and an appraiser and evaluator of the need for further intervention.

Adult and Older Adult. Adults assume many roles, including career, intimacy, marriage, and parenthood. Although these categories help structure our thinking, the patterns of resultant roles and relationships are not as clear-cut. Patterns of intimacy and parenting are not predictable or set. Although physical intimacy is required for the bearing of biologic offspring, intimacy is not always linked with parenting. Parenting may be deferred in favor of establishing a career, parenting may be inhibited because of infertility or lack of a mate, or the person may make a choice not to parent.

For middle and older adults, the loss of relationships through relocation, divorce, death, or illness is equally challenging. The middle-aged person may have elderly parents who require care, and death of parents often occurs in middle age. Middle age is also a time of evaluation and reflection, which may lead to role conflict and altered relationships. Older adults experience loss of the work role, reduced mobility and activity, which may limit social contacts, and changes in family roles and relationships.

Nurses can be helpful by offering support and referring community resources. Parents of young children can be counseled regarding parenting skills and sources for improving and reinforcing them. Middle-aged adults can be reassured that midlife review is a normal developmental process and that there are resources available to assist them in sorting through feelings and conflicts that arise. Preparing for retirement years through development of new interests and activities helps to minimize the adjustment to the various role losses and changed relationships that most older adults experience (Fig. 16-6). This is discussed further in Chapter 49.

Sexuality and Reproduction

Newborn and Infant. Gender is determined at the time of fertilization. In the first weeks of embryologic life, sexual differentiation is determined by exposure to hormones. Gender is established at birth based on the

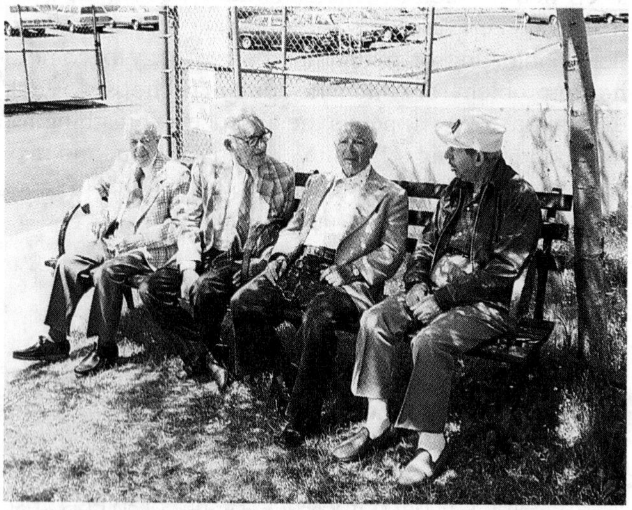

Figure 16-6 • Maintaining social contacts and activities are important in later life.

physical sexual appearance. Gender identity seems to depend primarily on biologic characteristics; however, some theorists believe environmental factors exert some influence. Health problems can occur if gender cannot be established by unambiguous physical characteristics. The nurse can encourage parents to provide love, comfort, intimacy, and nurturance, the bases for later sexuality.

Toddler and Preschooler. The exploratory behavior of toddlers includes exploration of the body, and preschoolers recognize physical differences between the sexes, identifying gender based on body parts and appearances. This age group often engages in exhibitionistic behaviors of removing clothing and discussing sexual organs, their own and others. Anticipatory guidance includes reminding parents that exploratory behavior and interest in sexuality is to be expected. The nurse can also communicate to parents the importance of affection and acceptance of the child as a basis for future sexuality and positive self-concept.

School-Age and Adolescent. Research suggests that by the time the children are 6 or 7 years of age, they have formed a stable concept of themselves as male or female (Cole & Cole, 1993). The school-age child has increasing curiosity about sexual function, although peer relationships and friendships are almost exclusively with children of the same gender. Sexual behavior becomes a problem only when the child seems to be turning to masturbation as a primary source of comfort.

Health problems for adolescents are associated with lifestyle activities of the adolescent and peer group. STDs and AIDS are significant potential problems for the sexually active adolescent, with drug use as a contributory factor. For numerous reasons, use of birth control methods is inconsistent among adolescents. One result is the increasing number of adolescent pregnancies.

Although most sexual activity occurs between heterosexual couples, homosexual experimentation during adolescence is not uncommon. Sometime during adolescence, the identification of oneself as heterosexual or homosexual occurs. Although the origins of homosexuality are poorly understood, this lifestyle demonstrates alternate patterns of sexual development that have not been clearly explicated (Greydonus & Shearin, 1990; Isay, 1990). Nurses can be supportive of adolescents who are coming to terms with their sexual orientation and are encouraged to be aware of community resources.

Children of any age are the potential victims of sexual abuse. Children who are preschool-age may demonstrate indications of anxiety, fear, sleep disturbances, and holding on to parents. School-age children exhibit similar clues, plus phobias and a decline in school performance. Adolescents may exhibit socially unacceptable behavior, sexual promiscuity, running away from home, and failing academic performance. The nurse needs to participate in teaching children of all ages to tell someone (friend, pastor, teacher) when they have been approached or touched in a way that makes them uncomfortable. The nurse encourages parents to listen carefully to their children and not discount what the parents might term as "imaginative."

Adult and Older Adult. Reproduction is a prime concern of early adult years, with the major related health problems being infertility, STDs, and specific sexual dysfunction. During the middle years, menopause occurs in women and may present health problems related to decreased estrogen production (eg, hot flashes, osteoporosis). STDs and AIDS remain as potential problems throughout adulthood.

Body structure and function, sexual expression, and intimacy are primary aspects of human function in the older adult. Sexuality, which is more than the act of intercourse, is still important. In normal aging, decreased mobility and energy production may limit sexual activity. Health problems are related to interference with sexual expression that may be the result of illness (eg, stroke), death of a spouse, or environment (eg, nursing homes).

The nurse who works with infertile couples needs to be sensitive to their feelings and support their efforts to seek therapies to correct the problem. Encouraging couples to maintain their personal intimacy as well as sexual intimacy is essential. Preventing STDs and AIDS is a continuing problem with which the nurse is concerned. Nurses can also help older adults to understand that age alone is not a barrier to sexual function and can counsel (or refer to counselors) older people on alternate forms of sexual expression. Sensitivity on the part of nurses in anticipating privacy needs for older adults in healthcare settings is a valuable nursing function. For further information, see Chapter 52.

Coping and Stress Tolerance

Newborn and Infant. Infants are not immune to stress. Thomas and Chess (1977) have used the concepts of adaptability and rhythmicity to describe infant behaviors and have classified infant temperament styles as easy, slow to warm up, and difficult. Sources of stress in infancy involve satisfaction of basic needs within the context of the caregiving or parental relationship. The major stressor of infancy and early childhood is separation, reflecting the impact of attachment (Karen, 1994). A limited understanding of time and the absence of the parent or caregiver during this period of trust development are the sources of this anxiety.

Anticipatory guidance includes counseling with parents and caregivers regarding the reason for separation anxiety and the range of normal for this response. Within the context of the early parent–infant interaction, coping behaviors are established. Infants employ

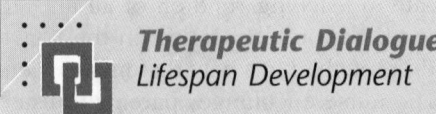

Therapeutic Dialogue
Lifespan Development

Scenes for Thought

Mr. Rifkin is a 70-year-old man whose wife died 3 years ago. He owns his own home and lives alone. He enjoys the company of a companion, Mrs. Alcott, and she enjoys taking care of him. Mr. Rifkin's only daughter and her family have moved to another state. When he visits his daughter, Mrs. Alcott comes along. Daughter Carol feels that she now has an "intruder" in her relationship with her father and doesn't know what to do. When Carol comes in for her yearly physical, she begins to discuss this situation with you, Shawnna Weber, her RN.

Effective

Client: *I'd like to tell my Dad that he should leave the woman at home so we can talk together without her butting in all the time.*
Nurse: *She gets in the way of you and your Dad spending time alone? (Restating the client's words.)*
Client: *Yes, she does. And she can't take a hint, either. I suggested Dad and I take a walk together and she immediately jumped in and came too.* Client looks frustrated.
Nurse: *Sounds like she's afraid of being left out. (Observation of behavior.)*
Client: *That's what I'd like to do, leave her out. But I don't want to alienate my Dad or make him choose between her and me or make myself look like a jealous daughter, either. I just want . . . what do I want?*
Nurse: *Good question. (Allowing client time to think and come up with her own solution.)*
Client: *I want time with my Dad alone. Now I have to figure out how to get it without hurting anyone.* Client looks determined and a bit more sure of herself.

Less Effective

Client: *I don't know what to do about my Dad's girlfriend. She seems to be taking over a bit too much and getting in the way of our relationship.* Client looks frustrated and annoyed.
Nurse: *He's 70 and has a girlfriend? Good for him! I think it's so cute when old folks can get together and take care of each other. Helps them live longer, I hear.*
Client: *Well, that may be but I can't get a word in edgewise when she's around. Sure is different from what it used to be.* Continues to look and sound frustrated.
Nurse: *Why don't you talk to her about it? I'm sure once you've let her know how you feel she'll be much more sensitive to you.*
Client: *Sure she will.* Begins to ask questions about her cholesterol levels.

Critical Thinking Challenges

• Based on Erickson's theory of development, analyze what stage Carol is in. • Determine stages for Mr. Rifkin and Mrs. Alcott. • Detect the losses Mr. Rifkin has experienced and state how he is coping. • Consider the losses Carol has experienced and what she is doing about them. • Appraise the advice given to Carol. Also critique the lack *of advice.*

self-regulating and soothing behaviors, such as sucking, crying, motor activity, or withdrawal. The responsiveness of the caregiver is an important determinant in how the infant learns to cope.

Toddler and Preschooler. The stressors of toddlerhood include separation and loss as well as dealing with increasing autonomy. Death, divorce, and illness of a family member can affect toddlers (Behrman, 1994). In addition, birth of a sibling is a common stressor, not only during the toddler years, but throughout childhood. With the birth of a sibling, the toddler loses his or her place as the center of the parents' concern. Illness and hospitalization are especially stressful for toddlers and preschoolers, not only because of the separation, but because they lack the cognitive ability to understand what is happening.

Cognitive development includes changes in memory. The role of memory in coping is twofold. First, the child can relate to previous stressful events, learning from such experiences; this learning can be positive or negative, depending on the coping behaviors used and the outcome. Second, memory sensitizes the child to stressors. A child who is bitten by a dog may become afraid not only of dogs but of all furry animals. Fears and fantasy are also characteristic of preschoolers and cause related stress. Motor development increases the possibilities for coping behaviors. Mobility can be used to avoid or exit a stressful situation, to change the situation directly, or for aggression.

Nurses can assist parents in recognizing the stressors their toddlers or preschoolers encounter and in nurturing their children by teaching them coping skills for managing these stressors. Learning coping styles helps the young child manage similar situations in the future.

School-Age and Adolescent. Performance expectations, academic pressures, and widening interpersonal contacts are characteristic sources of stress in the school-age child. Although performance is the primary stressor at this age, many of the stressors that were problematic as a preschooler may continue to some degree in the school-age child. The school-age child has, over the years, developed many coping skills as well as the ability to learn more. The nurse who has assessed coping skills should be supportive of coping abilities. Children can be helped to understand pressures they are encountering. School nurses are in an excellent position to teach children effective cognitive coping strategies.

Academic demands, conflicts over issues of independence, threats to identity, and peer pressures dominate adolescent stress. Substance use and abuse become common means of coping. The increased suicide rate among adolescents reflects the seriousness of the effects of stress on this age group. Parents can be guided to observe for signs of excessive stress and dysfunctional coping mechanisms in their adolescent. Adolescents need to feel supported and accepted regarding their stress experiences, and nurses are often in the best position to participate in this.

Adult and Older Adult. The various roles of adulthood involve specific kinds of stressors. Balancing these roles is a further form of stress. The underlying features in stressful events are change and loss. Coping is a function of both the stressors or demands posed by the environment as well as the person's or family's capabilities and vulnerabilities (Woods et al., 1993). Health problems related to stress include cardiac, nutrition, sleep, and substance use disorders. Chapter 51 presents a complete discussion of stress, coping, and adjustment. The nurse can encourage the person to learn a variety of methods for managing stress, including exercise, relaxation, imagery, and biofeedback.

Values and Beliefs

Newborn and Infant. Infants have a limited understanding of right and wrong and do not appreciate the cause–effect relationship between their actions and punishment or reward. The nurse can help parents understand that, because the infant is not defying them deliberately, punishment is not appropriate.

Toddler and Preschooler. At this age, egocentricity results in a self-centered approach to right and wrong—whatever the child wants is deemed right. Punishment and reward guide behavior, and authority figures, external to the child, determine and dispense rewards and punishment. Toddlers and preschoolers learn religious practices through family activities and imitation, although without understanding. The nurse's role is to help parents use this stage to enhance positive behavior through rewarding desired behavior. Encouraging parents to include their child in their religious practices fosters spiritual beliefs and development (Cole, 1991).

School-Age and Adolescent. The school-age child tends to follow orders to gain the approval of others. Because of the desire for conformity and the wish to fit in, the will to do right guides behavior and there is less emphasis on punishment and rewards. Religious beliefs reflect a beginning appreciation of the existence of a "god" or deity. Because doing right is associated with reward, the school-age child may engage in making "deals" with the deity figure. Parents can be influenced to reinforce desired behavior in their child. Being aware of the child's spiritual development enhances the parents' ability to further development.

Adolescents learn to make moral judgments that are situation-specific, to transfer moral judgments across situations, and finally to make autonomous decisions regarding moral issues. Problems occur when the adolescent tries out various activities and behaviors, such as substance use and promiscuous sexual behavior. At this time, faith and religious beliefs are questioned and challenged as the adolescent develops a personal identity and expands independence from the family. The nurse can assist the adolescent and parents in awareness of the developmental aspects of this stage.

Adult and Older Adult. Values and moral development are at the level of autonomous decisions, in which principles are applied to differing situations. Moral reasoning is bound less by rules, and actions are guided to a greater extent by personal values. Spiritual beliefs evolve and are applicable across a variety of situations. Health problems occur when there is disharmony between spiritual beliefs and events in the adult's life (Reed, 1991). Chapter 53 has a complete discussion of spirituality and alterations in spirituality.

Key Concepts

- Growth and development occur throughout the lifespan.
- Development is the process of ongoing change, reorganization, and integration occurring throughout a person's life, and includes body structure and function, psychosocial behaviors, and cognition.
- Genetics and environment are the two primary factors driving development.
- Principles of growth and development are drawn from biologic and psychosocial sciences and express commonalities in the process.
- Theorists have attempted to explain growth and development within various contexts, such as psychodynamics, cognitive development, human needs, developmental tasks, and moral development.
- There are progressive, sequenced aspects of development for various stages of life on which future development expands.

- The nurse's primary role in growth and development is understanding the person's position in the process, being aware of expectations in terms of functional health, and recognizing functional health problems related to development.

Critical Thinking Challenges

Now you have added information about growth and development across the lifespan to your knowledge base of nursing. Turn back to the situation at the beginning of this chapter and consider the following questions.

1. *Determine what the mother may feel that she has not expressed verbally.*
2. *Identify the concepts of growth and development that are pertinent to this situation.*
3. *Relate these components to this child and this situation.*
4. *Clarify what additional assessment you will need of the mother and her child.*
5. *List some appropriate nursing considerations and interventions.*

References

Ainsworth, M. D. S., Blehar, M. C., Waters, E., et al. (1978). *Patterns of attachment.* Hillsdale, NJ: Erlbaum.

Barratt, M. S., Roach, M. A., & Leavitt, L. A. (1992). Early channels of mother–infant communication: Preterm and term infants. *J Child Psychol Psychiatry, 33,* 1193–1204.

Behrman, R. E. (1994). Children and divorce: Overview and analysis. *Future of Children, 4,* 4–14.

Betz, C., Hunsberger, M., & Wright, S. (1994). *Family-centered nursing care of children* (2nd ed.). Philadelphia: W. B. Saunders.

Beyer, J. E., Denyes, M. J., & Villarruel, A. M. (1992). The creation, validation, and continuing development of the Oucher: A measure of pain intensity in children. *Journal of Pediatric Nursing, 7,* 335–346.

Bronfenbrenner, U. (1979). *The ecology of human development.* Cambridge, MA: Harvard University Press.

Cole, R. (1991). *The spiritual life of children.* Boston: Houghton Mifflin.

Cole, M., & Cole, S. (1993). *The development of children* (2nd ed.). New York: Scientific American Books.

De Casper, A. J., & Fifer, W. P. (1980). Of human bonding: Newborns prefer their mothers' voices. *Science, 208,* 1174–1176.

DuPont, H. (1994). *Emotional development: Theory and applications.* Westport, CT: Praeger.

Erikson, E. (1963). *Childhood and society* (2nd ed.). New York: W. W. Norton.

Freiberg, K. L. (1987). *Human development: A life-span approach.* Boston: Jones & Bartlett.

Gilligan, C. (1982). *In a different voice.* Cambridge, MA: Harvard University Press.

Greydonus, D., & Shearin, R. (1990). *Adolescent sexuality and gynecology.* Philadelphia: Lea & Febiger.

Hamburger, V. (1975). Cell death in the development of the lateral motor column of the chick embryo. *J Comp Neurol, 160,* 1121–1125.

Havighurst, R. J. (1972). *Developmental tasks and education* (3rd ed.). New York: David McKay.

Isay, R. (1990). *Being homosexual: Gay men and their development.* New York: Farrar, Strauss, Giroux.

Johnsen, E. P. (1991). Searching for the social and cognitive outcomes of children's play: A selective second look. *Play and Culture, 4,* 201–213.

Karen, R. (1994). *Becoming attached: Unfolding the mystery of the infant–mother bond and its impact on later life.* New York: Warner Books.

Kohlberg, L. (1976). Moral stages and moralization: The cognitive–developmental approach. In T. Lickona (Ed.), *Moral development and behavior.* New York: Holt, Rinehart, & Winston.

Kohlberg, L. (1984). *The psychology of moral development: The nature and validity of moral stages* (Vol. 2). New York: Harper & Row.

Kurtines, W. M., & Gewirtz, J. L. (Eds.). (1991). *Handbook of moral behavior and development: Vol. 1. Theory.* Hillsdale, NJ: Erlbaum.

Lobo, R. (Ed.). (1994). *Treatment of the postmenopausal woman: Basic and clinical aspects.* New York: Raven Press.

Lynch, M., & Lynch, C. (1991). Self concept development through adult life cycle. *Journal of Research in Education, 1,* 13–17.

Murray, R., & Zentner, J. (1993). *Nursing assessment and health promotion: Strategies through the life span* (5th ed.). Norwalk, CT: Appleton & Lange.

Mussen, P. H. (1990). *Child development and personality* (4th ed.). New York: Harper & Row.

Nemeroff, R., & Colarusso, C. (Eds.). (1990). *New dimensions in adult development.* New York: Basic Books.

Newport, E. (1991). Contrasting concepts of the critical period for language. In S. Carey & R. Gelman (Eds.), *The epigenesis of mind: Essays on biology and cognition.* Hillsdale, NJ: Erlbaum.

Nino-Murcia, G., & Keenan, S. (1987). Enuresis and sleep. In C. Guilleminault (Ed.), *Sleep and its disorders in children* (pp. 1–16). New York: Raven Press.

Peterson, M. (1994). Physical aspects of aging: Is there such a thing as "normal?" *Geriatrics, 49,* 45–49.

Piaget, J. (1952). *The origins of intelligence in children.* New York: International Universities Press.

Reed, P. G. (1991). Spirituality and mental health in older adults: Extant knowledge for nursing. *Family and Community Health, 14,* 14–25.

Sasser-Coen, J. R. (1993). Qualitative changes in creativity in the second half of life: A life-span developmental perspective. *Journal of Creative Behavior, 27,* 18–27.

Schulz, R. (1993). *Adult development and aging: Myths and emerging realities* (2nd ed.). New York: MacMillan.

Schuster, C. S., & Ashburn, S. S. (1992). *The process of human development* (3rd ed.). Philadelphia: J. B. Lippincott.

Spitz, L. A., Ventural, S. J., Koonin, L. M., et al. (1993). Surveillance for pregnancy and birth rates among teenagers by state—United States, 1980—1990. *MMWR, 42*, 1–27.

Thomas, A., & Chess, S. (1977). *Temperament and development*. New York: Brunner/Mazel.

Thompson, J. E. (1990). Maternal stress, anxiety, and social support during pregnancy: Possible directions for prenatal intervention. In I. R. Merkatz & J. E. Thompson (Eds.). *New perspectives on prenatal care* (pp. 319–335). New York: Elsevier.

Turner, J., & Helms, D. (1987). *Lifespan development* (3rd ed.). San Francisco: Holt, Rinehart & Winston.

Woods, N. F., Haberman, M. R., & Packard, N. J. (1993). Demands of illness and individual, dyadic, and family adaptation in chronic illness. *Western Journal of Nursing Research, 15,* 25–30.

Worthington-Roberts, B. S., & Klerman, L. V. (1990). Maternal nutrition. In I. R. Merkatz & J. E. Thompson (Eds.). *New perspectives on prenatal care* (pp. 235–271). New York: Elsevier.

Bibliography

Davis, R., & Truesdale, M. (1993). Creative approaches to promoting parent–infant bonding. *Journal of Pediatric Nursing, 8*, 201–202.

Donley, R. Sr. (1991). Spiritual dimensions of health care: Nursing's mission. *Nursing and Health Care, 12*, 178–183.

Fisher, J. (1993). A framework for describing developmental change among older adults. *Adult Education Quarterly, 43*, 76–89.

Kohlberg, L., & Ryncarz, R. (1990). Beyond justice reasoning: Moral development and considerations of a seventh stage. In C. Alexander & E. Langer (Eds.), *Higher stages of human development: Perspectives on adult growth*. New York: Oxford University Press.

Konner, M. (1991). *Childhood: A multicultural view*. Boston: Little, Brown, & Co.

Scarr, S. (1992). Developmental theories for the 1990's: Development and individual differences. *Child Dev, 63*, 1–19.

Schaie, K. W. (1994). The course of adult intellectual development. *Am Psychol, 49*, 304–313.

Spencer, M. B., & Markstrom-Adams, C. (1990). Identity processes among racial and ethnic minority children in America. *Child Dev, 61*, 290–310.

Whitman, J., & Sweeney, T. (1992). A holistic model for wellness and prevention over the life span. *Journal of Counseling and Development, 71*, 140–148.

Individual, Family, and Community

Key Terms	Learning Objectives
Community *Developmental stages* *Family* *Feedback loop* *Systems theory*	*Upon completion of this chapter, the student will be able to do the following:* • *State interactions among individuals, family, and community.* • *State the key concepts of two different conceptual frameworks used to study the family.* • *Describe three methods a nurse can use to assess a family.* • *Discuss family responsibilities for healthy function of the family.* • *Describe the components that could be included in a definition of community.* • *Define family and community.* • *Compare various types of community.* • *Discuss the implications of different types of communities for nursing care.* • *Discuss community responsibilities for healthy function and the nurse's participation in community.*

17

Mrs. Benoli is a 78-year-old Italian-American who came to the United States as a young bride. Devoutly Catholic, she and her husband have three grown children, six grandchildren, and two great-grandchildren. Mrs. Benoli enjoys gardening and sewing. She never finished high school. She retired at the mandatory age despite her desire to continue working as a seamstress in a small dress shop in her neighborhood. Before her illness, she went to the dress shop daily to visit her friends. Mrs. Benoli states that she has lived in the same neighborhood since her arrival in the United States. She has never had a reason to leave the neighborhood except to visit relatives in Italy.

Mrs. Benoli, who is hospitalized, has passed the acute phase of a cerebrovascular accident. Plans are being made for her discharge. A primary concern is her support system, and the nurses are concerned about Mrs. Benoli's attitude. She expresses no motivation to walk. She prefers to skip meals to avoid the embarrassment of "eating as babies do." Her speech is slurred, so she would prefer not to talk. At present she cannot continue her hobbies. Her one interest is to continue to go to church whenever possible. Her husband is frail, spends most of his time sitting on the porch, and has never participated in household chores. Mrs. Benoli believes she would be least burdensome to her husband if she remains quietly in bed and eats only when necessary.

In previous chapters you learned about holistic health, assessment, and planning for care. This chapter expands your knowledge base of nursing management, including consideration of the individual, the family, and the community function in nursing care. Mrs. Benoli will need the assistance of her family and community to regain as high a level of function as possible. You will need to integrate what you learned about holistic health, assessment, and care planning with this new knowledge of the relationship between individual, family, and community. Critical Thinking Challenges at the end of the chapter will help you apply what you have studied in this chapter to Mrs. Benoli's care.

Earlier in this century, healthcare focused on the client as the recipient of care. It is now known that care is enhanced when the client is understood as an individual in the context of a family and community. For example, much of Mrs. Benoli's physical and psychosocial support will have to come from outside herself. The renewed interest in family and community emerged in the 1970s and was reflected in the American Nurses Association's Standards of Nursing Practice description of nursing practice as "a direct service, goal oriented and adapted to the needs of the individual, the family and the community during health and illness" (American Nurses Association, 1973, p. 2).

The beliefs and values individuals hold and the support they receive come in large measure from the family and are reinforced by the community. Understanding family dynamics and the community context assists the nurse in planning care that, because it is compatible with the client's everyday life, has the greatest chance of success. This chapter explores the interactions of the individual, family, and community.

The Individual

Individuals are not isolates. They both influence and are influenced by other people and the environment. Other chapters in this unit address issues related to the individual: lifespan considerations, culture and ethnicity, values, and nurse–client communication. Some basic needs can be met independently, whereas some require interaction with family and community, and others may require the interventions of a nurse to be met (Fig. 17-1). Nursing care can be organized around the unmet basic needs in Maslow's hierarchy (Maslow, 1968). These are prioritized, as discussed in Chapter 2, and one must be able satisfactorily to meet the lower-level need to meet the next-level need fully.

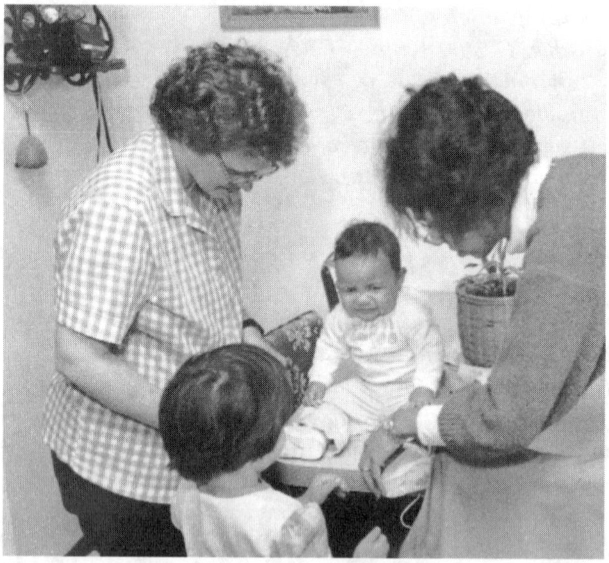

Figure 17-1 • *The nurse assesses individuals and the family functions in relation to each individual. Different developmental levels need different types and amounts of care from the family and nurse. (Courtesy of Seattle University.)*

Individual Responsibility for Healthy Function

The ideal goal of healthcare is for individuals to be responsible for their own health. Instead of nurses and physicians being solely responsible for the client's health, a partnership is developed between healthcare providers, who teach and assist, and healthcare consumers, who ask for specific information or general guidance. This text presents such healthcare concepts. A variety of self-help evaluations are available to individuals who want to assess and apply "do-it-yourself" tactics. Sample questions appear in the accompanying display.

The Family

Traditionally, the family has been considered the basic unit of human society and has played a central role in the organization of social relations. Although there is debate among social scientists about the universality of the functions of the family, the consensus among anthropologists provides a useful perspective on this issue. Most agree that the family provides for the following needs: sexual, reproductive, economic, nurturing, educational, socialization, caring, status, and political. Several, if not all, functions seem to be necessary to designate a group as a family. This is not to say that these functions cannot be carried out by other individuals or institutions, but that over time, the family has proven to be a successful social institution in fulfilling these functions. Family functions and structures are discussed in Chapter 49.

For the purposes of this chapter's discussion of the **family**, the following general definition is offered:

> The family is a social group whose members share common values, occupy specific positions, and interact with each other over time. Adults bear and rear children, engage in economic and political cooperation, and care for the elders.

Family Conceptual Frameworks

Conceptual frameworks provide useful guidelines for organizing family information. Each framework ana-

Nursing Assessment

Suggestions to Elicit Information Related to Individual Function

Health Perception and Health Management

- How would you rate your own health?
- Tell me about the last time you were sick.
- Do you have routine physical exams? If yes, how often?
- In the past year, how many times have you seen a healthcare provider? For what reason(s)?

Nutrition and Metabolism

- Describe what you ate last night for dinner. Was that a typical dinner for you?
- What are your favorite foods? How often do you eat them?
- Do you eat between meals? If yes, when and what do you usually eat?
- Who prepares your food, and how is it usually prepared?

Elimination

- Do you have any problems with elimination? If yes, describe them.
- Do you move your bowels regularly? How often?
- Have you ever been taught exercises to strengthen your urinary tract sphincter? If yes, when, and describe the exercise(s).

Activity and Exercise

- Are you currently doing any regular exercises? If yes, how often?
- How do you spend your leisure time?
- What hobbies are you engaged in now? Are there others you would like to pursue?

Sleep and Rest

- How many hours of sleep do you get a night?
- Do you take nap(s) during the day?
- Do you have a regular bedtime routine?

Cognition and Perception

- How honest can you be with yourself?
- What happens when you set a goal for yourself? Do you usually meet it?
- Have your perceptions of an event ever varied widely from those of others? If yes, what did you think of that?

Self-Perception and Self-Concept

- Have you ever been described in a way you never thought of yourself? How did that make you feel?
- State five adjectives you feel describe you most accurately.
- Finish the following statements:
  My self-concept is most positive when ___________ .
  My self-concept is most negative when ___________ .

Roles and Relationships

- Describe your relationship to each of the other members of your family.
- List your various roles at this time in your life.
- How easy is it for you to be the decision maker?

Sexuality and Reproduction

- How do you express tenderness and affection?
- Do you have any questions or concerns about fertility or family planning?
- Do you engage in any high-risk sexual practices?

Coping and Stress Tolerance

- Describe a stressful event for you.
- How do you resolve conflicts?
- How satisfied are you with the way you resolve conflicts?

Values and Beliefs

- How do you define illness?
- Would you rank health at the top, middle, or bottom of what you consider important?
- What do you believe makes a person healthy?

lyzes the family from a different perspective. No one framework is inherently right or wrong, but each framework requires the nurse to obtain somewhat different pieces of information. There are many frameworks, and it is not the intent of this chapter to acquaint the nurse with all of these but rather to show briefly the implications of their use.

By comparing two frameworks, the nurse can see how each framework guides nursing care. The two frameworks chosen for this chapter are a developmental framework and a systems framework.

Developmental Framework

The developmental framework is popular in the study of families. In the early 1950s, Duvall (1962) directed a

Nursing Research
Family

Selected Nursing Research Studies

D'Avanzo, C. E., Frye B., & Froman, R. (1994). Stress in Cambodian refugee families. *Image, 26*(2), 101–105.

Horowitz, A., & Reinhard, S. (1992). Family management of labeled mental illness in a deinstitutionalized era: An exploratory study. *Perspectives on Social Problems, 4,* 111–127.

McCubbin, H. I., Thompson, E. A., & Thompson, A. I., et al. (1993). Culture, ethnicity, and the family: Critical factors in childhood chronic illness and disabilities. *Pediatrics, 91,* 1063–1069.

Reinhard, S. C. (1994). Perspectives on the family's caregiving experience in mental illness. *Image, 26*(1), 70–73.

Possible Topics for Nursing Inquiry

- What is the relationship between a family's perception of an illness and an individual's collaboration with nursing interventions?
- What kinds of support will family members accept during a relative's terminal illness?
- Does viewing a problem from a systems perspective versus an individual perspective increase the probability of resolution of the problem?
- Do nurses who use a theoretical framework to collect family assessment data provide more individualized nursing care than nurses who do not?

group that studied the concept of family developmental tasks. This research focused on developmental tasks and role expectations of parents and children throughout a life cycle. The framework was meant to allow for biologic and cultural differences as well as differences in values.

Duvall's framework, essentially based on the individual life cycle, demonstrated that families move through a series of eight **developmental stages**. These stages are based on the developmental stage of the oldest child in the family, and address marriage, childbearing, preschool years, school years, adolescent years, young adulthood, middle-aged parents whose children have left home, and aging parents. The critical family developmental tasks for these stages include learning to be a marital partner, adjusting to parenthood, stimulating the curiosity of preschool children, adapting to other school-age families, assisting adolescents to balance independence and autonomy, launching young adults into the work world, redefining the marital dyad without children, and coping with loss (Duvall, 1977). Tasks not completed at any one developmental stage produce chronic difficulties as the family struggles to master tasks at the next stage. Carter and McGoldrick (1980) refined this framework to reflect the changing times and make it applicable to divorced families.

In 1959, anthropologist Meyer Fortes noted in the introduction to *The Developmental Cycle in Domestic Groups* (1971) that the family life cycle consisted of three phases: expansion, dispersion or fusion, and replacement. The papers in that collection point out the universality of the family developmental cycle, describing families in Southeast Asia, Africa, and the Western Pacific.

The developmental cycle of the family, combining the work of Duvall, Fortes, and Carter and McGoldrick, is shown in Table 17-1. At each stage, Duvall and Carter and McGoldrick identified specific tasks for the family to accomplish.

Systems Framework

First described in the social science context by the biologist von Bertalanffy (1968), systems theory has become popular because it takes a holistic approach and tries to encompass all data collected at all levels of abstraction. **Systems theory** looks at the interaction of the parts that make up the whole. There is input to the system, throughput (input from one member in the system to another), and output from the system. When the system is under stress, it tries to regulate itself by use of **feedback loops**, in which some of the output is rerouted back to the system as input, which in turn affects subsequent output. This response restores the system's balance, or homeostasis.

Because there are many feedback loops, some of which overlap, systems theory describes a circular process, not a deterministic one. When feedback to the system causes the system to move away from homeostasis, it is called positive feedback; when the feedback causes the system to maintain homeostasis, it is called negative feedback. Systems are also considered to be either open or closed. These terms refer to the amount of exchange that takes place between a system and its environment. In a closed system, no exchange occurs, whereas in an open system, exchange occurs readily.

Families are basically open systems; however, the degree to which they are willing to exchange resources with other systems varies greatly. Healthy, functioning families exchange to a greater degree than dysfunctional families (Fig. 17-2).

Within the systems perspective there are many different schools of thought. Systems theorists include Virginia Satir (1988), Murray Bowen (1978), Salvador Minuchin (1974), Salvador Minuchin and H. Charles Fishman (1981), and Jay Haley (1971). Wright and Leahey (1994) are nurses whose family nursing theory is based on systems theory.

Several concepts are important for the nurse to

Table 17-1 • Developmental Cycle of the Family and Task Accomplishment

Family Developmental Stage	Developmental Task
Preexpansion	
Unattached adult	Stabilize image Develop independence
Expansion	
Unit formation	Develop mutual satisfaction Develop independence
Having children (by birth or adoption)	Adjust to child expectation Adjust to birth or adoption of child Establish a home for family
Raising children Newborn through preschool School-age child	 Nurture growth and development Adjust to less privacy Encourage education of children Develop community socialization
Adolescent	Balance freedom and responsibility Promote adolescent's independence
Dispersion	
Assist children to move on Readjust unit	Release children with appropriate assistance and stable home base Reestablish own interests and careers Readjust the relationships
Replacement	
Aging Death Children become adults	Maintain connection with other generations Cope with loss of job, significant other, friends, home Adjust to altered living space

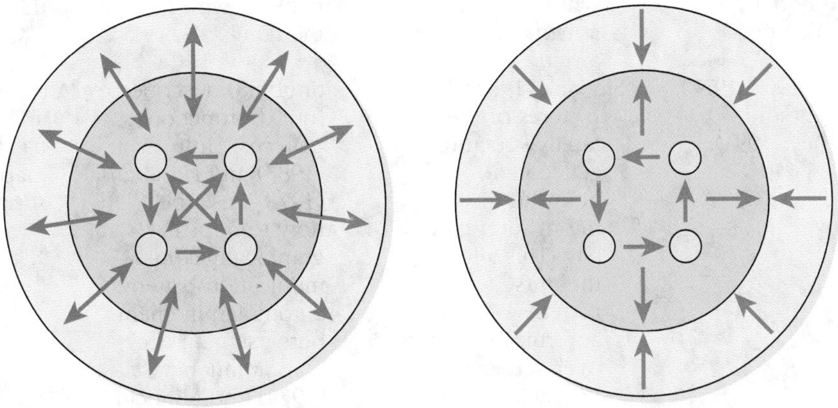

Figure 17-2 • *In a simple systems framework, the family and its members are in the center, and feedback loops interlap. The outer circle is the environment, or, in this chapter, the community: ethnic group, school, church, places of employment, institutions. According to systems theory, the whole is greater than the sum of the parts. In other words, there is no identified person at the center; rather all are equal and interrelated. All systems are acting, reacting, and interacting at the same time. Holistically, everything counts. The functional family (left) has interaction among all systems. The boundary between family and community is a broken circle, allowing for input and output between family and community. The dysfunctional family (right) has limited interaction that goes in only one direction, with a boundary between family and community that does not allow for input and output between those two systems.*

understand when viewing a family as a system. These concepts are wholeness, circular interaction, lack of an identified client, and holistic thinking and are defined as follows:

- Wholeness means that the whole is greater than the sum of its parts. Wholeness includes family values, beliefs, themes, and the rules by which the themes are carried out.
- Circular interaction means that all parts of the system are acting, reacting, and interacting at the same time.
- There is no identified client in systems thinking.
- From a holistic perspective everything—the biologic, psychological, social, and cultural aspects of the family's life—counts.

Family Assessment

Once the nurse has a framework for understanding the family, it is important to know how to assess the family. For each framework, the nurse will collect slightly different data and organize the data according to the

Table 17-2 • Family Assessment Based on Four Specific Frameworks

Areas to Assess	*Developmental Stage*	*Wholeness*	*Communication*	*Support*
Observe	Family behavior is consistent with their developmental stage.	Family themes and rule are explicit and implicit.	Family interaction and patterns of communication between members are recognized.	Types of support (such as emotional or financial) family members give each other.
Compare	Family behavior is similar to that of other families at the same stage of development.	Family rules derive from themes and fit a community standard.	Differences and similarities of interaction and communication patterns are noted among different families.	Family members are able to give and receive the amount of support needed for self and each other.
Interview	Tasks and stage of development the family is working on are clear and understood by members.	Members can articulate what is important in their family and what happens if a member breaks a rule.	Members can state functional and dysfunctional communication patterns within the family.	Members can state if they are receiving sufficient support from others in the family.
References	Duvall (1962, 1977), Wright and Leahey (1994).	Smoyak (1982) uses pictures of the family structure called genograms to display information graphically. This allows the nurse to see patterns of themes and rules repeated over generations. Wright and Leahey (1994) also use an ecomap to depict visually family members' relationships to the larger system.	Satir (1988) describes four dysfunctional patterns. Holman (1983) and Hartman (1978) describe how to depict graphically communication patterns among family members using an ecomap. Minuchin (1974) and Minuchin and Fishman (1981) describe techniques to establish family and communication boundaries. Wright and Leahey (1994) assess emotional, verbal, nonverbal, and circular communication patterns.	Attneave (1975, 1976) and LaFargue (1984) use family network maps to assess family support.

focus and principles of the selected framework. It is beyond the scope of this chapter to discuss various assessment tools; the reader is referred to the references for additional information. At the beginning level, a basic family assessment can be done by observation, comparison, and interview. The areas to be assessed depend on the framework the nurse chooses. Basic areas the nurse might assess are developmental stage, wholeness, communication, and support. These areas can be assessed by observation of behavior in the family, comparison of family behavior to the literature and to other families in similar circumstances, and interview (Table 17-2).

Nursing process in relation to the family is discussed further in Chapter 49.

Family Responsibility for Healthy Function

Family members share responsibility with each other for the functional health of all members. For example, the family should discuss health issues and how to lead

Nursing Assessment

Suggestions to Elicit Information Related to Family Function

Health Perception and Health Management

- What is your perception of your family's state of health?
- Are you able to cope with family health problems?
- Name one thing you do to promote healthy living for yourself and for each member of the family.

Nutrition and Metabolism

- Describe your family's eating patterns.
- What are typical meals and when are they served?
- Do you have any special way of preparing family meals?
- Who is the best cook in the house? Why?

Elimination

- Is garbage disposal a problem for your family?
- How is waste and, specifically, human excrement disposed of in this family?
- What hygiene practices are followed by members of this family after using the toilet?

Activity and Exercise

- How would you characterize the activity level in this family?
- What types of activities does the family engage in as a group? How often does this occur?
- What are the favorite leisure-time activities of this family?

Sleep and Rest

- What is the general sleep pattern in this family?
- What happens when this pattern is disturbed?

Cognition and Perception

- How are decisions made in this family?
- Are your decisions more concrete or more abstract, related more to the past, present, or future?

Self-Perception and Self-Concept

- What does each member like and dislike about being part of this family?
- How would each member describe the family?

Roles and Relationships

- Do you consider the relationship among and between family members to be healthy and supportive? Please explain.

Sexuality and Reproduction

- Is it acceptable to discuss issues of sexuality openly in this family?
- When, how, and what are children told about sexuality? Are you satisfied with your expression of sexuality within the family?
- Have there been any reproductive problems in the family? Please explain.

Coping and Stress Tolerance

- Name a stressful event in the family. What was each member's perception of the event? How did each member cope with it?

Values and Beliefs

- What are important beliefs this family holds? How does each member carry out such beliefs?
- How valued are the activities in which members of the family are engaged?

more healthy lives. The Benoli family is in the *replacement* stage of development; they have grown children. Maintaining a healthy lifestyle in their family might include gardening, walking together, or planning simple activities that include some exercise. The Benoli family eats a healthy Mediterranean diet. The younger generations read labels and discuss the nutritional values of the foods they cook. The accompanying display suggests questions the nurse can ask to elicit information on the interaction of the individual and family as it relates to functional health.

The Community

Nurses in every setting must be aware of their clients' interactions with and within the community. For beginning nursing students, the focus is on resources that exist within the community. The student is encouraged to see clients as individuals within a family within a community. This means that nursing care incorporates the interaction of clients with family members and with other institutions such as employer, religious institution, school, or other social group. As the student progresses through the nursing curriculum, this foundation will be built on so that the nurse can focus appropriate nursing care on any level of need (individual, family, or community) while not losing sight of the relationships between all three levels (Fig. 17-3).

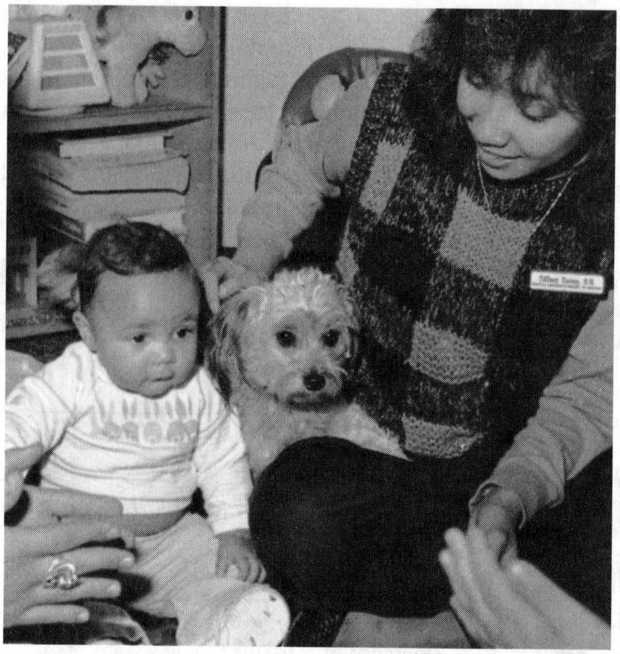

Figure 17-3 • *The nursing student learns about the individual, family, and community during a family healthcare visit. (Courtesy of Seattle University)*

Nursing Research
Community

Selected Nursing Research Studies

Kimball, F. J. (1994). Does an on-site satellite laboratory reduce surgical delays? A study of delays in a same day surgical center. *AORN, 59*(6), 1275–1290.

Molchany, C. A., & Peterson, K. A. (1994). The psychosocial effects of support group intervention on AICD recipients and their significant others. *Progress in Cardiovascular Nursing, 9*(2), 23–29.

Rosenbaum, J. N. (1990). Cultural care of older Greek Canadian widows within Leininger's theory of culture care. *Journal of Transcultural Nursing, 2*(1). 37–47.

Turner-Henson, A., Holaday, B., & O'Sullivan, P. (1992). Sampling rare pediatric populations. *Journal of Pediatric Nursing, 7*(5), 329–334.

Possible Topics for Nursing Inquiry

- Does a person's definition of community make a difference in his or her recovery from an illness?
- Do nurses who assess community data write more individualized Visiting Nurse Service referrals than nurses who do not assess community data?
- Is early discharge of hospitalized clients related to resources within their community?
- Are active community participants as likely to become ill as those who are passive?

Definition of Community

A definition of community and knowledge of types of communities form the foundation for understanding more advanced concepts of community. Much has been written about community, but there is no agreement on a single definition. Each attempt at a definition has had a particular focus, the one most appropriate to the community in question. A brief overview of how the definition of community has been summarized gives the nurse a sense of this variety.

Archer (1985) describes three general types of communities: emotional, structural, and functional communities. These community types are similar to Tucker's view of community "as a spatial unit, as an ethnic group with a common culture, and as an aggregate of people with shared values, interests and goals" (Tucker, 1983, p. 173).

Rubin and Rubin (1986) summarize the sociologists' perspective on community as the integration of linkages between individuals. They place these characteristics on a continuum, along which eight forms of community emerge. At one end is the "highly affective" or traditional community, such as a rural village, and at the opposite end is the "strictly interest group" or community of interest, such as the American Nurses Association.

Higgs and Gustafson (1985) believe that communities are social units and, like individuals, have a hierarchy of needs. They developed a community typology analogous to Maslow's hierarchy of individual needs. Because they view the community as the client, they do not discuss types of communities but rather enumerate functions of a community (1985, p. 12):

- Use of space
- Means of livelihood
- Production, distribution, and consumption of goods and services
- Protection of its members
- Education
- Participation
- Linkage with other systems

For the purposes of this chapter, **community** is defined as a social group whose members may or may not share common geographic boundaries, yet who interact because of common interests or shared values to meet their needs within a larger society.

Types of Communities

A list of the types of communities with examples gives the nurse an awareness of the scope of communities. The purpose in doing this is to make the nurse aware of resources that can be used for clients.

The early work of Warren (1963) still provides a useful approach to ways of examining types of communities. His six types of communities (space, people, institution, interaction, distribution, and social system) are discrete and provide useful guidelines for nursing care. Definitions previously discussed combine several of the types described by Warren. Archer's emotional community and Rubin and Rubin's affective community are not addressed in Warren's list, however. These can be combined into a seventh category: emotional security. Table 17-3 summarizes the seven types of communities.

Community Assessment

When the nurse is able to understand a client's community, nursing care and discharge planning are enhanced through the use of appropriate community resources. The case of Mrs. Benoli illustrates this point. The nurse might ask Mrs. Benoli to describe her community. Such assessment focuses healthcare planning on two points: a method the client finds acceptable, and a method that uses community resources to a maximum. The implications for Mrs. Benoli's nursing care, based on the type of community, are summarized in Table 17-4. This matrix shows possible goals on which the nurse and client could agree. The table is by no means exhaustive but is meant to show the nursing student a preliminary way to think of resources based on client needs and types of communities.

Community Responsibility for Healthy Function

The community environment affects the well-being of the individual and the family. Government, educational, recreational, and healthcare services affect all phases of function. One community may have suitable grocery stores with fresh produce and meats at a reasonable price, whereas another neighborhood may sell questionable products at a higher price. One community

text continues on p. 296

Table 17-3 • *Types of Communities: Their Focus and Selected Examples*

Type	*Focus*	*Example*
Space	Geographic boundaries	Town; hospital; unit of a hospital
People	Characteristics of people	Cajun population in New Orleans; group of adolescent diabetic campers
Institution and Shared Values	Common beliefs and values of a group and their behavior based on those values	American Jesuit Universities; support groups for the caretakers of Alzheimer victims
Interaction of People	Usually centered around interest	Parent–teacher association of a specific school; local nurses association
Distribution of Power	When influence is exerted over others so that, despite resistance, a favorable outcome is obtained	American Association of Retired Persons, American Medical Association
Social System	Interaction between systems	Family–school–hospital–church system
Emotional Security	Emotional ties between people and emphasis on ascribed characteristics	Prenatal classes; ethnic neighbors

Table 17-4 • Implications for Specific Nursing Interventions for Mrs. Benoli by Types of Communities

	Nursing Needs				
Types of Communities	*Mobility*	*Nutrition*	*Communication*	*Interests*	*Spirituality*
Space					
Neighborhood	Set walking criteria within neighborhood boundaries	Eat frequent small meals alone or with one trusted friend	Start with face-to-face communication and a one-to-one interaction with a trusted friend	Engage in gross motor activities around light gardening	Allow priest to come to home while planning how to get to church
People					
Friends in dress shop	Walk to dress shop to meet with friends	Eat with friends; allow them to assist periodically	Communicate first face-to-face, then in writing, and eventually by phone	Accept suggestions from friends to start new hobbies with them	Allow friends to take to church
Values					
Do for self	Walk short distances alone versus longer ones with assistance	Use assistive feeding devices	Use electric typewriter or computer where no assistance is needed and message is clear	Remain with known hobbies and learn to readjust to limitations	Go to church rather than have priest come to home
Interaction					
Stroke support group	Do what others in same circumstances suggest	Do as suggested by leader of the stroke support group	Read and keep abreast of what is new for members of the stroke group, try various methods of communication as encouraged within the group	Consider hobbies other members of the stroke support group can do successfully	Use resources of group to get to and from church

Power					
Italian female elders in the neighborhood	Sees very little need to walk because others will come to her; must walk to maintain independence	Eat with family to maintain public image of being in control	Speak within small sphere of other elderly women	Select a hobby that reflects status and can be mastered	Be physically present at church to act as a role model for the younger generation
Social System					
Interaction between family–dress shop–neighborhood–church–hospital–elders	Walk outdoors daily to carry out necessary chores	Eat a balanced diet daily with family	Contact two people daily: this can be done either face-to-face, in writing, or by phone	Select one hobby that can be done either alone or in a group	Set aside one hour a day for spiritual reflection; allow neighbors to take to church
Emotional Security					
Place of birth: Caravaggio, Italy; ethnic group: Italian	Walk as much as possible; would like to visit Caravaggio once again	Eat the foods her grandmother fixed, which she felt had a therapeutic value	Speak Italian and English; make contact with relatives in Italy	Select a hobby that centers around "the old days," and "the old country"	Pray, which takes a large part of the day; going to church is not as meaningful as it once was

may provide free smoke detectors and teach people how to check batteries, whereas another community ignores the issue of fires and safety. Conversely, some communities may be more prone to fires, such as run-down, crowded, inner-city areas with boarded-up houses and litter-strewn fire hazards.

Systems theory suggests that the community has responsibilities toward the family, but the family also is responsible for taking part in community activities and promoting good services. In the same vein, the community is responsible to the healthcare system for providing adequate facilities and resources. Healthcare workers participate in a feedback loop by volunteering in community activities, acting as resources, and assessing community needs and services.

The display covering family health in the community lists questions to be asked of individuals, community representatives, and nurses. The questions apply to the community at large or, on a smaller scale, to institutions such as hospitals, schools, and factories.

Advanced Community Concepts

One way communities may improve the health of people within their community is by addressing the goals of *Healthy People 2000* (Public Health Service, U.S. Department of Health and Human Services, 1990). Three overall goals targeted for the year 2000 are

- Increase the span of healthy life for Americans
- Reduce health disparities among Americans
- Achieve access to preventive services for all Americans.

This can happen if the community organizes itself. One strategy is to organize based on the typology of *community as a social system.* The community needs to maintain communication among its various social systems such as transportation, health, family, education, finance, safety, religion, and industry. Involvement of all people at some level in the system increases the likelihood of achieving the goals of *Healthy People 2000.*

Organizing and intervening at a community level are advanced concepts that are beyond the level of the beginning nursing student. These concepts require the nurse to conceptualize community as the unit receiving care. There are several approaches to studying community in this way. Higgs and Gustafson (1985), for example, discuss community assessment and diagnosis from four perspectives: epidemiologic, descriptive, systems, and adaptive.

The concept of "at risk" also is a useful concept because it targets the group most likely to encounter health-related problems. In so doing, preventive measures can be taken to stop those problems either before they occur or in the early stages. Research and health programs in the community target "at-risk" communities.

The Functional Approach to Individual, Family, and Community

Looking again at assessments and care being planned and implemented for Mrs. Benoli at the beginning of the chapter, the team planning for her discharge and care realize that an individual's needs are sometimes met in the family or community. The following section plans her care around individual, family, and community participation in functional health.

Health Perception and Health Maintenance. Mrs. Benoli considers herself "sick." As a sick person, she feels she should be cared for and that nurses and physicians should make her well again. The nurse needs to explore the whole area of chronic illness with Mrs. Benoli, focusing on functions she can control. The local Easter Seal Society has agreed to build a ramp with handrails from the sidewalk to the front door. Mrs. Benoli's oldest son will install grab bars in the bathroom to facilitate her independence.

Nutrition and Metabolism. Mrs. Benoli can no longer shop for groceries, cook, or feed herself. The nurse will assess who among family members and friends can do which of these chores. For instance, Mr. Benoli can be taught to shop for groceries, and Mrs. Benoli's friends can take turns with other family members in preparing food. The nurse will pay special attention to teaching Mrs. Benoli to feed herself. The nurse will also teach Mrs. Benoli to evaluate the nutritional values of food so that she makes wise choices about the foods she eats.

Elimination. This is an area Mrs. Benoli is motivated to control. Recently she experienced success with her bowel program, which delighted her. The nurse can capitalize on Mrs. Benoli's motivation in this area to praise her and to point out the relationship between input (food and fluids) and output (stool and urine). Mrs. Benoli can limit her fluid intake to morning and afternoon so she will not have accidents at night.

Activity and Exercise. Mrs. Benoli is hesitant to start walking; she is afraid she will fall and cause more problems. The nurse might build Mrs. Benoli's confidence with exercises to demonstrate to Mrs. Benoli her abilities. Together the nurse and Mrs. Benoli can set goals and destinations for activities Mrs. Benoli would enjoy. One destination Mrs. Benoli would like to reach is her church, so she can attend mass.

Sleep and Rest. Mrs. Benoli feels she gets plenty of rest because she spends so much time in bed. Mrs. Benoli rests frequently during the day, but is fitful at night and hardly ever sleeps more than 2 hours at a time. This is an area of concern, and the nurse has to make a careful assessment.

Nursing Assessment
Suggestions to Elicit Information Related to Community Function

Health Perception and Health Management

- Is your community a safe community in which to live? Why?
- What are the major health problems in your community?
- What health problems are on the decline/increase in this community? Why has this decline/increase happened?
- Review morbidity and mortality statistics for the community.

Nutrition and Metabolism

- Do residents seem well nourished in your community?
- Are there any specific nutritional programs in your community?
- Observe specific groups in the community such as children, pregnant women, and the elderly. What does their nutritional status appear to be?

Elimination

- How is hazardous waste disposed of in your community?
- Does your community have a recyclng plan? How does it work?
- How is household waste disposed of in your community?
- What infectious diseases in your community can be traced to improper waste disposal?

Activity and Exercise

- How efficient is the public transportation system in your community?
- What are the recreational activities in your community? Who plans them?
- Are there parks, and bike and hike paths?
- What are the cultural activities in your community?

Sleep and Rest

- What is the noise level like in your community at night?
- Do noises in the community interfere with your sleep and rest?

Cognition and Perception

- Are the schools providing a good education?
- How are decisions made in this community? Who participates in decisions that affect all community members?
- Observe the process used by any one group to make their voice heard in the community.

Self-Perception and Self-Concept

- Is there a sense that the community "cares for" its residents?
- Are residents proud of their community? Are they fearful?

Roles and Relationships

- Do community institutions collaborate with each other?
- Can individuals access agencies easily in terms of health-related issues?

Sexuality and Reproduction

- What is the attitude toward sex education in your community? Who should be teaching this material? Are they?
- Review the marriage and birth statistics for the community. Note birth rate, age of mother at pregnancy, abortions, and adoptions.

Coping and Stress Tolerance

- What are the issues causing stress in your community? (Examples drawn from other communities are racial tension, child molestation, AIDS, and noise pollution.)

Values and Beliefs

- How effective are the local media (newspaper, radio, television)? Who makes decisions on programming?
- Do people feel strongly about local government? Do they vote?
- What health-related issues would your community spend money on? What issues would they not?
- How would you complete this sentence related to health issues in your community? We believe that health ______________________ ______________________.

Cognition and Perception. Mrs. Benoli is alert and mentally sharp. As her speech improves, it is easier to understand her. The nurse is both affirming and empathetic by talking *to* the client and not *through* the client. In the meantime, her children and husband speak openly and honestly in front of her. They try to include her in all decisions.

Self-Perception and Self-Concept. Mrs. Benoli sees herself as a burden. She says she has regressed in her abilities, causing others to attend to her needs. Her concept of a positive self is one that does not inconvenience others. The nurse can help build Mrs. Benoli's self-concept with honest praise for her accomplishments. Her family, under Mrs. Benoli's direction, will take care of her garden and encourage her to participate as she is able. The Community Garden Club plans to honor her for a hybrid rose she grew just before becoming ill.

Roles and Relationships. The Benoli children say their mother has changed since the stroke. She has become a timid, retiring woman who expects her children not only to take over her care but to take care of their father as she did. The nurse can help Mrs. Benoli understand the changes that have taken place and help her find a satisfactory role to play in her family. As Mrs. Benoli's confidence and independence improve, she can become responsible for much of her own care. Her husband will learn to participate in simple household

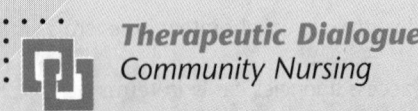

Therapeutic Dialogue
Community Nursing

Scenes for Thought

The following conversations are based on the care of Mrs. Benoli, who is discussed at the beginning of the chapter. You are the community health nurse and are making a visit to Mrs. Benoli to see how she is at home. You find her sitting in a chair on the front porch in the sunshine with her husband.

Effective

Nurse: *Buongiorno, Signora e Signore Benoli. How are you both today?*
Mrs. Benoli: *Ah, hello Susan. You remembered what we taught you last week. Bene, bene!* Smiles broadly and motions you to sit with them.
Nurse: *How are you both doing?*
Mrs. B: *Oh, we're okay. It's good to be home from the hospital.* Looks sideways at her husband.
Nurse: *And how are you, Mr. Benoli?*
Mr. B: *I'm fine now that my wife is home. I worried so much about her when she had the stroke. And I'm glad to have her here, even though she can't do much around the house.* Mrs. B. frowns at him.
Nurse: *You don't look too happy about what your husband said, Mrs. Benoli. What's on your mind?*
Mrs. B: *Well, I can't help it if I can't do what I used to. He gets his meals and our daughter comes in to clean once a week.* She looks insulted.
Nurse: *Perhaps you could talk a little more about what you meant, Mr. Benoli.*
Mr. B: *All I meant, Susan, was that she can't get around as much as she used to. This is one busy woman! And I know it bothers her not to do everything she used to. It bothers me, too. We're just getting old, cara mia, we'll just have to face it.* Pats his wife's hand. She smiles at him, sadly.
Nurse: *Maybe we three can talk about ways you could continue to do what you want to, Mrs. Benoli. I have some ideas that maybe would work out for you.* The couple look at each other and then lean forward a little, watching Susan pull pamphlets out of her bag.

Less Effective

Nurse: *Buongiorno, Signora e Signore. How are you both doing today?*
Mrs. Benoli: *Hello, Sally. You remembered what we taught you last week. Bene, bene!* Motions you to sit down.
Nurse: *So how is it going for you?*
Mrs. B: *Oh, we're okay. It's good to be home from the hospital.* Looks sideways at her husband.
Nurse: *Good for you! I wanted to check with you about how you're getting your meals and who's helping you with the housework. (Takes out notebook to record information.)*
Mrs. B: *My daughter comes once a week to clean and then my daughter-in-law brings us our meals or we go over to her house to eat.*
Nurse: *Sounds like you have it all organized. Are you getting out of the house at all? I remember you liked to go to church as often as you could. (Continues writing.)*
Mrs. B: *Yes, our children take us every Sunday.* Husband and wife look at each other.
Nurse: *Terrific! I think you're doing great, Mrs. Benoli. I'll stop in again next week. Hope the week goes well for you. Bye.*

Critical Thinking Challenge

Analyze who the client is in the above situation. • Identify what Susan observed. • Summarize what Sally missed. • Determine which nurse had the better eye contact and explain why. • Critique the questions each nurse asked.

chores. The community will send a housekeeper once a week for heavier chores.

Sexuality and Reproduction. Intimacy has always been an essential part of the Benolis' relationship. They have managed to maintain this throughout Mrs. Benoli's illness. Often Mr. Benoli sits beside his wife, holding her hand, and singing old Italian love songs to her. She smiles in response. The Benolis function well in this aspect of their lives and do not need help in fulfilling basic needs in these areas.

Coping and Stress Tolerance. In the past, Mrs. Benoli confronted problems head-on. Now her old coping strategies no longer work. The nurse can help her identify and prioritize her stresses. New coping strategies can be developed or old ones adapted to her current abilities.

Values and Beliefs. Mrs. Benoli sees her condition as "old age," and therefore has a resigned attitude toward her present condition. The nurse will learn what Mrs. Benoli values and believes before intervening. The nurse will refocus Mrs. Benoli on her likes, abilities, and accomplishments. The nurse will use the priest and a nun from the nearby convent as sources of strength for Mrs. Benoli's daily life.

The nurse, after assessing which areas need to be addressed and which do not, helps the team develop a plan of care. For example, intervention is not needed in the area of sexuality. On the other hand, the area of values and beliefs is fundamental to understanding Mrs. Benoli's perceptions of health, and need to be addressed early in the nurse–client relationship. Strengthening these areas will help motivate Mrs. Benoli to participate in her own care and restructure her image of herself as a burden.

Key Concepts

Nursing care for the individual is best developed in the context of the client's family and community. An individual can meet some basic activities of daily living independently but often needs the help of family and community.

- The concept of healthy function is useful at individual, family, and community levels.
- Conceptual frameworks provide useful guidelines for organizing family information.
- Developmental frameworks focus on developmental tasks and role expectations of parents and children throughout the life cycle.
- Family systems frameworks look at the interaction of the parts, such as individual members, that make up the whole, the family.
- Different types of communities offer different types of resources to their residents.
- The federal government has established goals to be met by communities by the year 2000.
- Nurses should find a means of participating in the community.

Critical Thinking Challenges

Now that you have studied this chapter, you should be able to apply what you have learned about individuals, families, and communities to the nursing care of Mrs. Benoli. Turn back to the situation at the beginning of the chapter and consider these problems.

1. *Identify the strengths of Mrs. Benoli that will help her cope in her adjustment to her illness.*
2. *Using your information about Mrs. Benoli, analyze her needs and how she can be supported by her family and community.*
3. *Summarize how each member of the healthcare team (eg, physician, nurse, nutritionist, social worker, physical therapist, speech therapist) can participate in planning for Mrs. Benoli's discharge.*

References

American Nurses Association. (1973). *Standards: Nursing practice.* Kansas City, MO: Author.

Archer, S. E. (1985). Selected concepts and process for client-centered community health nursing. In S. E. Archer & R. P. Fleshman (Eds.), *Community health nursing* (3rd ed.) (pp. 96–130). Monterey, CA: Wadsworth Health Sciences.

Attneave, C. L. (1975). *Family network map.* Available from The Boston Family Institute, 315 Dartmouth Street, Boston, MA 02116.

Attneave, C. L. (1976). Social network as the unit of intervention. In P. Guerin (Ed.), *Family therapy: Theory and practice* (pp. 220–231). New York: Gardner Press.

Bowen, M. (1978). *Family therapy in clinical practice.* New York: Janson Arson.

Carter, E. A., & McGoldrick, M. (Eds.). (1980). *The family life cycle: A framework for family therapy.* New York: Gardner Press.

Duvall, E. M. (1962). *Development* (2nd ed.). Philadelphia: J. B. Lippincott.

Duvall, E. M. (1977). *Marriage and family development* (5th ed.). Philadelphia: J. B. Lippincott.

Fortes, M. (1971). Introduction. In J. Goody (Ed.), *The developmental cycle in domestic groups* (reprint) (pp. 1–14). Cambridge: The University Press.

Haley, J. (1971). Approaches to family therapy. In J. Haley (Ed.), *Changing families: A family therapy reader* (pp. 227–236). New York: Grune & Stratton.

Higgs, Z. R., & Gustafson, D. D. (1985). *Community as a client: Assessment and diagnosis*. Philadelphia: F. A. Davis.

Hartman, A. M. (1978). A diagrammatic assessment of family relationships. *Social Casework, 59*, 465–476.

Holman, A. M. (1983). *Family assessment tools for understanding and intervention*. Beverly Hills, CA: Sage Publications.

LaFargue, J. P. (1984). Application of cultural concepts to nursing care: Working with family networks. In J. Uhl (Ed.), *Proceedings of the Ninth Annual Transcultural Nursing Conference* (pp. 14–26). Salt Lake City, UT: The Transcultural Nursing Society.

Maslow, A. H. (1968). *Toward a philosophy of being* (2nd ed.). New York: Van Nostrand Reinhold.

Minuchin, S. (1974). *Families and family therapy*. Cambridge: Harvard University Press.

Minuchin, S., & Fishman, H. C. (1981). *Family therapy techniques*. Cambridge: Harvard University Press.

Public Health Service, U.S. Department of Health and Human Services (1990). *Healthy People 2000*. Washington, DC: Government Printing Office.

Rubin, H. J., & Rubin, I. (1986). *Community organizing and development*. Columbus, OH: Merrill.

Satir, V. (1988). *The new peoplemaking*. Mountain View, CA: Science and Behavior Books.

Smoyak, S. (1982). Family systems: Use of genograms as an assessment tool. In I. W. Clements & D. M. Buchanan (Eds.), *Family therapy: A nursing perspective* (pp. 245–250). New York: John Wiley & Sons.

Tucker, W. H. (1983). The nature of a community. In M. J. Fromer (Ed.), *Community health care and the nursing process* (2nd ed.) (pp. 173–198). St. Louis: C. V. Mosby.

von Bertalanffy, L. (1968). *General system theory: Foundations, development, applications*. New York: George Braziller.

Warren, R. L. (1963). *The community in America*. Chicago: Rand McNally.

Wright, L. M. & Leahey, M. (1994). *Nurses and families: A guide to family assessment and intervention* (2nd ed.). Phiadelphia: F.A. Davis.

Bibliography

Thompson, M. K. (1984). Family development theory. *Nurse Practitioner, 9*(6), 54–58.

Uphols, C. R., & Strickland, O. L. (1989). Issues related to the unit of analysis in family nursing research. *Western Journal of Nursing, 11*, 405–417.

Culture and Ethnicity

Key Terms

Belief
Culture
Culture change
Cultural diversity
Cultural relativity
Cultural sensitivity
Culture shock
Ethnicity or ethnic identity
Ethnocentrism
Key informant
Minority
Race
Racism
Ritual
Stereotype
Subculture
Transcultural nursing

Learning Objectives

Upon completion of this chapter, the student will be able to do the following:

- *Discuss characteristics of culture.*
- *Define concepts related to culture.*
- *Build an understanding of people by viewing human responses in a cultural context.*
- *Identify patterns of behavior that reflect cultural and ethnic influences.*
- *Communicate effectively with people of diverse orientations.*
- *Increase awareness of personal culturation and its influence on nursing practice.*
- *Recognize and discuss cultures and ethnic groups, including one's own, that are represented in one's community of practice.*

18

You work in a rehabilitation facility where you are the primary nurse for 6-year-old Spencer. When Spencer was 3 years old, he was in an automobile accident in which he broke his neck at the first cervical vertebra. He is alert and intelligent, but he is immobile from the neck down, breathes by means of a respirator, and requires total care. His parents are Samoan. They have stated that Spencer will come home for future care. The staff wants to send him to another long-term care facility. How will these two different opinions be resolved?

In earlier chapters, you studied about the interrelationships among the individual, family, and community. This chapter expands your knowledge base with information about culture and ethnicity. As you study the chapter, you will learn how the family and its culture are woven together and affect nursing care. The Critical Thinking Challenges at the end of the chapter will help you apply your body of knowledge to Spencer's care.

Nursing is concerned with human responses to actual or potential health problems (American Nurses Association, 1980). In this chapter, the student is encouraged to think about how those responses might be affected by Spencer's and the nurse's cultural backgrounds. Understanding culture and ethnicity helps improve the quality of nursing care in several ways: by increasing the diversity of people with whom nurses communicate effectively; by enabling nurses to attend more accurately to the integrity of the client as a socially and culturally connected person; and by preventing nurses from imposing, however unintentionally, their own culturally shaped presuppositions on clients and peers.

In the first part of the chapter, theoretical interpretations of culture and related concepts are examined. Related concepts include culture change, ethnicity or ethnic identity, minority, race, racism, ritual, subculture, and stereotype. In the second part of the chapter, the relationship of culture and ethnicity to nursing care is discussed. Particular emphasis is placed on nursing assessment and intervention.

What Is Culture?

Nursing derives the concept of culture and methods for studying it from anthropology. The anthropologic concept of culture is relatively new; it was first defined in print only in 1871 (Tylor, 1871). Since then, various schools of thought about culture have waxed and waned, but most anthropologists would agree that "culture controls behavior in deep and persisting ways, many of which are outside of awareness and therefore beyond conscious control of the individual" (Hall, 1959). In this chapter, the following definition of culture is explained:

> **Culture** is a belief system that the culture members hold, consciously or unconsciously, as absolute truth. That belief system guides everyday behavior and makes it routine; it provides answers to the unanswerable questions of life, sickness, and death; and it makes the world make sense. In fact, it may explain or comprise common sense. Culture thus enables a person to behave reasonably in contexts that she or he shares with members of the same culture.

There are many other definitions of culture. *Culture* can imply qualitative enrichment: the intellectual and aesthetic content of civilizations is called *culture*, and people become *cultured* by engaging in the fine arts such as painting, drama, and opera; bees, fish, and oysters are *cultured* to increase their supply. Culture is also thought to make humans qualitatively distinct, distinguishing *Homo sapiens* from other orders of being. Both psychological and sociologic characteristics have been found in plants (Goetschs, 1937; Rhoades, 1985; Tompkins & Bird, 1972) and in animals (Darling, 1937; Goodall, 1986), but neither is thought to have and create culture. This is because other animals and phylogenetically lower forms of life are believed not to have the capacity that humans do to communicate in symbols. Construction and use of symbols as effective and powerful vehicles of human communication reflects the unique human capacity for culture (Douglas, 1973).

Almost anything can carry symbolic meaning. Colors, for example, tend to do so universally, but their meaning varies across cultures and by context (Berlin & Kay, 1969). Black signifies death and mourning among Westerners, but white does the same for Chinese. Westerners color-code sex (pink and blue) and movement (red and green), but not time or social status. The Thai color-code time and social status, but not sex or movement: they designate a specific color as auspicious for each day of the week and reserve blue for royalty and yellow-gold for monks and the king. Christians clothe their priests in black and white; Mahayana Buddhists clothe their monks in gray; Mien* clothe their shamans in red. The traditional white of hospital nurses' uniforms symbolizes the cleanliness and purity of nursing. Physicians, in contrast, wear white jackets or coats that convey the same symbolic meaning, but with dark pants or skirts, the dark color signifying authority.

Nurse anthropologists generally concur that "whatever a person believes to be true or right about any aspect of his [sic] life stems from his culture" (Brink, 1990). Culture patterns ways of perceiving, interpreting and evaluating, and responding to life and the world (Andrews & Boyle, 1995). It provides a blueprint for reacting, feeling, behaving, and interacting socially. People who grow up or live together in the same community of thought and communication share a culture. Their experiences are carved by a shared cultural heritage. That heritage shapes their behavior just as grammar shapes a language: it provides rules that are so well known to a native that they are followed automatically.

In Western society, for example, spitting in public is considered dirty and aggressive, but exposing the nude body for physical examination by nurses or physicians is a generally accepted protocol. In Moslem societies, in contrast, spitting during ritual ablutions is understood as a religious act of cleansing, and exposure of the bare body, particularly to people of the opposite sex, is highly embarrassing and offensive because it violates strong cultural mores associated with intimacy. Such different interpretations of the same behaviors indicate that culture is learned and taught within a society. Culture is the accumulated "common sense" shared and generated among members of a group. It provides solutions to common problems of living that have been handed down through generations (Leininger, 1970, p. 49).

In Western society, spitting was not disparaged for centuries. Spitting became an unattractive behavior in the West only when public health science changed the understanding of the world by showing that bacteria cause disease and that sputum carries bacteria. What triggered the reversal of Westerners' attitude toward spitting was the association of spitting with tuberculosis, which in the late nineteenth century was highly prevalent and feared. This example shows that culture is created by people, often unconsciously, when their old common sense does not work, as when they attempt to deal with new knowledge, situations, challenges, or threats.

There are two reasons why it is vital for nurses to understand how culture affects behavior and what functions it serves. First, nurses are accountable for observing and assessing clients' responses; second, culture influences all learned human responses. *Culture is, consequently, an integral component of the knowledge base*

*The Mien are a people who live a seminomadic lifestyle of agricultural self-subsistence in the hills of Laos and surrounding countries. Some of them fought with the CIA against the Communists in the 1960s and 1970s in the Vietnam War. With the 1975 takeover of the Laotian government by the communists, many Mien fled as refugees, and some have resettled in the United States.

of nursing. Culture makes communication highly efficient among people who share the same culture, but it can seriously distort and squelch communication among people who do not understand each other's cultures. Culture enables people of similar cultural heritage to understand the meanings of each other's words as part of the particular context in which they are expressed, to "read" each other's nonverbal behavior fairly accurately (often so well that they are barely aware they are doing so; Hall, 1969), and to communicate through symbols.

It has been estimated that at least *two thirds of the meaning of a social interaction is communicated nonverbally,* that is, in gestures, vocalizations (sighs, throat clearing, laughter, grunts, whistling, and so forth), and use of space and distance (Birdwhistell, 1970). This means that even when a nurse cares for a client who speaks English, if the nurse and the client do not understand each other's cultures, they may misconstrue at least two thirds of each other's messages or information.

Characteristics of Culture

Characteristics of culture are discussed here and summarized in the accompanying display.

Culture Is Learned. By sustained contact between groups and by repeated observations of and participation in a group, culture is learned (Fig. 18-1). It takes time to learn a culture. Some of the learning is purposeful, and some is absorbed without awareness. When the culture one has learned is different from the culture learned by the people in one's environment, one can become radically disoriented and stressed. The acute experience of not comprehending the culture in which one is situated is called **culture shock** (Oberg, 1954). Culture shock is a stress syndrome that normally progresses through a series of recognizable stages (honeymoon, disenchantment, beginning resolution, and effective function) to its resolution (Brink & Saunders, 1990). Clients from other cultures or countries where healthcare systems are not as technologically complex as in North America are at risk for culture shock if they are suddenly hospitalized here. Resolution of culture shock requires time, opportunity to observe and participate in the new setting, and careful anticipatory guidance that introduces people, behaviors, and events of the new environment as they affect daily routine.

Culture Is Shared Unequally by Its Members. Because culture is unequally shared by its members, not all members of the same culture act and think alike. Knowing a cultural norm does *not* enable one to predict a person's response. It is particularly inappropriate to generalize about cultural norms in contemporary urban societies because people belong to more than one subcultural group and are influenced uniquely by multiple and diverse reference groups. There are always exceptions to cultural norms. For example, Americans pride themselves on being generous and altruistic and admire others who are the same. Yet millions of people and families with children are homeless on U.S. streets, or do not get basic healthcare because they cannot afford it. Much of American international

Characteristics of Culture

Culture Is

- *Learned from other people*; not innate
- *Learned over a period of time*
- *Shared* by people who communicate with each other over time
- *Shared unequally* by its members: some learn and use more of it than others, and some have and use more access to it or to other cultures than others
- *Dynamic*; it is always changing at variable rates
- *Diversified*; it increases ideas and opinions
- *Reasonable* from the perspective of the members of the culture; it makes good sense to them
- *Implicit*; it is habit and habitated assumptions
- *Not easily described by its own members*
- *Stabilizing;* it makes human responses generally predictable
- *Ethnocentric*; it uses one's own culture as the correct standard
- *Relative* to socioecologic context
- *Pervasive and holistic*
- *Ritualistic*
- *Recognizable* in patterns at many levels

Culture Is Not

- Predictable at the level of the individual
- Necessarily logical or reasonable to the outside observer
- A set of traits

Culture Functions To

- *Guide behavior* by providing a "blueprint" for action
- *Interpret or give meaning to experience*
- *Explain what is otherwise unknowable*: why we are born; why we are born into the families we are; why we suffer our afflications, dream our dreams, die our deaths, and have experiences different from others'

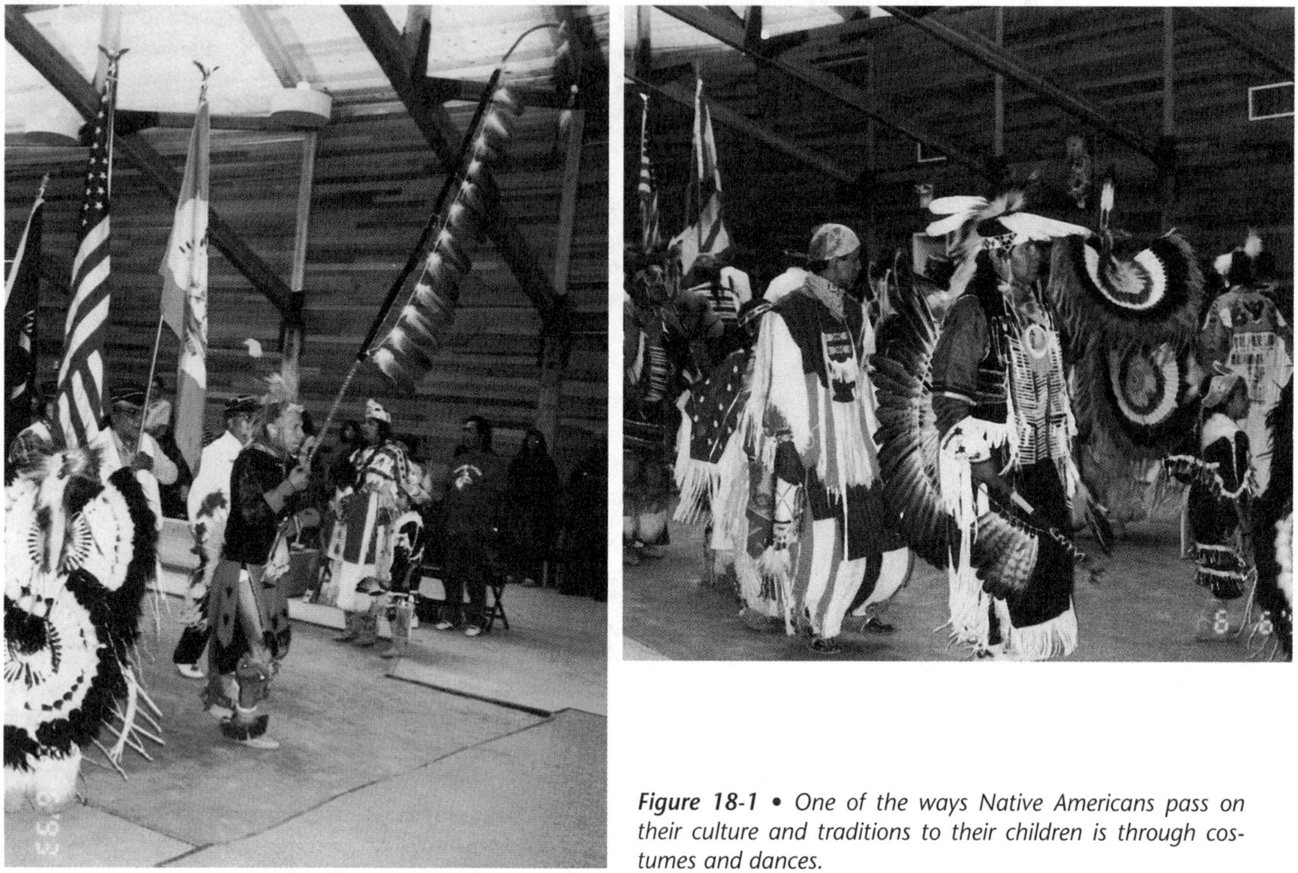

Figure 18-1 • *One of the ways Native Americans pass on their culture and traditions to their children is through costumes and dances.*

aid is actually disposal of surplus or obsolete material that otherwise would not be used. Americans also think of themselves as friendly, yet people from other cultures may view this friendliness as insensitively intrusive or aggressive; and clients waiting in public hospital and clinic waiting rooms are not likely to find the atmosphere there friendly.

People who know certain aspects of their culture better than others are called **key informants**. Usually, key informants not only have an especially rich base of cultural knowledge, they are reflective, like to talk, and have consciously considered their culture so that they can discuss it. Nurses, for example, often make excellent key informants on hospital culture (Germain, 1979; Muecke, 1993).

Culture Is Dynamic. Culture is dynamic. It changes as people come into contact with new beliefs and ideas. Culture change is much more rapid in the twentieth century than ever before because of the vast reduction in distances between different peoples that the communication and transportation industries have achieved. Immigrants and refugees from developing countries who resettle in North America change their cultures quickly (Fig. 18-2). Consciously or not, they revise their culture by blending those things from their original culture that seem to work in their new surroundings with new behaviors, attitudes, or beliefs that they find, often by trial and error, work and make life easier for them. Simultaneously, North American society is changed by the introduction of cultural ideas from refugees, immigrants, foreign business, and media from abroad. For example, there has been a rise in demand for and use of (Chinese) acupuncture in medicine and a surge in popularity of "ethnic" food and restaurants, clothes, and music.

Culture Provides Diversity. The cultural diversity of a population increases the plurality of ideas and options for behavior to which people are exposed, and so adds to the texture and complexity of their society's human resources and potential for well-being and achievement.

Culture Is Reasonable From the Perspective of Its Members. Members of the culture in question find their culture reasonable, even though it might seem illogical, counterproductive, or insensitive to an outsider. People such as spouses in cross-cultural marriages, resettling refugees, clients who come from abroad for specialized healthcare, or those who for whatever reasons move quickly from one culture to another, tend to act according to the rules of their culture of origin. When those rules do not make a reasonable fit with cultural rules in their new setting, they are culturally stressed, at risk for culture shock. Ways in which the culturally informed nurse can minimize this stress are addressed in

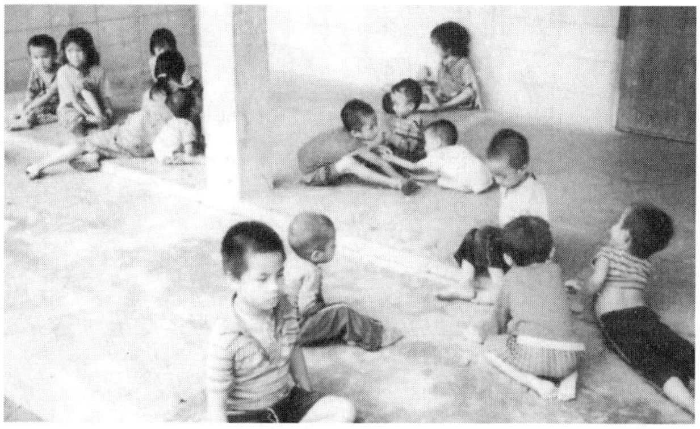

Figure 18-2 • The cultural exposure and understanding of physically disabled children in a refugee camp, Thailand, may be different from other members of their own culture. Further changes occur as they settle in the United States or Canada. (Photo courtesy of Marjorie A. Muecke.)

the section of this chapter on Nursing Assessments Based on the Client's Perspective.

Culture Is Not Easily Described by Its Members. Much of culture is implicit, a combination of habit and habituated assumptions about the world. Habits are enacted without reflection in the daily course of living. Thus, asking clients directly "What do you believe about (for example) prenatal care?" proves a less productive approach than reading about a cultural group or talking with a key informant about it.

Culture Is Habituated Assumptions. Culture is habituated assumptions that people learn through socialization as they grow up and become deeply involved in different subcultures. Cultural habituation is advantageous in that it reduces the extent to which we have to take environmental cues into account—it allows us to respond to routine situations almost without thinking. This is a key element in expertise. Benner (1984) differentiates the expert nurse from the novice nurse on the basis of being able to take in a large number of cues rapidly; to scan, assess, and prioritize them; and to respond appropriately and effectively in unusually short order. To the extent that culture is shared with others in our community, cultural habituation makes our world familiar and predictable. Having a predictable environment, being able to perceive the world as coherent, is essential for our functioning. Without it, we suffer extreme mental stress (Antonovsky, 1980), a mild form of which is culture shock.

Culture Is Ethnocentric. Because much of culture usually is generally learned from authority figures (such as parents, clergy, or celebrities), one tends to hold cultural beliefs as truth. The use of one's own culture as the only correct standard by which to view people of other cultures is **ethnocentrism**. It reflects a fear of difference from one's belief system, and consequent derision or disqualification of people and practices that do not conform to one's own view. Because cultural habituation makes us unaware of many of our cultural assumptions, we are not always aware of our cultural biases. This is why, for example, some whites have difficulty accepting the charge of white supremacy that may be leveled against them by blacks, or why some men have trouble understanding charges of their being male chauvinists by women.

Culture Is Relative. The example of variation in the meanings of colors across cultures given earlier demonstrates the principle of cultural relativity. Another example is the handshake. Westerners attribute trust and agreement to the handshake, and view it as a positive social act. Asians may avoid handshaking because it involves touching a stranger or touching hands that may be dirty. A cultural interpretation of the difference is that the handshake by itself is meaningless; when carried out by Westerners it is invested with one meaning, and when enacted by Asians it has another. At its extreme, the principle of cultural relativity would assume that there is no absolute, that nothing has meaning by itself, that the meaning or significance of any act or symbol is created and assigned by human groups. It has been argued that such an extreme position is untenable because it is amoral. Most nurses accept the principle of cultural relativity only up to a certain (but variable and debatable) degree in order to preserve moral standards.

Culture Is Pervasive. A culture is a systematic way of interpreting people, behaviors, and events holistically. The holistic nature of culture is congenial with nurses' concern that nursing care be holistic, individualized, and safe. Both the cultural and nursing approaches regard people in their entire humanity, and both direct attention to the total context of a person or group (Leininger, 1970, pp. 21-22). Culture links a wide variety of disparate behaviors and events in unique ways. For example, for Western nurses, autopsy is culturally linked to medical beliefs (that cause of death can be discovered or validated by examination of the internal organs and tissues; and that by learning organic causes of death of one person, the deaths of others can be postponed or prevented); to the Cartesian belief in the separation of the body and soul; and to the Judeo-Christian belief that the body ultimately decomposes into "dust" or generic organic matter. Peoples of other cultural heritages may link autopsy with other belief systems and practices. For example, Hmong† who have not converted to Christianity tend to link autopsy to their recent experience of genocide in Laos and to their

†Like the Mien, the Hmong have resettled in Western countries as refugees from the Vietnam War.

Therapeutic Dialogue
Culture

Scenes for Thought

Spencer, whose situation was described at the beginning of the chapter, is being prepared for discharge. Plans are being made for the next step in Spencer's care. A discharge planner at the hospital is having difficulty discussing Spencer's future care with his parents, who are Samoan. The discharge planner asks you, the primary nurse, to speak with them.

Effective

Nurse: *Hello, Mr. and Mrs. Lewis. I appreciate your coming in today. It seems that there has been some difficulty determining where Spencer will go to be cared for next month after his discharge from here. Could you tell me what you see as the problem with placement?*
Mr. Lewis: *We can't let him go to another hospital.* He looks at his hands in his lap. His wife stares straight ahead, her teeth clenched.
Nurse: *You don't seem very comfortable about that decision. Could you tell me more? (In a relaxed manner, seeks more information.)*
Mr. Lewis: *It isn't my decision to make. It doesn't matter what we think.* He looks ashamed and his wife's eyes fill with tears.
Nurse: Trying not to look surprised. *I don't understand. Could you explain that to me?*
Mrs. Lewis: Breathlessly interrupts. *We don't want you to think we're bad parents. We think he should go to another hospital. He needs so much care and we don't know how. . .! Crying.*
Mr. Lewis: *It's because my father is in charge of our family and he makes the decisions for all of us. Especially for Spencer, because I was driving the car and my father thinks I was at fault and shouldn't make decisions for him. He thinks we should take care of him at home.* Looks miserable.
Nurse: *(Nonjudgmental) Thank you for telling me. I understand better now. I have an idea on how we might work this out, but you need to tell me if this will work with your father. (Shows consideration for both the parents' feelings and the cultural conventions.) Suppose we ask him to come to a special team meeting with the doctor and me and all the others who care for Spencer and show him what we do with him all day. Perhaps we can then ask his advice about Spencer's placement. What do you think?*

Mr. and Mrs. Lewis talk this over together and decide that Mr. Lewis Senior would feel important and included. They decide it would be a good idea. They look hopeful.

Less Effective

Nurse: *Hello again. Thank you for coming in this morning. I wanted to talk to you about where to place Spencer after he gets discharged next month. I understand that you want to care for him at home, is that right?*
Mr. Lewis: *Yes.* He looks miserable, his wife stares straight ahead with her teeth clenched.
Nurse: *Do you really think that's a good idea? He has a ventilator, has to be fed three meals a day, exercised with the standing board, turned all the time so his skin stays healthy. Do you think you can handle that?*
Mr. Lewis: *Yes.* His wife is crying quietly beside him and he looks as though he's going to cry, too.
Nurse: Trying not to act exasperated. *Okay, if that's your decision, we'll be happy to work with you on that. When do you want to come here to start learning how to take care of him? I think we can do it in a week and then have you practice for a couple of weeks before we send him home with you.*

Mr. and Mrs. Lewis take deep breaths and start to arrange for each of them to come in and learn about Spencer's care.

Critical Thinking Challenge

Describe the tone each nurse sets at the beginning of the discussion. • Determine who did most of the talking in each of the examples. • Judge if either nurse knew anything about the Samoan culture, and give a reason for your answer. • Examine the method the first nurse used to determine how this particular family operates. • Propose places you could learn about the family structure of the various South Pacific cultures.

beliefs in reincarnation, multiple souls, and the inseparability of body and spirit. They tend to interpret autopsy as preventing the continuation of their society by preventing the union of a person's soul with its body after death, thereby making it impossible to be reborn.

Culture Has Common and Observable Rituals. Rituals are a common and observable expression of culture in the hospital, clinic, home, school, and work settings. Clients and their families practice rituals that are intimately important to them, particularly during illness and hospitalization. For the client and family, observance of rituals in times of stress and uncertainty helps restore a sense of control, competence, and familiarity, and, to the extent it does so, is a desirable adjunct to nursing care. Nurses' observance of professional rituals helps standardize practice and ensure efficiency. Nurse–client misunderstanding, however, may arise unintentionally when the nurse's rituals are incompatible with the client's. For example, a common home remedy for fever among Southeast Asians is to keep the body well covered with clothes or blankets to keep it warm. This secular ritual of caring conflicts with nurses' rituals or procedures of caring for febrile clients, which are designed to cool rather than to warm the body.

Nursing Research
Culture and Ethnicity

Selected Nursing Research Studies

Botash, A. S., Kavey, R. W., Emm, N., et al. (1992). Cardiovascular risk factors in Native American children. *New York State Journal of Medicine, 92*(9), 378–381.

Carroll, M. C., Carter, S. V., & Hayes, E. R. (1993). Attributional theory applied to a baccalaureate nursing community experience. *Journal of Nursing Education, 32*(4), 163–169.

Gilbert, T. J., Percy, C. A., Sugarman, J. R., et al. (1992). Obesity among Navajo adolescents: Relationship to dietary intake and blood pressure. *American Journal of Diseases in Children, 146*, 289–295.

Leininger, M. (1994). Quality of life from a transcultural nursing perspective. *Nursing Science Quarterly, 7*(1), 22–28.

Meleis, A. I., Lipson, J. G., & Paul, S. M. (1992). Ethnicity and health among five Middle Eastern immigrant groups. *Nursing Research, 41*(2), 98–103.

Neves-Arruda, E. N., Larson, P. J., & Meleis, A. I. (1992). Comfort: Immigrant Hispanic cancer patients' views. *Cancer Nursing, 15*(6), 387–394.

Seideman, R. Y., Williams, R., Burns, P., et al. (1994). Culture sensitivity in assessing urban Native American parenting. *Public Health Nursing, 11*(2), 98–103.

Possible Topics for Nursing Inquiry

- What are cultural variations in use of immunizations among parents for their school-age children?
- How does the health–wellness concept of a specific ethnic group affect adherence to treatment programs?
- How does use of prenatal care services relate to cultural identity?
- What cultural factors in a specific ethnic group have a relationship with access to healthcare?
- How does cultural background influence response to pain?

Culture Is Recognizable at Many Levels. The easiest level of culture to recognize is *material*—in artwork, drama, tools, clothes, food, buildings, rituals. Generally, we think of rituals as events such as Thanksgiving dinner, weddings, funerals, and parades; however, there are also nursing rituals—report, handwashing, gowning, nursing rounds, annual professional meetings, and so forth. Harder to recognize are *values and beliefs*. Sometimes they can be accessed by asking about items of material culture. For example, interested, nonjudgmental inquiry about a tattoo on a client's arm could lead to explanations about the person's religious background (from a Coptic Christian), belief in magic (from a Thai), or occupational history (from an American sailor). Sometimes understanding a people's values and beliefs requires long-term contact with careful observation and inquiry about patterns in behavior. Although this is the approach of anthropologists, it takes too long for most nurses. Its results are available to nurses in books, journals, documentary movies and videos, lectures, and coursework.

Concepts Related to Culture

A number of concepts are so closely related to the concept of culture that each may sometimes be used synonymously with culture, but each also carries some specific connotation. The concepts to be discussed are ethnicity or ethnic identity, minority, race, racism, subculture, and stereotype. In North American society, African Americans, Chinese, Hmong, Mexican Americans, whites, and similar categories of peoples may be legitimately referred to as ethnic groups, minorities, or subcultures, depending on context, but each group may also be misleadingly described or stereotyped.

Ethnicity or Ethnic Identity

Ever since Erik Erikson published his "Reflections on the American Identity" in *Childhood and Society* (Erikson, 1950), ethnicity has implied a culturally informed identity (Petersen, et al., 1980). **Ethnicity** or **ethnic identity** refers to a *self-conscious, past-oriented form of identity* that is based on a notion of shared cultural and perhaps ancestral heritage, and current position in larger society. Whites in North America, for example, have an ethnic identity that is grounded in a sense of common European heritage and the associated migration to the land where they were free to develop frontiers. The ethnicity of African Americans in North America is linked to a belief in common descent from African peoples and a history of having been brought from there against their wills as slaves to a land where white supremacists dominated.

What distinguishes ethnic identity from culture is that ethnic identity is self-conscious about select symbolic elements that are taken as the cynosure or emblem of group social identity. In one context, an ethnic group might use native language as its cynosure, as Hmong or Mien do to distinguish themselves from other ethnic groups in North America. In another context, the group might draw on other ethnic indicators, such as style of dress (as when Hmong of one tribe encounter Hmong of another tribe) or religion (as when animist Hmong exclude Christian Hmong from the ranks of "true" Hmong) to stress within group differences.

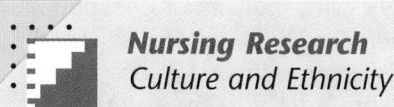

Ethnicity involves the selection of certain shared cultural characteristics as symbols of a common group origin, history, or descent. That selection may be made by the ethnic group or by the larger society to which it is subordinate. Some European American families have adopted children from a race or ethnic group different from their own (Fig. 18-3). This has led to controversies regarding raising children in such a home. For instance, will African American children or Korean children lose their roots? Will they have problems assimilating as they enter adolescence if their predominant community is European American?

Margaret Mead (1982, p. 175) has documented a history of change in North Americans' images of Native Americans:

> The early explorers in the south painted the portraits of the southeast Indians as royalty and nobles, placing on their impressive physiognomy the mark of European aristocracy and dressing them in the clothing of the courts. Faced with a need to come to terms with those who possessed the land and knew how to live on it, the settlers elevated them to petty princes before whom it was no shame to ask for help or to admit failure, in the disease-ridden, inexpertly managed colonies of the southeast.

And, after several centuries of subjection, ruthless pillage, and exile into remote reservations, the ethnic emblems of Native Americans remained ambiguous status symbols:

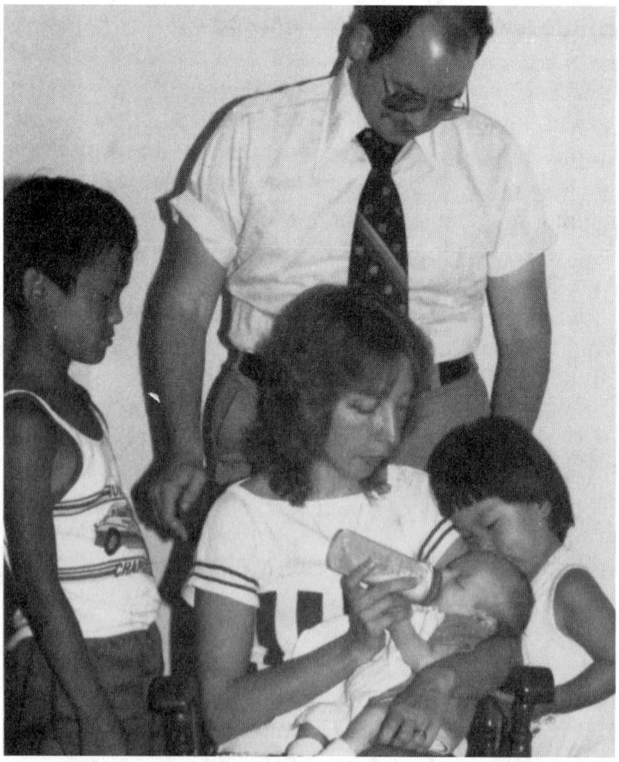

Figure 18-3 • *A European American husband and wife with their newborn. Adopted Korean children are part of the family.*

> Thus, in the 1930s the Indians of Oklahoma who were oil rich used to go to New York and buy theatrical Indian costumes for the poorer members of other tribes to wear in local rodeos. In Florida the remnants of different tribes gathered into an artificial synthesis, costumed in European materials, and set themselves up in tourist-oriented Seminole villages.

Ethnic emblems preserve and create a sense of special social identity (eg, the valuable Indian head nickel), but even such romanticized images as those described by Mead deny regard for the integrity of ethnically badged groups as human beings.

Minority

Several parameters define the term **minority**: social power, size of the population, and ethnicity. Generally, the term refers to a disadvantaged or less powerful group rather than to a numeric minority (Wirth, 1945). A minority does not have the preeminent authority over the society's value system and the allocation of its resources that the dominant segment does (Schermerhorn, 1978, pp. 12–14). People in ethnic groups are usually considered minorities because more ethnic groups are in subordinate than dominant positions in society. Thus, the term emphasizes the political dimension of cultural identity in a pluralistic society such as the United States or Canada, each of which has numerous ethnic groups.

Race

Although the terms *race* and *ethnic group* sometimes refer to the same people, **race** takes biologic characteristics as the markers of separate social status, and ethnic group takes them as markers of cultural identity. The biologic features used to differentiate racial groups are easily identifiable only in the extreme or at the level of large population groups such as Asians, blacks, or whites. They include blood type, bone length, and the size, shape, and number of teeth. There are *no* true or readily identifiable physiologic boundaries between races, however, because interracial marriages have made countless people part of more than one racial heritage. Because criteria for identifying race are so loose, the U.S. Census Bureau no longer uses standardized criteria to identify racial heritage; rather, it asks each person to identify his or her own race or racial mix without regard for the criteria for doing so. This practice equates race with ethnic identity.

Racism

Since the Renaissance, European expansion occurred at the expense of peoples whose skin was of darker hue.

As a result, skin color has become the symbol of both social status or power and cultural difference. **Racism** takes skin color as the primary indicator of social value. In Euro-American society, racism reserves legitimate dominance for those with white skin and penalizes the rest by minimizing their value. This form of racism defines peoples with darker skin as inferior on the basis of accidents of history that denied them resources and privileges of the elite. It is also racist to define people as somehow naturally inferior on the basis of skin color. Racism may be an ideology of the elite who use it to legitimate and perpetuate their dominance and their oppression and exploitation of peoples of different skin color (Schermerhorn, 1978, pp. 73–77). Or racism may be any negative belief or action that stereotypes another person on the basis of skin color.

Subculture

A **subculture** is a holistic belief system that is marginal and subordinate to the belief system of a culture, and that is held most expertly by a recognizable portion of the larger population (Fig. 18-4). The beliefs and standards of a subculture are active only when a person or group acts in a particular social capacity, such as an occupational group or an ethnic group (Harwood, 1981b).

Nursing is a middle-class subculture of Western society, particularly of Western medicine. It epitomizes the valued role of nurturers and caregivers. Nurses reflect many values of the dominant group: they generally adhere to the work ethic, whereby work is seen as a reward, independent of other compensation; they spend much talent and time on planning for the future; they are keenly sensitive to use of time. Nurses are recognizable as a subgroup in numerous ways: by their legally sanctioned authoritative stance vis-à-vis clients and the general public; by their dress; by their language ("nursese" includes a large vocabulary of acronyms specific to healthcare professions, as well as its own subcultural lingo); and by the rituals and ritualized behaviors into which nurses are socialized as nurses. Nurses who are aware of their own subcultural values and behaviors can see how their own cultural make-up might distance, confine, or threaten persons from other cultural backgrounds.

Subcultural identity, like ethnic identity, can be a source of social support, or it can be a target for stigma and exploitation (see Fig. 18-2). For example, in the 1960s, Oscar Lewis' work (Lewis, 1966) spread the misleading notion that poverty is a subculture. He thought that family disorganization made people poor (Harrington, 1962). The theory that culture accounts for poverty blames the poor for being poor: it implies that if people were not fatalistic and if they pulled themselves up by their bootstraps, they would not be poor. Critics disproved this theory by demonstrating that societal mechanisms such as the dependency-making welfare system and the lack of adequate day care for children maintain people in poverty. They have noted that many of the features said to be characteristic of the culture of poverty, such as unemployment and low wages, are characteristic of poverty, not of culture (Stack, 1974; Valentine, 1968). Informed professionals no longer adhere to the notion of a subculture of poverty.

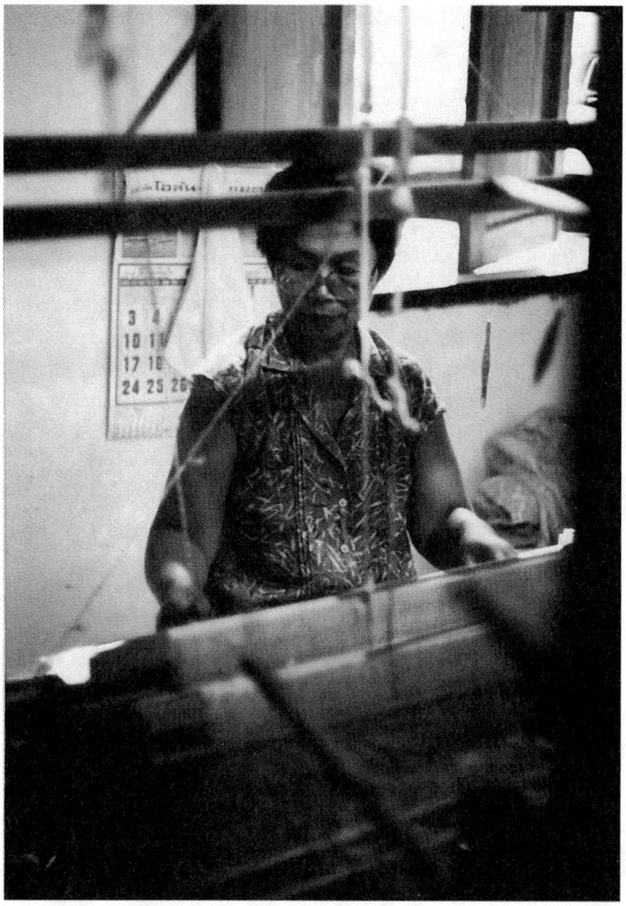

Figure 18-4 • *Cultural traditions are maintained through crafts of members of the cultural group.*

Stereotype

Assigning people to specific categories because of their culture, race, or ethnic emblems is stereotypic thinking. **Stereotypes** are preconceived and untested beliefs about people. They are exaggerated descriptors of character or behavior that are commonly reiterated in the mass media, idiomatic expressions, and folklore. They may be denigrating ("people on welfare are lazy, just living off handouts"; "the rich are greedy and selfish") or idealizing ("Vietnamese are the valedictorians"; "nurses are client people"; "physicians are gods on feet"). Either way, they mislead the hearer and deny the individuality of the person.

Use of stereotypes in nursing results in wrong assessments and, consequently, inappropriate and potentially harmful and unethical interventions or nonaction. For example, acting on the stereotype that "Orientals are stoic" could result in the nurse's failure to assess pain and to undertake nursing measures to alleviate pain in a client who looks "Oriental."

Concepts of Culture and Nursing Care

Culture shapes all learned human responses. Clients have the right to receive care that is culturally acceptable to them. Because nursing focuses on human responses to actual or threatened health problems, nurses increase the quality and safety of their care insofar as they take account of cultural influences on their own, a client's, family's, or community's responses to illness. Culture is an integral component of the knowledge base of nursing.

The field of **transcultural nursing**, described as a synthesis of anthropology and nursing, has been gaining ground in recent years. The focus of transcultural nursing centers on the cultural dimension of care and recognizes that health and illness states are both influenced and determined by the cultural background of an individual (Andrews & Boyle, 1995). Figure 18-5 illustrates the components of transcultural nursing.

Culturally Sensitive Nursing Care

The culturally sensitive nurse is alert to the possibility of cultural influences on behavior as part of routine assessments of clients, families, and communities. Common cues to subcultural or ethnic identity that should be assessed include religion, native language or language spoken at home, strong food preferences, characteristic body adornments (including tattoos, amulets, head coverings, and jewelry), and communication style (including decision making, relationship to authority figures, and relationships to the same and opposite sexes). Once identified, the culturally sensitive nurse arranges to adapt nursing *and* medical care to respect the client's subcultural characteristics to the extent that puts the client at greatest ease while ensuring medical safety. The nurse should expect to find cultural variation in client responses to pain, hygiene practices and exposure of the body, food preferences and eating styles, gestures (eye contact, touch), the sex and age of the healthcare provider, isolation and quiet, and need for visitors, among other areas (MacGregor, 1989).

The cultural assessment should identify not only cultural characteristics of the client to take into account

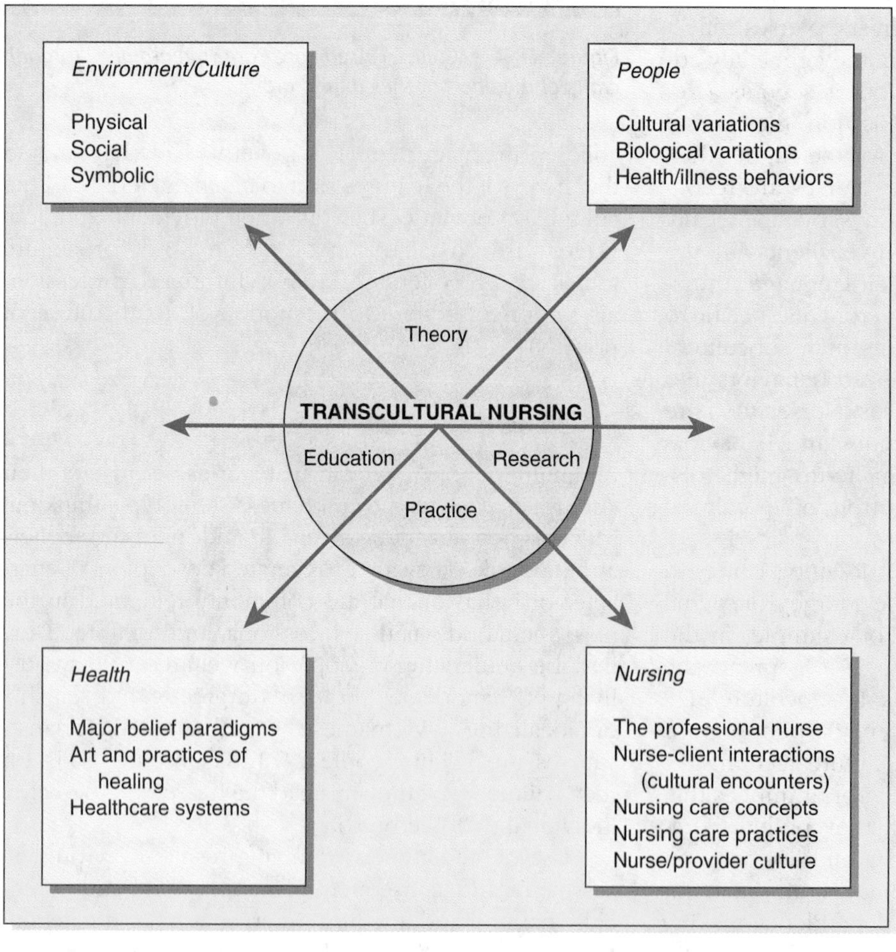

Figure 18-5 • *Model for components in transcultural nursing. (From Andrews M. M. & Boyle J. S. (1995). Transcultural concepts in nursing care [2nd ed]. Philadelphia: J. B. Lippincott)*

for nursing care, but areas of discrepancy between the client's culture and the culture of the nurse and healthcare setting. Areas of discrepancy indicate the need for providing anticipatory guidance and for clarifying nursing and medical expectations for the client. This clarification might require the assistance of a trained interpreter. Culturally informed case management prevents or minimizes culture shock for the client who is embedded in the subculture of a hospital or healthcare agency. It also reinforces the client's sense of competency, thereby promoting learning for self-care.

It is becoming increasingly important for nurses to exercise cultural sensitivity. Demographic trends, such as the rise in average age of the population and the increasing ethnic heterogeneity of the population, expand the proportion of clients for whom primary prevention, health education, and long-term care are fundamental intervention strategies. If these interventions are to result in effective outcomes, the nurse must understand the client's lifestyle, living environment, and values and beliefs. An example is given in the display on Cultural Variation in Health.

Other major but more recent changes in society—the emergence of the AIDS pandemic and the practice of early discharge from hospital—also demand that the nurse take account of the client's cultural orientations. The stigma and emotional responses attached to HIV/AIDS require that nurses be skilled in eliciting the meanings of the illness from their clients and their support persons, and from the public at large *before* undertaking health education about AIDS prevention and control. The shift in site of nursing care away from hospitals to clients' natural environments (homes, workplaces, schools, ambulatory care settings) changes the nurse–client power balance in favor of the client. In the hospital, the client was the guest/visitor in the nurse's domain; outside the hospital, the nurse is the guest of the client. When caring for clients outside the hospital, the nurse needs to learn more from his or her clients.

Cultural Variation in Health: Birthweight and Infant Mortality

People of the same cultural background share some learned standards of behavior that may be reflected in characteristic morbidity, mortality, and fertility patterns. For example, in the United States, the proportion of low-birthweight (<2500 g) infants among total births is lower among Chinese (4.9%) than among other groups for whom figures are available: whites (5.6%), Mexican Americans (5.7%), Hmong (9.9%), and African Americans (12.4%). Similarly, infant mortality rates (per 1000 live births) are lowest among Chinese (5.9), almost twice as high among whites (11.4), and over three times higher among African Americans (21.8).

From Hahn, R. A., & Muecke, M. A. (1987). The anthropology of birth in five populations: Implications for obstetrical practice. *Curr Probl Obstet Gynecol Fertil, 10*(4), 133–171.

Biocultural Variation

People's adaptation to different econiches over the years, group in-marriage, and the transmission of cultural traditions across generations together probably account for much of the genetic variation that occurs among different ethnic and racial groups. Nurses need to take account of the variation in assessing clients. The discussion here is limited to noting variations in growth and development, nutritional tolerance, body odor, and skin color.

Growth and Development. Populations differ in their average adult size, their tempo of growth, and their shape because of complicated interactions of genetic and environmental factors (Fig. 18-6). At the level of population comparisons, there is some racial difference in size, with Asian children distinctly smaller than African or European children, even when all children compared are raised in well-off environments. This difference in standing height should be taken into account when evaluating growth curves of children, whether in well-child screening or for pediatric assessment of response to treatment. Asian and African children also have a faster tempo of growth than Europeans (eg, on average, girls reach menarche at a younger age), but African children are more advanced in skeletal maturity and motor development than Europeans from birth on to adolescence (Tanner, 1978, pp. 137–141). Nutritional status has a strong influence on growth; however, even though disease may cause some growth retardation among children with inadequate diets, the growth usually catches up after the disease is cured. Socioeconomic status also affects growth, most likely because it is associated with type of diet available to the child. In every society studied, children in the upper socioeconomic sector are larger and grow more rapidly (Tanner, 1978, pp. 141–153).

Nutritional Tolerance. Dietary tolerance is associated with both cultural food preferences and biologic variation. White people, for example, have inherited the ability to continue digesting milk sugar after weaning through adulthood, but most of the rest of the world's population become lactose intolerant after the age of 5 years. Symptoms of lactose intolerance are dose dependent; they include bloating, cramps, flatulence, and sometimes diarrhea after the ingestion of milk. Because of the associated poor absorption, milk should be with-

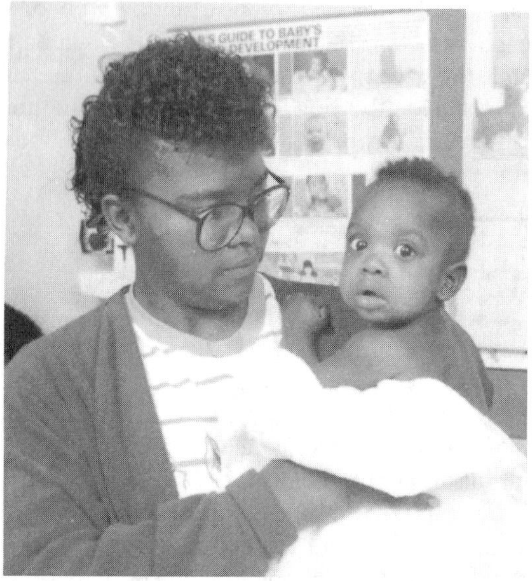

Figure 18-6 • Fostering the parent's understanding of growth and development contributes to family health. (Photo courtesy of the University of Washington School of Nursing.)

held. It is hard to obtain adequate calcium, however, unless milk and milk products are used or unless the diet is high in other calcium-rich foods (nuts, peanut butter, canned fish, cracked roast meat bones in soups, dark green leafy vegetables, and so forth).

There is also a racial difference in reaction to the ingestion of alcohol and alcoholic beverages. Enzymatic differences (lower levels of alcohol dehydrogenase and acetaldehyde dehydrogenase) account for the finding that most Asians and Native Americans experience a rapid onset followed by a slow decrease of blood acetaldehyde levels when alcoholic beverages are consumed. This leaves them with a long period of exposure to the substance that is thought to cause many of the symptoms of alcohol intoxication (facial flushing and other vasomotor symptoms) that are found much less often among blacks and whites (Overfield, 1985).

Body Odor. Both body odor and the ways people respond to it vary among populations. Body odor results from deterioration of apocrine sweat, particularly in the axillary area. Populations that have less body odor include Asians and Native Americans (Andrews & Boyle, 1995). In other populations, cultural patterns determine the extent to which the body odor is disguised, ignored, or enhanced.

Skin Color. Skin color darkens with greater amounts of melanin. Melanin protects the skin from the sun's ultraviolet rays; its presence accounts for the low prevalence of skin cancers found among blacks and Native Americans. *Mongolian spots* are clusters of melanocytes that commonly appear (80% to 90% prevalence) among Native American, Asian, and black newborns as poorly circumscribed, macular, blue-black areas of pigmentation, particularly on the lower back around the buttocks. The pigmentation usually disappears by early childhood. Assessment of oxygenation of the tissues by examination of people with darkly pigmented skin requires practice. Color changes, as in anemic pallor, cyanosis, and jaundice, are most easily observable in the areas that are least densely pigmented: the sclera, conjunctiva, nailbeds, buccal mucosa, tongue, palms and soles. It is normal for some blacks to have bluish pigmentation of the gums and deposits of brown melanin in the sclera.

Nursing Assessments Based on the Client's Perspective

Accurate nursing assessments require that the nurse minimize ethnocentric tendencies and maximize cultural sensitivity. Cultural assessments identify patterns of behavior over time from the same person and from people of similar background. They are fundamental ways to "locate" culture in carrying out the nursing process.

> Subjective data represent the client's/family's view of themselves, their health, their patterns of daily living, demands that are made on them, their usable and unusable resources, and their values and goals. In the subjective data realm the interviewee is *the expert*. It is his [sic] life, his experience, his responses, his resources, and his world as he sees it. In the domain of nursing, gathering and recording subjective data without adulterating it is critical (Carnevali, 1983).

There are several ways to obtain an understanding of the client's perspective. Usually combining several of the methods yields more complete and accurate results than relying on any single one. The most effective methods are open-ended interviewing, a variant of which is the ethnographic interview; the use of key informants; and observation over time (Buchwald, et al., 1993).

Open-Ended Interviewing

A variety of techniques are used in open-ended interviewing to elicit responses from the interviewee that are as free from influence by the interviewer's comments as possible. Open-ended questions require that the respondent use his or her own words to answer. Silent pauses are sometimes useful because they give the respondent time to think about more things to say. Prompts, such as "Could you tell me more about

_______?," encourage the client to elaborate on a point of interest to the nurse.

The Ethnographic Interview

The ethnographic interview is a structured way to elicit the respondent's concepts and understandings (Spradley, 1979). The nurse-interviewer asks questions, the client answers; the nurse-interviewer asks for repeated clarification of the client's responses. Highly skilled nurse-interviewers conduct ethnographic interviews that sound so much like a friendly conversation that the respondent does not feel he or she is being interviewed. In effect, the nurse-interviewer guides the client to teach about the subject at hand. The nurse does this by expressing interest in the topic, incorporating the client's own words, and using hypothetical examples. Asking the client to clarify words reveals their individual meaning. Most important is the sense of mutual effort to gain understanding of the client's perspective that the nurse conveys.

There are three parts to an ethnographic interview.

1. It begins with an open-ended, general question such as "How have you been feeling since I saw you yesterday?" or "I'm wondering about your family . . . ."
2. From the client's response, the nurse selects some *key terms* and asks for clarification. For example, "You felt 'hot in your throat'? I'm not sure what you mean, would you tell me more?" or "You said your 'absent father'—what did you mean by that?" Note the nurse repeats exactly the words and phrases that the client used. The terms are clues to what is important to the client, so the nurse asks the client to talk more about them.
3. The last part of the ethnographic interview is documentation. Information on the client's view of himself or herself or of the issue discussed should be recorded as soon as possible after the interview to retain it as accurately and completely as possible.

Key Informant Technique

The key informant technique is a method in which the interviewer looks for, locates, and interviews people who have expert or a native's knowledge about a culture the interviewer needs to know. They must be willing to discuss it with the interviewer, and there must be rapport. The optimal key informant about a client is the individual client, but medically or culturally compromised clients might not be able to fill the role. Nurses' direct, regular, and ubiquitous (in hospital, clinic, home, school, or workplace) contact with their clients enables them to observe and assess client behaviors, social support system, and environmental constraints and resources. But without an understanding of the cultural meaning of what is observed, the nurses' observations have little value.

For most clients with limited English-speaking ability, the most useful key informants in the hospital or clinic situation are bilingual, bicultural, *trained* interpreters (Putsch, 1985; U.S. Department of Health and Human Services, 1985). Unfortunately, only a small proportion of healthcare agencies have hired such experts. Others who might make useful key informants for nurses include the ethnic herbalist or druggist and the religious official (particularly on matters relating to preparation for death, emotional disturbances and social crises, and for explanations of illness; Muecke, 1987). The role of the religious official in health is often overlooked. It is important, however, because people usually interpret life–death and health–illness issues in terms of their cultural heritage of religious beliefs.

The following examples indicate the diversity of religious practitioners who might serve as key informants for different ethnic groups in the United States. For *African Americans*, ministers and church mothers can be excellent informants because the church plays a strong central role in many African American communities (Jacques, 1976). Church mothers are particularly well informed about pregnancy, childbirthing, and women's health in general. For *Haitian Americans*, a voodoo priest is the expert in the mythology of spirits and the use of plants for home remedies (Laguerre, 1981). For *Mexican Americans* who are Roman Catholic, the priest as well as the *curandera* (secular folk healer; Kiev, 1968) may be useful informants on people's self-diagnoses and self-care practices. Many Mexicans are Protestant; a minister of the client's particular sect should be sought because there is a vast difference between the nonpossessional sects (those that do not believe in spirit possession, such as Baptist, Methodist, Seventh-Day Adventist) and the possessional sects (Pentecostals believe in spirit possession and the healing power of prayer, and oppose the use of medicines and biomedical services; Clark, 1970; Kay, 1977; Rubel, 1966; Schreiber & Homiak, 1981). For *Native Americans*, candidates for key informants vary by tribe. *Navajo* practice a wide diversity of religious practices: on the reservation, a peyote leader would be an important informant on health-related problems and behavior; other informants would be ministers of evangelical groups (Baptist, Nazarene, Pentecostals; Kunitz & Levy, 1981). The *Apache* and *Pueblo* of the Southwest rely heavily on medicine men (Joe, Gallerito, & Pino, 1976). For *Puerto Ricans*, both spiritist healers (people who are said to lend their bodies to spirits who communicate through them) and Pentecostal ministers may be helpful informants for conditions not recognized or curable by biomedicine, such as emotional disturbances, incurable chronic or terminal illness, intractable somatic symptoms, and life crisis adjustments (Garrison, 1977; Harwood, 1981a).

Language Differences Between the Client and the Nurse

A deliberate search for the meaning behind client responses enables the nurse to plan and provide safe and individualized client care. Language differences between the nurse and client compound cultural differences between them, however, and can keep the nurse from getting at the client's point of view (Berkanovic, 1980). When the client does not speak the same language or does so only to a limited extent, the nurse may decide to act in the client's best interests—without actually knowing what the client thinks those interests are. For example, when a client from an ethnic minority is alert but nontalkative or responds only with affirmatives, healthcare providers might conclude that the client does not understand English. If there is no interpreter at hand, they might do what they think is best or necessary for the client even if they do not have the subjective data normally required to guide clinical decision making. The result can be tragic in terms of client welfare and loss of trust with a subcultural community (Fink & Yang, 1983).

For example:

An international client of limited English-speaking ability underwent major surgery and recuperated without complications in the intensive care unit (ICU) of a tertiary care hospital. The staff liked him very much. After he was transferred to a regular care unit, his behavior changed dramatically: he exhibited anxious and paranoid behavior. When a psychiatric consultant and interpreter were brought in to handle the problem, they became the first healthcare providers to attempt to access the client's point of view. They found that the transfer from the ICU to a regular unit did not signify recuperation to the client at all. In fact, he interpreted it as meaning the hospital had given up on him because they thought he was so sick that he was no longer worth caring for. In his view, he had been moved from an environment of expert care and the best of technologic assistance into an old part of the hospital that was practically devoid of technologic props and wanting in staff to tend to him. The healthcare team's belief that the transfer was a self-explanatory demonstration of recuperation is a classic example of medical/nursing ethnocentrism, because they neglected to assess the client's perspective.

The client's confusion, fear, and isolation were all preventable: they could be considered iatrogenic, that is, caused by hospitalization. Cases such as this could be defined as negligent in today's healthcare system because an interpreter should have been obtained to explain to the client what the plans for him were before transferring him to another unit. *Hospitals are obliged to provide trained language interpreters for "the client who does not speak or understand the predominant language of the community"* (Joint Commission on Accreditation of Hospitals, 1985). Furthermore, hospitals that receive Medicare or Medicaid reimbursement are subject to Title VI of the Civil Rights Act, which prohibits recipients of federal funds from discriminating or denying benefits on the basis of race, color, or national origin: hospitals that fail to provide trained interpreters for non- or limited-English speaking people, or for deaf people who use sign language, are in violation of the law (U.S. Department of Health and Human Services, 1982). The nurse who is frustrated in efforts to communicate with a client owing to language differences or impaired hearing or speech, and unable to provide the quality of care deemed appropriate, has legal recourse *to urge a hospital to provide a trained interpreter to resolve the difficulty* (U.S. Department of Health and Human Services, 1985).

It is important to secure trained interpreters rather than bilingual members of the client's family or friends, however well intentioned or convenient the latter might be. Much of the vocabulary of the medical world is difficult to translate into some languages. For example, the phrase "the lab tech dialed the wrong number" could not be translated into a language of a culture that did not have telephones or scientific laboratories (Werner & Campbell, 1973). Furthermore, should the client's condition deteriorate, the emotional burden of responsibility could be overwhelming on someone close to the client.

For example:

A Vietnamese woman was hospitalized with cancer; her 20-year-old daughter was in a nursing home with leukemia. The husband–father spoke little English. The hospital staff relied on the 12-year-old daughter–sister to interpret for them. First the sister died, then the mother. The 12-year-old, suffering from a sense of complicity in their deaths because of her influence on their care owing to her role as translator, had an acute psychotic episode for which she had to be institutionalized. Perhaps this tragic outcome could have been prevented by using a professional interpreter.

A person's need for an interpreter should be established at first contact with the healthcare agency. An interpreter should be provided whenever requested, and definitely at any time when plans for the client are being made or a change in procedure inaugurated. The occasions that an interpreter should be involved include during admission, for consent for treatment, during treatments, for discharge planning, for client education, and so forth. Tips for communicating through an interpreter are given in the accompanying display.

Nursing Care Guidelines
Communicating Through an Interpreter

- Speak *to the client* rather than to the interpreter: this enables the client to "read" your nonverbal language.
- Watch the verbal and nonverbal interactions between the interpreter and client: "read" their nonverbal language.
- *Speak slowly.*
- Use simple sentences.
- Rephrase a question in different words or ask it indirectly if the answer you received is inappropriate or inconsistent with other indications.
- Avoid using metaphors: they are too hard to translate (eg., "Have you been feeling down?", "Once in a blue moon," "Does it feel like pins and needles?").
- Expect that it might take an interpreter much longer to say or explain something in another language than in English. This is particularly true when the concept is a medical one for which there is no equivalent in the other language or culture, or when the topic is considered taboo or embarrassing in the other culture.
- When unsure how to bring up a delicate subject, ask the interpreter for advice; use the interpreter as a key informant on the culture of the client.
- Try to work consistently with the same interpreter; with practice, you both can learn to communicate better with each other.
- Relate to the interpreter as a professional colleague; your nursing care depends on the interpreter's skill.

Increased Effectiveness of Client Education

The culturally sensitive nurse looks for patterns in the occurrence of unusual behavior in a client from a subculture or ethnic group other than his or her own. The nurse who understands the principle of cultural relativity expects that there is an underlying explanation for behavior, particularly for behavior that is repeated by different people of the same culture or ethnic group. When refugees from rural and mountainous areas of Southeast Asia first arrived in the United States, health-care and social service providers had many stories of the "funny" and "bad" things they did. Analysis of these stories identified clusterings of similar tales, each cluster representing unfamiliarity with Western ways. Nurses interpreted the unfamiliarity as areas of poor previous communication and, therefore, as the starting points for health education. Some of the frequent problems were:

When women who were taking birth control pills forgot to take a pill, they either took two pills the next day, or gave the extra pill to their husbands.

A large number of newborns in families of non–English-speaking refugees were brought into the emergency room with dehydration.

Many refugee households with newborns put the heat on in their apartments even during the hot summer, and they swaddled infants and toddlers who had fevers in layers of clothing.

By using the ethnographic interview, observing in clients' homes, and consulting key informants, the nurses discovered the following rationales for the refugee behaviors:

The women who forgot to take a birth control pill were trying to compensate for its omission. Because they did not know the principles on which the pills work, they made legitimate guesses about how to overcome their oversight. Also, their cultural heritage had taught them not to ask questions of authority figures lest they be considered rude and offensive.

The mothers of dehydrated babies had followed infant feeding instructions that they had been given in the postpartum unit. A hospital nurse who researched the problem discovered that the mothers had learned their lesson well. The problem was that the method they were taught was correct only for the ready-to-use formula for which the hospital gave out free samples. Once those samples were used up, the women began using formula from the Women, Infants, and Children (WIC) Program. The WIC milk was dry powder. Because the women could not read the English language directions on the labels, they guessed how to mix the dry formula. Many guessed wrong, resulting in dehydrated babies.

The households that turned the heat up and overdressed children with fevers were exercising their belief in the humoral theory of physiology that is prevalent in Southeast Asia (Muecke, 1976). According to this theory, blood is "hot." Because women lose blood during delivery, they lose heat; to keep them from getting sick, their bodies must be kept so warm that they regain the "heat" they have lost. Similarly, children, who tend to have higher fevers than adults, are thought to lose "heat" when they have a fever; dressing them warmly is thought to prevent "heat" from leaving their bodies.

The culturally sensitive nursing assessments that revealed these rationales for untoward self-care practices provided a highly valid basis for nursing diagnoses and related client education. The health education that resulted from these assessments increased the clients' and their ethnic communities' trust of nurses and of health-care agencies.

Key Concepts

- Culture is defined as a belief system that the culture members hold, consciously or unconsciously, as absolute truth.
- This belief system guides everyday behavior and makes it routine; provides answers to the unanswerable questions of life, sickness, and death; and makes the world make sense.
- Culture enables a person to behave reasonably in contexts that the person shares with members of the same culture.
- Culture is an integral component of the knowledge base of nursing.
- Accurate nursing assessments require that the nurse minimize ethnocentric tendencies and maximize cultural sensitivity.
- Physical assessment skills require knowledge of biocultural variation in such areas as growth, nutritional tolerance and preference, skin color, and body odor.
- Client assessments that take account of the client's perspective are most likely to yield diagnoses and interventions appropriate to the client.
- Methods to gain the client's perspective include open-ended interviewing, a variant of which is the ethnographic interview; the use of key informants; observation over time; and use of the client's language.

Critical Thinking Challenges

Now that you have studied this chapter, you should be able to apply what you have learned. Turn back to the situation involving Spencer at the beginning of the chapter and consider these issues.

1. *Determine the major problems Spencer's parents would have if they cared for Spencer at home.*
2. *Considering your own cultural background, analyze how you would feel if you were Spencer's parent and indicate how you would respond in this situation.*
3. *Analyze how your cultural background affected your thinking (1) when you originally read about the family, and (2) after you studied the chapter.*

References

American Nurses Association. (1980). *Nursing: A social policy statement* (p. 9). Kansas City, MO: Author.

Andrews, M. M., & Boyle, J. S. (1995). *Transcultural concepts in nursing care* (2nd ed.). Philadelphia: J. B. Lippincott.

Antonovsky, A. (1980). *Health, stress and coping.* San Francisco: Jossey-Bass.

Benner, P. (1984). *From novice to expert: Excellence and power in clinical nursing practice.* Menlo Park, CA: Addison-Wesley.

Berkanovic, E. (1980). The effect of inadequate language translation on Hispanic's responses to health surveys. *American Journal Public Health, 70,* 1273–1276.

Berlin, B., & Kay, P. (1969). *Basic color terms: Their universality and evolution.* Berkeley: University of California Press.

Birdwhistell, R. L. (1970). *Kinesics and context: Essays on body motion communication.* Philadelphia: University of Pennsylvania Press.

Brink, P. J. (Ed.). (1990). *Transcultural nursing: A book of readings* (p. 3). Prospect Height, IL: Wavel and Press.

Brink, P. J., & Saunders, J. M. (1990). Culture shock: Theoretical and applied. In P. J. Brink (Ed.), *Transcultural nursing: A book of readings* (pp. 126–138). Prospect Height, IL: Wavel and Press.

Buchwald, D., Caralis, P., Gany, F., et al. (1993). The medical interview across cultures. *Patient Care, 27,* 141–166.

Carnevali, D. L. (1983). *Nursing care planning: Diagnosis and management* (3rd ed.) (p. 93). Philadelphia: J. B. Lippincott.

Clark, M. (1970). *Health in the Mexican-American culture* (2nd ed.). Berkeley: University of California Press.

Darling, F. F. (1937). *A herd of red deer.* London: Oxford University Press.

Douglas, M. (1973). *Natural symbols.* Middlesex, England: Penguin Books.

Erikson, E. H. (1950). *Childhood and society.* New York: W. W. Norton.

Fink, J., & Yang, D. (1983). *Peace has not been made: A case history of a Hmong family's encounter with a hospital* (video). Rhode Island Office of Refugee Resettlement.

Garrison, V. (1977). Doctor, *espiritista* or psychiatrist: Health-seeking behavior in a Puerto Rican neighborhood of New York City. *Medical Anthropology, 1*(2), 54–180.

Germain, C. (1979). *The cancer unit: An ethnography.* Wakefield, MA: Nursing Resources.

Goetschs, W. (1937). *The ants.* Ann Arbor: University of Michigan Press.

Goodall, J. (1986). *The chimpanzees of Gombe: Patterns of behavior.* Cambridge, MA: Belknap Press.

Hall, E. T. (1959). *The silent language* (p. 35). Greenwich, CT: Fawcett Premier.

Hall, E. T. (1969). *The hidden dimension.* Garden City, NY: Anchor Press/Doubleday.

Harrington, M. (1962). *The other America*. New York: Macmillan.

Harwood, A. (1981a). Mainland Puerto Ricans. In A. J. Harwood (Ed.), *Ethnicity and medical care* (pp. 397–481). Cambridge, MA: Harvard University Press.

Harwood, A. (Ed.). (1981b). *Ethnicity and medical care* (p. 27). Cambridge, MA: Harvard University Press.

Jacques, G. (1976). Cultural health traditions: A black perspective. In M. F. Branch & P. P. Paxton (Eds.), *Providing safe nursing care for ethnic people of color* (pp. 116–134). New York: Appleton-Century-Crofts.

Joe, J., Gallerito, C., & Pino, J. (1976). Cultural health traditions: American Indian perspectives. In M. F. Branch & P. P. Paxton (Eds.), *Providing safe nursing care for ethnic people of color* (pp. 81–98). New York: Appleton-Century-Crofts.

Joint Commission on Accreditation of Hospitals. (1985). Rights and responsibilities of patients. In *AMH-85 Accreditation manual for hospitals* (p. xi). Chicago, IL: Author.

Kay, M. A. (1977). Health and illness in a Mexican-American barrio. In E. Spicer (Ed.), *Ethnic medicine in the Southwest*. Tucson, AZ: University of Arizona Press.

Kiev, A. (1968). *Curanderismo*. New York: The Free Press.

Kunitz, S. J., & Levy, J. E. (1981). Navajos. In A. J. Harwood (Ed.), *Ethnicity and medical care* (pp. 337–396). Cambridge, MA: Harvard University Press.

Laguerre, M. S. (1981). Haitian Americans. In A. J. Harwood (Ed.), *Ethnicity and medical care* (pp. 172–210). Cambridge, MA: Harvard University Press.

Leininger, M. M. (1970). *Nursing and anthropology: Two worlds to blend*. New York: John Wiley & Sons.

Lewis, O. (1966). The culture of poverty. *Sci Am 215*(4), 19–25.

MacGregor, F. C. (1990). Uncooperative patients: Some cultural interpretations. *Am J Nurs 67*(1), 88–91 [Reprinted in Brink, P. J. (Ed.). (1990). *Transcultural nursing: A book of readings* (pp. 36–43). Prospect Height, IL: Wavel and Press

Mead, M. (1982). Ethnicity and anthropology in America. In G. De Vos & L. Romanucci-Ross (Eds.). *Ethnic identity: Cultural continuities and change* (pp. 175–177). Chicago: University of Chicago Press.

Muecke, M. A. (1976). Health care systems as socializing agents: Childbearing the North Thai and Western ways. *Soc Sci Med, 10*, 377–383.

Muecke, M. A. (1987). Resettled refugees' reconstruction of identity: Lao in Seattle. *Urban Anthropology 16*(1), 273–290.

Muecke, M. A. (1993). On evaluating ethnographies. In J. Morse, (Ed.), *Critical issues in qualitative research methods*. Newbury Park, CA: Sage.

Oberg, K. (1954). *Culture shock*. Indianapolis: Bobbs-Merrill.

Overfield, T. (1985). *Biologic variation in health and illness: Race, age, and sex differences* (pp. 80–81). Menlo Park, CA: Addison-Wesley.

Petersen, W., Novak, M., & Gleason, P. (1980). *Concepts of ethnicity* (pp. 56, 116). Littleton, MA: Harvard University Press.

Putsch, R. W., III. (1985). The special case of interpreters in health care. *JAMA, 254*, 3344–3348.

Rhoades, D. F. (1985). Pheromonal communication between plants. In G. A. Cooper-Driver, T. Swain, & E. E. Conn (Eds.), *Chemically mediated interactions between plants and other organisms* (pp. 195–218). New York: Plenum.

Rubel, A. J. (1966). *Across the tracks: Mexican Americans in a Texas city*. Austin: University of Texas Press.

Schermerhorn, R. A. (1978). *Comparative ethnic relations: A framework for theory and research*. Chicago: University of Chicago Press.

Schreiber, J. M., & Homiak, J. P. (1981). Mexican Americans. In A. J. Harwood (Ed.), *Ethnicity and medical care* (pp. 264–336). Cambridge, MA: Harvard University Press.

Spradley, J. P. (1979). *The ethnographic interview*. New York: Holt, Rinehart & Winston.

Stack, C. (1974). *All our kin: Strategies for survival in a black community*. New York: Harper & Row.

Tanner, J. M. (1978). *Foetus into man: Physical growth from conception to maturity*. Cambridge, MA: Harvard University Press.

Tompkins, P., & Bird, C. (1972). *The secret life of plants*. New York: Avon Books.

Tylor, E. B. (1871). *Primitive culture*. London: Murray.

U. S. Department of Health and Human Services. (1982). *Your rights under Title VI of the Civil Rights Act of 1964 in Health and Human Service Programs, HHS 391*. Washington, DC: Author.

U.S. Department of Health and Human Services, Office for Civil Rights. (1985, February). *How to establish effective communication procedures for people with limited English proficiency and for people with impaired hearing, vision, or speech*. Region X, Seattle, WA: Author.

Valentine, C. A. (1968). *Culture and poverty: Critique and counterproposals*. Chicago: University of Chicago Press.

Werner, O., & Campbell, D. T. (1973). Translating, working through interpreters and the problem of decentering. In R. Naroll & R. Cohen (Eds.), *A handbook of method in cultural anthropology* (pp. 398–420). Irvington-on-Hudson, NY: Columbia University Press.

Wirth, L. (1945). The problem of minority groups. In R. Linton (Ed.), *The science of man in the world crisis*. New York: Columbia University Press.

Bibliography

Adams, R., Briones, E., and Rentfro, A. (1992). Cultural consideration: Developing a nursing care delivery system for a Hispanic community. *Nurs Clin North Am, 27*(1), 107–117.

Andrews, M. M. (1992). Cultural perspectives on nursing in the 21st century. *J Prof Nurs, 9*(1), 1–9.

Campinha-Bacote, J., and Ferguson, S. (1991). Cultural considerations in childrearing practices: A transcultural perspective. *Journal of the National Black Nurses Association, 5*(1), 11–17.

Leininger, M. (1991). *Culture care diversity and universality: A theory of nursing*. New York: National League for Nursing.

Reeb, R. (1992). Granny midwives in Mississippi. *Journal of Transcultural Nursing, 3*(2), 18–27.

Wenger, A. (1992). Transcultural nursing and health care issues in urban and rural contexts. *Journal of Transcultural Nursing, 3*(2), 4–10.

Values

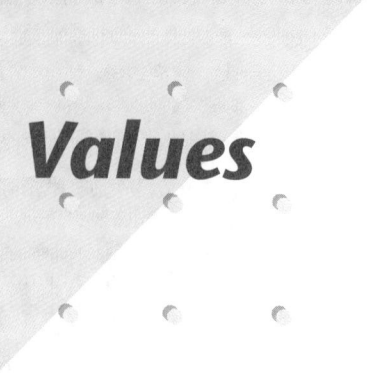

Key Terms	Learning Objectives
Attitudes Action values Behaviors Beliefs Choice values Cultural value orientation Hierarchy of skills Imaginal skills Instrumental skills Interpersonal skills Moral values Operative (means) values Systems skills Terminal (ends) values Values Value system Vision values World view	Upon completion of this chapter, the student will be able to do the following: • Define values. • Identify sources of professional nursing values. • Apply developmental and cultural perspectives when identifying values. • Relate values with functional health patterns. • Examine values conflict and resolution in nursing care situations. • Integrate values assessment into nursing care. • Appreciate the impact of values in situations such as the initial nursing assessment and healthcare planning.

19

You are a nurse volunteer in a program serving homeless women in the downtown area of a large city. One of the women with whom you have talked before approaches you after a health class. She asks you to look at her abdomen. It is the size of a soccer ball. You also notice that she has swollen legs and ankles. She says she has had fibroids for several years and that the medical center where she goes for healthcare has encouraged her to have surgery. If she were to have surgery, she would have to sign a release that says a hysterectomy can be performed if it is necessary as part of the surgical procedure. She describes her family of origin as very child focused, and she says she will not agree to have any surgery that would make it impossible for her to have children.

In this unit, you have been learning about concepts essential for human function. You now have a knowledge base that includes health and wellness; development across the lifespan; individual, family, and community functions; and cultural and ethnic factors. In this chapter, you will study the importance of attitudes, beliefs, and values. These factors will increase your knowledge base to work with people such as the woman in the volunteer program. The Critical Thinking Challenges at the end of the chapter will increase your awareness of your own values and the values of people with whom you come in contact.

What is really important in your life? How do you decide what actions to take? On what do you base your decisions? The answers to these questions are found when you examine your attitudes, beliefs, and values. People who do not take time to reflect on these issues often are unclear in their purpose in life. They may find that decision-making is difficult because they cannot effectively articulate or defend their position. They lack an awareness of their inner self or being.

As beginning students of nursing, you have decided that you want to work with people and help them improve their health. If you examine the thoughts and feelings connected with this decision, you will find that you have a positive attitude toward people, that you like to be with people. You also probably like the study of the biologic and social sciences. There may have been a variety of other influences on your choice to become a nurse, such as other family members who are healthcare professionals. Perhaps you understood the critical need for caring nurses in a world of pain and suffering. Your decision to become a professional nurse is deep, reflecting your core attitudes, beliefs, and values. Ultimately, these values, beliefs, and attitudes will emerge in the way you care for clients and their families.

Just as you have core attitudes, beliefs, and values, so do the clients, their families, and the healthcare organizations with which you will be working. Clients and families will demonstrate their values by their behaviors, whereas healthcare organizations demonstrate values in mission statements and policies.

Usually, the conflicts that nurses observe or deal with have a value base. These value conflicts represent a variety of preferences and levels of development, and they can lead to ethical dilemmas for nurses and clients. Whatever the conflict, it is important for nurses to understand their own attitudes, beliefs, and values and be sensitive to others' value systems to be effective healthcare providers.

Value and Belief Patterns

Values are standards for decision-making that endure for a significant time in one's life (Hall, Kalven, Rosen, & Taylor, 1982). Values have four parts: thinking, choosing, feeling, and behaving (King, 1984). The first aspect of a value is that it is an abstract idea, for example "truth." The word "truth" means little until one makes a choice about being honest and consequently behaves in a truthful manner. Unless a person has thought about the concepts of truth and honesty, these values remain unchosen and would not be easily articulated unless behaviors or choices were questioned or explored.

A **value system** is an enduring set of principles and rules organized into a hierarchy (Rokeach, 1973). When choosing between alternative actions and making decisions, one must decide which value is the most important. To use the example of truth and honesty, suppose a nurse believes in truth and honesty, and a client asks what the medical diagnosis is. The nurse might not want to give an answer immediately, especially if the diagnosis were unusual, complicated, or a disease that usually causes death. Other values against which the nurse might balance truth could include caring, harmony, duty, or responsibility. The situation might be further complicated if the nurse knew that the family or other healthcare team members had different preferences. This scenario represents an internal, personal values conflict and a conflict within the family and healthcare team.

Attitudes, beliefs, and behaviors are often linked with values but are not the same as values (Hall, et al., 1982). An **attitude** is one's disposition toward an object or a situation; it can be a mental or emotional mind-set, and it may be positive or negative. Attitudes can be seen in behaviors or opinions. **Beliefs** are ideas that are accepted as true; they may be expressed by such things as decisions, opinions, or creeds. **Behaviors** are observable actions. To continue with the example of truth telling and the medical diagnosis, a nurse's attitudes and beliefs about the medical diagnosis would influence the valuing process. The ultimate behavior, however, would demonstrate the value that held priority. Attitudes, beliefs, and behaviors are value indicators, and if the nurse is encouraged to take time to reflect on them, his or her values and value system will be realized and articulated.

Major Categories of Values

There are several ways of categorizing values. For the purpose of this discussion, three categories are considered: operative (or means), terminal (or ends), and moral values. **Operative values** are indicated by a specific behavior, which may be a response or a preference (Hall, et al., 1982). For example, honestly sharing observations indicates that honesty is valuable to that person. **Terminal values** are regarded as good in themselves; they transcend immediate needs and shape long-term goals (Rokeach, 1973). Truth is an ends value, while honesty is a means value. **Moral values** involve correct behavior, such as having some sense of right and wrong or "oughtness" (Rokeach, 1973). They deal with such issues as how to treat life and people; truth and honesty are moral values. Nonmoral values serve a personal preference or purpose or make a contribution. They do not involve right and wrong behavior. For example, a healthy lifestyle is good, but if people choose not to take care of their health, it is not considered immoral unless their habits and decisions affect others (eg, driving while intoxicated).

Professional Values in Nursing

Professional nursing values can be traced in the history and traditions of nursing. Beginning with the Nightingale Pledge in 1893 (see the display) through to the current American Nurses Association's (ANA's) Code for Nurses (see Chap. 3), nurses have endeavored to identify and define standards of practice. These standards are based

Nightingale Pledge

"I solemnly pledge myself before God and in the presence of this assembly to pass my life in purity and to practice my profession faithfully. I will abstain from whatever is deleterious and mischievous, and will not take or knowingly administer any harmful drug. I will do all in my power to maintain and elevate the standard of my profession, and will hold in confidence all personal matters committed to my keeping and all family affairs coming to my knowledge in the practice of my calling. With loyalty will I endeavor to aid the physician in his work, and devote myself to the welfare of those committed to my care."

on universal moral principles or values, the central one being respect for people, or human dignity. Other values based on human dignity include self-determination, doing good, avoiding harm, truth telling, respecting privileged information, keeping promises, and treating people fairly. When one enters nursing, however, one also "inherits a measure of both the responsibility and the trust that have accrued to nursing over the years"; thus, one becomes a part of the nursing tradition of service.

A second statement of values, advanced by the American Association of Colleges of Nursing (AACN) in *Essentials of College and University Education for Professional Nursing* (AACN, 1986), identifies seven core values for nurses: altruism, equality, esthetics, freedom, human dignity, justice, and truth. The AACN stresses that it is especially important for nurses to adopt these essential values to have a sense of commitment and social responsibility, a sensitivity and responsiveness to the needs of others, and responsibility for themselves and their actions.

Although the ANA and the AACN both have statements on the importance of values (Table 19-1), how do nursing students develop these values? There are at least three ways values are developed in nursing: socialization, classroom study, and clinical study.

Socialization

Based on some beginning nursing research, it appears that prenursing students already have values similar to those of nursing faculty (Thurston, 1989). For example, the top four means values selected by faculty and students were to be responsible, honest, loving, and forgiving. One explanation for this is that our society already has some accurate perceptions about values basic to nursing, despite the distortions of the television image. Thus, the process of socialization to nursing begins long before nursing education programs.

Classroom Study

Several different approaches to values education have been adopted by nurse educators: values clarification, values inquiry, and applied ethics (King, 1984). Requisite to any study of values is an understanding of growth and development and, in particular, moral development. Because children and adults view the world differently, they make different moral choices when deciding what is right and wrong behavior toward other human beings. Children and adults also have different needs or motivators that influence their value choices.

Clinical Study

The major learning experience in clinical study is client care. After the nurse becomes proficient in giving basic client care, he or she often begins to examine whether the care was effective, what made it effective, and whether it was acceptable to the client. When answering these questions, what is important to the client and the nurse becomes apparent. The whole care-planning process is a value-rich situation: The questions asked during the nursing assessment, the prioritizing of nursing diagnoses, and the establishment of client goals all reflect values.

If the care-planning process is mutual and the client's values are taken into account, the nursing care will support the client's unique qualities; "if a person's values are ignored or replaced with the values of others, the person ceases to exist as a singular human being" (Curtin & Flaherty, 1981, p. 90). Therefore, if the client's values are affirmed during the caring process, the client also is affirmed as a worthwhile person. Thus,

Table 19-1 • Values in Professional Nursing

ANA Code of Ethics (Ethical Values)	AACN Essentials (Professional Values)
Human dignity	Altruism
Autonomy	Equality
Doing good	Esthetics
Avoiding harm	Freedom
Truth-telling	Human dignity
Confidentiality	Justice
Keeping promises	Truth
Justice	

From American Nurses Association (1985). *Code for nurses with interpretive statements.*. Kansas City, MO: Author; American Association of Colleges of Nursing (1986). *Essentials of colleges and university education for professional nursing.* Washington, DC: Author.

the study of client care includes a consciousness of the client's values and the nurse's values and how these interact in the caregiving process.

Values Clarification

Values clarification is "a method of self-discovery by which people identify their personal values and their value rankings" (King, 1984, p. 25). This process does not evaluate the values as such, but helps people identify their own values. According to Raths, Harmin, and Simon (1966), there are three phases to this process (choosing, prizing, and acting) and seven steps (as listed in the display).

This process can be used in several ways:

- To examine past situations and decisions
- To conduct a general case study
- To explore how time is spent by listing activities in a typical 24-hour period

Whatever the vehicle for examination of values, certain assumptions underlie the process. First, for people freely to choose beliefs and behaviors, they must have a sense of who they are, or a sense of self (King, 1984) (Fig. 19-1). This generally begins to occur in late childhood, and individuation is well developed by young adulthood. If individuation has not occurred to some degree, the chosen values will reflect others' values and be externalized rather than internalized. Second, people need to have basic self-esteem to be confident in relying on their feelings, beliefs, and behaviors as guides for decisions (King, 1984).

The prizing and cherishing of one's beliefs and behaviors tend to affirm self-worth and contribute to a sense of inner harmony, purpose, and meaning (King, 1984). These feelings are rewarding and enable one to act more easily on the indicated choices. As the beliefs are acted on repeatedly and consistently in a variety of situations, they become values, and a mature, self-conscious, personal value system begins to emerge.

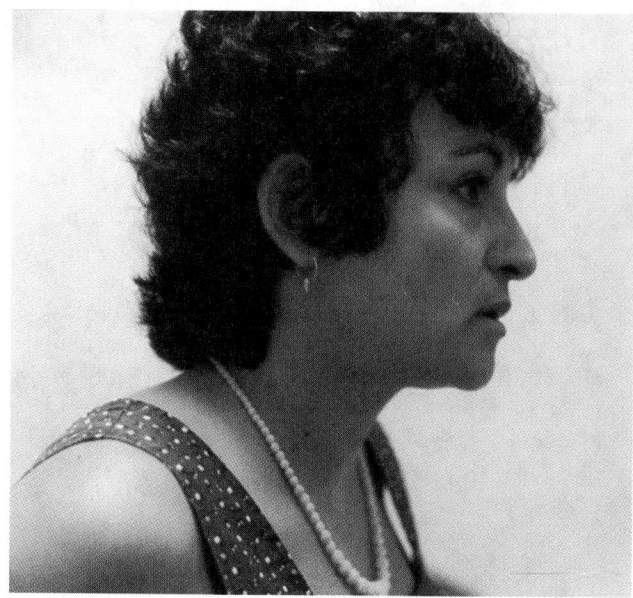

Figure 19-1 • *Values clarification helps people identify their own values and gives them a sense of who they are.*

Phases and Steps in Values Clarification

Choosing One's Beliefs and Behaviors

1. Choosing freely
2. Choosing from among alternatives
3. Choosing after consideration of the consequences

Prizing One's Beliefs and Behaviors

4. Prizing and cherishing
5. Affirming

Acting on One's Beliefs

6. Acting on choices
7. Repeating

Adapted from Raths, L. E., Harmin, M., & Simon, S. B. (1966). *Values and Teaching* (2nd ed.). Columbus, OH: Charles E. Merrill.

Values Inquiry

Whereas values clarification is a method of self-discovery of personal values, values inquiry (King, 1984) is a method of examining social issues and the values that motivate human choice. Case studies and issue-laden incidents provide ways to facilitate the inquiry process. A predetermined series of questions aids in discussing the issues. One set of questions follows:

1. What are the facts?
2. What can be inferred from the facts?
3. What can be inferred from the person's value system?
4. What evidence supports these inferences?

Another set of questions useful in assisting with values inquiry is based on problem-solving:

1. What is the problem?
2. What other alternatives were options?
3. What are the possible consequences of each alternative?
4. What was the evidence that these consequences might occur?
5. What are the advantages and disadvantages of each consequence and why?

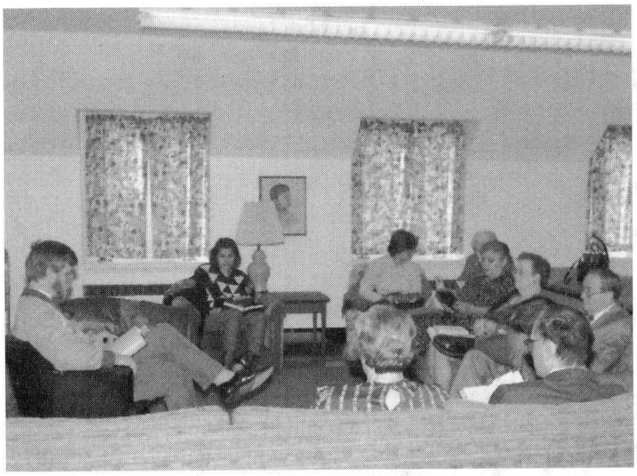

Figure 19-2 *• Values inquiry uses group discussion to examine social issues and values that motivate human choice.*

6. What would you do if you were in this situation and why?

Unlike values clarification, which can be an individual or a group experience, values inquiry lends itself more exclusively to group discussion (Fig. 19-2). The process increases understanding and enhances empathy within a broader social context and increases communication skills and the ability to verbalize one's position.

Applied Ethics

Nurses must acknowledge and be aware of their personal and professional values when they confront ethical dilemmas. Of particular importance are moral values, or those that deal with right and wrong behavior toward other human beings. Analyzing and critiquing case studies assists in applying certain ethical principles, or values, such as respect for people, honesty, and justice. Consideration of case studies also aids in developing moral reasoning skills, and if done in a group discussion, develops communication skills (King, 1984).

Sources of Values

Values come from many sources. Some authors, such as Fromm and Maslow, believe that values are rooted in the conditions of human existence, intrinsic in the structure of human nature, both genetically and culturally (Fromm, 1959). Kidder (1994), a long-time columnist for the *Christian Science Monitor*, explored the proposition that some values are so fundamental to humans that they transcend cultural boundaries. He interviewed 24 articulate, thoughtful people from all over the world to discover their core values and whether there were commonalities. His goal was to explore the possibility of a global code of values. Through an analysis and synthesis process, he identified eight core, universal values: love, truthfulness, fairness, freedom, unity, tolerance, responsibility, and respect for life. Though these values were elicited from visionary people and not, the author points out, the universal core values, it does demonstrate that humans share a basic understanding of how to live together.

Why do cultural values seem so different? Two ideas are helpful; one is *world view,* and the other is *cultural value orientation.* **World view** (Walsh & Middleton, 1984) is an unquestioned framework or predominant set of assumptions through which people view life; it is a perspective, an outlook, or an image of reality. A world view also guides our actions and determines our values. For example, a people's world view may be more easily captured in a story or a myth, which explains how they came to be and how they ought to live. The American dream captures a whole range of values, such as individualism, equality, freedom, privacy, change, progress, achievement, and materialism. **Cultural value orientation,** a theory originated by Kluckhohn and applied to nursing by Brink (1984), can be seen as a subset of world view. There are four general orientations with three ways of responding: nature, time, activity, and relationships.

A combination of Kluckhohn's cultural value orientations and Hall's value list (Table 19-2) is another way to understand the similarities and differences between groups. For example, if one believes that humans are masters of nature, then one values problem-solving and intervention. If one believes in harmony with nature, however, then one values balance. The subjugation-to-nature view values wonder, awe, or fate, focusing more on safety and survival. Time orientation refers to past, present, and future. A person with a future orientation values goals and planning, whereas a person with a past orientation values order, ritual, and tradition. Present orientation values include sensory pleasure, wonder, play, flexibility, and sharing. Activity orientation expresses the type of involvement with life. For example, a person whose orientation is toward "doing" values productivity as a measure of succes or happiness, whereas a "being" person values self-acceptance, and a "being-in-becoming" person values self-development or self-actualization.

The three relational responses or styles are individual, collateral, and linear. The main distinctions between these styles revolve around the value of the individual versus group well-being or goals. Collateral relationships emphasize such values as duty, mutual accountability, responsibility, and membership and focus on the group rather than the individual. Linear relationships value hierarchical group relationship based on authority, order, discipline, and tradition. Thus, by accepting the premise of universal values identified by Kidder (1994), along with the concepts of world view and cultural values orientations, one can

Table 19-2 • Cultural Value Orientations With Associated Values From Hall

Orientations	Associated Values		
Nature	**Mastery**	**Subjugation**	**Harmony**
	Control	Fate	Equilibrium
	Order	Awe	Balance
	Planning	Survival	Integration
Time	**Future**	**Present**	**Past**
	Management	Wonder	Tradition
	Achievement	Flexibility	Ritual
	Research	Sensory pleasure	Obligation
Relational	**Individual**	**Collateral**	**Linear**
	Independence	Mutual accountability	Authority
	Competition	Belonging	Discipline
	Success		Hierarchy
Activity	**Doing**	**Being**	**Being-in-Becoming**
	Productivity	Being self	Self-actualization
	Efficiency	Expressiveness	Wholeness
	Profits	Celebration	Search/meaning

From Brink, P. J. (1984). Values orientation as an assessment tool in cultural diversity. *Nursing Research, 33*, 198–203; Hall, B., (1980). *The personal discernment inventory*. New York: Paulist Press.

have some general guidelines for interpreting variation in meanings of behavior. In addition, values are codified in such social institutions as the family, school, and religion.

Children learn values in several ways: Parents reward and punish behavior; language colors thinking and perception; significant others model behavior; the media floods us with a variety of images; and unspoken expectations direct behavior (Hall, et al., 1982). During adolescence and young adulthood, people are likely to encounter a variety of values and become more aware of value differences. The process of value refinement continues throughout life. It may be a result of a planned self-conscious discovery process or it may be a matter of living and dealing with life situations as they are encountered. Lifespan considerations are discussed later in this chapter.

Two more phenomena that make it possible to become more conscious of different values manifest themselves in adolescence: social perspective taking and formal reasoning. Both of these abilities enable a person to understand and have empathy for another's thoughts, feelings, and points of view. In addition to these abilities, several other critical factors enhance values development, and various social institutions, particularly colleges, plan their programs in view of these factors: community, peer culture, role models, interactions with people of differing values and viewpoints, experiences that challenge one's way of thinking, and decision-making (Dalton, 1985).

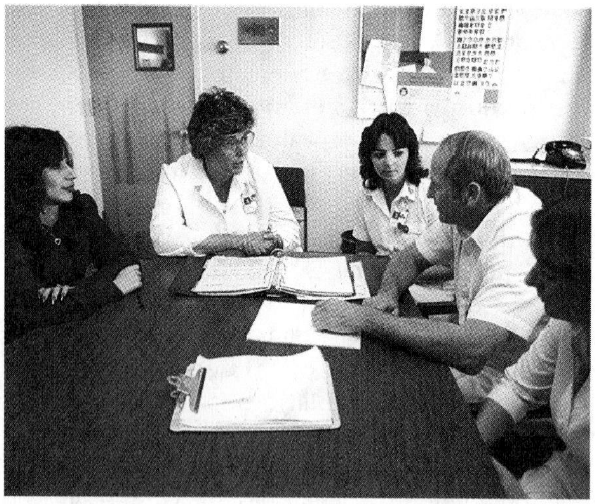

Figure 19-3 • *A community experience supports values and goals.*

Community

A sense of community is formed in an institution (eg, college) by fostering values and goals that are consistently integrated into the various classroom and extracurricular activities. It is further enhanced when people are treated with consideration, according to the stated values. The experience of community also provides a supportive environment in which one can experiment more freely with different attitudes, beliefs, and behaviors (Dalton, 1985) (Fig. 19-3).

Peer Culture

Although a sense of community has a strong influence on value development, the attitudes, beliefs, and behaviors that grow out of peer group relationships are powerful. Peer groups define themselves by common interests, needs, and problems. Out of these similar interests and bonds, values are clarified (Dalton, 1985).

Role Models

Effective role models demonstrate values in which they believe. Affirming values in this manner has a more powerful impact than "preaching." Young adults, quick to recognize incongruities between talking and doing, respond to more mature adults who make an effort to live the difference. Unfortunately, many role models fail to reflect on their own values and thus model conflict and confusion (Dalton, 1985).

Interaction With People of Differing Values and Viewpoints

Values development is promoted when one interacts with others of differing values and viewpoints (Fig. 19-4). "Such experiences tend to encourage and even demand reflectiveness and re-examination of what one may know or believe" (Dalton, 1985, pp. 55–56). In addition to being challenged by different values, which often stem from lifestyle, ethnicity, age, religion, or rural or urban living, one is also challenged to become more reasoned and articulate when defending one's own values. Dealing with people from different backgrounds also creates an awareness of larger social issues and values. Finally, people learn to disagree with others without necessarily rejecting them (Dalton, 1985).

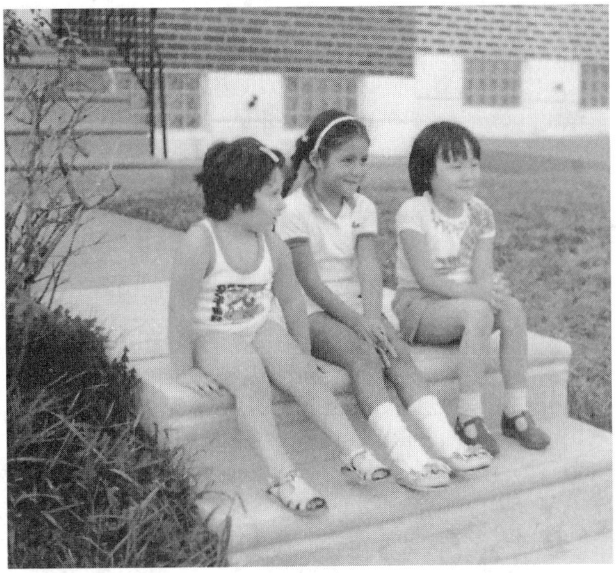

Figure 19-4 • *Interaction with peers from other cultures enriches one's values and viewpoints. The children are enriched by sharing their heritages: Italian, Hispanic, and Chinese.*

Experiences that Challenge A Way of Thinking

The move from adolescence into young adulthood often brings with it environment changes from home to college, the armed forces, or an independent living situation.

> This [new] environment often imposes new patterns of daily living and a variety of new relationships and social interactions. These changes in the individual's environment often force new adaptations and adjustments in one's values (Dalton, 1985).

These environmental changes are so potent that some institutions plan them to create a sense of disorganization in their new members and then provide a climate for reintegration. This promotes more mature and consistent values.

Decision-Making

Choosing one of several alternative behaviors, either real or hypothetical, creates an awareness of personal values. The awareness can be heightened if the choice occurs in a discussion in which various individual decisions can be compared and contrasted (Dalton, 1985). This process shares aspects with the values clarification and values inquiry processes.

Manifestations of Values

As discussed previously, values are reflected through attitudes, beliefs, and behaviors. Behavior, however, demonstrates whether or not a person truly holds and lives out a value. Brian Hall (1991), a researcher in the area of values, identified three levels of valuing: foundation, focus, and future (Fig. 19-5).

In this schema, two kinds of behavior indicate a held value. One kind is habitual; the person does not have to think about it. For example, such health practices as brushing and flossing teeth can become a routine part of morning care; this habit would indicate a **foundation value.** Another type of behavior relies on choice; this behavior is done only when the person sets it as a goal. For example, the dentist also recommends the use of a water-spray oral hygiene device. To add

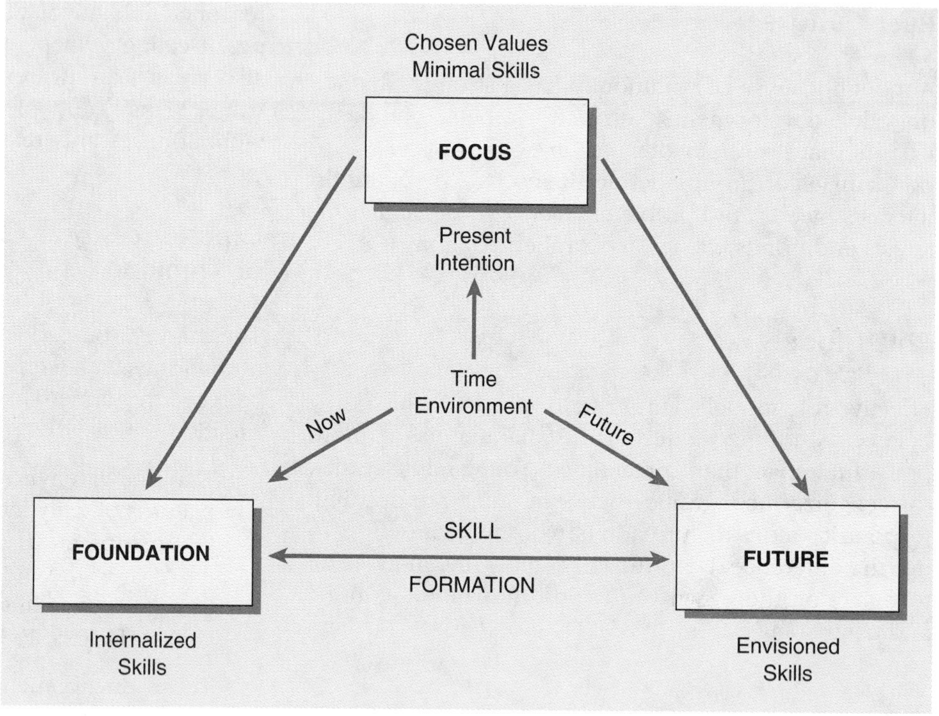

Figure 19-5 • Three levels of valuing: Focus, Foundation, and Future. (From Hall, B. (1980). The personal discernment inventory (p. 36). New York: Paulist Press.)

this procedure to the morning routine, the person would need to purchase the equipment and allow additional time to use it. It might also entail setting the alarm to get up earlier. Until these additional behaviors become habits, the extra dental care would remain a choice or **focus value.** If the person only thought about buying a water-spray device, however, telling the dentist that he or she thought it was a good idea, the value of additional dental care would remain a vision or **future value;** this value will not become "real" until the person acts. Vision values are those we ultimately would like to hold, but for which we momentarily lack the knowledge or skills necessary to integrate them into our lives.

Effect of Values on Functional Health

When assessing values related to functional health, the nurse needs to be aware of three levels of information: general human needs, social and culture-specific needs, and individual or personal needs. These needs are discussed in detail in Chapters 2, 17, and 18. These three levels of need determine client behaviors and indicate the values that influence health status.

The nursing profession has identified 11 functional health patterns that represent general, basic human needs. For example, the preceding discussion about values and dental care comes under the second pattern, nutritional and metabolic patterns.

> All human beings have in common certain functional patterns that contribute to their health, quality of life, and achievement of human potential. These patterns are the focus of nursing assessment. Description and evaluation of health patterns permits the nurse to identify functional patterns (client strengths) and dysfunctional patterns (nursing diagnoses) (Gordon, 1987; 1993).

The culture or social group also defines how the client views health. The culture may promote specific beliefs about health, the body, and the cause and cure of illness, which dictate certain behaviors and indicate values. For example, in a Southeast Asian culture, the top of a person's head is sacred; if something covers this area, the person's spirit is harmed. Thus, certain diagnostic procedures, medical treatments, or surgeries are frightening and cause conflicts between values of spiritual well-being and medical care.

Finally, each client is unique, expressing personal preferences and values. For example, some clients like touch, whereas others do not.

When understanding and being sensitive to client values and their interactions with functional health patterns, the nurse should move from the perspective of general human needs to cultural or social needs and finally to unique individual needs. The following briefly reviews the 11 health patterns, relating values issues to each. The values identified with each pattern are taken from the list of 120 values (as shown in the accompanying display) identified by Hall (1980).

Health Perception and Health Management

Personal health is a value. The basis of this value resides in people's value to themselves, usually expressed

Hall's Value List With Skills

Values	Skills
1. Accountability/mutual	IS
2. Achievement/success	I_2
3. Adaptability/flexibility	IP
4. Administration/control	I_2
5. Affection/physical	IP
6. Art/beauty as pure value	IM
7. (Self) assertion	IP
8. Being liked	IP
9. Being self	IS
10. Care/nurture	IP
11. (Self) centeredness	IP
12. Communications	I_2
13. Community/personalist	IS
14. Community/supportive	IS
15. Competition	I_2
16. (Self) competence/confidence	I_2
17. Congruence	IP
18. Construction/new order	IS
19. Contemplation/asceticism	I_2
20. (Self) Control	IP
21. Control/order/discipline	I_2
22. Convivial tool/Intermediate	IS
23. Cooperation	IS
24. Corporation/construction/new order	IS
25. Courtesy/respect	IP
26. Creativity/ideation	IM
27. Criteria/rationality	I_2
28. (Self) delight	IM
29. Decision/initiation	IP
30. Design/pattern/order	I_2
31. Detachment/solitude	IS
32. (Self) directedness	IP
33. Discernment/communal	IM
34. Discovery/delight	IS
35. Duty/obligation	IP
36. Economics/profit	I_2
37. Economics/success	I_2
38. Ecority/beauty/aesthetics	IM
39. Education/certification	I_2
40. Education/knowledge/insight	I_2
41. Efficiency/planning	I_2
42. Empathy	IP
43. Equality/liberation	IP
44. Equilibrium	IS
45. Equity/rights	IP
46. Ethics/accountability/values	I_2
47. Evaluation/skill self system	IP
48. Expressiveness/Freedom	IM
49. Faith/risk	IP
50. Family/belonging	IP
51. Fantasy/play	IM
52. Food/warmth/shelter	I_2
53. Friendship/belonging	IP
54. Function	I_2
55. Generosity/service	IP
56. Growth/expansion	IS
57. Harmony/system	IS
58. Health/personal	IS
59. Hierarchy/property/order	IS
60. Honor	IS
61. Human dignity	IS
62. Independence	IP
63. Instrumentality	I_2
64. Integration/wholeness	IP
65. Interdependence	IS
66. Intimacy	IP
67. Intimacy and Solitude as Unitive	IP
68. Justice	IS
69. Knowledge/discovery/insight	I_2
70. Law/guide	IS
71. Law/rule	I_2
72. Life/self-actualization	IP
73. Limitation/celebration	IP
74. Loyalty/respect	IP
75. Macroeconomics	IS
76. Management	I_2
77. Membership	I_2
78. Mission/goals	IS
79. Obedience/duty	IP
80. Obedience/mutual accountability	IS
81. Objectivity	I_2
82. Ownership	IP
83. Patriotism/esteem	IP
84. Pioneerism/innovation/progress	IS
85. Play/leisure	IP
86. Poverty/simplicity	IS
87. Pluriformity	IS
88. Power/authority/honesty	IP
89. Presence/dwelling	IP
90. (Self) preservation	IP
91. Prestige/image	IP
92. Productivity	I_2
93. Property/control	I_2
94. Recreation/freesence	IM
95. Relaxation	IS
96. Research/originality/knowledge	IM
97. Responsibility	IP
98. Ritual/meaning	IS
99. Rule/accountability	I_2
100. Safety/survival	I_2
101. Search/meaning	IM
102. Security	IP

(continued)

Hall's Value List With Skills (continued)

Values	Skills	Values	Skills
103. Sensory pleasure/sex	IP	112. Truth/wisdom/intuitive insight	IM
104. Service/vocation	IS	113. Unity/solidarity	IP
105. Sharing/listening/trust	IP	114. Wonder/awe/fate	IM
106. Simplicity/play	I_2	115. Wonder/curiosity	IM
107. Social affirmation	IS	116. Word	IS
108. Support peer	IP	117. Work/labor	I_2
109. Synergy	IS	118. Workmanship/craft	I_2
110. Tradition	IS	119. Worship/duty/creed	I_2
111. Transcendence/global confluence	IS	120. (Self) worth	IP

I_2, instrumental skills; IP, interpersonal skills; IM, imaginal skills; IS, systems skills; (Adapted from Hall, B. (1980). The personal discernment inventory. New York: Paulist Press.)

as self-esteem or self-acceptance. Health values also reflect beliefs about the nature of health and health practices; most of these beliefs and practices are culturally or socially defined. For example, good health may be seen as an indicator of balance in life or of being a good person. To maintain health as a value, additional values are necessary to carry out health practices; these might include discipline, planning, responsibility, education, and cooperation. When working with specific people, nurses need to assess how the clients experience health and what they do to maintain health, all within their cultural and social environment. The client's level of self-esteem, which also is a value, will reflect their ability to incorporate new health behaviors into their lifestyle.

Nutrition and Metabolism

The essential value represented by the nutrition and metabolism pattern is survival; however, the various attitudes and beliefs about nutrition represent cultural and personal preferences. The presentation of food may reflect esthetic values, such as art and beauty, and socialization values, such as family, work, service, or ritual. For example, some cultures consider color, texture, and design as part of food preparation; others may emphasize the social interaction at meal time.

Elimination

Values associated with excretory functions of the bowel, bladder, and skin may include sensory pleasure, control, discipline, and self-competence. Practices associated with these functions are learned within cultural and family frameworks. For example, adolescent Americans learn to be self-conscious regarding body odor and body hair, whereas those from other parts of the world may not.

Activity and Exercise

The activity and exercise pattern deals with a person's energy level. People who have a sensory orientation to the world tend to be more physically active. Values associated with this pattern might include sensory pleasure, competition, image, play, leisure, relaxation, and recreation. For example, in American society values of knowledge and research are a priority; physical fitness (especially through aerobic exercise) has been shown to reduce risks of heart disease. Not all people at risk exercise, however; they might give priority to other values or they might not have the time management skills to incorporate an exercise program into their schedule.

Sleep and Rest

Survival is the value basic to the sleep and rest pattern, but culture and family also support practices related to sleep and rest; siestas and coffee breaks are examples. Also, the manner of sleeping varies across cultures and families; family members might sleep in separate beds and bedrooms or in a large family room on mats on the floor. Generally, all people need 6 to 8 hours of sleep per day, but much variability occurs with age, occupation, and individual needs.

Cognition and Perception

The cognition and perception pattern involves the five senses, language, memory, and decision-making. Values associated with this area include sensory pleasure, expressiveness, communication, rationality, evaluation, and intuition. Language is probably the most important of these aspects, because it reflects cultural patterns of thinking in such areas as time, space, and world view. Within that culture, a person's sentence structure indicates the thinking process, reality orientation, and sensory preference.

The four value orientations (human nature, time, activity, and relationships) have numerous implications for thinking and perceiving. They affect the understanding of the illness process, intervention in the process, the decision as to which people are to be involved in the process, and acceptable treatments. One way to understand this pattern is to read Tony Hillerman's detective novels, set in the Navajo culture of the southwestern United States (Hillerman, 1990). He successfully captures the value orientations of "present," harmony with nature, collateral or tribal relationships, and "doing" as the investigation unfolds. Because there is usually a murder involved, one should pay particular attention to the understanding of the body and the spirit.

Self-Perception and Self-Concept

Values underlying this pattern are self-preservation, self-delight, self-worth, self-competency, self-assertion, self-actualization, integration, and being oneself. Initially, the family and larger society prescribe how to think and feel about oneself. In American culture, where individuality and independence are valued, the emphasis is on a unique sense of self apart from the group.

Roles and Relationships

How people relate to others is often defined by their function or role. Some of the values associated with the many possible role relationships include belonging, social affiliation, support, work, duty, ownership, membership, education, service, power, authority, cooperation, and intimacy. The major roles in our society are family roles, student or work roles, and social roles (Fig. 19-6).

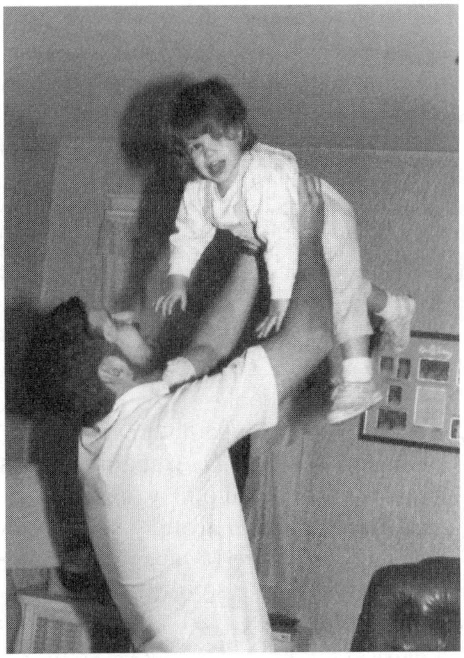

Figure 19-6 • *Values are displayed through roles and relationships in the family. The child learns values through time spent with the parents.*

Sexuality and Reproduction

The pattern of sexuality and reproduction is closely associated with self-concept and role relationships. Self-delight, self-control, belonging, sharing, wholeness, being oneself, and intimacy are values associated with this pattern. Participation and levels of satisfaction are usually defined within the society and culture. For example, the focus of sexuality may be primarily on reproduction, or it may be on intimacy and pleasure.

Coping and Stress Management

Though people respond to stress in many ways, the basic values underlying this pattern are self-preservation, safety, and survival. Other values related to this pattern reflect various coping styles; some of these values include support, competition, equilibrium, control, planning, management, flexibility, assertion, relaxation, sharing, listening, education, creativity, detachment, cooperation, and insight.

Values and Beliefs

The values and beliefs pattern reflects a person's overall attitude or feeling about life and is associated with hope, meaning, and purpose. It may involve spiritual and religious issues that support the person's world view and his or her attitudes about the importance of life and the meaning of death. Values typical of this pattern include wonder, duty, loyalty, tradition, worship, design, law, unity, service, search, human dignity, intimacy, justice, mission, faith, truth, and transcendence.

Manifestations of Nurses' Values

Nurses demonstrate their values in their attitudes and behaviors. For example, a nurse may say that he or she values family and belonging. Observation of the nurse's interaction with families—supporting them, sharing information with them, and consulting them for discharge planning—might indicate a discrepancy between what the nurse says and does. The nurse's value of family and belonging might be questioned. When a nurse claims to value family and belonging but does not demonstrate this when caring for clients, the nurse might be deficient in communication skills or not understand family dynamics. Thus, this value would be a vision value or an ideal not yet committed to behavior.

In Hall's schema, values also can be organized in a **hierarchy of skills** (Hall, 1980). These skills are instrumental, interpersonal, imaginal, and systems. **Instrumental skills** comprise the first level of skills and are associated with basic physical and intellectual competencies that enable one to shape ideas and the external environment. A nursing example of instrumental skills would be the knowledge and clinical application necessary to provide basic client care (ie, skin care, wound care, range of motion, vital signs). **Interpersonal skills** determine the ability to relate happily and productively with others. Communication skills, such as listening and sharing; problem-solving skills; teaching; and counseling are some of the interpersonal skills necessary in nursing (Fig. 19-7). **Imaginal skills** bring imagination and creativity into play, enabling the nurse to envision a plan for adapting and personalizing client care. The values that support imaginal skills are esthetic; esthetics also is an essential value of nursing, as identified by the AACN (1986). **Systems skills** are those that help a person see the whole picture and how various parts relate. As nurses initiate changes in one aspect of client care, they need to be aware of how this may affect other departments in the hospital, such as housekeeping, pharmacy, physical therapy, and x-ray or laboratory services.

Returning to the example of the nurse whose vision value is family and belonging, knowledge of family dynamics and communication are instrumental skills. Understanding the process of the nurse–client relationship and being able to form relationships built on trust are interpersonal skills. For the value of family and belonging to become a behavioral reality, the nurse sets goals to use family dynamics knowledge and to practice communication. That is, this value is a choice value until the nurse does the behaviors automatically.

One of the essential values of the nursing profession is human dignity. Knowledge of family dynamics and communication are values that support the higher value of human dignity. In Hall's schema, human dignity is a systems skill, the most complex of all the skills. It requires incorporation not only of instrumental and interpersonal skills, but also imaginal skills. When these skills are integrated, the nurse can move beyond a particular family and begin to think of family health programs in the larger healthcare system. At this level, human dignity for all families becomes an action value. This hierarchy of instrumental, interpersonal, imaginal, and systems value skills and other concepts in Hall's theory have implications for growth and development.

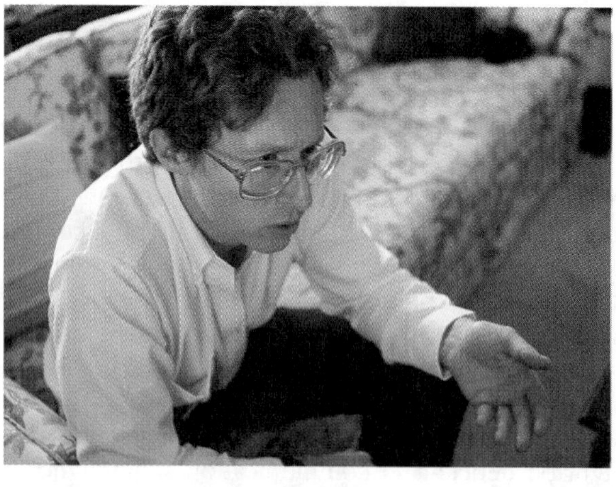

Figure 19-7 • Interpersonal skills are an expression of values and attitudes.

Lifespan Considerations

Values also can reflect the person's age and stage of development. Although not everyone automatically develops all values, most people's values change or are refined by various life experiences. Table 19-3 illustrates key values during different stages of life, combining Erikson's (1982) and Hall's theories of development.

Infant, Toddler, and Preschooler

At the most basic level, an infant begins value development with the evolution of trust and autonomy. Moral development and cognitive ability are closely related. As the child progresses to toddlerhood, moral and values development begin with the child identifying which behaviors elicit reward or punishment. Kohlberg (1964) refers to this as the first-level preconventional stage; the child learns to distinguish right from wrong and understand the choice between obedience and punishment.

The preschooler learns that rules are unchanging and are imposed by parents and adults. In this later stage of development, the child recognizes and accepts fairness and cooperation, although these are limited by the child's self-interest and self-will. Children are concerned when the situation seems "unfair" to them, yet do not have enough maturity to project that same sense of fairness to their peers.

Child and Adolescent

The school-age child is industrious, recognizing the need for moral codes and social rules. The younger child maintains a strict understanding and application of the rules, seeing things in clearly dichotomous ways (ie, right or wrong). As the child grows into preadolescence, he or she becomes more flexible. The threat of discipline becomes less important than social expectations. Kohlberg (1964) refers to this as the second-level or conventional stage, characterized by conformity to expectations and behaviors of others.

For the adolescent, the influence of peer identification reaches its greatest persuasiveness. Although this

Table 19-3 • Stage of Human Development: Parallels

Eras	*Erikson's Eight Stages*	*Hall's Four Phases of Consciousness*
Infancy	**Trust** (Hope)	**Phase I**
		Security
	Autonomy	Survival Pleasure
Early Childhood	(Will) **Initiative** (Purpose)	Wonder
Childhood	**Industry** (Competence)	**Phase II**
		Belonging Work Self-competence
Adolescence	**Identity** (Competence)	Belonging Work Self-competence Self-worth
Young Adulthood	**Intimacy** (Love)	**Phase III** Independence Service/vocation
Adulthood	**Generativity** (Care)	Creation Being self
Maturity	**Integrity** (Wisdom)	**Phase IV** Harmony Interdependence Intimacy Esthetics

period of development is often characterized by rebellion, the adolescent has a high level of moral judgment with a law-and-order orientation. The adolescent understands that morality is derived from principles of conscience and that rules are cooperative agreements that can be modified. As the person reaches late adolescence, he or she begins to move away from the strong peer influence based on individual principles, and peer group values decrease in importance.

Adult and Older Adult

The adult focuses on generativity and intimacy as careers and families are formed. The primary moral concerns are now directed to meeting the expectations of employer, family, and adult social group. Values that were taught and caught in childhood generally develop into what the adult will accept as guiding principles for life.

The older adult's attention is on personal integrity and the wisdom that he or she has accumulated over a lifetime. Values are firmly ingrained, yet the older adult is often more accepting of values of others that may be different from his or her own.

Hall's Value Development Theory

Hall's theory of values and value development is complex and draws on many sources, two of which are Freire's work on "conscientization" and Maslow's hierarchy of needs (Hall, 1986). Building on these sources, Hall outlines a potential natural growth process for a values hierarchy. In this framework, needs are the basis of values that flow from different stages of life.

Table 19-3 identifies Hall's four phases of consciousness or world views (Hall, 1980; 1986; Hall, et al., 1982). The perspective in Phase I is that of the infant or child with the self as center, focusing on physical existence; the world is a mystery over which the self has no control. The basic needs or values are food, shelter, and pleasure. Phase II, the time from adolescence through young adulthood, sees the world as a problem to be solved. The self copes by doing and learning and by belonging to a social or peer group. The basic values are social acceptance, affirmation, approval, and achievement. At the Phase III level of consciousness, the self, similar to Maslow's self-actualizer, views the world as a project and invention. The basic values include personal authority, freedom, dignity, and integrity. The self seeks to satisfy the personal need of independence. In Phase IV, the world view is one of mystery, but unlike the child, the self reaches out to care. This caring is in the global sense, beyond the immediate environment. The values are truth, community, harmony, and interdependence. This stage is possible from adult midlife through old age; however, not everyone is able to reach this level of function.

These phases of consciousness or levels of development are significantly different from other developmental theories in that they are not necessarily related to age but to experience and self-reflection (Hall, 1986). For example, in the first few years of life, a child experiences the world as a mystery over which he or she has no control but also perceives it with wonder, awe, curiosity, and self-delight. If the child's survival needs are not met, however, then as an adult, the experience of the world will continue in Phase I as the self struggles to survive in an environment perceived as hostile, alien, oppressive, and capricious. In this example, the adult continues to struggle with basic needs or values. If the environment is supportive, however, the young adult emerges secure and competent. Then, as a midlife adult, the person is able to move toward self-actualization.

The nurse can apply these phases of consciousness and values in the initial assessment; however, the client's life experience and reflection on this experience determine the actual level of values development.

Value Conflicts

Whenever there is human interaction, value conflicts are likely to occur. These conflicts can be resolved if the nurse is aware of his or her own values and the client's values. Resolving these conflicts may entail a clarification of values and an appreciation and acceptance of value differences. Because value conflicts may affect compliance with nursing care, the nurse's appreciation and acceptance of value differences can be the basis of negotiation and compromise, leading to acceptable care for the client.

Client and Family Conflicts

Value conflicts between family members arise from developmental differences, experience differences, and personal preference differences. One fairly common ex-

Therapeutic Dialogue
Values

Scenes for Thought

Mrs. Haverford, a 42-year-old woman, is in the hospital with an acute episode of her chronic rheumatoid arthritis. Her husband of 20 years has come to visit. He asks to speak to you because you are her primary nurse, and he has some questions. He meets you in the hallway.

Effective

Nurse: *Hello, Mr. Haverford. I'm Darla Jessup, your wife's primary nurse. You wanted to talk to me?*
Husband: *Yes, Ms. Jessup. I wanted to ask you some questions about the care my wife is getting, and they said you'd be the one to ask.* Looks serious.
Nurse: *How can I help? (Offering self.)*
Husband: *Well, I don't know if you can. I've seen my wife through many of these flare-ups of her arthritis, the joint operations and the changes in medicines, but I don't remember her ever being this sick before. I'm thinking it might be the new medicine her doctor put her on. What do you think?* Continues to look worried.
Nurse: *I can see that this is troubling you. What have you been told about why she's in the hospital? (Observation and seeking information.)*
Husband: *Not much, but I want to know more. She's a very independent woman, and I don't want her to get so sick that she won't be able to be as independent as she was. That would bother her a lot.*
Nurse: *It sounds as though you would like some information and that your wife might like it, too. How about setting up a time when we can talk together about this? (Offering information.)*
Husband: *Fine. Millie will be pleased, but let me ask her. She's still not feeling too good yet.*
Nurse: *Okay. I'll be coming to her room soon to give her some medication and see to her comfort. I'll see you then.*

Less Effective

Nurse: *Hi, Mr. Haverford. I'm Vicki Driessen, your wife's primary. You wanted to speak to me?*
Husband: *yes, my wife is looking awfully sick this time around, and I wondered what was going on. I've seen her through a lot of flare-ups of the arthritis, but...(interrupted by Vicki).*
Nurse: *I understand that you're worried about your wife's condition. You know we're doing everything we can for her. When she's home, you work hard to care for her, but now it's time for you to relax and let us take over. I'll be down to her room in a little while to see how she's doing. We can talk more then.*

Critical Thinking Challenge

- *From Hall's Value List (see the display), record the values that the husband exhibits while talking to the nurses about his wife. Make a similar list for each nurse. Compare the difference between Ms. Jessup's and Ms. Driessen's list of values.*
- *Examine what kind of effect this difference might have on the client and her husband.*

ample is when one spouse refuses to take the time to have a health checkup. Depending on how the healthcare system was experienced in early life or interpreted by the culture, the person refusing care may have values of tradition, self-control, competition, self-directedness, independence, fate, and risk that counter values of regular preventive healthcare. These values may reflect an underlying struggle with other values, such as security, self-competence, or self-worth. The nurse's role might be to help the spouses explore their personal health history and needs rather than continuing the argument about the health checkup. Ideally, the nurse could assist each spouse in setting some attainable personal health goals, helping them realize the values of sharing, listening, trust, accountability, and responsibility.

Client and Healthcare Conflicts

Areas of conflict between clients and healthcare providers can evolve around values related to knowledge, cultural differences, developmental differences, and personal preference. For example, in the case of an American family in which the grandmother has died, the parents may prefer that the children not go to the funeral, stating that the children do not understand death, and it might be difficult for them. The nurse, who values communication, support, and the research findings on children and death, might disagree with the parents. Realizing that death is a traumatic event for the survivors and that the parents' protection of the children is really a protection of their own feelings, the nurse might explore other ways in which the children's grief and loss needs could be met. Depending on the ages of the children, these might include stories, drawing, or playing with a doll house family that includes a grandmother (Cook & Oltjenbruns, 1989).

Resolving Value Conflicts in the Healthcare System

Three main issues that arise regarding the resolution of value conflicts are the perception of conflict, the meaning of resolution, and the values underlying the resolution process. When nurses face value conflicts, it is important for them to examine their own values regarding conflict. If the nurse views conflict as negative, he or she might feel threatened; his or her own values of self-competence, duty, success, authority, and esteem are questioned. If the nurse views conflict as positive, however, the values of respect, communication, care, equilibrium, harmony, service, and creativity are enhanced. These two views of conflict are based on the nurse's life experience and level of values development. For example, to a nurse who was raised in a dysfunctional family, conflict is threatening and should be avoided; the core value is security. For the nurse who has experienced more functional patterns of family interaction, the core value might be interdependence or innovation.

Several definitions of the word "resolution" apply to resolving value conflicts. One definition is that it is a clarifying or explanatory process. For example, many people have not reflected on their values, so when conflicts occur, they are not able to articulate their position. Therefore, one of the first goals for the nurse is to assist the client in exploring and defining the relevant issues, attitudes, and beliefs. This clarification or explanation may be the resolution, or it may be the first step in a resolution process.

A second definition of resolution is that it occurs by answering questions. Clients have many questions related to their care. What nurses take for granted as routine care may be strange to the client. Encouraging questions by saying something like, "I have asked you a lot of questions; now do you have some that you would like to ask?" can be helpful. For example, an adolescent woman is admitted for a suicide gesture; she cut her wrist. After a lengthy assessment, the nurse asks her if she has any questions. Her question is, "How is the food here?" Although a suicide attempt indicates that the client is dealing with survival issues, this question also is a concrete demonstration that the client is in the Phase I value development mode or basic survival mode, focusing on food and shelter. She is not able to focus on setting goals related to communication skills, assertiveness, or dealing with loss and grief, although the nurse has mentioned that these are some areas she might work on during her hospitalization. The first nursing intervention is getting the client something to eat. If the nurse insisted on focusing on the counseling goals of communication or assertiveness in the ensuing 24 hours, there would have been a values conflict. The client is not ready to deal with feelings on a verbal level.

Another kind of resolution involves coming to a decision or a determination for future action. For example, a client may have several treatment options. Even after examining all the facts and getting a second opinion, a client decides to take a course of action that the nurse does not like. If the nurse were to impose his or her decision on the client at this point, it is highly likely that a value conflict would arise, and the client might not comply with any treatment.

A fourth definition of resolution involves breaking up the issue or problem into its elements. Perhaps there are some elements of the situation on which the nurse and client can agree, thus facilitating care. This is especially important with clients from different sociocultural backgrounds. The client often has a different belief system regarding the cause of illness, resulting in different values regarding prevention and cure. For example, a male refugee from Africa becomes psychotic because of major losses and culture shock. He is hospitalized for several months, discharged, and then rehospitalized because he did not take the prescribed psychotropic medications. Exploring the client's belief system reveals that he believes that his problems are due to displeasing his family and being a coward. Mental illness is viewed as a punishment. Rather than focusing on the scientific explanation supported by Western values of knowledge, the nurse assists the client in learning about the community by taking him to various activities and facilities. The client likes this approach, finding that a prayer meeting held at a church of his ethnic group was especially helpful.

It is useful to view conflict and its resolution as part of an ongoing process in human relationships. Value conflict resolution based on respect involves a process that includes understanding one's perception of conflict, clarifying values, answering or encouraging questions, making decisions, and finding elements for agreement or negotiation and compromise.

Values Assessment

Values assessment occurs in the nursing history, but any interaction with a client may give the nurse value indicators. The following discussion identifies how the nurse can assess a client's values.

Nursing Research
Values Assessment

Selected Nursing Research Studies

HiHunen, E. (1994). Validation of decisional conflict by critical care nurses. In R. M. Carroll-Johnson & M. Pacquett (Eds.), *Classification of nursing diagnoses, proceedings of the tenth conference.* Philadelphia: J.B. Lippincott.

Rozmus, C. L., & Edgil, A. E. (1993). Values, knowledge, and attitudes about acquired immunodeficiency syndrome in rural adolescents. *Journal of Pediatric Health Care, 7*(4), 167–173.

Peter, E., and Gallop, R. (1994). The ethic of care: A Comparison of nursing and medical students. *Image The Journal of Nursing Scholarship, 26*(1), 47–51.

Possible Topics for Nursing Inquiry

- What changes in values occur during the nursing education process?
- What are the value differences at various levels of nursing education and nursing service?
- Define nursing values assessment.
- Test values as they relate to functional health.

Level of Values Development

The age and experiences of a client may indicate the primary values associated with the four phases of consciousness. For example, young adults are concerned with family and belonging, self-worth, and self-competence, whereas adults at midlife may be more concerned with life and self-actualization, service, and vocation. Asking the client to share a major turning point in his or her life or a life-changing experience may clarify the phases. If the client has had some traumatic experiences or is facing a life-threatening illness, he or she may temporarily focus on values of self-preservation and security typical of the Phase I level of consciousness.

View of Hospitalization and Illness

Useful initial openings for a nursing assessment are "What brought you in for the hospitalization?" (if the person has been in several times), and "What is your understanding of your condition (illness)?" These questions clarify the client's perception of health and illness and elicit information on the client's world view (defined in the section, "Sources of Values") (Brink, 1984). These views indicate the client's probable acceptance of therapy; for example, a client who sees the illness as a problem to be solved might be more open to the problem-solving process and goal setting than the client who sees the illness as fate.

Activities of Daily Living

When the nurse asks clients questions about how they spend their time (ie, how a typical day or week is), he or she is gathering information related to operative or action values. The behaviors clients describe indicate their value commitments. Many of these action values can be identified as functional health is assessed. These include nutrition and metabolism, elimination, activity and exercise, sleep and rest, roles and relationships, sexuality and reproduction, and coping and stress management. How the clients describe their day indicates the patterns of health perception and health management, self-perception, and values and beliefs.

Healthcare Planning

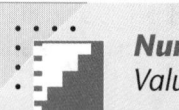

Healthcare planning should be integral to all contacts with the client and the client's family. Nurses cannot assume that all the care planning is done in the clinic or at the time of discharge. For example, the short-stay surgery experience usually entails prehospital orientation, brief hospital care, and follow-up care or home care. In the prehospital phase, the clients and families are usually given a "map" or an expected trajectory of their care. In this setting, the nurse may act as the case coordinator to teach self-care skills, evaluate living arrangements, and meet with the family to assess their abilitities in home care. During this process of interaction, the nurse will continue to identify client and family values. Three value orientations are particularly useful in assessment at this time: role relationships, activity modes, and time orientation (Brink, 1984).

In terms of role relationships, the nurse must assess the client's view of himself or herself and his or her relationships to family and friends. If the client comes from the general American culture, he or she is more likely to have a smaller nuclear family and value individualism. This client will want more say about his or her own healthcare unless he or she is a dependent child or elderly. If the client comes from a larger extended family, the group opinion is more valued. If the extended family is hierarchical, the senior group members may have more decision-making power. Thus, it is important to understand these role relationships and how they may affect the discharge planning process.

Goal setting will be influenced by the activity values orientation. For example, clients who like to "do" things might be more involved in a physical rehabilitation program, because it is concrete and measurable. By contrast, those who have a "being" orientation might be less planned or more sporadic. When working with the being-oriented person, the nurse might assist the client and family to find a variety of ways to meet the physical rehabilitation needs, thus allowing for more spontaneity.

The goal-setting process is influenced by the client's time orientation values. Clients who are future oriented can think more easily of goals than those who are past or present oriented. For clients who have tradition as a value, the nurse may explore ways to relate some of these rituals to new healthcare regimens. Present value orientation clients may need activities that are fun, stimulating, and calming and that give immediate feedback or sensation.

Healthcare planning also may be a time when clients discuss the need for behavior change, which concerns their focus or future values. To help accomplish these changes, the nurse could assist clients in assessing additional skills and values they need. For example, a newly diagnosed diabetic client who values independence might be concerned about the impact of the illness on his or her family. To maintain independence, he or she might become involved in the instrumental skills of learning how to manipulate a glucose-monitoring machine, self-administering insulin, and managing his or her diet, but the client might avoid talking about feelings or concerns with his or her family. The nurse could help the client explore his or her feelings about the diagnosis. The nurse could then discuss the values of sharing, listening, and trust as they relate to the well-being of the family. In this example, the future values would be interdependence, expressiveness, and intimacy.

Values are an integral part of all human interactions. An understanding of values and their influence on nurse–client–family interaction is vital for acceptance of healthcare and for integration of the value of personal health into the lives of clients and families (Uustal, 1987).

Key Concepts

- All human interactions are value based.
- Nurses must clarify and respect the values of others and examine their own values.
- Sources of values for professional nursing are parents, family, and significant others; they are absorbed through observation and experience throughout a lifetime.
- Values are enhanced and refined by experiences that cultivate values development, such as interactions with people of differing values and viewpoints and experiences that challenge one's way of thinking.
- The *Code for Nurses* by the ANA is a set of standards based on universal moral principles or values.
- The AACN identifies seven core values for nurses.
- Values in nursing are developed through socialization, classroom study, and clinical study.
- Values clarification is a method of self-discovery by which people identify their personal values without evaluating the values.
- Hall's developmental theory of values can be related to functional health patterns, how clients and nurses manifest their values, values conflict and resolution, and values assessment.
- An understanding of values and their influence on the nurse–client–family interaction is vital for acceptance of healthcare and the integration of the value of personal health into the lives of the client and family.

Critical Thinking Challenges

Now that you have added the concept of values to your knowledge base, you are better able to address the concerns of the homeless woman. Turn back to that situation, and consider the following questions.

1. *Describe your initial thoughts and feelings concerning the woman and her situation.*
2. *Compare your responses with what the woman appears to be telling you.*
3. *As you explore this situation, identify your values, and determine their origin.*
4. *List and group potential common grounds and potential conflicts as you imagine working with this woman.*
5. *Name some values that might be key in building a common ground.*

References

American Association of Colleges of Nursing (1986). *Essentials of colleges and university education for professional nursing*. Washington, DC: Author.

American Nurses Association (1985). *Code for nurses with interpretive statements*. Kansas City, MO: Author.

Brink, P. J. (1984). Values orientations as an assessment tool in cultural diversity. *Nursing Research, 33,* 198–203.

Cook, A. S., & Oltjenbruns, K. A. (1989). *Dying and grieving: Lifespan and family perspectives.* New York: Holt, Rinehart and Winston.

Curtin, L., & Flaherty, M. J. (1981). *Nursing ethics: Theories and pragmatics.* New York: Appleton-Lange.

Dalton, J. C. (1985). Promoting values development in college students. *NASPA Monograph Series, 4,* 47–59.

Erikson, E. (1982). *The life cycle completed.* New York: W.W. Norton & Co.

Fromm, E. (1959). Values, psychology and human existence. In A. Maslow (Ed.), *New knowledge in human values.* New York: Harper and Row.

Gordon, M. (1987). *Nursing diagnosis process and application* (2nd ed.). New York: McGraw-Hill.

Gordon, M. (1993) *Manual of Nursing Diagnosis, 1993–1994.* St. Louis: Mosby Yearbook.

Hall, B. (1980). *The personal discernment inventory.* New York: Paulist Press.

Hall, B. (1986). *The genesis effect.* New York: Paulist Press.

Hall, B., Kalven, J., Rosen, L., & Taylor, B. (1982). *Readings in value development.* Ramsey, NJ: Paulist Press.

Hall, B. (1991). *Spritual connections: The journey of discipleship and Christian values.* Dayton, OH: Values Technology Inc.

Hillerman, T. (1990). *The coyote waits.* New York: Harper & Row.

Kidder, R. M. (1994). *Shared values for a troubled world.* San Francisco: Jossey-Bass Publishers.

King, E. C. (1984). *Affective education in nursing.* Rockville, MD: An Aspen Publication.

Kohlberg, L. (1964). Development of moral character and moral ideology. In M. L. Hoffman & L. N. W. Hoffman (Eds.), *Review of child development research, Vol. 1.* New York: Russell Bage Foundation.

Raths, L. E., Harmin, M., & Simon, S. B. (1966). *Values and teaching.* Columbus, OH: Charles E. Merrill.

Rokeach, M. (1973). *The nature of human values.* New York: The Free Press.

Thurston, H. I. (1989). Values held by nursing faculty and students in a university setting. *Journal of Professional Nursing, 5,* 199–207.

Uustal, D. B. (1987). Values: The cornerstone of nursing's moral art. In M. D. M. Fowler & J. Levine-Ariff (Eds.), *Ethics at the bedside.* Philadelphia: J.B. Lippincott.

Walsh, B. J., & Middleton, J. R. (1984). *The transforming vision, shaping a Christian world view.* Downers Grove, Illinois: InterVarsity Press.

Communication: The Nurse–Client Relationship

Key Terms	Learning Objectives

Key Terms

Advocacy
Circle of confidentiality
Communication channel
Empathy
Encoding
Feedback
Metacommunication
Nonverbal communication
Therapeutic communication

Learning Objectives

Upon completion of this chapter, the student will be able to do the following:

- *Define various types of communication.*
- *Discuss elements of the communication process and their relevance to nursing.*
- *Discuss the relationship of language and experience to the communication process.*
- *Explain the nature of the nurse–client relationship.*
- *Distinguish between a professional and a social relationship.*
- *Name the elements of an informal nurse–client contract.*
- *Discuss four key aspects of therapeutic communication.*
- *Give examples of areas of assessment applied to nurse–client communication.*
- *Define and give examples of a variety of therapeutic communication techniques.*
- *Name key nontherapeutic responses and explain how these interfere with therapeutic communication.*
- *Describe some special situations that affect communication.*

20

While you are visiting your client in his retirement apartment, you begin to discuss his recent hospitalization and the fall that occurred during his recovery period. Your concern is for his safety and for preventing further falls. When you ask him why he thinks the fall occurred, you notice that his posture changes. He becomes more erect, and his facial expression is guarded and resolute. He tells you curtly that he simply "lost [his] balance and fell." He goes on to remind you his career has been that of a banker. He continues, "I still advise family and friends, and I am very capable." He does not need "bars" on his bed or little "alarms" to wear like they put on him in the hospital. Thank you for inquiring, but he understands how to be safe and how to protect himself. You feel that he has no further interest in discussing what you believe is a significant problem.

In previous chapters you learned about nursing process and its application to your care of clients. You learned about individuals and their response to healthcare. This chapter expands your knowledge base with information about the importance and the art of establishing good communication with the client. You will learn how to apply a new skill in the therapeutic relationship. Critical Thinking Challenges at the end of the chapter will help you apply your body of knowledge to the care of the man living alone in his retirement apartment.

Effective communication within the nurse–client relationship is not so much a natural process as it is a learned skill. It is a way of being helpful to clients that differs from the way a clerk in a grocery store is helpful, or the way friends are helpful to each other. For example, when the grocery clerk gives a courteous answer to a question about a product, the result is a satisfied customer. In a conversation between two friends who are sharing their problems, each friend feels cared for and understood. Although nurse–client communication may include some of the elements in these examples, it differs considerably.

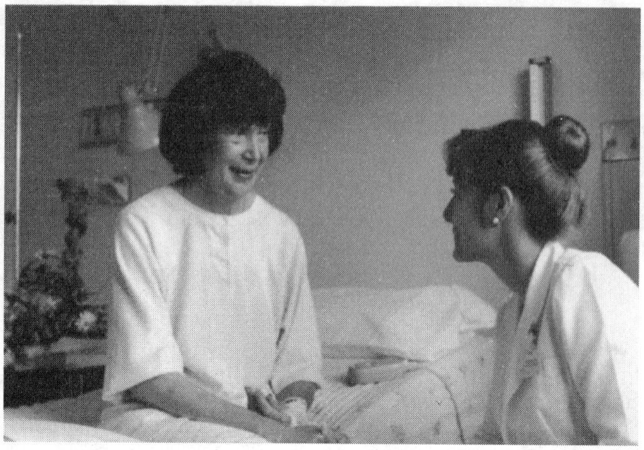

Figure 20-1 • Listening and investigating are ways to address client concerns. This occurs in all aspects of care and is the purpose of therapeutic communication.

The main subject of communication in the nurse–client relationship is the *client* and his or her experiences and problems. The results are directed toward improving coping skills related to the client's health status and well-being. Thus, **therapeutic communication** is a way of being helpful by facilitating interactions that are focused on the client and the client's concerns. The purpose of therapeutic communication is to help the client express and work through feelings and problems related to his or her condition, treatments, and nursing care (Fig. 20-1).

What kind of a process is therapeutic communication, and how does it fit into the context of nursing practice? Because nursing is a practice based on the sciences, nurses master many scientific principles and technical skills. Nursing is an interpersonal process also. Interaction between the nurse and the client has a great deal to do with the outcomes of care. The following happens during the communication process:

- The nurse and client work together to solve problems centered around the client's healthcare needs.
- The client feels cared for and understood.
- The family is included in the care.
- Health teaching is conducted.
- Preventive care is delivered.

Peplau, a psychiatric nurse and nurse theorist, considered nursing to be a "significant therapeutic interpersonal process" and defined nursing as a "human relationship between an individual who is sick or in need of health services and a nurse especially educated to recognize and respond to the need for help" (Peplau, 1952). In short, communication is at the heart of all nursing care.

To understand therapeutic communication, we must first understand the communication process and the importance of language and experience. Specific ingredients and techniques of communication, and knowledge about the nurse–client relationship, contract setting, advocacy, confidentiality, and developmental issues related to communication are important as well. This chapter gives an overview of these and other concepts related to therapeutic communication. Communication as a social interaction is discussed in Chapter 48.

The Communication Process

There are many definitions of communication. To communicate means to impart information, to exchange ideas, to express ourselves in such a way that we are understood. Communication can be defined as a system of sending and receiving messages that forms a connection between the sender and the receiver (Fig. 20-2). It is a process for giving and receiving information, a form of interaction or transaction.

Communication is a continuous function of human life, much like breathing or cardiac functioning. The process goes on all the time. In many ways, the saying "You cannot NOT communicate" is true. For example, when a person decides not to share information, or one person stops talking to another person because of hurt or anger, communication has still taken place.

Communication is basic and essential to being human. Through communication, people relate to their environment and to each other. Without it, we would be unable to learn, to direct our lives, and to work together cooperatively in families, organizations, and communities. Communication is basic to human feeling and intellect; without it, we could not survive (Berlo, 1960; Thayer, 1968).

Types of Communication

People communicate in a variety of ways. *Verbal communication* involves the spoken or written word. It is an exchange using the elements of language (see Chapter 48). Equally important is **nonverbal communication**. A person communicates by gestures, facial

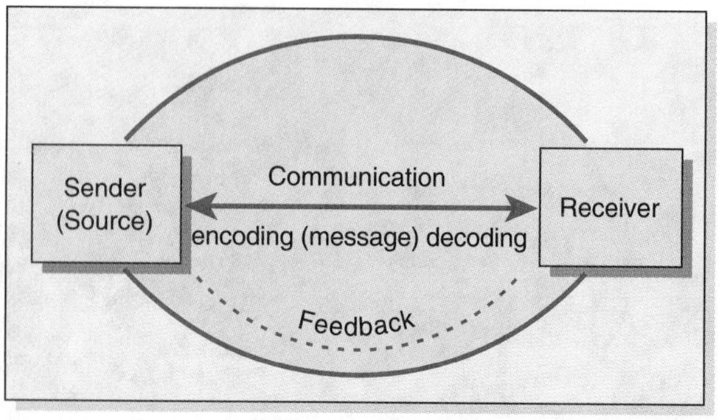

Figure 20-2 • Communication is a process in which information is sent and received. It is a form of interaction that is continuous and ever-changing.

Examples of Types of Communication

Verbal	*Nonverbal*
Written	Touch
Spoken	Eye contact
Television and radio	Facial expression
Movies	Body posture
Magazines	Gestures
Books	Physical appearance
Computers	Voice tone
Posters	Rate of speech
Brochures	Neatness
	Movement

expressions, posture, body movement, voice tone, rate of speech, and even dress. Silence is a form of nonverbal communication. Verbal and nonverbal communication are discussed more fully in Chapter 48. Examples of types of communication are listed in the accompanying display.

Another kind of communication, **metacommunication**, is a message *about* a message. It looks beyond the literal level of communication (that is, beyond just the words of the message). Metacommunication includes anything that is taken into account when interpreting what is happening, such as the role of the communicator, the nonverbal messages sent, and the context of the communication taking place (Crowther, 1991).

Relationship of Types

The relationships between these kinds of communication (verbal, nonverbal, and metacommunication) are important. The way they fit or do not fit together reflects just how complex communication is. The following two examples illustrate this.

Incongruence. A client and a nurse have been working together on diabetic teaching. After the teaching session is completed, the client says to the nurse, "Yes, I understand my diabetic diet and how to take my insulin." On the surface, this seems to be a straightforward communication indicating that the client understands the components of care needed to deal successfully with diabetes. If, however, the words of the message were said with an irritated facial expression and a harsh tone of voice, the nonverbal and metacommunication aspects of the message do not "fit" with the verbal message; they are incongruent. The metacommunication in this example may be conveying, "I am tired of being told how to run my life. I am angry about having a chronic illness." Furthermore, if the client is later seen sneaking a candy bar, this nonverbal communication may convey the message that the client has not yet accepted the illness. In this example, recognizing incongruence between kinds of communication informs the nurse about the client's experience.

Congruence. A nurse makes rounds on her assigned primary clients at the beginning of the shift. She explains her role to each client, confers with them about their nursing care needs, and schedules with them the care tasks to be done on that shift. The nurse is dressed in a professional manner and wears a name tag and hospital identification badge. She speaks in a well-modulated voice and listens carefully to what each client says.

In this example, each kind of communication conveys messages that are congruent. The messages say, "I am your professional nurse. We will work together to meet your nursing care needs. I respect you." There is a "good fit" between verbal, nonverbal, and metacommunication.

Elements of the Communication Process

As shown in Figure 20-2, communication is a continuous operation, dynamic, ongoing, and ever-changing. Although it is somewhat artificial to break down communication into components, doing so can be useful. Knowing the individual elements of a process can be helpful in identifying where in the process a problem is occurring. The elements of the model presented here are based on the work of Berlo (1960), a communication theorist.

All communication has a *sender* (a person or group with a purpose for the communication). The sender's purpose must be translated into a code. This is done with language or nonverbal signals such as gestures, facial expressions, or body cues. The process of getting the purpose translated into the code is called **encoding**. Encoding results in a *message*. Another element in the communication process is the **communication channel**, the medium or carrier of the message. Television is a channel; the voice or written word are channels; touch can be a channel.

If the communication process were to stop at this element, no communication would have taken place because there must be someone at the other end of the channel, the *receiver*. The receiver is the target of the communication, and must be able to understand or decode the message. Once messages are decoded and received, feedback occurs. **Feedback** means that the source and the receiver use one another's reactions to produce further messages.

Knowledge about the elements of the communication process can be useful to the nurse because sometimes specific difficulties in communication can be traced to one or more of the elements identified. A basic example is the client who speaks a different language.

In this case, the nurse needs to attend to the communication channel. An interpreter may be needed to help the client decode the nurse's messages. Pictures may also be used to convey messages.

Problems in the encoding process may occur as well. These problems can occur in clients with thought disorders or certain forms of brain damage. The client has an intent to communicate, but impairment in encoding results in a garbled message. A frightened client whose thoughts are disturbed may say, "The FBI is after me," when he really means, "I am very frightened and out of control." In the case of a client suffering from a stroke, the client may understand communication directed at him, but cannot encode a returning message because of brain damage. Chapter 48 provides more specific information about altered communication due to brain damage.

Importance of Language and Experience

The importance of language and experience to the process of communication cannot be overestimated. Language distinguishes humans from other animals. It is used not only to communicate but to develop the person's view of life and the world. Thus, language and experience are closely related. This idea was developed by Brandler and Grinder (1975), and the following discussion is based on their work.

A person's view of the world is developed through several kinds of filters. One such filter consists of the neurologic receptor systems: sight, hearing, touch, taste, and smell. Stimuli processed through these receptor systems enable the person to experience the outside world, and through language such experiences can be compared with others' experiences. Alterations in sensory perceptions can change the person's view of the world. A person with poor hearing or vision, for example, experiences the world differently from someone with perfect hearing and vision.

Another filter through which a person experiences the world is the particular language system into which the person is socialized. Words and sentences give meaning to things and events. Language allows us to conceptualize the world. If a language has only three words for all the color distinctions possible to see, for example, then a person would conceptualize colors differently from someone whose language offered more choices. Someone with a limited vocabulary has more difficulty describing experiences than does someone with a rich, diverse vocabulary. In fact, limitations in language skills may actually limit the person's choices in life.

A third filter through which a person experiences the world is his or her unique personal history. Every human has a set of experiences that are unique. Cultural background enters into personal history, as do family relationships, the person's place in the sibling ranking, the type of parenting received, the genetic makeup of the person, and other factors.

Both nurse and client bring their backgrounds into the communication that occurs between them. Some aspects of their background are shared and some are different. Consider, for example, the image of "a nurse" that is brought to a nurse–client situation. Nursing may be viewed by some as a female profession, and may invoke certain stereotypes about female behaviors and roles. In many societies, women are defined as subservient to men and their work is devalued. Often, the "caring" image of nursing overshadows the knowledge and decision-making and technical abilities of the nurse. Campbell-Heider and Hart (1993) point out that the language and dress of the nurse reflect not only society's view of the nurse but the nurse's view of self. Professional presentation, in turn, influences how the client perceives and responds to the nurse.

The interaction of the nurse and the client is productive when communication is aimed toward a common understanding. To communicate effectively, the nurse understands and appreciates his or her own background, while at the same time acknowledging different perspectives held by the client.

In the clinical setting, the extent to which clients and nurses successfully exchange information is affected by the degree to which their realities are mutually compatible. The very system in which most nurses work produces barriers to communication. For example, technical language can be a barrier to communication. Studies have shown that the inability of working-class clients to understand technical language intimidates them and prevents them from asking questions on their own behalf. Other barriers include talking about the client in front of him or her, withholding information from the client, and being too busy to spend time with the client (Matthews, 1983).

In her classic work on the nurse–client relationship, Peplau (1952) identified two overriding principles that guide communication: clarity and continuity. Table 20-1 illustrates the concepts of clarity and continuity.

Clarity refers to words and sentences used to help a client clarify events. Meaning is established or made understandable as a result of the joint and sustained effort of everyone involved in the communication. Clarity is facilitated when the client's perceptions are expressed and discussed.

Continuity in communication occurs when language is used to promote coherence or connections of ideas expressed. Continuity occurs when the nurse picks up threads or cues of conversation offered by the client. A conversational thread or cue is a vaguely expressed word, phrase, or idea that hints at a problem or concern. The nurse helps the client focus on and elaborate on these cues. By doing so, the client is helped to express underlying problems or concerns.

Table 20-1 • Examples of Clarity and Continuity

Clarity	Continuity
Client: I am having pain. ("Pain" can mean many things.) Nurse: Where is the pain? Client: In my stomach. Nurse: What kind of pain is it? Can you describe it to me? (Client describes exact nature and place of pain.) Outcome: Nurse and client come to a common understanding about the client's experience.	Client: This place is crazy. Things are confusing here. ("Crazy" and "confusing" are conversational cues.) Nurse: Confusing? Client: Yes, I can't tell what is going on. ("Going on" is a cue.) Nurse: "Going on" in what sense? Client: About my condition. No one is explaining it to me. Outcome: Client is helped to focus on the real problem because the nurse helped him elaborate on conversational cues.

The Nurse–Client Relationship: A Helping Relationship

Within the nurse–client relationship, the nurse assumes the role of a professional, a helper. The client is the one seeking help. This kind of relationship differs from a social or intimate relationship. The nurse–client relationship is focused on the client, is goal directed, and has defined parameters. Another important way that the nurse–client relationship differs from a social one concerns the nurse's self-assessment. In the professional relationship, the nurse learns to assess his or her own role, communication skills, personal history, and values in terms of how these may be affecting the nurse–client relationship and interactions. Table 20-2 compares the nurse–client relationship with a social relationship.

Phases

The nurse–client relationship can be thought of in terms of three phases: orientation, working, and termination. The *orientation* phase consists of introductions and an agreement between nurse and client about their mutual roles and responsibilities. In the psychiatric setting, the orientation phase of the relationship represents

Table 20-2 • Comparison of Professional With Social Relationship

	Nurse–Client	Social
Key Focus	Client	Both participants
Goals	Meeting client's needs. Help client identify feelings and concerns; problem-solve, cope, and adapt in relation to healthcare situation.	Meeting own needs. Mutual companionship, enjoyment, and interaction. May lead to intimacy and commitment.
Parameters	Limited primarily to the needs incurred by the healthcare situation. Nurse self-discloses only what is appropriate for the client's benefit. Relationship is terminated when goals are met and service no longer needed.	Sharing of life's events, activities, or other aspects of self. May stay superficial or lead to long-term relationship. Relationship may be terminated when own needs are no longer met.
Self-Assessment	Nurse assesses own role, communication skills, values, and so forth, and how these affect the professional relationship.	Each person assesses how own needs for enjoyment, affection, and sharing, or love and intimacy, are met in the relationship.

the first phase of therapeutic work. The nurse and client get to know each other and trust is developed (Forchuk, 1992; Trojan & Yonge, 1993).

During the *working* phase, the nurse and client participate together in nursing care activities. During this period the client "uses" the nurse's expertise and abilities on his or her behalf. The nurse functions as the client's advocate, caring for his or her physical and emotional healthcare needs. With psychiatric clients, the working phase consists of problem solving around emotional, behavioral, and interpersonal issues.

Termination is the closure of the relationship. The nurse reviews with the client aspects of care and how they have dealt with physical and emotional responses. Discharge planning is a key component in the termination process. Termination can take various forms. For example, the nurse–client relationship can end when the client is discharged or the nurse is reassigned. It is important for the nurse to be clear about termination. Continued contact beyond professional responsibilities usually is not good practice.

In psychiatric nursing, the nurse–client relationship tends to be more structured, with the nurse functioning as a therapeutic counselor. The nurse is actually using the relationship itself to help the client develop better coping skills and improve relationships. In the more general nursing setting, the nurse–client relationship tends to be more clinical in nature. Nurse–client contact is shorter and revolves around brief treatments (Morse, 1991). Other nurses and professionals often share in the care of the client. The nurse's days off interrupt the continuity of the relationship. Even though the professional relationship may lack some continuity, however, it is still important that the relationship retain some structure. Attention needs to be given to the appropriate roles and functions within each phase of the relationship.

Contract Setting

The professional relationship can take various forms. Generally, the nurse–client relationship is based on an informal contractual model. In the contractual relationship, clients are seen as having control over the significant decisions affecting their lives (Aroskar, 1980; Smith, 1986). Aspects of care, goals of treatment, and necessary adaptations are discussed with the client, and the nurse takes no major action without consulting the client or a family member representing the client. The basic attitude in the contractual relationship is one of collaboration. The nurse discusses his or her role with the client, as well as the client's condition, treatment, and nursing care. Decisions about nursing and healthcare are made collaboratively.

The contractual relationship between nurse and client is an informal one, which means that contracting is done verbally and is an assumed attitude toward the relationship. In the area of psychiatric nursing practice, contracts tend to be more formal, sometimes even written, and tend to be used as a therapeutic tool to help a client develop more insight and control over his or her own behavior (Loomis, 1985).

Elements of an Informal Nurse–Client Contract

Nurse and client know each other's names
Roles and responsibilities are clarified
Parameters of the professional relationship are clear
Mutual expectations are agreed on
Circle of confidentiality is respected

The elements of an informal contract between nurse and client are summarized in the accompanying display. The usual way for a nurse to establish an informal contract with a client is to make a verbal agreement as to how they are to work together. A nurse might approach a client as follows: "I'm your primary nurse while you are a client here. This means I'm responsible for planning your care. On the evening and night shifts, other nurses will care for you according to the plan we decide on together. This afternoon we'll review your care plan together and decide how we can best meet your nursing care needs. How does that sound to you?"

An important advantage to the informal contractual relationship has to do with values and rights. The nurse maintains his or her own rights while respecting those of the client. For instance, what if a nurse disagrees with abortion, but the client under her care is considering having one? She can contract with the client to provide the information, but she need not participate in the procedure. The nurse must respect the client's rights. Because abortion is a legal procedure, she cannot restrain the client from having one. Indeed, she is obligated to provide the client with information so that the client can make a decision based on such information. The nurse, however, has every right to participate in organized protests against legalized abortion. She may also decide not to work for an institution that performs abortions.

Advocacy

Nurses are the most constant professionals in the client's environment. The ideologic orientation that nursing as a profession holds toward communication is one of **advocacy**, or taking the client's side. Advocacy holds that clients have a right to information so that they can make their own decisions about treatment options and nursing care. Clients need information about their health status and the course of illness so that they can make the necessary adjustments in their lives. Nursing believes that sharing information reduces anxiety and is an integral part of being therapeutic (Matthews, 1983).

Being an advocate for the client means that nurses must avoid taking a *maternalistic* approach (Taylor, 1985). Maternalism is the female counterpart of paternalism, but either men or women can be paternalistic or maternalistic in their relationships. The paternalistic approach is taken by professionals in authority, such as physicians. This approach assumes that the professional will make the decisions for the client ("father knows best"). The maternalistic approach takes the attitude of wanting what is best for the person by laying out consequences, not alternatives. The client is led to choose between "hurting" and "caring" or "being selfish" and "being responsible."

An example of a maternalistic approach is telling a child, "I cooked this dinner especially for you, and now you aren't going to eat it." The underlying message is "because you did not eat the dinner, mother is hurt and you are selfish." When used in child-rearing situations, maternalistic approaches are often appropriate because the child learns how his or her behavior affects another. But in the nurse–client relationship, the maternalistic approach is inappropriate and manipulative. Table 20-3 compares paternalistic and maternalistic approaches with the advocacy approach.

Open communication between the nurse and client sometimes conflicts with the physician's viewpoint (Barry, 1984; Matthews, 1983). Physicians tend to see the physician–client relationship as primary and exclusive, and tend to see themselves as in control of information. The best approach to this problem is for the nurse to develop a collaborative working relationship with the physician so that open communication and information sharing can occur between physician and nurse (Fagin, 1992). The nurse can also help the client become more assertive with the physician.

For instance, a client may confide in the nurse that she believes she is not receiving enough information about her condition. The client complains that the physician does not spend enough time with her, and she feels left out of the decisions made about treatment. If the nurse provides the information to the client without conferring with the physician, the nurse has intruded into the physician–client relationship; after all, the client's perception is that more information is needed from the physician.

In this instance, the nurse can do several things. He or she can discuss the problem with the client and help the client assert herself through such means as writing a list of questions to ask the physician. With the client's permission, the nurse can seek out the physician and share the client's perceptions with him or her. By handling the situation in this manner, the nurse has not interfered in the physician-client relationship but has acted on the client's behalf. This action is true to the role of advocacy.

Circle of Confidentiality

Every client has a right to privacy, but it is important for client information to be shared with all the professionals involved in his or her care. The people with whom client information can be shared can be thought of as a **circle of confidentiality**. This circle includes all the people in a nursing unit who have responsibility for the client. It usually includes the family, unless the client objects.

The nurse should clarify with the client that he or she is part of a team. Consider, for example, a nurse who has been caring for a client with a serious prognosis.

Table 20-3 • Comparison of Paternalistic, Maternalistic, and Advocacy Approaches

Clinical example: Surgery has been recommended but the client is reluctant to have the operation.

	Paternalistic	Maternalistic	Advocacy
Approach	No choice	Choice based on consequences of actions	Choice based on information and examination of alternatives
Response	"Surgery is your only choice. You need this operation."	"If you don't have the surgery, you may not live to see your grandchildren. Your family needs you."	"Whether or not you have the surgery is your choice. It is your body. What is your understanding of the situation?"
Underlying Message	The professional knows best and should make the decisions for you.	If you don't do what the professional recommends, you and others will get hurt.	The professional is here to help you make informed choices about your health and well-being.

The client says to the nurse, "If I tell you something, will you promise to keep it in the strictest confidence? Don't tell anyone else, not even my family." The nurse agrees. Then the client says that he plans to kill himself after he is discharged, stating that he has a loaded gun at home.

The nurse in this example failed to adhere to the concept of the circle of confidentiality. The proper response would be to tell the client that the nurse is part of the healthcare team, and important information is shared with the team if the nurse believes that to be in the client's best interest. This protects both nurse and client.

Transmitting information beyond the nursing unit, however, needs to be carefully considered. It is best to obtain written permission from the client before information is given out. The client's right to privacy is important. A client may not want others to know about his or her hospitalization, for example, or may not want anyone to know the nature of his or her illness. This is especially true in the case of stigmatized condition such as AIDS, substance addiction, and psychiatric illness. Nurses need to consider client confidentiality in such mundane situations as talking about clients at lunch or at home.

Ingredients of Therapeutic Communication

Up to this point, we have presented theory related to the communication process and the nurse–client relationship. Now we move on to therapeutic communication. What makes communication therapeutic, and how is it different from other forms of communication? For this discussion, we turn to the work of Carl Rogers (1961), who studied the process of therapeutic communication.

Rogers believed that a person cannot be separated from the techniques of communication he or she uses. Based on his research, the characteristics of a therapeutic, "helpful" person were identified. Empathy, positive regard, and a comfortable sense of self were among the key ingredients.

Empathy

Empathy is the ability to enter into another person's experience to perceive it accurately and to understand how the situation is viewed from the client's perspective. Empathy includes the ability to respond receptively to the other person's experience while still maintaining objectivity, and the ability to communicate to the person that they are understood (Williams, 1990; Morse, et al., 1992). This is done through the process of reflective or "active" listening, which is explained in the Intervention section of this chapter.

Empathy is a complex process. The nurse must

- Have enough knowledge and experience accurately to perceive the client's perspective
- Feel secure enough not to be intimidated if the client experiences a situation differently
- Feel comfortable enough with himself or herself to be able to imagine what a situation might be like for someone else, while remaining outside that situation to maintain objectivity
- Know how to let the client know that the nurse perceives the client's feelings, thoughts, and experiences accurately.

Empathy can be communicated to the client both verbally and nonverbally (Fig. 20-3). In two studies (Hardin & Gerace, 1983; Hardin & Halaris, 1983), researchers videotaped nurse–client interactions. The clients in the study and objective raters were asked to rate how empathic they thought the nurses were. Raters were then asked to identify behaviors they thought were empathic or nonempathic. After this, the researchers analyzed the identified behaviors by looking systematically at the behaviors on the videotapes. The results are summarized in Table 20-4.

It can be seen that focusing on feelings and being warm and nonjudgmental play an important role in empathic communication. Body orchestration, in terms of looking comfortable, is important as well. Moderate amounts of movement, such as tilting the head toward the client, smiling, leaning forward, and keeping the arms open, seem to communicate empathy. But looking away, stabbing gestures, closed or leaning-away body posture, sitting too still, or moving too much were experienced as nonempathic.

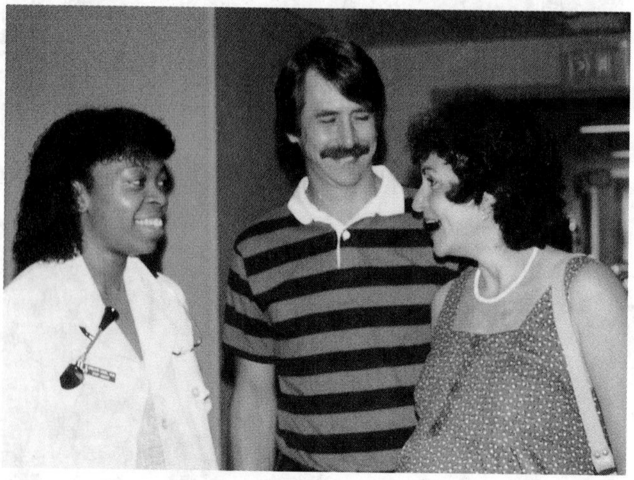

Figure 20-3 • The nurse communicates positive regard in interactions with clients.

Table 20-4 • Emphatic and Nonemphatic Behaviors

Emphatic	Nonemphatic
Verbal	
Focus on feelings	Ignore feelings
Reflect feelings	Closed (yes-no) questions
Open-ended questions	Judgmental attitude
Nonjudgmental attitude	Flat vocal tone
Warm vocal tone	
Nonverbal	
Eye contact	Looking away
Head nods	Nods too much
Some smiling	Picking at clothing on body
Smooth gestures	Too few smiles; inexpressive
Open arms	Laughs too much
Leaning toward	Stabbing gestures
Looking comfortable	Crossed arms
Movement synchronized	Leaning away
	Looking uncomfortable
	Movements not synchronized with client

From Hardin, S., & Gerace, L. (1983). Verbal and nonverbal counterparts in nurses' emphatic communication. Paper presented at Midwest Nursing Research Society, University of Iowa.

Positive Regard

Positive regard means warmth, caring, interest, and respect for the person. It is a way of seeing the person unconditionally or nonjudgmentally. Respect for the person does not depend on the person's behavior; instead, the person is regarded as worthwhile simply for being human.

How can this work? What if, for example, the nurse cares for a person who has been convicted of a serious crime? Does that mean that the nurse condones the things this person has done?

Positive regard does *not* mean that the nurse accepts all aspects of a person's behavior. The nurse does not condone or encourage behavior that is socially inappropriate or abusive. However, the nurse must separate that behavior from the person. The assumption is that the person is worthwhile and has value and dignity.

Positive regard also means that the professional avoids unnecessarily labeling clients. The focus of healthcare professionals on disease tends to label the client as an object (for example, a diabetic, an amputee, or an alcoholic). As a result, the client is seen as someone who is defective. There is an undeniable tendency to see clients not as if they *have* a disease but rather that they *are* the disease (Remen, 1980). This attitude can interfere with seeing the person behind the label and tends to come through in the communication process. When the person is ignored, it becomes more difficult to know and understand his or her response to health and illness and to use his or her strengths and potential.

Comfortable Sense of Self

Before a nurse can communicate therapeutically, it is important for him or her to have a comfortable sense of self. The nurse should be aware of his or her own personality, values, cultural background, and style of communication. Rogers (1961) used the term "becoming a person" to mean dropping the false fronts we sometimes assume in our professional roles and becoming the people we are inside.

A person with a comfortable sense of self is open to experiences and is aware of his or her feelings and attitudes. Doing so allows the person to take a more flexible view of life. For example, the nurse may notice that not all clients respond the same way to a similar surgical procedure, and that not all people in a given culture fit those cultural stereotypes. The differences between the nurse and client can be seen as interesting or challenging, not as threatening or "bad."

A person's sense of self is made up of a collection of characteristics. For example, a nurse may be a professional, a parent, and a sibling, and may be overweight, tall, athletic, or a host of other characteristics. How the nurse experiences these characteristics influences how he or she sees others.

The nurse with a comfortable sense of self can evaluate his or her strengths and weaknesses. For example, one nurse may say, "I work well with postoperative clients, but I have less aptitude for working with rehabilitation clients because I like things to happen more quickly." Another nurse might enjoy working with psychiatric clients because he finds working on interpersonal goals rewarding.

Self-evaluation also means taking responsibility for our actions as professionals. For example, a nurse might think, "I could have said something more supportive," or, "I should have included the family in the planning phase." Through this process, the nurse grows in professional competency.

The professional with a comfortable sense of self feels separate from others. This is an important aspect of being therapeutic, because it is easy for a nurse to overidentify with clients. A nurse who becomes too involved in the suffering of clients soon burns out and lacks the objectivity it takes to be therapeutic. A comfortable sense of separation from others also means that the nurse does not seek gratification by promoting excessive client dependence. The nurse gives appropriate support and care but has confidence in clients' abilities to make choices about their health and lives.

Having a comfortable sense of self is in part acomplished by having a well rounded life. Nursing is demanding work, and can be emotionally draining and physically tiring. To maintain professional enthusiasm and job satisfaction, nurses must attend to their needs as people. They should get enough rest and exercise and should eat a balanced diet. They must take care of themselves emotionally by having supportive relationships, interesting activities, and time to relax and enjoy themselves. Being therapeutic with ourselves is necessary before we can be therapeutic with others.

Communication and Nursing Process

The nurse–client relationship and therapeutic communication are instruments used to implement the nursing process. The nursing process can also be applied to the communication that takes place between nurse and client, as well as the professional relationship. There are specific things to assess about the client's communication, and specific therapeutic communication techniques are part of nursing intervention. Also, developmental considerations affect communication with different age groups.

Assessment

Because therapeutic communication takes place within the nurse–client relationship, the first area of assessment concerns the goals of the relationship. Goals vary depending on the client's needs, the area of nursing practice, and the specific role of the nurse in each particular clinical situation.

For example, a nurse works on a postpartum unit where the average length of stay is only 2 days. Each nurse cares for an average of eight clients per shift. The nurse's role is primarily to care for the mother's physical needs, facilitate mother–infant bonding, and assess and conduct whatever teaching is necessary to help the family care for and adjust to the newborn. In this situation, the nurse–client relationship is short-term and focused. The nurse renders little direct physical care, working instead as an adviser and health teacher. The nurse and client move through each phase of the nurse–client relationship quickly.

In contrast, another nurse works for a hospice program and gives care in the homes of terminally ill clients. The nurse spends 2 hours three times a week with the client and family. Her role is to give direct physical care, to support the client and family, and to teach the family how to care for the client. This relationship is intense and demanding. During the orientation phase, the nurse needs to establish a working relationship with the family and the client. She talks with the client and family about how they will communicate and work together, thus establishing a verbal contract. In this situation the nurse works as a direct caregiver, teacher, and therapeutic counselor.

After the nurse has established appropriate goals for the nurse–client relationship, the nurse introduces herself and calls the client by name. The nurse then clarifies the nature of their relationship and the purpose of the interactions to take place. An agreement is made that includes the frequency, length, and goals of nurse–client contacts.

During this initial phase of the relationship, the nurse assesses the client's communication, using the theoretical base presented earlier in this chapter. Some key areas of communication assessment are summarized in the display. Are verbal and nonverbal communications congruent? What are the feelings and themes conveyed by the client? What emotions are expressed? What are the client's communication patterns? Does he or she speak slowly or rapidly? Does he or she get caught up in minute details? Are there long silences? Can the client express himself or herself openly and ask the questions he or she needs to ask? When messages are sent by the nurse, does the client return feedback that is precise, pertinent, and directed toward the goals of the nurse–client relationship?

Assessing the environment in which communication takes place is also important. The external environment must be conducive to communication. How are the nurse and client positioned in relation to each other? How far apart are they? Noise is another important consideration. Telephones, televisions, radios, and

Communication Assessment Tool

Name__________ **Age**______ **Sex**______ **Diagnosis**______

I. Sender or receiver impairments

- Structural deficit ______
- Sense deficits: hearing, sight, smell, touch, taste ______
- Loss of functions ______
- Disease ______
- Drugs ______
- Other ______

II. Message variables

Nonverbal communication

1. Facial expression ______
2. Gestures ______
3. Body movements ______
4. Affect ______
5. Tone of voice ______
6. Posture ______
7. Eye contact ______
8. Voice volume, quality, pitch ______
9. Other ______

Verbal communication

1. Content of message ______
2. Themes ______
3. Emotions ______

Communication patterns

1. Blocking ______
2. Slow ______
3. Rapid ______
4. Quiet ______
5. Halting ______
6. Aphasic ______
7. Continuity ______
8. Excessive ______
9. Detailed ______
10. Stammering ______
11. Circumstantial ______
12. Tangential ______
13. Long silences ______
14. Other ______

III. Noise

IV. Communication skills

- Openness, spontaneity ______
- Use of clarification ______
- Request for feedback ______
- Tolerance of silence ______
- Acceptance of confrontation ______
- Other ______

V. Setting ______

VI. Feedback

- Precise ______
- Pertinent ______
- Goal-directed ______
- Informative ______
- Solicited ______
- Positive ______
- Negative ______
- Clarified ______
- Opportune ______

VII. Environment

External influences

1. Temperature ______
2. Physical arrangement ______
3. Personal space ______
4. Lighting ______
5. Noise level ______
6. Privacy ______

Internal influences

1. Beliefs ______
2. Experiences ______
3. Thoughts ______
4. Attitudes ______

VIII. Cultural influences

- Health practice ______
- Religious implications ______
- Language barriers ______
- Food preferences ______
- Other ______

Adapted from Johnson, B. S. (1993). *Psychiatric mental-health nursing: Adaptation and growth.* (3rd ed.) Philadelphia: J. B. Lippincott.

machines, such as ventilators, cardiac monitors, and suctioning machines can be distracting. Privacy is another important factor. The presence of other clients and employees can interfere with comfortable communication.

The client's internal environment is made up of his or her cultural background, beliefs, and experiences. Assessing how these affect nurse–client communication is important. For example, do the client's religious beliefs pervade all aspects of his or her life and decision making? If so, this will affect communication, especially if the nurse has a different belief system. Language and cultural practices also should be assessed.

Many of the same factors assessed in the client pertain to the nurse as well. The nurse needs to consider his or her voice tone, quality, and pitch, body language, facial expressions, and verbal fluency, and should know how anxiety may affect them. The nurse must constantly assess his or her communication and feedback skills, and must also examine how his or her cultural beliefs and personal history affect his or her perception of the client (Cravener, 1992; Murphy & Clark, 1993).

Intervention

Once communication has been assessed, how does the nurse use communication as a therapeutic intervention? Specific techniques to facilitate therapeutic communication are summarized in Table 20-5. The therapeutic communication skills highlighted in this section are considered basic to any therapeutic relationship. More advanced skills are usually studied in psychiatric nursing, especially at the advanced practice (master's degree) level.

Helping the Client Get Started

Generally, nurses are involved in informal therapeutic relationships, which can be important to the client (Barry, 1984). In the acute cure setting, the nurse often combines physical care with a discussion about the client's concerns. One of the most important things a nurse can do to encourage a client to express concerns is to sit down. Clients do not feel like expressing themselves to someone who is always in a hurry or seems too busy. It helps to draw the curtain between beds, and to see that the client faces away from any roommates and toward the nurse.

The nurse should call the client by name, asking if the client prefers to be called by the first or last name. Many adults find being called by their first name intrusive or rude. The nurse should convey interest and readiness to listen. By leaning toward the client, making eye contact, and assuming a relaxed, open posture, the nurse offers himself or herself to the client. General principles for facilitating communication appear in the accompanying display.

Open-Ended Questions. An *open-ended question* is one that elicits more than a "yes" or "no" answer. Such questions ask how, what, where, and when. Examples of appropriate questions are "How are things going for you at this point?" or "What have your experiences been like?"

Opening Remarks. Other ways to help a client get started include *opening remarks* based on observations and assessment about the client. Having assessed the communication and behavior of the client, the nurse can make statements such as, "You've been having a pretty rough time," "I notice you're going through some important changes," or "You seem to be feeling better."

These questions and statements must be neutral and tentative, not probing or interrogating. "Why" questions usually are not considered therapeutic because they are too intrusive; newspaper reporters and schoolteachers ask "why" questions. For example, asking a client why they are upset is more threatening than just noting that they seem upset.

Table 20-5 • Therapeutic Communication Techniques

Technique	Definition
Offering self	Making self available to listen to the client
Open-ended questions	Neutral questions that encourage the client to express concerns
Opening remarks	General statements based on observations and assessments about the client
Restatement	Repeating to the client the main content of his or her communication
Reflection	Identifying the main emotional themes contained in a communication and directing these back to the client
Focusing	Asking goal-directed questions to help the client focus on key concerns
Encouraging elaboration	Helping the client to describe more fully the concerns or problems under discussion
Seeking clarification	Helping the client put into words unclear thoughts or ideas
Giving information	Sharing with the client relevant information for his or her healthcare and well-being
Looking at alternatives	Helping the client see options and participate in the decision-making process related to his or her healthcare and well-being
Silence	A pause in communication that allows nurse and client time to think about what has taken place
Summarizing	Highlighting the important points of a conversation by condensing what was said

Nursing Care Guidelines
Facilitating Communication

- Speak in a normal tone.
- Do not raise your voice or shout unless the client is deaf.
- Realize that speaking louder does not increase comprehension.
- Speak to the client on an adult level.
- Remember that impaired communication does not indicate impaired intelligence.
- Avoid carrying on more than one conversation at a time.
- Ask simple questions that require simple answers.
- Keep the atmosphere quiet and relaxed.
- Reduce or eliminate environmental noises.
- Make sure you have the client's attention before you speak.
- Maintain eye contact with the client throughout the conversation.
- Assume clients can understand you. Do not discuss their cases or other inappropriate topics in front of them.
- Do not rush the client. Give him or her adequate time to respond.
- Do not correct mistakes.
- If you do not understand, ask the client to repeat what he or she said.
- Praise clients for their attempts at speech.

Active Listening

Nurses often underestimate the value of listening and the skills needed to listen well (Gibbons, 1993). The nurse must be able to focus on the client and what the client's messages are about. Listening actively means that the nurse conveys back to the client an accurate picture of what the client is expressing (Fig. 20-4).

Listening actively means that the listener must constantly decode the messages sent. The nurse listens for both content and feeling. The content part of the message includes thoughts, words, opinions, and ideas; the feeling part refers to the client's emotions. Emotions may be described verbally but usually are manifested more accurately through nonverbal means such as facial expression, body posture, laughter, or crying. Noting congruence or incongruence between these messages helps the nurse understand how clients are experiencing the things they are discussing.

The nurse must also observe what is behind the message sent by the client. For example, is the client conveying an attitude of helplessness, rejection, or aggression toward the nurse?

As the nurse decodes the conversation, he or she listens actively by using two important techniques: restatement and reflection. These key techniques are used to help a client feel listened to and understood.

Restatement refers mainly to the content portion of the communication. The nurse listens carefully to the client and restates the content of the communication back to the client, to verify the nurse's understanding with the client. When the content is restated, the client has the opportunity to hear himself or herself, and to gain understanding of his or her own communication.

Reflection means identifying the main emotional themes contained in a communication and directing them back to the client. The nurse listens for the underlying feeling that a client is conveying, then states his or her understanding of that feeling in a neutral, open manner. The purpose is to verify the feelings that are being heard and to check what is being heard with the client. As a result, the client gains a clearer understanding of the feelings being experienced.

The following example shows how these might be used in an informal therapeutic relationship:

Client: I can't sleep. It's too hot in here and the noise is bothering me.
Nurse: You can't sleep because it's uncomfortable in here. (*Restatement*)
Client: That's right. All I can think about is having that operation in the morning. (Sounds irritable, looks anxious.)
Nurse: The thought of having surgery is keeping you awake. (*Reflection*)
Client: Yes. I'm really scared.

In this situation, the nurse listened carefully and found that it was not really the environment but the anxiety about having surgery that was keeping the client awake. By communicating back to the client in a

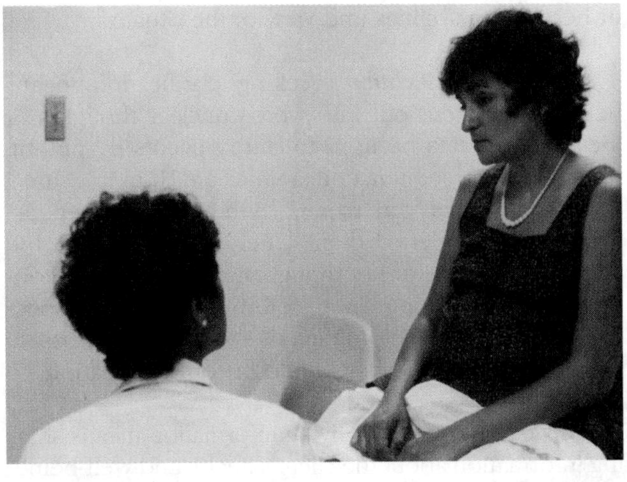

Figure 20-4 • *Waiting silently and attentively is an effective means of therapeutic technique.*

careful way the things she was hearing, the nurse opened up an opportunity to clarify concerns and misperceptions about the impending surgery.

Exploring

Exploring is a way of communicating therapeutically without giving direct advice. Instead, the nurse helps clients express their concerns and solve their own problems by exploring the situation, how the client feels about it, and what some alternatives might be.

Focusing. Focusing means asking goal-directed questions that help the client stay on the topic and talk more about it. The questions should still be open-ended, but are directed toward the key concerns. An example of focusing is, "We were talking about how people will respond to your mastectomy. Can you say more about that?"

Asking focused questions helps the client to discuss the main issues of concern. It keeps the conversation on target by not changing the subject or becoming too generalized. By staying on the subject, the nurse is conveying that he or she will stay with the clientand help explore concerns.

Sometimes helping a client express things of importance can be frightening. The nurse encounters a variety of suffering when working with ill and dying clients. To be therapeutic, a nurse must develop maturity and a sense of perspective about life. This takes time and experience.

Encouraging Elaboration. Encouraging elaboration is a technique used to help the client describe more fully the concerns or problems under discussion. By nodding one's head, using an attentive demeanor, and making comments such as "go on" or "I see," the nurse encourages the client to keep talking and to express himself or herself more thoroughly. This helps the nurse to learn about the client's emotional state and his or her coping abilities and view of the situation.

Seeking Clarification. Seeking clarification means helping the client put into words unclear thoughts or ideas. It can also be used to clarify events by putting them in a time sequence. Examples are, "I'm not sure I understand what you mean," "What else happened?" and "What happened then?" Such questions help the client to order his or her thoughts, put events into context, and place things in a more manageable perspective. By clarifying the problem or event being discussed, the client gains new insight into his or her situation.

Giving Information. Giving information means sharing information about the client's health and well-being. This must be done in a timely manner and should be based on what is currently known about the client's condition. Giving information can mean sharing what is known about a client's illness, treatment, and recovery. It can also mean correcting misperceptions.

For example, a young woman is brought to the emergency room after she was raped. After medical care is completed, police reports filled out, and her family notified, the nurse sits with her for a few minutes while she waits for a family member to come. The client says, "I should have been more careful. I was wearing a short skirt. Maybe that caused the rape."

Based on what the nurse knows about rape victims' perceptions, a timely intervention might be for the nurse to say, "When people are raped, it is usual for them to look for the cause within themselves. But the rape is not your fault. You are the victim in this situation." This information is based on research showing that rape victims commonly assume that they provoked the rape. In addition to giving this information, the nurse might also refer the client to a rape counseling center in the community.

Giving information is a skill used by nurses in health teaching and is often done while the nurse is giving physical care. Information must be distinguished from suggestions or advice. A typical way to give advice is to start by saying, "Why don't you?" or "You should." Such advice-giving reinforces the client's dependence on the nurse. A more useful strategy is to give the information the client needs so he or she can make a decision.

Looking at Alternatives. Looking at alternatives means exploring options for the client's consideration. When more options are identified, the client's perceived choices are increased (Fig. 20-5). The nurse does not always need to present the alternatives; the client can be asked for them instead. Examples of questions to use are as follows:

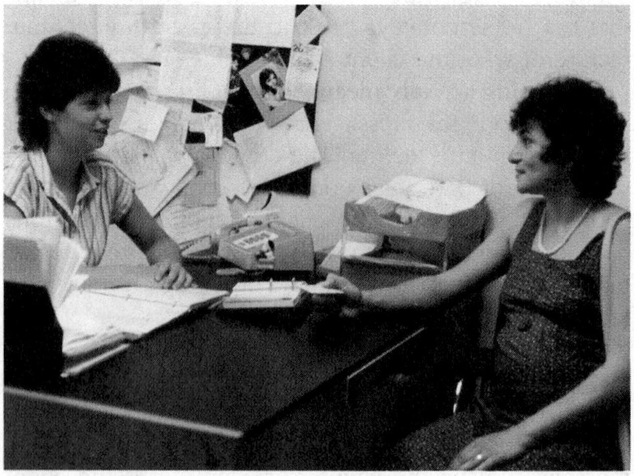

Figure 20-5 • Examining alternatives increases the client's perceived choices.

- What are some of your ideas about how to handle this?
- Have you thought about (alternate courses of action)?
- What else could you do?
- If you met someone in the same situation as you, what would you advise him or her to do?
- What are some advantages (disadvantages) of (alternatives)?

Alternatives should not be discussed too early or before the client has a clear understanding of the current situation. Sometimes the client must first express feelings such as grief or anger before he or she can explore how to deal with the situation.

Silence. Another useful therapeutic technique is using silence, a pause in communication that allows the nurse and client to reflect on what has taken place. By waiting quietly and attentively, the nurse encourages the client to initiate and maintain conversation.

Summarizing. Summarizing means highlighting the important points of a conversation by condensing what was said. This is useful toward the end of a therapeutic conversation. Summarizing helps both nurse and client review the main themes of the conversation and gives a sense of closure. It also enables the nurse and client to think about what else needs to be thought or talked about in the future. It emphasizes the progress made toward self-understanding and problem solving. Examples of summarizing include, "Today it seems that you've thought about . . ." and "Let's review what we've talked about today."

Developing Communication Skills

These and other therapeutic techniques are helpful in maintaining the boundaries of the nurse–client relationship. Communication between nurse and client in the clinical setting is based on client needs, not on personal or social interests. By maintaining a professional approach and being client centered, the nurse maintains a focus on the client's health and well-being.

It takes time and experience for the nurse to become skilled at using therapeutic communication. One way to develop this skill is to study one's interactions, either by tape recording a therapeutic conversation (after obtaining the client's permission) or by recreating the conversation from memory. Once a transcript of the conversation is made, the nurse can then analyze his or her skill. The nurse should look at what techniques were used, their timing and appropriateness, and how the client responded to the nurse. The nurse's own thoughts and feelings should also be noted, because these affect how he or she responds to the client. An example of a process recording is shown in Table 20-6.

Nontherapeutic Responses

Nontherapeutic responses are those that interfere with or block therapeutic communication. Often such responses are the more natural ones that might be made in social situations. Nontherapeutic responses may prevent the nurse from functioning as a professional and a therapeutic agent in the client's care.

The nurse's own needs must be met outside the therapeutic context. A nurse might, for example, become overly involved with clients because he has not developed his social life in a way that meets his needs. Another nurse might be uncomfortable with clients who express feelings because she has never been allowed to express her own. The nurse must engage in self-evaluation to determine his or her own strengths and weaknesses.

Inexperienced healthcare workers may believe that serious problems can be easily solved. After all, on television, dire problems are solved in half an hour. But in real life this is not always the case, and presenting quick solutions and unwarranted cheerfulness blocks the therapeutic process. Some people have incurable illnesses. Others must adapt to situations for which there are no quick or simple answers. Through experience, nurses learn that they can help, but cannot always provide perfect solutions. It is important to maintain a supportive presence and to provide competent care while the client struggles through a difficult situation.

A variety of nontherapeutic responses block the therapeutic communication process.

Rescue Feelings. A nurse has rescue feelings when he or she feels essential to the client's welfare. The nurse thinks that he or she has exceptional abilities to help the client, and expectations for the client will be high.

Some rescue feelings may be useful, because having confidence in one's abilities to be helpful is part of being therapeutic. Strong rescue feelings, however, impede the therapeutic process. The nurse may believe that only he or she can meet the client's needs, alienating himself or herself from the healthcare team. The nurse may also raise the client's expectations too high; when these expectations are not met, the client is disappointed.

False Reassurance. False reassurance means giving reassurance that is not based on fact. It is a way of minimizing the client's situation. For example, saying, "Don't worry, everything will be fine," minimizes the client's concerns. Other forms of false reassurance include telling a client not to dwell on his or her problems, or saying that an injection will not hurt. Although the intention of such comments is to reassure the client, they actually serve to diminish trust in the professional.

Real reassurance must be based on fact. For example, telling a client that there will be postoperative pain

Table 20-6 • Sample Process Recording

Situation: The client is a 35-year-old man who sustained burns on his face and upper body due to a car accident. He was transferred from the burn unit to the rehabilitation unit 2 days ago.

Verbal and Nonverbal Interaction		Analysis
Nurse:	When I left you yesterday things weren't going very well for you. How are you doing today? (Nurse sits down, facing patient.)	Opening remark establishes that nurse remembers events from previous day. Indicates working phase of relationship. Open-ended question to help client get started. Nurse offers self.
Client:	It has been a rough 2 days.	Client makes a general statement.
Nurse:	. . . rough 2 days . . .	Restatement.
	SILENCE	Nurse allows silence so that client can collect his thoughts.
Client:	I've come to the realization that I'm not going to look the same as I did . . .	Client begins to clarify what he means.
Nurse:	. . . and . . .? (Remains attentive.)	Encouraging elaboration.
Client:	It's hard. (Becomes tearful.)	Client showing feelings nonverbally.
Nurse:	(Gently) It is upsetting to deal with the after-effects of your burns.	Reflection. The nurse reflects the client's feelings so he can own them.
Client:	I shouldn't cry. (Appears embarrassed.)	Nurse assesses that client's past experiences and personal history have led him to the conclusion that men should not cry.
Nurse:	You think men shouldn't cry when they have a really difficult adjustment to make?	Reflection of metacommunication (embarrassment about crying). The nurse shows the patient what he feels about his feelings.
Client:	(Laughs slightly.) I guess it's okay for me to cry. My situation isn't easy to deal with.	The client gained understanding of his feelings and his metacommunication.
	SILENCE	
Client:	(Looks sad. Remains thoughtful.)	
Nurse:	Some of what you are experiencing is a natural grieving process that people in your situation go through. You have lost part of your former self, and that is a painful experience.	Giving information. The nurse is experienced and well read in the rehabilitation of burn clients. She shares this information in a timely manner. The nurse realizes that there is no easy solution for this client's problem. She provides support.

Table developed by Laina Gerace, Ph.D., R.N., Associate Professor, University of Illinois at Chicago, College of Nursing.

and how it will be controlled is much more reassuring than saying, "There's nothing to this operation. We do it all the time." A procedure may seem routine to the nurse, but to the client it is a major event. The client will feel much more supported if allowed to express anxiety and ask questions.

Giving false reassurance violates the client's trust. If the nurse tells a client not to worry when the client actually is worried, or that something does not hurt when it does hurt, how can the client have confidence in the nurse? It is much better to supply any needed information and give reassurances based on facts.

Giving Advice. Giving advice is another common nontherapeutic response. Giving advice focuses exclusively on the nurse's experiences and opinions. Examples of giving advice include statements that begin, "I think you should . . .," "Why don't you . . .," and "The same thing happened to me and I . . ." The problem with giving advice is that it diminishes the client's responsibilities and choices and tends to be controlling. Clients may feel that they must do what the nurse says, even though the advice might not work well for them.

Giving advice is different from giving a suggestion, an alternative idea for the client's consideration. If carefully done, a suggestion increases the client's perceived options. Usually, however, it is better if the client comes up with his or her own ideas. A helpful way to give a suggestion is to frame it tentatively, such as, "I wonder if you have thought about (an alternate course of action)?"

Changing the Subject. Changing the subject is a nontherapeutic response that usually indicates anxiety on the nurse's part. It is a way of resisting hearing about a client's distress, sadness, and difficulties. The nurse might change the subject in an attempt to cheer the client up or to distract the client from painful thoughts; however, changing the subject can be a way to avoid listening to what the client has to say.

Being Moralistic. Being moralistic means seeing a situation in terms of goodness or badness, or right or wrong. It is a judgmental approach. The nurse must become aware of how he or she uses the word "should." Talking to clients in terms of "shoulds" means the nurse has a preconceived idea about the "right" thing to do. For instance, a nurse would be moralistic by saying to an unwed mother, "I think you should keep the baby." Many factors go into making a decision of this magnitude. What might work for one person may not work for another.

Another way of being moralistic is to give approval or disapproval by judging the client's actions as good or bad. Everyone has moral attitudes, and being moral is part of being human. Nurses have a right to their own values, but in the clinical situation they must transcend them and view their clients in more objective terms.

Nonprofessional Involvement. Nonprofessional involvement means being overly social or trying to be the client's friend or buddy (Burgess, 1990). Although it is sometimes appropriate, too much social chit-chat points to a nonprofessional relationship. Nurses who talk too much with clients about themselves and their own goals and problems are nonprofessional. Sometimes the nurse may chat briefly with the client about the weather or a major news event. But if most of a nurse's relationships with clients are social or overly friendly, this is a red flag that the nurse's involvements are nontherapeutic.

Being nontherapeutically involved has pitfalls for both nurse and client. The client is receiving nursing care because of a need for professional services. The nurse must maintain a professional attitude to remain objective in clinical decision making. The client wants to feel confident that a professional is in charge of nursing care. If the nurse becomes a friend to the client, he or she has abdicated the professional role.

Special Situations

Several situations call for particular communication techniques. Communication with the person with sensory dysfunctions is discussed in Chapter 48. Communication techniques and skills for the unconscious client and special lifespan considerations are presented in Chapter 48.

Children and Adolescents. Children and adolescents present unique challenges to effective communication. These age groups are undergoing many changes that make clear communication more difficult.

> **Nursing Research**
> *Therapeutic Communication*
>
> ***Selected Nursing Research Studies***
>
> Astrom, S., Nilsson, M., Norberg, A., et al. (1991). Staff burnout in dementia care—relation to empathy and attitudes. *International Journal of Nursing Studies, 18*(1), 65–75.
>
> Reid-Ponte, P. (1992). Distress in cancer patients and primary nurses' empathy skills. *Cancer Nursing, 15*(4), 283–292.
>
> Reisch, S. K., Tosi, C. B., Thurston, C. A., et al. (1993). Effects of communication training on parents and young adolescents. *Nursing Research, 42*(1), 10–16.
>
> ***Possible Topics for Nursing Inquiry***
>
> - What are nonverbal communication cues in the intensive care client?
> - What are nonverbal confirmations of verbal communication in the client in pain?
> - What nurse responses promote communication with the preschool child?

Children are responsive to nonverbal communication, such as body movements, voice tone, and eye contact. The nurse should talk to a child at the child's eye level in an effort to minimize intimidation. Speaking gently and calmly and using quiet body movement engenders greater trust.

When children first learn words, it is sometimes difficult to understand what they mean. The way words are combined does not always convey the exact meaning intended. The nurse should clarify meanings with the child until the message can be understood, using restatement and clarification.

Child: "Baby socks."
Nurse: "You have little socks?"
Child: No response.
Nurse: "You have socks?"
Child: Shakes head to indicate "no."
Nurse: "You want your socks?"
Child: Smiles and nods head to indicate "yes."

Young children are more attentive to simplified speech. The nurse should use language the child can understand. When speaking to a child who does not respond, the nurse should rephrase the communication. For example:

Nurse: "It's time for your dinner now."
Child: No response.
Nurse: "Time to eat now."
Child: Takes nurse's hand to go to dining area.

The nurse can use play to help children deal with the stress of hospitalization. For example, having children play with dolls representing physicians and nurses can help them enact their fears. By observing play, the nurse can identify a child's concerns. By participating in such play, children can develop feelings of mastery over the situation. Many hospitals caring for young children provide structured play to help clients deal with their illnesses and treatments.

Hospitalization for physical problems in this age group is anxiety producing. Children and adolescents often feel embarrassed about their bodies, and they feel vulnerable to the control of adults. Therefore, it is important that the nurse be considerate of the child or adolescent's personal space, and not be too intrusive. Touch should be judicious, and the client's modesty maintained. Adolescents are particularly conscious of the need for privacy and modesty in communication situations with health professionals.

Information about procedures and treatments needs to be given in a straightforward manner, and it is especially important not to give false reassurance. For example, if a procedure might be painful, it is best to share this in a matter-of-fact way.

To work effectively with children and adolescents, the nurse needs a sense of give-and-take. The nurse might be a little less formal than with an adult, but still maintains some professional distance. Limit setting is a key factor in working effectively with children and adolescents, and to set limits the nurse must be seen as authoritative. Being *authoritative* means being in charge but permitting freedom within reasonable limits (Hetherington and Parke, 1986). This is different from being *authoritarian*, which means exerting power over another person. Being authoritative means the nurse clearly communicates the limits of behavior and elicits participation in their reinforcement.

Adults and Older Adults. It is difficult to specify communication strategies for any phase of development, especially for adulthood. Adulthood is an ongoing developmental period, not the end of growth and development. As people grow and age, they must constantly adapt to many changes, and less is known about adulthood than any other phase of development.

Hospitalization can create a period of transition in which adults question the progress of their lives, their goals, and even life's meaning. Their responsibilities are interrupted by the illness, and feelings of vulnerability may overwhelm them. It can be difficult for an active, achieving adult to be dependent on the nurse, and the adult may sometimes behave in ways that are difficult for the nurse to manage.

The nurse also may experience a range of feelings in relation to various adult clients. For example, an elderly male client may remind a nurse of her grandfather. She may relate to him as she does to her grandfather, or may treat him as if he is helpless and cannot make any decisions. If the client is a physician or a wealthy or well-known person, the nurse may feel intimidated. Numerous complex situations come into play when communicating therapeutically with adults. Nurses must recognize their feelings and share them with fellow professionals, because these feelings affect the way in which communication takes place.

Communication strategies with adults draw on all the concepts discussed in this chapter. The contractual approach provides an opportunity to work out with the client how communication will take place. For example, whether to call an adult by his or her first or last name can be discussed at the outset. It helps to remember that all human beings, no matter what their job, social status, or wealth, at some point in their lives are vulnerable and suffer anxiety and worry. The therapeutic communication skills presented in this chapter will facilitate expression and problem solving with any adult.

The Person Who Speaks a Foreign Language. The nurse should learn what non–English-speaking groups live in the community and should become familiar with common phrases related to nursing care (eg, identity, bathing, eating, eliminating, walking). A dictionary of common conversational phrases in the other language is helpful.

Remember that the non–English-speaking client has a language barrier, not a hearing problem (unless one exists). The nurse should speak clearly and distinctly in a normal tone of voice, using hand motions and demonstrations when appropriate. But even with the most careful efforts, misunderstandings may occur, and in healthcare it is particularly important to avoid them. Therefore, an interpreter should be used whenever possible. The interpreter can also provide insight into cultural meanings and nuances of the language and the related culture that may have a bearing on the client's healthcare needs.

The Person in the Intensive Care Unit. The intensive care unit (ICU) is an environment designed to help maintain the lives of seriously ill clients. It is characterized by unfamiliar sounds and noises, artificial lighting, and undefined colors (Williams, 1989). Being admitted to the ICU is a stressful event: the client fears the diagnosis and the extent of the injury and may be unable to communicate. Communication is hindered if the client does not know or understand the severity of the illness, feels a lack of control over what is being done, does not know the reason for therapies, receives care from several different providers, and loses contact with the outside world, including a sense of day and time (Chyun, 1989).

It is easy for the nurse to get caught up in the complexities and technology of the unit and as a result have minimal communication with the client. The nurse must be constantly aware that the client in this life-threatening situation is a person for whom communication is more important than ever. Even when the client cannot answer (because of decreased level of consciousness, intubation, or other reasons), the nurse should assume that the client can hear. The nurse should talk to the client about what is being done as he or she would with any other client. Nonverbal communication, such as touch and facial expressions, is especially meaningful for ICU clients.

To give cues about day and time, the nurse can provide clocks and calendars where the client can see them. For clients who can use their hands but cannot speak, note pads or magic slates aid in communication. Call bells within easy reach help the client to communicate his or her needs.

Once the client has been stabilized, the nurse can help the client understand the illness and the reason for various therapies. Explanations must be clear, direct, and simply stated. Because of the client's state, the nurse should expect to repeat them. When the client is able, discussing his or her perceptions and understanding enhances the client's sense of control and decreases stress. Nurses in the ICU have a valuable opportunity to facilitate communication between the client and the healthcare system.

Key Concepts

- Effective communication within the nurse–client relationship focuses on the client and the client's experiences and results in improved health status and well-being.
- Communication is a system of sending and receiving messages that forms a connection between the sender and the receiver.
- Verbal communication involves language; nonverbal communication includes gestures, facial expressions, body posture, body movement, voice tone, rate of speech, and dress.
- The elements of communication are the source, the message, and the receiver, with the processes of encoding, decoding, and feedback.
- The nurse–client relationship is focused on the client, is goal directed, and has defined parameters.
- The three phases in the nurse–client relationship are orientation, working, and termination.
- Empathy, positive regard, and a comfortable sense of self are among the key ingredients of the nurse–client relationship.
- The nurse–client relationship and therapeutic communication are instruments used to implement the nursing process.
- Skillful use of therapeutic responses is essential to accurate assessment and interventions.
- Ineffective communication can be avoided if the nurse is aware of nontherapeutic responses.
- Clients in special situations need modified communication techniques.

Critical Thinking Challenges

Now that you have studied this chapter, you should be able to apply what you have learned about effective communication to the situation at the beginning of this chapter. Turn back to the situation and then answer the following questions.

1. *Analyze what might have triggered your client's response to your inquiry and identify how you as the sender of the message may have contributed to his response.*
2. *Outline the threats that your client may perceive from this interaction.*
3. *Assess the incongruencies between verbal and nonverbal communication in this visit.*
4. *Based on your analysis of the above responses, identify the blocks to communication that may be occurring.*
5. *Construct some options for how you might proceed to improve communication and accomplish your nursing plan of care.*

References

Aroskar, M. A. (1980). Ethics of nurse–patient relationship. *Nurse Educator,* March–April, 18–20.

Barry, P. D. (1984). *Psychosocial nursing assessment and intervention.* Philadelphia: J. B. Lippincott.

Berlo, D. K. (1960). *The process of communication: An introduction to therapy and practice.* New York: Holt, Rinehart & Winston.

Brandler, R., & Grinder, J. (1975). *The structure of magic: A book about language and therapy.* Palo Alto, CA: Science & Behavior Books.

Burgess, A. W. (1990). *Psychiatric nursing in the hospital and the community.* Englewood Cliffs, NJ: Appleton & Lange.

Campbell-Heider, N., & Hart, C. A. (1993). Updating the nurse's bedside manner. *Image,* Comments in: *25*(2), 133–139; *25* (4), 362–363.

Chyun, D. (1989). Patients' perceptions of stressors in intensive care units. *Focus on Critical Care, 16*(3), 206–211.

Cravener, P. (1992). Establishing therapeutic alliance across cultural barriers. *J Psychosoc Nurs Ment Health Serv, 30*(12), 10–14.

Crowther, D.J. (1991). Metacommunications: A missed opportunity? *J Psychosoc Nurs Ment Health Serv, 29*(4), 13–16.

Fagin, C. M. (1992). Collaboration between nurses and physicians: No longer a choice. *Academic Medicine, 67*(5), 295–303.

Forchuk, C. (1992). The orientation phase of the nurse–client relationship: How long does it take? *Perspect Psychiatr Care, 28*(4), 7–10.

Gibbons, M. B. (1993). Listening to the lived experience of loss. *Pediatric Nursing, 19*(6), 597–599.

Hardin, S., & Gerace, L. (1983). Verbal and nonverbal counterparts in nurses' empathic communication. Paper presented at the Midwest Nursing Research Society, University of Iowa.

Hardin, S., & Halaris, A. (1983). Nonverbal communication of patients and high- and low-empathy nurses. *J Psychosoc Nurs Ment Health Serv, 21,* 14–20.

Hetherington, E. M., & Parke, R. D. (1986). *Child psychology: A contemporary viewpoint.* New York: McGraw-Hill.

Loomis, M. (1985). Levels of contracting. *J Psychosoc Nurs Ment Health Serv, 23*(3), 9–14.

Matthews, J. J. (1983). The communication process in clinical settings. *Soc Sci Med, 17,* 1371–1378.

Morse, J. M., Anderson, G., Bottorff, J. L., et al. (1992). Exploring empathy: A conceptual fit for nursing practice? *Image, 24*(2), 273–280.

Morse, J. M. (1991). Negotiating commitment and involvement in the nurse–patient relationship. *J Adv Nurs, 16,* 455–468.

Murphy, K., & Clark, J. M. (1993). Nurses experiences of caring for ethnic-minority clients. *J Adv Nurs 18,* 442–450.

Peplau, H. E. (1952). *Interpersonal relations in nursing.* New York: G. P. Putnam's Sons.

Remen, N. (1980). *The human patient.* New York: Doubleday.

Rogers, C. (1961). *On becoming a person.* Boston: Houghton-Mifflin.

Smith, L. (1986). Talking it out. *Nursing Times,* March 26, 38–39.

Taylor, S. (1985). Rights and responsibilities: Nurse–patient relationship. *Image, 17*(1), 9–13.

Thayer, L. (1968). *Communication and communication systems in organization, management and interpersonal relations.* Homewood, IL: Richard D. Irwin.

Trojan, L., & Yonge, O. (1993). Developing trusting, caring relationships: Home care nurses and elderly clients. *J Adv Nurs, 18,* 1903–1910.

Williams, C. A. (1990). Biopsychosocial elements of empathy: A multidimensional model. *Issues in Mental Health Nursing, 11,* 155–174.

Williams, M. A. (1989). Physical environment of the intensive care unit and elderly patients. *Critical Care Nursing Quarterly, 12*(1), 52–60.

Essential Assessment Components

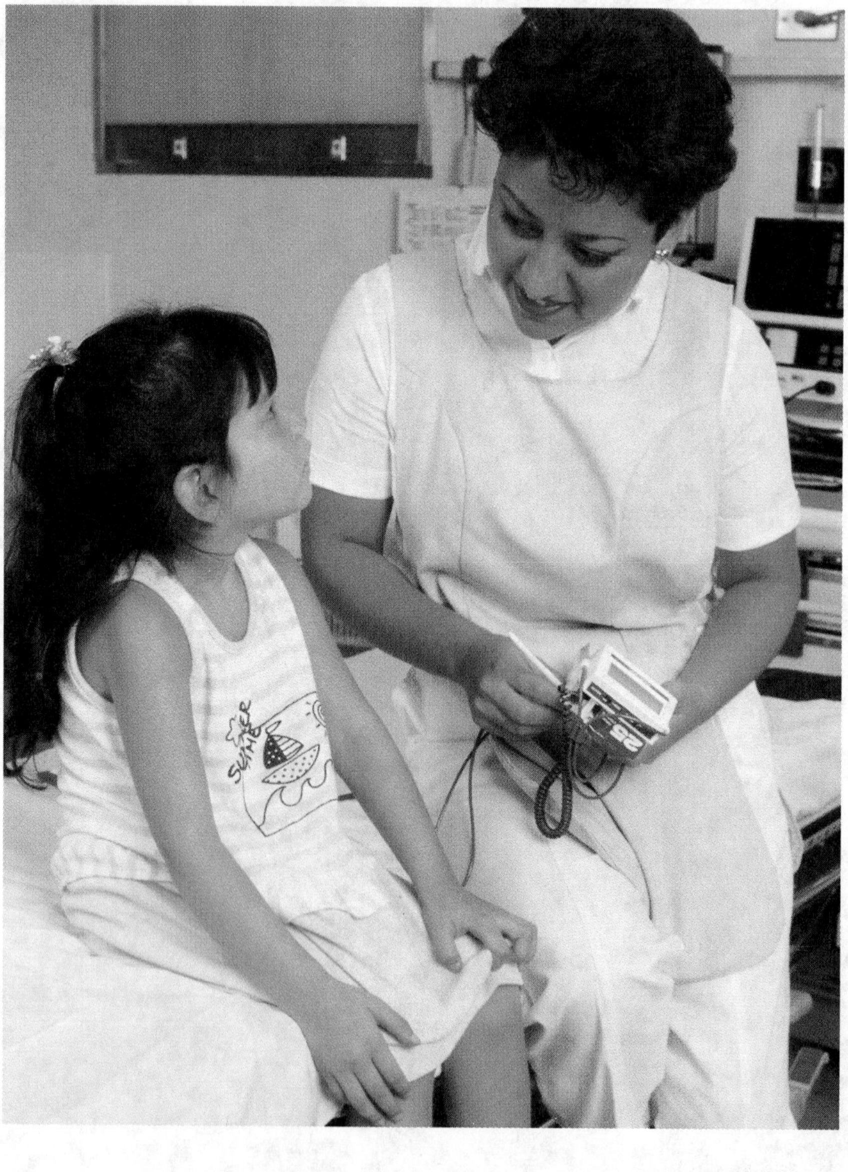

UNIT V

Unit V details the fundamental skills and knowledge needed to carry out each component of health assessment. The information gathered during health assessment and vital sign assessment, combined with information from diagnostic tests and procedures, forms a database from which many nursing care decisions are made.

The chapter on health assessment of human function describes the systematic and continuous gathering of subjective and objective data, beginning with a health history and physical examination. Along with discussing normal or acceptable findings, this chapter provides a knowledge base that is basic to identifying client strengths and responses to health problems. Chapter 22 presents the knowledge and skills required for accurate and timely vital sign measurement, along with a discussion of normal parameters and variations; an awareness of both is essential for nursing practice. The final chapter in this unit discusses the role of the nurse in assisting with or performing diagnostic tests and procedures and describes how the data from laboratory and diagnostic tests factor into the client's overall health assessment.

Unit V focuses on how and why the nurse gathers data from and about a client. These chapters provide a composite picture of essential assessment components, the first phase of the nursing process, thus providing a strong foundation for the remainder of the nursing process.

Health Assessment of Human Function

Key Terms	Learning Objectives
Auscultation *Bruits* *Comprehensive health assessment* *Dermatomes* *Functional health assessment* *Health history* *Inspection* *Murmur* *Objective data* *Ophthalmoscope* *Otoscope* *Palpation* *Percussion* *Physical examination* *Stethoscope* *Subjective data* *Tangential lighting*	*Upon completion of this chapter, the student will be able to do the following:* • *Organize a nursing assessment using a functional health framework for data collection.* • *Discuss preparation of the client and the environment to foster data collection* • *Differentiate between objective and subjective data.* • *Discuss methods to obtain subjective information using the client interview.* • *Describe the techniques of inspection, palpation, percussion, and auscultation used in the physical assessment.* • *Individualize the nursing assessment based on lifespan considerations.*

21

The chart describes your client as a 38-year-old woman, married, and the mother of two children in the sixth and eighth grades. She works full-time as a paralegal professional. Her past medical history is listed as a tonsillectomy at age 8 and a urinary tract infection at age 14 years (none since then). She has sought healthcare at this clinic for the last 2 years, and had a comprehensive assessment when she entered the system. Her husband says that she has been fatigued for the last 2 weeks, and that she gets short of breath on exertion. The client's reason for seeking care is "stabbing chest pain on my right side when I take a deep breath or cough." Her height is 67 inches, weight is 160 pounds, and she is alert and oriented. Her vital signs are temperature 102.2 °F.; pulse 120 and regular; respirations 32 per minute and regular; and blood pressure 152/80. She is coughing up moderate amounts of thick, yellow sputum. A pleural friction rub is present.

In Unit III you studied about critical thinking and nursing assessment. In this chapter you will add more detailed information about client assessment and examination to your knowledge base. You will prepare yourself to provide holistic care to the functional health needs of your clients and their families. The Critical Thinking Challenges at the end of the chapter will help you apply this knowledge base to the situation above.

A **comprehensive health assessment** encompasses the physical, psychological, social, and spiritual dimensions of living. *Physical health* includes basic functions such as breathing, eating, and walking, as well as complex functions such as learning, reproducing, and sensing. *Psychological health* involves intellect, self-concept, emotions, and behavior. The *social dimensions of health* encompass relationships and interactions among family, friends, and coworkers. *Spiritual health* is influenced by belief in a higher being, personal interpretation of the meaning of life, and attitudes toward moral decisions and personal conduct. In performing a comprehensive health assessment, the nurse considers all of these dimensions.

This chapter discusses how nurses can perform assessment using a functional health framework as a structure for data collection. The organization of and information on how to conduct the health assessment are included in this chapter. Significant additional information is included in clinical chapters in the second section of this textbook. Using information provided in this chapter and the subsequent clinical chapters, the nurse selects the most important interviewing questions or assessment techniques for each client. Selection often depends on time constraints or the client's current health status.

A *comprehensive* functional health assessment may be performed routinely as a client makes initial contact within the healthcare system. Usually such an assessment includes collecting subjective data through interviewing the client and obtaining objective data by physically examining the client. A comprehensive functional health assessment should take approximately 45 minutes, but can vary in length depending on the specific client. Although a comprehensive assessment is ideal, it may not always be practical or feasible. The nurse must often select the most important interviewing questions or assessment techniques to use, and perform a *focused* health assessment based on the client's problems.

Purpose of the Assessment

The purpose of a health assessment is to establish a database for the client concerning normal functional abilities, risk factors that can contribute to dysfunction, and actual alterations in normal function. A clear description of health status and identification of health-related problems are the desired outcomes of a functional health assessment.

From this information, the nurse and the client together can plan strategies to encourage continuation of healthy patterns, prevent potential health problems, and alleviate or manage existing health problems. Assessment data are used to individualize client care in promoting optimum health for the client. A detailed initial database has long-term usefulness in measuring a client's progress toward health-related goals.

Frameworks for Health Assessment

There are three major frameworks for organizing assessment data. These include the head-to-toe framework, body systems framework, and functional health framework. Each framework organizes the information collected and helps ensure that important assessment data are not inadvertently omitted. Usually the interview is conducted to elicit subjective information first, followed by the physical examination. Each framework of assessment begins with observing the client's general appearance and obtaining vital signs. Historically, medicine has used a body systems approach to assessment. Practitioners of nursing and medicine have commonly used a head-to-toe approach. Increasing numbers of nurses are using Gordon's functional health patterns to organize the collection of assessment data. Regardless of the sequencing of data collection, information obtained can be organized within functional areas for analysis of data in a meaningful manner. This is especially important for the nurse, whose practice revolves around the human response to health and illness rather than medical conditions or diseases. Developing a consistent, comprehensive method for assessment is more important than which specific framework a nurse decides to use.

Head-to-Toe Framework

The head-to-toe framework is a system for collecting data in an organized manner, starting from the head and proceeding systematically downward to the toes. This framework is used to improve efficiency and expedite the actual physical examination. The organization for head-to-toe assessment is outlined in the accompanying display. The interview is conducted at a separate time, usually before the physical examination, to guide and focus data collection. A typical outline of data collection is head (hair, scalp, eyes, ears, oral cavity, and cranial nerves), neck, upper extremities, chest, abdomen, lower extremities, pelvis, genitals, and rectum.

Body Systems Framework

Body systems is a framework that is commonly used by medicine, and focuses on the pathophysiology involved within specific body systems (eg, cardiovascular, genitourinary) (Table 21-1). A body systems approach may be used during the focused assessment of an acutely or critically ill client. It is also commonly used when the purpose of the examination is to determine function of a particular body system (Fuller & Schaller-Ayers, 1994). For example, after orthopedic surgery, a musculoskeletal assessment may be important to assess impact on mobility and activity.

Functional Health Framework

A **functional health assessment** is an evaluation of mind, body, and environment and their effect on a person's ability to perform the tasks of daily living. The functional health framework for assessment organizes data collection around Gordon's 11 functional health patterns: health perception–health management; nutrition–

Physical Assessment Collection Using Head-to-Toe Framework

General

General health state
Vital signs

Head and Neck

Inspect hair, scalp, cranium
Inspect eyes, examine eyes with ophthalmoscope
Test vision
Inspect ears, examine ears with otoscope
Test hearing
Inspect oral cavity and teeth
Test cranial nerves
Palpate thyroid gland
Palpate and auscultate carotid arteries
Inspect neck veins

Upper extremities

Inspect skin and nails
Evaluate muscle strength and tone
Evaluate range of motion
Brachial and radial pulsations
Bicep tendon reflexes

Chest and Back

Inspect and palpate breast
Inspect and palpate axillae and nodes
Inspect, palpate, and auscultate lungs
Inspect, palpate, and auscultate heart
Inspect spinal alignment

Abdomen

Inspect, auscultate, palpate four abdominal quadrants
Palpate and percuss specific organs (eg, bladder, liver)

Genitals and Pelvis

Inspect external genitalia
Palpate for hernias
Testicular examination
Inspect vagina and cervix
Inspect rectum and perform rectal examination if indicated

Lower extremities

Observe gait and muscle strength
Inspect skin and toenails
Test deep tendon and plantar reflexes
Palpate popliteal, posterior tibial, and pedal arteries

Table 21-1 • Physical Assessment Using the Body Systems Model

Body System	Criteria
Sensory–perceptual	Mental status Vision and appearance of eyes Hearing Touch Taste and smell
Skin	Condition (color, turgor, character) Lesions Edema Hair distribution Breast
Respiratory	Rate, character Breath sounds Cough
Cardiovascular	Pulses (rate, quality, rhythm) Apical Radial Carotid Dorsalis pedis Brachial Posterior tibial Femoral Blood pressure Circulation (mucous membranes, nailbeds)
Neurologic	Pupillary reactions Orientation Level of consciousness Grasp strength
Gastrointestinal	Mouth, gums, teeth, and tongue (color and condition) Gag reflex Bowel sounds Presence of distention, impaction, hemorrhoids (external)
Genitourinary	Presence of retention Discharge (vaginal, urethral) Uterine response (pregnancy, postpartum) External genitalia
Musculoskeletal	Muscle tone, strength Gait, stability Range of motion

From Carpenito, L. J. (1993). *Nursing diagnosis: Application to clinical practice* (5th ed.). Philadelphia: J. B. Lippincott, p. 56.

metabolic; activity–exercise; elimination; sleep–rest; cognitive–perceptual; self-perception–self-concept; roles–relationships; sexuality–reproduction; coping–stress tolerance; and values–beliefs (Gordon, 1994). Gordon's functional health patterns, which are outlined more completely in Chapter 10, will provide the organizing framework for this assessment chapter. Nurses may collect subjective information using functional health patterns, but conduct the physical assessment using a head-to-toe approach. After all data have been gathered, the nurse can use a functional health framework to organize and analyze the data obtained. Table 21-2 compares data collection using the functional health framework versus the head-to-toe framework or body systems framework.

Using Diagnostic Reasoning

The functional health framework for health assessment enables the nurse to organize data into meaningful groupings, identify missing data, and draw significant conclusions. One piece of data is not used in isolation, but is used in combination with other data to provide a holistic view of the client. The functional assessment framework provides an adequate database to help formulate a conclusion or a problem statement, such as a nursing diagnosis. By comparing the client's assessment findings with the defining characteristics for the diagnosis, the nurse can determine if enough data have been obtained to label the diagnosis, if further data should be gathered, or if another diagnosis is more appropriate. Thus, an accurate assessment provides an essential foundation for the care of the client.

Conducting a Health Assessment

Reviewing General Information

Usually it is possible to obtain some general information about the client using *secondary data sources* before introducing yourself to the client. If the chart is available, the nurse notes the client's name, age, primary language, health history, and current medications or treatment. Notes will give the nurse an idea of previous problems and items on which to follow up. This promotes efficient communication with the client, and prevents several people from asking the same questions over again. Other healthcare providers may express their concerns and plans for the client. Collaboration among providers of care shows concern for the individual client's well-being. If friends or family are available, they may be able to provide information about the client's symptoms and history.

During the initial stage of the assessment, the vital signs are taken to obtain a general overview of the client's status and detect any conditions that require immediate intervention. The vital signs may be performed by a health assistant or by the nurse. The techniques for accurate vital sign measurement are discussed in Chapter 22.

Considering Culture

Cultural sensitivity is important in conducting a health assessment. Often, the client's language, customs, beliefs, and values are different from those of the nurse

Table 21-2 • Comparison of Functional Health Framework to Body Systems Framework and Head-to-Toe Framework

Functional Health Pattern	Body System	Head-to-Toe
Health perception and health management	Breast exam Testicular exam	Breast
Activity and exercise	Respiratory Cardiovascular Musculoskeletal	Upper and lower extremities (pulses and circulation) Precordium and anterior thorax, posterior thorax
Nutrition and metabolism	Gastrointestinal Integumentary Endocrine	Hair and scalp, head, oral cavity, thyroid, nails, abdomen
Elimination	Genitourinary Gastrointestinal	Abdomen, pelvis, anus, and rectum
Sleep and rest	—	—
Cognitive and perception	Neurologic Sensory	Eyes, ears, cranial nerves
Self-perception and self-concept	Psychosocial	—
Roles and relationships	Psychosocial	—
Coping and stress tolerance	Psychosocial	—
Sexuality and reproductive	Endocrine Reproductive	Breast, testicles, pelvic exam, genitalia
Values and beliefs	Psychosocial	—

performing the assessment. Interpretation of data can be influenced by preconceived biases held by the nurse. For example, if the nurse is very verbal and freely expresses discomfort and pain, misinterpretation may occur when assessing a stoic man who feels it would be a loss of face if he verbalized his pain.

Special arrangements may be made when assessing a client who does not speak English. Interpreters may be used. Family members are sometimes helpful, but staff or official translators provide a more objective translation and do not breach confidentiality. Even if a client has a good command of English, specific medical terms may need to be explained, or different terms may be used to describe body functions. In some cultures, the husband is the family spokesperson and often requires that he be present during the health assessment of his wife.

Nurses need to be sensitive to physical differences among different races. For instance, cyanosis and color changes may be difficult to detect in dark-skinned people, and screening for specific health problems such as sickle cell anemia among blacks is important to include in health assessment.

Preparing the Client and Environment

Thoughtful preparation of the client and the environment is advantageous for both the client and the nurse. Understanding the process and knowing what to expect ensures the client's physical and emotional comfort. The nurse who is well organized and competent is efficient and reassuring to the client.

Most clients undergoing a health examination are anxious. Pain, fear, and embarrassment may all contribute to a client's distress. By thoughtfully preparing the client and environment before the assessment, some of the controllable sources of anxiety for the client can be eliminated.

Introduction to the Client

The nurse should introduce himself or herself to the client and explain the nature and purpose of the health assessment. Assessment can be described as a series of questions about the client's past and present state of

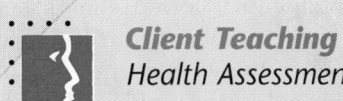

Client Teaching
Health Assessment

Instruct the client as follows:

- *Understand what the nurse is planning to do and how you can assist him or her.*
- *All information collected will be used to help plan and individualize your nursing care and will be kept confidential.*
- *Alert the nurse if you are becoming fatigued or uncomfortable during the assessment.*
- *Slowly exhale during palpation. This prevents tensing muscles, which can make palpation difficult and cause you discomfort.*
- *Perform self-assessment (such as breast self-examination) following the technique used by the nurse during assessment.*

health, followed by a physical examination. The nurse should explain that information obtained in the assessment will be used to understand the client's current state of health and illness, to monitor progress, and to determine ways to make treatment more effective and comfortable. During this introductory phase, the nurse should tell the client approximately how long the assessment will take. The client should also be assured that information obtained during the assessment process is confidential and will be shared only with other health-care professionals participating in provision of care.

Environment

The environment should be comfortable for both nurse and client. A warm, quiet, well-lit room is ideal. All necessary equipment should be gathered in advance and fully functional. Leaving the client to find equipment is distracting and time consuming.

Privacy and confidentiality are important concerns for the client who is about to share personal information and submit to a physical examination. The client should feel confident that he or she will not be viewed or overheard by others during the interview or physical examination. This can be a challenge if the client shares a room with another client. Family members and visitors may be asked to leave, depending on the client's preference. Pull the curtains around the bedside and position yourself so that you are away from others in the room.

The client should be as physically comfortable as possible during the assessment. A relaxed client is more attentive and can provide more accurate and complete information. Ask the client if he or she needs to use the bathroom before beginning the assessment, especially if an abdominal assessment is anticipated. Occasionally, the nurse may be unable to provide comfort to the client in acute pain or distress *until* an assessment of the client's condition has been accomplished. When this occurs, the nurse should acknowledge the distress and promptly begin the assessment, focusing immediately on the client's primary problem. Physical examination usually takes priority over obtaining a detailed client history when a client is uncomfortable or acutely ill.

Positioning and Draping

One way to provide privacy is to draw the curtain or close the door of the examining room. Draping is another method to help ensure privacy. During the examination, the nurse covers the client's body parts not included in the specific examination taking place, exposing only the part of the body being examined. As the nurse examines another part of the body, the client is redraped. Draping also keeps the client warm during examination. Draping materials include paper sheets, special cloths, or bed linens.

The client may need to assume various positions for the physical examination (positions are discussed and illustrated in Chapter 33). Clients may need assistance with positioning and, if in pain, should not remain in any position for an extended length of time. Organization and planning of the assessment should take positioning and the client's current status into consideration.

Organizing and Documenting

The major portion of the client interview is usually conducted before the physical examination is performed, but dialogue with the client is continued throughout the assessment as more information is gathered and new questions are formulated.

During most health assessments, a preprinted form is used to record information. An example of a completed health assessment is given in Figure 21-1. Health assessment forms vary in title and format, depending on the institution, the client population, and the purpose of the assessment. Some common titles for health assessment forms include Nursing History, Nursing Admission Form, Client Data Base, and Nursing Assessment Form. The format may be structured, using specific questions and lists of required data, or the format may be unstructured, defining broad areas of health. Following a printed form is useful, particularly when the nurse is learning to perform health assessment, because it provides a structure for moving logically from one health area to another. It also helps to prevent the omission of any pertinent information.

Types of Data Collection

The information (or data) acquired in a health assessment falls into two categories: subjective and objective. **Subjective data** are the information that only the client can provide. They refer to internal events, private feelings, and experiences, none of which can be observed by an outsider. Subjective data include the client's descriptions of bodily sensations (such as pain, nausea, dizziness, fatigue) and perceptions, experiences, and feelings about past and present health problems. Interviewing is the technique used for acquiring subjective data. This process is commonly called taking a nursing history. The nursing history is also discussed in Chapter 10 as part of the nursing process.

The second category of information obtained in an assessment is objective data. **Objective data** are tangible, observable facts that an outsider can obtain. They include observations (such as the presence of a rash, a limp, or excessive perspiration) and measurements

Nursing Assessment Form Based on Functional Health Patterns

Client Profile

Name ______ Birthdate ______ Sex ______
Ethnic origin ______ Religion ______
Medical diagnoses ______
Present treatment ______
Past treatments ______
Past hospitalizations ______

Current Medications

Name	Dose	Purpose	Problems

Subjective

Health Perception-Health Management Pattern
Reason for seeking health care ______
______
______
Health rating 1 Poor 2 Fair 3 Excellent
Perception of illness ______
______
Effect of illness on ADLs ______
Use of alcohol ______
tobacco ______
drugs ______
Special health habits ______
______
Last immunizations ______
Compliance with treatments ______

Objective

Appearance ______
Grooming ______
Posture ______
Expressions ______
Ht ______ Wt ______
P ______ R ______ T ______
(oral, axil., rectal)
BP sitting R ______ L ______
standing R ______ L ______

Subjective

Nutritional-Metabolic Pattern
Daily Food and Fluid Intake
B.F. ______
Lunch ______
Supper ______
Snacks ______
Food intolerances ______
Difficulty chewing ______
Dysphagia ______
Sore gums ______
Sore tongue ______
N and V ______
Abd. pains ______
Antacids ______
Laxatives ______
Skin condition ______
Hair condition ______
Nail condition ______
Ideal wt. ______ Difficulty gaining ______
losing ______
Cold/heat intolerances ______
Voice changes ______
Difficulty with nervousness ______

Objective

Skin: Color ______
Lesions ______ Texture ______
Temp ______ Moisture ______
Turgor ______
Hair: Color ______
Amt. ______ Texture ______
Scalp lesions ______ Dry ______
Nails: Color ______
Shape ______ Condition ______
Texture ______ Tenderness ______
Oral Mucosa: ______ Teeth No. ______
Condition ______
Lesions ______
Gums ______ Tongue ______

Figure 21-1 • *Example of a health assessment form organized by functional health patterns. (From Weber, J. [1992]. Nurses' handbook of health assessment, 2nd ed. Philadelphia: J. B. Lippincott.)*

Elimination Pattern
Bowel habits
Frequency ________ Color ________ Pain ________
Consistency ________ Laxatives ________
Enemas ________ Suppositories ________
Ileostomy ________ Colostomy ________
Bladder habits
Frequency ________ Amt. ________ Color ________
Pain ________ Hematuria ________
Incontinence ________ Nocturia ________
Retention ________ Infections ________
Catheter ________ Type ________

Abdomen
Contour ________
Lesions ________ Umbilicus ________
Striae ________ Veins ________
Bowel sounds char. ________
Frequency ________
Size of liver dullness ________
Masses palpated ________
Liver palpated ________
Spleen palpated ________
Rectum
Rashes ________
Lesions ________ Tenderness ________

Subjective

Activity-Exercise Pattern
Daily Activities
Hygiene ________
Cooking ________
Shopping ________
Housework ________
Yard work ________
Eating times ________
Dyspnea ________ Palpations ________
Chest pain ________ Stiffness ________
Weakness ________ Aching ________
Leisure activities ________
Exercise routine ________
Occupation ________
Effect of illness on activities ________
____

Sleep-Rest Pattern
Sleep time ________ Quality ________
Difficulty falling asleep ________
Difficulty remaining asleep ________
Sleep aids ________
Sleep medications ________
Sexuality-Reproduction Pattern
Female: Menstruation
Date began ________ Last cycle ________
Length ________
Problems ________
____
____

Objective

Musculoskeletal
Gait ________ Posture ________
Extremity swelling ________
Symmetry ________ ROM ________
Crepitus ________ Tone ________
Strength ________
Respiratory
Thorax shape ________
Symmetry ________ Retractions ________
Tenderness ________
Diaphragmatic level ________
Breath sounds ________
Adventitious sounds ________
Cardiovascular
Jugular venous pressure ________
Pulsations ________ Heaves ________
Lifts ________
PMI ________ S_1 ________ S_2 ________
S_3 ________ S_4 ________ Murmurs ________

Peripheral Vascular Pulses
Carotids ________ Radial ________
Ulnar ________ Brachial ________
Popliteal ________ Femoral ________
Pedal ________ Posterior tibial ________
Bruits ________

Appearance ________
Yawning ________ Irritability ________
Short attention span ________

Breasts
SBE ________ When ________
Shape ________ Symmetry ________
Nipples ________ Discharge ________
Masses ________ Lymph nodes ________

Figure 21-1 • *Continued*

(such as blood pressure, cholesterol level, and pupil size). Objective data are obtained by physical examination and diagnostic testing. Diagnostic testing includes an array of laboratory, x-ray, and special procedures, as discussed in Chapter 23.

Obtaining Subjective Data: The Interview

The **health history**, or interview, is a goal-directed conversation between nurse and client. Goals may include the following:

Subjective

Sexuality-Reproduction Pattern (cont'd.)
Female: Menstruation (cont'd.)
Gravida ______ Para ______ Abortions ______
Current pregnancy ______
Infertility ______
Male-Female ______
Contraception used ______
______
Undesirable side-effects ______
Problems with sexual activities ______
______
______
Effect of illness on sexuality ______
______
______
Sexually transmitted diseases ______
______
Pain ______ Burning ______
Discomfort during intercourse ______
Discharge ______
Sensory-Perceptual Pattern ______
Perceptions of: Vision ______
Hearing ______ Taste ______
Smell ______ Sensation ______
Pain ______
Aids for vision ______
Aids for hearing ______

Objective

Male Genitalia
Testicular exam ______ When ______
Masses ______ Swelling ______
Texture ______
Penile exam ______
Masses ______ Growths ______
Lesions ______ Discharge ______
Foreskin retraction ______
Urethral opening ______
Inguinal masses ______
Lymph nodes ______
Female Genitalia
Labia ______ Color ______
Swelling ______ Symmetry ______
Urethral opening ______
Discharge ______
Vaginal opening ______
Lesions ______ Discharge ______
Hymen ______ Inflammation ______
Muscle tone ______

Visual Acuity: OD ______ OS ______
OU ______ Visual fields ______
EOMs ______
PERRLA ______
Fundoscopic Exam: Red reflex ______
Optic disc ______ Macula ______
Arterioles/venules ______
Hearing: Weber ______ Rinne ______
Ext. canal ______
Tympanic membrane ______
Sensations: Superficial ______ Deep pressure ______
2 point discrimination ______
Cranial Nerves
I. Olfactory ______
II. Optic ______
V. Trigeminal ______
III, IV, VI. Oculomotor, Trochlear, Abducens ______
VII. Facial ______ Acoustic ______

Subjective

Value-Belief Pattern
Values ______
Goals ______
Source of hope/strength ______
Significant religious person ______
Religious practices ______
Relationship with God ______

Objective

Presence of religious articles ______
Religious activities ______
______
Visits from clergy ______

Figure 21-1 • *Continued*

- Obtain the client's history and perceptions of past experiences.
- Identify factors that either positively or negatively influence health status.
- Describe how functional abilities are influenced by health status.
- Identify what changes have been made to adapt to the health status.

The interview component of a health assessment is often the client's first encounter with the nurse, and therefore the first step toward establishing a trusting and therapeutic nurse-client relationship. The nurse should be professional, concerned, and attentive throughout the interview. When the client responds to a question, it is important to convey interest by maintaining eye contact, occasionally nodding, or verbally responding to remarks made. Nonverbal behavior, particularly the nurse's body language, can convey a strong message during an interview. The nurse who sits at eye level with the client, appears unhurried and alert, and takes notes conveys to the client that the information being shared is important and deserves attention. In contrast, the nurse who stands over a client during an interview communicates that the nurse's stay will be brief, and the client may feel powerless or conclude that the nurse is in a hurry or has more important tasks to do. The nurse who sits on the bed may invade the client's personal space or appear unprofessional. Throughout the interview, the nurse should be aware of his or her verbal and nonverbal messages. These messages can either promote or discourage the client's trust and confidence.

Questioning clients about their health is a skill that requires study and practice to achieve competence. Before the first assessment and interview, the nurse should prepare questions in each health area. Some questions, such as those about allergies, can be asked with a closed-ended, or yes/no, question. Open-ended questions are preferable in other areas of health concern. For example, the question, "Describe what you eat on a normal day" will yield more valuable information than "How is your appetite?" Follow-up or probing questions should be asked when a problem area is discovered or suggested. Further detail can be solicited by statements such as, "Tell me more about that" or "That seems to concern you." After the planned interview questions have been covered, it is important to ask the client, "Is there anything you would like to discuss that I have not yet mentioned?" This question invites the client to add information that was overlooked or was not anticipated by the nurse.

Special techniques may be necessary to control the interview if a client is overly talkative, particularly in relation to unrelated information. Many clients have difficulty staying on a topic or limiting their answers to significant points. A sensitive yet effective method for directing the client might be, "Because our time is limited, we won't be able to discuss that in detail now. I would like to hear more about. . . ." The ability to skillfully, yet sensitively control the interview is essential for obtaining pertinent information in a timely manner.

Reason for Seeking Healthcare

The first subject usually discussed in a client interview is the client's specific reason for seeking care. This subject is often called the client's "chief complaint" or "chief concern." The nurse should listen carefully to the client's description of the primary problem and document it, quoting the client's exact words. In-depth questioning and discussion of this problem should follow. Information obtained during the interview alerts the nurse to areas of pain or probable abnormality so that the examination of the affected areas can be more careful, thoughtful, and thorough.

Health History

During the interview, the nurse obtains information about the client's health history and family health history. Health history information should include known allergies, childhood illnesses, previous surgeries, and chronic health conditions. It is important to ascertain what, if any, medications the client is currently taking. After the client's initial concerns have been addressed and the health history obtained, the nurse should proceed with a systematic survey of each functional health pattern.

Obtaining Objective Data: The Physical Examination

Physical examination involves the use of one's senses to obtain information about the structure and function of an area being observed or manipulated. The four basic techniques of physical examination are inspection, palpation, percussion, and auscultation. It is often suggested that beginning students practice newly learned physical assessment skills on fellow students or willing friends. This helps to acquire some skill, confidence, and organization before approaching a client. Expertise in the techniques of physical examination can only be learned through practice.

Inspection

Inspection is used to make specific observations of physical features and behavior. The eyes and nose are sensitive tools for this part of the examination. Inspection is the natural beginning to physical examination because it starts immediately on meeting the client. These initial observations provide an overall impression of the client's present state of health and when immediate interventions are indicated. General inspection of a client focuses on the following areas:

- Overall appearance of health or illness (Does the client appear weak, frail, or older than the stated age?)
- Signs of distress (Is the client grimacing, as if in pain? Is breathing labored? Is the skin color blue or pale?)
- Facial expression and mood (Does the client appear anxious, depressed, angry, or uninterested?).
- Body size (Does the client appear thin and malnourished or overweight?)
- Grooming and personal hygiene (Are the client and his or her clothing clean and neat? Is there an unusual odor?)

If it is determined that the client is in acute distress, the functional health assessment should be deferred, assistance should be obtained, and a focused assessment should be performed.

In addition to the role of inspection in the general survey of a client, inspection is the first method used in examination of a specific area. The chest and abdomen, for example, are inspected before palpation, percussion, or auscultation are performed.

The optimal conditions for effective inspection are full exposure of the area and adequate lighting. Removal of clothing and bed linen is necessary. In respect for the client's modesty and comfort, however, only the specific area being examined should be exposed. A well-lit room is essential for good visualization. **Tangential lighting** is provided by indirectly shining light with a lamp or flashlight so that a shadow is created over the area being examined. The shadow brings out subtle differences in contour and movement.

Palpation

Palpation usually follows inspection. **Palpation** uses the hands and fingers to gather information through touch. Palpation is used to discriminate position, texture, size, consistency, masses, and fluid. For client comfort, the hands should be warm and the touch should be gentle and respectful. This "laying on of hands" takes on special significance and may be therapeutic for many clients.

Different parts of the hand are more suitable during palpation for different tactile sensations. The fingertips are concentrated with nerve endings and can sense fine differences in texture and consistency. The fingertips are used to discriminate a raised versus a flat skin lesion or to evaluate an arterial pulse. The skin over the dorsum of the hand is sensitive to temperature because this skin is thin and nerve density is great. Skin temperature over a specific area may be evaluated by comparing its temperature to adjacent areas or opposite sides of the body. The palm of the hand is sensitive to vibration and is useful in locating a vibration associated with a heart murmur.

In addition to this superficial palpation, light or deep palpation can be used. These two latter types of palpation require client relaxation because tensed muscles block access to underlying tissue. The client's ability to relax is enhanced if the actions are explained to the client before he or she is touched.

With *light palpation*, three or four fingers of the dominant hand depress an area of the client's skin approximately 0.5 to 1 inch, as in Figure 21-2. The fingers evaluate the skin temperature and moistness. The hand is moved in a gentle, circular motion to detect abnormal masses and locate areas of discomfort. Using a systematic pattern, the examiner lightly palpates and then releases. Discomfort is best monitored by observing the client's facial expression while palpating (Fuller & Schaller-Ayers, 1994). A ticklish client may place his or her hand on top of the examiner's to reduce ticklish sensations. This pattern of light palpation always precedes deep palpation. If discomfort is elicited, deep palpation of that area is avoided. If the client experiences rebound tenderness, discomfort is greater when pressure is released as the hands are removed.

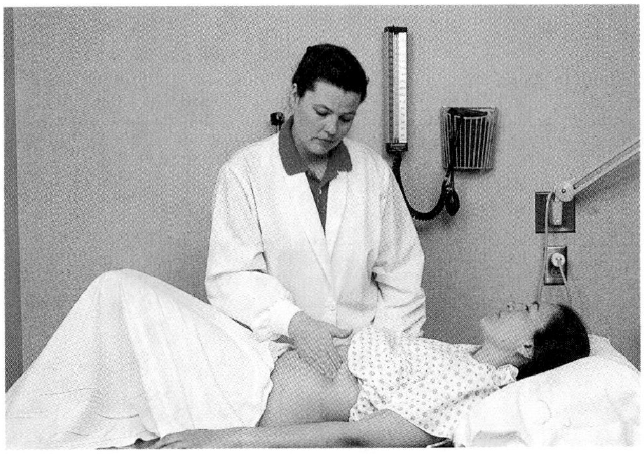

Figure 21-2 • *Light palpation. The fingertips move in a circular motion, depressing the body surface 0.5 to 1 inch.*

Deep palpation involves compression of an area to a depth of 1.5 to 2 inches and requires significantly more pressure than light palpation (Fig. 21-3). In addition, the fingers are placed at a greater angle to the body than in light palpation. One or both hands may be used, depending on the structure being examined. When both hands are used, the fingers of one hand are placed over the fingers of the other hand. The top hand presses and guides the bottom hand (Fuller & Schaller-Ayers, 1994). The purpose of deep palpation is to locate organs, determine their size, and to detect abnormal masses.

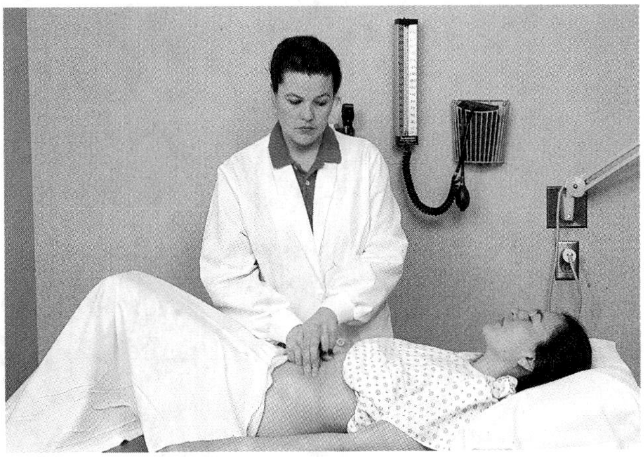

Figure 21-3 • *Deep palpation. The fingers are held at a greater angle to the body surface than in light palpation, and the skin is depressed 1.5 to 2 inches.*

Table 21-3 • Characterictics of Percussion Tones

Tone	Quality	Pitch	Intensity	Location
Flatness	Extreme dullness	High	Soft	Sternum, thigh
Dullness	Thud-like	Medium	Medium	Liver, diaphragm
Resonance	Hollow	Low	Loud	Normal lung
Hyperresonance	Booming	Very low	Very loud	Emphysematous lung
Tympany	Musical, drum-like	High	Loud	Air-filled stomach

Percussion

Percussion, which uses the sense of hearing, involves using the fingers and hands to tap an area on the client to produce sound. The type of percussion tone is determined by the density of the medium through which the sound is traveling. Smaller hands generate less sound, which may make hearing difficult (Fitzgerald, 1991). Percussion provides information about the nature of an underlying structure. It is used to outline the size of an organ, such as the bladder or liver. Percussion is also used to determine if a structure is air-filled, fluid-filled, or solid. This has application in percussion of the lungs and abdomen.

The degree to which sound propagates is called *resonance*. Sound propagates through air; therefore, air-filled spaces are resonant, whereas solid tissue is not. Five characteristic tones are produced by percussion: tympanic, hyperresonant, resonant, dull, and flat (Table 21-3). Characteristically, percussion of the abdomen is *tympanic*, hyperinflated lung tissue is *hyperresonant*, normal lung tissue is *resonant*, the liver is *dull*, and bone is *flat*. The sound is also characterized in terms of the intensity, or loudness. The more dense the medium, the quieter the percussion sound. Tympanic is the loudest and flat is the quietest.

Percussion may be performed directly or indirectly (Fig. 21-4). *Direct percussion* is accomplished by tapping an area directly with the fingertip of the middle finger or thumb. *Indirect percussion* interposes a finger between the area to be percussed and the finger creating the vibrations; indirect percussion usually is used. The steps for indirect percussion are

1. Rest your nondominant middle finger flatly against the client's skin over the area to be percussed. The rest of this hand should not touch the client. Identify the interphalangeal joint of this middle finger because it is the striking area for your opposite hand.
2. Poise your dominant hand about 4 to 5 inches above the striking area, and slightly flex the fingers. Snap this wrist downward, and with the tip of the middle finger, sharply tap the striking area.

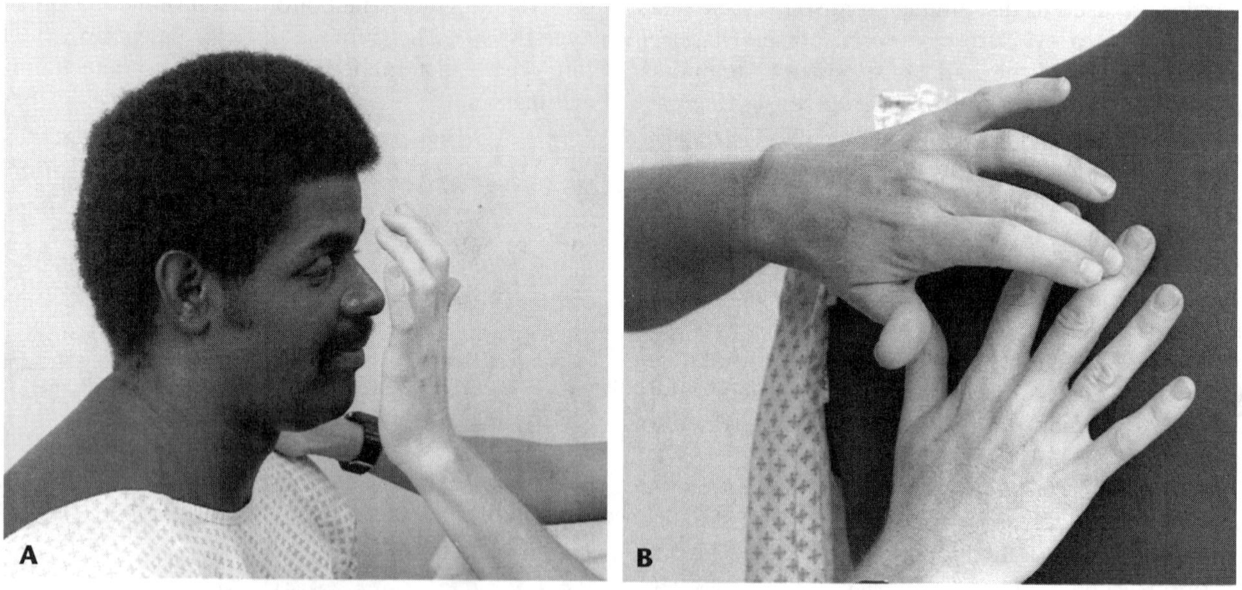

Figure 21-4 • Two percussion methods. (A) Direct percussion is performed by using the fingers of one hand to strike the surface. (B) Indirect percussion is performed with two hands, using the finger of one hand to tap on the finger of the other hand.

(The fingernail should be short to facilitate percussing with the tip, not the pad, of the finger.)
3. Deliver several sharp successive blows, rapidly withdrawing.
4. Identify the percussion sound (see Table 21-3).
5. Proceed to the next area, moving from more resonant to less resonant areas.

Perfecting the percussion technique is often difficult; repetition and practice are essential. Begin by refining the technique over a tympanic area such as the stomach. Once the percussion sound is clearly audible, move to another area and listen for changes in the tone and intensity. Try to label the tone and intensity in this second area. Work from areas of tympany to areas of dullness, and repeat the percussion until the tone and intensity are clear.

Auscultation

Auscultation is listening for sounds of movement within the body. The heart and blood vessels are auscultated for the sound of moving blood; the lungs are auscultated for moving air.

The **stethoscope** collects and transmits sound, selects frequencies, and screens out extraneous sound. The head of the stethoscope applied to the skin collects the sound from beneath it. Most stethoscopes have two types of heads, a diaphragm and a bell (Fig. 21-5). The *diaphragm* is a flat piece that is applied firmly against the skin and responds best to high-frequency sounds and excludes low-frequency ones. The *bell* is funnel- or cup-shaped and allows high-frequency sounds to escape while collecting low-pitched sounds. The bell should simply be allowed to rest on top of the skin. If too much pressure is applied, the skin is stretched and a diaphragm effect is produced. Table 21-4 contrasts the bell and diaphragm.

The ability to auscultate clearly also depends on transmission of sound. The tubing should be short (12 to 18 inches) to avoid distortion. The rubber should be thick and heavy to conduct the sound optimally. It is essential that the room be as quiet as possible during auscultation. Extraneous noise can come from bed linen

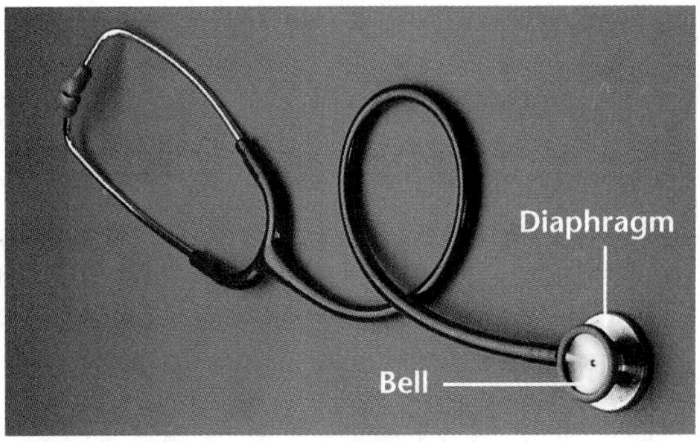

Figure 21-5 • The bell of the stethoscope is used to auscultate low-frequency sounds, and the diaphragm is used to auscultate high-frequency sounds.

or clothing, rubbing against the stethoscope, bumping the stethoscope tubing, or moving the head of the stethoscope. The head of the stethoscope must be completely sealed by the client's skin over the area of auscultation. If a client has body hair over the area of auscultation, wetting it with water reduces the crackling sound that hair creates. The earpieces of the stethoscope should fit snugly, occluding the ear canal and screening out environmental noise. Stethoscopes with angled earpieces should be worn so that the angle points toward the nose, thereby directing sound toward the tympanic membrane.

Four properties are used to describe sound: frequency, intensity, duration, and quality. *Frequency* is the measure of vibration, expressed in cycles per second, which is heard as *pitch.* Many cycles per second or a high frequency produces a high-pitched sound; few cycles per second produce low-pitched sounds. *Intensity* describes the loudness of sound. Breath sounds over the trachea are loud, whereas most heart sounds are soft. The length of the sound is the *duration.* An abnormal heart sound is described according to its duration within the cardiac cycle. Timing of the sound may also be described, such as during inspiration or expiration. *Quality* reflects the musical characteristic of a sound. Blowing, squeaking, and humming are adjectives frequently used in describing the quality of a sound.

Table 21-4 • Stethoscope Diaphragm and Bell Usage

	Technique	Purpose	Example
Diaphragm	Press firmly against the skin	Detects high-pitched sounds	Breath sounds, normal heart sounds, bowel sounds
Bell	Lay lightly on the skin	Detects low-pitched sounds	Abnormal heart sounds, bruits

Assessment Using a Functional Health Framework

The remainder of this chapter discusses the information and skills needed to conduct a basic client assessment, organized according to functional health. Each functional pattern describes an aspect of human performance or ability that contributes to the overall health of the person. The nurse's goal in assessing each pattern is to identify

- Client's normal functional pattern
- Risk factors for dysfunction
- Presence of any dysfunction
- Client's satisfaction with functional abilities
- Client's adaptation to limitations or dysfunction
- Effect of dysfunction on performance of daily activities.

Assessment skills described in this chapter are intended as an overview of a general health assessment. If an area of dysfunction is observed, a more in-depth assessment should be performed. Chapters in Section II of this text address assessment of each functional-health pattern in depth.

Assessment of Health Perception and Health Management

The major health problem in the United States and Canada is chronic disease, such as heart disease, cancer, and stroke. Control of these health problems depends directly on modification of a person's behavior and habits of living. Prevention necessitates eliminating activities that many people enjoy: overeating, overindulgence in alcohol, and use of nicotine. Prevention also implies doing things that require special effort: exercising regularly, eating a healthy diet, seeking regular health examinations, and striving for a harmonious life. Assessment of a person's health perception and health maintenance reveals knowledge, behavior, and attitudes toward preventing disease and living a healthy lifestyle. The chapters in Unit V of this text are concerned with health maintenance and health management.

Subjective Data

Client interview is the primary method of gathering information about the client's perception of his or her health and methods used to maintain health and wellness. The major focus includes the client's perception of health status, preventive health practices, compliance with medical treatment, and client safety.

During a health assessment, the nurse should discuss the client's health-promotion activities, such as exercise, nutrition, routine preventative examinations (eg, dental, vision, hearing), immunization history, safety precautions (eg, child safety seats, bicycle helmets), and stress management. The nurse should inquire about nicotine (eg, chewing tobacco, pipe, cigar, nicotine gum or patches), alcohol (amount, frequency, type), and drug use (recreational and prescription). The client's overall willingness and ability to follow health-related advice should be assessed, such as taking medications on schedule or following a prescribed diet. Other sources of health advice, such as an acupuncturist, herbalist, or naturopath, should be elicited.

A detailed allergy history should be obtained for every client, including medication, food, pollen, insect, and any environmental allergens. The nurse should inquire about the *specific type of reaction* that was experienced. Some clients may confuse a medication side effect, such as nausea, with an allergic reaction. Severe allergic reactions should be documented and communicated to others.

Selected sample interview questions for eliciting the client's perception and management of health include

- Describe the problem with your health.
- Why did you come to seek care? What do you hope treatment will accomplish?
- How would you describe your health?
- When was your last dental, eye, or physical examination?
- Do you use tobacco, alcohol, or recreational drugs? What type? How often?
- What safety practices to you follow (eg, safety belt, bicycle helmet)?
- What do you do to keep healthy or prevent disease progression?

Objective Data

Although direct observation of a client's health practices usually is not possible, some objective data reflecting effort toward health promotion may be found through specific measurable consequences of health behavior. Examples of such behavior include the blood sugar level of a diabetic client; the number of pounds lost by an overweight client; blood pressure measurement of a hypertensive client; the number of clinic appointments a client has kept or canceled; or the number of hospital admissions for a health problem. Some nurses count a client's pills to estimate if medications are being taken correctly.

Assessment of Activity and Exercise

Activity and exercise describe the wide range of physical activities that people initiate and perform to maintain life, health, and well-being. Physical activity is necessary for many functions in daily living, including the ability to care for oneself, to work, to maintain a home, to obtain resources, and to engage in social and recreational activities. In addition, physical exercise is important for promoting health and preventing complications associated with inactivity.

Collection of subjective and objective data concerning musculoskeletal function, respiratory function, and cardiovascular function is important in the assessment of activity and exercise. Body movement depends on the normal functioning of the bones and muscles of the body, and how well movement is coordinated by the nervous system. The respiratory and cardiovascular systems work together to supply the muscles of the body with oxygen and energy and to ensure that waste products produced during activity can be transported to other parts of the body for removal. For clarity in discussing assessment of activity and exercise, the assessment has been divided into musculoskeletal and mobility assessment, respiratory assessment, and cardiovascular assessment.

Musculoskeletal and Mobility Assessment

Mobility, the ability to move about freely, is an important component of activity and exercise because it affects independence and self-care ability. For clients with no deficits, only a brief discussion of mobility and self-care is necessary. Many other clients, however, experience mild to severe deficits. For such clients, a detailed evaluation is needed.

Subjective Data

A program of regular physical activity is important at every age and should be discussed with every client. Participation in sports and recreational activities contributes not only to physical but to psychological wellbeing. The nurse should determine if the client has any pain or discomfort associated with exercise, and if there are desirable activities that the client is unable to participate in. Energy level also affects the desire and ability to be physically active. Fatigue is frequently associated with cardiac and respiratory disease, anemia, and cancer.

When a client's mobility or self-care functions are compromised, a daily living assessment should be performed. A daily living assessment includes evaluation of the ability to perform self-care skills (bathing, toileting, dressing, grooming, and eating) and simple motor activities (sitting, standing, walking, climbing stairs, and opening doors). Depending on the client's living situation, an assessment of some home maintenance skills may also be appropriate. These skills include cooking, shopping, housekeeping (making a bed, cleaning, vacuuming, washing dishes), doing the laundry, paying bills, and using the telephone. The architecture of a home, particularly the presence of stairs, can complicate independent activity and should be considered.

Table 21-5 • Self-Care Abilities Scale

0	Full self-care, independent
I	Needs to use equipment or device
II	Needs supervision
III	Needs equipment or device and supervision
IV	Unable to perform, dependent

A scale is used to rate these self-care abilities (Table 21-5). The daily living assessment provides key information about a person's ability to live independently or the amount of assistance that is required to do so. If major disabilities are present, an occupational therapist may be consulted for further evaluation. More information on daily living assessment is provided in Chapter 31.

Mobility assessment is preventive as well as descriptive. Clients with impaired mobility are at risk for accidents and injury. Older people, particularly those who have fallen in the past, are most susceptible. A thorough assessment of risk factors can determine the risk for falling, and appropriate safety precautions may be instituted.

Suggested client interview questions related to mobility and self-care include

- Describe your usual activities in a normal day (or week).
- What limitations in ability do you have (eating, toileting, walking, dressing, bathing)?
- Have you recently fallen or consider yourself to be at risk for falling?

Objective Data

Objective data useful in evaluating a client's musculoskeletal and mobility status include gait and balance, muscle strength, joint mobility, and assessment of acute injury.

Gait and Balance. Gait describes the manner of walking. Balance refers to stability and equality between both sides of the body. An evaluation of gait and balance contributes to the assessment of a client's mobility as well as risk for injury due to falling. Gait and balance abnormalities may also indicate dysfunction or disease in other body systems, particularly the brain, spinal cord, muscles, and skeleton. A client may acquire a slowed, cautious, or unnatural gait as an unconscious means of protection from pain, weakness, or loss of balance.

Gait and balance may be observed during many activities that naturally occur in the course of a health assessment. The nurse should assess the client's balance as he or she walks into the room, moves around in bed, rises from the sitting position, or rolls onto his

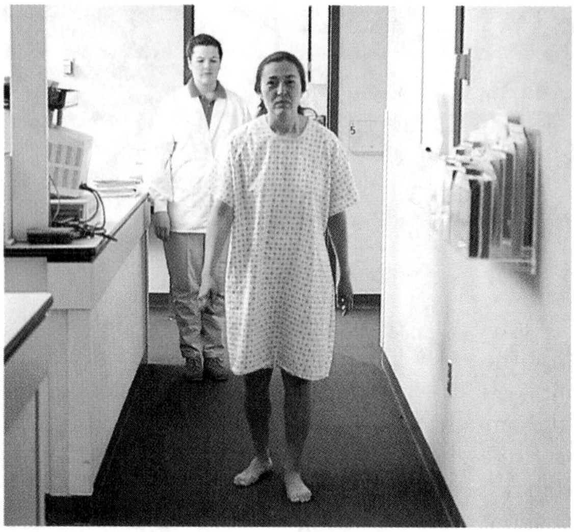

Figure 21-6 • The examiner observes gait as the client walks.

or her side. To assess gait further, the nurse asks the client to walk a distance of about 10 feet down a hallway (Fig. 21-6). A normal gait is quick, springy, and rhythmic, with the arms naturally swinging back and forth. Characteristics of abnormal gait include the following: slow, measured steps; limping; leaning to one side; shuffling of the feet; shorter steps taken on one side compared to the other; wide outward swinging of one leg; a wide gait or stance; leaning the trunk forward; lifting the knee higher than normal with each step; and short, hurrying steps.

Foot pain is a common cause of decreased mobility. The client's feet should be inspected for the presence of bunions, corns, calluses, ingrown toenails, spurs, and ulcers.

If the client uses any assistive devices for ambulation, such as a cane, crutches, walker, prosthesis, or brace, he or she should be assessed while using the aid. The nursing assessment should focus on coordination, stability, comfort, and safety. For additional information on assessing mobility status, refer to Chapter 33.

Muscle Strength. A nurse should perform a simple screening of motor function in the arms and legs because limb movement and strength are essential for many self-care activities. A simple method is to measure hand strength by having the client squeeze the nurse's wrists, and measure foot strength by having the client push the ball of the foot against the nurses's hand. Muscle strength may also be observed by evaluating the amount of strength against resistance or gravity. For clients able to participate in the examination, have the client move the limb against your resistance. Other clients may be asked to hold a limb in a position, with gravity acting as the resistance. The response is then graded (Table 21-6).

Symmetry of strength is evaluated. It is expected that muscle strength is slightly greater in the dominant arm. Notable differences in strength or overall difficulty in performing these tests reveal problems with movement or weakness in the arms. Deficits should be reported to the physician or a nurse specialist for a more comprehensive and detailed assessment of muscle function.

Joint Mobility. Joint movement is also important to activity and exercise function. All joints should have appropriate range of motion. Often the nurse can observe this by watching the extent and ease with which a person moves extremities. If the client complains of stiffness or does not move an area of the body, the nurse should evaluate joint mobility by moving each joint through full range of motion and noting any limitations in movement. Generally, greater than 20% reduction in the normal range is abnormal. A physical therapist may be consulted for further evaluation. Refer to Chapter 33 for additional information on assessment of joint mobility.

Circulation, Movement, Sensation. When an acute problem with the limb is suspected, circulation, movement, and sensation (CMS) are evaluated. Circulation is assessed by color, temperature, pulses, and capillary refill. Movement is assessed by asking the client voluntarily to move the extremity. Sensation is assessed by asking the client to say when they feel the nurse touch them. Also question the client about paresthesias, or numb and tingling sensations. CMS is normal if the skin is pink and warm, pulses are present, and capillary refill takes place within 3 seconds. The client should be

Table 21-6 • Grading Scale for Muscle Strength

0—No detectable muscle contraction
1—Barely detectable contraction
2—Complete range of motion or active body part movement with gravity eliminated
3—Complete range of motion or active movement against gravity
4—Complete range of motion or active movement against gravity and some resistance
5—Complete range of motion or active movement against gravity and full resistance

able to wiggle the toes or fingers, and he or she should be able to report when the nurse touches him or her. No paresthesias should be present.

Respiratory Assessment

Assessment of general respiratory status occurs every time you interact with the client. A survey of skin color, respiratory difficulty, and position taken to breathe is important to determine the acuity of the client's problem. For acute respiratory distress, immediate assistance should be obtained so that appropriate interventions can be made.

Subjective Data

Functional respiratory assessment should focus on four major areas: risk factors for lung disease (such as smoking or occupational exposure to pollutants); signs and symptoms of respiratory dysfunction (such as cough, sputum production, and dyspnea); impact of respiratory status on activities of daily living; and adaptive measures for any respiratory dysfunction. Suggested interview questions that can help to elicit this information include:

- Have you been exposed to environmental or occupational materials that have affected your breathing? What are they?
- Have you had allergies, asthma, bronchitis, emphysema, tuberculosis, or other lung problems?
- How often do you cough? Describe the sputum.
- Are there any breathing difficulties that limit your activity? What are they?
- What position do you assume for sleeping?

Objective Data

Anatomic Landmarks of the Chest and Lungs. Anatomic landmarks and imaginary reference lines are used during the assessment of structures that lie within the thorax (chest) (Fig. 21-7). The lines and landmarks of the chest are used during lung auscultation and percussion to define the specific area of the lung being examined. These landmarks and reference lines also provide a standard vocabulary for use in describing and documenting assessment findings.

Inspection. Inspection related to the respiratory examination focuses on four general areas: configuration of the thorax; breathing patterns; signs of labored breathing; and observation of the skin and nails. The shape of the thorax is best examined by having the client sit upright with the chest area unclothed. The *anterior-posterior (AP) diameter* is a term used to describe the distance between the sternum and the vertebral column, drawn as a straight line through the thorax. In the normal adult, the AP diameter is approximately one-half of the lateral diameter (or width) of the chest.

One of the most common abnormalities of thorax configuration is seen in clients with chronic obstructive pulmonary disease. These clients exhibit a "barrel-shaped" chest in which the AP diameter is enlarged and approximately equals the lateral diameter. Other thoracic abnormalities include kyphosis, an exaggerated convex curve of the spine; scoliosis, a lateral deviation of the spinal curve; and kyphoscoliosis, a combination of abnormal lateral and convex curvature of the spine. The presence of any of these conditions may deform the rib cage, impede lung expansion, and interfere with breathing.

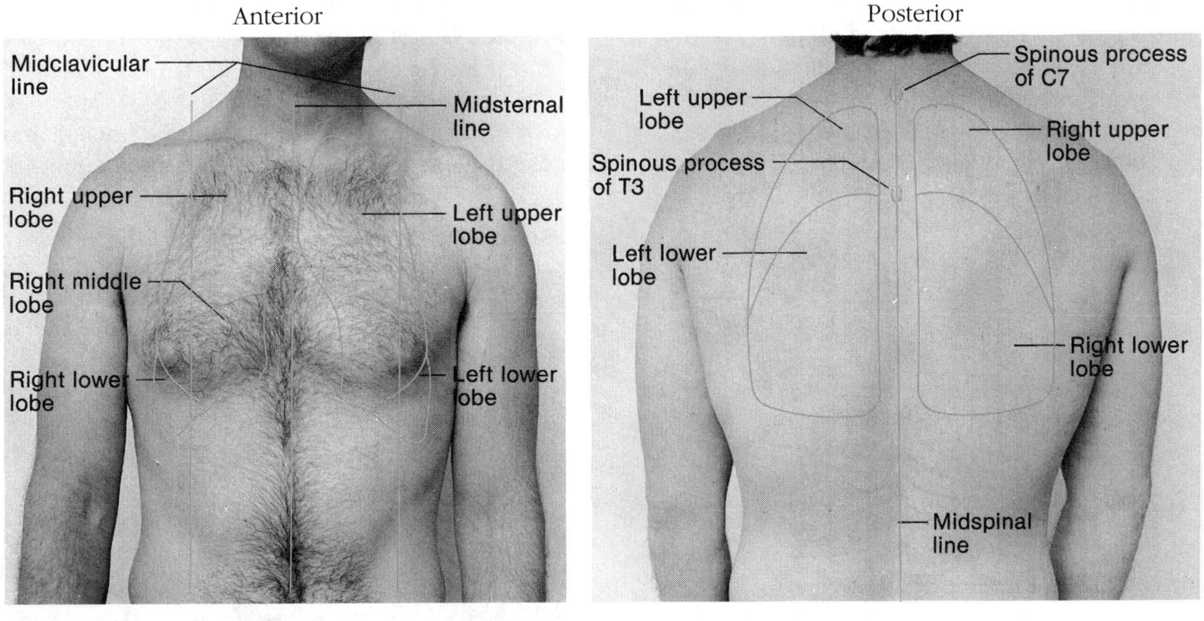

Figure 21-7 • *Landmarks of the anterior and posterior chest wall.*

Normal breathing is silent, effortless, and occurs at a rate of 12 to 20 times per minute in adults. Careful observation of the client's breathing should normally reveal a pattern that is smooth, regular, symmetric, and rhythmic. Conditions to observe for include too fast (tachypnea), too slow (bradypnea), too shallow (hypoventilation), too deep (hyperventilation), or irregular (Cheyne-Stokes) breathing. Abnormal breathing patterns are discussed in Chapter 22.

While observing the client's breathing pattern, the nurse should look for indications of respiratory distress or increased effort in breathing, noting the position that the client has assumed to breathe. Clients with difficulty will be sitting, and may be leaning forward or need a pillow for support. Symptoms such as nasal flaring, facial straining, and pursed-lip breathing indicate abnormal respiratory effort. Abnormal effort during inspiration is evidenced by active, visible use of the scalene and sternomastoid muscles of the neck and shoulders. These muscles are called accessory muscles. Contraction of the abdominal muscles, which assists upward movement of the diaphragm, may also be observed. During inspection of the client's breathing, observe the intercostal space. Airway obstruction or decreased lung compliance may result in retraction of the intercostal spaces during inspiration, whereas some respiratory diseases (such as emphysema) can cause bulging of the intercostal spaces during expiration.

The color and appearance of the skin and nails may reflect insufficient delivery of oxygenated blood to the tissues because of respiratory dysfunction. With normal supply of oxygen, the nailbeds, the tongue, and the lips appear pinkish-red in color. Hypoxia (decreased supply of oxygen to the tissues) changes this color to a grayish, bluish, or purplish tone. When this change in color is confined to the nailbeds and lips, it is called peripheral cyanosis; when it progresses to the tongue and mucous membranes of the mouth, it is called central cyanosis. Central cyanosis indicates a significant problem with oxygenation of body tissues and can be caused by respiratory, cardiac, or metabolic problems. Chronic bronchitis may also cause the skin to become reddish and leathery, which appears as ruddiness.

Clubbing of the nails is a sign of chronic hypoxia. To determine if nail clubbing is present, the nurse examines the contour of the nail and adherence of the nail to the nailbed. When viewed in profile, normal fingernails present an angle of 160 degrees between the nailbed and the finger (Fig. 21-8) With clubbing, swelling flattens the angle to 180 degrees or less. With advanced clubbing, the nail becomes less adherent to the base of the nail and feels spongy. The nails and fingertips appear large and swollen, and are sometimes described as "drumstick-like."

Palpation. Palpation is used in respiratory assessment to evaluate painful or abnormal areas on the chest wall, to test for symmetry of chest expansion, and to detect tracheal deviation. To examine any areas on the chest where the client has complained of discomfort, or where visible abnormalities are present, lightly palpate the area and surrounding area. Note tenderness, masses or bulges, or a crackling feeling (crepitus) that may indicate an air leak into the subcutaneous tissue.

Normal chest expansion during inspiration is symmetric, indicating equal expansion of both lungs. To evaluate chest symmetry, the nurse stands behind the client, places his or her thumbs at the level of the 10th rib, and wraps the hands around the lateral rib cage (Fig. 21-9). The client is asked to inhale deeply, and the nurse observes his or her thumbs for equal, outward movement.

The trachea is normally in a straight, vertical position. Some lung disorders, such as large masses and pneumothorax, can cause a shift in the trachea from its normal midline position. The nurse may stand behind the client and reach across the client's shoulders, placing the index finger on each side of the trachea in the suprasternal notch. Alternatively, the trachea may be palpated anteriorly by placing the index finger along one side of the trachea and noting the space between it and the sternomastoid (Fig. 21-10). The trachea and surrounding area are palpated; the other side is compared. The space on either side of the trachea and the ends of the suprasternal notch should be equal (Bates, 1995).

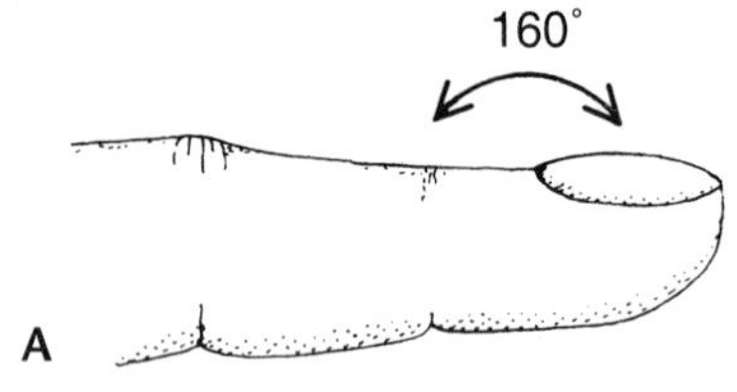

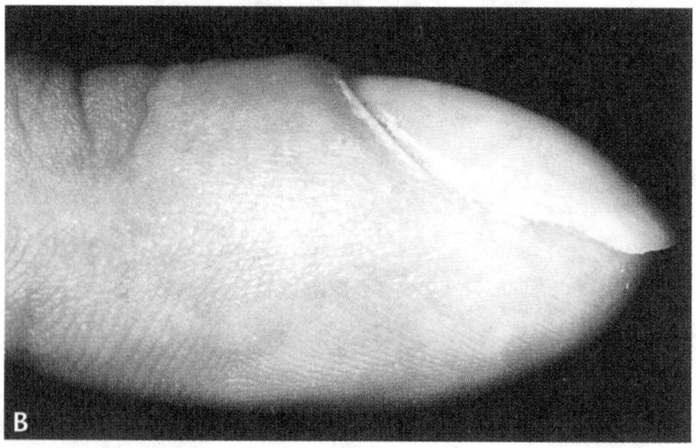

Figure 21-8 • Clubbing of the nails. (A) Normal nail. (B) Clubbing of nail and finger.

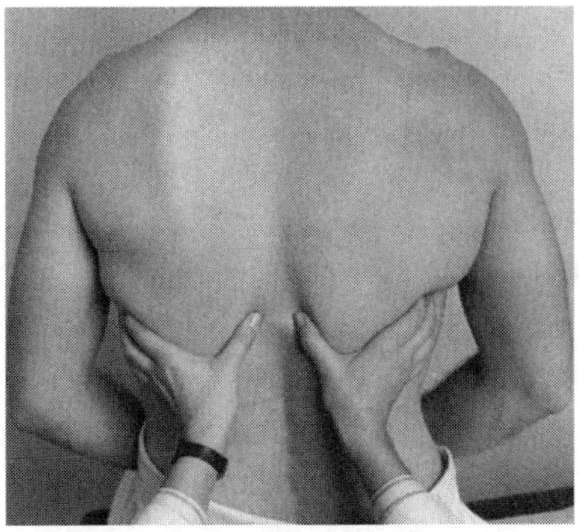

Figure 21-9 • *Palpation of thoracic excursion. In the posterior approach, the nurse's hands are placed at the level of the 10th rib and observed for equal outward movement as the client inhales.*

Percussion. Percussion of the lung normally reveals a hollow, loud, low-pitched resonant sound because the lung is air-filled. Percussion that reveals dullness or reduced resonance may indicate masses, fluid, or tissue-filled lung space. Percussion that is hyperresonant indicates hyperinflation of the lung, such as with the air trapping that occurs with emphysema. Diagnostically, chest percussion has largely been replaced by examination of the chest x-ray.

Auscultation. Lung auscultation involves listening with a stethoscope over the anterior and posterior chest wall for variations in breath sounds. Breath sounds are created by the movement of air in and out of the airways with each inspiration and expiration. Auscultation of the lungs reveals direct, objective data about the client's ventilatory status. Data gathered through auscultation provide important clues to underlying pathophysiology. Lung assessment should be systematic, and takes time and practice to perfect. Refer to Procedure 21-1 for the steps in pulmonary auscultation.

Normal Breath Sounds. Normal breath sounds are classified as bronchial, bronchovesicular, and vesicular. They are described according to location, ratio of inspiration to expiration, intensity, and pitch, as summarized and illustrated in Table 21-7.

Bronchial breath sounds are loud and high-pitched, with a hollow quality often compared to the sound of air blowing through a pipe. Expiration is longer and louder than inspiration with bronchial breath sounds. They are normal when heard over the trachea but indicate a lung abnormality when heard elsewhere. Abnormal bronchial sounds may be associated with pneumonia, pleural effusion, tumor, or atelectasis.

Vesicular breath sounds are normally heard over all areas of the lung except over or near the major airways. Vesicular sounds are described as soft and breezy, with inspiration markedly longer than expiration.

Bronchovesicular breath sounds are intermediate in character between bronchial and vesicular sounds. They are described as breezy, but softer and lower pitched than bronchial sounds. Inspiratory and expiratory times are approximately equal. Bronchovesicular sounds are normally heard in two areas only: on the anterior chest over the bifurcation of the main bronchi in the first or second intercostal spaces, and posteriorly between the scapulae. Like bronchial sounds, bronchovesicular sounds should not be detected elsewhere over the chest.

Adventitious Breath Sounds. Adventitious breath sounds are abnormal sounds that occur from air passing through narrowed airways or fluid, or from an inflammation of lung pleura. The major adventitious breath sounds are crackles, wheezes, and friction rubs (Fig. 21-11). These sounds are often superimposed over normal breath sounds and take much practiced listening to discern. Adventitious breath sounds are described in detail in Chapter 34.

When abnormal breath sounds are detected, continue to listen, requesting the client to say words or sounds. When consolidation or atelectasis is present, the words (such as "ninety-nine") will sound louder and clearer than they usually do. This is known as bronchophony. Also, if the client says "ee," the sound will transmit as "ay"; this is called egophony (Finesilver, 1992).

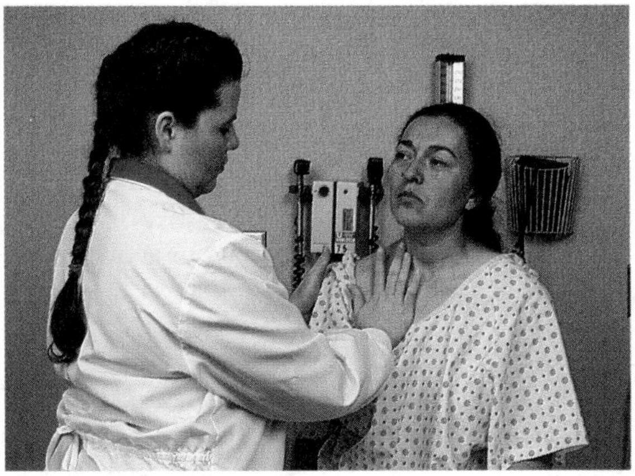

Figure 21-10 • *The nurse may examine for tracheal deviation anteriorly by placing the index finger along side the trachea, noting bilaterally the space between the trachea and sternomastoid muscle.*

Cardiac Assessment

Activity and exercise are impeded when the heart cannot work effectively to pump blood, or when the vasculature is unable to supply the perfusion of blood needed by the body's tissues. Assessment of cardiac and peripheral vascular status provides clues about circulation and oxygenation to every part of the body.

Table 21-7 • Normal Breath Sounds from Anterior Location

Location	Description	Ratio of Inspiration to Expiration	Intensity	Pitch
Bronchial	Blowing, hollow sounds over the trachea 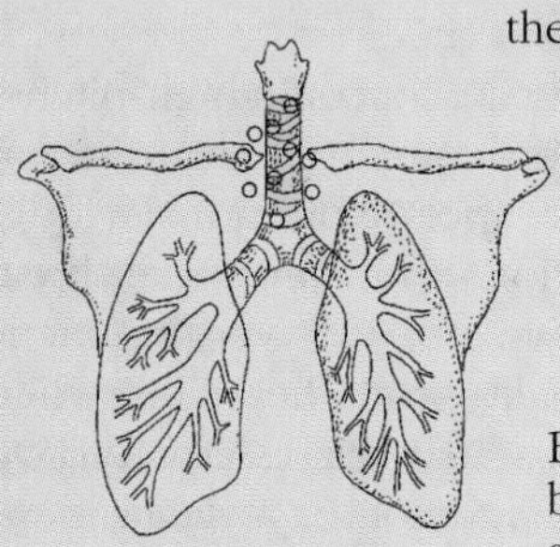	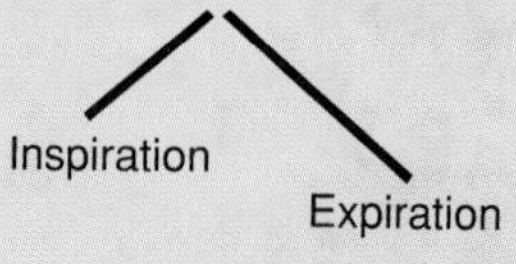	Expiration is longer and louder	Expiration is higher
Bronchovesicular	Intermediate sounds over first and second anterior intercostal spaces and posteriorly between scapula 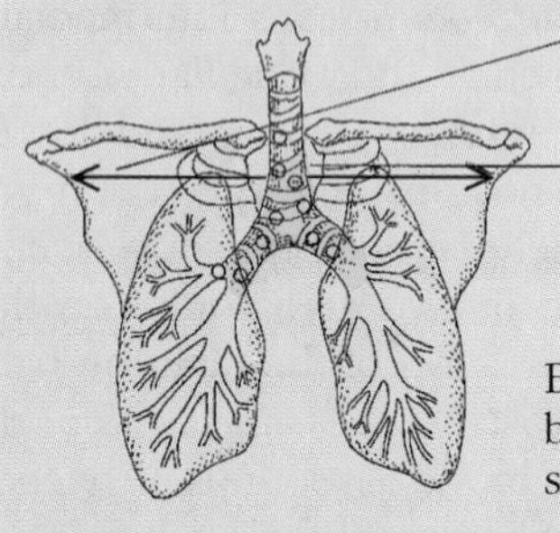	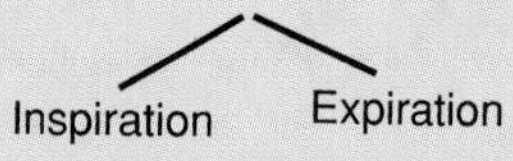	Medium and similar	Medium and similar
Vesicular	Soft and breezy sounds over all lung area except airways 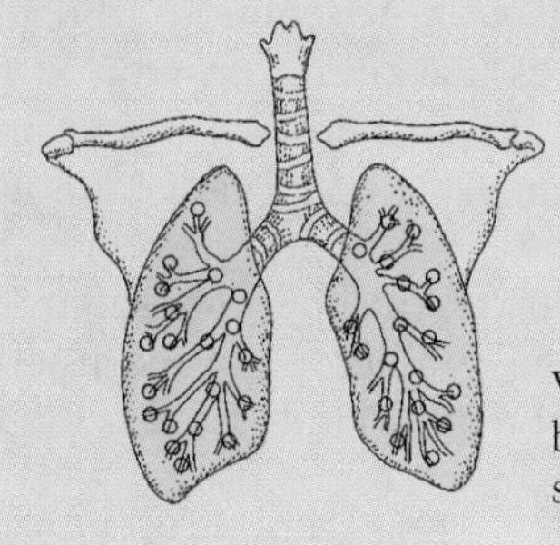	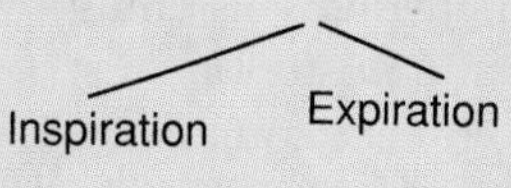	Inspiration markedly longer and louder	Inspiration is higher

Subjective Data

The major thrusts for assessment of cardiovascular function include risk factors for cardiovascular disease (such as hypertension, elevated cholesterol, or smoking); signs and symptoms of cardiovascular dysfunction (such as pain, dizziness, or palpitations); the impact of cardiovascular dysfunction on activities of daily living; and specific adaptations to cardiac or circulatory impairment.

Interview questions to help elicit this information might include

- Describe your normal diet or exercise pattern.
- Do you have a history of heart attack, heart rhythm problems, high blood pressure, or high blood cholesterol?
- Have you had any chest pain, shortness of breath, cough, swelling in the legs, leg or calf pain, fluttering in the heart, or fatigue?
- How has this problem limited your activities?

Objective Data

Objective data about cardiovascular status are obtained by assessing vital signs, assessing the heart, and assessing arteries and veins. In most cases, assessment of the client's vital signs is the first objective information gathered in a health assessment. Significant deviation from normal heart rate and blood pressure may be the first indicator of a serious problem in circulatory function.

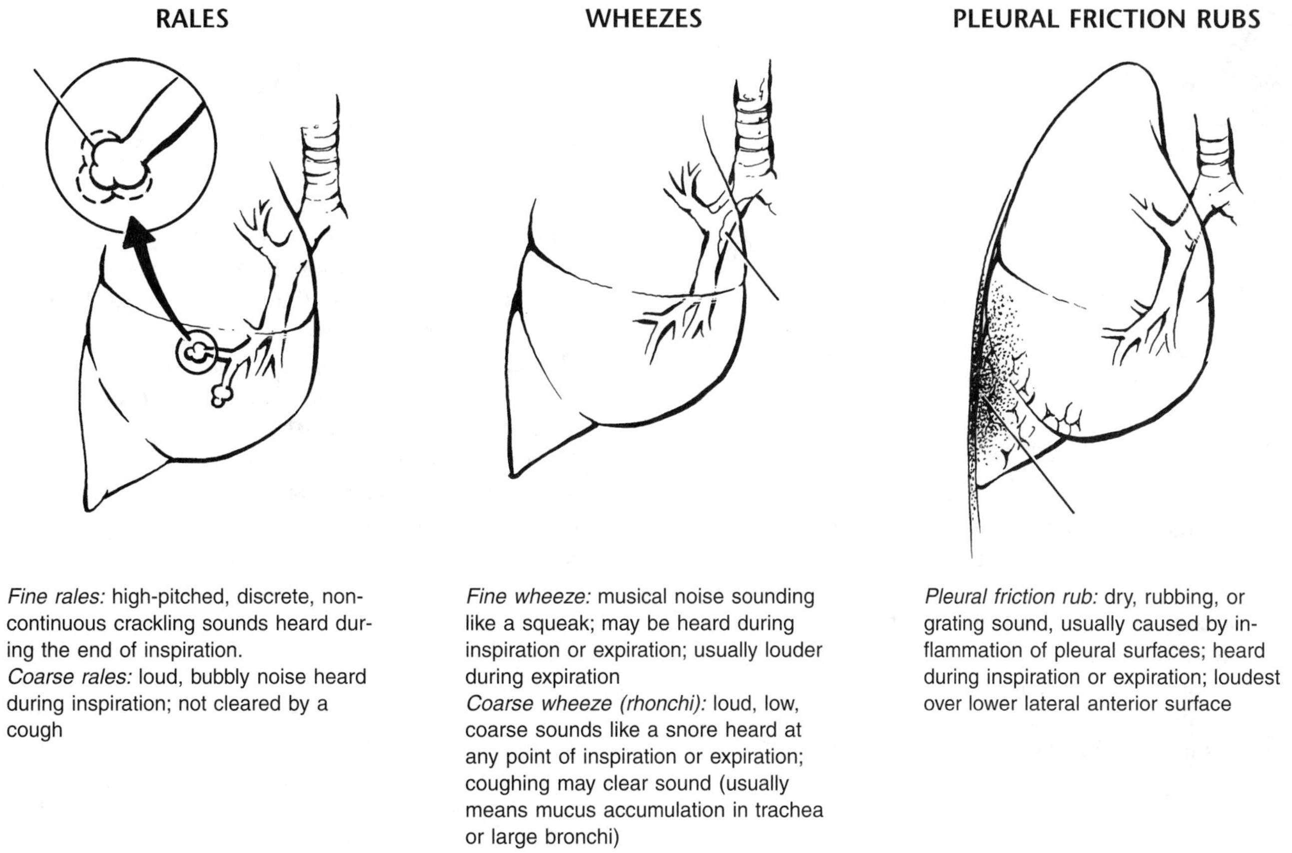
RALES
WHEEZES
PLEURAL FRICTION RUBS
Fine rales: high-pitched, discrete, noncontinuous crackling sounds heard during the end of inspiration.
Coarse rales: loud, bubbly noise heard during inspiration; not cleared by a cough
Fine wheeze: musical noise sounding like a squeak; may be heard during inspiration or expiration; usually louder during expiration
Coarse wheeze (rhonchi): loud, low, coarse sounds like a snore heard at any point of inspiration or expiration; coughing may clear sound (usually means mucus accumulation in trachea or large bronchi)
Pleural friction rub: dry, rubbing, or grating sound, usually caused by inflammation of pleural surfaces; heard during inspiration or expiration; loudest over lower lateral anterior surface

Figure 21-11 • *Adventitious breath sounds.*

Landmarks for Cardiac Assessment. The *precordium* is the area on the anterior chest overlying the heart and its great vessels. Knowledge of the location of structures within the precordium is necessary to perform effective cardiac assessment.

There are four major areas on the precordium for examining the heart (Fig. 21-12). Each area corresponds to one of the heart's four valves and is located as follows:

- Aortic area—second intercostal space to the right of the sternum
- Pulmonic area—second intercostal space to the left of the sternum

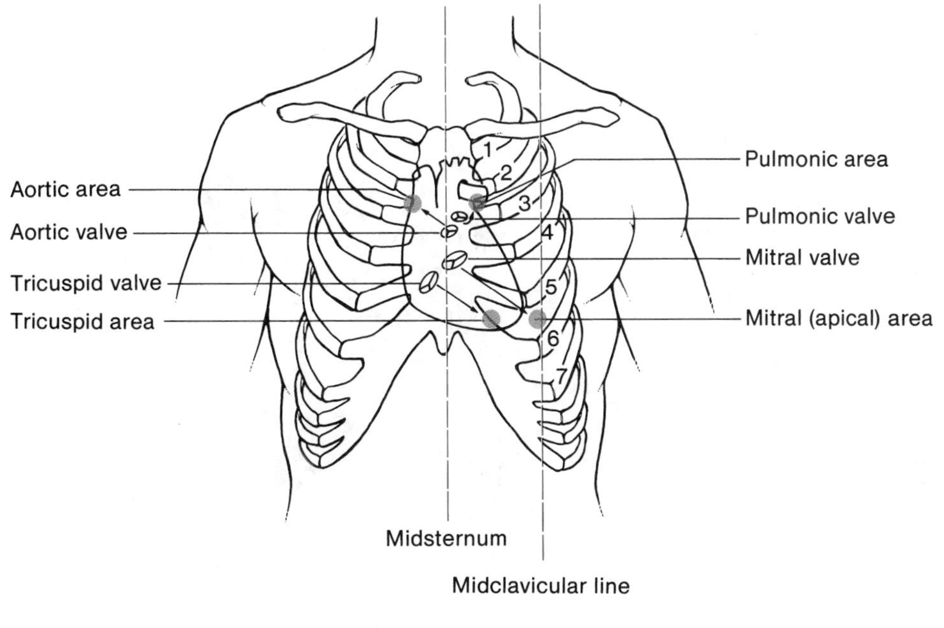

Figure 21-12 • *Heart sounds are referred from valvular points of origin to the auscultatory or precordial landmarks. Sound travels in the direction of blood flow and may be heard some distance from the valve.*

Procedure 21-1
Auscultating Breath Sounds

Purpose

1. To listen for variations in breath sounds that may indicate the presence of airway obstruction or disease process.
2. To assess the effectiveness of medications or therapies in opening or clearing airways.

Assessment

- Determine if the client is distracted by an immediate need (eg., pain, need to void, and so forth). Attend to that need first.
- Explain to the client what you plan to do and approximately how long it will take.
- Provide for privacy so client is not concerned about being viewed or overheard. Visitors and family members may be asked to leave the room.
- Ensure that the room is warm and quiet.

Equipment

Stethoscope

Procedure

1. Wash hands.
   Note: Moderately warm water increases circulation to warm your hands; this decreases discomfort to client during examination.
2. Assist the client to an upright sitting position. Remove client gown to expose chest.
   Rationale: Upright position improves chest excursion. Breath sounds are distorted or muffled if assessed through clothing.
3. Warm diaphragm of stethoscope by holding between hands for a short time.
   Rationale: A warm stethoscope is more comfortable for the client and helps put the client at ease.
4. Ask client to breathe deeply through the mouth. Client should breathe slowly.
   Rationale: Mouth breathing enhances volume of breath sounds; nasal breathing decreases volume and can simulate adventitious sounds. Slow breathing rate is necessary to avoid hyperventilation.

Auscultate Anterior Chest

5. Place diaphragm of stethoscope about 1 inch below the middle of the right clavicle, making sure it lies between the ribs. Listen to one full inspiration and exhalation. Repeat the process at the corresponding site on the left side.
   Rationale: Placement of stethoscope over intercostal space improves sound quality. Representative sounds of the right and left upper lobes are audible here.
6. Note normal and adventitious breath sounds at each point on the chest as you proceed.
   Rationale: Movement of air through airways produces characteristic sounds. Abnormal sounds are indicative of airway disturbances.
7. Move stethoscope downward about 1.5 to 2 inches along midclavicular line. Note sounds; move scope laterally to opposite side.
   Rationale: Air movement through other (larger) airways of upper lobes can be heard here. Listening to sounds at corresponding points on opposite sides of sternum allows you to compare similar lung fields.
8. Move stethoscope downward another inch or two along midclavicular line to fifth intercostal space. (This space lies just below the nipple line on males, approximately across from the head of the xiphoid process of the sternum.) Note sounds, then move to same spot on opposite side.
   Rationale: Right middle lobe and corresponding segments on left can be heard here.

Auscultate Posterior Chest

9. Instruct client to lean forward and cross arms in front.
   Rationale: This position separates scapulae and facilitates listening to posterior breath sounds.
10. Begin by auscultating the area about 2 inches below the shoulders and 2 inches to the right of the spine. Note sounds, and move to corresponding point on left.
    Rationale: These positions allow the nurse to compare breath sounds of posterior segments of upper lobes.

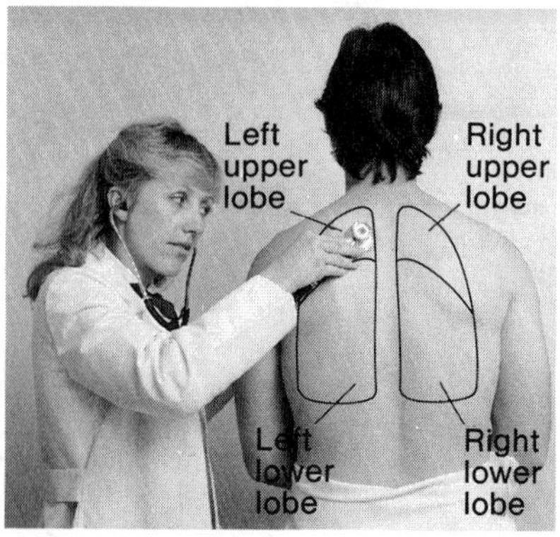

Step 10 • *Auscultating the upper posterior chest.*

11. Move stethoscope directly downward 2 or 2.5 inches; note sounds, then move stethoscope laterally and listen on right.
    Rationale: Superior segments of lower lobes are audible here.
12. Repeat process, moving downward 2 to 2.5 inches; listen to corresponding opposite side.
    Rationale: Each placement of stethoscope allows you to hear sounds of different segments of lung.
13. Move stethoscope downward to area just below scapula. Listen on right and left. Listen also to areas laterally along lower rib cage.
    Rationale: Lower lobes end at level of 10th thoracic vertebra (about 1.5 inches below scapulae) and follow the contour of the lower ribs. Their large size and the fact that many clinical problems can affect the lower lobes make lateral assessment essential.
14. Replace client's clothes and assist to comfortable position.
15. Discuss your findings with client.
    Rationale: Discussion provides an opportunity for client feedback on effectiveness of therapies. Provides directions for client teaching if new therapies are to be initiated (eg, cough, deep breathing, incentive spirometry).
16. Record assessment findings. Be specific as to description and location of adventitious sounds.

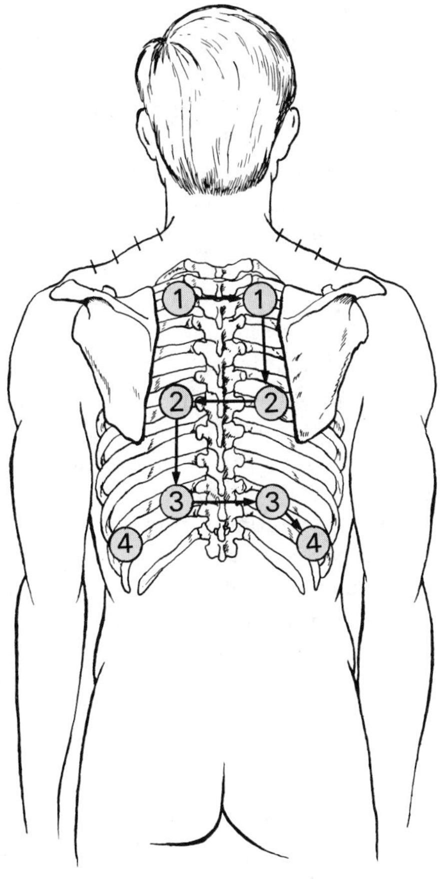

Steps 10–13 • *Sequence for posterior chest auscultation.*

Lifespan Considerations

Newborn and Infant

- Newborns have difficulty maintaining body temperature. Uncover only body area that you are directly assessing.
- At 8 to 12 months of age, infants become fearful of strangers. Spend several minutes becoming acquainted with the child before examining.

Toddler and Preschooler

- Children 2 to 5 years of age are often afraid of examining equipment. Letting them handle the stethoscope and using a "This is a game" approach often helps allay the fear.
- Auscultate breath sounds before performing any invasive examination, which may cause the child to cry.

Child and Adolescent

- Older children are modest. They may or may not want a parent to be with them during the examination; give the child the choice. Protect modesty through use of gowns or drapes.

Older Adult

- A lengthy physical examination may be exhausting for the older adult and may need to be completed in phases.
- The older adult may become easily chilled. Provide warmth through adequate draping or gowning.

- Tricuspid area—fifth intercostal space, left of the lower sternal border
- Mitral (or apical) area—fifth intercostal space, just medial to the midclavicular line

Inspection, palpation, and auscultation are the three basic techniques used to assess the precordium and vasculature. Percussion may be used to estimate the size of the heart, but this method has generally been replaced by x-ray examination.

Inspection. The entire precordium should be inspected for movement. Inspection can be enhanced by using tangential light across the chest and by observing the heart at eye level. Normally, the only movement seen is in the mitral valve area. A visible pulsation occurs with ventricular contraction as the left heart strikes the anterior chest wall. This pulsation is called the *point of maximal impulse* (PMI). It is not abnormal if the PMI is not seen, as often occurs in clients with thick chest walls or large breasts. Abnormal movements over the precordium include forceful movement around the area of the PMI, called a *heave*; anterior movement of the sternum, called a *lift*; or small areas of pulsation in the intercostal spaces or around the sternum.

Palpation. Palpation follows and complements inspection. The nurse should palpate in each of the four precordial areas, noting any vibrations (termed *thrills*) or pulsations. The fingertips are the most sensitive to pulsation; the heel and ulnar surfaces of the hand are most sensitive to vibration. The nurse should feel for the PMI in the mitral area and note its exact location and size. The normal PMI is a light tap, located at the medial to midclavicular line, confined to the area of one intercostal space. A PMI lateral to this may indicate an enlarged heart. Pulsations or vibrations over the aortic, pulmonic, or tricuspid areas may indicate problems with those heart valves.

Auscultation. Valuable information can be acquired by listening to heart sounds. Learning the basic techniques of cardiac auscultation is enhanced by using a consistent pattern for auscultating the precordium and by concentrating on one heart sound or phase in the cardiac cycle at a time. Steps in auscultation are given in Procedure 21-2.

Normal Heart Sounds. Normal heart sounds include S_1 and S_2. Systole (ventricular contraction) is the period of time from the beginning of the first heart sound (S_1) to the beginning of the second heart sound (S_2). Diastole (ventricular relaxation) is the period of time from the beginning of the second heart sound to the beginning of the next ventricular contraction.

The first heart sound coincides with the beginning of systole, when the mitral and tricuspid valves close. When an audible difference in closure of the two valves is detected, the first sound is said to be *split*. Because the force generated in the left ventricle is much greater than that in the right ventricle, the first heart sound is dominated by the mitral valve and is best heard in the mitral (apical) area. The second heart sound coincides with the beginning of diastole, when the aortic and pulmonic valves close. Aortic valve closure slightly precedes and dominates the second heart sound, and therefore the second heart sound is best heard in the aortic area.

The first and second heart sounds are high-pitched sounds heard best using the diaphragm of the stethoscope. When the heart rate is slow, it is easy to differentiate the two sounds. Systole is shorter than diastole, so two "paired" sounds (S_1 then S_2) are heard, followed by a pause. When the heart rate is faster, the pause is less distinctive or even absent. To clarify S_1 from S_2 in this situation, the nurse feels the client's carotid pulse

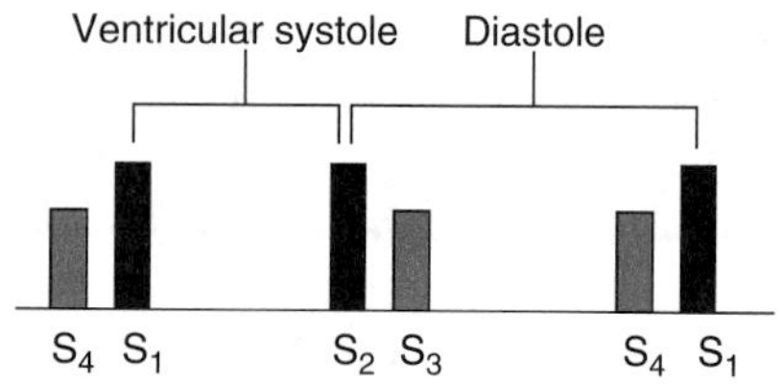

Figure 21-13 *• Occurrence of S_3 and S_4 heart sounds in the cardiac cycle.*

when listening to the heart. The carotid pulse and S_1 occur almost simultaneously.

Extra or Abnormal Heart Sounds. The third heart sound, also referred to as S_3, is an *extra sound* occurring early in diastole as the ventricle rapidly fills. It can be normal in healthy children or young adults, but in older people it often signifies congestive heart failure. The presence of a third heart sound is an important clinical finding that should be sought if a client is at risk for congestive heart failure. The fourth heart sound, also referred to as S_4, is an extra sound occurring late in diastole, just before the first heart sound. It coincides with atrial contraction when blood is actively propelled into the ventricle. The fourth heart sound is thought to result from a stiffened left ventricle and is frequently associated with hypertension and coronary artery disease. The development of an S_4 is not as serious as an S_3 and does not necessarily indicate heart failure. Auscultation of the third and fourth heart sound is clearest at the apex when the client is positioned on his or her left side (Yacone-Morton, 1991). Figure 21-13 illustrates where the third and fourth heart sounds, commonly called *gallops*, occur in the cardiac cycle.

A **murmur** is vibrating sound produced from turbulent blood flow through the heart, especially across the valves. The more common causes for a murmur include partially obstructed flow through a valve opening (stenosis), increased blood flow across a normal valve, backward (regurgitant) blood flow due to a leaky (incompetent) valve, blood flow into a dilated chamber, and blood flow through an abnormal opening between heart chambers (Boorse-Fabius, 1994). Murmurs resemble a blowing or swishing noise and may occur during systole or diastole. They may be low-pitched or high-pitched, so both the bell and diaphragm of the stethoscope are appropriate for detecting murmurs. When a murmur is heard, it should be noted whether it occurs during systole (between S_1 and S_2) or during diastole (after S_2) and where it is heard on the precordium. Figure 21-14 illustrates where systolic and diastolic murmurs fall in the cardiac cycle. Diastolic murmurs are almost always caused by heart disease; systolic murmurs may be related to heart disease but are frequently benign.

Clicks, abnormal, sharp, high-pitched sounds, can occur in the presence of mitral value prolapse, aortic or pulmonic valve disease, or in the presence of a mechanical heart valve (Boorse-Fabius & Stunkard, 1994).

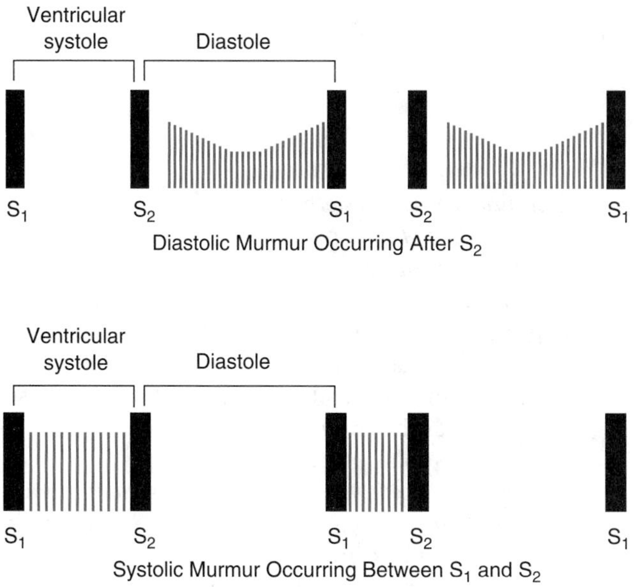

Figure 21-14 • *Location of heart murmurs in the cardiac cycle.*

Peripheral Vascular Assessment

Subjective Data

Subjective data can be collected concerning adequate peripheral (arm and leg) circulation, evaluating arterial and venous blood flow. Use of vasoconstricting agents such as nicotine should also be evaluated. Possible interview questions include

- Do you experience leg pain or cramping with exercise?
- Do you have edema or a sore that won't heal in your lower extremities?

Objective Data

Inspection. Inspection can be used to assess peripheral circulation. Skin should be examined for color and temperature. Poor peripheral circulation may be associated with hair loss and skin discoloration or scaling. Observed varicosities (swollen, twisted veins) can indicate venous problems. Edema, or fluid, may also be detected through inspection. Arterial problems are associated with pallor, dependent rubor, shiny, cool, hairless skin, weak or absent pulses, decreased capillary refill, and sharp pain with increased activity. Venous problems are associated with edema, warmth, bluish discoloration when legs are dependent, brown pigmentation, flaky dermatitis, achy, chronic pain, and ulcers that heal slowly (Gehring, 1992).

Palpation. Palpation is important in peripheral vascular assessment. Skin temperature is best evaluated using the back of the hand. Symmetric coolness or warmth may be normal; unilateral coolness may indicate decreased blood flow; unilateral warmth may indicate local infection. Generalized cool skin accompanied by pallor and moistness may indicate peripheral vasoconstriction due to circulatory shock. Arterial pulses should also be palpated, noting rate, rhythm, amplitude, and symmetry. The brachial, radial, ulnar, femoral, popliteal, posterior tibial, and dorsalis pedis pulses are used (see Fig. 22-5). A grading scale is used to compare the strength of the pulses (Table 21-8).

Table 21-8 • *Grading Scale for Pulses*

0	=	Absent
1 +	=	Diminished; thready; easily obliterated
2 +	=	Normal; not easily obliterated
3 +	=	Increased; full volume
4 +	=	Bounding; hyperkinetic

Palpation is also used to assess capillary refill. Capillary refill time is a simple test of circulatory status using the nailbeds. The nurse presses down on the nailbed until it turns white and notes how quickly the color returns when pressure is released. Normal refill time is 3 seconds or less; prolonged capillary refill indicates poor circulation (see Fig. 35-4).

Edema is evaluated through palpation. Edema is fluid accumulation in the tissues. The degree of edema is estimated by noting how long the tissue remains indented when pressed. Edema is assessed in dependent areas such as the hands, feet, ankles, and lower legs. The nurse should press firmly with the thumb, for at least 5 seconds, behind the medial malleolus, over the dorsum of the foot, and over the shin. When a client is bedridden, the dependent areas are the back and sacrum. A grading system, ranging from +1 to +4, is often used to record edema (Table 21-9). Lower limbs

Table 21-9 • *Grading Scale for Edema*

1 + Edema	• Slight indentation (2 mm) • Normal contours • Associated with interstitial fluid volume 30% above normal
2 + Edema	• Deeper pit after pressing (4 mm) • Lasts longer than 1 + • Fairly normal contour
3 + Edema	• Deep pit (6 mm) • Remains several seconds after pressing • Skin swelling obvious by general inspection
4 + Edema	• Deep pit (8 mm) • Remains for a prolonged time after pressing, possibly minutes • Frank swelling
Brawny edema	• Fluid can no longer be displaced secondary to excessive interstitial fluid accumulation • No pitting • Tissue palpates as firm or hard • Skin surface shiny, warm, moist

Procedure 21-2
Auscultating Heart Sounds

Purpose

1. To assess normal and abnormal functioning of the heart valves.
2. To detect cardiac problems.

Assessment

- Determine if the client is distracted by an immediate need (eg, pain, urge to urinate). Attend to that problem first.
- Explain to the client what you plan to do and approximately how long it will take.
- Provide for privacy so client is not concerned about being viewed or overheard. Visitors and family members may be asked to leave the room.
- Ensure that the room is warm and quiet.

Equipment

Stethoscope with a bell-shaped and flat-disc diaphragm.

Procedure

1. Wash hands.
   Note: Moderately warm water increases circulation to warm your hands; this decreases discomfort to client during examination.
2. Assist the client to supine position. You may want to reexamine the client in the upright sitting position and a left lateral position. Lift the client's gown to expose the chest.
   Rationale: Some heart sounds may be accentuated in certain positions.
3. Warm diaphragm of stethoscope by holding between hands for a few moments.
   Rationale: A warm stethoscope is more comfortable than a cold stethoscope.
4. Listen in the mitral area using the diaphragm (see Fig. 21-12). Identify the first and second heart sounds. Count the heart rate, noting whether the rhythm is regular or irregular. If the rhythm is irregular, count the heart rate for a full minute. Also note whether the irregularity has a pattern, or whether it is totally unpredictable.
   Rationale: Auscultation is performed systematically, concentrating on one sound at a time in each area.
5. Listen in the aortic area using the diaphragm. Concentrate first on S_1, then S_2, noting if splitting occurs. Shift your concentration to systole and then diastole; listen for extra sounds, such as murmurs.
   Rationale: The diaphragm of the stethoscope transmits the high-pitched sounds of S_1 and S_2. Murmurs are best heard over the valvular areas in the direction the blood is flowing through the heart.
6. Listen in the pulmonic area, still using only the diaphragm. Repeat the sequence described in step 5, concentrating on S_1, S_2, systole, and diastole. Compare the loudness of S_2 in the aortic and pulmonic areas.
   Rationale: Loudness of S_2 in the aortic area relates to the systemic arterial blood pressure and can be louder than normal in adults with hypertension. Loudness of S_2 in the pulmonic area relates to the pulmonary artery pressure and may be louder than normal in patients with chronic obstructive pulmonary disease. It is abnormal for the pulmonic S_2 to be louder than the aortic S_2 in adults older than 40 years of age.
7. Move the diaphragm and listen to the tricuspid and mitral areas.

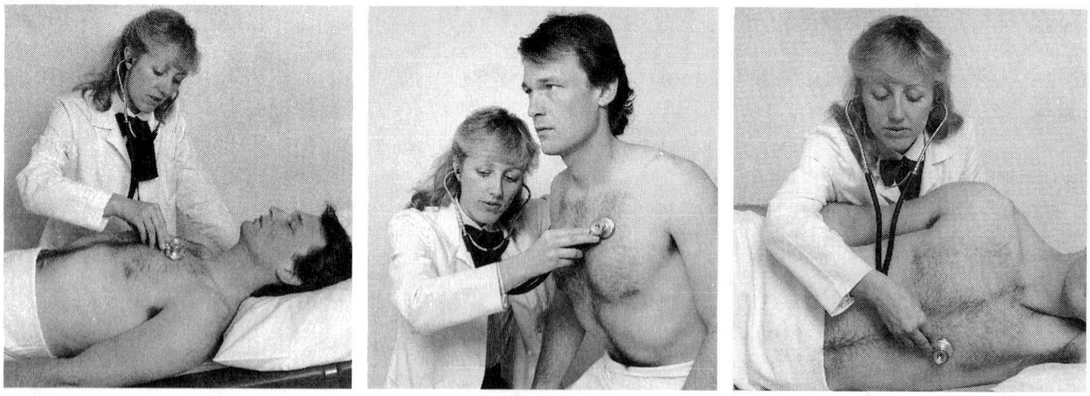

Supine | Forward Sitting | Left Lateral

Step 2 • *Precordial positions for heart auscultation.*

8. Return to the aortic area, this time using the bell of the stethoscope. As before, concentrate individually on S_1, S_2, systole, and diastole.
9. Repeat the same process, using the bell, in the pulmonic, tricuspid, and mitral areas. Especially in the mitral area, concentrate during diastole to detect the presence of a third or fourth heart sound.
   Rationale: The lower-pitched sounds of the mitral and tricuspid valves, as well as an S_3 or S_4, are best transmitted through the bell of the stethoscope.
   Note: To increase your ability to hear an S_3 or mitral murmur, have the client lie on the left side while you auscultate with the bell. An S_3 often disappears when the client sits up.
10. Replace the client's clothes. Assist to a comfortable position.
    Rationale: The nurse provides comfort and warmth before leaving.
11. Record your assessment findings, describing the intensity, quality, and location of the sounds.

Lifespan Considerations

Newborn and Infant

- Newborns have difficulty maintaining body temperature. Uncover only body area that you are directly assessing.
- At 8 to 12 months of age, infants become fearful of strangers. Spend several minutes becoming acquainted with the child before examining.

Toddler and Preschooler

- Children 2 to 5 years of age are often afraid of examining equipment. Letting them handle the stethoscope and using a "This is a game" approach often helps allay the fear.
- Auscultate heart sounds before performing any invasive examination, which may cause the child to cry.

Child and Adolescent

- Older children are modest. They may or may not want a parent to be with them during the examination; give the child the choice. Protect modesty through use of gowns or drapes.
- An S_3 is normal in children and young adults.

Older Adult

- An S_3 may indicate heart failure in older adults. An S_4 may be present with coronary artery disease or hypertension.
- A lengthy physical examination may be exhausting for the older adult and may need to be completed in phases.
- The older adult may become easily chilled. Provide warmth through adequate draping or gowning.

may also be measured for circumference to evaluate for changes in edema and symmetry.

Auscultation. Auscultation is used to detect **bruits**, abnormal arterial sounds similar to murmurs, caused by increased turbulence of blood flow. Bruits can be detected by placing the stethoscope over major blood vessels, such as the renal artery, iliac artery, femoral artery, carotid artery, or the abdominal aorta. Bruits occur when an artery is partially obstructed or distended, which prevents blood flow from moving straight through the vessel.

Assessment of Nutrition and Metabolism

Assessment of nutrition and metabolism collects data concerning dietary habits and metabolic needs. Information reflects how well the body is able to ingest, digest, absorb, and metabolize food, and use it to maintain tissue integrity and fluid and electrolyte balance, and to fight infection.

Subjective Data

Assessment of nutrition and metabolism requires specific information about the client's normal diet and careful observations of the physical features that reflect nutritional state. The nutrition-metabolism assessment should focus on normal food and fluid intake, alterations in normal eating patterns, how dietary changes have affected daily living, and the development of medical problems secondary to altered nutritional status.

Interview questions to focus a nutrition-metabolism assessment might include some of the following:

- Tell me what you've eaten in the last 24 hours.
- Do you have any problems with getting groceries, or preparing or cooking food?
- Do you have any problems with tasting, chewing, or swallowing food?
- Do you have dentures? partials? bridges? plates?
- Do you have problems with nausea, vomiting, constipation, or diarrhea?
- Do you have any skin lesions, itching, infections, or skin changes in the last year?
- What is your usual weight? Has it changed in the past 6 months? How much?

Objective Data

Objective data are used to validate subjective information obtained during the client interview. Objective data collected for nutrition and metabolism pattern include height and weight measurement, assessment of the mouth and teeth, assessment of the abdomen, and assessment of the skin.

Height and Weight. Weight measurement can provide important information regarding nutritional status. Standardized tables have been developed (eg, Metropolitan Height and Weight Tables for Men and Women, Ages 25 to 59) that recommend ideal body weight for men and women. Standardized tables are also available to evaluate growth in children. Such tables provide a baseline for evaluating the client's weight. Deviations from normal body size, ranging from obese to severely underweight, can influence not only nutritional state but other health patterns, such as exercise, activity, and self-concept.

Use of the standardized weight tables to evaluate nutritional status has recently been questioned because the tables fail to consider individual and group (eg, cultural, ethnic) variances. A percentage of weight change, which uses the client's usual weight as the standard, may be more meaningful. Using the following formula, the nurse can calculate the percentage of weight change:

$$\frac{\text{Current weight} - \text{Usual weight}}{\text{Usual weight}}$$

Generally, a change in weight of 10% over the last 6 months is considered to be abnormal. A dietitian should be consulted for further evaluation.

Weight measurement can also be used to evaluate fluid status or the response of the client to medical treatment (eg, diuretic therapy to treat congestive heart failure). Rapid weight gain or loss (eg, 10 pounds in 2 weeks) is usually caused by the gain or loss of body fluid rather than body fat.

Weight measurement can be done on a variety of scales; the choice depends mainly on the status of the client. An upright scale is appropriate for the client with normal mobility who can step onto a platform and maintain balance while weight is determined. A chair scale is used when a client can transfer to a chair but is unable to support the body in a standing position for accurate weight measurement. A bed scale is used for the client who is too weak or immobile to use other scales safely. Special infant scales are used to determine the height and weight of babies.

Scales can be calibrated in terms of pounds or kilograms, with some scales providing both measures of weight. To convert from pounds to kilograms, divide by 2.2; to convert from kilograms to pounds, multiple by 2.2. For most clients, height and weight measurements are obtained on admission to a healthcare agency. When daily or frequent weights are required to evaluate client progress, weight is measured at the same time each day (usually before breakfast), using the same scale. Procedure 21-3 outlines steps in measuring weight.

Height is measured with a measuring stick attached to a standing scale. The client stands erect without shoes on the scale, and the height is determined by lowering the sliding arm until it rests on the client's head.

Height can be measured in inches or centimeters. To convert inches to centimeters, multiply by 2.54; to convert centimeters to inches, divide by 2.54.

Assessment of the Mouth. Examination of the mouth includes the buccal mucosa (cheek), teeth, lips, gums, and tongue (Fig. 21-15). The lips should be evaluated for color, moisture, cracks, or lesions. A bright light and a tongue blade are used to inspect the mucous membranes, teeth, and gums. Mucous membranes should appear pink and moist. The nurse should observe for lesions in the mouth or on the gums. Dental appliances should be removed for inspection, especially if the client complains of pain or has ill-fitting dentures. The teeth should be inspected for stability and overall hygiene. The bite should be evaluated. A major concern when examining the mouth is to detect any abnormalities that might impede the client's ability to taste, chew, swallow, or enjoy food.

Abdominal Assessment. Basic abdominal assessment consists of inspection, auscultation, and palpation. Abdominal assessment provides clues to general gastrointestinal function and any related problems.

Landmarks for Abdominal Assessment. The abdomen is divided, for descriptive purposes, into four quadrants. The upper and lower quadrants are separated by an imaginary horizontal line through the umbilicus. The right and left quadrants are separated by an imaginary vertical line between the xiphoid and symphysis pubis. Structures underlying each of the four quadrants are listed and illustrated in Table 21-10.

Inspection. During inspection, the contour, skin, and movement of the abdomen are noted. The client is observed at eye level from the side, from the foot of the bed, and from directly over the abdomen. Tangential lighting is used across the abdomen to accentuate subtle changes. The contour of the abdomen can be evaluated by placing the client supine and viewing at eye level from the side. It is described as flat, rounded, protuberant, or scaphoid (boat shaped or hollowed). Ascites is the accumulation of serous fluid in the peritoneum. This fluid may cause the shape to become protuberant, or distended and firm. A distended abdomen may also be measured to provide more specific data.

The abdominal skin should be similar in color and texture to skin on other areas of the body. Note the presence and location of scars, rashes, lesions, petechiae (small, red, hemorrhagic spots), or striae. *Striae* are streaks from rapid or prolonged stretching of the skin.

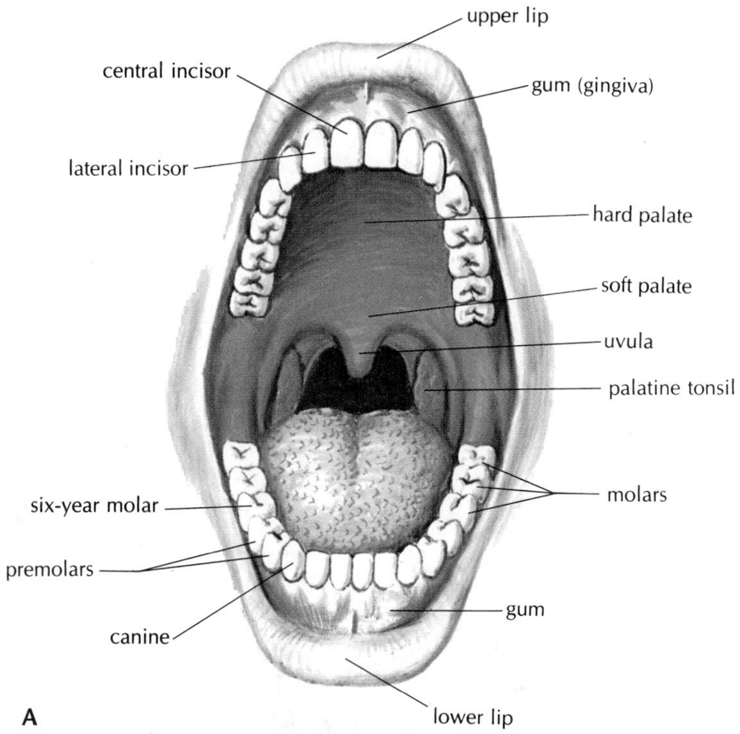

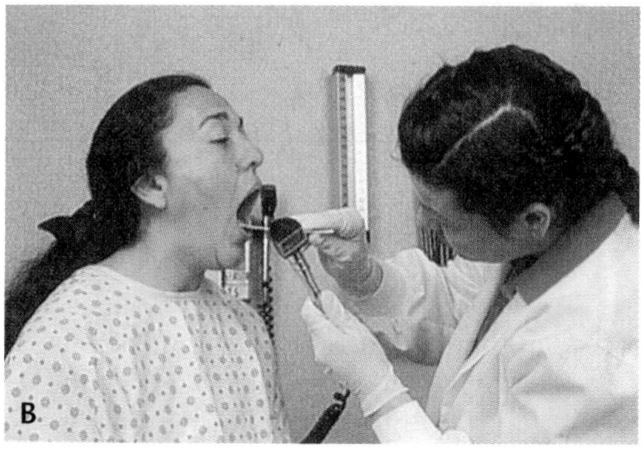

Figure 21-15 • *Examination of the mouth. (**A**) Structures of the mouth. (**B**) Examining the oral cavity.*

Recent striae are pink or blue; they turn silvery white with age. Pregnancy, ascites, and weight loss are common causes of striae. Fine veins may normally be visible on the abdomen, especially in the inguinal area; distended, prominent veins are abnormal and are frequently associated with liver disease. Scars provide clues about previous surgeries.

Visible movement over the abdomen is not uncommon. Wave-like movements of intestinal peristalsis may be seen in thin clients. A normal aortic pulsation

Table 21-10 • *Organs in the Four Abdominal Quadrants*

1—Upper Right Quadrant	***3—Upper Left Quadrant***
Liver	Left lobe of liver
Gallbladder	Stomach
Duodenum	Spleen
Head of pancreas	Upper lobe of left kidney
Right adrenal gland	Pancreas
Upper lobe of right kidney	Left adrenal gland
Hepatic flexure of colon	Splenic flexure of colon
Section of ascending colon	Section of transverse colon
Section of transverse colon	Section of descending colon
2—Lower Right Quadrant	***4—Lower Left Quadrant***
Lower lobe of right kidney	Lower lobe of left kidney
Cecum	Sigmoid colon
Appendix	Section of descending colon
Section of ascending colon	Left ovary
Right ovary	Left fallopian tube
Right fallopian tube	Left ureter
Right ureter	Left spermatic cord
Right spermatic cord	Part of uterus (if enlarged)
Part of uterus (if enlarged)	

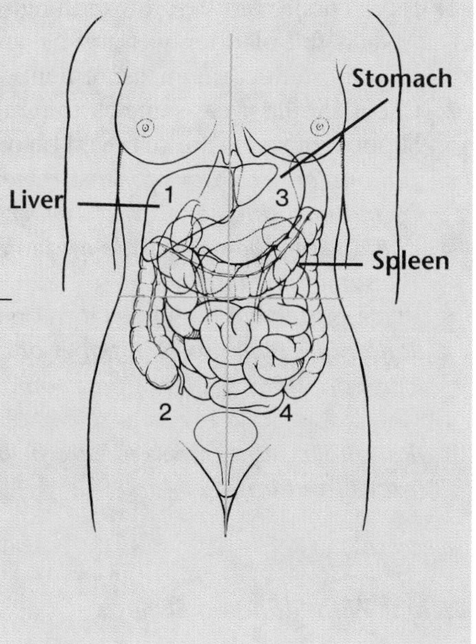

The uterus and urinary bladder fall in the lower midline.

Procedure 21-3
Measuring Weight

Purpose

1. To provide baseline data from which to assess total fluid balance or nutritional status.
2. To provide baseline data to determine drug dosages or information for diagnostic testing with dye or radioactive injections.

Assessment

- Assess necessity for baseline, daily, or weekly weight measurements.
- Review previous weight measurements, if available.
- Identify time of day previous weights were measured. Weights can vary considerably during a 24-hour period so it is important that serial weights be done at the same time each day. Most hospitals weigh clients in the early morning. Check hospital policy.
- Assess client's mental and physical status to determine if a standing, sitting, or bed scale is appropriate.

Equipment

An appropriate scale.
Note: Use the same scale each time you weigh the client.
Protector towel or plastic sheet

Procedure

1. Have client void before weighing.
   Note: A full bladder, wet gowns, and saturated dressings affect the measurement.
2. Client should wear same clothing for each weight. Slippers or shoes are removed before measurement.
   Rationale: Accuracy of measurement is increased by maintaining consistency. Other measures include using the same scale and taking weights at the same time of day.
3. Place protective paper or cloth on scale.
   Rationale: Placing clean paper or cloth on scale helps prevent transfer of microorganisms.
4. Check that scale registers zero. Adjust as necessary.
   Rationale: Adjustments to zero help ensure accuracy of readings.

Procedure

Weight With Standing Scale

1. Assist client onto scale. Client must stand in *center* of platform and not lean or hold onto supports.
   Rationale: Depending on type of equipment, movement may cause inaccurate weight.
2. Read digital display or adjust counterweights to determine client's weight.

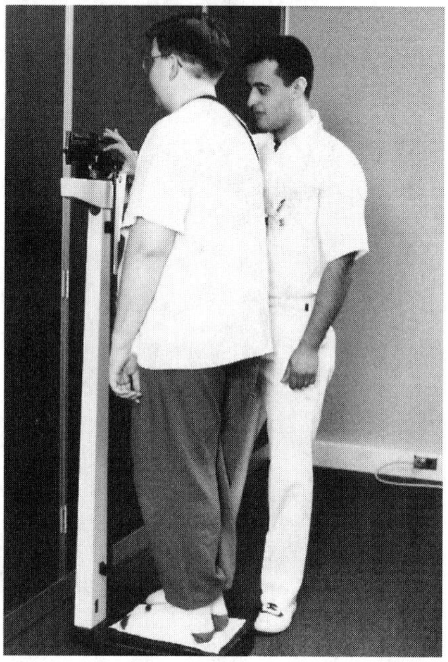

Step 2 • Adjust counterweights on the balancing arm.

3. Assist client from scale. Dispose of protector sheet if used.
   Rationale: This action helps prevent transfer of microorganisms.

Procedure

Weight With Chair Scale

1. Place scale beside client and lock wheels.
   Rationale: An easier transfer helps prevent accidental falls.
2. Transfer client onto chair.
   Note: If arm of chair is removable, unlock and remove before transfer. Lock back into place after transfer to provide security and prevent accidental falls.
3. Read digital display or adjust counterweights to determine client's weight.
4. Transfer client back to bed or wheelchair.
   Rationale: The nurse provides for client's safety and comfort.

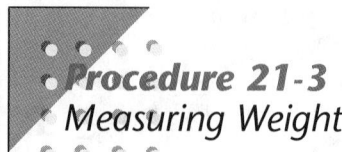

5. Clean the scale according to agency policy.
   Rationale: A clean scale helps prevent transfer of microorganisms.

Procedure

Weight With Bed Scale

1. Elevate client's bed to level of stretcher scale.
2. With one or two assistants, turn client with back toward the scale.
3. Roll scale toward the bed, lock wheels in place, and lower stretcher onto bed.
   Rationale: Provides for safe transfer of client to bed scale.
4. Position folded stretcher under client. Roll client onto stretcher.
5. Attach stretcher arms to stretcher and gradually elevate stretcher about 2 inches above mattress surface.
   Note: Inform client before elevating. Reassure that he will not fall but his head may feel lower than his body.
   Rationale: Decreases client's anxiety and improves cooperation.

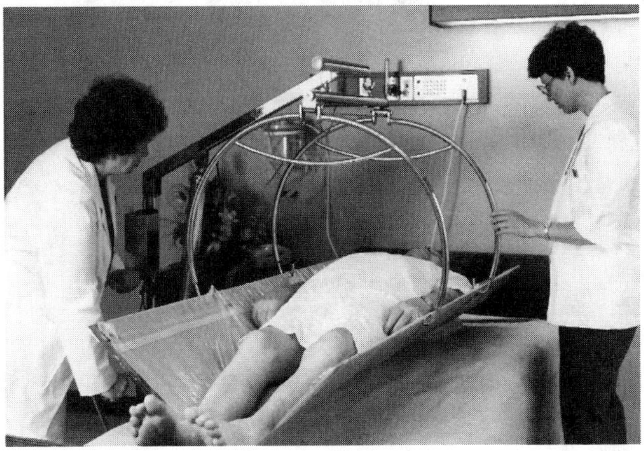

***Step 5** • Elevate client on stretcher, approximately 2 inches off bed surface.*

6. Determine that stretcher is not touching any equipment. Lift all drains and tubing away from stretcher.
   Rationale: Equipment alters measurement and affects accuracy.
7. Read digital display for client's weight.
   Note: This is a good time to change client's linen as he or she is elevated off the bed.
8. Gradually lower stretcher to the bed. Remove stretcher arms and transfer client off stretcher. Remove stretcher.
   Rationale: Ensures safe transfer of client.
9. Unlock bed scale wheels and move away from bed.
10. Assist client to comfortable position.
11. Clean stretcher and scale according to agency policy.
    Rationale: Prevents transfer of microorganisms.
12. Record weight and note any extra linen or equipment weighed with the client.

Lifespan Considerations

Infants

- Infants are usually weighed nude. Be careful that room temperature is warm because infant's body temperature can fluctuate severely because of their immature thermoregulatory system.
- Infants often roll and kick. The nurse's hand should always be within 1 to 2 inches of the child's body to prevent accidental falls.

Home Care Modifications

- Clients requiring serial weights are encouraged to keep a written log of their weights.
- If visual problems restrict the client's ability to read the scale, family members may be able to assist.
- Clients are instructed to weigh at the same time each day, usually in the morning before breakfast, and to wear similar-weight clothing for each measurement.

is frequently visible in the epigastrium. Rise and fall of the abdomen synchronized with respiration is frequently seen, especially in men.

Auscultation. The nurse should always auscultate the abdomen before palpating or percussing, because movement or stimulation may alter motility of the bowel and increase the sounds. Bowel sounds are created as air and fluid mix in the intestine. Procedure 21-4 outlines the method of abdominal auscultation.

Normal bowel sounds are tinkling, gurgling noises that occur between 5 and 34 times per minute (Holmgren, 1992). Only after listening to a quadrant for 5 minutes and hearing no sounds can the nurse conclude absence of bowel sounds. Clinically, this becomes impractical because some bowel assessments could take up to 20 minutes. Most nurses listen for 1 to 2 minutes in each quadrant. If bowel sounds are not detected after this time, bowel tones are charted as hypoactive. Increased frequency and loudness of bowel sounds are called borborygmi, or hyperactive. Borborygmi reflect increased intestinal peristalsis, which may be related to diarrhea, laxatives, emotional upset, or intestinal obstruction. Borborygmi heard before a meal are better known as "stomach growling."

Palpation. Light palpation is performed to obtain information about pain or discomfort. The nurse should pal-

Procedure 21-4
Auscultating Bowel Sounds

Purpose

1. To determine the presence or absence of intestinal peristalsis.

Assessment

- Plan to auscultate the abdomen before palpating or percussing if performing a complete abdominal examination. Stimulation of the abdominal wall may alter bowel mobility.
- Determine if the client is distracted by an immediate need (eg, pain, urge to urinate). Attend to that problem first.
- Provide for privacy so client is not concerned about being viewed or overheard.
- Ensure that the room is warm and quiet.
- If the client has a nasogastric tube with suction, turn off the suction during auscultation because the sound will confuse your assessment.

Equipment

Stethoscope

Procedure

1. Wash hands and warm stethoscope diaphragm.
   Rationale: Cold hands or stethoscope may cause contraction of the abdominal muscles, which may be heard during auscultation.
2. Ask the client when he or she last ate.
   Rationale: Bowel sounds may be increased shortly after eating or if a meal is long overdue.
3. Have a client urinate before the examination.
   Rationale: An empty bladder enhances validity of observations and promotes client's comfort.
4. Assist client to a supine position with abdomen exposed.
   Rationale: Supine position prevents tension in the abdominal muscles.
5. Visually divide the abdomen into four quadrants using the umbilicus as the central crossing landmark (see Table 21-10).
   Rationale: Consistent landmarks facilitate accurate description of assessment findings.
6. Place the stethoscope diaphragm in each of the four quadrants. Listen for pitch, frequency, and duration of bowel sounds at each site.
   Rationale: Active bowel sounds are irregular, gurgling noises, occurring every 5 to 20 seconds.

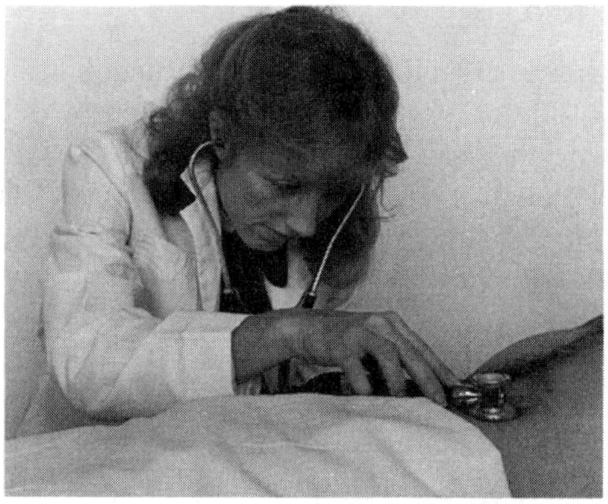

Step 6 • *Auscultate bowel sounds with diaphragm of stethoscope.*

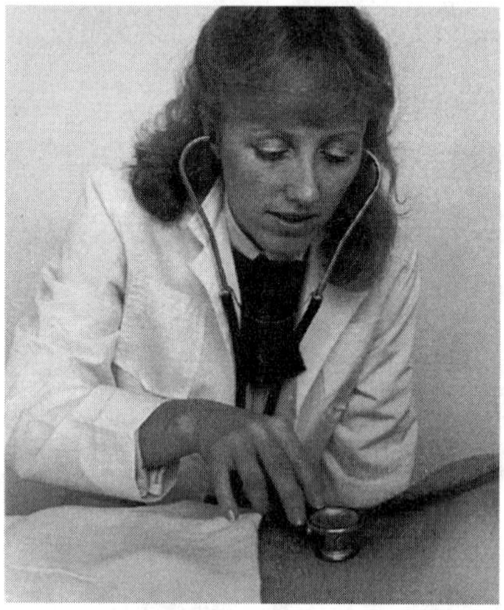

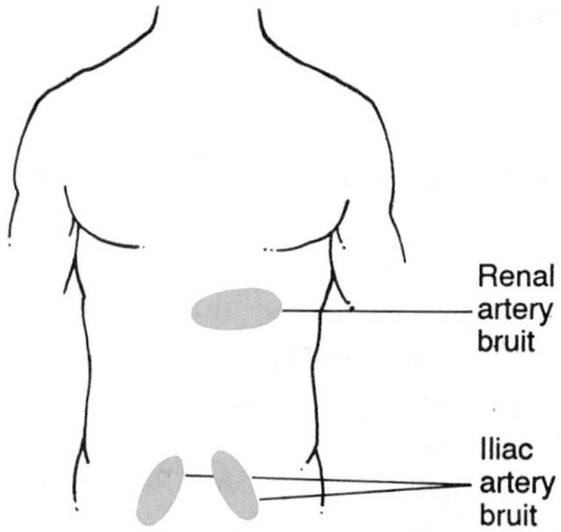

Step 8 • *Auscultate for bruit with stethoscope bell over the epigastrium. Renal artery and iliac artery bruit may be heard over these areas.*

7. If bowel sounds are not heard, listen for 3 to 5 minutes in all quadrants before concluding that they are absent.
Rationale: Bowel sounds are very irregular and require assessment to continue longer to confirm that they are absent and not hypoactive. Absent or hypoactive bowel sounds indicate inhibited intestinal motility.
8. Place stethoscope bell over the epigastrium. Listen for sounds associated with pulse rate.
Rationale: A bruit is created by blood flow through the arteries. It may be normal or associated with irregularities of the arterial system.
9. Proceed with the rest of physical examination or cover the client's abdomen and assist to a comfortable position.
10. Document your findings.

Lifespan Considerations

Newborn and Infant

- Newborns have difficulty maintaining body temperature. Uncover only body area that you are directly assessing.
- At 8 to 12 months of age, infants become fearful of strangers. Spend several minutes becoming acquainted with the child before examining.

Toddler and Preschooler

- Children 2 to 5 years of age are often afraid of examining equipment. Letting them handle the stethoscope and using a "This is a game" approach often helps allay the fear.
- Auscultate bowel sounds before performing any invasive examination, which may cause the child to cry.

Child and Adolescent

- Older children are modest. They may or may not want a parent to be with them during the examination; give the child the choice. Protect modesty through use of gowns or drapes.

Older Adult

- A lengthy physical examination may be exhausting for the older adult and may need to be completed in phases.
- The older adult may become easily chilled. Provide warmth through adequate draping or gowning.

pate all four quadrants, reserving the area of suspected pain or abnormality until last. Relaxation of the abdominal wall is necessary for an accurate assessment. The nurse can promote relaxation by positioning the client with knees slightly flexed and arms to the sides or across the chest. Areas of pain found through light palpation are avoided during deep palpation. With deep palpation, masses of stool may normally be palpable in the abdomen. The liver border may be assessed during palpation, although it is normally not palpable at the midclavicular line in adults. The location and approximate size of any abnormal masses or enlarged organs should be noted.

Percussion. Percussion is used to detect the location of organs not normally palpable, and to give clues about the characteristics of the masses underlying the skin. Generalized tympany is present over the intestines, although varying degrees of tympany will be heard depending on the location of food and stool masses. The liver is percussed at the right midclavicular and midsternal lines, and the sound elicited is dull. The gastric bubble in the left lower rib cage is normally very tympanic. The spleen is found at the left 10th rib posterior to the midaxillary line, and is dull (see Table 21-10).

Skin Assessment. The skin is examined through inspection and palpation. It is assessed for color, moisture, temperature, texture, and hygiene. Normal skin color may be pink, tan, brown, or yellowish. The skin is normally dry; extreme dryness or excessive sweating (diaphoresis) are abnormal. Temperature is normally warm; hot may indicate fever and cool may indicate poor circulation. Texture is usually soft, and rough over the elbows, knees, and heels of the feet. Hygiene is described as well groomed or poor personal hygiene.

The skin should also be observed for past injuries: calluses, stains, scars, needle marks, and insect bites. The location of rashes should be noted. Frequently a diagram is helpful in identifying the location of lesions. The scalp and hair are inspected for color, quantity, distribution, texture, hygiene, nodules, and lesions. Hair color may range from pale blonde to deep black; graying begins normally in the third decade of life. Texture may be straight, curly, or kinky, fine or coarse. The base of the hair follicle should be examined for pest infestation and dandruff. The nails are inspected for shape, color, and texture.

Skin Turgor. The amount of fluid in the tissues is assessed by checking skin turgor. The nurse can check for skin turgor by pinching a small area of skin and noting how quickly it returns to position when released. If skin turgor is poor, the skin remains elevated (tenting) or slowly resumes position. Poor skin turgor may indicate dehydration, but may also occur with normal aging or with weight loss.

Skin Lesions. A skin lesion is an abnormality in the structure of the skin as a result of injury or disease. Every lesion should be described in terms of size, color, type, and location. Lesions may be measured with a metric ruler to ensure accurate size determination. Take note of the appearance of the border of the lesion and surrounding skin. It is also important to palpate the lesion to distinguish between flat and raised. Lightly press the lesion to determine if it blanches with pressure. These steps will assist in labeling the lesion and identifying the cause. A lesion that exhibits asymmetry, irregular borders, uneven color, a raised surface, or a recent change in size may indicate malignancy, and should be referred for evaluation (Flory, 1992). Refer to Chapter 38 for a complete description and graphic representation of different types of lesions.

Wounds. Wounds may be caused by accidents, pressure, or surgeries. It is especially important to note the wound color. Yellow or green coloring may indicate infection. A black, brown, or gray color may indicate necrotic (dead) tissue. Pink is the color of the tissue, and bright pink or red is the color of new granulation tissue. Be sure to note the color, character, and amount of any drainage (exudate) from the wound. Creamy, colored drainage indicates infection. Bright red drainage indicates blood. A watery, clear drainage is serum. Refer to Chapter 38 for a complete description of different characteristics of wounds and exudate.

Assessment of Elimination

Elimination is the excretion of waste products from the body through the gastrointestinal and urinary systems. Elimination assessment focuses on determining the adequacy of bowel and bladder function, observing characteristics of feces or urine, identifying risk factors that may contribute to problems in elimination, assessing the impact of bowel or bladder dysfunction on daily living, and understanding the client's methods of management and coping for any bowel or bladder dysfunction.

Urinary Elimination

Subjective Data

The collection of subjective information should focus on the client's normal urinary pattern and any recent changes in this pattern. Questions the nurse may use to elicit this information from the client include

- Describe your normal voiding pattern.
- Have you had a change in your usual voiding pattern?
- Have you had any discomfort, pain, frequency, incontinence, or difficulty starting the urine stream?

Objective Data

Objective data concerning urinary elimination are obtained through inspection of the urine and the lower abdomen, and light palpation and percussion of the urinary bladder.

Nursing Research
Health Assessments

Selected Nursing Research Studies

Bulette, M., Macaluso, S., & Palumbo, D. (1994). Assessment of same-day-admit patients with a patient-completed assessment form. In R. M. Carroll-Johnson & M. Paquette (Eds.), *Classification of nursing diagnosis: Proceedings of the ninth conference, North American Nursing Diagnosis Association* (pp. 369–370). Philadelphia: J. B. Lippincott.

Lant, K. (1992). Physical assessment by nurses: A study of nurses' use of chest auscultation as an indicator of their assessment practices. *Contemporary Nurse, 1*(2), 93–7.

McNaull, F., et al. (1992). A comparison of educational methods to enhance nursing performance in pain assessment. *Journal of Continuing Nursing Education, 23*(6), 267–271.

Monninger, E., Padgett, D., Fleeger, M. E. (1994). Functional health pattern assessment for BSN students. In R. M. Carroll-Johnson & M. Paquette (Eds.), *Classification of nursing diagnosis: Proceedings of the ninth conference, North American Nursing Diagnosis Association,* (p. 341). Philadelphia: J. B. Lippincott.

Nielsen, L. (1994). An interview study of nurses' assessment and priority of post surgical pain experience. *Intensive and Critical Care Nursing, 10*(2), 107–114.

Possible Topics for Nursing Inquiry

- How often do staff nurses use percussion to determine bladder distention on postoperative clients?
- How does client's perception of nurse interviewer differ when nurse sits rather than stands during the collection of subjective data?
- What role does intuition play in directing advanced practitioner versus beginning practitioner in interviewing technique during admission assessment?
- What is the significance of privacy in obtaining subjective data during a client interview?
- How does the functional health approach compare with the body systems approach to nursing assessment in obtaining accurate information to support nursing diagnoses?
- How effective is clinical simulation in refining physical assessment techniques?

Inspection. Assessment of the bladder for distention due to urinary retention is warranted when a client complains of lower abdominal (or bladder) discomfort or reports a history of difficulty urinating, or when a prolonged time has elapsed since the last voiding occurred.

The bladder is inspected for signs of distention, which appears as a swelling of the lower abdomen, just above the symphysis pubis. Observation of urinary distention may be difficult in the obese person. When the bladder contains less than 500 mL of urine, no bulge is present on inspection.

Inspecting the client's voided urine provides additional data concerning urinary elimination status. Urine is normally pale yellow to colorless, aromatic, clear, and without sediment. Urine that is cloudy or foul-smelling may indicate infection. Urine that is dark yellow may indicate fluid volume deficit. The normal amount is 250 to 400 mL for each void, approximately four to six times per day. For additional information about assessment of urine, refer to Chapter 41.

Palpation. Light palpation can provide additional data when bladder distention is suspected. The nurse palpates from the umbilicus to the symphysis pubis, using the fingertips of both hands. With light palpation, a firm ridge or mass is felt as the bladder is located. Often the client exhibits signs of sensitivity or discomfort when the full bladder is being palpated. Palpation can stimulate voiding.

Percussion. Percussion of the lower abdomen follows inspection to determine the presence of a distended bladder. Percussion begins at the umbilicus and proceeds toward the symphysis pubis. When the bladder is empty or contains only a small amount of urine, a tympanic note is heard when the bladder is percussed; percussion over a full bladder produces a duller sound.

Bowel Elimination

Assessment of bowel elimination completes data collection for the elimination pattern. Collection of subjective and objective data should focus on normal bowel habits, risk factors for bowel dysfunction, and the impact of bowel dysfunction on daily activities.

Subjective Data

Bowel function is considered a private matter, but it is important for the nurse to develop comfort in asking clients questions regarding their bowel status. Interviewing the client can elicit information concerning normal bowel habits and any current or past problems in bowel status, as well as the impact of the elimination on daily living. Sample questions to elicit this information include:

- Tell me your normal bowel pattern.
- What things do you do to stay regular?
- Have you had any changes in your normal bowel pattern?
- Have you had any problems with discomfort or control with bowel movements?

Objective Data

Inspection of the feces, abdominal examination, and rectal examination provide objective data concerning bowel elimination. Abdominal assessment has been previously outlined.

Inspection. In relation to elimination, the abdomen is observed for distention, which can signify decreased peristalsis in the intestines. When distention is present, the abdomen appears larger than usual, and in severe distention, the skin appears stretched and taut. The client may be able to verify that the abdomen appears larger than usual, or that clothes are tighter. Inspection of the perirectal area should reveal smooth, intact skin without stretching or shininess.

Inspection of normal stool reveals soft-formed, light or dark brown, aromatic feces. The frequency of elimination varies widely among individuals; from one to two times daily to once every 2 to 3 days is within the normal range. *Changes* in the normal pattern are more significant than variations between individuals. Stool that is hard may indicate *constipation.* Stool that is watery indicates *diarrhea.* Stool that is foul-smelling may indicate infection. Stool characteristics and tests for the presence of blood are presented in detail in Chapter 42.

Palpation. In addition to the abdominal assessment, palpation is used to evaluate the rectum for abnormalities or the presence of stool. To palpate the rectum, a lubricated, gloved index finger is inserted in the rectum and directed toward the umbilicus (Fig. 21-16). The presence of internal or external hemorrhoids, polyps, or abnormal masses should be documented. Frequently, a rectal examination is performed to detect the presence and consistency of stool in the rectum. Hard, dry stool may indicate the presence of a fecal impaction, which may require manual removal.

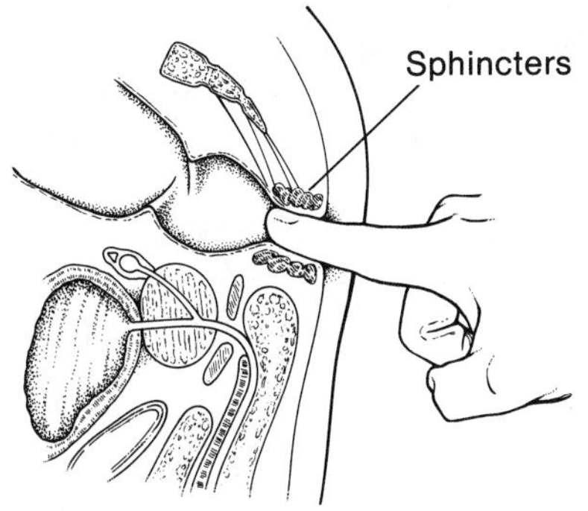

Figure 21-16 • *During a rectal exam, the nurse inserts a gloved, lubricated index finger into the rectum to detect stool or abnormalities.*

Assessment of Sleep and Rest

The assessment of sleep and rest focuses on normal sleep patterns of the client, alterations from the normal pattern, and satisfaction with quality of rest and sleep.

Subjective Data

Information is collected from the client concerning sleep habits, problems with obtaining adequate rest or sleep, and any aids that are used to induce sleep. Suggested questions to elicit this information include

- Tell me when you usually go to sleep. Tell me when you usually wake up. Do you awaken during the night?
- Can you easily fall asleep? What do you do to promote sleep?
- Do you feel rested on awakening?

Objective Data

Most of the data indicating a dysfunctional sleep pattern are subjective, although a few objective signs may support subjective data. Frequent yawning, decreased attention span, and dark circles or puffiness around the eyes may be related to sleep deprivation. Continual dozing during the day may also occur when the amount or quality of sleep is inadequate.

Assessment of Cognition and Perception

Perception involves acquiring information about the environment through the senses (sight, hearing, touch, taste, and smell). Cognition involves intellectual abilities such as memory, reasoning, thinking, and motivation. The goal in assessment of cognition and perception is to identify impairments in sensory function and to evaluate cognitive function, comfort, pain, language, and communication. Deficits in any of these areas may increase the person's susceptibility to injury and interfere with the ability to live independently.

For assessment purposes, cognition and perception are divided into three areas: cognitive function, sensory function, and pain. Each of these areas affects the others, so the interrelationships among data must be considered, as well as specific subjective and objective information.

Cognitive Function

Cognitive function refers to a person's ability to think, which is primarily evaluated through written and verbal communication. Factors that contribute to cognition include awareness, thought processes, memory, language, judgment, and attention span. Whereas significant impairment in cognitive abilities is readily noticeable on first interaction, it often requires repeated assessments over a period of time to detect subtle changes or minor deficits in cognitive ability.

Subjective Data

Subjective data for appraising mental abilities are gathered throughout the health assessment, from the context of a client's conversation and the degree of cooperation given during the physical examination. The nurse assesses whether the client has difficulty understanding or answering questions or following directions. The client's responses to questions are evaluated in terms of clarity and appropriateness. The client should be able to express any health concerns in a coherent, clear manner.

Possible questions to elicit further information concerning a person's cognitive and communication ability include

- Tell me how your memory is. Have you had any recent changes?
- Do you have problems with speaking? reading? writing?
- Describe the last experience you had learning something. How do you believe you learn best?

If deficits in cognition are present, ask

- Tell me your full name. What is today's date? Where are you right now?

Objective Data

Objective data concerning the cognitive abilities of the client are obtained through the neurologic examination.* This examination also obtains information on sensory function. The neurologic examination is a systematic method of assessing the integration of brain function and motor response. Abnormalities often reflect impairment to the brain or spinal cord. If a client is fully alert and oriented, the nurse may perform a full neurologic assessment to obtain a baseline. In many agencies, comprehensive detailed neurologic testing is performed by advanced practitioners. See Procedure 21-5 for a detailed description of how to perform a neurologic assessment.

Level of Consciousness. Consciousness is awareness of and responsiveness to the surrounding environment.

* The neurologic system is responsible for numerous functions such as memory and consciousness, reception of sensory impulses, coordination, and initiating muscle movement. A complete neurologic assessment comprises an integration of assessments of cognitive-sensory and activity-mobility patterns. Deficits in any of these functional areas may increase the client's susceptibility to injury and interfere with the ability to live independently.

Impairment in consciousness is evaluated on a continuum. At the highest level of consciousness, a person responds to environmental stimuli with appropriate verbal and motor activity. The person is attentive, cooperative, and completely oriented to self, time, and place. Impaired consciousness may initially be demonstrated by loss of orientation and inability to follow simple commands. At the lowest level of consciousness, the comatose state, painful stimuli are necessary to induce a verbal or motor response.

The Glasgow Coma Scale (Table 21-11) provides the nurse with a standardized assessment tool, with which subtle changes in consciousness states can be detected quickly. This tool is used when serial assessments are done for high-risk clients (eg, brain tumor, after brain surgery, after a cerebral vascular accident). The nurse is able to detect subtle changes in consciousness state by reviewing the scale and noticing deviations from baseline. In addition, this tool evaluates the best verbal response and the best motor response so that increased intracranial pressure can be detected and treated quickly. The client is scored according to the best response given, and the results are documented appropriately in the client's record.

Orientation. Orientation is evaluated by asking simple, direct questions about time, place, and person. Orientation × 1 indicates person orientation, orientation × × 2 indicates person and place, and orientation × 3 indicates person, place, and time. If the client is not oriented, information provided may not be accurate. Asking family for additional information or to be present during the assessment may help verify data provided by the client (Barker & Moore, 1992).

Mood. Abnormalities of mood may indicate psychological or neurologic problems. Normal mood is described as happy or pleasant. A client who is unusually overjoyous may be described as elated or euphoric. Depression is being overly sad. Clients easily provoked or annoyed are described as irritable. Those with a rapid change of emotions may be described as labile. A client whose affect is clearly out of context with the situation may be described as inappropriate. Flat affect describes the client who expresses few emotions.

Language and Memory. Communication and memory are specific aspects of cognitive functioning that are important to effective client teaching. Speech deficits may take on a variety of appearances. It is important to differentiate between problems in receiving the communication (receptive aphasia) and problems in expressing communication (expressive aphasia). With receptive aphasia, clients are unable to understand simple directions. With expressive aphasia, the client understands and follows directions but is unable verbally to communicate effectively with the nurse. Problems with articulation of words may be caused by mechanical, muscular or sensory problems.

If impaired reading ability is suspected, the nurse should ask the client to read aloud a short passage from the newspaper or a client education pamphlet and paraphrase what was read. Some clients, however, may be unable to read for reasons other than neurologic deficits, such as illiteracy or speaking a different primary language. Writing ability involves a complex series of tasks, and can simply be evaluated by having the client write his or her name.

Short-term memory can be evaluated by asking the client to recall events in the day, such as activities, visitors, or meals eaten. Cues to short-term memory loss include if the client forgets to use the call bell, loses direction easily, or is unable to remember discussion that took place earlier in the conversation. Long-term memory is reflected in the ability to provide historic information about family, health problems, or hospitalizations.

Sensory Function

The purpose of assessing the client's sensory status is to determine functioning of the five senses: vision, hearing, touch, taste, and smell. Assessment should also include the impact sensory deficits have on daily activities and any devices the client uses to cope with sensory impairment.

Sensory losses may be congenital but are often associated with the aging process. Older clients should be assessed carefully for sensory deficits because many adaptive techniques are available to improve the safety,

Table 21-11 • Glasgow Coma Scale

Best Eye-Opening Response		Best Verbal Response		Best Motor Response	
Purposeful and spontaneous	4	Oriented	5	Obeys commands	6
To voice	3	Disoriented	4	Localizes pain	5
To pain	2	Inappropriate words	3	Withdraws to pain	4
No response	1	Incomprehensible sounds	2	Flexion to pain	3
Untestable	U	No response	1	Extension to pain	2
		Untestable	U	No response	1
				Untestable	U

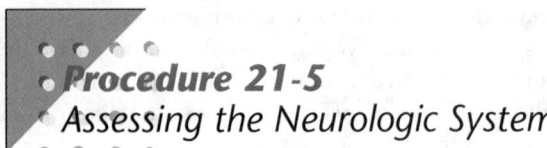

Procedure 21-5
Assessing the Neurologic System

Purpose

1. To obtain baseline information about the client's neurologic status.
2. To assess the client's orientation to his or her environment.
3. To evaluate the client's cognitive function and ability to make judgments.
4. To assess the integrity of motor and sensory pathways and the client's ability to ambulate safely.
5. To detect increased intracranial pressure.

Assessment

- Determine if the client is distracted by an immediate need (eg, pain, urge to urinate). Attend to that need first.
- Explain to the client what you plan to do and approximately how long it will take. A complete neurologic assessment can be very lengthy. The nurse must decide how extensive the assessment should be based on the client's diagnosis, level of consciousness, and physical disabilities. An efficient nurse learns how to integrate components of the neurologic assessment with other parts of the client's functional assessment (ie, cranial nerves assessed during head and neck examination, mental status evaluated during nursing history, and reflexes tested during musculoskeletal assessment).
- Ask significant others if they have noted memory loss or changes in behavior of client.
- Question client about presence of headache, seizures, dizziness, visual changes, or numbness/tingling of any body parts.
- Review medication history for any drugs that may alter level of consciousness or cause behavioral changes (ie, analgesics, sedatives, antidepressants, antipsychotics, or central nervous system stimulants).

Equipment

May need all or part of equipment depending on comprehensiveness of assessment.

Sterile safety pin or toothpick
Sterile cotton applicator
Vials of hot and cold water
Tongue blade
Penlight
Vials of coffee, vanilla, or clove extracts
Vials of salt, sugar, lemon solutions
Snellen chart
Tuning fork
Reflex hammer

Procedure

Cognitive/Sensory Assessment

1. Assess the level of consciousness by asking direct questions that require a verbal response. Note appropriateness of response and emotional state.
   Rationale: Alterations in mental status may be demonstrated by irritability, decreased attention span, inability or unwillingness to cooperate, and an abnormal perception of the environment.
2. Evaluate client's speech patterns.
   Rationale: Normally, speech should be clear, well paced, and coherent. Language should seem appropriate for educational and socioeconomic level.
3. Observe general appearance: hygiene, appropriateness of clothing to setting and weather.
   Rationale: Unkempt appearance or inappropriate clothing for weather conditions may give clues to client's altered mental status.
4. If client responses are inappropriate, ask direct questions related to person, place, and time (eg, "What is your name?" "Where are you right now?" "What city do you live in?" "What day is this?").
   Rationale: Measures client's orientation to immediate environment. As consciousness deteriorates, clients become disoriented to person, place, and time.
   Note: Be sure client's inappropriate response is not caused by a communication or language problem.
5. If client doesn't or inappropriately responds to orientation questions, give simple commands (eg, "squeeze my fingers" or "wiggle your toes"). If there is no response to verbal commands, test response to painful stimuli by applying firm pressure on client's sternum or finger nailbed with your thumb.
   Rationale: Level of consciousness can vary from fully alert and oriented, to unable to follow commands, to unresponsiveness to external stimuli.
   Note: Avoid pinching client's skin to elicit a pain response.
6. Document cognitive or sensory assessment objectively by stating specific client responses to verbal or tactile stimulation.
   Note: Use of Glasgow Coma Scale (see Table 21–11) helps charting of frequent level of consciousness testing. Assessments are more objective and consistent.

7. Assess function of cranial nerves as noted in Table 21–12.
   Note: An increase in intracranial pressure (ICP) puts direct pressure on the optic nerve (C-II). The osculomotor (C-III), trochlear (C-IV), the abducens (C-VI) exit the brain stem at the level of the tentorial notch. When ICP increases and the brain shifts downward, changes in the functions of these nerves are noted.
8. Assess sensory pathways:
   a. Client's eyes are closed during all sensory tests.
      Rationale: Tests are valid only if client doesn't see where stimulus strikes skin.
   b. Apply stimuli to skin in a random, unpredictable order while comparing one side of body to the other.
      Rationale: Sensations should be felt equally on both sides of the body. Random stimuli prevent client from anticipating and correctly guessing where stimulus is.
   c. Client should verbally state when he or she feels a particular stimulus. If an area of altered sensation is detected, note which spinal cord segment is affected by referring to a dermatone chart (Figure 21-20).
      Note: Boundaries of sensory dysfunction can be found by testing responses about every 2.5 cm in a localized area.

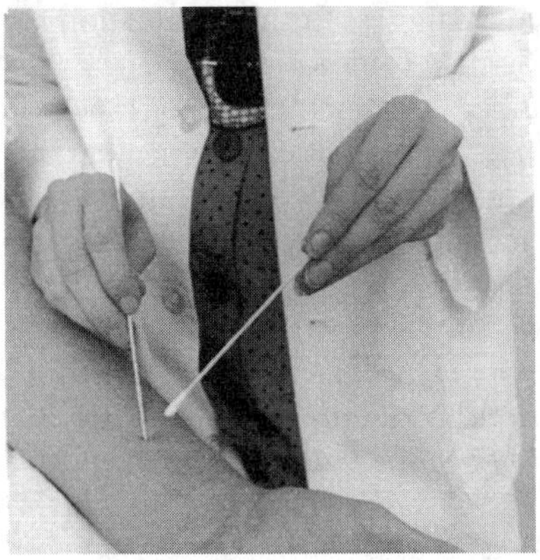

Step 8 • *Assessing light touch with a cotton applicator.*

9. Test pain sensation first by lightly touching pointed then blunt end of sterile pin to proximal and distal aspects of the arm and legs.
   Rationale: Assess intactness of spinothalamic tract. If pain sensation is intact, nurse may omit tests for temperature.

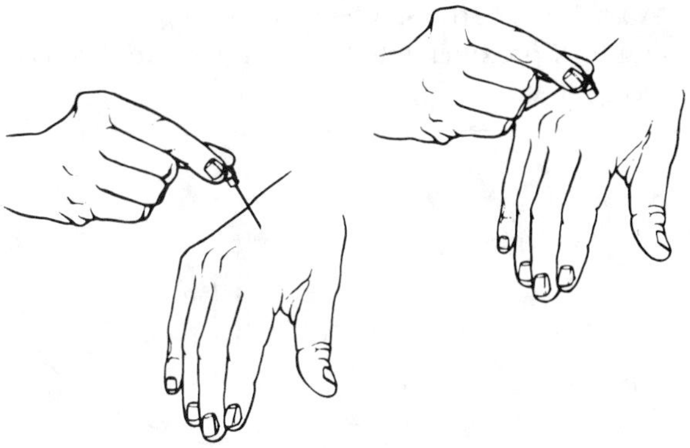

Step 9 • *Assessing pain sensation with a sterile pin.*

10. Test temperature sensation by touching skin with vials of hot, then cold, water.
    Note: Client should identify hot versus cold sensation.

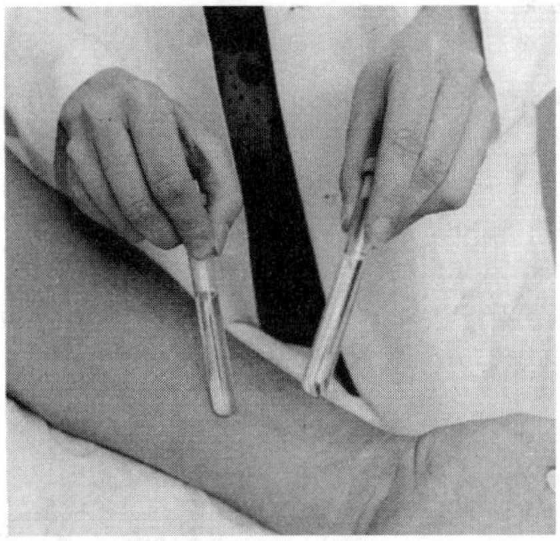

Step 10 • *Assessing temperature sensation.*

11. Lightly stroke proximal and distal aspects of client's arms and legs with a cotton ball. Ask client to tell you when and where each stroke is felt.
    Rationale: Testing the client's perception of light touch and the following tests of vibration and position assess intactness of the posterior column. Loss of any of these sensations may indicate a lesion of the posterior column on the same side as the loss.
12. Apply a vibrating tuning fork to the distal interphalangeal joint of fingers and great toe. Ask client to describe what he or she feels and when it stops.

(continued)

Note: If client doesn't feel vibration, move the tuning fork proximally to the next joint until sensation is felt.

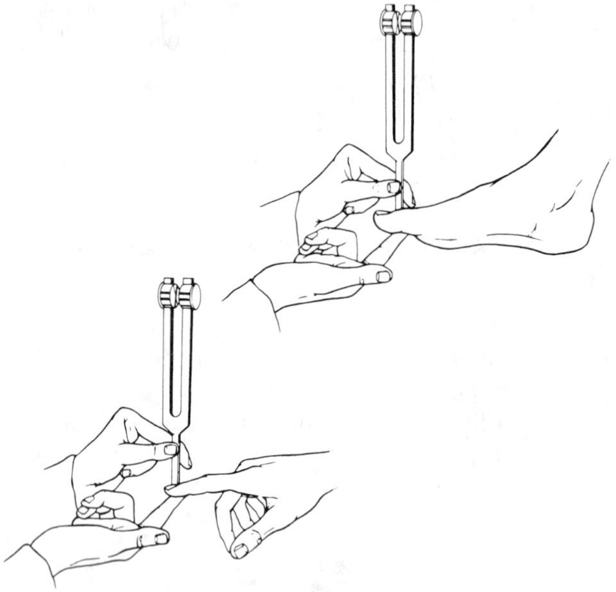

Step 12 • *Assessing vibratory sense with a tuning fork.*

13. Grasp client's finger. Move finger up and down, asking client to identify position. Repeat procedure with toes.
    Rationale: These actions assess kinesthetic sensation or sense of bodily position.

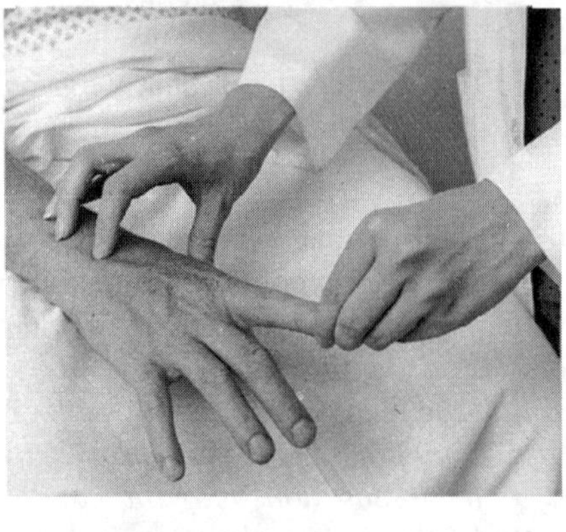

Step 13 • *Assessing sense of body position with client's index finger.*

Activity-Mobility Assessment

14. Inspect arm and leg muscles for atrophy, tremors, fasciculations, or other abnormal movements.
15. Assess strength of specific muscle groups by having client extend or flex individual joints against resistance provided by examiner's hands. Test biceps, triceps, wrist, leg muscles, and ankle. Evaluate for symmetry of same muscle groups.
16. Ask client to close eyes and hold arms in front of body with palms up. Hold position for 30 seconds and observe for pronation of hands or drifting of arms.
    Note: Notice of weaknesses are on one or both sides.
    Rationale: Detects presence of deformities, reduced mobility of joints, or decreased muscle strength. Upper and lower extremities of dominant side are usually stronger than nondominant side.
17. Evaluate coordination and balance by:
    a. Performing a series of rapid alternating movements (RAMS).
        1) Have client pat upper thigh by rapidly alternating his or her palm and the back of the hand.
        2) With dominant hand, have client touch his or her thumb to each finger on that hand as quickly as possible.
        3) Have client use his or her dominant forefinger to first touch your forefinger, then his or her nose. Instruct client to repeat this many times as fast as he or she can.
        Note: Difficulty performing any of these tests may suggest further evaluation for cerebellar disease is indicated.
    b. Romberg test: Ask client to stand with feet together, arms at sides. Have client maintain this position for 30 seconds with eyes open, then 30 seconds with eyes closed. Assess for swaying.
    Note: Stay close to client to assist in case he or she begins to fall.
    Rationale: Clients with cerebellar disease may not maintain balance with eyes open or shut; problems with proprioception cause difficulty only with eyes shut.
    c. Ask client to walk across the room. Observe gait for symmetry, rhythm, limping, shuffling, or other abnormalities.
    Rationale: Changes in gait may be characteristic of specific neurologic diseases.
18. Assess deep tendon reflexes (see Table 21-13).
    a. Compare symmetry of reflex on each side of body.
    b. Extremity to be tested should be completely relaxed and slightly extended.
    c. Reflex hammer should be held loosely and allowed to swing freely in an arc.

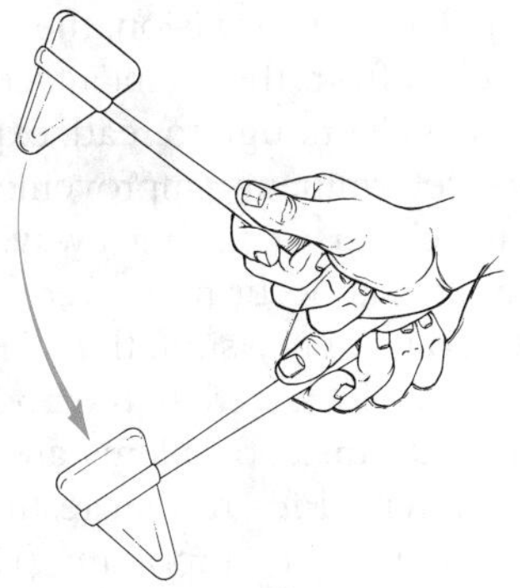

Step 18C • *Swing reflex hammer in an arc.*

d. Tap tendon briskly.
e. Document reflexes by grading 0–4 + on stickman.

Rationale: The quality of a reflex response varies among individuals and by age.

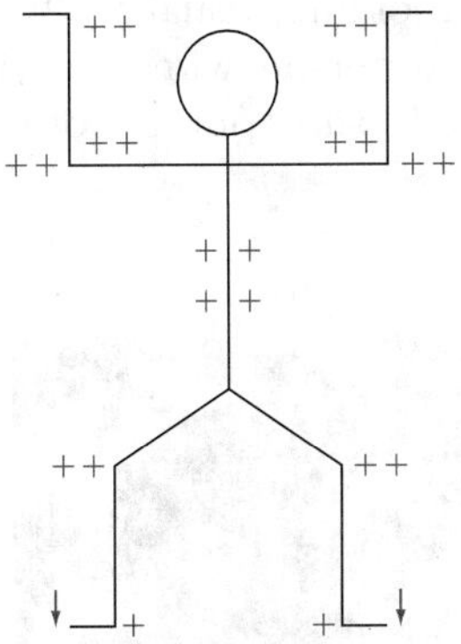

0 —no response
1+—diminished reflex (may be normal)
2+—normal
3+—brisker than normal (may be normal)
4+—hyperactive—upper neuron disorder suspected

Step 18E • *Document reflexes by grading 0–4 + on a stickman.*

Lifespan Considerations

Newborn and Infant

The infant at birth has little or no voluntary control over muscular movements. Much of the infant's motor activity is seen as mass responses to stimuli, and the infant has built-in reflexes as described below:

Rooting reflex
- Infant turns head toward a warm object placed against his or her cheek.
- Function is to help the infant locate the mother's breast when nursing.

Sucking
- Swallowing and gagging reflexes—well developed in healthy infants at birth.

Moro reflex
- In response to loud noise or sudden movement, infant extends arms in tense, quivering embrace and often cries.

Tonic neck reflex
- When relaxed or asleep on back, infant has head turned to one side with arm and leg of that side extended, while extremities of opposite side are flexed.

Toddler and Preschooler

- Children are often fearful of strangers and examining equipment. Spend several minutes becoming acquainted with the child. Allowing them to handle the equipment before examining and using a "This is a game" approach often helps allay the fear. There are several screening tools available such as the Denver Development Test, which is designed to evaluate cognitive and psychomotor skills of infants and children of varying ages.

Older Adult

- A lengthy examination may be exhausting for the older adult and may need to be completed in phases.
- Arthritic changes in joints may limit range of motion and physical mobility, and should be considered in evaluating assessment data.
- Some reflex responses may become less intense as a person ages. The Achilles reflex and the plantar reflex may be difficult to elicit.
- Short-term memory may be decreased in the older adult. Long-term memory is usually unaltered.
- Being in an unfamiliar place or situation can be stressful and promotes confusion.

pleasure, and independence of their lives. Physical examination of the senses usually is not performed in a basic health assessment, unless evidence of impaired function is uncovered during the client interview. Physical examination of the senses routinely is part of health screening examinations.

Subjective Data

Clients are usually aware of sensory loss and can verbalize specific deficits to the nurse when questioned. During the interview, the nurse should observe the client for signs of sensory impairment, such as asking questions to be repeated, watching lips closely during speech, squinting to improve vision, or holding reading material at arm's length. Questions concerning sensory status include

- How is your vision? Do you have glasses, contact lenses, or a prosthesis?
- How is your hearing? Do you use a hearing aid?
- Do you notice that it is difficult to feel in your hands or feet?
- Do you have any numbness or tingling in your hands or feet?
- Have you noticed any changes in your taste or smell?

Objective Data

Objective data that provide valuable information about sensory function include use of sensory aids, tests for visual acuity, tests for auditory acuity, cranial nerve assessment, and sensory assessment.

Sensory Aids. The use of glasses, contact lenses, hearing aids, and other assistive devices should be documented in the client's health assessment. The proper care of such devices should also be solicited and written in the client's record. This helps ensure proper use and care of expensive devices during the client's stay in a healthcare agency.

Visual Acuity. To test near vision, the nurse can hold newsprint 14 inches from the client's face. If the client is unable to focus well enough to read, experiment with the distance to determine if improvement occurs by moving the print closer or farther away. Visual problems with close objects occur more frequently after the age of 40 years. To test far vision, the client is asked to read the time on a clock across the room, or a sign across the hall or room. If problems are detected, the client should be referred for further testing.

Visual screening is an important part of routine health examinations. The Snellen "E" is used for assessing distant visual acuity.

The client is positioned 20 feet from the Snellen chart (Fig. 21-17*A*), which has been placed at eye level. Each eye is tested separately, and both eyes together. As one eye is covered, the client is directed to read the smallest line that can be seen. Young children who do not yet know the letters of the alphabet may be tested with another chart that has pictures. The client's distance from the chart (20 feet) is compared to the number by the line that the client can read. For example, if the client can read the 100-foot line, visual acuity would be reported as 20/100. Any person with less than 20/20 acuity should be referred to an ophthalmologist or optometrist for evaluation.

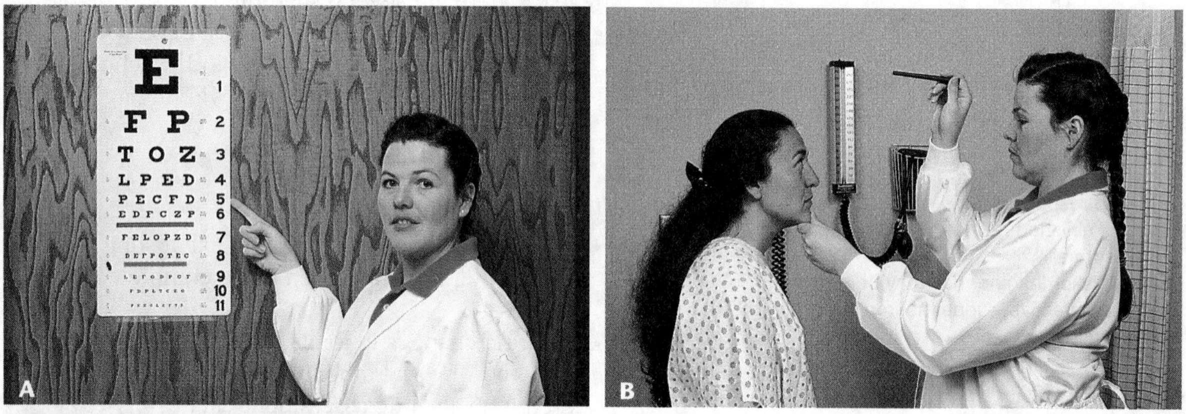

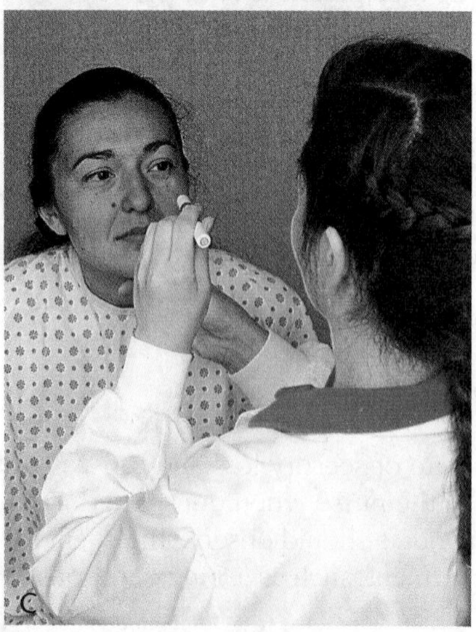

*Figure 21-17 • Eye and visual examination. (**A**) Test for visual acuity using the Snellen eye chart. (**B**) Extraocular eye movements (cranial nerves III, IV, and VI) are assessed by asking the client to hold her head still and follow a pen as it moves through the cardinal eye positions. (**C**) To test the pupil reflex, the nurse shines a penlight from the side into the pupil, observing the rate and amount of pupil constriction. The pupils should constrict briskly, both being equal in size after constriction.*

Extraocular Movement and Visual Fields. The oculomotor, trochlear, and abducens nerves control the horizontal, vertical, and diagonal movement of the eyes. Assessment of peripheral visual fields and six ocular movements is important in a comprehensive visual assessment. To evaluate extraocular movements, the nurse has the client follow an object (such as a pencil) through different positions (horizontal, vertical, and diagonal; see Fig. 21-17*B*). The head remains still as the eyes move to follow the object. At each position the nurse pauses to evaluate the presence of nystagmus (involuntary, rhythmic oscillations of the eyes) and evaluates whether the eyes can follow smoothly.

Peripheral vision can be tested in a similar manner. The nurse can have the client look straight ahead with one eye covered as a finger or object is brought within the field of vision. This can be repeated for each eye from different fields (temporal, upward, downward, and nasal).

Pupils and Pupillary Reflexes. As a beam of light is directed through the pupil and onto the retina, stimulation of the third cranial nerve causes the muscles of the iris to constrict. The nurse evaluates pupils bilaterally for size, shape, accommodation, and reaction to light. Normally pupils are black, round, and constrict briskly when exposed to a bright light source. To test pupils, the nurse first dims the light in the room. As the client gazes straight ahead, a penlight is shined into the pupil from the side of the head (see Fig. 21-17*C*) The nurse observes both pupils. The directly illuminated pupil should constrict briskly and the other pupil constrict consensually. Accommodation can be tested by having the client look at a close object (eg, a finger held approximately 4 inches from the nose) and then look at a distant object (eg, a picture on the wall). As the client is doing this, the nurse observes the client's pupils to see if they constrict to focus on the close object and dilate to see the distant object. Normal pupil assessment data are recorded as PERRLA, or pupils equal, round, reactive to light, and accommodation.

Pupils can appear cloudy when cataracts are present. Dilated pupils can occur when glaucoma is treated with drops or neurological impairment is present. Unilateral changes in pupil reflexes can signify increased intracranial pressure caused by tumor, trauma, or cerebral vascular accident. Changes in pupillary response should be reported to the physician.

External and Internal Eye Structures. External eye structures should be free of lesions or inflammation. A blink reflex should be present. An **ophthalmoscope** is the instrument used to assess internal structures of the eye. Such examinations are usually performed by advanced practitioners with additional training and practice. Ophthalmic examination permits visualization of the retina, optic nerve disc, macula, fovea centralis, and retinal vessels. As the fundus is observed through the ophthalmoscope, a round red glow (the red reflex) is noted (Fig. 21-18). Normal findings include uniform red reflex; round, white, or pink optic nerve disc; reddish retina; and bright red arterioles and dark red veins (Barkauskas, et al., 1994).

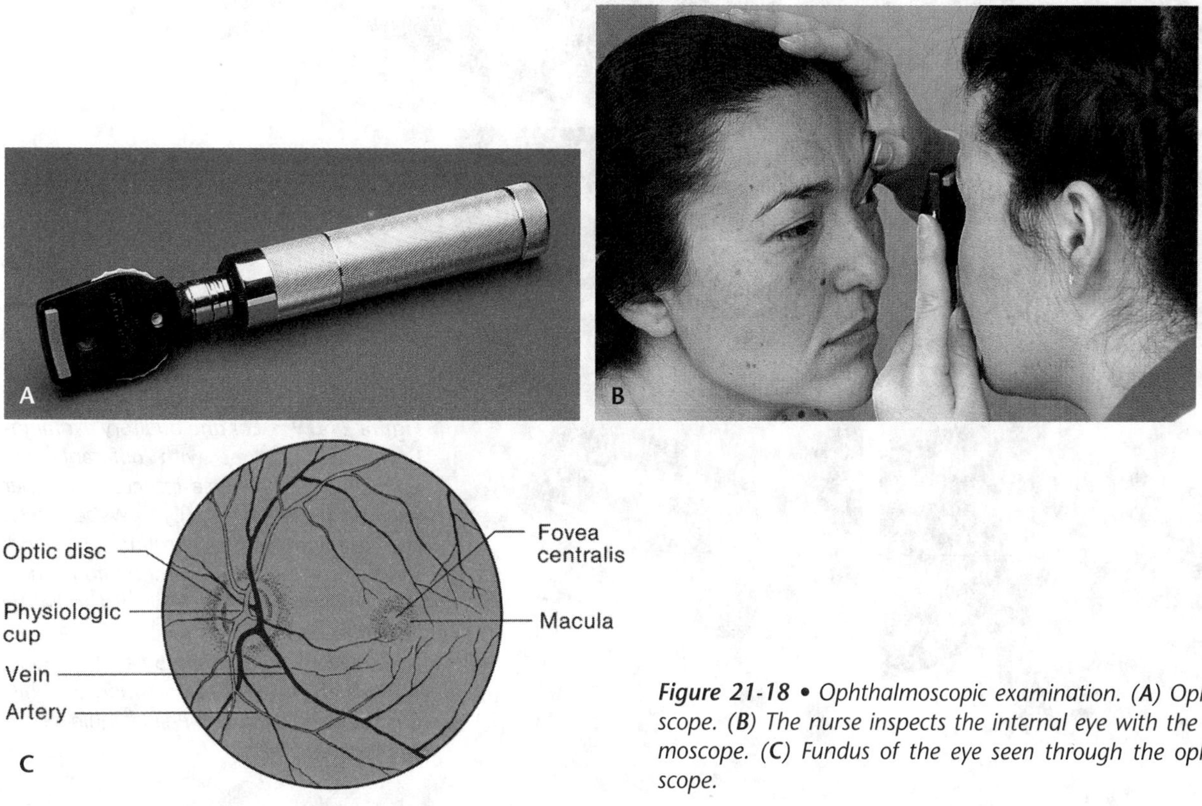

Figure 21-18 • *Ophthalmoscopic examination. (**A**) Ophthalmoscope. (**B**) The nurse inspects the internal eye with the ophthalmoscope. (**C**) Fundus of the eye seen through the ophthalmoscope.*

Auditory Assessment. Assessment of auditory function can occur simply during normal conversation. During the interview, the nurse should lower his or her voice to assess the client's ability to hear. Hearing loss is suggested in a client who turns a particular ear or leans toward the speaker, hears only when able to see the speaker's face (evidence of lip-reading), or speaks in a loud or distorted voice. People with hearing loss may avoid social settings because conversation is especially difficult in groups with background noise. Other physical symptoms associated with the ear are tinnitus (ringing in the ears) and vertigo (dizziness).

If hearing loss is suspected, the external ear canal should be inspected for inflammation or cerumen (ear wax). Using an otoscope (the instrument for examining the ear) the canal is visualized after the pinna has been pulled up, out, and back to straighten the ear canal (Fig. 21-19). A bulging, red, tight tympanic membrane is indicative of otitis media. A build-up of cerumen can also be detected with an otoscope. Because cerumen can temporarily impede normal hearing, it should be removed. If the ear canal appears open and noninflamed, the client may need to be referred for further testing.

Health screening, during annual physical examinations or routinely in the schools, may include hearing tests. The client wears headphones that are capable of transmitting sounds of different frequencies. The client indicates when a sound is heard by raising his or her hand. Such tests may also be administered to high-risk clients who are receiving medications (such as aminoglycoside antibiotics) that can cause hearing impairment.

The Weber's test and the Rinne test, in which a tuning fork is used, can be performed to evaluate hearing loss further. The Weber's test is used to evaluate lateralization of sound (see Fig. 21-19C). The tuning fork is activated and placed at the top of the client's head. Normally, vibrations can be heard equally in both ears, but in conduction deafness, the vibrations may be heard best in the affected ear, whereas in sensorineural loss, the sound lateralizes to the unaffected ear.

The Rinne test discriminates between bone conduction and air conduction of sound (see Fig. 21-19D). The tuning fork is struck, and its stem is placed in front of the ear and then firmly against the mastoid process. Normally, the person should hear the sound of the tun-

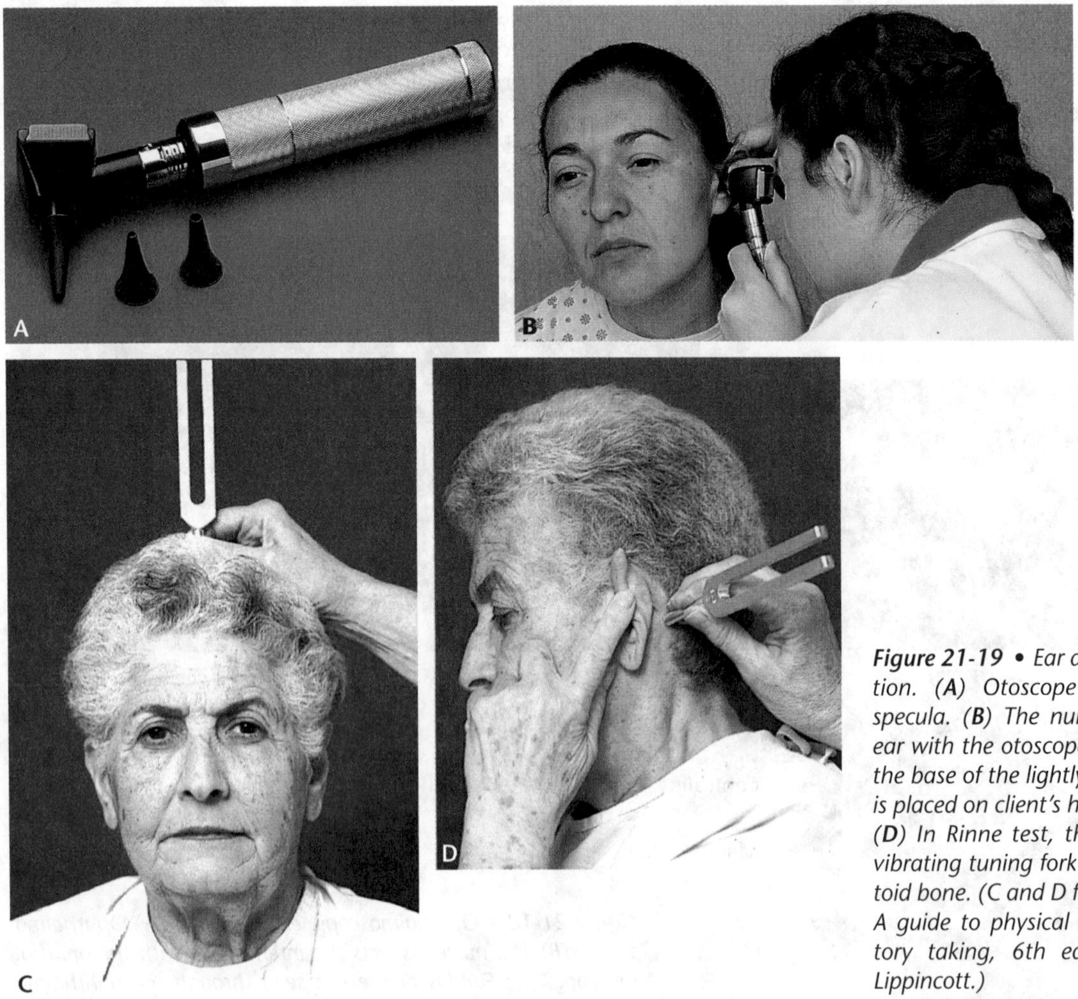

Figure 21-19 • *Ear and auditory examination. (**A**) Otoscope with different-sized specula. (**B**) The nurse inspects the inner ear with the otoscope. (**C**) In Weber's test, the base of the lightly vibrating tuning fork is placed on client's head (or midforehead). (**D**) In Rinne test, the base of the lightly vibrating tuning fork is placed on the mastoid bone. (C and D from: Bates, B. [1995]. A guide to physical examination and history taking, 6th ed. Philadelphia, J. B. Lippincott.)*

ing fork when it is placed in front of the ear, indicating air conduction of sound is greater than bone conduction. When the sound is not detected until the tuning fork is placed on the mastoid process, bone conduction of sound is greater than air conduction because of a conductive hearing loss.

Sensation Assessment. Loss of tactile sensation may occur with a variety of conditions such as diabetes, peripheral vascular disease, spinal cord injury and brain trauma, tumor, or vascular lesion. Clients with decreased tactile sensations are at risk for injury from heat or cold, prolonged pressure, or shearing force. Sensory function is also evaluated in clients recovering from surgery with spinal anesthesia, receiving epidural pain medication, or with spinal cord injuries. Function is evaluated in dermatomes around and below the suspected problem. **Dermatomes** are sensory fibers from a single spinal nerve that serve a particular skin surface (Fig. 21-20). Sensory perception is evaluated by observing the client's response to light touch, vibration, and pain. With the client's eyes closed, various areas of the body can be touched with a wisp of cotton to assess light touch, a tuning fork to test vibration, and a toothpick to test pain. Water of different temperatures can be used to assess temperature discrimination. Documentation should include the inability to sense stimuli and the affected location of the body. Any abnormal sensations such as paresthesias, numbness, or tingling also should be reported.

Cranial Nerve Assessment. Intact cranial nerve function is important for normal sensory functioning. Vision depends on normal functioning of cranial nerves II, III, IV, and VI. Cranial nerve VIII is important for hearing, and cranial nerve I is important for the sense of smell. Other cranial nerves are important in the coordination of facial movement or reflex activity. During an initial

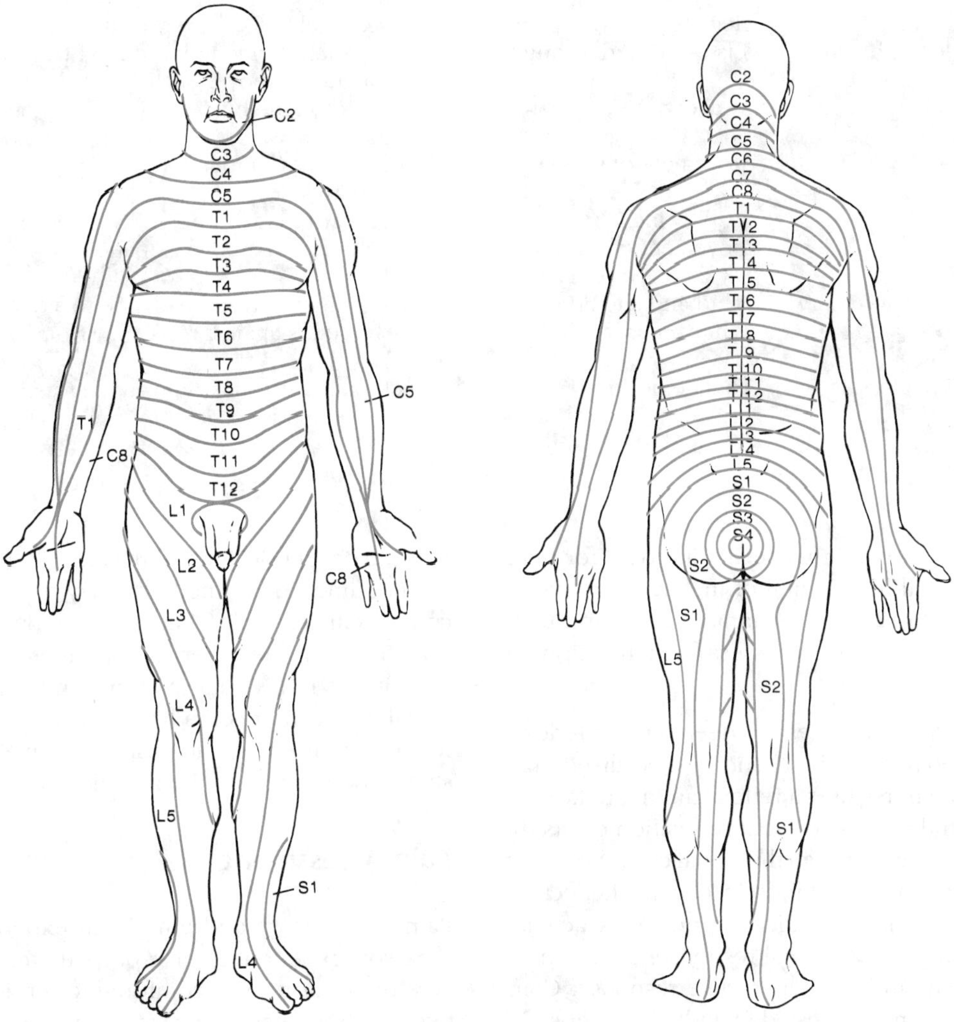

Figure 21-20 • *Dermatones are sensory fibers from a single spinal nerve that serve a particular skin surface. They are used to evaluate sensory function for high-risk individuals, eg, following epidural analgesia, spinal anesthesia, or spinal cord injury.*

Table 21-12 • Cranial Nerve Function and Assessment

Number	Name	Function	Method of Assessment
I	Olfactory	Sense of smell	Ask patient to identify different mild aromas, such as vanilla, coffee, chocolate, cloves.
II	Optic	Vision	Ask patient to read Snellen chart.
III	Oculomotor	Pupillary reflex	Assess pupil reaction to penlight.
		Extraocular eye movement	Assess directions of gaze by holding your finger 18 inches from patient's face. Ask patient to follow your finger up and down and side to side.
IV	Trochlear	Lateral and downward movement of eyeball	Assess directions of gaze. Test with cranial nerve II.
V	Trigeminal	Sensation to cornea, skin of face, nasal mucosa	Lightly touch cotton swab to lateral sclera of eye to elicit blink.
			Measure sensation of touch and pain on face using cotton wisp and pin.
VI	Abducens	Lateral movement of eyeball	Assess directions of gaze. Test with cranial nerve III.
VII	Facial	Facial expression	Ask patient to smile, frown, raise eyebrows.
		Taste—anterior two-thirds of tongue	Ask patient to identify different tastes on tip and sides of tongue: sugar (sweet), salt, lemon juice (sour).
VIII	Auditory	Hearing	Assess ability to hear spoken word.
IX	Glossopharyngeal	Taste—posterior tongue	Ask patient to identify different tastes on back of tongue as above.
		Swallowing	Place a tongue blade on posterior tongue while patient says "ah" to elicit a gag response.
		Movement of tongue	Ask patient to move tongue up and down, and side to side.
X	Vagus	Swallowing Movement of vocal cords Sensation of pharynx	Assess with cranial nerve IX by observing palate and pharynx move as patient says "ah."
XI	Spinal accessory	Head and shoulder movement	Ask patient to turn head side to side and shrug shoulders against resistance from examiner's hands.
XII	Hypoglossal	Tongue position	Ask patient to stick out tongue to midline, then move it side to side.

neurologic assessment, or at specific intervals for high-risk clients, normal functioning of the cranial nerves is checked. Table 21-12 lists the cranial nerves and techniques the nurse can use to assess their functioning.

Deep Tendon Reflexes. Testing deep tendon reflexes may be indicated in high-risk clients in specialized practice settings. The nurse uses a reflex hammer to tap various tendons in the body to see if this action elicits the appropriate reflex arc through the spinal cord. Normally, a brisk contraction of the muscle occurs. Reflect response can be graded, 0 indicating no reflex activity; +1 minimal activity; +2 normal response; +3 more active than normal; and +4 hyperactive response. Common reflexes that may be tested include the biceps, the triceps, the patellar, and the Achilles. These are illustrated and the procedure is explained in Table 21-13. Three significant variations from the normal reflex pattern can occur (McHugh & McHugh, 1990). First, reflexes on the same side of the body may be different. Second, cortical damage may affect reflexes on one side of the body and not the other. Finally, there can be a difference in the reflex pattern above and below the waist if spinal cord compression has occurred. As a person ages, reflex response may diminish. Abnormal reflex patterns should be brought to the attention of the physician.

Pain Assessment

Pain is a sensory and emotional experience in which a person experiences or reports the experience of severe discomfort or uncomfortable sensations. Pain has two components: a sensory component, which is neurophysiologic, and a perceptual component, which is cognitive and emotional. Theories of pain are discussed in depth in Chapter 44. Acute illness, chronic disabil-

Table 21-13 • Assessment of Deep Tendon Reflexes

Reflex	Procedure		Normal Response
Biceps	Flex patient's arm at the elbow with his or her forearm resting on the thigh, palm up. Place your thumb on the base of the biceps tendon in the antecubital fossa. Strike your thumb with the reflex hammer.	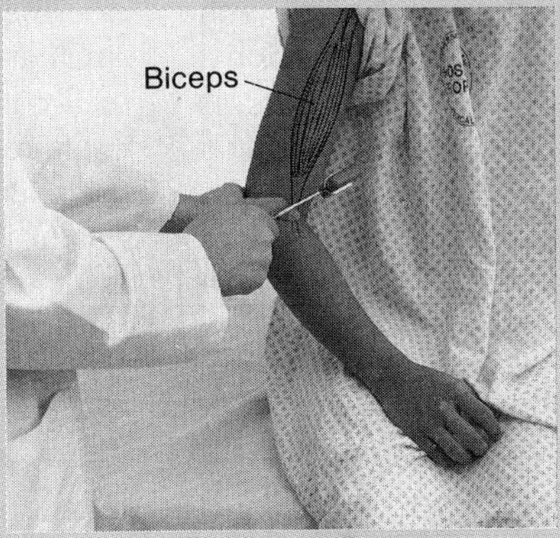	Flexion of forearm at the elbow
Triceps	Hold patient's arm across his or her chest, flexing the elbow at a 90-degree angle. Support wrist as patient allows forearm to become limp. Strike the tendon just above the olecranon process.	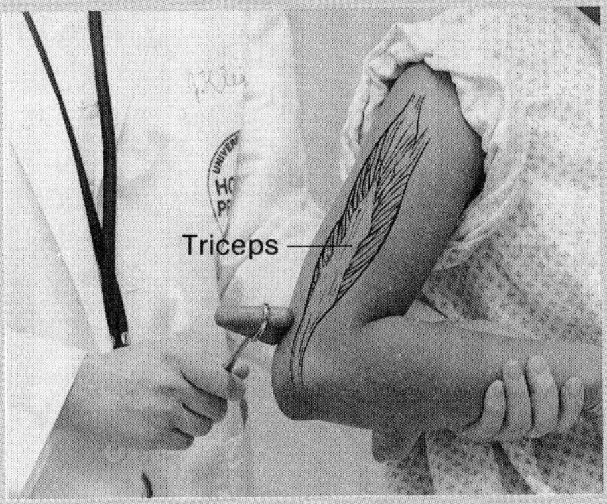	Extension at the elbow
Patellar	Patient sits upright with legs hanging loosely over side of bed. If patient remains supine, support back of knee while leg is flexed at a 45-degree angle. Strike patellar tendon just below patella.	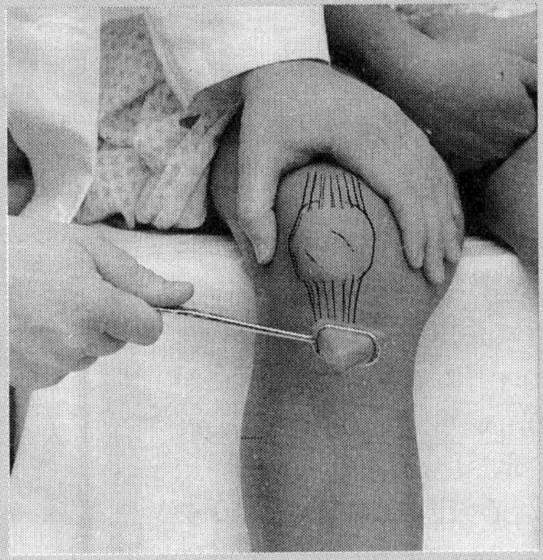	Extension of lower leg at the knee
Achilles	Patient's knee should be slightly flexed while foot is dorsiflexed. Strike Achilles tendon 1 inch above heel.	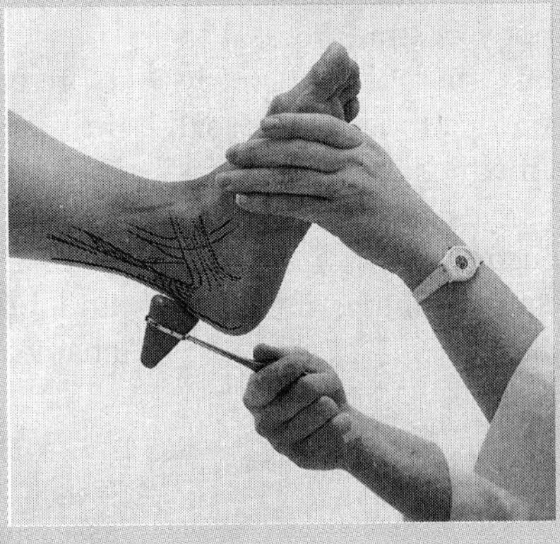	Plantar flexion

ity, surgical intervention, and treatment modalities can all cause the client pain. Pain can limit normal function and affect wellness in all health patterns. Accurate assessment of pain is necessary to identify and treat the underlying cause of pain. Assessment permits the nurse to better understand the client's pain experience.

Subjective Data

The pain experience is personal and subjective; thus, the client interview is the best way to collect information to assess pain. Pain assessment should include asking the client to describe the location, intensity, quality, onset, and chronology of his or her pain experience. Factors that influence the pain experience and methods of effective pain management should also be determined. Last, the impact the pain experience has on daily life and other health patterns should be explored. Some clients are reluctant to discuss and describe their pain experience because of personal beliefs or values.

Questions helpful in soliciting subjective information concerning the client's pain experience include

- Do you have any pain or discomfort? How long have you had it?
- If yes, tell me how bad it is on a 1 to 10 scale, with 10 being the worst.
- Show me where it is. Does it move or radiate anywhere?
- Describe what it feels like.
- When does it come on? How long does it last?
- What makes it better? What makes it worse?

Objective Data

Objective data are not always available to document the experience of pain. Acute pain stimulates the sympathetic nervous system and produces the following objective symptoms: increased blood pressure, increased pulse, increased respiratory rate, dilated pupils, and diaphoresis. This sympathetic response is not present in chronic pain states. Observing the client's body position and facial features also gives clues to the presence of pain. Grimacing, guarded positioning, tense body posture, refusal to move a body part, muscle spasms, or rubbing a body part can all indicate the presence of pain despite verbal denial. A "facial mask of pain," in which the client's facial expression is flat or fixed, the eyes appear dull, and fatigue is evident, commonly occurs in chronic pain. Emotional expression such as crying, moaning, or yelling also can occur during severe pain.

Assessment of Self-Perception and Self-Concept

The self-perception and self-concept pattern focuses on the content and feelings associated with a person's self-evaluation. The components of self-concept include one's self-knowledge, self-expectation, social self, and self-evaluation. Self-concept is influenced by the way others evaluate and interact with a person throughout the lifespan. Body image, the mental picture and feelings about one's body, is an important component of self-concept. Individual beliefs concerning locus of control are also important to explore. Some people believe that life events are self-determined (internal locus of control), whereas others view individual happenings as a matter of fate, luck, or the influence of others (external locus of control).

During a basic health assessment, the goal in assessing the self-perception is to describe the client's general view of self and his or her satisfaction with that image. Clients whose primary health problem directly relates to a disturbance in self-concept, such as psychiatric, chemically dependent, abused, or anorectic clients, require an extensive evaluation by a mental health specialist. However, many illnesses alter one's self-concept because of changes related to physical strength, appearance, and loss of control. For this reason, consideration of self-concept should be integrated into the health assessment of every client.

Subjective and supporting objective data should be collected concerning normal self-concept, recent changes in self-concept, and the presence of conditions (eg, burns, skin disorders, colostomy, mastectomy, or obesity) that could threaten or alter body image.

Subjective Data

Possible questions that help the client describe self-perception include

- What are you most concerned about in relation to your health?
- How would you describe yourself?
- How has being sick made you feel differently about yourself?

Objective Data

Nonverbal cues to a person's self-concept are reflected in eye contact, personal grooming and appearance, posture, body movements, mood, emotions, voice and speech pattern. Low self-concept may be reflected in poor eye contact, inattention to personal grooming, and body language that conveys embarrassment or shame.

Written Assessment Tools. Some paper-and-pencil tests have been developed to assist with self-concept assessment. Rosenberg's Self-Esteem Scale (Rosenberg, 1979), the Piers-Harris Self-Concept Scale (Piers & Harris, 1969), and the Locus of Control Scales (Wallston, et al., 1978) are examples.

Assessment of Roles and Relationships

Most people fill a variety of roles: husband or wife, parent, worker, student, colleague, friend, coach, and advisor. These roles may be rewarding and stimulating, or they may be overwhelming and stressful.

The goal in a basic health assessment is to identify the client's major roles in the family, at work, and in social life, and to identify the client's relative satisfaction or dissatisfaction with each role. The assessment should also indicate how health problems or hospitalization may interfere with a person's ability to fulfill role expectations and maintain relationships. Whereas this information normally is obtained from the client, it is often helpful (and sometimes necessary) to consult other members of the family unit to obtain meaningful data.

Information obtained in the assessment should focus on the client's family configuration and occupation, recent or anticipated changes in the roles or relationships of the client, and the client's level of satisfaction with current roles and relationships.

Subjective Data

Within the family unit, important information includes who shares the household, what responsibilities or dependencies each member has, and the presence of specific problems, such as issues related to parenting, caring for elderly parents, or marital discord. The illness of a family member may necessitate shifting responsibilities within the family, such as financial support, child care, cooking, and home maintenance. Chronic illnesses often involve the client in long and sometimes permanent dependence on others. It is important to evaluate the specific circumstances of that dependence, the client's attitude, and the client's coping ability.

Roles and relationships related to work are an important area to assess. Factors such as job-related stress, insufficient time for leisure activities, unsafe work environment, job insecurity, inadequate pay, or lack of recognition may negatively affect physical and psychological well-being.

A change in relationships may contribute to the cause or exacerbation of an illness. The nurse should explore areas in which recent change has occurred, such as divorce, death, or illness of a family member, loss of a job, change in job status or pay, increase in job responsibility, or transition from student to worker.

Suggested questions to help obtain this information from the client include

- Are you employed? retired? disabled?
- What do you see as your primary role at work? home?
- Who do you live with?
- Who do you ask for help when you need it?

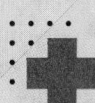

> **Safety Alert**
> *Health Assessment*
>
> - Always hold an infant on an examining table and restrain during invasive assessment procedures to avoid injury on sudden movement.
> - Never palpate the abdomen of a client complaining of sudden, severe abdominal pain because this could rupture an inflamed appendix, causing peritonitis.
> - When listening to breath sounds, give the client rest periods to avoid hyperventilation because this could cause dizziness and syncope.
> - Never palpate both carotid arteries at the same time because blood flow to the brain can be occluded.
> - Don't leave confused or unstable clients alone on an examining table because they may try to get down and fall.

- Are there any problems at work or home that influence your health?
- Do you have any insurance or financial concerns that you would desire help with?

Objective Data

Objective data are obtained by watching the interactions of the client with family members and others. Verbal interactions and nonverbal communication can support what the client has discussed in the interview. Observing visitors, cards, and flowers can help to validate that the client has positive relationships with others. Likewise, the absence of visitors and communication from others might suggest the lack of positive relationships.

Repeated unexplained injuries, such as bruises, burns, and fractures, should be noted with suspicion of possible abusive relationships. Frequently, people involved in abusive relationships verbally deny that abuse has occurred.

Assessment of Coping and Stress Tolerance

Stress is an event that disrupts or challenges a person's equilibrium. Although stress is most readily conceptualized as negative, positive life changes also challenge a person and therefore create stress. Examples of positive stressors include marriage, planned pregnancy, job promotion, and a long-awaited vacation. Serious illness, hospitalization, and surgery are universally perceived as stressful events.

Whether something is a stressor depends largely on a person's perception of the event. Each person's response to stress is unique. The way in which a person reacts, and, it is hoped, adapts to stress is called a coping behavior. Coping behaviors may be adaptive, producing relief from stress and even growth, or they may be maladaptive, leading to further disintegration and disorganization.

In assessing coping and stress tolerance, the goal is to identify and acknowledge current stressors the client is experiencing, determine how the client has handled stressful events in the past, and identify current methods the client is using to cope.

Subjective Data

Subjective data concerning coping and stress tolerance can be obtained through the interview, which can consist of open-ended or specific questions. Another technique is to ask the client to describe a stressful event that has occurred in the past and his or her response to it. Such a description can help the nurse to identify past stressors as well as how the client managed the situation. The manner in which past life crises were handled is often a good predictor of how present or future situations will be managed. Suggested questions for interviewing the client regarding coping and stress tolerance include

- Have there been any changes or stress recently in your life? What are they?
- How do you usually handle stress?
- Is there anything that the nurses can do to help you deal with the stress of being sick?

Objective Data

The nurse can collect objective data from the client by observing for symptoms indicating sympathetic stimulation or by having the client fill out a stress assessment tool, which objectifies the current stress level. Such tools include the Social Readjustment Rating Scale by Holmes and Rahe (1967) and the newer Everyday Hassles Scale by Lazarus (1981) and Stress Audit by Miller and colleagues (1991).

Sympathetic Stimulation. Stress activates the sympathetic nervous system, which produces certain physiologic effects. Sympathetic stimulation may increase the force and rate of the heart beat, increase respiratory rate and depth, decrease blood flow to the skin, resulting in pallor and diaphoresis, and increase blood flow to the muscles. These symptoms may be pronounced in the event of a sudden stressful event. When a person is exposed to chronic stress, the symptoms may be less sudden and less dramatic. The sympathetic response to stress is detailed further in Chapter 51.

Assessment of Sexuality and Reproduction

Sexuality is the behavioral expression of sexual identity. It may involve, but is not limited to, sexual relationships with a partner. Sexual expression is a complex integration of physiologic, psychological, and social aspects of human nature. Physical illness and its treatment may influence sexual function. For example, impotence is frequently associated with diabetes mellitus, alcoholism, chronic renal disease, and several drug therapies. Clients may question their own desirability after such surgeries as mastectomy, radical neck dissection, ostomy, and hysterectomy. Diseases that reduce tolerance, such as heart or lung disease, may limit physical endurance.

Although it is increasingly more acceptable in society to discuss sexual matters, many clients and nurses are hesitant in addressing this subject during a health interview. Sexuality is, however, such an integral aspect of human nature that to ignore it would be neglecting a vital component of health. The subject of sexuality should be introduced in the context of a comprehensive health assessment. Including sexuality in the initial client contact conveys to the client that sexual health is an appropriate, legitimate concern. The sexual assessment is not meant to illuminate nonexistent problems. Rather, the client is, in effect, given permission and encouragement to present sexually related questions.

The areas for assessment of sexuality and reproduction include reproductive functioning, sexual role and satisfaction with that role, and potential for alteration in sexual role or function. The impact of the client's current health status on sexual role and functioning should also be discussed.

Subjective Data

The best approach to obtaining a sexual history is to introduce subjects of least sensitivity first. The nurse should begin by focusing on chronologic events such as puberty, menstruation, menopause, and reproductive history. The nurse can invite the client to elaborate on any problems or expectations in these areas. The nurse can also determine the client's knowledge and compliance with preventive health practices such as breast self-examination, regular Papanicolaou smear, and testicular and prostate examination.

A sexual assessment is appropriate at every age and should be adapted to correlate with the client's developmental level. Many adolescents are concerned with changes in their bodies and early sexual experience. The nurse can use this opportunity to educate, support, and guide the adolescent in matters involving sexuality. Married people may have concerns about their own sexuality, as well as concerns related to parenting and sex education for their children. Many elderly clients enjoy sexual relations throughout their lives and may desire acknowledgment and discussion of their concerns.

Selected questions to elicit information concerning the sexual-reproductive pattern include (individualize for each client):

- What method of contraception do you use? Is this method acceptable to you and your partner?
- Have you ever been diagnosed as having a sexually transmitted disease (gonorrhea, genital herpes, chlamydia, or AIDS)?
- Many (men, women) in your situation have questions about how their illness or surgery will affect the sexual aspects of their lives. What questions do you have?
- Has your illness interfered with your being a (mother, wife, husband, father)?
- Has anything changed your ability to function sexually?
- Adolescents: Many (boys, girls) at your age have questions about dating, becoming intimate, contracting a disease, or getting pregnant. What questions do you have?
- Women: At what age did you begin menstruating? How long is your typical menstrual cycle? What was the date of your last menstrual cycle? Do you have any problems related to menstruation? How many times have you been pregnant? How many children do you have? Do you examine your breasts? How often?
- Men: Do you examine your testicles? How often? Do you have any concerns about sexual function?

Objective Data

Objective data concerning sexual-reproductive function can be obtained through examination of the breasts and the reproductive organs. Examination of these "private" areas is not usually performed unless the client has problems in that area, or as part of a preventive health examination. Breast examination is important in early detection of breast cancer. Breast examination should be conducted as a joint activity of the client and the nurse, with the nurse's primary role as educator. Although breast cancer is rare in men, a brief examination of the male breast is also appropriate. Examination of the testicles in men is important for early detection of testicular cancer. As with women, the examination should be undertaken as a joint activity, with the nurse as educator.

Examination of female internal reproductive organs is not commonly part of the basic health assessment unless the nurse is working in a specialized area such as a gynecology clinic or labor and delivery. Frequently the nurse is present with the client during a pelvic examination. The following can assist relaxation and comfort (Barkauskas, et al., 1994):

- Assist the client to assume the lithotomy position and drape to maintain privacy and warmth
- Warm the speculum
- Have a mobile or pictures on the ceiling to focus attention
- Encourage rhythmic breathing, breathing deeply and slowly through the mouth
- Concentrate on relaxing body muscles with each exhalation
- Remind client not to hold her breath

Inspection. The client should be taught to do a breast self-examination while the examiner is performing the breast examination (Fig. 21-21). Teaching related to self-examination of breasts is outlined in Chapter 52. Normal breasts appear rounded and essentially symmetric, although one breast is often slightly larger than the other. The skin should be smooth and intact with the areola darker in color, round, and symmetric. The nipple should be everted and without discharge or lesions. Abnormal findings with inspection include flattening, bulges or changes in breast size, marked asymmetry, redness, dimpling, and edema.

Inspection of the female external reproductive organs includes the labia minora, labia majora, clitoris, and vaginal opening. The color of these organs should be pink, with some blue or brown pigments occasionally seen. Bright red color or obvious areas of excoriation are abnormal and often occur in the presence of infection. Normal vaginal secretions, which are white, colorless, and odorless, may be noted. Foul-smelling, purulent drainage is abnormal.

Inspection of the external male reproductive organs includes the glans, foreskin and shaft of the penis, and the scrotum. The man may be circumcised or uncircumcised. If uncircumcised, the foreskin must be gently retracted during the examination to inspect the glans and the urethral opening. The foreskin is replaced to the previous position after the inspection. Inspection of the penis should reveal no lesions or abnormal discharge. Smegma is a normal white discharge that may collect around the glans, especially in the uncircum-

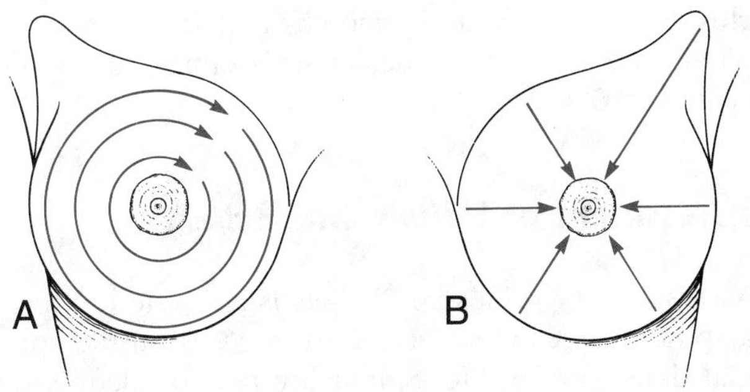

Figure 21-21 • *Breast examination. Begin at the outer edge and gradually work toward the nipple. (**A**) Clockwise approach. (**B**) Spoke approach.*

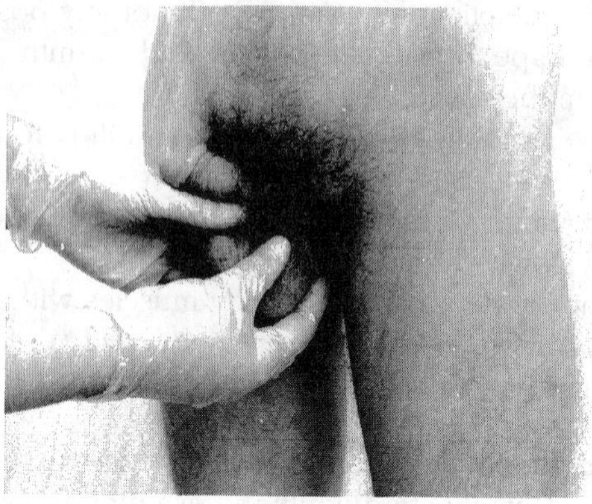

Figure 21-22 • Palpate the testicle by grasping the scrotum gently and rolling the testicle between the thumb and forefinger.

cised man. The scrotal sac is wrinkled in appearance, with the left scrotal sac usually hanging lower than the right.

Palpation. Palpation is used in examining the reproductive structures to determine possible underlying abnormalities in the breast or scrotum. The breast should be palpated with the client in the supine position with hands behind the head. Palpate each breast for tenderness, nodules, or masses. The nurse should use three or four fingers, pressing the flat part of the fingers in small circles, moving the circles slowly around the breast. A sequential pattern of palpation should be followed so that all areas in the breast are included. Begin at the outer edge of the breast, gradually working toward the nipple. The area between the breast and the axilla also should be examined. The final step in breast examination is gentle squeezing of the nipple to check for discharge. Again, during the palpation the examiner teaches the woman how to perform breast self-palpation.

Palpation of the male genitalia is performed to detect the presence of the testicle in each scrotal sac and the absence of pain, swelling, or growths. One scrotal compartment is palpated at a time by grasping the scrotum gently between the thumb and forefinger. The testicle is rolled gently to palpate (Fig. 21-22). The testicles should feel round, smooth, and freely movable within the scrotum. Testicular self-examination is discussed in Chapter 52.

Assessment of Values and Beliefs

Assessment of values and beliefs is also referred to as a spiritual assessment because it focuses on the spiritual dimension of life. Spirituality may be defined as the quality that transcends the physical world, permeates and unifies a person's entire being, and gives life purpose, meaning, and importance. Spirituality usually, but not always, involves a belief and relationship with a higher being. Values and beliefs emerge from a person's sense of spirituality and guide the opinions about what is right, good, proper, and meaningful. Values help determine choices about the conduct of one's life, including health-related decisions concerning personal practices, treatments, and even life or death. The spiritual realm is one aspect of being human that often comes into focus during illness or crisis.

Illness, injury, loss, aging, and disability are spiritual as well as physical and emotional experiences. Serious or life-threatening illness often triggers a person's first encounter with mortality. Crisis often provides the motivation to question one's life, goals, and what is important.

Because body, mind, and spirit are intertwined, distress in any one area affects the health of the whole person. Spiritual distress can adversely affect a person's response to illness and treatment, and the ability to cope effectively with the crisis. Conversely, spiritual contentment can have an equally positive influence. Prayer and other religious practices are stabilizing forces in many people's lives. A nurse who understands a client's spiritual beliefs is better prepared to support coping strategies and provide the resources that are spiritually helpful to the client.

Assessment of values and beliefs focuses on the significance of religious affiliation and religious practices; the spiritual needs of the client and the resources available to meet those needs; and the relationship between spiritual beliefs and the current state of health.

Subjective Data

By this time, the nurse has become established as a sensitive, helpful professional and has a sense of the client's willingness to share personal information. Mention of spiritual beliefs may arise during the discussion of coping-stress tolerance pattern. If this occurs, the nurse can smoothly direct the conversation toward the values-beliefs pattern.The following interview questions may be used to discuss the values-beliefs pattern:

- Are there any religious or spiritual practices that are significant to you?
- Have any of these practices or beliefs been affected by this illness?
- Is there a religious person or practice that you would like during this illness?

Objective Data

Assessment of the values-beliefs pattern depends primarily on subjective data. However, visible expression of spiritual values is sometimes present. The nurse may notice religious articles such as a Bible, Buddha, Koran, or rosary in the room of a hospitalized client. The nurse may also observe the client in prayer, either alone or with family, friends, or clergy.

Concluding the Assessment

The nurse should bring formal closure to his or her interaction with the client when the assessment is completed. The nurse summarizes the findings and evaluates the client's primary problems and concerns. The client may want to add to or correct the nurse's conclusions. Sharing this information validates the nurse's impressions and clarifies any misunderstandings between the nurse and the client. The nurse may want to validate what the most important problem is at this time. The nurse should explain, particularly to the hospitalized client, that assessment of his or her condition and needs is ongoing. The nurse should encourage the client to volunteer additional or new information as changes occur. Assessment findings should be documented in the client's chart by the nurse in a legible, concise fashion according to agency protocol.

Lifespan Considerations

Developmental age and other age-related factors are important in planning, focusing, and performing a functional health assessment. The nurse should be knowledgeable about common problems of each age group, so that appropriate screening measures that permit early detection can be included. It is also important to be aware of the cognitive development of the person so that questions can be phrased appropriately. Under-

Therapeutic Dialogue
Health Assessment

Scenes for Thought

You are the nurse practitioner in an HMO's pediatrics clinic. Your client, Georgie Stevens, is 5 years old. He was brought in by his mother because he has a fever of 2 days' duration. He says he is feeling "bad."

Effective

Nurse: *Hi, Georgie, remember me from last time?*
Georgie: *Yeah, you're Theresa. Can I play with the hearing tube again?*
Nurse: *Sure you can. You can warm it up before I use it to listen to your breathing. I'm going to talk to your mom now.*
Georgie: *Okay. (Plays with stethoscope contentedly.)*
Nurse: *How long has he had this fever?*
Mother: *Two days. And sniffles and coughing all night long and wheezing. I'm worried it might be pneumonia.* She looks tired.
Nurse: *I can see it's been a long 2 days for both of you. I'm going to examine him and then see what I can recommend so he and you can get some rest. Georgie, here's what my plan is. (Tells child how she'll proceed with the exam and then explains each step of the way. Georgie is cooperative and "assists" Theresa by holding the tongue depressor, warming the stethoscope, and so forth.)*
Nurse: *Okay, Georgie, you've been a great help to me today. You have a cold, my friend, and here's what you need to do. (Proceeds to tell Georgie and his mother about the importance of fluid intake, getting rest, using cough medicine appropriately, and the like. Includes Georgie in decisions about what kind of fluids he likes and the flavor of the cough syrup they should buy, as well as agreeing to wash his hands before he eats or drinks anything and after going to the bathroom.)*
Georgie: *I'll do everything you say, Theresa, because I want to get better and go back to school.*
Nurse: *Georgie, you're a smart person and I know you'll get better soon. Call me if you have any questions, Ms. Stevens.*

Less Effective

Nurse: *Hi, Ms. Stevens, how's Georgie doing? I see he's had a fever lately. (Looking at the chart.)*
Mother: *Yes, and coughing all night and sniffles and wheezing.* She looks weary.
Nurse: *Let's see what we can find out here. (Examines Georgie while talking to his mother. Keeps all equipment out of his reach. Doesn't explain what she's doing.)*
Mother: *Is it pneumonia?* Looks worried. Georgie looks worried, too, when he sees his mother's face.
Nurse: *No, it's just a bad cold. I'll give you some prescriptions for over-the-counter medications you can buy at the pharmacy, and then give him lots of fluids and get him to wash his hands before he eats and after going to the bathroom so the rest of the family doesn't catch it, too. Okay, Georgie?*
Georgie: He stopped paying attention when you said it wasn't pneumonia. He's playing with the paper on the examining table, making little decorative rips in it. He looks up guiltily. *Uh-huh. Can we go home now, Mommy?*
Nurse: *Bye, Mrs. Stevens. See you next time, Georgie.*

Critical Thinking Challenge

- *List the subjective data each nurse had at her disposal.*
- *Based on her behavior toward him, detect what Theresa knew about Georgie that the second nurse did not know.*
- *Explain the benefit in including Georgie in decisions.*
- *Judge if Theresa could treat all her 5-year-old clients this way, and give your reasons.*

standing the emotional development of the client helps the nurse plan the examination to be less traumatic and anxiety provoking. The accompanying Therapeutic Dialogue gives examples of nursing care during assessment and planning.

Newborn and Infant

Nursing assessment is made shortly after birth and at 24 hours of age. If parents are present during the assessment, the nurse should explain what the examination includes and why it is being performed. Whenever possible, parents should be reassured about findings that are normal. Permitting parents to see their newborn and participate can help parent bonding and allay fears.

During the first year of life, the infant is frequently examined by a nurse for well-baby examinations. This is a wonderful opportunity to educate the parents on a variety of infant care topics. It is important to assure parents of the wide range of normal growth and development and to allow time to discuss any concerns they may have about their child.

Keeping the newborn and infant properly covered during the physical examination is important to prevent a drop in body temperature. During the first year of life, head and chest circumference are measured, the infant is weighed, and reflexes are tested. Inspection and auscultation are finished before doing any invasive procedure. Such techniques can frighten the infant or cause pain, which may cause the infant to cry. The nurse should encourage the parent to hold the infant during the examination to decrease fear and help the child feel more secure. The infant should never be left on an examining table without being properly guarded. Infants can move quickly and fall. The infant must be properly restrained when the nurse is looking into his or her ears, eyes, nose, or throat, so that quick movements do not result in injury.

Toddler and Preschooler

The young child is often afraid to be examined and may associate physical examination with the discomfort of invasive procedures or getting injections. Encouraging the parent to assist by holding and comforting the child during the examination can be helpful. The nurse should explain in simple terms what he or she plans to do. Demonstrating how equipment works can help alleviate some anxiety in toddlers and preschoolers (Fig. 21-23). Allowing the child to touch the stethoscope or see the shining light of the otoscope can help prepare the child for examination procedures. For some children, it may be helpful to use a puppet (see Fig. 21-23) or allow them to role play examining a doll or stuffed animal. It is important to be honest with children. If the child is going to experience pain, it is best to say, "This will hurt for a while, but I'll try and make it quick."

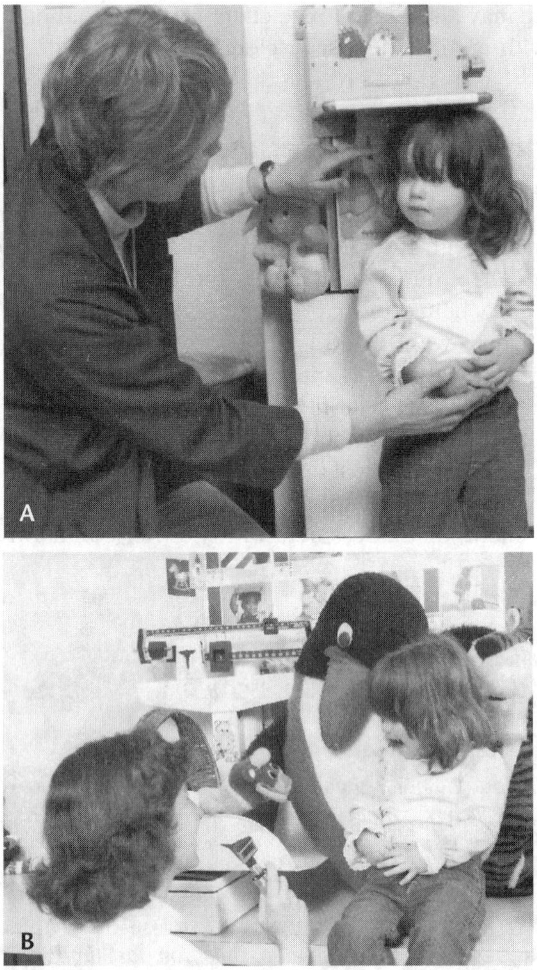

Figure 21-23 • *Physical assessment of the toddler. **(A)** Even the simple activity of weighing or measuring a child should be explained first in terms the child can understand. The nurse holds a protective hand in front of the child in case the child should move suddenly. **(B)** The nurse uses a hand puppet to explain procedure to the young child.*

Plan uncomfortable procedures toward the end of the examination. Then, the nurse should perform uncomfortable procedures immediately after the explanation so that anxiety does not escalate.

Child and Adolescent

As the child ages, more of the assessment questions can be directed specifically to the child. The nurse should use vocabulary that the child can understand when asking questions or explaining procedures. The nurse should encourage the child to ask questions. Whenever possible, the child should be given simple choices. The child can be distracted during the examination through conversation or playing simple games. Some children are ticklish, especially when the abdomen is examined. Children at this age can be modest, so proper draping and measures to ensure privacy are important.

Adolescence is a period of rapid physical and emotional development. During this time period, the youth is often examined alone, unaccompanied by a parent. Sensitive questioning and honestly answering any questions the teen asks help develop good rapport. Because sexual maturation occurs during this period of time, the examination includes examination of sexual organs and appropriate health teaching. Be aware of the sensitivity of adolescents about their body during this time. The nurse should discuss any concerns the adolescent has about the maturation process.

Adult and Older Adult

By the time the person has reached adulthood, multiple exposures to physical examination and assessment have occurred. Some adults still are apprehensive and feel invasion of privacy during assessment procedures. It is important to prepare the client for all procedures and provide for privacy. Health teaching regarding desirable screening measures, such as breast self-examination, testicular self-examination, and routine gynecologic examinations, should be included in the health examination for the adult.

During later years of adulthood, a person may have chronic health problems that necessitate adaptation of the physical assessment. Arthritic joints or decreased mobility may make getting onto an examination table more difficult. Holding various positions required for examination, especially for long periods of time, may be tiring. Lengthy examinations may be fatiguing and should be planned when the client is well rested, if possible. Hearing loss may necessitate speaking more loudly and clearly to facilitate communication. The elderly person can easily become chilled, so proper draping in a warm examination room is important for client comfort.

Key Concepts

- A functional health assessment is the collection of subjective and objective data concerning functional ability.
- Adequate psychological and physical preparation of the client is important for effective assessment.
- The nurse uses interviewing techniques to obtain subjective (client perception) data concerning each functional health pattern.
- Objective data are collected through the techniques of inspection, palpation, percussion, and auscultation during the physical examination.
- The focus of a functional health assessment by the nurse is to determine normal and abnormal aspects of function, the client's degree of satisfaction with function, the client's adaptation to dysfunction, and the effect of function on performing activities of daily living.
- Assessment of health perception and health management should focus on the client's perception of health status, preventive health practices, compliance with medical treatment, and safety.
- Assessment of activity and exercise should focus on mobility, self-care, energy level, activity tolerance, oxygenation, and circulation.
- Data are collected concerning musculoskeletal function in the areas of gait and balance, muscle strength, joint mobility, independence in self-care activities, and any assistive devices that are used.
- Respiratory and cardiac function are evaluated through inspection, palpation, percussion, and auscultation using normal landmarks of the thorax and pericardium.
- Assessment of nutrition and metabolism should focus on food and fluid intake in relationship to metabolic demands, skin integrity, and wound healing.
- Assessment of elimination should focus on normal excretory function (bowel and bladder) and specific management to assist normal function.
- Assessment of cognition and perception should focus on cognitive functions such as memory, language, reasoning, problem-solving, pain level, and sensory–perceptual capabilities such as vision and hearing.
- Assessment of sleep and rest involves eliciting the client's perception of sleep, rest, and relaxation.
- Assessment of self-perception and self-concept focuses on the client's perception of self, such as body image and sense of worth.
- Assessment of roles and relationships describes the quality of a person's family, work, and social roles.
- Assessment of coping and stress tolerance describes current stressors the client is experiencing, past coping methods, and the effectiveness of current coping methods.
- Assessment of sexuality and reproduction describes reproductive function, sexual role, and the impact of current health status on sexual role function.
- Assessment of values and beliefs includes the significance of religious affiliation and religious practices, resources available to meet the spiritual health needs of the client, and the relationship between spiritual beliefs and the current state of health.
- Lifespan considerations are important in individualizing assessment techniques to obtain important information from the client.

Critical Thinking Challenges

You have now added the concepts and skills of a functional health assessment to your knowledge base of nursing assessment. To understand better the details of these examinations, turn back to the situation at the beginning of the chapter and consider the following:

1. *Construct a list of which data presented in the situation were primary data and which were secondary data. Determine which data were subjective and which were objective.*
2. *Develop the order in which you would collect your assessment information about the client.*
3. *Using either a functional or a systems framework, cluster the data into meaningful groups.*
4. *Using this framework, select which groups of data are priority data and which data are irrelevant at this time.*
5. *Identify gaps in the priority data. List what further data you should gather. Summarize the procedures that you would use to obtain these data.*
6. *Determine if you are able to make a nursing diagnosis at this time. If yes, identify the diagnosis. If not, explain why.*

References

Barkauskas, V., Stoltenberg-Allen, K., Baumann, L., & Darling-Fisher, C. (1994). *Health and physical assessment.* St. Louis: Mosby.

Barker, E., & Moore, K. (1992). Cranial nerve assessment. *RN, 55* (5), 62–69.

Bates, B. A. (1995). *Guide to physical examination and history taking* (6th ed.). Philadelphia: J. B. Lippincott.

Boorse-Fabius, D. (1994). Solving the mystery of heart murmurs. *Nursing94, 24* (7), 39–44.

Boorse-Fabius, D., & Stunkard, J. (1994). Uncovering the secrets of snaps, rubs, and clicks. *Nursing94, 24* (7), 45–50.

Carpenito, L. J. (1993). *Nursing diagnosis: Application to clinical practice* (5th ed.). Philadelphia: J. B. Lippincott.

Flory, C. (1992). Skin assessment. *RN, 55* (6), 22–27.

Finesilver, C. (1992). Respiratory assessment. *RN, 55* (2), 22–29.

Fitzgerald, M. A. (1991) Perfecting the art: The physical exam. *RN, 54* (11), 34–39.

Fuller, J., & Schaller-Ayers, J. (1994). *Health assessment: A nursing approach* (2nd ed.) Philadelphia: J. B. Lippincott.

Gehring, P. (1992). Vascular assessment. *RN, 55* (1), 40–48.

Gordon, M. (1994). *Nursing diagnosis: Process and application* (3rd ed.). St. Louis: Mosby.

Holmgren, C. (1992). Abdominal assessment. *RN, 55* (3), 28–33.

Holmes, T. H., & Rahe, R. H. (1967). The social readjustment rating scale. *J Psychosom Res, 11,* 213–218.

Lazarus, R. (1981). Little hassles can be hazardous to your health. *Psychology Today, 15* (7), 58–62.

McHugh, J., & McHugh W. (1990). How to assess deep tendon reflexes. *Nursing90, 20* (8), 62–64.

Miller, L., Smith, A., & Mehler, B. (1991). *The stress audit.* Brookline, MA: Biobehavioral Associates.

Piers, E. V., & Harris, D. B. (1969). *Piers-Harris children's self-concept scale.* Nashville: Counselor Recording and Tests.

Wallston, B. S., Wallston, K. A., & DeVellis, R. (1978). Development and validation of the health locus of control (HCL) scales. *Health Education Monograph, 6,* 160–170.

Yacone-Morton, L. A. (1991). Cardiac assessment. *RN, 54* (12), 28–35.

Bibliography

Benner, P. (1993). The phenomenology of knowing the patient. *Image, 25* (4), 273–280.

Beyea, S., & Matzo, M. (1989). Assessing elders using the functional health pattern assessment model. *Nurse Educator, 14* (5), 32–37.

Brigdon, P., & Todd, M. (1990). In search of the perfect assessment. *Professional Nurse, 5* (4), 181–184.

Calloway, C. K. (1990). Zeroing in on chest pain. *Nursing90, 20* (4), 44, 45.

Derdiarian, A. K. (1990). Effects of using systematic assessment instruments on client and nurse satisfaction with nursing care. *Oncology Nursing Forum, 17* (1), 95–101.

Flannery, J., & Korcheck, S. (1993). Use of the levels of cognitive functioning assessment scale (LOCFAS) by acute care nurses. *Applied Nursing Research, 6* (4), 167–169.

Jarvis, C. (1992) *Physical examination and health assessment.* Philadelphia: W. B. Saunders.

Kaufman, J. (1990). Nurse's guide to assessing the twelve cranial nerves. *Nursing90, 20* (6), 56–58

Lant, K. (1992). Physical assessment by nurses: A study of nurses' use of chest auscultation as an indicator of their assessment practices. *Contemporary Nurse, 1* (2), 93–97.

McConnell, E. A. (1990). Assessing abdominal pain in a post-operative client. *Nursing90, 20* (3), 86–88.

McNaull, F., et al. (1992). A comparison of educational methods to enhance nursing performance in pain assessment. *Journal of Continuing Nursing Education, 23* (6), 267–271.

Neilsen, L. (1994). An interview study of nurse's assessment and priority of post surgical pain experience. *Intensive and Critical Care Nursing, 10* (2), 107–114.

Reed, J., & Watson, D. (1994). The impact of medical model on nursing practice and assessment. *Int J Nurs Stud, 31* (1), 57–66.

Vital Sign Assessment

Key Terms	Learning Objectives

Key Terms

Apnea
Auscultatory gap
Blood pressure
Bradycardia
Bradypnea
Core temperature
Dyspnea
Hypertension
Korotkoff sounds
Orthostatic hypotension
Pulse deficit
Tachycardia
Tachypnea

Learning Objectives

Upon completion of this chapter, the student will be able to do the following:

- *Describe the procedures used to assess temperature, pulse, respirations, and blood pressure.*
- *Describe factors that can influence temperature, pulse, respirations, and blood pressure.*
- *Identify equipment routinely used to assess vital signs.*
- *Identify rationales for using different routes for temperature assessment.*
- *Identify the location of commonly assessed pulse sites.*
- *Define and describe how to assess orthostatic hypotension.*
- *Recognize normal vital sign values among various age groups.*

22

A middle-aged couple are shopping in a mall. A health fair is set up in the mall, and you are participating as a nurse at a booth where blood pressures are checked. After much coaxing, the woman persuades her husband to have his blood pressure taken. You obtain a reading of 168/94. The wife reacts strongly, saying, "I told you that your lack of exercise and overeating would catch up with you one day. How am I going to manage being a widow at such an early age?" The husband responds by saying, "Don't worry about me. I'm just as healthy as ever, and I plan to live until I am 99 years old. I'm sure there is something wrong with that machine." Both of them turn to you. The wife says, "Tell him it's not the machine and that he isn't taking care of himself!"

In previous chapters you learned about assessment, functional health concerns across the lifespan, and therapeutic communication. This chapter expands your knowledge base about specific assessment findings called vital signs. The previous situation gives you an opportunity to apply your knowledge about the importance of vital signs at specific age levels. Therapeutic communication allows you to share that information in a helpful manner. The Critical Thinking Challenges at the end of the chapter help you apply your knowledge base to the care of the couple at the health fair.

Vital signs—body temperature (T), pulse (P), respirations (R), and blood pressure (BP)—indicate the function of some of the body's homeostatic mechanisms. The blood pressure reading of the man in the previous situation is more than a number; it can reflect many things about his health status. One important component of assessment involves measuring and interpreting the vital signs. Client teaching concerning vital signs is part of nursing intervention.

Typical or normal values for vital signs have been established for clients of various ages (Table 22-1). During initial measurement of a client's vital signs, the values are compared with the normal ranges to determine

Table 22-1 • Normal Vital Sign Ranges Across the Lifespan

	Pulse	Respirations	Temperature (°F)	Blood Pressure (mm Hg) Systolic	Diastolic
Newborn (> 96 h)	70–190	30–60	96–99.5	60–90	20–60
Infant (> 1 mo)	80–160	30–60	99.4–99.7	74–100	50–70
Toddler	80–130	24–40	99–99.7	80–112	50–80
Preschooler	80–120	22–34	98.6–99	82–110	50–78
School-age	75–110	18–30	98–98.6	84–120	54–80
Adolescent	60–90	12–20	97–99	94–140	62–88
Adult	60–100	12–20	97–99	90–140	60–90
Older adult (> 70 y)	60–100	12–20	96–99	90–140	60–90

any variation that might indicate illness. When several sets of vital signs have been obtained, this information forms a baseline with which subsequent measurements can be compared. Isolated vital sign values are not as helpful; the nurse should evaluate a series of values and establish trends for the client. Vital sign trends that deviate from normal are much more significant than isolated abnormal values.

The tasks involved in measuring vital signs are simple and easily learned, but interpreting the measurements and incorporating them into ongoing care and assessment requires knowledge, problem-solving skills, and experience. Although vital signs are often part of routine care, they provide valuable information and should not be taken lightly.

The frequency with which vital signs are assessed should be individualized for each client. Healthy individuals may have vital signs checked only during their annual physical. Very ill hospitalized clients may have their vital signs monitored more frequently than hospitalized clients who are less ill. Very young clients and elderly clients usually have their vital signs checked more frequently. Clients seen in ambulatory settings, wellness clinics, or psychiatric institutions may require infrequent vital sign checks. Most inpatient settings have a policy regarding the minimum frequency of vital sign assessment. In addition, physicians order vital signs to be checked at specific intervals based on the client's condition. Ultimately, however, the nurse caring for the client is the best judge of how often vital signs should be obtained.

Body Temperature

Humans are warm-blooded creatures, which means they can maintain internal body temperature without regard to the outside environment. The body's tissues and cells are best able to function within a relatively narrow temperature range. The body's surface or skin temperature can vary widely with environmental conditions and physical activity. Despite these fluctuations, the temperature inside the body, the **core temperature**, remains relatively constant, unless the client develops a febrile illness. The body's organs require this constant internal temperature for optimal functioning.

Although the normal adult temperature ranges from 36.1°C to 37.2°C (97°–99°F) taken orally, body temperature can fluctuate with exercise, changes in hormone levels, and extremes of external temperature. Rectal temperatures are usually higher than oral temperatures by 0.6°C (1°F), and axillary temperatures are usually lower than oral temperatures by 0.6 C (1°F) (Guyton, 1991).

Regulation of the body temperature requires the coordination of many body systems. For the core temperature to remain normal, heat production must equal heat loss. The hypothalamus, part of the central nervous system, is the body's built-in thermostat. It can sense small changes in body temperature and stimulates the necessary changes in the nervous system, circulatory system, skin, sweat glands, or shivering mechanism to maintain homeostasis. Chapter 40 describes the regulation of body temperature in detail.

Factors Affecting Body Temperature

Understanding the factors that can affect body temperature helps the nurse accurately assess the significance of body temperature variations.

Age. Newborns have unstable body temperatures because their thermoregulatory mechanisms are immature. Temperature instability continues into adolescence and then stabilizes. Normal temperature drops as a person ages; it is not uncommon for an elderly person to have a body temperature as low as 35°C (95°F), especially in cold weather (Darowski, Weinberg, & Guz, 1991). When evaluating low-grade temperatures in the elderly and identifying those at risk for hypothermia, remember that older age is associated with lower temperatures.

Environment. Ordinarily, changes in environmental temperatures do not affect core temperature because of our internal regulatory mechanisms, but exposure to extremely hot or cold temperatures can alter body temperature. The degree of change is related to the temperature, humidity, and length of exposure. It also is influenced by the body's thermoregulatory mechanisms; for example, infants and the elderly often have diminished control mechanisms (Darowski, Weinberg, & Guz, 1991). When the body is exposed to temperatures below 33°C (91.4°F), its ability to adjust is impaired, and the body cannot maintain a normal temperature. If the core temperature drops to 25°C (77°F), death may occur.

Time of Day. Body temperature normally fluctuates throughout the day. Temperature is usually lowest from 1 to 4 AM and highest from 4 to 6 PM. A person's body temperature can vary by as much as 2°C (1.8°F) from early morning to late afternoon (Samples, et al., 1985). In the past this variation was attributed to variations in muscle activity and digestive processes, which are usually minimal in the early morning while people sleep. However, no absolute relationship has been found between circadian rhythm and body temperature (Vick, 1985). In some humans, the situation is reversed, and body temperature is increased at night and decreased during the day. There is even greater variation in body temperature at various times of the day in infants and children.

Exercise. Body temperature increases with exercise because exercise increases heat production as carbohydrates and fats are broken down to provide energy. Strenuous exercise, such as running a marathon, can temporarily raise the temperature as high as 40°C (104°F) (Guyton, 1990).

Stress. Emotional or physical stress can elevate body temperature. When stress stimulates the sympathetic nervous system, circulating levels of epinephrine and norepinephrine are increased. As a result, the metabolic rate is increased, which in turn increases heat production. Stressed or anxious clients may have an elevated temperature without underlying pathology.

Hormones. Women usually have greater variations in their temperature than do men. Progesterone, a female hormone secreted at ovulation, increases body temperature by 0.3°C to 0.6°C (0.5°–1°F) above baseline. By measuring their temperature daily, women can determine when they ovulate; this is the basis for the rhythm method of birth control. Following menopause, mean temperature norms are the same for men and women (McGann, Marion, Camp, & Spangler, 1993). Thyroxine, epinephrine, and norepinephrine also elevate body temperature by increasing heat production (Shaver, 1991).

Factors Affecting Body Temperature Measurement

Smoking. If body temperature is measured orally immediately after a client has been smoking, the measurement may be altered by −0.2 ± 0.2°F (Woodman, Perry, & Simms, 1967). This small difference is not usually clinically significant.

Oxygen Administration. For years it was thought that the increased air current directed at the nasal pas-

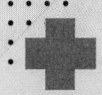

Safety Alert
Taking Vital Signs

- Do not take oral temperatures in infants, young children, or unconscious or irrational clients, because they cannot follow directions and may bite down or choke on the thermometer.
- Do not take rectal temperatures in infants because rectal perforation or mucosal damage may occur.
- If a glass thermometer accidentally breaks, avoid contact with the mercury, and call environmental services (or the designated group) for safe disposal.
- To prevent trauma when taking a rectal temperature, lubricate the thermometer generously and insert gently, especially if hemorrhoids are present.
- Palpate the carotid artery in the lower half of the neck to avoid stimulating the carotid sinus, which can result in bradycardia and syncope.
- Do not palpate bilateral carotid pulses simultaneously since this can seriously impair blood flow to the brain.
- When checking for orthostatic hypotension, assist the client from a lying to a sitting to a standing position, and monitor carefully for dizziness or difficulty maintaining balance. If the client appears unsteady, return the patient to the supine position immediately.
- When using an automatic blood pressure device for serial blood pressure readings, check the cuffed limb frequently to ensure adequate arterial perfusion and venous drainage between measurements.

sage decreased the temperature of the mouth. However, numerous studies have found minimal differences (−0.4 ± 0.69°F) in clients receiving oxygen by mask or cannula (Dressler, Smejkal, & Ruffolo, 1983; Lim-Levy, 1982; Yonkman, 1982).

Drinking Hot or Cold Liquids. Drinking hot or cold liquids may cause slight variations in oral temperature readings; the most marked variation is found after drinking ice water (−0.2° to −1.6°F) (Woodman, Perry, & Simms, 1967). Cole (1993) recommends waiting only 15 minutes after iced water ingestion to retake oral temperature, because 80% to 90% of individuals have returned to baseline.

Assessing Body Temperature

Temperature measurement is a routine part of vital sign evaluation. This establishes a baseline so that comparisons can be made as a disease progresses or therapies are instituted. The reliability of a temperature value depends on choosing the correct equipment, selecting the most appropriate site, and using the correct procedure. The nurse must ensure that the thermometer is placed correctly and is left in place the appropriate length of time.

Sites

Nurses should use their judgment when selecting the route by which temperature is measured. The four sites most commonly used are the mouth, ear, rectum, and axilla. In most clinical situations, any of these sites is satisfactory if proper technique is used and normal variations are considered for the different sites. Additional sites are the esophagus and pulmonary artery, both of which are considered core temperatures. Normal temperature varies within a person, from person to person, and from site to site (Table 22-2).

Oral. The most common site for temperature measurement is the oral route. Advantages of this route include easy access and client comfort. Because the temperature measurement could be affected if the person has had hot or cold liquids, the nurse should wait 15 minutes before placing the thermometer in these situations. This allows the mouth temperature to return to baseline.

The oral route is contraindicated in some situations. It should not be used in people who cannot follow instructions to keep their mouths closed, who are mouth breathing, or who might bite down and break the thermometer. Oral temperature assessment, especially with a glass thermometer, may not be prudent or safe in infants, young children, unconscious clients, irrational clients, or clients with seizure disorders.

Rectal. The rectal route is believed to be the most reliable, because few factors can artificially influence the reading. Rectal temperatures are recommended for clients who cannot have their temperatures taken orally or when an oral temperature changes quickly or unexpectedly. Care should be taken to avoid placing the thermometer into fecal material, because this may falsely elevate the temperature reading. This route is contraindicated in clients with diarrhea, those who have undergone rectal surgery, those with diseases of the rectum, or those with cancer who are neutropenic. It also is contraindicated in infants, because it may cause trauma to the rectal mucosa. Some adult clients may be uncomfortable having their temperature taken rectally, so careful explanation of the rationale for this route is important.

Ear. Since the development of the tympanic membrane thermometer, the ear has been added as a site where temperature can be easily and safely measured. The tympanic membrane receives its blood supply from the same vasculature that supplies the hypothalamus; thus, tympanic temperature readings reflect core body temperature (Baird, White, & Basinger, 1992). Cerumen in the ear canal or the presence of otitis media does not significantly alter temperature readings (Chamberlain, et al., 1991). Measurement also is not affected by smoking, drinking, or eating, which slightly alter oral temperature measurement. The ear is readily accessible and permits rapid temperature readings in very young, confused, or unconscious clients. Because the ear canal has fewer pathogens than the oral or rectal cavities, infection control is less of a concern.

Axillary. The axillary route is considered the least accurate and least reliable of all the sites because the temperature obtained using this route can be influenced by a number of factors. For example, if the client has recently bathed, the temperature may reflect the temperature of water used. If friction was used to dry the skin, the friction may influence the temperature. The axillary route is recommended for infants and children and is the route of choice in clients who cannot have their temperatures measured by other routes.

Table 22-2 • Normal Temperatures for Adults Obtained From Different Sites

Oral	Axillary	Rectal	Esophageal/ Pulmonary Artery
37°C 98.6°F	36.5°C 97.6°F	37.5°C 99.5°F	37.3° 99.2°F

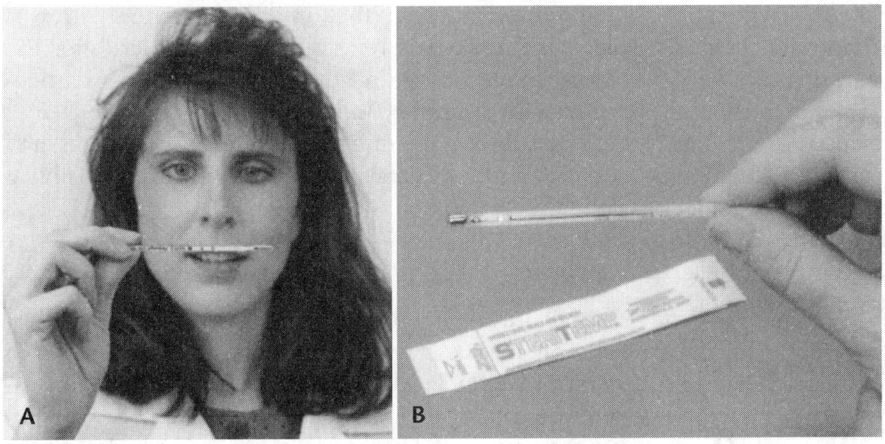

Figure 22-1 • *To read a glass thermometer correctly, the person holds it at eye level (**A**) and turns it to note the location of mercury on the scale (**B**).*

Equipment

Several types of thermometers are available. Traditionally, all temperature monitoring was done using a glass mercury thermometer, but advances in technology have provided quicker, more sanitary methods.

Glass Mercury Thermometer. The glass thermometer is still used in many homes. It is a slender glass tube that is sealed at one end and has a bulb of mercury at the other end. It should be handled only at the sealed end because touching the mercury bulb could influence the temperature reading. The tube is calibrated in degrees, using the Celsius or Fahrenheit scale. Exposing the bulb to heat causes the mercury to expand and rise to a point on the scale. The mercury stabilizes at this point and does not fall unless the thermometer is shaken vigorously. The temperature is read by holding the thermometer at eye level and noting the location of the mercury on the scale. Figure 22-1 shows the correct way to hold a glass mercury thermometer to obtain an accurate reading.

The tip of the oral glass thermometer is slender and allows for maximal exposure to the oral mucosa. The rectal glass thermometer tip is blunt to decrease the risk of trauma to the rectal mucosa. Often the tips are color-coded (blue for oral and red for rectal) to avoid mixups. The oral thermometer also may be used for axillary temperature measurement.

Electronic Thermometers. The electronic thermometer is widely used in healthcare facilities. There are many types on the market, but all have similar characteristics (Fig. 22-2). The thermometer consists of a battery-powered display unit and a temperature-sensitive probe connected to the display unit by a thin cord. When used, the probe is covered by a disposable plastic sheath to prevent the transmission of infection. These thermometers provide a reading in less than 60 seconds and are thought to be most accurate if placed in the sublingual pocket (Erickson, 1980). Results may be displayed in Celsius or Fahrenheit; some thermometers can display both. The electronic thermometer is ideally suited for use with children because the sheath is unbreakable and the time necessary for accurate measurement is relatively short.

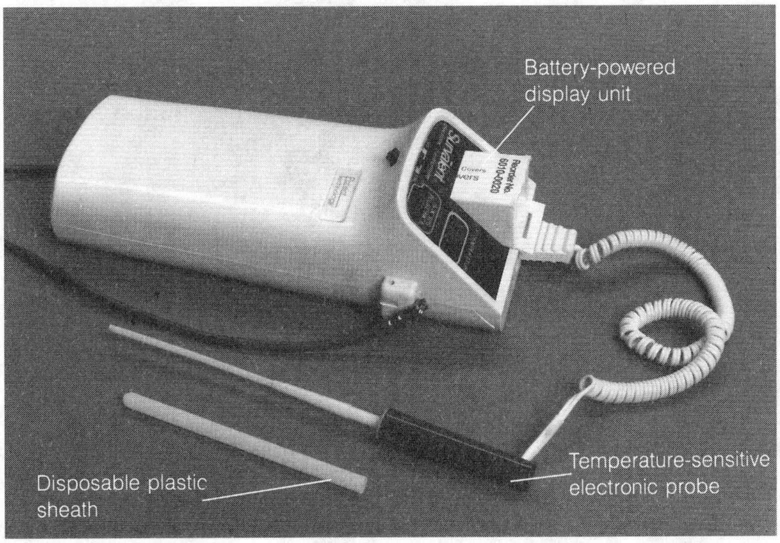

Figure 22-2 • *Electronic thermometer.*

Tympanic Membrane Thermometer. The tympanic membrane thermometer is a portable, hand-held device resembling an otoscope that recharges using a battery pack. It is illustrated in Procedure 22-1 later in the chapter. It records temperature through a sensor probe that is placed in the ear canal to detect infrared radiation from the eardrum. The tympanic membrane thermometer can record temperature in either Fahrenheit or Celsius, with some models providing both readouts. Studies indicate good correlation of tympanic temperature readings with core body temperature (Shinozaki, et al., 1988; Kenney & Fortenberry, 1990; Baird, 1992; Erickson & Meyer, 1994).

The tympanic membrane thermometer is especially appropriate in infants or very young children who may have difficulty remaining still while the temperature is recorded using other methods. Because recordings are obtained in 2 seconds or less, the tympanic membrane thermometer is often preferred in emergency rooms or other areas where assessments must be made quickly. Tympanic thermometers should not be used on individuals with ear drainage or a scarred tympanic membrane (Pransky, 1991).

Disposable Paper Thermometers. Single-use paper thermometers (Fig. 22-3) are thin strips of chemically treated paper. They have raised dots that change color to reflect the temperature, usually in less than 1 minute. These thermometers are available in Celsius or Fahrenheit scales and are reported to be accurate (Pontious, et al., 1994).

Temperature-Sensitive Strips. Temperature-sensitive strips can be used to obtain a general indication of body surface temperature. They are usually placed on the forehead or abdomen; the skin under the strip must be dry. After a specified length of time, the strip changes color. On one brand, a green "N" indicates a normal temperature, a brown "N" indicates a transition phase, and a blue-green "F" indicates an elevated temperature. The transition phase reflects the onset of a high temperature in the area where the strip was placed. The strip is removed and discarded after the color change has been noted. This method is particularly useful at home. Because children younger than 2 years still have immature thermoregulatory systems, any variation from normal should be confirmed using a standard thermometer.

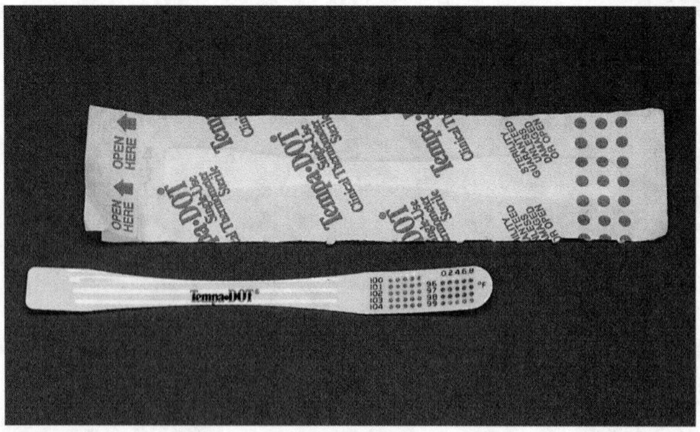

Figure 22-3 • *Disposable paper thermometer. The dots change color to indicate temperature.*

Scales

Temperature can be measured on the Celsius or Fahrenheit scale (Fig. 22-4). The scale used varies from agency to agency. Nurses do not routinely have to convert from one scale to the other. However, if conversion is necessary, simple formulas can be used. To change Celsius into Fahrenheit, multiply the Celsius reading by $\frac{9}{5}$ and add 32 to the result.

$$F = (9/5 \times C^\circ) + 32^\circ$$

For example:

$$F = (9/5 \times 37^\circ) + 32^\circ = (66.6^\circ) + 32^\circ = 98.6^\circ F$$

To change Fahrenheit into Celsius, subtract 32 from the Fahrenheit reading and multiply the result by $\frac{5}{9}$.

$$C = (F^\circ - 32^\circ) \times 5/9$$

For example:

$$C = (102^\circ - 32^\circ) \times 5/9 = (70) \times 5/9 = 38.8^\circ C$$

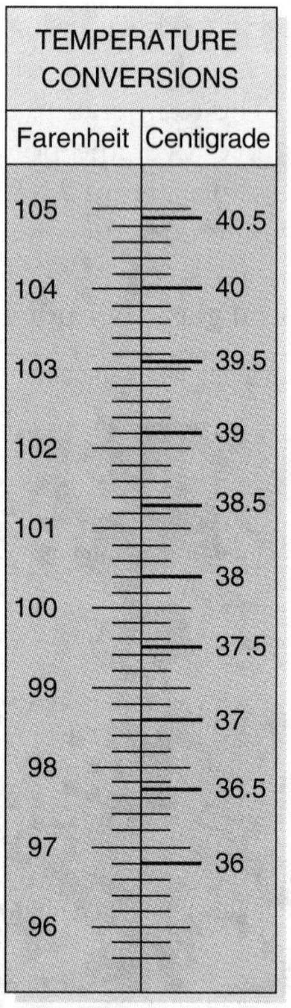

Figure 22-4 • *Temperature conversion chart.*

text continues on p. 433

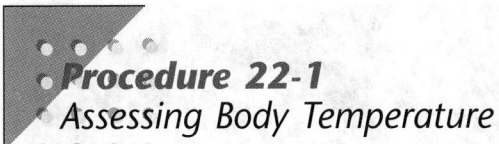

Procedure 22-1
Assessing Body Temperature

Purpose

1. Obtain baseline data with which future measurements can be compared.
2. Screen for alterations in temperature.
3. Evaluate temperature response to therapies.

Assessment

- Identify client's baseline temperature.
- Assess for clinical signs and symptoms of temperature alteration.
- Assess for factors that influence body temperature:
  - Ingestion of hot or cold foods or liquids in last 15 minutes
  - Smoking within last 15 minutes
  - Recent exercise
  - Age, hormones, drugs that cause variations in body temperature.
- Determine site most appropriate for temperature measurement.

Equipment

Appropriate thermometer
Plastic thermometer sheaths or tissues to wipe thermometer
Water-soluble lubricant and disposable gloves (for rectal temperature)
Pen and vital sign documentation record
Gloves

Assessing Oral Temperature With Glass Thermometer

Procedure

1. Wash hands. Explain the procedure to the client.
2. When using a mercury thermometer, put on disposable gloves.
   Rationale: Gloves protect nurse's hands from body secretion contamination. Unnecessary with electronic thermometer because nurse never touches oral probe.
3. Remove thermometer from storage container, and rinse in cold water. Wipe dry with tissue.
   Rationale: Storage solution is irritating to mucosa. Cold water is used to rinse thermometer because hot water would cause mercury to expand and break thermometer.
4. Hold thermometer at eye level.
   Rationale: Reading at eye level ensures accuracy.
5. Check temperature reading on thermometer. If reading is not below 35°C, shake down by holding thermometer at end away from bulb between thumb and forefinger, and snap wrist sharply.
   Rationale: Thermometer must be at eye level to accurately read mercury. Mercury must be below client's body temperature before use to register accurately.
6. Place thermometer probe in client's mouth in the posterior sublingual pocket (at the right or left of the frenulum at the base of the tongue).
   Rationale: Sublingual pocket has large superficial blood vessels that reflect heat of core body temperature.
7. Ask client to maintain thermometer position with lips closed.
   Rationale: This position maintains correct placement of thermometer in sublingual pocket.
8. Leave in place 3 to 5 minutes. Check agency policy regarding recommended time interval.
   Rationale: Research results vary as to amount of time needed to register accurate temperature.
9. Remove the thermometer. Wipe any secretions from the thermometer with a paper tissue. Holding the thermometer at eye level, rotate slowly until mercury column is visible. Note upper end of column as the temperature reading.
   Rationale: Clear visualization is necessary for accurate temperature determination.
10. Wash thermometer in soapy, tepid water, and return to storage container.
    Rationale: Proper care prevents breakage.
11. Record temperature on vital sign documentation record. Discuss finding with client if appropriate.
    Rationale: These actions ensure proper documentation and envourage client's understanding of health status.

Assessing Axillary Temperature

Procedure

1. Wash hands. Explain the procedure to the client.
2. When using a nercury thermometer, put on disposable gloves.
   Rationale: Gloves protect nurse's hands from body secretion contamination. Unnecessary with electronic thermometer because nurse never touches oral probe.
3. Remove thermometer from storage container, and rinse in cold water. Wipe dry with tissue.
   Rationale: Storge solution is irritating to mucosa. Cold water is used to rinse thermometer because hot water would cause mercury to expand and break thermometer.
4. Hold thermometer at eye level.
   Rationale: Reading at eye level ensures accuracy.

(continued)

5. Check temperature reading on thermometer. If reading is not below 35°C, shake down by holding thermometer at end away from bulb between thumb and forefinger, and snap wrist sharply.
   Rationale: Thermometer must be at eye level to accurately read mercury. Mercury must be below client's body temperature before use to register accurately.
6. Close bedroom door or unit curtains; assist client to comfortable position, and expose axilla.
   Rationale: This provides privacy.
7. Insert thermometer into middle of axilla; fold client's arm down, and place across chest.
   Rationale: This position maintains correct position of thermometer against blood vessels in axilla.
8. Hold thermometer in place 9 minutes in adults, 5 minutes in children.
   Rationale: Research now indicates there is no significant difference in accuracy between axillary and rectal temperature if the thermometer is left in place for the recommended period of time.
9. Remove the thermometer. Holding the thermometer at eye level, rotate slowly until mercury column is visible. Note upper end of column as the temperature reading.
   Rationale: Clear visualization is necessary for accurate temperature determination.
10. Wash thermometer in soapy, tepid water, and return to storage container.
    Rationale: Proper care prevents breakage.
11. Record temperature on vital sign documentation record. Discuss findings with client if appropriate.
    Rationale: These actions ensure proper documentation and encourage client's understanding of health status.

Assessing Oral Temperature With Electronic Thermometer

Procedure

1. Wash hands. Explain the procedure to the client.
2. Remove electronic thermometer from the battery pack, and remove the temperature probe from the unit, noting a digital display of temperature on the screen (usually 34°C or 94°F).
   Rationale: The electronic thermometer is stored in a battery pack to ensure that it is always charged and ready for use. Removing the temperature probe prepares the machine to measure and record temperature. The digital display of temperature indicates that it is charged.
3. Securely attach the disposable cover over the temperature probe.
   Rationale: Disposable cover prevents the transmission of microorganisms.

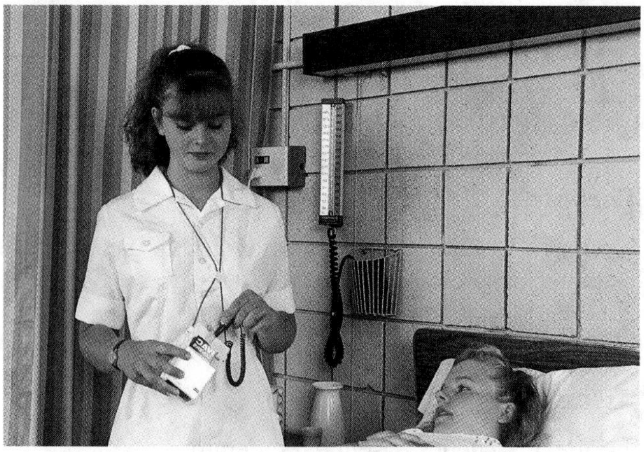

Step 3 • Cover temperature probe with disposable cover (© B. Proud)

4. Hold the probe in the sublingual pocket of the client's mouth.
   Rationale: The sublingual pocket obtains the most accurate temperature. The weight of the probe will displace it from the sublingual pocket if left unsupported.

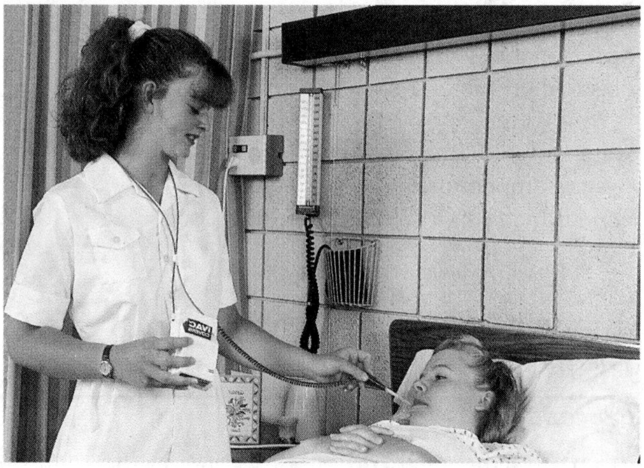

Step 4 • Hold probe in sublingual pocket (© B. Proud)

5. Wait for a beep (usually 10–20 seconds) and then remove the probe from the client's mouth, noting the temperature displayed on the unit.
   Rationale: Beep indicates maximum temperature has been reached, and this temperature should be recorded.
6. Displace the probe cover by pressing the probe release button as you hold the probe over a waste container.
   Rationale: The contaminated probe cover can be removed without touching the nurse's hands, thus preventing the transmission of microorganisms.

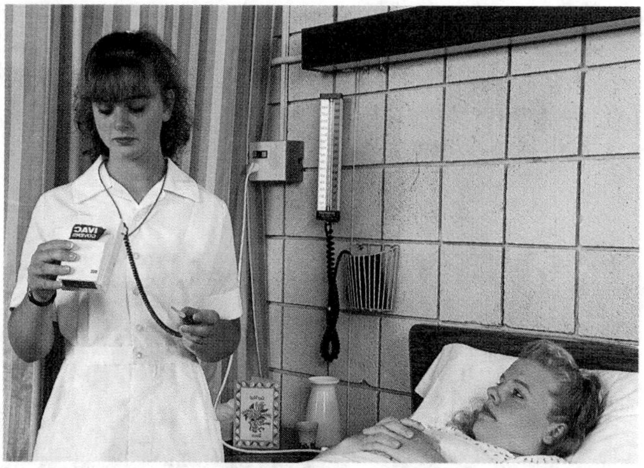

Step 5 • After beep, obtain reading (© B. Proud)

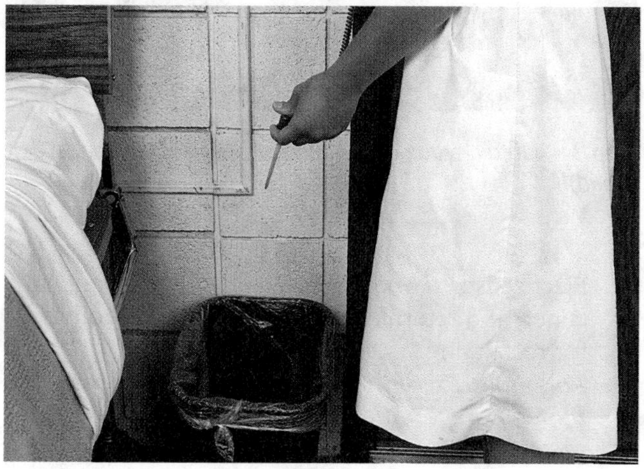

Step 6 • Release probe cover into waste receptacle (© B. Proud)

7. Return the probe to the storage place within the unit and the thermometer to the battery pack.
   Rationale: Proper storage prevents damage to the sensitive temperature probe and ensures that the unit will be recharged and ready for use.
8. Record temperature on vital sign documentation record. Discuss findings with client if appropriate.
   Rationale: These actions ensure proper documentation and encourage client's understanding of health status.

Assessing Rectal Temperature With an Electronic Thermometer

Procedure

1. Wash hands. Explain procedure to client.
2. Remove rectal (red) electronic thermometer from battery pack and remove the temperature probe from the unit, noting a digital display of temperature on the screen.
   Rationale: Removing the temperature probe prepares the machine to measure and record temperature. Ensure that rectal (red) probe only is used for monitoring rectal temperature to prevent cross-contamination of oral probe with rectal bacteria.
3. Securely attach the disposable cover over the temperature probe.
   Rationale: Disposable cover prevents transmission of microorganisms.
4. Close bedroom door or bed curtains. Assist client to Sims' position with upper leg flexed. Expose only anal area.
   Rationale: Privacy is essential to reduce embarrassment from exposing buttocks. Lateral position exposes anal area for thermometer placement.
5. Apply water-soluble lubricant liberally to thermometer probe tip.
   Rationale: Lubricant facilitates insertion of thermometer without irritating or traumatizing the rectum.

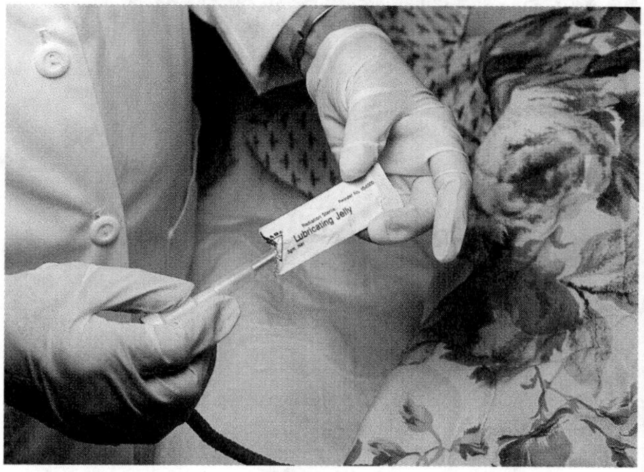

Step 5 • Lubricate thermometer probe (© B. Proud)

6. Separate client's buttocks with one gloved hand.
   Rationale: Exposure of anus ensures visualization for accurate placement of probe.
7. Ask client to take a deep, slow breath. Insert thermometer into anus in direction of umbilicus, for an infant ½ in, for an adult, 1 ½ in. Do not force.
   Rationale: Deep, slow breath allows client to relax external sphincter. Insertion depth allows adequate exposure of probe against blood vessels in rectal wall.
8. Hold in place until beep is heard. Obtain reading.
   Rationale: Holding thermometer prevents rectal damage or perforation from client moving with thermometer in place.

(continued)

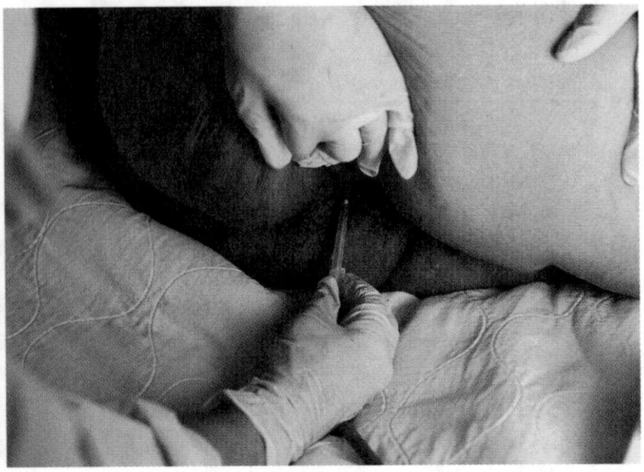

Step 7 • Gently insert into anus (© B. Proud)

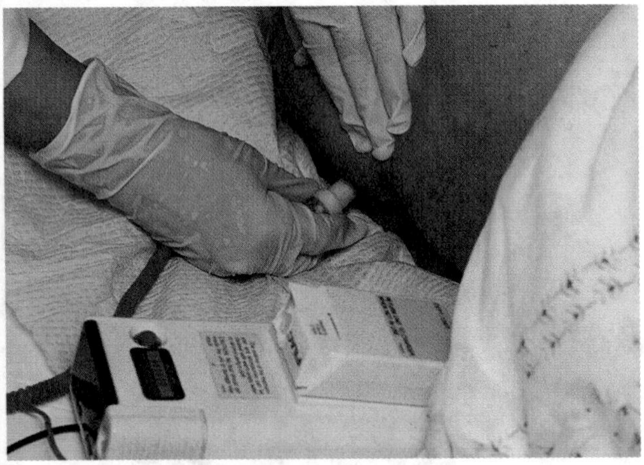

Step 8 • Hold thermometer in place (© B. Proud)

9. Follow steps 6–8 in Assessing Oral Temperature with Electronic Thermometer.

Assessing Temperature Using a Tympanic Membrane Thermometer

Procedure

1. Remove tympanic thermometer from recharging base, and attach tympanic probe cover to sensor unit.
   Rationale: Probe cover keeps unit clean and prevents the transfer of microorganisms.
2. Insert probe into ear canal, making sure the probe fits snugly. Avoid forcing the probe too deeply into the ear. Pulling on the pinna may help to straighten the ear canal, which permits better exposure of the tympanic membrane.
   Rationale: Snug fit into the ear canal is necessary for accurate temperature detection. Forceful deep insertion could result in injury to the ear drum.
3. Activate the thermometer, and watch for the temperature readout, which is usually displayed within 2 seconds.
   Rationale: Temperature assessment occurs very quickly with the tympanic membrane thermometer.

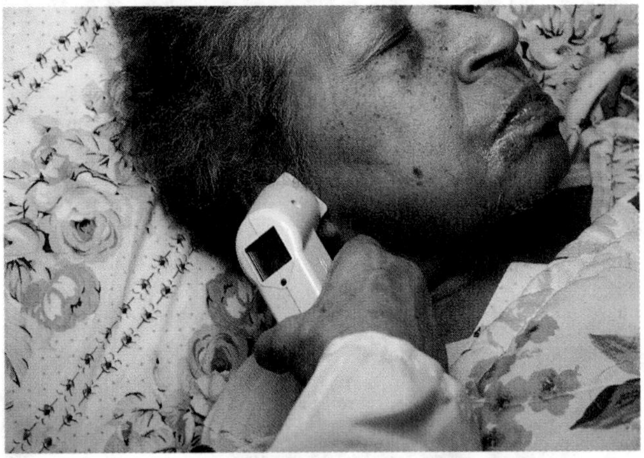

Step 3 • Obtain reading with probe inserted in ear canal (© B. Proud)

4. Eject sensor probe cover directly into waste container, and return tympanic thermometer to base for recharging.
   Rationale: Preventing contamination of nurse's hands is important. Recharging tympanic thermometer will prepare thermometer for use.
5. Record temperature on vital sign documentation record. Discuss findings with client if appropriate.
   Rationale: These actions ensure proper documentation and encourage client's understanding of health status.

Lifespan Considerations

Infants and Children

- Neonates have ineffective and immature thermoregulation. They are greatly influenced by environmental temperatures.
- When taking rectal temperature in an older infant or child, do not allow the child to roll over or kick due to risk of thermometer advancing and perforating rectum. Have assistance if necessary, or select an alternate site for temperature evaluation.
- Tympanic or axillary temperature is the preferred site in infants and children because it is easily accessible, there is little danger of mercury poisoning from thermometer breakage in mouth, and there is no chance of rectal perforation and possible resultant peritonitis.

Older Adults

- Older adults may have difficulty flexing their legs and assuming the left lateral position. Thermometer may be inserted with both legs straight.
- Body temperature drops to an average of 36°C in the older adult.
- Alcoholic clients are at risk for hypothermia because of heat loss from vasodilation.

Home Care Modifications

If family members need to assess temperature of clients, they may need to know

- How frequently to monitor temperature
- When to notify home care nurse or physician
- Not to measure temperature orally in children younger than 6 years, or in confused or unconscious clients
- To wash the thermometer in tepid, soapy water, and to store it dry

Methods

The nurse is responsible for taking temperatures, documenting the results, and reporting abnormal values. After selecting the most appropriate method of measurement, the nurse should gather the necessary equipment and explain the procedure to the client. Whenever possible, temperature measurements should be recorded at the same site so that interpretation of fluctuations is easier. See Procedure 22-1 for specific details on how to obtain a temperature measurement using each of the different routes and equipment.

Pulse

Contraction of the ventricles of the heart ejects blood into the arteries. The force of the blood entering the aorta from the left ventricle causes stretching or distention of the elastic aortic wall. As the aorta first expands then contracts, a pulse wave is created that travels along the blood vessels. The pulse wave or pulsation can be felt as a throb or tap where the arteries lie close to the skin surface.

Characteristics

Characteristics of the pulse include rate or frequency, rhythm, and quality. Rate or frequency refers to the number of pulsations per minute. Pulse rhythm refers to the regularity with which pulsation occurs. Pulse quality refers to the strength of the palpated pulsation.

The rate and rhythm of the pulse are established by specialized cells that make up the conduction system of the heart. The stimulus for contraction of the heart normally starts as an electrical impulse in the sinoatrial (SA) node of the right atrium. In adults, the SA node initiates the impulse 60 to 100 times per minute. The electrical impulse then spreads quickly through the conduction system to the remainder of the heart so that the heart muscle fibers contract in a synchronous fashion. Irregularities of heart rhythm usually indicate a failure in the conduction system or origination of an impulse in a site other than the SA node.

The quality of the arterial pulse is determined by factors such as the force with which blood is ejected from the ventricles, the amount of blood ejected with each heartbeat (the **stroke volume**), and the patency and compliance or elasticity of the arteries.

Factors Affecting Pulse Rate

Age. The average pulse rate of an infant ranges from 100 to 160 beats per minute. The heart rhythm in infants and children often varies markedly with respiration, increasing during inpiration and decreasing with expiration. The normal range of the pulse in an adult is 60 to 100 beats per minute. The normal pulse ranges for various age groups are shown in Table 22-1.

Autonomic Nervous System. Stimulation of the parasympathetic nervous system results in a decrease in the pulse rate. Normally there is a certain amount of parasympathetic control of the heart beat to maintain the pulse rate below 100 beats per minute. Conversely, stimulation of the sympathetic nervous system results in an increased pulse rate. Sympathetic nervous system activation occurs in response to a variety of stimuli, including pain, anxiety, exercise, fever, and ingestion of caffeinated beverages, and in response to changes in intravascular volume.

Medications. Certain cardiac medications, such as digoxin, decrease heart rate. Medications that decrease intravascular volume, such as diuretics, may cause a reflex increase in pulse rate. Other medications mimic or block the effects of the autonomic nervous system. For example, atropine inhibits impulses to the heart from the parasympathetic nervous system, causing increased pulse rate. Other medications, such as propranolol, block sympathetic nervous system action, resulting in decreased heart rate.

Assessing the Pulse

The pulse is an important part of vital sign measurements. The baseline pulse rate and rhythm are established during the initial nursing assessment and are used for comparison with future measurements.

Sites

The pulse can be assessed in any location where an artery lies close to the skin surface and can be compressed against a firm underlying structure, such as muscle or bone. The most commonly assessed pulses are the temporal, carotid, apical, brachial, radial, femoral, popliteal, pedal, and posterior tibial (Fig. 22-5).

Temporal. The temporal artery courses across the temporal bone of the skull. The pulsation of the temporal artery is most easily palpated just in front of the upper part of the ear.

Carotid. The sternomastoid muscles, which stand out when the jaw is forcefully clenched, run from below the ear to the clavicle and sternum. Beneath them lie the carotid arteries. The artery is most easily palpated along the medial border of the sternomastoid muscle in the lower half of the neck. Palpating the carotid arteries in the upper part of the neck may result in stimulation of the carotid sinus, which causes a reflex drop in pulse rate. The carotid pulse best represents the quality of pulsation in the aorta because of its proximity to the central circulation.

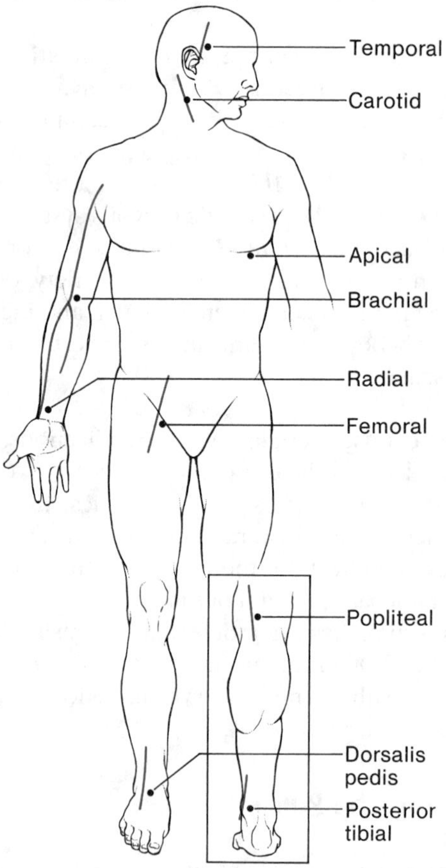

Figure 22-5 • *Pulse sites. The insert shows the left leg. The posterior tibial pulse is on the medial aspect of the ankle.*

Apical. The contraction or beating of the heart ventricles also can be palpated with the hand or auscul tated with a stethoscope placed over the area of the left ventricle. Normally this area is at the level of the fifth intercostal space at about the midclavicular line.

Brachial. The brachial artery lies between the groove of the biceps and triceps muscles in the inner aspect of the upper arm. The brachial pulse is most easily palpated with the client's arm flexed at the elbow and supported by the examiner to prevent muscle contraction, which may obscure the pulse.

Radial. The radial artery is the site most commonly assessed in the clinical setting. The radial pulse is palpated on the thumb side of the inner aspect of the wrist.

Femoral. The femoral pulse is palpated in the anterior, medial aspect of the thigh, just below the inguinal ligament, about halfway between the anterior superior iliac spine and the symphysis pubis. Deep palpation may be required to detect the femoral pulse beneath the subcutaneous tissue.

Popliteal. The popliteal pulse is palpable behind the knee in the lateral aspect of the popliteal fossa (the hollow area at the back of the knee joint). The pulse is best assessed with the knee flexed and the leg relaxed. The client may be supine or prone.

Pedal. The pedal pulse or dorsalis pedis pulse can be felt on the dorsal aspect of the foot (the area of the foot that is on top in a standing position). The pulse is palpated lateral to the tendon that runs from the great toe toward the ankle. The dorsalis pedis pulse may be congenitally absent in some clients.

Posterior Tibial. The posterior tibial pulse is located behind the malleolus (the rounded protuberance of bone) of the inner ankle. The pulse is palpated by hooking the fingertips behind the bone.

Methods

Palpation. The pulse is palpated with the first and second or second and third fingers of one hand. Light pressure is initially used to locate the area of strongest pulsation. More forceful palpation may then be used to count the rate, determine the rhythm, and assess the quality of pulsation. The number of pulses is counted for 15, 30, or 60 seconds and multiplied as necessary to yield pulses per minute. The time interval used to assess the pulse depends on the client's condition and the norms of the institution. Hollerbach and Sneed (1990) found the 30-second interval to be the most accurate and efficient, although in some areas when pulse needs to be monitored quickly, the 15-second interval is still used. Clients with irregular pulse rates or abnormally slow or fast pulse rates are best assessed for 1 full minute. Clients with a regular rhythm and normal rate may be assessed for a shorter time. Intervals of 15 seconds may be used when the pulse is assessed frequently, as during recovery from anesthesia.

Regardless of the time interval selected, the initial pulsation is counted as zero. Pulses at or after completion of the time interval are not counted. Counting the first pulse as one or counting pulses after the period of assessment results in overestimation of the pulse. The error is multiplied when intervals of less than 60 seconds are used to assess the rate. Counting even one extra pulsation in a 15-second pulse assessment results in overestimation of the pulse rate by four. Procedure 22-2 gives detailed instructions on taking a pulse.

Auscultation. The apical pulse provides the most accurate assessment of the pulse rate and is the preferred site whenever the peripheral pulses are difficult to assess or the rhythm of the pulse is irregular.

Apical pulse is assessed by placing the diaphragm of the stethoscope over the apex of the heart. The sounds heard are due to vibrations caused by the opening and closing of the cardiac valves. Each heartbeat consists of two sounds. The first, S_1, is caused by closure of the mitral and tricuspid valves separating the atria from the ventricles. The second sound, S_2, is caused by the closure of the pulmonic and aortic valves. The sounds are often described as a muffled "lub-dub." Together they constitute one heartbeat. To determine the apical pulse, the heartbeats are counted for 1 full minute.

Equipment

Stethoscope. Auscultation of the apical pulse requires a stethoscope. The stethoscope should have snugly fitting ear pieces and thick-walled tubing about 12 inches long for optimal sound transmission (Bates, 1995). The stethoscope should be equipped with a bell and a diaphragm.

Doppler. Peripheral pulses that cannot be detected by palpation may be assessed with an ultrasonic Doppler device. The transmitter of the device is placed over the artery to be assessed. A conductive gel is first applied to the skin to reduce resistance to sound transmission. High-frequency waves directed at the artery from the transmitter are disturbed by the pulsating flow of blood and are reflected back to the ultrasound device. The sound disturbances (Doppler shifts) are amplified and heard through ear pieces or a speaker attached to the device.

Doppler assessment of the pulse is generally used to determine the adequacy of flow to an area when occlusive vascular disease threatens the blood supply or for postoperative assessment where peripheral circulation can be occluded. The Doppler also may be useful in situations of cardiopulmonary collapse where peripheral vasoconstriction makes pulses difficult to palpate or when obesity makes palpation difficult.

Assessing Pulse Characteristics

The pulse is assessed for rate, rhythm, and quality. Pulse rate and rhythm are routinely assessed; pulse quality is assessed less often or in exceptional circumstances when abnormalities may be anticipated.

Rate. In adults, the normal rate is 60 to 100 pulsations per minute. Adult pulse rates above 100 beats per minute are called **tachycardia**. Sympathetic nervous system activation results in an increased pulse rate. Tachycardic rates also may occur when the impulse for cardiac contraction comes from an abnormal site in the heart that stimulates the heart to beat faster.

An abnormally slow pulse rate is called **bradycardia.** In adults, a pulse rate below 60 is considered bradycardic. Bradycardia may be the normal resting heart rate in a trained athlete. Disease of the SA node may result in bradycardia due to poor impulse formation. Bradycardia may be caused by enhanced parasympathetic nervous system activity, as occurs with stimulation of the carotid sinus.

Rhythm. Normally, cardiac contractions occur at evenly spaced intervals, resulting in a regular rhythm. Infants and children often have increased pulse rates during inspiration and decreased rates during expiration; this is called *sinus arrhythmia.* This tendency decreases with aging.

Heart disease, medications, or electrolyte imbalances may alter the normal rhythmic beating of the heart, causing an irregular pulse. An irregular pulse rhythm that still has a consistent pattern of pulsation is called *regularly irregular.* An example is pulsus bigeminus, in which a normal heartbeat initiated in the SA node is followed by a heartbeat initiated in a different part of the heart. The second beat is early and often weaker than the first, resulting in a regularly irregular pulse.

If there is no pattern to the pulse, it is called *irregularly irregular.* Irregularly irregular pulses may be detected in many conditions, for example a condition known as atrial fibrillation. In atrial fibrillation, the atria of the heart do not contract in a synchronous fashion, and the impulse for the heartbeat does not come from the SA node. Consequently, the time interval between successive ventricular contractions varies, and an irregularly irregular pulse is detected.

When an abnormal pulse rhythm is noted, the examiner should consider using the auscultatory method

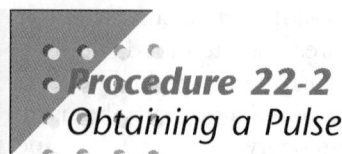

Procedure 22-2 Obtaining a Pulse

Purpose

1. Obtain a baseline measurement of heart rate and rhythm.
2. Evaluate the heart's response to various therapies and medications.
3. Peripheral pulse may be palpated to assess local blood flow to an extremity.

Assessment

- Review medical history to determine risk factors for alterations in pulse rate (heart disease, fluid or electrolyte imbalances, pain, hemorrhage).
- Assess for physical signs and symptoms of alteration in cardiac or vascular status (dyspnea, chest pain, palpitations, syncope, edema, cyanosis).
- Identify factors that influence pulse (age, medications, fever, exercise).
- Identify site most appropriate for pulse assessment.
- Review previous and baseline pulse assessments, if available.

Equipment

Wristwatch with second hand
Vital sign flow sheet and pen
Doppler and jelly (optional, for hard-to-palpate pulses)
Stethoscope

Obtaining a Radial Pulse

Procedure

1. Wash hands, and explain the procedure to the client.
2. Position client comfortably with forearm across chest or at side with wrist extended.
   Rationale: Relaxed position of lower arm with wrist extended allows easier artery palpation.
3. Place fingertips of your first three fingers along the groove at base of thumb, on client's wrist.
   Rationale: Fingertips are the most sensitive part of the hand for palpating pulses. Do not use the thumb to palpate: it has a strong pulse that may be confused with the client's.
4. Press against radial artery to obliterate pulse, then gradually release pressure until pulsations are felt.
   Rationale: Moderate pressure is needed to accurately assess rate and regularity of pulse.

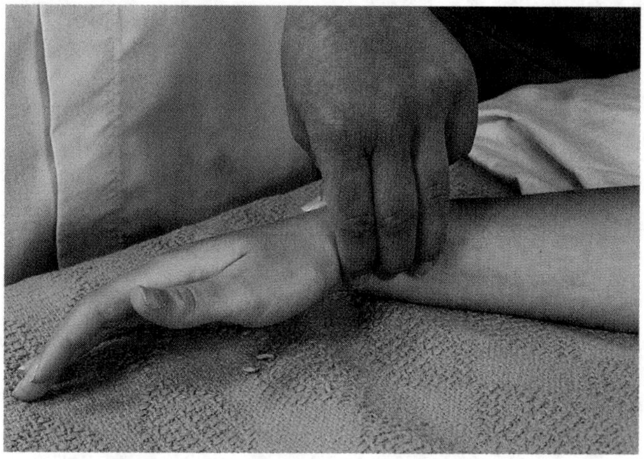

Step 3 • Obtaining a radial pulse (© B. Proud)

5. Assess pulse for regularity and strength.
6. If pulse is not easily palpable, use Doppler:
   a. Apply conducting gel to end of probe or to radial site.
      Rationale: Doppler works by ultrasound, which transmits sound better with the airtight seal provided by gel.
   b. Press "on" button, and place probe against skin on pulse site. Reposition slightly using firm pressure until pulsating sound is heard.
7. If pulse is regular, count pulse for 30 seconds, and multiply by two. If pulse is irregular, count for 1 full minute. Initial pulse is counted as zero.
   Rationale: Prevents overestimation of pulse. If pulse is irregular, a longer counting period ensures a more accurate pulse rate determination.

Obtaining an Apical Pulse

Procedure

1. Position client in supine or sitting position with sternum and left chest exposed.
   Rationale: Allows easy access for selection of auscultatory site. Rustling from clothing or bed linens will not distract from hearing pulse.
2. Warm diaphragm of stethoscope by holding in the palm of your hand for 5 to 10 seconds.
   Rationale: Cold metal or plastic diaphragm can startle the client when placed directly on the chest. This would possibly alter pulse rate.
3. Insert the ear pieces of stethoscope into your ears and place diaphragm over apex of client's heart.

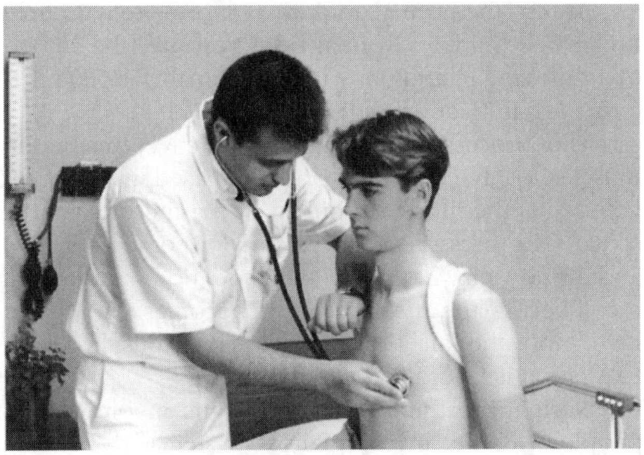

Step 3 • Obtaining an apical pulse

Rationale: The heartbeat is usually heard loudest at the fifth intercostal space, near the midclavicular line.

4. Assess the heartbeat for regularity and arrhythmias.
   Rationale: Frequent irregularities within 1 minute may indicate inadequate cardiac perfusion.
5. If rhythm is regular, count the heartbeat for 30 seconds, and multiply by two. Count for 1 full minute if the rhythm is irregular. Initial pulse is counted as zero.
   Rationale: Prevents overestimation of pulse. Heart rate is more accurate counted over a longer period if the rate is irregular.
6. Replace client's gown and assist in returning to a comfortable position.
7. Share results of assessment with client, if appropriate.
   Rationale: Promotes client's understanding of health and response to therapies.
8. Document pulse on vital sign record. Specify in documentation that an apical pulse was obtained (eg, A).

Lifespan Considerations

Infants and Children

- Newborns and children younger than 2 have weak radial pulses. Apical pulses are assessed for heart rate.
- The apex of the heart on an infant is at the third to fourth intercostal space, to the left of the midclavicular line.
- Crying greatly increases the pulse rate. Crying can be decreased by taking the pulse while the child sits in a parent's lap or by distracting the child with toys.

Older Adults

- If client is taking cardiac medications, such as digitalis preparations or beta-blockers or if patient has a history of cardiac arrhythmias, a more accurate assessment of heart rate and rhythm is obtained using the apical pulse site.

Home Care Modifications

- Pulse may need to be assessed at home if client is taking various cardiac medications. The caregiver or client must be taught how to locate and count the pulse, and to keep a diary of daily pulse rate to take to healthcare appointments.
- Digital pulse rate devices are available for home use.

to obtain an apical pulse rate. The examiner also must determine whether irregularity of the pulse is a new finding for the client. Many people have chronically irregular pulse rhythms, but a new finding of pulse irregularity requires immediate investigation to determine the causes and to assess the need for treatment.

Quality. Pulse quality generally refers to the strength of pulsation and may be rated on a numerical scale (Table 22-3). The normal quality of the pulse is described as full or strong and easily palpated. Weak pulses are easily obliterated by the examiner's fingers and may be described as thready. A bounding pulse is stronger than normal and difficult to obliterate. Pulse quality reflects the stroke volume, the compliance or elasticity of the arteries, and the adequacy of blood delivery. When stroke volume is decreased, as in severe hemorrhage, the pulse is often thready and may be difficult to palpate in the peripheral arteries. In cardiopulmonary failure, the pulse is usually palpated more easily in the central areas, such as the carotid or femoral arteries. With aging, the arteries lose elasticity, and the pulse becomes more bounding. The combination of rapid pulse rate and increased stroke volume with exercise results in a pulse that can be felt by the client and is sometimes called a pounding heart.

Peripheral pulses should be palpated bilaterally to compare quality. Equality of pulsation provides information about local blood flow. For example, partial occlusion of a right femoral artery would result in weaker femoral, popliteal, dorsalis pedis, and posterior tibial pulses on the right than on the left. Bilateral pulse comparison is used to monitor for complications after procedures invasive to the arteries, such as arteriography.

Table 22-3 • Scale to Rate Pulse Quality

0	No pulse detected
1+	Thready, weak pulse, easily obliterated with pressure; pulse may come and go
2+	Pulse difficult to palpate; may be obliterated with pressure
3+	Normal pulse
3+	Bounding, hyperactive pulse; easily palpated and cannot be obliterated

After an arteriogram, during which a large artery is punctured and injected with radiographic dye, the normal clotting to seal the artery may cause total arterial occlusion. Weakened or absent pulses distal to the puncture site would signal an occlusion.

Pulse Deficits. In some situations, stroke volume may vary from beat to beat during cardiac contraction, resulting in a pulse wave so weak that it cannot be perceived by palpation at a peripheral site. It is important to recognize this situation because it provides information about the heart's ability to perfuse the body adequately. When some of the ventricular contractions do not perfuse, there is a difference between the apical and peripheral pulses—a **pulse deficit.** The presence and magnitude of the pulse deficit can be determined by having two nurses simultaneously measure the apical and radial pulses. Procedure 22-3 gives details on determining pulse deficit. Both nurses should use the same watch or clock to count the pulse for 1 full minute. The difference between the pulses is then documented. When a pulse deficit is present, the radial pulse rate is always lower than the apical pulse rate.

Respirations

Respiration is a term used to summarize two different but related processes: external respiration and internal respiration. External respiration is the process of taking oxygen into the body and eliminating carbon dioxide from the body. Internal respiration refers to the use of oxygen, the production of carbon dioxide, and the exchange of these gases between the cells and the blood.

The respiratory system is made up of four parts, all of which must be functioning for the system to maintain homeostasis:

- The lungs, which are responsible for gas exchange
- The thoracic cavity, which includes the chest wall and the respiratory muscles
- The respiratory control center in the brain
- The nerves and nerve tracts that connect the brain and the muscles

At rest, the normal adult respiratory rate is 12 to 20 breaths per minute. Normal **tidal volume** (the amount of air moving in and out with each breath) is 500 mL or 6 to 8 L/min (Ganong, 1993).

The process of inspiration is active. Inspiratory muscles contract, resulting in increased intrathoracic volume as the lungs are pulled into a more expanded space. The pressure in the airway becomes negative, and air flows in. At the end of inspiration, natural lung recoil occurs, the airway pressure becomes slightly positive, and the air flows out as the muscles relax. Expiration is basically a passive process.

Normal breathing is automatic and involuntary. In people with healthy respiratory systems, the normal stimulus to breathe is hypercarbia, an increased carbon dioxide level. Chemoreceptors throughout the body sense changes in carbon dioxide levels and stimulate the respiratory center, which increases or decreases respiratory rate and depth accordingly. A decreased oxygen level also has the effect of increasing respiratory rate and depth.

There are two separate centers in the nervous system for control of breathing. Voluntary control of breathing is possible, and the center for voluntary control is in the cerebral cortex. Spontaneous, involuntary respirations are controlled by a rhythmic discharge of impulses from the brain to the nerves that innervate the respiratory muscles. The rate of these discharges is regulated by alterations in the arterial levels of carbon dioxide and oxygen. Breathing stops if the spinal cord is cut above the level of the phrenic nerve (Ganong, 1993). Chapter 34 provides an in-depth explanation of respiratory control.

Factors Affecting Respirations

Several factors can affect respiratory rate, rhythm, and depth, and familiarity with these factors allows the nurse to determine the significance of alterations.

Age. Normal growth from infancy to adulthood results in a larger lung capacity. As lung capacity increases, lower respiratory rates are sufficient to exchange air. As a person continues into older age, lung elasticity decreases. With this decrease in lung capacity, the respiratory rate once again increases to allow for the same exchange of air.

Medications. Narcotics can impair the ability to voluntarily inspire, and the respiratory rate and depth may decrease. Other drugs, depending on their action, may alter rate, rhythm, and depth in other ways.

Stress. Stress or strong emotions can change a person's respiratory pattern, because the sympathetic nervous system is stimulated. Stress increases the rate and depth of respirations.

Procedure 22-3
Assessing Pulse Deficits

Purpose

1. Evaluate the effectiveness of cardiac contractions by determining if there is a difference between apical and radial heart rates.

Assessment

- Identify clients at risk for unequal apical and radial heart rates (history of heart disease, elderly clients).
- Assess for physical signs and symptoms of altered cardiac status (dyspnea, palpitations, syncope, cyanosis).
- Review baseline pulse assessments, if available.

Equipment

Wristwatch with second hand
Stethoscope
Vital sign documentation sheet and pen
Second examiner

Procedure

1. Explain procedure to client. Introduce second examiner. Position client comfortably.
   Rationale: Ensures client comfort and cooperation.
2. Remove clothing as necessary to select stethoscope placement site. Warm diaphragm of stethoscope by holding in hand. Place stethoscope over apex of heart.
   Rationale: The heartbeat is usually heard best at the fifth intercostal space, near the midclavicular line.
3. Second examiner places fingertips over radial artery pulse site.
   Rationale: Accuracy in obtaining pulse deficit is improved by use of second examiner.
4. Place a watch where both examiners can clearly observe the second hand. Both examiners agree to start counting when the second hand reaches a predetermined number.
   Rationale: A pulse deficit will be accurate only if apical and radial heartbeats are counted simultaneously.
5. Count the apical and radial rate for 1 full minute.
   Rationale: Accuracy is increased by counting heart rate for 60 seconds.
6. Reposition client, and adjust clothing.
   Rationale: This provides comfort for the client.
7. Document the apical and radial heart rates.

Lifespan Considerations

Infants and Children

- Pulse deficit tends to be a problem in the older adult and is rarely evaluated in children.

Older Adults

- If radial pulse is weak and difficult to count, repeat procedure for a second minute to check accuracy of radial pulse.

Exercise. When people exercise, their tissues need more oxygen. Also, extra carbon dioxide and heat are produced and must be eliminated. The body responds to these needs by increasing the rate and depth of respirations.

Altitude. The oxygen content of the air decreases as the altitude increases. To compensate for the decreased oxygen content, the rate and depth of respirations at higher elevations increase to improve the supply of oxygen available to the body tissues.

Gender. Because men normally have a larger lung capacity than women, men may have a lower respiratory rate than women.

Body Position. When the body is slumped or stooped, gas exchange can become impaired. As a result, the rate and depth of respiration may be increased.

Fever. When a person has a fever, the respiratory system provides an avenue for the release of extra heat. Because heat can be lost from the lungs, the result is an increased respiratory rate. Also, as the metabolic rate increases with the temperature, the respiratory rate is affected. Respiratory rate can increase as much as four breaths per minute with every 0.6°C (1°F) increase in temperature above normal (Guyton, 1991).

Assessing Respirations

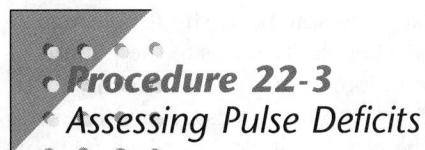

Respirations should be assessed in every vital sign evaluation. A normal baseline for each client should be established so that comparisons can be made. The assessment should include respiratory rate, rhythm, depth, and quality.

The respiratory assessment can provide valuable information, and a thorough assessment of a client's respirations is vital in gathering clues to his or her condition. When assessing a client's respiratory status, the nurse should keep in mind the client's normal pattern, the influence of any disease conditions, and the influence of any therapies that could affect the client's respiratory status.

Assessing Respiratory Characteristics

Rate. Respiratory rate changes with age. At rest, the normal respiratory rate for an infant is 30 to 60 breaths per minute, decreasing to 12 to 20 breaths per minute for an adult. **Tachypnea** is an abnormally fast respiratory rate (usually above 20 breaths per minute in the adult). **Bradypnea** is an abnormally slow respiratory rate (usually less than 12 breaths per minute in the adult). **Apnea,** the absence of respirations, is often described by the length of time in which there are no respirations (for instance, a 10-second period of apnea). Continuous apnea is synonymous with respiratory arrest and is not compatible with life.

Rhythm and Depth. Respirations should be regular in rhythm and depth. Regularity refers to the pattern of inspiration and expiration. Expiration is normally twice as long as inspiration. Depth is assessed by observing the movement of the chest wall. Several abnormal patterns may be found during the physical examination (Table 22-4).

Biot's respirations are a cyclic pattern of breathing in which periods of shallow breathing alternate with periods of apnea. This respiratory pattern is seen in clients with meningitis, encephalitis, head trauma, brain abscess, and heatstroke.

Cheyne-Stokes respirations are a cyclic pattern of breathing in which periods of respirations of increased rate and depth alternate with periods of apnea. Common conditions causing Cheyne-Stokes respirations include congestive heart failure, drug overdoses, increased intracranial pressure, and meningitis. Cheyne-Stokes respirations are the most common abnormal pattern assessed (Guyton, 1991).

Kussmaul respirations are a pattern of breathing characterized by respirations of increased rate (more than 20 breaths per minute) and increased depth. This abnormal pattern is most commonly associated with metabolic acidosis and renal failure.

Apneustic respirations are a pattern of breathing characterized by a long gasping inspiratory period fol-

Table 22-4 • Abnormal Breathing Patterns

Abnormal Breathing Pattern	Description	Conditions
Bradypnea 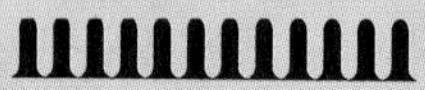	Respiratory rate below 12 beats per minute	Neurologic disturbances electrolyte disturbances, narcotic or barbiturate overdose, postanesthesia
Tachypnea 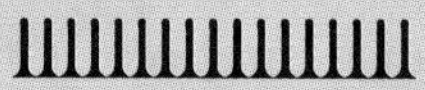	Persistent respiratory rate above 20 beats per minute	Trauma, injury, stress, pain; respiratory, cardiac, liver disease
Biot's Biot's 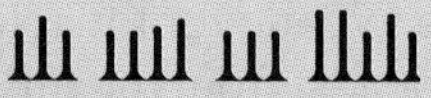	Cyclic breathing pattern characterized by shallow breathing alternating with periods of apnea	Neurologic problems (meningitis, encephalitis), head trauma, brain, abscess, heatstroke
Cheyne-Stokes 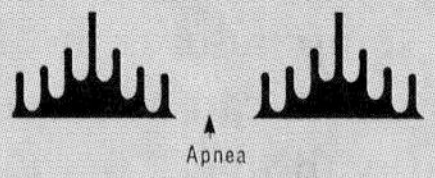	Cyclic breathing pattern characterized by periods of respirations of increased rate and depth, alternating with periods of apnea	Congestive heart failure, drug overdose, increased intracranial pressure
Kussmaul 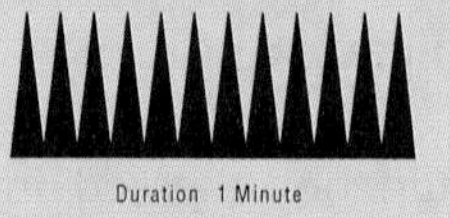	Increased rate (above 20 beats per minute) and depth of respirations	Metabolic acidosis, diabetic ketoacidosis, renal failure

lowed by a short expiratory period. This pattern is commonly seen in clients with central nervous system disorders.

Quality. Respirations are usually automatic, quiet, and effortless. When assessing respirations, the nurse should be attentive to changes from the normal quality. Abnormalities in quality are usually characterized as problems with effort or noise.

Dyspnea describes respirations that require excessive effort. Respirations can be painful and labored. Clients may report being unable to catch their breath. Dyspnea can occur at rest or with activity; dyspnea that occurs with activity is called exertional dyspnea. Healthy people who are not in good physical condition may experience exertional dyspnea.

Breathing also can be noisy. A number of terms are used to describe the different types of noisy respirations that the nurse can hear without a stethoscope.

Stridor is a harsh inspiratory sound that can sound like crowing. It may indicate an upper airway obstruction. It is commonly heard in children with croup or after aspiration of a foreign object.

Wheezing is a high-pitched musical sound. It is usually heard on expiration but may be heard on inspiration. It is associated with partial obstruction of the bronchi or bronchioles, as in asthma.

Sighs are breaths of deep inspiration and prolonged expiration. Everyone sighs, and sighing aids in the expansion of alveoli. However, more frequent sighing may indicate stress or tension.

Methods

Clients must be unaware that the nurse is doing a respiratory assessment, because if they are conscious of the procedure they may alter their breathing pattern or rate. Often, nurses assess the respiratory rate after taking the radial pulse, while still holding the client's wrist. If respirations are very shallow and difficult to visually detect, the nurse can count them while observing the sternal notch where respiration is more apparent. If the client is sleeping, a hand can rest gently on the chest so the rise and fall of the chest can be detected. With an infant or young child, respirations should be assessed before the temperature is taken so that the child is not crying, which would alter the respiratory status. See Procedure 22-4 for details on assessing respirations.

Blood Pressure

Blood pressure is the force that blood exerts against the walls of the vessels. The pressure in the systemic arteries is most commonly measured in the clinical setting. Blood pressure is stated in millimeters of mercury (mm Hg).

Physiologic Factors Determining Blood Pressure

The contractions of the heart result in a pulsating flow of blood into the arteries. The pressure is highest when the ventricles of the heart contract and eject blood into the aorta and pulmonary arteries. The blood pressure measured during ventricular contraction (cardiac systole) is the **systolic blood pressure**. During ventricular relaxation (cardiac diastole), blood pressure is due to elastic recoil of the vessels, and the measured pressure is the **diastolic blood pressure**. The mathematical difference between the measured systolic and diastolic blood pressures is the **pulse pressure**. For instance, a systolic pressure of 120 mm Hg and a diastolic pressure of 80 mm Hg results in a pulse pressure of 40 mm Hg.

Blood pressure is a function of the flow of blood produced by contraction of the heart and the resistance to blood flow through the vessels (Kaplan, 1988). The pressure, flow, and resistance relationship is described mathematically as pressure equals flow multiplied by resistance ($P = F \times R$).

Blood Flow

Blood flow is essentially equal to cardiac output. Cardiac output is the product of stroke volume (the amount of blood pumped from each ventricle with each heartbeat) and heart rate. A stroke volume of 70 mL and a heart rate of 72 beats per minute results in a cardiac output of 5,040 mL/min, or about 5 L/min. Average cardiac output in a resting man is 5.5 L/min (Ganong, 1993).

Decreased stroke volume due to poor cardiac pumping (as occurs with a failing heart) or reduced blood volume (as in severe hemorrhage) may result in decreased cardiac output. Bradycardia also may cause decreased cardiac output. Conversely, a rapid heart rate and larger stroke volumes would be expected to increase cardiac output. The magnitude of change in cardiac output created by increases or decreases in one of the factors (heart rate or stroke volume) is influenced by the concurrent response of the other factor. For example, if stroke volume falls to 40 mL, the cardiac output stays in the normal range if the heart rate simultaneously increases to 100 beats per minute ($40 \times 100 =$ 4,000 mL, or 4 L). A person with a heart rate of 50 beats per minute can maintain a normal cardiac output only if the stroke volume is 80 mL or more ($50 \times 80 = 4{,}000$ mL or 4 L). An increase in heart rate in response to a decrease in stroke volume to maintain a normal cardiac output is an example of a compensatory response.

Resistance

Resistance to blood flow is caused by the friction among the cells and other blood components and be-

Procedure 22-4
Assessing Respirations

Purpose

1. Assess respiratory status by evaluating rate and quality.
2. Evaluate the influence of medications and therapies on respiration.

Assessment

- Identify risk factors for altered respiratory status (chest trauma, respiratory disease, smoking history, respiratory depressant medications).
- Assess for physical signs and symptoms of altered respiratory status (cyanosis, clubbed fingers, reduced level of consciousness, pain during inspiration, dyspnea, coughing).
- Review pertinent laboratory studies (arterial blood gases, oxygen saturation, complete blood count).
- Determine baseline respiratory rate.

Equipment

Watch with second hand
Vital signs documentation sheet and pen

Procedure

1. After assessment of pulse, keep your fingers resting on client's wrist and observe or feel the rising and falling of chest with respiration. If client is asleep, you may gently place hand on chest so you can feel chest movement. *Do not* explain procedure to client.
   Rationale: Explaining procedure may make client self-conscious about respirations and could cause him or her to alter respiratory pattern.
2. When one complete cycle of inspiration and expiration has been observed, look at second hand of watch and count the number of complete cycles. If rate is regular in an adult, count 30 seconds and multiply by two. In children younger than 2 years or in adults with an irregular rate, count for 1 full minute.

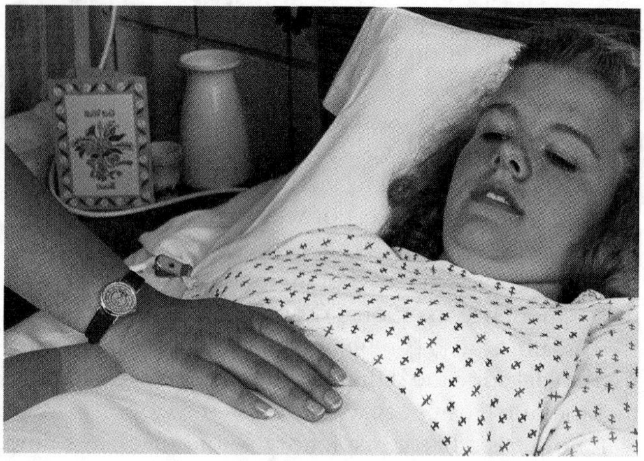

Step 1 • Assessing respirations while asleep (© B. Proud)

   Rationale: Children normally have irregular respiratory patterns.
3. If respirations are shallow and difficult to count, observe at the sternal notch.
   Rationale: Respirations are more visible at the sternal notch.
4. Note depth and rhythm of respiratory cycle.
   Rationale: Respiratory characteristics give additional data about alterations in respiratory status.
5. Discuss findings with client, if applicable.
6. Document respiratory rate, depth, rhythm, and character.

Lifespan Considerations

Infants and Children

- A crying child's respiratory rate cannot be accurately assessed. Count respirations when the child is sleeping, if possible. If the child is crying, attempt to quiet him or her before assessing respirations. If the child cannot be quieted, write "crying" on the vital signs documentation sheet.

tween the blood and the vessel walls. The friction within the blood components reflects the viscosity of the blood and is largely due to the number and shape of the blood cells. Normally, the number and type of blood constituents do not vary greatly, and viscosity is a constant factor when determining resistance.

Friction between the blood and the vessel walls varies with the dimensions of the vessel lumen. The most important luminal dimension is the diameter (Guyton, 1992). The diameter of the blood vessel is controlled by contraction and relaxation of the smooth muscle in the vessel walls.

Factors Affecting Blood Pressure

Age. Blood pressure gradually increases throughout childhood and correlates with height, weight, and age. This makes it difficult to identify abnormal blood pressure levels for children at various developmental stages, but it has been proposed that a diastolic pressure consistently above the 95th percentile for age indicates a need for diagnostic evaluation (Pruitt, 1987).

In adults, there is a trend toward gradually increasing systolic and diastolic blood pressure with aging. In part, this trend is due to increased systemic vascular resistance, reflecting arterial narrowing and decreased vessel elasticity due to atherosclerotic vessel disease. The increase in systolic blood pressure is proportionally greater than the increase in diastolic blood pressure; therefore, pulse pressure widens. Normal blood pressures for various age groups are shown in Table 22-1.

Autonomic Nervous System. The autonomic nervous system influences heart rate, cardiac contractility, systemic vascular resistance, and blood volume. Increased sympathetic nervous system activity results in increased heart rate, stronger contraction of heart muscle, changes in vascular smooth muscle tone, and increased blood volume due to retention of water and sodium. The cumulative effect is increased blood pressure. Therefore, factors that enhance sympathetic nervous system activity (such as pain, anxiety, fear, smoking, and exercise) result in increased blood pressure readings.

Exceptions occur when sympathetic nervous activity cannot keep up with a stressor. An example is a client with severely diminished blood volume resulting from hemorrhage. The sympathetic nervous system is activated to maintain adequate blood pressure, but this may not be enough to compensate for the volume loss. Measured blood pressure may be quite low, although sympathetic nervous system activity is markedly increased.

Circulating Volume. A decrease in circulating volume, either from blood loss or fluid loss, results in lower blood pressure. Fluid volume deficit can occur with abnormal, unreplaced losses, such as diarrhea or diaphoresis. Insufficient oral intake also can cause fluid volume deficit. Excess fluid, such as in congestive heart failure, can cause elevated blood pressure readings.

Medications. Any medication that alters one or more of the previously described determining factors may cause a change in blood pressure. Examples are diuretics, which decrease blood volume; cardiac medications, which affect the rate or contractile force of the heart; narcotic analgesics, which reduce pain and sympathetic nervous system activity; and specific antihypertensive agents.

Therapeutic Dialogue
Blood Pressure

Scenes for Thought

Mr. Richards is sitting up in bed with an IV in his left arm and EKG leads attached to his chest. Being careful to use his right arm, you, Cheryl Bianco, prepare to take his blood pressure.

Effective

Nurse: *Hi, Mr. Richards. I'm Cheryl Bianco, and I'll be taking care of you today. How's it going?*
Mr. R.: *Okay, I guess. Are you going to take my blood pressure again? (Looks irritated.)*
Nurse: *Yes, I am. You look irritated about that. Are you? (Exploring her observation.)*
Mr. R.: *Well, yes. I mean, I'm not annoyed at you, but ever since I had the heart attack, people have been taking my pressure every 10 minutes, it seems, and I don't like it. (Stopping to breathe).*
Nurse: *It feels like the staff is focusing on your pressure. (Restating.)*
Mr. R.: *Are they worried? Am I going to have another heart attack? Should I be worried? I'm confused. (Looking upset.)*
Nurse: *It sounds like you're looking for some information. Let's talk about it. (Opportunity to provide information and allay his fears.)*

Less Effective

Nurse: *Hi, Mr. Richards. I'm here to take your blood pressure.*
Mr. R.: *Again? They just took it 20 minutes ago. (Looks irritated.)*
Nurse: *Sure, we have to do that on heart patients. Just let me get this cuff on, and I'll be out of your way in a minute, okay?*
Mr. R.: *I guess so. Everyone else does. (Continues to look annoyed.)*
Nurse: *There, all done. I'll be back to change your bed and get you up in the chair in a little bit.*
Mr. R.: *'Bye. (Sinks back onto the pillows.)*

Critical Thinking Challenge

Analyze the significance of his blood pressure as Mr. Richards sees it. • Detect his feelings regarding the blood pressure readings. • Infer what his thinking might do to all of his vital signs if he is upset about frequent blood pressure readings.

Normal Fluctuations. Blood pressure fluctuates from minute to minute in response to a variety of stimuli. Increased ambient temperature causes blood vessels near the skin surface to dilate, decreasing resistance and blood pressure. Blood pressure also fluctuates with the respiratory cycle, increasing during expiration and decreasing during inspiration.

In addition to minute-to-minute fluctuations, there is a discernible circadian pattern to blood pressure. Investigators performing direct, continuous monitoring of blood pressure have documented a consistent variation in blood pressure throughout the day. One study revealed a peak pressure at about 10 AM, a plateau through the late afternoon, and a gradual fall in pressure during the night, with lowest pressures recorded at about 3 AM. Blood pressure then gradually rose during the early morning, with a sharp increase between 7 and 10 AM (Pruitt, 1987).

Assessing Blood Pressure

Blood pressure may be measured directly with a catheter placed into an artery. Direct measurement provides a continuous reading of blood pressure and is used in critical-care settings. However, blood pressure is usually measured by indirect methods, using an inflatable cuff to temporarily occlude arterial blood flow through one of the limbs. As the cuff is deflated and flow returns, the blood pressure can be determined by palpation, auscultation, or oscillations. Table 22-5 summarizes potential sources of error in blood pressure measurement. Procedure 22-5 gives detailed instructions for measuring blood pressure.

Sites

Upper Extremity. The blood pressure is usually measured in the arm with a cuff wrapped around the upper part of the limb and the flow auscultated or palpated at the brachial artery. Blood pressure also may be determined by auscultation or palpation of the radial artery in the wrist with an appropriate-sized cuff applied to the forearm.

Lower Extremity. The cuff may be wrapped around the thigh or above the ankle. Thigh pressure measurement requires a larger cuff. The client is placed in a flat, prone, or supine position with the cuff centered midthigh over the popliteal artery. Blood flow is auscultated or palpated at the popliteal fossa. A systolic blood pressure measured in the thigh is generally 20 to 30 mm Hg higher than that measured in the arm (Perloff, et al., 1993). To measure blood pressure in the ankle, the client is placed in a flat, supine position, and a standard arm cuff is placed just above the malleolus. The posterior tibialis or dorsalis pedis pulse may be auscultated or palpated as the cuff is deflated.

Equipment

Sphygmomanometer. A sphygmomanometer consists of an inflatable bladder enclosed in a nondistensible cuff. The bladder is connected to an inflating mechanism, such as a bulb or pump, a valve for deflation, and a manometer (Fig. 22-6). The manometer may be a gravity mercury or aneroid type.

Mercury manometers consist of a vertical glass tube marked in 2-mm increments. Cuff pressures are transmitted through the tubing into the manometer and force the mercury to rise in the glass tube. The surface tension of the mercury in the tube causes the top of the mercury column to be curved. The pressure reading is made from the top point of the curved surface, or meniscus, of the mercury. The manometer must be at eye level to ensure an accurate reading. Particulate matter or air bubbles in the glass tube distort readings. Enough mercury must be present in the reservoir to maintain the meniscus at zero with the cuff deflated. The air vent at the top of the glass tube must be clean and allow free passage of air, or the mercury will be unable to rise and fall smoothly in the tube.

Aneroid manometers have a circular gauge marked in 2-mm increments. The pressure transmitted from the cuff causes movement of a metal bellows within the manometer, and this movement is indicated by a needle on the gauge. Aneroid manometers require yearly calibration with a properly functioning mercury manometer or other pressure standard. Checks of manometer function should be made throughout the range of pressure measurement to ensure the device's accuracy. Aneroid manometers with a stop peg at the zero point or an external reset are not recommended,

text continues on page 448

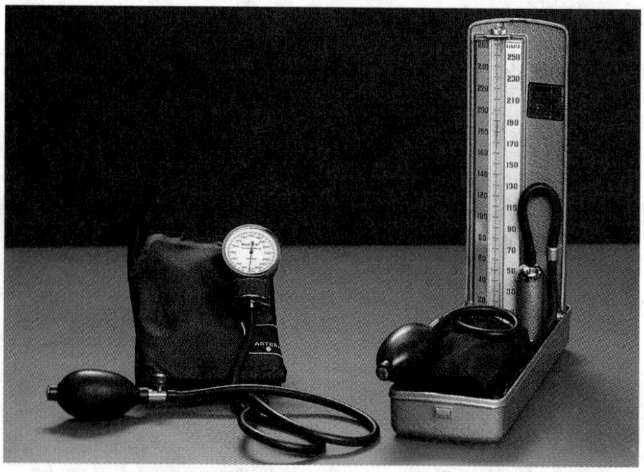

Figure 22-6 • *Sphygmomanometers. Left, aneroid; right, mercury.*

Table 22-5 • Potential Errors in Blood Pressure Measurement

Error	Cause	Recommendation
Falsely low readings	Environmental noise	Turn down TV or radio; stop talking; avoid moving stethoscope or tubing.
	Hearing deficit	Use hearing-amplified stethoscope or hearing aid.
	Ear pieces fitting poorly	Angle ear pieces forward to fit snugly into ear canal.
	Stethoscope tubing too long	Shorten tubing to 30–38 cm (12–15 in).
	Viewing meniscus from above eye level	Place meniscus at eye level.
	Failing to pump cuff up high enough	Palpate systolic pressure to avoid missing auscultatory gap.
	Cuff too wide	Measure arm circumference; bladder should be 80% of arm circumference.
	Arm above heart level	Reposition arm at level of heart, generally fourth intercostal space.
	Releasing valve too rapidly	Practice slow release of 2 mm Hg per second.
	Reading taken at inspiration (in selected high-risk clients, COPD, pulmonary embolus, hypovolemic shock)	Consistently try to record BP at end expiration.
Falsely high readings	Measuring BP when a client has just eaten, is in pain, is anxious, or has a full bladder	Try to assess BP during basal state, or adjust interpretation accordingly.
	Cold hands or stethoscope	Warm hands and stethoscope prior to measuring BP
	Viewing meniscus from below eye level	View meniscus from eye level.
	Cuff too narrow	Measure arm circumference; bladder should be 80% of arm circumference.
	Wrapping cuff unevenly or loosely	Rewrap cuff snugly.
	Deflating cuff too slowly	Practice steady deflation of cuff at 2 mm Hg per second.
	Venous congestion	Wait 2 min before reinflating cuff to retake BP; elevate arm to promote redistribution of blood.
	Unsupported arm	Support arm on table to prevent muscle contraction.
	Back unsupported, legs dangling	Provide support for legs and back.
	Arm below heart level	Reposition arm at heart level, usually at the 4th intercostal space.
Inaccurate readings	Meniscus or needle not at zero	Recalibrate or service.
	Faulty valves or leaky tubing	Replace equipment.
	Examiner digit preference	Do not round up or down.
	Forgetting measurement	Record immediately in the room.

Procedure 22-5
Obtaining Blood Pressure

Purpose

1. Evaluate the client's hemodynamic status by obtaining information about cardiac output, blood volume, peripheral vascular resistance, and arterial wall elasticity.
2. Obtain baseline measurement of blood pressure
3. Monitor the hemodynamic response to various therapies or disease conditions.

Assessment

- Assess blood pressure on initial client examination and whenever status changes.
- Identify factors that may alter blood pressure (medications, exercise, age, emotional conditions, smoking, postural changes).
- Assess best site for obtaining blood pressure.
- Review previous blood pressure readings, if available.

Equipment

Stethoscope
Sphygmomanometer with bladder and cuff
Documentation record and pen

Procedure

1. Wash hands; explain procedure to client; assist client to a comfortable position with forearm supported at heart level and palm up.
   Rationale: Variations in blood pressure can occur with client in different positions. Blood pressure increases when the arm is below heart level and decreases when above heart level. Diastolic blood pressure may increase 10% if arm is unsupported, secondary to isometric exercises used to support arm.
2. Expose the upper arm completely.
   Rationale: Accurate placement of cuff and stethoscope requires complete exposure of upper arm.
3. Wrap deflated cuff snugly around upper arm with center of bladder over brachial artery. Lower border of cuff should be about 2 cm above antecubital space (nearer the antecubital space on an infant).
   Rationale: Placing bladder directly over brachial artery ensures proper compression of artery during cuff inflation. Loose or uneven application can result in falsely high readings.
4. If using a mercury manometer, the manometer should be vertical and at eye level.
   Rationale: Prevents distortion and promotes accurate reading of mercury level.

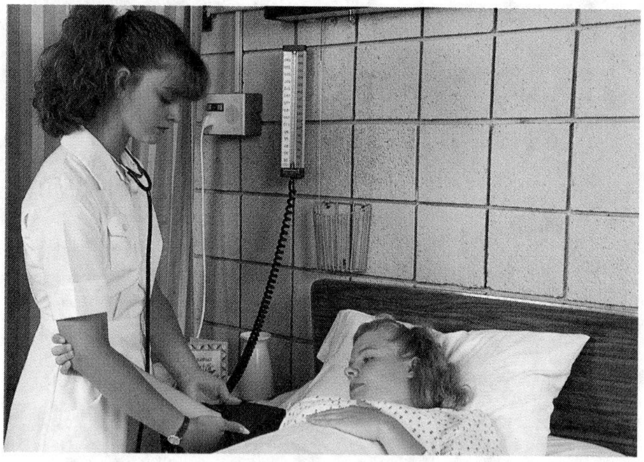

Step 3 • Snugly wrap cuff around upper arm (© B. Proud)

5. Palpate brachial or radial artery with fingertips. Close valve on pressure bulb and inflate cuff until pulse disappears. Inflate cuff 30 mm Hg higher. Slowly release valve and note reading when pulse reappears.
   Rationale: Identifies approximate systolic blood pressure reading, to prevent underestimating systolic blood pressure should client have an auscultatory gap.

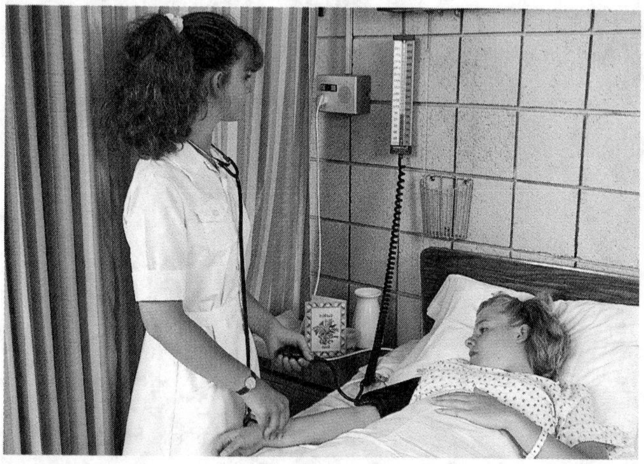

Step 5 • Palpate radial pulse to estimate systolic blood pressure (© B. Proud)

6. Fully deflate cuff, and wait 1 to 2 minutes.
   Rationale: Waiting period prevents falsely high readings by allowing blood trapped in the vein to be recirculated.
7. Place stethoscope ear piece in ears. Repalpate the brachial artery and place stethoscope diaphragm or bell over site.

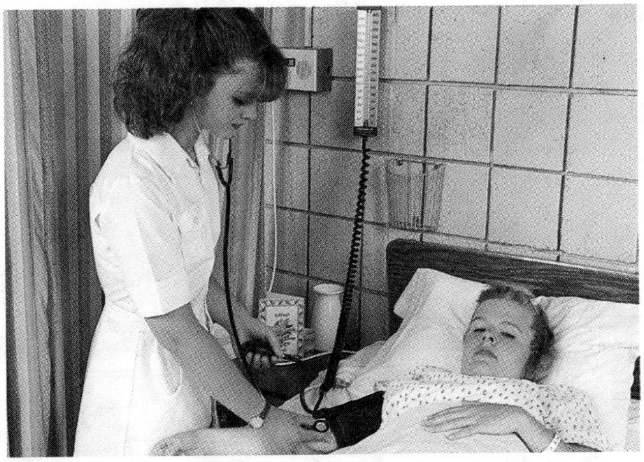

Step 7 • Place stethoscope over brachial artery and inflate cuff (© B. Proud)

Rationale: Blood pressure is a low-frequency sound and is best heard with the stethoscope bell, but the diaphragm is widely used because it is easily placed and more generally available.

8. Close bulb valve by turning clockwise. Inflate cuff to 30 mm Hg above reading where brachial pulse disappeared.
   Rationale: Ensures accurate assessment of systolic blood pressure.
9. Slowly release valve so pressure drops about 2 to 3 mm Hg per second.
   Rationale: Inaccurate measurements may occur if deflation rate is too fast or too slow.
10. Identify manometer reading when first clear Korotkoff sound is heard.
    Rationale: Indicates systolic pressure reading.
11. Continue to deflate, and note reading when sound muffles or dampens (fourth Korotkoff) and when it disappears (fifth Korotkoff).
    Rationale: American Heart Association recommends using the fifth Korotkoff sound as diastolic pressure in adults, fourth Korotkoff in children. In adults, if fourth and fifth Korotkoff are 10 mm Hg or greater apart, note all three readings.

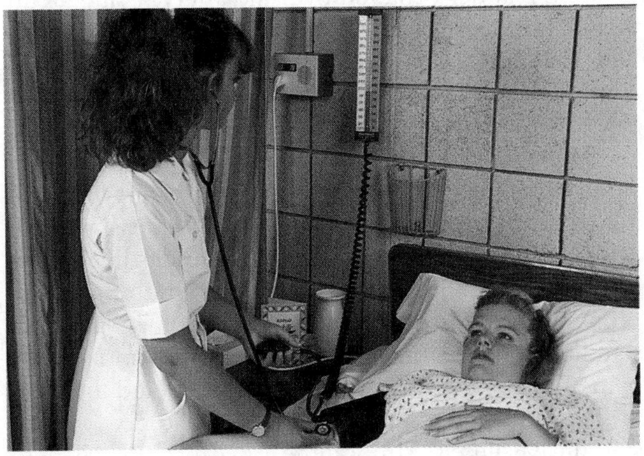

Steps 10 & 11 • Slowly release valve and note systolic and diastolic pressure readings (© B. Proud)

12. Deflate cuff completely, and remove from client's arm.
13. Record blood pressure. Record systolic (eg, 130) and diastolic (eg, 80) in the form 130/80. *Note: If three pressures are to be recorded, use the form 130/80/40 (40 is the fifth Korotkoff). Abbreviate RA or LA to indicate right or left arm measurement.*
14. Assist client to comfortable position, and discuss findings with client, if appropriate.
    Rationale: Encourages client understanding of health status and promotes compliance with therapies.

Lifespan Considerations

Infants and Children

- Selection of proper-sized cuff and bladder is important for obtaining accurate blood pressure measurements in children and adults. The bladder width should be 40% of the circumference of the limb.
- In infants, Korotkoff sounds may be too faint for accurate measurement. Accurate assessment of systolic pressure can be obtained using a Doppler ultrasonic device. Flush method may be used to estimate mean blood pressure.
- When blood pressure is monitored in children, take respirations and pulse rate first, because they are less invasive and least likely to cause the child anxiety. Temperature should be the last vital sign measured because it is the most invasive.

Older Adults

- Adults with hypertension are prone to auscultatory gaps in blood pressure. Estimation of systolic pressure using the brachial artery palpation technique will prevent inaccurate readings secondary to auscultatory gap.
- Diastolic pressure often increases with age as a result of decreased compliance of the arteries.

Home Care Modifications

- Clients with hypertension may be taught to monitor their blood pressure at home.
- A variety of monitors for home use are available. They include digital printouts with time and date for accurate record-keeping.
- Teach the client:
  - To avoid caffeinated beverages, smoking, and exercise for 30 minutes before measurement
  - To use the same arm and body position for each measurement
  - At what measurements the client should alert the nurse or physician.

because it is impossible to verify the accuracy of the manometer.

The tubing and hand bulb must be free of cracks or holes, and connections must be airtight to prevent leaks that cause poor transmission of pressure. The deflation valve must function smoothly to allow the operator to control the rate of deflation.

Stethoscope. A stethoscope is necessary for the auscultatory method of blood pressure measurement. The stethoscope should have snugly fitting ear pieces and thick-walled tubing about 12 in long for optimal sound transmission. The stethoscope should be equipped with a bell and a diaphragm.

Doppler. The Doppler method is useful during low flow states or when the blood pressure is difficult to auscultate by stethoscope. The method involves the use of an ultrasonic device that transmits and receives high-frequency sound waves (Fig. 22-7). A standard cuff is used to occlude an artery while the ultrasound transducer is placed over the artery distal to the site of occlusion. Arterial wall motion creates Doppler shifts in the ultrasonic frequency, which are received and amplified by the ultrasound unit. Systolic blood pressure is the point at which continuous pulsatile flow is heard. Diastolic blood pressure may be difficult to identify reliably with the Doppler but is considered the point at which continuous flow is heard.

Electronic Devices. Automated devices are frequently used to monitor blood pressure indirectly during anesthesia, in the critical-care area, postoperatively, or in ambulatory settings when frequent assessments are necessary. The electronic units determine blood pressure by analyzing the sounds of blood flow or measuring oscillations. In either case, a cuff attached to the machine is automatically inflated to occlude the artery. The sounds of blood flow are detected by a microphone in the cuff. Oscillatory devices measure blood pressure by microcomputer analysis of oscillations (the amplitude of the pulsations) transmitted from the artery to the cuff. Although absolute values detected with automatic cuffs may vary slightly, the overall trend in blood pressure can be safely monitored (Perloff, et al., 1993). Systolic, diastolic, and mean arterial blood pressure and heart rate are displayed on the monitor (Fig. 22-8). The machine can be set to record these values automatically at a preset interval (eg, every 15 minutes). The data obtained are stored in the machine and can be easily retrieved as needed.

Methods

Baseline blood pressure ideally is measured with the client in a resting state. Therefore, the client should be in a warm, quiet environment and at least 1/2 hour should elapse after smoking, exercising, or eating. Sometimes blood pressure must be measured when the client is anxious or in pain, but the readings may differ from those made if the client were in a basal state.

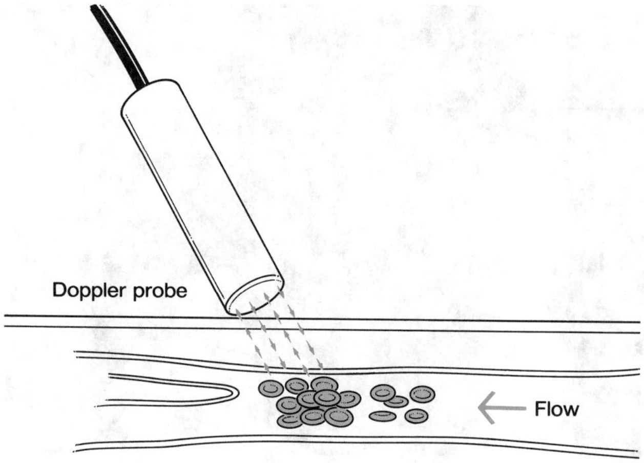

Figure 22-7 • *Doppler sound generation. The transmitting crystal emits an ultrasound beam through the skin to a vessel and moving red blood cells. The red cells reflect the ultrasound beam to the receiving crystal. (Adapted from Durbin, N. (1983). The application of Doppler techniques in critical care.* Focus on Critical Care, 1010*(3), 44–46.)*

Proper Cuff Size. The American Heart Association has made specific recommendations about cuff size and application (Table 22-6). Using an inappropriate size or placement may lead to an erroneous reading. This is a common error; one study documented that "miscuffing" occurred in 32% of blood pressure measurements (Manning, Kucherirka, & Kaminiski, 1983).

Cuff size is based on the circumference of the limb being used. The width of the cuff bladder should be 40% of the circumference of the midpoint of the limb. An average adult arm requires a bladder 12 to 14 cm wide. The bladder length should be 80% of the limb circumference, or about twice the bladder width.

The cuff should be applied snugly around the limb, with the bladder centered over the artery. Using a cuff that is too small or loosely applied results in spuriously high readings. Using a cuff that is too large results in spuriously low readings.

Proper Positioning. Blood pressure should be measured with the arm at heart level. Elevating the arm above heart level results in a falsely low measurement; positioning the arm below heart level results in a falsely high reading. When the client is flat, the arm is approximately at heart level. If the client is sitting or standing, the forearm should be supported horizontally at the level of the heart (generally considered the level of the fourth intercostal space, where the ribs join the sternum). Failure to support the arm causes the client to contract the arm muscles, elevating the blood pressure.

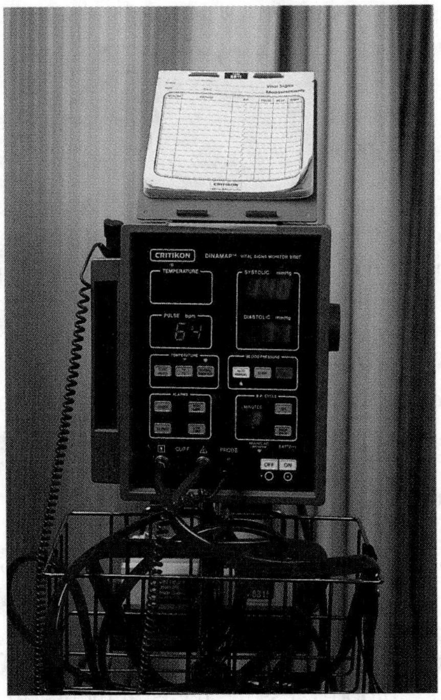

Figure 22-8 • Automated monitors measure blood pressure and heart rate. They can be set to record these values at certain intervals, and the information is stored for later retrieval.

Correlation with the Respiratory Cycle. The intrathoracic pressure changes that occur during a normal respiratory cycle affect the heart and great vessels. Consequently, blood pressure is lower during inspiration than expiration. Exaggerated decreases in systolic blood pressure with inspiration (called pulsus paradoxus or **paradoxical blood pressure**) occur in diseases such as cardiac tamponade, constrictive pericarditis, emphysema, hypovolemic shock, and pulmonary embolus (Braunwald, 1988). Consistently measuring blood pressure at end expiration eliminates variability of readings due to respiratory changes.

Proper Inflation and Deflation. An inflated cuff reduces venous blood return to the heart in the extremity. Increased venous pressures are transmitted back to the arterial side of the circuit, and arterial pressures are transiently elevated. Slow, prolonged, or frequent cuff inflation promotes venous congestion. The cuff should be inflated rapidly when taking a reading and deflated completely after measurement. At least 2 minutes should elapse before sequential cuff inflation on any one limb. Elevating the arm above the head between cuff measurements speeds venous return to the heart.

Auscultation. When the blood pressure is determined by the auscultatory method, an inflatable cuff is used to occlude flow through a limb temporarily. As the cuff is deflated and blood flow returns, the **Korotkoff sounds** can be heard with a stethoscope placed over the artery. Five distinct phases are identifiable, as shown in Figure 22-9 and Table 22-7. The onset of the Korotkoff sounds of phase I is the recorded systolic pressure. Diastolic pressure is indicated by the onset of phase V sounds in adults and phase IV sounds in children.

Because the Korotkoff sounds are low in frequency, the bell of the stethoscope is best used for auscultation, although most practitioners use the diaphragm because of its larger shape and ease of placement (Perloff, et al., 1993). If the sounds are inaudible with the diaphragm, the nurse can try the stethoscope bell. The head of the stethoscope must not be pressed too firmly against the skin, because this may partially occlude blood flow and alter the reading.

An **auscultatory gap** is the absence of Korotkoff sounds between phases I and II (Nelson & Egbert, 1984). Failure to identify an auscultatory gap may result in underestimation of the systolic blood pressure or overestimation of the diastolic pressure. An auscultatory gap can be detected by palpating the brachial or radial pulse while inflating the cuff. The cuff should be inflated about 30 mm Hg above the number where palpable pulsation disappears. In addition to detecting an auscultatory gap, palpation gives an initial estimate of systolic blood pressure and eliminates the need to inflate the cuff to extremely high pressures in people with normal or low blood pressure. When an auscultatory gap is detected, the systolic and diastolic pressures are recorded as usual, and the magnitude and range of the auscultatory gap are noted (eg, 196/90; auscultatory gap from 184 to 150).

Table 22-6 • Acceptable Bladder Dimensions (in cm) for Arms of Different Sizes*

Cuff	Bladder Width (cm)	Bladder Length (cm)	Arm Circumference Range at Midpoint (cm)
Newborn	3	6	≤6
Infant	5	15	6–15†
Child	8	21	16–21†
Small adult	10	24	22–26
Adult	13	30	27–34
Large adult	16	38	34–44
Adult thigh	20	42	45–52

*There is some overlapping of the recommended range for arm circumferences in order to limit the number of cuffs; it is recommended that the larger cuff be used when available.

†To approximate the bladder width:arm circumference ratio of 0.40 more closely in infants and children, additional cuffs are available.

From Perloff, D. et al. (1993). Human blood pressure determination by sphygmamonometry. American Heart Association in *Circulation 885*, Part I, p. 2469.

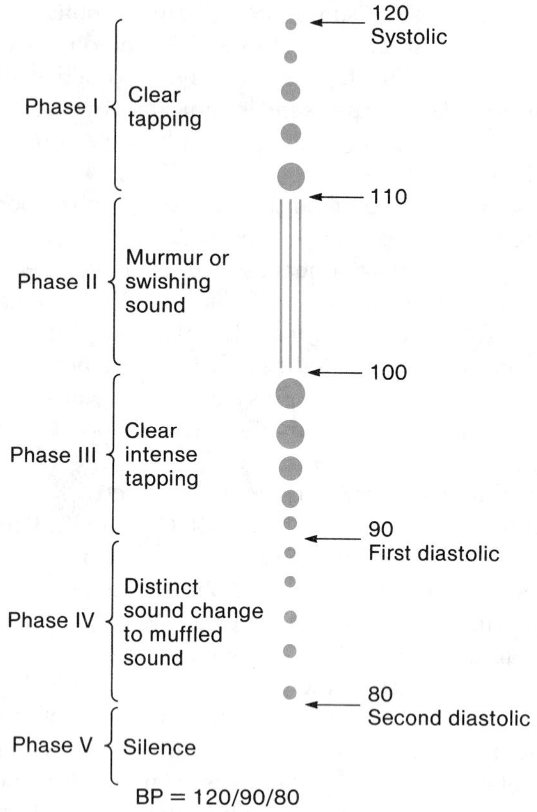

Figure 22-9 • *Korotkoff sounds.*

Palpation. When Korotkoff sounds are inaudible, blood pressure may be estimated by palpation. The cuff is applied and inflated as previously described and the brachial or radial artery palpated during cuff deflation. Systolic blood pressure is the point at which pulsation returns. Diastolic blood pressure is difficult to determine reliably with palpation but is indicated by a snap or whipping palpable vibrations. Palpated blood pressure is usually recorded as a systolic reading over "P" for palpated (eg, 110/P).

Table 22-7 • *Korotkoff Sounds*

Phase	Description	Recording
I	Initiated by the onset of faint, clear tapping sounds of gradually increasing intensity	Recorded as systolic pressure
II	Sound has a swishing quality	
III	Marked by crisper, more intense sounds	
IV	Characterized by muffled, blowing sounds	Recorded as diastolic pressure in children
V	Absence of sound	Recorded as diastolic pressure in adults

Abnormalities

Hypertension. **Hypertension** is the condition in which blood pressure is chronically higher than normal. Although the natural trend in industrialized societies is for increased blood pressure with aging, hypertension is a dangerous disease associated with increased risk of morbidity and mortality. Therefore, adults of any age with blood pressure above 140/90 mm Hg should be evaluated for hypertension. Hypertension is diagnosed on serial elevated values rather than a single measurement. Studies have shown that some clients demonstrate higher recorded blood pressure in the physician's office than in the home setting. Ambulatory blood pressure measurements refer to blood pressure values obtained away from the medical environment while the individual is engaged in normal activity (Perloff, 1993). Ambulatory blood pressure measurements are helpful to diagnose accurately and treat hypertension. Hypertension is covered in greater detail in Chapter 35.

Hypotension. **Hypotension** is blood pressure below 100/60. Low blood pressure readings can be normal for some healthy, young adults and are no cause for concern. A sudden drop in blood pressure, significantly below the normal range for an individual, causes an individual to experience hypotension. For example, a hypertensive client who usually has blood pressure readings of 180/94 would be considered hypotensive if the blood pressure fell to 120/80. Once again, a significant change from baseline values is more important than any one specific measurement.

Orthostatic Hypotension. In an adult, moving from a flat, horizontal position to a vertical position results in pooling of blood in the lower extremities. People with a healthy, intact autonomic nervous system reflexively compensate for the volume shift by increasing the rate and force of myocardial contraction and vasoconstriction, thus maintaining adequate blood pressure. Even with normal compensation, however, systolic blood pressure usually falls and heart rate increases with a position change.

Inadequate reflex compensation to position change results in **orthostatic hypotension.** Symptoms of orthostatic hypotension are those of decreased cerebral perfusion such as dizziness, weakness, blurred vision, syncope, and marked changes in blood pressure and heart rate. Orthostatic blood pressure changes may indicate failure of autonomic nervous system protective reflexes or hypovolemia. Hypovolemia or impaired vasoconstriction is signaled by decreased blood pressure and increased heart rate. Autonomic nervous sys-

Nursing Research
Vital Signs

Selected Nursing Research Studies

Bogan, B., et al. (1993). Nursing student compliance to standards for blood pressure measurement. *Journal of Nurse Educator, 32*(2), 90–92.

Cole, F. (1993). Temporal variations in the effects of iced water on oral temperature. *Research in Nursing and Health, 16*(3), 107–112.

Derrico, D. (1993). Comparison of blood pressure measurement methods in critically ill children. *DDCN, 12*(1), 31–39.

Erickson, R. & Meyer, L. (1993). Accuracy of infrared ear thermometry and other temperature methods in adults. *American Journal of Critical Care, 3*(1), 40–54.

Hollerbach, A., & Sneed, N. (1990). Accuracy of radial pulse assessment by length of counting interval. *Heart and Lung, 19*(3), 258–264.

Selfridge J, et al. (1993). The accuracy of the tympanic membrane thermometer in detecting fever in infants three months and younger in the emergency department setting. *Journal of Emergency Nursing, 19*(2), 127–130.

Possible Topics for Nursing Inquiry

- In clients who have no rectums, are temperatures obtained from the stoma accurate?
- What constitutes significant changes in systolic and diastolic blood pressure and heart rate when a client moves from a supine to a sitting position?
- How often do nurses use the palpation method for determining auscultatory gap when monitoring blood pressure in acute-care settings?
- What is the validity and accuracy of respiratory rate measurement in a typical acute-care setting?
- What is the effect of eating versus fasting on pulse rate?
- Is taking an apical pulse for 1 full minute more reliable for accurately measuring pulse rate when an irregularity of rhythm is noted?

tem dysfunction is indicated by decreased blood pressure without marked increases in heart rate (Skov & Underhill-Motzer, 1995). Orthostatic hypotension is a drop in systolic pressure of at least 25 mm Hg or a drop in diastolic pressure of at least 10 mm Hg (Skov & Underhill-Motzer, 1995).

The person experiencing postural hypotension is at risk for falling. Therefore, checking postural vital signs is one way of screening to ensure client safety. Clients with chronic orthostatic hypotension should be instructed to change positions slowly, moving from a lying to a sitting to a standing posture and allowing several minutes to elapse before proceeding to the next position.

Orthostatic blood pressure should be measured in clients exhibiting symptoms of dizziness, blurred vision, or weakness when changing position; clients taking diuretic medications; and those with a history of volume loss. Systematic, consistent technique in assessing blood pressure and heart rate response to position change provides the best data for determining and monitoring therapy. Procedure 22-6 gives a step-by-step description for assessing for orthostatic hypotension.

The initial measurement of blood pressure and heart rate is made with the client in a flat, supine position. The client should remain in this position for at least 10 minutes before the nurse measures the blood pressure and heart rate. The cuff is then left in place, and the client is assisted to a sitting position with his or her legs dangling over the side of the bed or examining table. Two minutes should elapse before the second measurement of blood pressure and heart rate. The client should be asked whether any symptoms of dizziness, lightheadedness, dimming of vision, or weakness are present. The client is assisted to a standing position, and after 2 minutes, blood pressure and heart rate are measured. Again, the client is asked to report symptoms of decreased cerebral perfusion.

Clients experiencing severe orthostatic hypotension may be unable to tolerate a standing position long enough for the nurse to obtain the blood pressure and heart rate. If the client becomes severely symptomatic while standing, he or she should return to bed without completing the measurements.

The blood pressure and heart rate values and the position of the client when the values were obtained are recorded. Any symptoms of diminished cerebral perfusion are documented.

Lifespan Considerations

Knowledge of developmental considerations is important for the nurse who is measuring and interpreting vital signs. Normal ranges for the vital signs across the lifespan are summarized in Table 22-1.

Newborn and Infant

Temperature, pulse, and respirations fluctuate widely in newborns. Thermoregulatory mechanisms are immature in newborns, and ambient temperature may markedly affect their body temperature. Pulse and respiration increase rapidly above resting values when a newborn is active, crying, or startled. The apical pulse is the most reliable method of assessing heart rate, because peripheral pulses are faint and difficult to palpate and accurately count. Healthy newborns may exhibit periodic

Procedure 22-6 Assessing for Orthostatic Hypotension

Purpose

1. Assess the compensatory status of the cardiovascular and autonomic nervous systems to changes in body position.

Assessment

- Identify clients at risk for postural drops in blood pressure:
  - History of volume depletion
  - Inadequate vasoconstrictor mechanisms secondary to prolonged bed rest
  - Autonomic insufficiency secondary to spinal cord injury or drugs (digoxin, beta-adrenergic blockers, calcium channel blockers)
- Assess client for complaint of dizziness or lightheadedness during position changes.
- Review serum electrolytes, if available, for imbalances.
- Review baseline blood pressure measurements, if available.

Equipment

Stethoscope
Sphygmomanometer
Watch or clock with second hand
Vital sign documentation record and pen

Procedure

1. Wash hands. Explain procedure to client.
2. Position client supine with head of bed flat for 10 minutes.
   Rationale: To allow blood pooled in lower extremities to reenter circulation.
3. Check and record supine blood pressure and pulse. Keep blood pressure cuff attached.
   Rationale: Provides baseline information with which to compare measurements after position changes. Pulse rate is assessed to help differentiate the cause of postural hypotension. During position changes, if pulse rate rises as blood pressure falls, secondary to sympathetic stimulation, the cause may be volume depletion. If the pulse does not increase when the blood pressure falls, the cause may be related to the lack of sympathetic response.
4. Assist client to a sitting position with legs dangling over the edge of the bed. Wait 2 minutes, and check blood pressure and pulse rate.

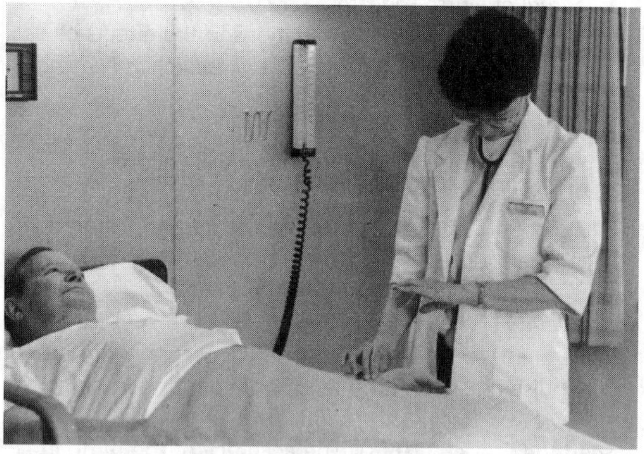

Step 3 • Obtain blood pressure and pulse in supine position

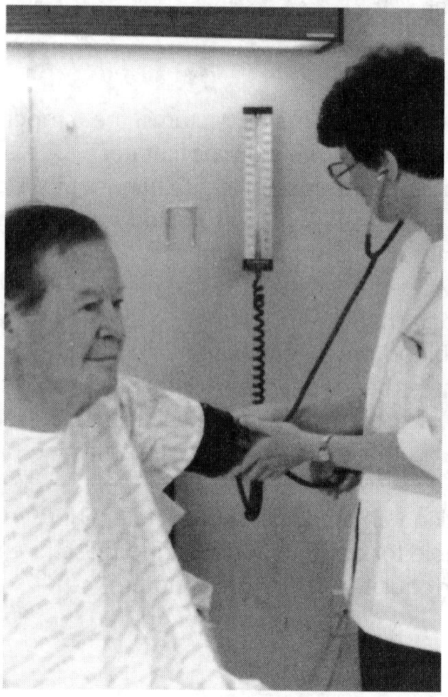

Step 4 • Obtain blood pressure and pulse in sitting position with legs dangling over bed

   Note: The waiting period is a convenient time to auscultate the client's lung fields.
   Rationale: 2 minutes provides adequate time for the autonomic nervous system to reflexively compensate for volume shifts in the normal person.
5. Assist client to standing position. Wait 2 minutes and check blood pressure and pulse rate. Be alert to signs and symptoms of dizziness.

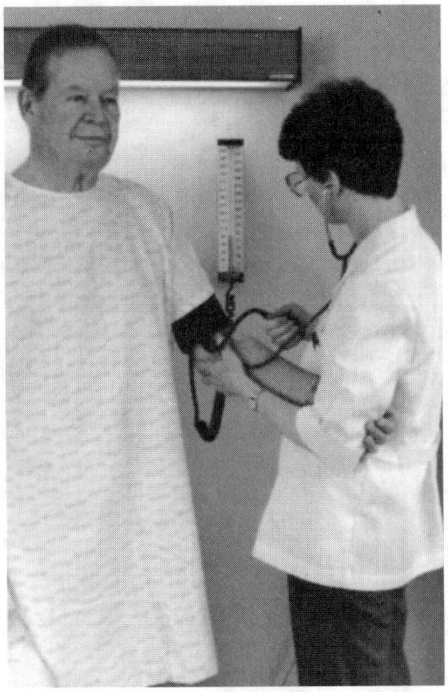

Step 5 • Obtain blood pressure and pulse in standing position

Rationale: If blood pressure drops significantly, the client may become lightheaded and may need to be returned to bed before test completion.

6. Assist the client back to a comfortable position.
7. Record measurements and any symptoms that accompanied the postural change.
   Rationale: A drop of 25 mm Hg in systolic pressure or a drop of 10 mm Hg in diastolic pressure should be reported.

160/92 82
154/90 82
150/86 84

8. Discuss findings with client, if appropriate.
   Rationale: If there is a significant postural blood pressure drop, advise the client to sit on the edge of the bed for several minutes before walking to avoid dizziness and possible falls.

apnea (Nelson, Behrman, & Vaughan, 1987). Blood pressure is not routinely assessed in the newborn or infant because the information obtained is unreliable.

Safety considerations are important when monitoring the vital signs of the newborn or infant. Tympanic or axillary temperatures are preferred, because rectal temperature monitoring can cause mucosal tearing or perforation, and an oral thermometer cannot safely be held in the infant's mouth. Infants move quickly, so it is important to protect them from falling or injury during vital sign monitoring.

Toddler and Preschooler

As a child enters the second year of life, vital signs fluctuate less. The pulse rate decreases to a normal range of 80 to 120 beats per minute, and respirations fall to 22 to 40 breaths per minute. Normal blood pressure ranges from a systolic pressure of 80 to 112 mm Hg over a diastolic pressure of 50 to 80 mm Hg. Blood pressure is routinely monitored after the age of 3 years.

Toddlers and preschoolers may become fearful of procedures involving vital sign measurement, and at this age verbal explanations do little to allay fears. Permitting the child to play with a stethoscope or to push the button on the electronic thermometer may help calm his or her fears. Having the parent hold and talk to the child can be comforting when the child is frightened.

Safety concerns continue to be important in this age group. Temperature should be monitored using the tympanic or axillary route until the child is 4 or 5 years old and can follow directions about holding the thermometer in the sublingual pocket. It is not safe to use an oral glass mercury thermometer in children in this age group, because inadvertently biting down on the thermometer could cause breakage, lacerations, and possibly mercury poisoning.

Child and Adolescent

The broad range of normal values reflects the wide variability in children's vital signs. In general, temperature, pulse, and respirations gradually decrease through childhood, but blood pressure increases and is correlated with height and weight (Nelson, Behrman, & Vaughan, 1992).

Children in this age group are familiar with vital sign assessment and seldom exhibit fear during monitoring. Health teaching about normal values and the reason for taking vital signs helps to educate the child. A child may try to experiment by putting the thermometer under hot water or near a light source, so any unlikely temperature readings should be validated.

Adult and Older Adult

Vital signs usually stabilize during young adulthood. As adults age, the effects of lifestyle and chronic diseases become evident in the vital signs. Respiratory rate and pattern are influenced by chronic respiratory disease and exposure to pollutants, such as cigarette smoke. Cardiovascular diseases may cause changes in the heart rate and rhythm. The incidence of hypertension increases with age: half of all adults older than 64 years have hypertension (Roben, 1993). Conversely, orthostatic hypotension is common in the elderly, although the actual incidence is unclear. It is also uncertain whether

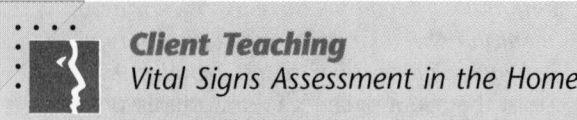

Client Teaching
Vital Signs Assessment in the Home

Instruct the client as follows:

- If you are monitoring your own vital signs, make sure you know and understand normal ranges and when it is important to contact a healthcare professional.
- Keep a chart of specific vital sign measurements so you can show it to your healthcare provider for identifying trends.
- Never leave a small child alone when taking his or her temperature. You may need to hold the child firmly to prevent injury and to obtain an accurate reading.
- Keep the thermometer in the sublingual pocket of the mouth when obtaining an oral temperature.
- When monitoring your pulse, palpate the radial artery for 1 full minute to determine rate and rhythm.
- If you plan to monitor your blood pressure at home, compare various types of monitoring equipment to determine the most cost-effective system for your needs.

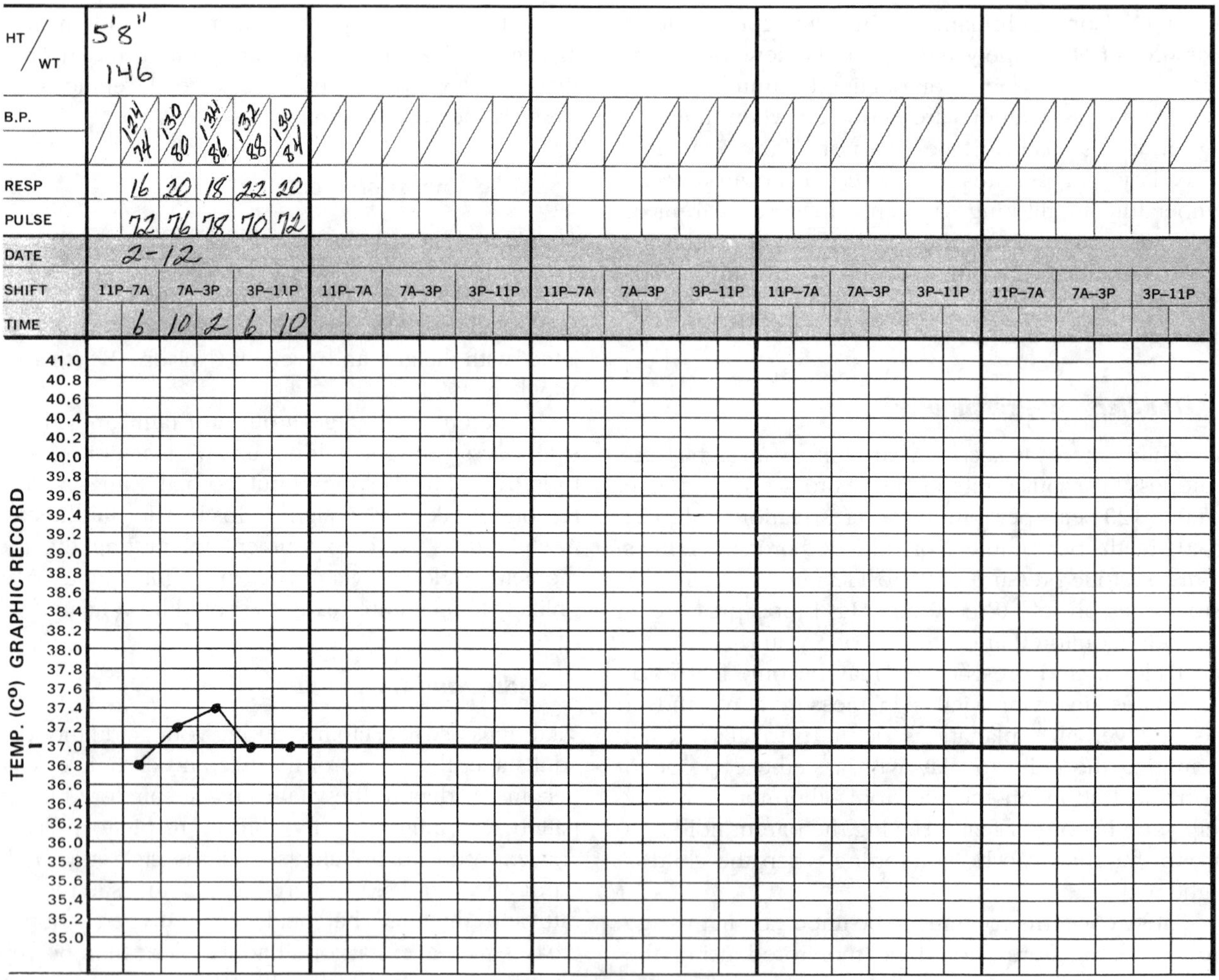
HT / WT
5'8"
146
B.P.
124/74 130/80 134/86 132/88 130/84
RESP
16 20 18 22 20
PULSE
72 76 78 70 72
DATE
2-12
SHIFT
11P–7A 7A–3P 3P–11P
TIME
6 10 2 6 10
TEMP. (C°) GRAPHIC RECORD
41.0 40.8 40.6 40.4 40.2 40.0 39.8 39.6 39.4 39.2 39.0 38.8 38.6 38.4 38.2 38.0 37.8 37.6 37.4 37.2 37.0 36.8 36.6 36.4 36.2 36.0 35.8 35.6 35.4 35.2 35.0

Figure 22-10 • *Vital signs graphic flowsheet.*

orthostatic hypotension occurs as a result of the normal aging process or is seen only in elderly people with existing disease states (Mader, 1989). Older adults also have lower normal ranges for body temperature. Often adults ask the nurse about the values obtained during monitoring. This is an excellent opportunity for client education.

Documenting Vital Signs

The nurse is responsible for documenting the vital signs that have been assessed and reporting any abnormalities to the physician in a timely fashion. Vital signs are often documented in a graph format, with time as the horizontal axis and the measured value as the vertical axis (Fig. 22-10). This allows trends to be seen easily. Trends may reflect normal variations or a change in response to disease or therapy. For example, the normal trend is toward a decreased body temperature in the early morning. If the graph shows increasing values during the night and early morning, this trend may indicate fever and would require further investigation.

Key Concepts

- Temperature, pulse, respirations, and blood pressure are considered the vital signs, because significant deviations from normal ranges are not compatible with life.
- Vital sign assessment is an important nursing function that permits the nurse to detect alterations from normal and evaluate client progress.
- Body temperature can be monitored easily in four sites: oral cavity, ear, rectum, and axilla.
- Factors that can affect body temperature include age, environmental conditions, time of day, exercise, stress, and hormone level.
- Equipment to monitor body temperature includes glass mercury thermometers, electronic thermometers, tympanic membrane thermometers, chemically treated paper thermometers, and temperature-sensitive strips.
- As the heart contracts and ejects blood into the circulation, pulsations can be palpated at various arterial sites in the body.
- Evaluation of the pulse should include rate, rhythm, and quality.
- Factors such as age, autonomic nervous system stimulation, and medications can affect the pulse.
- An irregular pulse should be counted for 1 full minute, preferably at the apical site.
- A pulse deficit occurs when a cardiac contraction creates a pulse wave that is weak and not palpable at peripheral sites.
- Respiratory rate, rhythm, and depth can be altered by age, medications, stress, exercise, altitude, sex, body position, and the presence of a fever.
- Abnormal breathing rates include tachypnea (more than 20 breaths per minute), bradypnea (less than 12 breaths per minute), and apnea (interval of absent respirations).
- Abnormal breathing patterns include Biot's respirations, Kussmaul respirations, and apneustic respirations.
- Blood pressure is a function of the flow of blood produced by the heart and the resistance to blood flow through the vessels.
- Systolic pressure occurs during ventricular contraction, and diastolic pressure occurs during ventricular relaxation. Pulse pressure is the difference between systolic and diastolic pressure.
- Factors that can affect blood pressure include age, autonomic nervous system input, circulating volume, medications, and circadian rhythms.
- Blood pressure is usually measured indirectly using a sphygmomanometer and a stethoscope.
- Auscultation of blood pressure reveals five different phases known as Korotkoff sounds. The first Korotkoff sound corresponds to systolic pressure and the fifth (fourth in children) to diastolic pressure.
- Selecting proper cuff size, keeping the arm at heart level, avoiding venous congestion, and detecting the presence of an auscultatory gap are important steps in obtaining accurate blood pressure readings.
- Orthostatic hypotension occurs when a person experiences a decrease in blood pressure when changing from a supine to an upright position.
- Normal variations in vital signs occur throughout the lifespan.

Critical Thinking Challenges

Now that you have studied this chapter, you should be able to apply what you have learned about the importance of vital sign readings to the situation posed at the beginning of the chapter.

1. *Identify possible interpretations of an isolated blood pressure reading of 168/94, and list factors that may have affected the accuracy of the blood pressure reading.*
2. *Analyze the man's reaction to this situation, and indicate health teaching concerning blood pressure that would be appropriate in this situation.*
3. *Outline possible ways to deal therapeutically with*

the wife's anxiety, describing possible verbal and nonverbal interactions.

References

Bates, B. (1995). *A guide to physical examination and history taking* (6th ed.). Philadelphia: J.B. Lippincott.

Baird, S., White, N., & Basinger, M. (1992). Can you rely on tympanic thermometers? *RN, 55* (8), 48–51.

Braunwald, E. (1988). *Heart disease: A textbook of cardiovascular medicine* (3rd ed.). Philadelphia: W.B. Saunders.

Cole, F. (1993) Temporal variations in the effects of iced water on oral temperature. *Research in Nursing and Health, 16*(2), 107–111.

Chamberlain, J., et al. (1991). Comparison of a tympanic thermometer to rectal and oral thermometers in pediatric emergency department. *Clinical Pediatrics, 30*(4), 24–29.

Darowski, A., Weinberg, J., & Guz, A. (1991). Normal rectal, auditory canal, sublingual, and axillary temperatures in the elderly. *Age-Aging, 20*(2), 113–119.

Dressler, D., Smejkal, C., & Ruffolo, M. (1983). A comparison of oral and rectal temperature measurements in patients receiving oxygen by mask. *Nursing Research, 32,* 373.

Erickson, R., & Meyer, L. (1994). Accuracy of infrared ear thermometry and other temperature methods in adults. *American Journal of Critical Care, (3)*1, 40–54.

Erickson, R. (1980). Oral temperature difference in relation to thermometer and technique. *Nursing Research, 29,* 157.

Ganong, W. F. (1993). *Review of medical physiology* (16th ed.). Los Altos, CA: Lange Medical Publications.

Guyton, A. (1991). *Textbook of medical physiology* (8th ed.). Philadelphia: W.B. Saunders.

Guyton, A. (1992). *Human physiology and mechanisms of disease* (5th ed.). Philadelphia: W.B. Saunders.

Hahn, G. D. (1985). Clinical monitoring in anesthesia: Applied technology in monitoring blood pressure. *AANA Journal, 53,* 149.

Hollerbach, A., & Sneed, N. (1990). Accuracy of radial pulse assessment by length of counting interval. *Heart and Lung, 3*(19), 258.

Kaplan, N. M. (1988). Systemic hypertension: Mechanisms and diagnosis. In E. Braunwald (Ed.), *Heart disease* (3rd ed.). Philadelphia: W.B. Saunders.

Kenney, R., & Fortenberry, J. (1990). Evaluation of an infrared tympanic membrane thermometer in pediatric patients. *Pediatrics, 85*(5) 856.

Lim-Levy, F. (1982). The effect of oxygen inhalation on oral temperature. *Nursing Research, 31,* 150.

Mader, S. L. (1989). Aging and postural hypotension. *Journal of the American Geriatric Society, 37,* 129.

Manning, D. M., Kucherirka, C., & Kaminiski, J. (1983). Miscuffing: Inappropriate blood pressure cuff application. *Circulation, 68,* 763.

McGann, K., Marion, G., Camp, L., & Spangler, J. (1993). The influence of gender and race on mean body temperature in a population of older adults. *Archives of Family Medicine, 2*(12), 1265–1267.

Moore, K. I., & Newton, K. (1986). Orthostatic heart rates and blood pressures in healthy young women and men. *Heart & Lung, 15,* 611.

Nelson, W. E., Behrman, R. E., & Vaughan, V. C. (1992). *Nelson's textbook of pediatrics* (14th ed.). Philadelphia: W.B. Saunders.

Nelson, W. P., & Egbert, A. M. (1984). How to measure blood pressure—accurately. *Primary Cardiology, 10,* 14.

Perloff, D., Grim, C., Flack, J., Frohlich, E., Hill, M., McDonald, M., & Morgenstern, B. (1993). Human blood pressure determination by sphygmomanometry. Circulation, (88)5, 2460–2470.

Pontious, S., Kennedy, A., Chung, K., Burroughs, T., Libby, L., & Vogel, D. (1994). Accuracy and reliability of temperature measurement in the emergency department by instrument and site in children. *Pediatric Nursing, (20)*1, 58–63.

Pransky, S. (1991). The impact of technique and condition of tympanic membrane upon infrared tympanic thermometry. *Clinical Pediatrics, 30*(4), 50–52.

Pruitt, A. W. (1987). Systemic hypertension. In W. E. Nelson, R. E. Behrman, & V. C. Vaughan (Eds.), *Nelson's textbook of pediatrics* (13th ed.). Philadelphia: W.B. Saunders.

Roben, N. (1993). Hypertension. In D. L. Carnevali & M. Patrick (Eds.), *Nursing management for the elderly* (3rd ed.). Philadelphia: J.B. Lippincott.

Robertson, D., & Robertson, R. M. (1985). Orthostatic hypotension—diagnosis and therapy. *Modern Concepts of Cardiovascular Disease, 54,* 7.

Samples, J., Van Cott, M., Long, C., et al. (1985). Circadian rhythms: Basis for screening fever. *Nursing Research, 34,* 377.

Schatz, I. J. (1984). Orthostatic hypotension: Diagnosis and treatment. *Hospital Practice, 19*(4), 59.

Shaver, J. (1991). Assessment of reproductive function. In M. Patrick, S. Woods, R. Craven, et al. (Eds.), *Medical-surgical nursing* (2nd ed.). St. Louis: J.B. Lippincott.

Shinozaki, T., et al. (1988) Infrared tympanic thermometer. Evaluation of a new clinical thermometer. *Critical Care Medicine, 16*(2), 148–150.

Skov, P. & Underhill-Motzer, S. L. (1995). History-taking and physical examination of the patient with cardiovascular disease. In S. L. Woods, E. S. Sivarajan, et al. (Eds.), *Cardiac nursing* (3rd ed.). Philadelphia: J.B. Lippincott.

Vick, R. (1984). *Contemporary medical physiology.* Menlo Park, CA: Addison-Wesley.

Woodman, E., Perry, S., & Simms, L. (1967). Sources of unreliability in oral temperatures. *Nursing Research, 16,* 276.

Yonkman, C. (1982). Cool and heated aerosol and measurement of oral temperature. *Nursing Research, 31,* 354.

Bibliography

Anderson, F., et al. (1993). Indirect blood pressure measurement: A need to reassess. *American Journal of Critical Care, (2)*4, 272–279.

Cooper, J. W. (1989). High blood pressure monitoring guidelines: Diuretics. *Nursing Homes, 38*(3), 7–9.

Hahn, W. K., Brooks, J. A., & Hite, R. (1989). Blood pressure norms for healthy young adults: Relation to sex, age, and reported parental hypertension. *Research in Nursing and Health, 12*(1), 53.

Hellmann, R., et al. (1989). The influence of talking on diastolic blood pressure readings. *National League for Nursing,* Publication #15-2232, 78–82.

Leigh, B., Guisinger, D., & Fech, J. (1989). Blood pressure screening in the workplace. *American Association of Occupational Health Nurses Journal,* *7*(1), 14–17.

Mathews, J. (1991). How to use an automated vital signs monitor. *Nursing '91, 16*(2) 60–64.

Neff, J., Ayoub, J., Longman, A., et al. (1989). Effect of respiratory rate, respiratory depth, and open- versus closed-mouth breathing on sublingual temperature. *Research in Nursing and Health, 12,* 195–202.

Sheehan, M. M. (1990). Blood pressure monitoring. *Nursing '90, 20*(4), 79–81.

Tifft, C. P. (1989). Management of orthostatic hypotension. *Hospital Medicine, 25*(3), 25–28.

Thomas, S, et al. (1993). Nursing blood pressure research, 1980-1990: a bio-psycho-social perspective. *Image, Journal of Nursing Scholarship, 25*(2), 157–164.

VanBuskirk, M. et al. (1993). Monitoring blood pressure in ambulatory patients. *American Journal of Nursing, 93*(6), 44–47.

Diagnostic Tests and Procedures

Key Terms	Learning Objectives

Key Terms

Angiography
Ascites
Barium
Biopsy
Blood gases
Coagulation studies
Culture
Endoscopy
Fluoroscopy
Hemoglobin
Leukocytosis
Leukopenia
Lumbar puncture
Mammography
Myelogram
Nuclear scan
Paracentesis
Radioisotope
Radiopaque
Roentgenogram
Thoracentesis
Thrombocytopenia
Thrombocytosis
Ultrasonography
Venipuncture

Learning Objectives

Upon completion of this chapter, the student will be able to do the following:

- *Discuss the nursing responsibilities before, during, and after laboratory and diagnostic procedures.*
- *Describe the collection of blood samples or other specimens for laboratory analysis.*
- *Discuss the significance of various laboratory tests.*
- *Identify common noninvasive viewing tests used to visualize body organs or functions*
- *Discuss how information gained from laboratory or diagnostic procedures can be used to individualize client care.*

23

A middle-aged man comes into the cardiology clinic for a cardiac workup. He experienced chest pain during a round of golf. He has never liked going to a physician or a healthcare facility; their procedures scare him. He feels that men should be able to handle any of their problems without help. Angiography is scheduled to determine whether surgery is needed. The physician discussed this procedure with the client and obtained his signature on the consent form. After the physician walks away, the client confides in you, the nurse, "The doctor said I have to have this procedure, but I don't know what to do. I'm afraid of needles and I have this friend who had a heart test and he ended up having a heart attack during the test! Tell me what to do."

In previous chapters you learned about ethical and legal concerns and holistic healthcare. This chapter expands your knowledge base about diagnostic tests and procedures, and the nurse's responsibility with the client having diagnostic procedures. The Critical Thinking Challenges at the end of this chapter will help you apply what you have studied in this chapter and what you have learned in previous chapters.

Diagnostic tests make use of specialized equipment designed to visualize or evaluate normal body function. Ultrasound, x-rays, or visualization of internal body organs through scopes are examples of diagnostic procedures. Laboratory tests include procedures that require the collection of specimens from the client (for example, blood, urine, or sputum). Once these specimens are obtained, they are studied in the laboratory for abnormalities.

Information obtained from diagnostic or laboratory tests is used to diagnose specific illnesses or conditions, or to follow the progress of treatment. The nursing role in diagnostic and laboratory testing has a broader focus, as shown in the situation at the beginning of the chapter. In addition to benefiting from the information obtained to assess a client's health status, the nurse facilitates diagnostic and laboratory procedures by obtaining samples, preparing and supporting the client, providing important teaching, performing postprocedure assessments, and sharing the results of the procedures with the physician. Finally, the nurse uses the data obtained in diagnostic or laboratory procedures to assess function and dysfunction, to identify clients at risk for dysfunction, and to help individualize nursing care.

This chapter provides an overview of common diagnostic and laboratory tests and outlines general rather than specific nursing responsibilities associated with the procedures. The chapter includes common nursing implications of the diagnostic and laboratory tests. Each clinical chapter in Section II provides specific information about important diagnostic and laboratory tests related to a particular area of function.

The Nurse as a Facilitator for Diagnostic Testing

Client Preparation

The nurse plays a key role in preparing the client for laboratory and diagnostic tests. The nurse may have responsibility for scheduling the procedure, for client teaching, for witnessing signatures for informed consent, for physically preparing the client, or for obtaining the supplies and equipment (see Procedure 23-1, Preparing the Client for Diagnostic Tests).

Client Scheduling

Appropriate test scheduling is important to optimize test results and promote client comfort. Each client should be considered individually when tests are scheduled. The nurse must consider that scheduling too many consecutive procedures may overtire the elderly, the severely ill, or clients with chronic health problems. Fasting may be difficult for clients with diabetes mellitus; tests should be scheduled early in the morning for these clients to avoid potential complications.

Whenever possible, tests involving the same specimens or similar procedures are grouped together. For example, tests involving a venipuncture for sampling of blood are ordered to be done at the same time to avoid unnecessary resampling. Tests requiring fasting are usually grouped together to avoid requiring the client to fast on numerous occasions. X-ray procedures also may be scheduled at the same time to avoid many trips to the x-ray facility.

Tests may need to be ordered in the proper sequence for optimal results. For example, tests using barium (a contrast medium used to visualize the digestive tract) can interfere with other internal body-viewing techniques and should be scheduled to take place after these other tests are completed.

Laboratory and diagnostic procedures often are performed on an ambulatory basis. In this situation, the client or the client's caretaker may do the scheduling. The nurse provides the client with details of the test, information about scheduling, and the telephone number to call to schedule the test, and documents information provided in the client's records. It is helpful to provide this information in written form; when clients encounter difficulties or become confused, they may neglect to have important tests done.

Client Teaching

Explanations about the testing procedure can help relieve the client's anxiety, ensure cooperation, and assist the client in coping with an uncomfortable or painful procedure. Often, diagnostic procedures are performed

Client Teaching
Diagnostic Testing

Instruct the client as follows:

- *NPO means nothing by mouth; determine from the nurse which meals to omit, whether water can be taken, how to take necessary medications, and when normal intake of foods or fluids can be resumed.*
- *If a sputum specimen is to be collected, avoid touching the inside of the sputum-collection container with your fingers, tongue, or lips when coughing the specimen into the container.*
- *Be sure you understand what is expected of you before all procedures, particularly if you must remain motionless during any part of the examination.*
- *Do not use deodorants, powders, perfumes, or creams on the day you are having a mammogram.*
- *Tests involving radioisotopes will not cause you to become radioactive.*
- *Keep the limb immobilized before and after angiographic examinations. It is also necessary to report numbness and tingling in the affected limb after the examination.*

Procedure 23-1
Preparing the Client for Diagnostic Procedures

Purpose

1. Decrease anxiety and increase client cooperation with a procedure.
2. Ensure that diagnostic test will provide good test results without complications.

Assessment

- Review client's history of drug or food allergies (especially important for dye injection studies or when procedures require premedication).
- Assess client's knowledge of the procedure.
- Assess client's ability to follow directions and cooperate before and during the test.
- Evaluate client's physical ability to tolerate the procedure.
- Assess need for nursing staff to accompany client to procedure.
- Obtain and document client's baseline vital signs.
- Identify correct name band on client's wrist.

Equipment

Signed permission for diagnostic procedure.
Pajama bottoms and hospital gown.
Patent intravenous access (if necessary for procedure).
Supplies and equipment specific to procedure.

Procedure

1. Identify the specific procedure or procedures to be performed.
2. Obtain a written consent for invasive procedures after the physician has explained the study to the client.
   Rationale: Clients should be informed of the reason for the procedure, what to expect during the procedure, and what are the associated risks. The client's signing of the consent must be observed and signed by a witness.
3. If more than one procedure is ordered, they should be scheduled in an order least traumatic to the client and which will produce the most accurate results.
   Rationale: Tests that need to be repeated owing to inaccurate results are traumatic and costly to the client, and can delay needed treatment. Rescheduled procedures can mean an extended hospital stay.
4. Identify specific preparations needed to be performed before the procedure (eg, enemas, NPO status, ingestion of contrast material)
   Rationale: Thorough preparations increase accuracy of test results.
5. Provide instruction to the client and significant others regarding the procedure and rationale for any special preparations or dietary/fluid restrictions required by the study.
   Rationale: Client understanding of the procedure increases client compliance and decreases anxiety.
6. Monitor dietary or fluid restrictions.
   Note: Clients who have NPO diagnostic procedures scheduled for several consecutive days may become dehydrated. Encourage them to eat and drink well when not NPO. Consider scheduling a rest day between procedures if possible.
7. Continue to provide psychological support to the client as needed.
   Rationale: Many clients are anxious about the test procedure as well as uncertain about test results.
8. When a client who routinely takes special medications (ie, cardiac medications, anticonvulsants, anticoagulants, diabetic medications) is NPO, obtain physician orders regarding the administration of his or her medications before the procedure.
   Rationale: Holding essential medications may alter therapeutic blood levels of the drug. Giving medications with a sip of water may not interfere with the outcome of the procedure.
9. Immediately before the procedure:
   a. Have patient urinate unless contraindicated by the study.
   b. Reidentify any client allergies and identiband.
   c. Remove hairpins, contact lenses, jewelry, and fingernail polish if required by procedure.
   d. Administer and document premedication if ordered.
   e. If transported with intravenous line, assess that IV is patent and remaining volume is sufficient.
   f. Supervise transfer from bed to wheelchair or gurney. If transported to gurney, side rails or safety belt should be fastened.
   g. Provide blanket.
   Rationale: All of these interventions are directed toward client safety or comfort.
10. Accompany client during transport if required by client's physical and emotional status.
    Rationale: Your presence provides for client's psychological and physiologic safety.

(continued)

Lifespan Considerations

Infants and Children

- It is often difficult to explain a procedure so a child can understand. Role-playing, puppets, or showing the equipment are useful techniques for client teaching.
- Children younger than 12 years of age should never be left alone in a strange department.
- Allow parents to accompany child to procedure, or have child bring a "security object" (eg, blanket, stuffed animal) to decrease his or her anxiety.
- Painful procedures should never be done at the bedside of children younger than 12 years of age. The bedside should be kept in a "safe place" for them at *all* times.

Clients With Mental or Sensory Impairments

- Clients who have mental or sensory impairments often have established a trusting relationship with their nurse. They may have difficulty communicating with or relating to people they don't know well. Accompany these clients to other departments whenever possible.

to determine what is causing the client's current symptoms. It is not unusual for the client to imagine the worst, fearing that the test may reveal a serious or life-threatening disease. Careful client teaching may help alleviate these fears. Conversely, the client also should be informed that not all questions can be answered by performing a specific test; some tests may raise as many questions as they answer.

Most client teaching occurs before the procedure, but some information can be offered during the testing session (Fig. 23-1). Explanations are made in terms the client can understand. Children present a unique situation, and methods such as role-playing or showing the equipment may be helpful. For all age groups, time is allowed for questions after explanations. When the client is anxious, information may need to be repeated several times before the client is able to process the important content. Explanations need to be age-appropriate, factual, and individualized for clients with special needs (eg, clients who are hearing or vision impaired). An interpreter should be used for clients who do not understand or read English.

The nurse should be prepared to answer such questions as: What will they do? Where will the test be done? Will it be painful? How long will it take? Will I be able to go to work (school, home) after the test is completed? When will I know the results of the test? Clear, direct answers to these questions will help to prepare the client emotionally and physically for the procedure.

In many agencies, printed information on common diagnostic procedures is available. After the client has had time to read the information, the nurse can clarify points and answer questions. When the nurse is not knowledgeable regarding a particular procedure, the department performing the test can be contacted for information.

Informed Consent

Before any diagnostic procedure, the client should possess adequate and accurate information to make the decision whether to have the procedure performed. Most clients agreeably submit to diagnostic studies because they hope to learn the reason for pain or discomfort. The client also expects that the test will provide information about how the problem can be treated and resolved.

When the client has been informed about what the procedure entails, the risks and benefits of the procedure, and the alternatives to the procedure, the client has received the information necessary for him or her to give informed consent for the procedure. (Informed consent is discussed in Chapter 3.) It is important to consult agency protocol to identify those procedures that require a *written* statement of informed consent.

If the adult client should indicate a lack of understanding about a procedure or is unsure regarding the decision to undergo the procedure, the nurse should not attempt to assist the client in making a decision; instead, the physician should be contacted. When the client is a child or is incapable of understanding the procedure, his or her representative should be the one to indicate understanding.

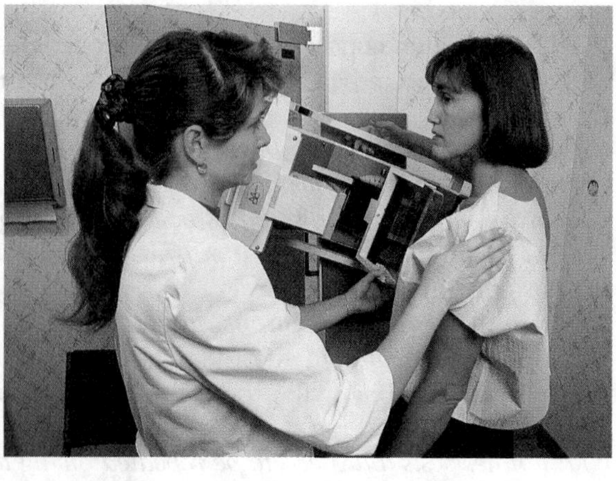

Figure 23-1 • *The nurse prepares the client for mammography. Teaching can take place before, during, and following the procedure.*

Physical Preparation

Many procedures require specific physical preparation of the client (preprocedure protocols) to ensure accurate test results. Frequently, the nurse explains preprocedure protocols to the client and conveys the importance that they be followed. The protocols are usually found in written form and will be available for many inpatient and ambulatory studies.

Fasting is commonly required before many examinations. The client receives a "nothing by mouth" (NPO) order for a specified period before the procedure (usually overnight or a period of hours). When an NPO client is receiving routine medication (eg, medication to control blood pressure or anticonvulsant medication), however, it is important to verify if the medications can be given with a small sip of water or by means of an alternate route.

Cleansing of the bowel is a common preparation when the gastrointestinal tract is the focus of the study. For some studies, the client may need to be "scrubbed" (involving a specific protocol for skin cleansing) or shaved before the procedure. Although it is desirable most of the time for the client to have an empty urinary bladder, some tests may require that the bladder be full. Medication, often a sedative, may be ordered to be administered at a specific time before the test.

Collection of Supplies

Some procedures do not require that the client be transported to another department; instead, the tests are performed at the bedside. In this situation, it is usually the nurse's responsibility to obtain the supplies and equipment. Often, supplies for a specific procedure are prepackaged, and only sterile gloves or local anesthetic agents may be needed in addition to the prepackaged kit.

Responsibilities During Testing

The nurse works collaboratively with the physician or the technician performing the diagnostic test. Setting up equipment, ensuring the maintenance of sterility, administering medication, and providing for client safety are some of the typical tasks that a nurse may perform.

Client Assessment

Client assessment is necessary to detect any changes in status during the procedure. Vital signs and observations such as the client's comfort level, skin color, and mental status are recorded before the procedure, and serve as baseline data. Allergies and laboratory data pertinent to the study are noted.

During the procedure, the client is observed for adverse effects. Vital signs and other observations are documented at specific intervals on flowsheets. Changes in vital signs or in other baseline parameters are reported promptly and treated.

Client Support

Supporting the client during the procedure is an important function that may be performed by the nurse and possibly a family member, especially if the client is a child. Activities such as holding the client's hand or quietly standing next to the client may be all that is needed. The distraction technique of visual imaging also can help decrease anxiety.

The nurse can offer emotional support with statements about what to expect (eg, "You may feel some stinging as the doctor injects the anesthetic," or "We are nearly finished"). Attending to the client's physical comfort by supporting a tired limb or by making sure that the client is warm enough also can be comforting.

Client Positioning

It is often the nurse's responsibility to position the client during diagnostic procedures. Positioning can be a matter of simply assisting the client into a position of comfort, or, in many situations, assisting the client into the specific position indicated for the test or procedure. Figure 23-2 illustrates some body positions that are used for selected diagnostic procedures.

Once positioned, the client may require assistance in maintaining that body position. Certain positions can cause fatigue, especially when limbs are not adequately supported. The nurse should support the client and use pillows to increase comfort and decrease fatigue. The elderly or other people with limited joint mobility may experience pain or discomfort when an extremity must be manipulated or held stationary. Some positions may cause breathing difficulties for those with respiratory problems. Infants and young children, who are unable to understand the necessity of remaining still, may need to be restrained to ensure safety during the testing procedure.

Responsibilities After Testing

Client Assessment

After the procedure is complete or the client returns from the procedure, the nurse continues to assess the client's status. Vital signs and other appropriate observations are monitored and compared with baseline data. It is important to be well informed about specific possible complications for each procedure. Observations will be directed at detecting such problems

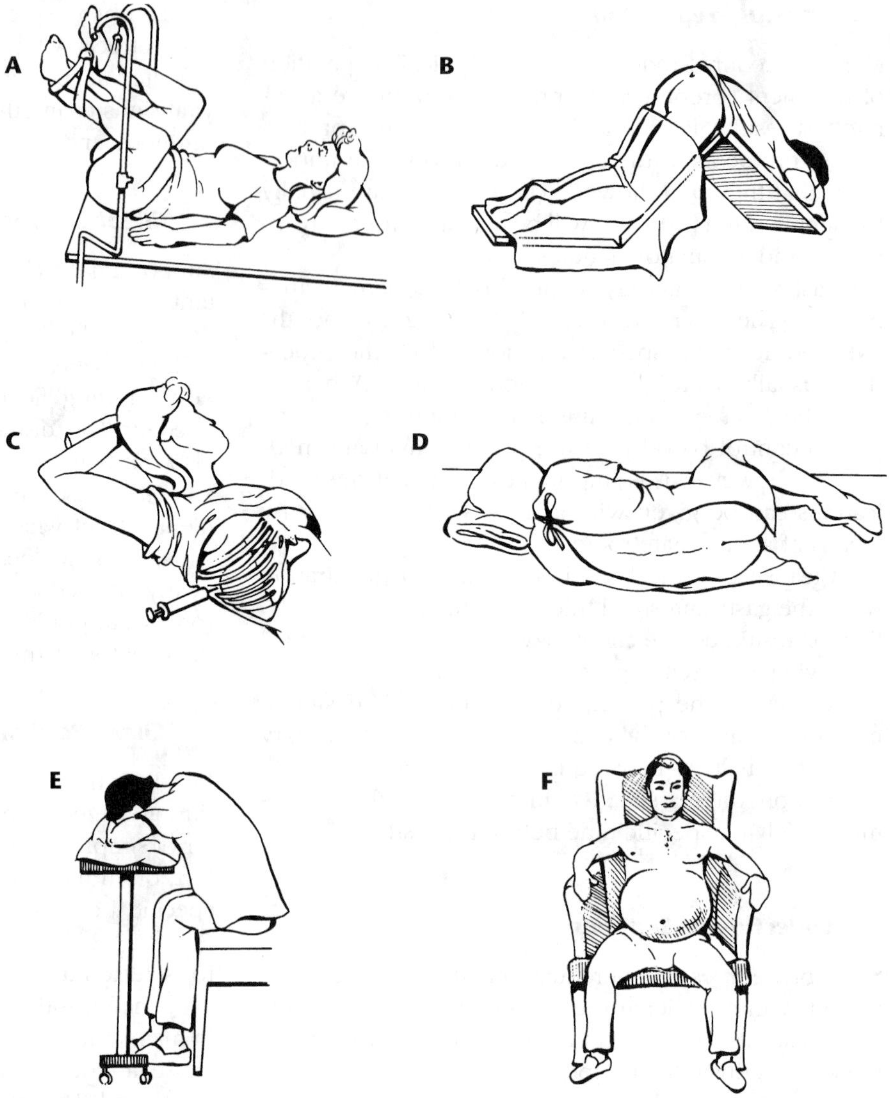

Figure 23-2 • Positions for selected diagnostic tests: **(A)** *cystoscopy;* **(B)** *sigmoidoscopy;* **(C)** *liver biopsy;* **(D)** *lumbar puncture;* **(E)** *thoracentesis;* **(F)** *paracentesis.*

promptly. The frequency of assessment may be determined by agency protocol. All significant changes from baseline data should be reported immediately to the physician.

Specimen Collection and Equipment

During many diagnostic procedures, specimens are collected and transported immediately to the laboratory for analysis. The nurse may be responsible for ensuring that the specimen is collected in the appropriate container, labeled properly, and transported to the laboratory. Universal precautions, which include the wearing of gloves, are followed to avoid contact with body fluids. It is wise to send the specimen to the laboratory before the area is cleaned to avoid inadvertent disposal of the specimen.

Cleaning the work area after a diagnostic procedure may be the responsibility of the nurse. Care should be taken to dispose of needles and other sharp objects in a designated receptacle to avoid accidental injury and exposure of other healthcare workers.

Documentation

It is important to document the diagnostic or laboratory test. The type of procedure, the name of the person performing the procedure, the date and time of the procedure, a summary of client assessments before, during, and after the procedure, and collection and disposition of specimens should be recorded. The client's response should also be documented, particularly any complications during or after the procedure (eg, pain, nausea, fatigue).

Client and Family Support

The time between performance of diagnostic tests and availability of test results can be very difficult for the client and family members. If possible, the nurse gives some indication of when test results are likely to be back. During this waiting period, the client is encouraged to keep as busy as possible. Spend time just sitting with the client so that concerns can be discussed. The nurse may need to request an order for antianxiety medications if anxiety is acute.

Using Data to Individualize Care

The nurse uses the information obtained through laboratory and diagnostic testing to assess the functional health of the client and to plan individualized care. The use of test results to help plan nursing care may be the most important aspect of diagnostic and laboratory testing. Selected examples are provided to illustrate this.

Chest x-rays are often obtained to diagnose and follow the course of treatment for pneumonia. The nurse is not expected to read or interpret the chest x-ray, or suggest changes in treatment based on the x-ray findings. Rather, the nurse uses the information obtained from the x-ray report to plan optimal positioning of the client. The x-ray report describes the portion of the lung affected by pneumonia and by poor air exchange. Knowing that both air flow and blood flow are gravity dependent, the nurse positions the client with the nonaffected side down to maximize air flow and blood flow to the healthy lung tissue (Yeaw, 1992). In this way, the nurse uses the x-ray information to promote oxygenation in a client.

Laboratory data also can be used to individualize care. When a nurse notes a low hemoglobin value (hemoglobin is the oxygen-carrying component of the red blood cell), the client's activity plans can be changed to include frequent rest periods. This planning ensures that the oxygen supply is sufficient to meet the demands of the body.

Blood tests may reveal that a client has dysfunctional urinary elimination because of kidney failure. In this situation, the nurse reviews the client's medications that are eliminated by the kidney and watches for signs of toxicity.

Another example of the nurse individualizing care based on test data is the identification of a client at risk for skin breakdown or poor wound healing, by noting a low serum albumin level; this client may require increased attention to nutrition or a pressure support mattress to ensure skin integrity and good healing of wounds.

Finally, a test such as cardiac catheterization may reveal extensive coronary heart disease (CHD). The nurse, aware of the potential problems with oxygenation, may appraise the client's heart rate during activity to assess the client's response to exercise. Table 23-1 lists selected laboratory and diagnostic tests for each functional health pattern.

Laboratory Tests

Although specimens for laboratory tests may be obtained either at the bedside or in the laboratory, the assay of blood, urine, and other body samples takes place in the laboratory. Protocols for sample collection ensure that specific amounts of samples are collected and analyzed under standard conditions. After laboratory assay, the nurse may be responsible for communicating any abnormal results to the physician. In addition, the nurse uses the information gathered through laboratory testing to plan the client's care.

Using Laboratory Reference Ranges

The nurse examines the client's records thoroughly each day for the results of diagnostic laboratory testing. Changes in the client's condition (deterioration or improvement) often are reflected in changes in laboratory values. For this reason, normal reference values for common laboratory tests are provided in the Appendix B. Caution should be exercised in comparing the client's values to the reference values. Normal values for some laboratory tests will vary between laboratories because of regional differences in client characteristics and differences in measurement technique. Comparison to previous values is also important in evaluating the significance of laboratory findings for a specific client.

Blood Specimen Collection

The sampling of blood for laboratory assay is performed by either laboratory phlebotomists or nursing personnel. Venous blood is most commonly used for blood tests. Venous blood can be obtained by means of a venipuncture or through an intravenous catheter placed into a central vein. Arterial blood is less commonly assayed; it can be obtained with arterial puncture or through an indwelling arterial catheter. Capillary blood is obtained using a lancet. Gloves are worn during all blood collection procedures in accordance with Universal Precautions for avoiding contact with body fluids (Centers for Disease Control and Prevention, 1994).

Venipuncture

The procedure for blood sampling, known as **venipuncture**, involves puncturing the vein with a needle for the purpose of blood withdrawal. Aseptic technique is used during the procedure to prevent the transfer of microorganisms into the bloodstream. The most common sites for venipuncture are the antecubital area (basilic, median cubital, or cephalic veins), or the

Table 23-1 • Relationship of Selected Laboratory and Diagnostic Procedures to Functional Health

Functional Area	Laboratory Tests	Diagnostic Tests
Health perception and health management	None	Mammogram Pap smear Biopsy
Activity and exercise	Hemoglobin Hematocrit Blood coagulation Blood lipid studies Serum enzymes Arterial blood gases	X-rays (chest; extremities) Lung perfusion scan Angiography Cardiac catheterization Thoracentesis Electrocardiogram Bronchoscopy
Nutrition and metabolism	Hematocrit White blood cell count White blood cell differential Sedimentation rate Electrolytes Protein (albumin) Blood glucose Blood lipid studies 24-hour urine collection	Barium enema Upper gastrointestinal series Abdominal ultrasound Endoscopy Liver biopsy Bone marrow biopsy Paracentesis Cholangiogram, cholecystogram, endoscopic retrograde cholangiopancreatography
Elimination	Urinalysis Urine culture and sensitivity Stool culture and sensitivity Blood urea nitrogen (BUN) Creatinine	Sigmoidoscopy Barium enema Pelvic ultrasound Renal biopsy Intravenous pyelogram (kidney x-ray with contrast) Cystoscopy
Sleep and rest	None	Electroencephalogram
Cognition and perception	Electrolytes Blood glucose Blood chemistries Arterial blood gases	Computed tomography Magnetic resonance imaging Cerebral angiography Electroencephalogram Lumbar puncture Myelogram
Self-perception	None—assessment of pattern based mainly on subjective data	
Roles and relationships	None—assessment of pattern based mainly on subjective data	
Coping and stress tolerance	None—assessment of pattern based mainly on subjective data	
Sexuality and reproduction	Hormone levels Pregnancy tests	Pelvic ultrasound Mammography
Values and beliefs	None—assessment of pattern based mainly on subjective data	

dorsal surface of the hand (the dorsal metacarpal, basilic, or cephalic veins).

To obtain a sample using venipuncture, the nurse applies an occluding tourniquet above the area where the sample will be drawn; cleanses the area with an antiseptic solution; pierces the skin with the bevel of the needle up; and withdraws the blood sample into a syringe or vacuum tube (Fig. 23-3). Pressure is applied to the venipuncture site for 1 to 2 minutes until the bleeding has stopped.

Arterial Puncture

Arterial sampling is performed to evaluate blood gases, which indicate the metabolic, oxygen, and ventilatory status of the client. In most agencies, personnel must receive special training to become certified for arterial puncture. The radial artery at the wrist is the preferred arterial site because it is superficial and easily palpable, but occasionally the brachial or femoral arteries are used. Pressure should be applied over the puncture site for at least 5 minutes to prevent bleeding and hematoma formation.

Capillary Puncture

Finger or heel pricks with a lancet or autolet can be used to obtain small samples of capillary blood for analysis. Most commonly, this method of blood sampling is used for blood glucose, hematocrit, or peripheral blood smear studies, or for phenylketonuria tests in newborns.

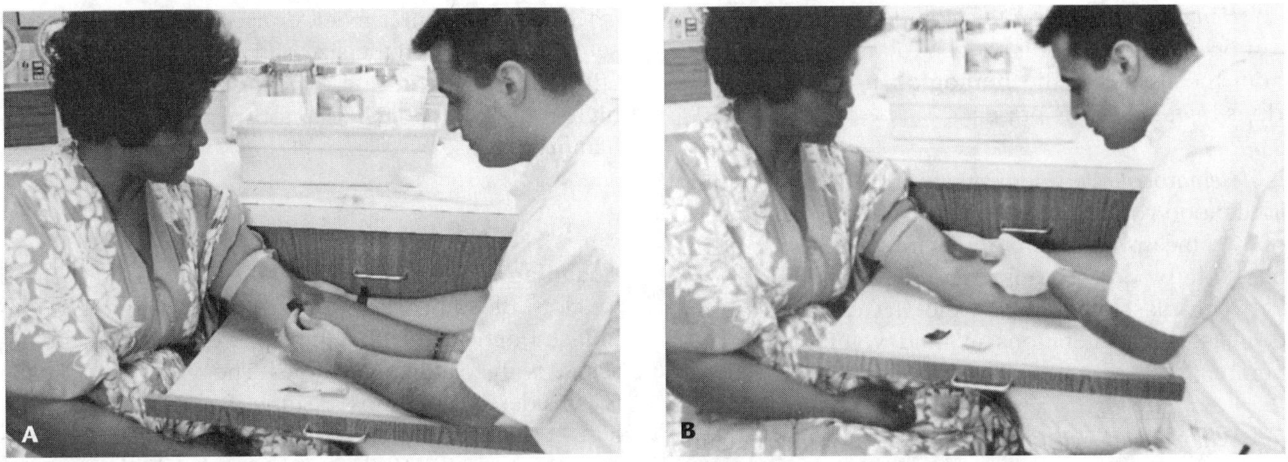

Figure 23-3 • Venipuncture. (A) Cleansing the site with Betadine. (B) Aspirating blood with a vacuum tube.

Obtaining a capillary sample can be aided by warming the finger or heel or placing the extremity in a dependent position to improve blood flow. To acquire the capillary blood sample, the skin is cleansed, usually with alcohol. Gloves are donned and the point of the lancet or autolet is briskly pierced through the skin (Fig. 23-4). If a finger is used, the side of the finger pad, rather than the center, is pricked; this is less painful for the client. Likewise, the side of the heel should be selected for infants.

Blood From a Central Venous Catheter

The use of a central venous catheter allows access to the client's blood supply for long-term intravenous infusions and for frequent blood sampling. This method of blood sampling avoids venipuncture and allows for frequent, speedy blood collection. Commonly, central venous catheters are used for clients with cancer who will receive chemotherapy and follow-up evaluation for an extended period of time, for clients on long-term antibiotic therapy, and for clients who are receiving total parenteral nutrition.

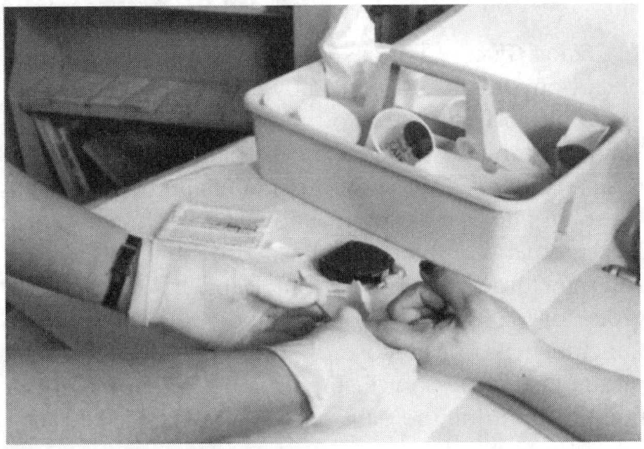

Figure 23-4 • In capillary puncture, the side of the finger is cleansed and pricked.

Hematologic Tests

Diagnostic laboratory tests for hematologic values are common. Anemias, bleeding or coagulation problems, hemolytic disorders, or nutritional disorders can be identified through assessment of blood values. A few of the most common hematologic studies—complete blood count (CBC), the erythrocyte sedimentation rate (sed rate; ESR), blood coagulation studies, blood chemistry and lipid studies, serum drug and enzyme levels, and arterial blood gases—are examined briefly in the following discussion. For more complete information, refer to Chapters 34, 35, and 36.

Complete Blood Count

The CBC is one of the most commonly performed laboratory tests. The components of the CBC are the blood cells, which are formed in the bone marrow and are suspended in plasma. The blood cells accounted for in a CBC are the red blood cells (erythrocytes or RBCs), the white blood cells (leukocytes or WBCs), and platelets. Also examined are the WBC differential, hematocrit (Hct), hemoglobin (Hb), the morphology (shape or structure) of the cells, and activity (appropriate function) of the blood cells. Appendix B contains CBC reference ranges.

Red Blood Cell Count. The RBC count is expressed in the number of RBCs per microliter (μL) of whole blood. Red blood cells are produced in the bone marrow in response to a chemical produced in the kidney (erythropoietin). Increased RBCs in the blood suppress the production of new RBCs.

Hemoglobin. The protein compound in RBCs that is responsible for carrying oxygen to and carbon dioxide from the tissues is the **hemoglobin** molecule. When Hb is low, anemia is present.

Hematocrit. The percentage of RBCs in 100 mL of total blood volume is the Hct level (consequently, a Hct of 39% means that there are 39 mL of RBCs in 100 mL of whole blood). Because Hct reflects the relationship between plasma and RBCs, the Hct can increase and decrease with alterations in fluid volume or in RBC number.

White Blood Cell Count. The WBCs defend against foreign substances in the body, such as bacteria, parasites, or other foreign substances. The WBC count reflects the number of WBCs per microliter of whole blood. An elevated WBC count (**leukocytosis**) usually indicates infection in the body, but can follow severe tissue injury. A low WBC count (**leukopenia**) can accompany diseases of the bone marrow, or immunosuppression (unresponsiveness of the body's natural immune system) due to chemotherapy or AIDS. Leukocytosis or leukopenia can be interpreted best through examination of the WBC differential.

WBC Differential. The differential count is a list of the relative number of each type of WBC in the blood. There are five different types of leukocytes that can be seen under the microscope when a peripheral blood smear is examined (see Appendix B). The most common type of leukocyte is the neutrophil, which responds to infection and inflammation in the body. Other types of leukocytes include eosinophils (seen in allergic reactions), basophils (which play a role during anaphylaxis), lymphocytes (seen in viral conditions), and monocytes (which migrate to areas of injury to ingest damaged cells and foreign particles). Refer to Chapter 39 for more information on interpreting WBC differential results.

Platelet Count. Platelets, like the red and white blood cells, also are formed in the bone marrow. The disk-like shape of these cells helps them to aggregate and form a plug at bleeding sites. A very low number of platelets (a condition known as **thrombocytopenia**) increases bleeding time; an excessive number of platelets (**thrombocytosis**) is found after some surgeries or hemorrhage, and is often associated with anemia or infection.

Erythrocyte Sedimentation Rate

The ESR measures the speed at which anticoagulated erythrocytes settle in a long, narrow tube. Inflammation and infection affect the protein content of the erythrocytes, making them heavier. Consequently, the speed of settling depends on the size of the clumps in which the affected cells aggregate. The faster the settling, the higher the ESR. The ESR is a nonspecific indicator of inflammatory disease.

Blood Coagulation Studies

Coagulation studies evaluate the ability of the blood to clot. Bleeding disorders, as well as medication-induced anticoagulation (clot prevention), can be assessed with coagulation studies. The type of test chosen is considered a diagnostic study if bleeding is a problem. If anticoagulation is the goal of medication therapy, tests specific to the particular anticlotting mechanism affected by the drug are chosen. Common blood coagulation studies include platelet count (see previous discussion), bleeding time, platelet aggregation, partial thromboplastin time (PTT or aPTT), and prothrombin time, and international normalizing ratio (INR) (see Appendix B).

Blood Chemistry Studies

Homeostatic mechanisms in the body are responsible for maintaining the body's stable state through regulation of cellular activity. Among the homeostatic mechanisms are the regulation of blood chemistries—the electrolytes and other chemical substances in the blood that affect cellular activity (see the Appendix for reference ranges for common chemistry studies).

Electrolytes. When electrolytes are ordered, a sample of blood is analyzed for sodium, potassium, carbon dioxide, and chloride levels. The levels of these constituents are stable in the healthy person but may become unbalanced in several disease states (including diseases of the lungs, kidneys, and heart), and in relation to the body's fluid-volume status. Because the electrolyte balance in the body can change rapidly, certain values may be measured several times daily.

Blood Glucose. Glucose is formed from the digestion of carbohydrates and is used by cells as a source of energy. Entry of glucose into the cells is facilitated by insulin, a hormone secreted by the pancreas. Blood glucose testing is used to detect disorders in the process of carbohydrate breakdown and glucose metabolism. Measurement of blood glucose can be done with a venipuncture sample or with capillary blood (see Procedure 23-2, Measuring Blood Glucose by Skin Puncture). Blood glucose analysis may be performed on the fasting person (fasting blood sugar) or at specified times during the day.

Chemistry Profiles. Frequently, blood chemistry tests are ordered in groups (profiles or panels) and use a

Procedure 23-2
Measuring Blood Glucose by Skin Puncture

Purpose

1. Monitor blood glucose levels at the bedside for clients who are at risk for hypoglycemia or hyperglycemia.
2. Monitor the effectiveness of insulin administration.

Assessment

- Review the physician's order to determine the time and frequency of glucose monitoring.
  Note: The procedure should be performed before meals because carbohydrate ingestion will alter blood glucose levels.
- Assess the client's medical history to determine if he or she is at risk for complications from skin punctures (ie, bleeding disorders, anticoagulant therapy, or low platelet count).
- Assess the skin area to be used for puncture (fingers, toes, heels). Avoid areas with open lesions or ecchymosis.
- Assess the client's understanding of the purpose of the procedure and his or her physical and emotional ability to learn the procedure and perform it independently.

Equipment

Alcohol or povidone–iodine swab
Sterile lancet or autolet
Cotton balls
Blood glucose reagent strip
Glucose testing meter
Disposable gloves

Procedure

1. Have the client wash hands with soap and warm water.
   Rationale: The fingertips are the most common skin puncture sites in adults. Washing not only decreases the chances of infection but, due to the warm water, promotes vasodilation of the puncture site.
2. Position client in a comfortable posture.
3. Remove the reagent strip from the container and handle according to the manufacturer's instructions.
   Rationale: The glucose meter may need recalibration or "rezero-ing."
4. Place the reagent strip with test pad up on a dry surface.
   Rationale: Moisture on the test pad could alter the final test results.
5. Choose the finger to be punctured, massage gently, and hold in a dependent position.
   Rationale: The dependent position and stimulation will help increase circulation to the puncture site.
6. Wipe the puncture site with alcohol (or a povidone–iodone swab). Allow the site to dry completely.
   Rationale: If tracked into the puncture site, alcohol may cause stinging and could hemolyze or dilute the blood sample, giving an inaccurate reading.

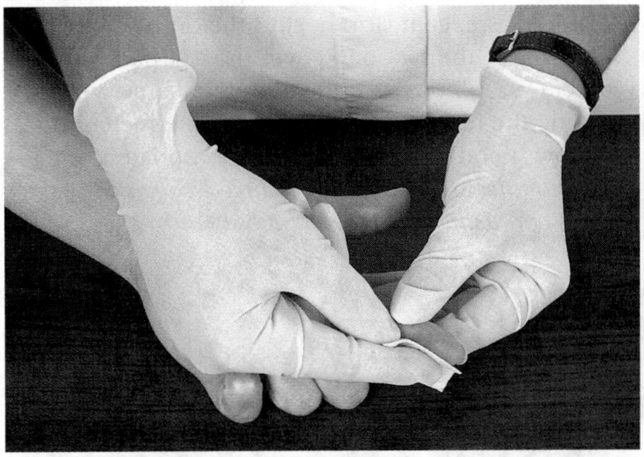

Step 6 • Wipe puncture site with alcohol, allowing site to dry before puncture. (© B. Proud)

7. Don gloves.
   Rationale: Gloving is the observance of Universal Precautions against transfer of microorganisms.
8. Remove the cover of the lancet or autolet. Place the autolet against the side of the finger and push the release button. If a lancet is used, it should be held perpendicular to the side and should pierce the site quickly.
   Rationale: Quick brisk puncture of skin is less painful.
9. Wipe the initial drop of blood with a cotton ball.
   Rationale: The first drop of blood may contain more serous fluid than blood cells and lead to a false glucose reading.

(continued)

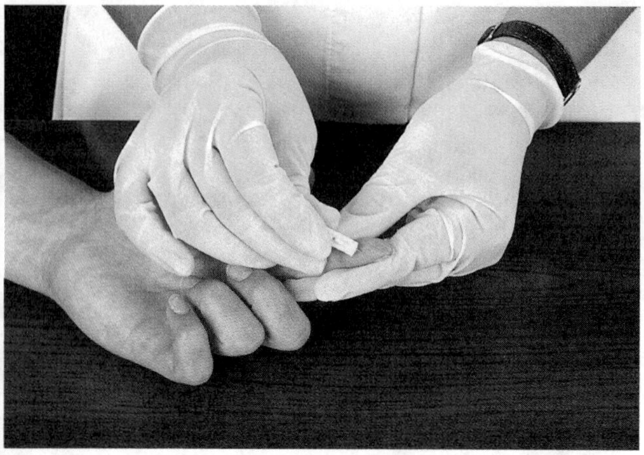

Step 8 • Puncture site to obtain the blood sample. (© B. Proud)

10. Squeeze the puncture gently or massage the skin toward the site to obtain a large drop of blood. Hold the reagent strip next to the drop of blood and allow the blood to cover the test pad completely. Do not smear the blood. In some meters, bring the finger to the test site on the meter and allow blood to drop onto the appropriate area.
    Rationale: Smearing or incomplete coverage of the test pad will lead to false glucose readings.

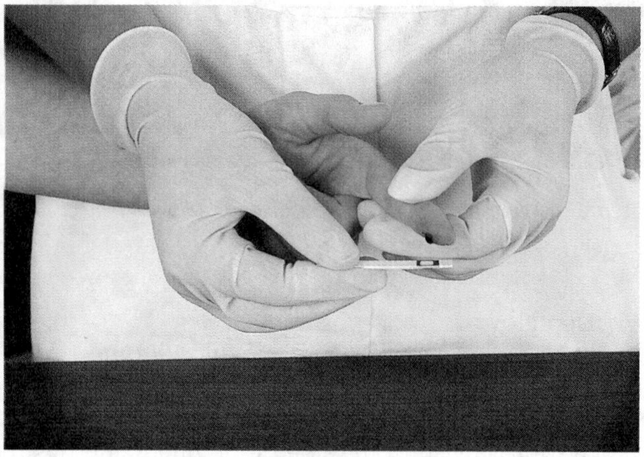

Step 10 • Cover the test pad completely with a large drop of blood. (© B. Proud)

11. Start the timing (usually less than 60 seconds) using the glucose meter, or a watch if the meter is not available.
    Rationale: Blood must be in contact with the test pad for the time period required by the manufacturer to ensure accurate results.
12. Following the manufacturer's instruction, wipe the blood from the test pad with a cotton ball after the specified period of time.
    Note: Slight variations may occur in the procedure between different manufacturers.
13. Place the reagent strip into the glucose meter. After the recommended period of time, read the results. *For meters on which blood is placed directly, read the results at the designated time.* If a glucose meter is not available, compare the color of the test pad with the color strip on the side of the reagent strip container.
    Rationale: Accurate timing of the test ensures a correct reading of the glucose level.

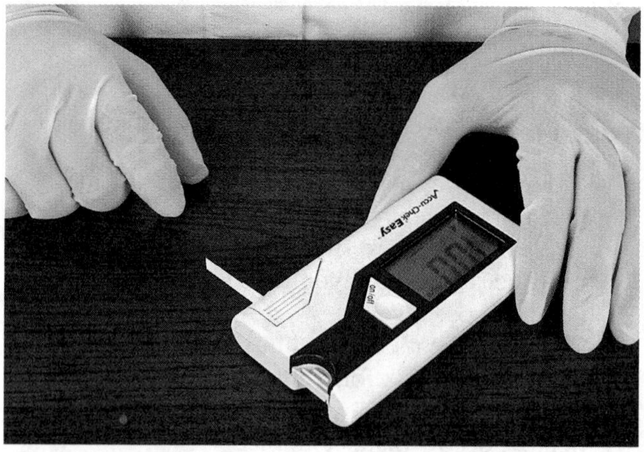

Step 13 • Place reagent strip into the glucose meter and after appropriate time read the results. (© B. Proud)

14. Turn off the glucose meter. Dispose of used equipment in the appropriate manner.
    Rationale: The lancet or autolet should be disposed of in a used-needle receptacle to avoid inadvertent punctures by others.
15. Share test results with client and record obtained values in the client's chart.
    Rationale: Encourages client participation and maintains appropriate documentation.

Lifespan Considerations

Infants

- The heel is the most common site for skin puncture. The nurse may want to use a heel-warming device or may wrap a warm, moist towel around the foot before the skin puncture to promote vasodilation.

Children

- Children are especially apprehensive about any type of skin puncture. The use of distraction techniques and allowing parents to be present may increase the child's cooperation with the procedure.

Home Care Modifications

- Handwashing alone before skin puncture is sufficient to cleanse the skin when the test is performed at home.
- Client should be instructed to keep a log of all blood glucose readings.

single venous sample. A typical profile may include the measurement of electrolytes, glucose, and blood urea nitrogen (BUN). Occasionally, larger panels are obtained and contain (in addition to the electrolytes, glucose, and BUN) results of calcium, magnesium, inorganic phosphate, creatinine, and protein values, including total protein, albumin, globulin, and the albumin/globulin ratio. Reference ranges for these tests are given in Appendix B.

Blood Lipid Studies

Blood lipid studies measure the level of fat in the blood. Evaluation of the amount of total cholesterol, low-density lipoproteins (LDL), and high-density lipoproteins (HDL) is important for accurate identification of people at risk for coronary heart disease (CHD).

Current guidelines identify an optimal cholesterol level as less than 200 mg/dL (National Cholesterol Education Program, 1988). Total cholesterol can be sampled in a nonfasting individual. If the total cholesterol level is found to be elevated, a second test may be done to evaluate LDL and HDL. Because LDLs carry blood cholesterol to the cells of the body, high LDL levels are directly related to an increased risk of CHD. On the other hand, increased levels of HDL may have a protective effect because HDL removes cholesterol from cells and transports it to the liver, where it is secreted in bile (Goe, 1995). See Chapter 35 for more information on blood lipid levels.

Serum Enzymes

Enzymes are protein substances that enter into energy-producing reactions within cells. When cells are damaged, either through disease or injury, enzymes are liberated into the blood, where they are detected through enzyme assay. The testing of blood for the presence of enzymes is useful for detecting abnormalities in the bones, liver, kidney, brain, muscles, and, most commonly, the heart. Isoenzymes (subfractions of enzymes) may be specific to certain organs and therefore a more specific indicator of where cell destruction has occurred. For example, the death of cardiac tissue after a myocardial infarction can be detected by evaluating serum enzymes.

Serum Drug Levels

Serum drug levels are obtained to determine the effectiveness of drug therapy or to identify toxic levels. Information about the serum concentration of drugs is most commonly used to monitor the blood levels of cardiac medications (eg, digoxin, quinidine, or procainamide), antibiotics (eg, gentamicin and tobramycin), or theophylline. It is important to remember that serum drug levels should be interpreted in the context of the client's signs and symptoms. When serum drug levels exceed therapeutic ranges, the physician should be notified.

Arterial Blood Gases

Arterial **blood gases**, obtained from an arterial sample of blood, are used to evaluate the metabolic and respiratory status of the client. The pH of blood as well as the partial pressure of oxygen and carbon dioxide are measured. The bicarbonate level is usually calculated from the results. These parameters can be altered by changes in respiratory pattern, changes in activity, changes in oxygenation, changes in renal status, or changes in other factors such as shock or an elevated blood glucose level. Blood gases are drawn when there has been no change in oxygen delivery or activity level for at least 15 minutes (see Appendix B for reference values for arterial blood gases; also see Chapters 34 and 36).

Urine Testing

The analysis of urine is an important indicator of a person's health status. Alterations in metabolism, infection, renal disease, and fluid volume problems can be confirmed by examination of the urine.

Urine Specimen Collection

Urine samples can be collected for routine analyses, for identification of bacteria, and for special 24-hour examination. Specimens are voided into a clean container for routine urinalysis. Once labeled, the specimen must be rapidly transported to the laboratory because any bacteria will multiply rapidly if the specimen is left at room temperature. When culture for identification of bacteria is desired, a clean-voided procedure or catheterization is performed. Specimens for urinalysis also can be taken from an indwelling urinary catheter by aspirating urine from a special port with a needle and syringe. Refer to Chapter 41 for details regarding different procedures for urine specimen collection.

Routine Urinalysis

Routine urinalysis is a common procedure performed on admission to the hospital and during physical examination. Reported information includes the urine color and turbidity; pH and specific gravity; presence of protein, glucose, or ketones; and the presence of bacteria, blood cells, and sediment. Any bacteria or more than five red or white blood cells (viewed in a high-power field) should be considered abnormal (Fischbach, 1992).

Safety Alert
Laboratory and Diagnostic Tests

- Use universal precautions for all tests involving collection of body fluids.
- Determine whether the client is allergic to iodine before cleansing the skin with a povidone–iodine antiseptic.
- Apply pressure over the puncture site after all venipunctures. If bleeding continues, have the client elevate the area and continue to hold pressure.
- When arterial puncture is performed, apply pressure over the puncture site for at least 5 minutes.
- Do not draw blood from an extremity into which intravenous fluids are infusing. Tests may not be accurate.
- Restrain an infant on an examination table during invasive procedures to avoid injury should the child move suddenly.
- Determine if client is allergic to iodine whenever a test involving contrast dyes is anticipated.
- Closely monitor vital signs and watch for bleeding after all invasive tests involving the vascular system.
- Ensure that all clothing with metal fastenings, all jewelry, and any metal hairpins have been removed before magnetic resonance imaging examinations.
- After angiographic examinations, including cardiac catheterization, monitor peripheral pulses distal to the catheter puncture site to ensure that arterial circulation has not been impaired. The temperature and color of the skin on the extremity should be compared with the opposite extremity.
- Encourage fluids after studies involving contrast dye unless fluids are contraindicated. Fluids will help the kidneys to excrete the dye.
- Do not leave confused clients alone on an examination table because of the possibility of fall should they try to get down unassisted.

24-Hour Urine Collection

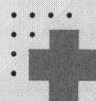

Occasionally, urine is collected for 24-hour analysis for urine metabolites to evaluate the client for abnormalities in metabolism, kidney function, or hormone activity. Catecholamines (epinephrine and norepinephrine), electrolytes, proteins, creatinine, cortisol, porphyrins, amylase, or vanillymandelic acid are most commonly assayed. Refer to Chapter 41 for specific information concerning 24-hour urine collection.

Culture and Sensitivity Testing

Culture refers to the growth of microorganisms in a specialized growth medium under precise conditions (heat, moisture, nutritive ingredients, oxygen). Sensitivity (susceptibility to specific antimicrobial drugs, eg, antibiotics) can be determined during the culturing process. Culture and sensitivity testing of collected specimens are performed when a microorganism is suspected during routine examination of a specimen, or after a **Gram stain** analysis, in which bacteria are stained to allow tentative identification of suspected organisms.

Testing for culture and sensitivity can be performed on a number of specimens, such as blood, urine, or sputum. These specimens are collected using techniques designed to prevent contamination of the specimen with other substances. Once collected, each specimen is labeled and transported to the laboratory immediately to prevent multiplication of bacteria within the specimen. See Chapter 39 for specific information on obtaining various cultures.

Diagnostic Tests

Diagnostic examinations may be performed for a variety of reasons, ranging from ruling out suspected disease to evaluation of current treatment modalities. A single diagnostic test or a series of tests may be required for complete evaluation of a particular client's symptoms.

This section includes a description of general categories of diagnostic tests. The discussion covers noninvasive viewing techniques, invasive viewing techniques, tests that entail the examination of body tissues or fluid, and tests that evaluate neural or muscle electrical conduction. Information included in this section about the procedures can be used by the nurse to teach and inform the client, for preparing the client, for supporting the client, and for assessing the client. Individualization of client care is based on information gained from the examination. Table 23-2 discusses ways in which diagnostic procedures can affect normal function.

Noninvasive Viewing Techniques

A number of noninvasive procedures have the capability of visualizing organs within the body and detecting structural abnormalities. The oldest and most common noninvasive procedure is the **roentgenogram**, or x-ray. Many new, more sophisticated diagnostic techniques such as computed tomography (CT), ultrasound, and magnetic resonance imaging (MRI) have been developed in the last decade to permit better visualization of internal structures. Occasionally, noninvasive viewing procedures are coupled with invasive techniques, such as the injection of dye to enhance visualization of internal structures.

X-rays (Radiography)

X-rays (radiographs) visualize internal structures on film by directing roentgen rays (short gamma rays) from an

Table 23-2* • *Potential Alteration in Normal Function Secondary to Diagnostic Procedures

Function	Potential Disruption
Nutrition and metabolism	NPO status may increase potential for inadequate nutrition or fluid volume deficit Bowel preparation may contribute to fluid volume deficit Invasive procedures increase risk for infection
Activity and exercise	Bed rest or restricted activity may be required postprocedure Fatigue is common Increased potential for shock with many invasive procedures
Elimination	Increased potential for constipation after using barium Bowel preparation before a procedure can cause diarrhea NPO and resulting fluid volume deficit can decrease urine output
Sleep and rest	Necessary preparation and anxiety can disrupt sleep
Cognition and perception	Pain or discomfort commonly occur with invasive procedure Confusion can occur when procedure prep causes fluid volume deficit electrolyte imbalances
Self-perception	Embarrassment common with some procedure (eg, sigmoidoscopy) Scars or invasive techniques may affect self-image
Roles and relationships	Testing may necessitate absence from work, school, or social activities Tests may interfere with ability to carry out normal activities as wife–husband or mother–father Expense of tests may be a burden on the family provider
Sexuality and reproduction	Some tests (eg, fluoroscopy) are unsafe during pregnancy Fatigue and anxiety may interfere with normal sexual response
Coping and stress tolerance	Anxiety concerning discomfort during the procedure and the test results is common for most diagnostic procedures Hospitalization may be necessary for some procedures
Values and beliefs	Some people may question the necessity or ethical validity of certain prescribed tests

x-ray machine toward body tissues. Underlying structures of differing densities permit varying amounts of the x-ray to penetrate the tissues and form an image on the x-ray film. Soft tissues, such as organs and muscle, visualize poorly and appear as gray forms. Dense tissues such as bone appear white and are the most clearly defined. Empty space, such as an empty bladder, appears black on film. Because x-rays are absorbed differentially, diagnoses can be made by noting abnormalities in the projected image on the film. X-rays are commonly used to identify fractures, abnormal growths, structural abnormalities, or the abnormal presence of fluid.

Radiology facilities are available in hospitals, clinics, physicians' offices, and some community diagnostic and laboratory centers. Frequently, x-rays are obtained on an ambulatory basis on a physician's direction. In the hospital setting, clients usually are transported to the radiology department for x-rays; however, if the client cannot be moved safely, some x-rays can be obtained with a portable apparatus in the client's room.

Nursing Considerations. Simple, routine x-rays (eg, chest x-rays or abdominal x-rays) take place in the radiology department and require no preparation other than removal of clothing, jewelry, or metal in the area to be examined. Female clients should be queried as to whether they are pregnant and the date of their last menstrual period so that the reproductive area can be protected from x-rays when pregnancy is a possibility.

All clients should be reassured that x-rays cause no pain or sensation as they pass through the body. In addition, most clients want to be reassured that the amount of radiation exposure will be minimal. The nurse may or may not accompany the client to the radiology department. During the procedure, all personnel leave the room during filming to limit their exposure to radiation.

The client will be positioned by the nurse or technician, depending on the view that is needed. It may be helpful if the nurse communicates any limitations in mobility or positioning to the radiology personnel. For example, some clients, particularly the elderly, may find it uncomfortable to assume necessary positions for extended periods of time. Finally, long waits in the x-ray department may be very fatiguing for some individuals.

X-rays Using Contrast Media. Frequently, a contrast medium, usually a **radiopaque** (opaque to x-rays) dye, is used to allow better visualization of soft tissues or to permit observation of organ motion. The procedure for administration of the contrast medium can vary according to the test being performed. When the gastrointestinal (GI) tract is being studied, the contrast medium **barium** can be swallowed for an upper GI series, or administered rectally for a barium enema examination.

Radiopaque dye also can be injected directly into the venous circulation. In this situation, the noninvasive x-ray procedure is coupled with an invasive technique. When circulating dye reaches the organ to be studied, the organ is clearly outlined, in contrast to the shades of gray normally produced on x-ray. To ensure that a concentrated amount of dye reaches the target organ, a catheter may be inserted into the venous circulation and advanced near the organ before dye is injected.

Nursing Considerations. Some contrast media are iodine based; consequently, sensitivity to iodine should be determined before the procedure. An allergy history should be taken by the nurse, especially noting allergies to fish or to iodine, and any past reactions to diagnostic procedures using contrast dyes. If the client has a possible allergy, the nurse should call the radiology department, as well as clearly indicate the allergy on the client's chart and wrist band. Reactions to iodine for sensitive people can be minor or severe, including itching, hives, pallor, wheezing, hypotension, and loss of consciousness (Stafford, 1987).

It is important to inform the client that some people may experience a burning sensation or a hot flush as the dye is injected. This reaction is normal. The client should also be informed to report all sensations to the personnel in the radiology department. Table 23-3 provides a list of diagnostic procedures using contrast media.

Fluoroscopy. **Fluoroscopy** is a type of x-ray procedure used to visualize movement within the body. Fluoroscopy can be performed at the bedside using portable equipment but usually takes place in the radiology department. Fluoroscopy may be used to permit continuous observation of the GI tract and is often used during placement of catheters (eg, pacemaker catheters; feeding tubes) to visualize organ structures and facilitate manipulation of the catheter.

Nursing Considerations. The client is placed on a specialized table through which x-rays can pass. The x-rays are projected "live" onto a fluoroscopy screen, much like the projection of a television image; recordings are made of the moving picture. Occasionally, the client is given contrast medium, which projects black on the screen.

The client should be informed that tests involving fluoroscopy are performed in a darkened room to permit better visualization. Fluoroscopy exposes the attending personnel as well as the client to more irradiation than a standard x-ray. Consequently, most tests or procedures will be performed rapidly to prevent unnecessary exposure; this may require that the client be asked to restrain movement for an extended period.

Table 23-3 • Diagnostic Procedures Using Contrast Media

Procedure	Area Visualized
Arteriography	Circulation through arteries
Arthrography	Joint cartilage and surfaces of the joint
Barium enema	Large intestines
Barium swallow	Pharynx and esophagus during swallowing
Bronchography	Bronchi and pulmonary tree
Cerebral angiography	Circulation to the brain
Cholangiography	Bile ducts
Cholecystography	Gallbladder
Endoscopic retrograde cholangiopancreatography (ERCP)	Pancreatic ducts, liver, and biliary tree
Intravenous pyelography (IVP)	Kidneys and ureters
Myelography	Spinal cord, spinal canal, and spinal roots
Upper gastrointestinal series (UGI)	Esophagus, stomach, and duodenum

Mammography. **Mammography** involves x-ray examination of the breast to screen for cancer and to evaluate palpable breast masses or cysts. Performed in the radiology department or on an ambulatory basis, mammography involves a specialized x-ray technique using xerographic plates instead of film. This method requires lower levels of radiation to obtain reliable images (Dodd, et al., 1987). Occasionally, tests requiring the injection of dye into the mammary ducts or scans that detect subtle variances in tissue temperature are performed after mammography.

Nursing Considerations. The client who is to have a mammogram should be instructed not to use creams, perfumes, powders, or deodorants the day of the examination; these products interfere with images. The nurse should also provide the client with information regarding the frequency of repeat mammography: currently it is recommended that women who are 35 to 40 years of age have a baseline mammogram; women 40 to 49 years of age should repeat mammography every 1 to 2 years; and women older than 50 years of age should have annual mammograms. High-risk women may have more frequent mammography. (American Cancer Society Recommendations, 1994). The importance of continuing monthly breast self-examination should be stressed. Cystic breast disease or very dense breast tissue can result in false-positive results.

Radioisotope Scanning. Some diagnostic radiology examinations scan the body after the introduction of radioactive isotopes. This type of examination, known as a radioactive or **nuclear scan**, may take place in the nuclear medicine or radiology departments, and can be helpful in evaluating organ function and identifying disease. Organ function, organ size, or the presence of abnormal structures in the thyroid, heart, brain, lungs, spleen, bone marrow, bones, and kidneys can be detected through nuclear scans.

The client can be informed that a **radioisotope** is a radioactive chemical that can be used safely in diagnostic testing. Some of these substances pass uniformly through normal tissue but collect in higher concentration in rapidly growing tissues such as cancerous tumors. Other radioisotopes have an affinity for certain body organs; for example, radioactive iodine is picked up by the thyroid. Still other radioisotopes gather in vascular areas of organs such as the heart while remaining conspicuously absent in areas that are ischemic and deprived of blood.

Very small quantities of radioisotopes are administered either orally or intravenously. Occasionally, agents also are administered to block the absorption of the substance by nontarget organs or tissues. After a short waiting period (minutes to 1 or 2 hours) while the isotope is assimilated, the body is scanned. The scanner visualizes the transit and uptake of the isotope in the body, and the image is recorded on a photographic plate.

Nursing Considerations. The client should be warned that some clients may experience anxiety and claustrophobia because the equipment is large, noisy, and placed close to the body. This poses no danger to the client. When explaining the procedure to the client, the nurse stresses that radiation exposure is minimal (usually no more than with a standard x-ray), and that there is no possibility that the client will become radioactive. The scanning itself is not painful, but some discomfort may be experienced because of the necessity to remain still for long periods of time. Most scans take between 30 and 90 minutes. Universal precautions are necessary only when handling any body secretions from the client who has had a nuclear scan.

Because of their potential for causing damage to developing fetuses, some radioactive scans are not recommended for pregnant women. When they are indicated, the pregnant woman has to sign a special consent. Nursing mothers need to stop breast-feeding until the isotope has cleared the body (McDonagh, 1991).

Computed Tomography. Computed tomography is performed in the radiology department. CT scans (also referred to as CAT scans) take multiple, thin, cross-sectional images of organs by directing a narrow beam of x-rays at the organ. A computer then generates a multidimensional image, which can reveal abnormalities. After initial scanning, a contrast medium may be used to improve imaging, and additional scans may be obtained.

CT scans are able to discern minor differences in the density of soft tissues. This information is used to diagnose such problems as tumors, benign growths, infarction, bleeding into tissues, and abscess formation.

Nursing Considerations. The client should be reassured that very low doses of radiation are used in CT scans; thus, radiation exposure is less than that with a normal x-ray, even when many images are obtained. The testing takes more time than an ordinary x-ray examination—up to an hour—and the client must remain still during the procedure. Children and restless adults may require sedation. Of concern to some clients is the feeling of claustrophobia experienced as the bulky CT scanner appears to "surround" the body during examination. Solid food is usually withheld on the day of the scan, and the client may be required to be NPO for a few hours before the test when radiopaque dyes are used.

Ultrasonography

Ultrasonography (ultrasound) is a noninvasive technique that uses high-frequency sound waves. Ultrasound procedures are performed both at the bedside and in specialized areas in the ultrasound or radiology department. During an ultrasound, a small instrument called a transducer converts electrical energy to sound waves, which are directed toward structures of the body and are then deflected back to the transducer and recorded. For this reason, ultrasounds are often called echograms (or "echoes"). Body tissues of differing densities deflect sound waves uniquely, enabling differentiation of tissues. The pattern of sound waves can be viewed on an oscilloscope, and a photograph can be made.

Ultrasound is used to provide information about the size, consistency, and shape of internal structures; abnormalities such as masses, edema, inflammation, stones, and free fluid are also identified. A number of body organs such as the heart, liver, gallbladder, and thyroid can be scanned using ultrasound. Ultrasound also is used frequently to evaluate the size of the fetus and placenta during pregnancy (Fig. 23-5). Because sound is poorly conducted by air, ultrasound is not very helpful in diagnosing lung abnormalities. A Doppler stethoscope can be used with ultrasound to detect blood clots or peripheral vascular disease (Massey, 1986).

Nursing Considerations. The ultrasound procedure requires no contrast medium, so allergic reaction is minimized. A coupling agent (mineral oil or gel) is used on the client's skin to facilitate good contact between the transducer and the skin. The client must lie still during the procedure; sedation may need to be ordered for the very young or restless. Consent forms usually are not required because ultrasound is noninvasive, involves no radiation exposure, and is associated with no complications or side effects.

Ultrasonography should be performed before any procedures that require contrast medium, or any procedures that involve the introduction of air or gas into an organ (eg, sigmoidoscopy); such tests could alter the clarity of the ultrasound. The client may be kept NPO for 8 to 10 hours before an abdominal ultrasound to reduce any gas present in the intestines. For some examinations, particularly those involving the pregnant uterus, the client may be asked to have a full bladder because this helps to elevate pelvic organs and provide better visualization. In this situation, the client should be asked not to void for 3 to 4 hours before the test.

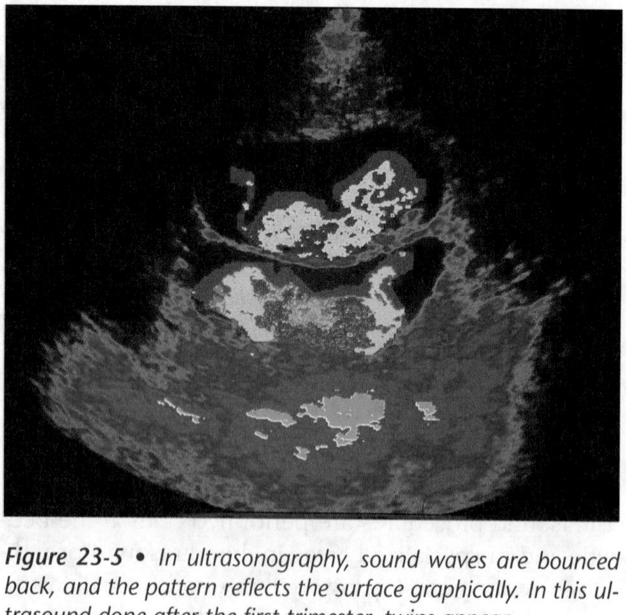

Figure 23-5 • *In ultrasonography, sound waves are bounced back, and the pattern reflects the surface graphically. In this ultrasound done after the first trimester, twins appear.*

Magnetic Resonance Imaging

Magnetic resonance imaging is the most recent technologic advance in noninvasive viewing techniques. The technique uses a bulky piece of equipment that usually is located in or adjacent to the radiology department. The MRI procedure uses a strong magnetic field and radio waves to produce images of bones, joints, muscles, and organs, and to evaluate blood flow. MRI can detect deviations in the pumping action of the heart, lesions or masses in fluid-filled soft tissue, or abnormalities in blood vessels. Tissues absorb and deflect electromagnetic energy differently depending on their physiochemical composition. Computers then detect and analyze abnormal findings.

There are two advantages of MRI: radiation is not used and contrast media are not necessary to clarify images. The expense of MRI and the necessity for cooperation from the client, who must remain motionless during the fairly lengthy scan time, are considered disadvantages. MRI also cannot be used on some clients with metal implants or cardiac pacemakers (Chernecky, 1993) because the strong magnet used in the procedure can actually dislodge metal within the body. Steel objects such as metal braces and some prostheses will not injure the client but will affect the clarity of the image obtained.

Nursing Considerations. Most MRI scans require minimal client preparation. Abdominal or pelvic scans require the client to be NPO for 4 to 6 hours before the procedure. All clients should have empty bladders. All clothing with metallic closures must be removed; all metallic objects should be removed from pockets and hair before the procedure. The nurse should inform the technician of any client prostheses. A consent form is required before the procedure. Like the CT scanner, the MRI machinery is large and encloses the client (Fig. 23-6); consequently, some clients may experience claustrophobia. It is also helpful to inform clients that a rhythmic knocking may be heard during the procedure.

Invasive Viewing Techniques

Directly accessing a body organ or cavity may be necessary to obtain information that cannot be obtained through noninvasive means. Common invasive diagnostic procedures include endoscopy, angiography, and cardiac catheterization.

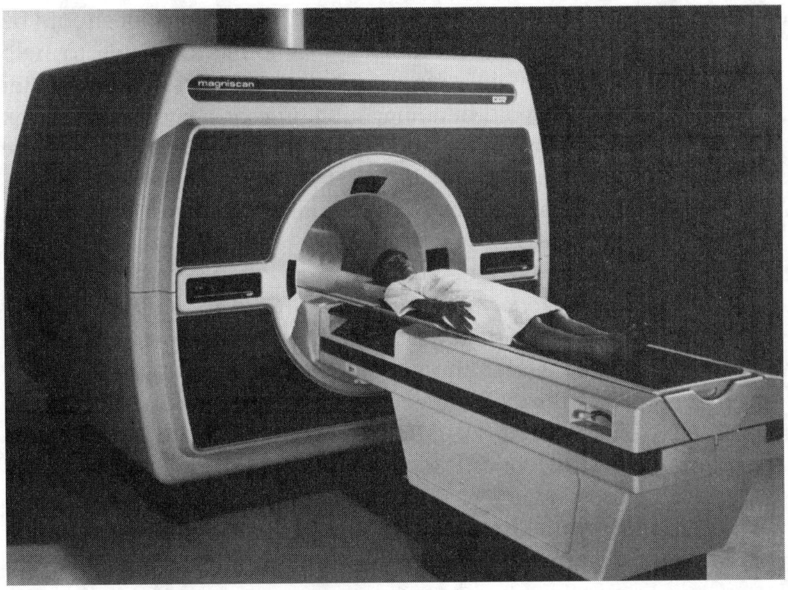

Figure 23-6 • *Client is shown on the gantry of a magnetic resonance imaging machine. (Courtesy of Thompson-CGR Corporation)*

Endoscopy

Visualization of a body organ or cavity by means of a scope is referred to as **endoscopy**. Endoscopy may be performed on an inpatient or an ambulatory basis, in a special treatment room located in the radiology department, or in surgery or, rarely, at the bedside. The physician examines areas directly through the scope, or views images on a television screen directly connected to a camera within the scope. Specific endoscopic examinations are named for the organ or part of the body visualized (eg, bronchoscopy visualizes the bronchus and sigmoidoscopy examines the sigmoid colon). Table 23-4 provides a listing of common endoscopic procedures. More specific information regarding endoscopic procedures is given in Chapters 37 and 42.

During the procedure, special instruments called endoscopes are used to visualize interior parts of the body. In the past, these instruments were rigid metal or plastic tubes. Fiberoptic scopes represent a tremendous advance over these earlier devices. The distal tip of the scope may have an opening through which anesthesia can be given or lavaging fluids infused and suctioned. Fiberoptic scopes can be inserted through normal body openings (eg, mouth or anus) or inserted through small surgical incisions. Endoscopic thoracotomy, which has been recently developed, permits diagnosis and treatment of some lung disorders (Tampinco-Golos, 1993). Endoscopy permits tissue to be removed for biopsy, bleeding sites cauterized, or foreign objects removed. Endoscopic examination is usually performed under local anesthesia, with most procedures lasting less than 1 hour.

Table 23-4 • *Endoscopic Procedures*

Procedure	Area Visualized
Arthroscopy	Internal structure of a joint
Bronchoscopy	Bronchus and bronchial tree
Colonoscopy	Large intestine (sigmoid through cecum)
Colposcopy	Cervix and vagina
Cystoscopy	Urinary bladder, urethra, and prostatic urethra
Endoscopic thoracetomy	Thoracic cavity
Endoscopic retrograde cholangiopancreatography	Common bile ducts and pancreatic ducts
Upper gastrointestinal endoscopy or esophagogastroduodenoscopy	Esophagus, stomach, and upper duodenum
Fetoscopy	Fetus in utero
Laparoscopy	Abdominal (peritoneal) cavity to visualize pelvis and adjacent organs
Mediastinoscopy	Mediastinal structures, organs, and lymph nodes
Sigmoidoscopy	Sigmoid colon, rectum, and anal canal

Nursing Considerations. Nursing care before and after endoscopic procedures can vary depending on the specific procedure performed. It is important that the nurse explain the procedure to the client before the examination. If the examination is to be performed on an ambulatory basis, the preparation for the examination must be discussed thoroughly, with provision of written material as available. Informed consent may be necessary for some examinations, and the agency policy manual should be consulted.

Before the actual examination, baseline vital signs and assessments are obtained. Frequently, the client is kept NPO; laxatives or an enema may be given for lower GI visualizations. Sedation may be administered before the procedure to help relax the client. Dentures or partial plates should be removed if the scope will pass through the mouth. Two positions for specific endoscopy procedures are illustrated in Figure 23-2*A* and *B*.

After the procedure, vital signs are monitored; any significant changes, complaints of pain, or abnormal bleeding are reported promptly, because endoscopy can cause perforation or other trauma to the visualized organ. After some endoscopic procedures, the ability to swallow must be assessed before the client eats or drinks; local anesthesia used in procedures involving the upper GI or respiratory tracts can temporarily paralyze the trachea or esophagus (Renkes, 1993).

Angiography

Angiography, performed in the radiology department, permits visualizations of the vascular system. Angiography is helpful in evaluating patency, blockage, or aneurysm (dilation weakness of a blood vessel). Angiography can allow studying of blood flow to the heart, brain, kidney, lungs, and lower extremities (Massey, 1986). Under fluoroscopy, an intravenous catheter is placed in either the femoral or brachial artery and is threaded to the area to be studied. After administration of a contrast dye, x-rays and cineographs are taken of the vessels being studied.

Nursing Considerations. Before the procedure, the client is usually kept NPO. Once the procedure is explained by the physician, informed consent is obtained. Allergies to contrast media or to iodine are assessed before the procedure.

Postprocedure care includes maintenance of a pressure dressing over the arterial access site for a period of 6 to 8 hours. Vital signs are monitored frequently, and frequent assessments are made of the access site and peripheral arterial pulses distal to the access site. Any bleeding, excessive swelling, or signs of decreased circulation or sensation to the extremity distal to the access site should be reported promptly to the physician. The client is kept on bed rest, and the extremity is kept immobile for 6 to 12 hours after the procedure. Because the dye is excreted by the kidneys, the client should be encouraged to drink large amounts of fluids to help eliminate the dye. Discharge instructions should include: avoid bending, squatting, or heavy lifting; drink plenty of fluids; and notify your physician if you have any bleeding at the incision site or experience pain, numbness, or tingling in your lower extremities (Dault, et al., 1992).

Coronary Angiography (Cardiac Catheterization). Cardiac catheterization is an angiographic procedure performed in the radiology department to assess blood flow through the coronary arteries, to evaluate congenital structural defects, or to evaluate heart valve dysfunction. After the angiographic approach under fluoroscopy, dye is injected into the coronary arteries, pressures in various areas of the heart are measured, and the flow of blood through the chambers of the heart can be observed.

Nursing Considerations. Before the procedure, all current laboratory work, particularly coagulation studies and hematocrit, should be recorded on the client's chart. Allergies should be assessed. Informed consent should be obtained after discussion with the physician. The client may be NPO or restricted to clear liquids before the procedure. After the procedure, nursing care is the same as that for other angiographic procedures. In addition to observing and reporting bleeding and changes in circulatory status, any chest pain should be reported to the physician immediately.

Aspiration Diagnostic Procedures

Aspiration diagnostic tests may be performed at the bedside or in the operating room. Aspiration is performed to obtain specimens for examination or to withdraw fluid that has collected abnormally in a body cavity. Usually, a special aspiration needle with a stylet and an outer, hollow-bore needle is used. The stylet is used to pierce the skin and then is withdrawn, leaving the outer needle in place through which tissue and fluid can be withdrawn. Biopsy, lumbar puncture, paracentesis, and thoracentesis are examples of aspiration diagnostic examinations.

The client undergoing aspiration diagnostic examination will experience discomfort associated with piercing the skin and obtaining specimens. Aseptic technique must be observed to prevent introduction of bacteria through the entry wound. Gloves should be worn during handling of body fluids.

Biopsy

Biopsy involves an excision of a small amount of tissue for microscopic examination. A biopsy may be performed to rule out or confirm cancer or to identify the nature of organ dysfunction. Frequently, biopsies are performed in surgery, but tissue for examination can be obtained by needle aspiration at the bedside. Liver biopsy, renal biopsy, and bone marrow aspiration are three biopsy procedures that may be done at the bedside.

Liver Biopsy. When liver dysfunction is suspected, a liver biopsy may be performed to identify cellular changes within the liver. Because blood clotting depends on proper liver function, any liver dysfunction can alter normal clotting and result in excessive bleeding. Consequently, blood coagulation studies are performed and evaluated before liver biopsy. If the laboratory results show an increase in bleeding time or prothrombin time, the physician may order vitamin K (AquaMEPHYTON) to be administered before the biopsy is performed.

Nursing Considerations. Before the procedure, an informed consent is signed. The client may be NPO. Sedation and a local anesthetic are used during the procedure; the client should be informed that some discomfort will be experienced as the local anesthetic is injected. The client assumes a supine position with the right hand under the head, which is turned to the left (see Fig. 23-2*C*). A biopsy needle is inserted aseptically, usually between the sixth and seventh ribs. A small amount of liver tissue is withdrawn (the client will experience some pressure as the specimen is removed). While the biopsy specimen is obtained, the client may be instructed to take a deep breath and hold it. The deep breath elevates the diaphragm and prevents chest wall movement, thus minimizing the risk of inadvertent trauma to the diaphragm or lung.

After a liver biopsy, it is important to check vital signs and assess frequently for signs of bleeding. A pressure dressing is applied to the biopsy site, and movement is limited to prevent bleeding. The client may be instructed to lie on the right side, often on a small towel, to provide extra pressure to the site. Potential complications of liver biopsy include hemorrhage, pneumothorax, and peritonitis.

Renal Biopsy. A renal biopsy is performed to verify abnormalities in the nephrons of the kidney. The procedure is similar to that for liver biopsy, but the biopsy needle is inserted through the flank (posteriorly, between the ilium and the lower rib area) and into the kidney.

Nursing Considerations. Because the kidney is highly vascular, postprocedural bleeding is a possible complication. Monitoring of vital signs, applying a pressure dressing, and careful assessment of the client are indicated. After renal biopsy, the urine is assessed for blood; the comparison of serial specimens will ascertain that any blood in the urine is decreasing in amount.

Bone Marrow Biopsy. Red and white blood cells and platelets are produced in the bone marrow. Should the client's hematologic studies reveal abnormal cell numbers or certain abnormalities in the structure of these cells, a bone marrow biopsy may be performed to rule out or diagnose anemias or cancer (eg, leukemia, multiple myeloma, Hodgkin's disease), or to evaluate the effectiveness of chemotherapy. The iliac crest or the sternum is commonly chosen for biopsy in adults. The tibia is the preferred site for biopsy in small children, because little marrow is found in the iliac crest or sternum of children.

Nursing Considerations. After explanation of the procedure and the signing of informed consent, the client is positioned in the supine position for a sternal puncture, or in the prone position for puncture of the iliac crest. Usual sterile procedures are performed, including draping of the area and preparation of the area with an antiseptic such as a povidone–iodine solution. The client should be informed that the aspiration of marrow is painful, but that it is important to remain still during the procedure. The bone is punctured with appropriate equipment and approximately 0.2 to 0.5 mL of marrow is aspirated. Concurrently, a venous blood sample is obtained.

After the biopsy procedure, the client is assessed for signs of bleeding or infection. Vital signs are monitored closely. Bed rest is usually maintained for an hour, after which normal activities may be resumed.

Lumbar Puncture

A **lumbar puncture**, or spinal tap, is performed to obtain samples of cerebrospinal fluid (CSF), to assess for infection, bleeding, or tumors, or to obtain CSF pressure measurements in situations where blockage of CSF circulation is suspected. The procedure can be performed at the bedside, in the radiology department, or in special procedure areas. A lumbar puncture also may be performed to administer anesthesia, antibiotics, chemotherapy, or to perform specialized examinations such as a **myelogram** (an x-ray examination of the spinal cord using contrast dye).

To gain access to the CSF, a needle within a stylet is placed between the vertebrae of the spinal column into the subarachnoid space. The space between the third and fourth lumbar vertebrae (Chernecky, et al., 1993) is usually chosen because it contains spinal fluid but is below the level of the spinal cord (Fig. 23-7). Once spinal fluid is obtained, it is evaluated for appearance and the presence of cells, protein, or glucose; CSF may also be cultured for the presence of bacteria.

Nursing Considerations. After the procedure is explained to the client, informed consent is obtained. Fasting is usually not required, but the client is encouraged to empty the bowel and bladder before the procedure. To separate the vertebrae as much as possible,

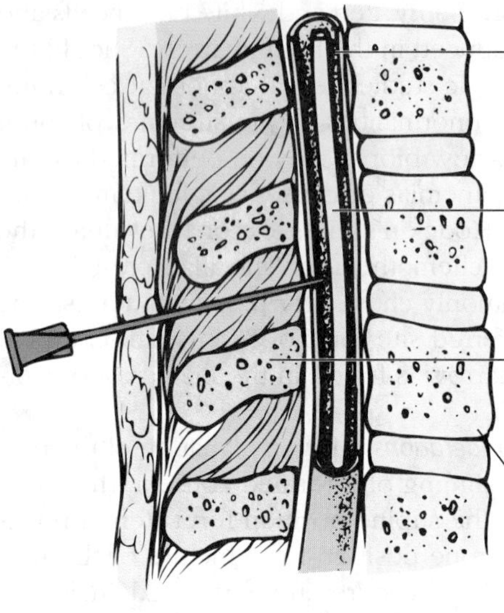

Figure 23-7 • *Site of the lumbar puncture.*

the client is positioned in a side-lying position with legs flexed and head bent toward the chest (see Fig. 23-2*D*). Aseptic technique is maintained throughout the procedure to prevent infection.

Once the procedure is completed, pressure is applied to the puncture site for a brief period; an adhesive bandage may be applied over the site. The site should be assessed for the leakage of CSF or any signs of inflammation. Assessment of vital signs and neurologic status should be performed according to agency protocol. Severe headaches can occur after the procedure if air was introduced at the time of the procedure or if a significant amount of CSF was lost. Occasionally, the client is instructed by the physician to lie flat for a specified period of time; other physicians may ask that the client's head remain elevated at a specified angle, usually less than 30 degrees (Chernecky, et al., 1993). The client may be encouraged to drink lots of fluids after the procedure to replace lost CSF and minimize discomfort from headache.

Thoracentesis

Thoracentesis, performed at the bedside, is a procedure performed to aspirate fluid from the pleural cavity surrounding the lungs. Normally, this space contains a minimal amount of fluid that lubricates the pleural lining around the lung; occasionally, more fluid can collect. A small amount of fluid can be removed from the pleural space for laboratory analysis. Larger amounts of fluid that have collected in the pleural space owing to infiltration or infection may be removed, restoring space for lung expansion and improving respiratory function.

Nursing Considerations. The procedure is explained to the client, and an informed consent is obtained. The client is positioned upright and asked to bend forward; leaning over a bedside table may be suggested (see Fig. 23-2*E*). This position widens the spaces between the ribs to permit easier access to the pleural space. The area is cleansed and draped, and a local anesthetic is administered. The aspiration needle is inserted, and fluid is withdrawn through a syringe or connected to a catheter and allowed to flow into a sterile, closed container. During the procedure, the client is observed carefully for alterations in pulse or respiratory rate, changes in skin color, or difficulty breathing.

After the fluid is aspirated, the catheter or needle is removed and a sterile dressing coated with petroleum jelly is applied firmly to the site. Vital signs continue to be monitored and the client is observed closely for changes in respiratory status. Breathing after the procedure is usually easier; however, pneumothorax can occur should the needle accidentally puncture the lung. Changes in respiratory pattern, bloody sputum, or severe coughing should be reported to the physician.

Paracentesis

Paracentesis is a bedside procedure intended to remove fluid from the peritoneal space in the abdomen. Like the pleural space, the peritoneal space normally contains only a small amount of lubricating fluid. Large amounts of fluid (eg, 1,000–2,000 mL) can accumulate in liver failure, renal failure, or cancer. The large accumulation of fluid, also known as **ascites**, can press on the diaphragm and make breathing difficult for the client. Pressure from ascites can also interfere with GI function.

Nursing Considerations. An informed consent is obtained from the client after explanation of the procedure. The client's weight is recorded before the procedure, and abdominal girth may be measured. The client is encouraged to void before the procedure because an empty bladder decreases the likelihood that accidental perforation of the bladder will occur.

The client having a paracentesis is placed in a sitting position with support for the back (see Fig. 23-2*F*). If the client cannot tolerate a sitting position, the bed should be placed in a high Fowler's position. The upright position allows most of the fluid to gravitate to the lower abdomen for easy removal. Strict aseptic conditions are used to puncture the abdomen at a site generally halfway between the symphysis pubis and the umbilicus. A large-bore abdominal paracentesis needle (sometimes referred to as a trocar) is used. Once the inner stylet is removed from the needle, a catheter is attached, which permits fluid to flow freely from the abdomen.

Once the procedure is completed, a bulky dressing may be applied to the puncture site because there usually is some leakage of fluid after the procedure. Vital signs are monitored after the procedure. In addition, electrolytes may be monitored frequently. If a very large amount of fluid is withdrawn, pressure changes can occur that will affect blood flow. In addition, because the fluid contains protein and electrolytes, the fluid and electrolyte status of the client may be affected. For these reasons, some physicians limit the amount of fluid withdrawn at any one time during paracentesis. Another possible complication is the possible puncture of organs during the procedure, so the client is observed for early signs of shock.

Diagnostic Procedures That Evaluate Electrical Conduction

Studies that evaluate electrical impulses supply information regarding the functioning of body organs, commonly skeletal muscle, the heart, or the brain. Electrodes (electrical sensors) are applied to specific areas of the body to measure the strength, tone, velocity, or direction of electrical impulses. These impulses are displayed on an oscilloscope or printed on a paper graph. The most common diagnostic procedures used to evaluate electrical conduction are the electrocardiogram (EKG or ECG) and the electroencephalogram (EEG).

Electrocardiography

The **electrocardiogram** is a recording of the electrical impulses generated by the heart. The ECG can be obtained on an inpatient or scheduled on an ambulatory basis. For hospitalized clients, the ECG usually is obtained in the client's room, using portable equipment. A technician usually obtains the ECG, although nurses with special training obtain tracings in some agencies.

The ECG is capable of identifying abnormalities such as arrhythmias (irregular disturbances in heart rhythm), injury from a myocardial infarction, enlargement of heart chambers, and, occasionally, electrolyte imbalance. Should a client complain of chest pain, an ECG is usually ordered to rule out the heart as a source of the pain. Nurses working in specialty units (eg, ICU, CCU) are responsible for detecting arrhythmias from ECG tracings (Fig. 23-8). See Chapter 35 for additional information on interpretation of the ECG.

Nursing Considerations. To obtain an ECG, the nurse applies electrodes to the arms, legs, and chest. Clothing is removed from areas where the electrodes are to be placed. A conducting medium, usually a gel, is applied to the skin surface underneath the electrode. The client will feel no unusual sensation as the recording is obtained. Occasionally a client may be asked to refrain from consuming food or beverages containing caffeine for 24 hours before a scheduled ECG, because caffeine is a stimulant and can affect heart rate and rhythm. The client should be asked for a list of all current medications because the ECG requisition may require specific information regarding the client's medications. After the procedure, the client should be assisted in removing any gel used on the skin before dressing.

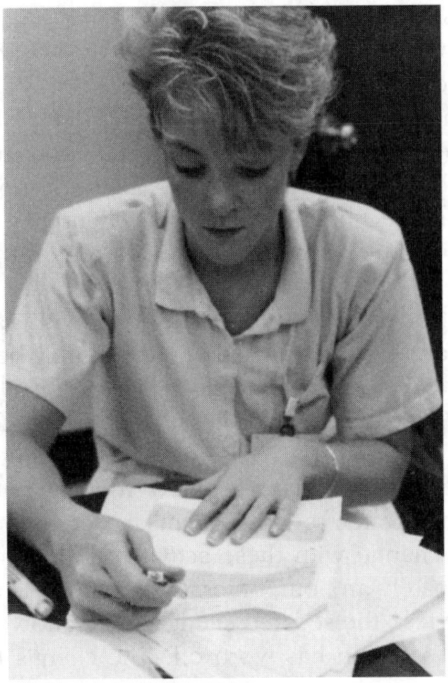

Figure 23-8 • Nurse interpreting ECG tracing.

Exercise Tolerance Testing. The maximal exercise capacity and functional impairment can be assessed through exercise tolerance testing (stress ECG). This test uses a wide, motorized belt (treadmill) on which the client walks. The speed and slope of the treadmill apparatus is adjusted every few minutes according to an established protocol. The client is monitored with a continuous ECG tracing and blood pressure determinations. The test usually lasts about 30 minutes.

Electroencephalography

An **electroencephalogram** is a recording of the electrical activity in the brain. The EEG can be scheduled on an ambulatory basis or obtained in the hospital. In the hospital, it is most desirable to obtain the EEG in a quiet area reserved for this procedure; however, with portable equipment, the EEG can be performed at the bedside when clients cannot be moved.

During an EEG, a regular pattern of waves is recorded with scalp electrodes and a multichannel, high-amplification recorder (electroencephalograph). The recording is particularly useful in identifying brain activity responsible for epilepsy, although between seizures clients often show normal electrical activity (Fischbach, 1992). The absence of electrical activity in the brain is used to support the diagnosis of brain death.

Nursing Considerations. Ideally, the client's hair should be free of oils, creams, or sprays when an EEG is to be obtained; however, this is not always possible. When the study is to be made during sleep, sleep may be limited the night before the test. Food and fluids should be ingested normally because hypoglycemic states can affect brain patterns. The client may be asked to avoid stimulants such as coffee or tea on the day of the test.

Electrodes are placed on the scalp with paste (tiny needles are sometimes used). Sedation may be ordered before the test to stimulate sleep. The test itself is painless and the client experiences no electric shocks or any unusual discomfort. Occasionally, the client will be asked to hyperventilate, to view moving patterns or cards, or to watch revolving lights to determine if brain patterns change with these activities. The study takes approximately an hour, unless a sleep EEG is required. After the test, the sedated client will be allowed to rest until the sedation has worn off. The client's hair may need to be washed to remove the electrode paste.

Nursing Research
Laboratory and Diagnostic Tests

Selected Nursing Research Studies

Crools, C., et al. (1993). Prediction and verification of a woman's intention to participate in a mammography screening program. *Journal of Health Education, 24*(4), 214–218.

Henrick, J., et al. (1992). Psychosocial factors and mammography use. *Journal of Women's Health, 1*(2), 123–129.

Johnson, J., et al. (1993). Difference in the evaluation of communication sources by women who have had a mammogram. *Journal of Psychosocial Oncology, 11*(1), 83–101.

Johnston, C., et al. (1993). The effect of the sight of blood and the use of decorative adhesive bandages on pain intensity rating by preschool children. *Journal of Pediatric Nursing, 8*(3), 147–151.

Klein, E. (1992). Premedicating children for painful invasive procedures. *Journal of Pediatric Oncology Nursing, 9*(4), 170–179.

Mansson, M., et al. (1993). The effect of preparation for lumbar puncture on children undergoing chemotherapy. *Oncology Nursing Forum, 20*(1) 39–45.

Shaw, C., et al. (1994). Information needs prior to breast biopsy. *Clinical Nursing Research, 3*(2), 119–131.

Possible Topics for Nursing Inquiry

- What difference in the client's perception of anxiety occurs when preprocedure instructions are given verbally rather than in writing?
- What is the variability in blood values in samples obtained with an evacuation collection tube rather than with a needle and syringe?
- What is the significance of privacy in a client's perception of dignity during procedures that expose body parts?
- Is bedtime blood glucose testing done most commonly before or after the evening snack?
- What is the effect of music during invasive procedures in reducing perceived pain or anxiety?
- What is the average length of time between collection of a urine sample and receipt of the sample in the laboratory?

Lifespan Considerations

At each stage of life, there are distinct ways of reacting to health-related issues. The age-related developmental stage of a client will affect the diagnostic and laboratory testing process. The needs of the client before, during, and after diagnostic and laboratory procedures must be considered. In addition, the age of the client may have an influence on the interpretation and individualization of the information obtained from the test.

Newborn and Infant

The newborn is entering the world with basic trust. The parents of the newborn are in the process of bonding and usually experience a strong sense of protectiveness. Parents should not be excluded from the testing environment unless their presence is deleterious to the process. When they are present, the nurse should explain why the test is being performed and what the test includes.

Some general principles apply to the newborn infant. If testing includes exposure of the infant to the environment, the procedure should be performed as quickly as possible to prevent excessive body cooling and a drop in body temperature. A heel stick is the preferred method of obtaining blood; occasionally, femoral artery samples are needed. If the test requires that the infant not be fed for a period of time, the infant should be observed for signs of dehydration.

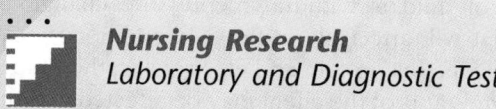

During the first year of life, the infant has learned to experience fear of strangers and strange environments. Conscious sedation is necessary for many diagnostic procedures, with chloral hydrate the drug of choice (Blevins & Benson, 1992). Parents should be encouraged to hold the infant whenever possible for the procedure. If this is not possible, the infant should be restrained on the examination table to prevent sudden, quick movements during the procedure. After the procedure, the parent should be allowed to hold the child warmly and closely. Because the skin is fragile, tape should not be used to secure dressings. Any observations to be made of the child after the procedure should be carefully explained to the parents.

Toddler and Preschooler

The toddler is becoming autonomous. Events are "processed" and assimilated into the child's world, and the parent is closely involved with the child's happiness. The toddler tends to resist external control, and may loudly proclaim unhappiness at being restrained. Consequently, it may be difficult for the parent to see the child restrained and struggling. Explanations about the test should be given completely and carefully to the parent, the test should be performed quickly, and the parent should be allowed to hold and comfort the child if possible. Adequate premedication is especially important in the young child undergoing painful procedures or procedures in which it is important to remain still (Klein, 1992). Pentobarbital seems to work better in children older than 2 years of age (Blevins & Benson, 1992).

The preschooler has more developed language skills. This child has become familiar with play and with fantasy. These skills can be useful in helping the child work through fears associated with testing procedures. Playing with doctor or nurse dolls or using dramatic play with role reversal (the child is the doctor; the parent the child) can help the child process feared or traumatic events. Allowing the child to keep a security blanket or favorite toy during the procedure may also be helpful.

Before the test, the child should be allowed to touch instruments if possible. If questions are asked, it is important to reply with simple, honest explanations. If the child asks if the procedure will hurt, the nurse should say something like, "Yes, it will hurt for a very short time, but it is alright if you yell as loud as you want." At this point, it is important to perform the procedure immediately and quickly so that the fear does not become overwhelming for the child. After the test the child should be comforted. Instruments and equipment should be removed from the environment immediately because these children want to explore their world and need to be protected from possible accidents.

Child and Adolescent

The school-age child is rapidly becoming less dependent on parents, but continues to "cuddle" in times of stress. During this developmental stage, the child learns right from wrong and has a strong sense of morality. It is also a period of rapid growth. Modesty may be evident.

Because language skills are developed, instructions and information about testing procedures should be directed at the child in easily understood language. Sometimes cooperation can be enhanced if the child is offered simple choices (eg, "which arm" or "when"). The parent should be encouraged to support the child. The natural modesty and privacy of the child should be protected.

The adolescent has entered a period marked by confusion. At the same time, the adolescent is searching for identity. Because this age group is very active, injury may lead to a number of diagnostic and laboratory tests. The youth may prefer to have tests done unaccompanied by a parent. Nevertheless, the parent must be responsible for giving informed consent for invasive procedures until the child is of "legal" age. Consequently, both must be involved in discussions.

Adult and Older Adult

By the time the person is an adult, a number of diagnostic and laboratory tests may have been experienced. Fear, pain, and anxiety, however, continue to be associated with tests for diagnostic purposes. Careful teaching and support from the nurse can help the client deal with these feelings.

Explanations of tests may be processed more slowly by the older adult. The significance of the test may be associated with fear of debilitating or chronic illness. Blood sampling may be difficult: an appropriate site for venipuncture may be difficult to find; veins are fragile and hematomas may form easily; and skin is fragile and easily torn with application and removal of tape. It may be difficult for the older adult to maintain a position for a very long period. Because some preparations require a period of abstinence from food or drink, dehydration is a potential problem. Some test results may vary with age, and careful interpretation should be made of results. Finally, preparations for tests may be fatiguing, and an opportunity for rest should be provided if possible.

Key Concepts

- The nurse facilitates diagnostic and laboratory testing by physically preparing the client, by scheduling the procedure, through client teaching, and by obtaining necessary supplies and equipment.
- The nurse may have responsibilities during the procedure that include offering support to the client, assessing the client, and collecting or assisting with collection of the specimen.
- After the procedure, the nurse may be required to offer additional support and to assess the client

for complications. Also at this time, the nurse documents the procedure, including the client's response to the procedure.

- Whereas information obtained from diagnostic and laboratory tests is used by the physician to diagnose specific illnesses or conditions, or to follow the progress of treatment for medical problems, the nurse will use this information to individualize client care.
- Adequate psychological and physical preparation of the client and support of the client during diagnostic and laboratory testing ensures the client's cooperation as well as adequate test results. The nurse should consider the client's age and developmental level.
- The physician is responsible for obtaining informed consent. The nurse may witness the signature of the client.
- Blood specimen collection includes venipuncture, arterial puncture, capillary puncture, and, occasionally, obtaining blood from central venous catheters
- Hematologic tests measure substances in the blood.
- Urine testing evaluates metabolic processes within the body.
- Diagnostic studies include procedures that allow organ systems or functions to be visualized and recorded. Some examinations are invasive and require entering a natural body opening or call for a puncture or an incision; other procedures are considered noninvasive.
- Noninvasive viewing techniques include radiographs (x-rays), fluoroscopy, mammography, radioisotope scanning, computed tomography, ultrasonography, and magnetic resonance imaging.
- Invasive studies include endoscopy, angiography, biopsy, and puncture of body cavities.
- Some examinations, such as electrocardiography and electroencephalography, measure the electrical activity within specific body organs.
- After diagnostic and laboratory testing, the nurse may be required to monitor the client closely for any signs of complications secondary to the procedure.

Critical Thinking Challenges

Now that you have studied this chapter, look back at the situation at the beginning of the chapter. You should be able to apply what you have learned about nursing responsibilities in diagnostic tests and procedures to the situation discussed there.

1. *Analyze the ethical and legal aspects to be considered in your response to the client's concerns and questions.*
2. *Plan two different ways of responding to this client, comparing and contrasting positive and negative aspects of each response.*
3. *Propose possible interactions with other health team members you feel would be helpful at this time.*
4. *Construct a telephone report to the nurse in day surgery if the client decides to have the procedure.*

References

Blevins, S., & Benson, S. (1992). A better way to get kids through scans. *RN, 55* (10), 40–44.

Centers for Disease Control and Prevention. (1994). Draft guidelines for isolation precautions in hospital; notice. *Federal Register, (59)* (214), 55552–55570.

Chernecky, C., Krech, R., & Berger, B. (1993). *Laboratory tests and diagnostic procedures.* Philadelphia: W. B. Saunders.

Dault, L., Groene, J., & Herick, R. (1992). Helping your client through cardiac catheterization. *Nursing, 22* (2), 52–55.

Dodd, G., Goodson, W., & Marchant, D. (1987). Optimizing Dx of breast lumps. *Patient Care, 15* (4), 43–58.

Fischbach, F. (1992). *A manual of laboratory diagnostic tests* (4th ed.). Philadelphia: J. B. Lippincott.

Goe, M. R. (1995). Laboratoty tests using blood. In S. L. Woods, E. S. Sivarajan Froelicher, et al. (Eds.), *Cardiac nursing* (3rd ed.) (pp 259–278). Philadelphia: J. B. Lippincott.

Jankowski, C. (1986). Radiation and pregnancy: Putting the risks in proportion. *Am J Nurs, 86,* 260–265.

Klein, E. (1992). Premedicating children for painful invasive procedures. *Journal of Pediatric Oncology Nursing, 9* (4), 170–179.

Massey, J. (1986). Diagnostic testing for peripheral vascular disease. *Nurs Clin North Am, 21,* 207–217.

McDonagh, A. (1991). Getting your patient ready for a nuclear medicine scan. *Nursing, 21* (2), 53–57.

National Cholesterol Education Program. (1988). Report of the National Cholesterol Education Program expert panel on detection, evaluation, and treatment of high blood cholesterol in adults. *Arch Intern Med, 148,* 36–39.

Renkes, J. (1993). GI endoscopy: Managing the full scope of care. *Nursing, 23* (6), 50–55.

Stafford, C. (1987). Reactions to drugs and diagnostic agents. *Postgrad Med, 82* (6), 179–183.

Tampinco-Golos, I. (1993). Endoscopic thoracotomy: How it can spare patients from major thoracic surgery. *Nursing, 23* (8), 62–64.

Yeaw, E. (1992) How position affects oxygenation: Good lung down? *Am J Nurs, (92)* 3, 27–29.

Bibliography

Clark, B. (1994). A new approach to assessment and documentation of conscious sedation during endoscopic examination. *Gastroenterological Nursing, 16* (5), 199–203.

Merrick, P. (1993). Nursing care for the patient undergoing IV conscious sedation for imaging studies. *Image, 12* (1), 1, 4–5.

Merritt, C. (1993). Bioeffects and the safety of diagnostic ultrasound. *Appl Radiol, 22* (1), 50–54.

Neilsen, B., et al. (1993). Pain with mammography: Fact or fiction? *Oncology Nursing Forum, 20* (4), 639–642.

Polis, S. (1993). Endoscopic procedures: Past, present, and future. *Today's OR Nurse, 15* (3), 7–14.

Tilkian, S. M., Conover, M.B., & Tilkian, A. G. (Eds.). (1991). *Clinical implications of laboratory tests* (5th ed.). St Louis: C. V. Mosby.

Selected Clinical Nursing Therapeutics

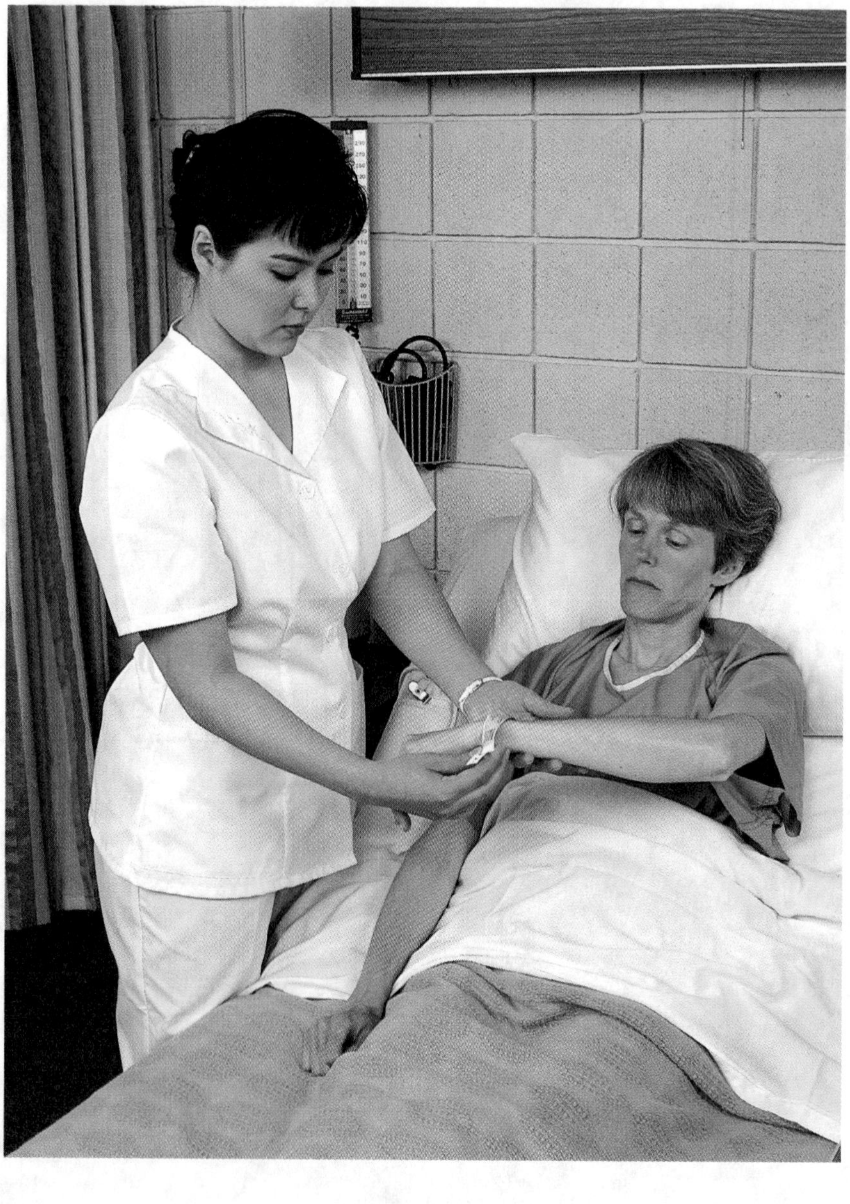

UNIT VI

Unit VI focuses on nursing responsibilities associated with common clinical situations that provide the basis for many aspects of nursing care: client teaching; asepsis; intravenous therapy; medication administration; and client care before, during, and after surgical procedures.

Client teaching, the subject of Chapter 24 and a fundamental nursing responsibility, has become even more important in modern healthcare provision. Nurses teach clients and families both formally and informally during almost every client encounter. The importance of asepsis has long been known. It is discussed in Chapter 25, with the latest information on infection control and aseptic practices. Knowledge of client teaching and asepsis is necessary for the description of care in the next three chapters. The nurse in his or her role in intravenous therapy, presented in Chapter 26, uses both client teaching and aseptic technique in giving intravenous fluids and medications, blood transfusions, and parenteral nutrition. Similarly, medication administration uses aseptic principles and often requires teaching the client about self-administration, drug actions, and side effects. Care of the surgical client involves much client teaching both before and after surgery and also requires application of the principles of medical and surgical asepsis. Additionally, Chapters 26, 27, and 28 involve nursing interventions resulting from physician orders as well as independent nursing actions.

Unit VI provides the knowledge base and skills needed for providing holistic nursing care in situations that are the basis for many client encounters and for clients at any point on the health–illness continuum.

Client Teaching

Key Terms	Learning Objectives

Key Terms

Affective
Androgogy
Cognitive
Compliance
Illiteracy
Learning
Motivation
Noncompliance
Pedagogy
Psychomotor
Return demonstration

Learning Objectives

Upon completion of this chapter, the student will be able to do the following:

- *Compare and contrast pedagogy with adult learning theory.*
- *Identify four purposes of client education.*
- *Describe important qualities of a teaching–learning relationship.*
- *Name and define factors that inhibit and facilitate learning.*
- *Discuss important assessment data used to individualize client teaching.*
- *Describe teaching methods and evaluation strategies.*
- *Explain the abilities, needs, and motivations of different age groups as they pertain to learning.*

24

A woman, accompanied by her husband, comes to the clinic for a blood pressure check. As they enter the office, you hear her husband speaking rapidly in Spanish, and it appears that he is upset. The wife does not respond but looks down and appears to withdraw. Because her blood pressure is elevated for the third consecutive visit, the physician decides to prescribe a blood pressure medication and a low-sodium diet. As the office nurse, you have 15 minutes to teach your client and her husband about the blood pressure medication and the new low-sodium diet.

Through the preceding chapters you have acquired a knowledge base of concepts and practical application related to nursing and client care. In this chapter, as you study about client teaching, you will expand your knowledge base of nursing therapeutics. You will learn how to apply the nursing process to teaching, which is important when caring for most of your clients. Critical Thinking Challenges at the end of the chapter will help you apply your knowledge to the care of the husband and wife in the clinic situation.

The well-known parable, "If you give a man a fish, you feed him for a day, but if you teach the man how to fish, you feed him for a lifetime," illustrates the importance of client education. Through the teaching–learning process, the client is empowered and often enabled to achieve higher level wellness or manage specific healthcare needs. Nurses frequently become the client's primary teacher; they also coordinate and reinforce information from other healthcare professionals.

Client education is an integral part of nursing practice. The American Hospital Association's *Patient Bill of Rights* (first published in 1975, updated in 1992, and printed in Chap. 3) addresses the issue that clients not only have the right to considerate, responsible care, but also to receive current information on diagnosis, treatment, and prognosis (American Hospital Association, 1992). The American Nurses Association's *Standards of Clinical Nursing Practice* include "educating clients about their illness, treatment, health promotion, or self care activities" (American Nurses Association, 1991) as a nursing responsibility for each client. Joint Commission on Accreditation of Healthcare Organizations (JCAHO, 1992) also has established standards for client education within healthcare agencies, which must be met for accreditation. *Healthy People 2000,* national health promotion and disease prevention objectives for the year 2000, have focused the entire nation on the need for education to promote optimum health for Americans (Office of the Surgeon General, 1990). Today, as the cost of healthcare is increasing dramatically and clients are discharged more quickly, research has demonstrated the cost effectiveness of client education.

Client teaching has always been a primary focus for the nurse regardless of the practice domain. The school nurse may talk with preadolescents about contraception and safe sex practices; the industrial nurse may conduct classes on plant safety; the clinic nurse may discuss with parents normal childhood development and age-appropriate activities; the ambulatory surgical center nurse may discuss postoperative care with a client prior to discharge; and the public health nurse may stress the importance of current immunizations to prevent the spread of illness.

A hospital stay seems to be an excellent opportunity for well-meaning healthcare professionals to impart as much wisdom as possible to the client. However, the stress of illness and hospitalization hinders learning. Even the most positive hospital experience (ie, the easy birth of a healthy baby) can be stressful. Because of this stress, the client may not hear or understand the teaching that is provided. Therefore, effective client education often involves follow-up after discharge.

Nurses can influence but not control their clients with education, because learning and changing are voluntary actions. Nurses encourage clients to improve their own health status, but no matter how important the nurse believes certain actions and attitudes are, the choice is the client's. The nurse never takes for granted that the client's beliefs are the same as his or hers; even beliefs that the nurse finds hard to understand must be respected.

Client education is seldom the formal process experienced in school. Much client teaching takes place informally during nursing care. During any client care activity, the client or family may ask questions, and this curiosity indicates a degree of motivation that must be honored. At these times, client education can be extremely effective.

Client education consists of more than handouts, pamphlets, and videotapes. It requires a therapeutic relationship, which was recognized by Florence Nightingale. Every time a nurse empowers a client toward autonomy and self-care, some autonomy and power is reflected to the nurse and the profession of nursing.

Teaching–Learning Process

Learning is the acquisition of a skill or knowledge by practice, study, or instruction. Learning theory has changed over the centuries. According to an early, teacher-centered theory, learning required a disciplined mind, and the goal was to memorize a great deal of facts. Later, student-centered theorists believed that learning could be completely intuitive; by encouraging self-direction, an active unfolding of knowledge would occur. Still others claimed that learning must build on prior knowledge and experience; the teacher actively imparts new ideas, while the learner passively associates them with related ideas to grasp principles (Rankin & Stallings, 1990). Different conceptual models of the learning process also view the role of the teacher differently, conceptualizing the teacher as director, designer, or programmer.

Nursing students have experienced all of these theories at work. It is impossible to learn anatomy without memorizing a great number of facts. Dealing with people, especially clients, always has an intuitive component. Pharmacology builds on the student's knowledge of pathophysiology, chemistry, anatomy, physiology, and mathematics.

Approaches to Learning

Early research on teaching and learning occurred in American classrooms, usually studying the learning process experienced by children or adolescents. Recently, a more complete understanding of learning has evolved as we study how adults learn. The term *pedagogy* is used to describe the approaches and assumptions about teaching as it usually applies to children or adolescent learners. *Andragogy,* first coined by Knowles, refers to his adult learning theory. Table 24–1 illustrates some of the differences between pedagogic and andragogic learning.

Pedagogy

The study of traditional classroom instruction of children focuses on the role of the teacher in ensuring that learning will occur. The teacher determines what will be taught and the methods that will promote learning. The teacher is responsible for providing motivation to learn and directing the process. The student's biologic and academic development also will influence the amount of learning that will occur. This conceptual picture of learning is one in which the teacher is in control and the learner passively participates.

Andragogy

Knowles theory of adult learning differs significantly from a passive pedagogic approach, with the locus of control as the teacher. Knowles (1990) views adult learning as based on the individual's need to know something, which is often influenced by a developmental task or a social role. The adult view of self often includes personal responsibility for decision-making and valuing independence. Rich previous life experiences assist in future learning for the adult. Andragogy assumes that adults learn better when learning directly relates to their lives or problems they anticipate will occur in the future. Andragogy focuses client teaching around the client's needs and personal goals.

Information Processing

Much research is being conducted to understand better how learning occurs. One such model concludes that learning involves a sophisticated method of information processing. This model begins with a sensory register, which determines whether an internal or external stimulus is noted or registered by the brain. Once registered, this information is stored in short-term memory, which is limited to five to seven thoughts at a time (Babcock & Miller, 1994). This limits the amount of data that can be processed at any one time.

While holding an idea in short-term memory, it is encoded by such factors as meaning, importance, or novelty so that transfer to long-term memory can occur. In the human brain, outlines of encoded information are thought to be stored as electrochemical deposits. When these deposits are stimulated, changes occur that can be reconstructed into memories. The more these pathways are accessed, the more stable the connection becomes and the more readily the memory can be retrieved (Babcock & Miller, 1994). Repetition in learning can help ensure that the memory is stored and can be retrieved more easily.

Domains of Knowledge

Knowledge can be acquired in three different domains: cognitive, affective, and psychomotor learning. These domains of knowledge were first described by Bloom in 1956. Frequently, learning does not occur in one domain alone, but encompasses all three domains.

Table 24-1 • *A Comparison of Assumptions of Pedagogic and Andragogic Approaches to Learning*

Assumptions About Learning	Pedagogy	Andragogy
Need to know	Established by the teacher; accepted by the learner	Must relate to the learners' need to know
Self-concept	Accepts direction from the teacher	Increasing need for self-direction
Role of experience	Happens to the learner	Integrally involved with self-concept; must be acknowledged
Readiness to learn	Biologic and academic development	Evolving social and life roles
Orientation to learning	Logic and system selected by the teacher	Life centered or task and problem centered
Motivation	External; approval of the teacher	Internal drives and life goals

From *The adult learner: A neglected species,* by Malcolm Knowles.

Cognitive

Cognitive refers to rational thought and is what we generally consider "thinking." Cognitive learning may involve learning facts, arriving at conclusions, making decisions, or drawing inferences. The nurse often participates in the teaching–learning experience in which the client assimilates new information to promote optimal wellness. During a cognitive teaching session, moving from the simple to the complex is likely to yield the best results. Ideally, the nurse starts with basic facts and concepts and moves to a discussion of how they are related. Finally, the client learns to apply the material correctly in different situations.

In the schoolroom, written examinations are an efficient and effective method of testing this sort of learning. Outside the schoolroom, written tests are often not the best evaluation tool because clients may feel intimidated by them. Verbal feedback can be effective. Ask the client questions that break down and reassemble the information. Give the client different theoretical situations in which to apply the information.

Teaching the new mother the anatomy and physiology of the breast as a mammary organ is an example of cognitive learning. When she can discuss the physiology of her milk supply, the let-down reflex, and the way these two work together, she has demonstrated her cognitive knowledge.

Affective

Affective refers to emotions or feelings. Affective learning results in changed beliefs, attitudes, or values. Sensitivity and emotional climate impact all learning, but they are especially important in the affective domain. Affective learning is more difficult to measure than cognitive or psychomotor learning because it is focused on thoughts and feelings. An example of affective learning might involve helping a new mother explore the possible benefits of breast-feeding for the health of her unborn baby and the mother–infant relationship.

Psychomotor

Psychomotor refers to the muscular movements that result from some sort of knowledge. Learning in this domain often means mastering a new skill or procedure. This is the easiest knowledge to measure because it can be physically demonstrated. Teaching a new mother to breast-feed is an example of psychomotor learning. When she can successfully and independently breast-feed her infant to the physical satisfaction of both, she has demonstrated her psychomotor learning. The nurse is often responsible for teaching a client to perform a certain skill independently (for instance, effective handwashing or good body mechanics). Principles are taught; the nurse demonstrates the skill; the client practices the skill; any questions are answered; and follow-up resources are identified. Because time is important, the process should be started as soon as the need is identified. A **return demonstration** is when the nurse observes the client performing the new skill; this is a valuable tool for evaluating psychomotor learning.

Learning Styles

The McBer Learning Styles Grid (McBer & Co., 1985) is one way to express **how** people prefer to learn and deal with ideas (Fig. 24-1). The horizontal axis represents the continuum of "doing" as opposed to "watching"; the vertical axis is the continuum of "feeling" (intuitive learning) as opposed to "thinking" (logical thought). A brief test is given, and for each of these two preferences, a number is assigned that expresses the degree to which the person prefers one or the other. Seldom does a person prefer solely one or the other, and under different circumstances, preferences may vary. However, the test indicates the person's general preferences and the personal style that he or she brings to the learning experience.

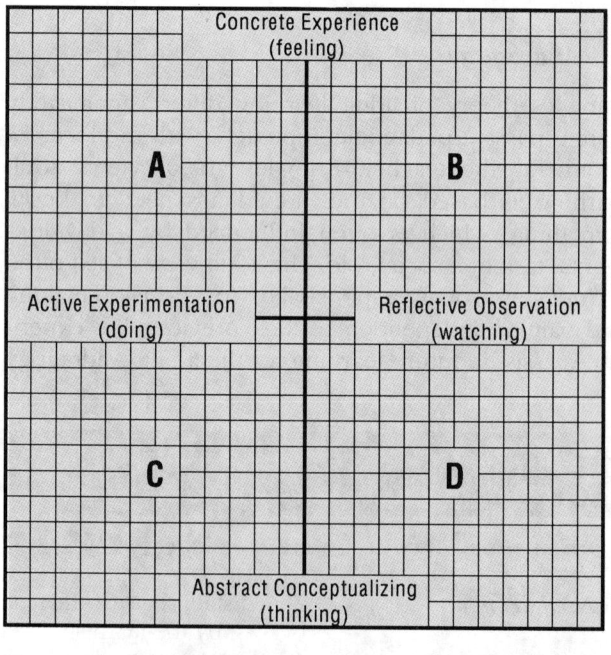

Figure 24-1 *• The McBer Learning Styles Grid plots how people prefer to learn. Learners are scored on two learning characteristics, a general preference to do or watch and a general preference to feel or think. People who score in Quadrant A are those who prefer to learn intuitively, with "hands on" experience. Quadrant B represents people who also prefer intuitive learning but would opt to observe rather than do. Quadrant C represents a "hands on" learner who prefers that information be given in an orderly way, for example, written instruction. Quadrant D represents the learner who prefers to learn by watching but likes data presented in an orderly, rational manner.*

Once these preferences are elicited, the learner is assigned to the corresponding quadrant:

Quadrant A learners enjoy "tinkering" (hands-on learning, generally without instruction).
Quadrant B learners prefer to see concrete situations, perhaps several times and from several points of view.
Quadrant C learners prefer hands-on experience and enjoy receiving information in a logical sequence (ie, written instruction).
Quadrant D learners enjoy watching step-by-step demonstrations. They can combine divergent ideas into a logical whole.

During client care, it is unlikely that the nurse will be able to explore the client's learning style in great detail, but the same material must be presented in different ways to different clients. For instance, if the nurse is demonstrating a psychomotor skill, and the client reaches over and takes the tools from the nurse's hands, the nurse should realize that this client has a "doing" learning preference. Another client may ask the nurse to demonstrate a skill repeatedly, reflecting a "watching" style. Whether the nurse chooses to talk the client through a procedure or to demonstrate many times depends on the client's preference.

Another clue to learning style is the client's response to written instructions. If the client responds positively by studying and asking questions, learning is probably occurring; however, if the directions sit on the bedside stand unread, the client may prefer a more intuitive, face-to-face approach. A possible opener could be, "I want to check out what you know about wet-to-dry dressings. Let's talk about it." Teaching the intuitive learner may take more time because he or she prefers human contact over written instructions.

Qualities of a Teaching–Learning Relationship

The interaction between a teacher and a learner is a special relationship characterized by mutual sharing, advocacy, and negotiation. Unlike some more traditional views, the teacher is not the expert who generously bestows knowledge onto the learner, nor should the nurse barter knowledge for compliancy. Both of these images represent the relationship as a power imbalance, in which the nurse, because of his or her knowledge and expertise, will control the situation. Effective learning occurs when the client and healthcare professional are equal participants in the teaching–learning process. At times, this means delaying teaching until the client desires to participate actively. Positive qualities that characterize the teaching relationship include client focus, negotiation, holism, and interaction.

Client Focus

Client education is a therapeutic relationship that should focus on the specific needs of the client. The client is living with whatever health issue necessitated treatment or involvement with a healthcare provider. The client also has unique values, beliefs, cognitive abilities, and learning styles that impact learning. Allowing a client to share enables the nurse to understand this uniqueness better so that teaching can be individualized to the needs of the client.

Holism

The teaching–learning relationship should consider the whole person, rather than focusing on the specific content being taught. This frequently requires a sharing process during which the client and nurse share feelings, beliefs, and personal philosophies. This sharing helps the nurse get a sense of the "big picture" of the client, which provides broad contextual meaning. Nurses also use their own experiential knowledge. For example, the nurse teaching insulin injections to a newly diagnosed client anticipates problems or questions other diabetic clients have had in the past; thus, the nurse is anticipating the impact of the diabetes on all areas of functioning.

Negotiation

Together the nurse and the client determine what is already known and what is important to learn. Once this has been determined, a plan can be developed with input from the client and the nurse. Sometimes negotiation is a more formalized process with a written contract to guide the learning experience. More often the process is informal and ongoing with continual checking and validating to guide the learning process.

Interactive

The teaching–learning relationship is a dynamic, interactive process that involves active participation from the nurse and the client. The nurse learns from the client, and the client learns from the nurse as content is introduced, specific points clarified or revisited, or new needs determined. This back and forth, nonlinear model is different from the simplistic model that many texts describe: presentation of content, learning, and evaluation of learning.

Purposes of Client Education

Nurses are involved in client education to promote wellness, prevent illness, restore optimal health and function if illness has occurred, and assist the client and family to cope with alterations in function and health

Table 24-2 • Examples of Client Teaching for Functional Areas

Health Pattern	*Example of Possible Teaching*
Health perception/ health management	Breast self-examination, importance of regular physical examinations and immunizations
Activity/exercise	Importance of regular exercise, how to use ambulation devices (eg, crutches, walker), deep breathing and coughing, leg exercises
Nutrition/metabolic	Healthy diet, dietary restrictions, wound care, how to monitor temperature, total parenteral nutrition at home
Elimination	How to maintain regular bowel function, Kegel exercises to decrease stress incontinence, self-catheterization
Cognitive/perceptual	Pain management (eg, how to use client-controlled analgesia), how to use memory aids, importance of regular eye and ear examinations
Sleep/rest	Importance of getting adequate rest, aids to promote sleep
Self-concept	Normal body changes, methods of promoting self-esteem
Role/relationship	Assertiveness training, parenting classes
Coping/stress	Biofeedback, relaxation techniques
Sexuality	Prenatal classes, contraception
Values and beliefs	Client's rights, "do not resuscitate" options

status. Such teaching includes all areas of function, as reflected in Table 24-2.

Wellness Promotion

The focus on health promotion has gained much momentum in recent decades. Nurses, irrespective of their practice arena, are involved in client education to promote optimum health and function. Knowledge and values are important when determining choices individuals make daily. Such things as food, rest, coping abilities, and hygiene and safety practices may influence optimal wellness. The motivation to change comfortable unhealthy habits is often lacking when an individual is feeling well. Health promotion is often aimed at the young so that bad habits will not develop. Figure 24-2 illustrates wellness promotion as nurses teach good nutrition to school-age children at a health fair.

Illness Prevention

Client education also focuses on teaching the knowledge and skills for early detection or prevention of disease or dysfunction. As research increases, the understanding of risk factors for disease improves. For example, studies have recently improved understanding of the link between some types of cancer and a high-fat diet. This knowledge enables the nurse to focus on dietary teaching to help decrease cancer risk. Studies also have proven the importance of early detection and support the teaching of testicular or breast self-examination on a regular basis. Research has better identified individuals at risk for specific illness, so resources and specific teaching programs can be directed at high-risk groups.

Restoration of Health or Function

When illness or dysfunction occurs, client education is important to help limit disability or restore function. In an acute care facility, much teaching is done with this aim. The client who is admitted for surgery receives instruction during the preoperative and postoperative period to help prevent possible surgical complications and ensure optimal recovery. In the ambulatory care setting, medications or diagnostic procedures are explained to

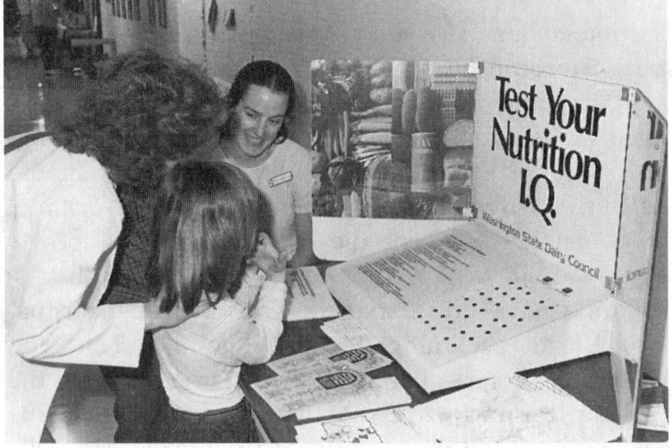

Figure 24-2 • Nurses teach people how to stay healthy by testing their knowledge of normal nutrition. (Courtesy of Overlake Hospital Medical Center, Bellevue, WA.)

Table 24-3 • Important Teaching Opportunities

Opportunity	Possible Learning Need
Admission	Unit policies, how to work call light and bed, specific treatments that have been ordered and why
New medication	Action of drug, possible side effects, frequency, and any special considerations
Diagnostic procedure	Preparation that is necessary before procedure, what will be experienced during procedure, any restrictions or special considerations after procedure
Surgery	Preoperative preparation, postoperative protocols (eg, deep breathing, leg exercises), pain control, how to get out of bed and turn easily
Discharge	Limitations on activity or diet, procedures such as wound care, when to call the physician

the client to reduce anxiety and assist the client in making informed healthcare decisions. During admission and before discharge also are important client teaching opportunities. Refer to Table 24-3 for common teaching opportunities.

Promotion of Coping

Client education is important for the individual or family who must cope with new and frightening procedures or adjust and continue to live with chronic illness or disability (Fig. 24-3). Teaching before surgery or a diagnostic procedure improves coping by decreasing the unknown (Davis, Maguire, Haraphongse, & Schaumberger, 1994). Adjusting to loss of function can be difficult for the client and family. Teaching may assist the individual to adapt by using new devices (eg, walker to assist with ambulation) or altering diet or activity. Some teaching assists with changes in body image or role expectations. Teaching may be necessary to prepare the caregiver for the technical and psychological challenges of caring for a loved one who has impaired function. Client education also is important for helping deal with grief, loss, and eventual death.

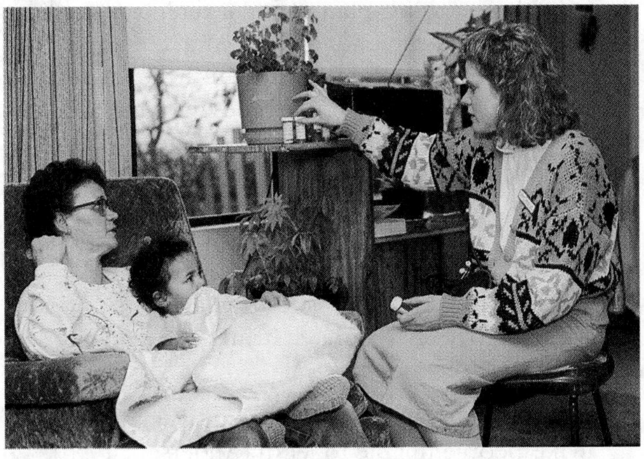

Figure 24-3 • *The nurse teaches about medication so the client can manage many chronic health problems. (Photo courtesy of Seattle University, School of Nursing.)*

Assessment for Learning

Nursing assessment in client education focuses on external and internal factors. External factors shape the nurse's perception of the client's learning needs, and internal factors show the client's readiness to learn. These assessments are usually simultaneous.

Assessing Learning Needs

The educational assessment begins with determining what the client needs to know or do to function more independently. An example is the need to gain knowledge or perform a certain skill before being safely discharged from the hospital or home care. For example, parents must demonstrate the ability to feed their infant with a new PEG tube before the infant can be discharged to their rural home. Another example is a couple who must show the visiting nurse that they can function independently with the wife's new paraplegia before routine nursing visits are stopped.

Baseline Knowledge

Often the client articulates specifically what learning is important and why this is so. Sometimes requests for knowledge come less directly; for example, a client may say, "I'm just not sure about all these new medications." The nurse must compare the client's knowledge, attitudes, and skills with those necessary for independent functioning. "Tell me what you know about (relevant topic)" can be a useful opener. If you feel this question might make the client feel tested, "When did your symptoms first appear?" may be a gentler lead, because most people are willing to talk about their symptoms; this can lead to further inquiry. For example, what the client did when the symptoms appeared can tell a great deal about baseline knowledge. Asking about family history may not only supply data about baseline knowledge, but also about cultural beliefs and attitudes. Finding out about previous client-education experiences may give some indication about where teaching can begin.

Cultural and Language Needs

Religion, health beliefs, language, and sex-role stereotyping are important factors to consider when planning client education. Cultural norms can influence beliefs about what constitutes illness and personal responsibility for one's own health (Falvo, 1994). Assessing a client's beliefs and ability to understand and speak English are important for effective teaching and learning. Not all groups share certain mainstream healthcare norms and values; for instance, Jehovah's Witnesses do not believe in accepting blood transfusions, most Islamic sects do not donate or receive organs, and many native Americans and Chinese people have folk medicine beliefs that they practice and trust. A Latino male may resist information about contraception if he feels it threatens his masculine identity. People who do not speak English require an interpreter. Working effectively with these people requires the nurse to have an open, accepting attitude (Fig. 24-4).

When a client from a different culture needs to be educated about nutrition, a registered dietitian may be able to help. Registered dietitians often are familiar with cultural food beliefs and can tailor a plan for that client's needs. In many cultures, women are the only ones to prepare food or care for the sick. Therefore, the nurse must identify and include these women in any dietary or health teaching.

Priorities

Clients often have many learning needs, so priorities must be set to help ensure that teaching will be effective. Priority setting may result in teaching a client basic skills in the hospital and arranging home nursing visits for follow-up teaching. Because time is usually the scarcest resource, assessment and priority setting should start early in the client–nurse interaction, whether it occurs in a clinic, a school, or an acute care facility.

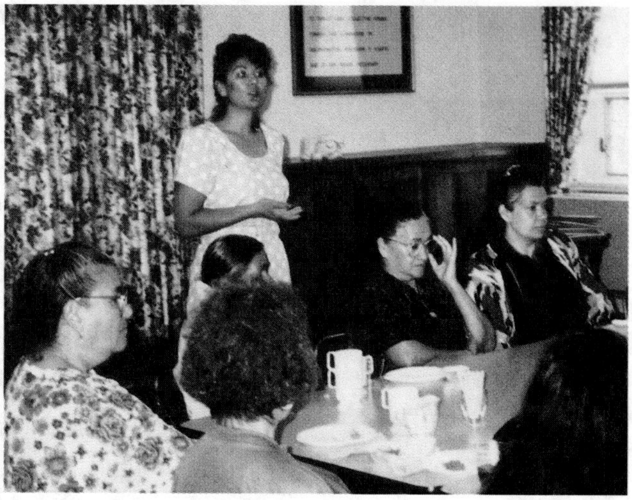

Figure 24-4 • *A nurse who is bilingual effectively teaches clients who do not use English as a first language.*

The client should be asked to identify his or her learning needs. The client may perceive a learning need when there is a desire to learn more to maintain or promote health or to fix a perceived problem that has occurred. For example, a routine physical examination may reveal an elevated cholesterol level. This information can increase the need and desire to learn how to make lifestyle changes to prevent heart disease. Teaching must occur when this learning is a high priority for the client. Sometimes the perceived need for health teaching comes from personal reflection, for example, a desire to exercise more and lose weight following the holidays.

In many situations, the nurse also shares with the client aspects that he or she feels are important to include in the teaching plan. After listening to a client who comes to the clinic for a urinary tract infection, the nurse shares that it might be helpful to learn how to prevent future infections and provides information about the medication that was just ordered. This process sets priorities and helps the nurse individualize teaching.

Realistic Approach

The nurse who takes a realistic approach sets priorities and tries not to teach too much in any one teaching session. Consider the following:

- The client's energy level. Physical weakness can make people unable to learn (Anderson, 1990).
- The client's age. Educational goals for children, adolescents, and adults are different, and these clients require different teaching styles.

- The client's lifestyle. If you foresee the need for follow-up care, will the client be able to gain access to it?
- The client's emotional state. The client may be too anxious or depressed to learn. It is not uncommon for those who have received an emotional shock (for instance, a diagnosis of cancer) to go through a period of denial, followed by painful periods of realization and depression.

Assessing Learning Readiness

Motivation

Motivation provides drive or incentive. It is a powerful determinant of success in client education and therefore is closely related to compliance. Motivation for learning starts with the client's recognition of the need to know. Motivation can be affected by financial problems, inconvenience, denial, lack of social support, nonacceptance of the disease, anxiety, fear, shame, or negative self-concept. Motivation can change from day to day. Some clients may be less motivated to learn ways to maintain optimum health or function independently if they derive important secondary gain from the sick role. Motivation can be affected by attitudes and beliefs. For instance, a middle-aged man who has started antihypertensive medications to control blood pressure may be less motivated to learn about them if a close friend confided that he became impotent when he took a similar medication.

When assessing motivation, it is important to learn what the client values. The client who associates a healthcare goal with something already valued will probably be more motivated. For instance, a pregnant diabetic woman is generally motivated to achieve good blood sugar control because her efforts increase the chances for a healthy baby.

Motivation is difficult to assess. There may be verbal cues (a client who says, "My wife takes care of all that") or nonverbal cues (lack of attention, missing appointments).

Compliance

Assessing the client's history of **compliance** or **noncompliance** (adherence or nonadherence to the recommended plan) is important. "What have you done in the past for your nausea?" may yield different answers from the client and family members. Unless a written record is available, past compliance may be hard to assess. "People often find it hard to take blood pressure pills twice a day, every day. Has this ever been a problem for you?" also can be a useful lead when assessing compliance. Giving the client an agenda can be useful:

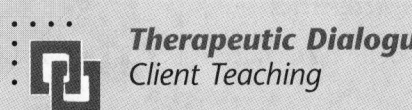

Therapeutic Dialogue
Client Teaching

Scenes for Thought

Jennifer Cohan is 14 years old and has been diagnosed with diabetes mellitus. She has said that she wants to learn to give herself her own insulin injections. You, the diabetes nurse specialist, have come to the clinic to talk to her.

Nurse: *Hi, Jennifer. I'm Lorraine Morris, the diabetes nurse. Your doctor told me you wanted to learn how to give yourself your shots. Is that right? (Making sure information is accurate.)*

Client: *Yeah, I told him that, but I don't know now.* Looks doubtfully at the equipment you've brought.

Nurse: *It's okay to be unsure. I see you're looking at the equipment I brought. Do you want to see it or talk about it first? (Assessment and giving choices.)*

Client: *Can I see it first? I know I need this insulin stuff, so I don't get sick like I did at school. That was so embarrassing! But I hate shots so I don't know how good I'll be at this.* Beginning to take out syringes, alcohol swabs, vials, and so forth.

Nurse: *(Sits and watches patient explore.)*

Client: *Look at those needles. They're so little!*

Nurse: *They do look small, don't they.*

Client: *Do we have to do this today?* Looks pleadingly at you.

Nurse: *I have a suggestion. How about if we go over the equipment today, and I'll give you some written stuff to take home and look at. Then we can reschedule the actual doing of it for next week. How does that sound?*

Client: *Okay. I like that better. Maybe if I read this for a week I'll get more courage.* Looks relieved.

Nurse: *That means that your Mom will have to give you the insulin until next week. Is that okay with you?*

Client: *Yeah, if that's okay with Mom. She hates shots, too! Laughs.*

(You and Jennifer look at the equipment together and make plans for next week. Then the parent comes in, and you teach her how to give the insulin while Jennifer watches.)

Critical Thinking Challenge

Determine how many of the three domains of learning Jennifer will use to acquire knowledge. • Calculate from the above information what kind of learner Jennifer might be. • Examine how the nurse assessed Jennifer's learning style. • Detect what the nurse did that makes you think she knew the principles of teaching adolescents. • Develop additional options the nurse might consider for teaching Jennifer.

"As I listen to you, it sounds like we need to talk about wound care and diet. What do you think?" Compliance is not just linked to inadequate knowledge. Many individuals decide not to follow conventional medical advice for many different reasons. This is often frustrating to the nurse and other healthcare providers, but the choice to follow advice is the client's and must be respected.

Sensory and Physical State

The client's sensory abilities and physical state affect his or her learning readiness, and the teaching plan must be modified accordingly. For example, a client with poor vision or compromised fine-motor skill may be unable to give a subcutaneous injection safely. A client with intermittent claudication (muscular pain brought on by exercise) may be unable to perform physical exercise. A woman who has just given birth may be too tired to participate actively in the learning session.

Literacy Level

One out of five Americans reads at or below a fifth-grade level (Falvo, 1994). They may not understand most written directions, videotapes, or even some audiotapes. Most client education materials are aimed at people who read at a high-school level or above, so a huge segment of the population is confused by this material but may be too ashamed to admit it. Also, the ability to interpret clocks and calendars is not universal, which can contribute to the inability to follow instructions and keep appointments (Vezeau, et al., 1991).

Illiteracy (inability to read or write) is found in every walk of life, among all races, and at all socioeconomic levels. A person's appearance and use of spoken language do not indicate his or her literacy. Many people with low literacy levels have average intelligence and can speak articulately. A roughly dressed laborer may be able to read well, but a professionally dressed person may be unable to read at a functional level. Educational level gives only a rough estimate of literacy.

How can the nurse determine the client's literacy level? Direct testing would be the most accurate way, but often this is impractical. Here are some less accurate, but expedient, methods:

- Check the level of the client's pleasure reading, if any.
- Give the client something to read, and later ask for a description of the contents in his or her own words.
- If possible, offer the client several options for learning methods (reading, watching, or listening). When in doubt, use the lower literacy material. When teaching stressed people, it is better to start with simpler material and add complexity later.

Nursing Diagnoses

It is wise to include at least one client education nursing diagnosis in the care plan. The most useful are Knowledge Deficit, Noncompliance, Ineffective Management of Therapeutic Regimen (Individual, Family, or Community), and Self Care Deficit. Knowledge Deficit, although approved by the North American Nursing Diagnosis Association (NANDA), has generated some disagreement in the nursing literature; for example, Jenny postulates that it is a related factor rather than a diagnostic label (Jenny, 1987). Client teaching also is incorporated under most other nursing diagnoses, because teaching is an integral part of nursing intervention planned for all problems. The nursing diagnosis should state the general area of knowledge deficit, which is more clearly delineated in the goals and outcome criteria sections of the care plan.

Diagnostic Statement: Knowledge Deficit

Definition

Knowledge deficit is the state in which an individual or group experiences a deficiency in cognitive knowledge or psychomotor skills regarding the condition or treatment plan.

Defining Characteristics

The following are defining characteristics of knowledge deficit:

- Verbalization of the problem
- Inaccurate follow-through of instructions
- Inaccurate performance of tests
- Inappropriate or exaggerated behaviors (hysterical, hostile, agitated, or apathetic) (NANDA, 1994)

Related Factors

Many factors can contribute to a knowledge deficit, such as lack of exposure, lack of recall, information misinterpretation, cognitive limitations, lack of interest in learning, and unfamiliarity with information resources (NANDA, 1994).

Outcome Identification and Planning

The planning phase of client education involves working with the client to develop a teaching plan, identifying appropriate teaching strategies, and developing a written plan to coordinate teaching among healthcare team members. Factors to consider in planning include client's assessed learning need and motivation level, learning style preference, literacy level, inclusion of

Nursing Research
Client Teaching

Selected Nursing Research Studies

Miller, B., & Bodie, M. (1994). Determination of reading comprehension level for effective patient health education materials. *Nursing Research, 43*(2), 118–119.

Owen, M. et al. (1993). Determination of the readability of educational materials for patients with cardiac disease. *Journal of Cardiopulmonary Rehabilitation, 13*(1), 20–24.

Reeber, B. J. (1992). Evaluating the effects of a family education intervention. *Rehabilitation Nursing, 17*(6), 332–336.

Young, R., et al. (1994). Effect of preadmission brochures on surgical patients' behavioral outcomes. *AORN Journal, 13*(3), 172–179.

Possible Topics for Nursing Inquiry

- What is the impact of shortened stays on teaching techniques used by nurses?
- How much do nurses know about written information available for clients from community agencies?
- How effective are return demonstrations as an evaluation tool for client learning?
- Is the McBer learning grid useful for individualized teaching to clients in a clinical setting?
- How significant is family involvement in client compliance after discharge?
- How effective is videotaped preoperative instruction on clients' learning of postoperative exercises?

family member or support persons, timing, and the appropriate amount of information to cover.

Outcome Identification

Client-centered, client-involved goals are the most effective. It is human nature to commit only to something in which we have some involvement or influence. Including the client in the planning process often shows the nurse clearly what the client is willing or unwilling to do, clarifying goals for the client and nurse.

Be brief and realistic when writing goals and outcome criteria. Do not promise overly optimistic outcomes. For example, make it clear to a pregnant diabetic that tight blood sugar control does not *guarantee* a healthy baby but definitely increases the odds. Create measurable goals with a time frame. Anderson (1990) suggests this form for writing a goal statement:

Who + Does + What + How + When = Goal.

For example;

Client + will demonstrate + dressing change + unassisted + before discharge.

Learning goals need to be evaluated and revised as necessary. If learning has been successful, new learning goals may be formulated. If outcomes have not been met, the time frame may be changed, or based on additional assessment data, the outcomes may be revised.

Planning Teaching Strategies

Availability of resources, learning style preference, and literacy level will help plan effective teaching strategies. Teaching sessions can be individual, small group, or large group sessions (Fig. 24-5). One-to-one teaching can be individualized. For this reason, it is often most effective but also most expensive in terms of money and time.

Choosing the right strategy for client education can make the experience more enjoyable for the nurse and client. If possible, use a variety of strategies to enhance learning and retention. Combining modalities such as seeing, hearing, and touching promotes better learning than using only one modality.

Lectures

A lecture involves a formal presentation of information by the teacher to a group of learners. This format is most effective when teaching facts (cognitive learning) but can be used for psychomotor or affective learning. A simple lecture (a one-way communication from teacher to learner) is much more effective when combined with discussion. Learners who are eager to contribute may be stifled by a lecture. Determine whether the client appears bored, anxious, or easily distracted.

Discussion

Discussion is an opportunity for the client to focus learning through exchange of ideas by exchanging information, clarifying feelings, or asking questions. It can be useful with individual clients or groups. Discussion involves learners more deeply in the learning process because it requires participation. Cognitive and affective learning can be enhanced by this strategy.

Demonstration

Demonstrations are particularly useful for psychomotor learning. Explaining the skill while slowly demonstrating it leads to talking the client through the procedure

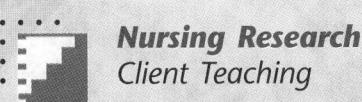

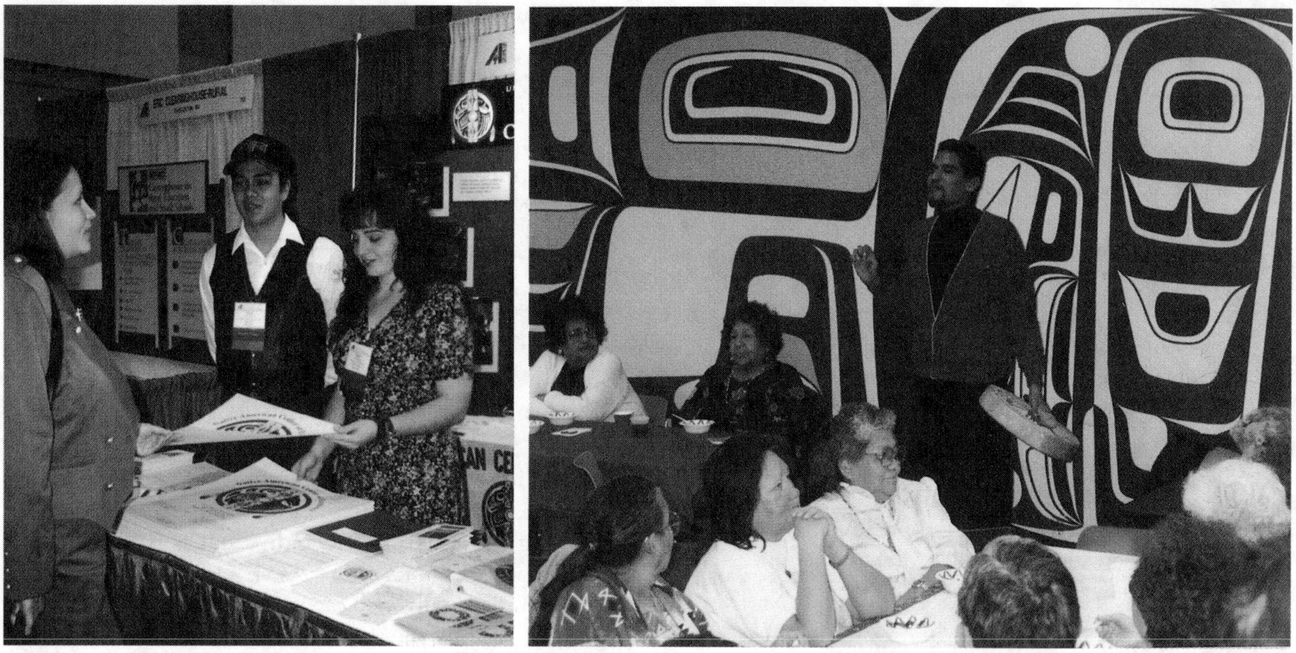

Figure 24-5 • *Teaching can take place in a variety of settings. At a health fair, a pregnant woman has individual teaching. Cultural gatherings can be used for health teaching.*

for the first few times. Videotapes or audiotapes can be used, but human contact is almost always preferable. Repeated practice can help the client move toward independent functioning. Return demonstrations help the nurse evaluate learning. Praise the client's learning while noting any areas for improvement.

Role Playing

Role playing, or acting out feelings or knowledge, is especially useful for teaching affective behavior to adults or children. It can be used to work through past, present, or anticipated feelings or new situations. The client reacts based on his or her experience, while the nurse stands by to offer guidance and feedback. Dolls can be used, especially when role playing is used with children. For example, a child may be asked to demonstrate how the illness in his or her mother has impacted all members of family by using a doll house and dolls representing each family member.

Values Clarification

Values clarification can be a useful tool for affective learning. A nonjudgmental discussion about people's perceptions of themselves and their world can help the client more accurately see the consequences of certain actions and articulate values. Values clarification does not focus on getting the client to adopt a prescribed way of thinking, but rather to better understanding his or her own values.

Teaching Aids and Resources

Teaching aids assist learning but are not a substitute for human contact. They are best used to supplement or reinforce face-to-face teaching.

Written Pamphlets

Access to written materials can assist the nurse in planning a teaching–learning session. Written materials are often prepared by agencies such as the American Cancer Society, American Heart Association, American Diabetes Association, or other health-related groups. Some written materials are prepared within the agency by a clinical nurse specialist or other nurses with a specialized teaching role. Being familiar with available written resources is important. The written material should pertain to the client's concern and should be written clearly, with up-to-date information that is consistent with what is taught verbally. The reading level of any written material must be screened for appropriateness for the individual client. Large print is important for clients with visual impairment. Frequently, written materials are provided in advance of a teaching session. This gives the client time to assimilate information and formulate questions or concerns. Whenever possible, encourage the client to interact with the materials immediately by circling important information or indicating important areas to review before the teaching session. It is best to select a few well-written materials rather than overwhelming the client with dozens of pamphlets.

Audiovisual Aids

Videotapes, slide-tape programs, and even computer-assisted instruction can be useful for subjects that are taught often, such as insulin injections or breast-feeding. Visual aids often increase learning during a formal lecture presentation. An overhead projector or chalkboard can be used. Some healthcare facilities have a special TV channel with programming to provide health education on a variety of topics. Let the client decide which aid might be helpful if more than one form is available. Audiovisual aids should not be used in isolation but are helpful when combined with discussion or one-on-one teaching.

Equipment and Models

Seeing and being able to practice on equipment promote learning. Whenever possible, the equipment that the client will actually use should be obtained. For instance, if you are a clinic nurse teaching a diabetic client glucose monitoring, the glucose monitor that the client will use should be used in the teaching demonstration. Models can be used to simulate actual conditions. For example, model breasts have been developed to assist teaching breast self-examination, permitting the client to palpate what a lump would feel like.

Use of Translators

When the client, family, or caregiver cannot speak English, a translator is necessary during the teaching session. When an interpreter is needed, the teaching session will take longer, because each message needs to be repeated twice. In addition to speaking the language, it is important for the translator to have knowledge of the culture and be able to interpret medical information clearly in a nonbiased manner (Falvo, 1994). Sometimes this is difficult when a family member or friend is used. Better choices would be bilingual staff members or professional translators (who may be available in large medical centers). Female translators may be able to communicate more freely with female clients without encountering cultural prohibitions.

When using a translator, the nurse should continue to talk to and look at the client. Information should be kept simple and direct. The translator should be instructed to translate the teaching word for word as much as possible. The name and number of the translator should be kept in the kardex or the client's record. A nod or "yes" from the client does not always indicate that understanding has occurred, because some people will agree just to avoid "losing face." Written translated material also should be provided.

Timing and Amount of Information

When planning a teaching session, factors to consider include amount of time available and amount of material to be covered. Often teaching sessions are brief and informal. For example, when you pass out medications, the nurse takes a few minutes to explain the newly ordered medication and possible side effects. This informal teaching should be reinforced whenever the medication is administered until the client can verbalize this information to you. When a more formal teaching session is necessary, planning the best time can help ensure teaching effectiveness. Things to consider include the following:

- The client is not tired
- The client is comfortable
- Family members or caregivers can be present
- Uninterrupted time is available so the teaching session is not interrupted by meals or necessary treatments
- Not just prior to an event, such as discharge or surgery

Hospital sessions should be limited to 20 to 30 minutes to avoid tiring the client. The nurse should warn the client about any time restraints. Saying "I have 20 minutes to talk" communicates clearly the nurse's time limit, minimizing the chance that the client will feel slighted.

Hospitalization is not the best time for teaching. Plan to cover essential material, but do not expect the client to learn all that is necessary when anxiety or pain is present. Outpatient education is often more effective than inpatient education for several reasons. Clients are generally less stressed and therefore are better able to learn when they are no longer in the hospital. They have lived at home with the change and bring practical, everyday questions to the session. Just attending an outpatient education session indicates a willingness to learn, and motivation is a strong indicator of educational success.

Appropriate Family and Friend Involvement

Whenever possible, plan to include family and friends in client education (Fig. 24-6). Their support is a strong indicator of client success. A statement such as, "I'm here because my wife made me come" may indicate denial on the client's part and tells the nurse about the wife's attitudes and influence. Never assume that because someone is a blood relative, he or she automatically wants to participate in client education or care. Friends are often as supportive as family members. For example, male homosexual acquired immunodeficiency syn-

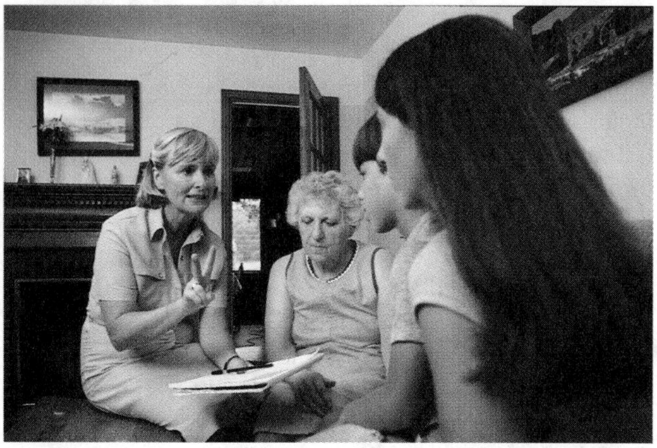

Figure 24-6 • Effective client teaching often includes the family.

drome (AIDS) clients are often cared for by partners and friends in family-like groups. When a family member or friend assumes the caregiver role, it may be necessary for that person to attend teaching sessions and demonstrate mastery of important skills and knowledge.

Written Teaching Plan

The development of a written teaching plan guides the teaching process and coordinates teaching among members of the healthcare team. Without a written plan, teaching is likely to be haphazard and ineffective. Having a written plan also serves as a useful reference for evaluation and fosters communication with other professionals so that they may take part in the teaching. A written teaching plan may be incorporated into critical pathways, indicating at what point in the care specific teaching should occur. The display shows the client education part of a sample plan of care.

Implementation of Client Teaching

Promoting client comfort, providing a comfortable environment, using repetition, relating new information to existing knowledge, organizing content, providing practice and feedback, and good communication skills facilitate learning.

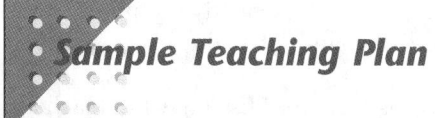

Sample Teaching Plan

Data	Initials	Nursing Diagnosis	Goals/Nursing Orders	Date	Initials	Outcome/ Evaluation
8/29	KM	Knowledge Deficit, wound care, related to inaccurate follow-through of instructions:	Mr. B. will demonstrate wound care independently by discharge, including:			
			1. Demonstrating wet-to-dry technique	9/1	KM	1. Demonstrated adequate technique
			2. Naming the signs and symptoms of wound infection	8/30	CJ	2. Named increased temperature, pain redness, and swelling
			3. Stating how to reach emergency resources	9/2	KM	3. Stated 555-1234 for consulting nurse, 911 for ambulance
			4. Stating the time and date of his first followup clinic appointment	9/2	CJ	4. Showed card data 9/5, 10 A.M., Dr. Smith

Meeting Priority Needs First

Prior to any teaching, it is important that the client is comfortable. Easing acute symptoms, such as pain, hunger, thirst, nausea, or dyspnea, allows the client to focus on learning. The client is given a chance to use the toilet. Pain medication is offered, and the nurse determines whether the client is comfortable.

Anger, fear, anxiety, worry, grief, and guilt also block learning. The nurse who is sensitive to client distress can modify the plan accordingly. Supportive body language and statements are useful. No matter how thorough planning has been, last-minute changes may be needed.

After assessing the client's sensory and physical state, the nurse may conclude that it is an inappropriate time to begin teaching, as demonstrated in the following example.

> *A young woman visits a diabetes education clinic, ostensibly to help get her type I diabetes under better control. During the interview, it becomes clear that the client has adequate knowledge to control her blood sugar. It becomes equally clear that she is under tremendous emotional stress: She was the victim of a date rape 6 months before. Apparently, she had been in a state of denial about the assault, and she could no longer sustain the denial. The emotional stress, not a lack of knowledge, rendered her unable to control her blood sugar. The nurse abandons the teaching plan. The most appropriate nursing intervention is to find appropriate, immediate mental health services for the client.*

Comfortable Environment

Anyone who has tried to study in a room that was too hot, cold, dim, bright, noisy, or distracting knows that environmental comfort affects learning. During client education sessions, the nurse tries to make the environment conducive to learning. If necessary, uninvolved visitors are sent away temporarily. Privacy is often important; closing the curtains in a semiprivate room, sitting close to the client, speaking quietly, and facing the client all contribute to a greater sense of privacy. The client's comfort is the most important factor. The client may feel more comfortable with certain belongings in sight or the heat at a higher temperature than the nurse would choose.

Individualized Teaching Sessions

Trying to teach too much at once can block learning (Anderson, 1990). It is important to be selective with information. Lecturing is appropriate only when addressing a group; discussion is much more effective when teaching a small group or one person (Fig. 24-7). Listening to the client's response gives excellent feedback about his or her progress.

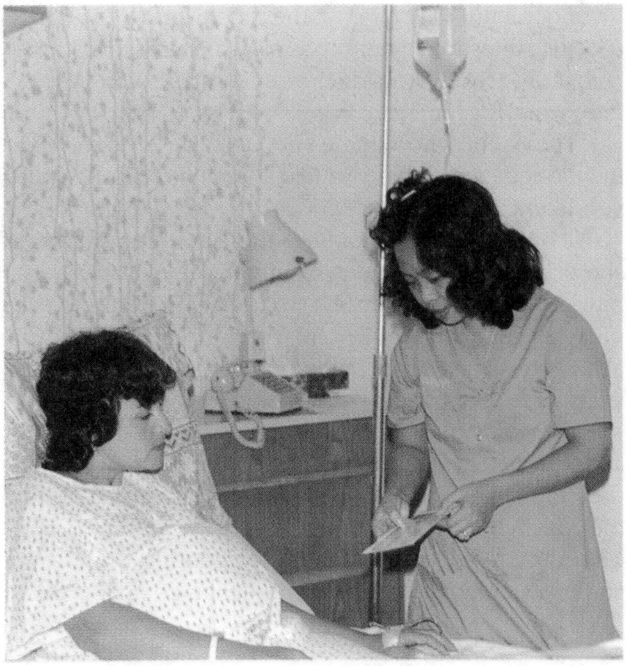

Figure 24-7 • *The nurse individualizes her teaching for the client, discussing her concerns, and answering her questions. (Photo courtesy of former Booth Maternity Center, Philadelphia PA.)*

People have different learning styles. Some prefer to do and others prefer to watch. When teaching a psychomotor skill, the nurse should be sensitive to those who like to do. A demonstration may have been planned, but if the client reaches out to touch the materials, the nurse may consider talking the client through the skill instead. Children learn through play and are generally energetic and eager "doers." However, if the child prefers to watch, a demonstration instead of instructive play may be best.

Communication

Good communication is necessary for effective client teaching. Chapter 20 discusses communication in the nurse–client relationship in more detail. Active listening requires the nonverbal communication techniques of silence, attending, and observing. If a client is comfortable and believes that he or she has the nurse's undivided attention, learning is greatly enhanced.

Participation is the best measure of involvement (Anderson, 1990). Getting a person to participate can occur by *leading*, making a pointed, specific statement, such as, "Your son has been readmitted to the hospital.

I wonder if this isn't hard on the whole family." Pointed, specific questions can accomplish the same thing: "What bronchodilators does your son take, and how do they work for him?"

The client who rambles needs to be *focused:* "You mentioned earlier that you fear going into labor. Would you like to talk about it?"

To *clarify* understanding, the nurse repeats what she or he hears the client saying and asks if it is accurate. To clarify with an AIDS client, for example, the nurse might ask, "Am I right? You've been hooking up all of your own total parenteral nutrition for the last year?"

Reflecting or *restating* (repeating the client's words) also can be a valuable communication tool. While expressing a great deal of personal feeling about death, the AIDS client could stop talking and begin to brood. The nurse could gently probe by quoting the client's earlier statement: "You'd rather die than go on like this?"

Repetition

The realities of today's healthcare—short hospital stays, limited home-care opportunities, and very ill clients—provide less time for client teaching. It is imperative to set priorities and repeat information. When cognitive or psychomotor learning is the goal, try repeating the information in different ways. For example, if the client has been learning a therapeutic diet, ask about appropriate food choices in different restaurants, on a picnic, or at a party. Have the client repeat the information several times. Ask the client how his or her daily routines will be affected by this new learning, and check to see if the new routines are being integrated into activities of daily living. Ask clients to practice and demonstrate psychomotor skills several times before discharge. Repetition may point out deficits in learning that would not be evident in a single evaluation session.

Because discharge instructions can be overwhelming to the client, the nurse should clarify important concepts, provide written instructions, review factual information, and have the client repeat the knowledge and practice the skills.

Teaching Methods

Methods of teaching differ in the three domains of knowledge. Principal teaching methods are listed in the display.

Principal Teaching Methods

Psychomotor (skill)

1. Skill demonstration
2. Talking the learner through the skill
3. Repeated practice

Cognitive (knowledge)

1. Lecture
2. Discussion (factual questions and answers)
3. Simulation (application of knowledge in different contexts)
4. Independent study
5. Tests

Affective (values)

1. Discussion and values clarification
2. Role-playing
3. Simulation
4. Discussion (factual questions and answers)

Cognitive

Because the cognitive domain of learning involves expanding knowledge, the material must be organized from the simple to the complex. Introduce the client to the basic concepts, and give definitions. Then help the client integrate these concepts into something meaningful and beneficial to health. Individuals do not learn isolated facts well. Learning is enhanced when information can build on previous knowledge. The most common error is to try to teach too much. It is better to teach some basic ideas well than to overload the client with many hard-to-remember facts.

Affective

When trying to modify an attitude or emotional response, the nurse must keep a nonjudgmental, nonthreatening attitude. Acknowledging the client's power to accept or reject the material can empower the client and lead to more healthy decision-making. The nurse who states emphatically the rightness of his or her position and the wrongness of the client's loses all credibility and influence. Listen carefully to what the client does value, and work from there.

For example, a nurse is trying to encourage a depressed, noncompliant paraplegic to join a support group. The client is too depressed to be involved in self-care but does seem to have a strong sense of contributing as a family member. Gently approach the client with the idea that better physical and mental health would enable him to contribute better to his family's well-being. The client may begin to assign a higher value to health when it is tied to better family functioning.

Psychomotor

Psychomotor methods involve the muscular motions needed to learn a skill. The nurse assembles the appropriate equipment (ie, dressings, syringes); having the necessary supplies at hand can save time and prevent interruptions. Written material, providing a step by step guide, can be a reference during the session and can be a reminder to the client the first few times he or she practices the skill independently. Approach the skill step by step, allowing for the client's questions and comments. Many adults are intimidated by learning a new skill, so encouragement and praise almost always improve performance. Comments such as, "Lots of people have that same concern" or "I've had many clients with that same problem" help the client feel less isolated.

Evaluation of Learning

Evaluation of learning is most effective when it is systematic, practical, and ongoing. Measurable, clearly stated goals and outcomes streamline evaluation. When the client actively participates in goal formation, he or she is likely to be able to do much of the evaluation.

This final phase depends heavily on what has preceded it. If evaluation becomes unclear, review the goals and outcomes. Were they realistic for the client's abilities, time frame, and resources? Were they clearly stated and measurable?

Evaluation occurs continually as the teaching proceeds, rather than waiting until the teaching is completed. In this way, the teaching session can be continually adjusted to meet the needs of the client. Feedback from the nurse to the client is most effective when it enhances the client's self-concept and motivates him or her to higher learning (Rankin & Stallings, 1990). Asking the client to repeat or demonstrate what has been learned to family members is one way to accomplish this, especially with children. Remind the client of the progress made rather than what is left to be done.

Evaluation can take several forms: written tests, questionnaires, oral tests, or return demonstrations.

Written Tests

Written tests are time consuming, intimidating, and not always specific to the client. They are useful only in the following situations:

- The client is literate (do not take this for granted).
- Clear educational objectives have been mutually decided.
- It is necessary to measure a broad sample of factual information.
- A skilled test writer has prepared the test.

As in the classroom, written tests are most useful for evaluating cognitive learning. Affective learning cannot be tested because no answer is right or wrong. Tests may be useful as assessment tools (pretests) or as evaluation tools to check the client's progress. A questionnaire may be used to evaluate how helpful an educational program has been for a group of learners, so positive changes can be made if the program is offered again.

Oral Tests

Oral tests are usually more expedient and less intimidating than written ones. Questions can be informally phrased, and the client usually gives immediate, specific, and useful feedback. It is best to stay as casual as possible, because the higher the client's anxiety about being tested, the less likely the evaluation will be accurate. Evaluation of the client's verbal response can be useful in testing cognitive learning, but affective learning in the form of an attitude change is more difficult to measure.

Return Demonstration

The return demonstration is a way of testing skill performance. How accurately and independently the client can perform a skill is almost always a clear indication of learning. Psychomotor skills can be evaluated with this method. The nurse should give feedback about parts done well, along with areas for improvement. Figure 24-8 shows how nurses use return demonstration to evaluate learning breast self-examination techniques.

Simulation

Simulation evaluates whether the client can apply learning in different situations. Offer a scenario to the client, and ask what the best choice(s) would be. For example, the nurse could evaluate dietary learning by asking the client about the best choices in various restaurants, or he or she could evaluate diabetic sick-day care by posing different sick-day scenarios.

Documentation of Learning

Documenting client education is as important as documenting any other aspect of client care. Documentation of client education serves several purposes (Anderson, 1990):

- It communicates the plan and progress to other healthcare professionals.
- It fulfills the nursing job description as delineated by local, state, and national licensing agencies.
- It provides a legal record.

Documentation must contain the subject matter, the client's response, and any necessary break in the process (for example, if after evaluation, the nurse found it necessary to return to the planning stage). Well-documented client education is a record of meth-

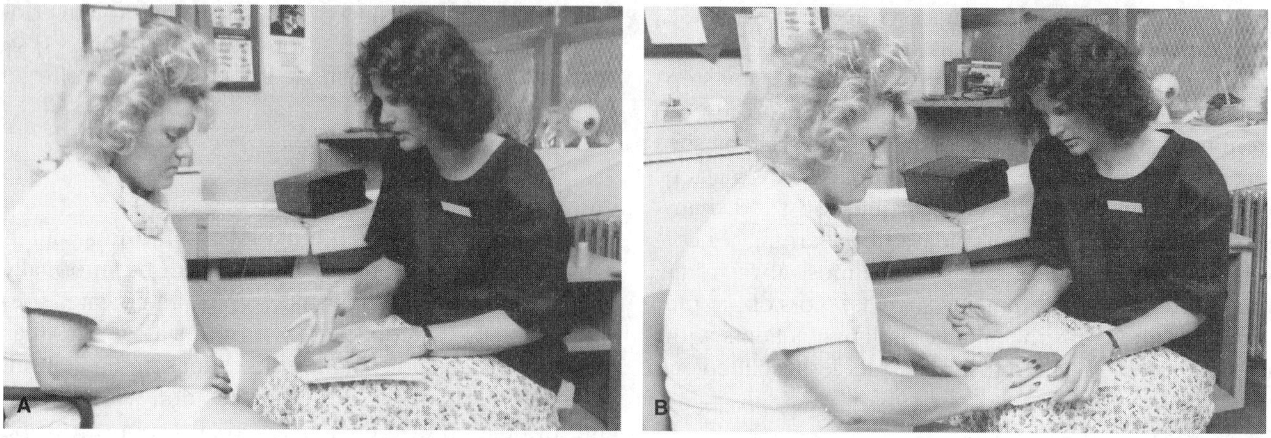

Figure 24-8 • (A) The nurse uses a visual aid to help her teach breast self-examination. (B) The client is asked for a return demonstration to evaluate skill attainment. (Courtesy of University of Washington School of Nursing, Seattle, WA.)

ods that did or did not work, and it can give some indication of client compliance over time.

Lifespan Considerations

Changes across the lifespan affect the client's learning needs and abilities. When planning client teaching, consider the client's developmental level to individualize the teaching and promote optimal learning.

Newborn and Infant

Newborns and infants learn by interacting with their environment. During this period of rapid development, the infant learns a great deal (for example, how to recognize his or her mother, how to follow objects as they move, how to hold toys). The nurse should encourage an environment rich in appropriate stimuli to foster normal cognitive development.

During this stage, the infant is not ready for formalized teaching; instead, any necessary teaching is given to parents and caregivers. Teaching the parents about various aspects of child care helps promote positive parent–child bonding.

Toddler and Preschooler

Because toddlers and preschoolers are accustomed to learning from and communicating with their parents, the parents are usually the most effective teachers. Children learn through play, so using dolls or toys as models can be effective and can be continued at home (Fig. 24-9). Learning is more successful if it can be continued at home and added to existing home routines (Anderson, 1990).

Children 2 to 5 years old like to be addressed with their parents listening. They are likely to have many questions and may ask the same ones many times. Their questions should be answered immediately, directly, and in language they can understand. Sometimes this means checking with the parent or caregiver concerning words that the child uses to describe body functions or important things. Preschoolers are generally energetic and restless, so try to limit the session to 10 minutes (Anderson, 1990). Let the child handle machines or supplies as soon as possible. Children of this age can understand some anatomy, so when possible, use models and correct anatomic names.

Trust is vital. If you tell a preschooler that a procedure will not hurt, but it does, you have lost credibility with the child, and learning is hindered.

Preschoolers, compared with toddlers, have learned to do many more things (using the toilet, eating, and dressing, for example), and they are usually proud of these things. Young children are extremely egocentric: They think the world revolves around them and that all events relate to them. Teaching should be related to the child's specific life experiences when possible.

Learning should be evaluated frequently to ensure that the child understands. A preschooler usually enjoys displaying new knowledge, giving the nurse the chance to praise the child repeatedly and offer rewards such as stickers, picture books, or rubber stamps.

Child and Adolescent

School-age children are usually eager to learn. They can understand cause and effect ("If I don't stay off my leg, it won't heal as quickly, and it'll be longer before I can play outside at recess"). Include children in educational planning, allowing them to help set goals. Being accustomed to a classroom atmosphere, they understand the scheduling of work and play.

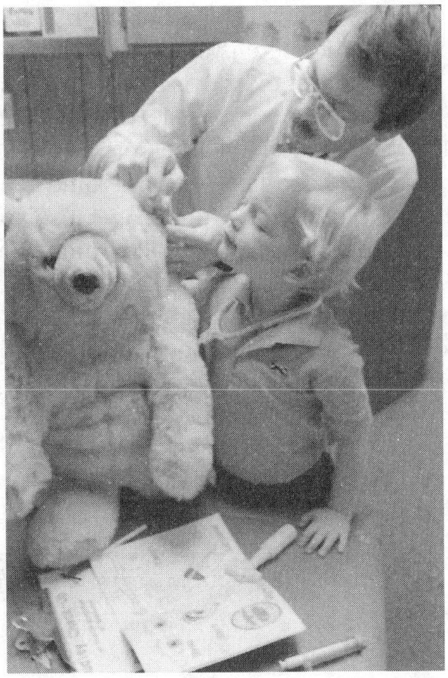

Figure 24-9 • Teaching should be individualized for the age of the client. Demonstrating on a friendly stuffed animal and using age-appropriate coloring books makes learning fun for this preschooler. Teaching used in the healthcare facility can be carried through in the home. (Courtesy of Overlake Hospital Medical Center, Bellevue, WA.)

All questions should be answered immediately and truthfully, or the nurse loses credibility. Trust is vital to learning and to establishing a relationship in which the child feels comfortable enough to express fears and concerns.

Educational content can be more sophisticated for this group than for the preschooler. Coloring books for teaching anatomy work well. Written material is fine at the proper reading level, keeping in mind that the hospitalized child may regress. Procedures must be explained directly to the child with the parents in the background. Sessions should be no longer than 30 minutes.

"Winning" is important for school-age children, so success is generally highly valued. Use of charts with stickers to mark progress is effective with this group.

Adolescents generally enjoy complete, open, and honest explanations to their questions. Their peers are usually more influential than parents, teachers, or nurses. It is fine to include peers in a teaching session; in fact, general healthcare information may be included for the benefit of these visitors. A sensitive, caring attitude is essential to educate adolescents effectively. To maintain the adolescent's trust, confidences must be kept; if a confidence must be broken, tell the client who you must tell and why.

Adolescents must be included in any educational planning because their struggle for independence makes them averse to having anything imposed on them. They are more likely to comply when alternatives and consequences are explained (Anderson, 1990). Ask the client what he or she needs to know. Find out the value system associated with the illness, and work from the youngster's point of view. Adolescents are generally sophisticated learners, able to understand broad concepts and assimilate much information. They are oriented to the present, however, and are more in tune with immediate advantages than with long-term results.

This age group is accustomed to teaching sessions of 45 to 50 minutes in school, and this is probably the maximum effective length. It may be better not to include parents in the session to encourage client autonomy and heighten self-concept; parents can be informed later. Literature to review between sessions can be useful with this group.

Adult and Older Adult

Adults tend to be motivated by activities that enhance or maintain their self-esteem. Self-direction and achievement generally boost self-esteem; dependence and error generally decrease it. Adults tend to take errors personally, thinking poorly of themselves if they think they are taking too long to grasp a concept.

Nursing Care Guidelines
Teaching the Older Learner

- Use a brightly lit, glare-free room.
- Use visual aids with large, well-spaced letters and primary colors.
- Eliminate extraneous noise.
- Face the learner.
- Speak in low, slow tones.
- Limit sessions to 20 to 30 minutes.
- Watch for cues indicating inadequate hearing, such as leaning forward, cupping an ear, frowning when trying to hear, or starting a separate conversation.
- Relate new material to the past or past experiences in a meaningful way.
- Supply one idea at a time. Use frequent summaries and positive feedback.
- Provide a written or recorded summary of the session.

Medication Teaching

- Be sure the client knows what each medication does, how many pills to take, and when.
- Discuss what to do if the patient misses a dose. (Containers that hold a week's worth of medications can be a boon to accuracy and consistency.)
- Be sure the client has written medication instructions in appropriate size, form, and language.

Adult learners respond well to a straightforward teaching approach and can apply the knowledge immediately. Try to provide a comfortable, informal, friendly learning environment where the client can feel appreciated.

Young adults usually have plenty of energy and take good health for granted. Learning must be practical, because these people generally lead busy lives. When setting educational goals with clients from this group, take a practical approach, if possible explaining how the change will improve daily life. Adults of this age are often motivated by the thought of maintaining their functioning to care for their children.

In general, middle-aged adults are more aware of health problems and do not take good health for granted the way younger adults do. Still capable of learning and changing, people in this age group sometimes lack the self-confidence to try something new. Middle-aged adults should be involved in all aspects of the teaching plan, because they are usually familiar with the concepts of goal setting and achievement. These people have a broad base of life experience, and teaching goals will more likely be met if they are given time to assimilate new knowledge into old. Approach learning directly, explaining all rationales fully. Try to keep sessions to less than 1 hour, and allow time for the client to practice skills in private.

Middle-aged people enjoy praise as much as anyone else. Evaluate the client in a supportive atmosphere, stressing how much progress has been made. Gently correct misconceptions, and be sensitive to the client's fears and anxieties.

Older adults are the fastest-growing segment of our population. General adult learning principles apply to this group; some special considerations are required, however.

Motivation to learn may be decreased if the client feels that life is near the end. Two motivational strategies to try follow:

- Show the client how the new knowledge will improve the quality of his or her life, regardless of its length.
- Show how the new knowledge could improve the client's independence.

A high quality of life and independence are usually highly valued by the older adult.

Physiologic changes that normally occur with aging may hinder learning. Vision may decrease because of cataracts; smaller, less-reactive pupils; or a decrease in color perception. The ability to hear high-pitched sounds usually decreases, although low-pitch hearing may be intact. Rapid speech may become unintelligible because older adults often take longer to process what they hear. Hearing loss can be a source of shame and frustration for the older learner, causing withdrawal and worsening feelings of isolation.

Older adults often suffer from *short-term memory loss*. Do not assume there is memory loss, but be sensitive to it. When it does exist, it is usually associated with meaningless learning, complex learning, or new information that has required a reassessment of old learning. If new information conflicts with old, time is needed to reexamine the old learning; this may cause some anxiety and may be a barrier to new learning (Babcock & Miller, 1994). The older learner has large stores of information, so scanning for recall may take longer.

Generally, older learners need more time to learn *psychomotor skills*. Often they compensate by putting a great deal of effort into accuracy.

Key Concepts

- Client education is a dynamic process used to empower the client toward autonomy and high-level wellness.
- For financial, legal, ethical, and humanitarian reasons, the responsibility for client education falls within the practice of nursing.
- The nurse, in collaboration with the client, assesses the client's learning needs and readiness to learn; he or she then forms a teaching plan. The plan is implemented, the learning evaluated, and the process documented.
- Determining whether the learning will be primarily psychomotor, cognitive, or affective affects the entire process.
- People have varying learning styles, and different age groups require different approaches.
- In client education, the nurse can influence but not control. Education must be client centered.

Critical Thinking Challenges

In this chapter, you have added the teaching–learning process and how to apply this process to client care. Now look again at the couple in the situation at the beginning of the chapter. Use your knowledge base to provide care for this couple by addressing the critical thinking challenges that follow.

1. *Prioritize important assessment data to collect from the couple so you can individualize your teaching.*
2. *Describe factors that might hinder or facilitate learning for the couple.*

3. *Role play how you might individualize teaching, focusing on three realistic goals.*
4. *Identify how you will evaluate learning and use this to revise future teaching.*

References

American Hospital Association (1992). *A Patient's* Bill of Rights. Chicago: Author.

American Nurses Association (1991). *Nurse's* Agenda for Healthcare Reform, (PR–12–91). Kansas City: Author.

Anderson, C. (1990). *Client teaching and communication in an information age*. Albany: Delmar Publishers.

Babcock, D., & Miller, M. (1994). *Client education: Theory and practice*. St. Louis: C.V. Mosby.

Davis, T., Maguire, T., Haraphongse, M., & Schaumberger, M. (1994). Understanding cardiac catheterization: The effects of informational preparation and coping style on patient anxiety during the procedure. *Heart & Lung, 23*(2), 140–50.

Falvo, D. (1994). *Effective patient education: A guide to increased compliance*. Gaithersburg, MD: Aspen Publishers.

Jenny, J. (1987). Knowledge Deficit: Not a nursing diagnosis. *Image, 19*(4), 184–185.

Joint Commission on Accreditation of Healthcare Organizations (1992). *Accreditation manual of hospitals*, Chicago: Author.

Knowles, M. (1990). *The adult learner: A neglected species* (4th ed.). Houston: Gulf.

McBer & Co. (1985). *Learning-style inventory*. Boston: Author.

NANDA. (1994). *Nursing diagnosis: Definition and classification 1995–1996*. Philadelphia: North American Nursing Diagnosis Association.

Office of the Surgeon General (1990). *Healthy People 2000*. DHHS Publication PHS #91–502130. Washington DC: U.S. Government Printing Office.

Rankin, S. H., & Stallings, K. D. (1990). *Client education: Issues, principles, and practices* (2nd ed.). Philadelphia: J.B. Lippincott.

Vezeau, T., et al. (1991). Literacy levels in a maternal child population. *Nursing Times, 87*(33), 48–54.

Bibliography

Barnes, L. (1992). The illiterate client: Strategies in teaching. *Maternal Child Nursing, 17*(3), 127.

Bernier, M. (1993). Developing and evaluating printed education materials: A prescriptive model for quality. *Orthopedic Nursing, 12*(6), 39–46.

Brownson, K. (1993). Patient handouts? We're wasting our time. *RN, 56*(7), 88.

Cunningham, D. (1993). Improving your teaching skills. *Nursing 93, 23*(12), 24.

Dellasega, C., Clark, D., McCreary, D., Helmuth, A., & Schan, P. (1994). Nursing Process: teaching elderly clients. *Journal of Gerontological Nursing, 20*(1), 31–38.

Doak, C. C., et al. (1985). *Teaching clients with low literacy skills*. Philadelphia: J.B. Lippincott.

Gaw-Ens, B. (1994). Informational support for families immediately after CABG surgery. *Critical Care Nurse, 14*(1), 41–42; 47–50.

Hussey, L. (1994). Minimizing effects of low literacy on medication knowledge and compliance among the elderly. *Clinical Nursing Research, 3*(2), 132–145.

Jubeck, M. (1994). Teaching the elderly—A commonsense approach. *Nursing 94, 24*(5), 70–71.

King, K. (1994). Preparing patients and families for health care procedures. *Heart Disease and Stroke, 3*(2), 95–97.

Meade, C., McKinney, W., & Barnas, G. (1994). Educating patients with limited literacy skills: the effectiveness of printed and videotaped materials about colon cancer. *American Journal of Public Health, 84*(1), 119–121.

Recker, D. (1994). Patient perception of preoperative cardiac surgical teaching done pre- and postadmission. *Critical Care Nurse, 14*(1), 52–58.

Redman, B. (1992). *The process of client education* (7th ed.). St. Louis: C.V. Mosby.

Schwartz-Barcott, D., Fortin, J., & Kim, H. (1994). Client-nurse interaction: Testing for its impact in preoperative instruction. *International Journal of Nursing Studies, 31*(1), 23–35.

Shaw, C., Wilson, S., & O'Brien, M. (1994). Information needs prior to breast biopsy. *Clinical Nursing Research, 3*(2), 119–131.

Wong, M. (1992). Self-care instructions: Do patients understand educational materials? *Focus on Critical Care, 19*(1), 47–49.

Asepsis

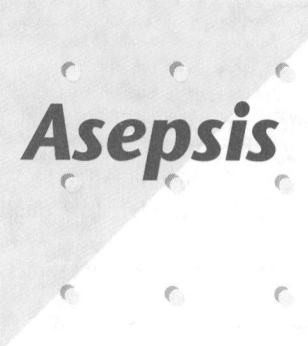

Key Terms	Learning Objectives

Key Terms

Antiseptic
Asepsis
Bactericidal
Bacteriostatic
Communicable disease
Contamination
Disinfection
Infectious disease
Isolation
Nosocomial infection
Pathogens
Sepsis
Sterilization
Universal Precautions
Virulence

Learning Objectives

Upon completion of this chapter, the student will be able to do the following:

- *Identify the chain of infection and give examples of ways infection can occur.*
- *Describe factors that increase infection in various settings.*
- *Discuss the role of various agencies and health personnel in infection control.*
- *Identify ways a caregiver can increase protection from infectious exposure.*
- *Identify ways a caregiver can decrease infection exposure for clients.*
- *Differentiate between medical and surgical asepsis.*
- *Incorporate good handwashing as an integral part of practice.*
- *Differentiate appropriate use of cleaning, disinfection, and sterilization.*
- *Discuss different systems of isolation.*
- *Identify age-related considerations in preventing the transmission of infectious disease.*

25

Your client, who had major abdominal surgery, has contracted a severe wound infection. As you enter the room, one of your coworkers is leaving. While you are washing your hands at the sink, the client says: "I wish all healthcare providers were as conscientious as you. Some poke around my wound without ever washing their hands."

In previous chapters you learned about ethical and legal concerns. This chapter identifies issues related to infection and infection control. Some of these issues involve ethical and legal concerns as well as general concerns about making a healthy environment for your clients, yourself, and your coworkers. After you have studied this chapter you should be able to apply your knowledge to the care of the client in the situation above. The Critical Thinking Challenge section at the end of the chapter will help you direct your knowledge to the care of this client.

Regardless of where they practice, preventing the transfer of microorganisms is a concern of every nurse. In homes, schools, clinics, industry, hospitals, and extended care facilities, nurses strive to teach about, prevent, and treat infections. Promoting healthy lifestyles and preventive health practices is an important focus.

A sea of microorganisms live and multiply on every surface we touch and in the air we breathe. They grow on our skin and flourish in our digestive tracts. Often microorganisms help produce food and maintain the ecology of the planet. Most of the time, humans and microorganisms live in harmony. When this balance is upset, however, microorganisms are capable of causing infection. **Asepsis** means to make free from disease-producing organisms.

Infectious disease is the most common reason people contact a healthcare provider and accounts for more clinic and physician office visits than any other cause. Preventable infectious diseases are common worldwide, resulting in great suffering and the loss of many lives. The economic costs of preventing and treating infection are great. Recent years have shown an alarming increase in resistant organisms, such as tuberculosis and *Staphylococcus aureus*-caused disease, that can no longer easily be eradicated by antibiotics. Recent outbreaks of *Escherichia coli* through undercooked hamburger sold at a national fast-food chain, and an outbreak of hantavirus in the Southwest causing a pulmonary disorder with 50% mortality, underscore the need for precise infection control practices.

This chapter discusses nursing practices aimed at providing a safe and therapeutic environment designed to protect clients, family members, and healthcare providers from acquiring infections. Chapters on skin integrity and wound healing (see Chapter 38) and infection (see Chapter 39) provide additional information on specific infectious diseases as well as diagnostic and treatment procedures.

Role of Microorganisms in Infection

Microorganisms that are capable of harming people are called **pathogens** or pathogenic; they produce disease. When these organisms enter and multiply within body tissues, they disrupt normal physiologic body processes. The organisms or their toxins disrupt normal cell function or kill the cells entirely. **Sepsis**, a term that means poisoning of tissues, is often used to describe the presence of infection. An infection or the products of infection carried throughout the body by the blood is known as *septicemia*. *Aseptic* is the opposite of septic—that is, to be without disease-producing organisms.

Infection (in the strictest sense of the word) means the process of causing to become diseased. Unfortunately, in common usage "infected" and "septic" are used interchangeably. In most instances when a client is said to be infected, it means he or she has a disease caused by microorganisms. When the client is referred to as septic, it means he or she is displaying the manifestations of microbial destruction of tissues, such as high fever or hypotension.

Infectious disease refers to the pathology or pathologic events that result from the invasion and multiplication of microorganisms in a host. Toxins and enzymes produced by the microorganisms cause tissue injury. This injury produces manifestations of infection, namely, fever; rashes; malaise; nausea and vomiting; diarrhea; purulent discharge from wounds; a hot, red, tender area around wounds or puncture sites; aches and pains; or total body collapse.

A major portion of the healthcare practitioner's time, energy, and talent is devoted to developing and maintaining good practices to control the spread of microorganisms. These practices, known as aseptic techniques, are used in the broader context of infection control.

Aseptic techniques start and end with handwashing. They include the processes of cleaning, disinfection, and sterilization. The use of barriers against the spread of microorganisms, such as gloves, masks, hair coverings, and gowns, as well as client isolation, is part of aseptic practice.

Agents Causing Infection

There are four groups of microorganisms potentially pathogenic to humans. They include bacteria, viruses, fungi, and parasites. Brief descriptions are given here. (For more information, see Chapter 39.)

Bacteria. Bacteria are single-celled, independent-living microorganisms, some of which are capable of causing disease in humans. Bacteria may be airborne, foodborne or waterborne, soilborne or vectorborne, or sexually transmitted. They differ in size and shape, in growth and replication requirements, and the method by which they inflict harm to the host. Some are capable of producing metabolic toxins, which they secrete into the host organism's system (exotoxin producers). Others can produce poisons that are contained in their cell walls and released after the death of the microorganism (eg, gram-negative endotoxin producers). In addition, all bacteria are capable of causing diminished organ function by invading tissues and initiating inflammation.

Viruses. Viruses are particles of nucleic acid and protein that are often membrane-bound. They reproduce inside living cells and cause a variety of diseases. Some infections are acute and controlled by the host's defense mechanisms; others spread throughout the body and cause severe tissue damage or result in chronic illness.

Fungi. Fungi are single-celled organisms that include molds and yeasts. *Candida albicans*, present in normal human flora, can cause a yeast infection of the mouth, skin, vagina, and intestinal tract in the immunocompromised adult. Fungal infections of the hair, skin, and nails also frequently occur in humans. Fungi also infest and destroy plant life and cause fermentation in food and milk.

Parasites. Parasites are multicellular organisms that live on another organism without contributing anything to the host. Examples of parasites include protozoa, helminth, and arthropod species. Protozoa are free-living microorganisms that commonly thrive in water and often are contracted by humans through unsanitary conditions surrounding food preparation or handling. Sexual contact, insects, and domestic animals can also carry parasites to humans. Malaria and sleeping sickness are examples of diseases caused by protozoa. Helminths are worms that infect the gastrointestinal tract or other body tissues of humans. Examples of helminths include tapeworms, hookworms, and trichinae (or porkworm). Arthropods include mites, fleas, and ticks, which often are responsible for skin diseases and systemic disease.

Drug-Resistant Microbial Strains

Microbes, just like humans, adapt to an ever-changing environment to vie for survival. In the 1940s, strains of staphylococcus emerged that were immune to the antimicrobial activity of penicillin. New penicillins were developed to effectively treat these drug-resistant strains. In the last few decades, increasing numbers of microbial organisms have developed drug-resistant strains. These drug-resistant strains pose a considerable health risk to the general population and specifically to healthcare workers, because the infections they cause are increasingly difficult to treat, and in some cases cannot be effectively destroyed by any known antibiotic. Infection control practices and breaking the chain of infection are critical in these instances.

Factors that have contributed to resistant microbial strains include:

- Overprescription of antibiotics
- Use of antibiotics not specific for an infecting organism
- Incomplete use of an antibiotic prescription as symptoms subside
- Harboring and spreading resistant organisms by carriers who remain symptom free, often not knowing that they have been infected
- Increased use of antibiotics in farming, thus contaminating milk and meat

Specific resistant microbial strains causing a significant challenge to healthcare providers include methicillin-resistant *S. aureus* (MRSA), *Streptococcus pneumoniae, Mycobacterium tuberculosis, Neisseria gonorrhoeae*, and enterococcus species (Boutotte, 1993a; Begley, 1994; Coll, et al., 1994).

Nursing Research
Asepsis

Selected Nursing Research Studies

Bauer, B., & Kennedy, J. (1993). Adverse exposures and use of universal precautions among perinatal nurses. *J Obstet Gynecol Neonatal Nurs, 22,* 429–435.

Chen, S., et al. (1994). Evaluation of single-use masks and respirators for protection of health care workers against mycobacterial aerosols. *Am J Infect Control, 22*(2), 65–74.

Goldrick, B., et al. (1994). Assessment of infection control programs in Maryland skilled-nursing long-term care facilities. *Am J Infect Control, 22*(2), 83–89.

Parras, F., et al. (1994). Impact of an educational program for the prevention of colonization of intravascular catheters. *Infection Control Hospital Epidemiologist, 15*(4), 239–242.

Piaskowski, P., et al. (1992). Results of CHICA-Canada survey of long term care infection control practitioners...Community & Hospital Infection Control Association. *Canadian Journal of Infection Control, 7*(4) 116–119.

White, M., et al. (1993). Infection control in home care agencies. *Am J Infect Control, 21*(3), 146–150.

Possible Topics for Nursing Inquiry

- Does handwashing practice increase in frequency when signs are displayed in prominent locations reminding caregivers to wash their hands?
- Do caregivers customarily provide clients with materials to wash their hands after toileting or before meals?
- Does the institution of isolation procedures increase the client's perception of social distance from significant others?
- Does the use of barrier precautions diminish the caregiver's attention to improving host defense mechanisms in the client?
- How do various recapping devices compare in preventing needle stick injuries?

Chain of Infection

The life cycle of pathogenic organisms frequently is described as an uninterrupted chain of events. For organisms to spread disease, they must grow, reproduce, and

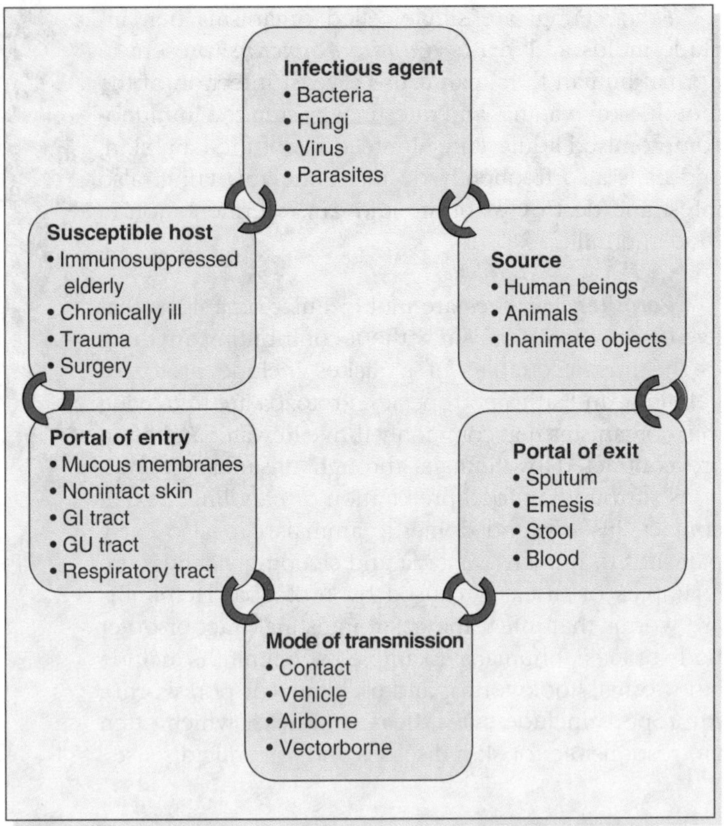

Figure 25-1 • *The chain of infection.*

move from one source to another. Nursing interventions are directed at stopping the transmission from the source to the client, and at controlling other links in the chain, thus controlling infection. The "chain of infection" includes the infectious agent, the source, the portal of exit, the mode of transmission, the portal of entrance, and a susceptible host (Fig. 25-1).

Infectious Agent

The first link in the chain of infection is the microbial agent, which may be a bacterium, a virus, a fungus, or a parasite. Characteristics that affect the ability of the infectious agent to cause disease include pathogenicity, virulence, invasiveness, and specificity. *Pathogenicity* is the ability of the organism to harm and cause disease. *Virulence* relates to the vigor with which the organism can grow and multiply. *Invasiveness* describes the ability of the organism to enter tissues, whereas *specificity* refers to the attraction of the organism to a specific host, which may include humans. The more pathogenic, virulent, and invasive the organism is, the more likely that normal body defenses can be overcome, causing an infection to occur.

These capacities are determined by the structure or chemical composition of the microorganisms, which include the organism's ability to attach to skin and mucous membranes, the production of enzymes that counteract the immune system's response to invasion, and the production of toxins.

Source

The sources of organisms, also called reservoirs, are elements in the environment. Inanimate objects, human beings, and animals are sources. Inanimate objects may include medications, air, food, water, blood, or any other material in which organisms can find nourishment or lie dormant and survive. Human sources include other clients, healthcare personnel, visitors, or the clients themselves. Clients may become infected from people who have active disease, people in the incubation portion of their own disease, or people who harbor the pathogens but have no symptoms of disease (known as carriers). A person's own bacterial flora may cause contamination. Endogenous microorganisms from the client's gastrointestinal tract cause disease if they become established in the lungs or a wound. Animals are often sources of disease for human beings. Insects and rats have been responsible for historic epidemics in the past and continue to spread disease today.

Portal of Exit

Portals of exit provide a means for the microorganism to leave the source. Sputum, emesis, stool, urine, blood, wound drainage, or secretions from genitals all permit microorganisms to exit from the source. Animal discharge or bloodborne organisms carried by mosquitoes can also provide a means of escape.

Mode of Transmission

The four main routes of transmission are contact, vehicle, airborne, and vectorborne. Contact transmission is the most frequent means of transmitting infections in healthcare facilities.

Contact Transmission. Contact transmission is by direct, indirect, or droplet contact. *Direct contact* involves physical transfer of organisms between a susceptible host and an infected or colonized person. Hospital personnel can transfer organisms to clients during client care such as bathing, dressing changes, and inserting invasive devices. *Indirect contact* occurs when a susceptible host is exposed to a contaminated object such as a dressing, a needle, or a surgical instrument. *Droplet contact* occurs when mucous membranes of the nose or mouth or conjunctiva are exposed to secretions of an infected person who is coughing, sneezing, or talking. It is considered contact instead of airborne transmission because droplets seldom travel more than 3 feet.

Vehicle Transmission. Vehicles are contaminated items that transmit pathogens. Food can carry *Salmonella*, water can carry *Legionella*, drugs can carry bacteria from contaminated infusion supplies, and blood can carry hepatitis.

Airborne Transmission. Airborne transmission occurs when fine particles are suspended in the air for a long time, or when dust particles contain pathogens. Air currents widely disperse organisms, which can be inhaled by or deposited on the skin of a susceptible host.

Vectorborne Transmission. Vectors are living animals, such as rats or insects, that carry pathogens. This type of transmission is of great concern in tropical areas where mosquitoes transmit diseases such as malaria.

Portal of Entry

The portal of entry permits the organism to gain entrance into the host. Pathogens can enter a susceptible host through orifices of the body such as the mouth, nose, ears, eyes, vagina, rectum, or urethra. Breaks in the skin or mucous membranes from wounds or abrasions increase opportunities for the organism to enter the host. Modern medicine's practice of placing tubes for long-term intravenous or gastric feedings and drainage of body cavities further increases the number of potential routes of entry into the body, thus increasing susceptibility to infection.

Susceptible Host

A host is a person whose own body defense mechanisms are unable at the time of exposure to withstand the invasion of pathogens. The body has numerous defense mechanisms that naturally resist entry and multiplication of pathogens. These factors are discussed in detail in Chapter 39. When infectious disease occurs in humans, the agent of infection has overcome the ability of the body to resist infection. A primary focus of nursing practice is identifying clients with compromised defenses and working to enhance their defenses.

Progress of an Infection

When the signs and symptoms of a disease are apparent, the disease is said to be clinical. Many infections are subclinical, in that the client and other observers note no symptoms of disease even though the organism is present in the body and causes antibodies to be formed and immunity gained (Alcamo, 1991).

The course of an infection that results in a disease state is a dynamic series of events that express competition between the host and the invading organism. Disease is usually a result of the organism's growth and multiplication inside the host. The exception to this is when the disease is caused by the release of toxins, such as in food poisoning and botulism. The pattern for most diseases follows a predictable course, which includes the incubation period, the prodromal period, acute illness with symptoms, and the convalescent period. The time frame during which a disease can be passed from one person to another is known as the communicable period. Figure 25-2 illustrates the progress of infection in the case of measles.

Incubation Period. The incubation period is the time between entrance of the pathogen and the appearance of symptoms. The length of this period varies depending on the number of organisms absorbed, the time they require to grow and multiply, their virulence, and the resistance of the host. The point of entry may also be a factor.

Prodromal Period. The prodromal period is characterized by nonspecific symptoms such as nausea, fever, general weakness, or aches and pains. Although prodromal symptoms are nonspecific, the cluster of symptoms and their order of appearance often help in the diagnosis of the disease.

Acute Phase of Illness. The acute phase of an illness occurs when specific symptoms appear. Depending on the pathogen, there is a cluster of symptoms, and often laboratory analysis can identify the disease. The period during which the symptoms subside is included in this

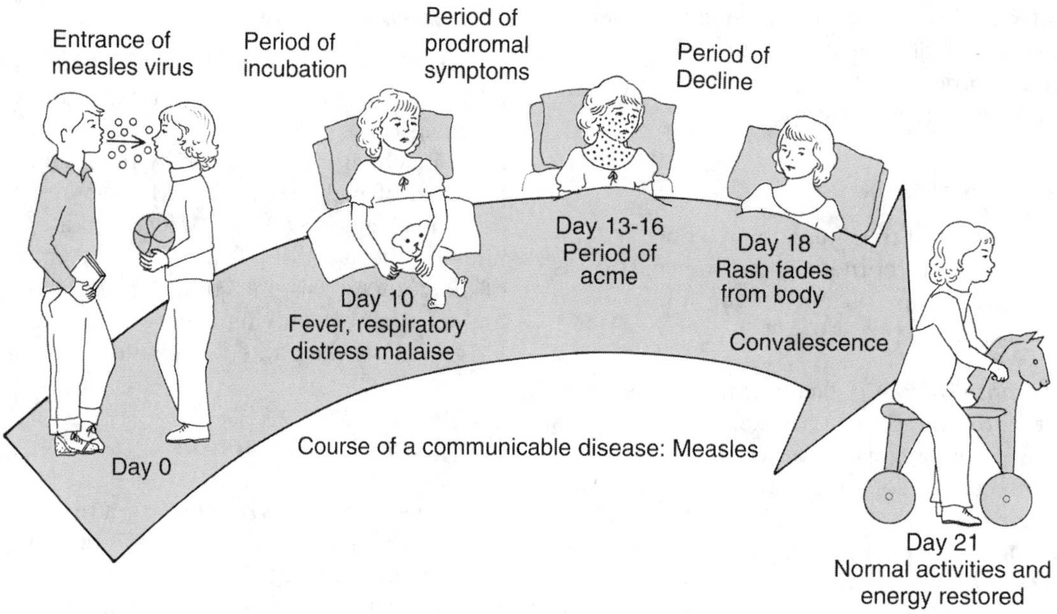

Figure 25-2 • *Course of a communicable disease: Measles. Day 0: Entrance of virus by absorption of respiratory droplets from another child's sneeze and incubation begins. Day 10: Fever, respiratory distress, and malaise. Day 13: Period of acme begins with appearance of the body rash. Day 18: The rash begins to fade. Day 21: Normal activities and energy restored. Period of communicability is from 4 days before rash to 4 days after rash disappears. (Modified from Alcamo, I.E. (1991).* Fundamentals of microbiology, *3rd ed. Menlo Park, Ca: Benjamin/Cummings Publishing Co.)*

phase. The acute phase of an illness may be preceded by a crisis period, followed by rapid recovery or a slow recuperation.

Convalescent Period. Convalescence is a period that completes the progress of an infection. The body systems return to normal, and appetite and energy return. Antibodies begin to be present in the person's blood.

Communicable Period. If the causative agent of the disease is transmissible between one person and another, the disease is said to be a **communicable disease**. If the agent passes with ease from one host to the next, it may be called a *contagious disease.* Not all diseases are contagious. For example, tetanus can be contracted in an isolated event when a person sustains a puncture wound. Childhood diseases (measles, mumps, chickenpox) are classic examples of communicable diseases. Infections in clients in healthcare agencies are not necessarily contagious, but because of the large number of clients with lowered host defenses, such infections are more easily transmitted in the facility than they would be in the community.

An infected person may be contagious during the incubation period, the acute phase, or the convalescent period, depending on whether organisms are being shed into the environment. When the agent is not present in body secretions, but hidden within the host's cells, the infection is called *latent.* When the agent is being shed from the host's body in respiratory secretions, feces, blood, or urine, or is cultured from body tissues, the infection is communicable. The period of communicability begins after the agent has multiplied sufficiently for shedding to begin and lasts as long as the level of shedding is sufficient for transmission. Diseases spread more rapidly if they have a short latent period. Unfortunately, the latent period is almost always shorter than the incubation period; thus the person usually is shedding microorganisms before any signs and symptoms are apparent. Periods of communicability vary with each disease and the control of microorganisms within the infected person's tissues. Because of the uncertainty of the period of communicability and the lack of identifiable infection in some people, all body secretions should be considered as potentially containing infectious agents.

Nosocomial Infections

Nosocomial infection is infection associated with healthcare delivery. The term is most commonly applied to those infections acquired in acute-care hospitals, although extended-care facilities, psychiatric institutions, and ambulatory care facilities are included in the scope of this definition. At times, the client is exposed to the infection while in the agency, but the disease itself does not become apparent until after discharge.

The urinary tract is the most common site for nosocomial infection, accounting for 40% of hospital-acquired infection. Other common infections are surgical wound infections (25%), respiratory tract infections (15%), infections of the skin and subcutaneous tissues (15%), and infections from intravascular infusion or monitoring devices (5%) (Schaffner, 1992).

Risk Factors in Nosocomial Infection Development

The longer the client is in a healthcare facility, the greater the risk of infection. Exposure to the facility's environment changes the client's own body flora. The risk factors that contribute to the development of nosocomial infections can be grouped into three categories: environment, therapeutic regimen, and the resistance of the client. They interact in varying patterns of importance, but all must be considered when attempts are made to decrease the client's risk. Figure 25-3 illustrates sources of microbial contamination.

Environment. Although modern facilities have come a long way since Lister and Nightingale, they still are reservoirs of organisms that pose a threat to an increasing number of clients who have decreased resistance. The sources of these organisms include the air, other clients, families and visitors, contaminated equipment, food, and personnel.

Therapeutic Regimen. Multiple factors that are part of the therapy used to cure the client can also contribute to the client's risk of infection. Steroids, immunosuppressive drugs, cancer therapy, and prolonged antibiotic use predispose the client to infection. Equipment such as arterial or venous catheters and indwelling urinary catheters invades body orifices and provides routes for bacterial invasion into the body. Prolonged intravenous and gastrointestinal tube feedings are also invasive and may become contaminated with improper use. Inadequate dressing techniques for wounds can provide media for bacterial growth. Identifying treatments that pose risk and discontinuing their use as soon as possible decrease the chance of nosocomial infection.

Client Resistance. Changes in the physical or psychological status of the client can affect resistance to infection. Any break in the integrity of the skin or mucous membranes increases the chance of infection. Stress, fatigue, poor nutrition, and chronic illness can also decrease the client's ability to ward off infection. Adequate

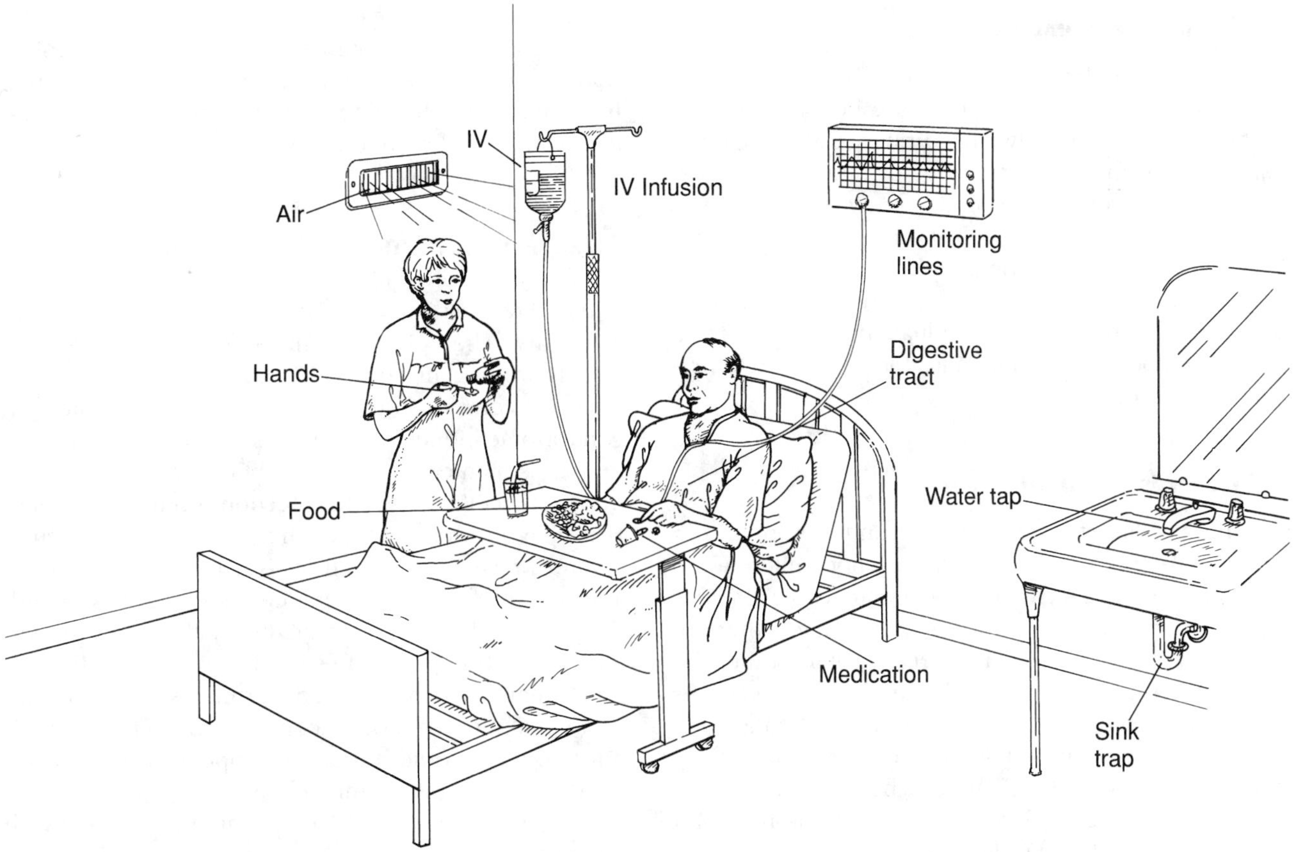

Figure 25-3 • *Potential sources of microbial contamination in the hospital environment. Transfer of contamination by hands of hospital personnel is the most frequent cause of exposure.*

hygiene is important to decrease microorganisms on the skin that could contribute to infection risk.

Hazards in Acute-Care Settings

About 6% of all hospital clients get nosocomial infections. The incidence has not changed in the last 15 to 20 years (Castle & Ajemian, 1987). There have been declines in some types of infections, but they have been replaced with increases in infections seen in compromised clients. As people live longer and more extensive surgeries are performed and more technology is used, rates could be expected to rise in the future.

Hazards in Ambulatory Care Settings

Clients come to ambulatory care settings for diagnosis or treatment of health problems. Such procedures frequently involve invasive techniques that increase the risk of infection. Waiting rooms may contain people with active infections; this is especially true of pediatric populations. Infection risk is increased because children frequently play with office toys or interact with one another. All equipment such as thermometers and devices used to examine body orifices must be cleaned and disinfected after each use to avoid cross-contamination.

Hazards in Home Care

Clients discharged to home care can be seriously ill, and sophisticated invasive treatments are being performed in the home setting. Indwelling urinary catheters, intravenous infusions for medications or nutrition, and extensive open wounds and drainage collection systems are seen more frequently in the home setting. The nurse is responsible for teaching people in the home how to perform prescribed procedures in an aseptic manner. The nurse often teaches individuals how to care for a family member with a communicable illness and to prevent its spread.

Hazards in Schools

Classrooms, athletic departments, and school health clinics pose the risk of infection to schoolchildren and their teachers. The incidence of communicable illness is high among children who are grouped together for study and play. Children are often unaware of their illness and have not yet learned good hygiene practices to prevent infection transmission. Schools often employ nurses to teach health classes and to develop and monitor infection control practices. The school nurse is often the first one to identify a potential outbreak of a communicable disease. Responsibility also includes evaluating children who may be infectious to help ensure their proper treatment.

Hazards in the Workplace

Employees in the workplace are exposed to, and can expose their coworkers to, infections. Working conditions and materials that workers use may have infectious risks. Farmers and other people who work with animals have a high risk of contacting diseases carried by animals. Sinks, bathrooms, lunchrooms, and food utensils may be sources of infection in the workplace. Many industries employ nurses who screen employees for communicable diseases and who collaborate with building maintenance personnel to maintain hygienic conditions and supervise waste disposal.

Hazards in Extended-Care Facilities

Nursing homes, psychiatric care facilities, drug and alcohol treatment centers, and group homes for the mentally or physically impaired are associated with a high risk for infection. Often such institutions are understaffed, and the available personnel do not have extensive training in infection control. Their residents may be incapable of maintaining their own personal hygiene and frequently are debilitated from chronic medical or psychiatric conditions. Communicable diseases are common in these facilities, and the clients' underlying medical problems often place them at risk for delays in early recognition of infections. Elderly clients often do not mount a febrile response to infection, and their increasing agitation or confusion in response to an infection may be dismissed as a sign of old age. Immunization status of the elderly and other facility residents may not be kept up to date.

Infection Control

Acute care hospitals have organized infection control programs. The Joint Committee on Accreditation of Healthcare Organizations (JCAHO) mandates an active infection control program and an appointed infection control practitioner who surveys the institution for active cases of infection and documents the occurrence of nosocomial infections. The infection control practitioner is usually a nurse with advanced training in infection control practices and methods for tracking the source and spread of infections (epidemiologic studies). In addition, each department in the hospital must have written policies and procedures for the control of infection. The caregivers in individual departments as well as support personnel (eg, housekeepers, transport personnel) must have periodic educational updates on infection control, usually on an annual basis.

Several studies have demonstrated cost saving with good infection control (Beyt, et al., 1985; Dixon, 1992). Approximately one-third of nosocomial infections can be prevented with effective infection control programs.

Safety Alert
Avoiding Infection

- Never recap a needle or other sharp instruments after use on a client. This could cause an accidental finger stick and expose a healthcare worker to infection.
- Place sterile objects on dry surfaces and avoid splashing liquids when pouring. Moisture may cause contamination.
- Never assume that an object is sterile. Always check the integrity of the packaging and the label for an expiration date.
- Discard sterile supplies if not used immediately. Opened, unused sterile objects do not remain sterile.
- Develop a habit of frequent handwashing whenever appropriate. Unwashed hands are the most frequent mode of transmission of microorganisms in healthcare settings.
- Wear gloves for contact with all body substances from any client. To avoid possible infection exposure, touch nothing wet that comes from a body surface with bare hands.
- Provide clients with washcloths and soap to wash their hands after toileting and before eating to prevent self-contamination with endogenous flora.

None of these studies begin to quantify the benefits of increased quality of life that result when infection is avoided.

Regulatory Agencies

Several agencies are involved in the control of institutional safety designed to protect the client, staff, and community from infectious disease. Local, state, regional, provincial, and national groups require reporting of specific infections. Physician's offices, school nurses, health clinics, extended-care facilities, and various acute care facilities must report episodes of infection to these agencies. Agencies compile statistics on the incidence of the disease in the area and provide the practitioner with information on control and treatment.

Both the Centers for Disease Control and Prevention (CDC) and JCAHO publish guidelines for storage, cleaning and disinfection, and use of equipment and supplies. JCAHO sets requirements to which healthcare agencies must adhere to obtain accreditation. The CDC does basic research on infectious disease and conducts large multicenter studies on data gathered by local centers. The CDC's *Morbidity and Mortality Weekly Report* outlines statistics on infectious disease. The World Health Organization receives information about communicable disease from all countries and compiles this information into periodic reports.

Infection Control Committee

The infection control program of the agency, compelled by JCAHO regulations, requires the existence of an infection control committee. The committee is composed of members from various departments: physicians, nurses, and personnel representing the laboratory, housekeeping, central supply, diagnostic imaging, and quality-assurance officers. The committee annually reviews all policies and procedures of all departments for current information on infection control. A person from the committee, usually a nurse, is appointed to be in charge of surveillance, analyzing, and reporting infectious diseases. This person, called the infection control practitioner, gathers all data on the occurrence of infections, reports required information to the local health department, and brings the information to the committee for review. The committee makes recommendations for changes in policies, revises procedures as necessary, and reviews individual practitioner infection rates. In addition, the infection control nurse is often involved in employee education programs.

Reporting Infectious Disease

The infection control practitioner is responsible for reporting diseases to appropriate agencies as required by law. The guidelines as to what is a reportable disease vary from location to location and from time to time. These variations are based on differences in the occurrence of disease in various climates, the consequences of the disease in terms of morbidity and mortality, and interest about the results of current control efforts. Health departments can mandate how urgently the reports are needed. Each local board designates whether the report must be made by a "same day as discovery" phone call or by written report. Good communication and rapport between clinical agencies and regulatory agencies are necessary to optimize infection control and prevent severe outbreaks of infectious disease.

Employee Health

Millions of people work in healthcare agencies. Some agencies have started personnel health service programs as part of their infection control program or employee benefits package. The objectives of the program include stressing maintenance of sound habits of personal hygiene, good health practices in diet, exercise, and rest, and individual responsibility in infection control; monitoring and investigating potentially harmful infectious exposures and outbreaks of infections among personnel; providing care to personnel for work-related illnesses or exposures; identifying the infection risks related to employment and instituting appropriate preventive measures; and containing costs by preventing infectious disease that results in absenteeism and disability.

Monitoring and Counseling of Personnel

People often have to provide an immunization and health history and undergo a screening physical examination for employment. Laboratory testing may also be required. Almost all institutions require a personal health and safety education lecture as part of the orientation process and on an annual or semiannual basis. Some institutions require laboratory screening for high-risk diseases and offer their employees routine immunization programs. A mechanism for prompt diagnosis and management of job-related illnesses and provision for prophylaxis of preventable diseases is important to ensure health of all employees.

Access to health counseling about infections is especially important for women of childbearing age. Personnel who are or who might become pregnant need to know about potential risks to the fetus due to work assignments and about preventive measures that reduce those risks. Pregnant nurses may not be allowed to care for clients who have diseases that pose risks to the unborn baby. Among the diseases that pose particular risk to the fetus if contracted by the mother are rubella, hepatitis B, varicella-zoster virus, cytomegalovirus, and human immunodeficiency virus (HIV) (Valenti, 1993).

Transmissible Diseases

The CDC Committee on Infection Control in Hospital Personnel has divided infections that commonly occur in hospitals and are transmissible between clients and staff into two groups. Category I infections are transmitted both to and from personnel and clients. Category II infections are transmitted primarily from infected clients to personnel. CDC guidelines include preventive measures, diagnostic and epidemiologic methods, and recommendations for prophylaxis after exposure, as well as guidelines for work restriction because of illness.

Because hospital personnel are at risk for contracting and transmitting vaccine-preventable diseases, maintaining current immunization status is a good health practice. Employees who work in high-risk areas, such as pediatric wards, dialysis units, or transplant units, can be required to prove that their immunization status is current as a condition of employment. Chapter 39 contains a list of available vaccines and their effectiveness. The cost of vaccination may be borne by the institution or by the employee, depending on individual personnel policies and benefits.

Significant Exposure

Institutional policies and employee restrictions are designed to prevent exposure to and contracting of an infectious disease. Any "significant" exposure is investigated to protect the employee, the client, and the institution. The significance of an exposure is determined

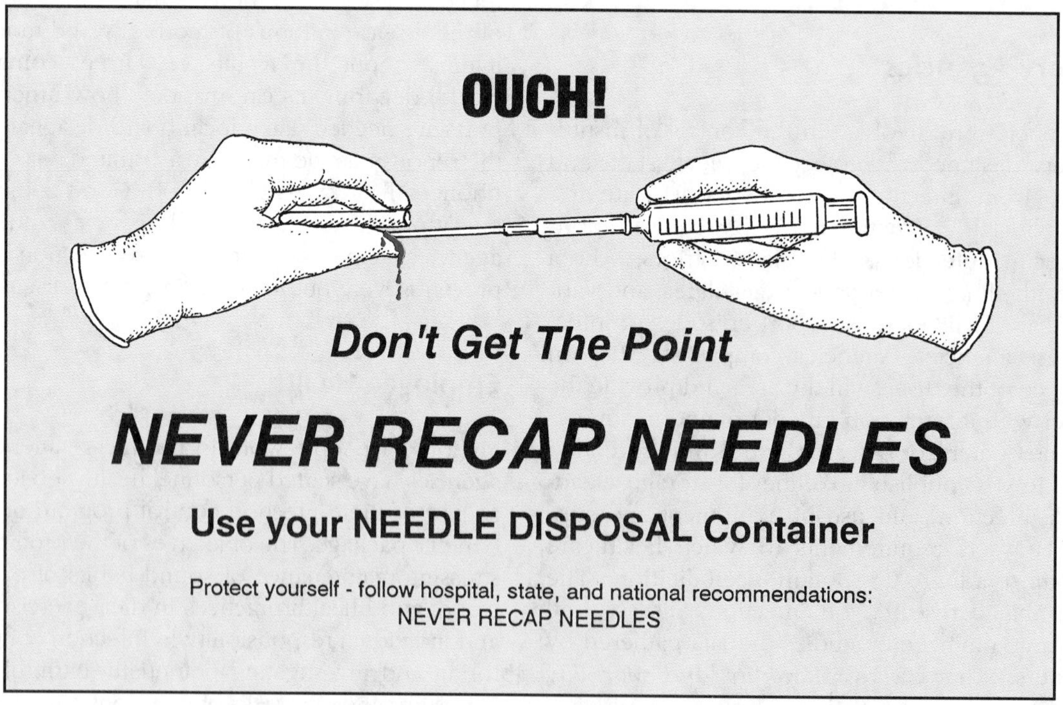

Figure 25-4 • Sample needle stick hazard poster.

by the type and duration of exposure, with consideration of the mode of transmission, whether the host was susceptible, and whether precautions were taken. Exposures to hepatitis, rubella, meningococcal meningitis, tuberculosis, varicella (chickenpox), and acquired immunodeficiency syndrome (AIDS) are commonly investigated by the infection control nurse. Most exposure requires timely reporting, by way of an incident or report filled out by staff members, to expedite prophylaxis (if any is available) and to qualify for labor and industry insurance coverage if an illness results. If an employee contracts an infectious disease, it must be reported to the local health department.

Needle Sticks. One of the most frequently occurring, potentially serious exposures for healthcare personnel is from needle stick injuries that may carry organisms that cause bloodborne diseases, such as hepatitis or AIDS. Accidental needle sticks account for nearly one-third of all healthcare accidents. Liability and treatment for infected personnel costs billions of dollars annually for employers and insurers (Baxter Healthcare Corporation, 1988). Every year, 18,000 healthcare workers contract hepatitis B from occupational exposure, resulting in 250 deaths annually (Grau, 1991).

Approximately 40% of all needle stick injuries result from recapping needles after their contact with blood from a client (eg, after an injection, drawing blood, or starting an intravenous line). In the past, used needles were recapped or bent or broken after use to prevent accidental contamination by housekeeping personnel. The CDC strongly advises all institutions to educate their employees as to the dangers of these practices (Fig. 25-4). Puncture–proof, plastic units (Fig. 25-5) into which needles can be safely deposited (uncapped) immediately after their use are provided in all client care areas. Needle-housing systems or new needleless systems have been developed within the last decade to decrease the incidence of needle sticks (Fig. 25-6).

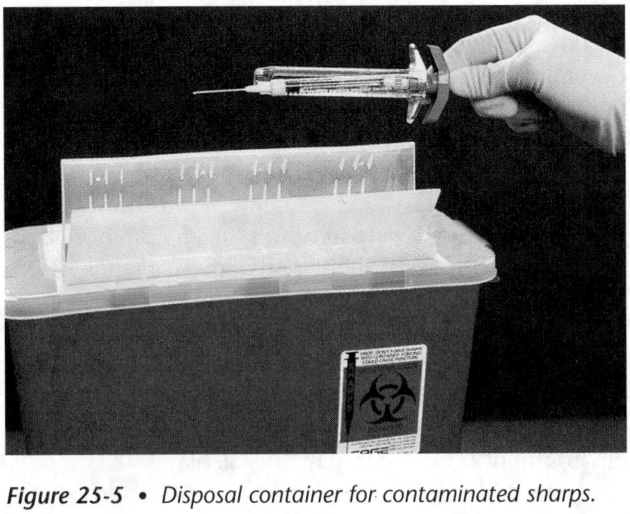

Figure 25-5 • *Disposal container for contaminated sharps.*

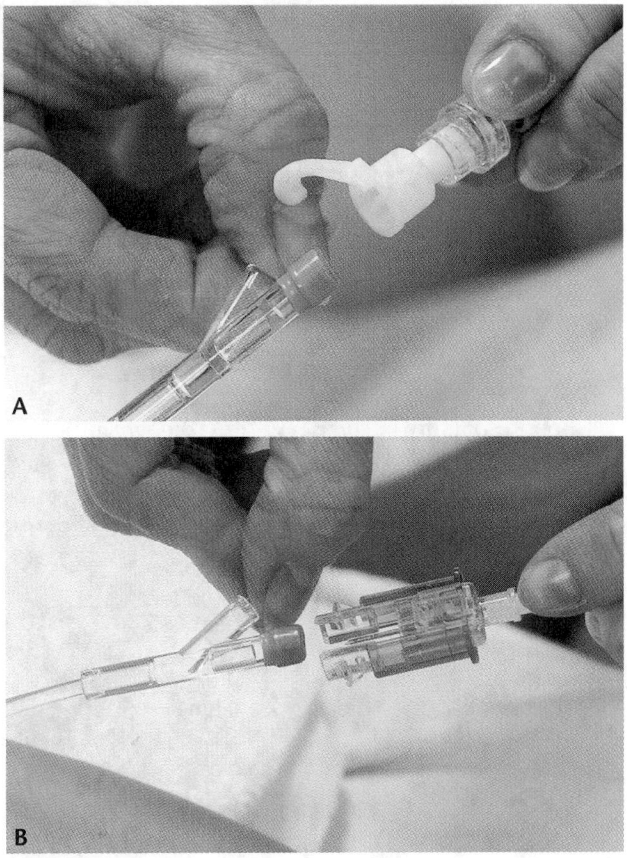

Figure 25-6 • *New IV systems have been developed to prevent needle stick injuries.* **(A)** *Needleless system—no needles are used, therefore, stick injuries are avoided.* **(B)** *Needle-housing system keeps the needle within a sheath to limit needle sticks.*

Studies document that infection risk from needleless systems is no greater and in some cases is less than that from traditional intravenous systems (Adams, et al., 1993).

Gloves. Gloves cannot protect all personnel in every situation, but increased use of gloves for contact with all mucous membranes, nonintact skin, and moist body substances, in combination with good handwashing practices makes a difference in cross-contamination between clients and staff. Gloves must be discarded and reapplied between clients to avoid spreading microorganisms from one client to another.

Work Restriction

An ill healthcare employee should not be in contact with clients if that illness poses a threat to the client or other personnel. Caregivers with diseases characterized by profuse coughing, sneezing, or frequent diarrhea should probably stay home from work and care for themselves. Agencies should have well-defined policies directed at restricting or limiting work for personnel with a potentially transmissible disease. Table 25-1 lists

Table 25-1 • Infectious Conditions Requiring Work Restriction

Condition	Infection	Duration of Restriction
Skin lesions that are infected or draining	Impetigo Infected sebaceous cysts Boils Hangnails	Until lesions resolve
Purulent discharges	Sinusitis Conjunctivitis Pharyngitis	Until discharge ceases
Gastroenteritis	Causing: Diarrhea Vomiting	Until stool is formed or vomiting has stopped
Upper respiratory tract infections	Accompanied by: Fever Purulent sputum	Until acute symptoms resolve
Diagnosed communicable disease	Chickenpox	Until all lesions dry and crust
	Hepatitis	Until antigenemia resolves
	Measles	Until 7 days after the rash appears
	Mumps	Until 9 days after onset of parotitis
	Pertussis	From the beginning of the catarrhal stage until 7 days after start of therapy
	Rubella	Until 5 days after the rash appears
	Shingles	Until lesions dry and crust
	Tuberculosis	Until sputum shows no growth on smears. Approximately 2 weeks after start of therapy
Herpes simplex	With open lesions excluded from: Nursery Delivery room Operating room Burn units Transplant unit Oncology unit	Until lesions heal

the conditions requiring relief from direct client contact or partial work restriction.

Healthcare Workers With AIDS. Personnel considered to have any of the clinical features associated with the AIDS spectrum should be counseled about the risks they pose to clients and to themselves in the work environment. There is no evidence that any healthcare worker infected with the AIDS virus has transmitted the infection to a client; however, there is potential risk. Healthcare workers who perform invasive procedures in which a needle stick or scalpel injury would expose their blood to that of the client's pose the greatest risk. All personnel with AIDS should wear gloves for direct contact with mucous membranes or nonintact skin of all clients. Any healthcare worker with AIDS and exudative lesions or weeping dermatitis should refrain from all direct care and handling of client care equipment until the lesions clear (CDC, 1988).

HIV impairs the immune system, making people with AIDS more likely to acquire infectious diseases or experience more serious complications. These staff members should be counseled about potential risks to themselves and may be counseled against working in acute-care settings.

Waste Disposal

Healthcare facilities produce tons of waste daily. Several regulatory agencies are involved in identifying and directing acceptable practices for collecting, transporting, and disposing of wastes. Rules and regulations are set by the JCAHO, the Department of Social and Health Services, the Environmental Protection Agency (EPA), the Occupational Safety and Health Administration, and local health departments. All of these agencies have partial jurisdiction over waste disposal.

Local health agencies and the JCAHO require hospitals to develop programs to dispose of wastes categorized as infectious, injurious, or hazardous to employees, clients, visitors, the general public, and the environment. The accompanying display lists common materials within each category of institutional waste for

Categories of Institutional Waste

Infectious Waste

Blood and blood products
Pathology laboratory specimens
Laboratory cultures
Body parts from surgery
Contaminated equipment (eg, dialysis materials and suction receptacles)
Food
Unrinsed infant and adult diapers

Injurious Waste

Needles
Scalpel blades
Lancets
Broken glass
Pipettes
Aerosol cans

Hazardous Waste

Radioactive materials
Chemotherapy solutions and their containers
Caustic chemicals

which proper waste disposal protocol must be followed. Hazardous waste from healthcare facilities comes from radiology, the laboratory, and pharmacy, in addition to nursing units. Most of the waste produced by hospitals is not infectious, injurious, or hazardous. Safe waste includes paper, plastic, metal, or glass products used for a multitude of purposes within the healthcare agency.

There is a great deal of controversy about hospital waste products, much of it caused by the public's fear of HIV infection. The CDC has maintained that hospital waste in general is no more infective than residential waste. There is no current evidence that hospital waste has contributed to disease in the community (CDC, 1987a). Public concerns about the disposal of hypodermic syringes, blood, and fecal material, however, have provoked board of health reviews of institutional policies. It is to be anticipated that there will be more consistent and rigid regulations in the future. Current CDC recommendations are for incineration or autoclaving of infective waste before disposing in a sanitary landfill. Liquid body fluids (blood, urine, aspirated body fluids) can be flushed down a drain connected to a sewer system. This practice has been questioned recently by the media and some political bodies.

Another public health concern is the use of disposable diapers for infants and geriatric clients. Although most commercial packages advise rinsing the diaper in the toilet before disposal into garbage containers, it is known that there is little institutional or residential compliance with this advice. The result is millions of tons of carefully wrapped feces lying in sanitary landfills in nonbiodegradable plastic.

Studies continue to assess the potential health risks of medical wastes. As a result, new regulations will emerge. The staff member who handles this waste conscientiously at the bedside by bagging and labeling all waste and who transports it to the proper receptacle in the dirty utility room saves others from potential harm and contributes to controlling the considerable cost involved in waste disposal.

Aseptic Practices

Aseptic practices are those techniques used to keep objects or people free from microorganisms. The dramatic reduction in the incidence of disease that occurred during the late 1800s and early 1900s was largely the result of understanding that microorganisms caused disease and that these organisms could be controlled. The established control methods include physical agents, such as disinfectants, which are used on agents outside the body; chemical agents, such as antiseptics, which are used on inanimate objects as well as on the body surface; and chemotherapeutic agents, such as antibiotics, which are used to combat microorganisms on body surfaces and inside the body.

Categories of Asepsis

The two major categories of aseptic practice are medical asepsis and surgical asepsis. Nurses practice these techniques to ensure client safety and comfort and to prevent the spread of infection. Regardless of the type, asepsis begins and ends with effective handwashing.

Medical Asepsis

Medical asepsis refers to measures taken to control and reduce the number of pathogenic organisms present. It is also known as "clean technique." Aseptic measures used to prevent the spread of organisms from place to place include handwashing, gloving, gowning, and disinfecting to help contain microbial growth.

Surgical Asepsis

Surgical asepsis refers to "sterile technique." To be sterile, an object must be free of all microorganisms. Sterile technique is used to prevent the introduction or spread of pathogens from the environment into the client. Sterile technique is employed when a body cavity is entered with an object that may damage the mucous membranes, when surgical procedures are performed, and when the client's immune system is already compromised. Procedures that require sterile technique include insertion of intravenous catheters, giving injections, urinary catheterization, dressing changes, irrigation of drainage tubes that enter sterile parts of the body, and all operative procedures.

Clients whose immune systems are compromised may require the use of sterile technique and supplies more than clients with adequate host defenses. Premature newborns, burn clients, transplant recipients, and clients receiving chemotherapy or radiation are examples of groups for whom sterile technique may be used more frequently.

Handwashing

Even with the emphasis on gloving for contact with client secretions, nothing is more effective in preventing the spread of infections than handwashing. It is also the least expensive method of decreasing the risk of infecting oneself or others.

Contact transmission is the most common form of contamination in client care. Contact is often from the hands of personnel or the clients themselves. Any client contact poses the risk of contamination of the caregiver's hands with microorganisms that become transient flora until the hands are washed. Caregivers' hands are common vehicles for transfer of pathogens from client to client, from contaminated articles to clients, and from their own body flora. Experts say that proper handwashing can reduce nosocomial infection rates by 50%, yet studies have demonstrated that handwashing is the least practiced infection control measure (Larson, 1992; Meengs, et al., 1994).

Equipment necessary for handwashing (soap, running water, and paper towels) is inexpensive and should be readily available to all healthcare providers. High-risk areas, such as the nursery, critical care, transplant or burn units, and operative suites, may also require the use of antiseptic cleansing agents, nail files or sticks, and antiseptic-impregnated scrub brushes.

Hands should be washed before and after every client care contact. The use of gloves during client care does not eliminate the need for handwashing. Hands should be washed in the following situations:

- At the beginning and end of shift of work
- Before contact with a client
- Between contact with different clients
- Before and after contact with wounds, dressings, specimens, or bedclothes
- Before performing any invasive procedures
- Before administering medications
- After contact with any client secretion or excretion
- After using the bathroom
- After sneezing, coughing, or blowing nose

Medical and surgical asepsis vary in the technique for proper handwashing. Handwashing for surgical asepsis is longer and more methodic. Usually special antimicrobial agents are used. These variations are usually defined by institutional protocols. During a surgical scrub of the hands, the hands are held higher than the elbows to avoid contamination from water running back from the forearms to the hands. This is not required when the handwashing is done to ensure medical asepsis, as described in Procedure 25-1. Antiseptics should be used during surgical scrubs before invasive procedures and routinely in some high-risk areas. Studies have demonstrated that effectiveness of handwashing is determined by adequate friction, thoroughness of surfaces cleansed, and minimum duration of use, rather than the particular cleansing agent employed (Larson, 1992; Sheldon, 1994).

Most long-term flora on the hands reside in the nailbed and under the fingernails. Special attention is required for these areas, and soft sticks or fingernails from the opposite hand may be used to clean them. Fingernails should be kept short, and nail polish should be avoided because cracked or chipped nail polish can harbor bacteria that cannot be reached by ordinary handwashing. Artificial fingernails present a similar reservoir for infectious agents. Ideally, rings should be removed before handwashing and placed in pockets or pinned to the uniform during client care so that potential places harboring bacteria can be minimized. Nurses who wear a thin wedding band may slide it up on the finger so the area under the ring can be properly cleansed.

If hands become dry or cracked or develop dermatitis, the caregiver is less apt to wash his or her hands as often as necessary. This is a frequent complication for people with sensitive skin. Switching to another soap or antiseptic solution, thorough drying after every washing, and using skin lotion may help. Gloves should be worn during client care when the nurse's skin is abraded.

Handwashing technique should be learned by all caregivers, the client, and their family members. Clients should be provided with materials to wash their hands after toileting, and all visitors should be instructed to wash their hands before contact with the client and before leaving the client's room. The paramount importance of adequate handwashing cannot be stressed too often, no matter how unsophisticated it may seem, if infection is to be controlled.

Cleaning, Disinfection, and Sterilization

Three methods used to control microorganisms include physical methods, chemical methods, and chemotherapeutic agents. Physical methods for controlling microorganisms include cleaning by scrubbing surfaces, the use

Procedure 25-1
Handwashing

Purpose

1. Reduce the numbers of resident and transient bacteria from the hands.
2. Prevent transfer of microorganisms from the hospital environment to the client and from the client to hospital personnel.

Assessment

- Inspect hands for breaks or cuts in skin or cuticles.
- Identify appropriate times for handwashing before and after client contact.
- Identify need to repeat handwashing if hands become contaminated during a procedure.

Equipment

Warm, running water
Soap. Most hospitals supply liquid soaps, containing a germicidal agent, in dispensers at each sink.
Paper towels.

Procedure

1. Remove all rings except a plain wedding band. Push watch 4 to 5 inches above wrist.
   Rationale: Microorganisms lodge in the irregular surfaces of jewelry.
2. File nails short. Refrain from wearing nail polish or artificial fingernails.
   Rationale: Microorganisms harbor under long nails, which are hard to clean. Microorganisms may hide in cracked nail polish crevices or along adhesive edges of paste-on nails.
3. Turn on the water and adjust temperature to warm. Do not splash water or lean against the wet skin.

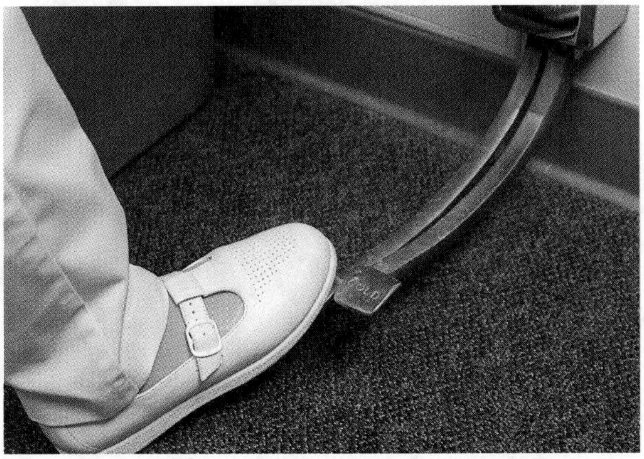

Step 3 • *Foot pedals may be available to turn on water.*

   Note: Faucets may be controlled by your hands or may be operated by knee levers or foot pedals.
   Rationale: Warm water removes less protective oils from the skin than hot water and reduces chapping of hands from frequent handwashing. Microorganisms need moisture to thrive. Avoid water splashing and sink contact on clothing to prevent contamination of uniform.
4. Hold hands lower than elbows and thoroughly wet hands and lower arms under running water.
   Rationale: Hands are more contaminated than lower arms; water should flow from least to most contaminated areas.

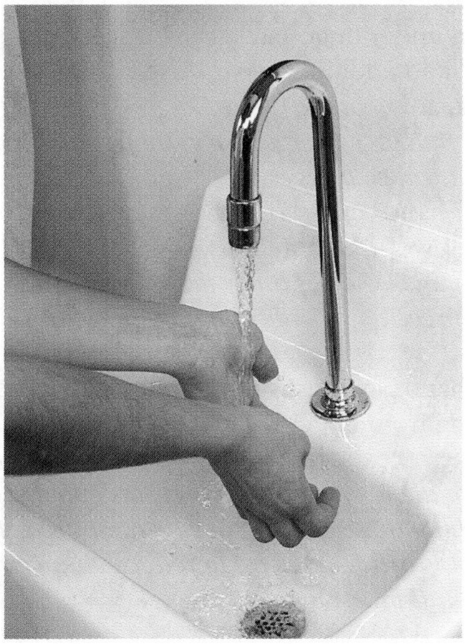

Step 4 • *Wet hands, holding wrists below elbow.*

5. Apply soap. If bar soap is used, rinse bar before lathering and rinse bar again before returning it to the dish.
   Rationale: The number of surface bacteria is to be reduced on the soap bar.
6. Rub palms, wrists, and back of hands firmly with circular movements. Interlace fingers and thumbs, moving hands back and forth. Continue using plenty of lather and friction for 15 to 30 seconds on each hand.
   Note: Timing of scrub may vary depending on purpose of wash.
   Rationale: Mechanically loosens and removes dirt and microorganisms on all hand surfaces.

(continued)

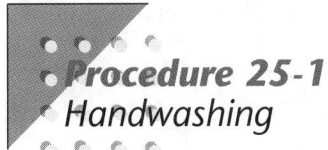

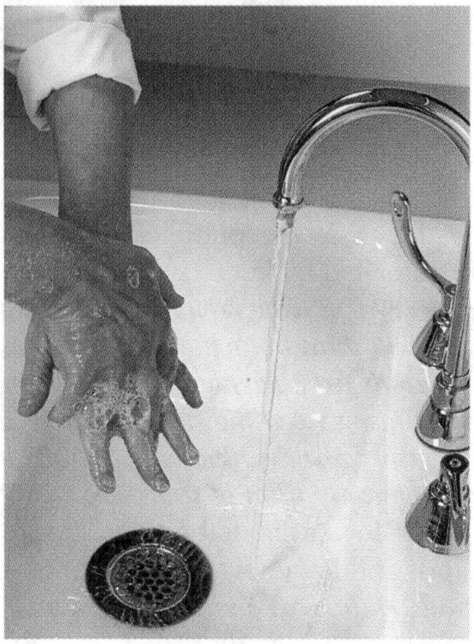

Step 6 • *Lather soap using friction.*

7. Clean under fingernails using fingernails of other hand and additional soap. Use orangewood stick if available.
   Rationale: Microorganisms are frequently harbored under nails.
8. Rinse hands and wrists thoroughly with hands held lower than forearms.
   Rationale: Washes away microorganisms and dirt and prevents recontamination of clean skin surfaces.
9. Dry hands and arms thoroughly with paper towel, wiping from fingertips toward forearm. Discard in proper receptacle.
   Rationale: Drying hands prevents chapping and cracking of skin. Dry from cleanest area (fingertips) toward least clean to reduce chances of contamination.

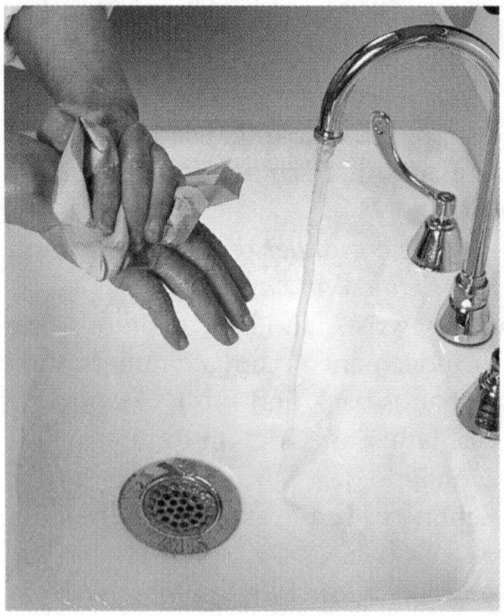

Step 9 • *Dry hands with paper towel.*

10. Turn off water using clean, dry paper towel on faucets.
    Rationale: Prevents transfer of microorganisms from faucet to hands.

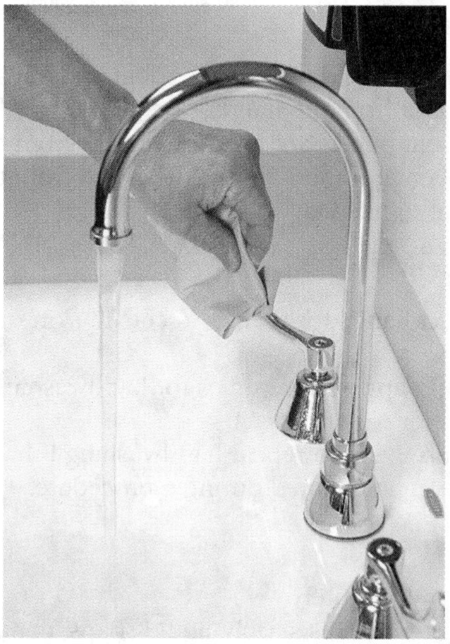

Step 10 • *Turn off faucet with clean paper towel.*

Home Care Modifications

- Visiting nurse should bring to client's home bactericidal soap in a plastic container and paper towels.
- If running water is unavailable, disposable washcloths or alcohol may be used as an alternative to handwashing. Both these agents are drying to the hands if used often.

Table 25-2 • Common Disinfectants and Antiseptics

Agent	Kills	Uses
Disinfectants		
Alcohol	Bacteria, not spores, virus, fungi	Thermometers, endoscopes, medication vials
Chlorine	Most microbes	Countertops and floors
Formaldehyde (formalin)	Bacteria, spores, fungi, virus	Hemodialysis units
Glutaraldehyde	Bacteria	Endoscopes, anesthesia and respiratory equipment
Antiseptics		
Povidone–iodine	Bacteria	Skin decontamination, wound packing, and irrigation
Sodium hypochlorite (Dakin's)	Bacteria, yeasts	Wound irrigation and packing
Chlorhexidine gluconate (Hibiclens)	Gram-positive organisms	Skin scrubs and irrigation
Acetic acid	*Pseudomonas*	Cleaning, packing, irrigating wounds
Hydrogen peroxide (3%)	Decomposes necrotic tissue	Irrigates wounds, cleans pus and necrotic tissue
Alcohol	Bacteria	Skin prep before injections
Hexachlorophene	Bacteria	Handwashing, skin prep; wash off to avoid neurotoxicity

of heat and cold to exceed the growth temperature of the organism, and the use of ultraviolet light, ionizing radiation, or ultrasound vibration. Chemical methods use solutions in various strengths to kill the organisms or prevent their growth and multiplication. Chemotherapeutic agents, such as antibiotics, also kill or retard the growth of pathogens after their administration.

A chemical used on lifeless objects is called a *disinfectant.* If the object is living, the chemical is called an **antiseptic**. Solutions that are disinfectants at higher concentrations may be diluted to be used as antiseptics on living objects. A chemical is **bactericidal** if it kills microorganisms; an agent that prevents bacterial multiplication but does not kill all forms of the organism is called **bacteriostatic.**

The method used for a particular procedure depends on characteristics of the object and the organism. To be useful, the method chosen must kill or retard growth of the pathogens without damaging the material or person being treated. Additional factors in method selection include the amount of time required to kill the organism and the stability of the agent being used.

Cleaning

Cleaning refers to the physical removal of visible dirt and debris by washing, dusting, or mopping surfaces that are contaminated. Soap is used for mechanical cleaning. It is manufactured from fats and chemicals that cause it to form a lather that emulsifies fats and lifts off dirt and other materials that can be rinsed away.

Contamination refers to an unclean condition where microorganisms are actually or potentially present. *Decontamination* refers to the removal of potentially pathogenic microorganisms using a process that makes the item safe to handle before other procedures are performed. Cleaning precedes disinfection and sterilization.

After client discharge, all client rooms should be cleaned as though the client were infected. Furniture and floors should be cleaned with a disinfectant detergent. Walls, blinds, and curtains should be washed if they are visibly soiled. Disinfectant fogging is no longer recommended. Terminal cleaning of client rooms should also be directed toward all items that were in direct contact with the client. All nondisposable items should be bagged, labeled, and sent for decontamination. All disposable items should be discarded even if unopened (Lynch & Cummings, 1987).

Disinfection

Disinfection refers to the processes used to reduce the numbers of potential pathogens from the surface of an object, usually by chemical or physical means. These processes do not necessarily remove all potential of infection, because spores may remain that may grow at a later time. Agents used in chemical disinfection are registered and regulated by the EPA. Chemical disinfectants used in the healthcare setting include alcohol, chlorine and chlorine compounds, formaldehyde, glutaraldehyde, and hydrogen peroxide. **Antiseptics** are used to retard bacterial growth on living organisms. Most commonly, antiseptics are used for handwashing, as skin preparation before invasive procedures, and to pack or irrigate wounds. Antiseptics used commonly for skin and wound care include povidone–iodine, sodium hypochlorite (Dakin's), chlorhexidine gluconate (Hibiclens), acetic acid, hydrogen peroxide, and alcohol. Table 25-2 lists common disinfectants and antiseptics along with their common uses. The CDC has published information on the use of these chemicals in relation to objects and humans and the level of disinfection they produce.

Sterilization

Sterilization is the complete destruction of all microorganisms, leaving no viable forms of organisms, including spores. Sterilization processes are caustic because they require extremes of heat, potent chemicals, or gas that cannot be used on body tissues. Any process used to sterilize equipment must be effective in killing organisms, but not destructive to the equipment.

The two most popular methods are steam sterilization and gas sterilization with ethylene oxide. Other sterilization methods include dry heat and ionizing radiation.

Steam Sterilization. Supersaturated steam under pressure—autoclaving—is the most widely used and dependable method of sterilization. It is nontoxic, inexpensive, and sporicidal, and it rapidly penetrates fabrics. Moist heat destroys microorganisms by the irreversible coagulation and denaturation of enzymes and structural proteins. Chemical indicators, which change color when the object being sterilized has been exposed to steam penetration for a specific period of time, are placed on the outside and inside of the object's package. This enables the healthcare worker to know when sterilization of an object has been effective (Fig. 25-7). Contamination can occur at a later time, so packaging should be checked for integrity.

Gas Sterilization. Ethylene oxide is used to sterilize medical products that cannot be steam sterilized. It is a colorless gas that can penetrate plastic, rubber, cotton, and other substances. Articles must be left to release the gas through aeration before they are used. Liquids may not be sterilized using this process because ethylene oxide is absorbed and not released. Disadvantages of this type of sterilization include expense and the length of time (2–5 hours).

Levels of Disinfection and Sterilization

There are different levels of disinfection of body sites and equipment. Agency policies identify whether cleaning, disinfection, or sterilization is to be used based on an item's intended use and factors such as cost. Many equipment items used in client care have the potential of harboring microorganisms that cause disease. It is impractical and unnecessary to sterilize all such items. Items can be grouped in categories to help identify proper methods of disinfection or sterilization. Modifications may be necessary in any of the categories when these items are to be used for high-risk clients.

Any item entering sterile tissues or the vascular system must be sterile. This category includes surgical instruments, cardiac and urinary catheters, implants, intravenous fluids, and needles. Most of these items are purchased as sterile or are sterilized by autoclaving. If the items could be destroyed by heat used during autoclaving, ethylene oxide gas or chemical solutions may be used.

Any item that may come in contact with mucous membranes or skin that is not intact must be free of all microorganisms, with the exception of spores. Intact mucous membranes in general are resistant to bacterial spores but are susceptible to viruses and tubercle bacilli. Respiratory therapy and anesthesia equipment, thermometers, and gastrointestinal endoscopes are included in this category. These items can be disinfected with high-level disinfectants. It is usually necessary to rinse items thoroughly to decontaminate them before they are disinfected; after disinfection, they are dried and wrapped to prevent dust exposure.

Because intact skin is an effective barrier to most microorganisms, items that come in contact with intact skin need not be sterile. Items such as blood pressure cuffs, linens, bedside tables, and room furniture can be cleaned and reused.

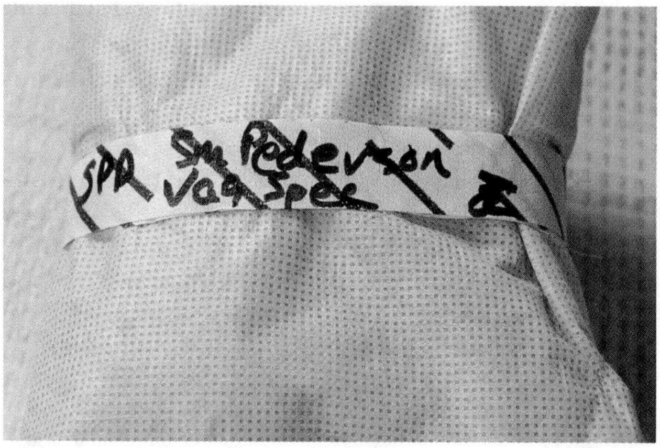

Figure 25-7 • *Color indicator strips change color, indicating sterilization has occurred.*

Use of Barriers

Techniques that prevent the transfer of pathogens from one person to another are referred to as "barrier nursing"; their aim is to contain pathogens by establishing aseptic barriers around the client and personnel. The most commonly used barriers are masks, gowns, gloves, private rooms, waterproof disposal bags for linen and trash, labeling and bagging of contaminated equipment and specimens, and control of airflow into sterile areas and out of contaminated areas. With the advent of AIDS, goggles have been added to the list, as well as check valves on masks used in mouth-to-mouth resuscitation. The most important aspect of barrier methods is the awareness of the staff about the need to prevent cross-contamination of people, equipment, and supplies.

Some research facilities are testing the effectiveness of laminar flow units, which totally isolate immune-suppressed clients from the environment. Plastic curtains are assembled in a box around a client's bed and connected to a system that filters the air entering the enclosed space. Ports with sleeves for covering the caregivers' arms are built into the sides of the unit.

Masks

Masks prevent transmission of infectious agents through the air. Masks protect the wearer from inhaling large-particle droplets, which are transmitted by close contact and usually travel only a short distance (up to 3 feet), and small-particle droplets that remain suspended in air and may travel further. Masks lose their effectiveness when they are wet or worn for long periods of time. They also are ineffective when they are not changed after caring for each client.

Disposable particulate respirators are indicated whenever working with a client who has, or is suspected of having, tuberculosis or other airborne diseases. Respirators look like masks, but fit the face more tightly and are able to filter out organisms as small as 1 micron (Boutotte, 1993b). Individual mask fitting is recommended because a tight seal must be maintained. Nurses working in communities with high-risk populations need to carry respirators and use them whenever indicated. In the hospital setting, when working in direct contact with tuberculosis clients, battery-operated respirators that cover most of the face can be used.

Gowns, Caps, and Shoe Coverings

Gowns should be worn when the caregiver's clothing is likely to be soiled by infected material. Gowns should be changed when they become moist and should be worn only once and discarded. Caps are used to cover the hair, and special covers are available for shoes. New products are being developed to be used in high–risk areas (eg, labor and delivery, emergency room) to shield body parts from accidental exposure to contaminated body secretions. Procedure 25-2 outlines the proper method for donning and removing a gown.

Gloves

Gloves protect personnel from acquiring infective organisms on their hands. They also reduce the likelihood that personnel will transmit their own or other clients' microbial flora from their hands to the client. Gloves are a major barrier to contact transmission when they are changed between clients, and when hands are washed and dried before and after gloving. Clean, nonsterile gloves should be worn when direct contact with moist body substances from any client is anticipated. Gloves should be changed between clients or when they become torn or grossly soiled. Gloves should not be washed and reused.

Latex and vinyl gloves are two categories of gloves that are widely used clinically. Latex gloves are made of natural rubber and are more flexible and durable. Although they are more expensive, latex gloves are preferred when lengthy exposure is anticipated or fine motor skill is required (Korniewicz & Garzon,1994).

Latex allergy has been noted in the literature, so it is important to be sure that neither the nurse nor the client is allergic to latex when this type of glove is used. Vinyl gloves, made of polyvinyl chloride, a synthetic rubber, fit loosely and offer less protection but are usually adequate for routine client care activities such as emptying bedpans, handling specimens, or providing hygiene. Using latex gloves for routine care activities is unnecessary and adds to the cost of care (Korniewicz, et al., 1992). Double gloving is indicated during activities when gloves may tear or puncture (Korniewicz & Garzon, 1994).

Private Rooms

Separation of clients into private rooms decreases the chance of transmission of infection by all routes. Airborne infections always require private rooms. Special negative-air-flow rooms are indicated for tuberculosis and protective isolation. Clients with poor hygienic habits or those who are incontinent should be placed in private rooms. High-risk groups include children younger than 5 years of age, clients with altered mental status, and clients with large, draining wounds or blood loss that cannot be contained in dressings.

Transporting clients with infections necessitating private rooms should be avoided whenever possible. If transport to other departments is necessary, the client's gown and dressings should be changed before leaving the room. If the infection is transmitted via the airborne route, the client should wear a mask and the transporters should be immune to the disease.

Equipment and Refuse Handling

Special handling of articles and linen soiled by all bodily fluids is indicated. These articles should be placed in im-

Procedure 25-2
Donning and Removing a Mask and Gown

Purpose

1. Prevent spread of microorganisms from the nurse to the client.
2. Prevent contamination of the nurse's clothing from the client.
3. Prevent spread of airborne microorganisms from the client to the nurse.

Assessment

- Identify when gowning or masking is appropriate.
- Examine uniform for obvious soiling.

Equipment

Clean, dry gown and mask. Gowns are to be used once and discarded for laundry or disposal.

Procedure

Donning Mask

1. Wash hands.
   Rationale: Washing hands prevents spread of microorganisms.
2. If required, position mask over mouth and nose. Bend nose bar over bridge of nose. Secure strings or elastic.
   Note: Mask should never be allowed to hang around neck. Mask should be changed if used longer than 30 minutes because effectiveness is dramatically reduced after that time.

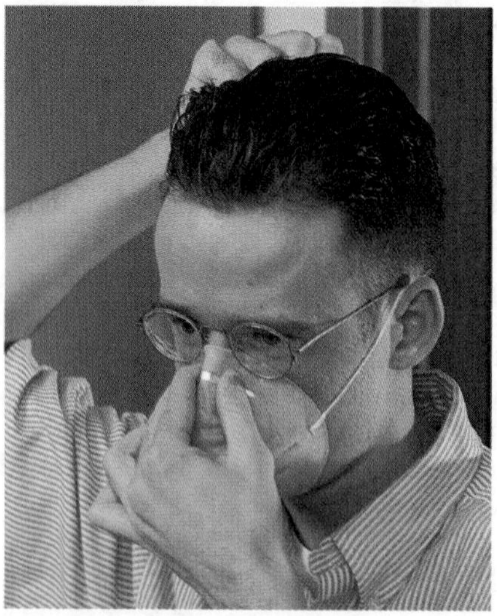

Step 2 • *Position mask, shaping nose bar for snug fit.*

Procedure

Donning Clean Gown

1. Grasp gown by collar allowing it to unfold.
2. Place arms through sleeve and pull gown over shoulders.

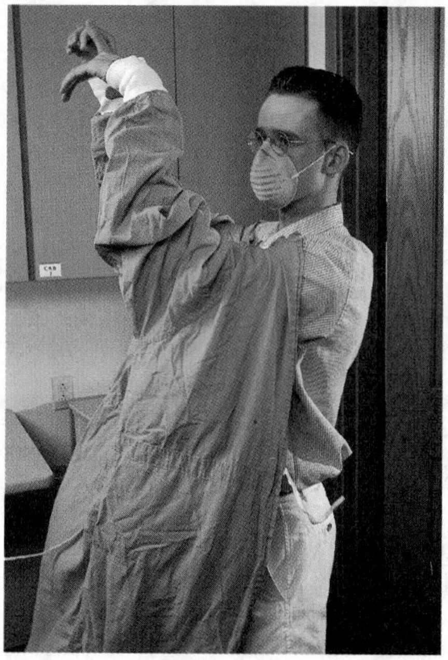

Step 2 • *Place arms in sleeves of gown.*

3. Fasten neck ties. Overlap the gown at the back and fasten waist ties.
   Rationale: Overlapping back ensures uniform is completely covered at the back.

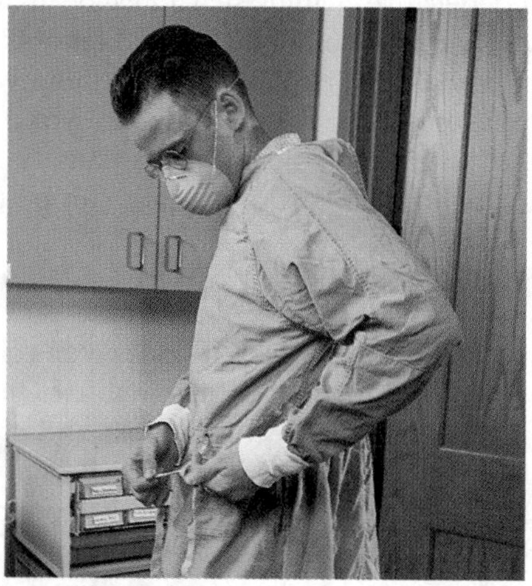

Step 3 • *Fasten ties.*

Procedure

Removing Contaminated Gown

1. Untie waist ties and let hang freely.
2. Wash hands.
3. Untie neck ties and let gown fall forward off shoulder.
4. Slide arms out of gown, working from the inside.

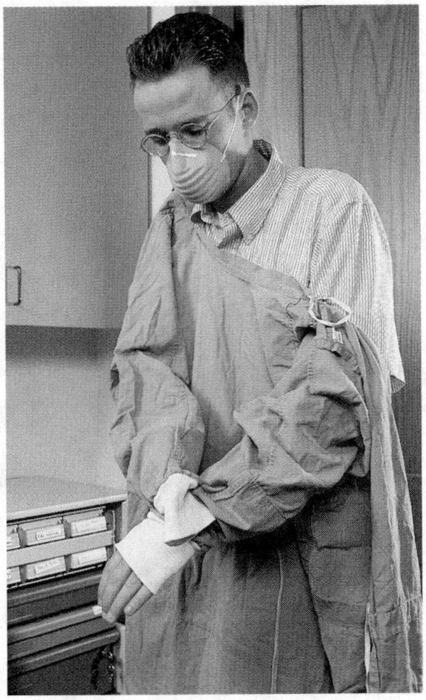

Step 4 • *Holding cuff, slide sleeve forward.*

5. Holding gown away from your body, fold contaminated side of gown toward the inside.
   Rationale: Turning gown inside out reduces spread of microorganisms and protects uniform from contamination.

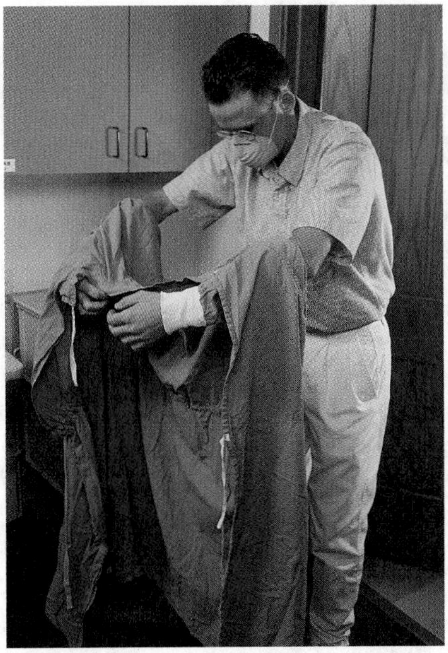

Step 5 • *Fold gown so that contaminated outside faces inside.*

6. Discard in appropriate receptacle
7. Remove and discard mask.
8. Wash hands.

pervious bags before they are removed from the client's bedside. Bagging in watertight containers is indicated to prevent exposure of personnel and to prevent contamination of the environment. The outside of the bag should not be contaminated when placing the articles inside it. Each hospital has procedures for labeling and decontaminating exposed articles. Items visibly soiled with body substances should be rinsed and placed in plastic bags or clearly marked containers in dirty utility rooms before returning them to the central processing areas.

Double bagging, a system of having all contaminated linen and waste placed in another bag for all clients in isolation, is no longer indicated. Studies show that bacterial contamination is not significantly decreased by using double-bagging techniques, yet this practice significantly increase the cost and nursing time required (Weinstein, et al., 1989).

Isolation Systems

Isolation refers to techniques used to prevent or limit the spread of infection. Some form of isolation has been used for centuries, whether to protect a high-risk person from exposure to pathogens or to prevent the transmission of pathogens from an infected person to others.

The first two manuals published by the CDC recommended only category-specific isolation. Increased episodes of nosocomial infections (especially among immunocompromised clients) and the AIDS epidemic in the 1980s fostered the development of two new systems. The CDC called for universal precautions related to blood and certain body fluids to protect healthcare workers from clients possibly carrying human immunodeficiency virus (HIV), hepititis-B virus, and other bloodborne pathogens. Body-substance isolation, developed at Harborview Medical Center of Seattle and at the University of California in San Diego, recommended barriers to provide protection from *all* moist body secretions.

In 1994, the CDC introduced draft guidelines for a new Two-Tiered System of Isolation Precautions that includes Standard Precautions and Transmission-Based Precautions. The new system is an attempt to synthesize different systems and to improve adherence to appropriate infection-control practices. These systems are discussed here.

Isolation systems are costly in terms of equipment, supplies, and the time required by caregivers. Even more expensive are breaks in isolation technique that result in infection. All personnel, physicians, nurses, technicians, students, and housekeepers are responsible for complying with isolation precautions. All personnel are responsible for tactfully calling observed infractions to the attention of those who do not comply. Compliance is best obtained by using a consistent, simple system; educating the staff; and instilling a sense of

Table 25-3 • Comparison of Category-Specific, Disease-Specific, Body Substance Isolation Precautions, and Standard (SP) and Transmission-Based Precautions (TBP)

	Category-Specific	Disease-Specific	Body Substance	Standard Precautions/ Transmission-Based Precautions
Isolation precautions	Seven categories, each with a different set of precautions	Individualized for each disease	Universal precautions for all moist body substances	SP—Universal Precautions and body substance isolation for all clients TBP—Clients with documented or suspected highly transmissible organisms
Instruction card for door or cubicle	Separate, preprinted, color-coded card for each category	All-purpose black and white card to be individualized for each client	All-purpose red, black, and white sign for all clients. In addition, STOP sign cards are used to identify rooms of clients with airborne diseases.	Yet to be developed by the Centers for Disease Control and Prevention
Advantages	Simpler system; less diagnostic information needed to assign precautions Less decision-making needed to assign precautions	Minimizes unnecessary precautions; may reduce cost of placing client on isolation precautions May encourage compliance, especially by physicians	Recognizes the potential colonization of all body substances No decision-making is necessary for the use of barriers other than recognition of the potential for exposure to body substances. Cross-contamination between clients is minimized because gloves are changed between clients and no surface touches two people.	Decreases transmission risk from recognized and unrecognized sources Permits individualization of isolation precautions for individuals with or suspected of having highly transmissible organisms Simplifies older category-specific isolation based on modes of transmission
Disadvantages	Unnecessary precautions taken for some diseases May increase cost of isolation	Requires more skill and responsibility to assign precautions Requires more diagnostic information about disease to assign precautions	None currently recognized. Cost is not acknowledged as a factor. No barriers are used other than those indicated to avoid soiling by obvious body secretions.	New system will require education among healthcare professionals

personal responsibility in all caregivers. The infection control committee usually examines all systems of isolation and decides which system is to be used throughout the agency. The different systems of isolation are compared in Table 25-3.

Universal Precautions

Universal Precautions are precautions universally applied to blood or body fluids containing traces of blood from all clients regardless of their diagnosis (CDC, 1988). The accompanying display summarizes actions in Universal Precautions. Healthcare providers are directed by the CDC to consider all clients as potentially infected with bloodborne pathogens such as HIV (AIDS) and hepatitis B virus. The CDC recommends that Universal Precautions also apply to semen and vaginal secretions as well as tissue extracted by biopsy or during operative procedures. Cerebrospinal fluid, synovial fluid, peritoneal fluid, and amniotic fluid require precautions because they may have been contaminated by the client's blood during needle insertion while obtaining the specimen. The CDC excludes feces, nasal secretions, sputum, sweat, tears, urine, and vomitus from the high-risk category of carrying bloodborne pathogens unless they contain visi-

Universal Precautions:

Prevention of Transmission of HIV, HBV, and Other Bloodborne Pathogens in Healthcare Settings

Under Universal Precautions, blood and certain body fluids of all clients are considered potential infectious for human immunodeficiency virus (HIV), hepatitis B virus (HBV), and other bloodborne pathogens. Blood is the single most important source of HIV, HBV, and other bloodborne pathogens in healthcare settings. Infection-control efforts for HIV, HBV, and other bloodborne pathogens must focus on preventing exposure to blood as well as delivery of HBV immunization.

Epidemiologic evidence has implicated only blood, semen, vaginal secretions, and possibly breast milk in transmissions. Although the risk is unknown, Universal Precautions also apply to tissues and to cerebrospinal fluid, synovial fluid, pleural fluid, peritoneal fluid, and amniotic fluid. Universal Precautions do not apply to feces, nasal secretions, sputum, sweat, tears, urine, and vomitus unless they contain visible blood.

Healthcare workers must consider *all* clients as potentially infected with bloodborne pathogens and must adhere rigorously to infection-control precautions for *all* clients.

General Precautions

- Consider all clients as potentially infected.
- Wear gloves when touching blood, body fluids containing blood, and body fluids to which Universal Precautions apply; for handling items or surfaces soiled with blood or applicable fluids, and for performing venipuncture and other vascular access procedures. Change gloves after each contact with a client.
- Use protective barriers (ie, wear masks, protective eyewear or face shields and gowns or aprons) when performing procedures that may produce blood or body fluid droplets or splashes.
- Wash hands and skin surfaces immediately and thoroughly if contaminated with blood or other body fluids to which Universal Precautions apply.
- Take precautions to prevent injuries from needles, scalpels, and other sharp instruments during procedures, when cleaning instruments, during disposal, or when handling. To prevent needle stick injuries, needles should not be recapped, purposely bent or broken by hand, removed from disposable syringes, or otherwise manipulated by hand. After they are used, disposable syringes and needles, scalpel blades, and other sharp items should be placed in puncture-resistant containers for disposal.

Special Considerations

- Healthcare workers who have exudative lesions or weeping dermatitis should refrain from all direct client care and from handling client care equipment until the condition resolves.
- Pregnant healthcare workers are not known to be at greater risk of contacting HIV infection than healthcare workers who are not pregnant; however, if a healthcare worker develops HIV infection during pregnancy, the infant is at risk of infection resulting from perinatal transmission. Because of this risk, pregnant healthcare workers should be especially familiar with and strictly adhere to precautions to minimize the risk of HIV transmission.

Precautions for Invasive Procedures

(Here an invasive procedure is defined as any surgical entry into tissues, cavities, or organs or repair

(continued)

Universal Precautions: *(continued)*

of major traumatic injuries.) General blood and body fluid precautions listed above, combined with the precautions listed below, should be the *minimum precautions for all such invasive procedures.*

- All healthcare workers who participate in invasive procedures must routinely use appropriate barrier procedures to prevent skin and mucous membrane contact with all clients' blood and other body fluids.
- Gloves and surgical masks must be worn for all invasive procedures.
- Protective eyewear or face shields should be worn for all procedures that commonly result in generation of droplets or splashing of blood, body fluids containing blood, or other applicable body fluids.
- Gowns or aprons made of materials providing an effective barrier should be worn during invasive procedures likely to result in the splashing of blood or other pertinent body fluids.
- All healthcare workers who perform or assist in vaginal or cesarean delivery should wear gloves and gown when handling the placenta or the infant until blood and amniotic fluid have been removed from the infant's skin. Gloves should be worn until postdelivery care of the umbilical cord.
- If a glove is torn or a needle stick or other injury occurs, the glove should be removed and a new glove used promptly as client safety permits; the needle or instrument involved in the incident should also be removed from the sterile field.

This information is originally from the Centers for Disease Control and Prevention (1987). Recommendations for prevention of HIV transmission in health care settings. *MMWR, 36* (Suppl), 25; and Centers for Disease Control and Prevention (1988). Universal Precautions for prevention or transmission of human immunodeficiency virus, hepatitis B virus, and other bloodborne pathogens in health-care settings. *MMWR, 37,* 24. This information agrees with the newest guideline proposals published in Centers for Disease Control and Prevention (1994). Draft guideline, for isolation precautions in hospitals: Notice. *Federal Register,* 59(214), 55552–55570.

ble blood. Saliva and human breast milk require precautions when there is intensive exposure, as in dentistry and breast milk banks.

Universal Precautions recommend gloves when exposure to blood or body fluids containing blood is anticipated. Masks and goggles should be worn when any splattering of blood or body fluids is anticipated during procedures. Gowns should be worn to avoid soiling of uniforms and the exposure of the caregiver's skin when gross contamination is possible (CDC, 1988a).

Category-Specific Isolation

Category-specific isolation protocol groups infections into seven categories according to their routes of transmission; the seven groups include most infectious conditions that have similar epidemiology. The advantage of this system is simplicity. It can be applied early in the hospital stay before an exact diagnosis is known. Because it is more general, this system is easier to implement. Its main disadvantage is that the system may lead to overisolation because more precautions are employed than are necessary for every disease in the category. This can add to hospital costs and may decrease caregiver compliance with the prescribed precautions.

The seven isolation categories are described below. A category ending in the term "isolation" is used when a private room is necessary, whereas the term "precaution" is used when a private room is optional. Cards for each category are commercially printed in specific colors with instructions for those who care for the client or are entering their room. Figure 25-8 shows an example of the card providing directions for respiratory isolation.

Strict Isolation. Strict isolation is designed to prevent transmission of very contagious or virulent infections that are spread by both air and contact. All barriers are used every time the room is entered.

Contact Isolation. Contact isolation is designed to prevent transmission by close or direct contact with a client who has a highly transmissible disease.

Respiratory Isolation. Respiratory isolation is designed to prevent transmission by droplet transmission through the air.

Tuberculosis Isolation. Tuberculosis isolation is designed to prevent small-particle transmission of microorganisms suspended in the air from clients with active cases of tuberculosis.

Enteric Precautions. Enteric precautions are designed to prevent the transmission of infections by direct or indirect contact with feces.

Drainage–Secretions Precautions. Drainage–secretions precautions are designed to prevent transmission of infections by direct or indirect contact with purulent secretions or body cavity drainage.

Blood–Body Fluid Precautions. Blood–body fluid precautions are designed to prevent transmission by infected

Respiratory Isolation

Visitors—Report to Nurses' Station Before Entering Room

1. **Private Room** – *necessary*; door must be kept closed.
2. **Gowns** – not necessary.
3. **Masks** – must be worn by all persons entering room if susceptible to disease.
4. **Hands** – must be washed on entering and leaving room.
5. **Gloves** – not necessary.
6. **Articles** – those contaminated with secretions must be disinfected.
7. **Caution** – all persons susceptible to the specific disease should be excluded from patient area; if contact is necessary, susceptibles must wear masks.

Figure 25-8 • *Category-specific sign for respiratory isolation.*

blood or body fluids. Body fluids include saliva, semen, peritoneal fluid, tears, and other body cavity aspirates.

Disease-Specific Isolation

More than 160 specific diseases are listed in the CDC guidelines for disease-specific isolation. These diseases are considered likely to occur in U.S. healthcare agencies. Disease-specific isolation depends on accurate identification of the infective organism. These precautions are aimed at interrupting the mode of transmission by identifying which secretions, excretions, body fluids, or tissues are or might be infective. Each specific disease is identified as to whether a gown, gloves, mask, or private room is required. Cards are available for posting outside client rooms with spaces available to write in directions for caregivers and visitors. The healthcare provider is required to make decisions based on the client's age, mental status, and overall status concerning minimum precautions necessary to prevent transmission of the organism. It is presumed that young children require more precautions than adults because often they are not toilet trained and may not comply with instructions. Similar adjustments may be necessary for people who become confused.

Disadvantages of disease-specific isolation precautions include the increased responsibility of decision-making by the healthcare provider; isolation also may be delayed until the organism is identified by laboratory means. This delay may actually exceed the period of greatest infectivity of the client. It may also presume that body fluids are sterile when they may also harbor pathogens. Advertising the diagnosis of the client outside the client's room, especially in the event of AIDS or sexually transmitted diseases, may breach client confidentiality.

Body-Substance Isolation

Infection control practitioners were aware of the shortcomings of both of these major isolation systems and were concerned about noncompliance of caregivers with infection control measures, unacceptable rates of nosocomial infections, and the appearance of an epidemic of AIDS infection.

Two basic premises underlie the body-substance isolation method of infection control. First, infection may be present before a diagnosis is made. Infection control measures often are initiated too late to prevent transmission. Second, the highest risk of transmitting or contracting infection from most organisms lies in direct contact of the organism with the caregiver's hands, or with equipment that has been soiled by potentially infectious bodily secretions. These premises lead to the conclusion that all body substances may harbor pathogens, and contact with them must be avoided. The cardinal rule of body-substance isolation is never to touch with bare hands anything wet that comes from a body surface or body cavity. Gloves are worn for all contact with mucous membranes, nonintact skin, and moist body substances at all times. Body substances include blood, urine, feces, sputum, saliva, wound drainage, or aspirated body fluids. Gloves are not necessary for contact with unsoiled articles or intact skin.

Gowns are worn when personal clothing may be soiled with the client's body fluids. Masks are worn for anticipated contact with respiratory droplet secretions, or while suctioning. Protective eyewear is added when secretions are likely to splash. Cards are available to remind staff of Universal Precautions, and can be located in all client rooms (Fig. 25-9). In addition, "STOP" cards are used to identify rooms of clients with airborne communicable diseases. Body-substance isolation has the advantage of being simple, and there is no delay in instituting this form of isolation until the causative agent is found.

Two-Tiered System of Isolation Precautions

The Two-Tiered System of Isolation Precautions employs two levels of precautions (CDC, 1994):

1. Standard Precautions for all clients to protect against blood and body fluid transmission of potential infective organisms
2. Transmission-Based Precautions to protect against the spread of highly transmissible or epidemiologically significant pathogens in clients with documented or suspected infections

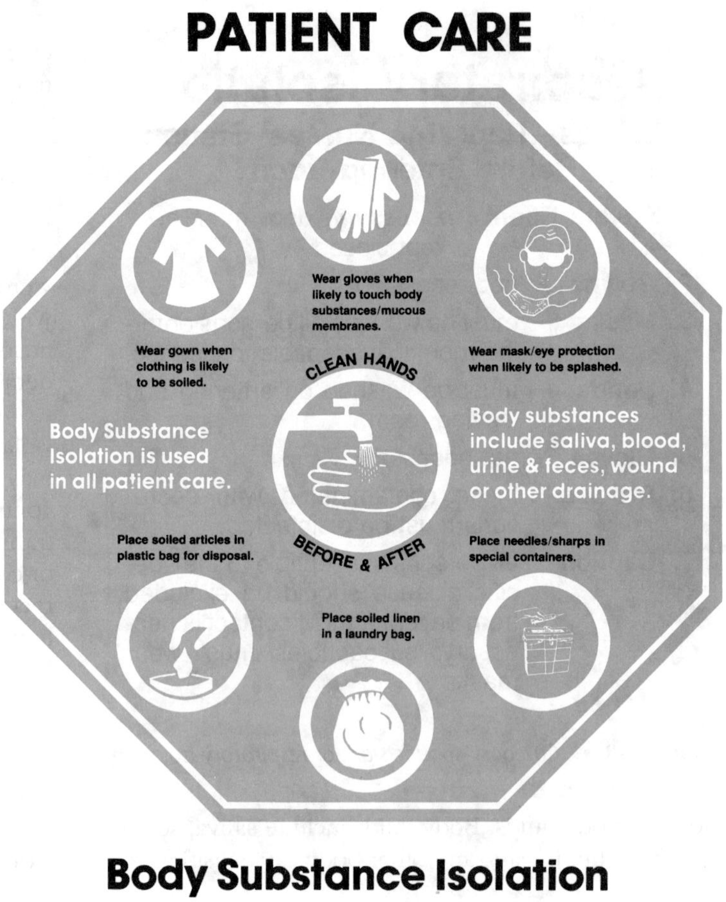

Figure 25-9 • Body substance isolation sign.

Standard Precautions. Standard Precautions synthesizes the major features of Universal Precautions (decreasing risk of transmission from bloodborne pathogens) and body substance isolation (decreasing risk of transmission from moist body substances). This protects against the transmission of undiagnosed infections as well as those that have been identified. Standard Precautions protects the healthcare provider as well as clients accessing healthcare services (Table 25-4).

Transmission-Based Precautions. When highly transmissible or significant pathogens have been identified, additional isolation may be required to prevent the spread of infection. Depending on the organism identified and its mode of transmission, Airborne Precautions, Droplet Precautions, or Contact Precautions may be instituted. Combined protocols may be used if the organism has more than one mode of transmission.

Airborne Precautions are used for microorganisms transmitted by small-particle droplets that can remain suspended and become widely dispersed by air currents. The client should be cared for in a private, negative-air-flow room, masks should be worn by caregivers, and the client should wear a mask if transport out of the room is necessary.

Droplet Precautions are used for microorganisms transmitted by larger-particle droplets, which disperse into air currents. For Droplet Precautions, the client should be in a private room, or with an individual who is infected with the same microorganism. A negative-air-flow room is not required and masks are used when working within 3 feet of the client. The client should wear a mask when outside of the room.

When clients are known to be infected with significant organisms (eg, drug-resistant pathogens), extra care is required to prevent transmission, and thus Contact Precautions are instituted. The client is cared for in a private room or has a roommate that is infected with the same organism, gloves are used and changed when exposed to potentially infected material during care delivery, and gowns and protective barriers are used when contamination is likely.

Protective (Reverse) Isolation

Protective (reverse) isolation is used to prevent infection for people whose body defenses are known to be compromised. Clients who are neutropenic (neutrophils 500/mm^3) as a result of chemotherapy, radiation therapy, or immunosuppressive medications are prime candidates. Clients with extensive burns or dermatitis are also at high risk. Such a client is placed in a private room, ideally one with a laminar flow unit, which directs airflow outward and away from the client. All people coming in contact with the individual must wear gowns, gloves, and masks. Meticulous handwashing is

Table 25-4 • Standard Precautions and Transmission-Based Precautions

	Precautions	Indications
Standard Precautions	Use Universal Precautions and Body Substance Isolation to protect against known or unknown exposure from blood, body fluids, or mucous membranes	All clients in all situations
Transmission-Based Precautions		
Airborne	Private, negative airflow room with adequate filtration; mask; client wears mask if transported out of room	Transmission via airborne route (small particle droplets); tuberculosis, measles, varicella
Droplet	Private room or cohabitation with client infected with same organism; mask required when working within 3 feet of client; mask used during transport	Transmission of large droplets through sneezing, coughing, or talking. *H. influenzae,* multidrug-resistant strains. *Neisseria meningitidis,* diphtheria, *Mycoplasma pneumoniae*
Contact	Private room or cohabitation with client infected with same organism; gloves at all times and change after exposure to organism; gown and protective barriers when direct contact with organism occurs	Serious illness easily transmitted through direct contact. Any multidrug-resistant strains, *C. difficile, Shigella,* impetigo, and others

also employed by everyone entering the room. Food and equipment coming into the client's room are treated at the highest level of disinfection. All of these measures help to ensure that the client's environment stays as free from pathogens as possible, thus decreasing the chance that infection occurs in these high-risk people.

Psychological Effects of Isolation

Psychological effects of being separated from staff and loved ones occur when isolation is used. Clients spend more time alone. The bodies, hands, and faces of caregivers are covered. Clients may mistakenly feel they are dirty or untouchable, especially if they have diseases that are considered socially unacceptable. Lack of social interaction can be psychologically injurious, especially to children and their parents. Nursing goals should be directed at preventing the spread of microorganisms while maintaining the client's social support.

Surgical Asepsis

Surgical asepsis, or sterile technique, is defined as those practices that produce or maintain equipment and areas that are free from all microorganisms. The purpose of sterile technique is to prevent the introduction of microorganisms from the environment into the client. Surgical asepsis is used during:

- Surgical procedures
- All procedures that invade the bloodstream
- Procedures that cause a break in skin or mucous membranes (eg, intramuscular injections)
- Dressing changes and wound care
- Procedures involving inserting catheters or devices into sterile body cavities (eg, bladder)
- Care for high-risk groups (eg, transplant recipients, burn clients, or immunosuppressed clients)

When all organisms and their spores are destroyed, the item is deemed sterile. These items are clearly labeled as sterile on their packaging. The packaging must not be torn, punctured, wet, or outdated. During any sterile procedure, care must be taken to keep all sterile equipment sterile.

Principles of Surgical Asepsis

Surgical asepsis starts with thorough planning and preparation of the environment, supplies, and personnel. Although surgical asepsis is carried out in many settings, the operating room is an area where surgical asepsis is carried out extensively. Staff members in the operating room require special training in maintaining aseptic technique for various operative procedures.

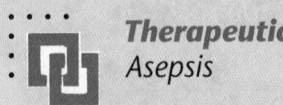

Therapeutic Dialogue
Asepsis

Scenes for Thought

Arnie McKellan is 43 years old and admitted to your unit for treatment of the complications of cancer therapy. This is his second admission to the hospital but the first time he has been in protective (or reverse) isolation. You, his primary nurse, are meeting him for the first time and have on the appropriate mask, gown, and gloves.

Effective

Client: *Well, well, another astronaut entering the forbidden planet. And who are you, spaceperson?!* Client looks annoyed, depressed and sounds cheerful all at the same time.
Nurse: *I'm Susan O'Shea, Mr. McKellan, your primary nurse. You sound cheerful today. Are you? (Standing next to the bed)*
Client: *Of course! Wouldn't you be, getting to spend all this time alone and spacepeople coming to see you every five minutes?* He says this with great sarcasm.
Nurse: *No, I'd be lonely and annoyed. (Says this quietly and seriously.)*
Client: He looks away and stays quiet for awhile. So does Susan. *I don't want to feel depressed about this admission, Susan. I know it's going to be one of many. So I guess I've been a little loud and sarcastic. I can tell you won't let me get away with it.* Smiles.
Nurse: *(Laughs) We can get loud together later, but we have other work to do first. Maybe I could start with the reason for the "spacesuits," and then we could go on to a short history and physical. How does that sound? (Making an alliance with the client, making sure to laugh rather than smile, which is hidden by the mask.)*
Client: *Okay, okay. Especially the part about the masks and everything. I'm not used to it. Makes me feel terminal already!*
Nurse: *Sounds like we have a lot to talk about. Let's get to it. (Explains about the reason for the isolation, what's involved, how long it will go on, and so forth. Mr. McKellan listens carefully, asking questions, making a few jokes, but appearing more relaxed.)*

Less Effective

Client: *Well, well, another astronaut entering the forbidden planet. And who are you, spaceperson?!* As above.
Nurse: *Well, I'm Sally Ride, the first woman astronaut! How's it going with you today? (Very cheerful, answers with the same tone of voice.)*
Client: *Couldn't be better with all the spacepeople coming in here. I get lots of company and nobody's done anything awful to me yet. How can I complain?* He looks strained, and his eye contact begins to slip.
Nurse: *Well, I'm not here to change that part yet. I'm really Sheila Evans, your primary nurse and I need to take a history and do a nursing assessment. It won't take long, I can see you're tired. (Sits down in the chair next to the bed, opens his chart and begins to write.)*
Client: *Yes, I really am. I'd appreciate it if you'd make it quick.* Continues to look strained.
Nurse: *Sure, no problem. (Proceeds to ask about functional health patterns. Client makes jokes, answers questions shortly, often with sarcasm.) You know, I can't tell if you're serious or joking sometimes! Makes it hard to fill out this assessment.*
Client: *Well, I'll try my best to be serious all the time from now on! Are you done yet?* Sounds irritated.
Nurse: *Yes, I am, for now. I'll let you rest now and I'll be back with your dinner tray. We can talk some more then. (Leaves the room thinking, "Just what I need. An angry client in isolation!")*
Client: Turns to the wall and sighs.

Critical Thinking Challenges

• List behaviors indicating the client is angry, afraid, apprehensive, annoyed. • Compare and contrast how Susan and Sheila responded to these behaviors. • Identify the concerns of each nurse. • Appraise your emotional reaction when you're confronted by an irritated, sarcastic person, and describe what you do. • Examine the aspects of communication that are lost with a mask.

Operative suites are specially constructed rooms that provide for no-touch handwashing at sinks controlled by foot pedals, have special airflow patterns, and control traffic into and out of areas.

Good personal hygiene is basic behavior for all personnel. Staff members who are ill with respiratory infections or who have conditions that cause diarrhea, vomiting, or skin lesions should not participate in sterile procedures. Street attire is not worn in the operating room or other hospital areas where sterility is important. Shoes can be covered with shoe covers, and beards and hair can be covered by caps and masks. Jewelry should not be worn on the hands. General principles of surgical asepsis are discussed in Table 25-5.

Skin Preparation

Skin preparation reduces microorganisms present on the skin. The skin cannot be sterilized, because chemicals used to sterilize objects would kill dermal cells. Skin is disinfected by chemicals in a procedure called *degermation.*

Bacteria on the skin include both transient and resident flora. The transient microorganisms are held in place by sweat, oil, and debris. They can be removed

Table 25-5 • Principles of Surgical Asepsis

Technique/Principle	Rationale
Moisture may cause contamination. • Handle liquids carefully near sterile fields to prevent splashing. • Place wet objects on sterile, water-impermeable surfaces, such as sterile basins.	Microorganisms travel more easily through moist environments. When a sterile surface becomes moist, microorganisms may be transmitted from an unsterile surface by capillary action.
Never assume that an object is sterile. • Check to see that it is labeled as sterile. • Always check the integrity of the packaging. • Always check the expiration date on the package. • If there is any doubt about the sterility of an object, it should be considered unsterile.	Commercially prepared products are labeled as sterile on their packaging. Special indicators are used to show that objects have completed their sterilization process, such as tapes on the outside of packages or chemically impregnated paper inside containers. Packages that are torn, punctured, or moist cannot be considered sterile. All packaging materials should have clearly visible dates that indicate when sterility cannot be guaranteed. Items that have passed that date cannot be used.
Always face the sterile field.	The area defined as sterile for the purposes of the procedure is the "field." Objects that are out of the line of vision may be inadvertently contaminated and their sterility is never guaranteed.
Sterile articles may touch only sterile articles or surfaces if they are to maintain their sterility.	Anything considered unsterile may transfer microorganisms to the sterile object it touches. An object used on an unsterile surface, such as swabs used in cleaning the skin, must be used once and then discarded because skin cannot be sterilized. Keep unsterile objects away from the field.
Sterile equipment or areas must be kept above the waist and on top of the sterile field. • Drapes hanging over the edge of the table are not considered sterile.	Waist level is the limit of good visual field. By defining only the top of the field as sterile, maximum visibility of all sterile objects used in the procedures is ensured.
Prevent unnecessary traffic and air currents around the sterile area. • Close doors. • Unfold drapes or wrappers slowly. • Do not sneeze, cough, or talk excessively over the sterile field. • Do not reach across sterile fields.	Microorganisms cannot be completely excluded from the air even with the best filtration and air flow designs. Movement creates air currents that circulate organisms in the air. Masks do not contain all organisms expelled from the oral or nasal cavities and become moistened more quickly from talking. Move around a sterile field or turn the field slowly by reaching under the drapes if an object is not convenient to a sterile person.
Open, unused sterile articles are no longer sterile after the procedure.	Once the protective wrappings have been removed, the article is being contaminated by the air. Even if it is untouched and resting on a sterile surface, it must be discarded or resterilized before it is used. Liquids opened during the procedure that remain in their original container are also considered to be contaminated.
A person who is considered sterile who becomes contaminated must reestablish sterility.	If a "scrubbed" person punctures the gloves or is contaminated accidentally by touching an unsterile object, he or she must change the contaminated article. If a scrubbed person leaves the area of the sterile field, he or she must go through the procedure of rescrubbing, gowning, and gloving.
Surgical technique is a team effort. • A collective and individual "sterile conscience" is the best method of enhancing sterile technique.	Staff members must rely on one another to maintain sterile technique. Persons who are considered sterile must have access to sterile supplies delivered to them by circulators in the operating room or prepared by themselves at the bedside. Team members must be open to critiques by other members about their technique and respond to their suggestions that objects of their clothing have been contaminated or that they have contaminated an object. Periodic review of procedures and infection control surveillance reports enhance everyone's sterile technique.

easily with soap and water, and by the friction of scrubbing. Resident flora adhere to epithelial cells and extend into hair follicles and glands in the skin. Resident flora vary according to different locations on the body.

Antiseptic agents are used in skin preparation and surgical scrubs to reduce the number of transient microorganisms. They do not penetrate into the dermis, nor are they able to remove all resident flora. The mechanical action of scrubbing and rinsing with water helps remove organisms from deeper layers of the skin, but a portion of these bacteria remains. When surgical gloves are worn, especially for extended periods, resident flora grow and replicate from deeper skin layers. Any puncture or tear of gloves during sterile procedures allows these organisms to contact an open wound. Torn gloves must be immediately changed to reduce the chance of contamination.

The objective of surgical scrubs and skin preparation of the client is to remove dirt, oil, and microorganisms from the skin; to reduce bacterial counts to a minimum; to avoid abrading the skin; and to leave a layer of antimicrobial material on the skin that inhibits the growth of microbes for an extended period of time.

Preparation of the client's skin consists of several steps. The first is a bath or shower or washing with soap and water before the planned procedure. Removal of hair with depilatory creams, clipping with sterile scissors, or shaving may be necessary. If shaving is ordered, it should not be performed more than 2 hours before the surgical procedure because tiny nicks in the skin may predispose the client to infection. After the skin is cleansed and hair has been removed, the skin is scrubbed with an antimicrobial agent. For surgical procedures, this may take place in the operating room.

Surgical Handwashing

Surgical hand scrubs differ from general handwashing that the nurse performs during most client encounters in both technique and length. A disposable scrub brush or sponge is usually used, but some agencies use equipment that can be resterilized. Sterile nail cleaners made of plastic or metal should also be available. Antiseptic soap containers that dispense the solution by knee or foot pressure must be located above or next to a splashproof sink. Some of the disposable brushes are impregnated with antimicrobial scrub solutions. The solution of choice in most institutions is an iodophor solution.

Before starting the scrub, all nail polish should be removed. Fingernails should be short and without sharp edges that can puncture surgical gloves. The hands should be free of lesions, cuts, or abrasions because traumatized skin can harbor bacteria. Hands should always be held higher than the level of the elbows and away from the body to allow water to run off at the elbows. Water running down the arms to the hands can cause contamination. Hands must be thoroughly dried. This procedure for surgical hand scrubbing should be written, well illustrated, and prominently posted in the scrub area.

Sterile Gloves

Sterile gloves are mandatory for all procedures that require surgical technique. Gloves are worn to prevent contamination of wounds, equipment, supplies, and the site of invasive procedures. Sterile gloves are donned after the hands have been thoroughly cleaned.

In the operative suite or during invasive procedures, the practitioner may use either a closed method or open method for donning gloves. The closed method is preferred when sterile gowns are used for the procedure. In this method the sterile gown is donned, the hands are slid into the sleeves until the cuff seam is reached, and the dominant hand is used to pick up a cuffed glove for the other hand. The glove is drawn over the nondominant hand, and the sleeve is pulled onto the wrist. The dominant hand is gloved in the same manner using the sterile glove on the other hand. For procedures performed at the bedside, it is more common to use the open method of gloving (Procedure 25-3).

Sterile Field

A sterile field is an area free of microorganisms on which sterile items can be placed. This provides a work surface to facilitate maintaining sterility during a sterile procedure. Drapes or sterile wrappers can be used to create a sterile field. Sterile items are transferred to the surface by peeling back packaging and dropping the item onto the field without contact with anything nonsterile. Refer to Procedure 38-1 (Changing a Dressing) for guidelines.

Lifespan Considerations

Age-related factors are important to consider in preventing the transmission of infection. Age affects the immune system, making some age groups more susceptible to infection. Activities also vary among different age groups, changing exposure patterns to infection. The groups people associate with at various ages harbor different organisms that pose risk to those who do not yet have immunity.

Newborn and Infant

Prevention of infection of the newborn begins by protecting the fetus from infection exposure during pregnancy. Maternal infections can be transmitted to the fetus during pregnancy. The result may be minor or

Procedure 25-3
Applying and Removing Sterile Gloves

Purpose

1. Prevent transfer of microorganisms from hands to sterile objects or open wounds.

Assessment

- Identify appropriate time to wear sterile gloves.
- Inspect glove package to determine whether it is dry and intact.
- Assess that nails are filed short and all jewelry is removed from hands.
- Examine ungloved hands for presence of open cuts or lesions, which may harbor microorganisms and prevent the nurse from participating in a procedure.

Equipment

Packaged sterile gloves in correct size
Flat working surface

Procedure

Applying Gloves

1. Wash hands.
   Rationale: Clean hands reduce the number of microorganisms that could be transferred if gloves accidentally puncture or tear.
2. Remove outside wrapper by peeling apart sides.
   Rationale: This protects inner package from inadvertently opening and contaminating the gloves.

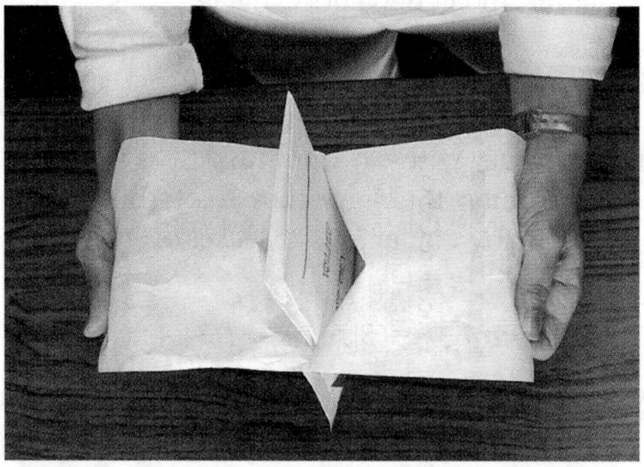

Step 2 • *Peel down to remove outside wrapper.*

3. Lay inner package on clean, flat surface about waist level. Open wrapper from the outside, keeping gloves on inside surface.
   Rationale: Objects below waist level are considered contaminated. Inner surface of wrapper is considered sterile.

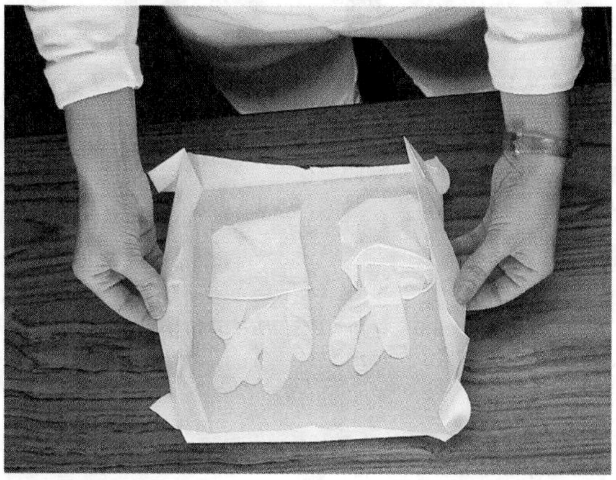

Step 3 • *Open inner wrapper, providing sterile field for glove application.*

4. Grasp inside edge of right cuff with thumb and first two fingers of left hand. Holding hands above waist, insert right hand into glove. Adjust fingers inside glove after both gloves are on.
   Rationale: Inner edge of cuff unfolds against skin of hand and is not sterile once applied. Contamination occurs if ungloved hand contacts gloved hand.

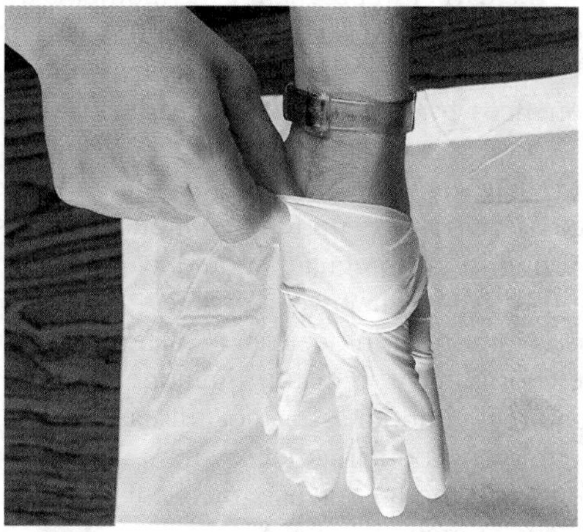

Step 4 • *Grasp first glove by inside edge of cuff and slide on.*

(continued)

5. Slip gloved hand underneath second gloved cuff still in package, and pull over left hand.
Rationale: Sterile cuff protects fingers of gloved hand from becoming contaminated.

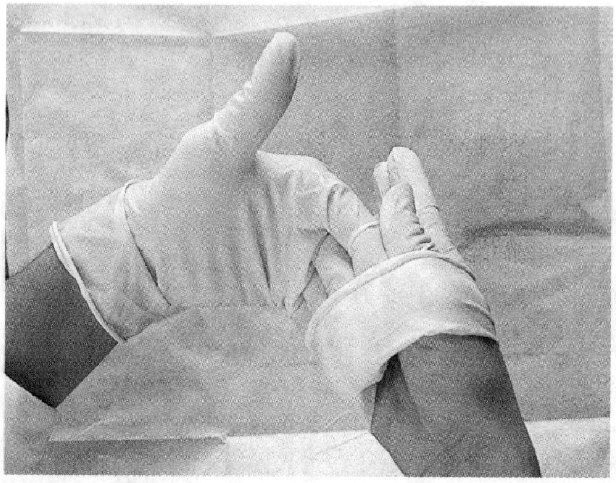

Step 5 • *Slip gloved fingers underneath cuff of other glove and pull over hand.*

6. Keeping hands above waist, adjust glove fit, touching only sterile areas.
Rationale: These actions prevent potential contamination while ensuring a smooth fit over fingers.

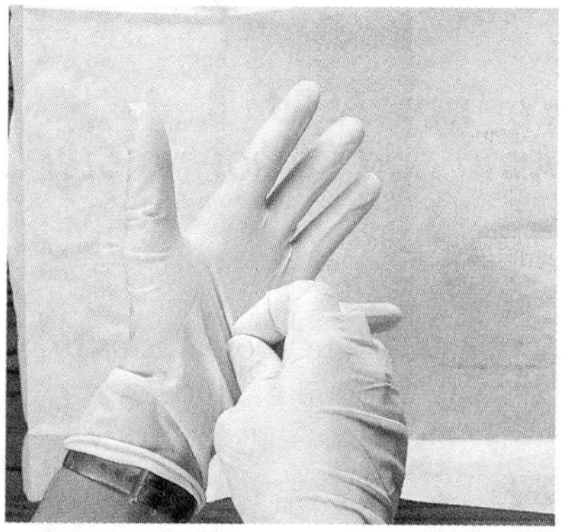

Step 6 • *Adjust gloves as necessary, taking care to keep both gloves sterile.*

Removing Gloves

7. With right hand, grasp outer surface of left glove just below thumb. Peel off without touching exposed wrist.
Rationale: After use, outer surface of gloves is contaminated and could transfer microorganisms to the nurse's wrist.
8. Place ungloved hand under thumb side of second cuff and peel off toward the fingers, holding first glove inside second glove. Discard into appropriate receptacle.
Rationale: Folding contaminated glove surfaces toward the inside minimizes the chances of contacting microorganisms.
9. Wash hands.

major congenital anomalies or fetal death, depending on the time of exposure and the organism involved. In general, the earlier in pregnancy the mother is infected, the more severely the fetus is affected. A very mild or asymptomatic infection in the mother may have serious consequences for the fetus. Very early in pregnancy, when exposure is most dangerous, the mother may be unaware that she is pregnant. All women of childbearing age should have up-to-date immunizations, and those trying to get pregnant should avoid exposure to infectious disease whenever possible. Adequate prenatal care is important in decreasing maternal infection.

Newborns have immature immune systems. They lack maternal antibodies for most diseases and are not yet capable of producing their own. At about 2 months of age, some body defense mechanisms appear to begin developing in infants. At 6 months of age, infants start to produce their own gamma globulin (that fraction of blood protein that contains antibodies), and they become more resistant to some organisms. The most frequent mode of transmission of organisms is from direct contact with the skin and hands of caregivers and, to a lesser extent, through contaminated infant formula. Teaching all caregivers the importance of scrupulous handwashing and general good hygiene has been shown to decrease infection in this age group (Donowitz, 1992). Immunizations are begun during infancy and continue on through childhood. It is important to provide parents with an immunization schedule and to teach parents the importance of this method of preventing many contagious diseases.

Toddler and Preschooler

Body defenses continue to develop as the infant reaches toddlerhood. Despite better defenses against infection, young children frequently become infected because normal behavior at this age fosters transmission of microorganisms. Children of this age often are not yet toilet trained and have poor personal hygiene. Playing on the floor, continually putting objects in their mouth, and even playing with their bodily secretions all contribute to exposure to potential pathogens. Increased exposure to groups of children in a day-care or

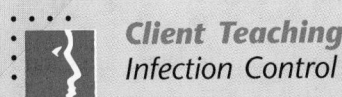

Client Teaching
Infection Control

Instruct the client as follows:

- *Cover your mouth when coughing or sneezing and properly dispose of paper tissues to avoid the transmission of infection through respiratory secretions.*
- *Wash your hands carefully and thoroughly, especially after using the bathroom or before eating.*
- *Boil items for 10 minutes or use a dilute solution of bleach to decrease bacteria counts when necessary.*
- *Learn the signs of infection so you can contact your healthcare provider promptly, this avoiding unnecessary spread of infection.*
- *Symptoms of infection may be less pronounced as you age so that an infection may be present without a significant increase in temperature.*
- *Traveling to a foreign country or to a different location (primitive woodlands and mountains) may increase your risk for some infections, and precautions such as boiling drinking water may be necessary.*
- *Preserve your intact skin because this provides the best barrier to invasion of pathogens into the body.*
- *Be sure to keep informed regarding required immunizations, so you and your family can keep up to date.*
- *Wash fruits and vegetables before eating.*
- *Store meat properly and cook fully before eating.*

preschool setting is another factor affecting the spread of infection. Upper respiratory tract and subsequent ear infections are common among this population.

In the very young child, it is important to begin teaching hygiene practices that help to limit infectious exposure during their entire lifetime. Proper handwashing after using the bathroom and before meals is an important habit for the young child to develop. When children of this age are exhibiting signs of infection, they should be isolated from other children so that infection transmission can be minimized.

Child and Adolescent

During the middle school years, the incidence of many infections decreases. Direct contact and airborne infections are more common in the winter months because children crowd into school rooms and engage in indoor recreational activities. Skin eruptions such as impetigo and infestations of lice occur in this age group because personal hygiene aids, clothing, and sports equipment are shared.

Adolescence brings new elements of exposure. Athletic injuries are common and pose infectious risk. Accidents become more frequent and often predispose a person to infection. Sexually transmitted diseases and mononucleosis begin to rise when adolescents begin sexual activity. Respiratory infections and viral diseases are common because many group activities keep adolescents in close quarters.

The school nurse plays a significant role in detecting and preventing the spread of infections among older children and adolescents. Health teaching is also important in preventing injury and sexually transmitted diseases among this population group.

Adult and Older Adult

By adulthood, most people have acquired immunity to many communicable diseases. Infection as a complication of injury and sexually transmitted diseases continue to be threats. As adults increase their independence and travel, especially to foreign countries, they may be exposed to new infectious organisms.

As the adult ages, the incidence of infection as a complication of chronic disease increases. The effects of long-standing cardiovascular disease, diabetes, drug and alcohol abuse, and cancer can predispose the adult to infection. Elective surgical procedures can also pose an infection risk. In working with adult populations, the nurse can stress preventive health practices to reduce the risk of chronic disease states and thus decrease potential infection risk. Monitoring to ensure current immunizations for the adult is also important because adults frequently forget to update immunization as necessary.

The risk of infection is greatly increased in elderly people owing to an increase in debilitating chronic diseases, malignancy, and waning immunologic responses in this age group. The elderly are predisposed to serious infections because of decreased nutritional status, decreased activity level, poor circulation, frequent breaks in skin integrity, and impaired mechanical clearance mechanisms. Sometimes old diseases such as tuberculosis and herpes zoster can be reactivated, and there is an increased incidence of staphylococcal and streptococcal infections among the elderly.

Severely disabled elderly people are at particular risk because they are often unable to perform their own personal hygiene. Immobility and incontinence also greatly increase infection risk. Approximately 5% of those older than 65 years of age are in extended care facilities. Clients are often housed in crowded rooms, and they frequently have invasive devices such as Foley catheters. Limited staffing as well as high staff turnover make it difficult to institute infection control programs. Accidents, especially falls, are more common as a person's functional abilities decrease. Medications, such as sedatives, can also indirectly contribute to increased infection risk.

Hospitalized elderly clients incur nosocomial infections at two to five times the rate of younger clients. They have higher rates of pneumonia, urinary tract infections, bacteremia, and surgical wound infections during the hospitalization, where they are often treated with vigorous courses of antibiotics. They are often returned to their nursing facilities on continuing antibiotic regimens. This can lead to the development of antibiotic-resistant organisms in nursing homes. When these clients, who are potential reservoirs for transmission to other clients in their nursing home, are readmitted to acute-care hospitals, they become reservoirs for the new facility. Thus, they may require several acute-care admissions and pass on more virulent organisms with each round trip (Garibaldi & Nurse, 1986; Gross & Levine, 1992).

Key Concepts

- Agents that cause infection are everywhere in the environment—on body surfaces, in food, and in products used in normal activities of daily living.
- Intact skin and mucous membranes are major barriers against organisms and infection transmission.
- A communicable disease is caused by an organism that is transmissible from one person to another.
- Infections in clients in hospitals are not necessarily easily passed from one person to another (contagious); but because of the large number of clients with lowered host defenses, diseases are transmitted more easily than in the community.
- Because of the uncertainty of the period of communicability and the lack of identifiable infection in some clients, all body secretions should be considered contaminated.
- The chain of passage of infectious organisms from person to person, from object to person, and from reservoirs in the environment can be broken with infection control practices.
- The incidence of infections associated with healthcare delivery (nosocomial infections) can be decreased with good infection control practices.
- Regulatory agencies at local, state, regional, and national levels are involved in the control of infection and institutional waste to protect clients, staff, and the community.
- The infection control committee, with the aid of the infection control practitioner, is responsible for developing and administering the infection control program of healthcare facility.
- Employee health programs to monitor and counsel personnel are important components of institutional and community infection control programs.
- Effective infection control measures have a favorable cost-benefit ratio.
- Contact transmission of infectious organisms on the hands of caregivers is the most frequent mode of transmission of infection in healthcare facilities.
- Handwashing is the single most important infection control practice. Handwashing techniques should be learned by all caregivers, the client, and family members.
- Institutional waste disposal methods are important factors in infection control programs.
- Aseptic practices are those techniques used to keep people or objects free from microorganisms.
- Isolation procedures and barrier nursing practices are important in preventing the spread of infection.
- Gloves should be worn whenever there could be contact with the client's body secretions.
- Cleaning, disinfection, and sterilization can be accomplished by various methods and agents.
- Sterile technique is used to prevent the introduction of microorganisms from the environment into the client.
- An item is sterile when all organisms and their spores are destroyed on the object.
- Manufacturers' instruction manuals must be consulted to ensure adequate exposure to the appropriate concentration of an agent to produce sterility of objects and to prevent damage to costly equipment.
- Infectious exposure and risk of contracting infectious disease change during a person's lifespan.

Critical Thinking Challenges

You have added asepsis to your knowledge base of important actions in nursing care. Now turn back to the situation concerning asepsis at the beginning of the chapter and consider the following questions.

1. *Identify individuals who are at risk for infection if the client's allegations are true. State your reasons.*
2. *Reflect on possible ways to respond to this client. You want to acknowledge the client's concern yet not act unethically.*
3. *Determine whether other members of the healthcare team need to be notified at this point. Describe factors you need to consider in making such a decision.*
4. *Plan measures you could use to help all members of the healthcare team adhere to infection control standards.*

References

Adams, K., Zehrer, C., & Thomas, W. (1993) Comparison of a needleless system with conventional heparin locks. *Am J Infect Control, 21*(5), 263–269.

Alcamo, I. E. (1991). *Fundamentals of microbiology* (3rd ed.). Reading, MA: Addison–Wesley.

Baxter Healthcare Corporation (1988). *A point of concern.* Product information. Mission Viejo, CA: ICU Medical, Inc.

Begley, S. (1994). The end of antibiotics. *Newsweek CXXI*(4), 47–51.

Beyt, B. E., Troxler, S., & Cavaness, J. (1985). Prospective payment and infection control. *Infect Control, 6*(4), 161.

Boutotte, J. (1993a). TB The second time around and how you can help to control it. *Nursing93, 23*(5), 42–49.

Boutotte, J. (1993b) Protecting yourself against TB. *Nursing93, 23*(10), 64.

Castle, M., & Ajemian, E. (1987). *Hospital infection control: Principles and practice* (2nd ed.). New York: John Wiley & Sons.

Centers for Disease Control and Prevention. (1986). Update: Universal precautions for prevention and transmission of human immunodeficiency virus, hepatitis B virus and other blood–borne pathogens in health–care settings. *MMWR,* November.

Centers for Disease Control and Prevention. (1987). Recommendations for prevention of HIV transmission in health–care settings. *MMWR, 36*(2S), 3S–17S.

Centers for Disease Control and Prevention. (1987). Reports on AIDS. *MMWR.*

Centers for Disease Control and Prevention. (1988). Recommendations for prevention of HIV transmission in health–care settings. *MMWR,* August.

Centers for Disease Control and Prevention. (1994). Draft guidelines for isolation precautions in hospital: Notice. *Federal Register, 59*(214), 55552–55570.

Coll, P., Crabtree, B., O'Connor, P., et al. (1994). Clinical risk factors for methicillin–resistant *Staphylococcus aureus* bacteriuria in a skilled–care nursing home. *Archives of Family Medicine, 3,* 357–360.

Dixon, R. E. (1992). Costs of nosocomial infections and benefits of infection control programs. In R. P. Wenzel (Ed.), *Prevention and control of nosocomial infections* (2nd ed.). Baltimore: Williams & Wilkins.

Donowitz, L. G. (1992). Infection in the newborn. In R. P. Wenzel (Ed.), *Prevention and control of nosocomial infections* (2nd ed.). Baltimore: Williams & Wilkins.

Garibaldi, R. A., & Nurse, B. (1986). Infections in the elderly. *Am J Med, 81*(Suppl 1A), 53–58.

Grau, P. (1991). Are you at risk for hepatitis B? *Nursing91, 21*(3), 45–46.

Gross, P. A., & Levine, J. F. (1992). Infections in the elderly. In R. P. Wenzel (Ed.), *Prevention and control of nosocomial infections* (2nd ed.). Baltimore: Williams & Wilkins.

Korniewicz, D., Cresci, K., & Larson, E. (1992). In-use comparison of latex gloves in two high–risk units: Surgical intensive care and acquired immunodeficiency syndrome. *Heart Lung, 21,* 81–84.

Korniewicz, D., & Garzon, L. (1994) Combating infection: How to choose and use gloves. *Nursing94, 24*(9), 18.

Larson, E. (1992). Skin cleansing. In R. P. Wenzel (Ed.), *Prevention and control of nosocomial infections* (2nd ed.). Baltimore: Williams & Wilkins.

Lynch, P., & Cummings, M. J. (1987). *Body substance isolation.* Information packet. Seattle, WA: Harborview Medical Center.

Meengs, M., Giles, B., Chisholm, C., et al. (1994). Handwashing frequency in an emergency room department. *Journal of Emergency Nursing, 20*(3), 183–188.

Schaffner, W. (1992). The global impact of hospital–acquired infections. In R. P. Wenzel (Ed.), *Prevention and control of nosocomial infections* (2nd ed.). Baltimore: Williams & Wilkins.

Sheldon, J. (1994). Combating infection: 25 tips on hand washing. *Nursing94, 24*(1), 20.

Valenti, W. (1993). Infection control and the pregnant health care worker. *Nurs Clin North Am, 28*(3), 673–686.

Weinstein, S., Gantz, N., Pelletier, C., et al. (1989) Bacterial surface contamination of patients' linen: Isolation precautions versus standard care. *Am J Infect Control, 17*(5), 264–267.

Williams, W. W., & Garner, J. S. (1986). Personnel health services. In J. V. Bennett, & P. S. Bachman (Eds.), *Hospital infections* (2nd ed.). Boston: Little, Brown & Co.

Bibliography

Centers for Disease Control and Prevention. (1988). *What to do to stop disease in child day care centers: A kit for child day care directors.* HE 20.7008:C 43/kit.

Crawford, N., & Pruss, A. (1993). Preventing neonatal hepatitis B infection during the perinatal period. *J Obstet Gynecol Neonatal Nurs, 22,* 491–497.

Crow, S. (1993). Sterilization processes: Meeting the demands of today's health care technology. *Nurs Clin North Am, 28,* 687–695.

Fedson, D. S. (1992). Immunization for health care workers. In R. P. Wenzel (Ed.), *Prevention and control of nosocomial infections* (2nd ed.). Baltimore: Williams & Wilkins.

Ford, C. D. (1990). Disposal of sharps: Implications and control. *Journal of Intravenous Nursing, 13*(1), 42–47.

Ford–Jones, E. L. (1992). The special problems of nosocomial infection in the pediatric client. In R. P. Wenzel (Ed.), *Prevention and control of nosocomial infections* (2nd ed.). Baltimore: Williams & Wilkins.

Hoeprich, P. (1994). *Infectious diseases: A modern treatise of infectious processes* (5th ed.). Philadelphia: J. B. Lippincott.

Hurt, N. (1993). The role of the infection control nurse in the quality management in the ambulatory care setting. *Journal of Healthcare Quality, 15*(3), 43–44.

Larson, E. (1989). Handwashing: It's essential—even when you use gloves. *Am J Nurs, 89,* 934–941.

Lovitt, S., et al. (1992). Isolation gowns: A false sense of security? *Am J Infect Control, 20*(4), 185–191.

McFarlane, A. (1990). Why do we forget to remember handwashing? *Professional Nurse, 5*(5), 250, 252.

Morita, M. (1993). Methicillin–resistant *Staphylococcus aureus*: Past, present, and future. *Nurs Clin North Am, 28,* 625–637.

Nadzam, D. (1992). Infection control indicators in critical care settings. *Heart Lung, 21,* 477–481.

Pottinger, J., et al. (1989). Bacterial carriage by artificial versus natural nails. *Am J Infect Control, 17*(6), 340–344.

Presdorf, K. (1993). Infection control: Regulatory impact on the home care setting. *Journal of Home Health Care Practice, 6*(1), 60–68.

Smith, J. (1991). Risk management: An aspect of infection control in an acute care hospital. *Canadian Journal of Infection Control, 6*(3), 74–76.

Steelman, V. (1994). Infection control: Quality assessment, improvement. *AORN J, 59,* 476–482.

White, M. (1992). Infection and infection risk in home care settings. *Infection Control and Hospital Epidemiology, 13*(9), 535–539.

Intravenous Therapy

Key Terms	Learning Objectives
Air embolism Colloid Crystalloid Cycling Hypertonic Hypotonic Infiltration Intravenous therapy Isotonic Parenteral nutrition Phlebitis Thrombophlebitis Total parenteral nutrition Venipuncture	Upon completion of this chapter, the student will be able to do the following: • Explain the purpose of infusion therapy. • Identify types of solutions administered intravenously. • List equipment used to administer peripheral and central therapy. • State principles of site selection in venipuncture. • Outline the nursing role in initiating, monitoring, maintaining, and discontinuing intravenous therapy. • Describe appropriate nursing interventions concerning blood transfusions. • Discuss components of total parenteral nutrition and commonly used additives. • List complications associated with infusion of total parenteral nutrition and describe appropriate nursing interventions. • Identify principles of client and family education.

26

You are assigned to care for an older man who is receiving intravenous (IV) therapy. The solution is isotonic saline (0.9% saline) and is being administered through a microdrip system. While counting the drops per minute, you notice that it is dripping slower than ordered and that opening the flow clamp does not increase the rate. You must decide what to do.

In previous chapters, you learned the application of the nursing process to client situations. In this chapter, as you add IV therapy to your knowledge base, you will learn how to apply nursing skills to care for the client receiving IV therapy. When you complete this chapter, you should be able to address the Critical Thinking Challenges at the end of the chapter.

People who cannot take fluids or nutrition orally may need support through alternate means. IV therapy and parenteral nutrition are such therapies. **IV therapy** is infusion of a fluid into a vein to prevent or treat fluid or electrolyte imbalance or to deliver medications or blood products.

Venipuncture is the technique that permits insertion of a needle or catheter into a vein. Because the integrity of the skin is broken, venipuncture is a sterile procedure. In most facilities, the nurse is responsible for starting IV therapy in this manner. In some agencies, a special IV team is responsible for all IV starts and, in some cases, general IV maintenance. Usually the IV team is composed of nurses with specialized training and extensive experience with venipuncture. In hospitals that do not employ IV teams, nurses usually are certified in venipuncture technique by the institution.

Options for venipuncture are peripheral veins (veins in the extremities) and central veins (veins in the central portion of the body). Peripheral veins are used commonly for most fluid infusions. Central veins are used for infusion under certain circumstances, such as infusion of hypertonic solutions. Central venous catheters are inserted by physicians.

IV therapy is initiated for a variety of reasons:

- To provide the client with fluids when adequate fluid intake cannot be obtained through oral intake
- To provide the client with electrolytes to maintain normal electrolyte balance
- To provide the client with glucose to use as an energy source
- To provide an access route to administer medications intravenously
- To provide a venous access to administer blood products
- To provide a venous access so that treatment can be administered promptly if an emergency situation occurs

Types of Intravenous Solutions

IV solutions are classified as **crystalloid** (fluids that are clear) or **colloid** (fluids that contain proteins or starch molecules). Crystalloids can be subclassified as isotonic, hypotonic, or hypertonic, depending on the tonicity of the fluid. Specific client fluid and electrolyte needs will determine which solution is prescribed.

Crystalloid Solutions

An artist's conception of the relationship of osmotic pressure to isotonic, hypotonic, and hypertonic solutions is presented in Figure 26-1.

Isotonic Fluids. **Isotonic** fluids have the same osmotic pressure as that found within the cell. Isotonic fluids are used to expand the intravascular compartment and thus increase circulating volume. Because these solutions do not alter serum osmolarity, interstitial and intracellular compartments remain unchanged. An isotonic solution would be helpful for hypotension caused by hypovolemia. Examples of an isotonic solution include normal saline (0.9% NaCl) and lactated Ringer's.

Hypotonic Fluids. **Hypotonic** fluids have less osmotic pressure than the cell. When a hypotonic solution is infused, it lowers serum osmolarity, causing body fluids to shift out of the blood vessels and into the cells and interstitial space. For this reason, hypotonic fluids are administered when a client needs cellular hydration. One-half normal saline (0.45 NaCl) is an example of a hypotonic solution. Five percent dextrose in water, although an isotonic solution before administration, quickly becomes a hypotonic solution once in the body, because the dextrose is quickly metabolized, leaving only the water.

Hypertonic Fluids. **Hypertonic** fluids have greater osmotic pressure than the cell. When a hypertonic solution is infused, it raises serum osmolarity, pulling fluid from the cells and the interstitial tissues into the vascular space. Hypertonic solutions are often administered to the postoperative client to maintain circulating volume and prevent edema. Examples of hypertonic solutions include 5% dextrose in normal saline, 5% dex-

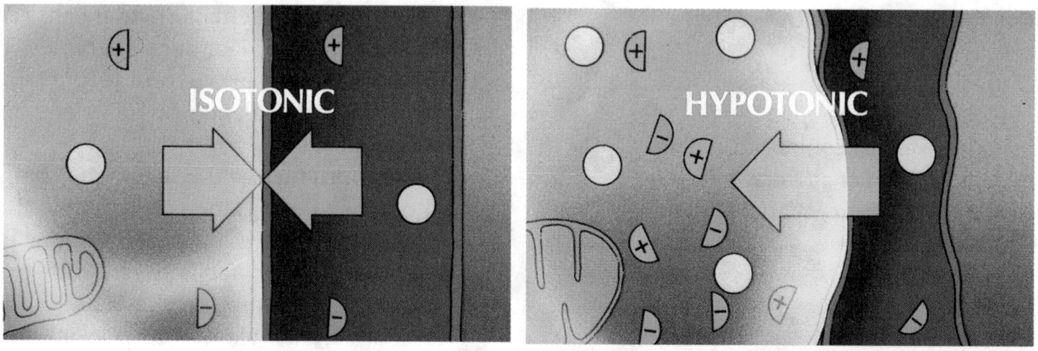

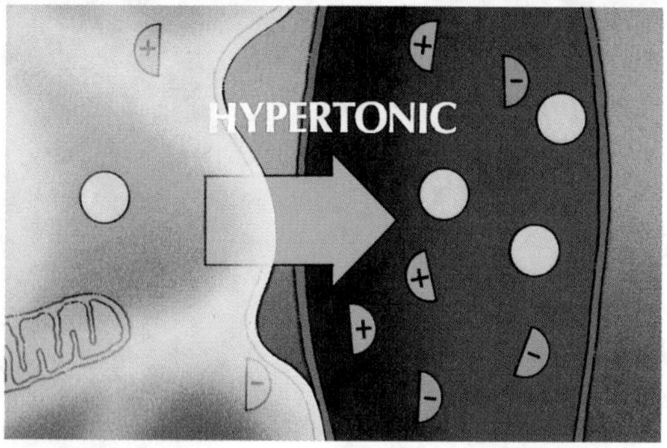

Figure 26-1 • Isotonic, hypotonic, and hypertonic solutions. In isotonic fluids, cells maintain normal size because of fluid balance. In hypotonic solutions, the body fluids shift out of the blood vessels and into cells and the interstitial space. In hypertonic solutions, the fluid is pulled from the cells and the interstitial tissues into the vascular space.

Therapeutic Dialogue
Intravenous Therapy

Scenes for Thought

On your nursing rounds this evening, you enter the room of Delores Davis, a 65-year-old social worker with a wide smile, hypertension and renal insufficiency, and an IV in her left arm. She greets you warmly as you assess the IV site, drip rate, and IV pump function.

Effective

Client: *Hi there. How are you this evening?* Big smile.
Nurse: *I'm just fine, Ms. Davis. How's it going for you this evening? (Gently palpating the area around the IV site.)*
Client: *Don't touch that, please.* She winces and pulls back.
Nurse: *(Standing still, your hand moving to rest on her hand gently.) Is the IV bothering you?*
Client: *Well, yes it is, actually.* Her face now looks worried, her eyes searching yours.
Nurse: *Tell me a little more.*
Client: *It started this evening after supper. I'm afraid I pulled on it when I was reaching for my tea. The other nurse put the tray where I couldn't reach it, and I didn't want to bother her for such a silly thing, so I just reached for it, and then the skin felt a little sore there. Did I do something wrong?* Face is still worried.
Nurse: *Well, let's see what the area is like. (Talking to Ms. Davis while examining everything.) I don't see any redness or swelling where the needle enters your skin, the pump seems to be functioning fine, and the fluid is dripping in at just the right rate. I think everything is working properly. One thing I can do is untangle the tubing a little so you'll have more room to move. How's that?*
Client: Looks more relieved. *Better. I'm pleased to hear that I didn't do any damage. I've never had one of these before.* Smiles but not as widely as before.
Nurse: *Sound like you're still a little worried about it. Anything I can help with?*
Client: *No, I'm fine.* Smiles bravely. *But could you come back and check it again later when you get the chance? It would put my mind at ease.*
Nurse: *I'd be delighted. I was going to suggest that myself. By the way, it isn't a bother to set your tray up more comfortably for you. Please ask next time. We're here to make you feel better, not to make you struggle!*
Client: *Thank you so much. I appreciate it.* Big smile.

Less Effective

Client: *Hi there. How are you this evening?* Big smile.
Nurse: *I'm just fine, Ms. Davis. How's it going for you this evening? (Gently palpating the area around the IV site.)*
Client: *Don't touch that, please.* She winces and pulls back.
Nurse: *(Standing still; your hand moving to rest on her hand gently.) Is the IV bothering you?*
Client: *Well, yes it is, actually.* Her face now looks worried, her eyes searching yours.
Nurse: *Let me check everything out now. (Thoroughly examine the site, pump, drip rate, tubing.) I can untangle this tubing a bit for you, but I don't see anything else wrong. Tell you what, I'll be back later on this evening to check on it again, and if there's something wrong we'll fix it. Okay? (Patting her hand reassuringly and smiling as you leave.)*
Client: *Okay. I guess.* Face has no expression except for two frown lines between her eyes.

Critical Thinking Challenge

• Analyze how the first nurse reassured Ms. Davis that everything is okay. • Explain how you can tell from behavior that a person is reassured. • Determine when reassurance becomes patronizing. • Assess what was missing between the nurse and client in the second dialogue.

trose in one-half normal saline, and 5% dextrose in lactated Ringer's.

Colloid Solutions

Blood products and parenteral nutrition are two colloidal solutions.

Blood Products. Whole blood or specific components of blood may be infused directly into a person's circulatory system. Some of the components of blood include packed red cells, white blood cells, platelets, plasma, albumin (as a volume expander), and cryoprecipitate. Nursing responsibilities associated with transfusion therapy are discussed in greater detail later in this chapter.

Parenteral Nutrition. **Parenteral nutrition** refers to nutritional elements supplied through an IV route, usually a central vein. **Total parenteral nutrition** (TPN) is a hypertonic solution containing dextrose, proteins, vitamins, and minerals that is injected into the venous circulation. TPN, also known as hyperalimentation, is indicated when there is interference with absorption of nutrients from the gastrointestinal tract or when complete bowel rest is necessary for healing. Parenteral nutrition is discussed later in this chapter.

Equipment for Intravenous Infusion

A diversity of equipment is available to provide IV therapy to clients; brands may vary slightly among different manufacturers. Essentially, IV setups contain the following:

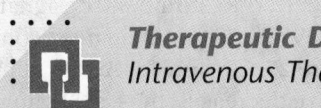

- An access device that gains entry to a vein
- A bag or bottle containing the IV solution
- An administration set that connects the IV bag with the access device

IV equipment is sterile, and sterility is maintained during use to prevent potentially life-threatening infection.

Access Devices

Peripheral Insertion Devices

Access devices most commonly used for peripheral IV therapy include winged infusion needles and over-the-needle IV catheters. *Winged infusion needles* are short, beveled needles with plastic flaps or wings. They may be used for short-term therapy or when therapy is given to a child or infant. Winged infusion needles also are referred to as scalp vein needles. *Over-the-needle catheters* are plastic catheters that are placed over metal stylets or introducer needles (Fig. 26-2). The metal stylet is used to pierce the skin and enter the vein, after which the plastic catheter is threaded into the vein, and the metal stylet is removed. (An inside-the-needle catheter was more commonly used in the past, but the over-the-needle catheter is preferred today.)

Both the winged infusion needle and the over-the-needle catheter come in a variety of sizes. The lumen size is measured in gauges; odd numbers designate winged infusion needles (19, 21, 23), and the most common adult catheter sizes are 22, 20, and 18. As the numbers increase, the lumen size decreases; thus, a 22-gauge needle is smaller in diameter than an 18-gauge needle. The length of the catheter also is significant. Usually the shortest length possible is appropriate. Most catheters are 1 or 1¼ in long.

Intermittent Infusion Devices

Intermittent infusion devices are available as winged needle sets or as over-the-needle catheters, each with an attached latex cap (Fig. 26-3). These are used when the client is to receive solutions or medications intermittently. Intermittent infusion devices also are called heparin locks. They are filled with saline to prevent blood clot formation, then they maintain venous access without requiring the client to receive continuous infusion, minimizing danger of fluid overload and electrolyte imbalance. Any type of peripheral venipuncture device can be converted, however.

Central Venous Catheters

Access to central veins is often necessary for infusion of concentrated medications or TPN. The placement of most of these lines is the physician's responsibility.

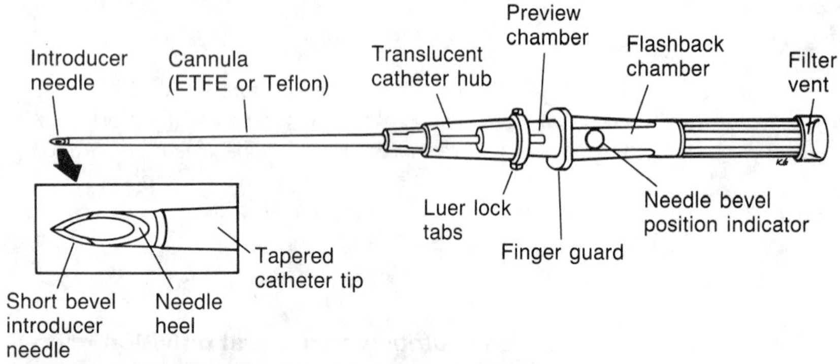

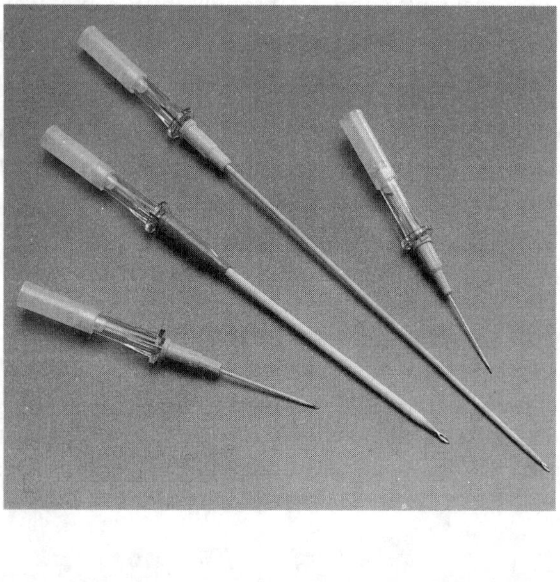

Figure 26-2 • *Parts of the over-the-needle catheter (courtesy of Terumo, Inc., Somerset NJ) and examples of the ANGIOCATH (registered) IV catheter (courtesy of Becton-Dickinson Vascular Access, Sandy UT).*

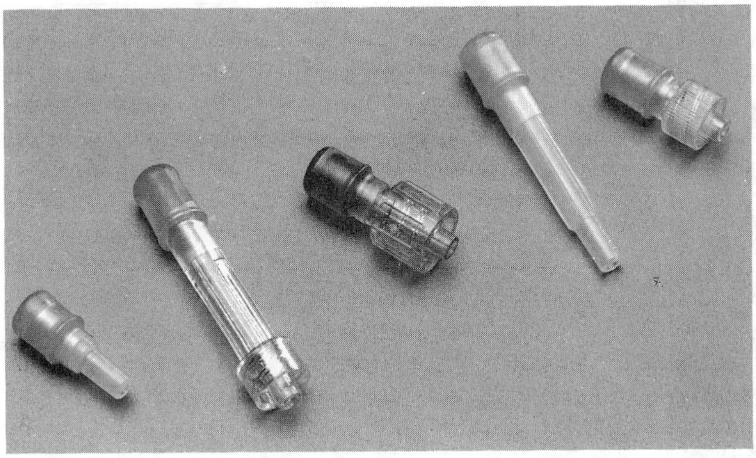

Figure 26-3 • Adapters used to convert indwelling IV catheters or infusion sets to intermittent infusion devices. (Courtesy of Becton-Dickinson Vascular Access, Sandy UT.)

When central access is necessary, a wide assortment of products may be used to facilitate cannulation of the central vein. Products used most frequently include the basic single-lumen central venous catheter or the multilumen catheter, which is dual or triple lumen and made of nonthrombogenic Silastic materials (Fig. 26-4). With multilumen catheters, more than one drug can be administered at the same time without incompatibility problems, and there is only one insertion site for care.

Tunneled Central Venous Catheters

When IV therapy is needed for a long time, a more permanent type of catheter can be used, such as a tunneled line. Hickman and Broviac are two common brand names of these catheters. The catheters, which may be single lumen or multilumen, are approximately 90 cm in length and contain a Dacron cuff. A tunneled catheter is implanted in the operating room through an incision made in the deltopectoral groove, isolating the subclavian vein. The term "tunneled" comes from the subcutaneous tunnel that is gently formed with a long forceps to a point between the nipple and the sternum (Fig. 26-5). The Dacron cuff is positioned between the skin incision and the vein. The catheter is threaded into the lower part of the vena cava at the entrance to the right atrium. Dressings, placed at both incision sites, require simple cleaning, application of an antimicrobial agent, and a sterile occlusive dressing. The catheter should be taped to the person's chest to lessen tension and tugging on it. Eventually, fibrous tissue grows around the Dacron cuff, which stabilizes it in place, decreases infection rates, and permits use as a long-term venous access route. Tunneled catheters may be used for months for continuous or intermittent therapy. For intermittent therapy, the catheter will be fitted with an intermittent infusion device to allow access as needed and to keep the system closed and intact. Patency of the catheter may be maintained with heparin flush as determined by the indvidual situation, with the exception of Groshong catheters, which require only normal saline instillation because of the unique catheter design.

Peripherally Inserted Central Catheters

Peripherally inserted central catheters (PICC) are a newer access device (Fig. 26-6). They are being placed successfully by nurses specialized in IV therapy. The basilic vein is usually used, but the median cubital and cephalic vein in the antecubital area can be used also.

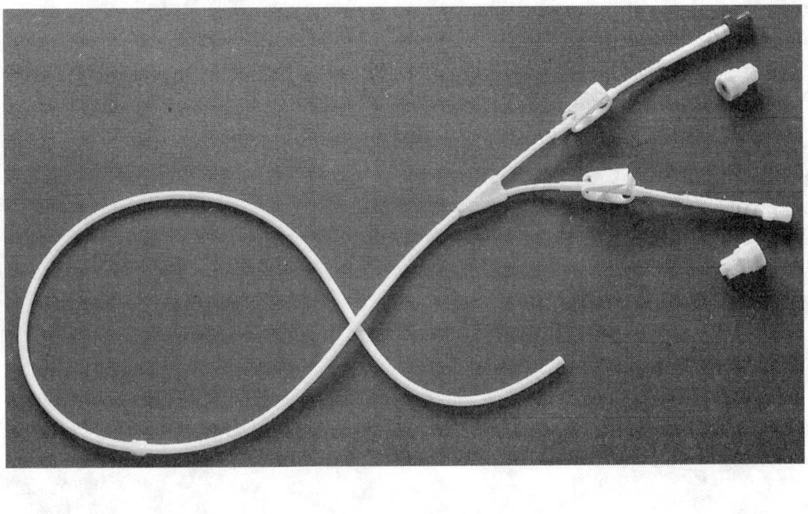

Figure 26-4 • Dual-lumen Hickman catheter showing the two ports and clamps. The Dacron cuff is on the lower left of the photograph. (Courtesy of Davol, Inc., subsidiary of CR Bard Inc., Salt Lake City UT.)

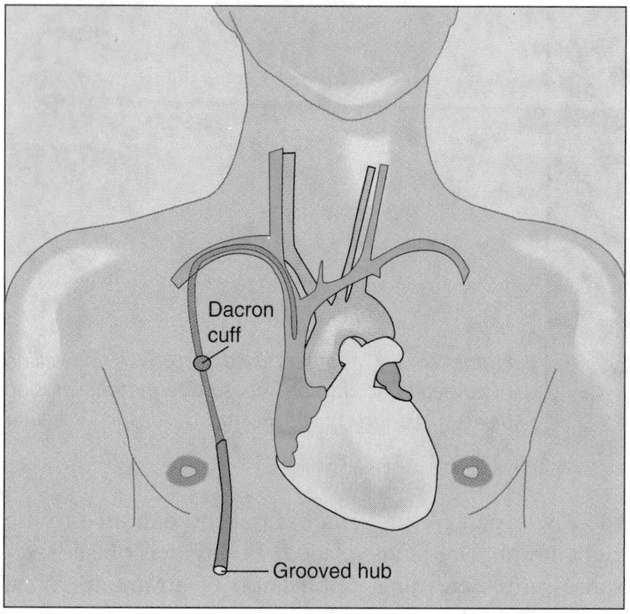

Figure 26-5 • *Insertion technique of indwelling tunneled catheter. A tunnel is formed from the vein to an area between the sternum and the nipple. The catheter tip is placed in the superior vena cava.*

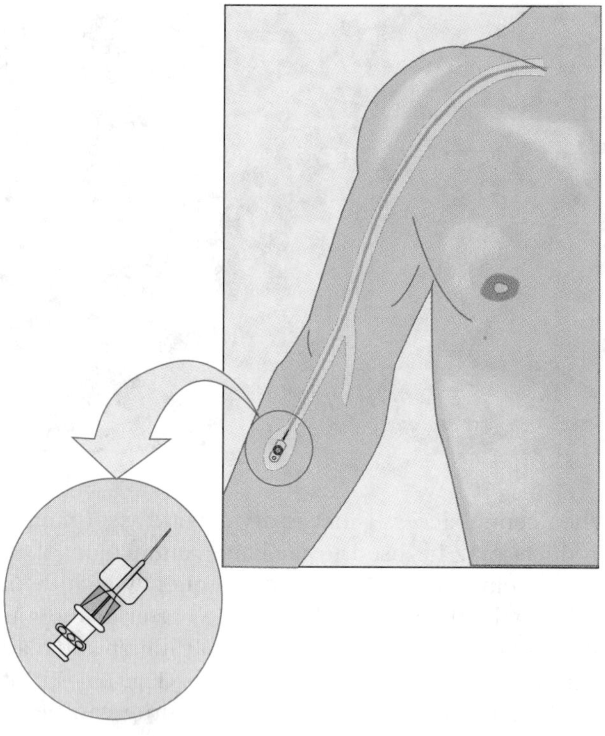

Figure 26-6 • *PICC access device.*

PICC lines are threaded so that the catheter tip may terminate in either the axillary or subclavian vein or the superior vena cava. The purpose of the PICC line and the therapy determine the actual site and termination point. PICC has gained wide acceptance in nursing and medical communities.

Implanted Vascular Access Devices

To allow long-term access without having a catheter protruding from the skin, totally implantable access devices have been developed (Fig. 26-7). The components of the system include the subcutaneous injection port and a Silastic catheter. The device has a self-sealing septum or port, allowing the access device to be used repeatedly. With the client under local anesthetic, the system is implanted subcutaneously (see Fig. 26-7*A*). When access is desired, the location of the injection port must be palpated. The system is then accessed with a noncoring needle, such as a Huber point needle (see Fig. 26-7*B*). As with other systems, patency is maintained by periodic flushing with a diluted heparin solution.

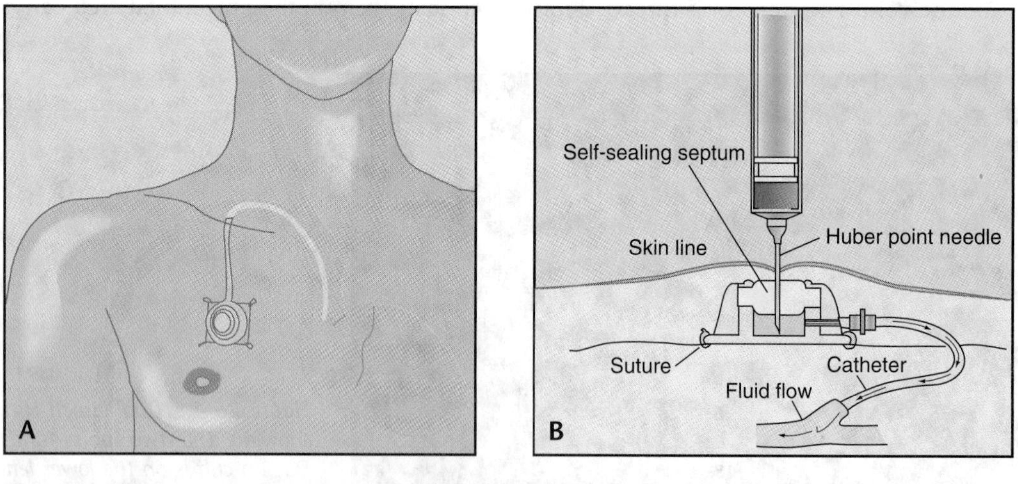

Figure 26-7 • *Implantable access system.* ***(A)*** *Placement of the implantable system beneath the skin.* ***(B)*** *Access to the system with a noncoring needle.*

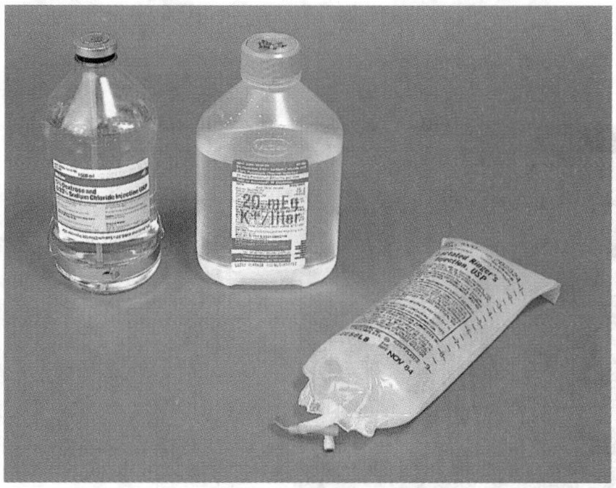

Figure 26-8 • Examples of solution containers.

Solution Containers

Containers for IV fluid include glass bottles and plastic bags, as shown in Figure 26-8. Plastic bags have become the standard in the industry, unless a particular infusate is unstable in plastic. Plastic bags collapse as they empty and therefore require no vent to equalize pressure. The amount of fluid remaining in the bag may be difficult to measure accurately, however, because of the semirigid nature of the bag. One other disadvantage of plastic bags is that certain drugs (eg, insulin) bind with the plastic, making IV administration of these drugs in plastic bags difficult.

Bottles and bags come in a variety of sizes. Usually 1,000-mL containers are used for normal hydration purposes. Smaller bags (eg, 250–500 mL) may be used for children or when fluid is infusing at a very slow rate. Smaller containers (50, 100, or 250 mL) also are used to dilute and dispense medications.

Administration Sets

IV administration sets connect the IV bag or bottle to the access device through tubing. Parts of the administration set are shown in Figure 26-9. Normally, IV tubing includes the following features:

- A piercing pin or spike permits the tubing to access the IV container.
- An inline filter traps any particles and prevents their entry into the client's bloodstream.
- A drip chamber allows the nurse to visualize and count the drops of IV fluid as they enter the system.
- Injection sites or ports permit the administration of medications, blood products, or other IV therapies.
- A needle adaptor is used for connection to the needle or cannula.

In addition to these features, a vent must be included in the drip chamber when an unvented bottle system is used. Individual manufacturers produce tubing with different drop factors. Two general classifications of tubing are macrodrip and microdrip (Fig. 26-10). Macrodrip tubing delivers 10, 15, or 20 drops/mL, depending on the manufacturer. Macrodrip tubing is generally used for adult clients, especially when large volume replacement may be required (eg, during surgery). Minidrip tubing delivers 60 drops/mL. Minidrip tubing is used for infants, children, or when fluids are infused slowly. Volume-controlled sets also may be used and provide greater accuracy and safety in controlling the volume of fluids (Fig. 26-11).

Needleless System. To eliminate the potential for breaks in the line and subsequent potentiation of blood-

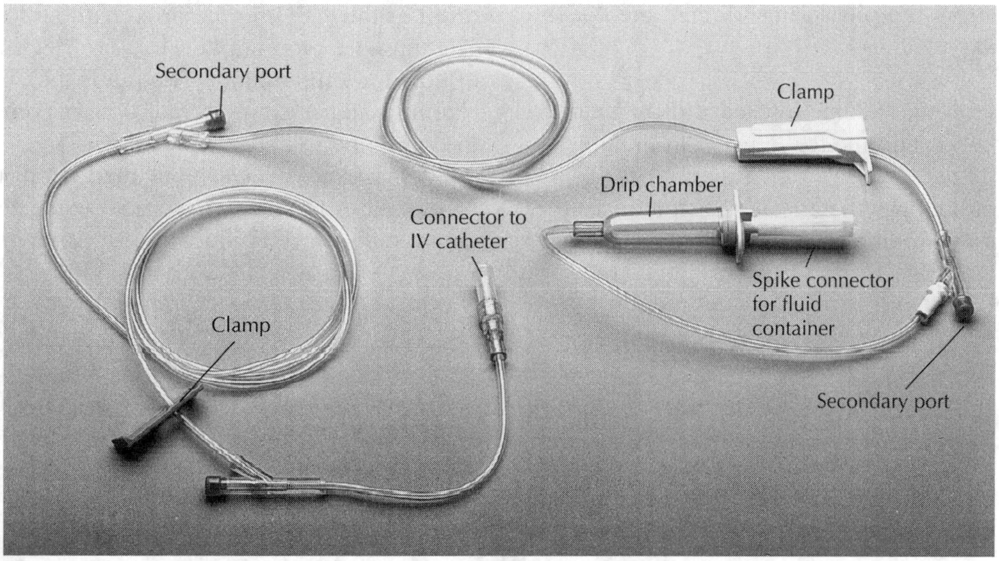

Figure 26-9 • Administration set. (Courtesy Abbott Laboratories, North Chicago, IL).

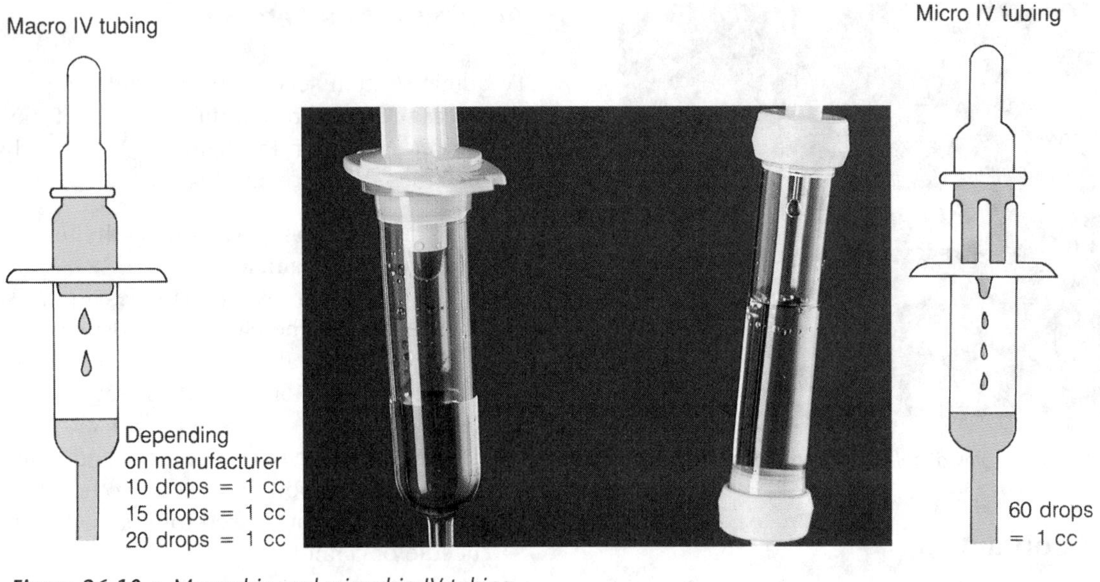

Figure 26-10 • *Macrodrip and microdrip IV tubing.*

borne bacteria, manufacturers have provided needleless systems. These systems enable the user to connect an adapter plug to a female luer of an administration set without using a needle because of the presence of an integral blunt fitting (Fig. 26-12). Many manufacturers make these products, some of which are set-specific and require the use of a manufacturer's products; others are universal.

Intravenous Flow Rates

Calculating Flow Rate

Calculating flow rate is the first step in ensuring the proper infusion of IV fluids. After the administration set is selected or known, the drip rate of the infusion can be calculated from the physician's order using the following formula:

$$\text{Drops/min} = \frac{\text{Total volume infused} \times \text{drop factor}}{\text{Total time for infusion in minutes}}$$

The size of the drop that the administration set creates is known as the drop factor, which can be found on the packaging of the administration set. This factor may change with different manufacturers, because macrotubing can deliver 10, 15, or 20 drops/mL. To calculate the drip rate of an IV that is to infuse 1,000 mL in 8 hours using tubing that has a drop factor of 10, the nurse would use the previous formula, obtaining a rate of 20 to 21 drops/min:

$$\text{Drops/min} = \frac{1{,}000 \times 10}{8\text{ h} \times 60} = \frac{10{,}000}{480} = 21\text{ drops/min}$$

Regulating the Flow Rate

The infusion can be regulated manually once the IV drip rate has been calculated. A roller clamp is used to adjust the rate of flow. The nurse usually counts the drops as they fall into the drip chamber for 15 seconds. This number is multiplied by 4 to determine the rate of flow for 1 full minute. The nurse then uses the roller clamp to adjust the flow rate until it corresponds with the prescribed rate of flow.

A *time strip*, which can be made from adhesive tape or purchased commercially, also can help ensure accurate infusion of IV fluids. An example of an IV time

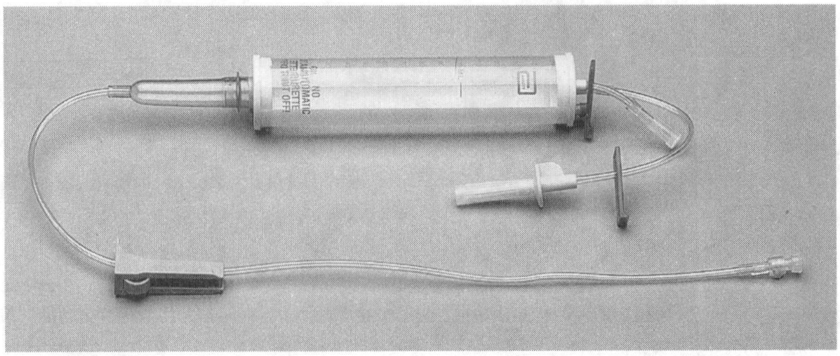

Figure 26-11 • *Volume-controlled set. (Courtesy Abbott Laboratories, North Chicago, IL).*

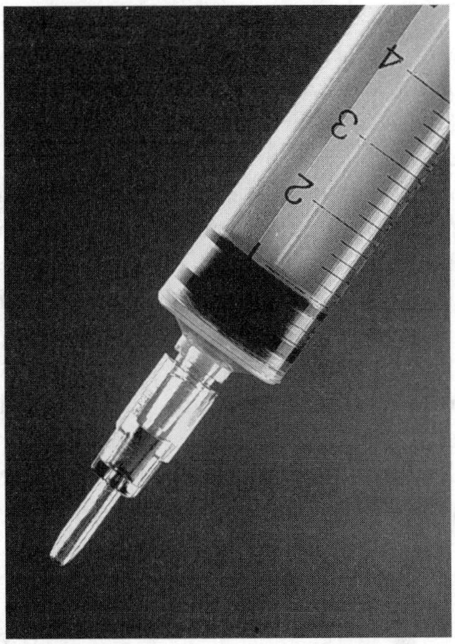

Figure 26-12 • *Needleless system.*

tape is illustrated in Figure 26-13. The time strip is placed along the IV bag or bottle next to the calibrated numbers that indicate the volume remaining in the container. The strip is marked in hourly increments, indicating where the fluid level will be at specific times. This device permits the nurse to assess at a glance when the IV is getting behind or ahead of schedule. It is important that the nurse check IV infusions every hour to ensure proper infusion of fluid.

An IV *electronic infusion device* (EID) may be used to regulate accurately the infusion rate. This is especially useful if fluid administration must be watched very carefully, such as when infusing fluid to an infant or administering certain medications. Various types of EIDs are available commercially. In general, a pump uses positive pressure to deliver the prescribed volume of fluid, whereas a controller depends on gravity to maintain a precise flow rate (Fig. 26-14).

The pump regulates the flow by volume, whereas the controller senses the drops infusing. Most newer models of pumps and controllers can be electronically programmed. The nurse enters the amount of fluid (eg, 1,000 mL) and the rate at which it is to infuse in cubic centimeters per hour. The instrument displays how many cubic centimeters have infused and how many are remaining in the IV container at any given time.

Most regulating devices have alarms that indicate when fluid cannot be delivered at the prescribed rate for any reason (eg, the container is empty; the tubing is kinked; air is in the line; the vein is clogged). Infiltration will not necessarily trigger the alarm. The nurse can troubleshoot to identify the cause of the problem and correct it to ensure proper infusion of fluids. Because many different types and models of these devices are used, the nurse must be knowledgeable about specific operating guidelines for the machine being used. Instructions for use also are permanently affixed to the particular EID. Alarms must not be turned off until the underlying problem has been discovered and resolved.

Factors Affecting the Flow Rate

Careful assessment of the IV infusion is necessary routinely after the IV is adjusted because many factors other than drop factor can affect the rate of infusion. Such factors as the height of the IV bottle, the position of the extremity, the position of the catheter within the vein, the patency of the catheter, a constriction or kink

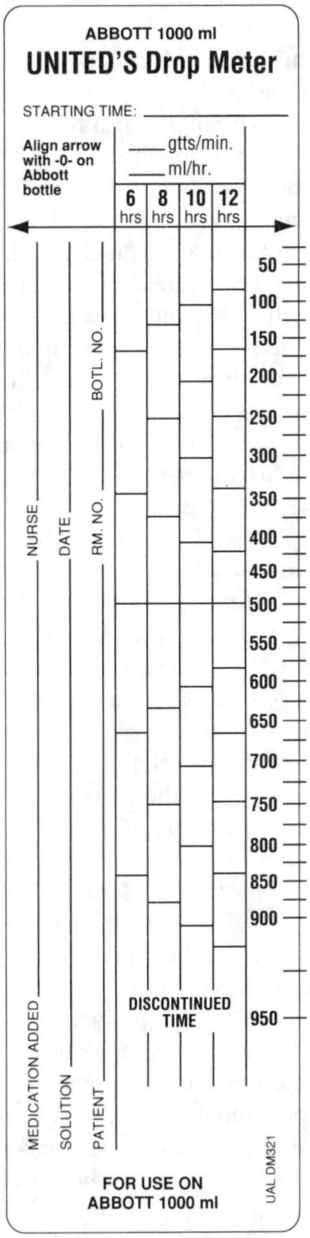

Figure 26-13 • *Sample time tape.*

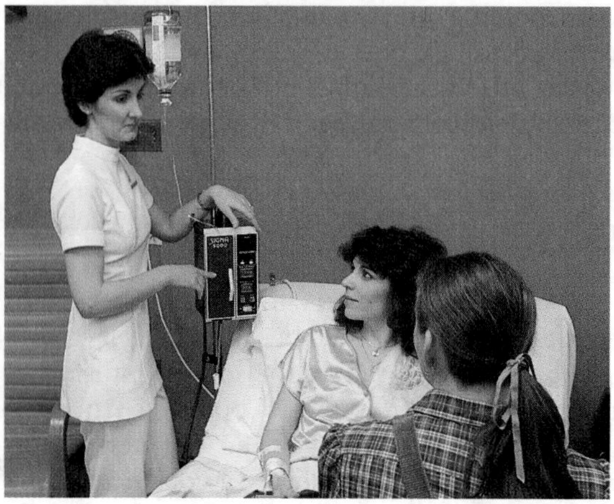

Figure 26-14 • *The nurse teaches the client about the electronic infusions device (EID).*

in the tubing, and clogged air vents can affect the flow rate of an IV infusion.

Height of the IV bottle can affect the rate of infusion because IV infusions are affected by gravity. As the height of the container from the infusion site is increased, the gravitational force will be greater and the fluid will flow in faster. Conversely, as the distance between the bottle and IV site decreases, the fluid will infuse more slowly. This often occurs when the client gets up and walks in the hall, pushing his or her IV pole with the hand in which the IV is flowing. In such a case, the drip rate slows and often stops altogether, and blood may flow back into the tubing. The nurse must watch for this and readjust the rate of flow so that the infusion is not disrupted. After ambulation, the rate should be reregulated if necessary to ensure timely delivery of the fluids.

The *position of the extremity* can affect the rate of flow. When the extremity is elevated, the fluid will infuse more slowly. Also, bending the extremity at a point of flexion, such as the wrist or the elbow, or leaning on the arm can slow the rate of infusion. Clients should be cautioned not to raise their arm over their head or sleep on the side where the IV is infusing.

Constriction or kinking of IV tubing also can contribute to altered flow rates. Tubing can become kinked if it is placed inadvertently under the client. Tubing also can be obstructed if tape is applied too tightly or if edema develops when the tape interferes with venous blood return in the extremity.

The *position of the needle* within the vein can affect the rate of flow. Sometimes position changes can cause the needle bevel to rest against a vein wall; this is known as a positional IV. Care must be taken to monitor an IV frequently that appears to be positional. When the IV slows down, the nurse should adjust the rate, but if the client moves again and the bevel becomes free of the vein wall, the rate of infusion will once again increase. Armboards are somewhat helpful in immobilizing the joint and decreasing the chance of needle movement.

Patency of the catheter also is important to ensure proper infusion of fluids. A blood clot can form at the end of the catheter and stop the infusion. If the clot does not completely obstruct the lumen of the catheter, the flow rate may slow and become sluggish. Whenever flow of fluids is interrupted for any reason (eg, bending at a joint, kinking of tubing), clotting can occur. This is often a problem when IVs are infusing very slowly to keep the vein open (TKO [to keep open] or KVO [keep vein open]). When a KVO rate is ordered, the nurse may increase the flow rate to flush the catheter and prevent clot formation (Metheny, 1992). If the flow has stopped completely, the catheter may be gently aspirated. It should never be irrigated because irrigation pushes the clot into the circulation, which can cause an embolus or systemic infection.

Clogged air vents can slow the rate of IV flow. If the air vent on a solution bottle or volume control chamber becomes clogged, fluid cannot leave the system because air is unable to enter to replace it. Changing the tubing may be necessary to correct this problem.

Role of the Nurse in Intravenous Therapy

Nurses are responsible for initiating, monitoring, maintaining, and discontinuing the IV infusion and for client teaching related to the infusion. While many clients who receive IV fluids are admitted to healthcare facilities, it is increasingly common for clients to receive IV fluids at home or in special ambulatory or short-stay settings. The type and amount of IV fluid and electrolyte replacement are ordered by the physician. Components of an IV order are the following:

- Type and amount of solution
- Any other solutions or medications to be added and their concentrations
- Rate or volume of infusion
- Length of time for infusion to be given

Initiating Intravenous Therapy

IV therapy is initiated on the order of a licensed physician. The nurse is responsible for checking the order to determine the correctness (eg, the volume of solution to be infused, the rate of flow per hour, any additives to the solution). When the solution has been prepared consistent with the physician's order, the nurse gathers all needed equipment and prepares the client for venipuncture.

Preparing the Client

A major component of client preparation is teaching the client about the type of therapy ordered and the role

> **Client Teaching**
> *Intravenous Therapy*
>
> *Instruct the client as follows:*
> - *Explain the purpose of the IV therapy.*
> - *Describe the type of equipment being used, including the location of the port of entry for fluids and where the tip of the catheter is located.*
> - *Identify the kind of fluid and what, if any, substances it contains.*
> - *Explain the care required at the entry site.*
> - *Identify what the client can or cannot do when fluid is being infused.*
> - *Remind clients of signs to observe: burning above the site of entry, redness, swelling, or pain at the entry site; unusual sensations.*
> - *Clarify precautions about site dressings or positioning.*

that he or she will play in maintaining therapy. These client teaching features are summarized in the accompanying display. Curtains are drawn for privacy, and visitors are asked to leave the room during the procedure. The client is positioned comfortably with the arm on a flat surface.

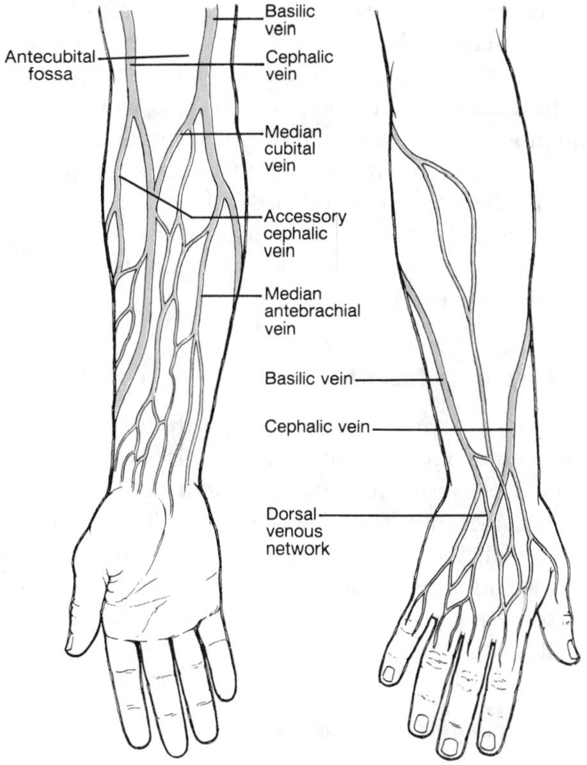

Figure 26-15 • *Site for insertion of the IV needle in adults. (Courtesy of Becton-Dickenson Vascular Access, Sandy, UT).*

Selecting the Site

In the adult, the veins of the hand and forearm are commonly used for IV infusion (Fig. 26-15). When the basilic or cephalic vein is used, the ulna and radius act as natural splints, which allows the client greater freedom of movement. Any vein selected should be free of sclerosis, pain, or hematomas. Whenever possible, larger veins are used. The distal portion of the vein is punctured first, leaving the more proximal sites for later venipunctures. Because infants and young children have very small veins, scalp veins in the temporal region are often used (Fig. 26-16). Veins located directly over movable joints should be avoided because their use increases the possibility that the IV will dislodge and infiltrate or that the client will develop phlebitis. Veins of the lower extremities should be avoided whenever possible because they limit mobility and increase the incidence of thrombophlebitis.

Various techniques are used to help locate and visualize veins before venipuncture. First, the nurse determines the type and duration of therapy and visually

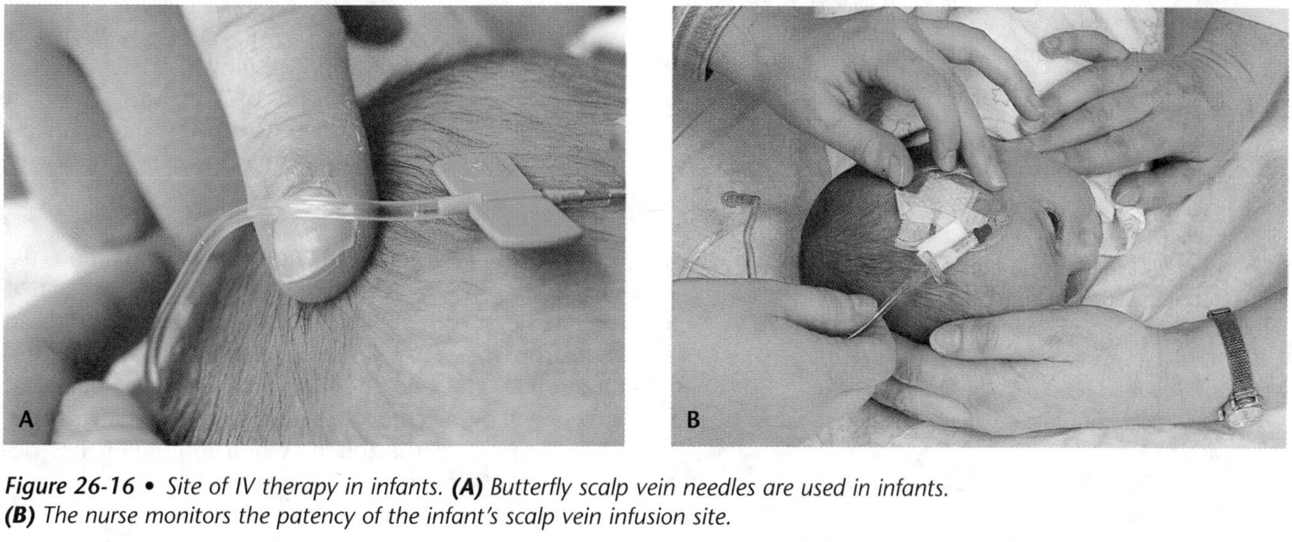

Figure 26-16 • *Site of IV therapy in infants.* ***(A)*** *Butterfly scalp vein needles are used in infants.* ***(B)*** *The nurse monitors the patency of the infant's scalp vein infusion site.*

inspects the client's veins, avoiding any areas that appear bruised or sclerosed. A tourniquet is placed on the extremity 4 to 6 in above the intended venipuncture site to distend the vein with blood. This will make the vein more visible. Additional tips that can help fill veins are to lower the extremity below the level of the heart, ask the client to open and close his or her fist several times, tap lightly over the selected vein, or use warm soaks for 5 minutes before venipuncture to vasodilate the selected vessel.

Preparing the Site

Adequate site preparation is necessary to avoid infection. Hair around the site may be clipped. Shaving is avoided because small microscopic nicks or abrasions can provide entry for microorganisms. The site is prepared with 70% alcohol or a povidone-iodine (Betadine) solution. Povidone-iodine is a better bactericide, but some people are sensitive to this preparation, and an allergic response is possible.

Performing the Venipuncture

All equipment should be assembled prior to attempting venipuncture. Tape is cut and all equipment placed within reach. Gloves are worn, as in any invasive procedure. The skin is stretched taut over the intended venipuncture site with the thumb and index finger. With the bevel up, the needle enters the skin at a 45-degree angle. As the skin is pierced, the angle of the needle is decreased to 30 degrees. This will permit entry into the vein at an angle and decrease the likelihood of accidentally puncturing the posterior vein wall. The needle is inserted 1/2 in into the vein. A blood return will ensure access to the vein. When an IV catheter is used, the plastic catheter must be threaded into the vein, usually after the needle and cannula have been inserted 1/2 in. The stylet is then removed while the catheter is fully inserted within the lumen of the vessel. When placement of the needle or catheter in the vein is ensured, the nurse attaches the tubing and releases the tourniquet.

Securing the Venipuncture Device

The cannula is taped flush with the skin with 1/2-in wide tape. Another strip of tape is placed under the hub, adhesive side up. One end is placed tightly and diagonally over the cannula. This is repeated with the other end of the tape, crossing the first. This secures the cannula and prevents sideways movement. The tubing is then looped and anchored with tape and a transparent dressing over the infusion site.

An armboard is used to help immobilize the extremity when motion can lead to infiltration or phlebitis. Armboards are useful when clients are uncooperative or disoriented, in children, or when the cannula is inserted in the dorsum of the hand. Care must be taken in using the armboard that function of the hand is not impaired.

Monitoring Intravenous Infusions

The nurse is responsible for monitoring IV infusions to ensure that the fluid infuses at the proper rate and that complications of IV therapy are detected promptly. The steps in monitoring the IV infusion are outlined in Procedure 26-1.

Assessing for Complications

An important nursing responsibility is monitoring the client for possible complications of IV therapy. The most significant complications of IV therapy include infiltration, phlebitis, infection, air embolism, and fluid overload.

Infiltration. When fluid enters the subcutaneous tissues, it is called **infiltration.** Infiltration can occur if the needle or catheter slips out of the vein or if IV fluid leaks from the vein into subcutaneous tissue. When infiltration occurs, the client may complain of pain and have swelling around the infusion site, which usually becomes cool to the touch. When infiltration has occurred, the IV usually infuses more slowly because of

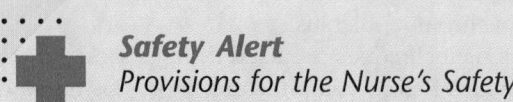

Safety Alert
Provisions for the Nurse's Safety

- Wash your hands before and after using IV equipment.
- Wear gloves when working with IV equipment; discard gloves appropriately after use.
- Use disposable needles when possible.
- Do not manipulate needles by hand (ie, do not bend or break them, attempt to recap them, or separate them from the syringe).
- Place used needles in the appropriate dispenser immediately after use.
- Wash your hands immediately if they come in contact with blood or other body fluids.
- Wear appropriate protective barrier equipment if there is a possibility of being splashed with blood or body fluid.
- Receive an immunization with hepatitis B virus vaccine.

Procedure 26-1
Monitoring an Intravenous Infusion

Purpose

1. Provide a dependable, patent route for infusion of IV therapy
2. Protect the client from introduction of air or microorganisms into the vascular system

Assessment

- Review client's chart for diagnosis and medical plan for IV therapy.
- Assess client's treatment schedule to identify times for drug administrations and laboratory sampling.
- Assess client for clinical signs of fluid or electrolyte imbalances.

Equipment

May need:

3-mL sterile syringe
Heparinized NaCl
Sterile NaCl
Alcohol or Betadine wipe (according to hospital policy)
Clean, disposable gloves
Dressing supplies

Procedure

1. Compare IV fluid currently infusing with the ordered solution.
   Rationale: Comparison ensures prompt recognition and correction of errors.
2. Inspect the rate of flow at least every hour. Check actual flow rate of 15 seconds and compare with prescribed rate of flow. If the infusion is ahead of schedule, slow it so the infusion will complete at the planned time. If infusion is behind schedule, review hospital policy before increasing flow rate. Many agencies require a physician's order to increase the rate of flow.
   Rationale: IV therapies that are not on schedule can be detrimental to the client. Fluids that are infused too rapidly may cause circulatory overload with resultant pulmonary edema and cardiac failure. Fluids that are behind schedule deliver insufficient fluids and nutrients.
3. Inspect the system for leakage, and if present, locate the source. Tighten all connections within the system. If leak is still present, slow IV flow rate to keep vein open and replace tubing with sterile set.
   Rationale: IV therapy is a sterile procedure. A break or leak in the tubing allows microorganisms to enter and contaminate the entire system.
4. Inspect the tubing for kinks or blockages. The tubing should be loosely coiled and placed on the bed.
   Rationale: Blockages in the tubing impede the flow of solution, and the client may not receive the necessary fluids and nutrients.
5. Observe the fluid level in the drip chamber. If it is less than half full, squeeze the chamber gently to allow more fluid in.
   Rationale: If the fluid level in the drip chamber is too low, turbulence from the fluid dripping into the chamber may create air bubbles that may enter the tubing.
6. Inspect the infusion site for infiltration. This occurs when the needle becomes dislodged from the vein and IV fluid flows into the interstitial tissue. The signs of infiltration are decreased rate of flow, swelling, pallor, coolness, and discomfort at or above the needle insertion site. If present, the IV site must be changed. If a large amount of fluid infiltrated, elevate the arm above the heart on several pillows.
   Rationale: Prompt detection is important to promote client comfort and permit early treatment. Elevation facilitates venous and lymphatic drainage.
7. Inspect arm above the insertion point for phlebitis, inflammation of the vein. The signs of phlebitis include redness, swelling, warmth, and pain along the vein above the IV insertion site. If present, the IV must be discontinued and restarted in another area.
   Rationale: This may occur as a result of trauma or chemical irritation secondary to intravenous additives or solution pH.
8. Inspect the insertion site for bleeding.
9. Monitoring IV therapy is a nursing responsibility, but if the client is able to comply, teach him or her to contact the nurse if the following occur:
   - The flow rate changes suddenly.
   - The fluid container is almost empty.
   - Blood is in the tubing.
   - The site becomes uncomfortable.
10. Chart any findings indicating complications of IV therapy (eg, infiltration).

(continued)

Lifespan Considerations

Infants and Children

- Children change position frequently, and their tubing can easily become kinked or disconnected. Taping all connections and protecting the insertion site with a medicine cup and rigid armboard may prolong the efficacy of the IV.

Additional

- Armboards and soft wrist restraints or mitt restraints may be used to protect the IV site in any client, regardless of age, who is at risk for purposefully disrupting the IV system.

Home-Care Modifications

- Client or caregiver must be taught the following:
- Inspect the insertion site at least four times daily through the transparent dressing.
- Assess for infiltration, phlebitis, or obvious dislodged catheter. If any of these situations occur, the caregiver should clamp the IV tubing, remove the catheter, and call the nurse.
- Observe flow rate for sluggishness or lack of dripping. Should this occur, the caregiver should open roller clamp and look for kinked tubing. If problem continues, contact healthcare provider.

the increased pressure within the subcutaneous tissues. Absence of blood return into the tubing as the IV bag is lowered below the level of the infusion supports the possibility that infiltration may have occurred. Absence of a blood return is not diagnostic, because some catheters do not readily permit the back flow of blood, and the location of the bevel of the needle may make back flow difficult.

Nursing intervention when infiltration occurs is to discontinue the IV and restart it in a new location. Elevation and application of a warm soak may help reduce edema. The nurse also should consider preventive measures, such as stabilizing the joint with an armboard and making sure the needle or catheter is adequately secured.

Phlebitis. **Phlebitis** refers to an inflammation of a vein. If a blood clot accompanies the inflammation, it is referred to as **thrombophlebitis**. Factors that contribute to the development of phlebitis include increased length of time the catheter is in a vein; infusion of irritating substances, such as potassium chloride or antibiotics; and using small veins or veins of the lower extremities where blood flow is relatively sluggish. Clinical manifestations of phlebitis include complaints of discomfort and a vein that appears red and feels warm and hard (almost cordlike) when palpated. The IV will be sluggish, especially if a clot is present. The IV should not be irrigated because irrigation could push the clot into the systemic circulation, thus contributing to systemic infection.

Nursing interventions for phlebitis include discontinuing the IV and restarting it in a different site and applying a warm compress to decrease inflammation. Phlebitis can be reduced if large veins are used for venipuncture, needles are used rather than catheters, irritating substances are diluted properly and infused slowly, and IV sites are changed per agency protocol (the Centers for Disease Control recommends every 72 hours; Metheny, 1992).

Infection. Infection can occur at the IV infusion site or systemically. The longer an IV is in one site, the greater the chance for infection; thus, IV sites often are routinely changed according to guidelines given in agency policies (eg, every 72 hours). Signs and symptoms of infection can be local (redness, warmth, or purulent drainage at the site) or systemic (fever, chills, general discomfort). If infection is suspected, the physician should be notified; he or she may order the IV to be discontinued and restarted and the IV catheter to be cultured.

Air Embolism. **Air embolism** refers to air entering the blood system and moving in the vessel. Air emboli are more common when central veins or infusion pumps are used. A significant amount of air (usually more than 5 mL) must enter the peripheral venous circulation before it poses a significant health risk for the client. Smaller amounts of air are significant when a central venous catheter is used for IV therapy. A few bubbles entering the system are not harmful but may worry the client. When large amounts of air enter the system, the client may become hypotensive, tachycardic, cyanotic, and actually lose consciousness. The classic sign of pending air embolism is a churning sound over the precordium. Treatment for air embolism includes placing the client on the left side with head down. This will allow the air to rise into the right ventricle and allow blood to pass into the lungs.

Fluid Overload. Fluid overload may occur if the client receives IV fluid too rapidly. Older people, especially those with poor cardiac function, and very young people are prone to fluid overload. Fluid overload can occur if the nurse tries to "catch up" when the IV infusion gets behind. The client may complain of headache and have neck vein distention, increased blood pressure, increased respiratory rate, and dyspnea. The nurse should slow down the IV to a KVO rate (30–50 mL/h) and contact the physician. The client should be placed in a semi-Fowler's position, and oxygen may be administered. Prevention of fluid overload is possible by careful monitoring of all IVs and placing high-risk clients on controllers or pumps.

Maintaining Intravenous Therapy

Policies specify expectations for site care. Frequently, semipermeable, transparent dressings are used to cover the IV site. The nature of these dressings permits continual viewing so that the site can be assessed frequently. These dressings also reduce the frequency of dressing changes and the incidence of infection (Shivnan, et al., 1991). Some agencies still prefer gauze dressing for IV site care. Whenever site care is performed, the nurse must take extra care not to dislodge the catheter.

Changing Intravenous Bottles and Tubing

The nurse is responsible for changing the IV bag or bottle as needed and changing IV tubing according to institutional policy. The IV bag or bottle is changed when the previous container is empty, when there is a change in IV orders, or when the IV container has been hanging for more than 24 hours.

All IV bag and tubing changes must be done under strict aseptic technique to prevent infection. Most facilities have policies that indicate the frequency and protocol for these procedures. Procedure 26-2 outlines changing IV solution and tubing.

> ***Safety Alert***
> *Provisions for the Client's Safety*
>
> - Wash your hands before and after using IV equipment.
> - Wear gloves when working with IV equipment.
> - Clip the client's hairs at the venipuncture site.
> - Clean the venipuncture site with 70% isopropyl alcohol or povidone-iodine solution.
> - Apply iodophor ointment after the site dries.
> - Check IV equipment before initiating the therapy.
> - Assess the client before beginning the IV therapy.
> - Never reuse a needle or catheter.
> - Cover the venipuncture site with a sterile dressing.
> - Change the dressing as often as needed or as agency policy requires.
> - Change administration sets as agency policy requires.
> - Discard gloves appropriately after use.
> - Use disposable needles when possible.
> - Do not manipulate needles by hand (ie, do not bend or break them, attempt to recap them, or separate them from the syringe).
> - Place used needles in the appropriate dispenser immediately after use.
> - Wash your hands immediately if they come in contact with blood or other body fluids.
> - Wear appropriate protective barrier equipment if there is a possibility of being splashed with blood or body fluid.
> - Receive an immunization with hepatitis B virus vaccine.

Intermittent Flushing of an Intravenous Lock

An existing intravenous catheter may be converted to an intermittent infusion device or heparin lock by the removal of the administration set and placement of a "plug" in which dilute concentration of saline solution or heparin in saline will be instilled. The locks are flushed constitent with institutional policy, usually once daily when medications are not being given. Procedure 26-3 outlines steps in flushing with both a needle-type system and the needleless system. Intermittent injection caps or ports may also be used to plug an unused line of a multiple lumen central line catheter. In each case, the quantity of flush solution instilled depends on the manufacturer's recommendation.

Discontinuing an Intravenous Infusion

An infusion is discontinued when all ordered fluids have infused or when complications develop. Before discontinuing an infusion, it is important to don disposable gloves, because contact with blood can occur. The flow of fluid is stopped by moving the roller clamp to the off position. Tape is carefully removed, while supporting the catheter. A gauze pad is placed over the venipuncture site as the catheter is withdrawn, and then pressure is applied over the site. A bandage can be applied if necessary, but it does not take the place of pressure. Documentation includes the amount of fluid infused, the time the infusion was discontinued, complications of therapy that occurred, and any nursing measures taken (such as application of a warm compress).

Blood Transfusions

Blood transfusion refers to the introduction of whole blood or blood components (packed red cells, plasma, platelets) directly into a client's circulatory system. Transfusions are given primarily to restore circulating blood volume, restore coagulation factor deficiencies, improve oxygen-carrying capacity of the blood, and in-

(text continues on page 565)

Procedure 26-2
Changing Intravenous Solution and Tubing

Purpose

1. Maintain sterility of IV system
2. Continue ordered therapeutic regimen

Assessment

- Determine if IV catheter needs to be restarted in a new site.
- It is recommended that peripheral IV sites should be changed every 72 hours. Review the policy of your agency.
- Inspect IV site for signs of infiltration, sluggish flow, or phlebitis.
- Determine what time next solution container is due. Prepare next solution 1 hour before it is due. Plan to change container when less than 50 mL remains.
- Review physician's orders for current IV fluid orders.
- Check label on currently infusing solution and tubing for the date and time they were hung.
- IV solutions are not considered sterile if they are open longer than 24 hours.
- It is recommended that IV tubing be changed every 48 hours to ensure sterility of system. Review the policy of your agency.
- Inspect IV system to determine type of tubing required. Many different administration sets are available. Some infusion pumps use specially designed cassette tubing. Review the policy of your agency and manufacturer's recommendations.

Equipment

Sterile container of ordered amount and type of solution
An appropriate sterile tubing administration set
Adhesive tape or premarked strips for labeling and timing solution container and tubing
Tape for securing tubing
Clean, disposable gloves (for tubing change)
Dressing material and antiseptic solution if IV site dressing is to be changed (follow agency procedure)

Procedure

Changing Solution Container

1. Wash hands.
2. Compare solution with physician orders.
3. Remove IV bag from outer wrapper.

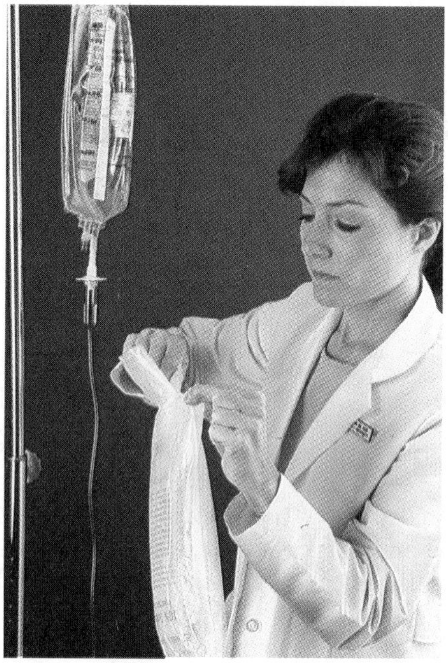

Step 3 • *Remove IV bag from outer wrapper.*

4. Label solution container with client's name, solution type, additives, date, and time hung. Time label side of container. Record solution change.

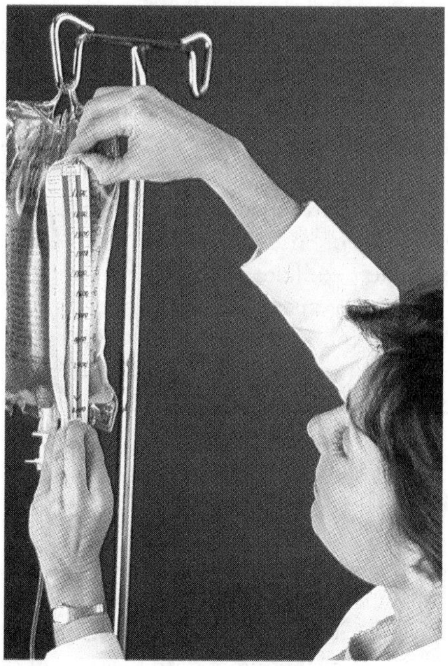

Step 4 • *Place time label on side of IV container.*

5. Prepare container for spiking:
   a. If solution is in a plastic bag, remove plastic cover from entry nipple. Maintain sterility of nipple end.
   b. If solution is in a bottle, remove metal cap, metal disk, and rubber disk. Maintain sterility of bottle top.
   Rationale: Sterility prevents transmission of microorganisms into container when spike is inserted.

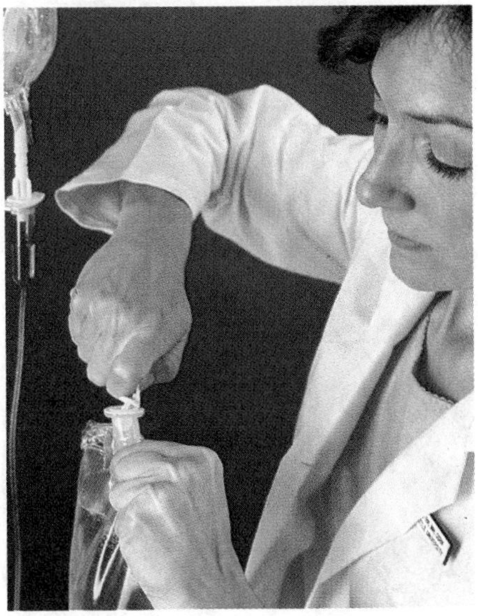

Step 5 • *Remove plastic cover from entry nipple.*

6. Close the clamp on the existing tubing.
   Rationale: Clamping prevents fluid in drip chamber from emptying and air entering tubing during changing procedure.
7. Take old solution container from pole and invert it.
   Rationale: Work is at eye level, and this position prevents fluid remaining in container from emptying onto floor when tubing is removed.
8. Remove spike from used container, maintaining its sterility. Spike new IV container with firm push/twist motion.

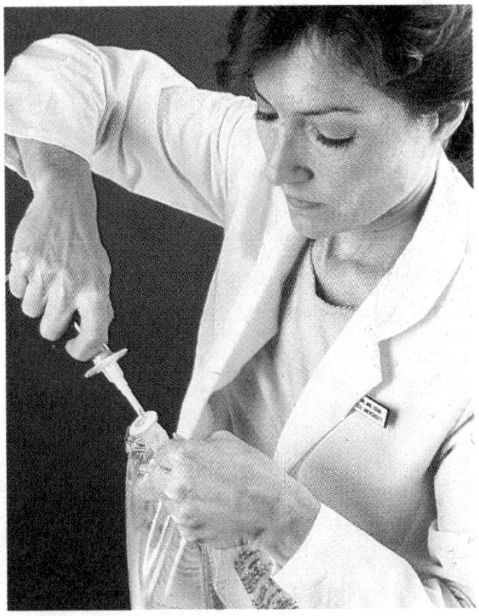

Step 8 • *Insert spike into IV bag.*

9. Hang new container on IV pole.
   Rationale: This action allows gravity to augment fluid filling drip chamber.
10. Inspect tubing for air bubbles, and assess that drip chamber is one-half full of solution.
    Rationale: Nurse takes actions to reduce risk of air embolis.
11. Adjust clamp to regulate flow rate, according to orders.
    Rationale: IV fluids are delivered as ordered to restore fluid balance.

Procedure

Changing Solution and Tubing

1. Follow first three steps of *Changing Solution Container* only.
2. Open new tubing package, keeping protective covers on spike and catheter adapter.
   Rationale: Sterility of new tubing set must be maintained.
3. Adjust roller clamp on new tubing to fully closed position.
   Rationale: Closed clamp prevents fluid spillage when new solution container is attached.
4. Prepare new solution container as directed in *Changing Solution Container.*
5. Remove protective cover from spike, maintaining sterility, and spike into new solution container.
6. Hang container and "prime" drip chamber by squeezing gently, allowing to fill one-half full.
   Rationale: This action prevents air bubbles from entering tubing with the solution.

(continued)

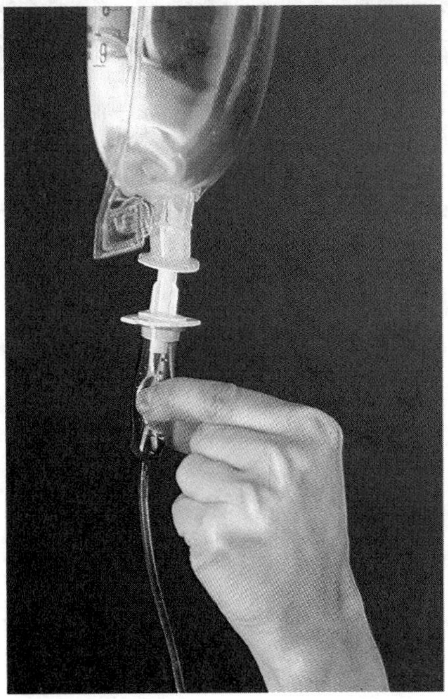

Step 6 • *Squeeze drip chamber gently to "prime."*

7. Remove protective cap from catheter adapter, and adjust roller clamp to flush tubing with fluid. Replace protective cap.
   Rationale: Air removal from tubing protects client from risk of air embolus. Protective cap maintains sterility of system.
8. Adjust roller clamp on old tubing to close fully.
   Rationale: Fluid leakage should be prevented when tubing is disconnected.
9. Don clean, disposable gloves.
   Rationale: Nurse is protected from transfer of microorganisms if blood inadvertently gets on hands.
10. Hold catheter hub with fingers of one hand (may use hemostat). With other hand, disconnect tubing using gently twisting motion.
    Note: The dressing may have to be removed.
    Rationale: Holding catheter hub firmly maintains needle position in the vein.
11. Grasp new tubing, remove protective catheter cap, and insert tightly into needle hub, while continuing to stabilize catheter hub with other hand.

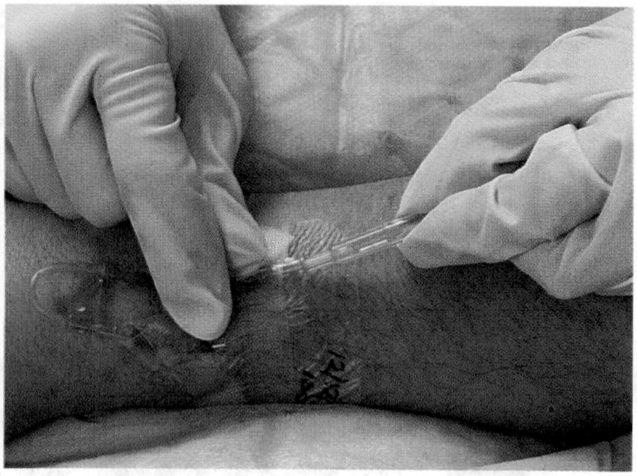

Step 11 • *Stabilize IV catheter hub while connecting new tubing tightly.*

12. Adjust roller clamp to start solution flowing according to physician's order.
13. Discard gloves.
14. Secure tubing with tape.
    Rationale: Secure tubing prevents accidental dislodging of catheter in the vein.
15. If dressing was removed, apply new dressing to IV site according to agency policy.
16. Label new tubing with date and time and your initials.

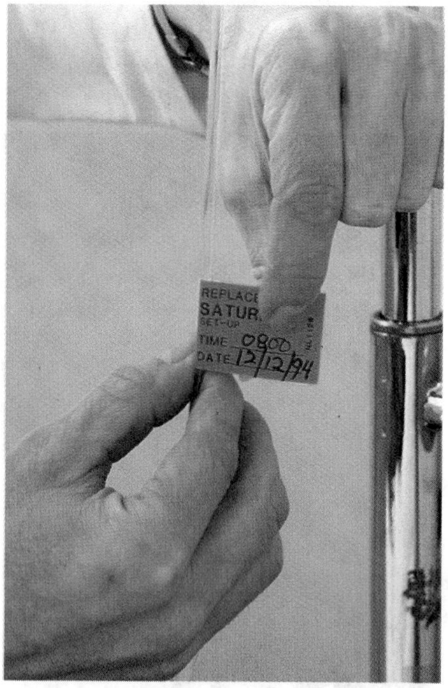

Step 16 • *Attach date and time label to new tubing.*

17. Label solution container with client's name, solution type, additives, date and time hung. Time label side of container. Record solution and tubing change.
    Rationale: Documentation facilitates monitoring by other staff members.

Lifespan Considerations

Infants and Children

- Infants and children are at risk for circulatory overload if IV fluids are accidentally infused too rapidly. IV solutions are available in 250- and 500-mL containers to guard against such accidents. Volume control administration sets also are available to allow only a preset amount of fluid to be infused. All children younger than 2 years should have this type of safety device during IV therapy.

Nursing Research
Intravenous Therapy

Selected Nursing Research Studies

Smith, C. E. (1993). Quality of life in long-term total parenteral nutrition patients and their family caregivers. *Journal of Parenteral and Enteral Nutrition, 17*(6), 501–506.

Savino, S. R., & Napolitano, B. (1994). A comparison between two intermittent intravenous systems without needles. *Journal of Intravenous Nursing, 17*(5), 256–260.

Adams, K. S., Zehrer, C. L., & Thomas, W. (1993). Comparison of a needleless system with conventional heparin locks. *American Journal of Infection Control, 21*(5), 263–269.

Smith, C. E., Giefer, C. K., & Bieker, L. (1991). Technological dependency: A preliminary model and pilot of home total parenteral nutrition. *Journal of Community Health Nursing, 8*(4), 245–254.

Reynolds, J. (1993). Comparison of percutaneous venous catheters and teflon catheters for intravenous therapy in neonates. *Neonatal Network, 12*(5), 33–39.

Possible Topics for Nursing Inquiry

- What type of dressing provides the most effective protection against infections for peripherally inserted central lines?
- What variables are associated with the client's and caregiver's quality of life when long-term total parenteral nutrition is used?
- Compare two systems of fluid infusion to determine the cost-effectiveness with the infusion efficiency.

crease white blood cells to decrease the chance of infection.

Blood Components

The client does not always need all components of whole blood, so certain blood components can be selectively transfused depending on the clinical needs of the client. Common blood products for transfusion include whole blood, packed red cells, white blood cells, platelets, plasma, albumin, and cryoprecipitate. The nurse should be knowledgeable regarding the indications and nursing considerations for each product.

Whole blood contains all blood components and is usually transfused to people who need both blood cells and volume replacement, such as after significant blood loss. A unit of whole blood is approximately 500 mL.

Packed red cells contain a concentration of red cells with most plasma removed. A unit of packed cells is approximately 250 mL. Packed red cells provide the same oxygen-carrying capacity, without the volume, as whole blood. They are especially useful in the treatment of chronic anemia. Problems of fluid overload and electrolyte imbalances can be avoided because packed cells contain less volume and less sodium and potassium. To prevent an allergic response, the packed red cells can be washed to remove most antibodies from the cell.

White blood cells, or granulocytes, can be administered to clients with a low or abnormal white blood cell count. Infusion of white cells is helpful in fighting infection. They are frequently given to cancer clients who have low white cell counts due to chemotherapy or the effects of the cancer.

Platelets may be administered in fresh blood, platelet concentrates, and platelet-rich plasma. The major function of platelets is to initiate blood clotting and hemostasis.

Whole plasma is the fluid component of the blood in which the corpuscles are suspended. Plasma consists of organic and inorganic substances dissolved in water. Whole plasma can be used to correct hypovolemia due to selective loss of plasma, such as occurs in extensive burns. Electrolyte solutions and albumin often replace the need for plasma infusions.

Albumin is a plasma protein contained within the plasma. It is used as a volume expander, because fluid is pulled back into the vasculature due to the oncotic force the protein exerts. Another advantage of albumin is that it, unlike whole plasma, carries no risk of hepatitis transmission.

Cryoprecipitate is a plasma fraction rich in fibrinogen and blood clotting factor VIII. Cryoprecipitate is concentrated from many units of blood and administered to hemophiliacs, who are predisposed to bleeding problems because genetically they lack factor VIII.

Blood Compatibility

The donor blood must be compatible with the blood of the client. To ensure this, the blood of the client and the donor is tested to determine ABO and Rh compatibility. Blood typing refers to testing the person's blood type, and crossmatching is the process of ensuring that it is compatible with the donor blood.

ABO blood groups can be determined by testing for antigens on the erythrocyte. The population can be divided into four ABO blood groups: types A, B, AB, and O. The erythrocytes of a person in group A have the A antigen; group B, the B antigen; group AB, both A and B antigens; and group O, neither A nor B antigens. In addition to antigens, each blood group also

(text continues on page 568)

Procedure 26-3
Providing Intermittent Flush of an Intravenous Lock

Purpose

Maintain patency of intermittently used intravenous lock.

Assessment

- Check medication orders for types of medications, dosage, and time scheduled to be administered via the heparin or saline lock.
- Assess for compatibilities of medications with solutions to be flushed through lock.
- Identify all pertinent allergies.
- Assess site for signs of erythema, pain, tenderness, edema.
- Assess label and documentation for date and time of IV device placement.
- Review procedure manual for specific policies regarding flushing locks with saline or heparin.

Equipment

Medication documentation sheets
Gloves
Antiseptic swab
Sterile 3-cc syringe with 21–25 gauge-needle (use high-risk needles if available)
Many facilities are promoting needleless equipment for procedures. If available will require sterile end protectors.
Vial of heparin flush solution, concentration dependent on agency policy: (1 mL= 10 units sodium heparin or 1 mL = 100 units sodium heparin) or vial of sterile normal saline
(Saline and heparin flush solutions may be available in prefilled syringes.)

Beginning the Procedure

Procedure

1. Wash hands.
   Rationale: clean hands help prevent spread of microorganisms.
2. Explain procedure to client.
3. Prepare syringe with heparin flush solution or saline solution according to facility policy and manufacturer's recommendations for the type of device in place (may use between 0.5–1 mL [peripheral], 2.5–3 mL [central line] heparin flush, or 1–3 mL normal saline).
   Note: If flushing lock after administering a prescribed medication, a saline flush may be required, followed by a heparin flush in order to completely clear the medication from the catheter to prevent incompatibilties with heparin.
   Rationale: Heparin is incompatible with many medications. Normal saline has been shown to be as effective as heparin in maintaining patency of peripherally inserted intravenous locks. Most central lines require patency to be maintained by intermittent heparin flushes.
4. Don gloves.
   Rationale: Gloves are worn to prevent transmission of microorganisms.
5. Inject the saline or heparin flush according to the following procedures for flushing with a needle-type system or a needleless system.

Flushing With Needle Type System

Procedure

Perform Steps 1 to 4 above.

5. Swab injection port with antiseptic swab and allow to dry.
   Rationale: This prevents introduction of microorganisms during needle insertion.

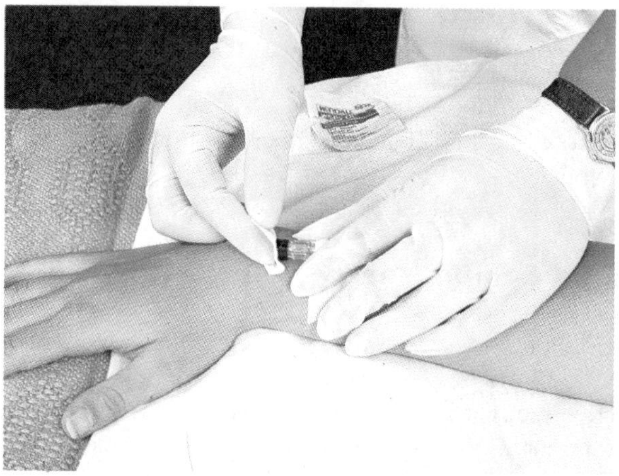

Step 5 • *Swab the injection port. (©B. Proud.)*

6. Insert the needle into the port and aspirate gently for evidence of blood return.
   Rationale: Clear aspiration determines if IV catheter is correctly positioned in the vein. Intravenous locks occasionally do not yield a blood return even when they are correctly positioned in the vein.

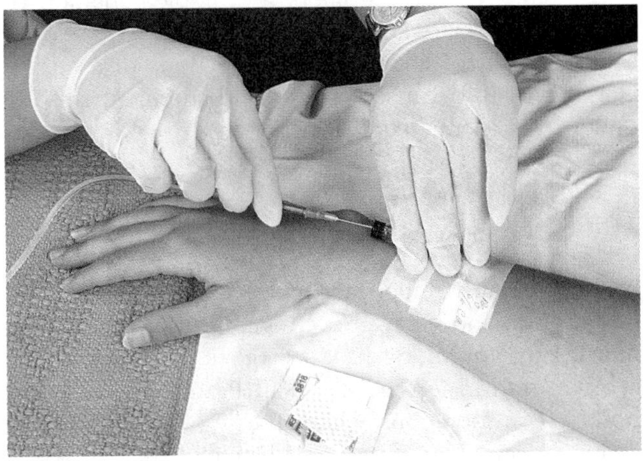

Step 6 • *Aspirate while assessing for blood return. (©B. Proud.)*

7. Inject the recommended amount of saline or heparin flush
   Rationale: Flushing blood out of intravenous catheter aids in assessing and maintaining patency of catheter.
   Note: This procedure must be done at least every 8 hours or after each use of the catheter for IV medications to ensure catheter patency. Most agencies recommend changing intravenous locks every 72 hours to ensure patency and to prevent commonly associated complications of IV therapy, ie, phlebitis.

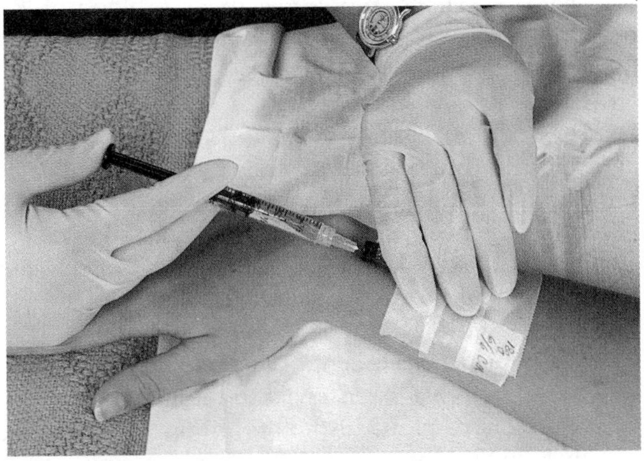

Step 7 • *Inject the recommended amount of saline or heparin flush. (©B. Proud.)*

8. Dispose of uncapped needles and syringes in proper container.
   Rationale: Accidental needle sticks are to be prevented.
9. Wash hands.
10. Document date, time, route, amount, and type of flush solution. Also document assessment of site.

Flushing With Needleless System

Procedure

Perform Steps 1 to 4 above.

5. Remove protective wrapper from device.
6. Attach syringe, with needle removed, to intravenous catheter.
   Rationale: Needleless systems are rapidly replacing syringes with needles in an effort to prevent inadvertent needle sticks and unnecessary exposure of healthcare providers to blood-borne pathogens.
7. Aspirate gently, observing for a blood return in the catheter.
   Rationale: Catheter is assured of correct placement in the vein.
8. Slowly inject the saline or heparin flush into the catheter.
   Rationale: Patency can be ensured when blood is flushed from the intravenous catheter.
9. Remove syringe from catheter and cap end with a new, sterile end protector.
   Rationale: Sterility of IV catheter prevents infection.
10. Wash hands and document date, time, route, amount, and type of flush solution. Also document assessment of site.

Lifespan Considerations

Infants and Children

- Check unit policy and physician orders carefully to determine type and required amount of flushing solution to be used.

Home-Care Considerations

- Clients requiring long-term intravenous access usually have devices placed that are especially designed for long-term use (ie, tunneled catheters such as the Hickman or Groshong, and implantable catheters, such as the Port-a-Cath). Each of these catheters has unique flushing requirements and procedures. Refer to manufacturer's recommendations or agency protocols for use.

contains naturally occurring antibodies (agglutinins) in the serum. Group A has anti-B antibodies, group B has anti-A antibodies, group AB has no A or B antibodies, and group O has anti-A and anti-B antibodies in the serum. Anti-A antibodies destroy A antigens, and anti-B antibodies destroy B antigens; this results in red cell destruction, known as hemolysis. People with type O blood are often referred to as universal donors, because the blood has neither A nor B antigens, and it can safely be given to people with other blood types. Likewise, AB blood is often referred to as the universal recipient, because the lack of antibodies enables accepting transfusions from other blood types.

Rh factor also is important to determine before transfusion to prevent blood incompatibility. Five antigens in the Rh system, the most important of which is D, are located on the surface of the erythrocyte. The presence of D antigen determines that a person is Rh positive (85% of Caucasian people), whereas the lack of this antigen designates an individual as Rh negative (15% of Caucasian people). Antibodies against Rh factor do not occur naturally. Such antibodies form only when Rh-negative blood is exposed to Rh-positive cells. After antibodies form, it is only on subsequent exposure to Rh-positive blood that a reaction (agglutination) occurs, in which there is hemolysis of cells. Rh factor is especially important in obstetrics. If an Rh-negative mother carries an Rh-positive fetus, antibodies can form in the mother's blood. If the mother should become pregnant again with an Rh-positive fetus, Rh agglutinogens can enter the circulation of the fetus and cause a hemolytic reaction. RhoGam, a commercial name for antibodies directed against Rh factor, is given to the mother after the first miscarriage, abortion, or pregnancy to prevent future problems.

Selection of Blood Donors

Nurses are frequently responsible for screening prospective blood donors and overseeing the process of blood collection. The nurse is responsible for ensuring the safety of the blood donor and the recipient of the blood. To do this, the nurse interviews the prospective donor to rule out any history of hepatitis or recent hepatitis exposure, recent infectious exposure, syphilis or malaria, recent immunizations, recent reception of any blood product transfusion, and exposure to human immunodeficiency virus (HIV) or risky behaviors, such as IV drug abuse or homosexual or bisexual activities. Screening for these factors is important to identify and prevent high-risk people from donating blood, thus ensuring the safety of the blood supply (Baranowski, 1992). To protect the blood donor, people are not permitted to donate if they are pregnant, anemic, do not fall within weight restrictions, have abnormal blood pressure, or have donated whole blood within the last 56 days.

Blood is tested for antibodies to HIV and hepatitis B. At this time, there is no way to test blood for non-A, non-B hepatitis, and transmission of this form of hepatitis can occur with blood transfusions. The chance of contracting acquired immunodeficiency virus (AIDS) through blood transfusions has been significantly reduced since the development and implementation of testing all blood for antibodies to HIV. The blood donor is not at risk for acquiring any infectious disease, including AIDS, because all blood procurement is done under strict aseptic conditions.

Transfusion Technique

The nurse must understand correct technique for administration and be aware of complications before administering any blood product. Steps in administering a blood transfusion are given in Procedure 26-4. Important considerations when infusing blood products include proper identification of the client and the blood, using a large enough access device (usually 18-gauge or larger) to avoid damage to the blood cells as they infuse, and using only compatible IV solutions of normal saline to prevent cell hemolysis. The nurse also frequently assesses the client for signs of a transfusion reaction (Querin & Stahl, 1990).

Complications of Blood Transfusion

The administration of blood or blood products involves a number of risks. The nurse should monitor the client carefully for any untoward effects. The major risks include febrile reaction, circulatory overload, septic reaction, allergic reaction, and acute hemolytic reaction.

Febrile Reactions. Febrile reactions to blood products can occur because of the recipient's hypersensitivity to the donor's blood cells. In this reaction, the client develops a fever and chills and complains of headache and malaise. Sometimes an antipyretic, such as aspirin, is ordered before blood administration to prevent a febrile reaction. If symptoms occur after the infusion has been started, the infusion should be stopped and the IV kept open with normal saline. The physician should be notified and vital signs monitored.

Allergic Reactions. Allergic reactions may occur because the client has a sensitivity to the plasma protein from the donor's blood. Symptoms of an allergic reaction include flushing, urticaria (hives), wheezing, and a rash with itching. Once again, the infusion must be stopped, the IV kept open with normal saline, and the

Procedure 26-4
Administering a Blood Transfusion

Purpose

Replace blood volume or blood components lost through trauma, surgery, or a disease process

Assessment

- Review physician's order for transfusion.
- Review chart for pertinent, baseline laboratory values (ie, CBC, platelets).
- Review chart for previous transfusion history, noting if client has ever had a transfusion reaction.
- Inspect client's current IV for patency and intactness. Assess that IV catheter is an 18- or 19-gauge cannula, which will facilitate transfusion flow and prevent hemolysis of red blood cells. Restart if necessary.

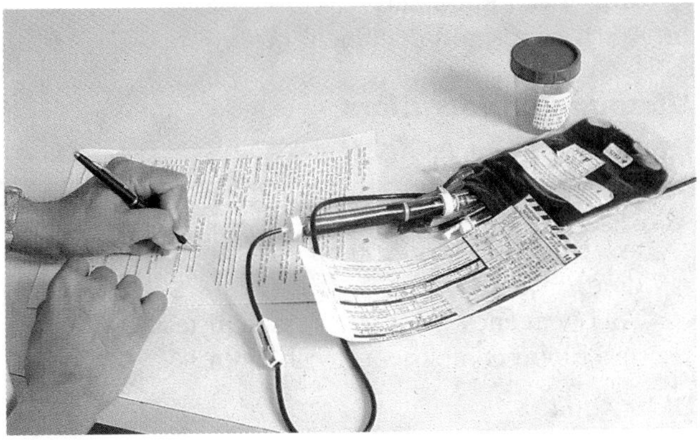

Equipment

Packaged blood component from blood bank according to agency protocol
250-mL IV container of sterile 0.9 normal saline
Blood administration set with filter
Blood warmer and pressure bag (optional) may be used if infusing large volumes of blood rapidly
Alcohol swabs and tape

Procedure

1. Explain procedure to client. Have client sign consent form if required by hospital policy.
2. Obtain client's vital signs to include temperature.
   Rationale: Baseline pretransfusion vital signs can be compared against vital signs taken during and after transfusion.
3. With another RN at the client's bedside, verify the blood product *and* the client's identity by comparing the laboratory blood record with:
   a. The client's name and identification number both verbally and against client's wrist band.
   b. The blood unit number on the blood bag label.
   c. The blood group and RH type on the blood bag label.

   Also verify the type of blood component and the expiration date noted on the blood label. Document verification by both RN signatures on transfusion record.
   Rationale: Strict adherence to verification prior to blood administration greatly reduces the risk of infusing the wrong blood type.

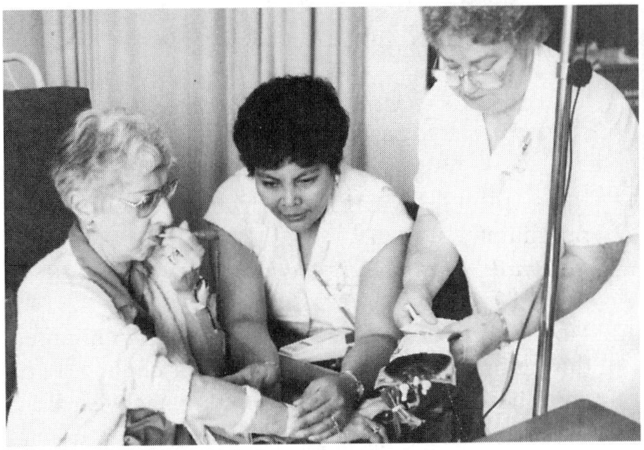

Step 3 • *Verify client's identity, blood product, and laboratory record with a registered nurse.*

4. Wash your hands.
5. Open Y-type blood administration set, and clamp both rollers completely.
   Rationale: Clamping prevents spilling and wasting blood.
6. Spike 0.9% NaCl container. Prime drip chamber and tubing with saline.
7. Spike blood or blood component unit with second spike. Keep roller clamp shut.
8. Remove primary IV tubing from catheter hub, and cover end with sterile protector.
   Rationale: If sterility of IV is ensured, it can be reconnected following transfusion.
9. Attach blood administration tubing to catheter hub, and secure with tape.

(continued)

10. Close clamp to 0.9% NaCl container. Open clamp to blood product. Open roller clamp below drip chamber and begin transfusion.

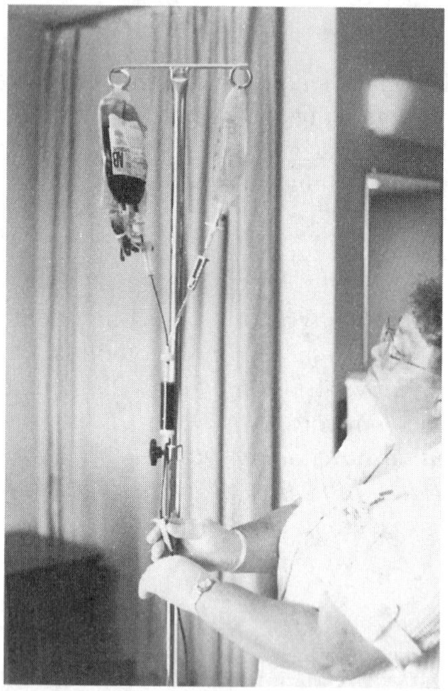

Step 10 • *Open roller clamp below drip chamber to begin transfusion.*

11. Infuse blood slowly for first 15 minutes (10 drops per minute).
Rationale: Most blood reactions occur within first 15 to 20 minutes of transfusion.
12. Monitor and document vital signs every 5 minutes during first 15 minutes, assessing for chilling, back pain, headache, nausea or vomiting, tachycardia, hypotension, tachypnea, or skin rash.
Rationale: Altered vital signs or other adverse reactions are early indications of a transfusion reaction. Infusing blood slowly during this period limits the amount of blood the client receives if there is a reaction.
Note: If any adverse reactions occur, close clamp to blood, open clamp to 0.9% NaCl, and notify physician immediately. Follow agency policy for laboratory notification and obtaining blood and urine specimens.
13. If no adverse reactions occur after 15 minutes, regulate clamp to increase infusion according to physician's orders. Monitor vital signs hourly until transfusion is complete.
Rationale: Altered vital signs may indicate transfusion reactions or fluid volume overload.
14. When blood transfusion is complete, clamp roller to blood and open roller to 0.9% NaCl. Infuse until tubing is clear.
Rationale: This action prevents wasting blood product and prevents hemolysis of cells from noncompatible Iv solutions.
15. Obtain and document post-transfusion vital signs.
16. If second blood component unit is to be transfused, slow 0.9% NaCl to keep vein open until next unit is available. Follow verification procedure and vital sign monitoring for each unit.
17. If transfusion orders are complete, disconnect the blood administration tubing from the catheter hub. Reconnect the primary IV solution and tubing and adjust to desired rate.
18. Wash hands and document procedure.

Lifespan Considerations

Infants and Children

- Many blood banks have "pedi-packs" of blood available in 50 and 100 mL for infusing to children.
- Follow agency protocol for administering blood and blood components to children.

Older Adult

- If the client has cardiac failure, careful assessment to prevent fluid overload is necessary. Packed red blood cells are frequently infused to limit the volume being infused. The infusion of 0.9% NaCl may be limited to the minimum needed to irrigate the tubing. The infusion time may be increased to decrease the load on the heart.

physician notified. An antihistamine may be ordered to decrease the severity of the reaction and make the client more comfortable. If hives are the only manifestation, the physician may elect to continue the infusion at a slower rate. The nurse must then monitor the client carefully for manifestations of a more severe reaction that could cause respiratory difficulty.

Hemolytic Reactions. Hemolytic reactions, the most serious of the acute complications, can be life-threatening. A hemolytic reaction occurs when the donor's blood is incompatible with the recipient's blood. This can occur if the wrong blood is mistakenly administered to a client. Hemolysis, or destruction of red cells, occurs when the antibodies in the recipient's blood quickly react to the donor's blood cells. Symptoms are immediate and include facial flushing, fever, chills, headache, low back pain, tachycardia, dyspnea, hypotension, and blood in the urine. Prompt intervention is essential to decrease mortality in hemolytic reactions. Vital signs should always be monitored before starting the infusion and during the first 5 minutes when the blood is infused slowly. If the nurse suspects a hemolytic reaction, the blood administration should be stopped and the IV kept open with normal saline. The physician will order drugs to treat the hypotension and have the client monitored closely. Blood from the donor and recipient will be tested to assess whether a hemolytic reaction has occurred. A urine specimen also is collected to determine if renal involvement is present.

Circulatory Overload. Circulatory overload can occur when blood products are infused too quickly or too much volume is infused. Circulatory overload is more likely to occur in the very young or older person with poor cardiac function. Symptoms of circulatory overload include increased venous pressure, distended neck veins, dyspnea, coughing, and abnormal breath sounds. Circulatory overload can be prevented by infusing packed cells rather than whole blood for high-risk clients and carefully monitoring the infusion rate of blood products. If the nurse suspects circulatory overload, he or she should slow the infusion of blood, position the client in an upright position with feet dependent, and notify the physician.

Septic Reactions. Septic reactions can occur if the blood products have been contaminated with bacteria. The client will likely have a rapid onset of fever and chills and perhaps vomiting, diarrhea, and hypotension. The transfusion should be stopped and the physician notified. Septic reactions can be minimized if blood products are kept refrigerated until used and infused in less than 4 hours. The longer blood products remain at room temperature, the more likely bacteria will grow and multiply.

Parenteral Nutrition

When assessment reveals the client has a condition that interferes with absorption of nutrients from the gastrointestinal tract, when diarrhea or vomiting is persistent and does not respond to treatment, or when complete bowel rest is necessary to promote healing, the physician may order parenteral nutrition. TPN is initiated when parenteral nutrition will be needed for more than 5 days (Taylor, 1994a; 1994b). With the addition of lipid emulsion to the TPN solution, a nutritionally complete diet (total nutrient admixture [TNA]) can be delivered intravenously, as shown in Procedure 26-5.

Because it is a highly osmotic solution, TPN must be infused through the central veins. Irritation and sclerosing of the vein and sudden fluid shifts are less likely when the hypertonic solutions are mixed adequately with blood. Common vessels used for central catheter insertion are the subclavian and jugular veins. Nonsurgical insertion can occur when a standard central venous line is inserted into a vessel and advanced to the appropriate site. When TPN is anticipated for an extended period, a more permanent catheter (eg, Hickman, Broviac) or vascular access device may be surgically placed, as shown in Figure 26-7.

Peripheral parenteral nutrition (PPN) supplies the client's full caloric needs without the risks associated with central venous access. PPN, however, requires a greater fluid volume for infusion. The client receiving PPN must be able to tolerate a large amount of fluid volume.

The largest available vein is used in PPN. Care involves the same actions taken for any client receiving peripheral IV infusion. Because most clients needing parenteral nutrition receive TPN, the rest of this discussion concerns TPN.

TPN Solutions

All TPN solutions contain essential nutrients, including protein, carbohydrates, electrolytes, vitamins, water, and trace elements. The proportion of each ingredient is individualized based on the client's clinical condition. The carbohydrate source is often a 50% dextrose solution, and protein is provided as synthetic crystalline amino acids. The client's caloric need is carefully assessed to provide the number of calories needed to maintain an anabolic state. Electrolytes, vitamins, and trace elements are added based on laboratory assays.

To supply all necessary nutrients, fat in the form of 10% or 20% lipid emulsion is often given with TPN. These isotonic solutions, which are milky in appearance, are compatible with TPN and can be infused simultaneously or in combination with dextrose and protein. TNA, which combines lipid emulsion with amino acid and dextrose, is frequently used in all clinical settings. This permits all necessary nutrients to be given in a single container, decreasing expense and possible infection risk (Taylor, 1994a; 1994b).

Continuous Versus Cyclic Infusions

Often TPN is given continuously and monitored using an EID to prevent inadvertent sudden infusion. **Cycling**, or the interruption of infusion for a period of time, is routinely used for clients receiving home infusion therapy. It permits increased freedom, because nutrition is delivered during the sleeping hours, and the client is able to continue with activities of daily living during "off" hours. When instituting cyclic infusions, rates should be increased gradually to avoid sudden fluid shifts or hyperglycemia.

Complications of TPN

Many potentially serious complications, such as pneumothorax and air embolism, associated with central line placement are associated with TPN. Other TPN com-

(text continues on page 574)

Procedure 26-5
Administering Total Parenteral Nutrition

Purpose

1. Provide parenteral nutritional support to malnourished clients
2. Provide parenteral nutritional support to clients requiring bypass of the GI tract for prolonged periods
3. Provide parenteral nutritional support to clients who have excessive metabolic needs due to trauma, cancer, or hypermetabolic states

Assessment

- Assess nutritional needs of clients.
- Check pattern of weight loss or gain, and intake and output balance.
- Check physician's order for TPN, noting additives and rate of infusion.
- Compare container of TPN against physician's order to ensure that it is correct.
- Assess client's knowledge of TPN and need for client teaching.

Equipment

TPN solution (usually prepared by pharmacy)
Appropriate IV tubing with filter
Infusion control pump
TPN dressing kit as per hospital protocol (usually contains transparent dressing, acetone swabs, Betadine swabs)
Sterile gloves and mask
Blood glucose monitoring equipment

Procedure

Monitoring TPN Therapy

1. Schedule and assist client with chest x-ray after central catheter insertion.
   Rationale: X-ray documents that catheter is in correct position and whether pneumothorax occurred during insertion.
2. Confirm correct solution is running at ordered rate. Check expiration date of solution. Use infusion controller to monitor and regulate flow rate.
   Rationale: Careful checking helps prevent medication errors.
   Note: Solutions with more than 10% dextrose must be infused directly into the subclavian or internal jugular vein to rapidly dilute the solution and prevent thrombophlebitis. Constant flow rate helps prevent hyperglycemia and electrolyte imbalances.
3. Inspect tubing and catheter connection for leaks or kinks. Tape all connections. Change tubing every 24 hours according to hospital policy.
   Rationale: Leaks prevent client from receiving prescribed volume of solution and are a potential entry site for bacteria. Kinks in tubing can obstruct flow of solution and result in clotting of catheter. Taping connections prevents accidental disconnection.
4. Inspect insertion site for infiltration, thrombophlebitis, or drainage. If present, notify physician.
   Note: The physician may order the catheter to be removed. If infection is suspected, catheter tip may be placed in sterile specimen cup and sent to laboratory for culture.
5. Monitor vital signs, including temperature, every 4 hours.
   Rationale: Elevated temperature may indicate catheter-related sepsis.
6. Assess for symptoms of air embolism (ie, decreased level of consciousness, tachycardia, dyspnea, anxiety, "feeling of impending doom," chest pain, cyanosis, hypotension).
   Note: If suspected, lay client on left side with head in Trendelenburg position.
   Rationale: Lying on left side may prevent air from flowing into the pulmonary veins. Lying in Trendelenburg position increases intrathoracic pressure, which decreases the amount of blood pulled into the vena cava during inhalation.
7. Use the TPN line *only* for TPN. Do not use the line for any other reason.
   Rationale: Using equipment meant for specific use minimizes breaks in integrity of line to prevent infection.
8. Test urine every 6 hours for specific gravity and ketones.
9. Perform test for glucose every 6 hours. Notify physician if abnormal.
   Rationale: Hyperglycemia may be an indication that client needs insulin to help metabolize glucose or may be an early indication of sepsis.
10. Monitor laboratory tests of electrolytes, BUN, glucose, as ordered, and report abnormal findings.
    Rationale: Constant checking of various factors and reporting them is a means of preventing complications or treating them immediately.
11. Maintain accurate record of intake and output to monitor fluid balance.
    Rationale: Intake and output records are important documentation for observance of early occurrences of complications.

12. Weigh client daily and record.
Rationale: Consistent record keeping helps the nurse compare and observe for complications.
13. Inspect dressing once a shift for drainage and intactness. Change whenever loose or moist and at least every 48 hours.
Rationale: Intact and dry dressings help prevent infection and keep client comfortable.

Procedure

Changing TPN Tubing and Dressing

1. Wash your hands.
Rationale: transmission of microorganisms is reduced with clean hands.
2. Cross-check new hyperalimentation solutions with physician's order. Check expiration date.
Note: TPN must be used within 24 hours of preparation.
3. Attach sterile tubing and filter to new parenteral hyperalimentation solutions.
4. Prime tubing as you would a conventional IV.
5. Place client in supine position.
Rationale: Position decreases pressure in vena cava to reduce risk of air embolism when catheter is disconnected.
6. Don a mask. Instruct client to turn head facing opposite direction of insertion site and not to cough or talk during dressing change.
Note: Place mask on client if he or she cannot cooperate.
Rationale: Insertion site and catheter must be protected from microorganisms from the nurse or client's nose and mouth.
7. Don gloves.
Rationale: Gloves protect nurse from secretions.
8. Remove old dressing and discard carefully.
9. Inspect insertion site for redness, drainage, swelling.
10. Remove gloves.
11. Wash your hands.
12. Open sterile supplies and place on bedside table.
13. Put on sterile gloves.
Rationale: This is a sterile procedure.
14. Cleanse insertion site with gauze soaked in 10% acetone. Wipe in circular motion, moving from the insertion site outward.
Rationale: Acetone removes old adhesive tape and defats the skin.
Note: Keep acetone from contacting catheter, because it could break down the plastic.
15. Cleanse site with same circular motion for 2 minutes using povidone-iodine solution (Betadine). Allow to air dry.
Rationale: Betadine has antimicrobial properties to reduce the number of microorganisms at the catheter insertion site.
16. Cleanse connection of catheter and tubing with Betadine.
17. Hospital policy may dictate cleansing Betadine off skin with alcohol.
18. Apply Betadine ointment to insertion site.
Rationale: Betadine provides long-term antimicrobial action.
19. Loosen tubing at catheter hub.
20. Ask client to hold breath and bear down (Valsalva) while you quickly disconnect old tubing and attach new tubing to catheter hub.
Rationale: The Valsalva maneuver increases pressure on large veins in chest and reduces chance of air embolism when catheter is open.
21. Tape all connections.
Rationale: Taping prevents accidental disconnection of tubing.
22. Place transparent, semipermeable dressing over insertion site. Optional: Paint skin margins with tincture of benzoin before placing dressing to ensure a tighter seal.
Rationale: Transparent dressing is preferred so insertion site can be easily assess without disrupting or manipulating dressing.
23. Loop and tape tubing next to dressing.
24. Label dressing and tubing with date and your name.
Rationale: Coworkers must be able to double-check care provided.
25. Adjust flow rate per physician's order.
Rationale: Physician's order is specific to this client.
26. Discard used solution and tubing. Remove gloves. Document amount infused on intake and output record.

Procedure

Administering Intralipids

1. Check solution against physician's order. Inspect solution for separation of emulsion into layers or for froth. Do not use if present.
Rationale: Solution is spoiled if it does not appear normal.
2. Wash your hands.
Rationale: Clean hands help prevent spread of microorganisms.
3. Attach fat emulsion tubing to bottle. Prime tubing as for a conventional IV.
Rationale: Tubing has no in-line filter that would cause separation of the emulsion.
4. Place 19- or 21-gauge 1-in needle on distal end of tubing.
5. Identify client.
Rationale: Correct client identification is important in any nursing care.

(continued)

6. Identify Y-port on hyperalimentation tubing (below in-line filter).
7. Cleanse Y-port with antiseptic swab. Allow to dry. Insert needle into port. secure with tape.
   Note: Lipids can be infused into a peripheral IV.
8. Adjust flow rate to infuse at 1.0 mL/min for adults and 0.1 mL/min for children. Infuse at this rate for 30 minutes while you monitor the client and vital signs every 10 minutes.
   Note: If any adverse reactions occur, stop infusion and notify physician.
9. If no adverse reactions occur, adjust flow rate:
   a. Adults: 500 mL intralipid over 4 to 6 hours.
   b. Children: up to 1 g/kg over 4 hours.

Lifespan Considerations

Infants and Children

- TPN solutions for children generally start with a 10% dextrose solution, increased to 25% dextrose. Exogenous insulin is usually not needed, because a child's pancreas adapts easily to higher glucose levels. TPN solutions also usually contain higher concentrations of calcium, phosphorus, magnesium, and vitamins.
- Children are usually more active than adults and require frequent assessment of the tubing to prevent disconnections or obstruction during ambulation or play.
- Instruct parents on preventing accidental disconnection or obstruction of tubing.
- Soft restraints may be necessary to prevent the child from pulling out the catheter. Provide play therapy, books, and stimulation to distract the child.

Home-Care Modifications

- The healthcare team must determine that the client or a guardian is responsible and able to be present during therapy.
- Identify and consult with a home health nurse who can be available 24 hours a day to troubleshoot complications.
- A long-term infusion device, such as a Hickman or Groshung catheter, should be in place before the client's discharge.
- The client or caregiver must be taught how to initiate, monitor, and maintain an IV catheter and infusion according to the above protocol.
- The client usually is weighed daily. Intake and output are recorded. Blood values are monitored at least every other week.

plications include infection, fluid overload, and hyperglycemia.

Pneumothorax can occur if the lung is punctured during insertion of the central venous line. Presenting symptoms include chest or shoulder pain, sudden shortness of breath, tachycardia, and absence of breath sounds on the affected side.

Air embolism, or the introduction of air into the vascular system, can occur when the catheter is introduced or if air is introduced into the line at any time. Having the client perform the Valsalva maneuver when the line is inserted or whenever the system is disconnected reduces the risk of air embolism. Tubing should be connected with luer locks to prevent accidental separation, and the client should take care not to pull on or dislodge tubing when moving.

Infection is a potentially serious complication of TPN (Wickham, Purl, & Walker, 1992). TPN is a glucose-rich solution that rapidly supports microbial growth (*Candida*). Use strict aseptic technique during catheter manipulations, dressing changes, and tubing and bottle changes. Institutional protocol determines the frequency and technique to be used for routine care of the site and tubing. The insertion site is frequently assessed (Fig. 26-17). Inflammation at the site and presence of fever usually necessitate catheter removal. The catheter tip should be cultured after removal. Use of a multiple-lumen cannula enables the client to receive TPN simultaneously with other medications (ie, antibiotics).

Fluid overload can occur if the osmotic solution is infused too quickly, drawing fluid into the circulatory system. This risk is especially high for clients who have a history of congestive heart failure and cannot tolerate rapid fluid shifts. TPN infusion should always be

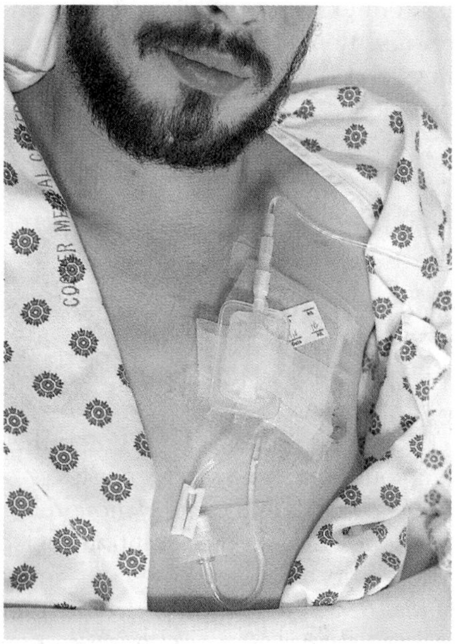

Figure 26-17 • *The nurse assesses the insertion site regularly for signs of inflammation.*

regulated by an EID to avoid sudden shifts in fluid rate. Monitor daily weights and intake and output.

Metabolic complications also may present a problem for the client receiving TPN. Metabolic complications, causes, prevention, and treatment are highlighted in Table 26-1.

Community-Based Nursing

Many clients continue treatment for fluid and electrolyte imbalances in the home (Wood, 1991). If so, the client and family members must be taught the principles of infusion therapy, including proper management of the fluids and how to use the equipment to regulate flow rate. It is important to teach the client and the family about potential complications of IV therapy. A plan for what to do if equipment malfunctions or problems with IV therapy develop should be in place, and telephone numbers for the supplier and nurse should be provided. Developing hypothetical problems that could occur and asking the client what could be done is a good method of evaluating problem-solving abilities and skills.

Clients on long-term TPN receive their solutions in the privacy of their place of residence with the support of home infusion providers (Smith, Moushey, Ross, &

Table 26-1 • Potential Metabolic Complications Associated With Total Parenteral Nutrition

Cause(s)	Prevention	Treatment
Hyperglycemia		
Carbohydrate intolerance → too rapid infusion of TPN Insulin resistance → stress, sepsis, diabetes	Urine S/A q8h. Accuchecks q6h. Be aware of meds that may cause glucose intolerance (ie, steroids). Start TPN infusion slowly.	Decrease TPN rate or dextrose concentration of solution. Add insulin to the solution or use sliding scale insulin coverage. Add lipids daily to prescription.
Hypoglycemia		
Interruption of TPN infusion Excessive insulin administration	Wean or slow down TPN infusion when stopping. Hang 10% D/W at same rate of TPN if unable to hang TPN. Maintain infusion rate; use an EID. Monitor urine/serum glucose levels.	Hang 10% D/W at same rate of TPN if unable to hang TPN. Give IV glucose STAT. 50% dextrose may be needed. Maintain proper flow rate.
Hyperglycemic Hyperosmolar Nonketotic coma		
Untreated glucose intolerance; which causes hyperosmolar diuresis, electrolyte imbalances, coma, death (40% mortality rate)	Monitor glucose appropriately. Perform frequent chemistry profiles to assess electrolytes, osmolarity.	Discontinue TPN insulin as needed. Correct electrolyte imbalances. Treat with hypotonic saline solution.
Hyperkalemia		
Excessive potassium replacement Renal disease—potassium cannot be excreted Leakage of potassium from cells following severe trauma	Monitor serum potassium. Anticipate that a sodium deficiency may lead to hyperkalemia. Start TPN in stable clients. Determine accurate I & O to evaluate fluid balance.	Stop or decrease potassium in solution. Monitor pulse for changes (bradycardia). In severe hyperkalemia, dialysis may be necessary.
Hypokalemia		
Excessive potassium losses (increase GI losses following diarrhea) Diuretic therapy Large doses of insulin	Monitor serum potassium. Anticipate potential potassium depletion with large GI losses. Monitor I & O. Be aware of drugs that cause excessive potassium loss. Be aware that clients severely malnourished are susceptible (refeeding syndrome).	Add potassium to TPN solution. May need additional IVPB potassium run over 4–6 h to correct severe deficiency. Monitor pulse for tachycardia or arrythmia. Monitor for metabolic alkalosis (potassium loss may cause retention).

(continued)

Table 26-1 *(continued)*

Cause(s)	Prevention	Treatment
Hypernatremia		
Dehydration Diarrhea Diabetes insipidus Excessive replacement	Continue monitoring I & O Monitor serum sodium. Be aware of drugs that cause sodium retention (ie, steroids).	Provide salt-free solution until corrected. Provide enough free water to meet needs. Treat or correct cause (ie, diarrhea).
Hyponatremia		
Diuretics GI loss (vomiting or fistula) Disease states (ie, renal failure/cirrhosis)	Determine accurate I & O. Determine urine-specific gravity. Perform accurate weights (to ensure fluid shifts).	Give 3%–5% sodium chloride IV. Add sodium to TPN solution. Minimize GI loss (ie, vomiting if possible with medication).
Hyperphosphatemia		
Renal insufficiency Excessive replacement	Determine accurate I & O. Determine specific gravity. Perform urine S/A help to access renal function.	Add low or nor phosphate. Switch to renal failure formula.
Hypophosphatemia		
Insulin therapy Disease states Alcoholism Respiratory alkalosis Renal problems Severe diarrhea Malabsorption associated with low calcium and low magnesium levels	Monitor chemistry profile. Be aware of potential disease states that cause low phosphate levels.	Replace phosphate in TPN. Replace calcium as needed (repletion may cause calcium to drop).
Hypercalcemia		
Pancreatitis in inactive/immobile client Excessive replacement	Monitor serum level. Be aware of potential problems in immobile client.	Decrease calcium replacement in TPN.
Hypocalcemia		
Vitamin D deficiency Insufficient replacement Pancreatitis Hypomagnesia hypophosphatemia	Monitor serum levels. Be aware of disease states, medications, malnutrition; can cause hypophosphatemia.	Replace by adding calcium to TPN; may require IVPB of calcium to correct severe deficiency; also must correct phosphate/magnesia to correct calcium.
Metabolic acidosis		
Renal insufficiency Diabetic ketoacidosis Diarrhea Ureteral diversions Lactic acidosis (shock) Potassium excess	Monitor CO_2, potassium, sodium. To assess kidney function, determine accurate I & O, specific gravity, urine S/A.	Give bicarbonate. Monitor vital signs. Decrease potassium in TPN solution to control diarrhea.
Metabolic alkalosis		
Body fluid losses (vomiting) Potassium deficit Chloride deficit	Monitor serum, CO_2, potassium, chloride.	Give ammonium chloride to replace chloride/potassium. Monitor vital signs. Control vomiting if possible.

S/A, sugar/acetone; I & O, daily intake and output; GI, gastrointestinal; IVPB, IV piggyback.
From Weinstein S. M. (1993). *Plumer's principles and practice of intravenous therapy,* 5th ed. Philadelphia, J. B. Lippincott.

Home Health Record

Guidelines For Patient TPN Home Health Record

This form will be available to the Home Health Nurse to help monitor patient's progress.

1. Patient's name.
2. Enter date daily.
3. Enter weight daily (same time).
4. Enter temperature reading twice a day.
5. Enter urine results (if appropriate) per physician's order.
6. Enter blood sugar value (if appropriate) per physician's order.
7. Enter amount of TPN infused.
8. Enter rate/amount of lipids infused.
9. Enter oral intake.
10. Enter urine output.
11. Enter other output.
12. Enter stool frequency/consistency.
13. Note dressing change by a check mark in the box. Indicate appearance of site by use of the key letter:
    C = clean/dry
    R = red
    D = drainage
    P = pain
    S = swelling
    L = loose
14. Enter information as noted in parentheses.
15. Enter any other situations/problems not addressed.
16. Save this record for Home Health Nurse.

Name:							
Date:							
Weight: _____lbs. _____kg.							
Temperature: a.m.							
p.m.							
Urine: A							
Sugar and acetone M							
P							
M							
Blood Sugar:							
Intake Rate/amount of TPN infused (cc's/24 hours)							
Lipids							
Albumin							
Antibiotics							
Oral fluid intake/24 hours (Total cc's)							
Output - Urine Other output (cc's) Type							
Stool frequency/ consistency L/F							
Dressing changed/site: C = clean/dry R = red D = drainage P = pain S = swelling L = loose							
General: (include problems, appetite, how you feel, foods eaten, supply problems, etc.)							

Figure 26-18. *Sample of a home health report to be used in TPN, with guidelines for use. (Courtesy of Midwestern Regional Medical Center, Zion IL.)*

Griffen, 1993). Clients are taught how to keep a record in their own home (Fig. 26-18). As with any IV therapy, a plan of action must be in place for inadvertent problems, and the name of the supplier and nurse must be readily available.

Explaining to the client during teaching the symptoms that need to be relayed to the physician is an important part of healthcare planning. For example, some physicians may want to be informed if the client gains more than 5 lb or has vomiting or diarrhea that lasts for more than 1 day. All client teaching is beneficial in preventing future occurrences of fluid and electrolyte imbalances.

Key Concepts

- Homeostasis of body fluids, electrolytes, and nutrition may need to be supported through the use of IV therapy or TPN.
- States of altered fluid balance include fluid volume excess or fluid volume deficit and can be managed through either short-term or long-term IV therapy.
- Important nursing interventions include client teaching and initiating, regulating, monitoring, and discontinuing an IV infusion.
- Height of the bottle, position of the extremity, position of the catheter in the vein, and patency of the catheter and tubing are all factors that can affect the infusion rate.
- Potential complications of IV therapy include infiltration, phlebitis, infection, air embolism, and fluid overload.
- Blood transfusions are administered to restore circulating volume, to improve oxygen-carrying capacity of the blood, to restore coagulation factors, and to increase white blood cell count to decrease the risk of infection.
- To prevent serious adverse reactions from blood administration, careful screening and matching of donor and recipient blood are necessary.

Critical Thinking Challenges

You have added IV therapy to your growing knowledge base of clinical skills and client care. Now turn to the situation at the beginning of the chapter, and consider the following.

1. *Describe further assessment steps you will take.*
2. *List the factors to check in the infusion system, and give rationale.*
3. *Identify other information you want to know about this IV therapy.*
4. *Outline potential problems that may exist in this situation.*
5. *Given your answers to the above, clarify how you will proceed.*

References

Baranowski, L. (1992) Current trends in blood component therapy: The evolution of a safer, more effective product. *Journal of Intravenous Nursing, 15*(3), 136–151.

Metheny, N. (1992) *Fluid and electrolyte balance: Nursing considerations* (2nd ed.). Philadelphia: J.B. Lippincott.

Querin, J. J., & Stahl, L. D. (1990). 12 simple sensible steps for successful blood transfusions. *Nursing, 20*(10), 68–81.

Shivnan, J. C., McGuire, D., Freedman, S., Sharkazy, E., Bosserman, G., Larson, E., & Grouleff, P. (1991). A comparison of transparent adherent and dry sterile gauze dressings for long-term central catheters in patients undergoing bone marrow transplant. *Oncology Nursing Forum, 18*(8), 1349–1356.

Smith, C. E., Moushey, L., Ross, J. A., & Gieffer, C. (1993). Responsibilities and reactions of family caregivers of patients dependent on total parenteral nutrition at home. *Public Health Nursing, 19*(2), 122–128.

Taylor, M. (1994a). Total parenteral nutrition (Part 1). *Nursing Standard, 8*(23), 25–28.

Taylor, M. (1994b). Total parenteral nutrition (Part 2). *Nursing Standard, 8*(24), 37–39.

Weinstein, S. M. (1993). *Plumer's principles and practice of intravenous therapy* (5th ed.). Philadelphia: J.B. Lippincott.

Wickham, R., Purl, S., & Walker, D. (1992). Long-term central venous catheters: Issues for care. *Seminars in Oncology Nursing, 8*(2), 133–147.

Wood, S. (1991) Extending the principle of self-care. Intravenous therapy in the community. *Professional Nurse, 6*(9), 543–549.

Bibliography

Corbett, K., Meehan, L., & Sackey, V. (1993). A strategy to enhance skills. Developing intravenous therapy skills for community nursing. *Professional Nurse, 9*(1), 60–63.

Dugger, B. (1993) Competency for intravenous nursing practice. *Journal of Intravenous Nursing, 16*(5), 293–298.

Green, S. L. (1991). Practical guidelines for developing an office-based program for outpatient intravenous therapy. *Review of Infectious Diseases 13*(Suppl. 2), S189–S192.

Intravenous Nurses Society, Inc. (1992). Revised standards of practice. *Journal of Intravenous Nursing*, September(Suppl.).

Paglione, M. A. (1991). Training home health nurses in IV therapy: A collaborative effort. *Home Healthcare Nurse, 9*(2), 23–27.

Porth, C. M. (1994). *Pathophysiology: Concepts of altered health states* (4th ed.). Philadelphia: J.B. Lippincott.

Ryder, M. A. (1993) Peripherally inserted central venous catheters. *Nursing Clinics of North America, 28*(4), 937–971.

Terrell, F., & Williams, B. (1993). Implementation of a customized needleless intravenous delivery system. *Journal of Intravenous Nursing, 16*(6), 339–344.

Woods, S., Sivarajan-Froelicher, E., Halpenny, J., & Motzer, S. (1995). *Cardiac nursing* (3rd ed.). Philadelphia: J.B. Lippincott.

Medication Administration

Key Terms	Learning Objectives

Key Terms

Absorption
Buccal
Distribution
Drug
Excretion
Intradermal
Intramuscular
Intravenous
Medication
Metabolism
Pharmacodynamics
Pharmacokinetics
Subcutaneous
Sublingual
Transdermal

Learning Objectives

Upon completion of this chapter, the student will be able to do the following:

- *Describe essential components in a drug order.*
- *Discuss pharmacokinetic principles of drug action.*
- *Describe variables that affect drug action.*
- *List the five rights of proper drug administration.*
- *Calculate proper drug dosage from different systems of drug measurement.*
- *Discuss important assessment information concerning medication to obtain from the client on admission and before medication administration.*
- *Individualize a teaching plan to improve client compliance.*
- *List two nursing diagnoses for the client managing self-medications.*
- *Describe recommended guidelines and procedures for oral, subcutaneous, and intramuscular medication administration.*

27

You are making a nursing visit to an older woman in her apartment in a retirement facility. She was recently discharged from the hospital where she was treated for a gastric ulcer secondary to the pain medications she was taking for arthritis. During your initial conversation, you inquire about her health. She appears distracted and seems to have difficulty following your questions and giving you answers. As you ask her about her current medications, her responses indicate that she is unsure about what they are for and how to take them. When you ask her to show you her medications, she produces a large plastic container with about 10 bottles: two bottles of a diuretic labeled "Take two tablets twice a day," three bottles of potassium chloride labeled "Take five tablets a day in divided doses," one bottle of a histamine blocker labeled "Take one capsule daily," one bottle of analgesic containing oxycodone to take "prn arthritis pain," one bottle of extra-strength acetaminophen, one bottle of stool softener capsules to take "as needed," and one bottle of another analgesic containing codeine. As you inquire again about which medications she takes and when, you learn that she has age-related macular degeneration and is legally blind.

In previous chapters, you learned about health and wellness, lifespan development, health assessment, and client teaching among other topics. Adding the medication administration information in this chapter to your knowledge base may better prepare you for thoughtfully and skillfully handling situations such as the older woman in the nursing home. Use the Critical Thinking Challenges at the end of the chapter to help you apply the new information.

The nurse's role in administering medications has become increasingly complex and diversified. Administering the correct medication and dosage by the specified route, using proper technique, and taking appropriate precautions was once all that was expected of the nurse. Today these important functions constitute only part of safe medication administration; the level of knowledge and skill now demanded of the nurse is much broader. In addition to delivering pills and giving injections, the nurse must observe and interpret the client's response to therapy and recognize medication incompatibilities and interactions. The nurse needs to know about the actions and side effects of medications and about the moral, ethical, and legal aspects of drug therapy. The nurse must be familiar with sources of medication information and know when and how to use them. Finally, the nurse must be able to recognize unsafe or unclear medication orders and know what to do when such an order is encountered.

This chapter discusses general principles of medication administration. Its purpose is not to provide information about specific drugs, but to identify the essential prerequisite knowledge the nurse must have to administer drugs safely to clients. Legal aspects of medication administration are considered, and a brief description of pharmacokinetics, or drug action, is presented. Finally, various aspects of assessment, preparation and administration of medications, and client teaching are discussed.

Drugs and Medications

The term drug is often used interchangeably with medication, but there is a specific difference between them. A **drug** is any substance that alters physiologic function, with the potential for affecting health. A **medication** is a drug administered for its therapeutic effects. Thus, all medications are drugs, but not all drugs are medications. To administer medications effectively and safely, the nurse must possess a broad range of general and specific knowledge.

Names of Drugs

Medications or drugs can be known by several names. The **chemical name** of a medication describes the constituents that make up its molecular structure. It describes in chemist's terms the placement of atoms or atomic groupings. An example of a chemical name is that of the anti-inflammatory agent ibuprofen, that is, 2-(4 isobutylphenyl) propinoic acid.

The **generic name** is the name assigned by the manufacturer before a new medication becomes official. This name is simpler than the chemical name, from which it is often derived. Examples of medications known by their generic names include morphine sulfate, cephradine, and ethacrynic acid.

The **official name** is the name under which a medication is listed in one of the official Food and Drug Administration (FDA) publications, such as the *National Formulary* or *United States Pharmacopeia*.

The brand name or **trade name** is a registered name assigned by the manufacturer. Brand names are proper nouns; their first letter is capitalized, and they are marked with a circled R. Some medications are manufactured by several companies and so may be known by several different brand names. An example is ampicillin sodium (official name); this drug is marketed under the names Omnipen-N, Polycillin-N, SK Ampicillin-N, and Totacillin-N.

Types and Forms of Drugs

Medications are classified in many ways, for example, according to their clinical composition, clinical actions, or therapeutic effect on body systems. For example, some agents used to fight cancer cells are known by the general classification, antineoplastic (ie, anticancer) agents. Drugs that open bronchial tubes narrowed by asthma are called bronchodilators. Each broad medication category has a set of characteristics common to all drugs within the classification. By understanding general drug classifications, it is easier to learn about the actions, side effects, and precautions needed for unfamiliar drugs. Table 27-1 lists classes of medications used to support or improve functional abilities.

Medications are prepared in various forms. Pills and powders, liquids for drinking or injection, suppositories, creams, ointments, and inhalants are some of the forms in which medications are manufactured. Table 27-2 lists different drug preparations.The most desirable form of medication for any client is determined by the disease process being treated, the age of the client, the ability of the client to swallow, the availability of personnel trained in special techniques of administration, and the amount of medication that must be delivered; these are only some of the factors that must be considered when deciding on appropriate medication forms. In addition, the same medication may be prepared in different dosage concentrations. Because of the wide range of available medication forms and dosages, the nurse needs to pay close attention to the medication order and administer the specified form.

Sources of Information About Medications

A fundamental rule of safe drug administration is "never administer an unfamiliar medication." Before giving any drug, the nurse must first understand the condition of the client for whom a medication is ordered. This knowledge combined with knowledge of the ordered medication explains why (and whether) the medication is appropriate for that client. The nurse should be familiar with dosage ranges of the medication being given, the expected therapeutic effects, and possible adverse actions.

Making a habit of consulting standard drug reference materials is a way to stay up-to-date on medications, dosage, purpose, administation, and side effects. Some standard references include drug manufacturer's package inserts or brochures, which provide detailed data on the product contained in a packaged unit.

The Physician's Desk Reference (Medical Economics, Montvale, NJ) details a medication or class of medications. *The American Medical Association Drug Evaluations* is a less comprehensive compendium of more than 1,300 monographs of separate medications and

Table 27-1 • Classes of Medications to Promote Normal Function

Health Pattern	Drug Class	Action
Activity and exercise	Antihypertensives	Decreases blood pressure
	Antiarrhythmics	Regulates heart rhythm
	Inotropes	Strengthens cardiac contraction
	Antianginals	Increases coronary blood flow
	Anticoagulants	Decreases clot formation
	Bronchodilators	Opens airways
Nutrition and metabolism	Antibiotics	Decreases or prevents infection
	Antiemetics	Decreases nausea
	Antacids	Decreases gastric acidity
	Insulin	Decreases blood glucose levels
	Corticosteroids	Decreases inflammation
	Thyroid	Regulates metabolic rate
	Vitamins and minerals	Supplements inadequate dietary intake
Elimination	Laxatives	Promotes stool evacuation
	Antidiarrheals	Decreases diarrhea
	Diuretics	Increases urine production
Sleep and rest	Sedatives, hypnotics	Induces sleep
Cognition and perception	Analgesics	Decreases pain
	Antipsychotics	Decreases psychotic symptoms (eg, hallucinations)
Coping and stress tolerance	Antianxiety agents	Decreases anxiety
	Antidepressants	Decreases depression
Sexuality and reproduction	Ovarian hormones	Provides hormone replacement Provides birth control

Table 27-2 • Drug Preparations

Type of Preparation	Description
Oral Preparations	
Capsule	Gelatinous container to hold powder or liquid medicine
Elixir	Liquid preparation of medication with alcohol base
Emulsion	Suspension within an oil base
Enteric coated	Coating that causes drug absorption in intestines rather than the stomach, which may be irritated by the drug
Lozenge (troche)	Tablet held in the mouth to be dissolved
Powder	Finely ground drug; frequently mixed with liquid before administration
Spansule	Timed-release drug capsule, which dissolves more slowly to provide an effect over a long period
Suspension	Medication in liquid, which must be shaken before administration because it separates
Syrup	Medicine dissolved in sugar and water
Tablet	Compressed hard disk of powdered medication; may be scored for easy breaking; may be sugar-coated or have film coating for cohesion
Tincture	Potent solution with alcohol base made from plants; dosage usually small
Topical Preparations	
Cream	Nongreasy, semisolid preparation for topical application
Gel or jelly	Translucent or clear semisolid substance that liquefies when applied to the skin
Liniment	Oily liquid used on the skin
Lotion	Emollient liquid; may be clear solution or suspension, which is applied to the skin
Ointment	Drug combined with oil base for external application
Paste	Thick ointment used for local application to the skin
Suppository	Medicine contained within a gelatinous base (shaped for easy insertion into the body), which dissolves at body temperature, slowly releasing the drug
Transdermal patch	Medicine in a patch, which, when applied to the skin, permits gradual, controlled absorption

compounds. *The American Hospital Formulary Service,* available by subscription from the American Society of Hospital Pharmacists, Washington, DC, publishes individual monographs on single generic medications and groups of medications. The drug information is organized by pharmacologic properties, and the medications are indexed by common brand names, generic name, and therapeutic class. Medication forms most commonly used by hospitals also are listed.

The latest developments in medication therapy are published in current journals, such as the *American Journal of Nursing* and *RN* magazine. In addition, monthly newsletters, such as *Nurses' Drug Alert* and *Medical Letter,* are useful.

Many hospital pharmacies also provide newsletters with up-to-date information about medication side effects and interactions and new medications. Information about specific medications that emphasizes nursing implications also can be obtained in nursing reference guides and textbooks, and computerized drug information systems and resources are becoming more available as well (Shumway, Jacknowitz, & Abate, 1990).

Medication Standards

Because medications may vary, the standards guiding medication quality are usually established and controlled by the government. The official list of medications in the United States is contained in two texts, the *United States Pharmacopeia* (USP) and the *National Formulary* (NF). The corresponding Canadian publication is the *British Pharmacopeia.* The USP and NF describe medication products according to their source, physical and chemical properties, tests for purity and identity, method of storage, category, and normal dosages. Both references provide invaluable information for practicing nurses.

Medications may vary according to their properties: purity, potency, bioavailability, efficacy, and safety and toxicity. Medication standards must provide an appropriate range of quality for these properties.

Systems of Medication Distribution

Three types of systems are used to ensure the safe storage and administration of medications: the stock supply, the unit dose supply, and the self-administered supply. Each of these distribution systems varies among institutions depending on their procedures and policies.

Hospitals have designated areas for medication preparation. Some institutions have a central room with locked cupboards containing supplies, whereas others may use mobile medication carts with locked drawers or locked wall cabinets near the clients' rooms. Other institutions have satellite pharmacy units that are located on a particular floor that serve several client-care areas. In accordance with narcotic control laws, narcotic medications are kept in locked drawers in all client-care areas.

Stock Supply. A stock supply system in a client-care area provides large quantities of frequently prescribed medications for that particular unit; these are stored in locked cupboards in a storage room. Individual doses are dispensed and administered by nurses, who measure individual doses from the large stock bottles or packaged containers. Examples of stock supply medications are narcotics and saline solutions.

Unit Dose. A unit dose system involves the pharmacy in prepackaging and prelabeling an individual client dose. This individual unit dose is a prescribed amount of medication dispensed at a specified time.

This type of system is gaining popularity because it provides a double-check mechanism, ensuring client safety. Pharmacists and nurses both participate in administering medications and evaluating their effects. The pharmacist can provide information to the nurse about potential medication interactions or contraindications. This system also saves valuable nursing time.

Self-Administered Medications. The self-administered medication (SAM) system supplies each client with his or her prescribed doses and quantities for a given period. Each medication is supplied in a separate container and is used for one client only. Medications can be stored at the client's bedside, allowing the client to administer his or her own medications. The SAM system can be used along with the stock or unit dose systems. For example, a client may have sublingual nitroglycerin supplied by the SAM system and other medications supplied by the unit dose system. This combination allows the nitroglycerin to be used immediately if chest pain occurs.

Moreover, this method of administration allows the client a greater opportunity to be involved in his or her own care. It also decreases the time the nurse spends administering medications.

Nonprescription and Prescription Medications

Nonprescription Medications. Many medications can be obtained without a written order (prescription) from a healthcare provider. They are sold over the counter (OTC) because they are generally regarded as safe enough for use without medical or nursing supervision. Common examples of OTC drugs include cold remedies and mild analgesics, such as aspirin. Control over the safety, effectiveness, and advertising of nonprescription medications is maintained by the FDA.

Nonprescription medications are considered safe when used as directed. The dangers of these readily available medications lie in their misuse, which can result in dangerous side effects. Overuse can cause cumulative drug effects. Some people persist in self-medicating with nonprescription drugs and delay seeking professional help, which can result in a minor problem developing into a major one because of early mistreatment. There also is danger of serious drug interactions. The nurse must determine which (if any) nonprescription medications the client has been taking and ensure that no medications are taken without the healthcare provider's knowledge.

Prescription Medications. For some clients, the narrow margin of safety between a therapeutic and toxic dose of a medication requires close monitoring. These medications require medical supervision and must be obtained with a formal written order. A prescription is a legal order for the preparation and administration of a medication. Healthcare providers and dentists are legally responsible for prescribing therapeutic agents. In some states, nurse practitioners and physician's assistants may prescribe some medications.

Components of a Drug Order

The healthcare provider conveys an order by specifying the name of the client, the name of the medication, amount and frequency of the dose, and the route of administration. Included with this directive is the date and time the prescription was written and the signature of the prescribing healthcare provider. In most hospitals or healthcare agencies, orders are written on a form specifically intended for the healthcare provider's orders. These orders are a permanent part of the client's medical record. The client's first and last name must be written with the medication order to avoid confusion between two clients with the same last name. The client's identification or admission number can be written with the order as further identification.

The month, day, year, and time also are part of the written order (eg, 1/19/95; 9 AM). The time should include the abbreviation AM or PM to eliminate confusion between morning and afternoon times. Some institutions use military time or the 24-hour clock (eg, midnight = 0000 hours, 6 PM = 1800 hours). Including the time on the written order also clarifies when certain orders (eg, narcotics) automatically terminate.

Abbreviations are commonly used in the medication order. Certain standard abbreviations indicate the amount and frequency of a medication dosage; these abbreviations are legal and can be used in the client's chart. The more commonly used abbreviations are listed in Table 27-3.

Medication Name. The name of the medication can be written in most settings using the generic or trade

Table 27-3 • Common Abbreviations Used in Medication Orders

Abbreviation	Meaning	Abbreviation	Meaning
a or a.	before	mg	milligram
a.c.	before meals	no.	number
ad lib	as desired	noct.	night
alt. h.	alternate hours	OD	right eye
AM	in the morning; before noon	os	mouth
A.D.	right ear	OS	left eye
A.S.	left ear	OU	both eyes
A.U.	each ear	oz	ounce
aq.	water	p or p.	after; per
b.i.d.	twice a day	p.c.	after meals
c̄	with	per os, PO	by mouth
cap., caps.	capsule	PM	afternoon; evening
cc	cubic centimeter	prn	as needed, according to necessity
d	day	q.	each, every
D/C, dc	discontinue	q.h.	every hour
dil.	dilute	q.i.d.	four times a day
dist.	distilled	q.1 h	every one hour
DS	double strength	q.2 h.	every two hours
EC	enteric coated	q.3 h.	every three hours
elix.	elixir	q.4 h.	every four hours
et	and	q.6 h.	every six hours
ext.	external, extract	q.8 h.	every eight hours
fl, fld	fluid	q.12 h.	every twelve hours
g	gram	q.o.d.	every other day
gr	grain	q.s.	as much as needed, quantity sufficient
gtt	drop	qt	quart
H	hypodermic	R. or PR	rectally, per rectum
h., hr	hour	Rx	take, prescription
h.s.	at bedtime	s	without
IM	intramuscular	sc	subcutaneously
inj.	injection	sol. or soln.	solution
IV	intravenous	SQ	subcutaneous
IVPB	IV piggy back	stat.	immediately, at once
kg	kilogram	tab.	tablet
L	liter	tbsp, T	tablespoon
lb	pound	t.i.d.	three times a day
liq.	liquid	tinct., tr	tincture
mcg, μg	microgram	tsp, t	teaspoon
mEq	milliequivalent	ung.	ointment

name. The name should be written clearly, because many medications are similar in spelling but different in drug action. When the medication name is not clear, the healthcare provider should be contacted for clarification.

Medication Dosage. Medication dosage can be written in the metric, apothecary, or household measurement systems. The strength and frequency of the dose also is indicated. If a medication is dispensed in only one dose, the healthcare provider may indicate the number of tablets or pills to be taken. Two examples of these directives are digoxin 0.25 mg once a day or Isocal (1/2 strength) 240 mL three times a day.

Route of Administration. The route of administration is commonly abbreviated as a part of the written order. Many medications can be given by several routes (eg, orally [PO], intravenously [IV], intramuscularly [IM]). If an order specifies a certain route for medication administration and the client's condition changes, making the ordered route inappropriate or possibly unsafe, the nurse must notify the healthcare provider so that the route of administration can be changed.

Signature. Because the written order is a legal request, the signature of the healthcare provider must follow the written order. An unsigned order is invalid and should not be carried out until the healthcare provider signs the order.

Types of Orders

Standing Order. The standing order is a directive that should be carried out for a specified number of days or until another order cancels it. In many hospitals or healthcare agencies, the standing orders must be reviewed and rewritten within a specified time frame, or they are canceled automatically.

PRN Orders. A prn (from the Latin *pro re nata*) order does not indicate a specific time for administering a medication; rather, it states guidelines so that the medication can be administered *as it is needed.* Pain medications, nausea medications, and laxatives are often ordered on a prn basis. This directive requires the nurse to use good judgment as to when a medication is needed and when it is safe to administer.

One-Time Order. The one-time or single order is written for a medication that will be given only once. A preoperative medication, to help calm the client and dry secretions before surgery, is an example of a one-time order.

Stat Order. A stat order (from the Latin *statim,* "immediately") is a single order for a medication that must be given immediately. An example of this order is furosemide 20 mg IV stat.

Telephone and Verbal Orders. At times the nurse and healthcare provider may discuss a client's condition over the phone and decide to change the client's medication regimen. Because the healthcare provider is not available to write and sign the order, the nurse may write the order on the healthcare provider's order sheet. This type of order is usually designated on the sheet as a "TO (telephone order) by Dr. –" and signed by the nurse. To ensure accuracy, the nurse needs to repeat the order to the healthcare provider before writing it down. The order must be cosigned by the healthcare provider within a specified time, usually 48 hours. Similar rules apply to verbal orders.

Systems of Drug Measurement

Calculation of medication dosages requires a knowledge of the three systems of measurement: metric, apothecary, and household. All three systems are used in North America, although the metric system is used with increasing frequency.

Metric System

Introduced in Europe in the late 18th century, the metric system is widely used throughout the world. The United States uses all three systems but has been committed to converting to the metric system since 1975. The USP uses only the metric system for weights and measures.

The metric system is based on the decimal system, which is organized in units of tens. The basic units can be multiplied or divided to form secondary units or subdivisions. Multiples are calculated by moving the decimal to the right and division by moving the decimal to the left.

The basic units used in the metric system include the liter (L), volume of fluids; the gram (g), weight of solids; and the meter (m), measure of length. The subdivisions of the metric basic unit, derived from Latin, are designated with prefixes as follows: deci (1/10 or 0.1 of the unit), centi (1/100 or 0.01 of the unit), and milli (1/1000 or 0.001 of the unit). Multiples of the metric basic unit, derived from Greek, are designated with prefixes as follows: deka (10 times the unit), hecto (100 times the unit), and kilo (1,000 times the unit).

Metric equivalents, in volume and weight, are used in medication administration and are listed in Table 27-4. The meter is not used to compute dosage of medication; rather, it is used for measurements related to the area of a client's body (abdominal girth, calf circumference), size of wounds, size of areas saturated with drainage, size of skin reactions to medications (tuberculin test), or size of the area to which medication is applied topically (nitroglycerin ointment).

In clinical practice, the subdivisions milligram (mg) and microgram (μg) and the multiple of the gram, the kilogram (kg), are used solely as measurements of weight. Secondary units of the liter are expressed in milliliters (400 mL) or as decimals (1.5 L) rather than fractions.

Apothecary System

Dating from 1617, the apothecary system is the oldest of the three systems of measurement. Although the apothecary system is slowly being replaced by the metric system, its units of measure are used in everyday life. In the United States, fluids, such as juice and milk, are bought in pints and quarts; gasoline is bought in gallons; distances are measures in inches, feet, or miles; and body weight is measured in pounds.

In the apothecary system, the basic unit of weight is the grain (gr), followed in ascending order by the scruple, the dram, the ounce, and the pound, although the scruple and the dram are seldom used for measurement. The basic unit of volume is the minim (m), followed by the fluidram, the fluid ounce (oz), the pint, the quart, and the gallon. Equivalent measures are listed in Table 27-4.

The symbol for the unit of measure usually is followed by the quantity, expressed by lower-case Roman numerals (eg, ii). An exception to this rule is in using fractions of a unit, where the fraction comes after the abbreviation or word but is expressed in Arabic numerals (eg, gr 1/4). When the unit of measure is written as a word or an abbreviation, the quantity is expressed in Arabic numerals and precedes the unit of measure (eg, 2 oz).

Table 27-4 • Approximate Volume and Weight Equivalents: Metric and Apothecary Systems

Metric		Apothecary
Volume		
0.06 milliliter (mL)	=	1 minim
1 milliliter (mL)	=	15 minims
5 mL	=	1 teaspoon
15 mL	=	1/2 fluid ounce or 1 tablespoon
30 mL	=	1 fluid ounce
240 milliliters (mL)	=	8 fluid ounces
500 mL	=	1 pint
1,000 mL or 1 liter (L)	=	1 quart
4,000 mL	=	1 gallon
Weight		
milligrams (mg) or 1/1,000 grams (g)	=	1/60 grain (gr)
60 mg or 0.06 g	=	1 gr
1,000 mg	=	15 gr
4 g	=	1 dram (3)
30 g	=	1 ounce (oz)
0.45 kilograms (kg)	=	1 pound (lb)
500 g	=	1.1 lb
1,000 g or 1 kg	=	2.2 lb

Household System

The household system is used primarily for measurements in the home, such as teaspoons, tablespoons, cups, glasses, and drops. Pints and quarts also are household measures but are defined as apothecary measures. The household system of measurement is the least accurate of the three systems.

Legal Aspects of Medication Administration

The power of various substances to promote healing or cause harm has been well known for ages, which is why many societies entrust the distribution and administration of these substances to a selected group or official body. In the United States, laws have been enacted to ensure that medications are safe, effective, and administered only by qualified people. Additional legislation has established agencies to enforce the laws.

Food and Drug Administration

In the United States, federal laws regulate and control how drugs are manufactured and marketed. Early federal action addressing drug safety resulted in the Pure Food and Drug Act of 1906, which prevented the marketing of many worthless and dangerous drugs. The act was later amended to require accurate labeling and to eliminate false and misleading claims. Although the law increased drug safety in many aspects, it was limited to enforcing safety only after a drug was marketed.

The law was again amended in 1937 after a drug manufacturer substituted the untested diethylene glycol for the elixir of sulfanilamide in a medication (Shlafer, 1993). The many deaths that resulted prompted congressional action, which established the FDA. Over the years, the FDA, a branch of the Department of Health and Human Services, has been assigned increasing responsibility for public safety related to medications.

The FDA regulates the manufacture, sale, and effectiveness of medications. It also requires drug testing in laboratory animals and in humans (through controlled, three-phase clinical trials) before approving the drug for use. The FDA also is charged with keeping an ineffective or unsafe drug off the market and recalling an inadequately tested or dangerous drug. Additional functions include identifying which medications can be obtained with or without a prescription, setting and enforcing standards of purity and potency, overseeing all antibiotics, and controlling drug advertising to the medical profession.

Other Watchdog Agencies

Other agencies, such as the Division of Biological Standards of the National Institutes of Health, a division of the Public Health Service, regulate biologic products, such as vaccines, antitoxins, immune serums, immunologic diagnostic aids, and blood derivatives.The Federal Trade Commission regulates the advertising of nonprescription medication to protect the public from false advertising and deceptive practices.

Drug Enforcement Agencies

As a result of rising drug abuse and increasing public concern in the late 1960s, Congress enacted the Comprehensive Drug Abuse Prevention and Control Act of 1970, which includes the Controlled Substances Act (CSA). The CSA categorizes controlled substances in five groups (I, II, III, IV, and V) based on their potential for abuse and their medical usefulness. Table 27-5 describes the five schedules. Some of these controlled substances include narcotics, amphetamines, barbiturates, and tranquilizers. Under this law, it is illegal to possess a controlled substance without a valid prescription, and the law limits the number of times the prescription can be

Table 27-5 • Five Schedules of Controlled Substances Categorized by the Controlled Substances Act

Schedule	Characteristics	Dispensing Restrictions	Examples*
I	• High abuse potential • No accepted medical use—for research, analysis, or instruction only	• Approved protocol necessary	Heroin, tetrahydrocanabinols, LSD, mescaline, peyote, levomoramide, racemoramide, benzylmorphine, and others
II	• May lead to severe dependence • High abuse potential • Accepted medical uses • May lead to severe physical or psychological dependence	• Written Rx necessary—only emergency dispensing permitted without written Rx • Only required amount may be prescribed • No Rx refills allowed • Container must have warning label	Opium, morphine, hydromorphone, meperidine, codeine, oxycodone, methadone, secobarbital, pentobarbital, amphetamine, methylphenidate, methaqualone
III	• Less abuse potential than drugs in Schedules I and II • Accepted medical uses • May lead to moderate or low physical dependence or high psychological dependence	• 34-day supply limit • Written or oral Rx required • Rx expires in 6 months • No more than 5 Rx refills allowed • Container must have warning label*	Preparations containing limited quantities of opium, codeine, hydrocodone, morphine, dihydrocodeine, or ethylmorphine, non-narcotic drugs, such as derivatives of barbituric acid except those that are listed in another schedule, glutethimide, methylprylon, chlorphentermine, mazindol, paregoric
IV	• Low abuse potential compared with Schedule III • Accepted medical uses • May lead to limited physical or psychological dependence	• Written or oral Rx required • 34-day supply limit • Rx expires in 6 months • No more than 5 Rx refills allowed • Container must have warning label†	Barbital, phenobarbital, chloral hydrate, meprobamate, fenfluramine, chlordiazepoxide, diazepam, oxazepam, chlorazepate, flurazepam, lorazepam, dextropropoxyphene, pentazocine
V	• Low abuse potential compared with Schedule IV • Accepted medical uses • May lead to limited physical or psychological dependence	• May require written Rx or be sold with Rx (check state law)	Medications, generally for relief of coughs or diarrhea, containing limited quantities of certain narcotics

Courtesy Winthrop Laboratories, New York, NY. Modified from Ruggieri, N. L. (1980). Drug therapy *10*(12) 58–64. and the DEA pharcist's manual—an informational outline of the Controlled Substances Act of *1970.* U.S. Dept. of Justice, Washington, D.C., June *1980.* (Data apply to federal CSA and Uniform Controlled Substances Act; state laws may differ.)

*The examples cited constitute a partial listing. Individual hospital counsel should be consulted for a complete list for a particular state.

†Caution: Federal law prohibits the transfer of this drug to any person other than the client for whom it was prescribed.

filled. The primary reasons for the CSA were to prevent drug abuse and dependence, provide treatment and rehabilitation for people dependent on drugs, and strengthen drug abuse laws.

In hospitals and other healthcare settings, narcotics are kept in a locked drawer or box as an additional safety measure. Narcotics may be ordered only by healthcare providers registered with the Department of Justice, Bureau of Narcotics and Dangerous Drugs. A record must be kept for each narcotic administered. Various types of narcotic control sheets are provided by individual hospital pharmacies; however, information generally required includes the name of the client receiving the narcotic, the date and hour the narcotic was given, the amount of the narcotic used, the name of the healthcare provider prescribing the narcotic, and the name of the nurse administering the narcotic.

A narcotic count is performed at specified times, for example, at each change of shift. The type and amount of narcotics issued by the pharmacy for that particular unit are counted, and any narcotic administered during the previous shift must be on the narcotic control sheet. Before administering a narcotic, the nurse should verify the count in the narcotics drawer and sign the narcotic control sheet to indicate that the medication has been removed. If all or part of a dose is discarded, a second nurse should witness the discarding of the dose and should countersign the control sheet. At the end of the shift, one nurse should record the amount of each narcotic on the narcotic control sheet while the other nurse counts the narcotics out loud. Any discrepancies must be identified and corrected before the nurse leaves the unit; if the discrepancy cannot be resolved, it must be reported to the nursing supervisor or pharmacy.

The Nurse's Role

Legal responsibilities for nurses administering medications include practicing within the scope of the state's nurse practice act and following the institution's medication administration policies.

Nurse Practice Acts

The administration of medications by nurses is controlled by nursing legislation. Nurse practice acts, established to describe legitimate nursing functions, vary from state to state. Nurses must be informed about how their state's nurse practice act defines the boundaries of their functions. Each nurse also must recognize individual limits of knowledge and skill.

Under current nurse practice laws, nurses are responsible for their own actions regardless of the healthcare provider's written order. If an order is ambiguous or inappropriate, it is the nurse's responsibility to clarify the medication order with the prescribing healthcare provider. If the nurse is not satisfied with the healthcare provider's response and believes the order is incorrect or unsafe, it is his or her responsibility to notify the charge nurse or head nurse. Nurses have the right and responsibility to decline to administer a medication if they feel it jeopardizes client safety.

Nurses also are expected to practice in a safe and prudent manner. Each nurse is responsible for being knowledgeable about the medication's actions, indications and contraindications, purpose, and any adverse effects of the drug. He or she must know appropriate dosages and dosage schedules, routes and methods of administration, and actions to take if the client has an adverse reaction.

Dispensing medications (ie, preparing a medication that someone else will deliver) is not a legal practice for registered nurses in most states. Whereas healthcare providers prescribe and pharmacists dispense therapeutic agents, it is the nurse's legal domain to administer medications in a safe and timely manner. For related information, see the accompanying Safety Alert display.

Institutional Medication Policies

Nurses work in various settings, including schools, hospitals, nursing homes, and private industries. Each institution develops and oversees its own medication administration policies, and these rules can vary widely.

Some institutions allow only registered nurses to administer medications. Others allow graduate nurses, licensed practical (or vocational) nurses, or nursing students to administer medications. Restrictions may be placed on the types of medications they can give or on the degree of supervision or experience required. Each institution is governed by its own policies and procedures, and it is the responsibility of the nurse and nursing student to be aware of the practice within their institution.

The Client's Rights

Often the client has little or no knowledge of pharmacology and medications and must trust the nurse's expertise for proper medication administration. Clients look to the nurse as a teacher: Many of them need to take medications at home, so an essential nursing function is teaching the client how and when to take home medications. The nurse is vested with tremendous responsibility.

The client has the right to expect safe and appropriate drug administration by the nurse (see the display "The Patient's Bill of Rights" in Chap. 3). To accomplish this, the nurse must observe "five rights": the right drug, in the right dose, at the right time, by the right route,

> ***Safety Alert***
> *Medications*
>
> - Clarify with the healthcare provider any drug order that is unclear or not seemingly appropriate.
> - Always adhere to the "five rights" (right client, right medication, right dose, right route and right time) when giving any medication.
> - Check a client's allergy history before administering any medication.
> - Always check a client's identification band against the medication record before administering any medication.
> - Do not administer any medication from an unlabeled or illegible container.
> - Assess whether client can swallow before giving any oral medication; if possible, have the person sit up.
> - Do not leave medications by the bedside, where they may be forgotten or inadvertently taken by another person.
> - Always use anatomic landmarks to locate the site for intramuscular injections to avoid potential nerve damage and injury.
> - Use aseptic technique when administering any parenteral medications.
> - Do not give any medication prepared by another nurse unless the unit-dose label clearly identifies the drug and the seal is intact.
> - Document medication administration immediately to avoid error.
> - Admit all drug errors promptly to limit all potential adverse effects to the client. Medication errors must be reported to the healthcare provider and documented according to agency policy.
> - In the home setting, all medications should be kept in child-proof containers to prevent accidental ingestion by young children.

to the right client. As simplistic as these general rules sound, full compliance with them requires great depth of knowledge. These rights are discussed more fully in the implementation ("Safe Medication Administration") section of this chapter.

In addition to these five rights, the client has the right to refuse to take medications. Under these circumstances, it is the nurses' duty to explain to the client as fully and clearly as possible the importance of taking the medication. When a client refuses to comply with prescribed medication therapy, the client's healthcare provider must be notified.

Substance Abuse

The illegal use of drugs by any health professional jeopardizes client welfare and professional credibility. Because the chemically impaired nurse cannot be trusted always to exercise optimal clinical judgment, he or she needs to be identified so that treatment can be obtained and client safety ensured. Stringent rules and procedures help to prevent diversion of client medications to healthcare personnel. It is the duty and legal obligation of each nurse to maintain accurate medication records and to report any discrepancies. Nurses are further required by law (and by concern for client welfare) to report any known diversion of controlled substances by colleagues.

Principles of Drug Action

Practicing nurses must have an understanding of the ways by which drugs and medications exert their effects. **Pharmacodynamics** refers to the physiologic and biochemical effects of a drug on the body, while **pharmacokinetics** is the process by which a drug moves through the body and is eventually eliminated. In addition to pharmacokinetics, many variables affect drug action.

Pharmacokinetics

Pharmacokinetics involves the absorption, distribution, metabolism, and excretion of a medication. Each medication has its own characteristic rate and manner by which it is absorbed by body tissues, delivered to reactive cells, transformed to harmless substances, and removed from the body. The effects and the effectiveness of all medications depend on these four primary factors.

Absorption

Absorption is the process by which a medication enters the bloodstream. The rate at which any drug is absorbed depends on several factors. First, the route of administration affects how quickly and how completely a medication is absorbed. For example, drugs injected directly into the bloodstream are absorbed almost immediately, whereas drugs taken orally can take longer to be absorbed. Drug solubility also is a factor affecting absorption; medications in solution are more rapidly absorbed than those in timed-release capsules.

The site of administration can inhibit or promote drug absorption. Tissues rich in capillary blood flow accelerate absorption. Conversely, poor circulation impedes absorption.

Finally, the acid–base environment of body fluids affects drug absorption. Acidic medications break down (or dissociate) more slowly in an acidic environment, such as the stomach, whereas alkaline medications dissociate more slowly in the small intestine. Slower dissociation causes slower absorption.

Distribution

Once the medication has entered the body and has been absorbed, it must be delivered to the target cells and tissues by the circulatory system, a process called **distribution.** The effectiveness of a medication depends on its concentration at the reactive site. Some medications are bound to plasma proteins, thus decreasing the total amount of medication available to the tissues. As with absorption, distribution depends on effective circulation.

Certain medications have greater affinity for a specific type of tissue than others. Iodine, for example, accumulates readily in the thyroid gland but minimally in other tissues. By contrast, alcohol is able to enter many types of tissue.

Metabolism

After the medication has been distributed to the cells and interacts with them, it undergoes chemical changes. These changes are necessary to convert it to a less active, more readily excretable form. The process by which the drug is deactivated is called biotransformation, or simply **metabolism.**

Metabolism of medications takes place mainly in the liver but also can occur in the blood plasma, kidneys, intestinal mucosa, and lungs. Alterations in liver function, including diminished liver function that occurs with aging, can affect the rate at which drugs are metabolized.

Excretion

Drug metabolic by-products are removed from the body by **excretion.** After a medication has been broken down, or metabolized, the resultant products are excreted from the liver in bile, which is dumped into the intestine. Some of the drug's metabolites are excreted in feces, but many are reabsorbed through the intestinal wall and reenter the circulation. Some drugs (such as alcohol and anesthetic gases) are excreted by the lungs. Most drugs are excreted by the kidneys, with the remnants of the original drug becoming components of urine.

Pharmacodynamics

Drug activity is the result of chemical interactions between a medication and the cells of the body to produce a biologic response. Drugs manipulate a body process. They can inhibit or stimulate a process, or they can replace a missing element. Most drugs interact with a cellular component to initiate a series of biochemical and physiologic changes that result in the drug's effect. The cellular component that interacts with the drug molecules is termed a receptor cite (Malseed & Girton, 1995). Drugs can affect a cell membrane, a cellular enzyme, or certain intracellular components.

Biochemical and physiologic effects can be local or systemic. Local effects can be seen in the application of moisturizing lotion to chapped skin. An example of systemic effects are those of some analgesics (pain medications), which can affect the nervous system, the heart, and the gastrointestinal tract.

Medication effects are monitored by changes in the client's clinical condition. Physical or psychological symptoms generally improve, or laboratory test results indicate improvement, when medications are effective. In addition to clinical observations, laboratory measurements of the concentration of medication in the blood are another indicator of effect.

Therapeutic Effects

The desired and intentional effects of a medication are called its therapeutic effects. These effects vary with the nature of the medication, the length of time the client has been receiving the medication, and the client's physical condition. Interactions with other medications also can affect a drug's therapeutic action. The onset of action of medications varies widely, so time needed for therapeutic effects to become evident also varies (Fig. 27-1).

Side (Adverse) Effects

Every medication is prescribed to accomplish a therapeutic goal, so each drug is carefully chosen for its therapeutic effects. Practically all medications produce effects other than their primary therapeutic effect. These additional effects are called side effects. Many of these effects are minor, essentially harmless, and can be ignored, but others are undesirable and potentially harmful. These adverse effects may result from the secondary effects of a medication, toxicity or cumulative medication effects, individual client sensitivity, or idiosyncratic reactions (Shlafer, 1993).

Secondary Reactions. Secondary reactions to a medication result from the multiple actions of a drug within the body. These effects vary in importance to the client. Minor secondary effects may be disturbing to the client who does not expect them. The client who has been

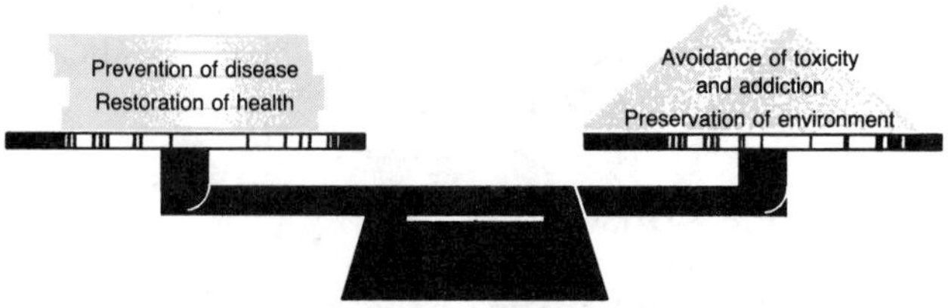

***Figure 27-1** • The proper use of medications attempts to strike a balance between risks and benefits.*

given phenazopyridine (Pyridium) to treat painful urination should be forewarned that the urine will turn red while the medication is being taken. Common side effects that may necessitate discontinuation of the medication include nausea and vomiting, changes in gastrointestinal activity (eg, gastric bleeding, diarrhea), and changes in level of consciousness, such as excitation or somnolence (Shlafer, 1993).

Sometimes unpleasant secondary effects may occur with initial doses of a medication, but they may subside with subsequent doses. A client may tolerate bothersome secondary effects of a medication if they are far outweighed by the therapeutic effects. In some cases, there may be little choice other than to accept secondary effects of a drug, especially when no alternative medication is available or when lack of treatment will result in death. Chemotherapeutic agents used to treat cancer are a prime example.

For some clients, the secondary effects of a medication may lead to life-threatening problems, such as liver or kidney damage or bone marrow suppression. If the healthcare provider and nurse are aware of medication side effects and if the client is closely monitored, important secondary effects of medications usually can be identified early and appropriate intervention instituted.

Medication Toxicity. Medication toxicity, a deleterious effect on various tissues of the body, results from overdosage, ingestion of a medication intended for external use, and a build-up of medication in the blood due to impaired metabolism and excretion. Careful attention must be given specifically to the dosage and to toxicity monitoring. Some medications can produce toxic effects almost immediately, whereas some do not produce toxic effects for days or weeks.

Cumulative Effects. Cumulative effects of a medication occur when the client cannot metabolize or break down a medication before the next dose is given. Unless the medication dosage is adjusted, the amount of the medication builds up in the client's body. In some cases, this cumulative effect is desirable, such as with medications used to prevent depression.

Tolerance. Tolerance to a medication occurs when a client develops a decreased response to a medication, requiring an increased dosage to achieve therapeutic effect. Some agents that produce tolerance include nicotine, ethyl alcohol, opiates, and barbiturates.

Hypersensitivity Reactions. Hypersensitivity reactions occur when a client is unusually sensitive to the therapeutic effects or to the secondary effects of a medication. An estimated therapeutic dosage of medication may be too large for the client and may result in a degree of action that is greater than desired. For example, a middle-aged man of normal body weight usually requires 75 to 100 mg of meperidine to relieve pain; rarely, a man of similar age and body size may respond with pain control of long duration and excessive somnolence. Usually, if the medication dose or the medication dosing interval is decreased, the medication may be administered safely.

Idiosyncratic Effects. Idiosyncratic effects are the unpredictable and inexplicable symptoms caused by a genetic defect in the client that alters the way in which he or she responds to a medication. The response to the medication is completely different from what is expected and may occur the first time a medication is administered. One genetic defect that results in idiosyncratic medication reactions occurs in African-American men who are given antimalarial medications. Between 5% and 10% of African-American men lack an enzyme that protects the integrity of the red blood cell membrane. When a susceptible man is given the antimalarial medication primaquine, his red blood cells undergo hemolysis (disintegration). When a client belongs to a known risk group, blood tests should be used to screen for a possible defect (Shlafer, 1993).

Allergic Reactions. Allergic reactions result from an immunologic response to a medication to which the client has been sensitized. A foreign substance or antigen has been introduced into the body, and the body responds by producing antibodies. Clients respond to certain medications as they would to this foreign substance and develop symptoms of an allergic reaction. These symptoms can be mild or severe.

Mild allergic reactions can produce hives (urticaria), pruritus, angioedema, rhinitis, nausea, vomiting, and diarrhea. Mild reactions can occur within minutes to 2 weeks after the administration of a medication. Skin reactions, including hives, rashes, and lesions, usually improve soon after discontinuing the medication (Shlafer, 1993). Severe allergic reactions produce symptoms such as wheezing, dyspnea, hypotension, and tachycardia and occur immediately after the medication is given. A severe allergic reaction is called an anaphylactic reaction and requires immediate medical intervention, because it can be fatal. Treatment includes discontinuing the medication responsible and administering IV fluids, steroids, and antihistamines.

Medication Interaction. Medication interaction occurs when the effects of a medication are altered by the concurrent presence of other medications or food (Fig. 27-2). This interaction of medications may result in potentiation or synergism, which increases a drug's effects. Interaction also can result in antagonism, by which drug effects decrease. In some cases, a drug will precipitate from solutions if mixed with other incompatible medications. Sometimes a drug is influenced by foods; an example of a food–drug interaction is the deactivation of the antibiotic tetracycline by dairy products.

The nurse must be aware of drug interactions with other medications and foods to protect the client from the harmful effects. Incompatibility charts and the hospital pharmacist are valuable resources for this information.

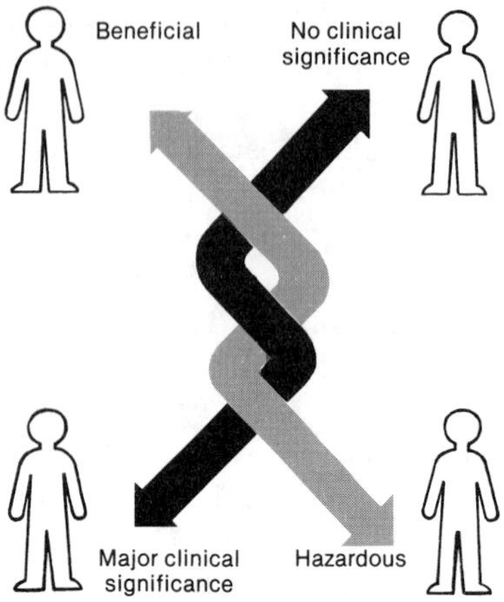

Figure 27-2 • *Drug interactions may vary.*

Factors Affecting Drug Action

Many variables can alter the effects of medications. Among them are the client's age, weight, height, gender, genetic factors, and environment. Others include time of administration, organ system function, and psychological condition.

Age. Developmental factors greatly affect the action of medications. During the first years of life, tissues, organs, and metabolic processes are developing. Factors in the infant that affect drug action include increased total body water volume, decreased body fat, decreased plasma proteins, relative lack of gastric acid, changing metabolic rate, and immature renal and hepatic function. An appropriate medication dose must be calculated for each infant, considering these variables. During this early period, medication also may affect developing tissues; for example, the antibiotic tetracycline causes permanent dental discoloration in very young children.

Many physiologic changes occur in older adults that affect their response to medications. Decreased lean body mass and total body water, increased body fat, more alkaline gastric secretions, and decreased gastric and intestinal motility all affect drug action in the body. In addition, many older people have chronic health problems involving the liver, the kidneys, or the cardiovascular system; the cumulative effect of these changes usually is that decreased doses of medications need to be administered at less frequent intervals. Side effects and adverse reactions are more common in older adults, usually because of physiologic changes, chronic disease, and multiple medications.

Weight. The client's body weight must be considered when administering any medication. The greater the body weight, the greater the mass of body tissues, and thus the larger the dose of medication required. A person's weight may be used to estimate the appropriate beginning dosage for a medication.

Height. Height and weight can be used to estimate body surface area. Drug and anesthetic dosages may be based on estimates of body surface area.

Gender. Men and women respond to medications differently because of differences in fat and water distribution and differences in hormones. Although women usually weigh less than men, they have proportionally more adipose (fatty) tissue, and men have more body fluid. Some medications are more soluble in fat, whereas others are more soluble in water. Generally, men absorb some medications more readily than women.

Genetic Factors. Because of genetic factors, a client may metabolize a medication differently or respond to a specific medication with abnormal sensitivity. These reactions, called idiosyncratic reactions, are discussed previously in this chapter.

Time of Administration. The time of administration of oral medications can affect their speed and duration of action. An empty stomach facilitates absorption of an oral medication, thereby enhancing its efficacy. Some medications, such as ferrous sulfate, irritate the gastric mucosa of the stomach and must be taken with or after meals.

Organ System Function. Predictable medication effects depend on properly functioning organs. Liver, kidney, or cardiovascular dysfunction and other organic or glandular conditions can seriously alter the effects of a medication. Because of their respective importance in medication metabolism and excretion, decreased liver or kidney function can result in cumulative drug effects. Decreased cardiac output, heart failure, or circulatory problems can alter delivery of medications to body tissues.

Glandular dysfunctions, such as thyroid disorders or diabetes, can have profound effects on medication action, and the nurse must be knowledgeable about the effects these types of disorders have on a wide variety of medications. The complexity of these effects makes drug reference resources a practical necessity.

Psychological State. The client's psychological status can affect the action of psychoactive medications. For example, if the person has confidence in the nurse and the expected effects of the medication, the effect of the medication is more likely to be positive.

Medication Assessment

To administer medications safely to any client, information must be collected during the initial assessment. In addition to this baseline data, a medication-specific assessment should be part of the ongoing nursing assessment to determine medication effectiveness and promptly identify side effects. Assessment also is necessary to plan appropriate client teaching to promote compliance with therapy.

Information Collected on Admission

Important information to elicit from the client during the initial interview focuses on a medications, allergies, medical history, and pregnancy and lactation status.

Medication History

During the initial interview, the nurse should learn the names, dosages, dosage schedules, and action of the medications routinely taken by the client before admission. Whenever possible, the nurse should discuss the medication history with the family. A family member may provide information that is not volunteered by the client, such as, "Mom doesn't take her water pill in the evening because she doesn't like to go to the bathroom at night." In the clinic or during home visits, clients should be encouraged to carry all of their medications with them (including nonprescription medications) so that the healthcare provider can assess whether the client needs to continue with these medications.

When hospitalized, the client must send all medications home or store them in a secure location until discharge. (Some agencies permit clients to keep their own medications at the bedside once they have been checked and labeled by the pharmacy department and an order has been obtained from the healthcare provider.) The healthcare provider should be alerted to all medications the client has been taking so that necessary medications can be ordered for the client. This is especially important if the client is taking antidiabetic agents, anticonvulsant medications, or cardiovascular medications.

The nurse also should discuss the client's use of any over-the-counter medications. A question such as, "What medications do you buy without a prescription?" may be helpful to elicit this information. A client may overlook common medications, such as aspirin, acetaminophen, or laxatives, when asked to list medications. In particular, eye drops, nasal sprays, skin lotions, and food supplements may not be considered medications by the client.

When clients are taking multiple medications, when they cannot remember the names of all the medications they are taking, or when their medication profile does not match their clinical status, the client or family should be asked to collect all medications for the nurse to evaluate.

Access to the client's medications allows the nurse to make a complete list of prescribed medications and to identify actual or potential medication problems. The nurse should note whether prescriptions have expired, whether all medications are stored separately in correctly marked containers, whether the prescriptions are actually this client's or another person's, and whether the number of pills in a bottle seems correct considering the date and directions of the prescription.

Allergies

During the initial interview, a client should be asked about allergies to any medication. If the client indicates any medication allergies, the nurse should ask follow-up questions about the allergic symptoms noted with each drug. This information allows the nurse to differentiate between a medication that caused a true allergic response and a medication that caused unpleasant side effects. In some situations, medications that caused unpleasant side effects, such as nausea, may be used.

All stated client allergies should be written on the client's record, on the cover of the client's record, and in any other locations mandated by agency policy. The record also should include the client's reaction to each medication. Clients in the hospital or long-term care should have all allergies listed on a wrist band and on all medication administration records.

Medical History

Before administering any medication to a client, the nurse should be aware of the client's medical diagnosis and general medical history. Any renal, hepatic, cardiac, respiratory, endocrine, or neurologic dysfunction is important to ascertain before administering any medication. The nurse can use this information to identify clients at greater risk for drug toxicity or those who may require extra care in drug administration.

Drug or alcohol abuse also is important to determine before medication administration. The client who has frequently used narcotics or alcohol may require higher doses of sedatives or narcotics to obtain the desired effect. Clients who have a history of drug abuse or addiction are more likely to become drug dependent when given narcotics, sedatives, or tranquilizers. Administering aspirin to an alcohol-dependent client may predispose the client to gastric irritation and bleeding, and normal dosages of acetaminophen in such clients occasionally may cause severe hepatic or renal dysfunction (Kumar & Rex, 1991; Dossing & Sonne, 1993).

Pregnancy and Lactation Status

A client's pregnancy or lactation status is important to determine before medication administration. Drugs known to cause birth defects are called teratogenic. Any drug that is known to be teratogenic or that has not been thoroughly evaluated should be avoided during pregnancy. Rarely (eg, a pregnant client with difficult-to-control epilepsy) using a potentially harmful drug during pregnancy may be indicated. The healthcare provider should discuss the risks and benefits of such treatment with the client before administering the drug, and this discussion should be documented in the medical record. Late in pregnancy, hepatotoxic medications should be avoided, because there is an increased risk of liver damage to the mother.

A medication may be excreted through breast milk and ingested by a nursing infant. Most medications are excreted in low dosages that do not affect a nursing infant, but some (eg, narcotics, antibiotics, anticoagulants, anticonvulsants, histamine antagonists, and tranquilizers) can be excreted in amounts great enough to affect the infant (Shlafer, 1993). If a woman must receive a medication that is excreted in large concentrations in breast milk, she should bottle-feed her infant.

Assessment Before Medication Administration

Before the administration of any medication, the nurse should assess the client's medication record, current diet and fluid orders, scheduled diagnostic tests or surgical procedures, and physical status.

Medication Record

Before giving a client any medication, the nurse should check the client's medication administration record. The client may have several medications ordered to treat the same problem. Checking the client's medication record allows the nurse to see which medication has been used most recently and whether it is time for the medication to be administered. Knowing a client's current medications also allows the nurse to avoid giving a medication that may interfere with or add to the effect of another medication the client has received.

Diet and Fluid Orders

A client may have fluids and food withheld in preparation for surgery or for a diagnostic test. When a client is ordered to have nothing by mouth (NPO), he or she should be reminded that most oral medications are usually not given. When the client is receiving important medications that should not be discontinued abruptly (eg, blood pressure medication, digoxin, anticonvulsants), the healthcare provider should be contacted concerning alternative orders for medication administration. In some situations, healthcare providers order that oral medications be administered with a small sip of water even though a client is NPO.

When a diabetic client is NPO, the nurse should contact the healthcare provider concerning specific orders for medications. Clients taking oral hypoglycemics still produce some endogenous insulin, so the healthcare provider may withhold these agents for short periods. However, the client's blood glucose level is monitored regularly, and insulin may be needed if blood glucose levels rise above normal.

When insulin-dependent diabetic clients are NPO, they should have their insulin doses adjusted and their blood glucose levels monitored frequently. If the insulin-dependent client is NPO for longer than 4 hours, infusion of IV dextrose solutions and continuous IV insulin may facilitate efficient, safe care. Clients receiving insulin must have scheduled tests or surgery on time to avoid glucose imbalance.

Laboratory Values

Laboratory tests may be used to monitor serum drug levels, medication effects, and medication side effects. Dosages of medications such as digoxin, gentamicin, phenytoin, and theophylline are evaluated by monitoring serum drug levels to determine proper dosage for the client. The nurse is responsible for assessing these serum drug levels and notifying the healthcare provider about values outside the therapeutic range. This permits the healthcare provider to change the medication dosage to ensure therapeutic effects without causing undesirable toxicity.

Laboratory tests also may be used to monitor the direct effects of a medication. Medications such as iron, potassium, and thyroid preparations that are given to maintain a body substance may be monitored by determining serum concentrations. Anticoagulants also are monitored for therapeutic effect by drawing venous blood to assess coagulation status.

Common or serious side effects of medications may be monitored using laboratory tests. Many diuretics are potassium-wasting, hence serum potassium levels are measured to detect hypokalemia. Many types of chemotherapy cause leukopenia (decreased numbers of white blood cells) or thrombocytopenia (decreased numbers of platelets); thus, blood counts are monitored before and after chemotherapy. When medications are known to cause kidney dysfunction, laboratory tests of kidney function (serum creatinine and blood urea nitrogen) are done at regular intervals. When medications can potentially cause liver damage, laboratory liver function tests (alanine aminotransferase [ALT], aspartate aminotransferase [AST]) may be ordered and evaluated (Shlafer, 1993).

Physical Assessment

Before giving a medication, the nurse should quickly assess the client's physical ability to take the medication. The ability to swallow and normal gastrointestinal motility are important considerations for oral medications; adequate muscle mass and venous access are important for parenteral medications. If the medication is likely to affect vital signs or the function of a body system, appropriate assessments are made before medication administration.

Ability to Swallow. Before administering an oral medication, the nurse must be sure that the client has an adequate swallowing reflex. If the nurse suspects that a client cannot swallow, he or she should give the client several sips of water. If the client coughs or chokes on the water, the medication should not be given, and the client's healthcare provider should be informed.

Gastrointestinal Motility. The client who has recently undergone major surgery or who has gastrointestinal dysfunction may be unable to absorb oral medications. If the nurse suspects that a client's gastrointestinal function is abnormal, he or she should perform a quick abdominal assessment before giving an oral medication. If the client's abdomen is distended and firm, and if bowel sounds are hyperactive or absent, gastrointestinal dysfunction is present. The client's healthcare provider should be contacted to check if oral medications should be given.

Adequate Muscle Mass. Premature infants or debilitated clients may have limited amounts of lean muscle mass. If an irritating medication is given into subcutaneous (SC) tissue or into a very small muscle, pain, inadequate absorption of medication, or tissue damage could occur. The client's healthcare provider should be contacted to determine if another route of administration could be used.

Adequate Venous Access. Before giving an IV medication, the nurse should be sure that the IV catheter is located in an adequate vein. The catheter insertion site should be checked for temperature, redness, swelling, and pain. If the catheter is being used to infuse IV fluids, the infusion rate should be calculated to deliver the IV medication in a time limit appropriate to the specific medication.

Vital Signs. Blood pressure, heart rate, and respiratory rate may be affected by medications. Before giving a medication that may affect one of the vital signs, the nurse should measure and record that value. Blood pressure should be measured before administering antihypertensive medications or before administering coronary vasodilators (nitroglycerin, isosorbide dinitrate). If the client's systolic blood pressure is low (usually less than 90 or 100 mg Hg systolic), the medication may be withheld. Counting apical heart rate is necessary before giving digitalis, a medication that slows the heart rate. If the heart rate over 1 minute is slow (usually less than 60 beats/min), the medication may be withheld. Respiratory rate should be counted before giving a medication, such as a narcotic, that may affect the rate.

Body System Assessment. Medications are often used to treat a dysfunctional body system. To assess the effect of a medication, the nurse needs to assess the appropriate body system before giving the medication. For example, bronchodilators can be inhaled by a client with chronic obstructive lung disease to treat bronchospasm. Before beginning the treatment, the nurse should assess the client's respiratory system. This quick assessment includes counting the respiratory rate, asking the client to rate his or her ease of breathing, noting the use of accessory respiratory muscles, and auscultating the client's breath sounds. After the treatment, the assessment is repeated. The nurse can judge the effect of the treatment by noting any changes in assessment findings and by noting the length of time the change lasts.

Assessment of Knowledge and Compliance

Many factors influence whether a client will comply with prescribed medication. Nursing assessment can provide a knowledge base to assist the nurse in better understanding whether the client is likely to comply with the healthcare provider's drug order. Assessment also can provide the basis for individualized client teaching to help ensure client compliance.

Knowledge

Client knowledge about a prescribed medication varies with the individual and depends on many factors. Some clients desire and receive detailed information about the medications they are taking, whereas other clients want and receive minimal information. The nurse should determine what the client needs to know to take the medication safely, and then ask questions to elicit this information. Inadequate knowledge or gaps in important knowledge areas should be clearly documented so that an individualized teaching plan can be formulated.

Assessing cognitive ability is important for individualizing the teaching plan and determining whether the client can independently manage self-medication. Cognitive impairment, confusion, and psychiatric disorders may increase the potential for noncompliance. Learning disabilities may necessitate creative teaching to help ensure understanding and compliance with therapy. It is often helpful to include family members or the caregiver in the teaching sessions. For confused or cognitively impaired clients, the nurse or caregiver may need to check the client's mouth to ensure that the pill has been swallowed.

Compliance

Compliance with a medication routine means that the client takes the medication as prescribed. Lack of compliance occurs in many ways, such as when the client fails to take any of the prescribed drug, fails to take the proper number of doses of the drug, takes extra doses of the drug, fails to follow the dosage schedule as prescribed, discontinues the medication prematurely, excessively uses a prn order, or takes medications that were ordered previously for another condition.

Compliance with a medication routine is more likely to occur when the client understands and agrees with the rationale for using the medication, the routine for taking the medications, and the desired effect of the medications. Simple medication routines that suit the client's lifestyle are more likely to be followed.

A client's attitude about medical care and about a specific medication can influence the client's compliance with drug therapy. The nurse can begin by asking general questions, such as "Do you feel that these medications will help you get better?" The nurse also should be alert to client comments indicating a lack of confidence in the prescribed drug treatment.

Lifestyle and financial considerations also affect compliance with drug therapy. The client with a regular income, health insurance, and a stable home situation is more likely to obtain medications and organize routines to remember to take them. When a client does not have a home, an income, or health insurance, buying, storing, and remembering to take medications regularly can be difficult.

Nursing Research
Medications

Selected Nursing Research Studies

Wolfgang, A. P., Jankel, C. A., & McMillan, J. A. (1993). Drug information and educational needs. A survey of rural home health care nurses. *Home Healthcare Nurse, 11(3), 20–23.*

Bliss-Holtz, J. (1994). Discriminating types of medication calculation errors in nursing practice. *Nursing Research, 43(6), 373–375.*

Minnick, A., Leahey, M. & Pischke-Winn, K. (1994). The impact of patient point-of-view pharmacy delivery on labor and quality. *Nursing Economics, 12(1), 45–50.*

Hentinen, M., & Kyngas, H. (1992). Compliance of young diabetics with health regimens. *Journal of Advanced Nursing, 17(5), 530–536.*

Possible Topics For Nursing Inquiry

- Do environmental factors, such as temperature or air quality, affect the absorption or effectiveness of medications?
- How is compliance with medication regimens affected by different types of client teaching?
- What is the rate of compliance with medications after client teaching by the home health nurse?
- How often is intravenous site care necessary to reduce risk of infection?
- What is the minimum amount of blood volume required to discard from a central venous catheter to obtain blood samples for laboratory tests?
- Does cleansing the skin with alcohol have an affect on infection rates after subcutaneous injections?

Health Promotion and Maintenance

The nurse can be effective in promoting and maintaining client health by encouraging clients who need medications to be proactive consumers. In such a role, the client develops an active understanding of medications, clarifies confusing information, insists on being consulted in every aspect of medication prescribing, and responsibly shares decision-making with the healthcare providers.

In many ways, the success of health promotion and maintenance planning depends on clients seeing themselves as healthcare participants with responsibility for choices about treatment and medications—whether alternative, prescribed, or over-the-counter. Health promotion and health maintenance are the domain of knowledgeable and responsible consumers encouraged by healthcare professionals, especially nurses.

Nursing Diagnoses

Noncompliance and Knowledge Deficit are North American Nursing Diagnosis Association (NANDA) nursing diagnoses commonly applied to the client who is managing self-medication. In addition, medication side effects can contribute to other significant problems for the client.

Diagnostic Statement: Noncompliance

Definition

Noncompliance is a person's informed decision not to adhere to a therapeutic recommendation (NANDA, 1994).

Defining Characteristics

Defining characteristics include behavior indicative of failure to adhere (by direct observation or statements by client or significant others), objective tests (physiologic measures, detection of markers), evidence of complications, evidence of exacerbation of symptoms, failure to keep appointments, and failure to progress (NANDA, 1994).

Related Factors

Related factors include client value system—health beliefs, cultural influences, spiritual values—and client–provider relationships (NANDA, 1994).

Diagnostic Statement: Knowledge Deficit

Definition

Knowledge Deficit is the absence or deficiency of cognitive information related to a specific topic (NANDA, 1994).

Defining Characteristics

Defining characteristics include verbalization of the problem, inaccurate follow-through of instruction, inaccurate performance of test, inappropriate or exaggerated behaviors (eg, hysterical, hostile, agitated, apathetic; NANDA, 1994).

Related Factors

Related factors include lack of exposure; lack of recall, information misinterpretation, cognitive limitation, lack of interest in learning, unfamiliarity with information resources (NANDA, 1994).

Related Nursing Diagnoses

Medication administration can increase the potential for the occurrence of many nursing diagnoses. Risk for Infection is an appropriate diagnosis when administering parenteral medications to some clients or when administering medications that decrease bone marrow function. Risk for Injury is an appropriate diagnosis when administering medications that can cause syncope or alter cognition. Many medications can alter normal bowel function, causing Diarrhea or Constipation, and some can cause Altered Sexuality Patterns, Sexual Dysfunction, and Sleep Pattern Disturbance. Impaired Home Maintenance Management may occur when medication regimens are complex and difficult to manage independently.

Safe Medication Administration

Knowledge and skill are important in ensuring client safety during medication administration. To administer medications safely, the nurse must do the following:

- Accurately interpret the healthcare provider's order.
- Accurately calculate the amount of drug to give for the prescribed dose.
- Develop a systematic and safe procedure, using the "five rights" for drug administration.
- Document medication administration according to agency policy.

Interpretation of the Order

The nurse is responsible for safe interpretation of the medication order. When a new order is written by the healthcare provider, the nurse must be able to read the specifics of the written order. When the order is illegible, the intended medication request can easily be misinterpreted. If the written order is not completely clear or contains unusual abbreviations, the nurse should consult the healthcare provider for clarification. Clarification of the written order also may be necessary if important information, such as the route or frequency, is omitted.

The nurse should evaluate whether the amount and route ordered are likely to be safe for the client. The nurse needs to know, or look up, the dosage range, the route of administration, contraindications, and side effects before giving any medication. If the nurse questions the safe use of any prescribed medication, he or she has the legal responsibility to consult with the healthcare provider rather than administer a medication that could potentially cause harm.

Calculating Medication Dosages

Medication orders are usually written in metric units of measure, and medications are usually supplied the same way. Occasionally, liquid medications or commonly used oral medications may be ordered in apothecary or household units of measure. If a medication is ordered in one unit of measure and supplied by the pharmacy in another unit of measure, the nurse must calculate the amount of medication needed in the measurement system ordered.

If the calculated dosage of a medication seems unusual (eg, if it consists of more than three tablets, a fraction of less than one-half tablet, or more than one unit dose of a liquid medication) or if the nurse has any doubts about the accuracy of his or her calculation, he or she should ask another nurse or a pharmacist to check the dosage calculation (Shlafer, 1993). Calculations of dosages of medications with important or toxic side effects (including heparin and insulin) also should be double-checked by another nurse or pharmacist.

Conversions Within a System. If the medication is ordered and supplied in the same measurement system, the nurse can use the following formula to calculate the amount of medication needed:

$$\text{Dosage ordered} \times \frac{\text{Volume on hand}}{\text{Dose on hand}} = \text{Volume to be given}$$

Conversions within the metric system can be calculated using this formula or by remembering that the metric system is based on units of ten. Equivalents are computed by multiplying or dividing, moving the decimal point to the right or left, respectively. There are only three basic units in the metric system used to calculate medication dosages: gram, milligram, and microgram. The equivalents among these three units are 1 g = 1,000 mg = 1,000,000 μg.

To change grams to milligrams, multiply the grams by 1,000 (because there are 1,000 mg in 1 g), or move the decimal point three places to the left. An example of this conversion in an equation is 800 mg = 0.8 g.

Conversions from One System to Another. Use of the metric is becoming more common, although the need to convert from one system to another continues to exist. For example, a client's order may specify, grains but the medication is dispensed from the pharmacy in milligrams. Nurses must have the knowledge of commonly used equivalents to help them convert from one system to another. Conversion from one system of measure to another system results in an approximate equivalent, not an equal answer. Referring to standard tables for common conversion equivalents is helpful. Knowledge of volume conversion may be necessary when using liquid medications.

Knowledge of approximate weight equivalents for the metric and apothecary systems is necessary when converting a client's body weight from kilograms to pounds or when converting grams and milligrams to grains and vice versa.

When converting units of weight from the metric system to the apothecary system, the nurse must remember that a milligram is smaller than a grain. When smaller units are converted to larger units, the result is a smaller number. If the healthcare provider orders the dose of medication in grains and the medication available is dispensed in grams, then the grams must be converted to grains. An example of this conversion is to change 15 mg to grains. Because 60 mg is approximately equal to 1 gr, the equation can be computed as follows:

milligrams : grains = milligrams : grains
60 : 1 = 15 : X
60 X = 15
X = 15:60 or 15/60
X = 0.25 grain or 1/4 grain

Conversely, when converting from a larger unit (grains) to a smaller unit (milligrams), the result is a larger number. An example of this conversion is to change 10 gr to milligrams. The equation is computed as follows:

grains : milligrams = grains : milligrams
1 : 60 = 10 : X
1/60 X = 10
X = 10 × 60
X = 600 milligrams (mg) or 0.6 grams (g)

These same rules apply when converting pounds to kilograms and vice versa. The pound is a smaller unit than the kilogram; therefore, the computation is made by dividing (so the result will be a smaller number). If a client weighs 180 lb, how many kilograms does this convert to? Because 2.2 lb is approximately equal to 1 kg, the equation is computed as follows:

pounds : kilograms = pounds : kilograms
2.2 : 1 = 180 : X
2.2X = 180
X = 180:2.2 or 180/2.2
X = 81.8 kilograms (kg)

To convert kilograms to pounds, the conversion is made by multiplying by 2.2 (so the result is a larger number). An example of this equation is as follows:

kilograms : pounds = kilograms : pounds
1 : 2.2 = 60 : X
2.2 X = 60
X = 60 × 2.2
X = 132 pounds (lb)

Calculating Children's Dosages. Children's dosages are most often calculated using the child's weight or body surface area. When necessary, they can be determined by several different formulas. Calculation of the adult dosage is reduced in proportion to the age or weight of the child. There is no one completely satisfactory method of computing a child's dose from an adult's; these formulas should be used as guides. Keep in mind that most drugs are ordered specifically for a child and are not computed from an adult dose. The nurse must take into account the many differences in sizes of children and the individual metabolic rate, which influences the therapeutic dose. Observing the child's response to the medication may determine if the dosage of the medication needs to be adjusted for the benefit of the individual child.

The most common formula for determining dosages for children is Clark's rule. This formula is based on the assumption that the average adult weighs 150 lb:

$$\frac{\text{Weight of child in pounds}}{150} \times \text{Usual adult dose} = \text{Child's dose}$$

Another method of determining medication dosages for children, called Young's rule, is based on the age of the child in years. This formula is stated as follows:

$$\frac{\text{Age of child in years}}{\text{Age of child} + 12} \times \text{Usual adult dose} = \text{Child's dose}$$

Intravenous Medication Calculations. IV medications are calculated to ensure the proper infusion rate for IV medications. For a thorough discussion, refer to Chapter 26. To infuse a medication for a set time, the nurse needs to calculate the appropriate rate of flow for the medication. IV flow rates are calculated in drips/min. To calculate IV drip rate, the nurse can use the following formula:

$$\frac{\text{mL of solution}}{\text{Hours to administer}} \times \frac{\text{Drops/mL (drip rate factor)}}{\text{60 (min/h)}} = \text{Drops per minute}$$

The amount, type, and infusion rate of IV medications are ordered by the healthcare provider. The drip rate varies with the type and brand of IV tubing. Two general types of IV tubing, macrodrip and minidrip, are available. Macrodrip (large-drop) tubing is often used to administer piggyback medications (see Chap. 26). Macrodrip tubing is made so that each drop of solution equals a fraction of a milliliter. The drip rate of macrodrip tubing varies with the brand of the tubing; most Cutter brand macrodrip tubing is made with a drip rate of 20 drops/mL; most Abbott brand macrodrip tubing is made with a drip rate of 15 drops/mL; and most Travenol brand macrodrip tubing is made with a drip rate of 10 drops/mL. The drip rate of macrodrip tubing is found on the outside of the tubing package. All brands of minidrip tubing have the same drip rate, 60 drops/mL. Because the drip rate per milliliter (60) is equal to the number of minutes per hour, the formula for calculating drip rate when using minidrip tubing may be simplified to mL/h = drops/min.

Administering Medications According to the "Five Rights"

After the nurse has validated the order and calculated the proper drug dose, accurate administration of a medication can be assured by following the "five rights" of medication administration (summarized in the display "Five Rights of Medication Administration"). Each time a medication is administered the nurse must be sure that the right client is given the right medication, in the right dose, by the right route, at the right time.

The Right Client. The first "right" of administering medications, the right client, means that the medication is given to the client for whom it is intended (Fig. 27-3).

Incorrect identification of clients can occur when a nurse is busy, when clients with similar names are located in the same areas of an institution, and when client identification procedures are not followed. Errors can be avoided if the nurse identifies the client by name and checks the name band against the client's medication record before giving him or her medications. The institution's "name alert" policy should be followed whenever clients with similar names are located in the same unit. Name alert procedures involve a special way of identifying clients with similar names and a way of alerting other departments of the clients' name similarity.

"Five Rights" of Medication Administration

- Identify the *right client.*
- Select the *right medication.*
- Give the *right dose.*
- Give the medication at the *right time.*
- Give the medication by the *right route.*

The Right Medication. The second "right" of administering medications, the right medication, means that the medication given is the medication that was ordered and that the medication ordered is appropriate for the client. Medication errors may occur as follows:

- When a pharmacist incorrectly dispenses a medication that is similar in shape and color to the ordered medication
- When a pharmacist or nurse incorrectly dispenses or administers a medication that has a smiliar name to the medication ordered (Cohen, 1994)

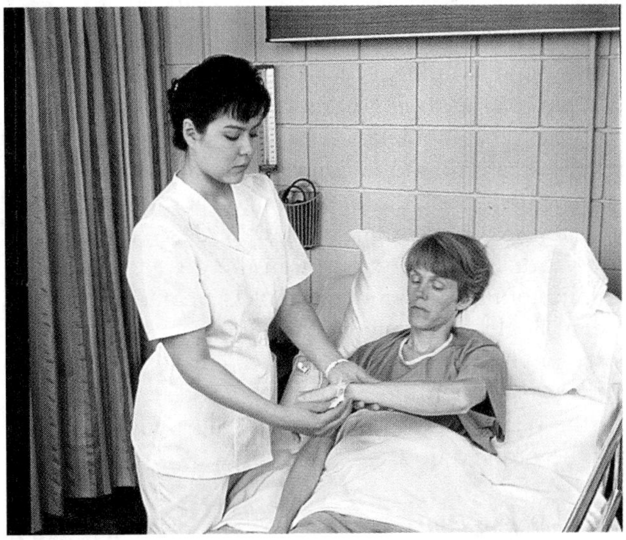

Figure 27-3 • No matter what the administration route, the nurse must always check that the right client will receive the right medication. The nurse checks the medication record, the unit dosage, and the client's identification bracelet. If the client is conscious, the nurse also asks the client to state his or her name. (Photo © B. Proud.)

- When the healthcare provider orders a medication that is not appropriate for the client
- When the nurse or healthcare provider administers a medication that they have not prepared
- When a nurse incorrectly identifies a medication

The risk of giving the wrong medication can be decreased by using a "unit-dose medication" system, by administering only medications that have been prepared and labeled by the nurse or by the hospital pharmacist, by checking the medication label with the medication order, by knowing the generic and trade names of a medication and the reason it is being given to the client, and by listening for client clues. Client clues include statements such as, "This doesn't look like the same pill I took before." If a nurse hears such clues, he or she should recheck the medication order.

The Right Dosage. The third "right" of administering medications, the right dosage, means that the medication is given in the dose ordered and that the dose ordered is appropriate for the client. Incorrect dosages may be given if a healthcare provider orders a dose that is inappropriate for a client; if a pharmacist dispenses or if a nurse administers an incorrect amount of medication; or if a pharmacist, nurse, or support staff transcribes an order incorrectly onto the client's medication record (Davis, 1993; Davis 1994a).

These errors may be avoided if the nurse and pharmacist are aware of the usual dosage ranges of medications; if the nurse double-checks with the healthcare provider whenever questions concerning the accuracy of a dosage arise; if the nurse and pharmacist correctly calculate the amount of medication required; and if the nurse double-checks medications transcribed onto a client's medication record with the healthcare provider's orders before administering a new medication and whenever a new medication record is started.

The nurse should double-check medication dosages whenever he or she encounters the following, which suggest that a medication dosage may be incorrect: whenever a client suggests that the dose he or she is used to taking is different from the dose the nurse is administering; when multiple tablets are needed to supply a single medication dose (Spencer, 1992); when large or abrupt changes in medication dosages are ordered; and when the amount of medication supplied by the pharmacist does not match the amount needed for the ordered doses.

The Right Route. The fourth "right" of administering medications, the right route, means that the medication is given by the ordered route and that the ordered route is safe and appropriate for the client. The healthcare provider's medication orders should always specify the route of administration. If a route is not specified or if the route ordered seems inappropriate, the nurse should check with the healthcare provider to clarify which route should be used (Davis, 1994b).

Other actions that help to ensure that a medication is given by the proper route include knowing the usual route(s) of administration of a medication, knowing the safety of administering a medication by the ordered route, and double-checking route of administration before administering a medication.

The Right Time. The fifth "right" of administering medications, the right time, means that the medication is given at the time ordered. Medication policies defining the meaning of "on time" vary with institutions; usually a medication is said to be given "on time" if it is given within 30 minutes or 1 hour before or after the dose is scheduled to be given.

Many factors influence the schedules used to administer medications, including the following: a medication may be more effective if given on an "around-the-clock" schedule when given in IV form but may be appropriate to give during waking hours in the oral form; a medication that interacts with food may need to be given before meals; a medication that causes gastric irritation may need to be given with meals; and routine medication administration schedules vary between institutions.

The nurse needs to be aware of the scheduling requirements of the medication he or she is giving and the routine scheduling times used at his or her institution. The nurse also should be aware of the situations in which medication scheduling problems frequently occur. Medication scheduling problems are more likely to occur when different units within an institution use different routine administration schedules, after the client transfers from one unit or facility to another, or when a limited number of doses of medication are ordered. Before giving a medication, the nurse should always check the medication record to note when the medication was last administered and, when necessary, the total number of doses administered.

Medication Errors

A medication error occurs when a medication is not administered as ordered; when the medication is administered according to the order, but the medication order is not safe or appropriate for the client; or when the documentation in a client's chart does not reflect that a medication was administered as ordered. The most common medication errors are related to documentation errors: The medication was given but not charted. Another documentation error is failure to note the site where a parenteral injection was given. Other common medication errors include an IV medication administered at the wrong rate, a dose of medication not administered in the dose ordered, a medication given at the wrong time, the wrong medication administered, and a medication charted but not given. Errors of medication substitution are more common with the increased use of generic medications, and the nurse must be sure that the name of the medication supplied is the same as, not just similar to, the name of the medication ordered. Less common errors include a medication given by the wrong route, a medication given to a client with a known allergy to that medication, and a medication given to the wrong client (Cohen, Senders, & Davis, 1994).

Documentation of Medication Administration

The medication policies of an institution define the time and type of medication documentation (charting) that is done. Documentation should be done immediately after a medication is given. Medication documentation includes the time, route, dosage, site of administration (for intradermal [ID], SC, or IM injections), and the nurse's initials and signature (Fig. 27-4).

Specific documentation also is required if a medication has not been given. In many agencies, the normal time of administration is circled when a medication has been withheld. It is important to indicate why the medication was not given; at times, this can simply be a matter of indicating NPO next to the designated time for administration. At other times, the reason is more complex, and an explanation needs to be written in other appropriate places in the chart.

Some medications (eg, insulin or heparin) may have separate flow sheets on the medication administration chart. Frequently, this flow sheet contains laboratory data or other pertinent information. Such a flow sheet permits a healthcare provider to visualize patterns of management over time. When numerous injections are administered, a chart documenting the location of each injection is provided to ensure adequate site rotation. Whenever injections are administered, the site used should be documented.

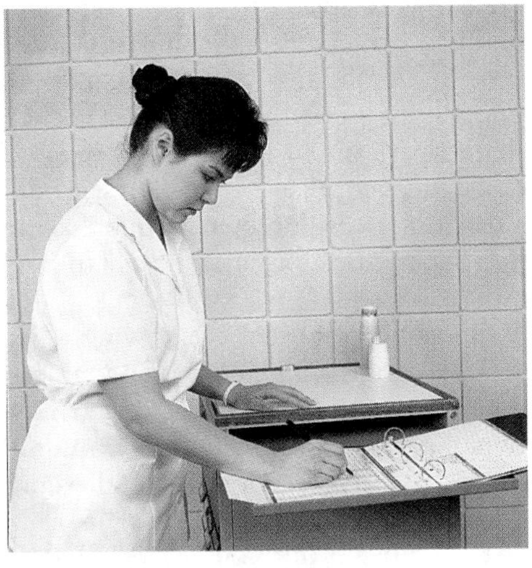

Figure 27-4 • Documentation of medication administration is an important nursing requirement. (Photo © B. Proud.)

The nurse also is responsible for documenting the therapeutic and side effects of any medication administered. For example, if a narcotic is administered for pain, the amount of pain relief the client obtains should be documented. If a client develops a rash after the administration of an antibiotic, the onset and type of rash should be described in detail.

A medication error is documented by charting the medication as it was given in the client's medication record, making note of the error in the progress notes, and filling out a quality improvement or unusual incident form.

Medication Administration in the Home

As technology advances, more medications are being administered in the home, and as more clients receive primary and follow-up care in the home, issues related to medication administration become increasingly complex.

Types of Medications

Oral medications, such as antibiotics and pain relievers, have always been prescribed for clients to take at home, and this practice continues to be common. In recent years, however, long-term antibiotic or antineoplastic medications are being administered in the home with a variety of portable IV drug infusion devices. Sometimes, home health nurses administer these medications at regular intervals, but more often, family caregivers must learn to give the medications.

In such situations, client education becomes a major nursing focus for maintaining accuracy and minimizing potential risks. Of equal concern is having help quickly available in case of an emergency. An additional nursing responsibility is ensuring that healthcare personnel are available on-call.

When supervising or administering medications in the home setting, the nurse needs to be sure that this nursing intervention is within the scope of the state's nurse practice act. Furthermore, if controlled substances are being administered in the home, the nurse must carefully comply with the law regarding appropriate drug storage, documentation, and disposal. Doing so protects the nurse from suggestions of improper diversion of the controlled substances and accounts accurately for controlled substances administered in the home.

In some areas, pharmacies may contract with the client to administer and manage medication administration within the home.

Organizing Medication Regimens in the Home

An important aspect of accurate home medication administration is ensuring a schedule, or regimen, that is easy to remember and fits the client's lifestyle. Arranging to take medications by linking them with normal events in the client's life (eg, meals or bedtime) promotes compliance and accuracy. The nurse does, however, need to assess the hours when these events occur so that medication administration is appropriately staggered.

For some clients, especially older ones, remembering to take medications and knowing which ones to take can present worrisome problems, as illustrated in the situation in the beginning of the chapter. When poor vision and lapsing memory are both factors, using a sectioned medication dispensing device may be helpful. This requires having someone set up the medications in the appropriate compartments, usually once a week for the entire week. The client then follows instructions to take medication from the appropriate compartment at the appropriate time. Using such a device may not prevent all errors, but medication administration with the device may be considerably safer than without it.

Oral Medications

Medications that are given by mouth are designed to be swallowed (oral route), to be held under the tongue until they dissolve (sublingual route), to be administered through tubes, or to be held in the side of the mouth until they dissolve (buccal route). Refer to Procedure 27-1, "Administering Oral Medications."

Advantages

Giving medications by mouth is usually the simplest and easiest way to take them. It minimizes client discomfort and is associated with the fewest side effects of any route. Oral medications tend to be less expensive and more widely available than medications given by other routes.

Contraindications

Medications should not be given by mouth when a client cannot swallow or is nauseated or vomiting. If the client cannot swallow water or fluids, oral medications should be discontinued or given by another route. Relative contraindications to giving oral medications include NPO status and gastric suction. If a client is NPO before a test or surgery, the healthcare provider may continue selected oral medications. These ordered medications would be given with sips of water. If the client is NPO after major surgery, oral medications are usually withheld or administered by another route until intestinal function resumes. Usually, in clients being treated with gastric suction, oral medications are withheld or given by another route. Occasionally, a healthcare provider may order a specific medication to be administered through a nasogastric tube and may order the gastric suction discontinued for a specified time (usually 30 minutes) after medication administration.

Forms of Oral Medication

Oral medications, commonly termed PO (from the Latin *per os,* "by mouth") are supplied in liquids, capsules, and tablets. Liquid medications are commonly used for small children or for adults who cannot swallow pills easily (see Table 27-2).

Routes of Oral Administration

Oral Administration. Methods of preparing and administering oral medications are designed to ensure that the medication moves to the back of the client's throat, moves down the esophagus, and is properly absorbed. Whenever taking any oral medications, the client should be standing or sitting, or should have the head of his or her bed elevated. If the client can swallow liquids, but cannot move liquids to the back of his or her mouth, liquid medications may be administered using a syringe with a piece of rubber tubing attached. The medication is drawn up through the tubing into the syringe; the tubing is inserted into the side of the client's mouth and the medication is slowly injected into the back of the mouth. Antifungal liquid medications, such as nystatin (Mycostatin), that work through contact with the mucous membranes in the mouth are given by the "swish and swallow" technique: The client puts the liquid in his or her mouth, moves the liquid back and forth in the mouth several times, and swallows it.

Several techniques may be used to administer medications to a client who can swallow soft foods but not whole capsules or tablets. A capsule can be opened and the contents added to a small amount of the client's food, such as ice cream or applesauce. Most tablets, except enteric-coated and sustained-release tablets, can be crushed and added to soft foods. Enteric-coated tablets should not be crushed, because this may allow the irritating medication to come in contact with the stomach and result in gastric irritation. If a sustained-release medication is crushed, all its medication will be absorbed at the same time, resulting in higher than expected initial levels of medication and shorter than expected duration of action.

Even clients with normal swallowing reflexes may have problems swallowing and moving tablets or capsules down the esophagus. Drug-induced esophagitis, an inflammation of the esophagus, may occur if a tablet or capsule lodges in the esophagus and begins to dissolve there. Several techniques help to aid movement of a tablet or capsule through the esophagus and to prevent drug-induced esophagitis. The client should be in a semi-Fowler's, sitting, or standing position when

Procedure 27-1
Administering Oral Medications

Purpose

1. Provide a safe, effective, economic route for administering medications.
2. Provide a sustained drug action with minimal discomfort.

Assessment

- Review medication orders for accuracy and completeness. An order should include client's name, drug name, dosage, route, and time.
- Consult drug package inserts, pharmacology textbooks, or other standard references about unfamiliar drugs.
- Assess client's allergy history.
- Assess client's ability to take oral medications:
  Level of consciousness, cooperativeness
  Active swallow reflex
  Nausea and vomiting
  Recent gastrointestinal surgery or bowel obstruction
  Nasogastric tube connected to suction
  Current diet order
- Identify and perform individual preadministration assessments of pulse, blood pressure, and so forth
- Ensure that correct medication and dosage are available at the time scheduled.

Equipment

Medication Kardex or medication administration record
Medication cart
Disposable medication cups
Water, juice, or milk
Mortar and pestle (optional for crushing pills)

Procedure

1. Wash hands.
   Rationale: Washing hands reduces transfer of microorganisms from hands to medication.
2. Arrange medication Kardex or cards next to medication cart or cabinet, medication trays, and cups.
   Rationale: Organizing work space saves time and reduces chance of errors.
3. Prepare medications for only one client at a time.
   Rationale: This prevents errors during preparation.
4. Remove ordered medication from cart or shelf. Compare label on medication with medication Kardex or card. If there is a discrepancy, recheck the client's chart and medication orders.
   Rationale: Cross-checking label against transcribed order decreases errors.
5. Calculate correct drug dosage if necessary.
6. Prepare medications.
   a. Unit dosage: Place packaged medication directly into medicine cup, or lay on tray without unwrapping.
   b. Medications from a multidose bottle: Pour tablets or capsules into the container lid, and transfer into medicine cup. Extra tablets can be returned to the bottle. Do not touch medications.
   Rationale: This maintains cleanliness of drugs.
   Note: If client has trouble swallowing tablets, grind with mortar and pestle until smooth. Mix powder in small amount of custard or applesauce. *Do not* crush enteric-coated tablets, because the contents are irritating to gastric mucosa. Consult pharmacist or physician.

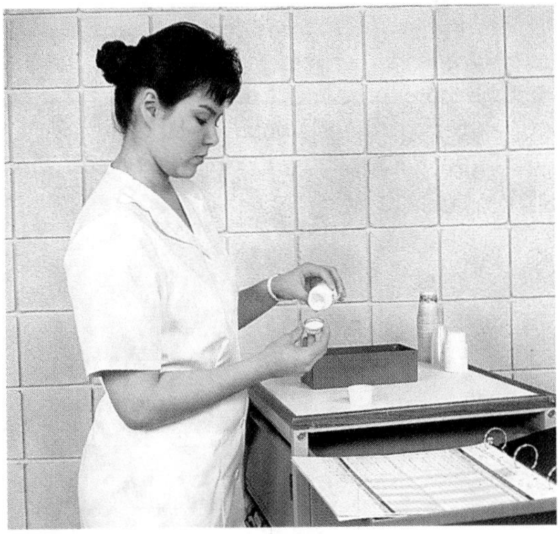

Step 6B • *Pour medication into medicine cup. (Photo © B. Proud.)*

   c. Liquid medications: Remove cap and place on counter top inside up to prevent contamination. Hold bottle so label is against palm of hand.
   Rationale: This prevents soiling of label when pouring medication.
   d. Hold medication cup at eye level, and fill until bottom of meniscus (the surface of the fluid that appears curved) is at desired dosage. Discard excess poured liquid from cup into sink. Do not pour back into bottle.

(continued)

Rationale: This permits accurate measurement and prevents contamination of medication in bottle.

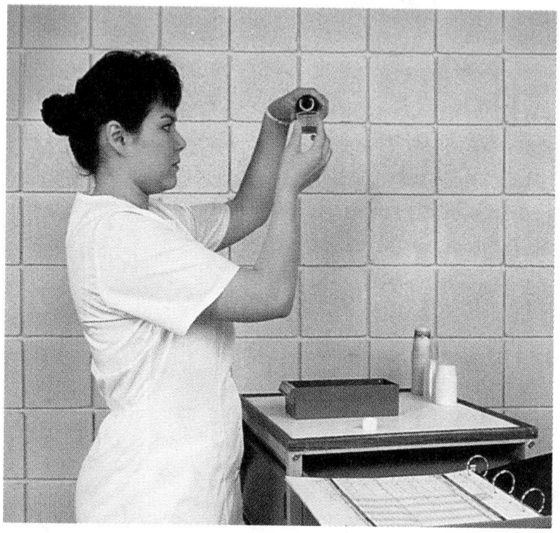

Step 6D • *Hold liquid medications at eye level to read dosage level at base of meniscus. (Photo © B. Proud.)*

e. Oral narcotic: Compare previous drug count on narcotic record with current supply. Place drug in medication cup, and record information on narcotic record.
Rationale: Strict monitoring is required of all controlled subtances.

7. Compare prepared medication with medication kardex (or card) and container label.
Rationale: Rechecking label reduces medication errors.

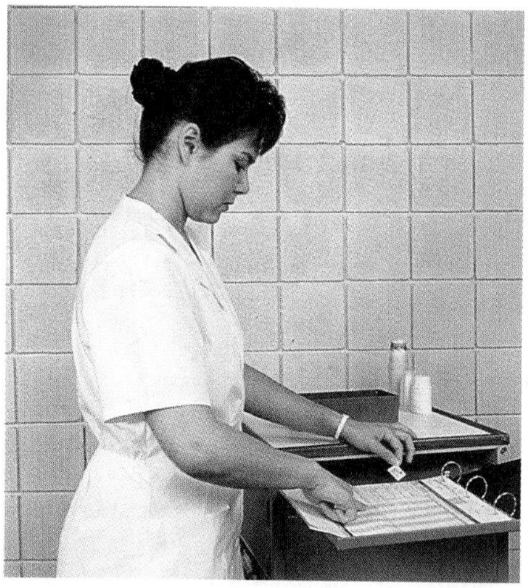

Step 7 • *Compare medication, container label, and medication record. (Photo © B. Proud.)*

8. Reread label, and place medication container or unused drug back on cart or shelf.
Safety Alert: Medications are checked three times before administering to the client:
   a. When removing container from the storage area
   b. After placing medication into cup
   c. Before returning container back to storage area (unless using unit-dose system)
9. Take medication directly to client's room. Do not leave unattended.
Rationale: Prevents medication errors.
10. Ask client to state his or her name, and compare name on medication card or record with name on client's identification band.
Rationale: Careful checking ensures administration of drugs to proper client.
11. Complete any preadministration assessment (ie, blood pressure, pulse) required by specific medication.
Rationale: Medications that have a direct action, such as decreasing pulse rate or blood pressure, require assessment to determine if medication can be given safely at that time.
12. Explain purpose of medication to client.
Rationale: This is in accordance with client's rights and will improve compliance.
13. Assist client to sitting position.
Rationale: This position assists swallowing and prevents aspiration.
14. If using unit-dose medication, read label, unwrap medication, and place in cup. Give medication cup and glass of water or juice to client.
15. If client is unable to hold the medication cup, place pill cup to lips and introduce medication into his or her mouth.
Rationale: Holding the cup prevents contamination of medication.
16. Stay with client until all medications are swallowed. You may need to look inside client's mouth to be certain.
Rationale: The nurse is responsible for client receiving ordered medications.

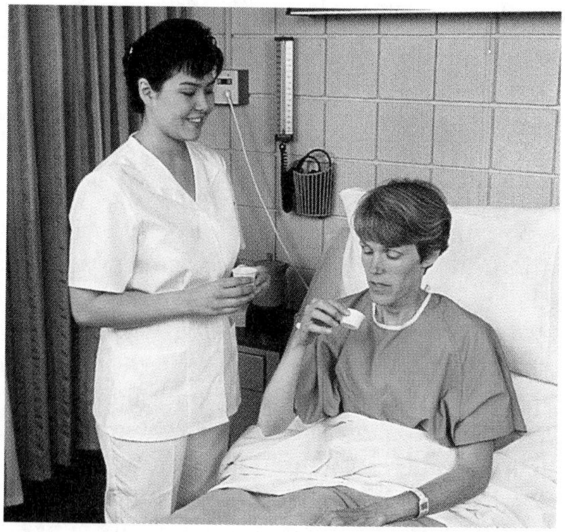

Step 16 • *Stay with client while medications are swallowed. (Photo © B. Proud.)*

Note: If tablet or capsule falls on the floor, discard and repeat preparation.

17. Dispose of soiled supplies, and wash hands.
18. Record time medication was administered and any preadministration assessment data that were collected.

Lifespan Considerations

Infants and Children

- Tablets and capsules are not recommended form of oral medication in children younger than 5 years because they may not be swallowed safely. Liquid preparations are available for most oral medications, and some come with a calibrated dropper for measuring small amounts of medication for infants. Do not interchange droppers among medications.
  Rationale: Different companies use different sized droppers, and medications may be inaccurately measured.
- Play techniques may encourage a child's cooperation in swallowing medications.
- Always let the child know that you have medicine, not candy.

Older Adults

- Normal physiologic changes with aging that may influence a client's ability to take oral medications include decreased salivation and elasticity of oral mucosa, resulting in a dry mouth and delayed esophageal clearance, which may impair swallowing. A liquid form of medication may be necessary.
- Additional changes with aging are decreased stomach peristalsis and gastric acidity and decreased colon motility.

Home-Care Modifications

- Assess client or family member's knowledge of drug therapy.
- Assess client's sensory function (sight, hearing, touch) to determine if special teaching or administration strategies are required. Have client wear eyeglasses or hearing aid during teaching sessions.
- Assess client's ability to read. Client may be unable to read prepared booklets or medication label.
- Client or family members should be instructed in purpose of medications, dosage schedule, common side effects, who to call with problems, and what to do about missed doses.
- Give guidelines for drug safety as appropriate: discarding outdated drugs, keeping drugs out of reach of children, refrigerating medications.
- Devise learning aids if needed. Examples include calendars for each week that contain separate ziplock bags with medications to take at specific times; egg cartons with color-coded sections for medications to take at specific times; and commercially available divided containers to provide 1 week of medication at a time.

taking medications and should not return to a flat, recumbent position for at least 1 minutes after taking a capsule or pill. Whenever possible, the client should drink about 100 mL of fluid after swallowing a capsule or tablet (Shlafer, 1993).

If a client senses that a medication is stuck in the throat, a small portion of a soft food, such as a banana, should be offered to help move the medication. If the feeling persists, the healthcare provider should be notified.

Hospitals or pharmacies provide calibrated medicine glasses and droppers for accurately measuring prescribed doses of liquid medications (Fig. 27-5). When measuring liquids, the nurse should hold the measuring container at eye level with one hand and use the other hand to pour the medication to the indicated level. An elliptical curve, called the meniscus, is produced because the solution clings to the side of the measuring container. The lower part of the meniscus should rest on the calibration line of the dose being measured (see Step 6 in Procedure 27-1).

Calibrated medicine droppers may be supplied with the medication. It is important to use the dropper supplied because the dose of the medication depends on the size of the opening in the dropper, the angle at which the dropper is held, and the viscosity of the solution.

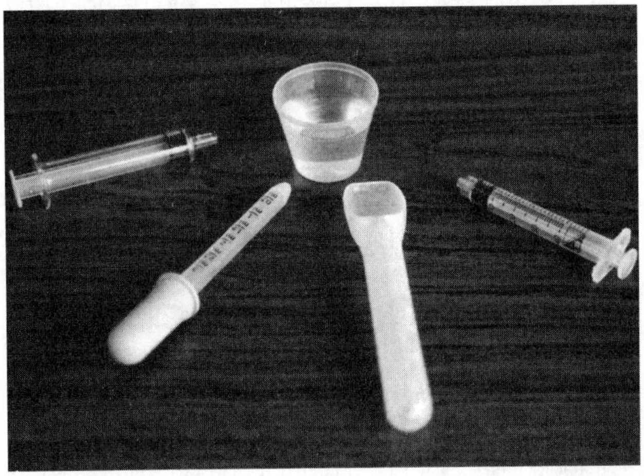

Figure 27-5 • *Devices used to measure liquid medications accurately:* (left to right) *oral syringe, dropper, medicine cup, spoonlike device, injection syringe without needle.*

Administration Through Tubes. Oral medications may be administered through nasogastric or gastric tubes or through nasointestinal or jejunal tubes. When giving oral medications through gastric or intestinal tubes, care should be taken to decrease the risks of client aspiration and a clogged feeding tube. The risk of aspiration (movement of matter into the lungs rather than into the stomach) decreases if the client is properly positioned, for example in a semi-Fowler's or Fowler's position, whenever receiving food or medications. Additionally, the head of the client's bed should remain elevated for at least 30 minutes after medications are administered (Shlafer, 1993). A feeding tube may become clogged if medications solidify in it. Hydrophyllic gels, such as Metamucil, should not be given through feeding tubes, because they tend to attract water and solidify within the feeding tube (Spencer, 1992).

Most liquid medications can be given through feeding tubes. Tablets may be given through a feeding tube if they can be crushed into fine particles and dissolved in water. Before and after administering a medication, the feeding tube should be irrigated with 15 to 30 mL of a saline solution or water. If it becomes difficult to instill fluid into the tube, the tube can be irrigated with 30 to 50 mL of warm water or carbonated beverage. These fluids may help to dissolve food or medication particles within the tube and may restore tube patency.

Sublingual Administration. The **sublingual** tablet is placed under the tongue and allowed to dissolve. If the client's mucous membranes are dry, 1 mL of normal saline solution or water should be used to wet the membranes underneath the tongue so that absorption can occur. Sublingual tablets should not be swallowed.

Buccal Administration. The **buccal** route is seldom used for medication administration, although recently, pharmaceutical companies have released a variety of medications for buccal administration, including sustained-release nitroglycerin, narcotics, antiemetics, tranquilizers, and sedatives. Buccal medications should be placed underneath the upper lip or in the side of the mouth. Buccal medications should not be chewed, swallowed, or placed under the tongue.

Topical Medications

Topical medications are placed on the skin surface or in body cavities.

Medications Applied to the Skin

Medications are usually applied to the skin to treat local (skin) or systemic conditions. Medications used to treat local skin conditions or infections are prepared in irrigation solutions or creams or lotions. When a transdermal medication is placed on the skin, it is absorbed through the skin, producing systemic (total body) effects.

Irrigation Solutions. Irrigation solutions, such as normal saline, Dakin's Solution (dilute bleach), or povidone-iodine (Betadine), may be used to clean a wound. These solutions should be applied using a large (50 mL) syringe and gentle pressure. Using a smaller syringe may generate pressure that is high enough to harm granulation tissue in healing wounds.

Creams and Lotions. Creams and lotions may be used to treat a skin or wound infection, to treat a skin disease, or to decrease symptoms of skin disorders.

Antibiotic creams, such as silver sulfadiazine (Silvadene) or Neosporin, may be applied to clean skin surfaces applied with a sterile swab, a sterile tongue depressor, or gloved fingers. Antibiotic creams should be applied in a thin layer; thick coatings increase cost and the likelihood of a systemic effect.

Transdermal Medications. **Transdermal** medications, those designed to be absorbed through the skin for systemic effects, are prepared in a medication patch or gel. The medication patches are made with special membranes that allow medication to be absorbed slowly. These patches allow controlled amounts of medication to be supplied over a 24- to 72-hour period. Clients should be cautioned to remove the patch and clean the skin underneath before applying another patch.

Nitroglycerin and scopolamine transdermal patches are commonly used (Fig. 27-6). Clients using scopolamine should be cautioned not to use more than one patch at a time; use of multiple scopolamine patches has resulted in death. Nitroglycerin gel is applied to nitroglycerin paper that is marked with half-inch increments, and the gel is applied to the measuring paper using a continuous motion. Large variations in dosage can result if thick bands of nitroglycerin are applied or if more than one layer of nitroglycerin is applied. The nitroglycerin and nitroglycerin paper are applied to a skin surface and secured to the skin with paper tape. If a dose of nitroglycerin ointment is applied before surgery, it should be placed on easily visible skin, such as that on the forehead or chest.

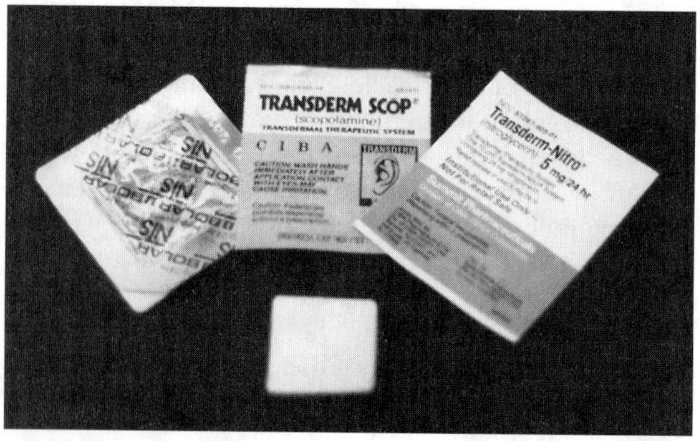

Figure 27-6 • Scopolamine and nitroglycerin transdermal patches.

Instillation of Eye Medications

- Assist client to sit in an upright position with the head hyperextended.
- Provide client with tissues to blot any medication or tears that spill from the eye during the instillation.
- Ask client to look toward ceiling.
- Place finger or thumb on lower bony orbit and gently pull the lower lid down (as shown).
- With other hand resting on the client's forehead, instill the required number of drops or the ointment on the lower conjunctival sac.
- Avoid touching the eyelids, lashes, or the eyeball with either hand or with the applicator.
- Avoid dropping a solution onto the cornea directly because it causes discomfort.
- Release the lower lid, and allow the client to close eye.
- If the client blinks and the medication is not instilled, repeat the steps.

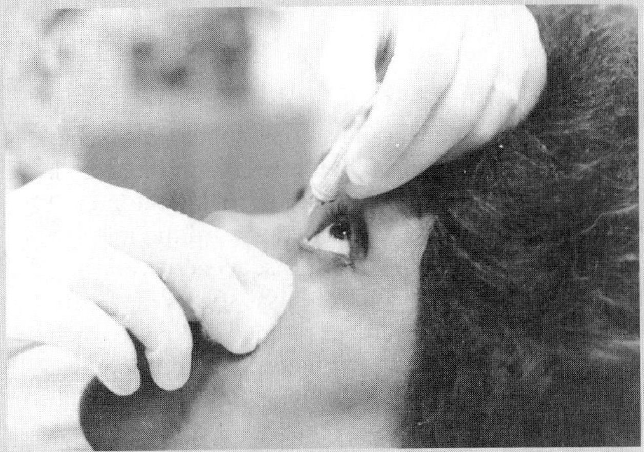

Ophthalmic Medications

Solutions or ointments may be placed in the eye to treat eye irritation, infections, and glaucoma. The lower eyelid is gently retracted, and the solutions or ointments are placed in the conjunctival sac (see the display "Instillation of Eye Medications"). Care should be taken to avoid touching the eye or eyelid with the tip of the ointment tube or dropper. The client should be instructed not to rub his or her eye after the medication is applied.

Otic Medications

Solutions may be dropped into the ear to treat external ear infections or to soften and remove ear wax. Solutions used in the ear should be at room temperature;

Instillation of Ear Drops

- Have client sit or lie with head turned to unaffected side.
- Warm solution to body temperature to prevent discomfort during instillation.
- Prepare appropriate amount of medication in dropper.
- Straighten the auditory canal by gently pulling the pinna (cartilaginous portion of outer ear) up and back in older children and adults (as shown) and down and back for infants and children younger than 3 years.
- Instill ear drops on side of the auditory canal to allow the drops to flow in and to continue to adjust to body temperature.
- Release the pinna, and gently massage tragus of the ear.
- If permitted, place a cotton ball or wick in the outer ear to keep medication in the canal.
- If drops are required in the opposite ear, wait a few minutes, and repeat the procedure in that ear.

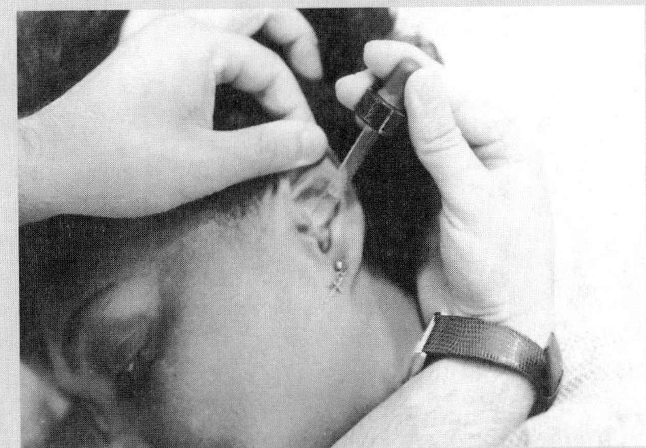

using hot or cold solutions in the ear may cause vertigo, nausea, and pain (Spencer, 1992). The client should lie on his or her unaffected side before the nurse instills the ear medication (see the accompanying display "Instillation of Ear Drops").

Nasal Medications

Solutions are usually sprayed into the nose to treat nasal congestion. The client should sit up and lean his or her head back. The medication bottle is held in one hand, with the top of the bottle placed just inside the nostril and the spray applicator top aimed toward the midline of the nose. The bottle should be squeezed while the client inhales. Over-the-counter nasal sprays may contain decongestant and adrenergic medications (which stimulate the sympathetic nervous system); frequent use can cause systemic effects, such as increased heart rate and increased blood pressure. Rebound nasal congestion, causing symptoms of nasal congestion that are as bad as or worse than original symptoms, commonly occurs if decongestant nasal sprays are used for longer than several days.

Rectal Medications

Medication in suppository form (medication incorporated into a small, cylindrically shaped, waxy base) may be placed in the rectum to treat systemic complaints or encourage bowel movements. Antiemetic suppositories may be used to treat nausea when other routes are not appropriate. The technique for placing suppositories is shown in Figure 27-7.

Liquid medications may be instilled into the rectum using an enema to encourage bowel movements or to treat clients with elevated potassium levels. Enema fluids are usually given in volumes of about 100 mL and are usually meant to be retained by the client for 10 to 30 minutes. An enema of resin-containing fluid may be used to remove potassium from the bowel of a client with an elevated potassium level. The procedure for administering small-volume enemas is discussed in Chapter 42.

Vaginal Medications

Medications given vaginally come in a variety of forms: foams, jellies, liquids (douches), creams, tablets, or suppositories. These medications may be used for contraception, to help kill any bacteria in the vaginal area before gynecologic surgery, to treat vaginal itching or infection, or to induce labor. Prostaglandin vaginal suppositories cause uterine contractions and induce labor in women after fetal demise (when death of the fetus occurs early in a pregnancy). The technique for instilling vaginal suppositories and tablets is shown in Figure 27-8.

Inhaled Medications

Inhaled medications may be used to induce anesthesia during surgery and to treat respiratory disorders. Anesthetic medications are administered by anesthesiologists or nurse anesthetists through a machine. Inhaled medications may be administered through a mechanical ventilator, a hand-held nebulizer, or a metered-dose inhaler. Liquid medications are added to a receptacle in the ventilator or the nebulizer and changed into a gas form when air or oxygen flows over them.

A metered-dose inhaler is a small hand-held device that a client presses before inhaling. Each time it is pressed, the metered-dose inhaler releases a set dose (metered dose) of medication. Inhaled medications have a rapid effect on the lungs and are rapidly absorbed by the systemic circulation. Bronchodilator medications, used to open lung airways and promote easier breathing, are frequently part of the therapy for clients with chronic obstructive lung disease. The client's respiratory status (reported ease of breathing, breath sounds,

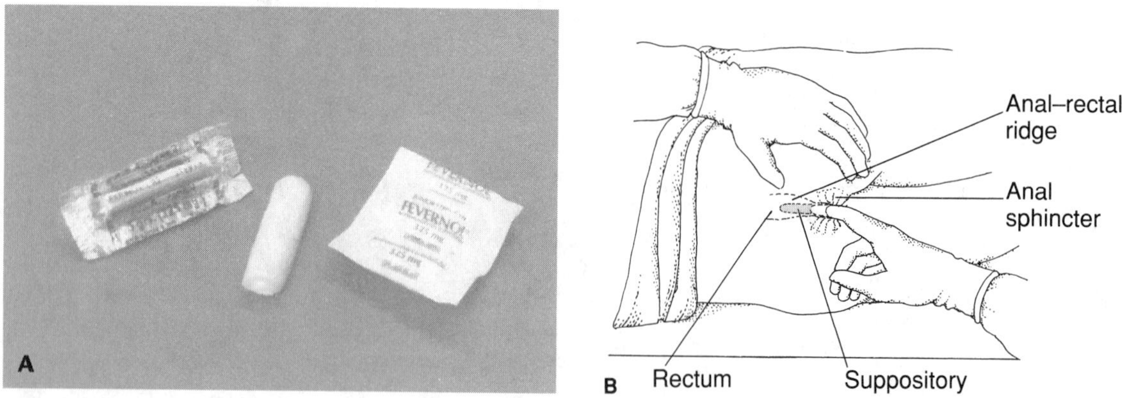

Figure 27-7 • *Insertion of rectal suppositories. (**A**) Prepackaged suppositories. (**B**) The suppository is inserted past the internal anal sphincter against the rectal wall.*

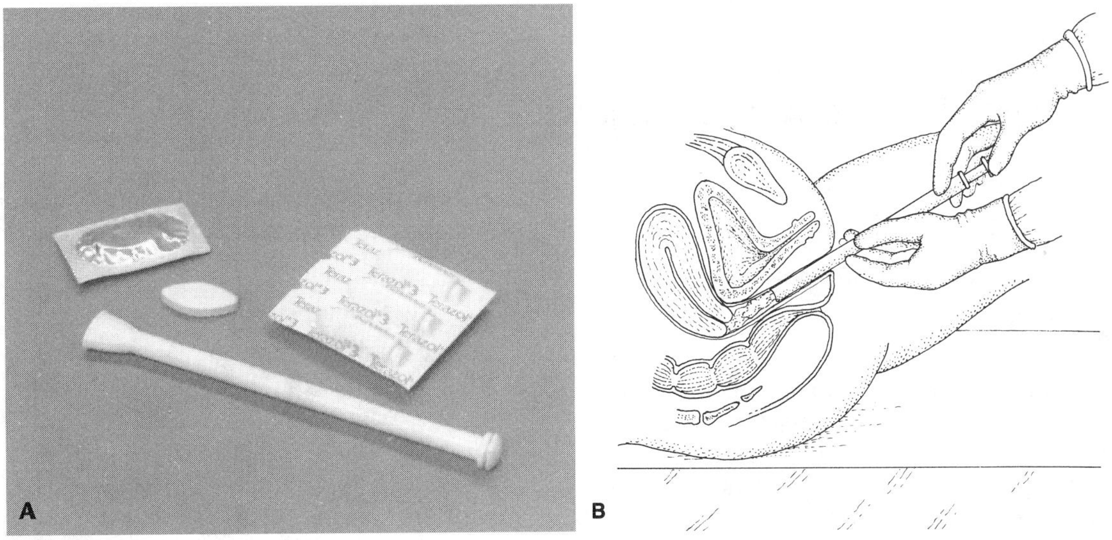

Figure 27-8 • *Insertion of vaginal medication. **(A)** Vaginal suppository and applicator. **(B)** Insertion of vaginal cream using applicator.*

respiratory rate, and use of accessory respiratory muscles) should be assessed before and after administering an inhalable medication.

Parenteral Medications

Medications that are given by injection or infusion are given by the parenteral route. Parenteral medications may be injected into ID, SC, IM, or intralesional tissue; into venous (IV) or arterial circulation; or into intraspinal or intra-articular spaces. The ID, SC, IM, and IV routes are discussed in this chapter.

Advantages and Disadvantages

Medications given by a parenteral route usually are absorbed more completely and begin acting faster than medications given by other routes. Parenteral medications are injected through the skin; bypassing the skin barrier makes infection more likely if aseptic technique is not used when preparing and administering parenteral medications. Complications may occur if parenteral medications are not given into the intended tissue site or space. Tissue damage may occur if the pH, osmotic pressure, or solubility of the medication is not appropriate to the tissue where the medication is given. Specialized equipment required for parenteral administration usually makes medications given by these routes more expensive than medications given by other routes.

Equipment

Equipment needed to administer parenteral medications includes a container for the medication and a system to deliver the medication. Medications used for ID, SC, or IM injections are usually supplied in vials, ampules, or prefilled syringes.

Vials. Vials are plastic or glass containers that may hold one or more doses of medication. The vial is opened by removing a plastic cap that covers a rubber diaphragm at the top of the container. A needle is used to pierce the center of the diaphragm, and the correct amount of medication is withdrawn into a syringe. See Procedure 27-2, "Withdrawing Medication from a Vial." Medications that are not stable for long periods may be supplied in a vial in powdered form. A diluent (sterile liquid specified by the drug manufacturer) is mixed with the powder to reconstitute it.

Ampules. Ampules are thin-walled glass containers that hold a single dose of a liquid medication. An ampule is shaped like a bowling pin; it has a wide base, narrow neck, and pointed top. Refer to Procedure 27-3, "Withdrawing Medication from an Ampule."

Filter Needles. Some agencies require the use of a filter needle to trap any rubber or glass fragments that may be drawn up with the medication in a vial or an ampule. For obvious reasons, the filter needle must be replaced by a regular SC needle before injecting the medication into the client.

Syringes. Syringes, usually made of plastic, consist of a barrel, plunger, and syringe tip (Fig. 27-9). The plunger fits snugly within the syringe barrel. Moving the plunger out of the barrel allows fluid or air to be moved into the syringe; pushing the plunger into the barrel allows fluid or air to be moved out of the syringe. A needle is attached to the syringe tip (the narrow end of the syringe); syringes may be packaged with or without an attached needle. Needle gauge (size)

Procedure 27-2
Withdrawing Medication From a Vial

Purpose

To withdraw a precise amount of medication from a vial without introducing contamination

Assessment

- Review physician's order, and assess the intended medication administration route (eg, SC, IM, IV) before selecting the needle and syringe.
- Inspect the ordered medication for clarity, crystals and expiration date.

Equipment

Medication order, card, or printout and medication record
Vial with medication
Alcohol wipes or antiseptic swabs for cleaning vial
Sterile syringe and needle
Optional: Solvent (sterile water or normal saline solution for reconstituting medication if it is in powder form); needle with filter if needed to prevent drawing solid matter into the needle and syringe

Procedure

1. Assemble equipment in one place or tray.
2. Check medication order (see Procedure 27-1 "Administering Oral Medications," Steps 1 to 5); compare the name of the ordered medication with the label on the medication vial.
3. Wash hands.
4. Assemble needle and syringe.
5. Pick up vial, and place it between the palms, rotating or rolling the vial back and forth.
   Rationale: The rolling motion mixes and disperses the medication.
6. Remove metal cap from vial.
7. Cleanse top of vial with alcohol wipe.
8. Remove guard from needle.
9. Pull back on barrel of syringe to draw in a volume of air equal to the volume of the ordered medication dose.
10. Holding the vial between the thumb and fingers of the nondominant hand, insert needle through the rubber stopper into the air space—not the solution—in the vial and inject air.
    Rationale: Injection of air into the air space in the vial prevents creation of negative pressure within the vial, allowing medication to be withdrawn easily. Injecting air into the solution creates bubbles and may interfere with withdrawing an accurate dose of medication.

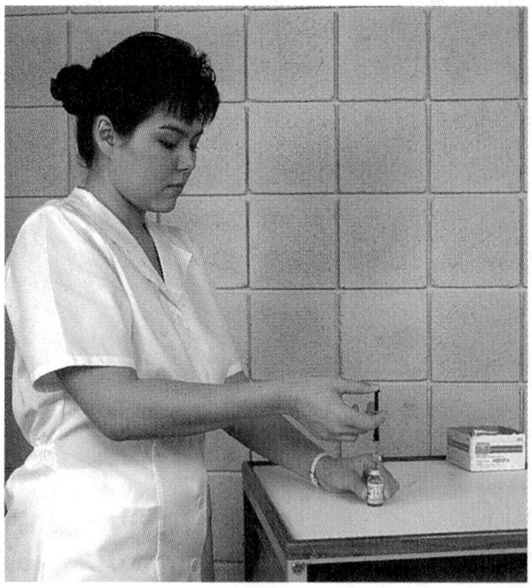

Step 10 • Add air to the vial. (Photo © B. Proud.)

11. Invert the vial and withdraw the ordered dose of medication by pulling back on the plunger.
    Rationale: Inversion of the vial brings the needle in contact with the solution in such a way that the needle and the bottle do not touch.

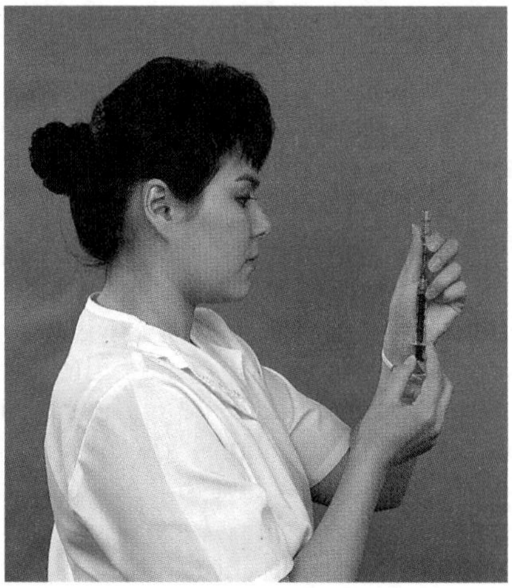

Step 11 • Withdraw medication from the vial. (Photo © B. Proud.)

12. Cover the needle with guard.
13. Wash hands.

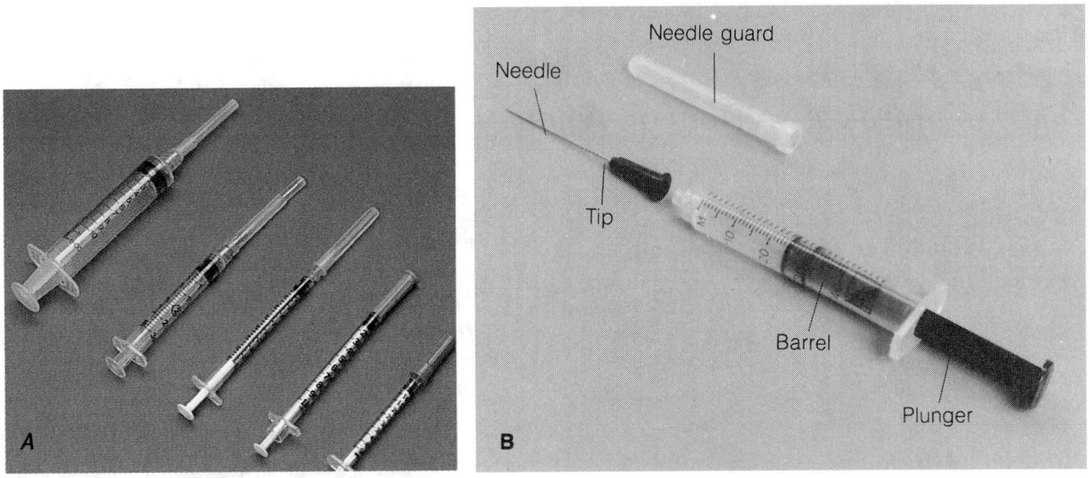

Figure 27-9 • *(****A****) Syringes (from top to bottom): 10 mL, 3 mL, tuberculin, insulin, and low-dose insulin. (****B****) Syringe parts and needle.*

varies from 14 to 29; the needles with the smallest gauge (that is, the smallest diameter) are labeled with the largest number. Needle length varies from 0.5 to 3 in (Fig. 27-10).

The three common types of syringes are tuberculin, insulin, and standard syringes. Tuberculin syringes are 1-mL syringes, calibrated with 0.1-mL markings, and supplied with a small-gauge (25- to 28-gauge), short (0.5- to 0.625-in) needle. Tuberculin syringes are used to administer tuberculin, rubella, or sensitivity (allergy) tests. Insulin syringes, calibrated in units of insulin (100 U of insulin per 1 mL), are used to administer insulin. Insulin syringes are made in ($^1/_3$-, $^1/_2$-, or 1-mL sizes, with very small-gauge needles (26- to 29-gauge) attached to them. Standard syringes are supplied in 3-, 5-, or 10-mL sizes. Standard syringes may be supplied without needles or with 18-, 21-, 23-, or 25-gauge needles that are 0.5 to 3 in long. IM injections are usually administered to adults using a 3- or 5-mL syringe with a long (1.5–2 in), medium-sized (21- or 23-gauge) needle. Larger-gauge needles are used to administer viscous medications or to mix IV medications.

Prefilled syringes, prepared by a medication manufacturer or by a pharmacy, may be used to supply medications. One system of prefilled syringes in widespread use is the Tubex system. Medications, such as narcotic analgesics and heparin, are supplied in a cartridge with an attached needle. The needle and cartridge fit into a metal or plastic injector device (Fig. 27-11). Air and any extra medication are expelled from the syringe, and the medication is injected. Because the needle is fused to the medication cartridge, needle gauge or length cannot be changed; the nurse must use the needle supplied, even if it is not the most appropriate size for the client. Another disadvantage of the prefilled syringe system is that the medications are usually more expensive than those supplied in vials.

Medication Preparation Techniques

Before a parenteral medication is administered, it may need to be drawn up into a syringe, reconstituted, or mixed with another medication.

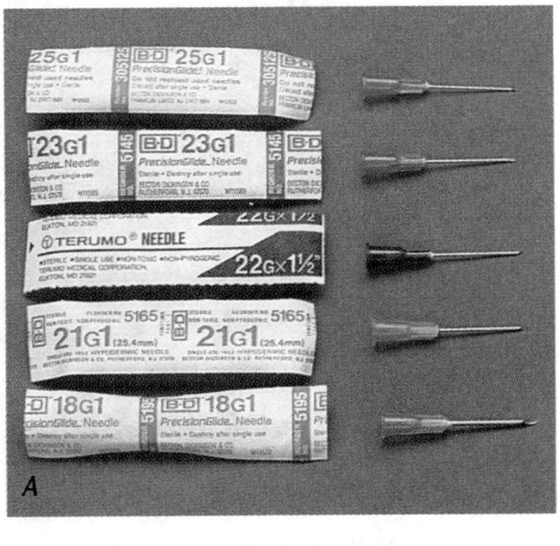

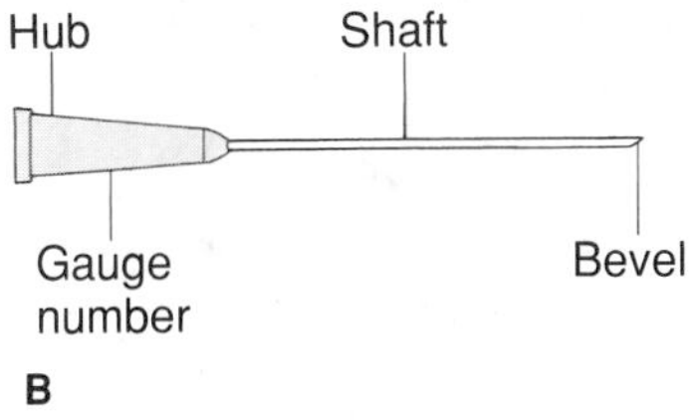

Figure 27-10 • *Needles. (****A****) Different gauges and lengths. (****B****) Parts of a needle.*

Procedure 27-3
Withdrawing Medication From an Ampule

Purpose

1. To withdraw the full dose of medication from an ampule safely and without introducing contamination

Assessment

- Same as Procedure 27-2.

Equipment

Medication order, card, or printout
Ampule with medication
Sterile syringe and needle (or a filter needle if indicated by agency policy)
Sterile gauze pad or alcohol wipe
Standard refuse container

Procedure

1. Check the medication order (see Procedure 27-1 "Administering Oral Medications," Steps 1 to 5), and make sure that the solution in the ampule matches the ordered solution.
2. Wash hands.
   Rationale: Safeguards against infection.
3. Gather equipment.
4. Assemble needle and syringe.
5. Pick up the ampule and flick its upper stem several times with a fingernail.
   Rationale: The sharp flicking motion releases medication trapped in the upper chamber of the ampule.

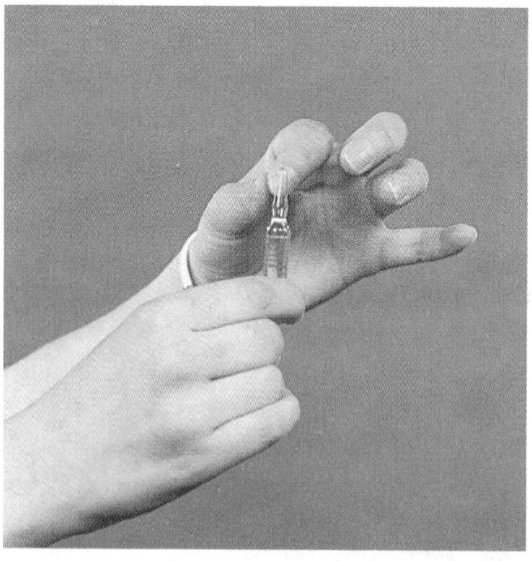

Step 5 • *Flick upper stem to release medication. (Photo © B. Proud.)*

6. Wrap a sterile gauze pad or alcohol wipe around the neck of the ampule before breaking the neck with an outward snapping motion.
   Rationale: The sterile gauze barrier protects the fingers from broken glass and may trap sharp fragments.

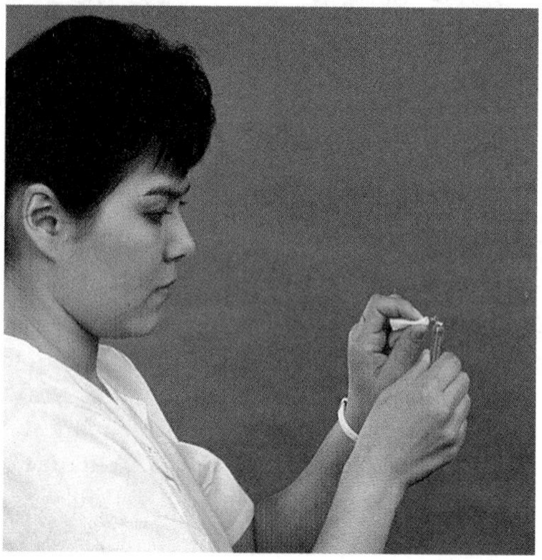

Step 6 • *Break neck of ampule. (Photo © B. Proud.)*

7. Discard the broken neck appropriately, and prepare to withdraw medication from the ampule using one or two methods.
   a. Place the ampule upright on a flat surface, insert the needle in the solution, and withdraw

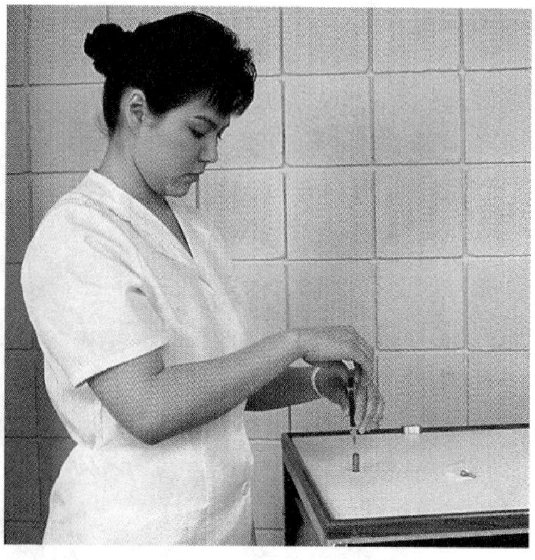

Step 7A • *Withdraw medication from upright ampule. (Photo © B. Proud.)*

the correct amount of medication by pulling up on the plunger. Do not touch the needle to the glass rim.
Rationale: Contact between the needle and the ampule contaminates the needle.

b. Inverting the ampule or tilting it sideways, insert the needle into the solution; pull back on the plunger, and withdraw the proper dose of medication.
Rationale: Keeping the needle in the solution keeps air out of the dose of medication.

8. Remove the needle from the solution. Hold the needle upright, inspect the syringe, and dispel any air that may have been drawn into the syringe. Make sure that the syringe contains the right amount of medication. Expel any extra into a container.
9. Discard ampule in appropriate container.
Rationale: Proper disposal of broken glass protects healthcare personnel from injury.
10. Wash hands.

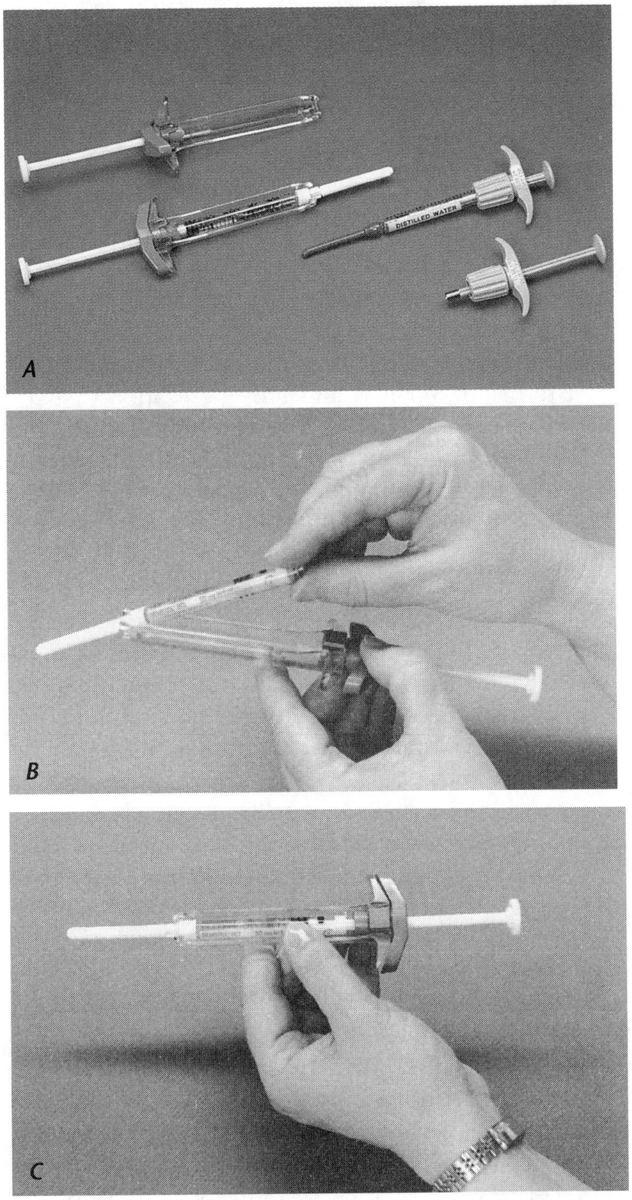

Figure 27-11 • *Prefilled syringes. (**A**) Prefilled medication cartridges and injector devices. (**B**) Inserting the cartridge into the injector device. (**C**) Ready for injection.*

Drawing up Medications. Drawing up medications is the process of moving medications from an ampule or vial into a syringe. When withdrawing medication from an ampule, the nurse first opens the ampule and then removes the needle cap from a syringe. The needle is placed directly into the open ampule, and the syringe plunger is pulled back until all the medication from the ampule enters the syringe. Air is usually drawn into the syringe along with the liquid medication. To dispel the air, the syringe is held with the needle pointed upward. If any medication has adhered to the top of the syringe in the air bubble, the barrel of the syringe is tapped until the liquid moves down the syringe barrel to rest of the medication. The air and any volume of unneeded medication should be expelled slowly.

Reconstituting Medications. Medications are reconstituted by adding the proper diluent to a powdered medication. Vials of powdered medications may be packaged along with vials of the proper type and volume of diluent. The manufacturer's directions printed on the medication box or vial should indicate the amount and type of diluent to add. To reconstitute the medication, the nurse first removes the caps from both the medication and diluent vials and cleans the tops of both vials with an alcohol wipe. The diluent is drawn into the syringe and injected into the medication vial. The nurse holds the medication vial and mixes the medication and diluent until the medication has dissolved. He or she then draws the reconstituted medication into a syringe, removes any air and unneeded medication from the syringe, and administers as directed.

Mixing Medications. Mixing medications in the same syringe may allow a client to receive fewer injections at a lower cost. Medications may be mixed if they are compatible with each other. The compatibility of medications (the ability to mix medications without their constituents or their actions being affected) is studied by pharmaceutical companies, and compatibility information is usually discussed in the package insert and in medication references. Medications are mixed in a syringe by first drawing up one medication into the syringe and expeling any air and unneeded medication from the syringe. The ordered volume of the second medication is slowly added to the syringe containing the first medication. If the medication is added rapidly, too much of the second medication may be drawn up. If too much of the second medication is added, the syringe and medications must be discarded. Refer to Procedure 27-4, "Drawing Up Two Medications in a Syringe."

Equipment Disposal. Discarding equipment carefully decreases the risk of inadvertent exposure to a client's blood. After administering an injection, the syringe and needle should be placed in a needle disposal box. Recapping a needle (placing the protective cap back onto the needle) or breaking the needle off increases the risk of an inadvertent needle stick injury. These practices should be avoided.

Intradermal Injections

ID injections are given into the dermis, the layer of tissue located beneath the skin surface (Fig. 27-12*A*). Allergy or tuberculin skin tests are administered by ID injection. Most frequently, ID injections are given into the inner forearm area, but sites in the upper chest, upper arm, and across the scapula also may be used. ID injections are usually administered using a 1-mL syringe and a small-gauge needle (25- to 28-gauge). The skin is cleaned with an alcohol wipe. The syringe is held with the bevel of the needle up, almost parallel to the skin. The needle is inserted until all of the bevel lies under the skin. Small volumes of medication (usually 0.25 mL or less) are injected slowly (Fig. 27-12*B*). The test site is documented; 48 hours after the injection is given, the site is examined.

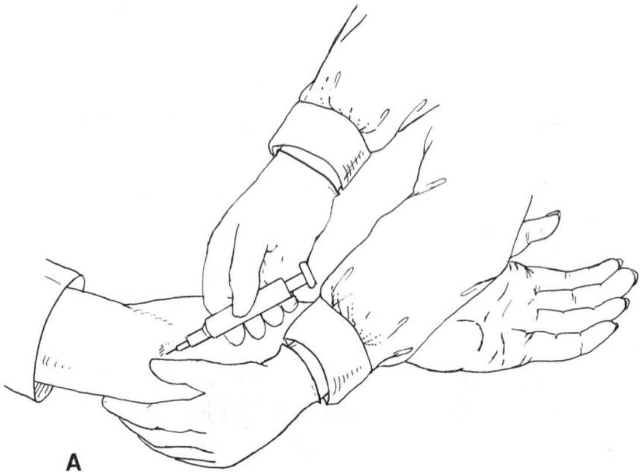

A

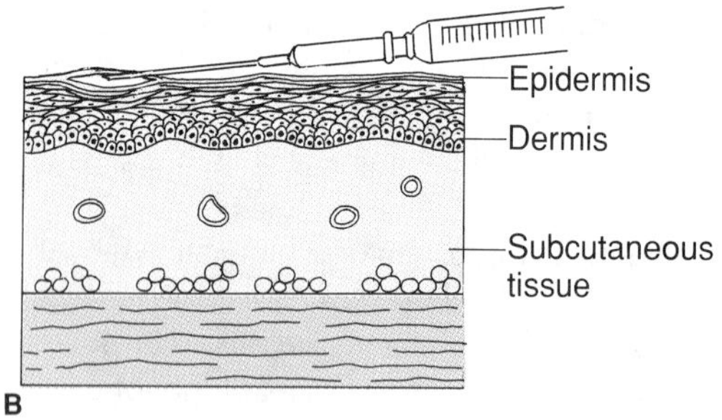

B

Figure 27-12 • *(A) For intradermal injection, the syringe is held almost parallel to the skin with the bevel up. (B) A small volume of medication is deposited right under the skin, forming a small bleb.*

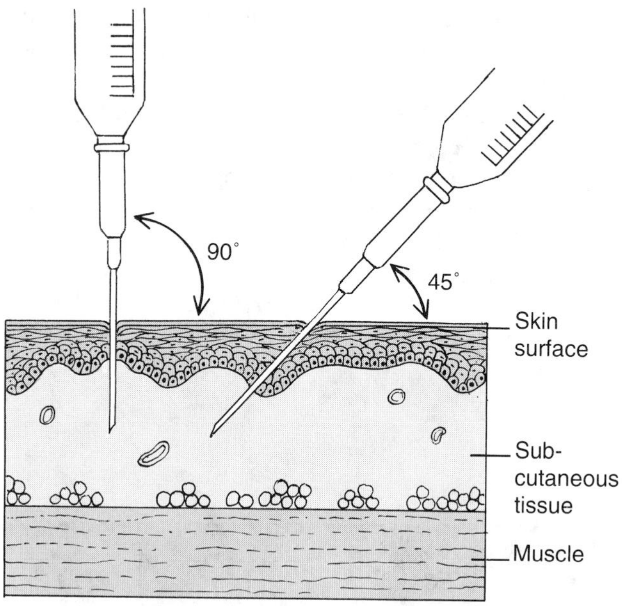

Figure 27-13 • *Subcutaneous injection deposits medication in subcutaneous tissue at a 45° or 90° angle.*

Subcutaneous Injections

SC injections are given into the SC tissue, the layer of fat located below the dermis and above the muscle tissue (Fig. 27-13). When a medication is injected into SC tissue, absorption is usually slow, sustained, and complete. Small amounts (0.5–1 mL) of medication may be injected subcutaneously using a syringe with a short (0.5- to 0.625-in), small-gauge (25- to 28-gauge) needle. SC injections may be given in the upper arm, the upper back, the abdomen, the upper buttocks, and the thigh (Fig. 27-14).

Speed of absorption varies with the site selected: Medications injected into the abdomen are absorbed most rapidly, those injected into the arms are absorbed at an intermediate rate, and those injected into the thigh are absorbed at the slowest rate. Sites of abnormal SC tissue, such as areas lying underneath burns, birthmarks, inflamed tissue, or scars, produce unpredictable medication absorption and should be avoided. Absorption may be slow or incomplete if SC medication is administered to a client with generalized edema, with severe peripheral vascular disease, or in cardiogenic shock

(continued)

Procedure 27-4
Drawing up Two Medications in a Syringe

Purpose

1. Minimize the number of injections a client receives.
2. Prevent contaminating one vial of medication with medication from the other vial

Assessment

- Review drug literature to ensure compatibility of the two medications.

Equipment

Medication order or card
Two vials of ordered medication
Sterile 1 to 3 mL syringe with appropriate gauge and length needle
Antiseptic swabs
Additional needle (optional)

Procedure

1. Wash hands.
2. Cleanse tops of both vials with antiseptic.
3. With syringe, aspirate volume of air equal to medication dose from first medication (Vial A).
4. Inject air into Vial A, being careful that needle does not touch solution.

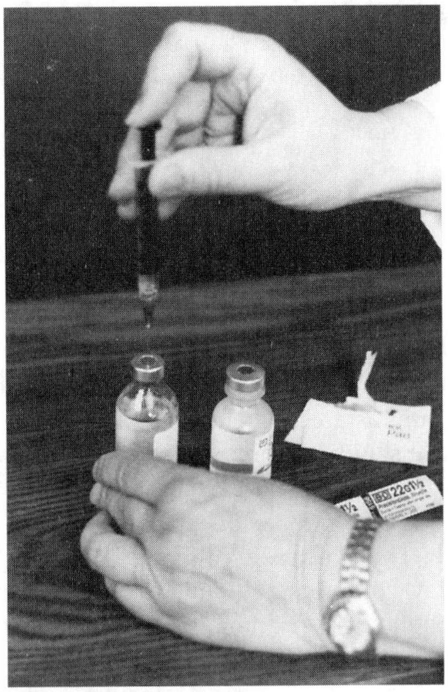

Step 4 • *Inject air into Vial A.*

Rationale: Air in vial creates positive pressure to facilitate solution withdrawal. The same needle will be used to withdraw medication from second vial, so it must not have medication from Vial A on it.

5. Remove syringe from Vial A.
6. Aspirate volume of air equal to the medication dose from second medication (Vial B). Inject air into Vial B.

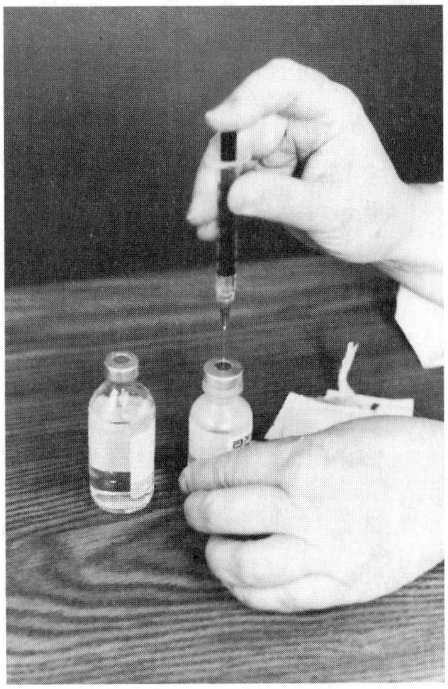

Step 6 • *Inject air into Vial B.*

7. Invert Vial B, and withdraw required volume of medication into syringe.
8. Expel all air bubbles, and withdraw needle from Vial B.
9. Attach new sterile needle to syringe.
   Rationale: This prevents medication adhering to needle from Vial B from contaminating medication in Vial A.
10. Determine what total combined volume of medication would measure on syringe scale.
    Rationale: This prevents accidental withdrawal of excess medication from Vial A.
11. Insert needle into Vial A, invert vial, and carefully withdraw required volume of medication (as in Step 7).

(continued)

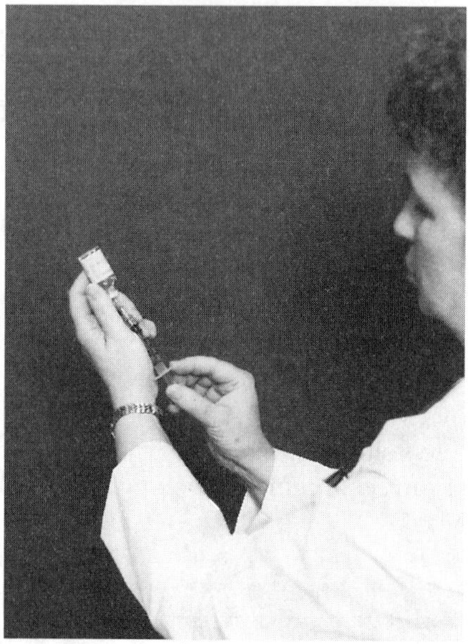

Step 7 • *Withdraw medication from Vial B.*

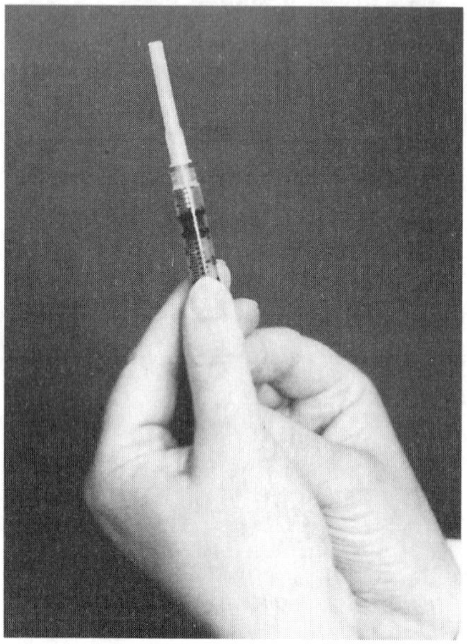

Step 9 • *Attach new sterile needle. (Photo © B. Proud.)*

12. Withdraw needle from Vial A.
13. Check medication and dosage before returning or discarding vials.
14. Wash hands.

Modification for Insulin

Equipment

U-100 insulin syringe
Vials of prescribed U-100 insulin

Procedure

1. Wash hands.
2. When preparing insulins in suspension, gently rotate vials between palms of hands to mix solution.
   Rationale: Medication separates from solution during storage. Mixing ensures accurate concentrations of medications throughout solution. Shaking vigorously causes frothing and may make accurate insulin measurement more difficult.
3. Follow Steps 2 to 7 above.
4. Regular insulin is the first insulin drawn into the syringe.
   Rationale: This ensures insulin will always be drawn up in the same order to prevent errors and prevents contamination of vial containing regular insulin, which may be used in emergency treatment.
5. Follow Steps 8 to 15 above. Extreme care must be taken to prevent contamination of regular insulin vials with insulins containing modifying proteins (intermediate or long-acting).
6. Have another nurse cross-check insulin dosage against healthcare provider's order while drawing up medication.
   Rationale: This prevents errors in insulin drug administration, which could potentially be serious.

(Spencer, 1992). Medications may be absorbed faster than expected when SC injections are administered to clients with little SC tissue, such as premature infants or cachectic adults. If a client has little SC tissue, abnormal SC tissue, or abnormal blood flow to SC tissue, the nurse should check with the healthcare provider to see if an alternate route of administration can be used.

Nonirritating, water-soluble medications, such as narcotics, may be administered by SC injection. Heparin and insulin are the most common medications given subcutaneously. See Procedure 27-5 for guidelines for administering SC injections.

Insulin Administration

Insulin is administered subcutaneously to regulate blood glucose levels. When administering insulin, an insulin syringe (1-mL syringe with 26- to 27-gauge, 0.5-in needle) is used. The needle on an insulin syringe is not detachable. The syringe is calibrated in units; most syringes today contain 100 U/mL and are referred to as U-100 syringes. When administering insulin, the number of units prescribed is measured in the syringe. It is important to use U-100 strength insulin with a syringe that has been calibrated 100 U/mL. Low-dose insulin

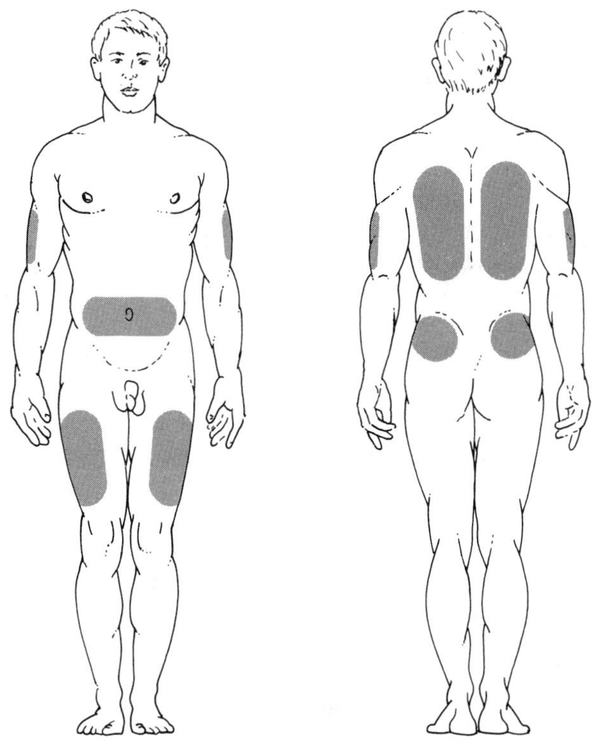

Figure 27-14 • *Sites used for subcutaneous injections.*

syringes (0.5 mL, 50 U) permit better visualization when small insulin doses (less than 10 U) are given.

If SC injections of insulin are given repeatedly into the same site, unpredictable insulin absorption and lipodystrophy (dimpling in the skin due to atrophy of SC tissue) may occur. Each injection should be given about 1 in. (the width of a thumb) from the previous injection site. Areas that feel numb or are located within 1 in of scars, burns, or irritated tissue should be avoided. Site rotation should be planned and well documented to prevent repeated use of the same site. Injection of cold insulin also has been linked to lipodystrophy formation; insulin need not be refrigerated for short-term use. It is helpful to observe clients injecting insulin because technique problems can affect dose administration and absorption.

Heparin Administration

Administering heparin subcutaneously may prevent deep vein thrombosis, which could cause pulmonary emboli. Because SC injections of heparin frequently cause hematoma formation, precautions are necessary. SC injections of heparin are given in the abdomen to avoid highly vascular areas (eg, arms and legs), which have an increased incidence of hematoma formation. Many techniques have been suggested to decrease the incidence of hematoma formation, including using an alcohol wipe to clean any heparin off the needle before injection, inserting the needle at a 90-degree angle to the skin, injecting heparin without aspirating to check for blood return, and using an air lock (0.2 mL of air) to prevent tracking of heparin through the SC tissue. None of these techniques has significantly decreased the risk of postinjection hematoma formation. Care should be taken not to cause trauma during or after the injection; thus, pinching the skin, moving the needle, or rubbing the site after the injection should be avoided.

Intramuscular Injections

IM injections are given into the muscle layer, beneath the dermis and SC tissue (Fig. 27-15). Medications administered by IM injection usually are absorbed at an intermediate rate, slower than IV administration but more rapid than SC. A larger volume of medication per injection and a wider variety of medications may be administered into IM sites than into SC sites. Medications in solution or suspension may be injected into IM sites; those given by this route include antibiotics, antiemetics, narcotics, and vaccines. IM injections are administered using a 3- to 5-mL syringe with a 19- to 25-gauge, 1- to 3-in needle. The larger-gauge needles are used when the medication solution is very thick; longer needles are used for larger adults. A 23-gauge, 1.25-in needle is commonly used for IM injections for average-sized adult clients. Procedure 27-6 discusses administering IM injections.

IM injections may be administered into sites in the upper arm (deltoid muscle), hip (ventral gluteal), thigh

(text continues on page 622)

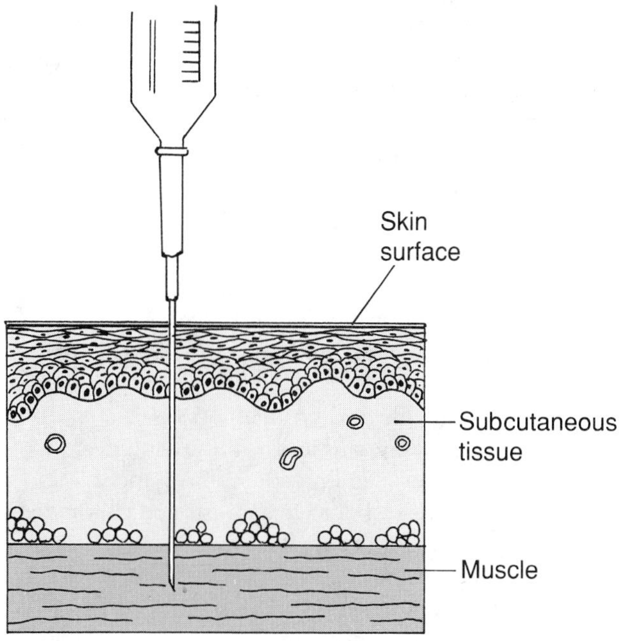

Figure 27-15 • *The intramuscular injection deposits medication into the muscle at a 90° angle.*

Procedure 27-5
Administering Subcutaneous Injections

Purpose

1. Ensure more rapid absorption and action of a drug than can be achieved orally
2. Administer drugs to clients unable to take oral medications (ie, unconscious, nausea/vomiting, NPO status)
3. Administer medications that are not active by the oral route or are inactivated by the digestive enzymes (ie, heparin, insulin)

Assessment

- Review client's medical history, medication history, and allergy status.
- Assess for contraindication to receiving subcutaneous injections. Circulatory shock or localized body areas of reduced tissue perfusion would interfere with drug absorption.
- Assess for anxiety related to fear of injections.
- Review chart for documentation of previous injection sites. Note rotation schedule when administering insulin or heparin.
- Inspect administration site for lesions, rash, ecchymosis, lipid dystrophy, and so forth.
- Refer to drug literature to determine appropriateness of medication and dosage, common side effects, and nursing implications.

Equipment

Medication card or order
Antiseptic swabs
Vial or ampule of ordered medication
Sterile gauze or cover for opening an ampule
Sterile syringe and needle: 1- to 2-mL syringe with 25- to 27-gauge ½-in needle
Gloves

Procedure

1. Check medication order. See Procedure 27-1 "Administering Oral Medications," Steps 1 to 5.
2. Wash hands.
3. Assemble needle and syringe.
4. Remove needle guard and withdraw medication from container (see Procedures 27-2 and 27-3).
5. Recheck drug and dosage against medication order or card for accuracy.
   Note: If administering insulin, cross-check with another nurse.
   Rationale: Cross-checking prevents drug errors.
6. Explain procedure to client, and identify client by name and identification bracelet.
7. Select injection site that is free from tenderness, swelling, scarring, inflammation.
   Rationale: Injection into skin areas with abnormal characteristics could impair drug absorption or increase change of abscess or infection.
8. Don gloves. Some authorities recommend gloving nondominant hand only.
   Rationale: Gloving maintains universal precautions in case blood leaks from injection site.
9. Cleanse site with antiseptic swab in circular motion from center toward outside. Allow area to dry thoroughly.
   Rationale: This cleanses site from cleanest toward more contaminated areas.

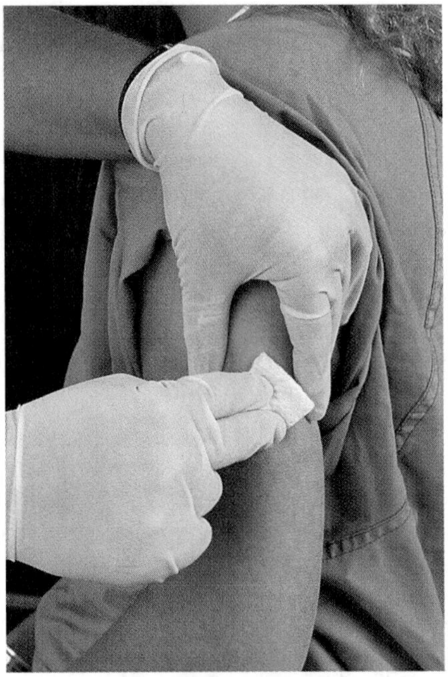

Step 9 • Cleanse site with a circular motion. (Photo © B. Proud.)

10. Remove needle cap, and expel air bubbles from syringe. Hold syringe in dominant hand.
11. Place nondominant hand on either side of injection site. Spread or pinch skin to stabilize site.
    Rationale: Pinching the skin is thought to lessen the pain of needle insertion by desensitizing the area. Spreading the skin creates a firmer surface for needle insertion. Recommendation to support either technique varies.
12. Hold syringe between thumb and forefinger of dominant hand. Inject needle quickly at a 45- to

90-degree angle depending on the amount of adipose tissue. Release pinched skin.
Rationale: Quick insertion minimizes discomfort.

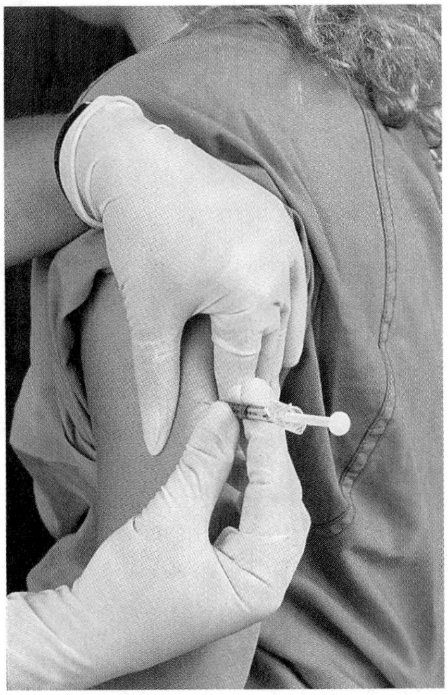

Steps 11 and 12 • *Inject at 45°–90° angle. (Photo © B. Proud.)*

13. Aspirate by slowly pulling back on plunger. If blood appears in syringe, withdraw needle, discard syringe, and prepare a new injection.

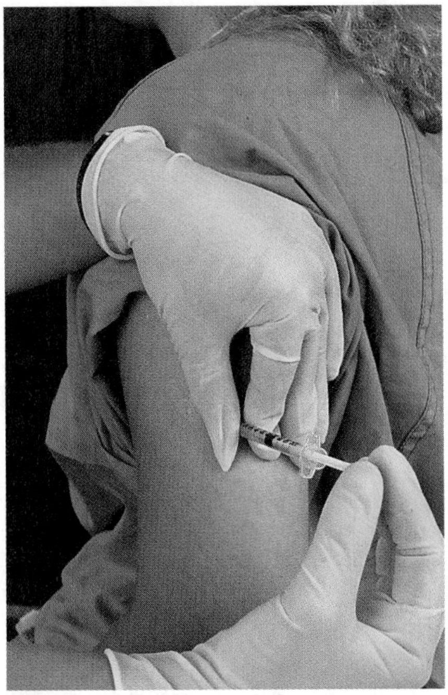

Step 13 • *Aspirate for blood return. (Photo © B. Proud.)*

Rationale: Aspiration of blood indicates needle is in a vein.

14. If no blood appears, inject medication with slow, even pressure.
Note: See "Variations for Administering Heparin."
Rationale: Subcutaneous medications are intended to be absorbed slowly from the subcutaneous tissues and may be dangerous if injected into the vein.

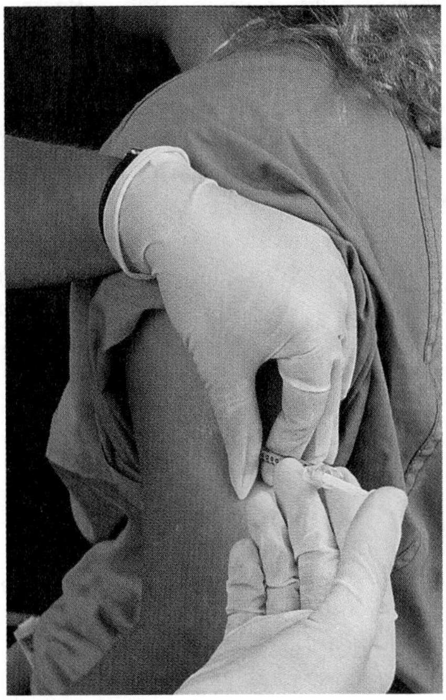

Step 14 • *Inject medication slowly. (Photo © B. Proud.)*

15. Remove needle quickly while pressing antiseptic swab over site.
Rationale: Client discomfort is minimized by supporting tissues while needle is withdrawn.
16. Gently massage site with antiseptic swab.
Rationale: Massage stimulates circulation to the injection site and may facilitate drug absorption.
Note: See "Variations for Administering Heparin."
17. Assist client to position of comfort.
18. Do not recap needle. Dispose of syringe and needle in appropriate container.
Rationale: This protects nurse and other healthcare workers from accidental needle injury.
19. Wash hands.
20. Record according to agency protocol.

Procedure

Variations for Administering Heparin

1. Select a site on the abdomen on either side of the umbilicus.
Rationale: The lack of major muscle groups or

(continued)

muscle activity in this area reduces the chance of hematoma.

2. Because heparin is an anticoagulant, pinching the site, aspirating for blood, and massaging the tissues are contraindicated.

Lifespan Modifications

Infants and Children

- Infants and children up to about 5 years of age should be restrained for injections. Quick movement by the child once the needle is injected could break the needle shaft. An assistant is usually required to help restrain the child. Tell the child, "I will help you to hold still," to convey you are asking for cooperation.
- Painful procedures should not be done in the child's bed, which is a "safe zone." Parents also are regarded as "safe protectors" and should not help restrain the child during a painful procedure. Let the parent comfort the child after the injection.
- Praise, bandages, and "good kid" stickers are effective rewards for children for a job well done.

Obese Adult

- Obese clients have a layer of fatty tissue above the subcutaneous layer. Select appropriate needle length to deliver medication to the subcutaneous skin layer. Pinching the skin at the site and injecting the needle below the tissue fold also may facilitate delivering medication to the subcutaneous layer.

Home-Care Modifications

- If a visually impaired client must self-administer injections, family members or the home health nurse can preload several syringes and place them in the refrigerator. This increases the client's independence.
- A client requiring multiple or daily injections should develop a pattern of site rotation to minimize trauma and scarring of body tissues.
- In some settings, the client may be taught not to cleanse the skin with alcohol or aspirate when giving self-injections.

(vastus lateralis or rectus femoris), and buttocks (dorsogluteal). Site choices are influenced by the age of the client, the medication to be injected, the amount of medication to be injected, and the general condition of the client. Injections should not be given into abnormal muscle tissue, such as tissue underneath burns, scars, or inflamed areas.

The Deltoid Site. The deltoid site has a small amount of muscle mass with little overlying subcutaneous fat; medication injected into this site is absorbed rapidly. The deltoid site is used infrequently because the muscle is small and it lies close to the radial nerve and the brachial artery. If the site must be used, the risk of injury to the radial nerve and brachial artery can be decreased if the site is located carefully, using anatomic landmarks.

The deltoid site is located by drawing an imaginary line two to three fingerbreadths (2.5–5 cm) below the lower edge of the acromion process of the scapula. The injection is given into the thickest area of muscle that lies over the midaxillary line (Fig. 27-16). To give the injection, the needle is angled slightly toward the acromion process or inserted at a 90-degree angle. Children younger than 18 months have poorly developed deltoid muscles and should not receive IM injections into this site. The deltoid muscle in children from age 18 months to 15 years is large enough to accommodate 0.5 mL of medication. Clients older than 15 years may receive injections of 0.5 to 2 mL into the deltoid (Shlafer, 1993).

Rectus Femoris and Vastus Lateralis Sites. Injection sites in the thigh, the vastus lateralis and rectus femoris sites, offer rapid rates of medication absorption. Because these muscles contain no large blood vessels or nerves, they are safe to use for IM injections for most clients.

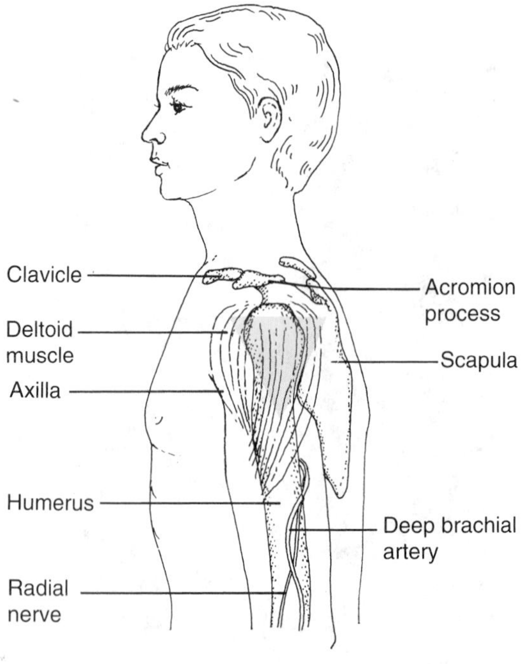

Figure 27-16 • *Deltoid muscle injection site. The site is located by imagining a line extending 2.5 to 5 fingerbreadths from the acromion process. A triangle is formed that indicates the injection site.*

Procedure 27-6
Administering Intramuscular Injections

Purpose

1. Administer medication deeply into muscle tissue, without injury to the client
2. Administer a medication that promotes absorption and onset of action quicker than the oral route and that may be irritating to the subcutaneous tissues

Assessment

- Review client's medical history, medication history, and allergy status.
- Assess for contraindications to receiving intramuscular injections: circulatory shock, reduced blood flow, or muscle atrophy.
- Assess for anxiety related to fear of injection.
- Review chart for documentation of previous injection sites, if client is receiving multiple injections.
- Refer to drug literature to determine appropriateness of medication and dosage, common side effects, and nursing implications.
- Assess adipose tissue and muscle mass of client to determine needle size.

Equipment

Medication card or order
Antiseptic swabs
Vial, ampule, or tubex of medication
Syringe or tubex: 2 to 3 mL for adult; 1 to 2 mL for child
Sterile needle 1.5- to 3-in, 21- to 23-gauge for adult; 0.5- to 1-in, 25- to 27-gauge for children

Procedure

1. Prepare needle, syringe, and medication by following the appropriate steps in Procedure 27-2 or Procedure 27-3.
2. If medication is known to be irritating to subcutaneous tissues, replace needle after withdrawing medication.
   Rationale: This prevents medication that adheres to outside of needle from irritating and burning subcutaneous tissues as needle passes into muscle.
3. Select appropriate injection site by inspecting muscle size and integrity. Consider volume of medication to be injected.
   Rationale: Larger muscles can absorb larger volumes of medication.
4. Assist client to a comfortable position, and expose only the area to be injected. Don gloves, especially on nondominant hand.
   Rationale: Exposing as little area as possible promotes comfort and privacy. Donning gloves maintains universal precautions if blood leaks from injection site.
5. Use anatomic landmarks (5*A*) to locate the exact injection site (5*B*) (see Figs. 27-16 to 27-20).
   Rationale: Injection into proper site prevents trauma to bones, nerves, or blood vessels.

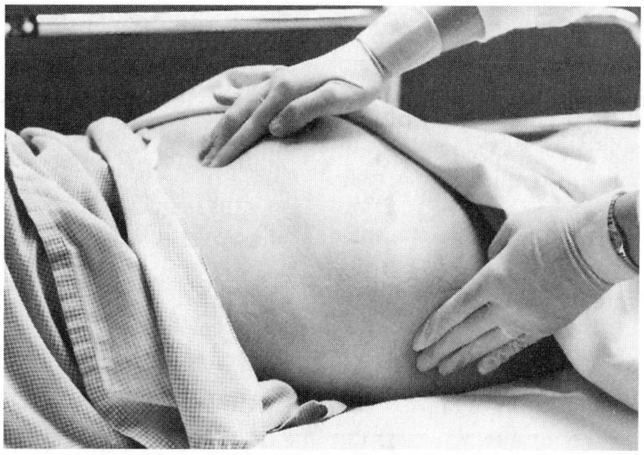

Step 5A • *Identify anatomic landmarks.*

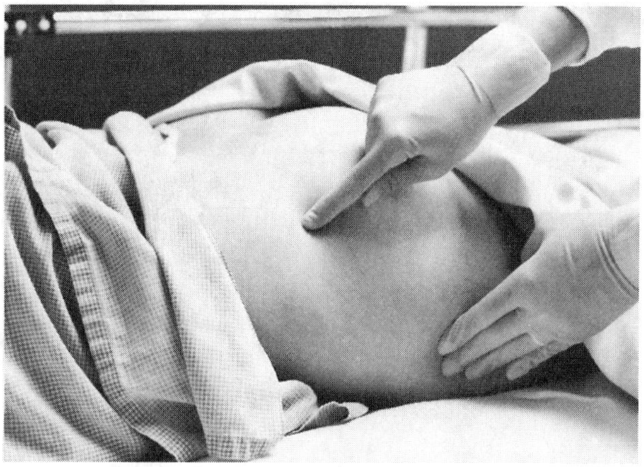

Step 5B • *Locate the exact injection site.*

6. Cleanse the site with antiseptic swab, wiping from center of site and rotating upward.
   Rationale: This cleanses site from cleanest to most contaminated areas.
7. Remove needle cover.
8. Expel air bubbles from syringe.

(continued)

9. Hold syringe between thumb and forefinger of dominant hand (like a dart).
10. Spread skin at the side with nondominant hand.
    Rationale: This facilitates needle insertion by firming skin surface and flattens tissue so needle penetrates into muscle.
    Note: If client has very small muscle mass, pinch muscle before insertion.

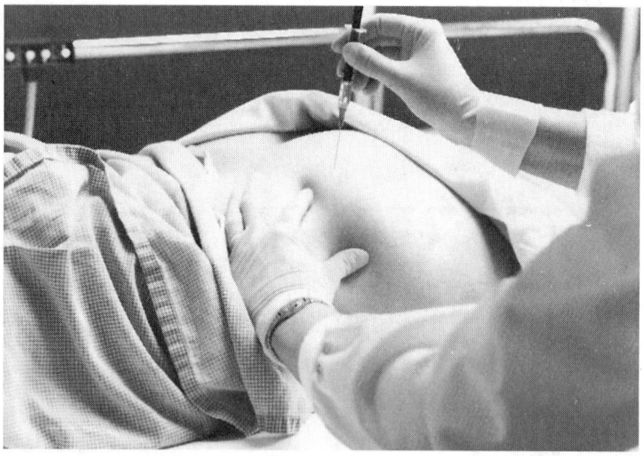

Step 10 • *Spread skin with nondominant hand.*

11. Insert needle quickly at a 90-degree angle.
    Rationale: 90-degree angle enables needle to reach deep muscle layers (see Fig. 27-15). Rapid needle insertion minimizes client discomfort.

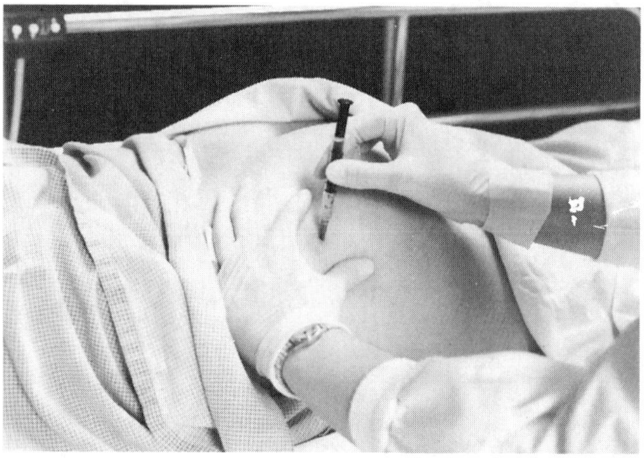

Step 11 • *Insert needle at 90° angle.*

12. Stabilize syringe barrel by grasping with nondominant hand.
    a. Aspirate slowly by pulling back on plunger with dominant hand.
    b. If no blood appears, inject medication slowly.
       Note: If blood appears in syringe, remove needle, dispose of syringe, and prepare new medication.

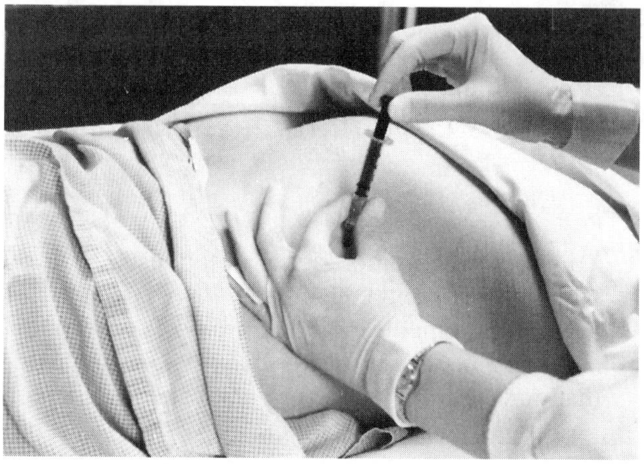

Step 12A • *Aspirate slowly for blood return.*

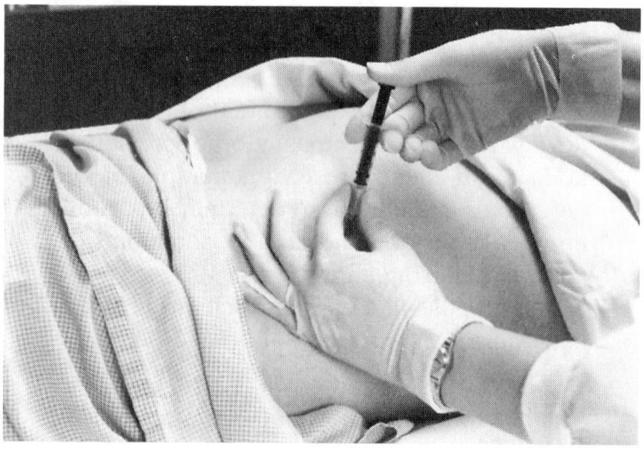

Step 12B • *Inject medication slowly.*

Rationale: Aspiration of blood indicates needle is placed intravascularly.

13. Withdraw needle while pressing antiseptic swab above site.
    Rationale: Minimize discomfort by supporting tissues during needle withdrawal.

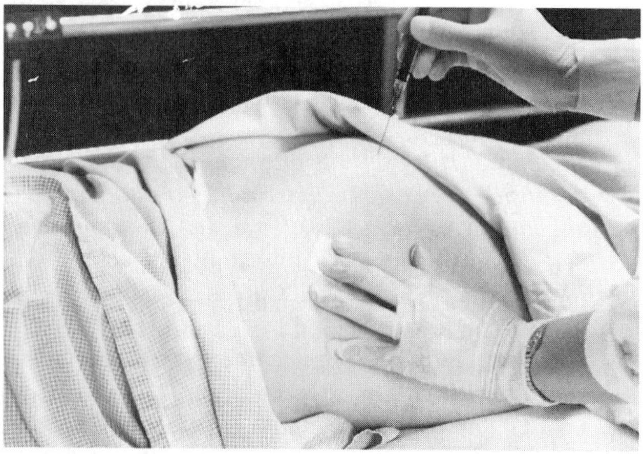

Step 13 • *Withdraw needle.*

14. Gently massage site.
    Rationale: Massage stimulates local circulation and speeds drug absorption.
15. Do not recap needle. Dispose of equipment in proper receptacle.
    Rationale: This protects nurse and healthcare workers from accidental needle injury.
16. Wash hands.
17. Record medication and client response according to agency protocol.

Procedure

Variations for Air Lock Injection Technique

1. If an airlock variation is selected:
   a. Withdraw desired volume of medication into syringe.
   b. Draw in an additional 0.2 ml (0.1–0.3 ml) of air.
   Rationale: It is believed that the air lock technique clears excess medication from the needle following injection. This technique is thought to prevent medication from leaking into the subcutaneous tissues and skin surface as the needle is withdrawn, preventing irritation and staining. This has been recommended particularly for use in combination with Z-track technique.
2. When preparing for injection, the needle must enter the client at a 90-degree angle to the floor.
   Rationale: This ensures that the air bubble follows the solution during the injection and maintains the "air lock" to protect the subcutaneous tissues.

Procedure

Variations for Z-track Injection

1. When preparing the injection site, pull the skin and subcutaneous tissues about 1 to 1.5 in to one side of the selected site (see Fig. 27-21).
   Rationale: This creates a zig-zag track through the tissues, which prevents back-leak of medication when needle is withdrawn.
2. Insert the syringe at a 90-degree angle.
3. Aspirate and administer medication while continuing traction on skin.
4. Leave needle inserted an additional 10 seconds.
   Rationale: This allows medication to disperse and muscle to begin absorption.
5. Remove needle, release traction on skin.
   Rationale: Zig-zag pathway seals medication into the muscle tissue.

The rectus femoris is the site of choice for infants and children, but also may be used for adults. The rectus femoris site is located one-third of the distance from the knee to the greater trochanter of the femur, in the center of the anterior thigh (Fig. 27-17). An injection is administered into this site by lifting the muscle away from the bone and inserting the needle at a right angle to the muscle. Short needles (not exceeding 1 in) should be used to administer injections into the rectus femoris site in children. Infants and toddlers can tolerate injections of 0.5 to 1 mL into the rectus femoris muscle; preschool-age children can tolerate injections of 1.5 mL into the rectus femoris site (Shlafer, 1993).

The vastus lateralis site is used for IM injections for older children and adults. In children, the vastus lateralis site is located in the middle third of the area between the greater trochanter and the knee on the medial outer aspect of the thigh. In adults, the vastus lateralis site is the area between one handbreadth above the knee and one handbreadth below the greater trochanter on the medial outer portion of the thigh (Fig. 27-18). Children younger than 15 years can tolerate injections of up to 2 mL into the vastus lateralis site; adults can tolerate injections of up to 5 mL into the vastus lateralis site (Shlafer, 1993).

Ventrogluteal Site. The ventrogluteal site on the lateral hip is free of major blood vessels, nerves, and fat.

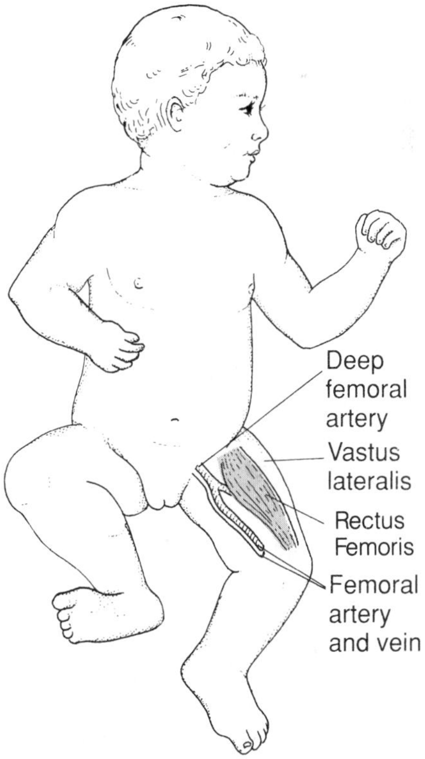

Figure 27-17 • Rectus femoris site used in children. It is located one-third of the distance from the knee to the greater trochanter of the femur in the center of the anterior thigh.

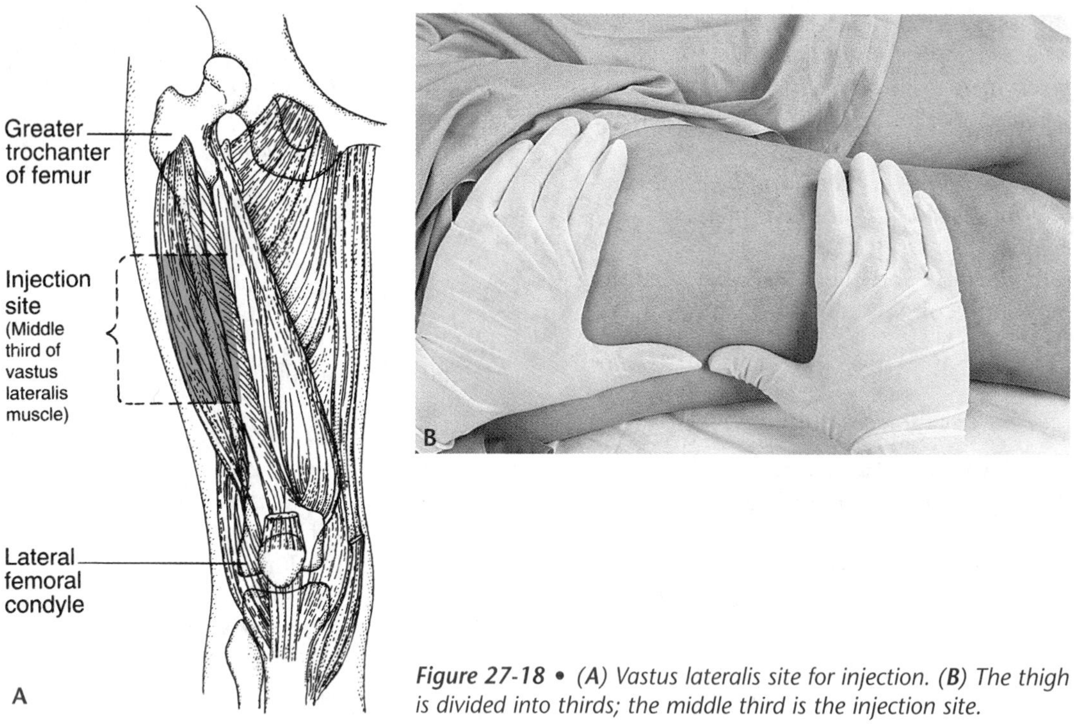

Figure 27-18 • *(A) Vastus lateralis site for injection. (B) The thigh is divided into thirds; the middle third is the injection site.*

To locate the ventrogluteal site, the heel of the opposite hand (for right hip, nurse uses left hand; for left hip, nurse uses right hand) is placed over the greater trochanter, with the index and middle fingers angled toward the anterior superior iliac spine and toward the iliac crest, respectively. The injection is given in the center of the triangular area thus formed, with the needle directed at a 90-degree angle to the skin or with the needle angled slightly toward the iliac crest (Fig. 27-19). Toddlers should not receive injections into the ventrogluteal site; muscles in this site are not well developed until a child begins to walk. After children are 3 years old, they can receive volumes of up to 1 mL in the ventrogluteal site; preschoolers can be given 1.5 mL; school-age children can be given 2.0 mL; and older children and adults can be given up to 2.5 mL (Shlafer, 1993).

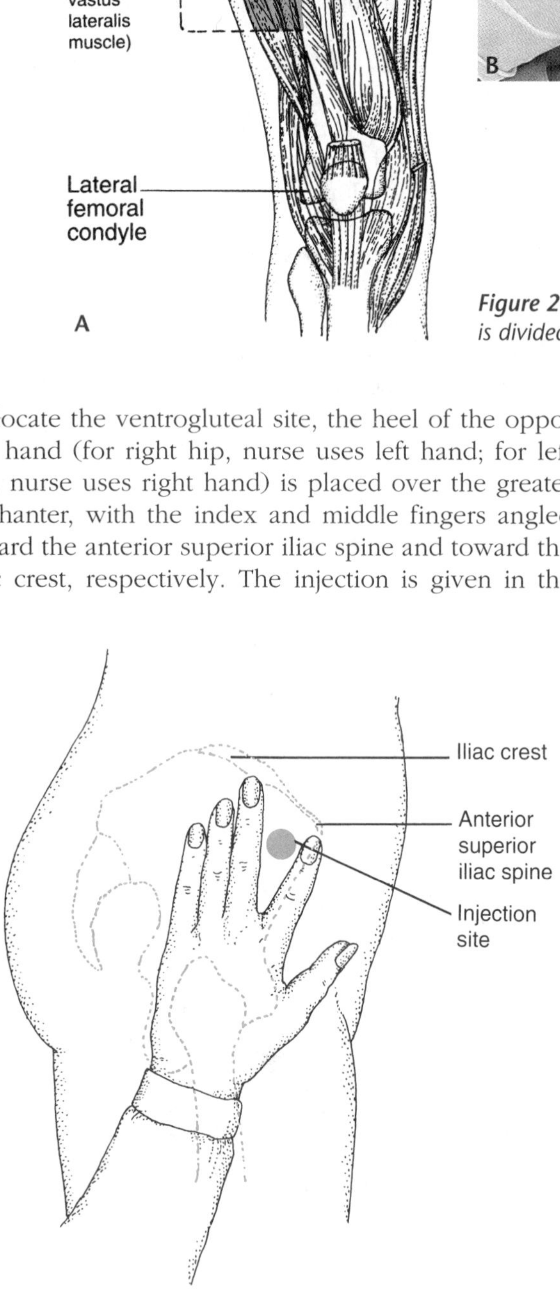

Figure 27-19 • *Ventrogluteal site injection. The heel of the hand is placed over the greater trochanter, and the middle fingers reach toward the iliac crest where the index finger is angled toward the anterior superior iliac spine. The injection is given in the center of the resulting triangle.*

Older and debilitated clients who have lost muscle mass elsewhere often have enough muscle in the ventrogluteal site to allow safe administration of IM injections. If adequate muscle mass is not visualized, the nurse palpates the ventrogluteal site. If adequate muscle mass is not felt, the nurse checks with the healthcare provider to see if medications can be administered by another route.

The Dorsogluteal Site. The dorsogluteal site of the buttocks has been used commonly for IM injections. To locate the dorsogluteal site, the nurse uses the index fingers to find the greater trochanter and the posterior superior iliac spine. An imaginary line is drawn between these landmarks, and the injection is given lateral and superior to the midpoint of this line (Fig. 27-20). The needle is inserted at a 90-degree angle to the skin. Problems with the dorsogluteal site include the following: Medication given into this site is slowly absorbed; the sciatic nerve and gluteal artery lie close to the site; infants younger than 18 months and debilitated adults may not have enough muscle mass to allow a safe in-

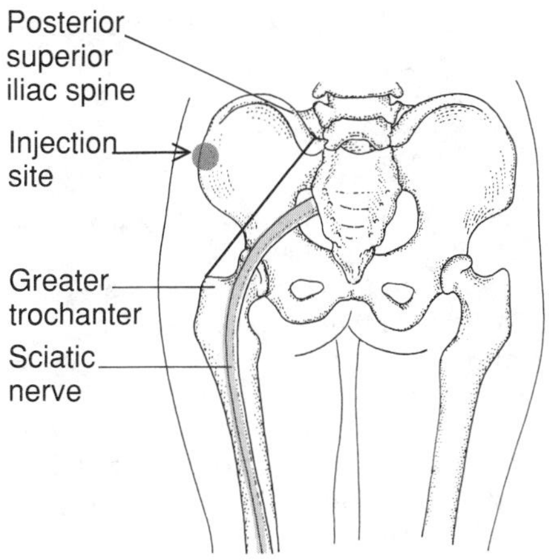

Figure 27-20 • *Dorsogluteal site for IM injection. The injection is given lateral and superior to the midpoint of an imaginary line drawn between the greater trochanter and posterior superior iliac spine.*

jection into this site; and the thick layer of fat over this site in many people may make it difficult to reach muscle tissue consistently. Some adult clients of normal size and weight who are given IM injections into the dorsogluteal site might receive the injection in SC fat. Researchers found that more than 95% of the women and 85% of the men they studied would have received IM injections into the SC fat if injections were given into the dorsogluteal site with 1.5-in needles.

Use of the gluteal site should be limited to medications that can be safely given into SC fat; irritating medications and medications that must be more rapidly and consistently absorbed, such as hepatitis B vaccine, should be given into the vastus lateralis or ventrogluteal sites. Children younger than 3 years can be given injections of up to 1 mL into the dorsogluteal site; children between 3 and 6 years can be given 1.5 mL; children from 6 to 15 years can be given 2 mL; and those older than 15 years and adults can receive injections of 2 to 4 mL into the dorsogluteal site (Shlafer, 1993). The pain and bleeding that may occur when injections are administered into the dorsogluteal site are less likely if the client is in the prone position with his or her toes pointing inward.

Most medications that are appropriate for IM injection can be given using the technique described in Procedure 27-6. Medications that irritate SC tissue (such as hydroxyzine) or that discolor SC tissue (such as iron) should be given by the Z-track method (Fig. 27-21), which is described in Procedure 27-6. Although the Z-track technique is generally used with medications that are irritating to the tissues, some authors suggest that it be used routinely for intramuscular injections (Hahn, 1991). The purpose of the Z-track technique is to administer the medication into the muscle tissue with no tracking of medications in the subcutaneous tissues. To ensure that medication does not leak back into the sub-

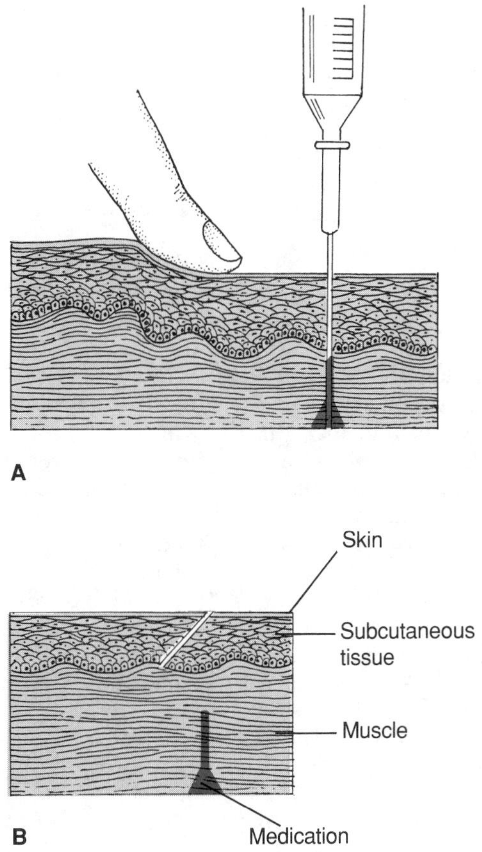

Figure 27-21 • *Z-track method. **(A)** Pull skin and subcutaneous tissue 1 to 1.5 inches to side of injection site while injecting medication. **(B)** Release traction to allow skin to fall back, sealing medication in site.*

cutaneous tissues, Hahn (1991) also recommends having an air lock of 0.4 ml that is above the level of the medication during injection. If these techniques are not followed or if site selection is not accurate, complications can occur; complications related to IM injections are listed in Table 27-6.

Intravenous Administration

IV medications are given in catheters inserted into veins. Advantages of using the IV route to administer medications include the following:

- The onset of medication action is usually rapid.
- Predictable, therapeutic blood levels of medications can be obtained.
- The route can be used when gastrointestinal dysfunction or compromised peripheral circulation make medication absorption unpredictable by oral or IM routes.
- Medications that cannot be given by other routes may be delivered IV.
- Larger doses of medications can be administered by this route than by IM injection.

Table 27-6 • Complications Associated With Administration of Intramuscular Medications

Complication (Signs/Symptoms)	Causes	Nursing Measures
Pain with injection (client reports discomfort)	Muscle tense during injection Medication irritates IM tissue Inadvertent tracking of medication or alcohol through SC tissue	Encourage client to relax muscles during injection. Use Z-track technique when administering medications that are irritating to SC tissue. Change needle after drawing up medication. Use an air lock when giving irritating medications. Let alcohol skin prep dry before giving injection.
Damage to SC or IM tissue, including sterile abscesses (collection of undissolved medication), SC tissue discoloration, hematomas, and muscle contractions (tissue nodules or indurations [indentations], bruising, brown discoloration, or pain in IM injection site; muscle contracture [in infants] characterized by difficulty crawling 4 weeks to 1 year after receiving IM injections)	Multiple injections given into same area Injection given into abnormal tissue Injection of drug that is not water-soluble (eg, dilantin or valium) IM administration of heparin IM route used for client with a low platelet count SC deposition of iron supplements (eg, Imferon)	Give an injection at least 1 in away from recently administered injections or from scars, burns, or areas of abnormal SC or IM tissue. Rotate injection sites (give injections at least 1 in away from recent injection). Record sites used for all injections. As soon as possible, change from IM route to another route. Be sure that medication is recommended for IM administration. Check with physician before administering IM injection to a client whose platelet count is under 30,000/mL. Do not administer IM injections into atrophied muscle. The risk of knee contractures for infants is decreased if passive range-of-motion exercises are done and if warm soaks and massage are applied to the thighs. Give iron supplements (eg, Imferon) using the Z-track technique.
Nerve injury (shooting pain down limb, temporary or permanent paralysis)	Nerve struck during injection Medication injected close to nerve	Use careful visual inspection and palpation to locate injection site. Avoid use of deltoid and dorsogluteal sites whenever possible.
Bone injury (pain or bone damage)	Bone struck during IM injection	Avoid use of deltoid site whenever possible. Use a short needle (1.25 in) when giving injections into the deltoid or ventrogluteal sites. Use visual inspection and palpation to locate injection sites.
Speed shock or rapid absorption of medication (unexpectedly rapid onset of action of medication; may lead to increased heart rate and respiratory rate, decreased level of consciousness, and cardiovascular collapse)	Medication administered directly into a vein or artery	After inserting needle into muscle, aspirate (pull back on plunger of syringe) to check for blood. If blood appears in syringe barrel, remove syringe and needle and discard. Draw up another dose of medication and administer in a new site.
Infection of muscle or bone (muscle or bone pain in injection site, skin redness or warmth, localized swelling)	Introduction of organism into tissue or bone during injection	Follow strict aseptic technique when administering IM injections.

Table 27-7 • Complications Associated With Intravenous Administration of Medications

Complication (Signs/Symptoms)	Causes	Nursing Measures
Speed shock (headache, tightness in chest, shock, cardiac arrest)	Medication administered more rapidly than intended	Know time period recommended for medication administration. If administering by IV bolus technique, time infusion with a watch with a second hand. If administering by continuous drip or intermittent drip methods, regulate drip rate accurately. Check rate of infusion of medication at least several times per hour. Infuse any medications with serious or toxic side effects using an infusion control device. Infuse all medications that are titrated at a consistent rate using an infusion control device.
Infection (redness, warmth, or pain at catheter insertion site; fever, increased leukocyte count, organisms present on blood culture samples, chills, shaking, increase in body temperature)	Break in aseptic technique when preparing or administering IV medications Contamination of IV catheter site when IV dressing is changed IV equipment changed infrequently Contaminated IV solution	Tape catheter securely to skin. Check catheter insertion site at least once per shift and before and after infusion of medications. Change IV tubing every 48 to 72 hours.
Extravasation during which medication leaks out of the vein lumen (pain, swelling at distal end of catheter, slowed rate of infusion, increase in size of one extremity [with IV] over the other extremity, severe tissue sloughing)	Catheter migrated out of vein during client movement	Avoid placing IV catheter close to client's wrist or elbow whenever possible. Tape catheter securely to skin.
Thrombophlebitis (redness and warmth along cannulated vein; burning pain; slow flow rate; when palpated, vein feels hard, cordlike)	Trauma to vein during catheter insertion or from catheter movement Irritation of vein resulting from medication administered	Tape catheter securely to skin. Inspect IV site at least once per shift. Whenever possible, avoid infusing irritating medications into the small veins of the hands and forearms. Whenever possible, avoid placing catheters near the wrist or elbow. If placement in these areas is necessary, decrease catheter movement by securing arm to an arm board. Check catheter insertion site at least once per shift and before and after infusion of IV medications.

The disadvantages of this route include the high cost of treatment, the difficulty of administering IV medications outside of healthcare settings, the difficulty of maintaining patent peripheral IV catheters in clients with limited adequate veins, and the increased risk of complications with this route. The complications related to IV administration of medications are given in Table 27-7.

IV medications should be prepared and packaged in a sterile manner and should not be prepared in an oil or aqueous suspension. IV administration of a medication that is not sterile, such as an oral medication, may cause an infection within the vein (phlebitis) or a generalized infection (sepsis). Medications prepared in oil or water suspension contain large particles suspended in a solution. If a medication suspension is given intravenously, the large medication particles may act as emboli and lodge in small veins. A wide variety of medications can be given intravenously. Categories of medications that are given commonly by the IV route are antibiotic, narcotic, antiarrhythmic, and antiulcer medications. IV catheters are placed in the peripheral or the central circulation.

IV medications can be administered directly into the vein or through various access devices that have been placed in a vein after venipuncture. Peripheral IV catheters or intermittent infusion devices (also known as "heparin locks" or "hep locks") are used for short-term therapy, whereas central venous access devices (Hickman or Groshong catheters) are selected for more long-term therapy. Venous access devices are discussed more completely in Chapter 26.

IV medications may be given by IV push (bolus), intermittent infusion (IV piggyback), or continuous infusion. IV pain medication maybe self-delivered by the client with equipment known as a patient-controlled analgesia (PCA) device (see Chap. 44).

IV Push Technique. The IV push technique is used to administer medications that must be given rapidly to have the desired therapeutic effect or those that are incompatible with IV fluids (eg, phenytoin). Most medications supplied by IV push can be administered following the steps in Procedure 27-7.

If a medication ordered to be given IV push is not prepackaged in a syringe, the nurse needs to draw up the medication into a syringe. A 3- or 5-mL syringe with a short (1-in), 20-gauge needle can be used for giving most IV push medications. If the total volume of a medication is less than 1 mL, it should be drawn up in a 1-mL syringe to allow more accurate measurement of medication volume. Some IV push medications may be ordered in volumes exceeding 5 mL. IV push medications may be given into a continuously infusing IV set or into a capped IV port (an intermittent infusion device or "heparin lock"). The infusion rate may be ordered by the healthcare provider; more commonly, the exact infusion rate is not specified, requiring the nurse to check a medication reference manual for the infusion time recommended by the pharmaceutical company. Once the nurse knows the recommended total infusion time, he or she can calculate the infusion rate by dividing the total volume of medication that is ordered by the recommended total time of infusion. Generally, IV push medications are given for at least 1 minute.

The Intermittent Infusion Technique. The intermittent infusion technique (also called IV "piggyback") is the most common technique for infusing IV medications. It is used to administer medications that need to be infused for an intermediate length of time (usually, 30 minutes to 1 hour) and for those that are not stable for long periods. Medications administered by intermittent infusion are supplied in bags that contain 50 to 250 mL of IV fluid. These bags of fluid contain the medication dissolved in normal saline solution or in 5% dextrose in water (D_5W). The pharmacist who prepares the medication labels the bag with the client's name, the name of the medication, the type of IV fluid, and the suggested infusion rate (see Procedure 27-8).

The nurse administering the medication is responsible for making sure that the medication supplied is the medication ordered; the medication, as ordered, is safe for the individual client; the IV catheter is patent (the catheter is still in the vein; the catheter is not clogged; the catheter site is not reddened or swollen); and the medication is infused at the proper rate.

Decisions about the safety of administering a medication to an individual client are based on the usual dose and dosage range of the ordered medication, the client's size and weight, the reason that the medication is ordered for the client, and any other conditions that might influence the way the medication affects the client.

Intermittent infusions of medications may be given when a client does not require continuous IV fluids. The client's IV catheter maybe converted to an intermittent infusion device or heparin lock. The heparin lock, a small, dead-end connector, is attached to the proximal end of an IV catheter. About 1 to 3 mL of solution are instilled ("flushed") through the heparin lock every 8 hours or after any medication is infused through the heparin lock. This maintains catheter patency. The fluid used to flush heparin lock catheters is usually a normal (isotonic) saline solution, although 10 U/mL heparin or more concentrated solutions of heparin (100 U/mL) also may be used, depending on the healthcare provider's orders and institutional policy. The use of heparin for flushing the intermittent infusion device is the source of the name—heparin lock.

The Continuous Infusion Technique. The continuous infusion technique is used to infuse medications that must be given continuously to achieve the desired effect (eg, heparin or theophylline) or medications that are toxic if given over short periods (eg, multivitamins or cisplatin). Medications ordered by continuous infusion are supplied in IV bags containing 250 to 1000 mL of IV fluid.

Macrodrip or minidrip IV tubing, with or without Luer-lock connections and in-line filters, are used to connect the IV medications and fluids to the IV catheter. Luer-lock tubing, made with connections that screw together, is usually used for administering medications or fluids into central catheters (IV lines placed in a central vein, such as the subclavian vein). Tubing made with an in-line filter is used to instill medications and fluids into central catheters. Before giving a medication through IV tubing with an in-line filter, the nurse should check whether the medication is affected by the filter. Some medications are filtered out of solution by an in-line filter; if one of these medications is infused through such a device, the client would not receive any medication.

If the client is receiving more than one continuously infusing IV, and if the ordered medication is compatible with other IV medications and fluids the client

Procedure 27-7
Administering Medications by Intravenous Push

Purpose

1. To achieve high blood levels of a medication in a short period
2. To achieve immediate and maximal effects of a medication

Assessment

- Check medication orders for type of medication, dosage, route, and time scheduled for administration.
- Assess for compatibilities of medications and solutions to be administered.
- Identify all pertinent allergies.
- Assess IV site for signs of erythema, pain, tenderness, edema.
- Collect all information to administer medication safely, including action, purpose, side effects, normal dosage, time of peak onset, pertinent laboratory work or vital signs if indicated, nursing implications.

Equipment

Medication documentation sheets
Antiseptic swab
Medication vial or ampule
Watch with second hand or digital display
Syringe; two 5 to 10-mL syringes (if medication is not compatible with IV solution)
Syringe of appropriate size for medication volume
Sterile #25-gauge needle
Gloves

Procedure

1. Wash hands and don gloves.
   Rationale: Handwashing and gloving prevent spread of microorganisms.
2. Prepare and draw up ordered medication from vial or ampule. Read package insert for proper amount and solution for dilution. Apply small-gauge needle to syringe or needleless adapter.
   Rationale: A small-gauge needle will prevent large puncture holes in the injection port.
   Note: Many facilities are promoting use of needleless equipment for IV procedures to prevent accidental needle sticks and decrease risk of infection. Refer to agency procedure manual for usage.
3. Explain procedure to the client.
   Rationale: Explanations allay client anxiety.
4. Identify the client by asking name, looking at nameband, and verifying with medication record.
   Rationale: The right medicine to the right client prevents medication error.

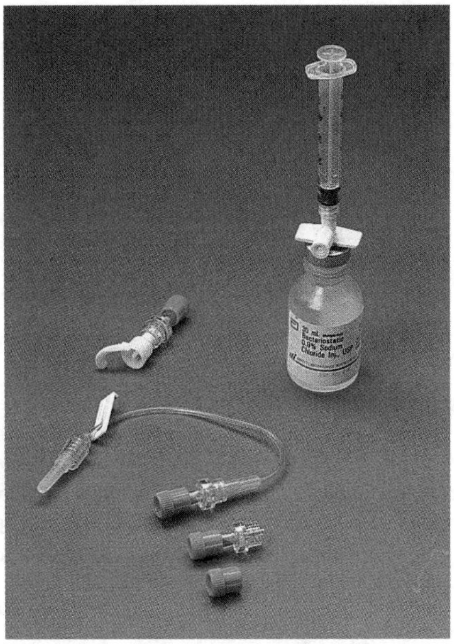

Step 2 • *Prepare ordered medication.*

Procedure

Administering Medication Into an Existing IV Line

1. Select injection port in IV tubing, closest to the IV insertion site.
   Rationale: This minimizes dilution of the medication and increases transit of medication into client's vascular system. Close proximity to the insertion site also makes it easier to assess catheter placement by blood return.
2. Cleanse injection port with antiseptic. Allow to dry.
   Rationale: Cleansing decreases transmission of microorganisms and prevents tracking wet antiseptic into the IV catheter.
3. Insert needle into the injection port.
4. Occlude the IV tubing above the injection port by pinching the tubing. Gently pull back on the syringe plunger until blood appears in the tubing.
   Rationale: Aspirating ensures that the IV catheter is correctly placed within a vein.
5. Inject the medication slowly into the IV port at the prescribed rate. Use a watch to time administration rate.
   Rationale: Timing ensures safe infusion of drug.
   Note: If IV medication and IV solution in tubing are incompatible, assess for blood return with a 10-mL syringe of sterile normal saline solution. After confirming IV catheter placement, flush line

(continued)

with normal saline solution while occluding catheter above port. Administer medication at prescribed rate; reflush with 10 mL of sterile normal saline solution, and release occlusion.

Procedure

Administering the Drug Into an Intermittent Injection Device or Heparin Lock

1. Swab the injection port with antiseptic. Allow to dry.
   Rationale: Cleaning the port prevents introduction of microorganisms into the IV catheter.
2. Insert needle of syringe with 1 mL normal saline solution into injection port. Gently pull back on syringe plunger to assess for blood return.
   Rationale: Assessment confirms correct IV catheter placement within vein.

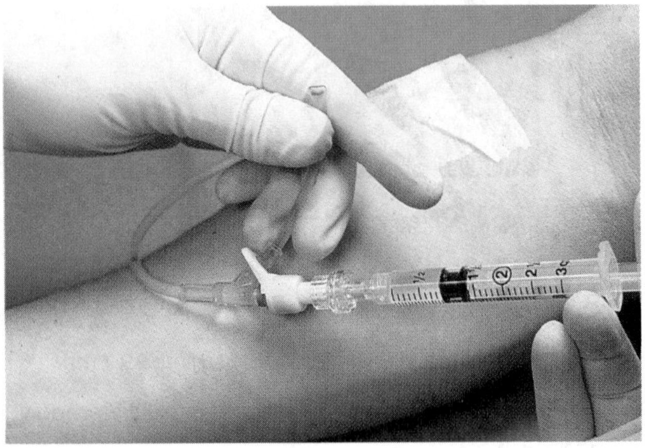

Step 2 • *Insert needle into injection port and assess for blood return.*

3. Flush IV lock with 1 mL normal saline solution. Remove syringe.
   Rationale: Flushing cleanses catheter and confirms patency of catheter.
4. Insert needle or connector of syringe with medication into injection port. Inject medication slowly at the prescribed rate. Use watch to time safe administration rate. Remove syringe.
   Rationale: Careful timing ensures safe medication infusion.
   Note: Too rapid injection of some IV medications can be fatal.

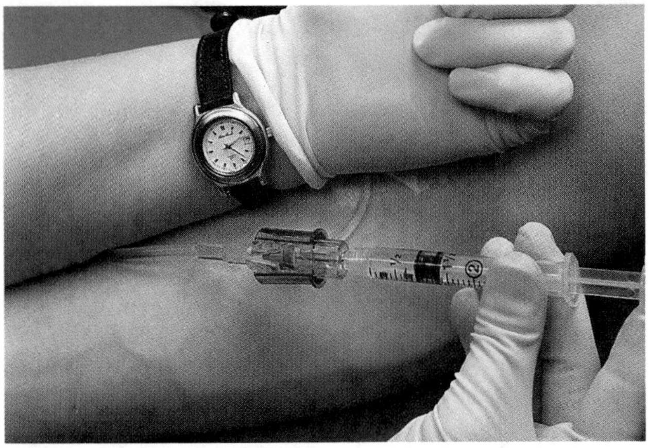

Step 4 • *Use a watch to time the slow injection of medication at the prescribed rate.*

5. Complete procedure by referring to Procedure 27-8, "Administering IV Medications Using Intermittent Infusion Technique."
6. Dispose of uncapped needles and syringes in proper container.
   Rationale: Careful disposal prevents accidental needle sticks.
7. Wash hands.
8. Document medication administration.
   Rationale: Accurate documentation is mandatory to prevent medication errors.
9. Evaluate the client's response to medication therapy.
   Rationale: Careful and timely assessment is necessary because medications given by IV bolus may have a rapid action.

Lifespan Considerations

Infants and Children

- Anticipate that medication dosages for newborns and children are greatly reduced and based on their body weight.
- Cross-check computations of weight-based medications with another nurse to maintain accuracy and prevent errors in administration.

is receiving, the second IV may be connected to a medication infusion port of the first IV so that the medications infuse into the same catheter. The ordered IV drip rate is calculated and the infusion rate regulated. An IV timing tape (a tape marked with the time that the IV is started, intermediate infusion times, and the time that the IV is ordered to be completed) can act as a quick reference to confirm that the infusion is progressing at the ordered rate. Refer to Chapter 26 for specific information concerning calculation and regulation of IV drip rates. The rate of flow of continuously infusing IV fluids should be checked at least hourly to ensure that it has not changed because of a change in the client's position or an alteration in catheter patency.

If an IV medication or fluid has infused at a faster or slower rate than ordered, a prompt correction may

Procedure 27-8
Administering IV Medications Using Intermittent Infusion Technique

Purpose

1. Maintain therapeutic levels of medication in client's blood
2. Dilute irritating IV solutions
3. Prevent complications associated with bolus administration by delivering medications over a longer time
4. Prevent combining incompatible medications

Assessment

- Review medication order, dosage, schedule, and if particular IV solution is needed.
- Assess patency of existing IV line.
- Inspect insertion site for infiltration or phlebitis.
- Determine client's drug allergy status.

Equipment

Medication Kardex or card
Medication prepared and labeled in a 50–250 mL sterile infusion container
IV infusion set
Needleless adapter set (21- or 23-gauge sterile needle) if needleless system not in use
Alcohol or povidone–iodine swab
20-mL syringe of sterile normal saline flush solution. (Optional: If medication is incompatible with primary infusing IV solution.)
Intermittent infusion device or heparin lock.
Two sterile syringes and needle with 3 mL normal saline solution each and a sterile syringe with
1 mL of normal saline or heparin flush solution (10 U heparin per mL).

Procedure

1. Wash hands.
Rationale: Handwashing reduces transmission of microorganisms.
2. Connect infusing tubing to medication container. (See Procedure 26-2, "Changing Intravenous Solution and Tubing.")
Rationale: Primed IV tubing prevents air bubble from entering client's vein.
3. If using a needle, connect capped, sterile needle to end of infusion set. If using a needleless system, connect the needleless adapter for the intermittent infusion device or port closest to the client.
Rationale: The cap on the needle or the cover on the adaptor maintains the sterility of the system prior to connection to the primary intravenous line.
(*There are many types of needleless systems available. Be sure to follow the manufacturer's instructions for use.)

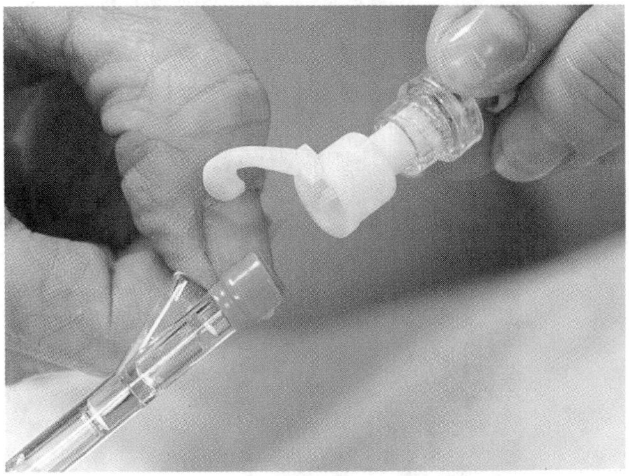

Step 3 • *Attach needleless adaptor to primary tubing port.*

4. Confirm client's identity by asking his or her name, and by looking at identiband.
Rationale: Identifying the client prevents administering medication to wrong client.

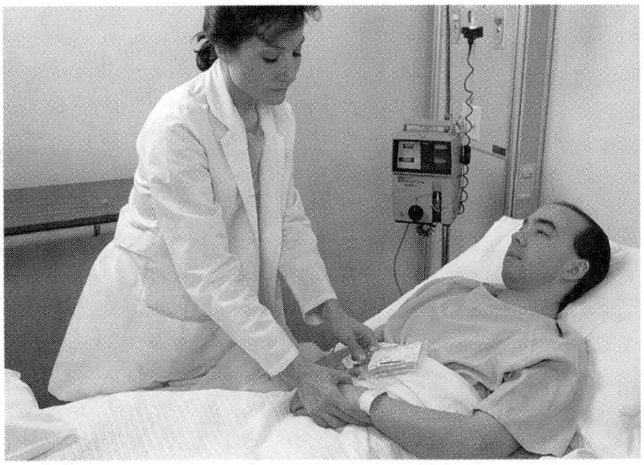

Step 4 • *Confirm client's identity verbally and by checking identification band.*

(continued)

5. Hang medication bag at or above level of primary IV solution.
   Rationale: Some infusion sets include backcheck valves that stop primary IV solution flow while medication infuses, then automatically open when medication infusion stops. When using these devices the primary bag is hung lower. If a backcheck valve system is not used, medications are infused simultaneously and hung at the same height.

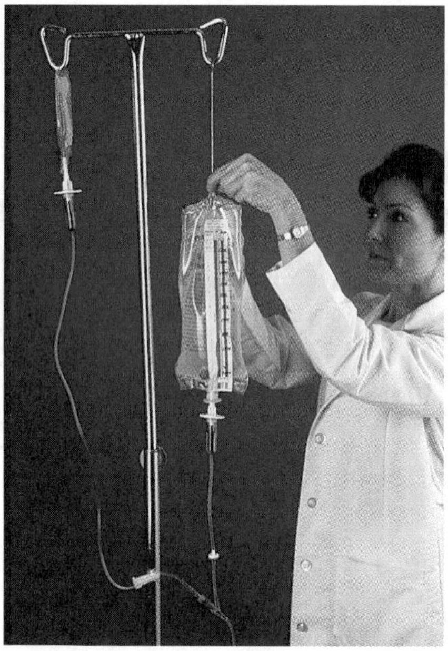

Step 5 • *Hang primary bag lower during IV piggyback administration when backcheck valve system is used.*

6. a. If using a needle, wipe injection port, nearest IV insertion site, on primary IV tubing with antiseptic and attach needle with needle protector.

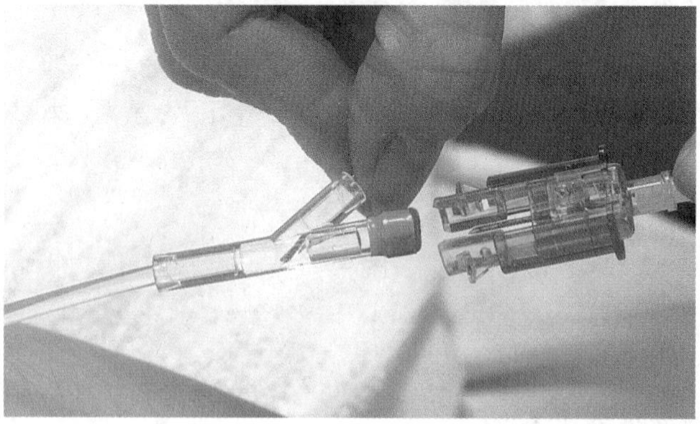

Step 6A • *Attach high-risk needle with needle protector into port on primary line.*

   b. If using a needleless system, insert secondary line into the needleless adapter port. A special needleless system may be used in situations where there is high risk (eg, the known presence of bloodborne pathogens).
   Rationale: Cleansing the insertion site prevents contamination with microorganisms during needle insertion. Using a needleless system prevents accidental needlesticks during the procedure.

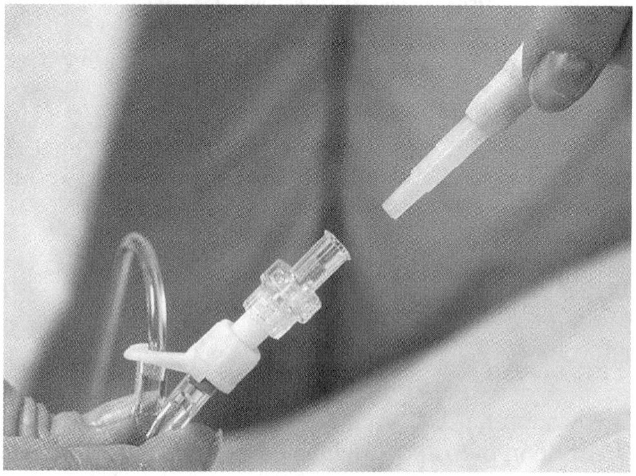

Step 6B • *Insert secondary tubing into adaptor.*

7. Check compatibility of medications to be administered with the IV solution being infused and any other infusing medications.
   Note: If medication is not compatible with primary IV solution, clamp primary IV tubing above injection port, insert needle with 20-mL syringe of normal saline flush solution and flush IV line.
   Rationale: Prevents reactions and precipitation of incompatible solutions.
8. Remove needle. Insert needle attached to medication tubing and secure with tape.
9. Regulate flow of medication solution. Most medications infuse over 20 to 60 minutes. Check pharmacy directives. Monitor periodically.
10. When medication has infused, turn off flow clamp. Regulate primary infusion as necessary.
    Rationale: Medication infusion may alter flow rate of primary solution.
11. Discard medication solution container, tubing, and needle or needleless adapter, or leave hanging with needle covered for future use, as dictated by agency policy.
    Rationale: Medication line establishes a potential route for microorganisms to enter the primary IV. Use protective covers and change tubing every 48

to 72 hours, according to agency policy in order to decrease the chance of contamination.

12. Wash hands.
13. Document medication administration and add IV volume to IV intake.

Procedure

Using an Intermittent Infusion Device (Heparin Lock)

1. Perform previous Steps 1 to 6.
2. Insert 3 mL normal saline flush solution into port with either a needle or needleless adaptor.
   Rationale: Blood return ensures that intravenous catheter is in the vein. Sometimes there is no blood return even though the catheter is patent.
3. Inject 2–3 mL of normal saline flush. Do not force solution.
   Rationale: Establishes patency of IV catheter and flushes heparin from the catheter.
4. Remove syringe and discard in appropriate receptacle.
5. Insert needle or needleless adaptor of medication tubing into ejection port. Secure and regulate flow as described above.
6. When medication has infused, turn off clamp and remove needle or adaptor.
7. Cleanse port.
8. Insert the second syringe of normal saline flush solution and inject 2–3 mL normal saline flush solution. Discard.
   Rationale: This action flushes remaining medication from the catheter and prevents incompatibilities with heparin.
9. In some situations a heparin flush solution is injected slowly. Remove and discard equipment.
   Rationale: Anticoagulant action of heparin prevents blood in IV catheter from clotting but is used less often today.
10. Wash hands.
11. Document medication administration and add IV volume to IV intake.

Lifespan Considerations

Infants and Children

- Infants receive much smaller volumes of fluid than adults. Intravenous medications should be infused through a volume control IV unit to avoid potentially serious fluid overload.

allow the actual infusion time to be close to the ordered infusion time. IV fluids or medications that infuse 1 to 2 hours earlier or later than ordered are generally considered to be medication errors. If a medication must be delivered at an exact rate or over a set period, an infusion controller pump may be used; these machines monitor and control the rate at which a medication is infused by counting the drops infused or by monitoring the IV volume infused.

Patient-Controlled Analgesia. PCA devices permit the client to administer narcotics intravenously as needed for pain control. A PCA device is programmed electronically to deliver a set amount of medication (usually a narcotic) through a prefilled syringe connected to IV tubing. Specific dosages and time intervals can be programmed into the machine to prevent overdosage; medication is delivered when the client pushes a control button (Cohen, 1993). Refer to Chapter 44 for more information on PCA.

Community-Based Care

Medication routines that are specific to the client and integrated into daily routine are more likely to be followed. To tailor medication routines and teaching plans to the client, the nurse should assess the client's physical and psychosocial status, financial situation, usual daily routine before the illness, and learning style and manner of coping with previous therapeutic regimens. This information can generally be gathered informally by talking with the client and family. By informing the client and family of an intent to make the medication routines practical so that they can work, the nurse is likely to elicit useful information.

The client's physical condition may influence his or her ability to take medications as prescribed. The physical senses of sight and hearing often deteriorate with disease or advancing age, evoking the question, "Does the client see and hear well enough to follow daily medication routines?" A diabetic client with retinopathy and blurred vision may be unable to draw insulin accurately into a syringe. The ability to perform fine motor movements also may change with illness or advancing age. Most people can learn the coordinated motor movements needed to administer injections, but the nurse should expect to spend more time teaching this technique to older clients.

Client assessments also involve making a judgment about the client's ability to comprehend, follow, and remember instructions. A neurologic deficit that may limit a client's ability to follow a medical routine may or may not be easy to recognize. Overt signs of aphasia (inability to speak or comprehend) or anomia (inability to remember the names of objects) can be easy to recognize; more subtle forms of neurologic dysfunction may be perceived as "vagueness" or "lack of attentiveness." When the nurse is concerned about a client's ability to comprehend and retain information, asking the client to restate instructions or demonstrate an activity several hours after hearing them may help clarify whether the client has the cognitive ability to self-administer medications safely.

The psychosocial condition of the client influences his or her ability to take medications correctly. People living in situations without supportive friends or family members may be less likely to follow medical regimens. If the nurse is aware of the situation, he or she can help the client problem-solve and get family support or counseling and simplify the medication routine to fit the client's situation.

The client's financial situation may limit his or her ability to obtain the medication or to take the medication as prescribed. Clients with limited resources should be placed on the least expensive, simplest medication routine possible. The nurse should make sure that the client understands the possible consequences of discontinuing medications.

The complexity of a medical routine may make compliance difficult for the client. Medication regimens that involve multiple dosing intervals of multiple medications or through-the-night dosing may be difficult to remember. The nurse should consider, given the client's abilities and limitations, whether medications can be self-administration safely. If the nurse has concerns about the client's ability to take medications safely, the client's healthcare provider should be consulted to see if the medication routine can be simplified or if help can be obtained for the client at home. After discussing the planned home medication routines with the client, it is helpful to ask the client his or her plan for taking the medications. If the client does not have a plan for taking the medications, useful techniques include prefilled medication boxes, calendars with the medications written on them, or storage of medications in places that prompt the client to remember them.

Priorities for teaching can be guided by determining what the client needs to know to take his or her medications safely. Information should be presented in everyday, nontechnical language, in written and discussion formats. Brief, practical information about the following topics is usually appropriate: the name of the medication; the reason for taking the medication; how and when to take the medication; how long to take the medication; the foods, drinks, and prescription or over-the-counter medications that may affect the action of the medication; any activities that may be affected when taking this medication; and the usual side effects of the medication and their treatment. (For more information, see the Client Teaching display.)

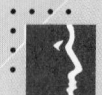

Client Teaching
Medications

Instruct the client as follows:

- *Learn the name, purpose, dose, and common side effects of any prescribed medications you are taking.*
- *Take every prescribed dose, even if you start to feel better before the medication is finished.*
- *Take only the prescribed dose of medication—increasing the dosage will not always increase the desired effect and in many cases may be dangerous.*
- *Study possible food or drug interactions to your prescribed medications. Find out whether the drug should be taken with meals or on an empty stomach.*
- *Learn symptoms that necessitate contacting a healthcare professional.*
- *Keep all medications in their original prescription containers, and store them according to specifications.*
- *Check expiration dates and discard when expired; old medications may lose potency and be ineffective.*
- *Never take medications prescribed for another individual. Never give your prescribed medications to anyone else.*
- *Do not take medications in the dark or when you are groggy, because drug errors may occur.*
- *If remembering to take prescribed medications is a problem, keep a chart or use a special dispensing unit to improve accuracy.*
- *Keep all medications out of reach and in child-proof containers to avoid accidental ingestion.*
- *Keep a list of all current medications, so accurate information can be given to any healthcare provider.*
- *Whenever possible, provide the client with written information on essential content for future reference.*

If a medication is being given to improve a bothersome symptom, for example, a metered-dose inhaler to treat shortness of breath, specific warnings about using more than the ordered dosage should be included. Without this warning, a client who thinks "if a little is good, more is better," may take excessive amounts of medication.

Begin teaching about medications as soon as possible. Teaching about administration techniques that require refining psychomotor skills, such as those used for injecting insulin, should begin at least 24 hours before client discharge. The client is unlikely to learn a complex psychomotor skill without frequent demonstrations and practice. Likelihood of compliance with medication routines can be difficult to predict. Clients who are unlikely to comply with medication routines can be easy to spot; included in this group are those with ongoing substance abuse problems or complex or unstable living arrangements.

Compliance with medication regimens is lower than one might expect among other groups of people. About

20% of people may not fill initial prescriptions; 40% to 60% of people may stop taking their medications early. Average long-term compliance with complication- preventing medication regimens (such as antihypertensive therapy) is about 50%. Matching medication routines and teaching materials to the individual client; ensuring frequent, ongoing follow-up; encouraging involvement of family or friends in assisting the person with medication compliance; and discussing compliance issues with the client may help increase rates of compliance.

Evaluation

Assessing the client's response to medications is an important function of the professional nurse. Evaluation should include therapeutic effects obtained from the medication, unexpected adverse effects from the medication, the client's compliance with the medication regimen, and the client's knowledge level concerning prescribed medications.

The nurse can ask the client if the prescribed medication seems to be working. Subjective feelings of improvement are important indicators of therapeutic effect for many medications. The nurse also can use physical assessments (eg, vital signs, lung auscultation) to identify physical improvements. Laboratory test values provide additional objective data useful in evaluating many medications.

The nurse should be knowledgeable about side effects for any drug administered. Signs of toxicity or unpleasant side effects should be documented and reported to the healthcare provider.

Assessment of the client's understanding and compliance with drug therapy is another important part of evaluation. Having the client describe the dose, frequency, action, and side effects of each medication is one way to evaluate knowledge level. Clients administering injections for the first time should demonstrate this skill before discharge. Clients should be able to explain how they plan to purchase, store, and take their medication after discharge.

Lifespan Considerations

Medication administration techniques are affected by developmental stage and age-related factors.

Newborn and Infant

Special considerations are important when giving oral, SC, IM, and IV medications to newborns and infants. Liquid oral medications should be used for newborns and infants; if these are not available, the medication should be crushed and dissolved in water. A syringe can be used to draw up and give oral medications. Medications should be given on an empty stomach unless otherwise noted; infant formulas may alter medication absorption, and the infant is less likely to spit up medications if given before feedings.

Parenteral medications should be given to newborns and infants with special care. The SC route is rarely used for administering medications to infants and newborns; SC injections can be difficult to administer to the newborn or premature infant who has little or no SC tissue. If this route must be used, the nurse should discuss technique concerns with the infant's healthcare provider. The healthcare provider may choose to have injections given into ID tissue. Once medication action, dosage, and length of action are determined, they will probably remain constant if the technique remains consistent.

IM injections of 0.5 to 1 mL of medication can be administered into the rectus femoris site in infants younger than 2 years.

Newborns and infants are given IV medications with the following guidelines:

- The smallest possible amounts of medication are used.
- Infusions are monitored using electronic flow devices.
- IV sites in the hand, scalp, forearm, foot, or central circulation are used.
- The catheter site is carefully monitored frequently.
- The catheter insertion site is protected, and the child is restrained, as needed.

Teaching concerning medication administration is geared toward caregivers. Teaching should encompass the reason the child is receiving the medication, the proper medication dosage, the method of measuring the dosage, the dosage schedule in relation to feedings, the amount of time to continue the medication, the desired effect of the medication, what to do if the child spits up the medication, and signs and symptoms of common important medication side effects. If an infant spits up a volume of medication that looks like the total dose within 5 to 10 minutes after receiving it, the medication should usually be repeated.

Toddler and Preschooler

Children in this age group are beginning to explore their world and learn about themselves and their environment. Because this is a time of exploration, accidental medication poisoning is a particular risk. Parents should be encouraged to store all medications in a protected area out of the child's reach; make sure that medications are packaged in containers with childproof caps; and make sure that children are aware that medications are not candy.

The toddler or preschool-age child who is given medication may have multiple concerns: a fear of the unknown or unfamiliar, pain, being separated from family, or loss of control. Procedures should be explained in simple terms, appropriate to the child's experiences and level of understanding. Attempts should be made to assure the child that the medication is not a punishment. Whenever possible, allow the child to make choices about therapy.

Effective teaching materials for toddlers and preschoolers include texts fashioned like coloring books and dolls or puppets. Dolls and puppets can be used to demonstrate a procedure, and if necessary, the child can return the demonstration on the doll.

Physical changes during this period also have implications for medication administration. Oral medications are still given in liquid form, or if necessary, tablets are crushed and mixed with food. Children younger than 3 years have straighter, stiffer external auditory canals than older children and adults. To administer ear drops to this age group, the pinna of the ear is pulled down and back before dropping medication into the ear canal.

The preferred site for administering IM injections to toddlers is the rectus femoris site; injections of up to 1.5 mL may be given. Preschoolers can receive injections of up to 0.5 mL into the deltoid site; up to 1.5 mL into the rectus femoris site, ventral gluteal, or dorso-

Therapeutic Dialogue
Medication Administration

Scenes for Thought

As you bring Mr. Abramson, aged 58, his cardiac pills, he turns his attention from the TV on the wall to you.

Effective

Client: *Christine, I don't want those pills. I told the doctor I don't need them. They give me headaches, and I don't want them.*
Nurse: *(Stop in surprise just inside the room. Settle your own heartbeat and sit in the chair next to his.) You sure seem upset about this. Tell me what happened.*
Client: *I just get headaches from them, that's all. And she said I'd have to take them for the rest of my life! I can't live with headaches for the rest of my life.* He looks angry and somehow powerless.
Nurse: *I can tell this is bothering you a lot. Did you mention the reason you don't want this medication to your physician?*
Client: *Yes. She said she'd change it.* Sounds irritated.
Nurse: *Let me check for you. (Checks the med order written that morning by the physician. The medication has been changed.) Well, she did change it, Mr. Abramson. This is the new medication she ordered. (Shows him the capsule.)*
Client: Takes it reluctantly. *How do I know this won't affect me the same way?*
Nurse: *I would like to come back and give you some information about it after I've given out the other medications on the unit. Would that help?*
Client: *Yes, indeed.* Looks relieved though still a little skeptical.
Nurse: *And maybe we can talk about your concerns that you'll have to take it for the rest of your life. That sounds like a separate issue but still important. Have I read that right?*
Client: *I think you have, Christine. I'll think about that while you're gone.* Gives you a small smile, almost sheepish.

Less Effective

Client: *Kirsten, I don't want those pills. I told the doctor I don't need them. They give me headaches, and I don't want them.*
Nurse: *(Stop in surprise just inside the room. Settle your own heartbeat and sit in the chair next to his.) You sure seem upset about this. Tell me what happened.*
Client: *I just get headaches from them, that's all. And she said I'd have to take them for the rest of my life! I can't live with headaches for the rest of my life.* He looks angry and somehow powerless.
Nurse: *I can tell this is bothering you a lot. Do you have a headache now?*
Client: *No, but after I take that little white pill, I always do.*
Nurse: *Which one is it? I don't seem to have one to give you right now. (Shows him the three capsules in the cup, two blue and one white with a yellow stripe.)*
Client: Looking in confusion. *It isn't there. Maybe she changed it already.*
Nurse: *I think that's what happened. There was a medication order change this morning after she made rounds, and the pharmacy just sent these new blue capsules up for you. Do you feel better about it now? (Pouring fresh water into a glass so he can take the medication.)*
Client: *Sure, sure. At least I won't have those headaches.* Looks somewhat relieved, but still skeptical.
Nurse: *Yes. I'm glad we got that straightened out! Call me if you need me. (Goes out to finish giving meds.)*

Critical Thinking Challenge

• *In both dialogues, the client received the correct medication. Detect what the client didn't receive in the second dialogue.* • *Explain what concerned Christine about Mr. Abramson's remark about having to take the medication for the rest of his life.* • *Look up the nursing diagnoses "Noncompliance" and "Knowledge Deficit" and consider their relationship.* • *Examine how they might apply to Mr. Abramson's concerns.*

gluteal sites; and up to 2 mL into the vastus lateralis site. Many young children fear injections, and the injection should be given as promptly as possible to avoid escalating anxiety and fear. The child must be carefully restrained, often by another person, to ensure safety during the procedure.

Child and Adolescent

As the child matures and develops, more teaching and responsibility for medication administration can be directed at the child. Most school-age children can swallow tablets and capsules. To increase compliance, the dosage schedule should avoid school hours whenever possible. When medication administration is necessary during school hours, most schools require that medications be deposited with the school nurse in the original prescription container.

Many school-age children are still fearful of injections and worry about crying or losing control when injections are administered in groups. Even though children of this age can understand the importance of remaining still during an injection, sudden movement often occurs as the needle pierces the skin. Support of the extremity or judicious positioning helps ensure safety during the injection. By the time a child has reached school age, all injection sites may be used, because all muscles have adequately developed.

Teaching during the adolescent years should emphasize the importance of not taking any prescription medication that has not been ordered specifically for the person. The adolescent's possible use of illegal drugs or alcohol may be explored because both usually interact with prescribed medications.

Adult and Older Adult

As adults age, the need for more medications to treat chronic health problems may become a reality. Compliance with complex medication schedules can be difficult, especially for the older person who has cognitive deficits. Most adults can swallow tablets, but neurologic problems may interfere with swallowing.

Physical conditions, such as cachexia or obesity, may influence which IM sites are chosen for adults. The cachectic adult may retain muscle mass in the ventrogluteal site longer than in other IM sites. The least desirable IM site for an obese adult is the dorsogluteal site, where a thick fat layer often causes the medication to be deposited in the SC tissue.

Visual deficits may make reading drug information and prescription labels more difficult. Decreased fine motor skill and tactile sensation may increase the difficulty of administering eye drops or insulin injections.

The older person is at increased risk for drug toxicity because of altered renal excretion and hepatic metabolism of drugs. Decreased circulation can affect absorption of ingested drugs. Older adults should be watched more carefully for drug toxicity, especially when renal or hepatic disease is present. Cognitive impairment in older adults is most commonly caused by adverse effects of medications (Miller, 1995).

Drug misuse can occur when medications are saved to be used at a future time; older people also may share their prescription drugs with a friend who complains of similar symptoms. Older clients on a fixed income may find that the expense of many medications stresses an already limited budget. Although these problems can occur among all age groups, they are more common among older people because of their increasing dependence on medications to improve health and functioning.

Key Concepts

- Medication administration is a significant nursing responsibility that requires a good understanding of pharmacologic principles, assessment skills, and ability to individualize client teaching.
- A drug is a substance that alters physiologic function, and a medication is a drug that is administered for its therapeutic effects.
- Medications can be identified by four different names: chemical name, generic name, official name, and brand name.
- Drug references are available to provide the healthcare professional with specific information on each medication. It is the nurse's responsibility to use drug reference resources to be knowledgeable about each drug administered.
- Medication distribution systems include the stock supply, the unit-dose, and SAM.
- A drug order must include the client's name, the date and time of the order, the name of the medication, the dose, the frequency, the route of administration, and the healthcare provider's signature.
- Types of drug orders include standing orders, prn orders, one-time orders, stat orders, and telephone and verbal orders. It is the nurse's responsibility to interpret accurately and carry out safely the healthcare provider's orders.
- Three systems of measure are used to calculate drug dosages: the metric, apothecary, and household systems. It is the nurse's responsibility to cal-

culate drug dosage accurately within a given system and from one system to another.
- Federal legislation controls the way medications are manufactured, marketed, and controlled. The nurse must practice within the state's Nurse Practice Act and the agency's policies and procedures concerning medication administration.
- To ensure client safety, the nurse must follow the "five rights" (the right drug, in the right dose, at the right time, by the right route, to the right client) whenever a medication is administered.
- Drug activity is the result of chemical interactions between a medication and the cells of the body, which produce a biologic or physiologic response. This response can be altered by drug absorption or distribution, metabolism, or excretion of the drug.
- Many factors, such as age, weight, gender, time of administration, and organ system function, can affect drug action.
- Therapeutic effects are the desired effects obtained from medication administration. In addition, side effects such as secondary effects, toxicity, cumulative effects, tolerance, hypersensitivity reaction, idiosyncratic reaction, allergic reaction, or drug or food interactions can occur.
- When the client first enters the healthcare facility, assessments are necessary to obtain baseline information concerning medications, before any administration of medications, and to individualize client teaching concerning medications.
- Nursing diagnoses related to medication administration may include Noncompliance or Knowledge Deficit.
- Many forms of medications, such as tablets, capsules, syrups, and elixirs are appropriate for oral administration. Oral medications may be swallowed, administered through gastric or intestinal tubes, or given by the sublingual or buccal route.
- Topical medications include those that are applied to the skin or inserted in a body cavity. Solutions, creams, lotions, and transdermal patches are applied to the skin. Topical medications can be inserted into the eye, ear, nose, rectum, and vagina.
- Parenteral medications are given by injection or infusion into ID tissue, SC tissue, IM tissue, or venous or arterial circulation.
- Sites commonly used for IM injections include the deltoid, ventral gluteal, vastus lateralis, rectus femoris, and dorsogluteal muscles. Anatomic landmarks must be used to identify each site properly.
- IV medications enter the venous circulation by IV push, intermittent infusion, or continuous drip. The client may self-deliver IV medications by using a PCA device.
- Developmental concerns are important for the nurse to consider when administering medications.

Critical Thinking Challenges

Using what you have just learned about medication administration techniques and their implications, refer to the situation at the beginning of the chapter. If you were the nurse visiting this older client, consider how you would respond to the following:

1. *Describe the direction that your assessment might take in this situation.*
2. *From the information the woman shared with you, identify the factors that you believe may present a threat to her health.*
3. *Propose a course of timely and appropriate nursing actions.*
4. *Describe the possible actions that you or the woman might pursue.*

References

Cohen, M. R. (1993). Preventing errors associated with P.C.A. pumps. *Nursing, 23* (4), 17.

Cohen, M. R. (1994). Second-guessing soundalike generic drugs. *Nursing, 24* (3), 29.

Cohen, M. R., Senders, J., & Davis, N. M. (1994). 12 ways to prevent medication errors. *Nursing, 24* (2), 34–41.

Davis, N. M. (1993). Misinterpreting written orders. *American Journal of Nursing, 93* (12), 18.

Davis, N. M. (1994a). Confusion over illegible orders. *American Journal of Nursing, 94* (1), 9.

Davis, N. M. (1994b). Clarifying questionable orders. *American Journal of Nursing, 94* (4), 16.

Dossing, M., & Sonne, J. (1993). Drug-induced hepatic disorders. Incidence, management and avoidance. *Drug Safety, 9* (6), 441–449.

Hahn, K. (1991). Brush up on your injection technique (published erratum). *Nursing, 20*(9), 54–58.

Kumar, S., & Rex, D. K. (1991). Failure of physicians to recognize acetaminophen hepatotoxicity in chronic alcoholics. *Archives of Internal Medicine, 151* (6), 1189–1191.

Malseed, R. T., & Girton, S. E. (1995). *Pharmacology: Drug therapy and nursing considerations* (4th ed.). Philadelphia: J.B. Lippincott.

Miller, C. A. (1995). Medications that may cause cognitive impairment in older adults. *Geriatric Nursing, 16* (1), 47.

North American Nursing Diagnosis Association (1994). *NANDA Nursing diagnoses: Definitions and classification 1995-1996.* Philadelphia: Author.

Shlafer, M. (1993). *The nurse, pharmacology, and drug therapy: A prototype approach* (2nd ed.). Menlo Park, CA, Addison-Wesley.

Shumway, J. M., Jacknowitz, A. I., & Abate, M. A. (1990). Analysis of physicians', pharmacists', and nurses' attitudes toward the use of computers to access drug information. *Methods of Information in Medicine, 29* (2), 99–103.

Spencer, R. T. (1992). *Clinical pharmacology and nursing management* (4th ed.). Philadelphia: J.B. Lippincott.

Bibliography

Abdoo, Y. M. (1992). Designing a patient care medication and recording system that uses bar code technology. *Computers in Nursing, 10* (3), 116–120.

Cargill, J. M. (1992). Medication complicance in elderly people: Influencing variables and interventions. *Journal of Advanced Nursing, 17* (4), 422–426.

Davis, N. M. (1994a). More patient education tips. *American Journal of Nursing, 94* (2), 16.

Davis, N. M. (1994b). Teaching patients to prevent errors. *American Journal of Nursing, 94* (5), 17.

Grant, A. (1994). Medication errors. *Canadian Nurse, 90* (8), 53.

Lilley, L. L., & Guanci, R. (1994). Getting back to basics. *American Journal of Nursing, 94* (9), 15–16.

Martin, P. J. (1994). Professional updating through open learning as a method of reducing errors in the administration of medicines. *Journal of Nursing Management, 2* (5), 209–212.

Parisi, S. B. (1994). What to do after a med error. *Nursing, 24* (6), 59.

Prince, K., Summers, L., & Knight, M. A. (1994). Needless i.v. therapy: Comparing three systems for safety. *Nursing Management, 25* (3), 80N, 80P.

Perioperative Nursing

Key Terms

Anesthesiologist
Certified registered nurse anesthetist
Circulating nurse
Conscious sedation
Elective surgery
Emergent surgery
Intraoperative phase
Local anesthetic
Malignant hyperthermia
Paralytic ileus
Postanesthesia care unit
Postoperative phase
Preoperative care unit
Preoperative phase
Regional anesthetic
Required surgery
Scrub nurse
Skin staple
Suture
Urgent surgery

Learning Objectives

Upon completion of this chapter, the student will be able to do the following:

- *Discuss three phases of perioperative client management.*
- *Discuss the impact of surgery on functional health.*
- *Identify lifespan considerations for the client undergoing a surgical procedure.*
- *Identify appropriate common North American Nursing Diagnosis Association (NANDA) nursing diagnoses for the preoperative, intraoperative, and postoperative phases.*
- *Describe appropriate perioperative client teaching.*
- *Discuss emotional support, safety, and asepsis during the intraoperative phase.*
- *Identify appropriate nursing assessments in the recovery facility and during the postoperative period.*
- *Identify common postoperative complications and appropriate nursing care to promote normal function.*
- *Develop an appropriate discharge plan for the surgical client.*

28

You are a nurse working in the preadmission surgical unit where preoperative assessment and teaching are performed. A young mother brings in her 2-year-old son, who is scheduled for a myringotomy (tubes inserted in the eardrums). You talk with the young woman about the surgery and then proceed to collect the following information:

- *A 12-month history of repeated ear infections, averaging usually between one and two per month*
- *No known drug allergies*
- *Currently on no medications*
- *Vital signs: temperature 37.9, pulse 108, respirations 22*
- *Tenacious, dark tan nasal drainage for last 48 hours*
- *Lungs clear on auscultation*
- *Rest of physical assessment within normal limits*

You observe that the mother-child interaction appears good, noting that the mother comforts the child when he begins to cry.

In previous chapters you learned about the nursing process, lifespan development, and health assessment.

In this chapter you expand your knowledge base to include perioperative nursing. Perioperative nursing is a specialty that draws on skills and knowledge from many areas, as you will find when reflecting on the case situation above. You may want to review concepts presented in previous units as you absorb the new content in this chapter. Critical Thinking Challenges referring to this situation are presented at the end of the chapter to help sharpen your critical thinking skills.

Surgery is a means of treating injury and disease. The goal of surgery is to return the client to the highest level of functioning and health possible, as soon as possible, within the limits imposed by the injury or disease state. In general, surgery is performed because other noninvasive treatments are not appropriate or have been unsuccessful. Surgery has been selected by the physician and the client as the best means to achieve the desired goal.

In modern culture, surgery has become a common method of treating disease and promoting health. In the last few decades the complexities of surgery have increased greatly, and entire organ systems can be transplanted to replace nonfunctioning body parts. All surgical procedures can potentially affect functional abilities of the person in every functional health pattern. The impact can be great and permanent or brief and temporary. Perioperative nurses provide specialized care to the surgical client, promoting the return to optimal function. As appropriate, family members and others are included in specialized care. The goal of perioperative nursing practice is to assist clients, their families, and significant others to achieve a level of wellness equal to or greater than that which they had before the procedure (adopted by the 1994 Association of Operating Room Nurses House of Delegates [AORN, 1995])

Perioperative nursing involves the period before, during, and after any surgical procedure. During this time, the nurse plays an integral role, using the nursing process to individualize care and meet the surgical client's specific needs.

Perioperative nursing is a continually challenging nursing specialty that requires knowledge, technical skill, creativity, leadership, and excellent communication skills. To meet the constantly changing needs of the surgical client in this age of ever-increasing technology, the professional nurse must continually upgrade knowledge and skill through self-education and participation in educational inservice opportunities. As with all professional nursing specialties, the importance of teamwork and cooperation among colleagues cannot be overemphasized. This spirit of teamwork is especially important and relevant for the perioperative nurse.

Surgical Intervention

Classification of Surgery

Surgery may be performed for many specific reasons: to investigate a problem or set of symptoms, alleviate pain, prolong life, improve mobility, provide vascular access for medications or nutrition, improve function, or improve appearance. General classifications of surgery according to purpose are provided in Table 28-1.

The urgency with which surgery must be performed differs for each situation (Applegeet, 1995). **Emergent surgery** is surgery that must be performed immediately to preserve function of a body part or the life of the client. An example of emergent surgery is the repair of a major blood vessel (ruptured aorta) to stop severe bleeding, or the repair of a perforated appendix. **Urgent surgery** is surgery that must be performed promptly within 24 to 48 hours. Examples of urgent surgery include incision and drainage of a wound infection or repair of fractures. The third category, **required surgery**, occurs when a decision for surgery is indicated for a health problem but the surgery does not need to be performed immediately to preserve life or function. Examples of required surgery include removal of a gallbladder or a cancerous growth. **Elective surgery** includes those surgical procedures that are performed to satisfy the desire of the client but are not needed to preserve life or function—for example, cosmetic surgery, such as a facelift.

Surgical Facilities

The facility chosen for surgery depends on the type and complexity of the procedure and the availability of necessary supplies and equipment. For example, if the planned surgical procedure requires laser or radiation technology, or if the client requires intensive care nursing, the chosen facility needs to have the required technical equipment and personnel available. Facilities where surgery is commonly performed include a clinic or physician's office, an ambulatory surgical center, or a hospital.

Clinic or Physician's Office

Surgery performed in a clinic or physician's office is usually limited to minor surgical procedures such as diagnostic procedures, oral procedures, gynecologic procedures, or removal of lesions from the skin. Procedures done in these facilities usually require either no anesthesia, local anesthesia, or regional blocks. Surgery performed in these facilities is the least expensive, because complex equipment is not used and inpatient recovery is not needed. As technology advances and pro-

Table 28-1 • Types of Surgery Based on Purpose and Urgency

Classification	Purpose	Examples
Purpose		
Diagnostic	Confirmation of suspected diagnosis	Biopsy, culture, endoscopy, fluid tap
Explorative	Confirms the type and extent of a disease process	Laparotomy, joint exploration
Reconstructive	Repairs physical deformities or improves appearance	Rhinoplasty, mammoplasty, skin grafting
Curative	Diseased or damaged body organ or structure is removed or repaired and the client is cured	Appendectomy, hysterectomy, fixation of fractures
Transplant	Diseased or damaged body organs and structures replaced with donated or artificial organs	Heart, kidney, cornea, bone, liver, lung, pancreas, or skin transplants
Palliative	Alleviates pain or other disease symptoms, slows progression of diseases but does not cure	Tumor debulking, nerve blocks, placement of feeding tubes
Urgency		
Emergent	Preserves function of body parts or life of client	Repair of major vessel to stop severe bleeding
Urgent	Requires prompt attention within 24–48 hours	Repair of fracture, incision and drainage of wound infection
Required	Indicated for health problem but immediacy not necessary to preserve function or life	Gallbladder removal, excision of cancerous growth
Elective	Satisfies client's desire but not needed to preserve life or function	Cosmetic surgery

cedures become less invasive, the number of surgeries performed in clinics and physicians' offices is growing.

Ambulatory Surgical Centers

Ambulatory surgical centers, also known as one-day surgical units and surgi-centers, have proliferated in an attempt to keep rising surgical costs down. These facilities admit clients for the day of surgery and may be affiliated with, and located in or near, hospitals.

Because ambulatory surgical centers can save time and money, many hospitals are increasing the number of surgeries performed. More than 50% of all surgery now performed is accomplished on an ambulatory basis, and this percentage is expected to continue rising (Parnass, 1993). The services provided by 1-day surgery centers are limited to procedures and clients suitable to this short-stay program. Clients must be assessed in terms of their anesthetic and surgical risk and in terms of their ability to safely care for themselves after discharge from the short-stay facility. Increasingly, cholecystectomies (gallbladder removal), appendectomies, and hernia repairs are being performed by laparoscope (a tubular optical and surgical instrument) in ambulatory surgical centers. Ambulatory surgery provides a special challenge to perioperative and postanesthesia nurses, who must provide optimal client care and teaching within a limited time.

Hospitals

Hospitals are comprehensive facilities for all types of surgery and postsurgical recovery. They have the necessary equipment and personnel available to perform surgeries requiring intensive monitoring, complex technology, and prolonged recovery. Hospitals provide a wide range of services and have extensive emergency backup systems, should these be necessary. However, they are in general more expensive than either the ambulatory surgery centers or clinics. Cost containment may prevent admission to a hospital for minor surgical procedures because insurance companies may not be willing to reimburse the cost of inpatient hospital care.

Phases of Perioperative Nursing

Perioperative nursing includes three distinct phases: preoperative, intraoperative, and postoperative. In each phase, the nurse plays an integral role, using the nursing process to individualize care and meet the surgical client's specific needs. Critical Pathways may be used in the perioperative surgical unit. A sample Pathway to be used with the abdominal surgical client is included here.

(text continues on page 648)

Collaborative Care Plan: Critical Pathway: TOTAL ABDOMINAL HYSTERECTOMY (TAH)

Patient Name:____________
Case Type: TAH__________ | Admit Date:____________ | Expected LOS: 4 – 5 days______ | Physician:____________
DRG:____________ | Date Path | Actual LOS:__________ | Case Manager:____________
ICD-9:____________ | Initiated:____________ | Discharge Date:__________

Outcome Criteria

	Pre-Op				Surg Day 1				PO Day 2–5			
Client Problems	Office/Pre Hosp	D	E	N	Surgery/PACU/Floor	D	E	N	Floor	D	E	N
Anxiety related to impending surgery, lack of knowledge of preoperative care activities, expectation of pain, & altered reproductive/sexual function	Verbalizes fears & concerns related to surgery Identifies previous coping mechanisms & support system				Verbalizes concerns related to hysterectomy, expectations for recovery, effects on sexual function				Acknowledges acceptance of surgery, changes in anatomy & function Participates in self-care Identifies concerns re: to body image, sexual function, menopause, hormone therapy			
Knowledge deficit related to lack of information about surgical procedure, sensations, pre & po care activities, effect on sexual function	Verbalizes understanding of surg. experience, pre & po activities Demonstrates po exercises (TCDB, IS) leg exercises States effects of surg on sexual function				Performs po exercises (TCDB, IS, splinting) leg exercises				Verbalizes activity restrictions (avoid heavy lifting, straining, prolonged sitting or standing, tub baths, douches) States S&S to report to MD (fever, chills, abn vaginal/wound drsg, br, red bleeding) States wound care & perineal hygiene Identify dietary needs			
Alteration in comfort related to surgical trauma to tissues & nerves	Verbalizes how to use pain rating scale of 0 – 10 Verbalizes knowledge when to notify nurse c̄ request for pain med				Rates pain <4 on scale of 0 – 10 15–30 min p̄ IV/IM pain med				Rates pain <2 on scale of 0 – 10 30 min p̄ po pain med Ambulates in hall without excessive pain (<2 pain rating)			
High risk for altered tissue perfusion related to trauma to tissues, blood loss, venous stasis, lithotomy position	Verbalizes rationale for po leg exercises.				Stable VS Peripheral pulses palpable: Bil Cap. refill < 3 sec Skin pink/warm Incision intact Sm amt vaginal bldg Adequate urine output > 30 CC/hr.				Hgb >10 Hct >30 Incision dry & intact without bleeding Scant vaginal bleeding p̄ packing DC No leg pain, edema, redness, pedal pulses palpable			
High risk for altered self concept related to loss of body part & sexual function	Verbalizes understanding of changes in sexual anatomy/function & effect of hysterectomy Verbalizes fears & concerns related to surgical procedure & effect on body image				Verbalizes feelings about hysterectomy Asks appropriate questions				Acknowledges acceptance of self related to inability to bear children, effect on sexuality & surgical menopause Participates in self care			
INTERVENTIONS												
Consult/Referral	Gynecologist/ H&P/consult								Follow up with gynecologist for Estrogen therapy, Pap smears			

	Pre-Op Office/Pre Hosp	D	E	N	Surg Day 1	D	E	N	PO Day 2–6	D	E	N
Client Problems		D	E	N		D	E	N		D	E	N
Diagnostic Tests	Schedule labs, CBC, lytes, coagulation profile, chemistry profile, chest x-ray, EKG, T&C X 2 units Pap smear/pregnancy test Ultrasound/CT scan				Validate lab/x-ray reports for chart				Hb & Hct as indicated			
Assessment	VS – Allergies H&P/past experience with surgery/hospital				Vital signs q 1–2 hr I&O q 1° Foley cath ECG rhythm Peripheral pulses O_2 sat Assess incision/vaginal bleeding				Vital signs q 8°/hr I&O q 8° – blood UA urine. DC Foley – cath PRN – Assess void prior to DC Peripheral pulses, Homan's sign, pain in calf, redness, edema, chest pain Assess bowel sounds, Abd distention, nausea, vomiting.			
Treatments	OR permit Surgical Scrub Hebiclens shown Foley cath				O_2 2–4 L/NC HOB ↑30° TCDB. IS q 1 hr IV fluids/blood products Antiembolism hose – remove q shift				DC O_2 if O_2 sat > 92% Wound care/perineal hygiene p̄ packing removed CDB/IS/leg exercises, DC IV – if sufficient po intake – Saline Lock Antiembolism hose – remove q shift Shower if incision intact			
Activity	UP ad lib				TCDB, q 1° HOB ↑30 – 45° Dangle – chair in P.M. Leg exercises (Calf pumps) Antiembolism Stockings/sequential compression device				Ambulate QID independently – Enc. freq. position changes Leg/foot exercises Anti-embolism stockings			
Diet	Diet as tol NPO p̄ mn prior to OR				Clear liquid as tol IV fluids Assess bowel sounds				Diet as tol DC IV fluids Assess bowel sounds prior to adv. diet			
Meds	Hypnotic HS Anti-anxiety agent as needed				Administer IV/IM pain meds as needed				Administer PO pain meds as needed (Tylenol, Percocet) (No ASA) Bowel care of choice			
Teaching	Pre/po teaching, related to surg. procedure, TCDB, sensation, pain rating				Teach SMI (sustained maximal inspiration) splinting while coughing, activity & diet progression				Discharge teaching re; wound care, vaginal bleeding, peri care, complications, signs of infection, activity progression, pain mgt Discuss misconceptions re: sexuality, menopause, Estrogen			
Discharge/Transfer Planning	Assess DC needs, home situation, support system, needs for assistance p̄ DC				Discuss home care needs/concerns re: to pt with family/sig. others Provide pt/family support				Discuss Estrogen, menopause, sexuality Discuss follow up care & when to report complication to MD Follow up appt c̄ MD			

(continued)

Critical Pathways *(continued)*

Initials/Signatures:	D=Day E=Evening N=Nite	Write "V" for variance in the box if expected outcome not met or staff intervention not performed. Patient variances must be explained in the progress note.

Preoperative Phase

The **preoperative phase** includes all the activities necessary to prepare the client properly for surgery. It begins when the decision for surgery is made and ends when the client is transferred to the operating room bed (AORN, 1995). Proper preoperative assessments by the nurse, anesthesia personnel, and the surgeon are essential to plan adequately for the designated procedure. This evaluation includes all functional health patterns. A thorough medical history is taken to ensure client safety.

The history and evaluations focus on the following areas: cardiac and respiratory assessments, medication history, previous anesthetic experiences, fluid and electrolyte status, allergies (especially to drugs, foods, and latex), mobility limitations, nutritional status, oral status, dental status, integumentary status, and emotional state. In addition, the client's learning requirements need to be assessed and preoperative teaching needs to be accomplished. The operative consent form is obtained in this phase. The client's psychological needs are also addressed at this point.

In the preoperative care area, the final preparations for the client's surgery are completed. The final assessment is accomplished and the intravenous (IV) access is established. These activities may be completed by the preoperative care nurse or the anesthetist, depending on the particular agency's protocol. A regional block (spinal, subarachnoid, or epidural) may be administered if this is the anesthetic of choice.

While these activities are taking place, the scrub nurse and circulating nurse are preparing the sterile instruments, supplies, and the remainder of the necessary equipment, medications, and nonsterile supplies that are required for the successful and efficient completion of the surgical procedure. All these activities require precise timing and cooperation among the people involved.

Intraoperative Phase

The **intraoperative phase** includes those activities that occur from the time the client is transferred to the operating room bed until the time the client is transferred to the postanesthesia area (AORN, 1995). During the procedure, the anesthetist or the monitoring nurse closely and frequently monitors the client's vital signs, IV fluids, urine output, medications, blood loss, and anesthetic agent being used for the particular procedure. Depending on the procedure, arterial blood gases and electrolyte values may also be frequently monitored.

The **scrub nurse** is responsible for maintaining the integrity, safety, and efficiency of the sterile field throughout the operation (Atkinson, 1992). The scrub nurse closely follows the procedure and provides the surgeons with the sterile instruments, sterile supplies and equipment, and the sterile sutures. The **circulating nurse** closely monitors and coordinates all activities in the operating room and manages the nursing care required for each client. This role, as the client's advocate, is critical to the safety and welfare of the client (Atkinson, 1992). In addition, the circulating nurse is responsible for maintaining accurate written records, and ensuring the continued sterility of the procedure and the safety of the client. At the end of the procedure, the circulating nurse, the surgeons, and the anesthetist provide for the safe and timely transport of the client into the recovery area (postanesthesia care unit, intensive care unit, or client unit).

Postoperative Phase

The **postoperative phase** involves those activities that occur from the time the client is transferred from the operating room until he or she has progressed beyond the acute phase of his or her recovery (AORN, 1995). This phase requires the nurse to monitor a number of parameters closely and frequently, including maintenance of an adequate airway, vital signs, blood gas and electrolyte values, level of consciousness, blood loss, IV fluid administration, level of regional block (if used), emotional state, level of pain control, and tolerance of the procedure. Further along in the recovery phase, the nurse continues assessing respiratory status, bowel status, incision status, and the client's tolerance of fluid and food.

The client's learning needs are also addressed in the recovery phase, and the client is encouraged to participate in care in preparation for self-care after discharge. As the client progresses in recovery, increased independence is anticipated. When the client is ready for discharge, complete discharge directions and instructions for follow-up care are given. These instructions are usually given to the client and a family member or another caregiver.

Impact of Surgery on Functional Health

Surgery can have a significant impact on a person's life. Changes resulting from surgery can influence many functional abilities. This section discusses these changes and how the nurse can make a positive contribution toward maximizing a client's health and function.

Health Perception and Health Maintenance

Frequently, the decision to have surgery is made jointly by the client and healthcare provider to promote health or improve function. This is an individual decision based on a person's perception of health and what actions are appropriate to manage current problems.

Many aspects of safety are involved in surgery. Safety considerations include both psychological safety and physical safety. Psychological safety is a feeling of comfort, security, and well-being, which can be enhanced by feelings of trust and confidence in the client's caregivers. Nurses can do much to promote these feelings. Providing emotional support and promoting an understanding of procedures greatly facilitate this process. When possible, family members and people the client chooses should be included in the explanation of surgical procedures. Physical safety considerations include safety with anesthesia, medications, chemicals, electricity, procedures, special equipment (such as lasers and radiation units), surgical positioning, and client transport.

Nursing Research
Surgery

Selected Nursing Research Studies

Avis, M. (1994). Choice cuts: An exploratory study of patients' views about participation in decision making in a day surgery unit. *International Journal of Nursing Studies, 31,* 289–298.

Poole, E. (1993). The effects of postanesthesia care unit visits on anxiety in surgical patients. *Journal of Postanesthesia Nursing, 8,* 386–394.

Redeker, N., Mason, D., Wykpisz, E., Glica, B., & Miner, C. (1994). First postoperative week activity patterns and recovery in women after coronary artery bypass surgery. *Nursing Research, 43,* 168–173.

Wynd, C., Samstag, D., & Lapp, A. M. (1994). Bacterial carriage on the fingernails of OR nurses: Does nail polish increase bacteria on fingernails? *AORN Journal, 60,* 796–805.

Zaza, S., Reeder, J., Charles, L., & Jarvis, W. (1994). Latex sensitivity among perioperative nurses. *AORN Journal, 60,* 806–812.

Possible Topics for Nursing Inquiry

- How does preoperative teaching retention compare when preoperative instruction occurred 1 week before surgery versus 1 day before surgery?
- How do antimicrobial showers compare with antimicrobial skin scrubs in preventing wound infections postoperatively?
- How effective is using music during the preoperative period in the surgical holding area to decrease patient anxiety?
- What is the incidence of compliance with leg exercises among postoperative clients?
- How useful is hypnotic suggestion in reducing postoperative nausea for clients having abdominal surgery?

Exercise and Activity

Depending on the nature of the surgery, the impact of surgery on exercise and activity levels can be significant. Such alterations in activity levels may be either temporary or permanent. The woman who is to have a breast biopsy in an ambulatory surgery center will probably need to curtail her regular activities for only a few hours, whereas the client who is to have an operation on a fractured leg will need to alter activity for several weeks to several months, depending on the extent of rehabilitation needed to return to a previous level of functioning. Both clients will experience relatively temporary changes in their activity levels.

However, permanent changes in a client's activity level may also occur as a result of surgery. A person who has a leg amputated secondary to trauma or peripheral vascular disease will need to make permanent changes in his or her activity patterns. All three of these clients will benefit from well-planned and well-implemented nursing interventions directed at returning them to their highest possible level of activity.

During the immediate postoperative period, respiratory and cardiovascular complications may result from immobility. Deep breathing and incentive spirometry are beneficial in preventing atelectasis (alveoli collapse) and pneumonia (Thomas & McIntosh, 1994). Leg exercises, antiembolitic hose, and sequential compression devices (SCD) help prevent deep vein thrombosis and subsequent pulmonary emboli. Accurate assessments, in-depth client preparation and teaching, excellent technical skills, and intensive follow-up care are important aspects of providing optimal care for the client to minimize the adverse effects of surgery on activity level.

Nutrition and Metabolism

Nutrition and metabolic function are additional areas that can be significantly altered by surgery. It is beneficial for the client to be in an optimal nutritional state to undergo surgery safely and successfully. Optimal nutritional status promotes wound healing, increases resistance to infection, promotes physical and psychological well-being, and maintains an adequate energy level and optimal fluid and electrolyte balance. After surgery, a diet with sufficient amounts of protein and vitamins A and C helps rebuild tissues and promotes wound healing. Adequate amounts of carbohydrates and fat are also important to avoid depleting protein stores. It is important to assess for metabolic disorders, such as diabetes mellitus, preoperatively. Such disorders need to be managed well to avoid intraoperative and postoperative complications.

Nausea and vomiting can occur during the postoperative period from the effects of anesthetic agents, pain medications, or manipulation of intestinal organs. During the postoperative period, oral fluid and food may need to be withheld until intestinal motility resumes. After positive bowel sounds have been detected, the diet is usually advanced as tolerated.

Infection. It is beneficial to detect and treat any infection before surgery. Doing so promotes healing and lessens the chance that the infection will spread or become systemic. Because the skin barrier is broken and trauma occurs during surgical procedures, the risk of infection increases. Meticulous intraoperative aseptic practices are necessary to prevent infection. Skin scrubs and bowel sterilization can decrease endogenous flora (microorganisms that normally live in the body), which might otherwise increase the infection risk. Antibiotic prophylaxis is especially important with intestinal surgery or joint replacement, but can be used for many other types of surgery or in high-risk clients. Usually a cephalosporin antibiotic is administered just before the surgical procedure so that the level of medication circulating in the client's blood will be high during surgery (Widdison, et al., 1993). During the postoperative period, the nurse monitors the wound for infection and institutes measures to prevent other infectious complications (eg, respiratory or urinary tract infections).

Thermoregulation. It is not uncommon for the surgical client to experience an undesirable alteration in body temperature regulation. Fever is often associated with an infectious process or trauma.

Hypothermia can occur secondary to a number of factors, including decreased ambient temperature in the operating room, vasodilation secondary to the use of certain anesthetic agents, blood loss, IV fluid administration, exposure of body surface area, cool skin preparation solutions, and decreased consciousness leading to a decreased ability to maintain body temperature. Hypothermia is greater in the very young and the very old. However, many interventions help alleviate body heat loss, including providing warm blankets, using electric warming devices, warming skin preparations and IV solutions, and minimizing body surface exposure.

Another problem of body temperature alteration is **malignant hyperthermia**, a hypermetabolic disorder of skeletal muscle that can be induced by some anesthetic agents, including certain inhalants and muscle relaxants (Donnelly, 1994). Because malignant hyperthermia has been identified as an inherited disease, clients who have a positive family history are particularly susceptible. This disease is manifested by masseter (jaw) muscle rigidity and ventricular dysrhythmias, which are associated with tachypnea (rapid respirations), cyanosis, skin mottling, and unstable blood pressure. These symptoms are followed by an increase in body temperature (possibly 1°C every 5 minutes if untreated), although fever may be a late sign of malignant hyperthermia. Consequently, in addition to identifying susceptible people, it is important to monitor muscle rigidity and body temperature closely during surgery for all clients and to have emergency medications and equipment immediately available.

Elimination

Both bladder and bowel elimination can be affected by surgery. Before surgery, the client usually receives no food or fluid orally (known as NPO status). This decreases urine production and bowel function.

Urinary Function. Adequate urine output usually indicates adequate renal function and cardiac output. Even in a client on NPO status, urine output should be at least 30 mL per hour (Wells, 1987). The client may have an indwelling urinary catheter placed in the bladder before surgery. If a urinary catheter is not in place, the client should void immediately before going to the operating room to help prevent bladder distention during or after the procedure. Emptying the bladder also helps to make the abdominal organs more accessible during abdominal surgery and prevents accidental injury to the bladder. During surgery, urine output is monitored closely for all clients with indwelling catheters. Clients who are undergoing shorter procedures (less than 2-4 hours) may not have a urinary catheter. For clients with urinary catheters and those without, blood pressure and fluid and electrolyte balance are carefully monitored intraoperatively, because these measurements provide information that helps evaluate the adequacy of renal function and circulation. The postoperative urine output should continue to be closely monitored. In this stage, inadequate output may indicate hypovolemia, hemorrhage, electrolyte imbalance, inadequate circulation, hypoxia, or impending shock. Clients without a urinary catheter should void within 8 hours of the surgical procedure.

Bowel Function. Bowel function may also be altered by the surgical experience. A client on preoperative NPO status has less active bowel function. In addition, the client may be required by the physician to have "enemas until clear" or to take laxatives. These help to clean the bowel of fecal material. This is especially important for clients undergoing gastrointestinal surgery, because it helps prevent the possible intraoperative spillage of bowel contents, which could lead to peritonitis.

In the postoperative phase, the bowel may take several days or longer to resume normal activity and function. This delay is caused by a combination of factors, including decreased intestinal peristalsis, decreased food and fluid intake, decreased dietary bulk, pain medications, decreased physical activity, stress, lack of a normal routine, and decreased privacy. Stool softeners frequently are prescribed after surgery, especially when the client is receiving large doses of opioid analgesics. Sometimes laxatives and enemas may be necessary.

A complication that can sometimes occur after surgery is **paralytic ileus**. Paralytic ileus is a condition in which there is significantly decreased bowel functioning. In some cases intestinal peristalsis may temporarily cease altogether. The bowel becomes distended and partially paralyzed. Bowel sounds are usually absent. This condition may result postoperatively from bowel manipulation during surgery and is especially associated with gastrointestinal surgery. A low serum potassium level, which can occur in the postoperative client, also contributes to paralytic ileus (Phippen & Wells, 1994). Paralytic ileus is very painful for the client and usually responds to treatment with a nasogastric tube, bowel rest, and IV therapy.

Sleep and Rest

The functional area of sleep and rest can be significantly affected when a person undergoes a surgical procedure. The surgical client may experience a disrupted sleep owing to preoperative preparation activities, changes in schedule, stress or anxiety related to the impending procedure, medication therapy, physical or emotional pain, separation from family and others, money worries and job uncertainties, and changes in normal diet and activity level. Nursing interventions that can help promote rest include providing a calm environment, relieving anxiety through client teaching and emotional support, making referrals to other health professionals as appropriate (mental health professionals, financial counselors, chaplains), and administering medications and treatments as appropriate. Sedatives or antianxiety agents are often administered the evening before surgery and during the postoperative period.

After surgery, adequate sleep and rest are important for wound healing and emotional well-being. Growth hormone, which promotes healing through protein synthesis and collagen formation, is released in greater amounts during periods of rest (Drain & Cristoph, 1987). The client who can rest sufficiently and maintain adequate amounts of REM sleep (rapid eye movement-dream sleep) can better handle the stress associated with surgery and recovery. Adequate periods of rest and sleep need to be planned, and a quiet, restful environment should be maintained.

Cognition and Perception

Pain perception, confusion, and sensory deficit are three of the areas in which alterations in cognition and perception may be manifested by the surgical client.

Pain. Pain may be experienced preoperatively and postoperatively. Pain, which has both a physical component and a psychological component, may occur before surgery secondary to a disease process or to a traumatic injury. It may also occur after surgery secondary to a surgical incision or procedure. Nursing interventions are vital in helping clients cope with pain. Some of these interventions may include administering medications, positioning, physical therapy, relaxation techniques, psychological support, distraction techniques, and appropriate referrals to other health professionals. It is also helpful to maintain a restful and comfortable environment. Administration of analgesics to control pain is often by the IV route, either IV push or by a patient-controlled analgesia (PCA) machine, or by epidural administration. These forms of administration are more successful in controlling pain than intramuscular or subcutaneous injections. Many hospitals now have a pain service or clinic that may be consulted.

Confusion. Confusion may be experienced by the surgical client secondary to medication therapy, unfamiliar surroundings and people, sensory overload, electrolyte imbalances, pain, anxiety, or sleep deprivation. Nursing interventions to assist confused clients include orienting and reorienting clients to unfamiliar surroundings and people, maintaining a safe and comfortable environment, promoting increased visual and auditory input (pictures of family and friends, calendars, radio, television) during waking hours, promoting a quiet and restful environment during the hours set aside for sleep and rest, and monitoring medication therapy.

Sensory Deficits. Sensory deficits also may contribute to a significant change in normal functioning for the surgical client. As discussed earlier, confusion may be associated with decreased sensory input. The client may become confused as to time of day, day of the week,

Therapeutic Dialogue
Postoperative Pain

Scenes for Thought

Alicia Martin, 52 years old, returned from the OR last evening. Her spleen had been removed after she was injured in a skiing accident yesterday afternoon. In addition to the splenectomy, the surgical team had reduced a comminuted fracture of her right leg and sutured a laceration of her right cheek. She has been awake and sitting up for the last few hours.

Effective

Nurse: *Hello, Ms. Martin, I'm Richard Hines, your primary nurse. How are you? (Good eye contact to indicate that the question is a real one.)*
Client: *Hello, Richard, you can call me Alicia. I'm okay, I guess.* Looks tired. Is leaning against the back of the chair.
Nurse: *You look tired. Do you want to get back into bed?*
Client: *Yes, please. Amazing how just sitting can tire you out.* Gets back into bed slowly, with help.
Nurse: *(Gets Alicia settled and comfortably positioned.) How does that feel? (*She smiles and nods okay.*) Good. I was wondering if I could talk with you for a while to see if you have any particular questions about the operation or your injuries.*
Client: *I don't have any questions. I just want to go home.* Looks like she's going to cry.
Nurse: *(Pulls up a chair.) Tell me a little more about that. (Leans forward.)*
Client: *I don't live here; I was just visiting with my husband and children, and I had the accident. And I hurt, a lot.* Crying while splinting the stitches on her left side. *I'm not used to being sick.*
Nurse: *How about if I get you some pain medication first, then we can talk about the rest after you're a bit more comfortable?*
Client: *I think that's a good idea. It's hard for me to think clearly with the pain.* Wipes her eyes.
Nurse: *I'll be right back. (Returns with pain medication, which he administers. Alicia reports relief after a few minutes, and they begin to discuss her questions, worries, and fears.)*
Client: *Thank you, Richard, I think I'll be able to rest now.*
Nurse: *I'm glad. I'll check back with you in an hour or so to see how you are.*

Less Effective

Nurse: Hello, Ms. Martin, I'm Robert Henderson, your primary nurse. How are you? *(Good eye contact to indicate that the question is a real one.)*
Client: *Hello, Robert, you can call me Alicia. I'm okay, I guess.* Looks tired. Is leaning against the back of the chair.
Nurse: *You look tired. Do you want to get back into bed?*
Client: *Yes, please. Amazing how just sitting can tire you out.* Gets back into bed slowly, with help.
Nurse: *(Gets Alicia settled and comfortably positioned.) How does that feel? (*She smiles and nods okay.*) Good. I was wondering if I could talk with you for a while to see if you have any particular questions about the operation or your injuries.*
Client: *I don't have any questions. I just want to go home.* Looks like she's going to cry.
Nurse: *I can understand that. Nobody likes to be in the hospital, especially in the middle of a vacation. (Puts hand on patient's arm in sympathy.) But I thought you might have some questions that I could help you with. You had quite a difficult accident, and I know it must be hard on you right now.*
Client: Starts to cry. *That's true, it is hard on me. And all I want to do is rest right now, I'm not feeling very well at all.*
Nurse: *Can I get you anything before I go?*
Client: *No, I'll be okay if I just rest a little.* Closes her eyes.
Nurse: *Okay, I'll check back with you in a little while.*

Critical Thinking Challenge

• Both nurses showed caring and sensitivity, but determine what the first nurse did that the second nurse did not. • Detect what information the first nurse gathered that the second nurse did not. • Using Ms. Martin's behavior, analyze the ways pain affects a person psychologically.

or what year it is. Clients may become forgetful or uncooperative from lack of stimulation. It is therefore desirable to promote sensory stimulation. Interventions may include diversional activities, reading materials, physical therapy, occupational therapy, exercise classes, informational classes, and various other stimulating activities appropriate to the client's condition.

Self-Concept

Self-concept reflects a person's sense of self-worth and involves attitudes, feelings, and beliefs. For many people, self-concept may be closely related to physical appearance. Physical appearance may be altered by a surgical procedure. This alteration may be minor, such as a small scar, or it may be major, such as a limb amputation or a radical neck dissection. The impact of surgery on self-concept depends on the client's perception of his or her value or image rather than a specific objective measure. Surgical alterations may also involve removal of certain organs (such as the uterus, breast or portions of the colon), which may result in significant emotional and psychological changes. Such alterations may extensively affect a person's self-concept, which may require intensive, long-term rehabilitation, both physical and emotional.

In addition to providing the client with the necessary technical care, teaching, extensive rehabilitation, and emotional support, nursing interventions may also include referral to agencies and support groups that can benefit the client after surgery and discharge from the acute care facility. Some of these groups include the American Cancer Society and its numerous affiliates, the American Heart Association, and the American Red Cross. These organizations sponsor support groups that can assist the client and family to cope with changes in self-concept. They may also assist with educational needs, financial and housing services, transportation services, and physical care needs.

Roles and Relationships

Another important area of health that can be affected by a surgical procedure is that of roles and relationships. Personal, family, and business relationships may all be affected by surgery and the separation that it may entail. Changes in relationships may be temporary or permanent. Procedures from which one quickly recovers usually allow a person to resume previous roles and relationships without any long-range changes or conflicts. Chronic illnesses and major procedures may, however, lead to long-lasting changes that require much adaptation. Surgery may directly affect energy level, so that fulfilling the role of provider, sexual partner, or parent may be more difficult. Moreover, a prolonged recovery period may create problems in a person's work relationships, which can have an impact on financial security.

The appropriate nursing interventions may depend on the specific role or relationship, values or beliefs, that are creating conflict. Providing the client and family members with emotional support and appropriate client teaching can positively affect role relationships. It also may be beneficial to refer the client to another healthcare team professional, such as a social worker, mental health counselor, or a chaplain.

Coping

Surgery, even minor procedures, entails significant stress. Coping behaviors and stress tolerance are closely related to how a person defines stress and how that person has managed stress in the past. It is important to identify stress management strategies that have been effective in the past, because these strategies may be effective again during the perioperative period. It is also important to keep in mind that stress tolerance and coping behaviors are an individual matter. What is effective for one person may not be effective for another. Nursing interventions to assist a person in coping and managing stress include identifying and promoting effective stress management strategies and coping behaviors, providing emotional support and instruction for the client and family, and making referrals to other health professionals as necessary.

Sexuality

Sexuality and reproduction may be temporarily or permanently affected by surgery. Separation, prolonged convalescence, and actual surgical alterations may all significantly affect a person's sexuality and sexual identity. The impact may be physical, psychological, or both. Physical changes that may affect a person's sexuality can result from surgeries that alter appearance, limit mobility, alter reproductive capacity, and limit physiologic functioning.

The accompanying display lists surgeries that may affect a person's physical appearance, mobility, and functioning. Some of these changes are permanent, whereas others are temporary. Although any of the surgeries listed may affect a person's psychological and physical functioning, some particularly affect sexual functioning. These surgeries include ostomies, urinary diversions, mastectomies, hysterectomies, and prostatectomies. In addition, some procedures may lead to impotence. These procedures include certain types of prostatectomies, orchiectomies (removal of the testes), and certain urinary diversion procedures. Although these procedures may leave a man impotent, surgically corrective procedures may be available to restore sexual functioning.

Surgical Procedures Affecting Appearance, Mobility, and Functioning

Physical Appearance

Radical neck surgery
Mastectomy
Amputations
Facial surgeries
Oral surgery

Mobility

Bone fusions
Dislocations
Spinal surgeries
Amputations
Joint replacement

Functioning

Vaginectomy
Hysterectomy
Prostatectomy
Ostomies (colostomy, ileostomy)
Oral surgeries

In terms of nursing interventions, it is important for the client to be fully informed of options regarding surgery or alternative treatments. Additional nursing interventions include performing a thorough assessment of the potential sexual or psychological impact and providing client teaching, technical skills, emotional support, and referrals as appropriate. It is also important for the client to understand clearly the depth and scope of any limitations imposed by the surgical procedure. Some clients feel uncomfortable discussing sexual matters with the nurse or physician. Therefore, it is important for the nurse or physician to create as open and comfortable an environment as possible and initiate discussion when appropriate.

Values and Beliefs

A person's value-belief system is a result of the culture in which that person is raised. As the population becomes more diverse, it is crucial that healthcare providers recognize and honor differences in cultures. The value-belief system is significant in that it guides personal choices and life decisions. Important aspects of the value-belief system are a person's cultural background, philosophy, and religious orientation. These aspects typically affect choices made with regard to surgery and treatment options. Of the many examples of how the value-belief system may affect surgical decisions, an outstanding one involves the decision whether to have an abortion. Another example involves blood transfusions. Some religions prohibit their members from receiving blood products. This is a significant factor for a person who has experienced major trauma, blood loss, or surgery.

Choices a person is required to make should be made only when the person is fully informed of the alternatives and the expected consequences of any decisions. After arriving at a decision, the person needs expert care, knowledgeable instruction, and emotional support. The services of a chaplain or other religious or cultural leader may be useful at this time. Even if the healthcare professional opposes or does not understand the person's decision, he or she needs to remain nonjudgmental and supportive.

Lifespan Considerations

People undergoing surgical procedures have different needs related to their age and developmental level. For each age group, the nurse must make appropriate assessments and then plan and perform the appropriate interventions.

Newborn and Infant

For the newborn or infant, the separation from his or her parents during a surgical experience may be a traumatic situation. The infant's ability to understand what is happening is limited, and he or she may perceive the experience as strange, frightening, and lonely. It is therefore important for the nurse to promote a calm, comfortable environment by holding the infant, keeping background noises to a minimum, and providing a stuffed animal, toy, or other diversion as appropriate. Research demonstrates that comforting behaviors (stroking, touching) shown by caregivers to postoperative neonates help improve settling (Morse, et al., 1993) It is also important to provide careful explanations to the parents and to include them in the care of the infant as much as possible.

Significant physiologic factors to consider when performing surgery on an infant include the infant's ability to tolerate blood loss and alterations in temperature. These are significantly less than an adult's (Phippen & Wells, 1994), making it mandatory to monitor these two factors closely and to make every attempt to minimize both blood loss and heat loss from the body. In addition, an infant's skin is sensitive. It is important to select skin preparation solutions, tape, and dressings that are gentle to the skin. Instruments, equipment, and medications are other important considerations; all of these items need to be appropriate to the infant's size and physiologic status.

Toddler and Preschooler

Many of the same factors that apply to the infant also apply to the toddler or preschooler. At this age, separation anxiety may be more pronounced because the child is more aware of his or her surroundings. Although the child has an expanded capacity to understand what is going on, the situation may still be perceived as frightening and lonely. It is important to provide careful explanations to the parents and to elicit their cooperation as needed. It is also useful to have all instruments and equipment ready in the operating room before the child arrives. This helps shorten the waiting time before anesthetic induction and helps to maintain a calm, quiet environment. It may also be useful to have the parents hold the child while medications are being administered, or a suppository may be prescribed to promote relaxation and anesthesia before the child is taken into the operating room. This causes sufficient relaxation so that other procedures are not perceived as quite so frightening. If possible, it is also helpful to remove the child's clothing, apply the grounding pad, and apply monitoring devices after the child is anesthetized. As with the infant, it is important to use instruments and equipment that are of appropriate size and medications that are of appropriate dosage. Again, as with the infant, minimizing blood loss and ensuring temperature control are significant factors in promoting a safe and efficient surgical experience.

Another important consideration for both the infant and the toddler is the planning of a safe recovery phase.

A crib with side rails provides a safe environment, and sometimes soft restraints may be useful. It is important to monitor the child's airway and vital signs carefully and to keep the child warm. It is also useful in many situations to have the child's parents in the recovery room as the child regains awareness of surroundings. This helps to keep the child calm and helps ensure cooperation with the necessary procedures.

Child and Adolescent

Older children, including school-age children and adolescents, may have an increased understanding of surgery and many of the activities that a surgical procedure will entail. These children usually benefit from a more detailed preoperative teaching program. Many hospitals include a tour of the operating room for school-aged children and adolescents and their parents, during the preoperative teaching period. The child who has seen the operating room, the operating room bed, the anesthesia machine, and the mask used to administer an anesthetic is usually not as frightened as the child who has not had this experience. The child can participate in the administration of anesthesia by holding the mask or counting as the anesthetic is administered. Simple choices (for example, selecting the arm for the IV line) may help give the child a sense of control. The older child is more likely to cope better with separation from parents than the infant or preschooler.

The adolescent having surgery also has special needs. Teenagers usually are concerned with body image and possible disfigurement. Adolescents may vary markedly in their ability to cope with the stress of the surgical experience. In striving for identity and independence, the adolescent may attempt to hide feelings. In addition to providing extensive teaching both to the adolescent and the family, it is important for the nurse to demonstrate support and acceptance of the adolescent's feelings and behavior.

For children of all ages, it is important to prepare instruments, supplies, and equipment with the size of the child or adolescent in mind. The dosages of medications to be given also depend on the young person's size and weight, and should be calculated accordingly.

Adult and Older Adult

Considerations previously discussed in the section on the impact of surgery on functional health patterns apply to many adults and older adults. Although surgical intervention is becoming more common for older adults, the risks of surgery and anesthesia are especially increased for older people with chronic illness (Litwack-Saleh, 1993). In addition, certain adults may require special considerations when having surgery because of alterations in vision, hearing, mobility, or the presence of chronic disease.

When the adult is visually impaired, it is helpful to leave the client's glasses on until just before an anesthetic is administered. Visual orientation helps to decrease fear and increase confidence. If the client is having a regional or local anesthetic, operating room personnel may allow the client to wear glasses or contact lenses during the procedure. Visual impairment should be noted on the chart, so that operating room personnel are aware of this significant deficit.

Older clients may also have hearing impairments. The operating room staff can speak loudly to this client or allow a hearing aid to be worn until the anesthetic is delivered. Being able to hear members of the health-care team helps alleviate fear, fosters successful teaching, and helps keep the client oriented to the environment. Clients with altered mobility may require individualized planning for positioning during the surgical experience. Special considerations may be necessary for the client with limited joint mobility, obesity, extreme thinness or fragility, or back problems. Specific positions necessary for surgical procedures (such as the lithotomy, prone, and lateral positions) may need modification or require special padding, positioning devices, or restraints to assist in maintaining required positions.

Alterations imposed by chronic illness, a common consideration in older adults, require specific planning and special monitoring during surgery. Respiratory insufficiency and cardiovascular problems may affect a person's ability to tolerate certain anatomic positions (eg, head-down positions may impede breathing for a person with respiratory problems). Kidney or liver dysfunction can affect excretion and metabolism of anesthetic agents. The elderly person with severe chronic organ dysfunction is a greater surgical risk, which usually permits only essential surgical procedures.

Preoperative Nursing

The preoperative phase begins when the decision for surgery is made and ends when the client is transferred to the operating room bed. The nurse uses the nursing process to individualize and provide safe care during this period.

Nursing Assessment

Nursing assessment during the preoperative phase is critical because it provides information that directly affects the client's safety and well-being throughout the entire surgical experience.

History and Physical Examination

The nurse assesses the client in each area of function. This data collection process includes obtaining subjective and objective information from a number of sources, including the interview and physical assessment of the client, information from diagnostic studies and laboratory reports, and information obtained directly from physicians, nurses, and other health professionals.

Some of the most significant assessment information in the client's medical record includes the hematology report, allergy history, chronic disease history, current cardiovascular and respiratory status, history of past surgeries and anesthesia, height and weight, and the results of diagnostic studies. The rationale for obtaining these data before surgery is given in the accompanying display. Current medication use, especially medications that can affect coagulation status (eg, warfarin, nonsteroidal antiinflammatory drugs, or aspirin), are important to determine and report to the surgeon.

The collection of physical data is an integral part of the preoperative assessment for many healthcare providers. The physician completes an in-depth medical history and physical examination of the client. The anesthesiologist, or in many cases the nurse anesthetist, completes a preanesthetic assessment form, such as the one shown in Figure 28-1. Data collected on this form are particularly important and useful to the anesthesia department in preparing to administer the selected anesthetic agents in a safe and prudent manner.

The nurse also completes an in-depth interview and physical assessment of the client during the preoperative period. This may be completed days or weeks before surgery during a preoperative visit, by telephone, or in the preoperative care unit just before surgery. With the increasing number of ambulatory surgeries resulting in decreased access to the client, completion of the preoperative assessment may be a challenge. However, the information obtained is critical. It provides the data needed to identify potential and actual nursing diagnoses and to individualize the perioperative nursing plan of care.

Allergies

Client allergies to medications, food, and latex must be assessed before the surgical procedure and clearly marked on the client record and on the client identification band. Allergies to tape and iodine-based solutions (eg, radiopaque dyes) are especially important to note, because exposure to these substances is common during surgery.

A recent increase in the number of clients (and staff) sensitized to natural rubber latex products is of concern throughout surgery. The sensitivity may be manifested by a mild Type IV allergic reaction (local inflammation, redness, and so forth) or it may cause a full-blown Type I anaphylactic response (Good Reis, 1994). The perioperative nurse needs to identify clients

Nursing Assessment
Preoperative Assessment Data and Rationale

Interview and Physical Assessment

- Proposed surgery: To individualize client teaching and preoperative preparation
- History of previous surgery: To recognize and avoid problems encountered in previous surgery
- History of allergies: To avoid exposing client to allergens that would elicit an allergic response (ie, medications, iodine, latex)
- Client preferences: To provide individualized care, decrease stress, and avoid potential problems
- Chronic disease history: To provide competent care and necessary medications for clients with chronic conditions, including diabetes, thyroid disorders, cardiac arrhythmias, cancer, respiratory insufficiency, renal insufficiency, and bleeding disorders
- Smoking history: To identify increased risk for postoperative respiratory complications
- Current respiratory and cardiac status: To assess for safe anesthetic and medication administration, to minimize postoperative complications
- Current height and weight: To determine body surface area for calculating proper drug dosage
- Vital signs: To detect abnormalities and provide baseline data
- Mobility restriction: To plan for client's surgical positioning needs and safe transport

Laboratory and Diagnostic Test Data

- Blood studies (hematocrit, hemoglobin, white blood cell count, sodium, potassium, coagulation studies): To evaluate client for actual or potential problems with anemia, infection, fluid and electrolyte imbalance, cardiac arrhythmias, or bleeding disorders
- Urinalysis: To evaluate for adequate renal function and the absence of urinary tract infection
- Electrocardiogram: To evaluate for normal cardiac function and the absence of cardiac arrhythmias
- Chest x-ray: To evaluate respiratory status
- Blood type and cross-match: To identify blood type and match with potential donor blood should a transfusion of blood be necessary

DATE	TIME	Inpatient Limited Stay / Out Patient AM	HT	WT (Kg)	BP	R	T	SaO2	Vital Signs Obtained By: (Print/Sign)

DIAGNOSIS	PROPOSED OPERATION	OPERATION DATE	SURGEON

ANESTHESIA EVALUATION

MEDICATIONS

ALLERGIES
Meds: Y N
Latex: Y N
Food: Y N
Tape: Y N
Prep Soln/Contrast: Y N

HABITS
ETOH: Y N
Drug Use: Y N
Smoking: Y N

RESPIRATORY No Yes Comments:

- Asthma/Bronchitis ☐ ☐
- COPD/Dyspnea ☐ ☐
- Productive Cough ☐ ☐
- Recent URI ☐ ☐

CARDIOVASCULAR

- Valve Dis/MVP ☐ ☐
- Exercise Tolerance ☐ ☐
- Abnormal EKG ☐ ☐
- CHF/Orthopnea ☐ ☐
- Angina/MI ☐ ☐
- Hypertension ☐ ☐

GASTROINTESTINAL

- Bowel Obstruction ☐ ☐
- Hepatitis/Jaundice ☐ ☐
- Cirrhosis ☐ ☐
- Hiatal Hernia/Reflux ☐ ☐

RENAL/ENDO

- Diabetes ☐ ☐
- Renal Failure ☐ ☐
- Thyroid Disease ☐ ☐
- Urinary Retention ☐ ☐
- Pregnancy/EDLMP ☐ ☐

NEUROMUSCULAR/SKELETAL

- Arthritis ☐ ☐
- Muscle Weakness ☐ ☐
- CVA/Stroke/TIA ☐ ☐
- Paresthesia ☐ ☐
- Headaches/ICP ☐ ☐
- Syncope/Seizures ☐ ☐

HEMATOLOGIC

- Anemia ☐ ☐
- Bleeding ☐ ☐

Told: ☐ NPO ☐ Ride Home ☐ AM Meds

PREVIOUS ANESTHETICS
General: Regional: Sedation:
Difficulties:

Family Anesthesia History:

AIRWAY EXAM
Mallampati I II III IV
Thyromental <6 cm >6 cm
Mouth Opening ________ cm
Prominant Incisors Y N
AO Extention 0 1/2 Full
Neck Mobility-Ext 0 < 2.5 cm > 2.5 cm
Flex 0 < 5 cm > 5 cm
Prior Difficult Intubation Y N
Anticipate Difficult Intubation Y N

DENTITION: Good Poor

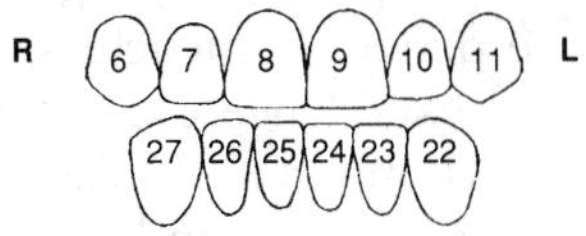

Chipped ________ Missing ________
Loose ________ Bridge ________
Capped ________ Denture ________
Patient Informed of Dental Risk Y N

PHYSICAL EXAM
Chest:
Cardiovascular:
Neuromuscular:

EVALUATOR SUMMARY CRITICAL ISSUES FOR THE ANESTHESIA TEAM

Physical Status	Evaluator Print/Sign

ANESTHESIA TEAM

ANESTHESIA TEAM EVALUATION AND PLAN

LAB/EKG/X-RAY RESULTS
Hb/Hct ________ Pregnancy Test ________
K+ ________ EKG ________
Chest X-ray ________ Other ________
PT/PTT

NPO: Y N RIDE HOME: Y N DENTURES: Y N
AM MEDS: Y N CONTACT LENSES: Y N CONSENT: Y N

PLANS & RISKS DISCUSSED WITH PATIENT: Y N
PATIENT CONSENTS TO PLAN: Y N
ANTICIPATE DIFFICULT INTUBATION: Y N

POSTOPERATIVE PLAN/PAIN MANAGEMENT

NAME	SIGNATURE

ANESTHESIA ATTENDING
☐ I have reviewed the evaluation and agree that the patient is an appropriate candidate for the planned anesthesia.

Signature of Attending Anesthesiologist

PT.NO.

NAME

D.O.B.

UNIVERSITY OF WASHINGTON MEDICAL CENTERS
HARBORVIEW MEDICAL CENTER - UW MEDICAL CENTER
SEATTLE, WASHINGTON
PRE-ANESTHETIC ASSESSEMENT

* U 0 0 0 4 *

UH 0004 REV MAY 94

WHITE - MEDICAL RECORD
CANARY - DEPT. COPY
PINK - RESIDENT COPY

Figure 28-1 • *Example of a preanesthetic assessment form.*

at risk; these include clients with many allergies, clients who have had multiple surgeries, clients with neural tube defects (eg, spina bifida, myelomeningocele), healthcare workers, and people with a stated intolerance to objects containing natural rubber latex (eg, latex balloons, condoms, gloves, underwear). Once a client is known to be at risk, the perioperative nurse will notify members of the operating room team and provide a latex-safe environment for the client.

Learning and Discharge Needs

Other important focuses of the preoperative assessment are the learning and discharge needs of the client and the family. Client teaching is begun during the preoperative period, but teaching is significant to a positive surgical experience during all perioperative phases of care. It is important to assess the client's and family's readiness to learn and their knowledge base so that teaching can be individualized. If the client will be discharged the day of surgery, it is important to identify someone who can take the client home and assist during the postoperative recovery.

Nursing Diagnoses and Outcome Identification

Preoperative nursing assessment allows the nurse to identify actual and potential problems for the surgical client. Common actual problems for the client before surgery include knowledge deficit, anxiety, pain, and sleep pattern disturbance. These problems, stated as nursing diagnoses, are listed in Table 28-2, along with appropriate outcomes.

Nursing Interventions

Nursing interventions in the preoperative period include client teaching, ensuring informed consent, adequate physical and psychological preparation of the client, and adequate preparation of the physical environment.

Client Teaching

Preoperative teaching helps clients understand what will occur during each phase of the surgical experience and how they can participate in their own recovery. Research has demonstrated that preoperative teaching helps decrease the client's anxiety and promotes recovery. Specific study findings show that preoperative teaching decreases medical complications, the need for postoperative medication, the length of hospital stay, and the amount of time until normal activity is resumed (Tarsitano, 1992).

Preoperative teaching should include a general orientation and explanation of the surgical experience. Discussion of preoperative activities to ready the client for surgery and postoperative care to promote optimal function and recovery should be included. Whenever possible, family members should be included in the preoperative teaching sessions.

Preoperative teaching can occur after the client has been admitted to the surgical unit. However, the client having ambulatory surgery may be instructed before admission. Usually, when the client is admitted the morning of surgery, there is little time available for client teaching. Moreover, the client may be anxious and unable to process the information given. Some surgical centers preadmit clients a few days or a week before the scheduled surgery. At this time, the nurse can begin preoperative teaching, while obtaining a nursing assessment and compiling necessary laboratory test results. Audiovisual material may be available for the client to view. Frequently, the client is sent home with written material explaining what will happen before, during, and after surgery, and what the client can do to participate in his or her own surgical recovery. When the client is admitted for surgery, any new questions can be answered and a review (reinforcement) of pre-

Table 28-2 • *Selected Preoperative Nursing Diagnoses and Client Outcomes*

Nursing Diagnosis	*Client Outcome*
Knowledge Deficit; regarding perioperative procedures related to verbalization of lack of knowledge	Client will verbalize understanding of perioperative care
Anxiety related to insufficient knowledge, separation from family, fear of death or disfigurement	Client will report decreased anxiety level regarding surgery
Pain related to disease process or injury	Client will experience adequate control of pain
Sleep Pattern Disturbance related to preoperative activities and anxiety	Client will achieve sufficient rest before surgery

Client Teaching
Perioperative Instructions

Instruct the client as follows:

- *Familiarize yourself with the following information: what time surgery is scheduled, how long it will take, how long you will be in the recovery facility, and where family members should wait during the surgery.*
- *Do not drink or eat anything after midnight of the evening before surgery (or as designated by the physician's order).*
- *Make sure you understand everything involved in preoperative preparation (eg, antimicrobial scrubs, enemas).*
- *Tell the nurse when you are uncomfortable or nauseous, because the physician will order something for pain and nausea as needed (PRN) after surgery.*
- *Have the nurse explain the reason for any tubes, drains or catheters (IVs, nasogastric tubes, hemovacs) that may be in place during the postoperative period.*
- *Before surgery, practice turning, deep breathing, coughing, leg exercises, and how to get out of bed.*
- *Practice (under the nurse's guidance) using any special equipment that will be used during the postoperative period (eg, incentive spirometer, patient-controlled analgesia machine).*

vious teaching can occur. The accompanying display provides examples of client teaching points.

Donation of autologous blood (one's own blood) for surgery is becoming a common practice, and the nurse can provide the necessary information for the client to donate blood if the client is seen a number of weeks before surgery.

General Information. A general orientation to the surgical experience should include

- The expected time at which the procedure will begin
- How long the procedure will take
- When the client will probably return to his or her room (or the waiting area in same-day surgery)
- Where the family and friends of the client can wait during the surgery
- How the client will be transported to the operating room
- What type of medications and anesthesia will be administered
- Other factors specific to the surgical procedure.

If the client will be transferred to an intensive care unit after surgery, some facilities offer a tour of the unit for the client and family.

Preoperative Protocols. The nurse should fully explain all preoperative activities and why they are important for a successful surgical outcome. Explanations should be provided for any procedure that must be performed preoperatively, such as bowel preparation, skin preparation, and the insertion of urinary or IV catheters or nasogastric tubes. The client should be informed of any dietary or fluid restrictions, including NPO status.

Postoperative Protocols. Preoperative teaching also provides the client with information concerning what conditions will be like after surgery. Frequently, clients have specific questions such as "How much pain will I have?" or "What will my scar look like?" It is usually better to ask clients what questions or concerns they have about their upcoming surgery and to deal with these issues before proceeding with the information that should be presented to each surgical client.

Before surgery, it is helpful to explain to the client what tubes (IV lines, catheters, nasogastric tubes) will be in place during the postoperative period, the size and location of the incision, which medications will be ordered to control pain and nausea, and activities that the client will participate in to promote recovery and prevent complications.

The client should be taught and given time to demonstrate turning, deep breathing, using the incentive spirometer, coughing, getting out of bed using good body mechanics, performing leg exercises, and (when appropriate) using a PCA device. Because these therapeutic procedures are used for a wide variety of clients besides the surgical client, specific guidelines are included in appropriate clinical chapters; these are listed in Table 28-3.

Informed Consent

The informed consent obtained before any surgical procedure is an important legal document. It is the responsibility of the surgeon to explain fully the proposed surgical procedure to the client and to obtain the client's informed consent. *Informed consent is part of the physician's legal responsibility, which involves providing the client with all the information needed to make the decision to undergo surgery.* This information needs to be discussed in language the client can understand. If the client does not speak or understand the physician's language, an interpreter should be used. The information that the surgeon usually discusses includes a description of the proposed surgery, the possible risks and benefits of the procedure, the reason why the surgery is indicated, the probability of success, the consequences of nonsurgical treatment or no treatment, and any other information that will help the client reach an informed decision. The client has the right to ask any questions and to withdraw consent at any point before the surgery begins. An example of a consent form appears in Figure 28-2.

The nurse may be involved in obtaining consent, usually by witnessing the signature of the client on the

Table 28-3 • Preoperative Client Teaching of Postoperative Protocols

Procedure	Rationale	Related Chapter
Turning, getting out of bed	Improve postoperative mobility to minimize impact of immobility	Chapter 33: Body Mechanics and Mobility
Deep breathing, coughing, use of incentive spirometer	Improve postoperative gas exchange and prevent respiratory complications	Chapter 34: Oxygenation: Respiratory Function
Leg exercises	Improve venous return and prevent deep venous thrombosis postoperatively	Chapter 35: Oxygenation: Cardiac Function and Tissue Perfusion
Using patient-controlled analgesia	Provide optimal pain control postoperatively	Chapter 44: Pain Perception and Comfort

consent document. The nurse should be knowledgeable about the healthcare agency's policy regarding informed consent and ensure that the policy is strictly followed. If the client seems unsure or indicates lack of understanding, the nurse should notify the physician so that more information can be provided. *It is the responsibility of the nurse to make sure that the consent form contains all correct, necessary information, is properly signed and witnessed, and is part of the client's medical record before the surgical procedure.*

In addition to the proposed procedure, the consent form also lists the name of the surgeon and assisting surgeons and the surgical site (eg, the left or right eye, knee, kidney, or ear). The consent needs to be signed and dated by the surgeon, the client, and a witness. If the client is a minor, or not mentally or physically competent to give consent, the consent needs to be obtained from the client's parents, spouse, legal guardian, or next-of-kin. It is important that the client not take any medications that might alter judgment or perception before signing the consent form. Many drugs that are commonly administered as preoperative medications, such as narcotics or barbiturates, can alter cognitive abilities and invalidate informed consent.

Client Preparation

The nurse is responsible for preparing the client physically and emotionally to ensure optimal condition for surgery. Client preparation includes the following, as prescribed by the physician or indicated by healthcare facility policy: placing the client on NPO status, starting an IV line, placing a nasogastric tube, preparing the intestinal tract, preparing the skin, and administering preoperative medications.

NPO Status. Food and fluids are restricted for any client receiving a general anesthetic. The client is usually put on NPO status after midnight of the evening before surgery, or, if the surgery is scheduled for late in the day, the client is NPO for 8 hours before the scheduled surgery. However, recent research is indicating that small amounts of clear liquids closer to the time of surgery may be acceptable (Hutchinson, et al., 1988). It is important that the client not have a full stomach to help ensure safe anesthetic administration and prevent vomiting and aspiration. If the surgical client is receiving necessary medications (such as antihypertensive, anticonvulsant, and antiarrhythmic agents) that should not be suddenly discontinued, the nurse should clarify with the physician how and if these medications should be administered. Some medications may be taken with a sip of water in certain situations, whereas others may need to be administered parenterally. Insulin orders for diabetic clients should also be clarified.

Intravenous Access. Intravenous access in any surgical client is important for providing fluid and electrolyte replacement and administering IV medications. Vascular access may be through a peripheral line or a central line. In certain situations both may be indicated. In other situations, for example, surgery requiring only local anesthesia, a heparin lock access device may be adequate. The IV line may be started in the preoperative period to ensure adequate hydration status. For those clients who are well hydrated, IV insertion may be delayed until the client is in the operating room. For any surgical client, a large-gauge (eg, 18-gauge) IV device should be used in case a blood transfusion is necessary during the surgical or postoperative period.

Nasogastric Decompression. For selected surgical clients, a nasogastric tube may be inserted to decompress stomach contents. Nasogastric decompression may be necessary for clients who have not been NPO before surgery—for example, those undergoing emer-

I HEREBY AUTHORIZE DR. J. M. Patrick, AND SUCH ASSISTANTS AS MAY BE DESIGNATED, TO PERFORM:

Appendectomy

(NAME OF TREATMENT / PROCEDURE)

AND ANY OTHER RELATED PROCEDURES OR FORMS OF TREATMENT, INCLUDING APPROPRIATE ANESTHESIA, TRANSFUSIONS THAT THEY DEEM NECESSARY FOR THE WELFARE OF:

Melissa A. Conroy

(NAME OF PATIENT)

I CONSENT TO THE ADMINISTRATION OF ANESTHESIA AND/OR SUCH DRUGS AS MAY BE NECESSARY. I UNDERSTAND THAT ALL ANESTHETICS INVOLVE RISKS OF COMPLICATION, SERIOUS INJURY, OR RARELY DEATH FROM BOTH KNOWN AND UNKNOWN CAUSES.

I CONSENT TO THE EXAMINATION AND RETENTION FOR EDUCATIONAL, SCIENTIFIC AND RESEARCH PURPOSES BY THE UNIVERSITY OF WASHINGTON MEDICAL STAFF OF ALL BODY FLUIDS, TISSUES AND ORGANS REMOVED DURING THE COURSE OF THE ABOVE TREATMENT/PROCEDURE WITH PRIVILEGE OF ULTIMATE USE AND DISPOSAL RESTING WITH SAID MEDICAL STAFF.

I UNDERSTAND THAT THE EXPECTED RESULTS OF SAID TREATMENT CANNOT BE GUARANTEED. THE PHYSICIANS, SURGEONS, OR DENTISTS OF THE UNIVERSITY OF WASHINGTON HAVE DISCUSSED TO MY SATISFACTION THE FOLLOWING:

A. THE NATURE AND CHARACTER OF THE PROPOSED TREATMENT/PROCEDURE.

B. THE ANTICIPATED RESULTS OF THE PROPOSED TREATMENT/PROCEDURE.

C. THE RECOGNIZED ALTERNATIVE FORMS OF TREATMENT/PROCEDURE.

D. THE RECOGNIZED SERIOUS POSSIBLE RISKS AND COMPLICATIONS OF THE TREATMENT/PROCEDURE AND OF THE RECOGNIZED ALTERNATIVE FORMS OF TREATMENT/PROCEDURE, INCLUDING NON-TREATMENT.

E. THE ANTICIPATED DATE AND TIME OF THE PROPOSED TREATMENT/PROCEDURE.

ADDITIONAL M.D. COMMENTS:

MY PHYSICIAN HAS OFFERED TO ANSWER ALL INQUIRIES CONCERNING THE PROPOSED TREATMENT/PROCEDURE. I UNDERSTAND THAT I AM FREE TO WITHHOLD OR WITHDRAW CONSENT TO THE PROPOSED TREATMENT/PROCEDURE AT ANY TIME.

WITNESS		SIGNATURE OF PERSON GIVING CONSENT
Joanne Soleski		Melissa A. Conroy
DATE SIGNED 1/20/96	TIME 7:00 ☒ A.M. ☐ P.M.	RELATIONSHIP TO PATIENT (IF APPLICABLE)

☐ PLEASE CHECK IF THIS IS A TELEPHONE MONITORED CONSENT.

NO TREATMENT WILL BE PERFORMED UNTIL THIS CONSENT HAS BEEN EXECUTED. THIS CONSENT WILL BE PERMANENTLY FILED IN THE PATIENT'S MEDICAL RECORD.

PT.NO.

NAME

D.O.B.

UNIVERSITY OF WASHINGTON MEDICAL CENTERS
HARBORVIEW MEDICAL CENTER
UNIVERSITY OF WASHINGTON MEDICAL CENTER
SEATTLE, WASHINGTON

SPECIAL CONSENT TO TREATMENT
(DIAGNOSTIC & SURGICAL PROCEDURES, ANESTHESIA, MEDICAL TREATMENT & OTHER PROCEDURES)

UH 0173 REV APR 92

Figure 28-2 • *Example of a consent form, which must be signed before surgery.*

gency surgery. Nasogastric decompression is also indicated when surgery is performed on the stomach or the intestines.

Bowel Preparation. Enemas, suppositories, laxatives, and oral antibiotics (eg, neomycin) may be given preoperatively to help clean and sterilize the colon. This is done to decrease the possibility of intraoperative bowel content spillage, which could lead to peritonitis and other complications. Bowel preparation is most important when surgery is performed on the intestines, but can be indicated for general abdominal surgery.

Skin Preparation. The purpose of preoperative skin preparation is to remove soil and transient microorganisms from the skin and to decrease the number of resident microbes and the chance of infection. Depending on the type of surgery, the healthcare policy, and the surgeon's preference, the client may need shaving, clipping of body hair, scrubbing of the surgical area, or showering with antimicrobial soap. Usually, the skin preparation focuses on the area that will be involved in the surgery itself and wide margins around that area. A surgical "prep," or shaving the hair in the affected area, was a common preoperative procedure a decade ago. Shaving hair on or near the surgical site is no longer recommended by most surgeons because tiny breaks in skin integrity can increase the risk of postoperative infection. There is much in the literature that supports leaving hair at the operative site. However, the necessity for hair removal depends on the amount of hair, the location of the incision, and the type of procedure to be performed. When hair removal is necessary, it should be performed by skillful personnel as close to the time of surgery as possible and done in a manner that preserves skin integrity. Hair clippers or chemical depilatory agents are less likely to disrupt skin integrity and are the preferred methods of hair removal when absence of hair at the operative site is desired (AORN, 1995).

Preoperative Medications. A sedative is often ordered the evening before surgery to help decrease client anxiety and induce sleep. Medications given just before surgery may have several purposes, such as promoting relaxation, decreasing nasal and salivary secretions, assisting anesthetic delivery, relieving pain, and promoting sedation. The trend in recent years has been to give fewer preoperative medications, except for antibiotics. However, it is important to administer any prescribed preoperative medication on time so that maximum effect can be coordinated with the time of surgery. Usually, preoperative medications are ordered to be given "on call" (when the operating room calls and says to administer the medication). The "on call" medication is usually made about 1 hour before the surgical procedure begins, so that optimal levels of the medication will circulate in the blood during the surgery (Meeker & Rothrock, 1994). Whenever medications that can impede cognition are administered, the client is kept in bed with the side rails up.

Assessment Checklist

Many hospitals use a preoperative assessment checklist on the day of surgery to summarize the client's preoperative preparation; provide such preoperative baseline measurements as level of consciousness, vital signs, and skin integrity; and ensure that all information is in the client's record before transport to the operating room. Figure 28-3 is an example of a preoperative assessment checklist. The checklist usually includes the information listed in the assessment display. Completing the preoperative checklist is a quick way to show that all client preparation activities have been accomplished and safety measures have been taken. The nurse usually checks off each item as it is completed, and then signs the form in the appropriate place.

It is important for the nurse to make sure that all activities requiring the client to be out of bed (such as

Nursing Assessment

Types of Information on a Preoperative Assessment Checklist, with Rationales

- Allergies: To decrease potential for allergic reactions
- Current vital signs: To provide vital sign baseline
- Units of blood available and kind (autologous or donor): To enable blood transfusion to take place in the event of blood loss
- Preoperative medications given: To ensure preoperative relaxation and decrease the risk of infection
- Jewelry removed or secured: Jewelry may be removed to prevent loss or damage and promote client safety during surgery
- Dentures or partial plates removed: To provide clear visualization during intubation if general anesthesia is delivered
- Skin preparation: To document the completion of antimicrobial scrubs and shaving to help prevent infection
- Availability of x-rays: To document availability because x-rays are used by the surgical team
- Availability of past records (old chart): To document availability because these records are often needed as reference by the surgical team
- Voided: To help prevent intraoperative or postoperative bladder distention
- Valuables secured: To prevent damage or loss of client's valuables
- Nurses' signature: To document the completion of all required preoperative activities

PATIENT CHECKLIST / INITIATING NURSE

NPO SINCE	BP	PULSE	RESPIRATION	TEMPERATURE	IV/LOCK ☐ EXISTING ☐ SEE PARENTERAL FLUID SHEET ☐ INITIATED - SEE BELOW
					GAUGE: SITE: LENGTH: SOLUTION: AMOUNT:

DENTURES/PARTIALS/BRIDGE WORK	☐ NONE	☐ REMOVED	☐ IN PLACE
HEARING AID/SPEAKING DEVICE	☐ NONE	☐ REMOVED	☐ IN PLACE
EYEGLASSES OR CONTACTS	☐ NONE	☐ REMOVED	☐ IN PLACE
JEWELRY/HAIRPINS	☐ NONE	☐ REMOVED	☐ IN PLACE
MAKE-UP/NAIL POLISH	☐ NONE	☐ REMOVED	☐ IN PLACE
OTHER PROSTHESIS	☐ NONE	☐ REMOVED	☐ IN PLACE

☐ GOWN ONLY
☐ DISPOSITION OF BELONGINGS ____________

☐ I.D. AND ALLERGY BANDS ON PATIENT
☐ ADDRESSOGRAPH
☐ CONSENTS SIGNED AND DATED
☐ LAB / EKG
☐ HISTORY AND PHYSICAL
☐ PHYSICIANS ORDERS
☐ INPATIENT FLOW SHEETS
☐ PROGRESS REPORT
☐ OLD CHART SENT
☐ VOIDED AT ☐ FOLEY

COMMENTS

PRE-OP MEDICATIONS	TIME	DOSAGE	INITIALS

MEDICATIONS SENT TO OR ☐ YES ☐ NO ☐ NONE ORDERED

ADDITIONAL NURSING NOTES
AUTOLOGOUS BLOOD DONATED: ☐ YES ☐ NO
AUTOLOGOUS ARMBAND IN PLACE: ☐ YES ☐ NO

FAMILY/SIGNIFICANT OTHER
NAME: RELATION: TELEPHONE NUMBER:
☐ PRESENT
☐ NOBODY AVAILABLE LOCATION: ☐ WILL CALL US ☐ WE NEED TO CALL TRAVEL TIME:

UNIT RN SIGNATURE DATE

PREOP CARE UNIT

TIME IN PREOP HOLDING AREA | VITALS ☐ NOT INDICATED BP PULSE O_2 SAT

INDWELLING LINES/TUBES:
☐ NONE ☐ DRAINS ☐ TRACH ☐ O_2 ☐ CHEST TUBE ☐ OTHER:

AWARENESS LEVEL
☐ ALERT ☐ DROWSY ☐ SEDATED ☐ UNRESPONSIVE ☐ ORIENTED ☐ CONFUSED ☐ OTHER:

ANXIETY LEVEL
☐ RELAXED ☐ COOPERATIVE ☐ NERVOUS ☐ TALKATIVE ☐ CRYING ☐ AGITATED ☐ WITHDRAWN ☐ OTHER:

COMMUNICATION LIMITATIONS
☐ NONE ☐ APHASIC ☐ UNCONSCIOUS ☐ HEARING IMPAIRED ☐ BLIND ☐ FOREIGN LANGUAGE ☐ INTERPRETER PRESENT ☐ OTHER:

ADDITIONAL NURSING NOTES
UNIT RN SIGNATURE DATE

OR ASSESSMENT

☐ I.D. AND ALLERGY BANDS ON PATIENT ☐ CONSENTS SIGNED AND DATED ☐ LAB / EKG ☐ CONFIRM CHECKLIST ☐ CONFIRM PLANNED PROCEDURE ☐ CONFIRM SITE

SKIN
☐ WARM/DRY ☐ COLD ☐ RASH ☐ MOTTLED ☐ BRUISED ☐ REDDENED ☐ OTHER:

MOBILITY LIMITATIONS
☐ NONE ☐ CAST ☐ TRACTION ☐ PARALYZED ☐ AMPUTEE ☐ OBESITY ☐ OTHER:

ADDITIONAL NURSING NOTES
AUTOLOGOUS BLOOD DONATED: ☐ YES ☐ NO
AUTOLOGOUS ARMBAND IN PLACE: ☐ YES ☐ NO
AUTOLOGOUS BLOOD HERE: ☐ YES ☐ NO
CIRCULATOR SIGNATURE DATE

PT.NO.

NAME

D.O.B.

UNIVERSITY OF WASHINGTON MEDICAL CENTERS
HARBORVIEW MEDICAL CENTER - UW MEDICAL CENTER
SEATTLE, WASHINGTON

PREOPERATIVE SURGICAL DATA / ASSESSMENT

* U 0 8 3 3 *

UH 0833 REV NOV 93

Figure 28-3 • *Example of a preoperative assessment checklist, which is completed by the nurse before the client is transferred to the operating room.*

showering and voiding before surgery) are accomplished before any medications that can alter the level of consciousness are administered. After such medications are given, the client should be instructed to stay in bed with the side rails up. When all the preparation for surgery has been completed, the preoperative checklist filled, and documentation completed according to protocol, the client is ready for transport to the preoperative care unit.

In the **preoperative care unit**, where the client remains until entering the operating room, final presurgical assessments of the client are completed. The preoperative care unit nurse and the operating room nurse will check the following: the client's name band; site and type of surgery; location of jewelry, eyeglasses, and dentures; allergies; appropriate dress of the client; surgical consent obtained; NPO status; appropriate records and paperwork; laboratory and diagnostic study results entered on the chart; blood availability; preoperative medication administration; and any additional physician's orders.

In the preoperative care unit, the nurse should provide a warm, caring environment and offer appropriate emotional support. In some facilities a limited number of family members may stay in the preoperative care unit with the client until the client's transfer to the operating room.

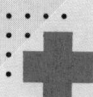

Safety Alert
Perioperative Care

- To avoid injuries from falls after preoperative medications that affect cognition have been administered, instruct the client to stay in bed with side rails up.
- Make sure all clients going to the operating room have the correct identification band, to avoid mistaken identity when the client is not alert.
- Make sure any allergies are clearly identified to avoid possible allergic reactions.
- Position clients carefully and pad bony areas well during surgery, to avoid possible nerve, muscle, or skin damage.
- Check postoperative circulation status frequently to detect impairment promptly, thus avoiding nerve and muscle damage.
- Check all equipment and monitors used in the operating room before each use, to ensure proper functioning and prevent potential client injury.
- Maintain strict surgical asepsis at all times in the operating room to prevent infection.

Evaluation

As the nurse performs interventions in the preoperative phase, continual evaluation of the client's response occurs and is documented in the client's chart. This information is essential for formulating an individualized plan of care in succeeding phases of the surgical experience. Selected outcome criteria are provided for each of the general preoperative client goals.

Goal

Client will verbalize understanding of perioperative care.

Possible Outcome Criteria

- During preoperative preparation, client asks questions about impending surgical procedure.
- During preoperative preparation, client describes what will happen during the surgical experience.
- After receiving instruction, client demonstrates effective turning, coughing, deep breathing, and leg exercises, and states why they are important in postoperative recovery.

Goal

Client will report decreased anxiety level regarding surgery.

Possible Outcome Criteria

- During preoperative teaching, client discusses fears and concerns regarding the surgical procedure.
- After client teaching, client verbalizes decreased anxiety.
- Client identifies support system and strategies to be used to reduce stress and anxiety imposed by surgical experience.

Goal

Client will experience adequate control of pain.

Possible Outcome Criteria

- Client reports an acceptable pain level during the preoperative period.
- Client completes presurgical activities without limitation caused by pain.

Goal

Client will achieve sufficient rest before surgery.

Possible Outcome Criteria

- Client verbalizes feeling adequately rested morning of surgery.
- Client sleeps restfully the night before surgery, as observed by the nurse during the night.

Intraoperative Nursing

The intraoperative phase begins when the client is transferred to the operating room bed and ends when the client is transferred to the designated recovery facility, for example, the **postanesthesia care unit (PACU)**, postsurgical unit, or intensive care unit. In the intraoperative phase, the nurse continues to individualize client care through use of the nursing process.

Nursing Assessment

Assessment is continual in the intraoperative period because of the dynamic status of the client and the potential for serious complications. Assessment begins when the client enters the **preoperative care unit**, the area where the prepared client waits to enter the operating room. Assessment continues throughout the surgical procedure. In addition to planning for the intraoperative needs of the client, assessment allows the nurse to begin planning for the recovery phase of the surgical experience. It is the responsibility of the operating room nurse to communicate specific assessment data to the recovery facility, so that the client's individualized needs can be anticipated.

When the client arrives in the operating room, the operating room nurse reviews the client's record and notes any new physician orders. A brief assessment is conducted to determine the client's physical and emotional status. Tubes such as IV lines and urinary catheter are checked for patency. The comfort and pain levels of the client are determined, as well as his or her communication ability, emotional needs, and ability to cope with the planned surgery. Any questions the client may have are identified and answered.

During surgery, assessment is continual. All clients will be monitored as appropriate to the procedure and the client's condition. Essential values include vital signs (blood pressure, heart rate, respiratory rate, temperature), oxygen saturation, electrocardiogram (ECG), arterial pressure, central line pressures, laboratory values (hematocrit, blood glucose level, sodium, potassium levels, arterial oxygen and carbon dioxide concentrations, blood pH, and clotting factors), urinary output, and blood loss. Vital signs, oxygen saturation, and ECG are monitored continuously and recorded on the client's chart. Continuous monitoring is necessary to detect and treat any abnormalities immediately.

Nursing Diagnoses and Outcome Identification

The nursing diagnoses and the client outcomes can be identified from the assessment data. Although diagnoses and outcomes vary depending on the client, some common problem areas during the intraoperative period include Risk for Injury, Risk for Infection, and Altered Tissue Perfusion. A new nursing diagnosis adopted in 1994 is Risk for Perioperative Positioning Injury. Possible nursing diagnoses and client outcomes for the intraoperative period are listed in Table 28-4.

Diagnostic Statement: Risk for Perioperative Positioning Injury

Definition. Risk for Perioperative Positioning Injury is a state in which the client is at risk for injury as a result of the environmental conditions found in the perioperative setting (NANDA, 1994).

Risk Factors. Risk factors include disorientation, immobilization, muscle weakness, sensory/perceptual disturbances due to anesthesia, obesity, emaciation, edema (NANDA, 1994).

Nursing Interventions

Nursing interventions during the intraoperative period focus on providing emotional support, ensuring a safe environment and preventing injury, providing anesthesia or monitoring the client during anesthetic administration, maintaining asepsis, and promoting wound healing. These interventions are carried out by both the scrub nurse and the circulating nurse.

The scrub nurse wears a sterile gown, mask, headgear, gloves, disposable shoe covers, and eye protection, and provides the surgeon with required instruments, sponges, drains, and other equipment, anticipating what will be needed throughout surgery (Fig. 28-4). Anticipation helps to minimize the time the client is anesthetized and the time the wound is open, which decreases potential complications. Other responsibilities include preparing the sterile tables before surgery. The scrub nurse must thoroughly understand the principles of asepsis, anatomy, and tissue care, as well as the surgical objectives. The scrub nurse also must have the knowledge and skills to anticipate needs of other members of the surgical team and the ability to make decisions and perform interventions in an emergency situation (Smeltzer & Bare, 1996).

Table 28-4 • *Selected Intraoperative Nursing Diagnoses and Client Outcomes*

Nursing Diagnosis	*Client Outcomes*
Risk for perioperative positioning injury related to length of surgery and obesity	Client will not experience positioning-related injury
Risk for Injury related to equipment, electrical, or physical hazards during surgery	Client will maintain injury-free status during the surgical procedure
Risk for Infection related to breaches in asepsis or individual risk factors	Client will maintain an infection-free wound site postoperatively.

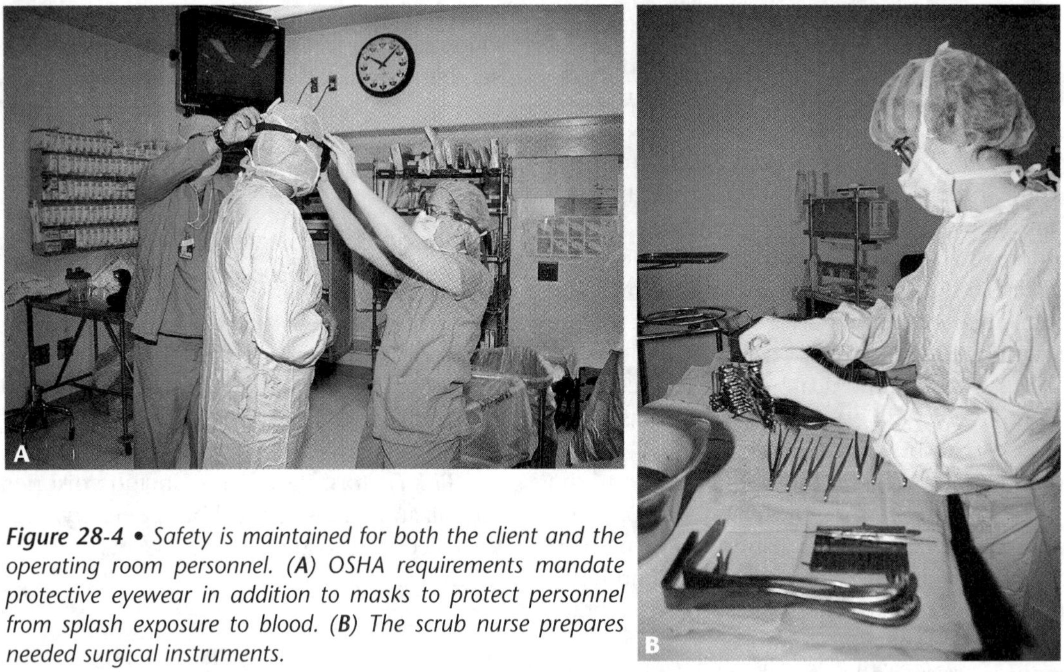

Figure 28-4 • *Safety is maintained for both the client and the operating room personnel. (**A**) OSHA requirements mandate protective eyewear in addition to masks to protect personnel from splash exposure to blood. (**B**) The scrub nurse prepares needed surgical instruments.*

The circulating nurse manages client care in the operating room environment and protects the safety and health needs of the client (Smeltzer & Bare, 1996). Protection involves controlling the environment for cleanliness, temperature, humidity, and lighting. The circulating nurse ensures that the client's rights are protected and coordinates client care in the operating room. Coordinating activities of related personnel (eg, laboratory, x-ray) and monitoring aseptic practices are also the circulating nurse's responsibilities (Smeltzer & Bare, 1996). The circulating nurse and the scrub nurse are responsible for accounting for all sponges and instruments at the close of surgery to ensure client safety.

Emotional Support

Providing emotional support for the client in the operating room can be vital to the success of the procedure. Although some clients may be awake only a short time (half an hour or less) before anesthetic induction, other clients are awake during the entire procedure. It is helpful to elicit the client's cooperation, and it is important to make the client as comfortable as possible. This allows the client to tolerate the procedure in a calmer, more relaxed manner, which should result in a better outcome. Providing appropriate information and explanations for each phase of the procedure helps prevent unexpected, stressful surprises for the client and promotes a more relaxed, cooperative environment. Usually, a relaxed client requires less medication during the intraoperative phase (Smeltzer & Bare, 1996).

Providing emotional support for the client's family is equally important. This is accomplished by answering the family's questions, providing them with information on the progress of the procedure, and giving more detailed information if indicated and if time permits. It also is important to let the family know when the procedure is completed, how long the client will be in the recovery facility, and where the client will go after discharge from the recovery facility. For ambulatory clients who are to be discharged home after their surgical procedure, the intraoperative nurse may also be involved in planning for discharge and in discharge teaching.

Client Safety

Although safety is important in all phases of the surgical experience, the following areas are particularly important in the intraoperative phase: equipment safety, electrical safety, chemical safety, radiation safety, client transport and positioning, and continuous asepsis.

Equipment Safety. The operating room nurse routinely checks and maintains equipment used during surgical procedures. Safety policies for client care equipment should include the following principles and activities:

- Establishment of written procedures for the use of equipment
- Institution of special classes and education for those people required to operate and care for equipment
- Establishment of routine, periodic maintenance programs for equipment that meet or exceed the manufacturers' recommendations
- Required inspection and testing of equipment (such as connectors, grounding pads, and settings) before each use

- Easily accessed, current, written instructional materials for all people required to use the equipment
- Rapidly available professional assistance if equipment problems should arise
- Written documentation for the use, settings, and care of special equipment.

Electrical Safety. One of the most significant potential hazards to the client in the operating room is electricity. Electrical equipment is used in many surgical procedures. Some of the more common devices that rely on electricity are lasers, x-ray machines, electrosurgical units (electrocautery), video equipment, physiologic monitors, microscopes, heart bypass machines, cell savers, blood warmers, heating-cooling blankets, ultrasonic devices, cryosurgery units, and surgical spotlights. Appropriate operating room personnel should know how to use the equipment safely, how to check the equipment for proper functioning, and how to report and handle problems, especially emergent problems such as fire or explosion. The most common potential threats to client safety related to electrical devices are electric shock and burns. Operating room personnel must know how to prevent these problems and how to activate the emergency system should they occur. The safety principles applicable to client care equipment should also apply to all electrical equipment. In addition, personnel using electrical equipment should be familiar with the safe use of backup systems should a power failure occur.

Chemical Safety. Chemical safety is another important area of client safety in the operating room. It is important that staff be aware of chemical hazards, read and follow warning labels, and heed all safety precautions. Common hazardous chemicals found in the operating room include ethylene oxide, used for sterilizing purposes (an eye irritant, also potentially explosive and flammable), alcohol, used as a disinfectant (flammable), methyl methacrylate, used as a bone cement (an eye and respiratory tract irritant, also potentially flammable and explosive), housekeeping products used for cleaning and disinfecting (potentially eye, skin, and respiratory tract irritants), and various gases (such as halothane, nitrous oxide, nitrogen, and carbon dioxide), used as anesthetics or fuels for gas-powered equipment (potentially combustible and asphyxiating) (Kneedler & Dodge, 1994). Personnel working with these chemicals must understand their potential hazards, how to use them safely, how to dispose of them safely, and what to do should an accident occur.

Because of the increase in the number of people sensitive to natural rubber latex proteins, perioperative nurses should constantly assess clients for potential risk factors. In addition, until it is mandatory for manufacturers to identify products containing latex, the perioperative nurse should continually assess the operating room environment for products that may contain latex so that they may be removed when a potentially sensitive client is undergoing surgery.

Radiation Safety. Radiation hazards in the operating room may come from the portable x-ray machine, fluoroscopic equipment, diagnostic radiologic devices, radiation implants, and other instruments and compounds used in radiation therapy. Radiation is potentially hazardous in that it changes or modifies body cells and can lead to genetic defects, thyroid disorders, and cancer. It is important that all personnel who work with radiation sources strictly adhere to the policies and procedures set forth by the healthcare facility's radiation safety officer. Such practices include wearing of monitoring badges, lead aprons, and other shielding devices. It is also important to stay a safe distance away from the radioactive source, because the amount of radiation exposure decreases inversely with the square of the distance from the source.

Positioning. The proper positioning of the client is another important safety consideration in the operating room. The responsibility for positioning is a shared one. The anesthesiologist, the surgeon, and the circulating nurse all participate in placing the client in the proper position for the surgical experience. The ideal position can be defined as the position that provides the best possible exposure for the surgeon, the best possible exposure for airway management and monitoring for the anesthetist, and the best possible position for the physiologic safety of the client.

Proper positioning helps prevent skin, nerve, and muscle damage, which can be temporary or lead to permanent dysfunction. Circulation is altered during surgery because anesthetic agents disrupt normal vasodilation and constriction, reducing perfusion to elevated or dependent limbs or to bony prominences (Walsh, 1993). It is important to use appropriate padding for all body prominences and joints to avoid excessive pressure on the skin and to ensure optimal functioning of the respiratory, nervous, and circulatory systems.

Some common surgical positions include supine, Trendelenburg, reverse Trendelenburg, lithotomy, sitting, prone, and lateral or side-lying. Illustrations of selected surgical positions are provided in Chapter 33. Clients in each of these positions require special padding or support devices to ensure physiologic safety.

Anesthesia Monitoring

Monitoring client status during and after anesthesia (the loss of feeling or sensation) is an important responsibility for the nurse in the operating room and in the recovery facility. Knowledge concerning specific anesthetic agents is important to focus assessment parameters.

Anesthesia may be classified as general, regional, or local. A **general anesthetic** effectively produces analgesia, relaxes muscles, and results in a sleep-like state. A **regional anesthetic** produces decreased sensation and pain in selected parts of the body via nerve blocks, intrathecal blocks, or epidural blocks. A **local anesthetic** depresses superficial peripheral nerves and blocks conduction of pain impulses from their site of origin.

The administration of general and regional anesthesia may be performed by an anesthesiologist or a **certified registered nurse anesthetist**. Both of these professionals have specialized education and skills in the administration of anesthetic agents and in monitoring clients during surgical and other procedures. An **anesthesiologist** is a physician who has specialized education in the administration of anesthesia. Similarly, a certified registered nurse anesthetist is a registered nurse who has specialized education and certification in the administration of anesthesia. Both professionals are also skilled in managing pain and in placing vascular access lines. Local anesthesia at the surgical site is usually administered by the surgeon.

General Anesthesia. General anesthesia may be administered either by the inhalation method or the IV method. Inhalation agents (gases) are delivered from the anesthesia machine and tubing by a face mask, endotracheal tube, or endonasal tube. Some commonly used inhalation agents include nitrous oxide, oxygen, halothane, enflurane, and forane. IV agents can also be delivered through an established vascular access. Some of these agents include barbiturates (thiopental), narcotics (morphine, meperidine, fentanyl), tranquilizers (diazepam), and phencyclidines (ketamine).

Muscle relaxants are also commonly administered during surgical procedures and are especially beneficial during wound closure. When an abdominal incision is to be closed with sutures, relaxed abdominal muscles allow the wound edges to be approximated (brought together) more easily than when muscles are tense.

Close monitoring of the client is necessary during induction, use of, and emergence from general anesthesia. The four stages of anesthesia are described in Table 28-5, beginning with induction of anesthesia or analgesia and ending with the toxic stage. Clients who are receiving general anesthesia normally go through the first three stages. The type of anesthesia may vary the transition. These stages are observed by the anesthetist; however, the nurse may assist by taking vital signs, applying cricoid pressure to occlude the esophagus and prevent regurgitation and aspiration of stomach contents, and assisting the anesthetist as needed to maintain the client's airway during intubation and extubation. As the client emerges from anesthesia, the sequence of stages is reversed.

Table 28-5 • Client Responses in the Stages of Anesthesia

Stage	Reflexes	Heart Rate	Respiration	Blood Pressure	Eyes
I. Analgesia amnesia	Present	Normal	Slow rate Increased depth	Normal	Some dilation Reacts to light
II. Dreams and excitement (frequently bypassed with intravenous induction agents)	Active	Increased	Irregular breathing Breath holding	Increased	Pupils widely dilated and divergent
III. Surgical Involves four planes: plane 2 and plane 3 best for surgery	In progression of loss: Lid reflex Pharyngeal (swallowing) Laryngeal (can tolerate oral airway, suctioning, and then intubation) Gag and corneal reflexes lost	Decreased	Progressively depressed until apneic	Normal to decreased	Early plane: constricted pupils, then slightly dilated and centrally fixed
IV. Toxic Extreme depression	No reflexes	Weak and thready	Completely flaccid	Decreased	Widely dilated pupils

From Patrick, M. L., et al. (1991) *Medical–surgical nursing: Pathophysiological concepts* (p. 376). Philadelphia: J. B. Lippincott.

Regional Anesthesia. Regional anesthesia can be a useful alternative to general anesthesia. Instead of placing the entire body in a sleep-like condition, regional anesthesia affects only selected parts of the body. This type of anesthesia can be used for surgeries of the lower extremities (feet, ankle, knees, hips) and other localized sites, such as the hands and arms. Regional anesthetics have the advantage of minimizing the pulmonary and gastrointestinal complications (pulmonary congestion, atelectasis, nausea, and vomiting) that sometimes occur with general anesthetics. A client receiving regional anesthetics usually recovers more quickly from the anesthetic than a client receiving a general anesthetic. If the client and the procedure are appropriate for regional anesthesia, it is usually considered the method of choice (Meeker & Rothrock, 1994). Regional anesthesia may also be used for postoperative pain control. Table 28-6 provides examples of regional anesthesia.

Local Anesthesia. Local anesthesia is actually a type of regional anesthesia. It is differentiated here by the people responsible for administering the agent and monitoring the client. Instead of the anesthetist, the surgeon is usually responsible for administering local anesthetics, and a perioperative nurse is responsible for monitoring the physiologic and psychological status of the client.

Methods used to provide local anesthesia include topical or direct application of an anesthetic agent to the skin or mucosal surfaces and injection of a local anesthetic agent into the areas surrounding the operative site. This type of anesthesia can be used for localized operations, such as breast biopsies, central line insertions, and surgery of the fingers, hands, nose, eyes, or ears. Clients who are candidates for local anesthetics are calm and able to cooperate with the surgical procedure and have no major systemic medical problems. Local anesthesia has the advantages of regional anesthesia, enhanced by decreased cost to the client because some healthcare facilities do not charge for local anesthesia services.

The choice of local anesthesia for a client has many implications for the perioperative nurse. In the absence of an anesthetist, the nurse is totally responsible for monitoring the client (Atkinson, 1992). This includes blood pressure, level of consciousness, respiratory rate, oxygen saturation, skin condition, cardiac rate and rhythm, and maintaining a patent IV access line.

Conscious Sedation. IV sedation may be administered during a surgical or diagnostic procedure to alter the client's conscious state, thereby allaying fear and anxiety (AORN, 1995). Frequently it is the nurse who is responsible for administering these agents and monitoring the client. Each client receiving IV conscious sedation should be assessed physiologically and psychologically and monitored for reaction to the drugs. The nurse monitoring the client should have a working knowledge of resuscitation equipment and monitoring equipment and should be able to interpret the data obtained (AORN, 1995).

Asepsis

Maintaining asepsis to avoid contamination of the surgical site by microorganisms is the responsibility of the nurse as well as all other members of the surgical team. The AORN, the professional organization for perioperative nurses, has established guidelines for maintaining asepsis and for sterilization of equipment, instruments, and supplies (AORN, 1995). These guidelines are highlighted in the accompanying display.

Table 28-6 • *Regional Anesthesia*

Type	*Definition and Uses*	*Examples of Use*
Topical	The direct application of an anesthetic agent to skin or mucosal surfaces (mouth, throat, nose, cornea)	Often used before injections (nerve blocks, epidurals) or endotracheal tube placement
Nerve or nerve bundle block (local)	The injection of a local anesthetic agent into a nerve bundle or the nerve supply of the operative site	Breast biopsy, lymph node biopsy, ear procedure, cataract extraction, or cornea transplantation
Epidural or peridural	The injection of a local anesthetic agent into the potential space outside the dura	Lower extremity surgery (foot, ankle, knee), lower abdominal procedures, or for postoperative pain relief
Spinal	The injection of a local anesthetic agent into the subarachnoid space	Useful for surgeries below the xyphoid process, or abdominal surgery

Nursing Care Guidelines
Maintaining Asepsis During Surgical Procedures

- All items within a sterile field should be sterile. Items of questionable sterility should be resterilized. All sterile packages should be inspected for damage to package integrity. They also need to be protected from moisture, tearing, sharp objects, or other threats to the integrity of the wrapping material. In addition, they must be unwrapped and dispensed according to acceptable sterile procedure.
- The gowns and gloves used by the scrubbed personnel should be sterile. They must be donned in the correct manner, and scrubbed personnel need to be cautious always to maintain the sterility of their gowns at the level of the sterile field and their gloves. Therefore, the arms and hands of the scrubbed personnel must be maintained between the level of the sterile field (table) and the scrubbed person's shoulder level.
- Tables and ring stands draped with sterile drapes should be considered sterile only at the table level. Drapes need to be impervious to moisture to remain sterile. Items dropping over the sides of the table need to be considered unsterile.
- Scrubbed personnel must remain close to the sterile field, and unscrubbed personnel must stay at least 1 foot away from the sterile field. Scrubbed personnel should move around a sterile field (never across it) in such a way as to maintain the sterility of the sterile field. Unscrubbed personnel should not move between two sterile fields.

Additional policies and procedures have been established in the operating room to ensure asepsis. Every operating room nurse should be familiar with policies concerning the surgical hand scrub, cleaning and preparation of the client's skin before surgery, special considerations for cleaning the operating room environment and disposing of waste products, procedures for sterilizing instruments and supplies, and methods for draping the surgical client and establishing the sterile field.

Draping. Proper draping helps to maintain asepsis by creating a sterile field, thus limiting exposure to microorganisms. Drapes are used to cover other areas of the body, exposing only the incisional area (Fig. 28-5). Drapes are woven (nondisposable) or nonwoven (disposable) and should resist penetration by blood and other liquids. In the past, disposable fabrics were thought to provide a better barrier, but newer woven fabrics now provide adequate barrier protection and at the same time reduce hazardous waste materials.

Wound Closure

The nurse often assists the surgeon in wound closure and may be directed to remove wound closure devices during the postoperative period. The type of material used for wound closure affects wound healing. In some situations, sutures or staples, or both, may be used. For example, a client may have absorbable sutures closing the viscera and staples approximating the wound edges.

Sutures. A **suture** is the material used to sew an incision together. Sutures can be absorbable (eg, catgut or chromic) or nonabsorbable (eg, synthetic nylon or polypropylene, or silk). Nonabsorbable sutures used for closing the skin must be removed after the incision has healed. When used internally, nonabsorbable sutures will remain in place. Absorbable sutures used in skin closure absorb into the skin, so that removal is not necessary. The type of suture used depends on the size and location of the wound being closed, how strong the suture material needs to be for the type of wound being repaired, the desired cosmetic result, and the surgeon's preference. In general, the less suture material used and the smaller the suture size, the better the wound closure. Sutures represent a foreign body that can potentially lead to infections, such as stitch abscesses.

Staples. The use of **skin staples** is also an effective wound-closure method. Skin staples are made of stainless steel, look like paper staples flat against the skin, and are inserted close to the incision with a staple gun. Skin staples are minimally reactive to the body as a foreign substance and therefore minimize the risk of infection. Using staples reduces tissue handling and accomplishes wound closure faster than sutures. Skin staples are usually removed with a staple remover within the first week after surgery, after the incision heals.

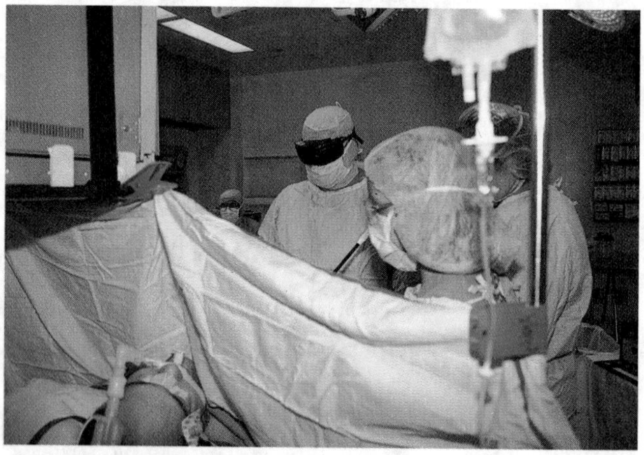

Figure 28-5 • Proper draping exposes only the surgical site, which decreases infection risk.

Transport to the Recovery Facility

When the intraoperative phase of the surgical procedure has been completed, the circulating nurse, the anesthetist, and the surgeon safely transport the client to the recovery facility, taking care to maintain the client's airway during this critical time. They each complete their written documentation and provide the recovery facility with these reports of the surgical experience. The nurses in the recovery facility have been notified of the client's impending arrival and have prepared for the client accordingly.

Evaluation

As the nurse performs interventions during the intraoperative period, the results are evaluated and revised as needed. Intraoperative evaluation focuses on the individual identified outcomes. Selected outcome criteria are provided, but the nurse should individualize surgical outcome criteria for each client.

Goal
Client will maintain injury-free status during the surgical procedure.

Possible Outcome Criteria
- Client will experience no skin injury due to electrical devices or chemicals used during surgery
- Client will experience no injury from defective or improper use of surgical equipment.

Goal
Client will not experience positioning-related injury.

Possible Outcome Criteria
- Client will maintain full range of motion and adequate sensation postoperatively.
- Client will not experience nerve or muscle damage from inadequate or improper padding or positioning during surgery.

Goal
Client will experience an infection-free wound site postoperatively.

Possible Outcome Criteria
- Client's wound site does not appear inflamed or have purulent drainage within 24 hours of surgery.
- Client's wound site appears well approximated and shows evidence of normal wound healing 24 hours postoperatively.

Postoperative Nursing

The postoperative phase begins when the client is transferred into the recovery facility and ends with a resolution of surgical consequences. This phase may be short (less than a day) or lengthy (several months or longer), depending on the nature and extent of the procedure and the client's ability to recover from it. Nurses in the recovery facility, nurses in the postsurgical unit, and nurses in extended care or home care settings use the nursing process during the postoperative period to individualize client care.

Nursing Assessment

Systematic assessment is essential during the postoperative period to detect quickly any complications and to individualize nursing care that promotes optimum recovery from the surgery (Fig. 28-6).

Assessment in the Recovery Facility

Assessments are made frequently during the immediate postoperative period. The PACU nurse usually obtains a verbal report from the operating room staff and reads the written documentation of the surgery and the physician's postoperative orders. To plan care, the nurse needs to know the following: the type and extent of the surgical procedure performed, the type of anesthesia used, the dosage and time medications were given, the amount of blood lost, whether the client is still intubated, and any surgical or anesthetic complications that may have occurred. It is also important to know whether the client will be an inpatient or will return home after recovery from anesthesia. Important assessments during the immediate postoperative period are listed in Table 28-7.

Assessment of cardiovascular function is necessary to detect bleeding promptly. Vital signs are usually monitored every 15 minutes, or more frequently if the client's condition warrants. The ECG is assessed for cardiac rhythm and rate. Both the blood pressure and pulse are evaluated for trends rather than absolute values. Decreasing blood pressure and an increased pulse rate in

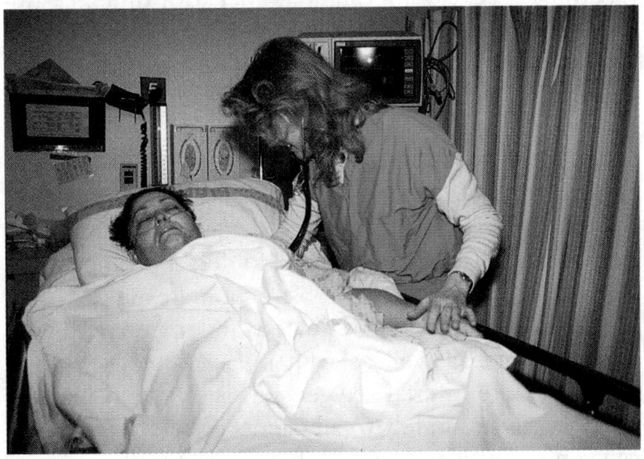

Figure 28-6 • *Close monitoring is needed in the recovery facility.*

Table 28-7 • Assessments in the Immediate Postoperative Period (Recovery Facility)

Focus Area	*Assessments*
Respiratory	Check airway patency and monitor respiratory rate and depth, breath sounds, skin color, and chest expansion
Cardiac	Monitor blood pressure and heart rate and rhythm at least every 15 minutes
Neurologic	Monitor pupillary response; monitor muscle strength to determine muscle relaxant reversal, if used
Dressings	Monitor for integrity of dressings and for hemorrhage or hematoma formation
Pain management	Monitor for both subjective and objective manifestations of pain, administer analgesics as appropriate
Renal function	Monitor amounts of urinary output for clients with indwelling catheter (at least 30 mL per hour); for clients without a urinary catheter, monitor for bladder distention

the postoperative client are significant because they may signify hemorrhage or shock. Certain anesthetic agents and muscle relaxants can also cause hypotension. The client's skin should be evaluated for color (eg, pale or cyanotic), temperature, and diaphoresis (perspiration). Pale, cyanotic, cool, or clammy skin can indicate impaired tissue perfusion, possibly from shock.

The dressing is inspected for bleeding. When present, the area of drainage may be circled on the dressing with a marking pen and a notation of the time. This provides the nurse with a baseline from which to track the amount of bleeding. When evaluating incisional bleeding, it is also important to check for drainage under the client, where bleeding may not be readily apparent. Catheters, drains, and chest tubes are also evaluated for the type of drainage and the amount of blood present. Laboratory values, such as hematocrit, may also be requested during this period to help evaluate circulatory status.

Respiratory function should be assessed during the immediate postoperative period to detect promptly any signs of hypoxia or airway obstruction. Respiratory rate and depth should be evaluated and compared with baseline data as well as with pulse oximetry values, which denote arterial oxygen levels. Oxygen may be administered routinely to all clients or selectively if the oxygen saturation level falls below 94% (DiBenedetto, et al., 1993). Hypoxia may be first detected as apprehension, anxiety, or restlessness. Loud, irregular respirations may indicate obstruction of the airway, possibly from vomit, accumulated secretions, or client positioning that allows the tongue to fall to the back of the throat.

The nurse performs neurologic assessments to evaluate recovery from the anesthetic agent. Return of reflexes, indicated by swallowing and gagging, occurs when the effects of a general anesthetic are ending. Level of consciousness changes also as the anesthetic agent wears off. Initially, the client is unconscious and does not respond to verbal or tactile stimuli. As the anesthetic agent begins to wear off, the client will respond to loud noises or to his or her name. Finally, the client becomes oriented to person and place. During this period, the client may still appear sleepy and will fall into a sleep when not stimulated. After regional anesthesia, the client should be assessed for the return of sensory and motor ability. Sensation can be plotted on a dermatome chart (see Fig. 21-20). Autonomic blockade may persist after regional anesthesia, causing severe postural hypotension when the client assumes an upright position (Rivellini, 1993).

The nurse also assesses the client's fluid balance, urine output, and pain level during the immediate postoperative period. Moreover, the nurse should ensure that all tubes and drains are patent and that all equipment works properly.

Assessment During the Postoperative Period

During the rest of the postoperative recovery period, the nurse performs systematic functional health pattern assessments. Table 28-8 lists possible postoperative complications and appropriate nursing assessments for each functional area.

The nurse individualizes each assessment based on the client and the surgery that was performed. Each assessment is also individualized based on the length of time since the surgery occurred. During the first few days after a major surgery, assessments may focus on pain, tissue perfusion, and respiratory function, whereas later in the postoperative course, the client's ability to perform self-care and manage at home after discharge may be more important. For an ambulatory client, self-care capability is a priority in the immediate postoperative period. More detailed information concerning assessment of each functional area is provided in clinical Chapters 29 through 53.

Nursing Diagnoses and Outcome Identification

Nursing assessment during the postoperative period facilitates identification of actual and high-risk postoperative problems. The general goal for any postoperative

Table 28-8 • Postoperative Assessment of Functional Health

Function	Potential Complication	Assessments
Health perception–health maintenance	Injury secondary to equipment or body positioning or inadequate recovery from anesthesia	Skin, CMS (color, movement, sensation), patent airway, safe environment (side rails up)
Activity–exercise	Hemorrhage/shock	Vital signs, color, bleeding from wound, hematocrit, urine output
	Atelectasis	Respiratory rate and depth, breath sounds, color, arterial blood gases, temperature
	Deep vein thrombosis	Circulation, calf pain or swelling
	Pulmonary emboli	Respiratory rate and depth and other vital signs, breath sounds
Nutrition–metabolism	Wound infection	Temperature and other vital signs, observe wound for redness, warmth, swelling, and purulent drainage
	Poor wound healing Dehiscence Evisceration	Observe wound
	Fluid volume deficit	Postural blood pressure and pulse, intake and output, weight, skin turgor
	Nausea/vomiting	Bowel sounds, abdominal distention
	Malignant hyperthermia	Monitor temperature and other vital signs
	Hypothermia	Monitor temperature
Elimination	Urinary retention	Urine output, (especially first 8 hours after surgery), bladder distention or discomfort
	Paralytic ileus	Absent bowel sounds, abdominal distention
	Constipation	Lack of stool, abdominal distention, hypoactive bowel tones
Sleep–rest	Sleep deficit	Sleep duration and quality
Cognition–perception	Pain	Pain level and pain relief after medication
	Confusion	Orientation to person, place, time; level of consciousness
Self-concept	Altered self-concept	Assess reaction to wound, drains tubes, etc.
Roles–relationships	Altered role relationship	Assess perception of alteration in roles or relationships
Coping	Ineffective coping	Assess anxiety, stress, and lack of coping
Sexuality	Altered sexual function	Assess impact on sexuality and sexual function
Values–beliefs	Spiritual distress	Assess surgery or recovery period effects on spiritual beliefs or values

client is to prevent or minimize complications and return to optimal functioning. Although the specific nursing diagnoses and goals vary from client to client, some of the more common nursing diagnoses and outcomes are listed in Table 28-9.

Nursing Interventions in the Recovery Facility

The primary responsibilities of the nurse in the recovery facility are assessment and continual monitoring of the client's condition until the effects of the anesthetic subside and the client's physiologic status stabilizes. The nurse provides a safe environment for the client so that injury does not occur. Family members usually are not permitted in the PACU, but some researchers have challenged this policy, especially for young children. In such cases, the anxiety of the client decreased when family members were permitted to visit in the PACU (Poole, 1993).

The PACU nurse maintains a patent airway for the client through positioning, suctioning, and care of the endotracheal tube, if it is still in place. Fluid replacement and blood administration may be necessary to maintain adequate circulating volume. Pain medications are frequently administered to control postoperative discomfort. As the client regains consciousness, the nurse begins to encourage deep breathing and moving to improve ventilation and circulation.

For the client to be discharged from the recovery facility to the postsurgical nursing unit, certain conditions must be met. These conditions usually include stable vital signs, patent airway, control of bleeding and wound drainage, normal thermal state, absence or control of any anesthetic or surgical complications, full or nearly full recovery from the anesthetic, adequate respiratory function, orientation to the environment, adequate fluid balance and urinary output, and ability to request assistance if needed (Drain & Cristoph, 1987).

After the client meets the recovery facility's discharge criteria, transfer to the postsurgical nursing unit

Table 28-9 • Postoperative Nursing Diagnoses and Possible Client Outcomes

Nursing Diagnosis	Client Outcomes
Risk for Aspiration related to anesthesia, decreased level of consciousness	Client will maintain a patent airway and not experience aspiration
Impaired Gas Exchange related to anesthesia, decreased mobility, pain, pain medications	Client will demonstrate adequate oxygenation of body tissues
Altered Tissue Perfusion related to loss of blood, postoperative edema, anesthetic agents, immobility	Client will maintain adequate circulation of blood to all body tissues
Risk for Fluid Volume Deficit related to loss of fluids during surgery, decreased oral intake, and abnormal postoperative drainage	Client will maintain adequate fluid volume
Risk for Infection related to surgical wounds, invasive lines, decreased nutritional status	Client will not develop postoperative infection
Ineffective Thermoregulation related to anesthetic agents	Client will maintain temperature within normal limits
Urinary Retention related to anesthesia, immobility, and edema	Client will void within 8 hours of surgery and without difficulty thereafter
Constipation related to anesthesia, pain medication, decreased mobility	Client will resume normal bowel function when normal diet resumes
Pain related to surgical trauma, inflammation, edema, and invasive procedures	Client will report that postoperative pain is well controlled
Risk for Impaired Physical Mobility related to pain, fatigue, and tubes, catheters, and drains	Client will maintain optimal state of mobility, progressively increasing activity daily
Anxiety related to pain and separation from family, job, and normal activities	Client will demonstrate adequate coping during the postoperative period
Knowledge Deficit related to lack of instruction in postoperative activities to prevent complications and promote return to normal function	Client will verbalize and participate in postoperative activities to prevent complications
Impaired Home Maintenance Management related to decreased mobility and decreased energy	Client will manage normal daily activities at home with necessary assistance from family and friends

may occur. The postanesthesia nurse gives a report to the nurse responsible for the surgical client. This report includes the following information: type of surgery performed and the client's tolerance of the procedure, the type of anesthesia used, vital signs, IV lines, blood loss, blood and fluid replacement, dressings, tubes and drains, urinary and drainage output, medications administered, level of pain and method of pain control, and any complications that occurred. If family members or friends are waiting in the surgery waiting area, they should be informed that the client is being transferred to another unit.

Discharge from The Ambulatory Surgical Center

Most ambulatory surgical centers have two recovery areas for surgical clients:

- A traditional recovery area where clients are kept recumbent on stretchers and monitored closely until significant effects of anesthesia have subsided
- An area with recliner chairs where clients are encouraged to ambulate, drink fluids, and eat some solids until they meet all the criteria for discharge

Recovery from anesthesia is usually much quicker when shorter-acting IV anesthetic agents, such as propofol (Diprivan), are administered. Before discharge from an ambulatory surgical unit, the client should

Void (after a spinal anesthetic)
Be able to ambulate
Be alert and oriented
Have minimal nausea and vomiting
Require no pain medication within the last hour
Exhibit no excess bleeding or drainage (Parnass, 1993).

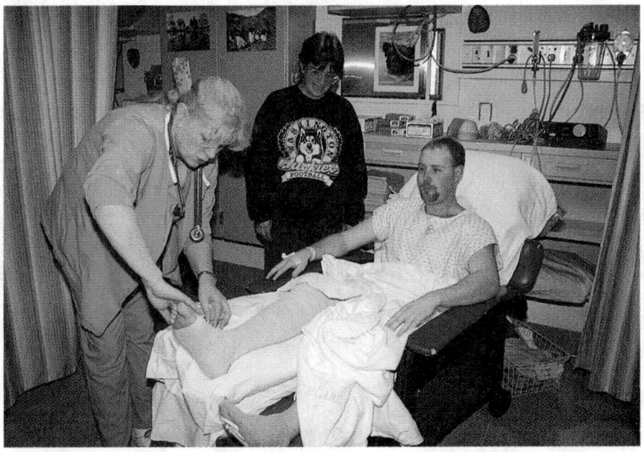

Figure 28-7 • *The client is assessed in ambulatory day surgery to determine if criteria for discharge have been met. Client and family teaching is an important part of care prior to discharge in the ambulatory surgery facility.*

Discharge teaching for the client also must be completed, and a responsible person must be available to accompany the client home (Fig. 28-7).

Nursing Interventions on the Surgical Unit

Nursing interventions are aimed at preventing postoperative complications and promoting optimal return to normal function. Nursing interventions build on the client teaching done in the preoperative period, and should be individualized for each surgical client. A brief overview of nursing intervention is provided here, but in-depth information is provided in selected clinical chapters throughout this text.

Mobility and Self-Care

During the early postoperative period the client may require assistance with mobility and self-care. Encouraging the client progressively to increase mobility and independence in self-care helps prepare the way for discharge. Early ambulation is indicated for most surgical clients to minimize potential complications. Activity orders are individualized for the client by the physician. The client usually sits in a chair or may even ambulate for a brief period on the evening of surgery. Administering pain medication before activity and providing instructions on how best to get out of bed will increase client comfort. The nurse should encourage the client to ambulate progressively longer distances each postoperative day. Standby assistance should be provided if the client is weak or unsteady when ambulating. If the client complains of dizziness or feels diaphoretic (faint) when ambulating, he or she should be returned to bed.

Adequate hygiene after surgery is important to ensure client comfort. If the client has many tubes and has had major surgery, a bed bath may be given on the first postoperative day. Any solutions used to prepare the skin before surgery (such as povidone-iodine) should be washed off. Compression devices and antiembolitic stockings should be removed at bath time and the skin inspected. The client should always be encouraged to perform as much self-care as possible. Usually the surgical client may shower if surgical dressings and IV sites are covered with a protective, waterproof barrier. Care should be taken when the client is showering, however, because the warm water can promote vasodilation and hypotension.

Respiratory Maintenance

Aggressive treatment, especially in the immediate postoperative period, is needed to minimize the risk of atelectasis and prevent possible respiratory complications. Deep breathing and coughing, turning and positioning, early and aggressive ambulation, and the use of incentive spirometry are all helpful in preventing postoperative respiratory complications. Refer to Chapter 34 for detailed descriptions of these interventions.

Circulatory Maintenance

Venous stasis resulting from immobility increases the incidence of blood clot formation in the lower extremities. If blood clots lodge in the pulmonary artery (a pulmonary embolus), gas exchange can be severely curtailed and death may occur. Leg exercises, frequent turning and positioning, the use of sequential compression devices (SCD) and antiembolitic stockings, adequate hydration, and early ambulation all decrease the risk of deep vein thrombosis.

Hydration and Nutrition

Intravenous fluids are provided during the postoperative period to ensure adequate hydration until the client can take fluids orally. Fluid volume deficit may occur because of excessive loss of fluids and inadequate fluid replacement. Postural blood pressure should be monitored on all postoperative clients to detect fluid volume deficits. How long IV fluids are required depends on the surgery and the client. Before IV fluids are discontinued, normal bowel sounds should be present, indicating that normal intestinal peristalsis has resumed after the surgery. Peristalsis may resume more slowly if surgery was performed on the gastrointestinal tract.

Progressive dietary intake is ordered postoperatively depending on the client's recovery. Frequently, the physician may order diet as tolerated (DAT), and the nurse orders the appropriate diet based on assessment of the client. After peristalsis resumes, a clear liquid diet is ordered, progressively followed by full liquids, a soft diet, and a regular diet. As the diet is advanced, the nurse continually assesses the client for nausea, vomiting, abnormal bowel sounds, or abdominal distention. Abnormal findings may necessitate a change in diet orders.

Elimination

Nursing interventions are important to promote normal urinary and bowel elimination. During the postoperative period, the client is expected to void within 8 hours of surgery. The postoperative client may be unable to void because of edema, trauma, medications, or the inability to ambulate to the bathroom. An order for intermittent catheterization may be necessary to treat urinary retention in the immediate postoperative period. An indwelling catheter may be indicated for clients having urologic or gynecologic surgery. Urine output should be at least 30 mL per hour during the postoperative period; urine volumes less than this should be reported to the surgeon. When low urine output occurs, challenging the client with increased IV fluid or administering diuretics may be necessary to ensure adequate urine output.

Bowel elimination may also be affected by the surgery. Normal bowel movements are not expected until normal intestinal motility resumes and the client has begun eating. Rectal tubes and return-flow enemas may be ordered to help relieve intestinal gas and promote the passing of flatus. Postoperative constipation may occur because of decreased activity, side effects of medication (especially pain medication), fluid volume deficit, and fear of painful evacuation. When the client has started eating, stool softeners are commonly ordered. The nurse should encourage activity, adequate fluid intake, and a diet that promotes normal bowel evacuation. If a bowel movement has not occurred 3 days after resuming normal dietary intake, laxatives, suppositories, and enemas may be necessary.

Wound Care

Wound assessment, aseptic care of the wound, and monitoring wound drainage systems are all important nursing interventions. The nurse inspects dressings regularly and notes the amount and type of wound drainage. Some surgeons prefer to change the first postoperative dressing, but if the nurse makes the first change, the dressing must be removed carefully to avoid inadvertent removal of drains. Increasingly, surgeons leave wounds undressed and open to the air to heal. Symptoms of wound infection (redness, warmth, or purulent drainage) should be reported to the physician. Finally, removal of sutures and staples is often the responsibility of nursing personnel.

Comfort and Rest

Pain management is an important nursing intervention during the postoperative period. The nurse uses nonpharmacologic interventions such as positioning, back massage, distraction, and emotional support to help the postoperative client feel more comfortable. The nurse also administers pain medications as needed to control postoperative discomfort. Teaching the client to recognize and report pain is an important part of pain management. If the dose, frequency, or medication ordered by the physician for pain control is ineffective, the physician should be notified. Many facilities have a pain service that routinely sees postoperative clients and assists physicians in determining appropriate pain management regimens.

Rest is important to promote healing. Hypnotics and barbiturates may be ordered to help ensure rest. The nurse can provide a quiet, comfortable environment that encourages sleep and rest. Whenever possible, nursing activities, especially during the night, should be grouped together to allow for uninterrupted periods of rest.

Community-Based Nursing

During the last decade, in-hospital recovery from surgical procedures has been significantly shortened, with an increasing number of surgeries being performed on an ambulatory basis. Much surgical recovery occurs in the client's home, with family or friends assisting in postsurgical care.

Discharge needs may vary depending on the surgical procedure and the individual client. Whereas many clients are discharged and recuperate in the home, other clients may need to be transferred to an extended-care facility. Some clients who have sufficiently recovered from their surgical procedure to be discharged home may need the assistance of home care nurses.

Many hospitals and surgical centers have developed special discharge procedures and forms that the nurse uses when preparing the client for discharge. Discharge concerns for the surgical client include pain management, wound care and dressing changes, monitoring for infection, dietary needs, bowel and bladder function, activity restriction, recommended sexual activity, and ability to perform self-care activities. The client or a responsible caregiver is taught to manage any special equipment that is required at home and perform necessary procedures (such as dressing changes) independently. The client needs to know where to buy needed supplies and how to obtain specialized equipment. A limited number of supplies may be given to the client to ensure continuing care until the client can obtain these necessary items.

The client's family or caregiver should be included in the client teaching session, as appropriate, and written guidelines should be given. Figure 28-8 provides an example of a written discharge teaching guide. Such guidelines usually include limitations on activity and diet, treatments, and medications necessary during postoperative recovery, as well as symptoms necessitating

CLIENT EDUCATION

POST-PROCEDURE DISCHARGE INFORMATION

Date ______________________

Procedure *Tonsillectomy*

Physician ______________________

Activity *Avoid excessive activity for 3–5 days.*

Diet: *Avoid harsh citrus fruit juices such as orange, lemon, pineapple or hot foods – nonacidic juices such as apple juice, flat soft ch water, popsicles, soft foods; like jello, custard, pudding, cooked cereal, soups, macaroni & cheese, mashed patatoes,*

Avoid red foods for 1st 24 hours – they may mask bleeding.

Avoid the use of aspirin or any aspirin containing products.

Pain *Expect some soreness for 5–10 days – often there is pain radiating to the ears. This does not represent infection. Gargling with mouth wash, coughing & excessive cleaning of the throat should be avoided.*

Symptoms to Report to the Physician *Fever greater than 100.6, severe pain that is unrelieved by pain medicine, or bright red bleeding that last more than 5 minutes.*

Calling the Medical Center

If you have any problems or questions, please call the Medical Center

ENT Clinic at *548-4022* (M-F 8:30 a.m. to 4:30 p.m.)

If after hours, call 548-6190 and ask them to page the resident on call for the *ENT* service.

Other: ______________________

Follow-up Appointment

Clinic ____________ Phone ____________

Date ____________ Time ____________

Figure 28-8 • *Home instructions for a client discharged following tonsillectomy.*

notification of the healthcare provider. Verbal and written instructions for any prescribed medications should be given and time provided to answer any questions. Instructions concerning a follow-up appointment with the surgeon, along with a phone number, should be given to the client.

The nurse should explore with the client what assistance he or she will have after discharge and how he or she plans to manage once home. Asking questions such as, "How do you envision your first few days at home?," may help to identify how the client will cope after discharge. When the identified plan does not seem realistic, the nurse can help the client explore alternative approaches or encourage the recruitment of family or friends for help.

Evaluation

During postoperative evaluation, the nurse determines whether goals have been met. Goals and outcome criteria relate to preventing postoperative complications and returning the client to optimal functioning. The more common postoperative nursing diagnoses and goals are listed in Table 28-9. Outcome criteria for four of these goals are presented here, but all postoperative care should be individualized for each client.

Goal

Client will experience normal bowel function when normal diet orders are resumed.

Possible Outcome Criteria

- Client verbalizes decrease in abdominal (gas) pain.
- Client reports normal bowel movement 24 hours after regular diet resumes.

Goal

Client will state that postoperative pain is well controlled.

Possible Outcome Criteria

- During postoperative period, client reports that pain does not interfere with turning, positioning, ambulating, or self-care activities.
- Client verbalizes good pain control on oral medications by time of discharge from acute care facility.

Goal

Client will obtain optimal mobility, progressively increasing activity daily.

Possible Outcome Criteria

- Client sits up in chair, with nurse's help, the evening of surgery.
- Client walks to bathroom, with nurse's help, by 24 hours after surgery.
- Client walks 24 feet in hallway on the day after surgery.

Goal

Client will manage postoperative treatments and normal daily activities in the home with assistance from family and friends

Possible Outcome Criteria

- Client can state discharge instructions before discharge from the hospital
- Client or responsible caregiver can demonstrate dressing change and wound drain management before discharge
- Client can satisfactorily complete activities of daily living with necessary assistance from a responsible caregiver during the first week after discharge.

Key Concepts

- Perioperative nursing provides individualized care for the surgical client during the preoperative, intraoperative, and postoperative phases of the surgical experience.
- Surgery may be performed in a variety of clinical facilities, including the physician's office, clinic, ambulatory surgical centers, or hospitals.
- Surgical procedures can affect all areas of function.
- Lifespan considerations are important when individualizing care for the surgical client.
- Preoperative teaching is important to minimize postoperative complications, increase client compliance, and decrease client anxiety.
- Informed consent must be obtained before any surgical procedure.
- Preoperative preparation of the client includes ensuring NPO status, starting IV access, initiating bowel preparation and skin preparation, administering preoperative medications, and at times, inserting a nasogastric tube.
- Nursing personnel in the operating room provide emotional support, ensure a safe client environment, and maintain asepsis.
- Anesthesia may be administered by an anesthesiologist or a certified registered nurse anesthetist.
- General anesthesia produces a sleep-like state, whereas regional anesthesia decreases pain and sensation in certain areas.
- Sutures or staples may be used to approximate wound edges and promote healing.
- Continual nursing assessment is important in the recovery facility to detect complications promptly and monitor recovery from anesthesia.
- Nursing care during the postoperative period focuses on preventing surgical complications and promoting optimum return of normal function.
- Complications that can occur during the postoperative period include hemorrhage, shock, atelectasis,

deep vein thrombosis, pulmonary emboli, wound infection, fluid volume deficit, nausea, vomiting, malignant hyperthermia, hypothermia, urinary retention, paralytic ileus, sleep deficit, pain, confusion, altered self-concept, altered role relationships, altered coping, and altered sexual function.
- To prepare for discharge, the client should be instructed regarding activity restrictions, incisional care, and symptoms to be reported to a physician.

Critical Thinking Challenges

Return now to the situation at the beginning of this chapter, and consider the following to synthesize material presented in the chapter that now is a part of your knowledge base, and to improve your critical thinking skills.

1. *Reflect on age-related considerations for a 2-year-old having surgery and how you will individualize care for this toddler and his family.*
2. *Reviewing the data that were collected, prioritize the most significant data, explaining why you think they are most significant.*
3. *Plan what teaching is appropriate at this time, and role play how you will individualize the teaching for this family.*
4. *Demonstrate how you will document or report this information to other team members by preparing a written or oral report to be shared, focusing on the most significant assessment data.*

References

Applegeet, C. (1995). Scheduling surgical procedures. *AORN J, 61,* 252.

The Association of Operating Room Nurses, Inc. (1994). AORN standards and recommended practices for perioperative nursing. *AORN J, 59,* 1190.

Atkinson, L. J. (1992). *Berry & Kohn's operating techniques* (7th ed.). St. Louis: C. V. Mosby.

DiBenedetto, R., Graves, S., Gravenstein, N., Konicek, C. (1993). Pulse oximetry monitoring can change routine oxygen administration in the postanesthesia care unit. *Anesthesiology Analgesia, 78,* 365–368.

Donnelly, A. (1994). Malignant hyperthermia: Epidemiology, pathophysiology, and treatment. *AORN J, 59,* 393–408.

Drain, C., & Cristoph, S. (1987). *The recovery room: A critical care approach to post anesthesia nursing* (2nd ed.). Philadelphia: W. B. Saunders.

Good Reis, J. (1994). Latex sensitivity: Controlling health care workers', patients' risks. *AORN J, 59,* 615–621.

Hutchinson, A., Maltby, J., Reid, R., & Crawford, R. G. (1988). Gastric fluid volume and pH in elective surgery patients: Part I. Coffee or orange juice versus overnight fast. *Can J Anaesth, 35* (1), 12–15.

Kneedler, J., & Dodge, G. (1994). *Perioperative nursing care: The nursing perspective* (3rd ed.). Boston: Blackwell.

Litwack-Saleh, K. (1993). The elderly patient in the post anesthesia care unit. *Nurs Clin North Am, 28,* 507–518.

Meeker, M., & Rothrock, J. (1994). *Alexander's care of the client in surgery* (9th ed.). St. Louis: C. V. Mosby.

Morse, J., Solberg, S., & Edwards, J. (1993). Caregiver–infant interaction: Comforting post-operative neonates. *Scandinavian Journal of Caring Science, 7* (2), 105–111.

North American Nursing Diagnosis Association (NANDA). (1994). *NANDA Nursing diagnoses: Definitions and classification 1995–1996.* Philadelphia: Author.

Parnass, S. (1993). Ambulatory surgical patient priorities. *Nurs Clin North Am, 28,* 531–545.

Phippen, M., & Wells, M. (1994). *Perioperative nursing practice.* Philadelphia: W. B. Saunders.

Poole, E. (1993). The effects of postanesthesia care unit visits on anxiety in surgical patients. *Journal of Postanesthesia Nursing, 8,* 386–394.

Rivellini, D. (1993). Local and regional anesthesia: Nursing implications. *Nurs Clin North Am, 28,* 547–572.

Smeltzer, S., & Bare, B. G. (1996). *Textbook of medical–surgical nursing* (7th ed.). Philadelphia: J. B. Lippincott.

Tarsitano, B. (1992). Structured preoperative teaching. In G. Bulecheck & J. McCloskey (Eds.), *Nursing interventions and essential nursing treatments* (2nd ed.). Philadelphia: W. B. Saunders.

Thomas, J., & McIntosh, J. (1994). Are incentive spirometry, intermittent positive pressure breathing, and deep breathing exercises effective in the prevention of postoperative pulmonary complications after upper abdominal surgery? A systematic overview and meta-analysis. *Phys Ther, 74* (1), 3–10.

Walsh, J. (1993). Postop effects of OR positioning. *RN, 56* (2), 50–58.Wells, M. P. (1987). *Decision making in perioperative nursing.* Philadelphia: B. C. Decker.

Widdison, A., Pope, N., & Brown, E. (1993). Survey of guidelines for antimicrobial prophylaxis in surgery. *J Hosp Infect, 25,* 199–205.

Bibliography

Avis, M. (1994). Choice cuts: An exploratory study of patients' views about participation in decision making in a day surgery unit. *Int J Nurs Stud, 31,* 289–298.

Carpenito, L. J. (1995). *Nursing diagnosis: Application to clinical practice* (6th ed.). Philadelphia: J. B. Lippincott.

Metzer, D., & Fromm, C. (1993). Laying out a care plan for the elderly postoperative patient. *Nursing93, 23* (4), 67–74.

Meyer-Pahoulis, E., Williams, S., Davidson, S., McVey, J., & Mazurek, A. (1993). The pediatric patient in the post anesthesia care unit. *Nurs Clin North Am, 28,* 519–530.

Oberle, K., Allen, M., & Lynkowski, P. (1994). Follow-up of same day surgery patients. *AORN J, 59,* 1016–1025.

Oetker-Black, S., & Taunton, R. (1994). Evaluation of self-efficacy scale for preoperative patients. *AORN J, 60(1),* 43–50.

Patrick, M. L. Woods, S., Craven, R., et al. (1991). *Medical-surgical nursing: Pathophysiological concepts* (2nd ed.). Philadelphia: J. B. Lippincott.

Redeker, N., Mason, D., Wykpisz, E., Glica, B., & Miner, C. (1994). First postoperative week activity patterns and recovery in women after coronary artery bypass surgery. *Nurs Res, 43,* 168–173.

SECTION II

Human Function and Clinical Nursing Therapeutics

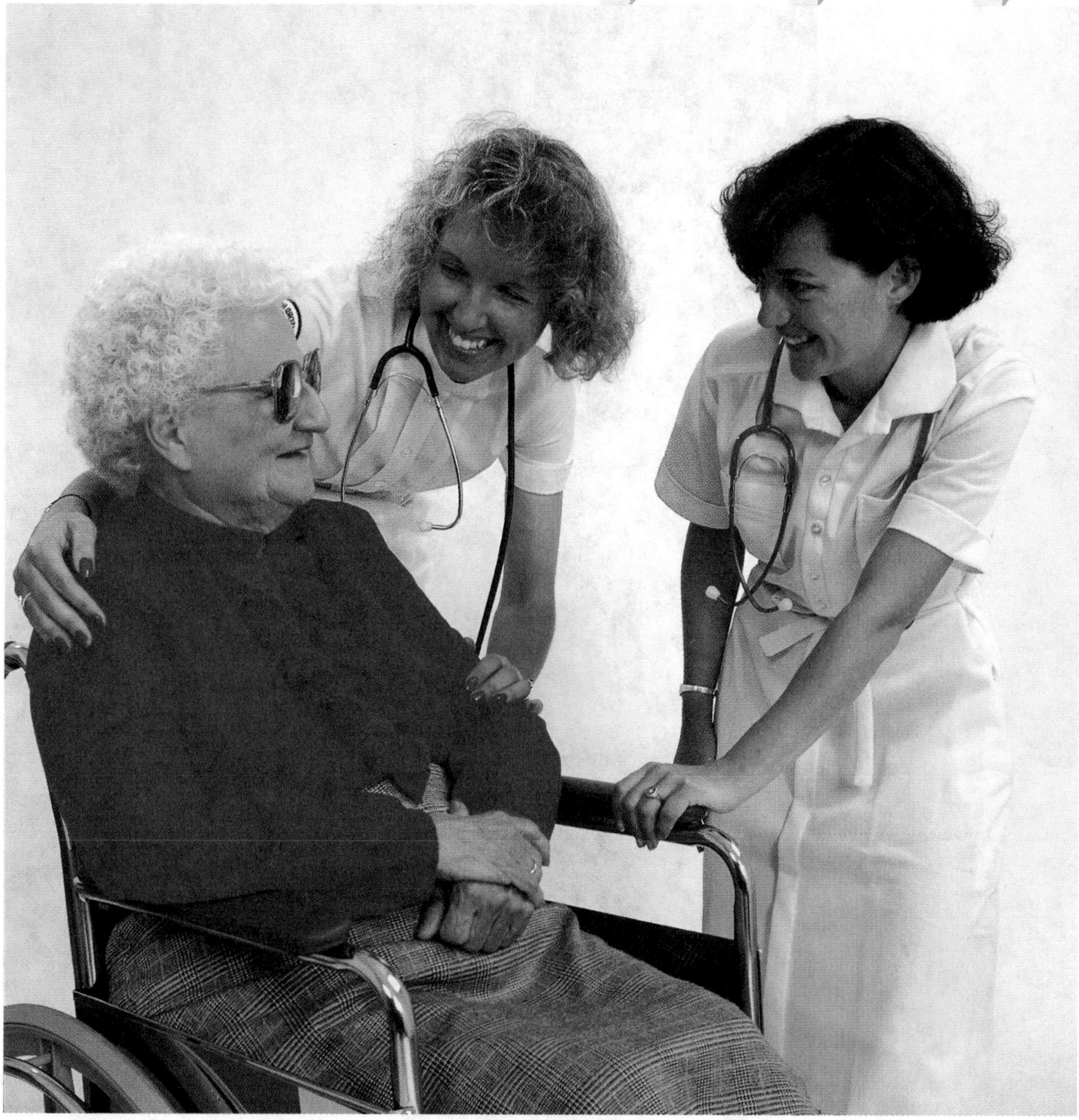

Health Perception and Health Management

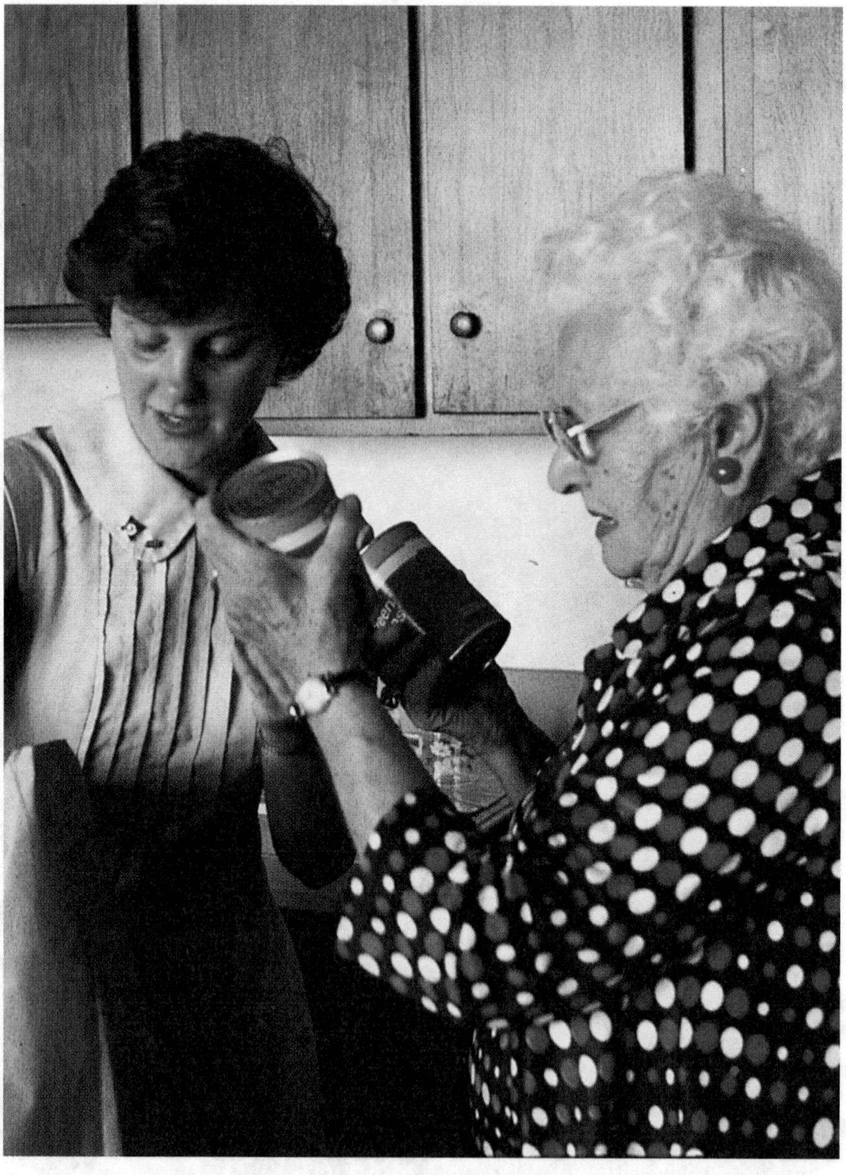

UNIT VII

A person's knowledge of and desire for health and safety affect the outcome of his or her care. Unit VII focuses on client's perceptions of their own health and their health-promoting practices. To take full advantage of client strengths, the nurse needs to know what a client has done or will do to maintain, support, or restore health and function.

Chapter 29 discusses the concepts and principles of safety and details nursing care for clients with safety needs. In addition to creating a safe environment within the healthcare facility, the nurse explores the safety of the client's own environment and identifies risks and hazards that represent a threat to the client's safety. The next chapter explores the client's health and wellness status. Health-promoting practices and resources are discussed so the nurse has a knowledge base from which to assess and intervene for clients with altered health maintenance. Client teaching is also emphasized for clients exhibiting health-seeking behaviors. The final chapter in this unit focuses specifically on the client's home environment. The concept of home management is explored, and assessment of the client's and family's ability to maintain the home is discussed. Finally, holistic nursing interventions for promoting or supporting home management are emphasized. Effective discharge planning is critical to home management. Planning elements for the client and nurse and levels of discharge planning are discussed. Other interventions include healthcare options and funding and meeting caregiver and family needs.

The chapters in this unit explore essential concepts and skills today's nurses need to provide safety, to maintain health, and to evaluate clients' ability to care for themselves at home.

Safety

Key Terms	Learning Objectives

Key Terms

Asphyxiation
Electrical shock
Ground
Nosocomial infections
Poisoning
Pollution
Restraints
Suffocation

Learning Objectives

Upon completion of this chapter, the student will be able to do the following:

- *Recognize the importance of safety in the home and healthcare environment.*
- *Identify factors that affect safety.*
- *Relate special safety considerations to developmental stages.*
- *Discuss factors that create a potential for altered safety.*
- *Describe common problems resulting from altered safety.*
- *Identify individual safety patterns through assessment.*
- *Using assessment, identify individuals at risk for safety dysfunction.*
- *Define and characterize the appropriate nursing diagnoses for altered safety.*
- *Discuss nursing interventions to promote a safe healthcare environment.*
- *List client teaching topics to promote safety.*
- *Identify nursing interventions for altered safety.*
- *Describe advantages and responsibilities in community-based nursing.*

29

You are a nurse in a pediatric primary care clinic conducting a well-child assessment for an active toddler and the young mother. As you discuss the home environment, the mother tells you that they live in a two-story house with the bedrooms on the second floor and the other rooms on the main floor. The mother tells you that the toddler climbs up and down the stairs, climbs on chairs, gets up on counters and table tops, and is very curious about boxes and bottles of all types. The mother seems tired and somewhat irritated as she tries to hold the toddler still on her lap. The toddler is fussing and struggling to get off her lap.

In previous chapters, you learned about conceptual foundations of nursing. This section of the book expands the practical clinical aspects of your nursing career. An important factor in nursing is safety: safety of clients in their home environment and safety within the healthcare environment. As you increase your understanding of safety, you will more fully understand holistic care of clients and their families. Critical Thinking Challenges at the end of the chapter will help you apply your body of knowledge to the care of the young mother and her active toddler.

Accidents are the fourth leading cause of death in the United States. In people aged 1 to 37 years, accidents were the leading cause of death in 1991 (National Safety Council, 1994). The leading categories of accidents resulting in death were motor vehicle accidents, falls, drowning, and fires and burns. Accidents also may result in injury, permanent disability, pain, emotional distress, and financial hardship.

Safety is important on every level of human interaction. It is an individual, community, national, and worldwide concern. Safety is a major focus of the National Health Promotion and Disease Prevention Objectives (1990), known as Healthy People 2000, a vision for improved health status for Americans by 2000.

A truly danger-free environment is rare. Consequently, the promotion of safety involves awareness and implementation. Traditionally, nursing's realm of safety care involved only the hospital environment. Nursing care today, however, is broad and specific. Not only does maintaining a safe healthcare environment remain one of the nurse's important roles, but also teaching the client and family about safety precautions at home, in the workplace, and in the community has become an important nursing action. Nurses work in many different environments, some hazardous. The nurse must minimize his or her own potential for injury. Safety habits for the client and nurse will ensure an optimal therapeutic environment and promote health.

Normal Safety Function

Safety and security are essential needs of basic human functioning. Safety and security are second in priority only to physiologic needs in Maslow's hierarchy of needs (Maslow, 1970). Safety not only prevents harm and injury, it allows a person to feel secure in his or her actions. Stress may be reduced, and general health is promoted. Safety allows other basic human needs, such as love, belonging, and self-esteem, to be met and personal goals to be accomplished. A positive outlook on life will result in better mental health and more effective functioning.

Characteristics of Safety

Characteristics of safety are illustrated in Figure 29-1.

Pervasiveness. Safety is pervasive; it affects everything. Subconsciously, people are concerned with safety in all their activities: eating, breathing, sleeping, working, and playing. Consciously, people take responsibility or neglect responsibility for their own safety.

Perception. A person's perception of safety and danger influences the incorporation of safety into life's activities. Safety measures are effective only as far as hazards are accurately perceived. Safety factors are not innately understood but are learned. Maturity brings a recognition of possible dangers and a realization of the importance of practicing safety. Parents, teachers, healthcare workers, and laws help in the perception process.

Management. Once a person recognizes dangers in the environment, he or she takes measures to prevent those dangers and thus practices safety. Prevention is a major characteristic of safety. Self-care is involved in safety practices, but safety for others should be provided as well.

Normal Functional Pattern

The complex physiologic and psychological systems of the human body work together to allow a person to avoid or minimize injury. Reflexes withdraw the hand from the flame before conscious thought can move the hand. A loud noise causes a startle reaction and an immediate increase in level of alertness. The sensation of pain provides important feedback that an activity or situation is dangerous. Normal functional patterns of safety involve the person's awareness of threats and conscious and unconscious responses to avoid harm.

Factors Affecting Safety

A person's full participation in safety promotion and avoidance of harm depends on a variety of individual and environmental factors. Examples of some safety features are pictured in Figure 29-2.

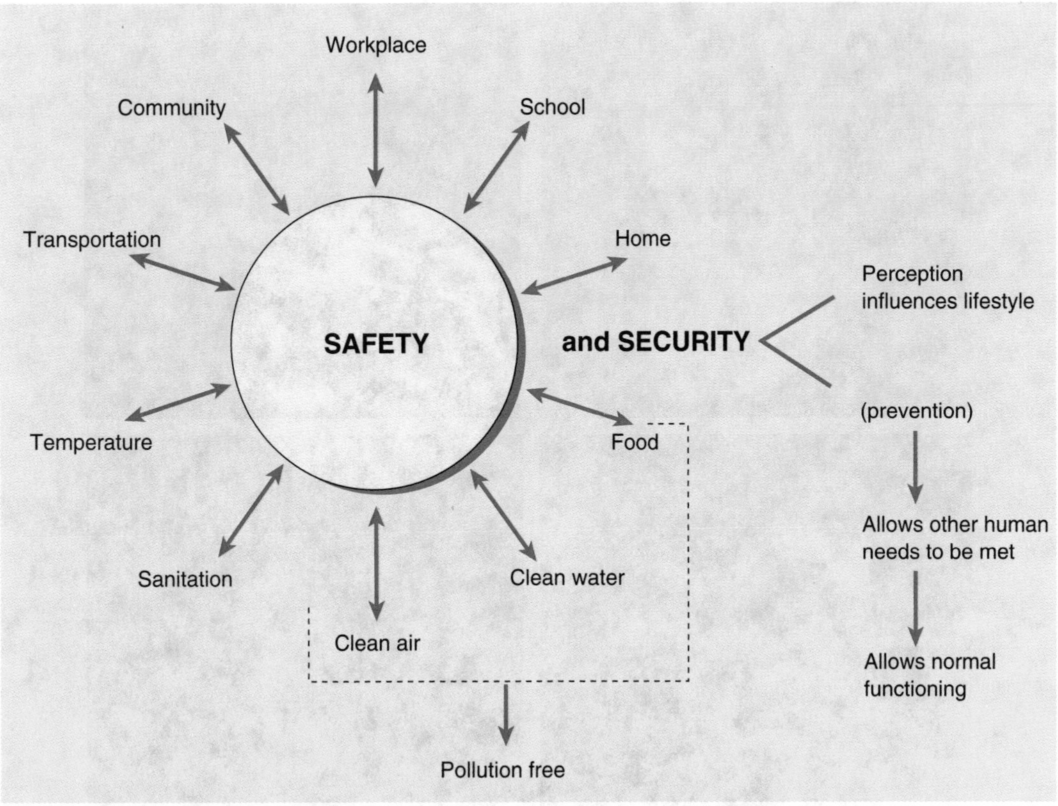

Figure 29-1 • *Characteristics of safety (pervasiveness, perception, and management) help the individual function normally.*

Cognition and Perception

Complex cognitive and perceptual functions, such as judgment, orientation, and socially appropriate behaviors, depend on the accumulation and accurate interpretation of information. The ability to think clearly, recall past problems and solutions, imagine feasible solutions to current problems, and solve problems are cognitive functions needed to promote safety. The perception of danger based on past experience and accumulated knowledge also is essential for promoting safety.

Activity and Exercise

Activity and exercise condition the body to react quickly in an emergency. Deficient activity and exercise may impair the ability to protect oneself from outside hazards.

Physiologic Factors

Promotion of safety depends on intact neurologic, cardiovascular, and musculoskeletal systems and on the proper functioning of many other physiologic processes. In terms of safety, a functioning neurologic system consists of peripheral nerves, which sense hazards in the environment; the spinal cord, which relays impulses that allow the reflex arc to function; and the brain, which coordinates activities, processes information, and initiates responses. A functioning cardiovascular system provides oxygen and nutrients to the rest of the body as needed for quick response. Musculoskeletal integrity is essential for normal posture and movement. Disruption inhibits mobility and the ability to respond to hazards, and it raises the risk of accidents.

Age and Developmental Level

Age and developmental level can affect safety because of knowledge and experience or because of physiologic abilities. Just as the very young do not possess the knowledge of potential hazards or the coordination to protect themselves from injury, the aged experience slowed cognitive functioning and slowed reflexes that put them at risk for falls and other accidents.

Previous Experience

Previous experience with danger and safety promotion will affect perception and behavior in future situations. A person who was injured in a fire in the past is likely to practice fire prevention in the home. Conversely, a person with little previous experience with danger or safety promotion may not share the concern for safety. For example, immigrants from warm climates may not

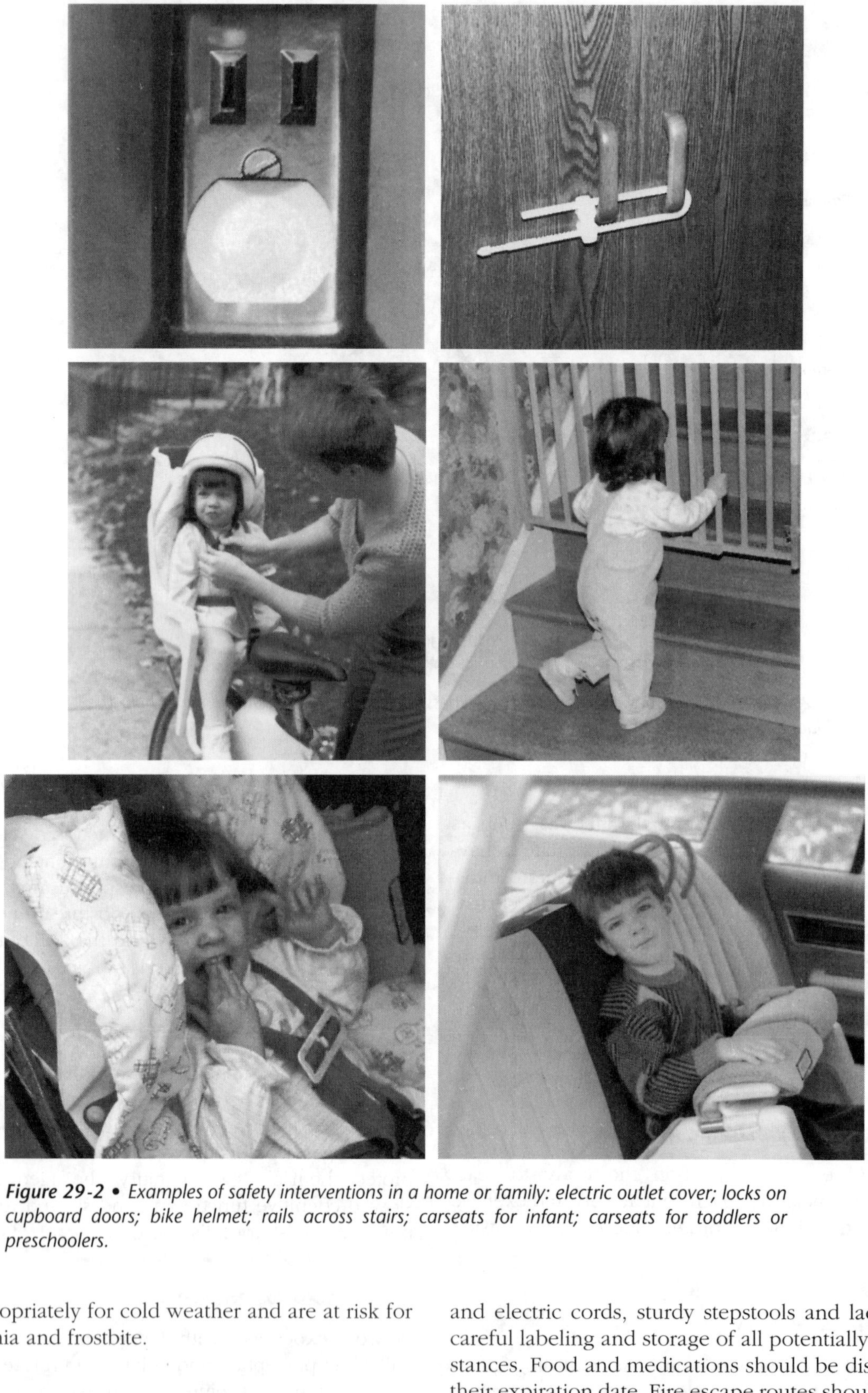

Figure 29-2 • *Examples of safety interventions in a home or family: electric outlet cover; locks on cupboard doors; bike helmet; rails across stairs; carseats for infant; carseats for toddlers or preschoolers.*

dress appropriately for cold weather and are at risk for hypothermia and frostbite.

Home Environment

The home environment may be safe or may contain many hazards. A safe home environment features adequate ventilation, a reliable heating system, a nonskid bathtub surface, well-maintained electrical appliances and electric cords, sturdy stepstools and ladders, and careful labeling and storage of all potentially toxic substances. Food and medications should be discarded on their expiration date. Fire escape routes should be practiced. Smoke alarms must be functioning and strategically located. Outdoor hazards may be corrected by having effective lighting, maintaining fences, and properly securing areas that may create potential hazards, such as swimming pools.

Workplace Environment

The workplace may include hazards that are obvious or invisible. From the secretary who works in an office with asbestos ceiling tiles, to the salesman driving long hours on the road, to the fisherman on an ice-coated ship deck, safety must be a concern of every worker. The Occupational Safety and Health Administration (OSHA) is required to investigate worker complaints (Stanevich & Stanevich, 1989), and many states have enacted worker right-to-know legislation that requires employers to notify workers of occupational hazards.

Safety concerns inherent to some occupations include noise, dust and air pollution, working at heights, dangerous machines, and exposure to toxic substances. These factors are dangerous when usual safety precautions, such as wearing protective gear, are not followed by the worker or the worker is unaware of the hazard.

Community Environment

The community in which one lives, works, shops, and plays may present safety concerns. Noise (eg, from trains and planes), crime, poor lighting, presence of landfills, busy intersections, dilapidated houses, cliffs, and unprotected creeks are hazards. The community should be free from most of these hazards to lend a feeling of safety and security.

Sanitation affects safety. Sanitation includes a clean water supply, sewage system, absence of insects and rodents, and refrigeration of food supply. Lack of sanitation may result in the danger of increased spread of disease and infection. Sanitation is often lacking in impoverished or less developed areas.

Thermoregulation

The temperature of the outdoor and indoor environments affects safety. Extremes in temperature or other climate conditions, such as wind, humidity, snow, rain, or ice, present a hazard. Inappropriate dress or protection increases the safety risk. Indoor thermoregulation problems may result from inadequate finances or lack of help maintaining a heating or cooling system in the home.

Lifespan Considerations

Safety concerns are individualized to fit developmental stages. The diverse physiologic and psychological capabilities across the lifespan put different age groups at risk for different injuries. Interventions are geared toward specific age-related concerns.

Newborn and Infant

Because they lack life experience and musculoskeletal and neurologic maturity, the newborn and infant may be susceptible to burns, falls, and accidents. Their ability to thermoregulate is immature (Freiberg, 1992), and their ability to satisfy basic needs depends on inarticulate cries and nonverbal communication. Without a clear means of communication and with limited ability to respond to environmental challenges, the newborn and infant depend on caregivers to create a safe environment in which normal growth and development can occur without injury. Safety in the environment is a major parenting task.

Infants are curious; they explore the environment by pulling things and placing almost anything in their mouths. Dangling cords, tablecloths, plastic bags, bottles, and cans are tempting objects for exploration. A safe environment for the newborn and infant should include a comfortable temperature range; nonrestrictive, nonflammable, adequate clothing; warm bath water; clean air; safe toys; guard rails at staircases and steps; protection with locked, padded rungs or rails for cribs or changing tables; covered electrical outlets; and appropriate car seats for automobile travel (see Fig. 29-2).

Toddler and Preschooler

Falls, bumps, and bruises are common at this age of exploration and exuberance. The increasing mobility

Nursing Research
Safety

Selected Nursing Research Studies

Schnelle, J. F., MacRae, P. G., Simmons, S. F., Uman, G., Ouslander, J. G., Rosenquist, L. L., & Chang, B. (1994). Safety assessment for the frail elderly: A comparison of restrained and unrestrained nursing home residents. *Journal of the American Geriatrics Society, 42*(6), 586–592.

Mahon, N. E. (1994). Positive health practices and perceived health status in adolescents. *Clinical Nursing Research, 3*(2), 86–101; 101–103.

Kidd, P., & Huddleston, S. (1994). Psychosometric properties of the Driving Practices Questionnaire: assessment of risky driving. *Research in Nursing and Health, 17*(1), 51–58.

Wilson, P. D., Testani-Dufour, L. (1993). Bicycle safety programs: Targeting injury prevention through education. *Pediatric Nursing, 19*(4), 343–346.

Possible Topics for Nursing Inquiry

- What factors contribute to the increased risk for falling in hospitalized elderly clients?
- What risk factors contribute to the potential for back injuries in caregivers?
- Do cultural factors have a relationship with usage of infant safety seats in motor vehicles?

of the toddler and preschooler and the lack of life experience and still immature neurologic and musculoskeletal systems are potentially hazardous. The parents of the toddler and preschooler must anticipate the wide-ranging interests of their explorer. Once upright, the toddler can reach up to a new source of interesting items. Curiosity still reigns; pets and other animals become new, moveable objects of exploration. Life experiences begin to accumulate, however, and learning of safe and dangerous behaviors begins. Setting a safe example is an important first step for the parents of the toddler and preschooler.

Improving eye–hand coordination, increasing strength, and increasing speed characterize the toddler and preschooler. This age group delights in opening and closing doors, turning knobs, climbing furniture, and engaging in all sorts of active play. Although these young children usually are able to communicate basic needs in words or actions, parents must still ensure a comfortable environmental temperature; adequate, nonflammable, nonrestrictive clothing; and warm bath water. The bathtub should have a nonskid mat or decals to prevent slipping when standing up.

Toddler toys must be sturdy, free of sharp or rough edges, and free of small, removable, or breakable parts that could be swallowed or could damage an eye. Tricycles, push cycles, rocking horses, and other active toys that use large muscle groups are enjoyed by toddlers and preschoolers but should be used under supervision until the child understands the safety limits of the toy.

Toddlers need guard rails at staircases and steps, but as the transition to preschool occurs, children begin to learn safety rules and gain motor control. Preschoolers usually can avoid bumps and learn to climb safely up and down stairs. Preschoolers also benefit from learning about safety zones; a safety zone is a safe place to stand or sit when a potentially dangerous activity is underway. For instance, a kitchen should have a safety zone where the child may watch activity but is out the reach of stove, oven, or knives.

Outside the home, toddlers and preschoolers initially need supervision but with caregiver guidance, will learn about playing out of the way of automobile traffic and avoiding strange animals.

The preschool years are marked by increasing social interaction. The rules of safe social interaction are often learned by trial and error, and striking out may occur. Usually the natural exuberance of this age is to blame rather than any malicious intent; however, parents may help their preschooler by teaching cooperation and sharing. This also is the age at which caution toward strangers should be encouraged. Identification bracelets, fingerprinting, and frequent photographs are recommended by some law enforcement agencies.

Fire safety is a family concern when children reach this age. Learning about matches, electric cords, stoves, and ovens is important for the curious preschooler who might be tempted to experiment. The whole family should regularly practice crawling on the floor, using escape routes in case of fire, and having a meeting place outside of the home. Local fire departments often have useful information about planning alternative escape routes and other safety procedures.

Child and Adolescent

Physiologic maturity is almost complete for the school-age child. Motor control of large muscles and rapidly developing fine motor control enable the school-age child to accomplish complex tasks. Learning occurs at an astounding rate. Life experiences accumulate and are used to make judgments about the appropriateness of behaviors. The expanding world of the school-age child demands flexible responses and presents opportunities for independent action.

Children in this age group can make their needs known verbally and often have reflexes that are quick enough to protect them from burns, falls, and other accidents. New activities will require new skills, and this age group may learn to ski, ride horseback, swim, bicycle, sail, or participate in team sports. Safety precautions are important. Helmets should be worn when cycling, riding, or playing contact sports; life jackets should be worn when sailing or boating. All children should be taught to swim or at least float and tread water. The buddy system is an important outdoor and water safety strategy to learn.

Safe examples set by parents continue to be a major influence on the school-age child. A home that uses alcohol in moderation; keeps guns, if any, locked away; and uses discussion rather than force to resolve conflict will demonstrate the safety habits needed for later years.

Growth and development spurt during adolescence. Physical maturity of the musculoskeletal system is nearing completion, and the nervous and cardiovascular systems are fully mature (Freiberg, 1992). While life experience is accumulating rapidly, so are new responsibilities. The autonomy of the adolescent develops in response to social and societal pressures. Driving a car, coping with drugs, beginning to explore sexuality, babysitting, working after school, and developing expertise are all adolescent activities that require judgment and independent action. As opportunities are explored, the adolescent may know a behavior is unsafe, but social pressure may persuade him or her to act against better judgment. Supportive parents who allow discussion and expression of conflict provide a home environment that is safe for the adolescent.

Adult and Older Adult

With physical maturity complete, the adult moves at will in a world full of potential dangers. Accidents at home, in the workplace, and during sports are too common. Safety habits may become rusty, and overconfidence or ignorance can still place the adult in the path of danger.

Traffic fatalities have dropped by one-third in the last decade and a half; however, motor vehicle accidents continue to be a major cause of adult deaths and were the leading cause of accidental death for people aged 1 through 78 years in 1991 (National Center for Health Statistics, 1990; National Safety Council, 1994). Use of safety belts with shoulder harnesses is mandatory in most states, as is the use of helmets when riding motorcycles. Many cars are equipped with air bags for increased safety. For the outdoor enthusiast, the buddy system is still the best safety measure. Boaters, hikers, skiers, hunters, and mountain climbers are lost every year when they travel alone. Every sport has experts who can share safety information with beginners, often through clubs or associations of enthusiasts.

Advancing age entails some loss in physical function and often in acuity of sensory–perceptual function. The older adult may have impaired eyesight, impaired hearing, decreased proprioception, and decreased sensitivity to touch. The ability to thermoregulate may be impaired; the elderly are at a higher risk than younger adults for hypothermia and heatstroke (Kane, Ouslander, & Abrass, 1989). Reflex responses slow, and the musculoskeletal system may lose flexibility and strength. Various conditions, such as arthritis, osteoporosis, or congestive heart failure, may limit the older adult's ability to endure sustained physical activity. Medications taken to control conditions such as high blood pressure or Parkinson's disease may result in orthostatic hypotension and the potential for falling. Some elderly experience cognitive impairment, with severity ranging from mild memory losses to a dementia that prevents safe independent living. The principles of a safe environment for the older adult follow the same general guidelines as for all ages: comfortable temperature range; adequate clothing; bath water of the right temperature (the setting on the hot water heater may need to be turned down); adequate ventilation; lighting that allows for safe navigation throughout the house at all times of day; nonskid surfaces on stairs, in the kitchen, and bathroom (throw rugs should be removed); and stable supports for climbing (firm stair rails, grab bars if needed).

Altered Safety

Potential for Altered Safety

Nurses at work, clients in institutional settings, families at home, or laborers on a job site are potentially compromised. They are at risk for hazards, invasive trauma, disease, and pollution.

Hazards

When hazards exist, the potential for altered safety function also exists. Hazards in the home include poorly lighted stairways, throw rugs, slippery floors, cluttered areas, and unstable ladders, all of which may lead to falls. The risk of falls is compounded when an aged person or person with impaired mobility encounters these hazards. Other hazards in the home include medications and household cleansers left within reach of children, careless smoking, and lack of supervision of infants and children at play. People are often unaware of hazards in the home until accidents occur. A summary of home hazards is listed in the accompanying display.

The healthcare environment contains many hazards as well. Falls, fires, and poisoning occur due to problems with equipment, procedural errors, and impairment of the client. Examples of equipment problems are a wheelchair with nonlocking wheels that causes a fall when a client attempts to sit down or a malfunctioning heating pad unit that causes a fire. The frequent use of oxygen in client care areas increases the risk of fire; therefore, smoking is prohibited wherever oxygen is in use. Many healthcare sites have adopted totally smoke-free environments to promote safety and health. Procedural errors, such as not checking client identification bands before administering medication or not monitoring intravenous infusion rates, may cause harm to clients as well. The client may suffer falls or burns because he or she is impaired by medication that causes central nervous system depression; sensory dysfunction, such as blindness or hearing loss; decreased mobility due to neurologic or musculoskeletal illness; language or other communication barrier; or confusion due to mental or physical illness.

Healthcare facilities have developed procedures and policies for client care and equipment operation to minimize hazards. They should be reviewed periodically to promote the safety of clients and staff. Nursing assessment of factors that put clients at risk for accidents should help identify safety concerns and the precautions necessary to minimize risks.

Invasive Trauma

Invasive trauma in the home may occur when electrical safety is ignored. Overloading outlets, using appliances with frayed cords, or allowing an infant or child to play with plugs or near electrical outlets may result in electrical shock or burns. New parents are often unaware of these household risks for their children and are amenable to safety education by nurses.

The healthcare environment contains electrical hazards for the nurse and client. With heavy use or misuse, equipment may develop flaws that result in excessive leakage of electricity. A potentially dangerous electrical

Summary of Hazards in the Home

- Poor lighting inside or outside
- Uneven walking areas
- Steps with broken concrete
- Steps without handrails
- Loose mats on steps
- Cluttered steps or clutter near head of stairs
- Slippery tub or shower
- Extension cords across open spaces where people may trip
- Throw rugs on slippery floors
- Chairs with wide legs at the base
- Folding chairs or outdoor chairs that topple easily when poorly balanced
- Insecure stools or stepladders
- Standing on chairs rather than stools or stepladders
- Items placed precariously on closet shelves
- Bookcases or heavy pieces of furniture that might topple
- Defective smoke detectors
- Oily or dirty rags bunched together, especially near heat
- Stacks of old newspapers or boxes in basement or garage
- Flammable liquids in illegal containers
- Items used often in the kitchen placed over the gas stove
- Loose-fitting clothes worn while cooking
- Water temperatures that are too hot and may burn
- Defective wiring
- Overloaded outlets or frayed cords
- Smoking in bed or alone at night in living room
- Electrical appliances in the bathroom, where they may fall in the bathtub or sink
- Obstructed doorways or pathways in case of fire
- Many medications, or unlabeled medications, in medicine cabinet
- Unlocked cupboards or cabinets with potential poisons
- Poisonous plants where children can reach them
- Unsafe sexual practices
- Pets that may harm children, the elderly, or visitors
- Cigarette smoking in a closed area in the presence of nonsmokers
- Plastic bags where children may find them
- Cribs near windows or near venetian blind cords
- Unsupervised children in the bathtub
- Poor hygiene, especially in the bathroom and kitchen
- Improper food preparation
- Rodents or insect infestation

circuit may be created by the nurse who simultaneously touches a damaged or ungrounded electrical appliance and the client with wet skin or a central intravenous line. The client with a skin surface broken by wounds, invasive lines, abrasions, or punctures or with wet skin is more vulnerable to electric current flow. Such clients should be considered electrically sensitive, and the nurse must avoid creating a potentially hazardous circuit. The use of faulty or ungrounded electrical equipment also increases the risk of electrical shock.

Clients and staff are at risk for invasive trauma in the form of radiation when safety function is altered. Radiation is used in diagnosis and treatment in many healthcare facilities. X-ray machines and pharmaceuticals for injection or implantation emit small doses of radiation into the environment. While the client receives the intended dose of radiation, nurses and x-ray technicians are exposed to small doses repeatedly. Safety precautions for staff include distancing and shielding themselves from the radiation source and measuring accumulated dose. Regular inspection and servicing of equipment and licensing of x-ray and pharmacy technicians help minimize risks to the clients and staff.

Disease

Disease is pervasive. An organism's ability to overwhelm the body's defenses is facilitated by injury or unsafe behaviors. Unsafe sex is associated with gonorrhea, genital warts, syphilis, and human immunodeficiency virus/acquired immunodeficiency syndrome (HIV/AIDS). Sharing of needles by intravenous drug abusers is associated with hepatitis B and HIV/AIDS. Use of contaminated water and food is associated with typhoid fever, hepatitis A, and parasite infections. Poor hygiene is associated with urinary tract infections, colds, and tuberculosis. Being bitten by an infected tick can result in Lyme disease.

Clients are exposed to microorganisms in the healthcare environment. Infection may result, especially if the client is compromised by fatigue, stress, poor nutrition, or other conditions that impair immunity. Clients are at risk for **nosocomial infection** (infection acquired in the healthcare environment) when safety precautions are not carried out. Medical and surgical asepsis are the primary safety precautions for preventing disease in the healthcare environment. Handwashing is the basis for medical asepsis (see Chap. 25). Nurses also are at risk for contracting infection.

Viruses, such as herpes, cytomegalovirus, and human T-lymphotropic virus, along with multiresistant bacteria and yeast, cause dangerous infections in susceptible people. To prevent the spread of these organisms in healthcare settings, the Centers for Disease Control and Prevention developed an approach entitled *Universal Precautions* (Centers for Disease Control, 1988). This approach considers any body substance—urine, stool, saliva, blood, sputum—contaminated. All healthcare staff must protect themselves and other clients from body substances by wearing disposable gloves when handling any of these substances. If aerosolization is suspected, goggles, mask, and gown must be worn. Nurses should be especially careful when bathing clients, because any open or fluid-filled lesion is a potential source of pathogenic organisms. Each healthcare agency will have an infection control manual to help guide the nurse in caring for clients in a safe, protective manner. Many agencies also are adopting special signs as a means of educating staff and the public (see sample signs in Chap. 25).

Dysfunction and Fatigue

Neurologic impairment, which may alter safety, can be caused by head injury, medications, alcohol and drugs, stroke, spinal cord injury, degenerative diseases (eg, Parkinson's disease and Alzheimer's disease), and brain tumors. Cardiovascular dysfunction that may impair safety can be caused by hypertension, congestive heart failure, congenital cardiac anomalies, or peripheral vascular disease. Musculoskeletal alteration that impairs safety can be caused by fractures, osteoporosis, muscular dystrophy, or arthritis.

Fatigue may be responsible for poor perception of danger, faulty judgment, and inadequate problem-solving. Careless driving, irresponsible taking of medication, and inadvertent overexposure to sunlight may result. Fatigue arises from poor sleep habits, lifestyle patterns, stress, or a variety of medical or other unknown conditions.

Coping and Stress Tolerance

Psychologic factors, such as anxiety and depression, alter the ability to perceive safety hazards, express concerns, and follow safety precautions. For example, a person may be anxious about a surgical procedure and not process information about postoperative procedures and home care; this could result in injury or complications following surgery. Coping mechanisms used in times of stress can have a direct relationship to safety. Personality factors may play a part in responsiveness. Impulsiveness, distrust, or shyness may affect safety promotion. Psychological factors may be inborn, learned, or the result of mental illness.

Pollution

Pollution is the presence of harmful or unnatural substances in air, water, or land. Toxic substances in the air, water, or ground, frequently the byproducts of manufacturing, increase the risk of cancer. Air pollution increases the risk for and severity of respiratory problems, such as asthma and chronic bronchitis. Allergy symptoms are often worsened by poor air quality due to pollution. Polluted water affects food supply and may lead to the spread of disease and infection. Noise pollution from airplanes, trains, heavy automobile traffic, loud music, or public stadiums may harm people by increasing stress and impairing hearing.

Pollution can affect safety for years. Radon, a gas resulting from natural radioactive decay processes, has been linked to lung cancer and may be present in excess in many homes (Loken & Loken, 1989). Increasing government and public awareness of environmental issues has led to many clean-up programs for known pollutants and safety guidelines to prevent further pollution. Safety risks from pollutants may be hidden for many years following their emission into the environment. Pollution results from ignorance about its risks or lack of concern for environmental safety (Fig. 29-3).

Disregard for Safety

Individuals or groups who disregard safety may jeopardize the safety of many. A person may engage in unsafe driving practices and potentially injure others in automobile accidents. Bicycle, skateboard, and other recreation and sports accidents also occur due to disregard for safety. Disregard may be intentional or due to ignorance of risks and safety precautions. Employers may disregard safety and cause harm to workers or the general population; this occurs when safety gear is not supplied for operating dangerous machinery, toxic waste is not disposed of properly, or a product is sold with potential safety flaws. Nurses can increase public awareness about automobile safety by talking with clients who have been involved in motor vehicle or bicycle accidents. Safety precautions, such as following safe driving speed for road conditions, using infant car seats, using seat belts, avoiding alcohol when driving, and using bicycle helmets, can minimize risk.

Some people are more prone to safety problems because of inherent lifestyle patterns and unhealthy habits. A person's lifestyle might involve risks or impulsive behavior, such as walking alone at night or high-speed driving. They may enjoy potentially dangerous sports, such as skydiving or mountain climbing, and may not follow usual safety precautions. Cigarette

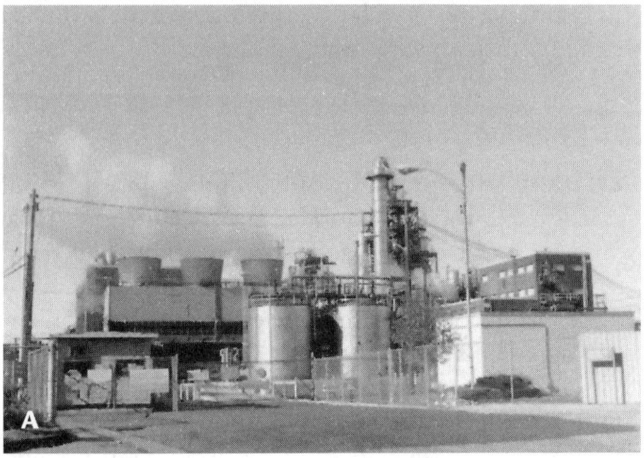

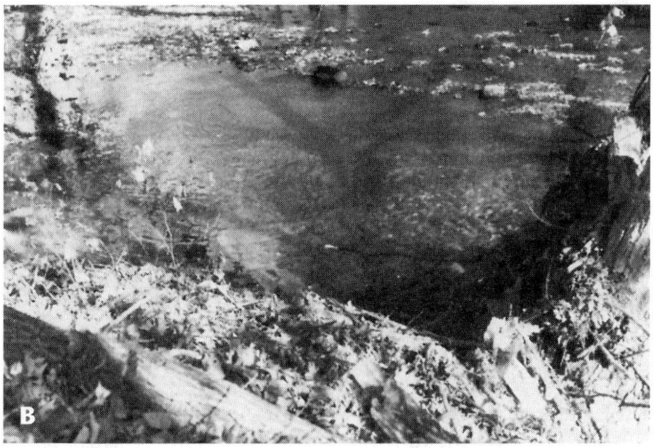

Figure 29-3 • *Two of the various types of pollution that alter safety conditions: air pollution **(A)** and water pollution **(B)**.*

smoking, use of alcohol and illicit drugs, sexual promiscuity, and poor dietary practices also impair safety. These practices may result from ignorance of risks, addiction, or lack of concern for health and safety.

Manifestations of Altered Safety

Altered safety is manifested in a variety of accidents and illnesses. Any accident or illness that causes harm and could have been prevented is a manifestation of altered safety. Accidents include falls, fires, burns, poisoning, suffocation, electrical shock, radiation exposure, infection, stress-related illness, and motor vehicle accidents. Illnesses attributed to altered safety include infection, respiratory problems, allergies, and the effects of pollution.

Falls

Falls are common inside and outside the healthcare environment and in very young, ill, or disoriented people. Falls often result in pain, permanent disability, and even death; in the elderly, they may result in hip fracture. Falls were the second leading cause of accidental death overall in the United States in 1991, and the leading cause of accidental death in people aged 79 and older (National Safety Council, 1994). Variables that increase a client's risk for falls include weakness, decreased mobility of the lower extremities, sleeplessness, incontinence, confusion, depression, and substance abuse (Easterling, 1990).

A common scenario for falls involves the elderly or impaired client who falls on the way to the bathroom at night. The client may be disoriented at night and not see obstacles cluttering the path from the bed to the bathroom. Falls at home commonly involve stairways. Poor lighting, obstacles on the stairs, or slippery or poorly repaired steps contribute to falls in the home.

Fires

Fires are potentially lethal in the healthcare environment and in the home. They may be caused by careless smoking practices, faulty electrical equipment, not attending to food cooking on the stove, the use of candles or kerosene heaters for heat, or children playing with matches. Clients in the healthcare environment are especially at risk for injury because they may be incapacitated and unable to flee the area without assistance.

Flammable gases, such as oxygen and anesthetic agents, contribute to the risk of fires in the healthcare environment. Commonly used electrical equipment, such as monitors, heating or cooling units, or respiratory therapy equipment, may malfunction or be used improperly, causing sparks that ignite linens easily in the presence of oxygen. Regular servicing of and education about electrical equipment and strict smoking policies in the healthcare environment may help reduce the risk of fires.

Grease fires originating from careless cooking practices are common in the home. Stoves in use may be left unattended and splattering grease may easily be ignited by a high flame. These fires may spread to curtains, kitchen cabinets, and clothing. Children left unsupervised near stoves contribute to the risk of kitchen fires.

Four classes of fires exist, based on the type of material burning:

- Class A: paper, wood, cloth
- Class B: flammable liquids, such as fuel oil, cooking oil or grease, paint, or solvents, and gases, such anesthesia gases
- Class C: electrical fires
- Class D: combustible metals

Firefighting measures, discussed later in this chapter, vary according to fire classification.

Burns

Burns are a major cause of injury and death in the home for infants and children (National Safety Council, 1994). Children may sustain burns in the home by playing with matches or candles, pulling a tea kettle off the stove, being fed formula that is too hot, or playing outdoors without sunscreen. Burns also occur in the healthcare environment due to scalds and fires. The person with sensory impairment is at risk for scalds from hot water or steam. A person with diabetic peripheral neuropathy may place hands under or step into very hot water and not feel the excessive temperature. Burns also may be sustained from cardioversion during resuscitation efforts.

Poisoning

Poisoning occurs by ingesting, inhaling, or absorbing potentially hazardous substances (Fig. 29-4). Poisoning compromises the cardiovascular, respiratory, central nervous, hepatic, gastrointestinal, or renal systems through chemical reactions. Toddlers and young children are at risk for poisoning, as are adults with sensory impairment and communication barriers.

In the home, children may ingest household cleansers or medicines, such as acetaminophen or aspirin. Adolescents and young adults frequently experiment with alcohol and drugs and may overdose inadvertently or attempt suicide. The older adult may ingest an overdose of medication because of mental impairment or difficulty reading the label from poor eyesight, illiteracy, or language barrier. Plants, pesticides, and paint products are potential household poisons. Improper storage and labeling of medications and household products contribute to poisoning accidents (see the display on common home toxins).

Poisoning may occur in the healthcare environment when pharmaceutical products are administered improperly. They may be given to the wrong client, in excessive dosage, or by the wrong route. Cardiac medications, narcotics, cancer chemotherapy, and intravenous medications are all potentially lethal. Short cuts taken when preparing and administering medications contribute to errors.

Suffocation

Suffocation or **asphyxiation** occurs due to drowning, smothering, strangling, airway obstruction, or entrapment in a confined space. Drowning was the fifth most common cause of accidental death in United States in 1991 (National Safety Council, 1994) and usually occurs in children.

Suffocations in the home include an infant suffocating in a pillow or blanket, toddlers strangling by a shoulder harness or clothesline, older adults choking on poorly chewed meat, a child trapped in an abandoned

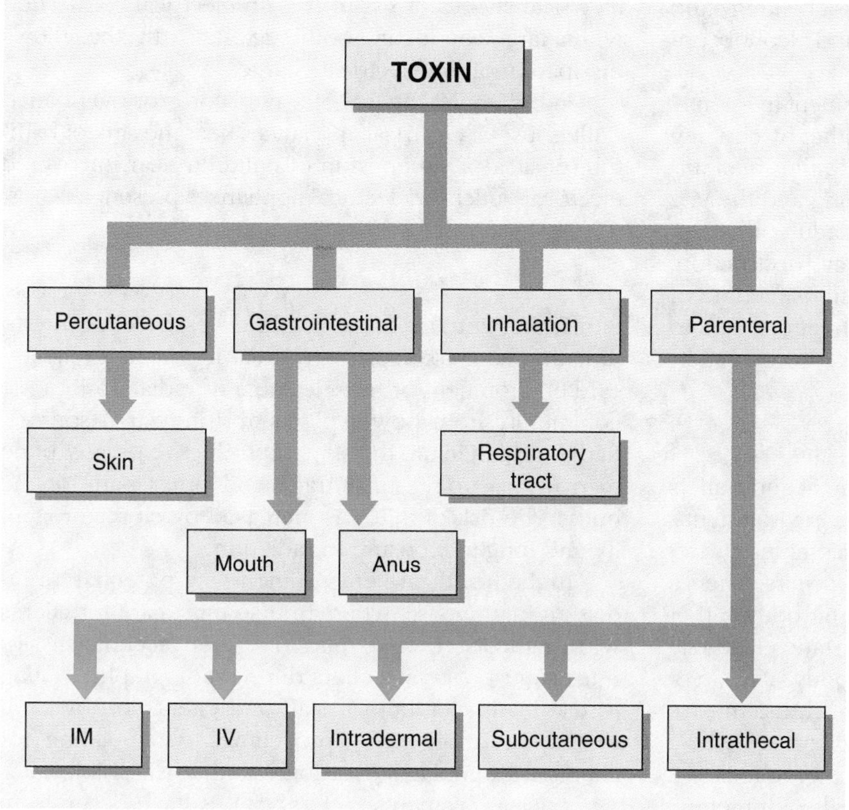

Figure 29-4 • *Routes by which toxins may enter the body.*

Common Home Toxins

Living Room/Den	Kitchen/Laundry
Air freshener	Scouring powder, ammonia
Glass cleaner	Oven cleaner, drain cleaner
Rug and upholstery shampoo	Dishwashing detergent
Houseplant insecticides	Moth balls
Flea collar, bomb	Bleach
Furniture polish	Metal polish
Permanent ink markers	Insect spray, rodent killer
Typewriter correction fluid	Laundry detergent
Carbonless copy paper	Spot remover
Bathroom	***Garage/Basement***
Toilet bowl cleaner	Latex, oil-base paints
Disinfectant	Paint stripper
Mildew remover	Wood preservative
Medicines	Adhesives, glues, epoxys
Hairspray	Herbicides, insecticides
Hair color	Insect repellents, poisons
Home permanent	Fertilizers
Nail polish/remover	Gasoline, fuels
Lice/flea shampoo	Other chemicals

refrigerator, and an infant drowning in a bathtub. Drownings occur in bodies of water, pools, bathtubs, and even large pails of water. Lack of supervision, hazardous swimming conditions, careless boating and water sports, and impairment by drugs and alcohol contribute to the risk of drowning.

Suffocation in the healthcare environment frequently occurs because of airway obstruction, either by choking on foreign objects or aspirating fluid into the small airways of the lungs. Impairment of chewing and the gag reflex, which usually occur in the older adult or neurologically impaired client, cause airway obstruction. Improperly fitting dentures and overzealous feeding of the elderly or neurologically impaired client can lead to choking and aspiration.

Electrical Shock

Electrical hazards from electrical equipment and outlets are common in the home and healthcare environments. Lighting and electric power lines in the community create a threat as well. **Electrical shock** occurs when a current travels to the ground through the body rather than through electrical wiring or from static electricity that builds up on the surface of the body. A macroshock may cause superficial and deep burns, muscle contractions, and cardiac and respiratory arrest.

In the healthcare environment, electrical shock is a danger because of the abundant electrical equipment in proximity to the client. Water from a spilled water pitcher, diaphoretic skin, or a leaking intravenous line increase the conduction of electricity. Three-pronged plugs that ground electrical equipment help prevent electrical shocks. A **ground** is an electrical connection with a large conducting body (eg, the earth) that allows dissipation of the electrical charge.

In the home, the use of frayed cords or overloaded outlets, use of electrical appliances near the sink or bathtub, or lack of supervision of children near uncovered electrical outlets or electrical appliances present hazards.

Radiation Injury

Radiation injury may occur from excessive exposure to radiation used to diagnose or treat illness in the heathcare environment or from leakage of radiation into the community from power plants and industrial sources. Radiation can injure the skin, reproductive organs, bone marrow, gastrointestinal tract, and other parts of the body. The risk of injury is increased by closer proximity and longer exposure to radiation.

In the healthcare environment, the potential for radiation injury exists when a nurse must care for clients with radioactive implants, or when technicians or nurses must restrain a client during radiography. Failing to use lead shielding for staff and clients and not following radiation safety procedures when caring for clients with implants contribute to the risk of injury.

Nuclear accidents and exposures have occurred in communities. In such cases, large groups of people are at risk for injury. Psychological stress may be incurred even if physical injury is avoided. Federal agencies, such as the Nuclear Regulatory Commission, are primarily responsible for establishing and enforcing guidelines for radiation safety.

Infection

Infection may occur in the healthcare environment or at home when safety against the transmission of microorganisms is altered. Infectious illnesses include gastroenteritis, hepatitis, tuberculosis, sexually transmitted diseases, and Lyme disease. Practices in the home that place a person at risk for infection are unsafe sex, lack of immunization, improper food preparation, and poor hygiene. Community problems, such as water supply contaminated by sewage or tick infestations near residential areas, also may cause infection. Nosocomial infections include urinary tract infections, pneumonia, hepatitis, and gastroenteritis. Debilitated clients, clients on mechanical ventilators, and those with chronic illnesses are at risk for nosocomial infection. Poor handwashing practices, lack of asepsis for invasive procedures, and lack of isolation precautions contribute to nosocomial infections.

Respiratory problems may result from unsafe air pollution levels in the community or occupational exposure to dust, asbestos, or other airborne substances. Passive smoke inhalation from living or working with those who smoke cigarettes is a recognized potential cause of respiratory disease. Cigarette smoking and asbestos exposure have been linked to lung cancer, and smog and dust worsen respiratory allergy symptoms and cause chronic bronchitis. Coal dust from mining causes fibrosis of the lungs, known as "black lung." OSHA has established guidelines to prevent injury to workers from pollutants.

Stress-Related Illnesses

Stress-related illnesses include peptic ulcer disease, anxiety, depression, and psoriasis.

Fear of the environment, caused by feeling unsafe and insecure at home and in the healthcare environment, can lead to stress-related illnesses. Unfamiliar surroundings, invasive procedures, and absence of close family members and friends contribute to client stress in the healthcare environment. Competent, caring nurses can alleviate much of the client's stress. Stress-related illnesses can develop outside the healthcare environment due to noise, crime in the community, and fear of environmental hazards. Community action groups help people work together to overcome these safety concerns and avoid undue stress.

Motor Vehicle Accidents

Motor vehicle accidents often occur because of hazardous driving practices. They may involve one or more drivers or passengers, bicycle riders, skateboarders, and pedestrians.

Motor vehicle accidents are the leading cause of accidental death in the United States, causing 49,000 deaths in 1991 (National Safety Council, 1994). Motor vehicle accidents also cause permanent disability, pain, and suffering. Factors that contribute to the risk of motor vehicle accident deaths include lack of defensive driving techniques, failure of bicycle riders and skateboarders to use helmets, and use of alcohol and other substances that cause impairment while driving. At least 24,000 people die and 534,000 are injured in alcohol-related motor vehicle accidents each year. More than half of the fatalities from motor vehicle accidents are alcohol-related (National Safety Council, 1994).

Impact of Safety Dysfunction on Activities of Daily Living

Many people, intentionally or as a result of physiologic dysfunction, behave in unsafe ways. Depending on the source of safety concern, the activities of daily living of the person and family will be affected correspondingly. A person's inability to complete activities of daily living safely indicates the need for nursing intervention. Interference with the ability to perform personal hygiene, prepare meals, participate in activities, and engage in usual vocational or career activities may be the outcome of altered safety. Loss of income or increased expenses may result from lost workdays and the need to purchase equipment or to hire people to assist with care or other activities of daily living.

Individual Considerations

The person who does not feel safe and secure may fear some of the activities essential for daily living. Fear of falls, fires, accidents on the job, or crime in the community may impair normal functioning. Fear may be generated from real or imagined safety hazards and may actually contribute to altered safety by increasing stress and anxiety. Emotional tension may impair perception and judgment, making a person accident-prone.

Altered safety may lead to social isolation. Rather than risk harm from potential safety hazards, the person may avoid activities and contact with others. Staying at home, where the person feels safest, isolates him or her from support systems.

Nutritional deficits may arise from contaminated food and water that are not safe to consume, fear of disease from polluted or contaminated food or water, or inability to shop for food due to fear of crime or falls outside the home. Many older adults have difficulty shopping for food and preparing balanced meals, resulting in weight loss and vitamin and iron deficiencies.

Altered safety may result in loss of sleep and rest due to anxiety and fear of potential danger. The person remains vigilant to safety hazards in the environment, preventing normal relaxation activities and proper sleep at night. Lack of sleep leads to poor job performance and loss of interest in recreation and sex.

Altered safety may impair self-concept. People may believe they are accident-prone, which is causing them to perform poorly at their job or sports activities; they may feel unworthy of enjoying usual activities. Problems in self-concept and self-esteem can lead to substance abuse and personality disorders (Freiberg, 1992).

Family Considerations

The family also fears that its family member may not be the person he or she was before the event that affected him or her. For example, if the event that endangered safety was related to employment, the family may fear that the person will not be able to return to work or find work due to the feelings of fear and the anxiety engendered by that memory or disability. This may disrupt the economy and financial support of the family.

If an injured person avoids activities and spends an inordinate amount of time at home, the family also will feel the effects of isolation. The family may assume greater responsibility for providing stimulation for the person, causing them to isolate themselves from their outside support systems.

Family members may help prevent nutritional deficits in the individual by providing the physical means of providing food and the social atmosphere to encourage eating. If, however, the affected individual has been the primary food provider and preparer, the family may face problems with ability to afford or obtain food and with preparation of meals.

If the sleep and rest of the affected individual is disrupted, the family's sleep and rest also may be interrupted, particularly that of the primary caregiver. If the caregiver does not get enough sleep and rest, taking care of the individual during the day becomes increasingly difficult and may predispose the caregiver to potential lack of safety.

The family may need to provide extra support and encouragement to the family member who has lost self-confidence. If the person is not or fears not performing well at work or in leisure activities, he or she may be reluctant to resume an active lifestyle. If poor self-concept progresses to depression, the family has a more serious problem to handle.

Assessment

Assessment of a person's ability to function safely involves careful investigation of individual and environmental aspects of their lives. Questions about safety reveal the ways people act in their home and in public. The nurse who builds trust by being nonjudgmental and supportive will elicit the most accurate information.

Subjective Data

Assessment of the person with a potential for altered safety begins with a careful investigation of the person's concerns or perception of hazards, including the accident and injury history. The accident-prone person often reports a history of falls, bruises, broken bones, burns, cuts, scratches, and restricted activity. The pattern of past injuries is important; accidents are often related to periods of emotional stress, fatigue, or diminishing health. People may share their fears about unsafe behaviors and concerns about the potential for injury. Many people are aware of their unsafe behaviors and will share this information if nonjudgmental assistance is offered.

Functional Pattern Identification

Current safety practices or plans for management of hazards are part of the assessment. The nurse may consider the following:

Does the person use appropriate restraints when in a car?
Can the person read traffic signs and danger warnings?
Does a child have a child-proofed home?
Does the person have up-to-date immunizations?

Keeping in mind the special concerns for each age group allows the nurse to direct questions appropriately. Recent changes in the environment (home, school, workplace), the support system (divorce, a change in caregivers, death of family member), or developmental stage (transition from infant to toddler) should alert the nurse to explore these areas. Data may need to be gathered not only from the client but also from his or her family, caregivers, referring health professionals, and others to obtain a clear picture of his or her safety. Data must be solicited from sources other than the client with the client's permission, unless he or she is underage or declared incompetent. This approach ensures client confidentiality and promotes trust.

Risk Identification

Current safety concerns must take into account the person's reason for seeking healthcare. A recent change in health status related to cognition, perception, sensation, or activity and exercise may have placed the person at risk for injury. The nurse should explore these areas fully and question the person about occupation, home environment, lifestyle, habits, and lack of knowledge of safety practices that may put him or her at risk. What

Therapeutic Dialogue
Safety Assessment

Scenes for Thought

Mrs. Jennie Adobo is 45 years old and has been your client for 6 months. During that time, you, Martha Davis, a community health nurse, have noticed that Jennie's small house has become increasingly cluttered with newspapers, saved paper bags, plastic bags, clean rags, and so forth. Everything is clean and orderly, but the piles seem to be growing at an alarming rate, especially since Jennie's husband left her and her two adolescent children. Jennie has controlled hypertension and is working with you on controlling her diabetes through diet.

Effective

Nurse: *Hi, Jennie. How are you this week? (Acknowledging patient by name.)*
Client: *Not too good, Martha. I can't seem to get enough sleep or enough to eat lately.* Fidgets with pieces of string she's winding into a ball.
Nurse: *Tell me more about that, Jennie. (Taking blood pressure, keeping an eye on Jennie's face.)*
Client: *It's just so hard for me to go to sleep at night. I hear noises and the sirens go off, and I just can't sleep.* Sounds annoyed.
Nurse: *Sounds difficult for you. How long has this been going on? (Putting away the cuff and sitting down facing her.)*
Client: *Since he went away.* Starts to cry.
Nurse: *That's been 2 months now, hasn't it? (Jennie nods.) Anything else you've noticed besides the sleeping problem? (Sits quietly watching Jennie.)*
Client: *I can't eat. I have no appetite.* Still fiddling with the string.
Nurse: *I noticed that you're looking a little thinner. How much weight have you lost?*
Client: *About 10 pounds. Actually, I needed to lose the weight, but not this way.* Crying.
Nurse: *Something else I've noticed, you've collected a lot more bags and stuff since the last time I was here. Can you tell me about that?*
Client: *I just can't throw them away. We may need them. He's not sending any money. We could sell them and get money to eat!* Sounds a little panicky.
Nurse: *You really do seem worried about a lot of things, Jennie. Would it help if we talked about them one at a time? I think we can work together on some resources to help you with the problems you're having.*
Client: *Okay.* Wipes her eyes. *I need some help; I can see that. I'm not used to having all these problems all at once.*

Less Effective

Nurse: *Hi Jennie, how are you this week? (Acknowledging patient by name.)*
Client: *Not too good, Martha. I can't seem to get enough sleep or enough to eat lately.* Fidgeting with string she's winding into a ball.
Nurse: *Let me just get your blood pressure and do a glucose test on you for a minute. (Does the procedures, concentrating on getting the readings correctly. Jennie watches fearfully.)*
Nurse: *Everything seems to be okay with your pressure and blood sugar. Especially since you seem to have lost some weight. How much would you say you've lost? (Putting the equipment away and smiling at Jennie.)*
Client: *About 10 pounds, I think. That is good, isn't it? My husband will be so glad when he comes back. He was always saying I should lose some weight.* Starts to cry and wring her hands.
Nurse: *Now, don't you worry. Everything will be just fine. Your pressure and sugar are down, you look much better than you did with the weight you lost, and I know your kids are helping out with jobs. You'll see. Is there anything else you'd like to talk about? (As she packs up the equipment bag.)*
Client: *No, I'll be fine. I just need to look on the bright side.* Smiles with her lips.
Nurse: *That's the ticket. I'll see you in a couple of weeks. Stay well!*

Critical Thinking Challenges

• Analyze intrinsic and extrinsic factors that are affecting Jennie's behavior with respect to the accumulation of bags, string, and so forth. • Detect the safety hazards associated with these items. • Determine what the first nurse attended to that the second nurse did not. • Identify with what common human emotion insomnia, anorexia, weeping, and sadness are associated. • Predict what the second nurse might discover when she returns in 2 weeks.

medications does the person take? Do side effects, such as drowsiness or dizziness, contribute to injury?

It also is the nurse's responsibility to assess for injuries related to abuse or neglect. This skill requires sensitivity and the ability to question the probability of explanations offered for injuries. Often it is essential to confer with other health professionals, and a diagnostic workup may be ordered (see section on Physiologic Assessment). If injuries seem disproportionate to the reported cause or occur with unexpected frequency, further investigation is warranted. No age group is immune to abuse or neglect, and people with higher dependency needs are at higher risk. The nurse should keep in mind that the highest risk groups include children, the elderly, the developmentally disabled, and the debilitated.

Dysfunction Identification

Nurses may determine dysfunctional patterns of safety when the person reports serious, preventable injury or a recent change in ability to participate safely in the activities of daily living. A dysfunctional pattern also may be evident in the presence of unsafe behaviors, observed by the nurse or described by the client. Using specialized knowledge, the healthcare team may determine that the person is at risk for injury, illness, or infection because of unsafe behaviors or physiologic dysfunction. Unless the client shares a concern for preventing injury, illness, or infection, there may be no agreement on the existence of a dysfunctional pattern. The nurse must help the client realize the importance of safety before safety dysfunction can be changed.

As part of the nursing health history, the nurse asks about previous injuries, accidents, and hospitalizations. The nurse should find out about the cause of these accidents and if any unsafe behavior or hazards have been rectified. For example, a client may report a history of burns from a fire. What was the cause of the fire? If smoking in bed contributed to the injury, have careless smoking practices been altered? If not, does the client realize the potential for further problems?

Objective Data

Objective data contribute to safety function assessment. Through physical assessment techniques, the nurse assesses for injuries and risk factors for injury. Physical assessment should focus on the neurologic system, skin integrity, and mobility.

Assessment of the Neurologic System

Assessment of the neurologic system includes determining mental status, sensory function, reflexes, and coordination. Assessment of mental status begins with observation of the client's appearance and general behavior. For the purposes of safety promotion, the nurse must focus attention on the client's ability to detect danger and rapidly avoid hazards. It is important to note any impulsive behavior or behavior that suggests impaired or unsafe judgment. Determine the client's level of alertness; orientation to time, person, and location; attention span; and basic cognitive function by asking simple questions. Decision-making can be determined by asking "what if" questions appropriate to the client's age and life experiences.

Examination of sensory function allows the nurse to verify the accuracy and quality of sensory input. Testing should at least include sensitivity to pinprick and light touch of the extremities. If sensation is impaired, the client is deprived of important information that may warn of danger or ongoing injury.

Nursing Assessment
Evaluation of the Healthcare Environment

Environmental Factors

- Is the bed in the lowest position?
- Are the bed wheels locked?
- Are the wheelchair brakes on?
- Is there a night light available in the room?
- Are there any obvious physical hazards in the room (wet floors, cords)?
- Are the items needed by the client within easy reach (water glass, tissues)?

Client Factors

- Can the client demonstrate correct use of the call light?
- Is the call light within reach of the client?
- What kind of footwear does the client use?
- Is the client aware of prescribed activity?
- Does the patient demonstrate physical or mental limitations (previously identified or new)?
- Is the client receiving medications that may have side effects contributing to falls (eg, hypnotics, sedatives, psychotropics, analgesics, diuretics)?
- Is the client receiving other medications or treatments that could potentially contribute to falls?

Assessment should include testing of the special senses—vision, hearing, taste, and smell. Impaired taste or smell may prevent the client from detecting spoiled food or a natural gas leak. Alterations in visual acuity may prevent the client from differentiating pills, detecting uneven terrain or stairs, and reading traffic signs or telephone numbers. Impaired hearing acuity has profound implications when it prevents the person from hearing cars, smoke alarms, or other warning sounds. The gag reflex also should be tested before feeding a client with decreased alertness or muscle strength. A review of important withdrawal reflex arcs will provide clues to the client's ability to respond reflexively to potentially harmful stimuli by pulling away from danger. Reflex arcs to test include biceps, triceps, knees, and ankles. Coordination is important to prevent falls. Coordination can be tested by observing the client's gait and repetitive motions.

In the healthcare environment, the nurse observes changes in the person's awareness and sensitivity to the environment. The person with delirium may have limited awareness of the environment and poor integration of information. He or she may move inappropriately to discontinue intravenous medication lines, feeding tubes, or ventilation tubing. Ongoing neurologic assessment of some clients is essential.

Assessment of the Integumentary System

A brief physical examination of the integument (see Chap. 21) provides important clues to the client's history of accidents or injury. The skin should be inspected for bruises, cuts, scratches, and scars. The location and distribution of the lesions should be carefully noted and correlated with the client's explanation of their origin. A bath is an excellent opportunity for the nurse to assess the integument while providing a refreshing comfort measure.

Assessment of Mobility

Mobility is assessed by inspecting and palpating the client's muscles, joints, and bones. Range-of-motion testing of joints, muscle strength testing of the extremities, and observation of ambulation are important for determining risk for altered safety. Any joint showing limited range of motion and any muscle group showing weakness places the person at a disadvantage when trying to avoid hazards. For example, the person with arthritis in the knees may be safely active on level surfaces but unable to use stairs in an emergency. Observation of posture and gait can provide valuable information about the stability of balance and the presence of sway.

Cardiovascular integrity as it relates to safety is assessed through determination of the person's mobility and activity tolerance and the presence of any conditions that impair function. If a person can walk only 50 feet before chest pain (exertional angina) becomes severe, the ability to accomplish many daily tasks is limited. If this person lives more than 50 feet from the emergency exit of his or her apartment building, escape during a fire may be impossible. Activity tolerance is usually stated as distance or duration of activity (walking, standing) before fatigue or other symptoms interrupt the activity; it is an important assessment in discharge planning for the person's safety outside the hospital environment.

Information about activities of daily living may be gathered from caregivers and family but should be supplemented by direct observation whenever possible. The nurse should observe the person moving from bed to chair or commode (and back) when appropriate; for more mobile people, the nurse should observe them walking from bedroom to bathroom, front door, kitchen, and telephone locations.

Toileting includes the ability to safely get on and off a toilet or commode. Weakness or pain in the hips may create a need for a raised toilet seat to make access safer. The nurse should assess for safe footing and transfers (position changes) in showers or at the sink and the need for grab bars or special benches if standing is difficult. Some people can get into the bathtub but are unable to get out without assistance.

Because assessment of the ability to dress safely is difficult when a person is allowed only a hospital-type gown, the nurse should observe the person dressing in street clothes before discharge. Putting clothes on in the correct sequence, maintaining balance, and avoiding pinching with zippers or shoelaces are assessed.

Nursing Diagnoses

The accepted nursing diagnosis involving alterations in safety is Risk for Injury. The nurse uses data from the subjective and objective assessments to determine if the client is at risk for injury.

Diagnostic Statement: Risk for Injury

Definition

Risk for Injury is a state in which a person is at risk for injury as a result of environmental conditions interacting with his or her adaptive and defensive resources (NANDA, 1994).

Defining Characteristics

The defining characteristics of Risk for Injury include presence of internal risk factors, such as changes in the biochemical or regulatory functions (eg, sensory dysfunction, integrative dysfunction, effector dysfunction, or tissue hypoxia); presence of malnutrition; an immune–autoimmune status; an abnormal blood profile (leukocytosis/leukopenia; altered clotting factors; thrombocytopenia; sickle cell, thalassemia; decreased hemoglobin). Physical alterations (broken skin, altered mobility) can contribute to the risk for injury by creating conditions conducive to infections or other agents that increase the potential for injury. Developmental age (physiologic, psychosocial) and psychological states (affective, orientation) can increase the risk for injury because of the possibility of errors in judgment or cognition (NANDA, 1994).

The environment can promote the risk of injury through biologic (immunization level of community, microorganisms), chemical (pollutants, poisons, drugs, pharmaceutical agents, alcohol, caffeine, nicotine, preservatives, cosmetics, dyes), nutritional (vitamins, food types), and physical (design, structure, and arrangement of community, building, or equipment) means. Additionally, the mode of transport or people or caregivers (nosocomial agents; staffing patterns; cognitive, affective, and psychomotor factors) contribute to the risk for injury (NANDA, 1994).

Related Factors

See the section Defining Charcteristics. Many factors can interact and interrelate, creating increased opportunities or risks for injury. For example, a person who is malnourished, has respiratory problems that alter the blood chemistry, and is exposed to large numbers of people with common respiratory infections will be at high risk for contracting a respiratory infection.

Related Nursing Diagnoses

Other nursing diagnoses may be evident in people at risk for safety or in those who have manifested safety dysfunction. Such nursing diagnoses include Risk for Aspiration, Ineffective Breathing Pattern, Fatigue, Risk for Infection, Risk for Poisoning, Risk for Suffocation, and Risk for Trauma. Safety dysfunction also affects the person's ability to perform activities of daily living. Nursing diagnoses in these situations may include Impaired Home Maintenance Management, Altered Nutrition: Less than body requirements, Situational Low Self Esteem, and Sleep Pattern Disturbance. Psychologic reactions may include nursing diagnoses such as Anxiety, Defensive Coping, Fear, and Hopelessness.

Outcome Identification and Planning

After the nursing diagnoses and related factors are identified, client goals and nursing interventions are identified. Common goals for the person at risk for injury include the following:

The client will identify actual and high-risk environmental hazards.
The client will demonstrate safety habits appropriate to selected environments (home, healthcare setting, workplace, community).
The client will experience a decrease in the frequency and severity of accidents.

These goals must be individualized to reflect the unique needs of the person at risk. Once individualized, goals are supported by specific nursing interventions.

Planning for nursing interventions to promote safety is based on the data gathered in the assessment and the resulting nursing diagnosis and client goals. Nursing interventions fall into two broad categories: providing a safe environment in the healthcare agency and providing safety education for the home. Nurses promote these safety interventions wherever they practice. Examples of nursing interventions commonly used to promote safety are listed in the accompanying display and are discsused in the following section of the chapter.

Implementation

The priorities of Healthy People 2000 (1990) address safety for the population by reducing unintentional injuries, improving occupational safety and health, and increasing environmental health through specific, measurable targets to be achieved by 2000.

Nursing Interventions to Promote Health and Safety

Nurses and clients interact in environments that contain some unique hazards. The nurse must provide for client safety in the healthcare environment and help the client develop personal safety habits. The Centers for Disease Control and Prevention and OSHA provide guidelines for promotion of safety. Each accredited healthcare setting must have an ongoing safety program.

Client Teaching

The same safety practices used in the healthcare environment can be used in the home. These include teaching about fire and electrical safety and prevention of falls, burns, accidents, and infectious disease.

Planning

Examples of Nursing Interventions Used in Common Safety Problems

- Provide client teaching regarding safety.
- Orient the client to the unit.
- Provide and plan for fire safety.
- Provide and plan for electrical safety.
- Provide and plan for radiation safety.
- Use infection control measures.
- Prevent falls with restraints and nonrestraint safety devices.
- Prevent falls in infants.
- Provide a safe environment at home and in the healthcare facility.
- Prevent burns.
- Prevent poisoning.
- Promote motor vehicle safety.
- Familiarize yourself with disaster plans. Be ready to participate in any emergency.
- Know how to use fire extinguishers for each type of fire.
- Be prepared to give emergency care in accidental poisoning.
- Be prepared to use cardiopulmonary resuscitation.
- File an incident report if an accident occurs.

Orientation to the Client Unit

The client is at risk for injury in the healthcare environment because of its unfamiliarity and the procedures the client undergoes. The nurse is responsible for protecting the client from environmental hazards wherever services are provided. It also is the nurse's responsibility to anticipate and minimize the adverse consequences of procedures and treatments. Many nursing policies and procedures are intended to protect the client, and a familiarity with these policies assists the nurse in the healthcare environment.

Initial nursing actions to promote safety and security in a healthcare agency are to introduce staff to the client and orient the client to the immediate environment. If the client is staying overnight, orientation includes instruction on the use of call-light system and bed controls, location of personal care supplies in the bedside stand, location of bathroom, operation of lights, and schedule of unit activities. The nurse should ensure that the room is uncluttered and free of obstacles between the bed and the bathroom. Use of a night light and bedside rails is standard. Each client should be instructed about activity limitations and assisted with ambulation as needed. The nurse who talks to the client and answers questions in a calm, confident, caring manner increases the security of the client.

Fire Safety

Healthcare agency safety programs emphasize reducing fire hazards by strictly limiting smoking, using nonflammable materials whenever possible, and practicing fire drills and firefighting skills. In the client care area, each nurse should become familiar with emergency phone numbers; the locations of fire alarms, fire extinguishers, and fire hoses; shut-off valves for oxygen and other flammable gases; evacuation equipment; and exits. Posted wall maps should show evacuation routes.

Fire extinguishers are designed to fight specific types of fires and are labeled appropriately. Table 29-1 describes the various classes of fires and the type of fire extinguisher used for each. Nurses can review these topics with children and adults as appropriate.

Electrical Safety

Nurses must protect themselves and clients from dangerous shocks by keeping hands dry when manipulating machinery, mopping up spilled fluid, ensuring all plugs are grounded (three-pronged), and reporting any equipment damage. Electrical equipment should be serviced regularly in the healthcare environment.

Radiation Safety

The area where radiation is used is marked by an international symbol (Fig. 29-5). Radioactive implants or ingestion of radioactive materials may make the client a source of radioactive contamination. Nurses routinely wear radiation detection badges to assist the institution's radiation safety officer in monitoring exposure levels. These badges are collected regularly and the exposure levels are calculated to ensure that staff are staying within safety limits of exposure. The three cardinal rules of radiation protection follow:

- Minimize time of exposure to the source.
- Maximize distance from the source.
- Use appropriate shielding.

Nursing care for radiation therapy clients must be well organized so that assistance and support are given efficiently without needless exposure of the nurse. Usually, lead shields or lead aprons are available if

Table 29-1 • Correct Fire Extinguishers to Use With Specific Classes of Fires

Class	Type of Material	Type of Fire Extinguishers
A	Paper, wood, cloth	Water (stored pressure, gas cartridge, soda acid, pump) Multipurpose dry chemical (stored) pressure, gas cartridge) Loaded stream
B	Flammable liquids, such as fuel oil, cooking oil or grease, paint, solvents; gases, such as anesthesia gases	Carbon dioxide Regular and multipurpose dry chemical (stored pressure, foam, loaded stream, gas cartridge)
C	Electrical fires	Regular and multipurpose dry chemical (stored pressure, gas cartridge) Carbon dioxide Liquefied gas
D	Combustible metals	Special dry powder

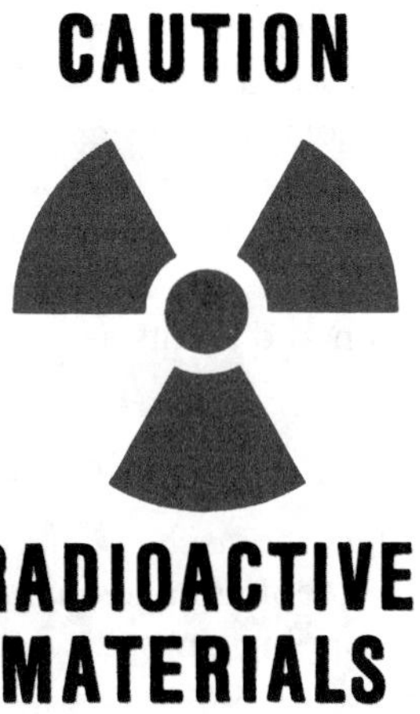

Figure 29-5 • *International Radiation Symbol.*

close contact with the client is required. Generally, gloves should be worn to prevent skin contact with any body substances (urine, stool, saliva, blood). Clients may be encouraged to do as much of their own care as possible. If admitted to a healthcare agency, a private room with private bath is essential to prevent accidental exposure of other clients. Linens should be kept in the room until the radioactive source is removed. Soiled linens, excreta, and other waste may require special labeling and disposal.

After cessation of therapy, the radiation safety officer will sweep the room with a radiation detector to assess for spills or contamination. After clearance, the room may be cleaned and linens sent to the laundry. If the client is to go home while receiving radiation therapy through an ingested substance (eg, iodine-131), the hospital radiation safety manual will list directions for protection of the family, caregivers, and home environment.

Although the risk of radiation injury in most communities is low, nurses should let the community know about the sources and effects of radiation. Greater public awareness and understanding of radioactive waste and nuclear power can lead to stricter regulation of radiation used in industry and a safer community.

Infection Control

Infection control is a high priority in the healthcare environment. Most healthcare agencies, particularly hospitals, have full-time staff, usually nurses, devoted to teaching and implementing infection control practices throughout the hospital. The principle of asepsis helps prevent the spread of microorganisms from place to place and person to person. Handwashing, disinfection, sterilization, isolation precautions, and immunization are carried out in the healthcare environment to control infection (see Chap. 25).

Immunization against infections (communicable diseases) is important for children, adults, and healthcare workers. Influenza and hepatitis B vaccines are frequently offered to healthcare employees working in close contact with clients or with clients' blood. Because there is no immunization for tuberculosis, healthcare workers are usually tested yearly for exposure. If a person has been infected with tuberculosis, treatment is implemented to prevent active illness and spread to others. With the increasing incidence of tuberculosis, this testing becomes especially important.

The nurse plays an important role in advocating timely vaccination of at-risk people. Childhood vaccination programs are mandatory in many states and should provide the child with protection from diphtheria, polio, measles, mumps, rubella, pertussis (whooping cough), and tetanus. Some of these vaccinations require booster doses throughout life. The recommendation for a tetanus booster is once every 10 years (Plotkin & Mortimer, 1988). Adults should be reminded of this, and tetanus status should be evaluated periodically, especially when a wound has been incurred. Vaccinations for influenza are generally suggested for the elderly and for people with underlying chronic disease. The influenza vaccine is changed annually to anticipate the most likely virulent strains and may need to be an annual event for those at risk. The pneumococcal vaccine is recommended for people older than 65 years or those between 2 and 65 years with asplenia, chronic illness, or immunosuppression due to illness or therapy (Plotkin & Mortimer, 1988).

Nurses also should teach sexually active adolescents and adults safe sex practices to prevent sexually transmitted diseases. These practices include abstinence, limiting the number of partners, using condoms and other barrier contraceptives, and using spermicide containing nonoxynal-9 (Burns, Robinson, & Scherger, 1988). Women should receive regular gynecologic checkups, and men and women should seek medical attention for possible exposure to or at the first sign of sexually transmitted disease.

Fall Prevention

In the healthcare environment, the nurse must ensure the client's safety from falls. The room needs to be free of clutter and well lit during transfers and ambulation, and side rails and grab bars must be firmly anchored (Fig. 29-6*A*). The floor must be nonskid, either carpeted or free of liquid. Wheelchairs, beds, commode chairs, or shower chairs must have working brakes (see Fig. 29-6*B*), be free of any sharp edges, and have a support surface that is comfortable. Clients with orthostatic hypotension should be taught to change position slowly to allow for blood pressure stabilization. Night lights are used, and the nurse should respond promptly to the call light. During daytime, the family should be encouraged to help the weak client to the bathroom, unless this is

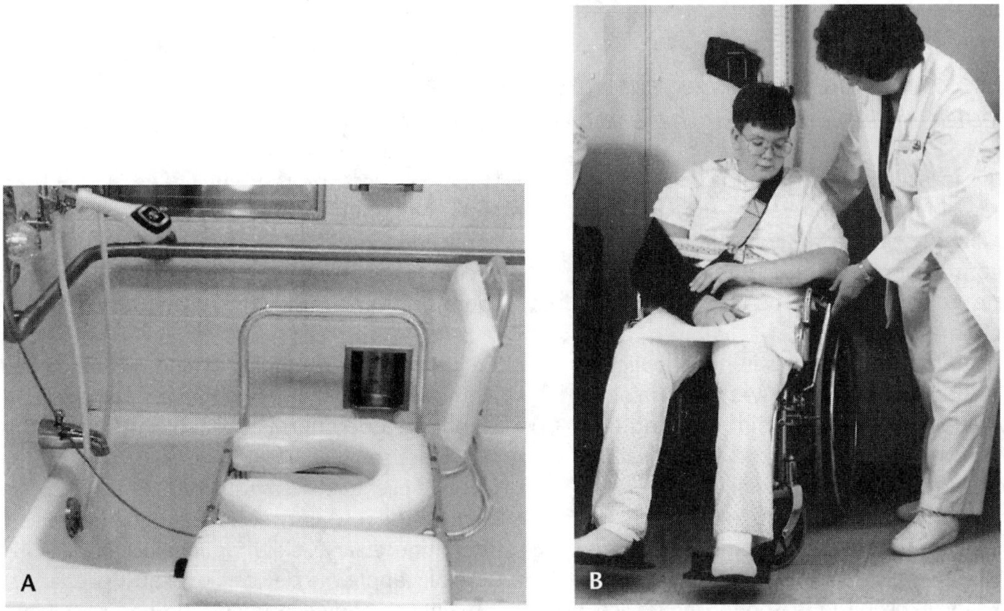

Figure 29-6 • *The healthcare facility must provide safety for the client.* ***(A)*** *This shower protects the client with grab bars, safety rails, shower seat, and transfer seat.* ***(B)*** *The nurse checks wheelchair brakes for safe use.*

not safe for the client. In some cases, two professionals are needed to support a very weak client.

Use of Restraints

A **restraint** is a protective device, material, or equipment, attached or adjacent to the person's body that restricts freedom of movement or normal access to one's body (Omnibus Budget Reconciliation Act [OBRA], 1989). Restraints may be physical, mechanical, or chemical. The latter involves medicine to relax or make a client sleep.

Generally, the use of physical restraints is not advocated; they are illegal if not used within the guidelines derived from OBRA. These guidelines require that restraints are part of the medical treatment; all less restrictive interventions are tried first; other appropriate disciplines have been consulted; and supporting documentation for their use is provided (Health Care Financing Administration, 1990). Restraints do not specifically prevent falls (Evans & Strumpf, 1990; Janelli, 1989; Powell, Mitchell-Pedersen, Fingerote, & Edmund, 1989), and in many instances, they can actually precipitate or exacerbate the risk of falls (Tideiksaar, 1993). The Food and Drug Administration (FDA, 1992) estimates that at least 100 deaths or injuries annually are associated with the use of restraints.

Restraints may be necessary, however, to limit physical activity of a client to prevent injury from a fall or to prevent movement that would disrupt therapy (eg, pulling out an intravenous line or mechanical ventilator tubing). Restraints must be used cautiously to prevent agitation, preserve dignity, prevent physical injury from the restraining device, and avoid abuse of a client's right to move freely. The accompanying display supplies information from the FDA regarding guidelines for the use of restraints. Healthcare institution guidelines should be followed regarding the use of restraints. The reason for their application must be described in the client's care record. Nurses may apply restraints in an emergency without a physician's order; however, an order should be obtained as soon as possible. The nurse also should use direct supervision and communication as much as possible to reassure and reorient the client. Use of restraints is not a substitute for vigilant nursing care, nor does it prevent falls or injuries.

Types of restraints include a jacket or vest restraint, which is worn on the client's chest and tied to the bed frame or legs of a chair, a belt restraint on stretchers or wheelchairs used in transporting, mitt or hand restraints that prevent confused clients from using their hands, wrist or ankle restraints that immobilize one or more limbs, and mummy restraints that are wrapped around a child's body to prevent movement during a procedure. Figure 29-7 gives some examples of restaints.

A common form of restraint is side rails, which are used on beds, stretchers, and other equipment. Side rails are a reminder to the client not to roll too far to the side, and they provide the client with bars to assist them when turning to the side. When used on beds, the bed must be in the lowest position with the wheels locked. Having side rails up does not replace careful and frequent observation of the client, because clients may still attempt to get out of bed by climbing over the side rails or over the foot of the bed. The need to go to the bathroom is the most frequent reason for clients trying to

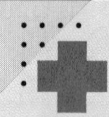

Safety Alert
FDA Recommendations To Decrease the Incidence of Deaths and Injuries With the Use of Restraints

- Assess the cause for which the restraint is being considered, develop alternatives to restraint use, and implement these alternatives before applying restraints.
- Allow the use of restraints *only* under the supervision of a licensed healthcare provider and for a strictly defined period of time.
- Define and communicate a clear institutional policy on the use of restraints (eg, alternatives to restraint use, appropriate conditions for restraint use, length of wear time). This written policy also should be available for any client/resident or any family member.
- Obtain informed consent from client/resident or guardian prior to use. Clients have the right to be free from restraints. However, if it is determined that a restraint is necessary, explain the reason for the device to the client/resident and guardian to prevent misinterpretation and to ensure cooperation.
- Display instructions for use in a highly visible location and interpret in foreign languages as necessary.
- Provide in-service training for staff as regularly as possible, which should include a return demonstration of proper application of restraints.
- Prior to use, read and follow the manufacturer's directions for use.
- Select the type of restraint that is appropriate to the client's condition.
- Use the correct size restraint.
- Note the "front" and "back" of the restraint, and apply correctly.
- Secure restraints designed for use in bed to the bed springs or frame, *never* to the mattress or the bed rails.
- Tie knots with appropriate hitches so that they may be released quickly.
- Emphasize good nursing, rehabilitative, and client care practices.
- Observe clients in restraints frequently.
- Remove the restraints at least every 2 hours and more often if necessary. Allow for activities of daily living.
- Carefully apply the device and adjust properly so that it maintains body alignment and ensures client comfort.
- Continue assessment even after a restraint is used, and discontinue use as soon as feasible. Restraint use should be considered a temporary solution to a situation.
- Clearly document in the client's record the medical reason for use of the restraint, the type selected, and the length of time for treatment.
- Follow local and state laws regarding the use of protective restraint devices.

From *Food and Drug Administration* (1992). *FDA safety alert: Potential hazards with restraint devices.* Rockville MD: Department of Health and Human Services.

get out of bed, no matter what kind of restraint may be in place. Anticipating the client's need to urinate is the primary safety measure that nurses can use.

Knots Used for Restraints. Many restraints require tying to an object: the bed, a chair, or a wheelchair. Any knot should be tied so the client cannot release it, but the healthcare provider can release it quickly in an emergency. Knots and restraints are tied to the movable part of the bed frame and not the side rails or mattress. Two basic types of knots can be used; they are both hitches. (A square knot is not used for restraints, but it is a useful knot in first aid and bandaging.) Directions for tying these knots are given here and illustrated in Figure 29-8.

Half-Hitch or Half-Bow Knot. A half-hitch is safer than a traditional knot. It may be used with wheelchairs or on beds. The strap is wrapped twice around the frame. A loop is made by folding the remainder of the strap in half. The middle of this loop is slipped under the part wrapped around the frame and tightened. A single knot will be formed which can be slipped open easily for release. The free end must be kept out of the reach of the client, especially children.

Clove-Hitch Knot. A clove-hitch may be used with limb restraints. A figure 8 is made with the free ends extending in each direction. The loops are picked up and brought together and then slipped over the padded extremity. Adjustments are made so there is one fingerbreadth between the extremity and restriant. Although it cannot be released as easily as the half-hitch, it can be cut easily in an emergency.

Nonrestraint Safety Devices

Increasingly, nonrestraint safety environments and devices are being developed and used to increase client safety without using typical restraints. These include alarm systems and pressure devices. Pressure devices are placed on the bed under the client's back. When the person sits up, an alarm is triggered to alert the staff that the client is attempting to get out of bed. Other alarm devices allow the person free movement in bed but trigger an alarm if the person is about to transfer from the

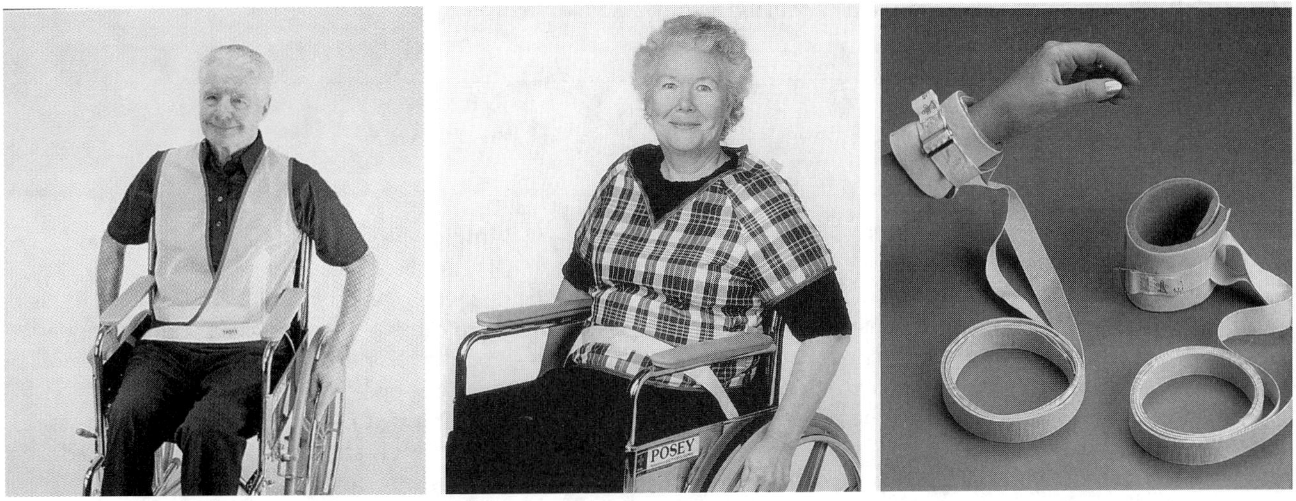

Crisscross vest *Jacket restraint* *Foam limb holder*

Examples of Pediatric Restraints

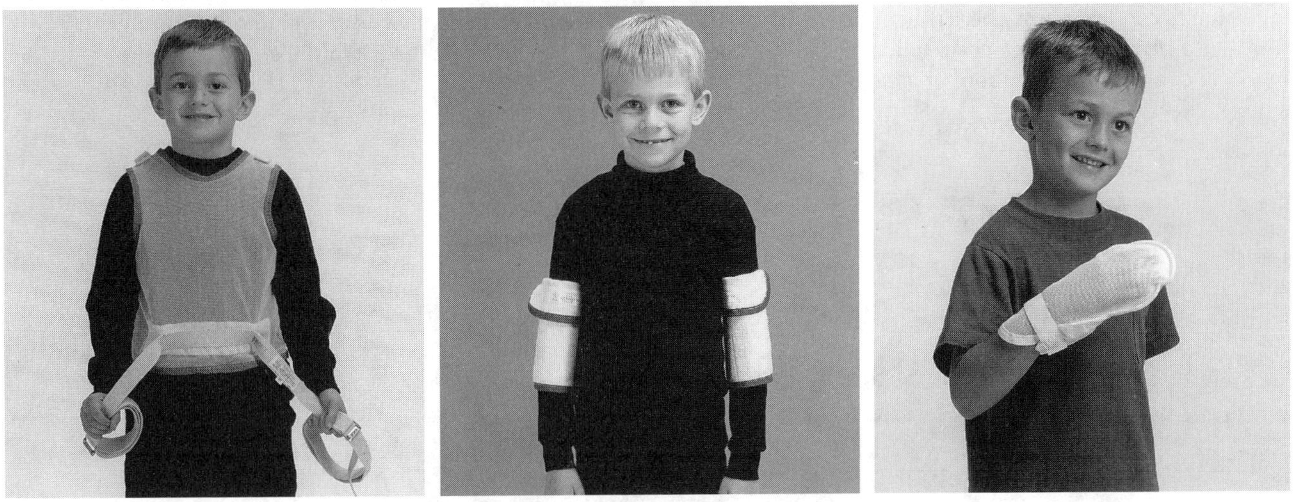

Jacket *Elbow* *Mitt*

Figure 29-7 *• Common restraints. (Product photos provided by Posey Company, Arcadia, CA.)*

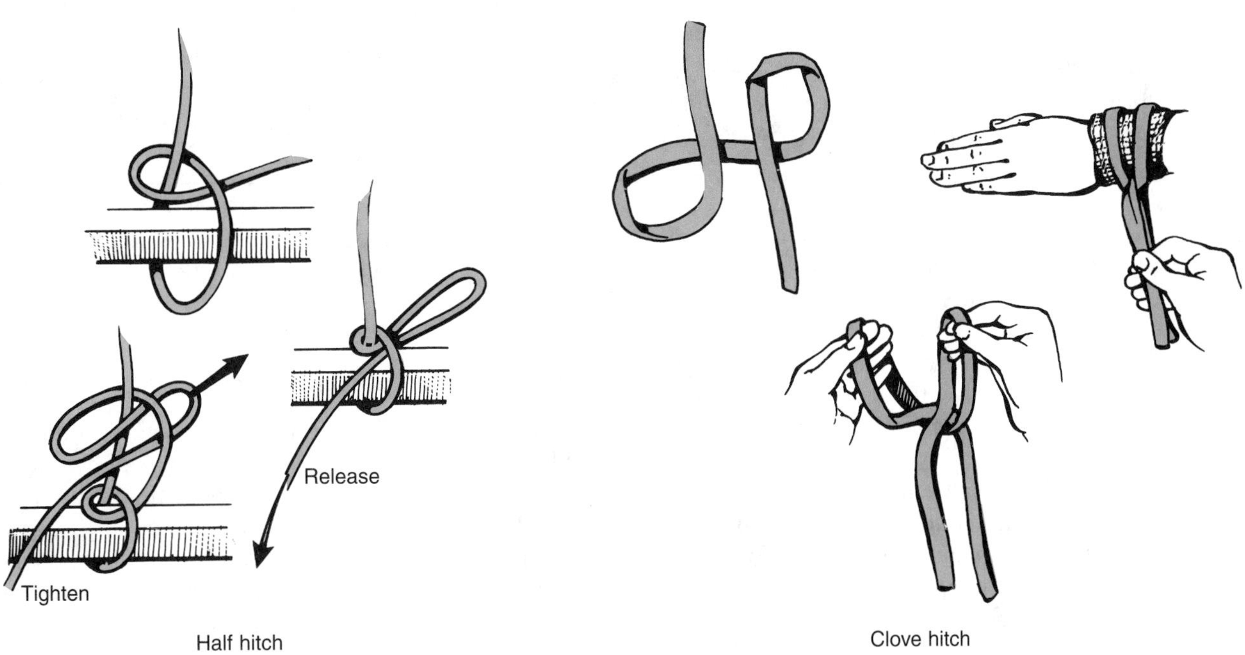

Figure 29-8 *• Two types of hitch knots used with restraints.*

Nursing Care Guidelines
Alternatives to Restraints

- Use alternatives to restraints (ie, less restrictive devices) before resorting to restraints.
- Assess and address reasons for agitation or confusion to find another solution to the problem.
- Keep the client's room orderly. The bed should be lowered and overbed table and chairs pushed out of the way so the client will not fall if he or she gets up during the night.
- Provide sufficient light so the client can see, especially when the surroundings are strange.
- Place the client in a room near the nurses' station if the client needs frequent observation or supervision. Nurses can take turns checking on the client.
- Use a barrier, such as a chair, to inhibit the client from wandering out of the room or area.
- Provide warm milk, soothing music, or a back massage to help the client relax and sleep.
- Use side rails when the client is in bed. However, if the client tends to climb over the rails, this can be unsafe.
- Provide a rocking chair during the day to help the client use up some energy.
- Use alarm systems that notify the nurse or nurses' station when the client is attempting to get out of bed or out of a chair.
- Use nonslip matting to hold cushions in place on chairs so the client will not slip off the chair.
- Use a pelvic-tilt wedge cushion to maintain proper seating alignment while preventing sliding by gently tilting the resident back in the chair.

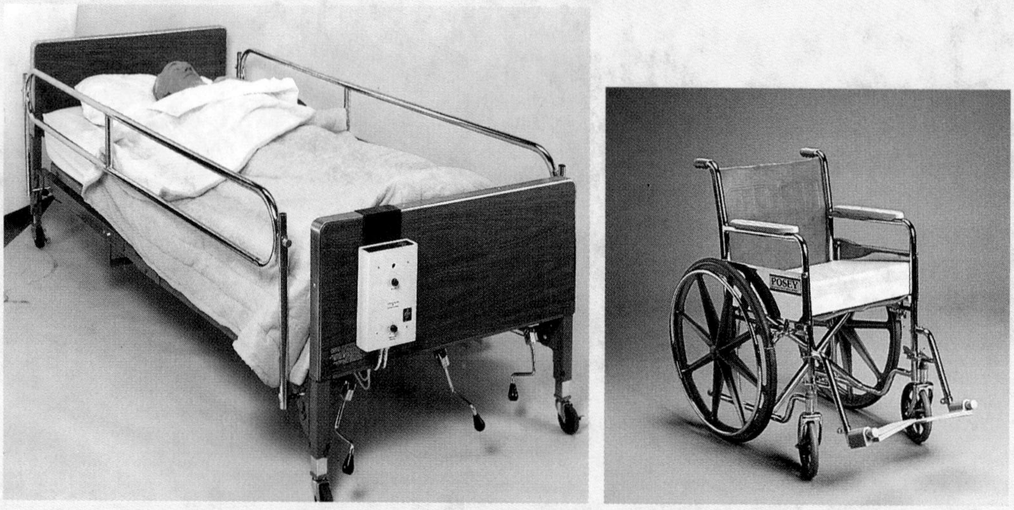

Side rails can be considered a restraint and a nonrestraint. A pelvic tilt (wedge) cushion helps maintain proper seating alignment and prevents sliding by gently tilting the client back. (Product photos provided by Posey Company, Arcadia CA.)

bed. Special cushions may be placed on chairs that are comfortable for the person to sit on, but because of the angle of the cushion and the material inside the cushion, it is extremely difficult for the client to rise without assistance. Both of these safety devices permit safety without restraints and involve the nurse or caregiver when the client ambulates, thereby improving the safety of the client.

With careful and imaginative attention to the client's environment, nurses can reduce environmental risks and improve safety. Anticipating client needs for assistance with transfers, responding to the need to go to the bathroom, or changing position or location are ways the nurse can help the client prevent falls and reduce the need for restraints (Brower, 1991; Haley, Nagy, & Roberts, 1991; Tideiksaar, 1993). Guidelines for using alternatives to restraints are listed in the accompanying display.

Prevention of Falls in Infancy

Nurses should educate parents about infants' potential for falling. Prevention includes not leaving an infant unattended in a bath, bed, or table where he or she may roll or fall off; keeping the crib side rails up; using guard rails or gates at the top and bottom of the stairs when the infant crawls; and supervising the child in a jumper, swing, or high chair. Walkers are particularly dangerous for toddlers, and many have been withdrawn from the market. Nurses should teach adults, especially older adults, to remove throw rugs, make sure stairways are well lighted and repaired, remove clutter from stairways and walkways, install handrails wherever needed, avoid use of unstable ladders and step stools, never attempt to do anything beyond reach or physical ability, and clean up damp areas promptly.

Childhood Safety

The care of children in the healthcare environment requires special safety precautions. High staff-to-client ratios, use of cribs and beds with side rails, carpeting on the floor, play areas with age-appropriate toys and furnishings, locked medications and supply rooms, and protected exits contribute to safety.

Parents should be made aware of the need to childproof the home and to supervise children in any potentially hazardous area outside the home (see Client Teaching display). Parents should be taught to use only cribs and other infant equipment approved by the U.S. Consumer Products Safety Commission or other regulatory agency. The use of older equipment that is worn or poorly designed may present a hazard. Figure 29-2 shows some safety features for raising children. Toys should be age appropriate. (Many of these factors are discussed in the section Lifespan Considerations.)

Nurses should make parents aware that drowning not only occurs in pools but also in bathtubs and other sources of water around the home. Pools should be fenced in, and children of all ages should be supervised at pools and beaches. Children should wear life jackets for boating and fishing and should be warned not to ice skate or play on ice unless ice thickness is proven safe. Infants and toddlers should never be left unattended in the bathtub or kiddie pools. Pails or basins of water should not be left in an infant's or toddler's reach.

Children should be taught bicycle safety. Helmets should be worn to protect against head injury in the event of a fall. Proper signaling and illumination of the child and bicycle at night are important for accident prevention. Parents should be taught to check for small children riding low vehicles before driving a car out of a driveway or parking space. Children should be warned about riding in streets or near driveways.

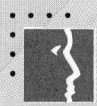

> **Client Teaching**
> *Childproofing the Home*
>
> *Instruct the client as follows:*
>
> - *Cover unused electrical outlets with safety plugs to prevent fingers from being poked into them.*
> - *Place electrical cords and handles of pots and appliances out of reach to avoid having appliances or substances pulled over.*
> - *Secure screens on all windows within reach of a toddler on a chair.*
> - *Place all plastic bags out of reach to avoid accidental suffocation.*
> - *Cover controls of appliances with tamper-proof locks or covers to prevent burns and other injuries.*
> - *Keep matches and cigarette lighters out of reach to prohibit fires caused by accident or curiosity.*
> - *Lock up potentially toxic substances to deter accidental swallowing.*
> - *Keep hot water temperature at less than 115°F to prevent scalds and burns.*
> - *Place nonskid mats in showers or tubs and bath mats on floor.*
> - *Remove doors from unused refrigerators and freezers to prevent entrapment and asphyxiation.*
> - *Fence yards for outdoor play within safe perimeters.*

Burn Prevention

Burns can be prevented in the healthcare environment by testing bath water for temperature when the client has sensory impairment; checking heating pads, heat lamps, and other electrical equipment to be sure they are functioning properly; assisting clients when handling hot beverages as needed; and not allowing clients to smoke in bed.

Nurses should teach clients with sensory impairment to monitor water temperature at home as well. The thermostat on the hot water heater may need to be adjusted. Parents should keep pot handles turned away from the front of the stove top where young children might reach. Young children should never be left to play unsupervised in the kitchen, near burning fireplaces, barbecue grills, or containers of gasoline. Parents should be reminded to apply sunscreen to children playing outdoors to prevent sunburn.

Adults should be taught never to smoke while using lighter fluid to start a charcoal fire or when filling lawnmowers with gasoline. Smoking in bed or late at night in a chair may be hazardous. Smoking materials should be properly extinguished.

Poison Prevention

Poison prevention in the healthcare environment can be accomplished primarily through safe medication preparation and administration practices. Nurses are responsible for checking that physician's orders for medications are signed and updated appropriately and that they have been transcribed accurately. The client must be identified by checking his or her identification band before administering any medication. Any significant side effects should be documented and reported to the physician.

Nursing intervention for poison prevention in the home involves education of parents (see Client Teaching display). All medications, including over-the-

Client Teaching
Prevention of Childhood Poisoning

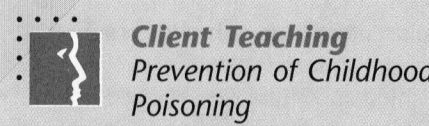

- *Maintain childproof caps on all medications and toxic products if children live in the home.*
- *Keep medications and toxic products in their original containers and out of the reach of children.*
- *Measure and give medications in well-lit areas to avoid errors in amount and type of medication.*
- *Read labels of medications carefully before administering.*
- *Destroy all medications not in use by flushing down toilet.*
- *Keep emergency drugs in the home (eg, syrup of ipecac).*
- *Have the phone number of the poison control center available.*
- *Keep cleaning products and garden chemicals out of the reach of children.*
- *Use chemical and cleaning products in well-ventilated areas.*
- *Do not mix chemicals or common household cleaning products.*
- *Remove or keep out of reach of children any houseplants or natural materials that may be poisonous to children.*

counter products, should be stored in childproof containers out of the reach of children. Parents should not treat medications as candy. Household cleansers and other potentially toxic products should be stored in childproofed or locked cupboards or on shelves out of children's reach. All household chemical products should be kept in their original containers with warning labels and emergency information intact.

All poisonous house plants should be kept out of young children's reach, and children should be supervised outdoors. Some poisonous plants include azaleas, buttercups, daffodils, mistletoe berries, philodendrons, poinsettias, potato sprouts, tomato greens, and tulip bulbs. Older children should be taught never to eat berries, mushrooms, seeds, or plants grown in the wild.

Nurses should teach people to keep poison control center phone numbers posted near telephones. An integrated system of local centers across the United States and Canada can provide emergency information whenever a substance is ingested, inhaled, or splashed in the eyes or on the skin.

Motor Vehicle Safety

Nursing intervention for motor vehicle safety involves client education about potential hazards and safety measures. Use of seat belts has greatly decreased morbidity and mortality on the highways (National Safety Council, 1994). Most states now have mandatory seat belt laws in effect.

Infants and children should be properly restrained in approved car seats when in automobiles. Infants weighing up to 18 lb need to be in a rear-facing car seat, semireclined with their heads well supported. Toddlers and preschoolers (20–60 lb) should be secured in a forward-facing car seat. Children weighing more than 60 lb need to wear a properly applied lap and shoulder harness (Slota, 1990).

Motor vehicle safety also includes maintaining a safe driving speed for road and weather conditions. Nurses have many opportunities to educate the public about the effects of alcohol on a driver. Any substance that can impair alertness and reaction time, such as antihistamines, should be avoided while driving motor vehicles.

Adolescents should be taught about the danger of riding with friends who are impaired by alcohol or drugs.

Nursing Interventions for Altered Safety

Harm to a person or group occurs when safety is not maintained. In the healthcare environment, specific nursing interventions are carried out when preventive measures fail. Nursing interventions for altered safety function include fire evacuation, emergency first aid for poisoning, administration of obstructed airway and cardiopulmonary resuscitation techniques, and filing an incident report.

Disaster Plans

Some areas of the country are prone to tornadoes, earthquakes, floods, and hurricanes. The nurse is responsible for knowing the disaster plans for such emergencies where he or she works. Understanding the plan and practicing it help the nurse remain calm in an emergency. There are two basic types of healthcare agency disasters: internal or external. Internal disasters are those in which the facility itself is in danger. Actions must be taken to protect employees and clients. In an external disaster, many people will be brought to a hospital or clinic for care after a large-scale emergency. Specific plans must be carried out when the healthcare agency or hospital is notified of any emergency.

Fire Evacuation

In the event of a fire in the client care area, nurses are responsible for determining which clients are in immediate danger. Ambulatory clients should be directed toward exits to wait in a safe area or enlisted to help evacuate bed-ridden clients. Stretchers and wheelchairs should be used, and if necessary, clients can be carried or dragged on sheets. Elevators should not be used in the event of a fire. The fire alarm should be activated and the healthcare agency's switchboard notified of the fire's location. The local fire department will be notified automatically. If the fire is small, a fire extinguisher can be used, but other interventions should not be neglected because small fires can quickly flare up out of control. Windows and doors should be closed and oxygen turned off in the area to reduce the fire's oxygen supply. Clients should be evacuated in surrounding areas, if necessary, and given wet washcloths to breathe through to reduce smoke inhalation.

Healthcare facilities are required to have fire evacuation plans with exits clearly marked. Additional staff from the facility and firefighters will respond quickly to help nurses evacuate clients. Nurses should never attempt to extinguish fires if the clients' or their own safety is in jeopardy. When evacuating clients requiring mechanical ventilation, an ambubag can be used for manual respiration. Tubes connected to suction must be clamped before disconnection, and intravenous fluids should be transported with the client.

Emergency Care in Accidental Poisoning

In the healthcare environment, ingestion of dangerous substances, overdosage, or incorrect medication can be treated as in the home. The client's physician should be notified, but if the substance is potentially toxic, the poison control center should be notified without delay. The center will require information about the specific poison (the ingredients section on the label may provide this information), quantity ingested, person's age and weight, and apparent symptoms. The nurse may be instructed to induce vomiting with syrup of ipecac if the client is not unconscious or convulsing or if the substance was not a strong corrosive or petroleum product. Doses are given in the accompanying display. The client should be positioned on his or her side or with the head placed between the legs to prevent aspiration. The nurse may gather urine, vomitus, or blood samples as instructed.

If poisonous substances have been instilled into the eye or on the skin, immediate irrigation with lukewarm water for 10 to 15 minutes may reduce harmful effects. Clothing should be removed from the skin. The person should be instructed to blink as much as possible during eye irrigation.

Nursing Care Guidelines

Doses for Inducing Emesis With Syrup of Ipecac

Pediatric

- 6–12 months—administer 10 mL orally.
- Over 1 year—administer 15 mL orally, followed by one to two glassfuls of whatever fluid the child will tolerate (ipecac is not effective on an empty stomach). Maintain activity level. Results should occur within 30 minutes.

Adult

- Administer 30 mL. The same procedure as above is applied to the adult victim.

Cardiopulmonary Resuscitation

If a client chokes, aspirates, or is found cyanotic and apneic, the nurse is responsible for initiating resuscitation efforts; see Chapter 35 for the procedure for obstructed airway and cardiopulmonary resuscitation. Electrical shock also may lead to cardiac arrest requiring cardiopulmonary resuscitation.

Filing an Incident Report

An incident report is filed when an accident occurs in the healthcare environment. It is a confidential document filed with the institution's legal, insurance, or quality assurance department for internal use only. In it, the nurse describes how an accident occurred, what the effects to the client were, and what was done for the client. Incident reports are commonly used for falls and medication errors.

In addition to filing an incident report, the nurse must enter on the client's medical record a description of the accident and effects on the client. The client's physician should be notified of the accident, and he or she will document the client's condition. The nurse does not make note of the incident report on the medical record because it is used internally. The incident report can be reviewed by the institution's attorneys in the event of a lawsuit, and it may be collected by the risk manager to see if trends of accidents in the workplace are developing.

Community-Based Nursing

Nurses promote safety interventions wherever they practice. For example, school nurses function as safety educators for school-age children. Children should be taught how to say no to drugs and how to tell anybody when they do not want to be touched. In many states, school nurses are required to report suspected child abuse. School nurses also may identify children who seem accident-prone. These children may have a neuromuscular or sensory-perceptual basis for their accidents and should be evaluated. Screening for problems with vision and hearing is especially important.

The occupational health nurse may be involved in safety education and accident prevention at the worksite. Adults often need to be taught the proper body dynamics for lifting heavy loads. For the sedentary worker, principles of body alignment and stretching may help prevent muscle strain from poor posture. Proper lighting may improve productivity and prevent eye strain. Occupational health nurses identify hazardous materials in the workplace and encourage appropriate worker protection (adequate ventilation, protective clothing and eyewear); they also develop instructional safety promotion programs to prevent back injury, on-the-job accidents, and illness.

All nurses may act as community activists and advocates for environmental safety in such areas as clean air and water; safe, well-lighted pedestrian walkways; and laws supporting seat belts, air bags, and helmet use.

Home Care Management

The nurse identifies areas in which the client is unsafe when performing essential activities of daily living. The nurse devises a plan that prepares the client, home caregivers, and the home itself for optimal safety. A display on hazards in the home is presented earlier in this chapter. Some guidelines for safety in the home are given in the accompanying display. Other health professionals, such as social workers, occupational therapists, and physical therapists, are involved in the planning process, but the nurse is often considered the most accurate source of information about the client's function in activities of daily living. The nurse observes the client engaging in transfers and mobility, toileting, hygiene, eating and feeding, and dressing. Observations made during assessments allow the nurse to anticipate the measures that need to be taken to promote safety in these activities at home (Fig. 29-9).

The nurse working with a newly disabled client in a rehabilitation facility helps the healthcare team anticipate environmental changes that may be needed after discharge. Often the client, family, or other caregivers are asked to draw a floor plan of the house, noting especially the width of doorways, configuration of the bathroom and kitchen, stairs approaching the home and within the home, and access to transportation from the home. Special equipment used during the hospitalization may need to be used in the home, and hospital beds, wheelchairs, tub benches, and mechanical lifts may not fit in the home. Early identification of the client's postdischarge equipment needs will help the family and caregivers to modify the home before the client is discharged.

Nursing Care Guidelines
for Home Safety

Throughout the Home

- Electrical cords in good repair
- Only one electrical fixture per plug
- Upholstered furniture away from heat sources: baseboards, space heaters, and so forth.
- Fireplaces screened
- Smoke detectors with operational power sources
- Adequate lighting
- Minimal clutter
- Loose carpeting tacked down
- Stair edges marked with tape or contrasting paint (especially in areas of poor lighting—basement, outdoors)
- Sturdy handrails by all stairs
- Safety glazing or glass in all glass doors and panels: visible decals will decrease chance of accidental collision

Bathroom

- Nonskid backing on bathmat
- Nonskid mat or decals for tub or shower
- Grab bars for toilet and tub if needed
- Expired medications discarded
- Hot water heated to less than 115°F

Kitchen

- Fire extinguisher in working order
- Adequate ventilation
- Liquid fuels stored away from heat sources (eg, charcoal lighter fluid)
- Expired foods discarded
- Refrigerator adequately cooled to prevent spoilage
- Pilot lights lit (gas stove or oven)

Miscellaneous

- Ladders in good repair with nonskid surface on feet and steps
- Bicycles in good repair with reflectors and brakes working
- Doors removed from unused refrigerators and freezers

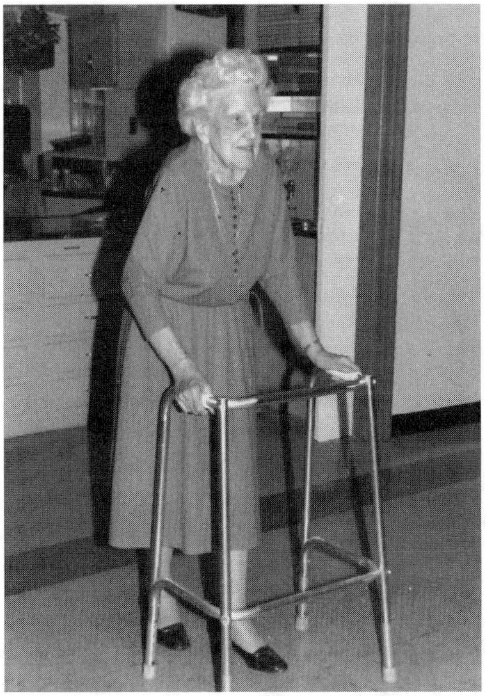

Figure 29-9 • Use of a walker promotes safety when walking. The nurse may observe the client and her ability to use the walker before she is discharged.

Support Systems for the Home

Essential to overall safety is the support system. Actively involved caregivers or supportive friends can provide assistance with assessing the availability of the caregivers, their level of desired participation, and their own capacity for safe judgment. The nurse should identify who will be providing care and whether they will be available occasionally, part-time, or 24 hours a day. The nurse must ask what care the caregivers can provide: assistance with mobility and transfers; with other activities of daily living (toileting, hygiene, dressing, eating); with laundry, shopping, and bill paying; or with supervision during inactive times. The nurse should determine what training the caregivers need to provide safe care. A home health referral may be needed to allow a home health nurse to visit the client and caregivers in the home and provide training there.

Community Services

Community health nurses may help the older adult safety proof his or her home against falls by removing loose rugs and obstacles in hallways and stairwells. Community health nurses often educate members of the community about safety promotion through health fairs and lectures. Some communities offer a service that will call the single older adult daily and will respond to a help signal activated by a medallion worn around the neck. This system or a buddy system of telephone calls can provide a quick response to accidents for the older adult.

Evaluation

The effectiveness of nursing interventions to promote safety is determined through nursing observation and feedback from client caregivers and healthcare professionals in the community. Nursing interventions have the long-term goals of identification of actual and potential environmental hazards, demonstration of safety habits, reduction in frequency and severity of accidents, and development of safe compensatory strategies for physical deficits. To measure the progress toward these goals, the nurse may question the client and caregivers (using "what if" and "what would you do if" questions), ask for and evaluate performance of selected safety habits (eg, transfers in and out of the bathtub), gather data on the frequency and type of accidents, and evaluate the effectiveness of compensatory strategies (are they using the suggested strategies; is the client satisfied; does the strategy make the activity easier, safer, faster to accomplish?). Any accident, fall, scrape, or bruise requires analysis by the nurse to identify the cause and the best means to prevent recurrence. The nurse has a fundamental responsibility to promote continuous client safety, and every opportunity for interaction with the client is an opportunity to promote and evaluate safety habits. Examples of outcome criteria that measure the achievement of client goals are given here.

Goal

- The client will identify actual and high-risk environmental hazards.

Possible Outcome Criteria

- Client verbalizes difficulty walking to bathroom in the healthcare facility within 24 hours of being admitted as a client or resident.
- Prior to discharge, client expresses fear of falling over obstacles at home.

Goal

- The client will demonstrate safety habits when performing activities of daily living and injury prevention.

Possible Outcome Criteria

- Immediately after instructions by the nurse, client uses nurse call light system for assistance each time he or she needs to use the bathroom.
- Client uses over-the-bed lights, nonskid slippers, and glasses when transferring to chair at first and subsequent times out of bed.
- Client identifies modification for home safety (removal of throw rugs, installation of handrails in hallway, better lighting of hallway and stairway) 24 hours after nurse's instruction about home safety.

Nursing Plan of Care
The Client at Risk for Injury

Nursing Diagnosis
Risk for Injury related to sensory and integrative dysfunction manifested by altered mobility and faulty judgment.

Client Goal
Client will demonstrate safety habits when performing activities of daily living and injury prevention.

Client Outcome Criteria
- Client uses nurse call light system for assistance at each need to use bathroom immediately after instruction by the nurse.
- Client demonstrates safety practices in dressing and hygiene.
- Client uses over-the-bed lights, nonskid slippers each time when transferring to chair or out of bed.
- Client identifies modification for home safety (removal of throw rugs, installation of handrails in hallway, better lighting of hallway and stairway) 12 hours after nurse's instruction about home safety.

Nursing Interventions	*Scientific Rationale*
1. Position bed in lowest position.	1. Low position minimizes distance to floor if client falls.
2. Place client call light within reach of hand, and give instructions.	2. A call light allows client to call for help.
3. Explain all safety modifications of the client's room: removal of clutter, providing a clear path to bathroom, use of a night light, brakes on bed and chairs, placement of call light.	3. Client and family will feel safer if they are aware of safety promotion strategies.
4. Perform frequent visual checks of client.	4. Client may attempt to get out of bed or chair without calling for assistance.
5. Use safety belt in all transfers if the client is unsteady or has difficulty with balance..	5. A safety belt allows for control/monitoring of client movement without trauma to any body part.
6. Evaluate the client's ability to use toilet; obtain raised toilet seat or grab bars if indicated.	6. Clients with hip muscle weakness may be unable to rise from low toilet seat. Grab bars may assist the weak person to move slowly and safely.
7. Assist client to perform hygiene at sink with large mirror; encourage client to scan the whole visual field.	7. Mirror provides client with visual reinforcement of activity.
8. Discuss floor plan of home with client and support person. Make suggestions for modifications that will lead to a safer environment.	8. Client and support person need to be involved in planning for client's safety in the home.

- Client demonstrates safety practices in dressing and hygiene.

Goal
- The client will experience decreased frequency and severity of accidents.

Possible Outcome Criteria
- Client practices safety precautions, as evidenced by absence of falls or accidents in 48 hours before discharge.

Key Concepts

- Safety is a basic human need essential in the healthcare environment, home, and community.
- Individual and environmental factors affect safety.
- Manifestations of altered safety include falls, fires, burns, poisoning, suffocation, electrical shock, ra-

diation injury, infection, allergies, respiratory problems, stress-related illness, and motor vehicle accidents.

- Infants, older adults, and those impaired by illness or medications are at risk for falls.
- Falls in the healthcare environment are frequently associated with walking to the bathroom.
- Nursing interventions to promote health and safety function involve client education and providing a safe healthcare environment.
- Nurses must educate parents about the developmental capabilities of infants and children and the special safety precautions needed for their care.
- Nurses must be familiar with emergency interventions for disasters, including fire evacuation and filing an incident report.

Critical Thinking Challenges

This chapter has emphasized the importance of safety in healthcare. Now turn to the situation at the beginning of the chapter. Apply what you have learned about safety across the lifespan and your knowledge of assessment and planning to the care of this mother and her toddler.

1. *List and analyze your immediate impressions of the family. Describe how you think the mother feels at this time.*
2. *Propose how you will proceed with your assessment of the mother, the toddler, and the home environment.*
3. *Summarize additional information you need to provide further anticipatory guidance to this mother and toddler.*
4. *Plan methods for improving safety for the toddler.*
5. *Reflect on how you can follow up with the mother and her coping strategies.*

References

Brower, H. T. (1991). The alternatives to restraints. *Journal of Gerontological Nursing, 17*(2), 18.

Burns, E. A., Robinson, J. C., & Scherger, J. E. (1988). Which barrier contraceptive for whom? *Client Care, 22*(15), 109–139.

Centers for Disease Control (1988). Update: Universal precautions for prevention of transmission of human immunodeficiency virus, hepatitis B virus, and other blood-borne pathogens in health care settings. *Morbidity and Mortality Weekly Report, 37*, 377–388.

Easterling, M. L. (1990). Which of your clients is headed for a fall? *RN, 53*(1), 56–59.

Evans, L. K., & Strumpf, N. E. (1990). Myths about elder restraint. *Image: Journal of Nursing Scholarship, 22*(2), 124.

Food and Drug Administraiton (1992). *FDA safety alert: Potential hazards with restraint devices.* Rockville MD: Author.

Freiberg, K. L. (1992). *Human development: A life-span approach* (4th ed.). Boston: Jones and Bartlett.

Haley, B., Nagy, M., & Roberts, S. (1991) Care versus control: the key to unlocking physical restraints. *Chart, 88*(4), 5.

Health Care Financing Administration (1990). *Federal Register, 54*(21), 1.

Janelli, L. M. (1989). Physical restraints: How little we know. *Nursing Homes, 38*(1/2), 10–12.

Kane, R., Ouslander, J., & Abrass, I. (1994). *Essentials of clinical geriatrics,* 3rd ed. New York: McGraw-Hill.

Loken, S., & Loken, T. (1989). Radon: Detection and treatment. *Nurse Practitioner, 14*(11), 45–46, 48, 51.

Maslow, A. H. (1970). *Motivation and personality* (2nd ed.). New York: Harper and Row.

National Center for Health Statistics (1990). *Health, United States, 1989 and prevention profile.* DHHS Publication #(PHS)90-1232. Hyattsville, MD: U.S. Department of Health and Human Services.

National Safety Council (1994). *Accident facts.* Itasca, IL: Author.

North American Nursing Diagnosis Association (1994). Official communication. Philadelphia: Author.

Omnibus Budget Reconciliation Act (OBRA). (1990). *Regulations and Interpretive Guidelines (draft).* Health Care Financing Administration: Washington.

Plotkin, S. A., & Mortimer, E. A. (1988). *Vaccines.* Philadelphia: W.B. Saunders.

Powell, C., Mitchell-Pederson, L., Fingerote, G., & Edmund, L. (1989). Freedom from restraint: Consequences of reducing physical restraints in the management of the elderly. *Canadian Medical Association Journal, 141*(6), 561–564.

Slota, M. C. (1990). Child passenger safety in the car: Are we involved enough? *Critical Care Nurse, 10*(4), 72–74, 77–79.

Stanevich, R. S., & Stanevich, R. L. (1989). Guidelines for occupational safety and health program. *American Association of Occupational Health Journal, 37*(6) 205–214, 242–244.

Tideiksaar, R. (1993). *Falls in older persons: Prevention and management in hospitals and nursing homes.* Boulder: Tactilitics.

U.S. Dept. of Health and Human Services, Public Health Service (1990). *Healthy People 2000: National Health Promotion and Disease Prevention Objectives.* DHHS Publication #(PHS)91-50213.

Bibliography

Finegan, J. M. (1994). Staff education can prevent OR fires. *Today's OR Nurse, 16*(3), 24–26.

Gellner, P., Landers, S., O'Rourke, D., & Schlagel, M. (1994). Communitry health nursing in the 1990's—risky business? *Holistic Nursing Practice, 8*(2), 15–21.

Halpern, J. S. (1990). Bicycle helmets for children. *Journal of Emergency Nursing, 16*(1), 36–40.

Hyer, K., & Rudick, L. (1994). The effectiveness of personal emergency response systems in meeting the safety monitoring needs of home care clients. *Journal of Nursing Administration, 24*(6), 39–44.

Kendrick, D. (1994). Children's safety in the home: Parents possession and perception of the importance of safety equipment. *Public Health, 108*(1), 21–25.

MacLeod J. A., Blazey M., Johnson F., & MacMullen J. A. S. (1994). It's not a drill, it's for real! *Journal of Nursing Staff Development, 10*(6), 293–299.

Sewell, K. H., & Gaines, S. K. (1993). A developmental approach to childhood safety education. *Pediatric Nursing, 19*(5), 464–466.

Spencer, R. T., et al. (1995). *Clinical pharmacology and nursing management* (4th ed.). Philadelphia: J.B. Lippincott.

Tideiksaar, R. (1989). Home safe home: Practical tips for fall-proofing. *Geriatric Nursing, 10*(6), 280–284.

Urton, M. M. (1991). A community home inspection approach to preventing falls among the elderly. *Public Health Report, 106*(2), 192.

Vandewater, D. A. (1990). Safety-proofing an elder's home: A checklist. *Perspectives, 14*(1), 5.

Veach, S. L. (1990). Advocating bicycle helmet use: A nursing issue. *Imprint, 37*(2), 141–142.

Watson, M. E., & Mayhew, P. A. (1994). Identifying fall risk factors in preparation for reducing the use of restraints. *MedSurg Nursing, 3*(1), 25–28, 30, 35.

Health Maintenance

Key Terms	Learning Objectives

Health-maintenance activities
Health-promotion activities
Health-protection activities
Illness-prevention activities

Upon completion of this chapter, the student will be able to do the following:

- *Describe characteristics essential for normal health.*
- *Give examples of health-promotion and illness-prevention behaviors.*
- *Describe important lifespan development considerations for health maintenance.*
- *Recognize major factors that affect motivation and health maintenance.*
- *Explain how environment, poverty, and unhealthy lifestyles or habits may alter health maintenance.*
- *Characterize manifestations of altered health maintenance.*
- *Obtain subjective data through a nursing history to assess health maintenance.*
- *Provide appropriate information about common illnesses that may result from altered health maintenance.*
- *List resources for client-teaching information on health maintenance.*
- *Value health-promotion concepts and act as a role model for clients.*

30

A college freshman comes to the clinic at the College Health Services, where you work, to ask for birth control pills. She tells you, the clinic nurse, that this is the first time she has been away from home. Her parents were "overly protective," and she was not allowed to date much in high school. She says she has engaged in sexual activity only since starting college 2 months ago. She has never had a pelvic examination and knows only superficial information about sexually transmitted diseases (STDs) and contraception. She also states that she has gained 15 pounds and spends most of her time attending classes, studying, and partying.

In previous chapters you learned definitions for health and wellness, you studied the concept of holistic health, and you developed an understanding of collaborative sharing of healthcare responsibilities. This chapter expands your knowledge base of health maintenance and illness prevention. The student in the situation above has much to learn about healthy attitudes. You have an opportunity to work with her in health promotion. Critical Thinking Challenges at the end of this chapter will help you apply what you have studied in this chapter to this client's care.

Florence Nightingale believed the following:

- Health is the ability to use well every power one has.
- Preventable disease should be a crime.
- It is cheaper to promote health than to care for illness.
- Goals of nursing should include health maintenance, health teaching, and disease prevention.

Contemporary nurses still address these issues. Nurses have the potential and the social responsibility to help people, families, aggregates, and communities maintain and improve their health. The nursing activities of health education and client teaching focus on enhancing a person's ability to engage in effective health behavior. Although nurses may promote healthy behaviors, it is the individual's option to accept or reject those behaviors. For example, you may teach the client in the situation above about sexuality, reproductive anatomy, and STDs, but she is the one who has to decide whether she will use the information she learned or ignore advice.

Health promotion and illness prevention have become increasingly popular concepts in healthcare reform and have contributed to the growth of health maintenance organizations (HMOs) and holistic healthcare. HMOs are based on the belief that it is easier and more economical to maintain health than to treat illness. Consumers of care in HMOs prepay for healthcare: regular examinations, immunizations, health teaching, and other health-related activities are a prime focus of the organization. There are several well-established HMOs that are free-standing organizations, and several health insurance groups have organized similar programs.

Normal Health Maintenance

Health-maintenance activities are the behaviors that a person in stable health uses to maintain or improve that state of health over time. To understand health maintenance, one must recall the concepts of health and wellness. Health and wellness involve assuming responsibility for oneself, making informed choices, feeling self-worth, and managing stress. Health maintenance, then, is the continuity and harmony of those beliefs and behaviors.

Health and wellness are defined in Chapter 15. Healthcare workers may define health and wellness in one way, but a client may define it differently. Ultimately, a person's understanding of health depends on how that person defines health. If a person believes that health means being free of disease, the parameters of health are narrow. If a person believes that health is the optimal functioning of biologic, psychosocial, and spiritual factors within the environment, the meaning of health becomes quite broad.

Characteristics of Normal Health Maintenance

To maintain our level of health and to strive for higher levels of well-being, we often must alter our health habits and our environment. This may involve seeking new support people. Normal health maintenance requires three characteristics (Fig. 30-1):

- Perception of health
- Motivation to change direction if necessary
- Adherence to management goals.

Perception

A person's ability to maintain a desired level of health depends on that person's perception of his or her current health status and the possession of knowledge to manage positive health behaviors. For example, many elderly people mistakenly believe joint pain is a normal part of aging and therefore do not seek medical attention. When asked about their health status, these people may say they are in good health, forgetting about or ignoring the joint pain.

The person who believes that health is a gift from God may believe there is little that can be done to improve health. The person's perception, then, influences how he or she rates personal health and influences the options available for management.

Motivation

The person's perception and understanding of health determines the accountability and responsibility that he or she assumes for health. This self-awareness reveals the person's level of motivation for changing his or her health behaviors. When a person is strongly motivated toward realizing an optimal level of wellness or maintaining current health status, the person will actively seek the health information, teaching, and activities that help achieve that goal. A person less strongly motivated may not succeed in achieving those goals and behaviors, no matter what the nurse counsels.

Because each person defines health in relation to personal expectations and values, the degree of motivation for change depends on those expectations and values. Motivation is internally generated; although the nurse can support and enhance motivation, the client is the ultimate determinant.

Biologic capabilities influence both the initiation of motivation in the person and the person's potential for success. For example, even a person who is highly motivated toward a healthy lifestyle with optimal nutrition, regular exercise, and stress management may not succeed in achieving wellness because of the limitations posed by his or her genetic inheritance or environmental exposure.

Management

Reducing health risks is not always easy. Reducing risks usually entails making a decision to change one's lifestyle and to break old habits (for instance, quitting

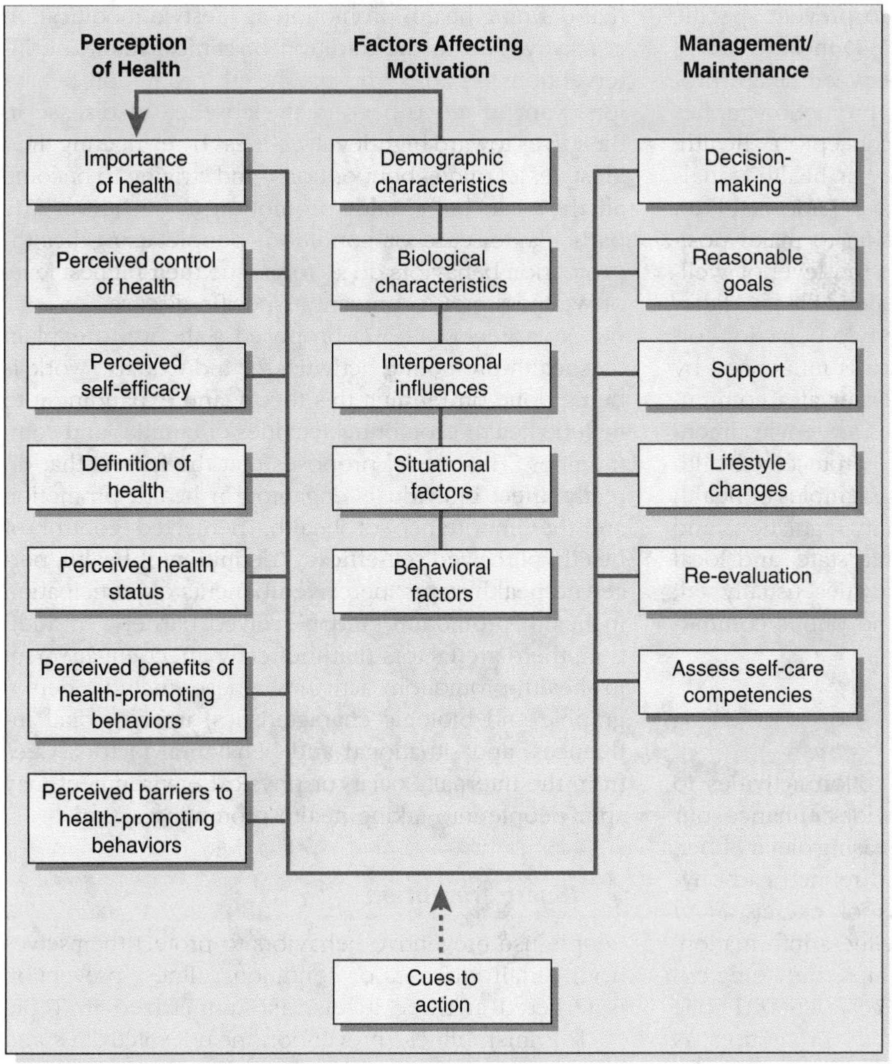

Figure 30-1 *• Characteristics of normal functional health maintenance. (Adapted from Pender, N. (1987).* Health promotion in nursing practice *(2nd ed.). Norwalk, CT: Appleton & Lange.)*

smoking, losing weight, controlling alcohol intake, and exercising regularly). Often it is far easier to continue the risky behavior, hoping the worst does not happen. Taking the initiative to change our lives is sometimes motivated by situational factors (such as marriage, pregnancy, or a friend's newly diagnosed lifestyle disease) or new awareness that a behavior is risky.

Once we make the decision and take the initiative to change, setting goals that are realistic and achievable is the next step. Momentary overenthusiasm may cause us to set goals that are unrealistic and difficult to achieve, and this may lead to failure. For example, a person who is 60 pounds overweight decides to lose 80 pounds within 6 months. For this person, the goal is unrealistic and unhealthy, and needs to be modified.

Adapting and adhering to new health behaviors can be trying and frustrating. During the transition, people may need social support to comply with their goals. Social support can be obtained from nurses and other health-team members, friends, family, and support groups such as Alcoholics Anonymous, Weight Watchers, Parents Without Partners, and Parents Anonymous. In some situations, changes maybe necessary in the person's social and physical environment. For instance, someone who takes illicit drugs probably has friends who do, too. The person who wants to stop using drugs may need to seek new friends as well as a new lifestyle and physical environment.

Managing health-maintenance goals is similar to the nursing process: an assessment of the need for change is completed, weaknesses and strengths are determined, goals are set, plans for intervention are made, and outcomes are evaluated and reconsidered. Selected health behaviors may be continued, or different health behaviors may be selected if the first selections are not useful or possible.

Normal Functional Health Maintenance

The basic components of health maintenance are health promotion and illness prevention. **Health-promotion activities** are approach behaviors that seek to expand the potential for health; **illness-prevention activities** are avoidance behaviors that seek to prevent specific diseases or conditions (Pender, 1987; Duncan & Gold, 1986). The focus of health differs between health promotion and illness prevention: health promotion implies a positive and multidimensional concept of health, whereas illness prevention implies that health equals the absence of disease (Stachtchenko & Jenicek, 1990). Approach behaviors require a decision to make positive changes in an effort to increase the level of wellness. We use avoidance behaviors to avoid illness, rather than to promote health per se. The two behaviors often overlap. Health maintenance also is influenced by **health protection activities** that occur at a community level. Health protection activities are environmental or regulatory measures that seek to protect the health of a community or large aggregates. Examples of health protection include air and water quality regulations and food and drug regulations by federal, state, and local governments. Health protection activities usually fall within the realm of public health and public/community health nursing.

Health Promotion

Put simply, people use health-promotion activities to feel better. Health-promotion behaviors enhance our overall well-being; examples are increasing dietary fiber, avoiding artificial food additives and refined carbohydrates, developing regular patterns of exercise and sleep, controlling stress, seeking wellness information, establishing and maintaining friendships, and being environmentally concerned. *Healthy People 2000* (Public Health Service, 1991) defines health promotion as lifestyle modification; however, others, such as Pender (1987) and Stachtchenko and Jenicek (1990), suggest that defining health promotion as lifestyle modification is narrow and in the tradition of clinical medicine interventions. People who use health-promotion behaviors want to move beyond the absence of disease in their lives toward high-level wellness by evaluating their lifestyle, learning about options, and striving to become all they can be. Health promotion is not about any particular disease or condition: people using health-promotion behaviors do so to pursue their highest level of wellness, not to prevent a specific disease.

Nola Pender (1987) proposed a theory to explain the health-promoting activities of individuals. Work is being done on refining this theory and expanding it to include health-promoting activities of families and communities. This model proposes that the factors that directly affect individuals engaging in health promotion are the importance of health, perceived control of health, perceived self-efficacy, definition of health, perceived health status, perceived benefits of participation in health promotion, and perceived barriers. In addition, there are factors that indirectly affect engagement in health-promotion activities; these include demographic and biologic characteristics, interpersonal influences, and situational and behavioral factors. Cues from the internal, social, or physical environment may spur people into taking health-promoting action.

Illness Prevention

People use preventive behaviors to protect themselves from certain diseases or conditions. Illness prevention is targeted at three levels, as summarized in Table 30-1. Primary illness prevention includes activities and lifestyle factors directed toward high-level wellness, such as adequate nutrition, adequate immunization sta-

Table 30-1 • Three Levels of Illness Prevention

Level	Description	Examples
Primary prevention	Seeks to prevent a disease or condition at a prepathologic state; to stop something from ever happening.	Immunizations, fluoride supplements, car seat restraints, oral contraceptives, education in elementary schools about drug addiction.
Secondary prevention	Seeks to identify specific illnesses or conditions at an early stage with prompt intervention to prevent or limit disability; to prevent catastrophic effects that could occur if proper attention and treatment were not provided.	Physical assessments, developmental screening, vision screening, breast and testicular self-examinations, pregnancy testing.
Tertiary prevention	Occurs after a disease or disability has occurred and the recovery process has begun. Intent is to halt the disease or injury process and assist the individual in obtaining an optimal health status.	Habilitation for handicapped children, support groups such as Reach for Recovery and Alcoholics Anonymous, cardiac rehabilitation, health education for a newly diagnosed diabetic.

tus, regular exercise, and stress management. Maintaining health is the primary mode for preventing illness.

Secondary prevention includes visiting screening clinics for well-child assessments and checks for blood pressure and cervical/uterine, breast, testicular, and prostate cancers. The goal of these clinics is to identify abnormalities within a population. The clinics tend to have one focus, and refer those with abnormal results elsewhere for follow-up.

Several theories have been proposed to explain why people do or do not participate in illness-prevention activities. These theories include the Health Belief Model (Becker, 1974), which is discussed in Chapter 15, the Theory of Reasoned Action (Fishbein & Ajzen, 1975), and the Theory of Care-Seeking Behavior (Lauver, 1992). Factors central to the Theory of Reasoned Action included attitude, subjective norm, and intention. Attitudes and social norms determine intentions, which in turn determine behavior. Subjective norms are determined by personal beliefs and perceived social standards regarding specific behaviors (Ajzen & Madden, 1986). In the Theory of Care-Seeking Behavior, the probability of engaging in health behavior is a function of psychosocial factors and facilitating conditions regarding behavior. Psychological factors include affect (the feelings associated with care-seeking behavior), expectations (belief of likelihood of desired outcome), utility (overall worth of care-seeking), norms (social and personal standards), and habits (how one usually acts). Facilitating conditions such as health insurance availability and a regular healthcare provider also have a direct effect on seeking healthcare. Finally, clinical factors such as having a symptom or a history of a health problem have been directly related to seeking healthcare.

Combination of Promotion and Prevention

Examples of health-promotion and illness-prevention activities are listed in the accompanying display. It may be difficult to differentiate between the two. For instance, daily jogging may be a health-promotion behavior for one person and an illness-prevention behavior for another. A person who begins to jog because of a risk of cardiovascular disease and then continues because she feels better may switch from illness-prevention to health-promotion behavior. A person may be involved with health promotion and all three levels of illness prevention. For example, a woman with diabetes mellitus may give herself insulin (tertiary prevention), perform a monthly breast self-examination (secondary prevention), brush her teeth daily (primary prevention), and exercise regularly to feel good (health promotion). Personal activities an individual or family can use to maintain health are listed in the accompanying display.

Factors Affecting Health Maintenance

Many factors influence health maintenance positively or negatively. These factors affect what people believe about health, as well as what healthy and unhealthy practices they perform.

Cognition and Perception. Cognitive and perceptual factors include what health means to a person, how important it is, and how the person perceives control over health, self-efficacy, health status, benefits, and barriers. The more we value health, the more likely we are to participate in health-promoting and health-maintaining behaviors (Orem, 1980; Lauver, 1992; Pender, 1987; Steiger & Lipson, 1985). Values are influenced by peers, family, and society. A person may believe that health is controlled primarily by himself or herself (internal) or by factors beyond his or her control (external). People with an internal perception of control are more likely to engage in health-seeking behaviors on their own, but people with an external perception of control are more likely to do so with social pressure (Steiger & Lipson, 1985; Pender, 1987; Zindler-Wernet & Weiss, 1987).

The person's belief about self-efficacy or the ability to accomplish a certain behavior affects his or her willingness to try the behavior. As the person's mastery of behaviors increases, he or she may be more likely to engage in additional activities. Success with one activity can motivate the person to try other activities (Bandura, 1977; Gillett, 1988; Sennott-Miller & Miller, 1987).

People may define health negatively (not being ill) or positively (an optimal state of well-being). That definition influences how the person perceives health and the mechanics of maintaining health (Murray & Zentner, 1993). People who see themselves as having a positive health status may be more likely to continue behaviors that promote and maintain that level of health. However, two people with the same health status may have different perceptions of that health status. Those who see the benefits of health behaviors are more likely to begin or continue those behaviors; those who see the effects as negative or neutral are less likely to do so (Murdaugh & Hinshaw, 1986).

People with a low perceived barrier to health behaviors are more likely to pursue healthy behaviors than those with a high perceived barrier. Barriers can be time, finances, access, convenience, attitude, culture, and social support (Murdaugh & Hinshaw, 1986).

Age and Developmental Level. Age may have a significant impact on the person's ability to manage his or her health status. A 17-year-old woman with arthritis or diabetes mellitus may perceive her health status as low and may not engage in proper health-maintenance practices, but an 80-year-old woman might see such conditions as acceptable and might carry out practices to promote optimum health.

Normal Functional Health Maintenance

Health perception and health maintenance

- Has a personal perception of health and all it entails
- Has a strong motivation for an optimal level of wellness
- Sets health goals and seeks help in managing them
- Has sufficient financial resources to maintain health
- Maintains a safe environment at home and work
- Performs activities of daily living

Nutrition and metabolism

- Has sufficient knowledge of nutrition
- Plans daily menu carefully
- Obtains and digests appropriate amounts of nutrients to promote optimal nutrition
- Protects body against infection
- Maintains homeostatic thermoregulation

Elimination

- Maintains a regular schedule for elimination
- Understands body processes in digestion and elimination
- Practices hygiene after elimination

Activity and exercise

- Maintains good hygiene through self-care
- Uses good body mechanics in activities of daily living
- Maintains optimum motor function
- Uses leisure hours in a healthy manner
- Uses oxygen efficiently

Cognition and perception

- Demonstrates optimum cerebral function
- Builds knowledge and skills
- Develops quality sensory perception

Sleep and rest

- Maintains a regular sleep pattern
- Maintains balance of work and rest
- Provides time for relaxation

Self-perception and self-concept

- Displays activities appropriate for developmental level
- Demonstrates positive self-concept
- Has a stable body image
- Recognizes and cherishes personal identity as unique
- Recognizes uniqueness of other people

Roles and relationships

- Demonstrates functional verbal and nonverbal communication
- Participates in social interactions
- Builds and maintains meaningful relationships
- Has intrinsic mechanisms or support people to help with coping during grieving

Sexuality and reproduction

- Has valid knowledge about sexual functioning and human sexuality
- Accepts sexual functions and sexuality as normal
- Recognizes and accepts personal sexual feelings
- Maintains healthy lifestyle during pregnancy

Coping and stress tolerance

- Makes decisions reflecting understanding of personal limitations
- Protects self against overwhelming situations and changes
- Manages to keep in touch with personal needs while balancing life's roles with minimal conflict

Values and beliefs

- Expresses respect for all life and the quality of life
- Maintains realistic goals for self based on value decisions
- Demonstrates a zeal for life
- Provides for spiritual sustenance

Developmental level also affects a person's ability to manage health. Although infants and young children must rely on their parents and guardians for health maintenance, school-age children can learn proper behaviors and may be able to carry them out independently or with little supervision. Common problems in older adults may also affect health maintenance. For example, loss of teeth may preclude proper nutrition, arthritis may affect the ability to exercise, or slowed cognitive processes may affect safety practices. In these cases, increasing age hinders health maintenance because of functional limitations.

Previous Experiences. A person's past experience with health and the healthcare system affects health maintenance. If a person had a negative experience with an agency or program, he or she may refuse to participate again even if no alternatives are available. If a particular health practice (for instance, a low-calorie diet) worked well for the person or a family member in the past, the person is likely to participate again. Also, a person's health maintenance may be affected by a relative's or friend's experience (for instance, a family history of cancer or a close friend who had a heart attack).

Lifestyle and Habits. A person's lifestyle and habits strongly affect health maintenance. For example, a student living in a dormitory may have a busy school schedule and may work part-time. She may find little time for regular exercise, a balanced diet, and adequate sleep; instead, she grabs vending machine snacks, stays up late studying, and spends her leisure time socializing with friends. A person whose lifestyle conveniently incorporates adequate sleep, exercise, and nutrition may more easily achieve good health maintenance.

Economic Resources. Economics plays a large role in health maintenance. People who live in poverty may be unable to afford nutritious food and adequate housing. They may not receive routine medical care and screenings and may seek healthcare only when a serious illness develops. Homeless children do not receive immunizations, dental care, or the usual safety and security required for health promotion. Wealthier people have greater financial access to medical care, nutritious food, and preventive programs such as aerobics classes and health lectures.

Culture, Values, and Beliefs. The culture in which a person was raised influences his or her health beliefs and practices, including diet, child-bearing and child-rearing customs, self-medication, and alternate therapies. A language barrier may prevent people from entering the healthcare system. Spiritual beliefs and personal or family values also affect health maintenance. Some people place great value on physical health to achieve spiritual health. Others may have religious beliefs that prohibit certain medical practices and treatments. A belief that health is solely God's will and cannot be altered may hinder health maintenance.

Roles and Relationships. People who are comfortable in their roles and relationships with others often form strong support systems and use available resources to promote health. Having role models and relationships with others who have good health-maintenance practices may benefit one's own health maintenance.

Coping and Stress Tolerance. Coping mechanisms people use to handle everyday events may help or harm their health. Stress-reducing techniques such as relaxation breathing or imagery promote health; other coping mechanisms, such as denial and use of alcohol, may lead to health problems.

Lifespan Considerations

Health-maintenance opportunities begin before conception and continue until we die. Characteristics of development at various stages call for specific health-maintenance behaviors.

Newborn and Infant

Health maintenance begins during the prenatal period. Low birth weight and congenital defects—which put infants at risk for additional health problems—have been linked to lack of prenatal care, poor nutrition, and use of alcohol, tobacco, and drugs during pregnancy. Because their immune systems are immature, infants are at risk for infectious diseases, so immunizations are of primary importance. The schedule of recommended immunizations is given in Chapter 39. The nervous system develops rapidly, and bones, muscles, and other organ systems grow during infancy, so proper nutrition and regular developmental and medical check-ups are important.

Toddler and Preschooler

Toddlers and preschoolers develop and learn through exploration and imitation. Curiosity and lack of experience predispose them to accidents and injuries. Exposure to other children in day-care centers, school, or play groups puts them at risk for infection. Safety practices, proper sleep and nutrition, avoidance of second-hand tobacco smoke, and regular immunization schedules are important for health maintenance. Toddlers and preschoolers begin to learn healthy and unhealthy practices by imitating their parents and other significant adults.

Child and Adolescent

School-age children begin to form beliefs about health. They are still influenced primarily by their parents, but teachers and friends become increasingly important. Peer influence is so strong for adolescents that they may adopt unhealthy practices, such as smoking or drinking. Peer pressure also can have positive influences when, for example, the peer group does not use tobacco or alcohol.

School-age children may begin to experience problems such as obesity, high cholesterol levels, and poor stress management that can become symptomatic in adulthood. Physical and intellectual development is rapid. Health-maintenance concerns include proper nutrition, sleep, and exercise; safety; and learning to deal with stress and frustration.

Adolescents must deal with sexual development and confirmation of their identity. Peer influence, a struggle for independence, and the physical changes accompanying sexual development make adolescence a time for experimenting with healthy and unhealthy practices. Safe driving, preventing STDs and pregnancy, avoiding drugs and alcohol, avoiding gang-related violence, and maintaining mental health are primary health-maintenance concerns during adolescence.

Adult and Older Adult

With rapid physical and intellectual growth completed and health beliefs ingrained, the adult should enjoy productive and satisfying years. The adult, however, may now become at risk for lifestyle chronic conditions, such as heart disease, hypertension, cancer, and stroke, depending on his or her health beliefs and practices and genetic factors. The responsibilities of raising a family, holding a job, and being a productive member of society may lead to addictions or stress-related illnesses. Health-maintenance concerns include exercise, nutrition, self-examinations, prenatal care for women, health screening, stress management, and reduction or cessation of alcohol and smoking.

Primary prevention continues in adulthood, however. Many adults have an inadequate immunization status because they forget or are unaware of necessary boosters and new immunizations such as influenza and pneumonia. Health maintenance with adults nevertheless focuses more on secondary prevention than the other levels of prevention, except during pregnancy. Exercise, nutrition, social stimulation, and regular medical check-ups are important because of the normal physiologic changes of aging and the increased risk of chronic illness in older adults. Using medications safely and identifying community resources and support groups are also important health-maintenance considerations.

Nursing Research
Health Maintenance

Selected Nursing Research Studies

Duffy, M.E. (1993). Determinants of health-promoting lifestyles in older persons. *Image: Journal of Nursing Scholarship, 25*(1), 23–28.

Foltz, A. (1993). Parental knowledge and practices of skin cancer prevention: A pilot study. *Journal of Pediatric Health Care, 7(5)*, 220–225.

Stuifbergen, A. & Becker, H. (1993). Predictors of health-promoting lifestyles in persons with disabilities. *Research in Nursing and Health, 17*(1), 3–13.

Underwood, S. (1992). Cancer risk reduction and early detection behaviors among black men: Focus on learned helplessness. *Journal of Community Health Nursing, 9*(1), 21–31.

Viverais-Dresler, G. & Richardson, H. (1991). Well elderly perceptions of the meaning of health and their health promotion practices. *Canadian Journal of Nursing Research, 23*(1), 55–71.

Possible Topics for Nursing Inquiry

- What are cultural indicators of health-seeking behaviors across the lifespan?
- What is the relationship between physical activity, age, and health-promoting behaviors?
- What macro factors (community availability) have a correlation with health-maintenance behaviors?

Altered Health Maintenance

Potential for Altered Function

Numerous factors, together or separately, may disrupt health maintenance.

Environment

Pollution, nearby highways, lack of safe play areas, inadequate housing, and unsanitary conditions lead to poor health maintenance and set the stage for illness. The work environment may lead to health-maintenance problems if conditions include long working hours, poor ventilation, poor lighting, loud noises, lack of nutritious food, and sedentary or repetitious tasks.

Poverty

Poverty is often associated with poor health maintenance. Poverty may cause homelessness or may force people to live in overcrowded conditions with poor sanitation and heating. Children may sleep poorly if they share beds with other family members. Nutrition may be inadequate, leading to poor school performance. Unemployment and dropping out of school cause boredom, and boredom and frustration about such conditions may lead to substance abuse and crime. A knowledge deficit about health maintenance, lack of motivation to improve practices related to unpleasant past experiences, and difficulty obtaining adequate resources are some of the reasons for increased morbidity and mortality rates in the lower socioeconomic group. Improving this group's access to resources may not be possible without social intervention.

Unhealthy Lifestyle and Habits

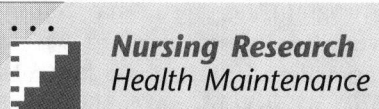

People with an unhealthy lifestyle and habits are considered to have poor health maintenance. Unhealthy habits include lack of exercise, poor diet (in terms of fiber, cholesterol, fat, mineral, vitamin, and protein content), use of tobacco, use of alcohol (except in moderation), use of illegal drugs or abuse of prescription drugs, multiple sexual partners, lack of sleep, lack of contraception, poor dental hygiene, and disregard for safety. Although most people can have some unhealthy habits without suffering health problems, all unhealthy habits carry some increased risk for illness. Repeated, multiple unhealthy habits usually lead to at least one preventable health problem and contribute to a foreshortened life.

Manifestations of Altered Function

Altered health maintenance may result in mental or physical problems. Common manifestations include chronic illnesses, childhood injuries and developmental problems, and psychosocial disruptions. Some manifestations are the result of prolonged exposure to poor health maintenance (for instance, smoking that leads to lung cancer). Other conditions, however, may be the result of a one-time exposure, such as the adolescent who becomes pregnant after failing to use contraception just one time.

Chronic Illnesses

Many chronic illnesses have been linked to altered health maintenance. Hypertension and cardiovascular disease are associated with diet, stress, tobacco use, and obesity. The Framingham Study identified risk factors for cardiovascular disease that are the basis for most cardiac prevention and rehabilitation programs (Dawber, 1980). Such risk factors as cigarette smoking, sedentary lifestyle, high-cholesterol diet, obesity, and stress can be modified, but family history cannot. People with multiple risk factors are at a much greater risk for coronary artery disease and myocardial infarction.

Cancer has been linked to a number of practices we now consider poor health maintenance, although the exact cause is unknown. A low-fiber diet is associated with colon cancer, tobacco smoking is directly related to lung cancer, chewing tobacco is related to oral cancer, and excessive exposure to ultraviolet light is related to skin cancer. A direct cause-and-effect relationship has not been established in many cancers, but continuing research will ultimately reinforce health-maintenance beliefs. Practices once considered healthy and desirable (such as eating large amounts of red meat and sunbathing) have now fallen out of favor because of research findings.

Gastrointestinal illnesses are also related to altered health maintenance. Stress contributes to the development of peptic ulcer disease and colitis. Gastritis may be caused by ingesting alcohol and other irritants. Obesity is considered an illness in itself because the person's general health is poor and the risk for other chronic conditions is increased. Obesity may have a genetic component but is directly related to diet and exercise patterns.

Musculoskeletal and dermatologic illnesses also result from altered health maintenance. Osteoporosis, which often occurs in postmenopausal women, has been linked to inadequate calcium intake during adulthood and lack of exercise as the woman ages. Psoriasis, eczema, and other rashes are aggravated by stress and dietary factors.

Accidents and Injuries

Many preventable accidents and injuries are caused by single episodes of altered health maintenance. They may result when safety practices are disregarded. Accidents, a leading cause of death and disability, include motor vehicle accidents, falls, drowning, and job-related injuries. Injuries include sprains, strains, fractures, lacerations, burns, and other trauma.

Unwanted pregnancy and transmission of STDs can be considered accidents as well because they may result when safe sex and contraception practices are disregarded. Adolescents who become pregnant are at higher risk for having babies with low birth weight, congenital defects, and additional health problems. Unwanted pregnancies and STDs can cause psychological distress and may isolate the victim from society.

Childhood and Developmental Problems

Problems that children experience because of altered health maintenance include tooth decay, infectious diseases, growth retardation, and learning difficulties. Tooth decay results from poor dental hygiene and ingesting sugary food and beverages. Infectious diseases such as mumps, measles, rubella, polio, diphtheria, and meningitis result from lack of immunization. The risk of bronchitis and asthma increases with exposure to second-hand smoke. Growth retardation and improper neurologic and musculoskeletal development may result from inadequate nutrition. Obesity may begin in infancy from an improper diet. Learning and intellectual development may be slowed by poor nutrition and lack of discipline and sleep.

Psychosocial Problems

Psychosocial problems may result from specific illnesses caused by altered health maintenance, or from a more general loss of well-being. Addiction is both a psychological problem and a physical illness. Behavioral changes often occur in the addicted person, including abusive and violent behavior, withdrawal, and mood swings. Other psychosocial manifestations of altered health maintenance include anxiety, depression, and social rejection. Anxiety often accompanies unhealthy lifestyles that include stress, excessive caffeine intake, lack of sleep, alcohol consumption, and tobacco use. These people worry about their health but do not improve their health maintenance. Depression may accompany obesity.

Family and friends may reject people who show disregard for their own health. Today, society values people who lead healthy lifestyles. Many smokers feel like outcasts in today's nonsmoking environments.

Impact of Dysfunction on Activities of Daily Living

Altered health maintenance may marginally or greatly affect activities of daily living (ADLs). The nurse must be able to identify the effect of altered health maintenance on both the individual and the family. Assessing the family's strengths as well as limitations can help them develop a realistic perspective for coping with the disruption accompanying the individual's altered health maintenance.

Individual Considerations

Poor sleep habits can affect a person's ability to work or a child's school performance. Poor nutrition reduces the energy a person has to carry out ADLs and affects normal growth and development. Ingesting alcohol impairs the drinker's cognitive and physical performance. Cigarette smoking can impair oxygenation and lead to frequent respiratory infections or chronic lung impairment, making ADLs more difficult to perform.

Any illness, injury, or other problem not prevented by health-maintenance activities disrupts a person's usual level of functioning. An athlete, for example, tries to maintain optimum health by getting enough sleep, not using tobacco, eating a nutritious diet, and doing physical conditioning. Any disruption in these health-maintenance activities would place him or her at a disadvantage in competition. Similarly, anyone with altered health maintenance does not perform ADLs optimally.

Family Considerations

Family functioning in ADLs becomes a significant focus as members alter their normal patterns to meet the person's altered health state. Family relationships change as usual roles are adapted. For example, someone must continue the household functions of cooking, cleaning, child care, and income production.

Assessment

The nurse's assessment of a client's health maintenance tends to be more abstract than other physical assessments. The objective of this assessment is to evaluate how well the client can manage his or her own health behaviors and those of the family (when appropriate), and to identify deficiencies, risks, potential for improvement, and motivation to change. Information about other functions, such as nutrition, mobility, and values, is used in the health-maintenance assessment. Much of this assessment is done through the health history interview, observations, and validation of self-assessment techniques.

Subjective Data

Subjective data are obtained in an organized interview. During the interview, the nurse should note the client's verbal and nonverbal communication and should use observation skills to guide the data collection. Subjective data identify the client's normal functional patterns of health maintenance, risk factors for altered health maintenance, and active health-maintenance dysfunction. Data are collected from sources such as the client, family members or significant others, parents (if the client is a child), and medical records.

Functional Pattern Identification

Clients in all settings should be assessed for health maintenance, even if no problems are suspected. Information on normal patterns of health maintenance helps reinforce the client's state of health, and information can also be gained on areas that need further work. For example, the nurse may learn while discussing exercise that the client walks three times a week for 20 minutes and places high value on cardiovascular health. This information could be used to encourage the client to reduce the amount of fat in the diet.

Questions the nurse must answer include (Gordon, 1993)

What is the client's perception of his or her health status?
How does the client define health?
What value does the client place on health?
How could the client's health be improved?
What is the client doing to maintain his or her health?
What prevents the client from engaging in a desired health behavior?
How much control does the client have over his or her own health?
What is the client's perceived ability to perform health behaviors?

The client's perception of his or her health and ability to manage health is important. The nurse should validate all information obtained in this area, because miscommunication can hurt the client-nurse relationship and can create barriers against health behavior.

Risk Identification

Cues from the nursing history can alert the nurse to risk factors, which are traits that increase the client's vulnerability to a certain condition or disease. Risk factors can be classified as genetic background, age, biologic characteristics, personal habits, and environment. They vary in intensity, and multiple risk factors may interact to develop additional risk factors (Pender, 1987). The intensity of the risk factor can be modified by behaviors such as dieting, exercising, avoiding tobacco, genetic testing, or leaving a particular environment or situation. The risk factor may be eliminated by abolishing the behavior. Risky behavior has been defined as any irresponsible behavior that leads to negative health outcomes. For example, the risky behavior of a sedentary lifestyle has health consequences of obesity, coronary heart disease, hypertension, and osteoporosis (McKie, et al., 1993).

Risk identification can be done with the help of several assessment tools. A computer program called *Healthier People,* developed by the Centers for Disease Control and Prevention and Emory University (Atlanta, GA), helps the client and nurse identify risk factors; another computer program, *Health Predict: Personal Health Analysis,* is available from Compuhealth Associates (St. Louis, MO). *The Health Hazard Appraisal* (Health Care Service, Inc., San Diego, CA, 1981) and *Lifestyle Assessment Questionnaire* (University of Wisconsin at Stevens Point, WI, 1981) are risk appraisals that are sent to the respective company for scoring. A self-test for risk appraisal is *Health Style: A Self-Test,* by the U.S. Department of Health and Human Services (Office of Disease Prevention and Health Promotion, 1981).

These risk appraisals are designed to help the client and nurse identify common threats to health and to motivate behavioral change. Some items are difficult for the client to answer, however; errors may result if the client cannot answer or selects an inappropriate answer. These appraisals are not a substitute for a nursing assessment (Berlin, et al., 1990).

Dysfunction Identification

A dysfunction is any behavior that alters health maintenance. In many cases, the client perceives the dysfunction and may or may not want to change, or the client may learn that a behavior is dysfunctional through health education. Many people are unaware of their dysfunctional behavior; for instance, someone immunized in 1965 for measles may not know that adequate immunity was not obtained. As researchers learn more about risks to health, nurses must transmit that information to clients.

Identifying dysfunction goes beyond identifying risk factors. The nurse assesses not only the risk factor but how that factor has altered the client's health maintenance. For example, when assessing the client's diet, the nurse might ask

How do you feel on your new diet? or, How would you evaluate your energy level since you have been on this diet?

Have you had your blood pressure checked since you stopped restricting your salt intake?

I see that you eat two or three eggs each morning for breakfast. Have you ever had your cholesterol level checked?

By asking such questions and having the client describe the possible effects of risky practices, the nurse identifies actual health-maintenance dysfunctions.

Objective Data

Objective data include results of the physical assessment and diagnostic tests that focus on general health management and prevention. Objective data are used to identify the client's health maintenance through screening techniques.

Physical Assessment

There is no specific physical assessment skill for health maintenance; instead, data obtained from other assessments are used (Fig. 30-2) The screening assessments in the accompanying health assessment display can be pooled to assess health maintenance comprehensively.

During the physical assessment, the client's self-examination skills (for example, breast or testicular self-

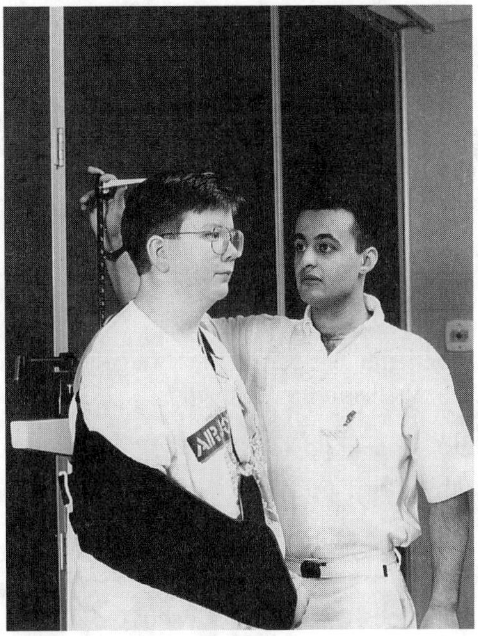

Figure 30-2 • *The adolescent undergoes a growth spurt, which the nurse monitors as a part of health assessment.*

Selected Health Assessment Across the Lifespan

Infant and Preschool Child (Birth–5 years)

Health history and family history: initially and then update as needed.

Vision: *Infancy*—follows objects, corneal light reflex, turn to light
Toddler—cornea light reflex, cover test
Preschool—Snellen E, screenings as for toddler

Hearing: *Infants*—startle reflex (birth), tracking sounds (3–6 months), recognizes sounds (6–8 months), location of sound (8–12 months)
Preschool—pure tone audiometry beginning at age 4 years. Inability to cooperate and understand instructions hinders this screening in younger children.

Speech: Assess in infancy and early preschool with Denver II and Denver Articulation Screening Examination for children 2.5 to 6 years.

General development: Denver II in ages newborn to 6 years can be done along with physical assessments.

Congenital hip dislocation: newborn though age 23 months

Blood pressure: before age 1 year, then yearly. Flush technique may be used.

Dental: *Infancy*—presence of teeth and oral care, screening by dentist at age 2 years and then every 6–12 months

General physical assessment: at ages 1, 2, 4, 6, 12, 18, 24 months, then yearly, including height and weight

Urine: phenylketonuria before age 4 weeks; glucose and protein at same time as physical assessment; between 2 and 5 years analysis for bacteriuria

Nutrition: same as for physical assessment

Blood: sickle cell if indicated at 6 months; hemoglobin or hematocrit at 9 months, and then every 6 months through 24 months, yearly thereafter

Tuberculin: baseline at 12 months if at risk, secondary to endemic status; repeat before beginning school year

Environment: ask parents about age-appropriate injury risks in environment

School-Age Child (6–12 years)

Health history: update

Vision: visual acuity every 1–2 years

Hearing: pure tone audiometry ages 6, 8, and 11 years

Dental: assessed by dentist every 6–12 months

General physical assessment: including blood pressure, general development, height, weight, and nutrition every year

Urine: glucose, protein yearly

Blood: hematocrit or hemoglobin every 1–3 years as indicated by nutritional status and history

Tuberculin: if in an at-risk environment, every 1–3 years

Environment: ask parents about age-appropriate injury risks in environment

Adolescent (13–18 years)

Health history: update; include tobacco and sexual practices

Vision: visual acuity every 1–2 years; usually odd year age (ie, 13, 15)

Hearing: pure tone audiometry ages 14 and 18 years

General physical assessment: including blood pressure, general and sexual development, height, weight, nutrition every 1–2 years

Scoliosis: age 11 and then yearly through age 14 or completion of growth spurts

Self-examination technique: *Girls*—breast at age 14–15 years. *Boys*—testicular at age 14–15 years.

Urine: analysis every 3 years

Blood: hemoglobin or hematocrit every 1–3 years, others as indicated

Dental: by dentist every 6–12 months

Emotional: be alert for depressive symptoms and need to screening

Young Adult (19–39 years)

Health history: update as needed

Vision: visual acuity every 1–5 years, glaucoma every 3 years beginning at age 35

Hearing: gross screening yearly

Physical assessment: including risk appraisal, height, weight, and nutrition every 3–5 years

Blood pressure: every 2–3 years

Dental: every 6–12 months

Self-examinations: *Women*—breast every month with professional evaluation every 1–2 years. *Men*—testicular monthly.

Mammogram: women, once between 35 and 39 years

Pap smears: women, every 3 years after two successive normal results

Urine: complete analysis every 5–10 years

(continued)

Selected Health Assessment Across the Lifespan *(continued)*

Blood: cholesterol every 5–10 years, blood glucose every 10 years, hematocrit—women every 3–5 years, men every 5–10 years
Tuberculin: establish baseline, repeat as needed if in high-risk environment

Pregnant Women

Initial assessment
History: genetic and obstetric; nutrition; tobacco, alcohol, and drug use. Risk factors for low birth weight, prior sexually transmitted diseases (STDs)
Physical assessment: height, weight, blood pressure, pelvic measurements, pap smear
Blood: hemoglobin and hematocrit, ABO/Rh typing, antibody screen, VDRL/PRP, hepatitis B surface antigens, human immunodeficiency virus (if at risk)
Urine: analysis for bacteriuria, protein and glucose
Other: gonorrhea culture and other STDs
Follow up
History: update
Physical assessment: blood pressure, weight, fetal heart sounds
Urine: analysis for protein and glucose
Other: may be necessary because of risks, including maternal serum alpha-fetoprotein, ultrasound, glucose tolerance, STD screening, hepatitis screening

Middle Adult (40–64) years

Health history: update as needed
Vision: visual acuity every 5 years, glaucoma every 3 years
Hearing: every 3–5 years, more frequently if in noisy environment
General physical assessment: every 2–3 years including height, weight, and nutrition
Blood pressure: every 2–3 years
Dental: every 6–12 months
Women only: breast self-examination monthly, with professional evaluation every 1–2 years, mammogram every 1–2 years, Pap smear every 1–3 years, bone mineral analysis after menopause
Urine: complete analysis every 5–10 years
Blood: cholesterol, blood glucose, hematocrit every 5 years
Other: stool guaiac yearly, sigmoidoscopy for bowel cancer every 5 years beginning at age 50, baseline electrocardiogram (EKG), and medication evaluation
Skin: yearly for malignant skin disorders

Older Adults (65 and over)

Health history: update as needed
Vision: acuity and glaucoma every 2–3 years
Hearing: every 3–5 years
Blood pressure: yearly
General physical assessment: every 2–3 years including height, weight, and nutrition
Cancer screenings: stool guaiac yearly, sigmoidoscopy every 5 years, skin for malignant tumors yearly. Women only—cervical/uterine every 1–3 years depending on risk, monthly breast self-examination, mammogram yearly until age 75, unless pathology found. Men only—prostate every 1–2 years
Urine: complete analysis every 2 years
Blood: chemistry, lipid, complete blood count thyroid function, and glucose every 2–3 years
Dental: every 6–12 months
Other: EKG as indicated or at risk, medication evaluation, especially for polypharmacy and drugs that may cause confusion or increase risk for falls

examination) must be validated to ensure that he or she is effectively performing each skill. Clients who engage in risky behavior should be assessed for their ability to spot potential abnormalities; for example, tobacco users should be able to perform oral screening, and intravenous drug users should be able to assess for phlebitis.

Many clients have health-assessment equipment at home, such as scales, thermometers, or machines to measure blood pressure or monitor blood glucose levels (Fig. 30-3). Inspecting the equipment for accuracy and assessing the client's ability to use the equipment safely increases the accuracy and reduces the risk of injury or incorrect data. The client should know what to do with the data obtained: does he or she know normal and abnormal readings? If abnormal data are obtained, when should a professional be consulted?

Diagnostic Tests

Many diagnostic tests can be used to assess health maintenance, including urine tests for protein and glucose, a complete blood count for hematocrit and hemoglobin, an electrocardiogram, a chest x-ray, a stool test for occult blood, and a mammogram (see the display on Selected Health Assessment Across the Lifespan). Some screening tests may be initiated independently by nurses; others require a physician or nurse practitioner's order. Some tests are performed on the nursing unit,

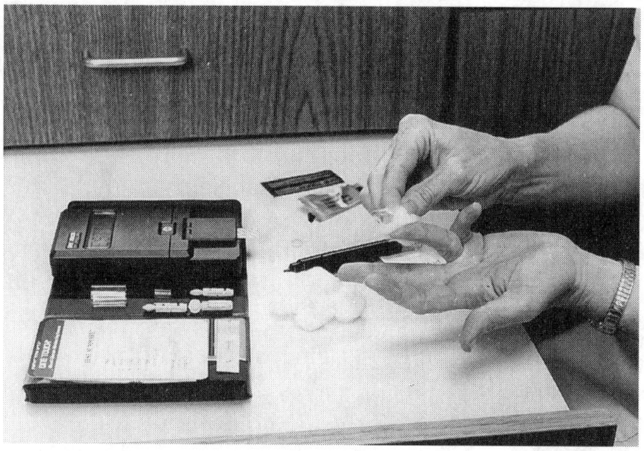

Figure 30-3 • Equipment for monitoring blood glucose increases the health-maintenance abilities of the person with diabetes.

some in the office or home, and still others in a laboratory. Some, such as cholesterol screening and mammograms, can be obtained in a community practice. Agency policies vary on physician's orders, written consent, and protocols. Nurses should review all diagnostic test results and incorporate them into the health-maintenance assessment.

Nursing Diagnoses

NANDA lists two diagnoses involving health maintenance: Altered Health Maintenance and Health-Seeking Behaviors.

Diagnostic Statement: Altered Health Maintenance

Definition

The inability to identify, manage, and/or seek out help to maintain health (NANDA, 1994).

Defining Characteristics

Of the defining characteristics or clinical cues that point to this nursing diagnosis, the following should be present:

- Demonstrated lack of knowledge regarding basic health practices
- Demonstrated lack of adaptive behaviors to internal or external changes
- Reported or observed inability to take responsibility for meeting basic health practices in any, or all, functional pattern areas
- Reported or observed lack of equipment, finances, or other resources for health maintenance
- Reported or observed impairment of personal support system
- History of lack of health-seeking behavior
- Expressions of interest in improving health behaviors

Related Factors

Numerous factors contribute to an individual's difficulty with health maintenance. They may include lack of or significant alteration in communication skills (written, verbal, and gestural), which may interfere with the ability to receive and process health information. The lack of ability to make deliberate and thoughtful judgments, and perceptual/cognitive impairment may interfere with the individual's ability to choose and participate in healthy behavior. Ineffective individual coping, dysfunctional grieving, ineffective family coping, and disabling spiritual distress also may interfere with the ability to make appropriate health behavior choices or consume the energy necessary to engage in healthy behavior. The lack of material resources may make some healthy behaviors difficult to perform, such as purchasing medication for chronic health problems, purchasing nutritious foods, and obtaining necessary immunizations (NANDA, 1994).

Diagnostic Statement: Health-Seeking Behaviors

Definition

A state in which an individual in stable health is actively seeking ways to alter personal health habits and/or the environment to move toward a higher level of health. (Stable health status is defined as age-appropriate illness prevention measures achieved; client reports good or excellent health; and signs and symptoms of disease, if present, are controlled [NANDA, 1994]).

Defining Characteristics

Of the defining characteristics or clinical cues that point to this nursing diagnosis, the following must be present:

- Expressed or observed desire to seek a higher level of wellness

Minor characteristics also may be present but are not required for this diagnosis

- Expressed or observed desire for increased control of health practice
- Expression of concern about effect of current environmental conditions on health status
- Stated or observed unfamiliarity with wellness community resources

- Demonstrated or observed lack of knowledge in health-promotion behaviors (NANDA, 1994)

Related Factors

There are several situational variables or changes in roles that generally increase an individual's desire to seek health information. These include marriage, parenthood, changes in living situations (children leaving home), and retirement. Health-seeking behavior can also be increased when the media brings to the individual's awareness the need for specific behaviors such as mammograms, testicular self-examinations, and immunizations. In addition, the advertisement of new resources such as exercise equipment in city parks piques interest in health-seeking behavior (NANDA, 1994).

Related Nursing Diagnoses

Nursing diagnoses closely related to health maintenance include High Risk for Infection, High Risk for Injury (trauma, poisoning, suffocation), Knowledge Deficit, and Noncompliance. Although Knowledge Deficit is an accepted nursing diagnosis, it more often is considered to be a related or contributing factor (Jenny, 1987). Noncompliance is a situation in which the client has expressed a desire to comply but does not do so because of barriers or an informed decision not to adhere to recommendations (Carpenito, 1992). This nursing diagnosis must be used carefully to ensure that the client is not labeled "noncompliant" before complete data collection is done.

Outcome Identification and Planning

After the nursing diagnoses and related factors are identified, client goals and nursing interventions are planned. Common goals in health maintenance include the following:

The client will identify areas for improvement in health maintenance.
The client will adopt appropriate health-seeking behaviors.
The client will maintain or improve current health status.

Planning will evolve around the client's motivation to be healthy. Did the client actively seek help, or was altered health discovered in an assessment or test? The client's cooperation is needed in planning and setting goals because it is the client who will manage appropriate care. Most nursing interventions for health maintenance are educational. Examples of nursing interventions commonly used in health promotion are listed in the accompanying display and are discussed in the next section of this chapter.

Planning

Examples of Nursing Interventions Used in Health Promotion

- Explore beliefs regarding health and the client's expectations.
- Encourage modification of lifestyle through smoking cessation and diet modification.
- Promote a regular program of exercise.
- Identify mechanisms for stress management.
- Teach client about common illnesses and risk factors appropriate to the age of the client.
- Encourage routine assessment of health maintenance practices, such as health screening and immunizations.
- Teach client self-examination techniques for early detection of dysfunction.
- Encourage contact with resources and support services to assist the client with health maintenance.
- Encourage safe sexual behavior.

Implementation

The nurse uses educational interventions to help the client explore alternatives in health practices. Such education can take place in acute-care settings, the home, school, workplace, or ambulatory clinics. The nurse uses the teaching-learning process to educate the client about self-care (Fig. 30-4). The nurse shares knowledge with the client and leads the client through the learning process. The nurse and client should assess the client's knowledge deficit and together set priorities, goals, and outcome criteria. The nurse lets the client set the pace and creates a supportive learning environment. Both nurse and client evaluate the process by observing progress toward goals.

Nursing Interventions to Promote Health and Function

Nursing interventions to promote proper health maintenance include

- Educating clients about common illnesses and how to prevent illnesses
- Teaching self-examination techniques
- Encouraging routine physical examinations, health screenings, and immunizations.

Education About Common Illnesses

Teaching clients about common illnesses can help improve health maintenance and prevent illness. Nurses

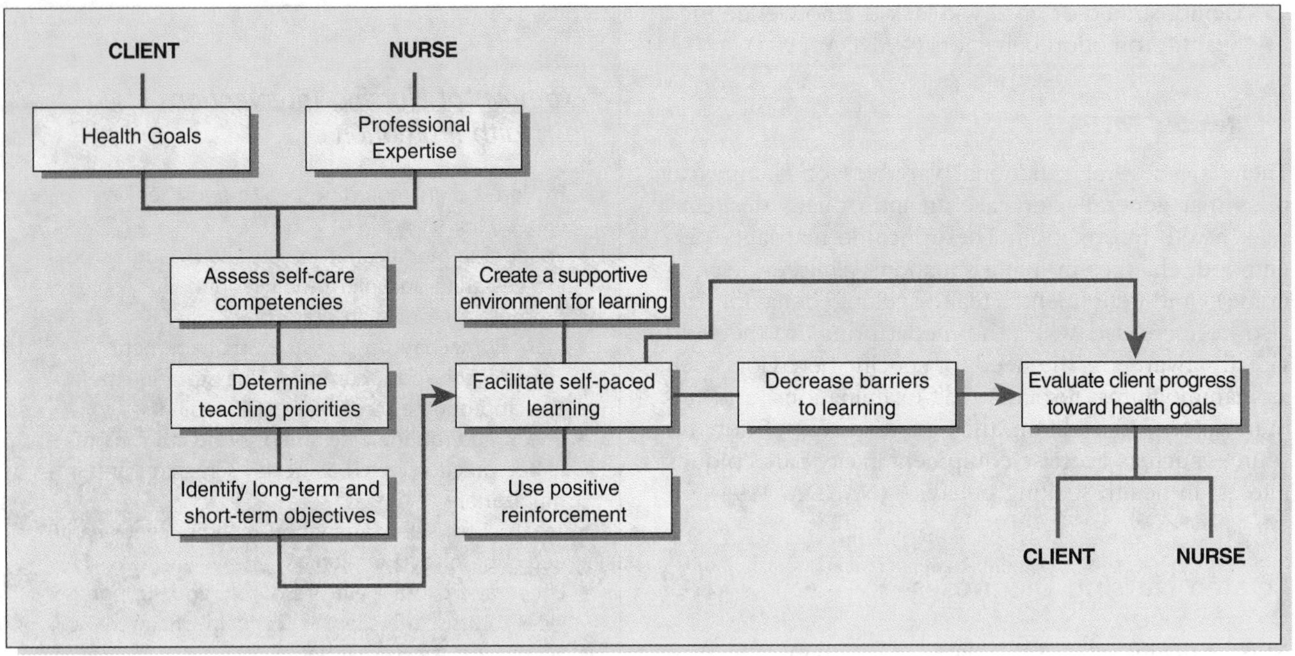

Figure 30-4 • The self-care education process. (Adapted from Pender, N. (1987). Health promotion in nursing practice *(2nd ed.). Norwalk, CT: Appleton & Lange, p. 195.)*

should know how to teach clients about hypertension, heart disease, cancer, osteoporosis, STDs, lung disease, and childhood infectious diseases. Client education involves teaching clients about risk factors for and warning signs of common illnesses, as well as ways to prevent these conditions. Information should be appropriate for the client's age and likelihood of contracting an illness. For example, adults and older adults should be taught about hypertension and heart disease; adolescents and sexually active adults who are not monogamous must be warned about STDs; young parents should be advised about childhood infectious diseases. Clients can also be referred to agencies such as the American Cancer Society for information.

Hypertension and Heart Disease. Hypertension and heart disease share some risk factors. Clients should be told that hereditary predisposition cannot be altered, but other risk factors can be altered and may aid in preventing such illness. Eliminating risky behaviors such as smoking, eating a high-fat and high-cholesterol diet, high sodium intake, being overweight, and lack of exercise may prevent subsequent illness. Healthy diet and exercise information should be given. Clients with one or two risk factors should learn the symptoms of myocardial infarction, as listed in the accompanying display. They should be advised to seek medical attention immediately if symptoms occur, because identification of early signs and prompt medical intervention reduce mortality. Teaching cardiopulmonary resuscitation to family members and close friends can be life-saving.

Cancer. Because cancer comes in many forms and can invade virtually any body tissue, there are many risk factors and warning signs (see display). Cancer education and screening programs have traditionally been age-related and gender-related. However, breast cancer does occur in men, and lung cancer, long considered a disease of men, recently has become the leading cause of cancer death in women. Therefore, the nurse must inform a wide variety of clients about the risks and warning signs of cancer; education should begin in childhood and carry on into old age. Risks include diet, sun exposure, tobacco use, exposure to asbestos, and pollution. Clients should be taught practices that are believed to prevent cancer, such as eating a high-fiber diet, using sunscreen, and avoiding chemical products associated with cancer.

Osteoporosis. Clients, especially women, should be taught that practices to prevent osteoporosis begin in childhood with adequate calcium intake. Calcium intake must be maintained throughout adulthood. Older women should learn the importance of weight-bearing exercise and estrogen replacement (for postmenopausal women) to decrease bone decalcification.

Self-Examination Techniques

Self-examination of the breasts, testicles, and skin is an important health-maintenance practice. It should be started by age 18 years in women and age 15 in men, but clients can be taught the techniques earlier if they want to learn. Education includes a demonstration by the nurse and a return demonstration by the client to ensure competency. Clients should know what they are looking for, and should learn that breast and testicular masses may be benign or malignant. Any mass, no mat-

Client Teaching
Health Promotion

Instruct the client as follows:
- *Reduce cholesterol intake by using low-fat dairy products and skim milk, fish, poultry with skin and fat removed, egg whites only, and unsaturated vegetable oils.*
- *Avoid red meat, egg yolks, fried foods, shellfish, cream sauces and soups, butter, lard, ice cream, and desserts made with whole milk and eggs.*
- *Avoid constipation by drinking at least eight 8-oz. glasses of fluid a day; increasing fruits, vegetables, and whole grains in diet; establishing regular exercise; and responding to the urge to defecate.*
- *If a balanced diet is eaten, don't take vitamin and mineral supplements; however, pregnant women and other clients with special needs should consult their physician.*
- *Perform relaxation breathing by inhaling deeply to the count of 4, holding your breath for 4 seconds, then exhaling to the count of 6. This exercise can be performed anywhere to relieve tension and can be repeated as needed.*
- *Exercise vigorously (raising the pulse rate) at least three times a week for 20 to 30 minutes to promote cardiovascular fitness. However, stop and consult a doctor for chest pain, dizziness, shortness of breath on mild exertion, or joint or muscle pains that persist.*

ter how small, should be brought to the physician or nurse practitioner's attention to aid in early diagnosis and treatment. Skin lesions that do not heal, are multicolored, or change color, shape, or texture are suspect. Skin cancers occur often in sun-exposed areas and in people with fair complexions, but everyone should carefully inspect all skin surfaces. See Chapter 52 for more information on breast and testicular self-examination.

Routine Healthcare

Part of health maintenance is the routine assessment by healthcare providers. Well-baby visits, yearly physicals, prenatal care, health screenings, and immunization programs are examples of routine healthcare. These visits can identify areas of strength and weakness in health maintenance, and education can be provided to improve health-maintenance practices, if necessary. The content of the physical examination may vary according to the client's age, family history, and previous health status. The nurse should encourage clients to comply with routine healthcare visits and to seek care sooner if problems arise.

Health screenings include blood pressure measurement, cholesterol screening, blood sugar testing, vision and hearing assessment, obesity screening, and stool testing for blood. There are additional screenings for pregnant women. Screenings are often aimed at high-risk populations, but all clients should be encouraged to participate. Screenings take place in hospitals, physicians' offices, clinics, schools, workplaces, community agencies, and even shopping malls. The nurse can provide information about screenings and the implications of their results.

Immunization programs are health-maintenance concerns for children and adults (Fig. 30-5). All new parents should be familiar with the immunization schedule for their children; adults often do not realize that children need periodic immunizations for protection from specific infectious diseases throughout their lifespan. The nurse should review immunization histories, particularly for tetanus, rubella, and measles, and advise clients appropriately (see Table 39-5).

Symptoms of Myocardial Infarction

Cardinal symptom is persistent chest pain. May be described as heaviness, squeezing, or crushing; may radiate to left side of jaw or neck or left shoulder or arm.

Other Symptoms

- Anxiety
- Dizziness
- Sweating
- Nausea
- Shortness of breath

Nursing Interventions for Altered Function

Nursing interventions for altered function also tend to be educational in nature and may include information about smoking cessation, diet modification, exercise programs, stress management, and alcohol and drug rehabilitation. The nurse may lead a program on smok-

Seven Warning Signs of Cancer

Changes in bowel or bladder habits
A sore that does not heal
Unusual bleeding or discharge
Thickening or lump in breast, testicle, or elsewhere
Indigestion or difficulty swallowing
Obvious change in wart or mole
Nagging cough or hoarseness

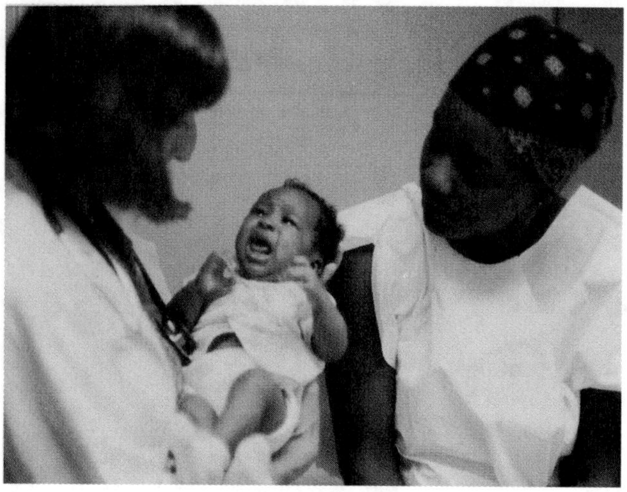

Figure 30-5 • Assisting the new mother in understanding her newborn's development helps prevent altered function.

ing cessation or diet modification, for example, or may simply provide background information and referrals to such programs.

The primary nursing goal is to help the client assume responsibility for self-care in these areas. To help a client assume responsibility, the nurse not only imparts knowledge, but may need to change the client's attitudes and instill motivation. Motivation to change may be increased by teaching the client the potential outcomes of altered health-maintenance practices. The nurse also provides emotional support to clients making changes in their health maintenance.

Interventions also address related and contributing factors as a way to correct the disruption in health maintenance practices. Barriers to health protection and promotion (such as misinformation or lack of transportation or health insurance) guide the type of interventions used. A client with financial problems can use a public clinic and the Department of Social Services. Giving the client information about public or volunteer transportation may solve transportation problems. Clients who cannot afford an exercise or diet program may borrow books and videotapes from a public library or attend free community lectures.

Safety Alert
Dieting and Exercise

- Advise clients beginning exercise programs to start slowly and proceed cautiously, never overexerting themselves. Pregnant clients and those with a history of cardiac problems, diabetes, arthritis, or hypertension should consult their physician before initiating an exercise program.
- Advise clients that dieting for weight loss must still meet the client's nutritional needs. Make sure meals contain foods from all five groups (meat, breads, fruits, vegetables, and dairy products) and that no meals are skipped.
- Warn clients against trying fad diets, exercise regimens, or other advertised "health" products or services that offer quick results. They are often a waste of money and may be dangerous.

Community-Based Nursing

The Nursing Plan of Care should reflect the client's educational needs. Goals are set and prioritized so that essential information is taught first and then reinforced. Nurses can enlist the help of other members of the healthcare team, such as a dietitian to help with meal planning or a clinical nurse specialist to provide information on smoking cessation. Family members and significant others should be included in the teaching so they can offer support after discharge. Reference materials such as printed menus for a low-cholesterol diet should be provided.

If the client needs extensive care or continuing help, additional interventions are indicated. For instance, the client may be referred to a home-health agency for inhome nursing assistance. Home-health nurses can help clients monitor their health status and manage diet and exercise. Often, clients can take responsibility for health maintenance with additional support and contact with the healthcare provider or referral agency on an ambulatory basis. A home-health nurse or public-health nurse may assist the client who is learning new skills or who needs reinforcement or continuation of learning.

Evaluation

Nursing interventions related to health maintenance are successful if the nurse and client agree that progress has been made toward the identified outcomes. Progress is easily measured by outcome criteria established in the planning phase. The following are general goals and outcome criteria for clients with altered health maintenance, although goals and outcome criteria are always individualized.

Goal

Client will identify areas for improvement in health maintenance.

Possible Outcome Criteria

Client identifies at least three problems in health maintenance (eg, overweight, sedentary lifestyle, cholesterol level above normal) by this afternoon.

Goal

The client will adopt appropriate health-seeking behaviors.

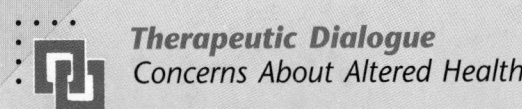

Therapeutic Dialogue
Concerns About Altered Health

Scenes for Thought

Abby Sinclair is 25 years old and has come to the community clinic for her annual physical. You, the nurse practitioner, have known her since she was 21. You know she is bright, has a good job, and is concerned about keeping healthy. She is sitting on the examining table when you come in, and quickly puts away the magazine she's reading.

Effective

Nurse: *Hi, Abby, I'm glad to see you. How's it going for you? (Giving recognition.)*
Client: *Um, fine, I guess.* She looks at her hands in her lap.
Nurse: *You don't sound too sure. What's up? (Sitting down next to the table and paying attention; exploring.)*
Client: *I've been having really bad cramps every month and sometimes in between my periods, too.* Looks worried.
Nurse: *How long has this been going on? (Asking for data.)*
Client: *For the last 3 months. Last month I couldn't go to work for 2 days, they were so bad. I take ibuprofen but sometimes it doesn't relieve the pain.* Begins to cry.
Nurse: *What worries you about this pain? (Requesting evaluation.)*
Client: *My mother had cramps like these and they found ovarian cancer. I'm so afraid I have it too.* Crying.
Nurse: *I remember you told me she died when you were 10 or 11.*
Client: *I remember her being in pain and having the operation and radiation, and then she died anyway.*
Nurse: *I know you're scared, Abby. But before you decide you have cancer, I'd like to examine you, get some more facts about your periods, and then we'll talk. (After further nursing assessment and confirmation by the gynecologist, endometriosis is diagnosed.)*
Client: *What a relief! But what do I do now? I can't miss any more work from this pain.* Now looking interested and ready to learn how to cope.
Nurse: *I have some pamphlets and articles on endometriosis. How about if you read them in the waiting room, and I'll come talk to you in about half an hour to answer any questions you might have. Do you have time today? (Offering teaching materials and self.)*

Less Effective

Nurse: *Hi, Abby. I'm glad to see you. How's it going for you?*
Client: *Um, fine, I guess.* Looks at her hands in her lap.
Nurse: *You don't sound too sure. What's up? (Looking through the chart while standing at the foot of the table.)*
Client: *I've been having really bad cramps every month and sometimes in between.* Looks worried.
Nurse: *I know you worry about your periods and cramps because your mom died of cancer when you were little. How long have these been going on? (Still reading the chart.)*
Client: *For the last 3 months.* Beginning to sound unsure of symptoms. *I even missed work because the pain was so bad.* Trying to convince you of how she suffered.
Nurse: *(Looks at client.) I'm going to examine you and then we'll see what we really have here. (Does further nursing assessment; diagnosis of endometriosis is confirmed by the gynecologist.)*
Client: *What a relief! What do I do now? I can't miss any more work from the pain.* Looks interested in learning more.
Nurse: *Don't worry too much about it; it's a pretty common problem, Abby. I have some pamphlets and articles you can take home with you. And there's a prescription for the pain and bleeding. We'll want to see you back here next month. Okay? (Doesn't wait for a reply. Abby takes the reading materials and slowly leaves the clinic.*

Critical Thinking Challenge

• Formulate the NANDA nursing diagnosis pertaining to Abby • Detect what the second nurse seems to be implying when she referred to Abby's worry of cancer. • Relate Abby's response to this • Compare and contrast the nurses' approaches to Abby before and after the medical diagnosis.

Possible Outcome Criteria

- Client asks for information about weight-loss programs at the next meeting.
- At the next meeting, client reports scheduling walks for 30 minutes four times a week.
- At the next meeting, client uses the stairs instead of the elevator and parks his or her car in the lot rather than using valet parking.
- Client and spouse read a complete book on low-cholesterol diets within the next week.
- Client says he or she will eliminate high-cholesterol foods from diet beginning immediately.

Goal

The client will maintain or improve current health status.

Possible Outcome Criteria

- Client loses 5 pounds in 3 weeks.
- Client says he or she feels better and has more energy in 3 weeks.
- Client reduces his or her cholesterol level by 10% in 1 month.

If no progress toward the goal occurs, the nurse and client need to reassess the goal. Conclusions may be

- The goal was too difficult to attain, and appropriate adjustments should be made.

Nursing Plan of Care
The Client With Health-Seeking Behavior

Nursing Diagnosis

Health-seeking behaviors as evidenced by lack of knowledge of testicular self-examination and a desire to learn.

Client Goal

Client will learn testicular self-examination techniques.

Client Outcome Criteria

- Client lists risks of and needs for regular self-examinations immediately after nurse's explanations.
- Client demonstrates effective self-assessment skills on return demonstration immediately after instruction.
- Client distinguishes normal from abnormal findings in discussion with nurse immediately after teaching session.
- Client performs monthly assessments as reported back to nurse at regular examinations.

Nursing Intervention	Scientific Rationale
1. Develop a teaching plan. a. Testicular cancer rates, risks, and survivor rates when treated early b. Skill c. Normal and abnormal findings	1. Individualized teaching plans meet unique learning needs as related to the diagnosis.
2. Provide written material for information.	2. This allows client to refer back to material and not rely on memory alone.
3. Demonstrate skill initially and on return.	3. Demonstration aids in learning of new skills, whereas return demonstration aids in validating proficiency of skill acquisition.
4. Assess performance with routine assessments.	4. Assessments reinforce need for health-promoting behavior.

- The client did not want the goal but agreed to it out of courtesy or because of intimidation or fear.
- Barriers exist, and interventions are needed to reduce them.
- The goal was established without the client's knowledge.
- The goal was established on insufficient information; additional information is needed to establish a desired goal.

After conclusions are reached, the client and nurse can then mutually decide whether to readjust previous goals, establish new goals, or terminate goals related to health maintenance.

Key Concepts

- Health-maintenance activities are those behaviors that the person in a stable state of health uses to maintain or improve that state of health over time.
- A person's ability to maintain health depends on his or her perception of health, motivation to change, and adherence to management goals.
- How a person perceives health depends on personal, cultural, and religious beliefs.
- Health promotion and illness prevention are components of health maintenance. Health promotion is characterized by approach behaviors, illness prevention by avoidance behaviors.
- Environmental factors, poverty, and unhealthy lifestyle and habits create a potential for altered health maintenance.
- The manifestations of altered health maintenance are chronic illnesses, accidents and injuries, childhood and developmental problems, and psychosocial problems.
- Two categories of altered health maintenance are approved by NANDA as nursing diagnoses: Altered Health Maintenance and Health-Seeking Behaviors.
- The nurse can diagnose and treat health maintenance alterations; most nursing interventions in-

volve client teaching of appropriate health behaviors and knowledge to manage self-care.

- Nursing interventions to promote health and function include education about risk factors for and warning signs of common illnesses.
- Routine healthcare, including prenatal care, well-baby visits, immunizations, yearly physical examinations, and health screenings can be nursing interventions to promote health and function.

Critical Thinking Challenges

Turn back now to the situation at the beginning of the chapter. After studying this chapter, you should be able to apply what you have learned about health promotion and illness prevention to your client's situation in the College Health Services. Consider the following:

1. *Reflect on the information you know about the freshman coed, your own values, and your initial impression of your client and her situation.*
2. *Formulate additional data you will need to make accurate diagnoses.*
3. *Analyze risky behaviors and health-seeking behaviors in your client's situation.*
4. *Based on your analysis of risky behaviors, recommend health information your client needs.*

References

Ajzen, I., & Madden, T. J. (1986). Prediction of goal directed behavior: Attitudes, intentions, and perceived behavioral control. *Journal of Experimental Social Psychology, 22*(5), 453–474.

Bandura, A. (1977). Self-efficacy: Toward a unifying theory of behavioral change. *Psychological Review, 84* (2), 191–215.

Becker, M. H. (Ed.). (1994). *The health belief model and personal health behavior.* Thorofak, NJ: Charles B. Slack.

Berlin, J., Thorington, B., McKinlay, J., et al. (1990). The accuracy of substitution rules for health risk appraisals. *American Journal of Health Promotion, 4* (3), 214–219.

Carpenito, L. (1992). *Nursing diagnosis: Application to clinical practice* (4th ed.). Philadelphia: J. B. Lippincott.

Dawber, T. R. (1980). *The Framingham Study: The epidemiology of atherosclerotic disease.* Cambridge, MA: Harvard University Press.

Duncan, D., & Gold, R. (1986). Health promotion: What is it? *Health Values, Achieving High-Level Wellness, 10* (3), 47–48.

Fishbein, M., Ajzen, I. (1975). *Belief, attitude, intention, & behavior: An introduction to theory & research.* Menlo Park, CA: Addison-Wesley.

Gillett, P. (1988). Self-reported factors influencing exercise adherence in overweight women. *Nursing Research, 37* (1), 25–29.

Gordon, M. (1993). *Manual of nursing diagnosis: 1993-1994.* New York: McGraw-Hill.

Jenny, J. (1987). Knowledge deficit: Not a nursing diagnosis. *Image, 19* (4),184–185.

Lauver, D. (1992). A theory of care-seeking behavior. *Image, 24* (4), 281–287.

McKie, L., Al-Bahir, M., Anagnostopoulou, T., et al. (1993). Defining and assessing risky behaviors. Journal of Advanced Nursing, 18, 1911–1916.

Murdaugh, C., & Hinshaw, A. (1986). Theoretical model testing to identify personality variables affecting preventive behaviors.*Nursing Research, 35* (1), 19–23.

Murray, R., & Zentner, J. (1993). *Nursing assessment and health promotion through the lifespan* (5th ed.). Englewood Cliffs, NJ: Prentice-Hall.

NANDA (1994). *Nursing diagnoses: Definitions and classification 1995–1996.* Philadelphia: North American Nursing Diagnosis Association.

Orem, D.E. (1990).*Nursing: Concepts of practice.* St. Louis: Mosby Year Book.

Pender, N. (1987). *Health promotion in nursing practice* (2nd ed.). Norwalk, CT: Appleton & Lange.

Public Health Service, U.S. Department of Health and Human Services. (1991). *Healthy people 2000: National health promotion and disease prevention objectives* (DHHS Publication No. 79–55071). Washington, DC: U.S. Government Printing Office.

Sennott-Miller, L., & Miller, J. (1987). Difficulty: A neglected factor in health promotion. *Nursing Research, 36* (5), 268–272.

Stachtchenko, S., & Jenicek, M. (1990). Conceptual differences between prevention and health promotion: Research implications for community health programs.*Canadian Journal of Public Health, 81* (1), 53-59.

Steiger, N., & Lipson, J. (1985). *Self-care nursing: Theory and practice.* Bowie, MD: Brady Communications.

Zindler-Wernet, P., & Weiss, S. (1987). Health locus of control and preventive health behavior. *Western Journal of Nursing Research, 9* (2), 160–175.

Bibliography

Edelman, C. & Mandle, C. (1986). *Health promotion throughout the lifespan.* St. Louis: C.V. Mosby.

Lierman, L.M., Powell-Cope, G., Benoliel, J.Q., et. al. (1994). Using social support to promote breast self-examination performance. *Oncology Nursing Forum, 21* (6), 1051–1057.

Pender, N. (1987). Health and health promotion: The conceptual dilemmas. In Duffy, M. & Pender, N. (Eds.), *Conceptual issues in health promotion: A report of proceedings of a wingspan conference.* Indianapolis: Sigma Theta Tau International.

Pender, N. & Pender, A. (1986). Attitudes, subjective norms, and intentions to engage in health behaviors. *Nursing Research, 35* (1), 15–18.

Smith, J. (1983). *The ideal of health: Implications for the nursing profession.* New York: Teachers College Press.

Wuorenma, J., Nichol, K., & Vonsternberg, T. (1994). Implementing a mass influenza vaccination program. *Nursing Management, 25* (5): 81–82, 84–85, 88.

Home Management

Key Terms	Learning Objectives

Key Terms

Activities of daily living
Anticipatory guidance
Caregiver
Case management
Continuity of care
Contract
Demands of daily living
Discharge planner
Facilitation
Homebound
Level of care
Medicaid
Medicare
Referral
Rehabilitation
Respite care

Learning Objectives

Upon completion of this chapter, the student will be able to do the following:

- *Define home management in terms of the balance and fit model.*
- *Identify factors that influence the ability to manage in the home.*
- *Describe assessment of the client, the family, the home, and community resources with regard to home management.*
- *Describe the client's, the family's, and the nurse's participation in the discharge planning process.*
- *Develop a plan for including a family member in the care of a person with impaired home maintenance management.*

31

You are a home health nurse and are making the first home visit to a single mother who gave birth to a premature baby 3 weeks ago. The baby was discharged yesterday with a gastrostomy feeding tube and an apnea monitor. The young mother arrives at the door, almost in tears, clutching the neonate. Two other preschool children are watching TV in the living room. The mother states "Why did you medical folks send my baby home? I just don't know if I can handle this all by myself. I was awake all night thinking my baby would stop breathing."

In Chapter 30, you learned the importance of individual responsibility in health maintenance. But most people live in a community. They have responsibilities to their family members and community, as you studied in Chapter 17. In Chapter 31, you will learn about home management and how the nurse helps individuals maintain optimal health and remain in their home environment. The Critical Thinking Challenges at the end of the chapter will help you apply this newly acquired knowledge to the situation of the single mother with a premature baby.

The last two decades have seen tremendous change in the area of healthcare delivery. More acute care management is taking place in the home than in the hospital. As the baby boom generation ages, and the focus of healthcare changes, home health nursing takes on greater significance. Home health nursing has expanded from home visits to chronically ill people to include managing care for individuals and groups to promote optimal wellness. Delivery of advanced technology has also become commonplace in the home setting.

All of us have a perception of ourselves in relation to the world and of our ability to maintain ourselves in that world. Independence is often linked to the ability to manage and care for ourselves at home. This involves the ability to care for our basic needs and to manage the complex activities necessary for independent functioning in our highly complex society.

The example of a young, single parent with two children living in a two-bedroom apartment in the suburb of a large Midwestern city will illustrate this concept. Many factors are important in enabling independent management for this parent. A safe, affordable shelter is required. Adequate financial resources are necessary to purchase food, clothing, and medical care and to pay for utilities. Household tasks such as cleaning and washing clothes are important in maintaining a healthy environment. The individual must be able to perform normal daily activities such as hygiene, cooking, dressing, and grooming, not only for himself or herself but for the children as well. Mobility, or the ability to move freely both within and outside the home environment, is important to perform many necessary tasks. The cognitive ability to understand how to organize work, manage financial responsibilities, and ensure safety within the home is essential. Transportation is necessary to purchase food, keep appointments within the community, and participate in social activities.

Alterations in health often affect a person's ability to manage independently at home. Sometimes independence can be maintained with adequate support from the family or the community. For example, a 68-year-old woman may be able to return to her home after surgery if her daughter stays with her for the first week after discharge. In more complex situations, many community resources may be needed to support a person in independent living at home. When home management is no longer feasible, the client may need to be placed in a facility to provide adequate support.

As a person moves or is moved from one environment to another, it is important to consider his or her ability to carry out functions of daily living in the new environment. Understanding the person in relation to the living environment is important in developing plans for care that maximize the person's ability to maintain himself or herself in a safe home environment.

Normal Home Management

A person's *environment* is his or her physical, psychological, or social surroundings. It may be the home, the hospital room, the neighborhood, the family, or a support system of friends. To maintain a safe, growth-promoting environment, the person must have adequate shelter, adequate nutrition, safe surroundings, and nurturing to allow for growth. Maintaining an optimum environment is a complex and dynamic process.

Normal Home Management Function

Normal management in the home occurs when a person can independently maintain a growth-promoting environment. The home is comfortable and safe, and the person performs self-care and hygiene tasks, interacts with others, meets financial obligations, and engages in activities from which he or she derives personal enjoyment and a sense of worth. Although some people may have deficits, they can adjust to their situation through their own resourcefulness or the assistance of others.

Characteristics of Normal Home Management

Balance

The ability to manage in the home environment is influenced by a balance between what the person *needs* to do and what the person *can* do for himself or herself. The person must be able to perform both **activities of daily living** (ADLs), such as bathing, grooming, dressing, feeding, and toileting, and **demands of daily living** (DDLs), such as responsibilities (self-imposed or imposed by others) for housing, pets, job, or home environment. Internal resources (eg, strength, knowledge, endurance, and motivation) and external resources (eg, friends, family, money, or professional services) are available to each person. Carnevali's balance model

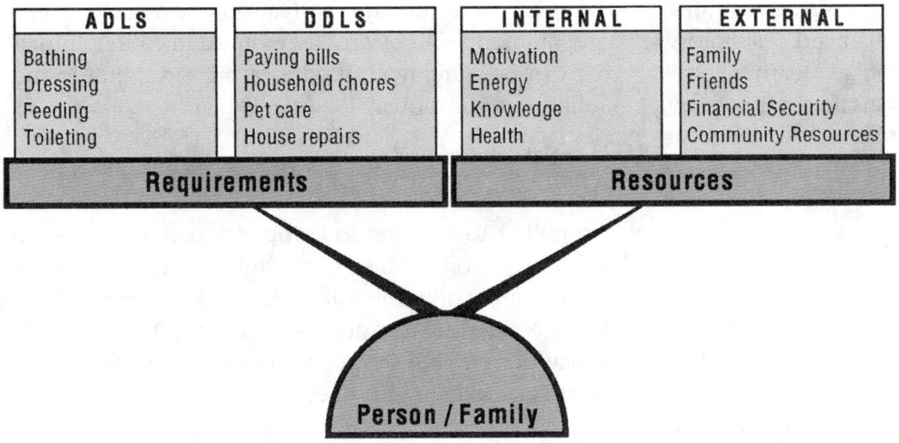

Figure 31-1 • *Balance model, showing the need to balance requirements (ADLs, DDLs) and resources (internal and external) to manage independently in the home.*

(Fig. 31-1) shows how ADLs and DDLs need to be balanced with internal and external resources (Carnevali, 1984). Also important to this balance is the relationship between the person's competence and the demands of an activity. For instance, does the person have the knowledge to perform ADLs? The strength?

Another model, the person and environment fit model, also helps us better understand home management (Fig. 31-2). This model emphasizes the importance of how well a person and his or her environment are matched. For example, a child in a friendly preschool environment is matched well with the activities and general surroundings.

Growth Promotion

A safe home environment provides basic needs such as shelter, nutrition, safety, and nurturing to allow growth. This growth includes all family members. Depending on the family, the environmental needs may vary: growth promotion for a toddler differs from growth promotion for a wheelchair-bound person. In some families, there may be a variety of needs over several generations.

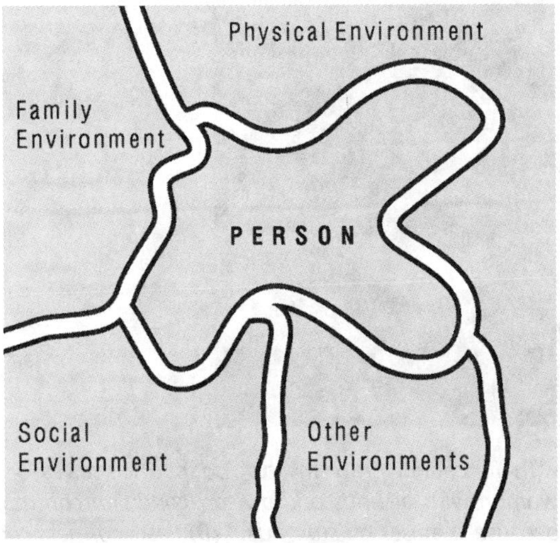

Figure 31-2 • *Person and environment fit model illustrates the importance of environment–person match for home management.*

Resources and Support Systems

Resources, both internal and external, are important for an individual to manage independently in the home. A homemaker, for instance, must have strength to lift and move objects; a knowledge of safety, cleanliness, and nutrition; physical and emotional endurance; patience; and motivation to perform ADLs and DDLs. External resources include family members who cooperate; friends for emotional support; money to buy food, clothing, cleaning materials, and transportation; and professional services as needed.

Support systems can include community agencies and organizations that provide needed services. Police and fire services are necessary for a safe community. Transportation to shops, medical services, and entertainment can be provided by public transport. Meals on Wheels brings food to the homebound and the elderly. Churches and synagogues provide a variety of support services.

Factors Affecting Home Management

Internal resources (a person's functional abilities) and external resources (family and social supports and community resources) affect a person's ability to manage successfully in the home. Each clinical chapter in the second section of this text describes how specific functional deficits affect a person's ability to perform ADLs and the support that may be necessary for the person to manage independently in the community.

Health Promotion and Safety

Living at home requires continual attention to promoting one's own health in whatever way is appropriate.

For a healthy adult, that may mean exercising three times a week; for a person with advanced respiratory disease, it may mean taking medication and learning new breathing techniques. Maintaining a safe environment by reducing the risk for injury is essential for living at home.

Cognition and Perception

The ability to interpret sensory cues and the ability to problem-solve appropriately are two tasks that are critical for living at home. Cognitive ability is needed to process the information presented in client teaching. Hearing, sight, touch, and smell are important in maintaining orientation and in interacting effectively with others and the environment.

Mobility

The ability to move within the environment is important in home management. Mechanical aids, such as wheelchairs or walkers, may be needed (Fig. 31-3*A*). The client must have enough strength and endurance to engage in those activities essential for daily functioning. The heart and lungs must be able to provide enough energy for normal activities.

Nutrition

A person's ability to buy, cook, and eat nutritious meals is another factor in independent home management. The ability to chew adequately and swallow so that aspiration does not occur promotes safe intake of food. The person's desire and motivation to eat and to follow a recommended diet are also important. Frozen meals that can be quickly cooked in a microwave help individuals eat nutritiously (see Fig. 31-3*B*).

Elimination

The ability to manage toileting independently (getting to the bathroom facilities, managing clothing, lowering oneself safely onto the toilet, cleaning the perineal area, and washing one's hands) is important. Lack of bowel or bladder control requires additional resources if the client is to remain at home.

Roles and Relationships

People need to be able to communicate needs and desires to others to meet many demands of living and to mobilize external resources. Communication is important within the family to foster positive relationships and promote self-esteem. Social isolation can occur when communication is limited.

Coping and Stress Tolerance

Coping ability is important, especially in our complex world. Think for a moment how a simple task such as shopping for groceries has grown in complexity, now that many stores offer dozens of choices in each food category and nutrition labels must be read for healthy choices. The ability to cope with day-to-day stresses in a way that promotes safety and growth fosters the ability to manage independently at home.

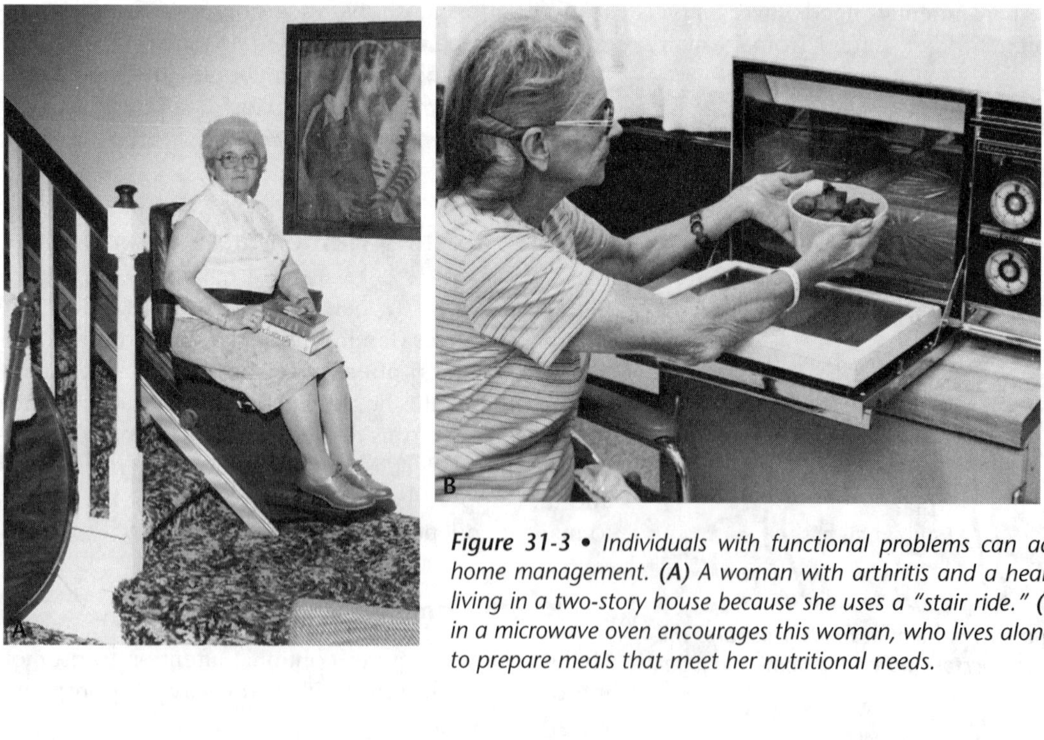

Figure 31-3 • *Individuals with functional problems can adapt themselves or their home management.* ***(A)*** *A woman with arthritis and a heart condition can manage living in a two-story house because she uses a "stair ride."* ***(B)*** *Fast, no-mess cooking in a microwave oven encourages this woman, who lives alone and has limited energy, to prepare meals that meet her nutritional needs.*

Lifestyle and Habits

There is great variability in expectations and values regarding independent home living. For example, one family may value a spotless home; another may feel more comfortable with clutter. One family may eat home-cooked meals together; another may eat out often or snack during the day. Some families have a traditional approach, in which the mother cooks and does housework and the father does home repairs, mows the lawn, and takes out garbage. Often these expectations are learned early in life from the family and community.

Economic Resources

Money is needed for such necessities as food, clothing, and shelter. Appropriate money management, such as paying bills on time and budgeting, is an important skill. A steady source of income offers security that allows planning and fosters living productively and managing in the home.

Family and Social Supports

Family and friends become important external resources for people with deficits in functional abilities. Family members or friends can volunteer to provide services: for example, young people may shop for an elderly relative, cut the grass, and do home repairs. When functional deficits are great, the support must increase. A family member may come every day to prepare meals and supervise daily activities.

Community Resources

The availability, accessibility, and acceptability of technical and professional resources in the community can affect the ability of those with limitations or special needs to remain in the home. Services such as hospice care, home healthcare, a crisis telephone line, a business that rents hospital equipment, and Meals on Wheels can provide needed support so that an individual can remain in his or her home. If functional deficits can be counterbalanced with appropriate community services, the ability to remain in the home is increased. A resource-rich community with, for example, support services for family caregivers and programs to transport wheelchair-bound people, provides extra support to allow individuals to remain in their homes.

Lifespan Considerations

Age and developmental level affect the ability to manage independently in the home setting. As people mature, they acquire the skills and abilities that permit greater independence.

Newborn and Infant

Newborns and infants depend on their caregivers for all their basic needs and for a safe environment in which they can grow and develop. The birth of a child can add stress to the family, making management more difficult for the parents. A mother coming home from the hospital with her newborn may be depleted of internal resources, limiting the energy she has to perform household chores and to care for herself and her neonate. This is a time when using external resources (such as the father, grandparents, or neighbors) can keep the house running smoothly and allow the mother to care for and nurture the baby properly.

Toddler and Preschooler

Tremendous physical growth occurs in the first few years of life, which allows the young child to move around more purposefully in the environment and communicate needs more clearly. Independence in a home environment is still not feasible for this age group. Children learn by actively exploring their surroundings, and their environment needs to be made safe so that injuries do not occur. Physical maturation permits the toddler, and especially the preschooler, to perform some ADLs independently, such as eating, toileting, and dressing. Assistance may still be needed with bathing, fastening buttons, doing up zippers, and tying shoes.

Some children in this age group are given increased responsibility around the house. Usually this starts with simple tasks such as putting away toys. Some parents also encourage young children to participate in household chores such as feeding pets or emptying wastebaskets. Such chores help set the stage for further responsibility for home management at later ages.

Child and Adolescent

The school-age child has independent self-care skills and usually assumes greater responsibility for household chores. In many families, everyone participates in tasks. Chores appropriate for a school-age child include keeping his or her room tidy, helping with the dishes or setting the table, vacuuming, sweeping, dusting, doing yard work, and caring for pets (Fig. 31-4). Some children show an interest in food preparation and may work with an adult to help prepare meals. Children can often independently prepare simple meals that do not need cooking, such as sandwiches. In some families, children receive allowances, which helps them learn how to manage money responsibly.

As the child approaches adolescence, greater independence is achieved. The preadolescent or adolescent may stay home alone while parents are away or working. The number of children left to manage independently has increased dramatically in recent years, as

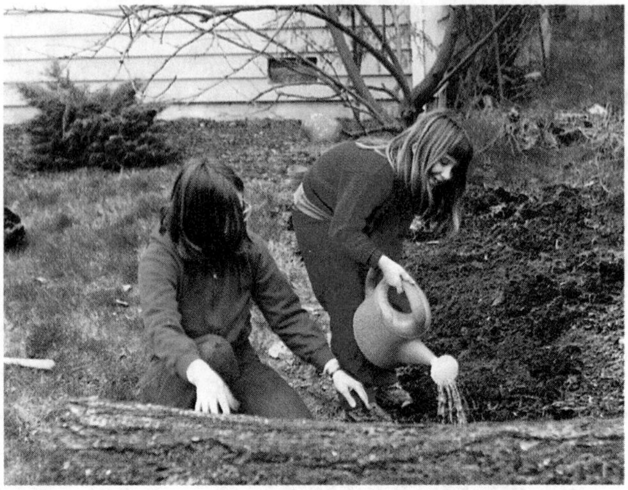

Figure 31-4 • *School-age children learn home maintenance tasks by working with their parents to perform chores.*

more mothers have joined the work force. Guidelines about what the child may do and how to handle emergencies should be made clear.

Adolescents may begin to work outside the home, often as paper carriers or babysitters. When babysitting, the adolescent is responsible for maintaining a safe environment for others. Getting a driver's license is another rite of passage that may increase the adolescent's responsibility, because he or she can run errands, go to a job, and get to appointments.

Some adolescents are legally emancipated and do not live with their parents. In such situations, several concerns arise. The adolescent's cognitive and developmental abilities may not be adequate to live independently. Family situations may support or hinder the adolescent's ability to manage. Often adolescents flee a negative home situation in which there was abuse and little opportunity to learn management skills, or a young woman who is pregnant may feel forced out of her parents' home. Those adolescents may find it impossible to stay in school and support themselves financially. With limited education, any jobs the adolescent may get are low-paying and do not offer benefits such as medical insurance.

Adult and Older Adult

A developmental task of early adulthood is emancipation from parents, which usually means moving away. Often this occurs for the first time when the young person leaves for college or the armed services, or gets a full-time job. The young adult must master many tasks, such as shopping for food, cooking, balancing a checkbook, and buying and maintaining a car. In recent years, there has been a trend toward delayed emancipation; some adults live with their parents into their thirties. Adult children often move back into their parents' home after a divorce or financial setback.

During early adulthood, marriage and the birth of children add to the complexity of home management. Buying a house also brings many new responsibilities. Because many young adults are healthy, home management is relatively easy and uncomplicated.

As children grow and leave home, middle aged parents may need to move to a smaller house or apartment to lighten their responsibilities. Retirement may cause financial burdens that affect the ability to remain in the home. As the adult ages, chronic health conditions that hinder the ability to manage independently become more common. Cognitive changes may impair safety, especially when the older person lives alone. Mobility deficits and problems with bowel and bladder control also significantly affect home management in the older adult.

Altered Home Management

Potential for Altered Home Management

Altered ability to function independently in the home may occur as a result of decreased functional abilities, insufficient family or social supports, or insufficient community resources.

Physical deficits or chronic debilitating diseases that decrease the client's ability to perform ADLs can lead to difficulty in managing a home. Factors affecting the ability to manage at home include the medical diagnosis of a chronic debilitating or limiting condition, the medical prognosis for the condition, and the need for treatments and complex medication regimens (Carpenito, 1995).

Health Promotion and Safety Deficits

Injury potential, altered health maintenance, and knowledge deficit regarding self-care procedures are important considerations in home management. Injury potential becomes a risk factor if the safety of any person is threatened; an example of this is a stairway without railings, on which children could fall and hurt themselves. Altered health maintenance due to health beliefs, a change in financial situation, or lack of supervision can also impair a person's ability to live at home. If a person cannot learn to manage necessary diets or treatments, his or her ability to promote health at home is impaired.

Cognitive and Sensory Deficits

Sensory loss, especially blindness, can hinder the ability to manage independently at home. The loss of sight can decrease independent functioning and can increase the risk for injury. Severe pain can also decrease the person's ability to carry out daily activities and functions.

An alteration in thought processes, if not responsive to treatment, can profoundly affect the ability to manage at home. Dementia (eg, Alzheimer's disease) is a progressive condition in which memory loss and confusion greatly affect the client's functional abilities. The severely confused person cannot live independently and may not be able to live safely with the family because of the care demand. Mental illness such as schizophrenia and substance abuse also may impair the individual's ability to manage at home with or without significant support from family or community resources.

Decreased Mobility

Many medical problems (eg, arthritis, neurologic impairments, fractures, respiratory disease, cardiovascular disease, cancer) can impair the client's mobility and alter self-care abilities. Minor mobility problems may make housework or home repairs difficult; limited mobility may also hinder the client's ability to get out of the house safely in case of a fire or emergency. The inability to do grooming, toileting, and personal hygiene tasks may impair the person's ability to live independently. The inability to maintain home hygiene and cleanliness may pose health and safety risks.

Altered Elimination

Inability to control bowel or bladder function affects the ability to manage independently in a home setting. Often such impairment occurs with other dysfunction such as mobility problems after a cerebral vascular accident, neurologic insult, or decreasing cognitive function.

Altered Nutrition

The inability to provide adequate nutrition impairs the client's ability to manage independently. Buying and cooking food and cleaning up require energy. Depression can decrease the desire to eat properly, especially when the person lives alone. Lack of financial resources may also hinder proper nutrition. Physical changes affect mastication and swallowing also contribute to the potential for impaired home management.

Insufficient Family or Social Supports

Family and social supports can compensate for functional deficits, and the extent to which family members and friends are interested or able to help is a crucial factor affecting home management. Their coping abilities and reserves, commitment and ability to be caregivers, and personal health are factors in the balance and fit equation. Busy adults may need their energy for their own home and family; they may not have time to meet the needs of an older person or a person with special needs.

Insufficient Community Resources

Community and service deficits—lack of community agencies that provide supportive health and social services to assist the client—will affect the person's ability to manage in the home. Some chronically mentally ill and developmentally disabled people cannot manage their finances or maintain hygienic living conditions without community assistance. Their environmental conditions may be stable, but without daily supervision from professionals or family they would be evicted and could become homeless.

Manifestations of Altered Home Management

Verbal Expression

Individuals often know when they cannot maintain an adequate, safe home environment. They may express this difficulty, or they may request advice or assistance. They may present financial difficulties and seek financial assistance. People with cognitive deficits may be unable to verbalize their concerns or remember their functional limitations. Sometimes the caregiver verbalizes an inability to continue to provide needed support.

Inability to Function Safely

Functional impairments, lack of family or social supports, or lack of community resources can hinder a person's ability to function safely at home. People living alone who have decreased functional abilities may manifest:

- Decreased ability for self-care or care of family members
- Decreased maintenance of safe and clean living space
- Decreased maintenance of economic obligations
- Decreased cognitive functioning and ability to respond appropriately to environmental stimuli.

Lack of External Supports and Resources

People with decreased family, social, or community resources and decreased internal resources may manifest altered or impaired home management in any of the following ways:

- Decreased ability or availability of caregivers to assist with or perform self-care activities
- Decreased assistance in meeting financial obligations
- Inability to reach available resources
- Unavailability of community resources or services specific to the client's needs.

Therapeutic Dialogue
Home Management

Scenes for Thought

Joyce Lewinski is a 42-year-old single mother of two preadolescents. Tim, the youngest, has cerebral palsy. He is in a wheelchair and, to this point, has been functioning well. When you, Matt Gunderson, come to the home for your monthly follow-up visit for the local clinic, you notice that the usually neat home is untidy, with newspapers on the floor and the dinner dishes still in the sink. Ms. Lewinski meets you at the door.

Effective

Nurse: *Hello, Ms. Lewinski, how are you today?*
Client: *Hi, Matt. Not too good, I guess.* Smiles weakly. Points to sofa to sit down.
Nurse: *What's up? (Sitting quietly and attentively.)*
Client: *Tim is up, that's what. He's hitting the teenager stuff hard, and I'm having a tough time handling him. Look at all this junk he threw around last night just because I told him he had to go to bed and not play with the computer anymore! He's been doing this for a week now.* Looks angry and embarrassed at the same time.
Nurse: *Sounds like a tough time for you. What do you think is going on all of a sudden?*
Client: *I don't know. I guess he's just being his age and rebelling. Lord knows he has it rougher than most kids his age. I guess I didn't see it coming.* Looks down at her hands.
Nurse: *(Listens quietly.)*
Client: *I guess I haven't been too attentive to him and Kristen lately. I have a new job.* Looks up and looks pleased. *I have to get more money since my ex isn't sending any. He's got another wife now, and she's been taking the money he's supposed to send to us. So I had to get another job that pays me more so I can afford the rent and my lawyer. But it's been more hours and I guess I haven't been here to oversee what's been going on with them.* Seems tired and overwhelmed.
Nurse: *You seem pretty tired and overwhelmed with all of it. What do you need help with?*
Client: Looks grateful at the question but unsure. *I'm not really sure. I know you're here to see Tim and check him. Maybe you could talk to him, and I could clean up a little? I never seem to have time anymore.*
Nurse: *Sure. And then maybe we can all talk afterward about what the kids can do about helping you around the house. And maybe what you all can do about spending more time together. I know he's in his room at the computer?*
Client: *Of course!* Laughs and goes around the room picking up papers and magazines.

Less Effective

Nurse: *Hello, Ms. Lewinski, how are you today?*
Client: *Hi, Matt. Not too good, I guess.* Smiles weakly. Points to sofa to sit down.
Nurse: *What's up? (Sitting quietly and attentively.)*
Client: *Tim is up, that's what. He's hitting the teenager stuff hard and I'm having a tough time handling him. Look at all this junk he threw around last night just because I told him he had to go to bed and not play with the computer anymore! He's been doing this for a week now.* Looks angry and embarrassed at the same time.
Nurse: *Kids can be tough at this age. I know, I have three of my own, remember.*
Client: *Yes, I remember you told me about them last month.* Silence. *Well, I guess you need to go see Tim now. I'll just clean up around here. I don't have much time to do that anymore.* Wearily begins to pick up papers in living room.
Nurse: *(Looks questioningly at Ms. Lewinski but decides she has dismissed him and goes to see Tim.) Okay, I'll get out of your way. Tim's in his room?*
Client: *Of course!* Laughs.

Critical Thinking Challenge

• Name the factors affecting Ms. Lewinski's usual home management style. Compare these factors with those affecting Tim's behavior. • Detect what cues Matt missed in the second dialogue • Organize your thoughts about what help the client received in the first dialogue that she didn't in the second • Examine what might have prevented Matt from following up his concerns regarding Ms. Lewinski's "dismissal" of him • Plan how Matt could follow up his concerns anyway, even after he had been in Tim's room and finished with him.

Family Stress

Family members of the person with functional health deficits may show signs of not being able to maintain the client or themselves at home. Caregivers responsible for round-the-clock supervision of the client may show signs of stress, reduced ability to cope, alterations in functional abilities, and financial loss. Physical or verbal abuse may signal severe family stress.

Poor Environmental Conditions

Unhealthy or unsanitary living conditions indicate impaired home management. Filth, rodents, infestation, or environmental hazards are visual cues to an unhealthy environment. Lack of running water, heat, or proper storage facilities for food also are seen in poor living conditions.

Homelessness

The homeless are people or families who have no regular shelter to live in and often move. Conditions contributing to homelessness include alcoholism, drug addiction, chronic mental illness, unemployment, personal crises leading to displacement from home, financial cuts in public assistance programs, and a decrease in available low-cost housing. Chronic mentally ill people who have been discharged from mental-health facilities and do not have access to adequate community services frequently become homeless. Increasing numbers of families with children are finding themselves homeless. Homelessness is also a problem in rural areas, where the exact numbers of homeless people are often hidden and governmental resource allocations are inadequate (Dahl, et al., 1993).

Homeless people subsist on public assistance, free shelters, food lines, or money obtained by begging. Because of the lack of shelters, homeless people are particularly vulnerable to assault and robbery, infectious and communicable diseases, and social isolation. Exposure to the elements, especially to extreme cold, can lead to severe health problems and death. In addition, homelessness has serious adverse affects on maternal and child health; homeless children are less likely to be fully immunized, and homeless women have a high incidence of low–birth-weight infants (Vermund, Belmar, & Drucker, 1987).

Assessment

Functional assessment of home management should encompass the functional abilities of the client, family, home, and community. Subjective information is collected to assess how the individual normally manages at home, what the home is like, and what family and community support is available.

Subjective Data

Interviewing the client, family, or other caregivers provides valuable information about the client's ability to manage at home, risk factors contributing to decreased ability to manage at home, and identification of actual home management problems.

Functional Pattern Identification

The client's competencies, capabilities, concerns, deficits, and limitations must be explored to understand how the person manages at home and what is desired by the individual and family. The accompanying display provides key questions that can be used to elicit this information.

Assessment starts by asking the client to describe his or her ability to manage self-care tasks such as bathing, dressing, grooming, and eating. Document the client's ability to carry out household chores independently or with assistance. The client can describe how functional limitations are handled at home and whether management has been satisfactory. Determine whether the client needs aids such as walkers, oxygen equipment, or a hospital bed. Assess medications and treatments and the client's compliance with the specified regimen.

> **Nursing Assessment**
>
> *Key Questions for Assessing Home Management*
>
> **Client**
>
> - How will you manage at home on a day-to-day basis?
> - What treatments will you be doing at home?
> - What medications will you be taking at home?
> - What do you want it to be like at home?
> - What kinds of problems do you think you will have at home?
>
> ***Family and Social Support***
>
> - How much can you rely on friends and relatives?
> - What help will you have at home?
> - How much do you think your friends and relatives understand your health and medical problems?
> - Whom would you like me to talk to about your health and medical problems?
> - How do you think your spouse and friends will handle or cope with your being home?

Family and social supports are also important to document. The client should verbalize adequate assistance from family members, neighbors, or community resources. The client should have a realistic plan in place should an emergency such as fire occur. Telephone numbers of emergency help should be posted near the telephone, and the client should know about appropriate community agencies.

Risk Identification

Rarely is a single factor the cause of impaired home management. The relationship between functional impairments and available internal and external supports determines the risk for impaired ability to manage at home. The greater the functional impairment, the greater the risk; the fewer available supports, the greater the risk. Common risk factors associated with impaired home management include:

- Multiple or catastrophic illnesses
- Limited social or physical functioning
- Repeated hospital admissions within 6 months
- Age older than 80 years, especially women
- Age older than 70 years with a disability
- Lack of social or family support and living alone.

The presence of these risk factors does not automatically indicate a problem; the importance of the risk factors for each client must be determined. During the entire assessment, it is important to be continually aware of cues that would indicate cognitive impairments, such as repeating the same question or giving vague answers that are not consistent. People with cognitive impairments are often unable to manage in the home but rarely are able realistically to identify their own limitations.

Community deficits also can contribute to decreased ability to manage at home. The incidence is greater in the following situations:

- Unsafe neighborhoods
- Inadequate housing for the disabled
- Refusal of agencies to accept difficult clients
- Inadequate home health services
- Lack of volunteer programs
- Long waiting lists for services (especially nursing homes)
- Lack of affordable housing

Dysfunction Identification

Assessment data about the client's functional abilities and the support available from family or others are important to diagnose impaired home management. A dysfunctional pattern can be identified when the client or family verbalizes the inability to perform daily tasks and manage at home. People have a deficit when they cannot perform self-care and hygiene tasks, do not engage in activities and interactions with others, and do not do things from which they would otherwise derive enjoyment and a sense of worth. Bills go unpaid; the house may be in disrepair.

It is important to assess family support to determine how well a person can function at home. Family assessment can be done with questionnaires covering a broad range of topics. The most significant factors to assess are barriers to home care and the ability of the family members to provide care. The display lists questions that can be used to obtain this information.

Assessing family support focuses on family characteristics that show decreased family involvement with or support for the client. To assess family involvement with the client, ask directly how much support family members are willing and able to provide. Observe for evidence of family visits. Look for evidence of family concern, such as cards and presents. Observe family communication patterns and dynamics. Families differ in their reaction to illness of a family member. The prognosis and severity of the illness can affect family interactions and subsequent involvement with the client. Chronic illness can lead to rejection of the client and can impair family dynamics (Levine, et al., 1985).

Assess the ability and willingness of the caregiver to perform, or to help the client perform, any therapeutic treatments. Caregiving often consists of bathing, dressing, toileting, transferring, feeding, housekeeping, shopping, preparing meals, managing finances, and providing transportation. Therefore caregivers must be assessed for their ability, willingness, and capability to carry out these activities. Wound dressing changes, ostomy care, home parenteral therapy, and physical therapy may require additional time and energy.

Other subjective data about the caregiver include the caregiver's comments about the emotional and physical strains of providing care or an overload of responsibility.

Objective Data

Objective signs of physical exhaustion, stress, and limited coping help to support such subjective data. Objective data can be collected from the client to support verbalized functional abilities. In addition, assessing the home and available community resources allows the nurse to individualize interventions. Medical records may be reviewed to determine past behavior (for example, compliance with prescribed therapies or keeping medical appointments).

Functional Deficits

General observation of the client can provide important information. Poor grooming, dirty clothing (especially with cigarette burns), or clothing inappropriate for the weather can indicate a self-care deficit. Clothing that hangs loosely, coupled with a gaunt appearance, may indicate difficulty providing appropriate nutrition. Note any inarticulate or difficult-to-follow stories, unusual emotional affect, inability to follow instructions, expression of self-harm, or display of anger or frustration.

Observing the client doing activities such as bathing, feeding, toileting, and walking provides objective data as to his or her ability to perform these tasks safely without undue fatigue. When complex procedures are necessary (eg, wound care, stoma management, glucose monitoring, insulin injections), observe the client or caregiver performing the task to determine his or her knowledge level and ability to manage necessary skills.

Braylock Risk Assessment Screen

Braylock developed a discharge planning screening tool to help quantify risk and amount of discharge planning required for different individuals (Braylock & Cason, 1992). Ten categories of risk factors are presented for scoring on the tool, including age, living situation/social supports, functional status, cognition, behavior pattern, mobility, sensory deficits, number of previous hospital/emergency room visits, number of medical problems, and number of medications. The higher the score, the greater the risk. The score helps identify those individuals that might require home care resources, extended discharge planning, or placement in a retirement or nursing home. (See display.)

Braylock Discharge Planning Risk Screen

Circle all that apply and total. Refer to the Risk Factor Index.*

Age
- 0 = 55 years or less
- 1 = 56 to 64 years
- 2 = 65 to 79 years
- 3 = 80 + years

Living Situation/Social Support
- 0 = Lives only with spouse
- 1 = Lives with family
- 2 = Lives alone with family support
- 3 = Lives alone with friends' support
- 4 = Lives alone with no support
- 5 = Nursing home or residential care

Functional Status
- 0 = Independent in activities of daily living and instrumental activities of daily living
- Dependent in:
  - 1 = Eating/feeding
  - 1 = Bathing/grooming
  - 1 = Toileting
  - 1 = Transferring
  - 1 = Incontinent of bowel function
  - 1 = Incontinent of bladder function
  - 1 = Meal preparation
  - 1 = Responsible for own medication administration
  - 1 = Handling own finances
  - 1 = Grocery shopping
  - 1 = Transportation

Cognition
- 0 = Oriented
- 1 = Disoriented to some spheres† some of the time
- 2 = Disoriented to some spheres all of the time
- 3 = Disoriented to all spheres some of the time
- 4 = Disoriented to all spheres all of the time
- 5 = Comatose

Behavior Pattern
- 0 = Appropriate
- 1 = Wandering
- 1 = Agitated
- 1 = Confused
- 1 = Other

Mobility
- 0 = Ambulatory
- 1 = Ambulatory with mechanical assistance
- 2 = Ambulatory with human assistance
- 3 = Nonambulatory

Sensory Deficits
- 0 = None
- 1 = Visual or hearing deficits
- 2 = Visual and hearing deficits

Number of Previous Admissions/ Emergency Room Visits
- 0 = None in the last 3 months
- 1 = One in the last 3 months
- 2 = Two in the last 3 months
- 3 = More than two in the last 3 months

Number of Active Medical Problems
- 0 = Three medical problems
- 1 = Three to five medical problems
- 2 = More than five medical problems

Number of Drugs
- 0 = Fewer than three drugs
- 1 = Three to five drugs
- 2 = More than five drugs

Total Score:

*Risk Factor Index: Score of 10 = at risk for home care resources; score of 11 to 19 = at risk for extended discharge planning; score greater than 20 = at risk for placement other than home. If the patient's score is 10 or greater, refer the patient to the discharge planning coordinator or discharge planning team.

†Spheres = person, place, time, and self.

Home Assessment

The client's house is important enough to be considered a separate assessment element. This assessment is often performed by a community health nurse. A comprehensive home assessment includes safety, sanitation, mobility, temperature, and personal space (Sargis, et al., 1987). The display summarizes home assessment.

- Learn whether the house is rented or owned, because this determines whether modifications are feasible.
- Look for smoke or fire alarms, adequate lighting, flat door sills, and adequate security.
- Determine whether the house is infested with vermin or rodents.
- Ask about sewer and garbage services.

Nursing Assessment
Assessment of Home Conditions

From Client

- Ownership: rent hotel room, apartment, or house; own; live with others
- Access: ground floor, stairs
- Condition:
  Utilities: heat, water, telephone, electricity
  Hygiene: housekeeping habits
  Sanitation: rodents, sewer, infestations
  Safety: handrails

From Home Visit

- Neighborhood: crime potential, located near environmental hazards
- Access: ground floor, condition of stairs and sidewalk, proximity to public transportation
- Utilities: type of utilities available and in service, cooking arrangements
- Hygiene: odors, facilities for cleaning, appropriateness of food storage
- Sanitation: presence or evidence of vermin or rodents
- Safety: short electrical cords, handrails, fire alarms, stable rugs
- Phone: private phone, accessibility, answering machine

- Determine the source of water and the condition of the plumbing.
- Assess for adequate and safe cooking and food storage equipment. Although rural and urban areas differ in the types of sanitation measures, sanitation should not be a source of disease.
- Assess for easy access throughout the house. Handrails on tubs and staircases, wide doorways for wheelchair access, and flat, even floors contribute to easy mobility. There should not be any scatter rugs, and halls should be uncluttered.
- Determine the adequacy of heating and cooling systems. Inadequate temperature control can lead to hypothermia or hyperthermia.

Do not overlook the personal aspects of a home. The presence of mementos, pictures, or religious items in a well-kept house reflects self-esteem. A nice garden, sewing equipment, or a workshop provides additional information on the person's home activities. A person may not be able to continue such self-actualizing activities. Being aware of the client's past gives the nurse a more complete understanding of the person and how the current health condition has changed the person's way of living. For example, an active 80-year-old man who gardens daily may interpret a broken hip as devastating, but a sedentary man who enjoys watching television and doing crossword puzzles may find the same situation a minor nuisance.

The nurse may recommend changes in the home based on a home assessment. Common physical changes include installing ramps and handrails, moving furniture to make room for a rented hospital bed, or installing equipment such as oxygen tanks and suction machines. If a severely disabled client is expected to return home, a home visit should be made before discharge.

Community Resource Assessment

The purpose of community assessment is to identify resources that can be used for people discharged with deficits to the home setting. A comprehensive community assessment is not needed to diagnose impairments, but being familiar with community resources allows the nurse to develop a more realistic and individualized nursing plan of care for the client. The nurse needs information about the economic stability of the community, the client's neighborhood, the social and health resources available in the community, and the community's cultural norms. An overview of community assessment is presented in the display in Chapter 17. The presence of services as recorded in service directories is one way to validate objectively what the client describes. Nurses should be familiar with available emergency care, equipment rental stores, and visiting nurse services, and should know where welfare and Medicare offices are located.

Nursing Diagnoses

The nurse uses data from the assessment to determine the presence of conditions that disrupt normal home management. Impaired Home Maintenance Management is a broad diagnosis that includes both management and maintenance aspects of living at home. Interdisciplinary professional communication is required for resolving this nursing diagnosis and assisting the client toward outcome goals. Other important North American Nursing Diagnosis Association (NANDA) nursing diagnoses include Caregiver Role Strain, Risk for Caregiver Role Strain, and Relocation Stress Syndrome.

Diagnostic Statement: Impaired Home Maintenance Management

Definition

Impaired Home Maintenance Management is the inability to independently maintain a safe, growth-promoting immediate environment (NANDA, 1994).

Defining Characteristics

Subjective characteristics are:

- Household members express difficulty in maintaining the home in a comfortable fashion
- Household requests assistance with home maintenance
- Household members describe outstanding debts or financial crises

Objective characteristics are:

- Disorderly surroundings
- Unwashed or unavailable cooking equipment, clothes, or linen
- Accumulation of dirt, food wastes, or hygienic wastes
- Offensive odors
- Inappropriate household temperature
- Exhausted or anxious family members
- Lack of necessary equipment or aids
- Presence of vermin or rodents
- Repeated hygienic disorders, infestations, or infections (NANDA, 1994)

Related Factors

Many factors can contribute to the development of Impaired Home Maintenance Management. Individual contributory factors might include individual/family member disease or injury, impaired cognitive or emotional functioning, and lack of knowledge. Family factors might include insufficient family organization or planning, insufficient finances, lack of role modeling, inadequate support systems, and unfamiliarity with neighborhood resources (NANDA, 1994).

Diagnostic Statement: Caregiver Role Strain

Definition

Caregiver Role Strain is defined as a caregiver's felt difficulty in performing the family caregiver role (NANDA, 1994).

Defining Characteristics

When Caregiver Role Strain is present, caregivers report they:

- Do not have enough resources to provide the care needed
- Find it hard to do specific caregiving activities
- Worry about such things as the care receiver's health and emotional state, having to put the care receiver in an institution, and who will care for the care receiver if something should happen to the caregiver
- Feel that caregiving interferes with other important roles in their lives
- Feel loss because the care receiver is like a different person compared with before caregiving began or, in the case of a child, was never the child the caregiver expected
- Feel family conflict around the issue of providing care
- Feel stress or nervousness in their relationship with the care receiver
- Feel depressed (NANDA, 1994)

Nursing Research
Home Management

Selected Nursing Research Studies

Helberg, J. (1993). Factors influencing home care nursing problems and nursing care. Research in *Nursing and Health 16*(5), 363–370.

Kammer, C. (1994). Stress and coping of family members responsible for nursing home placement. *Research in Nursing and Health 17*(2), 89–98.

Kelley, S. (1993). Caregiver stress in grandparents raising grandchildren. *Image, 25*(4), 331–338.

Lotas, M., et al. (1992). The HOME SCALE: The influence of socioeconomic status on the evaluation of the home environment. *Nursing Research, 41*, 338–341.

Mitchell, A., et al. (1993). Comparison of liaison and staff nurses in discharge referrals of postpartum patients for public health nursing follow-up. *Nursing Research 42*, 245–249.

Neundorfer, M. (1991). Coping and health outcomes in spouse caregivers of persons with dementia. *Nursing Research, 40*, 260–265.

Porter, E. (1994). Older widows' experience of living alone at home. *Image, 26*(1), 19–24.

Reinhard, S. (1994). Perspectives on the family's caregiving experience in mental illness. *Image, 26*(1), 70–74.

Possible Topics for Nursing Inquiry

- How can preventive healthcare services be provided to homeless families with school-age children?
- As caregivers become burned out and the client's health status deteriorates, what factors become important in their decisions about placement of the client?
- From the perspective of the client and caregiver, what community services are lacking in rural, suburban, and urban areas?
- How have nursing schools incorporated case management skills into their curricula?

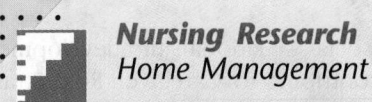

Related Factors

Physiologic, psychosocial, situational, and developmental factors all can contribute to Caregiver Role Strain. Physiologic factors include discharge of a family member with significant home care needs, illness severity, unpredictability or instability of the illness, addiction or codependency, premature birth, or congenital defects.

Psychological or cognitive problems in the care receiver, marginal family adaptation or dysfunction before the caregiving situation, marginal caregiver coping patterns, past history of poor relationships between the caregiver and the care receiver, or a care receiver who exhibits deviant, bizarre behavior all are psychological factors that can contribute to Caregiver Role Strain.

Situational factors related to Caregiver Role Strain include the presence of abuse or violence; the presence of stressors such as loss, disaster, crisis, poverty, or economic vulnerability; major life events (birth, divorce, retirement, hospitalization); duration of care required; inadequate physical environment for providing care; family/caregiver isolation; lack of recreational or respite care for the caregiver; inexperience with caregiving; caregiver competing role commitments; and complexity or amount of caregiving tasks.

Developmental factors, such as developmental delay or retardation of the caregiver or the care receiver, or a caregiver who is not developmentally ready for the caregiver role, can contribute to the development of Caregiver Role Strain (NANDA, 1994).

Diagnostic Statement: Risk for Caregiver Role Strain

Definition

Risk for Caregiver Role Strain occurs when a caregiver is vulnerable for felt difficulty in performing the family caregiver role (NANDA, 1994).

Risk Factors

The risk factors for this high-risk diagnosis, according to NANDA, are the same as the related factors given earlier for the actual diagnosis of Caregiver Role Strain.

Diagnostic Statement: Relocation Stress Syndrome

Definition

Relocation Stress Syndrome is physiologic and/or psychological disturbances as a result of transfer from one environment to another (NANDA, 1994).

Defining Characteristics

Major defining characteristics for Relocation Stress Syndrome include

- Change in environment/location
- Anxiety
- Apprehension
- Increased confusion (elderly population)
- Depression
- Loneliness.

Minor defining characteristics for Relocation Stress Syndrome include verbalization of unwillingness to relocate, sleep disturbance, change in eating habits, dependency, gastrointestinal disturbances, increased verbalization of needs, insecurity, lack of trust, restlessness, sad affect, unfavorable comparison of posttransfer with pretransfer staff, verbalization of being concerned or upset about transfer, vigilance, weight change, and withdrawal (NANDA, 1994).

Related Factors

Factors that can affect the development of Relocation Stress Syndrome include past, concurrent, and recent losses; losses involved with the decision to move; feeling of powerlessness; lack of adequate support system; little or no preparation for the impending move; moderate to high degree of environmental change; history and types of previous transfers; impaired psychosocial health status; and decreased physical health status (NANDA, 1994).

Related Nursing Diagnoses

Any nursing diagnosis indicating impaired functional capabilities, such as Activity Intolerance, Self-Care Deficit, Impaired Physical Mobility, Incontinence, Risk for Injury, or Altered Nutrition, can often be seen in the client who has impaired home maintenance management (Table 31-1). Also, the client's inability to care for himself or herself at home can increase Anxiety, Fear, Ineffective Individual or Family Coping, and Self-Esteem Disturbance. Noncompliance and Knowledge Deficit are also associated with Impaired Home Maintenance Management.

Outcome Identification and Planning

The basic goal for the client with impaired home management is to live in a supportive environment that has been agreed on by the client, family, and healthcare providers. Client goals can be written in terms of rehabilitation or restoration of independence. **Rehabilitation** goals should be written for people who are ex-

Table 31-1* • *Effects of Selected Nursing Diagnoses on Daily Life

Functional Cluster	ADL	DDL	IR	ER	Fit
Health Perception and Health Management					
Knowledge Deficit: treatments		X	X		
Knowledge Deficit: medications		X	X		
Risk for Injury	X		X		X
Altered Health Maintenance	X	X			X
Nutrition and Metabolism					
Altered Nutrition	X				
Altered Elimination	X	X		X	
Fluid Volume Deficit		X			
Activity and Exercise					
Impaired Mobility	X	X		X	X
Self-Care Deficit	X	X		X	X
Activity Intolerance	X	X			X
Pain		X	X		
Circulation and Respiration					
Impaired Gas Exchange		X		X	
Ineffective Breathing Patterns		X			X
Altered Tissue Perfusion		X			
Sensory/Perceptual					
Altered Vision	X				X
Altered Auditory Sense	X				X
Altered Tactile Sense	X				X
Roles and Relationships					
Impaired Social Interactions			X	X	X
Hopelessness		X	X		X
Powerlessness		X	X		X
Altered Thought Processes	X	X	X		X
Impaired Verbal Communication		X	X	X	

ADL, activities of daily living; DDL, demands of daily living; IR, internal resources; ER, external resources.

pected to regain some level of physical or cognitive functioning through training rather than through health improvement. In developing goals for the client, it is important to decide whether rehabilitation or independence is the best way to ensure a safe, nurturing environment.

When forming goals for the client, consider the following:

- The level of functioning to be achieved or maintained
- The extent of independence expected
- The level of family involvement
- The level of support services available to the client living in the community.

Possible goals for home management include:

The client will return to a safe home environment.
The client will continue to live at home.
The caregiver will care for the client at home.
The caregiver will obtain adequate support to continue in the role as caregiver.

The accompanying display outlines examples of some appropriate nursing interventions for Impaired Home Management planning.

Implementation

Nursing Interventions to Promote Health and Function

Client Teaching

Client teaching is a powerful tool to promote the client's ability to live safely at home. Teaching can focus on knowledge needed to improve functional abilities or limit dysfunction. Some teaching topics are:

Planning
Examples of Nursing Interventions Used in Home Management

Direct Care

- Administer parenteral medications
- Intravenous management
- Dressing changes and wound care
- Pain management
- Glucose monitoring and diabetic management
- Terminal care

Educational Needs

- Assess level of knowledge of disease and preventive behavior (rest, exercise, nutrition, mode of transmission of the disease, use of medications, aseptic technique).
- Provide simple written instructions.

Supplies and Equipment

- Evaluate insurance coverage.
- Refer to social services.
- Refer to volunteer organizations.
- Instruct in use of generic brands of medications.

Support in Altered Lifestyle

- Emphasize the positive aspects of increase in well-being.
- Set realistic goals with the client and significant others.
- Modify the plan of care to avoid conflict with religious beliefs or cultural practices by incorporating those behaviors that do not cause adverse effects.
- Enlist the support of other members of the family and social or religious group.

Supportive Social Network

- Give appropriate referrals to groups and agencies.
- Identify healthcare providers who will provide assistance.
- Counsel family members or significant others.

- When and who to call for help
- Medications
- Dietary modifications
- Medical equipment and procedures to be used at home
- Ambulation techniques to improve safety
- Community resources and how they can be reached
- Home safety measures (ie, removing clutter, installing handrails by tubs and stairs, improving lighting)
- Solving anticipated problems.

Client teaching is important and should not be left until just before discharge, when the client is anxious and may have difficulty learning. For additional information, see the Client Teaching display.

Anticipatory guidance is information given about a situation before the situation occurs so that the client can develop problem-solving and coping strategies. Anticipatory guidance is an important psychological intervention because it prepares the client for decisions to be made at home and for the extent of self-care required after discharge.

Discharge Planning

Discharge planning prepares for moving a client from one level of care to another within or outside the current healthcare facility. Traditionally, this has been viewed as discharge from the hospital to the home. But in the current healthcare system, discharge planning can occur from ambulatory surgical centers, rehabilitation units, drug treatment centers, or childbirth centers. Discharge can also occur within a facility as a client moves from one unit to another (client with a cerebral vascular accident moves from medical–surgical unit to the rehabilitation unit). Discharge planning is done *with* the client and family, not *for* the client and family. The **discharge planner** is the health or social services professional who is responsible for coordinating the transition and who acts as a link between the discharging facility and the community. Often, the discharge planner is a nurse.

Client Teaching
Home Management

Instruct the client as follows:

- *Familiarize yourself with community resources to help meet your needs after discharge.*
- *Learn about community support groups that may offer emotional support and assistance after discharge.*
- *Learn about new medications you will be taking after discharge. Ask for written information to which you can refer.*
- *Follow instructions and demonstrate procedure you will perform at home after discharge.*
- *Learn symptoms that are significant and warrant contacting the physician.*
- *Learn about any activity restriction or diet restrictions that must be followed after discharge.*
- *Familiarize yourself with new equipment you will be using at home after discharge.*
- *Learn how to contact help should an emergency arise. Have the number of your physician and the emergency room handy, and know how to contact emergency personnel (eg, 911), if necessary.*

Discharge planning does not solve all problems, but it can reduce readmissions, reduce residual effects of the health condition through continuity of care, and improve client and family satisfaction with healthcare.

Discharge Planning Elements for the Client. The key elements of discharge planning for the client are transition and continuity of care.

Transition. When people undergo transitions, their assumptions about themselves change, and they develop new assumptions that allow them to adapt (Schlossberg, 1981). As a nursing concern related to adaptation, transition is particularly obvious when a client moves between settings, such as from the hospital to home, or from home to a long-term care facility (Chick & Meleis, 1986). But the physical move is only one type of transition the client actually makes: the related change of assumptions may involve self-concept, role performance, mobility, self-care, or communication with family members. For example, a mother with terminal cancer may be experiencing the transition from her role as a caregiver to the role of a care recipient. Balance and fit change as the person makes the transition from old to new settings and assumptions.

Continuity of Care. Continuity of care is both an ideal and a necessity. **Continuity of care** is the provision of health services without disruption, regardless of the client's movement between settings. From the client's perspective, it involves having a home health nurse visit the day the client is discharged from the hospital or having the physician's office contact the local pharmacy about the client's medication needs. When health services are disrupted, the client may experience a relapse, requiring additional healthcare or hospitalization. Thus, continuity of care helps to maintain the client's health status and reduces healthcare costs.

Organizational policy and financial realities can work against achieving continuity. Communication between health professionals about a client's needs may not occur. Discharge plans started at admission can help ensure continuity of care through early, expedient referrals to community services and agencies.

Discharge Planning Elements for the Nurse. The nurse is responsible for ensuring that the client is prepared for discharge and that the family or caregiver has received necessary information and assistance. Safety is a factor in planning for the client in the home. Some safety features are listed in the accompanying display. The key elements of discharge planning for the nurse are coordination, facilitation, and negotiation.

Coordination. Coordination is the act of assembling and directing activities so that services are provided harmoniously. The result of coordination is a team working together with a unified purpose; health professionals work with the client and other health professionals (Fig. 31-5). Payment based on diagnosis-related groups has led to shorter hospital stays, and as a result, nurses must coordinate health and social services for postdischarge needs (Phillips & Cloonan, 1987). One way to coordinate services is to initiate and conduct team conferences and family conferences, preferably before the client is discharged or the client's problems have become too complex. At a team conference, discussion focuses on individualizing care for the client. At a family conference, professionals and the family gather to discuss family issues related to the client. Both types of conferences provide an opportunity for clients, family, and healthcare professionals to plan care and set goals.

Facilitation. **Facilitation** is making something easier and smoother, eliminating problems and barriers. To facilitate the client's transition, the discharge planner

Safety Alert
Home Management

Before discharging a client to the home setting, try to ensure a safe environment by

- Making sure fire alarms are in working order
- Removing obvious hazards, (eg, loose scatter rugs, loose handrailings, worn electrical cords)
- Ensuring that door locks are working
- Discussing use of security systems if advisable
- Installing needed devices to ensure safe mobility (eg, extra handrailings, especially around the tub or toilet; nightlights; ramps for wheelchair access)
- Displaying emergency numbers for *police, fire,* and *physician*
- Ensuring that heating system and refrigeration for food are in working order
- Developing a system in which a family member or neighbor calls or checks in on a person daily, if necessary

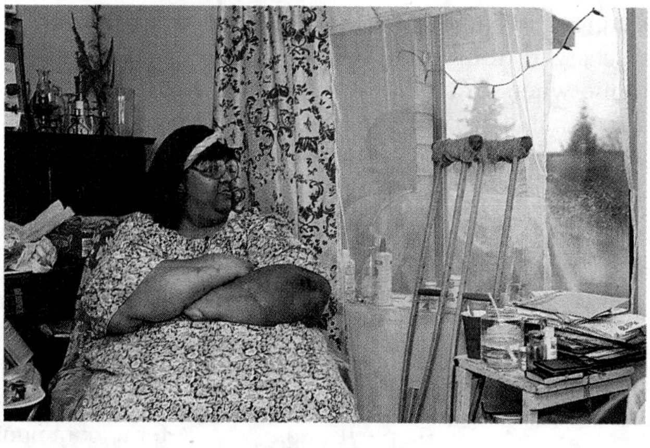

Figure 31-5 • *Clients with multiple chronic health problems need teaching, support, and coordination of health services to remain in the home. (Photo courtesy of Seattle University School of Nursing.)*

must anticipate client needs and plan ahead. Anticipation of discharge needs begins at admission. The nurse must take into account the different settings and client needs and available resources.

Negotiation. This is the process by which goals are determined between the client, the nurse, and the family. The most elaborate plan of care is doomed to failure if attempts to achieve the goals are hampered by the client, family, or a healthcare professional. Negotiation does not need be a formal process, but it must involve dialogue with the client and family to help articulate desires, values, and feelings about how realistic certain plans of care are for the client and family. For example, the home care priorities of a young mother with a respirator-dependent infant may differ from those of the nurse. Negotiating with the mother over which goals and objectives have priority has two effects: the mother will be more willing to work with the nurse to attain goals, and she will feel more in control of her situation.

At times, for clarification, a more formal process involving contracts may be necessary. A **contract** is a written agreement between the nurse and client that delineates the roles and responsibilities of each. Contracts help to limit the helplessness, stress, or disempowerment that the client and family often feel. The sense of control and empowerment achieved through the contract enhances the client's internal resources—specifically, motivation and commitment. The nurse and the client or caregiver discuss who will be responsible for what, and reach a consensus. The consensus on responsibilities is then written down so that each party can be held accountable.

Levels of Discharge Planning. Discharge plans vary depending on client needs and the nursing interventions required to assist the client after discharge. All client goals and nursing orders should be developed from the perspective that human responses to health and illness occur regardless of the healthcare delivery setting. Discharge planning is needed when a child is discharged from a day surgery center after a tonsillectomy, when an older woman leaves a clinic requiring additional diagnostic tests to rule out a diagnosis of cancer, or a young man with a long history of substance abuse is being discharged from a drug rehabilitation center. The level of discharge planning increases depending on the complexity of healthcare required and the complexity of the transition for the client. The three levels of discharge planning are summarized in Table 31-2.

Basic Discharge Plan. The least complicated and most common discharge plan is teaching the client about self-care. Client teaching may include teaching about medications, treatments, community resources, or energy conservation techniques. The teaching should anticipate problems the client may experience at home. For instance, when discharging a newborn with an apnea monitor to a home in which there are already three small children, the nurse should teach the parents to check that the monitor parameters have not been changed by the other children.

Simple Referral. The second type of discharge plan involves referring the client to community resources (eg, a smoker to a smoking cessation clinic, a high-risk mother to the local health department, a caregiver to a respite service). A **referral** is a request for a service that is outside the scope of the referring professional (Fig. 31-6). The nurse acts as the discharge planner and must know both the community resources and the client's ability to reach those resources. Knowledge of the community resources is based on the community assessment and on personal knowledge.

Complex Referral. The third and most complex type of discharge plan involves referring the client to the discharge planner. The nurse may choose to involve the discharge planner because the client situation is complex, so planning and referral to appropriate community resource would be too time-consuming or beyond the knowledge level or ability of the nurse. This type of discharge planning is particularly appropriate for clients with multiple risk factors for impaired home management.

This third level of discharge plan involves interdisciplinary collaboration and coordination. The discharge planner takes responsibility for coordinating the activities necessary to transfer the client from one setting to another. However, referring the client to the discharge planner does not absolve the nurse of responsibility. The nurse must follow up and evaluate if the discharge

Table 31-2 • *Levels of Discharge Planning*

Discharge Plan Level	Nursing Interventions	People Involved
Basic, universal	Self-care and illness teaching	Nurse, client, caregiver
Simple referral	Refer to community resources Coordinate for continuity	Nurse, client, caregiver
Complex referral	Refer to discharge planner Facilitate coordination	Nurse, discharge planner, family

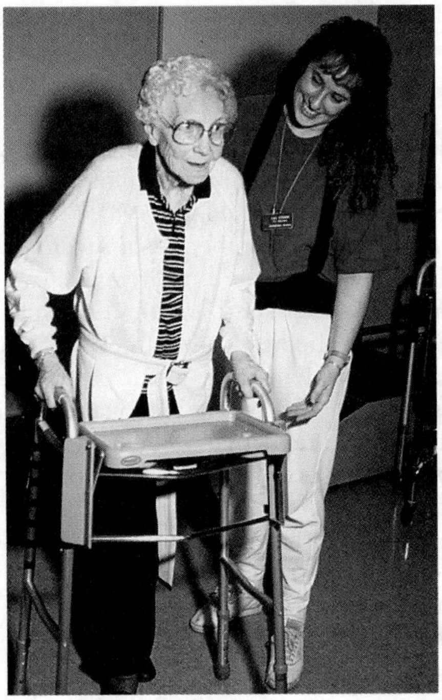

Figure 31-6 • A referral for physical therapy after discharge can help improve mobility, enabling a client to remain in the home.

planner has acted and if the client is satisfied with the discharge plan. The nurse may need to reinforce plans made by the discharge planner.

A referral to the discharge planner is appropriate for coordinating placement of the client in a skilled nursing facility or a long-term care facility. The discharge planner can also coordinate and initiate services the client will need if discharged to home (eg, a visiting nurse). Table 31-3 provides a list of healthcare providers often used as referrals during discharge planning.

Nursing Interventions for Altered Function

Healthcare Options and Placement

With each situation, a different level of deficit and support is manifested. The level of deficit determines the level of assistance needed with daily activities, which determines the level of healthcare required to stay at home. The **level of care** refers to the intensity and permanence of care required to maintain, restore, or promote health.

Levels of care range from minimal to extensive. Each level of care is related to a type of healthcare service. At the low end of the continuum is intermittent, temporary, or minimal care. Low-level care can be provided by temporary homemaker services to a healthy client recovering from hip surgery, for example; other low-level care services are adult or child day care centers. Moderate levels of care include home healthcare, residential care, and respite care. At the other end of the continuum is high-level care, which is continual, permanent, or intensive. An example of high-level care is 24-hour nursing care for a quadriplegic with a tracheostomy. High-level care services include hospice, high-technology home care, rehabilitation, long-term care, or skilled nursing facilities. If the client is homebound, moderate or high-level care may be appropriate depending on the client's abilities, external resources, and the home environment.

Table 31-3 • *Healthcare Providers Used in Discharge Referrals*

Healthcare Provider	*Role*
Home health nurse	Provides assessments, direct care, client teaching and support, coordinates services, evaluates outcomes
Home health aide	Provides hygiene care, cooking, supervision, and companionship
Social worker	Assists in finding and connecting with community resources or financial resources, provides counseling and support
Physical therapist	Assists with restoring mobility, strengthens muscle groups, teaches ambulation with new devices
Occupational therapist	Helps clients adjust to limitations by teaching new vocational skills or better ways to perform activities of daily living
Nutritionist	Teaches clients about meal planning and diet restrictions
Speech therapist	Assists clients to communicate better and works with clients who have swallowing problems
Respiratory therapist	Provides home follow-up for clients with respiratory problems including assessment, oxygen administration, and home ventilator care

Some clients may be so disabled and have such severely impaired abilities to manage independently that they cannot leave home. These clients are called **homebound**.

The specific type of service chosen is based on both the deficits manifested and the preferred place for receiving care. The interdisciplinary team of physician, nurse, and social worker work with the client and family to decide whether the client can remain in the home or placement in a healthcare facility is necessary. Placement decisions are affected by the presence or absence of family supports. The term "placement" reflects the attitude that a provider makes the decision and controls care, but ideally, placement occurs with the client and the family fully participating in the decision-making process. Widowhood, living alone, and childlessness are related to nursing home placement (Horowitz, 1985). The most common recipients of home and community services are very old women, people who have difficulty with several ADLs, people living alone, and Medicaid recipients.

Funding Sources. Although the physician, nurses, and social workers may prefer one type of service or level of care, the reality is that placement is often influenced by insurance coverage. **Medicare**, available to those older than 65 years of age, is a federally funded health insurance plan administered by the Social Security Administration. **Medicaid**, funded by the federal and state governments, provides financial assistance to the disabled or financially needy. Other constraints affecting placement are the limited number of nursing home beds and home health agencies. All these constraints force nursing plans of care to be both economically realistic and scientifically sound. For example, to qualify for Medicare-covered home healthcare, clients must be confined to their homes and must require skilled nursing care for an acute or postacute condition.

Family as Resource. Family supports and family decisions must be considered when placement options are considered. When a family member cannot provide self-care, other family members face a choice: they can help the person remain at home, or they can place the person in a healthcare facility.

The family member who cares for the client is called the **caregiver**. Often the caregiver is an adult child or spouse caring for a parent or spouse who has some degree of physical, mental, emotional, or economic impairment that limits independence and makes ongoing assistance necessary. The prevalence of caring for parents has increased and is discussed in the healthcare literature as "parentcaring." Caregiving includes providing emotional support, direct health services, and financial support; mediating with health and social service organizations; and sharing a household (Horowitz, 1985). It includes tasks such as bathing, toileting, feeding, preparing food, maintaining a home, and housekeeping. Another form of caregiving that has emerged in the last few decades involves grandparents raising grandchildren because their own children are unable to fulfill the role of parent (Kelley, 1993).

When one family member has a severe physical or mental disability, the strain on caregivers can be great (Neundorfer, 1991; Reinhard, 1994). The family may feel unable to provide the necessary care. Poor families with many existing problems may already be experiencing extreme stress and may be unable to take on the added responsibility of caregiving. A client in such a family would experience poor balance and poor fit with the family situation.

Each family must decide among different care options. The family, especially the caregiver, needs information on respite care, levels of care that are alternatives to home care, and realistic prognostic information. This information is important in making family choices. Those managing the affairs of an older person need to be aware of potential challenges.

Family dynamics vary widely, and the nurse must be sensitive to family patterns and facilitate the decision-making process without being judgmental. At times, families may make decisions that appear to the nurse as unloving, irresponsible, overly protective, or self-sacrificing. But the nurse must refrain from judging the decision while still taking action to meet the client's goals. Involving the family in the placement decision is as important as accepting their decision.

Family Preparation for Discharge

Social and family interventions are developed to meet social support and resource goals. Referrals may be made to social workers and the discharge planner. A social worker is trained to assess and help people regarding public assistance, social or family crisis, and access to social service programs. The social worker may be asked to see the client for financial or insurance matters or for counseling. A client may develop a fear of going home, especially if he or she lives alone or feels isolated; involving social supports in care is an important nursing intervention. Family conferences, another nursing intervention, can be held before the client is discharged.

The family and client should be told of any specific arrangements that have been made concerning referrals, appointments, or special equipment that is needed or ordered. Financial arrangements need to be clarified before discharge. It is helpful if the home health nurse can visit the client before discharge. When this is not possible, a telephone conference can permit exchange of information that will assist in individualizing care.

Physical Preparation for Discharge

The nurse, along with the family, helps prepare the client for discharge. Transportation arrangements should be made. If a family member is unable to pick up the client or the client is unable to go safely by automobile, an ambulance should be scheduled. The client should be dressed and ready, and all necessary paperwork completed before the ambulance is due to arrive, because most ambulance services charge for waiting time. An example of a Client Discharge Summary is provided in Figure 14-10. Before discharge, the client should be bathed and necessary procedures performed. Care should be taken not to overtire the client just before discharge because transfer to another setting can be physically and emotionally exhausting, especially for the client with limited energy reserves.

Community-Based Nursing

Much of this chapter is related to community-based support for the client and family. Two specific types of community-based nursing are discussed here: case management and home care.

Case Management

Case management is an approach to providing care in which the client's services are coordinated by one designated health provider. Case management can facilitate the continuity of care and also help provide necessary services in the most economic manner possible (Clark, 1992). Nurses are in ideal positions to be case managers of clients because they make home visits to provide care, make ongoing assessments of clients, and can act to coordinate services.

Coordinating client care is an important component of home healthcare. Clients today have complex coordination needs. Often they are discharged from the hospital or referred by their physician with acute medical conditions, many medication and treatment needs, unfamiliar equipment and supplies, and numerous therapists and agencies involved in their care. Consequently, client care coordination has become increasingly involved and time-consuming. Case management includes assisting clients to connect with community resources, evaluating the effectiveness of these resources in meeting the clients' needs, increasing family involvement, and participating as a health team member (Cloonan & Shuster, 1990). The case manager is not always involved in direct client care, but develops a plan of care for the client and delegates specific tasks to other members of the healthcare team. The case manager also evaluates the effectiveness of care through client outcomes. Areas that the case manager might include in planning are physical care needs, counseling needs, assistance with homemaking and other ADLs, nutritional needs, legal and financial assistance, transportation, medical and dental care, health education, and spiritual assistance (Clark, 1992).

Home Care

Home care feasibility depends on the client's condition, family and community support, and the home environment. Home healthcare is defined as "all the services and products that maintain, restore, or promote physical, mental, and emotional health that are provided to clients in their homes" (Spradley, 1990). Home care, even when extensive, is less costly than care within a healthcare facility. Home healthcare aims to support families and clients to prevent admission to a facility, provide respite care, maintain or restore impaired health, or provide follow-up services (Spradley, 1990). Home care has been found to play a role in recovery from illness and in permitting the very old person to continue living at home (Fig. 31-7).

Meeting Physical Needs. With relatively short lengths of stay in hospitals, clients are going home with increasingly complex health needs. As a result, there has been an increase in the use of high-technology equipment at home. Direct physical care is provided at home by visiting nurses and home health aides trained in the basics of personal care. Wound care, intravenous administration of antibiotics and hyperalimentation, and supervision of medications are common nursing activities in the home. Common high-technology therapies in the home are respiratory care, parenteral or enteral nutrition, intravenous therapy, dialysis, and biotelemetry.

Many clients who live at home cannot prepare meals owing to physical limitations. Meals can be delivered by Meals on Wheels. Table 31-4 shows that for

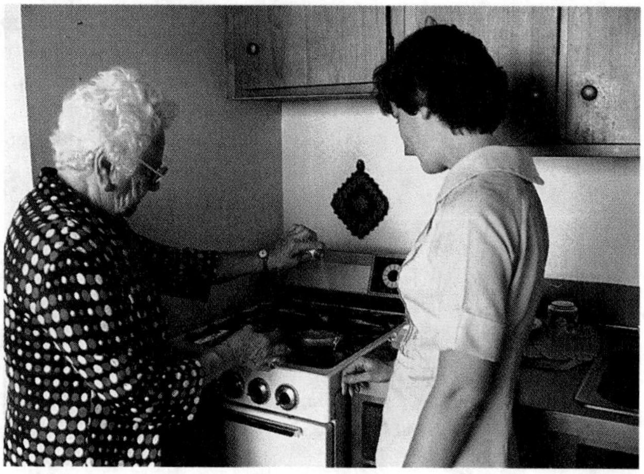

Figure 31-7 • *Home visits enable the nurse to assess whether the client can safely manage important tasks, such as cooking.*

Table 31-4 • Matching Community Resources and Impaired Home Maintenance Manifestations

Impaired Home Maintenance Manifestation	Possible Community Resources
Difficulty arranging transportation to employment, volunteer site, senior center, medical appointment, etc.	Carpools with neighbors, families of other older people, fellow volunteers or workers City provisions for older people: reduced bus fares, taxi scrip, "Trans-Aide" Volunteer services: Red Cross, Salvation Army, church organizations for emergency or occasional transportation
Living alone and fearing accidental injury or illness without access to assistance	Telephone checkup services through local hospitals or friends, neighbors, or relatives Postal alert: register with local senior center; sticker on mailbox alerts letter carrier to check for accumulation of mail Newspaper delivery: parents of the delivery person can be given an emergency phone number if newspapers accumulate Neighbors can check pattern of lights on/off
Needs assistance with personal care such as bathing and dressing	Private pay for hourly services: home aides from private agencies listed in phone book Visiting nurse association: services include aide services with nurses are used Medicaid/Medicare: provisions for home aides are limited to strict eligibility requirements, but such care is provided in certain situations Student help: posting notices on bulletin boards at nursing schools can yield inexpensive helpers Home sharing: sharing the home with another person who is willing to provide this kind of assistance in exchange for room and board
Needs occasional nursing care or physical therapy	Visiting nurse: services provided through Medicare or Medicaid or sliding-scale fees; must be ordered by a physician Home health services: private providers listed in phone book; also nonprofit providers, Medicare and Medicaid reimbursement for authorized services
Difficulty cooking meals, shopping for food, and arranging nutritious diet	Home-delivered meals: Meals on Wheels delivers frozen meals once a week, sliding fees Nutrition sites: meals served at senior centers, churches, schools, and other sites Cooperatives: arrangements with neighbors to exchange a service for meals, food shopping, etc.
Not enough contact with other people: insufficient activity or stimulation; loneliness and boredom	Senior centers: provide social opportunities, classes, volunteer opportunities, outings Church-sponsored clubs: social activities, volunteer opportunities, outings Support groups: for widows, stroke victims, and general support Adult day care: provides social interaction, classes, discussion groups, outings, exercise
Difficulty doing housework	Homemaker services for those meeting income eligibility criteria Service exchanges with neighbors and friends (ie, babysitting exchanged for housework help) Home helpers: hired through agencies or through employment listings at senior centers, schools, etc. Home sharing: renting out a room or portion of the home, reduced rent for help with housework
Forgetful about financial affairs; eyesight too poor for balancing checkbook and reading necessary information	Power of attorney given to friend or relative for handling financial matters Joint checking account with friend or relative for ease in paying bills Volunteer assistance available from the American Red Cross, Salvation Army, church groups, senior centers, other organizations
Needs assistance with will, landlord–tenant concerns, property tax exemptions, guardianship, etc.	Senior citizens' legal services Lawyer referral service offered by the county bar association City/county aging programs, hot lines for information and assistance in phone book

From Hooyman, N. (1983). Social support networks in services for the elderly. In J. K. Whittaker & J. Garbarino, (Eds.), *Social Support Networks: Informal Helping in the Human Services* (145–146). New York: Aldine de Gruyter Publishing Company.

many common physical limitations, there are community resources to assist the client to remain at home safely.

Other physical interventions may make small but important changes in the house. Color-coding medication bottles enhances the ability to self-medicate. Removing color can be equally important, however; for example, eliminating confusing color patterns in the home simplifies visual cues necessary to locate objects in a room (Schafer, 1985).

Ongoing education about self-care, treatment, and medications is a major psychocognitive intervention for homebound clients. Nurses should allow clients to express their frustrations due to lifestyle alterations. Communication is critical in making psychological interventions. Nurses with specialized education in psychological nursing manage cases of people with mental illnesses who live in the community.

Meeting Caregiver and Family Needs. Most commonly, social and family interventions are directed at the caregiver. Interventions include educational and support programs, burden-reducing programs, psychotherapeutic interventions, and self-help groups. Home health nurses must establish rapport and build trust with the client and the caregiver. The nurse encourages self-care and often assists clients and families in seeking and finding solutions for problems they are experiencing (McKenzie Stulginski, 1993).

A major and increasingly important family intervention is **respite care**, which provides a temporary break for the caregiver from the responsibility of caring for the client. Families must balance their caring, giving roles with meeting their own needs. For decreased social contacts and isolation, the nurse may refer the client to adult day care centers, group meals, church activities, senior centers, or support groups.

Evaluation

Clients with impaired home management often have a chronic illness or a progressive disease that leads to additional impairment. To evaluate the effectiveness of nursing interventions, goals must have been appropriately set for the client's condition and prognosis. Improvement may not be a realistic goal with chronic illness or progressive disease. For example, the physical health of a person with terminal cancer will not improve; thus, impaired home management will not resolve until death.

Meeting client goals can be taxing and frustrating for the nurse. Goals may not have been met because of factors outside the realm of nursing responsibility, such as medical complications that decrease the resources and abilities to perform ADLs. Other goals that initially seemed realistic and attainable may not be met owing to nurse-related problems. Unclear communication between the client and health and social service professionals is one such problem. Communication problems can result in decreased client compliance with medical and nursing treatments. Communication problems between nurses and other health professionals can result in decreased collaboration and coordination. Other problems include choosing inappropriate criteria for measuring nursing accomplishments, overinvolvement with the client, and general burnout. Table 31-5 lists some reasons for unmet goals.

The following is a list of sample goals and outcome criteria for clients with Impaired Home Maintenance Management.

Goal

The client/caregiver will overcome the functional deficit(s) that contribute or lead to Impaired Home Maintenance Management.

Possible Outcome Criteria

- Within 24 hours, client/caregiver expresses desire to maintain self or other at home.
- Within 24 hours, client/caregiver identifies the major factors that restrict self-care.
- By the third day, client expresses readiness and willingness to learn alternate ways to perform skills necessary for home living.
- By the third week, client demonstrates to nurse or occupational therapist the ability to perform tasks related to home living.

Table 31-5 • Some Reasons for Unmet Home Maintenance Goals

Client/Caregiver Community Factors	*Nurse-Related Factors*
Worsening medical condition	Poor communication with client
Constraints of the healthcare system	Poor communication with other health or social service professionals
Lack of insurance for needed services	Inappropriate goals or criteria selected
Lack of needed service in the community	Overinvolvement with client or family
Lack of client commitment to the care plan	Time constraints on developing plan and intervening
Caregiver stress and burnout	

- By discharge, caregiver eliminates major safety hazards from the home, as relayed to the nurse.

Goal

The client will return to a safe home environment.

Possible Outcome Criteria

- Within 1 week, client/caregiver agrees to perform responsibilities as outlined in the contract.
- By discharge, client/caregiver demonstrates ability to perform treatments or procedures correctly and confidently to be continued at home.
- By discharge, client expresses satisfaction with preparatory arrangements.
- By discharge, client/caregiver identifies at least two people or community service agencies who can answer questions and provide additional referrals.
- By discharge, client/caregiver expresses willingness to make financial arrangements for home care.
- After discharge, client/caregiver uses the home care support service needed and available, as described at next appointment.

Nursing Plan of Care
The Client With Impaired Home Maintenance Management

Nursing Diagnosis

Impaired Home Maintenance Management related to activity intolerance and living alone, as manifested by inability to perform instrumental activities of daily living (ADLs) and decreased ability to perform self-care.

Client Goal

The client will continue safely living in the home environment.

Client Outcome Criteria

- At initial interview, client expresses commitment to continued living at home.
- The client demonstrates how to contact emergency services before discharge.
- The client demonstrates an ability to meet financial obligations before discharge.
- During first month at home, client uses Meals-on-Wheels, home health aide, and church home visitation program on a regular basis, as reported to healthcare worker.
- The client demonstrates an ability to perform ADLs during regular home visits.

Nursing Intervention	*Scientific Rationale*
1. Discuss the options regarding living at home and the client's preferences. Develop a contract based on those preferences.	1. Client's participation in decision-making enhances the client's commitment to carrying out the contract. A contract facilitates communication and enhances efficiency for those involved.
2. Review financial obligations with the client and assess the client's ability to pay bills and keep records.	2. With the potential for impaired cognitive functioning and with the complexity of billing systems, the client's ability to keep financial records and to make financial decisions affects the client's ability to remain at home.
3. Refer to the community services necessary to support the client's living at home.	3. Referrals to community services are most successful if made by professionals with a client database and with a responsibility to coordinate the services provided to the client
4. Assess the client for social isolation, depression, or anxiety related to living alone. Refer to support groups as appropriate.	4. When people are unable to leave the home and have social contacts, affective disorders may develop.
5. Assess for specific client teaching needs related to living at home and then provide (or arrange to provide) that education. Periodically evaluate the knowledge retention.	5. Client teaching is most effective if it is tailored to the client's immediate knowledge needs. Knowledge retention may deteriorate with changes in physical status.

Goal

The client will continue to live at home.

Possible Outcome Criteria

- By 1 month after discharge, client/caregiver expresses desire for continued home living.
- By 2 months after discharge, client/caregiver continues to use available community resources that support continued living at home.
- By 3 months after discharge, client/caregiver demonstrates continued ability to carry out responsibilities as contracted.
- By 3 months after discharge, client/caregiver participates in learning and demonstrating new skills necessary for continued home living.
- By 3 months after discharge, client/caregiver seeks additional or alternative sources for financing home care.

Goal

The caregiver will participate in caring for the client at home.

Possible Outcome Criteria

- Within 1 week, caregiver lists at least three signs of stress he or she may experience as a caregiver and can name two ways to relieve stress.
- Within 2 weeks, caregiver participates in decision-making about care and placement of client.
- Within 2 weeks, caregiver demonstrates adequate physical strength to perform home care tasks.
- Two weeks before discharge, caregiver identifies physical barriers at home that must be changed before client arrives home.
- By discharge, caregiver lists signs or symptoms of changes in client status requiring immediate medical attention and describes steps to take in such an event.
- By discharge, caregiver describes alternate plans for client care if he or she cannot provide the necessary care or supervision.

Key Concepts

- Home maintenance management is the ability to maintain a safe, growth-promoting environment independently. Environment may be the hospital room, the home, the neighborhood, or the friend and family support system.
- It is stressful to change environments. The nurse considers whether the client can continue activities of daily living in the new environment.
- Impaired Home Maintenance Management is an imbalance between what the client *needs* for home maintenance and what the client can *provide* for himself or herself.
- The person and environment fit refers to the degree of match between the person's functional abilities and the resources within the client's environment.
- The ability to maintain a safe, nurturing home environment depends on the person's physical and emotional status.
- Discharge planning is done with the client and family to facilitate transition between different settings.
- Important in the discharge planning process are transition, continuity of care, coordination, facilitation, and negotiation.
- The family's needs must be considered in planning and implementing nursing interventions, because family members are often the primary caregivers for the client after discharge from the hospital.
- Assessment of the client, family, home, and community resources is important in individualizing a home management plan.
- Possible consequences of impaired home management include out-of-home placement, family strain, and homelessness.

Critical Thinking Challenges

Now you have added knowledge about the importance of discharge planning and home management to your knowledge base of nursing care. After you have reviewed the situation at the beginning of the chapter, consider the following.

1. *Role-play verbal and nonverbal interactions that will help establish rapport and trust with this family.*
2. *Prioritize assessments data you need to collect from the mother and neonate at this time, and describe what guidelines you used to prioritize assessments.*
3. *Prioritize immediate teaching needs and construct a plan to complete necessary teaching and evaluation during the 1-hour visit.*
4. *Propose possible supports and community resources that might be appropriate for this family.*

References

Braylock, A., & Cason, C. (1992). Discharge planning: Predicting patients' needs. *Journal of Gerontological Nursing, 18*(7), 5–10.

Carnevali, D. L. (1984). The nursing domain for diagnostic reasoning. In D. L. Carnevali, P. H. Mitchell, N. F. Woods, et al. (Eds.), *Diagnostic reasoning in nursing*. Philadelphia: J. B. Lippincott.

Carpenito, L. J. (1995). *Nursing diagnosis: Application to clinical practice* (6th ed.). Philadelphia: J. B. Lippincott.

Chick, N., & Meleis, A. I. (1986). Transitions: A nursing concern. In P. L. Chinn (Ed.), *Nursing research methodology: Issues and implementation*. Rockville, MD: Aspen.

Clark, M. (1992). *Nursing in the community*. Norwalk, CT: Appleton & Lange.

Cloonan, P., & Shuster, G. (1990). Care coordination: A resource intensive component of home health nursing practice. *Public Health Nursing, 7*(4), 204–208.

Dahl, S., Gustafson, C., & McCullagh, M. (1993). Collaborating to develop a community-based health service for rural homeless persons. *Journal of Nursing Administration, 23*(4), 41–45.

Haddad, A. M. (1987). *High-tech home care: A practical guide*. Rockville, MD: Aspen.

Hooyman, N. (1983). Social support networks in services to the elderly. In J. K. Wittaker & J. Garbarino (Eds.), *Social support networks: Informal helping in the human services*. New York: Aldine.

Horowitz, A. (1985). Family caregiving to the frail elderly. *Annual Review of Gerontology and Geriatrics, 5,* 194.

Kelly, S. (1993). Caregiver stress in grandparents raising grandchildren. *Image, 25,* 331–338.

Levine, H., Leventhal, E. A., & Nguyen, T. V. (1985). Reactions of families to illness: Theoretical models and perspectives. In D. C. Turk & R. D. Kerns (Eds.), *Health, illness and families: A lifespan perspective*. New York: John Wiley & Sons.

McKenzie Stulginski, M. (1993). Nurses' home health experience: The unique demands of home health visits. *Nursing and Health Care, 14,* 476–485.

Neundorfer, M. (1991). Coping and health outcomes in spouse caregivers of persons with dementia. *Nursing Research, 40,* 260–265.

North American Nursing Diagnosis Association (NANDA). (1994). *Nursing diagnoses: Definitions and classification 1995–1996*. Philadelphia: Author.

Phillips, E. K., & Cloonan, P. A. (1987). DRG ripple effect on community health nursing. *Public Health Nursing, 4*(2), 84–88.

Reinhard, S. (1994). Perspectives on the family's caregiving experience in mental illness. *Image, 26,* 70–74.

Sargis, N. M., Jennrich, J. A., & Murray, K. M. (1987). Housing conditions and health: A crucial link. *Nursing and Health Care, 8,* 335.

Schafer, S. C. (1985). Modifying the environment. *Geriatric Nursing, 6,* 157.

Schlossberg, N. K. (1981). A model for analyzing human adaptation to transition. *Consulting Psychology, 9*(2), 2.

Shapiro, E. (1986). Patterns and predictions of home care use by the elderly when need is the sole basis for admission. *Home Health Care Services Quarterly, 7*(1), 29–43.

Spradley, B. W. (1990). *Community health nursing: Concepts and practice* (3rd ed.). Boston: Little, Brown & Co.

Taylor, M. B. (1985). The effects of DRGs on home health care. *Nursing Outlook, 33,* 288.

Vermund, S. H., Belmar, R., & Drucker, E. (1987). Homelessness in New York City: The youngest victims. *New York State Journal of Medicine, 87*(1), 3.

Bibliography

Perlman, R., & Giele, J. Z. (1983). An unstable triad: Dependents' demands, family resources, community supports. *Home Health Care Services Quarterly, 3*(3/4), 12.

United States Department of Health and Human Services. (1990a). *Functional status of the non-institutionalized elderly: Estimates of ADL and IADL difficulties*. National Medical Expenditure Survey research findings (DHHS Publication No. [PHS] 90-3462). Washington, DC: Government Printing Office.

United States Department of Health and Human Services. (1990b). *Use of home and community services by persons ages 65 and older with functional difficulties*. National Medical Expenditure Survey research findings (DHHS Publication No. [PHS] 90-3466). Washington, DC: Government Printing Office.

Activity and Exercise

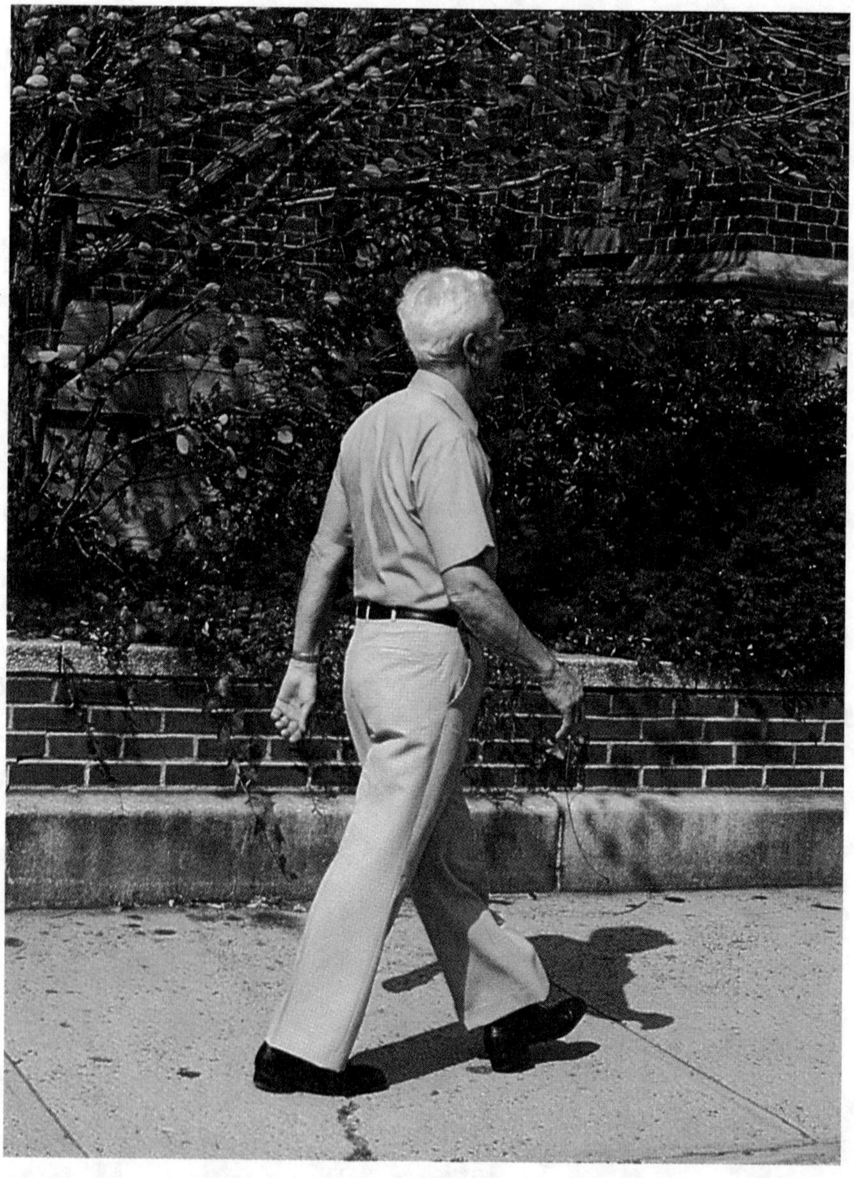

UNIT VIII

Activity and exercise are vital areas of human function that include both the ability and the desire to expend energy. Unit VIII discusses these areas of human function. The unit explores self-care, an area that involves activities that require energy expenditure; body mechanics and mobility; and respiratory and cardiac function.

Chapter 32 explores self-care and hygiene. Assessment focuses on how well the client can meet his or her own self-care needs. Holistic nursing interventions are aimed at assisting the client with self-care activities to the degree necessary to support independent function. The next chapter considers body mechanics and mobility, two major components of energy expenditure, as factors in client care from the perspectives of both the nurse and the client. The assessment emphasis is on evaluating a client's ability to move around in his or her environment to meet daily needs. Nursing interventions to promote health and function focus on helping the client engage in activity in safe, effective ways. The chapter also explores nursing interventions for clients with altered mobility. The last two chapters in this unit discuss respiratory and cardiac function. The ability to engage in energy-consuming activities is influenced by both areas of function. These chapters explore concepts and nursing care related to the basic human need for adequate oxygenation.

This unit considers client activity and energy use. These functions are essential for the client to maintain activities of daily living.

Self-Care and Hygiene

Key Terms	Learning Objectives
Alopecia *Caries* *Cerumen* *Commode* *Condom catheter* *Gingiva* *Hygiene* *Pediculosis* *Plaque* *Proprioception* *Self-care* *Tartar* *Urinal*	*Upon completion of this chapter, the student will be able to do the following:* • *Discuss the importance of self-care and hygiene in health and illness.* • *Identify factors that may alter self-care.* • *Discuss important subjective and objective areas of assessment when identifying self-care deficits and individualizing a plan for self-care.* • *Demonstrate basic self-care skills such as bathing, perineal care, foot care, back massage, toileting, and bedmaking.* • *Demonstrate proper care of eyes, ears, and teeth, including such aids as dentures, glasses, contact lenses, and hearing aids.* • *List beneficial client teaching for each of the four areas of self-care.*

32

You are caring for a 57-year-old bachelor, who is recovering from urologic surgery. He lived with his mother until her death a few years ago. He works independently as an accountant. This is your client's first surgery and, although the pathology reports are not back, there is some concern that your client may have bladder cancer. After your morning assessment, you tell your client you will help him get washed. He states he does not want to wash and just wants to be left alone. Your assessment reveals dirt under his fingernails, which are untrimmed and jagged; body odor and bad breath, which is easily detected; and dirty tissues all over his bed.

In previous chapters, you learned about legal and ethical concerns, critical thinking, the nursing process, and communication. These subjects may assist you in thinking through the bachelor's situation. This situation is not uncommon. As a nurse, you may often encounter clients who are not willing to participate in hygiene and self-care. Good hygienic practices are important in promoting optimal health, yet personal hygienic habits vary greatly among individuals. When you have completed this chapter and have added self-care and hygiene to your knowledge base, reflect on the Critical Thinking Challenges presented at the end of the chapter.

Self-care refers to a person's ability to perform primary care functions for himself or herself without the help of others; **hygiene** is the obervance of health rules, especially bathing, dressing, feeding, and toileting. Because these activities are so basic, they are often taken for granted. The ability to perform appropriate self-care and hygiene practices independently greatly enhances the client's health status and emotional well-being. When clients cannot perform these activities because of illness or injury, however, their health and well-being can be jeopardized. Proper nutrition and care of skin, teeth, hair, and nails promote good health by helping to protect the body from infection and disease and by allowing the person to feel good and have a positive self-image. The ability to perform self-care allows the person to remain independent, has a positive influence on self-concept and self-image, and gives him or her a sense of control.

The nurse can play a crucial role in helping clients learn or relearn self-care techniques. Because nurses focus on clients' responses to health and illness rather than on the disease itself, helping clients gain or regain independence in self-care is one of the most important goals of nursing. When illness or injury interferes with the ability to perform self-care, the nurse assists or performs tasks the client cannot manage or offers support to family members or other caregivers. However, the main focus is to help clients achieve as much independence in self-care as possible.

Benefits of Bathing

- Cleanses body secretions, microorganisms, debris, and perspiration from skin
- Stimulates circulation
- Improves joint mobility
- Provides relaxation, physical and emotional comfort
- Provides opportunity to evaluate skin status and observe for signs of physical problems or deterioration
- Provides opportunity for positive client–nurse interaction

Normal Self-Care

Characteristics of Normal Self-Care

Normal self-care is the ability to bathe and perform normal grooming functions and to dress, feed, and toilet oneself.

Bathing and Hygiene

The skin is the first line of defense against microorganisms and infection entering the body. This is why keeping skin intact and healthy is important. Increased perspiration interacts with bacteria on the skin to cause body odor, which can be offensive and promote bacterial growth. Regular bathing removes excess oil, perspiration, and bacteria from the skin surface. This is particularly important when the skin is compromised by an injury or illness (surgical wound or pressure sore), leaving the body more susceptible to infection.

Bathing also increases circulation (from the friction of a washcloth) and helps maintain muscle tone and joint mobility (from the movement of limbs during the bath). In addition, bathing provides relaxation and comfort and gives most people a sense of well-being. A warm or hot bath increases circulation by dilating blood vessels near the skin surface, allowing more blood to flow to the skin.

Bathing allows the nurse to assess the client's physical condition, noting injured areas, bruises, rashes, or any other unusual signs. Bathing also can promote conversation between the client and the nurse, facilitating a trusting, satisfying relationship.

Hair Care

Shampooing removes dirt and oil from the hair and scalp. It also increases scalp circulation. For most people, having their hair shampooed is relaxing. Clean hair makes clients feel good about their appearance and enhances feelings of self-worth. Daily brushing and combing of hair is important in maintaining the health of the hair by distributing oil across the hair shafts and massaging the scalp, which stimulates circulation. Neatly groomed hair also promotes a good self-image.

Feet and Nail Care

Healthy feet are crucial in helping people stand and walk. Feet are usually washed along with the rest of the body when showering or bathing. Nails are trimmed as needed. There are many tiny bones, ligaments, and muscles in the foot, and comfortable, properly fitting shoes are essential to healthy feet. Shoes should accommodate the size and shape of the foot and should be large enough so that toenails do not rub on the shoes, causing skin breakdown or ingrown nails.

Many people ignore their feet until problems occur. The feet are vulnerable to injury because of their increased exposure and susceptibility to skin breakdown. Mobility can be jeopardized by seemingly minor problems, such as ingrown nails, ill-fitting shoes, swollen feet, corns, or abrasions.

Parts of the exterior surface of the fingernail are shown in Figure 32-1. Fingernails are affected by the client's general condition and health habits. Brittle, broken nails may be caused by improper diet or fever. Some occupations affect the nails by staining them. Water and strong soaps or solutions dry nails. The cuticles around the edges of the nail can be a source of infection if they are torn. Dirt under the nails can spread infection.

Well-maintained nails are pleasing to see and give protection. Daily care involves cleaning beneath the nails and pushing back the cuticle. Fingernails should be filed rather than cut. Convalescing clients may be able to care for their own nails.

Eye, Ear, and Nose Care

Under normal conditions, the eyes require little care because the lacrimal fluid bathes them continually, and the lids and lashes prevent foreign material from entering the eye. Special care may be needed for clients who wear glasses, contact lenses, or prostheses; those who have other visual problems; or those who use eye medications.

Ears need little attention, although the external ear should be cleaned while bathing. Clients wearing hearing aids may need special care. Some people may have excess accumulation of ear wax (**cerumen**), which often requires careful removal. A sharp object, such as a hairpin or toothpick, should never be used to extract wax, because this can damage the tympanic membrane. Cotton-tipped applicators should not be used on the inner ear, because they can force wax further into the ear canal.

Nostrils can be cleaned by gentle blowing with both nostrils open. Closing one nostril while blowing can force foreign material into the eustachian tube or cause other damage to the inner canal.

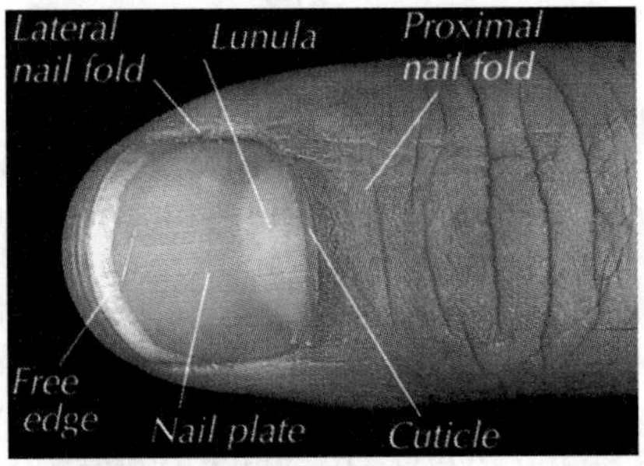

Figure 32-1 • *External fingernail surfaces. (Bates, B. [1995]. A guide to physical examination and history taking, 6th ed. Philadelphia, J. B. Lippincott.)*

Oral Care

The mouth and teeth play vital roles in the mastication (chewing) and digestion of food. The muscles in the cheeks aid in chewing. The tongue has taste buds for discerning different flavors of foods and helps mix saliva with food for food breakdown and digestion. The tongue also aids in swallowing by moving the food toward the pharynx.

Teeth (Fig. 32-2) are composed of the crown, the dentin, the pulp cavity, the neck, and the root. The crown, the hard surface exposed outside the gum, is covered with enamel. The dentin under the enamel covers the pulp cavity, which houses the blood vessels and nerves. The neck and root are below gum level.

Proper care of teeth and gums helps prevent gum deterioration and tooth loss. Cavities in the enamel (**caries**) are caused by deposits of **plaque,** a substance that forms and hardens on the teeth and is composed primarily of bacteria and saliva. Bacterial enzymes from the plaque combine with carbohydrates from food and organic acids to ferment and break down enamel. Caries form more often when food and plaque remain on the teeth for long periods. Plaque and food particles can be removed by daily brushing, flossing, and rinsing. When plaque remains on the teeth, it hardens into **tartar,** which cannot be removed by simple brushing; it must be scraped off by a professional with dental instruments.

Fluoride in small amounts strengthens teeth during their formation and helps prevent caries. Fluoride is added to most water-treatment systems at the appropriate concentration—1.0 parts per million (Valentine, 1988). Parents may want to ask the dentist how to give children appropriate supplements of fluoride until the age of 14 if their water system is not fluoridated.

Healthy gums are important because they provide support for the teeth. The gums are made up of the oral mucosa (**gingiva**), which covers the bone supporting the tooth; the alveolar bone, which forms sockets around the teeth; and the periodontal ligament, which joins the teeth to the bone. Inflammation in these tissues, called gingivitis or periodontitis, can be caused by local irritation from bacteria, plaque, tartar, food impaction, or mechanical, chemical, or thermal extremes.

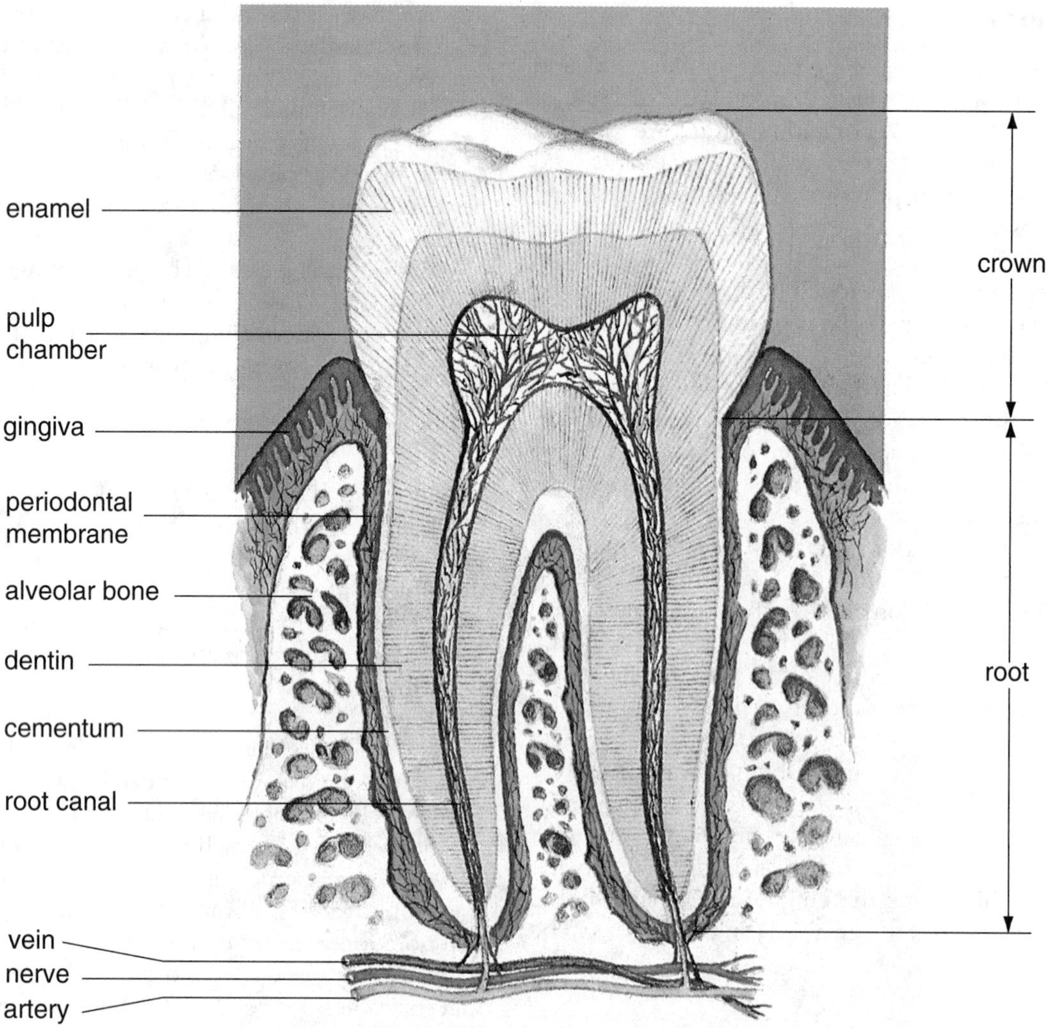

Figure 32-2 • *Parts of a tooth.*

Proper oral hygiene includes daily brushing, flossing, and rinsing of teeth and care of dentures or other appliances. Regular dental check-ups ensure the health of the teeth and gums.

Feeding

The ability to feed oneself may be the most important self-care skill in terms of independence. Independence or even partial independence in making food choices and being able to feed oneself can be immensely gratifying and can enhance self-concept for people of all ages. Feeding requires the desire to make food choices and eat, the energy and muscular coordination to move food from the plate to the mouth, and the ability to chew and swallow.

Toileting

Normal toileting includes feeling the urge to void and, independently or with assistance, moving to the toilet or bedpan, rearranging clothing, voiding, and effectively cleaning the perineal and rectal areas. Chapters 41 and 42 give detailed descriptions of normal urinary and bowel function.

Dressing and Grooming

Dressing oneself includes being able to get clothes from the closet or drawers, put them on, manage fasteners (such as zippers and buttons), and put on socks and shoes. Normal grooming patterns include the daily brushing and combing of hair. Depending on cultural or personal preferences, some women wear makeup and many shave underarms and legs as an important part of grooming. For men, shaving can be extremely important to their physical appearance and self-image. Some men feel as though they are not properly groomed without shaving every day, while others do not need to shave every day. Some men experience skin irritation if they do not shave daily. The amount of beard growth may dictate how often shaving is needed. Men with beards or mustaches may need to trim them periodically and must be careful to remove spilled food particles from them.

Normal Self-Care Patterns

Self-care and hygiene techniques vary depending on cultural or personal preferences, but in general, patterns include independence in eating and toileting; daily bathing or cleansing of the skin and perineal areas; daily brushing, flossing, and rinsing of the teeth; special care for dentures or other oral appliances; brushing or combing of hair; and other grooming preferences. Men may shave or trim facial hair; women may put on makeup. Some people prefer to bathe in the morning, whereas others bathe before going to bed.

Other areas that require attention and care are the hair, feet, and nails. The hair should be shampooed as frequently as needed to keep it clean, depending on its texture and oiliness. People with dry hair may need to moisturize it with conditioners or other commercial products. Shoes should be comfortable and fit properly. Toenails should be trimmed so that they do not rub against the shoes. Fingernails should be cleaned and trimmed periodically. Most people dress and groom themselves in the morning, soon after arising. Clothes may need to be changed during the day, depending on activities and weather.

Nursing Research
Self-Care

Selected Nursing Research Studies

Jirovec, M. M., et al. (1993). Predictors of self-care abilities among the institutionalized elderly. *Western Journal of Nursing Research, 15*(3), 314–326.

Kruger, S., et al. (1993). Foot care: Knowledge retention and self care practices. *Diabetic Educator, 18*(6), 487–490.

Muraki, T. (1993). Effect of respiratory and cardiometabolic response to tub bathing on elderly with cerebral palsy: A preliminary investigation. *Physical and Occupational Therapy in Pediatrics, 11*(2), 39–56.

Tombes, M. B., & Gallucci, B. (1993). The effects of hydrogen peroxide rinses on the normal oral mucosa. *Nursing Research, 42*(6), 332–337.

Possible Topics for Nursing Inquiry

- Do differences in self-care deficit exist between clients with acute problems and those with chronic problems with acute exacerbations?
- Does consistent help with bathing and toileting from the time of admission affect the level of self-care deficit at discharge?
- What interventions are effective in motivating clients toward independence in self-care?
- Have shorter hospital stays resulted in more or less independence in self-care at the time of discharge?

Factors Affecting Normal Self-Care

Many of us take self-care activities for granted because they seem simple and are accomplished on a routine basis throughout life. However, many factors influence whether a person can perform these tasks of daily living. Self-care requires adequate neuromuscular functioning, muscle strength, mobility, fine motor control, and energy levels and intact sensory capabilities. Cognitive functioning, psychological factors (motivation, mental status), and sociocultural factors (values, cultural grooming practices) also influence the performance of self-care activities.

Neuromuscular Function

Self-care activities, such as swallowing, getting to the toilet, and dressing, require a well-functioning neuromuscular system. To accomplish these tasks, the central nervous system sends messages to the peripheral nervous system and the muscle fibers to coordinate the necessary fine and gross motor activity. Normal muscle strength and normal contraction and relaxation of muscles also are needed.

Fine motor control allows the person to have command of small, precise movements (usually of the hands). Fine motor control requires coordination of muscle groups to facilitate activities, such as cutting food, opening a milk carton, buttoning a shirt, applying makeup, and wiping after toileting. *Gross motor activity* involves the coordinated movement of large muscle groups (eg, climbing in and out of the bathtub, walking or driving to the grocery store, carrying groceries home, getting on and off the toilet). Normal alignment, awareness of the body's spatial position (proprioception), and balance are needed to coordinate these large motor movements. Infants, in whom these motor skills are not developed, and people with compromised motor abilities from illness or injury cannot do these tasks without assistance.

Energy

Energy must be available at the cellular level for muscle movement. Adequate energy stores prevent fatigue during self-care. Adequate nutrition and the ability to break down food so it can be absorbed and used by the cells are important in providing energy for self-care. This process also requires adequate oxygen, so respiration plays a significant role. The circulatory system delivers nutrients, oxygen, and other substances to the cells to produce adenosine triphosphate, a nucleotide used to store energy and remove waste products produced by cellular metabolism.

Cognition and Perception

The ability to perceive and understand methods of self-care is important in achieving independence. People with normal cognitive and perceptive abilities are usually motivated to perform self-care. However, those with limited cognitive abilities may be unaware of the need for self-care, may not know appropriate methods of achieving it, or may be unable to assess what they can safely perform independently. They can be trained to perform some basic self-care skills, but the training requires a great deal of time, with much repetition of the skills and appropriate feedback. They can be taught to wash, dress, and toilet independently in a familiar setting, but they may require assistance with more complex tasks, such as shopping for groceries.

Intact Senses

Senses that function normally help a person to maintain independence in self-care activities. Sight is particularly important because it permits a person to locate and use objects. People with impaired sight can make adjustments to their environment to help them find objects and move around, but they may have difficulty in unfamiliar environments. Touch and taste can signal unsafe conditions, such as temperatures that are too hot or too cold. Hearing may not be essential to performing self-care activities, but impaired hearing can interfere with understanding verbal instructions and cues.

Motivation

Motivation can be a powerful factor in achieving independence in self-care. Even though a person is physically capable of self-care, he or she must be motivated to perform self-care and must feel that self-care is important. People with a positive self-image and those who perceive themselves as worthy of attention and care have a greater motivation to attend to self-care.

Culture, Values, and Beliefs

Self-care routines and practices are largely learned from the family and community. Habits formed around the frequency of bathing, brushing teeth, and changing clothes or eating patterns are usually learned early in life from family members, friends, and peers within the community. Such preferences may vary widely from person to person and culture to culture. For instance, many Americans do not feel clean unless they bathe daily and use a deodorant, but people in other cultures consider bathing once a week to be normal and do not feel the need to mask natural body odors. Some people are extremely sensitive regarding privacy during bathing; others are used to communal baths. Some people worry if they do not have a bowel movement each day; others are content with one every other day or even less frequently. There is a vast difference in family customs and personal preferences in relation to self-care practices.

Environment

The environment in which people learn and practice self-care activities greatly influences those practices. For example, in a household without running water, family members may bathe only once every 2 or 3 days, and the children may bathe together. Financial resources can influence diet and eating habits and grooming practices. Food buying can be greatly influenced by the availability of transportation (public or private) and the location of food stores in the community. Television and print advertising have a large impact on the products people use and consume and on their food-buying and grooming practices.

Lifespan Considerations

Normal developmental stages impact self-care throughout the lifespan. Considering the client's age helps the nurse understand self-care needs and plan appropriate interventions.

Newborn and Infant

Newborns participate in self-care only by crying and letting others know when they need to be fed or diapered. The feeding, bathing, dressing, and grooming are supplied by a caregiver. Newborns are born with sucking, rooting, and swallowing reflexes that allow them to ingest milk and liquids. They communicate hunger by crying and indicate satiety by falling asleep. By 3 to 4 months, infants begin to develop eye–hand coordination, and by 5 to 6 months, many children can grasp and eat pieces of food. As gross motor function develops around 7 to 9 months, children can hold a spoon or drink from a cup with help. At 9 to 12 months, children can usually pick up finger food and feed themselves, can hold and drink from a bottle, drink from a cup with some spilling, and spoon-feed themselves with quite a bit of spilling. Infants are totally dependent on caregivers for toileting. Urination may occur as frequently as 20 times a day, and the daily amount varies between 250 and 500 mL. Stools also are frequent and can be soft or liquid. Keeping the skin as dry and clean as possible helps preserve its integrity.

Changing an infant's diaper is relatively easy in early infancy and becomes more difficult as the child becomes more active. During a diaper change, an infant should never be left unattended where he or she could roll or fall.

Toddler and Preschooler

Self-care abilities increase considerably during this stage, particularly in feeding and toileting. As gross motor development increases in toddlers and preschoolers, they gain more mastery of their environment. Toddlers' eating patterns are erratic, but most can drink from a cup and use a spoon without spilling (Jackson & Saunders, 1993). Small portions of easy-to-handle food are appropriate.

Many children achieve daytime bowel and bladder control between 2 and 3 years. Staying dry through the night is usually achieved by 4 years, but some children still wet the bed at night until 5 years (Jackson & Saunders, 1993).

Preschoolers can manage most aspects of bathing and grooming with some support, but children younger than 4 years need support in wiping after toileting, handwashing, and dressing and undressing.

During illness or stress, most children regress in their toileting and feeding habits. Children who are toilet trained may revert to wetting their pants or the bed at night when ill or hospitalized. Older children who can feed themselves may want to be fed or drink from a bottle again. Regression is a common coping mechanism, especially for toddlers and preschoolers. During a stressful period, a child may revert from the most recently learned behavior to an earlier behavior that is more comfortable and satisfying. This "time-out" behavior permits the child to withdraw, conserve energy, and regain control. Regression is a normal reaction, and caregivers should understand and permit it.

Child and Adolescent

Although independent in self-care, some school-age children and adolescents may require reminders to bathe, brush their teeth, and change clothes appropriately. They still need direction and encouragement to eat healthy foods and use appropriate table skills. As the child approaches adolescence, self-care activities become more important as the body begins to mature, and physiologic changes start to occur.

Hormonal changes in adolescents result in the growth of body hair. Both sexes develop pubic and axillary (underarm) hair. Boys develop facial hair and may begin shaving. Sebaceous glands become more active and often produce excess oil on the skin. Many adolescents suffer minor skin problems, and some experience acne, which can be psychologically devastating to the adolescent's self-image. Sweat glands become fully developed and functional, and adolescents may need to begin using a deodorant or antiperspirant. Daily bathing and shampooing become important to counteract body odor.

Along with these physiologic changes, adolescents undergo extreme psychological and emotional changes. Adolescence is a time of burgeoning independence and self-discovery; adolescents begin to develop their own identity and define themselves. Girls and boys become interested in looking attractive to the opposite sex. Dressing and grooming practices are heavily influenced by the behaviors of peers, because adolescents want to be accepted by others. Adolescents also are influenced by magazine advertisements and television and often copy hairstyles or clothes worn by movie personalities or popular music celebrities.

Adult and Older Adult

Self-care is usually independently performed by young and middle-age adults. By this age, people have established self-care techniques that enhance their appearance and health. Busy lifestyles that include working and raising families may leave little time for self-care and health maintenance.

Special problems in self-care arise in the older adult. Skin becomes drier and less elastic and resilient because glands reduce their production of oil. The skin usually becomes discolored, and brown spots, called liver spots, may appear on the hands and feet. Hair becomes thinner and grows more slowly, and hair loss is common. Men and women experience changes in hair color. Teeth may gradually deteriorate from periodontal disease or caries, and many older people wear dentures. The oral mucosa tends to become drier as saliva

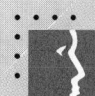

Client Teaching
Skin Care to Prevent Dryness

Instruct the client in the following:

- *Avoid bathing too frequently. Twice a week is usually sufficient.*
- *Avoid using harsh soaps and detergents on clothes.*
- *Use liquid, nondetergent cleansing agents rather than soap.*
- *Avoid astringents or alcohol-based solutions for cleaning the skin.*
- *Use lubricants containing lanolin immediately after washing or bathing to prevent moisture loss.*
- *Add oil to the rinse water for bed linens and underwear.*
- *Drink six to eight glasses of water per day.*
- *Maintain humid environment.*
- *Avoid linen that has been washed in harsh detergents or bleach. Chemical-free linen is available for sensitive skin.*
- *Pat dry with a cotton towel rather than rubbing.*

production lessens; some older people experience receding gums.

The feet of the older adult require special attention, because they generally are at risk for foot problems related to reduced peripheral blood flow from arteriosclerosis or poor circulation. Poor circulation makes the feet more vulnerable to infection and skin breakdown, particularly after trauma. Some older adults are not mobile enough to care for their feet and may be unable to inspect them easily.

Older adults may need to care for appliances, such as hearing aids, glasses, dentures, contact lenses, or artificial eyes. Reduced circulation and decreased muscular flexibility may impair the older person's agility and increase the time needed to perform tasks. Healing is often slower. Bones are often brittle and more vulnerable to fractures when falls occur. Older people generally are at greater risk for injury because of decreased perception and altered sensation. This age group has the greatest number of people with physically disabling chronic diseases that impact self-care abilities.

Altered Self-Care

Nurses often encounter people with deficits in self-care in the community and acute care setting. Problems with self-care range from short term and simple to long term and complex.

Potential for Altered Self-Care

Many factors can contribute to altered self-care. In addition to individual deficits, the attitudes of other people can affect self-care independence. A caregiver may want to do something "for" the disabled person that he or she can really do independently. The caregiver may do this to save time and effort, but performing a task independently to the fullest extent possible enables an individual to gain independence and self-confidence and bolsters self-concept.

Decreased Energy

Acute or chronic illness or injury can jeopardize independence in self-care by decreasing energy levels. Compromised respiratory or cardiac function reduces the body's ability to provide sufficient energy to the cells. An impaired cardiac system results in diminished delivery of nutrients and oxygen to the cells and removal of waste products of metabolism. Diseased lungs cannot provide adequate levels of oxygen to maintain cell metabolism. In both situations, the person's energy level declines, resulting in fatigue and decreased ability to carry out self-care. Decreased energy and weakness can result from disrupted diet, infection, disturbed gastrointestinal function, or fluid and electrolyte imbalance, or it can be a response to a medication.

Acute Illness and Surgery

People who have undergone surgery or who have been acutely ill often need assistance with self-care. The amount of help needed varies depending on the illness or surgery, the client's general health, and any sociocultural expectations. Drowsiness and confusion commonly result from analgesics, fluid and electrolyte imbalance, and hypoxemia. Nausea and vomiting add to the general malaise and produce a lack of motivation to perform self-care. Postoperative clients may experience weakness as a result of anesthesia, hypovolemia, lowered hematocrit level, and atelectasis, all of which may temporarily decrease cellular oxygenation. Weakness combined with pain also impedes self-care. Casts, splints, intravenous lines, incisions, urinary catheters, nasogastric tubes, surgical drains, and anxiety constitute encumbrances to mobility and interfere with the ability to perform activities of self-care.

Pain

Clients may experience so much pain that they are unable to care for themselves. The ability or willingness to move may be significantly curtailed. Caregivers should be aware that most analgesics given for pain also cause drowsiness and lightheadedness; therefore, clients taking such medications should be closely monitored during self-care activities to avoid falls. Some clients find bathing or being bathed a relaxing experience that can help distract them from the pain.

Neuromuscular Impairment

Conditions such as stroke, spinal cord injury, and some nervous system disorders (parkinsonism, cerebral palsy, myasthenia gravis, and muscular dystrophy) may cause permanent neuromuscular impairment and are serious threats to independent self-care. Many of these conditions produce muscle weakness, muscle atrophy, lack of coordination, spasticity, partial or total paralysis, and joint contractures that make walking, talking, eating, and using the extremities extremely difficult or impossible. However, many people with these conditions can progress to a high level of independence in self-care with the aid of appliances or other creative alterations.

Injury to upper or lower extremities can render a person unable to perform self-care functions because of immobility from casts, splints, or pain and weakness. These people need assistance from nurses or family members or special aids.

Sensorimotor Deficits

People who suffer sensorimotor deficits because of surgery, injury, or infection may need assistance in self-care. Those who have lost some sight may need help with eating or getting to the bathroom. If the visual impairment is prolonged or permanent, the client may learn to compensate by making adjustments to the environment. For example, placing food and utensils on a tray in a consistent manner makes it easier for a visually impaired person to eat independently. Furniture can be arranged so that the person does not bump into objects or fall on the way to the bathroom. Hearing-impaired people may have difficulty carrying out self-care activities because they cannot hear instructions or verbal cues. Devising alternate methods of cuing and communicating proper instructions can help them to perform self-care independently.

Cognitive Dysfunction

Clients with a decreased level of consciousness or confusion due to injury or illness must be carefully assessed to determine how much assistance will be needed for self-care. Although these clients may be physically capable of feeding, dressing, bathing, and toileting, they may not be alert enough to know when these activities need to be performed or how to perform them safely. The nurse plays an important role in helping such clients achieve and resume the highest level of self-care possible. The range of cognitive deficits is vast. Clients with minor deficits need to be reminded to provide self-care, but those with severe disabilities (such as severe head trauma or injuries) are often totally dependent on others and mechanical aids for self-care. Clients with cognitive deficits need to be carefully and individually assessed to determine what self-care skills they can accomplish or learn to accomplish with assistance.

Environmental Limitations

Some people, because of poverty or poor living conditions, may not have access to the facilities needed for appropriate self-care. Homeless people, migrant workers, and the rural poor often do not have access to proper resources, putting them at risk for self-care deficits. They may not have access to adequate bathroom facilities or running water to bathe properly and wash their clothes. They may not have enough food to ensure a proper diet or adequate cooking facilities to prepare a nutritious meal.

People in wheelchairs may have problems finding wheelchair-accessible facilities, putting them at risk for self-care deficits. For example, bathrooms must be designed so that wheelchairs can move in and out of stalls. Sinks must be at the right height for a wheelchair-bound person. Home alterations may be necessary to allow the person to perform self-care; see Chapter 31 for more details on home management.

Emotional Disturbance and Depression

Emotional factors can result in self-care deficits. The inability to perceive reality appropriately because of side effects of medication, an unfamiliar environment, psychosis, or schizophrenia may cause inattentiveness to the need for personal care. Such people are highly distractible and have short attention spans, making them unable to concentrate on such basic needs as eating, grooming, and toileting. Severe dysfunction may be reflected by wearing inappropriate or no clothes in public or refusing to eat due to a fear of being poisoned.

Autism is characterized by an inability to respond to external stimuli and preoccupation with inner thoughts, daydreams, delusions, and hallucinations. A person with such a severe disorientation to the environment requires a great deal of assistance or prompting to carry out self-care activities.

Depressed people may lack the energy or interest to care for themselves and may be poorly groomed, poorly nourished, or constipated. In addition, poor grooming may exacerbate feelings of depression. Self-care problems in older people may be greatly complicated by depression, disrupting self-care.

Manifestations of Altered Self-Care

Different degrees of deficit concerning ability to perform self-care can be seen in different people. Some deficits are temporary, whereas others are permanent. Indications that deficits are present are poor grooming and hygiene, inability to demonstrate self-care skills, or verbalization of reluctance to perform self-care.

Poor Hygiene and Grooming

Visual cues indicating poor hygiene and grooming are readily apparent. There may be an offensive body odor. The skin may be soiled, dry, or flaky or may have rashes and excoriated areas. Hair may be oily, unwashed, and uncombed. Nails may be dirty and broken. Clothes may be soiled, torn, or inappropriate. Inspection of the mouth may reveal sores, caries, inflamed gums, plaque build-up, and stained teeth. Mouth odor, or halitosis, is common. Soiling of pants with urine or feces may indicate difficulty in toileting.

Inability to Demonstrate Self-Care Activities

Inability to demonstrate gross and fine motor coordination needed for self-care activities indicates impaired

Therapeutic Dialogue
Self Care

Scenes for Thought

Rick Newfield is 32 years old and was admitted to the rehabilitation unit 2 days ago after being stabilized in the acute unit with a spinal cord injury. He had been in a motorcycle accident, and today is the first day you'll be meeting him.

Effective

Nurse: *Hello, Rick. I'm Susan Jacobs, your primary nurse. How's it going today?*
Client: *Just great! How do you think I am, Susan, I'm a paraplegic, or didn't you know this?!* Sarcastic tone of voice, swearing, angry face, glaring eye contact.
Nurse: *I knew. It sounds like you just found out. (Calm tone and body language.)*
Client: *Yeah, they told me yesterday that all the testing they did showed damage at L4 and L5. I won't be able to walk, go to the bathroom by myself, have sex with my wife, run with my little boy, none of that.* Turns his head to the wall.
Nurse: *(Sits in chair next to the bed.) Pretty devastated by it all right now, aren't you?*
Client: *Wouldn't you be? God, what a waste.* Lies back in the bed.
Nurse: *(Sits quietly and says nothing.)*
Client: *Well, what are you in here for? There's nothing I need right now. I'm not in pain; I don't need to be helped with anything.*
Nurse: *You're saying you want to be left alone? (Continues to sit quietly.)*
Client: Looks up in surprise. *What do you mean?*
Nurse: *It seems to me that you're pretty discouraged and angry right now and are having trouble seeing anything but the worst, and so you want to be left alone. Is that right?*
Client: Begins to cry quietly and tries to hide it. *No. I want someone to tell me I'm going to be fine.*
Nurse: *You will be fine, but you'll be different.*
Client: *Don't con me, whoever you are. I don't want to hear any of this.*
Nurse: *I wouldn't con you. You have lots of work to do on yourself, and some of it won't be easy. We'll be around to help and so will the other guys in the PG.*
Client: *What's that?*
Nurse: *It's a patient group called the Paraplegia Group. They help each other through the rehab you all have to go through, like the bowel and bladder training, upper body strength exercises, wheelchair races, skin inspection rounds, how to have great sex, and so forth.*
Client: *Sounds like fun.* Said sarcastically but with a spark of interest.
Nurse: *Jimmy Saguro will be by this afternoon to talk to you about it. Meanwhile, tell me a little about how your body* really *feels. You and I have to work together too, you know.* (Smiles.)
Client: *Smiles back.*

Less Effective

Nurse: *Hello, Rick. I'm Sarah James, your primary nurse. How's it going today?*
Client: *Just great! How do you think I am, Sarah, I'm a paraplegic, or didn't you know this?!* Sarcastic tone of voice, swearing, angry face, glaring eye contact.
Nurse: *I knew. It sounds like you just found out. (Calm tone and body language.)*
Client: *Yeah, they told me yesterday that all the testing they did showed damage at L4 and L5. I won't be able to walk, go to the bathroom by myself, have sex with my wife, run with my little boy, none of that.* Turns his head to the wall.
Nurse: *(Sits in chair next to the bed.) Pretty devastated by it all right now, aren't you?*
Client: *Wouldn't you be? God, what a waste.* Lies back in the bed.
Nurse: *Sure, I'd be devastated, but I wouldn't be so hopeless. There's lots of stuff we can do to help. (Still sitting quietly.)*
Client: *Sure, sure, I know. The doc told me all about the physical therapy and that stuff. Big deal. I'll still be crippled!* Angry face and voice.
Nurse: *We don't use that word around here. It means you can't do anything, and there'll be lots you can do. Just hang tight for a bit, and you'll begin to see a big change in yourself. (Smiles encouragingly.)*
Client: *Yeah, yeah.* Turns face to the wall again.
Nurse: *(Looks at his body language.) I can see you'd rather be alone right now. I'll be back in a bit to check on the incision from the operation and to see if you need anything.*
Client: Cries quietly with his face to the wall.

Critical Thinking Challenge

• Name obstacles that are in the way of Rick's self-care abilities. • Detect what Susan did that helped him change his perspective that he wouldn't be able to do anything. • Detect what Sarah did that did not change his perspective. • Critique timing and how each nurse used or ignored it.

ability to perform these functions independently. Gross motor abilities are needed to get to the bathroom, bathe, dress, and eat. Fine motor skills are required to fasten garments, apply makeup, open food containers, and cut food. The client should be able to perform self-care activities without cuing and without excessive fatigue.

Verbalization of Reluctance to Perform Self-Care

If the client expresses reluctance or fear to perform self-care activities, a deficit is present. Some clients may be reluctant due to depression, altered cognition, or dependent personality; others reasons may be fatigue or fear of pain. Some people may fear that they will be unable to perform the activity successfully. Other clients may lack interest in self-care because their value system does not attach significance to conventional grooming activities.

Impact on Activities of Daily Living

Individual Considerations

A self-care deficit by definition causes alteration in ability to perform activities of daily living. The impact of not being able to perform activities and demands of daily living independently is great for any individual. In a culture that values independence, the inability to perform personal care tasks for oneself has significant psychological and physical implications. Often, the individual has to depend on family or friends for physical help and psychological support. If needed assistance is not available within the client's support system, individuals may be hired to assist with basic daily needs. Finding qualified help is difficult and expensive, beyond the budget of many. Inability to perform self-care is a leading cause of inability to remain in the home setting.

Family Considerations

Family impact varies, depending on the level of self-care deficit. Often a female child or spouse is thrust in the role of caretaker. Willingness to perform these functions can vary, depending on many factors, including relationship with the client; comfort with such physical tasks; other obligations, such as work or children; and the degree and length of time that assistance is required. If self-care deficits are short term (eg, recovery from orthopedic surgery), family members can often arrange their schedule to provide care. If self-care deficits are extensive and long term (eg, caring for a ventilator-dependent child), demands placed on the family are great. If deficits are long term, the client may need to move to the designated caregiver's residence. Although at times this can be a positive experience for the entire family, it can create much strain and difficulty for every family member, including the client.

Assessment

To determine which self-care activities the client can perform, the nurse does a systematic assessment.

Subjective Data

By asking questions, the nurse can learn what the client considers normal self-care activity and in what areas the client perceives difficulties. These questions are designed to elicit the client's feelings about the problem, what he or she sees as the solution, and his or her level of motivation to alter self-care ability. If family members are present, they may give their perceptions of the client's self-care abilities.

Functional Pattern Identification

Interviewing the client permits the nurse to collect information about normal self-care patterns. Examples of questions to elicit this information are the following:

How do you manage bathing or hygiene (dressing, eating, toileting)? Are you satisfied with your ability to bathe (dress, eat, and toilet)?
Describe any factors that interfere with bathing (dressing, eating, and toileting)?
What goals and expectations do you have for these activities?
Do you foresee alterations in your ability to care for yourself?
Can you pursue important daily activities as much as you desire?
Is your desire for independence strong enough to withstand pain, inconvenience, and possible failure in performing self-care functions?

Such information helps to determine how the client normally manages self-care and what his or her feelings and values are about self-care. Determining normal self-care patterns permits the nurse to promote independence and optimal functioning.

This information can be used to individualize client care. Bathing can be scheduled in the morning or evening, according to client preference. Oral care can be provided before or after breakfast, with cold or warm water. Clients who sleep late may want to delay self-care activities, but others prefer to wash and apply makeup early in the morning, before seeing anyone.

Normal self-care patterns can be categorized according to the assistance required by the client; Table 32-1 summarizes the levels and give examples. Level 0 reflects complete independence; level 4 reflects complete dependence on others.

Risk Identification

As the nurse gathers self-care information from the client, she or he identifies factors that could put the client at risk for self-care deficits. The nurse should observe and interview the client for the following risk factors:

- Pain
- Immobility or limited use of an extremity
- Mental confusion or decreased mental alertness
- Decreased visual acuity or other sensory deficits
- Inability to control bowel or bladder function

Table 32-1 • Levels of Self-Care

Level	Description	Example
Level 0	Is independent in self-care activities	Healthy college student who lives in an apartment
Level 1	Uses equipment or devices to perform self-care activities independently	Elderly man who uses a cane for extra support during walking
Level 2	Requires assistance or supervision from another to complete self-care activities	Postoperative client who needs help in bathing first day after surgery
Level 3	Requires assistance or supervision from another and uses devices or equipment	Client who ambulates using a walker and needs contact supervision
Level 4	Is completely dependent on another to perform self-care activities	Comatose client who requires complete care by nursing staff

- Decreased energy levels or fatigue
- Socioeconomic factors that might impair self-care

The client's responses should be corroborated by a physical examination. For example, if the client says he or she does not have problems with bathing and shampooing, but the nurse observes skin breakdown, body odors, and dirty fingernails, this would indicate that the person is likely to be at risk for self-care deficits.

Dysfunction Identification

The nurse should be familiar with the signs indicating inability to perform self-care. The nurse can use an Index of Activities of Daily Living (Table 32-2), developed by Katz (1963; 1983), to aid in this assessment and determine the level of functional independence in self-care practices of feeding, continence, transferring, going to the toilet, dressing, and bathing. This standardized

Table 32-2 • Index of Independence in Activities of Daily Living*

ADL	Independent	Dependent
Bathing (sponge, shower, or tub)	Needs assistance only in bathing a single part (such as back or disabled extremity) or bathes self completely	Needs assistance in bathing more than one part of body; needs assistance in getting in or out of tub or does not bathe self
Dressing	Gets clothes from closets and drawers; puts on clothes, outer garments, braces; manages fasteners (act of tying shoes is excluded)	Does not dress self or remains partly undressed
Toileting	Gets to toilet, gets on and off toilet, arranges clothes, cleans organs of excretion (may manage own bedpan at night or may not be using mechanical supports)	Uses bedpan or commode or needs assistance getting to and using toilet
Transferring	Moves in and out of bed and chair independently (may be using mechanical supports)	Needs assistance in moving in or out of bed or chair; does not perform one or more transfers
Continence	Has self-control of urination and defecation	Has partial or total incontinence in urination or defecation; partial or total control by enemas, catheters, or regulated use of urinals or bedpans
Feeding	Gets food from plate into mouth; precutting of meat and preparation of food (as buttering bread) are excluded from evaluation	Needs assistance in feeding; does not eat at all or uses parenteral feeding

*Independence means without supervision, direction, or active personal assistance. This is based on actual status and not on ability. A client who refuses to perform is considered as not performing, even though he or she is deemed able.

assessment guide allows the nurse to compare self-care deficits with normal patterns. Katz believed that loss of self-care is a natural part of aging and proceeds in an orderly fashion, with more complex activities being lost first. He also argued that people regain functional self-care abilities in patterns similar to the development of these skills in children. For example, they achieve feeding and continence skills first, then transfer and toileting abilities, and finally dressing and bathing abilities.

Objective Data

The nurse can validate information obtained during the client interview by objectively observing the client as he or she engages in self-care functions. The nurse should look for several specific factors:

- Evidence of inability to manage self-care (ie, poor grooming, body odor, lice, skin lesions, poor nutrition)
- Ability to process sensory input by hearing, sight, smell, and touch
- Evidence of disabilities, such as weakness, cognitive deficits, immobility or spasticity, or mental lethargy
- Manual dexterity
- Use of sensory or mechanical aids (ie, glasses or contact lenses, dentures, hearing aid, cane or walker, condom catheter, raised toilet seat, or special eating utensils)

When activity intolerance or fatigue is suspected, the client's cardiopulmonary response is evaluated before, during, and after each self-care activity by assessing pulse rate, respiratory rate, and quality of breathing and observing for changes in skin color. At the same time, any alterations in the client's normal physical status (see display) are noted.

Nursing Assessment

Physical Assessment for Self-Care

- Body temperature, pulse rate, respiration rate (before, during, and after activity), breath sounds, blood pressure
- Height and weight
- Gait and posture
- Range of motion
- Muscle firmness
- Strength of hand grip
- Status of mouth and teeth
- Skin and nails (ie, bony prominences, lesions, color, temperature, texture)
- Food or fluid intake

To formulate realistic goals and interventions, the nurse must assess the resources available to the client. This can mean internal resources (psychological, intellectual, and emotional factors) and external resources (living arrangements, finances). The accompaying display lists external and internal resources and their influence on self-care.

Nursing Diagnoses

Self-care deficit is manifested as actual or potential problems with self-care. The nurse determines the existence and extent of self-care deficit through client assessment. Nursing diagnoses accepted by the North American Nursing Diagnosis Association (NANDA) are Bathing/Hygiene, Dressing/Grooming, Feeding, and Toileting Self Care Deficits. The diagnosis Self Care Deficit is broad and can be used for problems involving a variety of body systems.

Bathing/Hygiene Self Care Deficit

Definition

Bathing/Hygiene Self Care Deficit is a state in which the individual experiences impaired ability to perform or complete bathing or hygiene activities for oneself (NANDA, 1994).

Defining Characteristics

Defining characteristics are inability to wash body or body part, obtain water, or regulate temperature or flow of water (NANDA, 1994).

Related Factors

Related factors include intolerance to activity, decreased strength and endurance, pain, discomfort, perceptual/cognitive impairment, neuromuscular impairment, depression, and severe anxiety (NANDA, 1994).

Dressing/Grooming Self Care Deficit

Definition

Dressing/Grooming Self Care Deficit is a state in which the individual experiences impaired ability to perform or complete dressing or grooming activities for oneself (NANDA, 1994).

Defining Characteristics

Defining characteristics include impaired ability to fasten clothing or inability to maintain appearance at a satisfactory level (NANDA, 1994).

Nursing Assessment
External and Internal Resources and Influences

External Resources

- *Housing* (location, design, access by elevators/stairs, special equipment, kitchen and bathroom facilities, access to telephone, how many people share facilities)
  - Mobility around home
  - Ability to shop for and prepare food
  - Access to bathroom for self-care
- *Air and water*
  - Availability of water for bathing and drinking
  - Air quality for breathing
  - Hot water for bathing
- *Neighborhood* (proximity of shops, hospitals/clinics; available transportation)
  - Ability to obtain groceries
  - Access to healthcare and assistance
- *Financial resources*
  - Ability to purchase food and self-care products
  - Ability to afford healthcare
- *Support network and community resources* (family and friends, support groups and volunteers, such as Meals on Wheels, home healthcare)
- *Government and social services*
  - Help with shopping, getting to doctor's appointments, self-care, and meal preparation
  - Financial or material assistance for supplies and special equipment

Internal Resources

- *Inner strength*
  - Ability to handle physical, mental, and emotional work
- *Endurance*
  - Stamina or "staying power" to cope with physical, mental, or emotional difficulties
- *Sensory input*
  - Ability to attend to and process environmental stimuli to provide a safe environment when attending to self-care needs
- *Cognitive abilities*
  - Amount and use of knowledge regarding self-care
- *Desire*
  - Will or motivation to participate in self-care
- *Courage*
  - Willingness to take risks and bear hardship to achieve self-care independence
- *Skills*
  - Abilities regarding psychomotor functions, dexterity, or communication and interpersonal relationships
- *Communication*
  - Ability to make others understand and make needs known

Related Factors

Related factors include activity intolerance, decreased strength and endurance, pain, discomfort, perceptual/cognitive impairment, neuromuscular impairment, depression, and severe anxiety (NANDA, 1994).

Toileting Self Care Deficit

Definition

Toileting Self Care Deficit is a state in which the individual experiences impaired ability to perform or complete toileting activities for oneself (NANDA, 1994).

Defining Characteristics

Defining characteristics include inability to get to the toilet or commode, inability to sit on toilet or commode, inability to manipulate clothing for toileting, inability to carry out proper toilet hygiene, or inability to flush toilet or empty commode (NANDA, 1994).

Related Factors

Related factors include impaired transfer ability, impaired mobility, intolerance to activity, decreased strength and endurance, pain, discomfort, perceptual/cognitive impairment, neuromuscular impairment, depression, and severe anxiety (NANDA, 1994).

Feeding Self Care Deficit

Definition

Feeding Self Care Deficit is a state in which the individual experiences impaired ability to perform or complete feeding activities for oneself (NANDA, 1994).

Defining Characterics

Defining Characterics include inability to cut food or inability to bring food from receptacle to mouth (NANDA, 1994).

Related Factors

Related factors include intolerance to activity, decreased strength and endurance, pain, discomfort, perceptual/cognitive impairment, neuromuscular impairment, depression, and severe anxiety (NANDA, 1994).

Related Nursing Diagnoses

Other nursing diagnoses frequently exist along with Self Care Deficit, including Impaired Skin Integrity (related to inability to provide hygiene and clean oneself after toileting); Altered Nutrition: Less than body requirements and Fluid Volume Deficit (related to inability to feed oneself); Altered Oral Mucous Membrane (related to inability to manage mouth care and feed oneself); Ineffective Individual Coping (related to depression about limitation in self-care abilities); Anxiety (related to inability to reach the toilet reliably or perform other self-care activities); Powerlessness (related to difficulty in maintaining usual schedule); and Caregiver Role Strain and Altered Family Processes (related to stress).

Outcome Identification and Planning

After nursing diagnoses and related factors are established, the nurse and client plan outcomes and necessary interventions. The following general areas may be included when formulating goals for clients with the four self-care deficits:

Client will actively participate in hygiene measures.
Client will safely increase level of independence in eating.
Client will actively participate in dressing.
Client will manage toileting as independently as possible.

Examples of nursing interventions to help in planning are listed in the accompanying display and dis-

Planning
Examples of Nursing Interventions for Common Self-Care Problems

Bathing

- Plan hygiene when the client is well rested.
- Gather supplies before bath.
- Offer pain medication if necessary before hygiene.
- Encourage sitting by sink or in shower when endurance is limited.
- Work with occupational therapy to teach relearning of skills when new cognitive or physical impairments occur.
- Use verbal cuing if necessary; praise accomplishments.
- Assist with hygiene that cannot be performed independently.

Feeding

- Have client sit in chair or high Fowler's position in bed.
- Medicate as necessary for pain or nausea before meals.
- Provide opportunity for oral care, and make sure dentures are in place.
- Plan rest periods before and after meals.
- Provide an environment free from unpleasant odors or sights that may have a negative impact.
- Provide assistance with organizing food tray as needed (eg, open containers, cut meat, or verbally cue clients who are able to do so).
- Provide appropriate foods (eg, finger foods, thickened liquids) as needed.
- Provide utensils that aid feeding (eg, plates with rims, straws, special spoons and forks).
- Use verbal cueing and positive encouragement.
- Work with speech therapy or occupational therapy to individualize teaching plan for clients with new physical or cognitive impairments.

Dressing/Grooming

- Provide rest period before dressing or grooming activities.
- May need to space different grooming activities throughout the day to avoid fatigue.
- Assemble all necessary clothing or grooming aids.
- Clothing should be loose fitting and easy to fasten (eg, sweatsuits, Velcro fasteners).
- When possible, perform activities in sitting position.
- When client is unable to perform activities independently, ask for preferences so they can feel involved.
- Work with occupational therapy to individualize teaching for clients with new physical or cognitive impairments.

Toileting

- Encourage routine toileting to avoid urgent need to reach toilet facilities.
- Provide client with needed supplies (eg, bedpan, urinal, toilet tissue, washcloth for cleansing hands).
- Ensure clear access to toilet or bedside commode by removing clutter.
- Encourage clothing that is easy to remove.
- Provide equipment to ensure safety (call light, railings, raised toilet seat, adequate lighting).
- Provide ambulation aids or bedside commode if ambulation is difficult.

cussed in the following section. In practice, outcomes are highly personalized and specific. Because of their personal nature, outcomes reflect the wishes of the client and the stage of illness. For example, a chronically ill person who looks at death as a release may have a different response to working toward independence than a person who has a favorable prognosis for complete recovery.

Implementation

Nursing Interventions to Promote Health and Self-Care

Good hygiene is important in infection prevention. Frequently, the nurse is able to stress the relationship between good hygiene and optimal health. Such teaching can be done in preschools, where young children are taught the importance of proper hygiene following toileting or older children are taught how to detect and prevent the transmission of lice; in prenatal classes, where nurses teach how to bathe a newborn and prevent scalp problems; or in a community health center, where the nurse can teach proper foot care to an aging population. Teaching concerning dental health and regular visits to the dentist also is important.

Nurses can support community and governmental programs to promote self-care for high-risk groups. For example, promoting increased support for shelters or relief agencies so the homeless or mentally ill will have access to showers and bathroom facilities is one way a nurse might promote self-care on a community level.

> **Client Teaching**
> *Self-Care and Hygiene*
>
> *Instruct the client as follows:*
> - *Relearning self-care skills takes time and energy. Set realistic goals for yourself, and praise yourself when they are met.*
> - *If you have more energy in the mornings, plan to bathe, shampoo your hair, and put your makeup on then.*
> - *Plan a nap before you eat if eating makes you tired.*
> - *Keep a commode or urinal close to your bed for convenience.*
> - *Wear your glasses and dentures when eating.*
> - *Use a plate with a suction grip underneath. Push against the plate guard rim while eating.*
> - *Wear loose-fitting clothes if dressing is difficult. Pull-on pants and pullover tops are handy because you don't need to zip or fasten them. Shoes with Velcro closures or elastic laces are easier. Give yourself plenty of time until you get used to dressing yourself.*

Some communities with a large homeless population are encouraging the placement of portable toilets, so toileting can be private and sanitary. Free clinics need to be available and accessible to provide foot care for diabetic clients or dental care for low-income families.

The nurse also promotes self-care and hygiene by being a role model. The nurse should always report to work well groomed and verbalize the importance of hygiene measures. The image this presents is that hygiene is important to physical and mental well-being.

Nursing Interventions for Altered Self-Care

The nurse should emphasize to all clients the importance of increasing their independence in self-care. Client teaching is a cooperative venture that requires the nurse's knowledge, patience, and effort and the client's motivation to learn and offer information regarding personal preference. Some people have an innate desire to be independent and therefore have a willingness to learn. Others are inclined to be dependent and are less willing to learn or relearn how to care for themselves.

People with self-care deficits often must learn new skills or methods of overcoming or coping with difficulties. Rehabilitation involves many health team members working together to promote optimal functioning. Health team professionals who commonly work with clients to improve self-care abilities are listed in Table 32-3. The nurse works collaboratively with these health-care professionals, teaching and reinforcing skills and nurturing the desire for self-care independence. Careful assessment of client values and interests often reveals motivating factors that might encourage a client to achieve independence.

Careful communication is necessary when providing assistance or teaching clients self-care. Techniques are explained as simply as possible, avoiding technical or medical terms. Learning or relearning self-care skills often takes time and effort. The nurse should be patient, supportive, and reassuring. The client is not criticized when unsuccessful. When the client is successful, regardless of how small or insignificant the task may seem, reinforcement and encouragement are given. The nurse must not provide care for clients that they can perform for themselves, because this fosters dependence and a helpless role.

Nurses should be aware that some degree of regression in self-care is normal during illness, particularly in children and older adults. They may have temporary problems with incontinence or may not perform self-care due to weakness, fatigue, or anxiety.

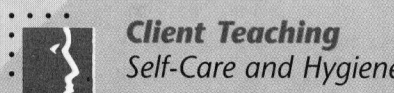

A study by Doyle and Stern (1992) demonstrates that negotiation with the client, rather than more aggressive tactics such as threatening, help promote independence in self-care. Ultimately, the client has con-

Table 32-3 • Collaboration to Promote Self-Care

Health Professional	Role
Registered nurse	Assesses abilities and deficits in self-care; coordinates and supports rehabilitation through individualized plan of care and client teaching
Rehabilitation physician	Directs rehabilitation and medical management of client enrolled in a rehabilitation program
Physical therapist	Assesses mobility, strengthens muscle groups, and works to improve motor function
Occupational therapist	Assesses ability to perform activities of daily living; helps clients relearn basic care skills and energy conservation methods
Social worker	Coordinates placement for clients unable to remain in the home, or identifies community resources to help client stay in the home despite deficits
Speech therapist	Evaluates swallowing, and retrains safe eating for clients with deficits
Home health nurse	Provides follow-up and coordination for self-care deficits in the home by accessing community resources, teaching, and providing support and direct care

trol over participation in self-care. Positive interventions to encourage self-care include coaxing, rewarding, and educating. Providing assistance with self-care activities gives the nurse an opportunity to develop a trusting, satisfying relationship with the client. Many of these activities, such as bathing, shampooing, or combing the hair, are relaxing and soothing to the client. Pleasant conversation during these activities can enchance feelings of comfort and self-worth. These activities give hospitalized or long-term clients a chance to interact with people.

Scheduled Care. Clients with self-care deficits may require the nurse's assistance in performing hygiene. For the client's comfort and the nurse's planning, specific types of hygienic care are given at regular inter-

Scheduling Hygiene Care

Early Morning Care

Comfort measures and preparation for the day

- Bedpan, urinal, or assistance to bathroom
- Preparation for diagnostic tests or early surgery
- Washing hands and face
- Oral care
- Preparation for breakfast

Morning Care (AM Care)

Morning hygiene and grooming

- Bedpan, urinal, or assistance to bathroom
- Bath, shower, or bathing
- Back massage
- Hair care and shaving
- Oral care
- Care for feet and nails
- Dressing
- Bed linen change
- Straightening bedside unit
- Positioning (bed or chair)

Afternoon Care

After tests, after lunch, and before visitors

- Bedpan, urinal, or assistance to bathroom
- Washing hands and face
- Oral care
- Bed linens and repositioning if needed

Hour-of-Sleep (HS) Care

Comfort measures and bedtime

- Bedpan, urinal, or assistance to bathroom
- Washing hands and face
- Oral care
- Back massage
- Bed linens (change soiled linens, fluff pillow, pull out wrinkles)
- Bedclothes
- Straightening unit (place needed night objects within reach)

vals. Routine times for providing hygiene care in an inpatient setting include early morning, morning, afternoon, or evening. Common measures provided are included in the display. Hygienic procedures should be individualized according to personal and cultural preferences. Because hospital stays are decreasing in length, client acuity is increasing, and staffing ratios are decreasing, the ability to provide complete hygiene care to all clients is challenged. The trend away from primary care nursing in many settings has resulted in the frequent delegation of hygiene measures to nursing assistants.

Bathing and Skin Care

The usual time of day for bathing varies greatly. Some people prefer to bathe in the morning; others find that an evening bath is relaxing and promotes a good night's sleep. It is not always possible to satisfy personal preferences, but clients appreciate the opportunity to wash their face and hands in the morning before breakfast and before going to sleep at night. The frequency of bathing should be determined by the client's needs. The comatose client or the client who has excessive body excretions or wound drainage requires bathing every day (sometimes more frequently) to avoid skin irritation, breakdown, and infection.

Some clients are anxious or embarrassed about needing assistance with bathing, grooming, dressing, and toileting. The nurse must be sensitive to the client's preferences and respect the client's sense of privacy and modesty. Curtains should be pulled around beds and doors closed when bathing or dressing clients to ensure privacy. Some clients are sensitive to having these activities performed by someone of the opposite sex.

The environment in the long-term care facility should promote self-care independence. Supplies or equipment should be available, such as a walker if the client needs support in getting to the bathroom.

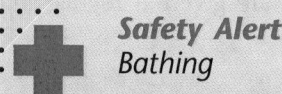

Safety Alert
Bathing

- Check and adjust water temperature to avoid burning.
- Use caution when moving in and out of the bathtub or shower. Use handrails and other means of support.
- Prevent chilling by closing the door to cut drafts, using warm water, and increasing the room temperature if possible. Dry exposed parts quickly and cover areas not being bathed during a bed bath.
- Monitor adults frequently when they are bathing or showering. If any doubt exists about a client's ability to tolerate the procedure while standing, use a shower chair or help the client bathe at the bedside.
- Avoid vigorous rubbing of dry skin, because this can facilitate skin breakdown in those with compromised circulation or with less elastic skin tone (ie, the elderly). Patting dry is best.
- Use nonslip surfaces and handrails in bathroom and shower stalls.
- Never leave infants or young children unattended in or near the bathtub or shower.

Types of Baths. There are two types of baths: cleansing baths and therapeutic baths. *Cleansing baths* are needed to keep the skin free of secretions, microorganisms, perspiration, and debris. All body parts should be cleansed, but areas requiring particular attention to prevent skin breakdown, odors, or discomfort are the face, hands, axillae, back, and perineum. *Therapeutic baths* soothe skin irritation or promote healing (Table 32-4).

Methods of Bathing. There are several methods of bathing, depending on the client's condition and abilities:

- Tub bath
- Stand-up shower
- Sit-down shower with shower chair
- Bed bath (partial or complete)
- Towel or bag bath
- Partial bath at a nearby sink or washbasin

Selecting the appropriate method should take into account the client's energy level and need to conserve energy for other activities, surgical dressings or body parts that may need to be kept dry, the client's preference, and the need to encourage independent self-care.

Some methods are easier for the client to perform independently or with limited assistance. If the nurse provides the needed equipment, some clients can bathe themselves, although assistance may be needed to reach the back and feet. When assessing which type of bath should be used, the nurse should take into account the client's abilities and the method that allows him or her the most independence in self-care. Tub baths or showers are more effective for cleaning and ensuring that the skin is thoroughly rinsed, but they require more mobility and agility. Oxygen requirements for showering are significantly greater than those for a tub bath or bed bath (Johnson, Watt, & Fletcher, 1981). Clients who suffer dizziness, weakness, or mental confusion should not be allowed to take stand-up showers. Obese clients may find it difficult to maneuver into a bathtub and might risk falling. For these clients, a shower may be more appropriate. Steps in assisting with a bath or shower are given on Procedure 32-1.

Table 32-4 • Types of Therapeutic Baths

Type	Purpose	Nursing Considerations
Sitz bath	To cleanse, soothe, and reduce inflammation of perineal or vaginal area after childbirth and vaginal or rectal surgery or from local irritation of hemorrhoids and fissures	Water temperature depends on the client's condition and personal preference but is usually 105°–113°F.
Hot-water bath	To relieve muscle spasms and soreness by total immersion	Water temperature should be 113°–114.8°F but may be individualized to client condition and preference. Be alert for vasodilation with resultant orthostatic blood pressure drop and for scalding of skin.
Warm-water bath	To cleanse, promote relaxation, and relieve tension	Water temperature is adjusted to client preference.
Cool-water bath	To relieve muscle tension or decrease body temperature in febrile clients	Water should be tepid (98.6°F), not cold. Avoid chilling; shivering may increase body temperature.
Soaks	To soften and loosen secretions during dressing changes or to reduce pain and swelling or itching of inflamed or irritated skin	Medications or topical agents may be added to the water. Hot, warm, or cold water is applied to an isolated body part.

Towel baths, sometimes referred to as bag baths, are given with a quick-drying solution (Septi-Soft) that evaporates from the body so rinsing is not necessary. Towels or multiple washcloths are placed in a plastic bag with the warmed solution and wrung out before being placed on the client. The damp towels are used to cleanse and massage body areas. Advantages of a towel bath include decreased bathing time, decreased energy expenditure by the client, and decreased skin drying because oil is contained within the solution. Clients report feeling clean and refreshed from this type of bath. Skewes (1994) also reports a decreased spread of gram-negative organisms when the bag bath or towel bath is used. Gram-negative organisms can proliferate when wet washbasins are stored between bed baths. The use of multiple washcloths ensures that organisms are less likely to be transferred from a contaminated area to a clean area, because a new cloth can be used for each area of the body.

Proper washing techniques to ensure asepsis include washing from clean areas to dirty areas when possible. Washing extremities from distal to proximal stimulates circulation and venous blood return. Preventing excess skin dryness is important for the health and integrity of skin. Dry skin is increased by inadequate fluid intake, too-frequent bathing with soaps or detergents, and the use of defatting solutions, such as alcohol, on the skin. Use practices that reduce skin dryness, and teach the client to do the same (see the display on client teaching earlier in the chapter).

Some clients are weak or comatose and cannot bathe themselves. Their weakness may necessitate the nurse bathing the client in bed. Steps for this are outlined in Procedure 32-2.

Perineal Care

If the client cannot perform adequate perineal and genital care, the nurse must do so. Cleaning the perineum and genitals is usually a part of the bath but may need to be done more frequently if the person is incontinent of urine or feces or has drainage in the perineal area. The nurse can teach perineal and genital care while bathing the client.

Perineal care for women involves cleansing the upper inner thighs, the labia majora, and the folds between the labia majora and minora. Wipe from front to back to avoid contaminating the vagina or urethra with microorganisms from the anus (Fig. 32-3*A*). For men, perineal care involves washing the upper inner thighs, the penis, and the scrotum; in uncircumcised men, the foreskin must be retracted and the glans penis washed (Fig. 32-3*B*). For both sexes, the buttocks are cleaned after the genitals, from a side-lying position.

Perineal tissue is more sensitive than other skin; therefore, temperature extremes are avoided. Pouring water over the perineum while the client sits on the toilet or a bedpan is a comfortable way of rinsing for the client who cannot use a tub or shower or between baths. Certain people are at greater risk for infection and irritation of these areas, including clients with indwelling catheters; those with perineal, rectal, or lower urinary tract surgery; incontinent clients; and women after childbirth. Perineal care is routinely performed frequently by or for these people.

Many clients can do their own perineal care with minimal assistance. A nurse giving perineal care to a client of the opposite sex should be direct and professional to help allay embarrassment. Gloves must be

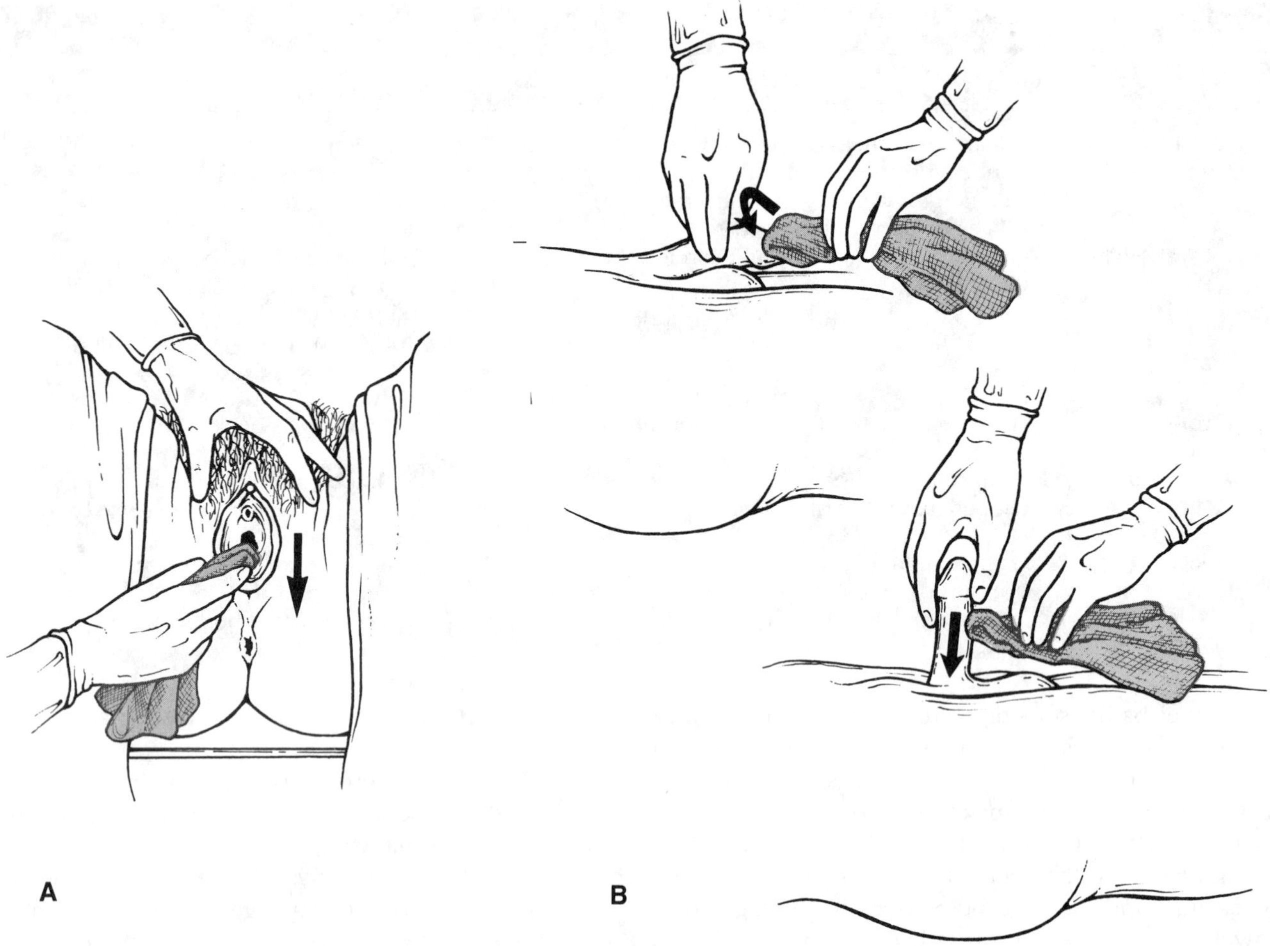

A B

Figure 32-3 *• Perineal care. (**A**) Female. The labia are spread to expose the urethral meatus and the vaginal orifice. The area is cleansed from the pubic area toward the anus in one stroke. This is repeated several times, always using a clean area of the wash cloth. (**B**) Male. The tip of the penis is cleansed from the urethral meatus downward in a circular motion. The penile shaft is cleansed from the tip downward toward the scrotum.*

worn during perineal cleansing of all clients and while handling items that may contain exudate from the perineal area, because organisms may enter the nurse's circulation through lesions (open sores, cuts, or burns).

Back Massage

Back massage is given to clients to enhance the blood supply to the skin and muscles, to promote comfort, and to promote relaxation. The degree of pressure used varies and should be determined by observing the client's response or verbal cues. For the most relaxing effect, both hands should maintain contact throughout the procedure. Avoid excessive pressure over bony prominences to avoid damaging the underlying tissue. A lubricant (cream or lotion) permits the hands to glide over the skin. Some young people with oily skin find alcohol a cooling and refreshing lubricant, but it is drying to the skin and can cause cracking and skin breakdown in dehydrated clients and older adults.

If possible, the client should assume a prone position for a backrub. If this is contraindicated or inconvenient, a side-lying position is used. With immobile clients, it may be effective to perform a partial backrub after turning him or her from one side to the other to enhance circulation to the lateral aspect of the hips. Procedure 32-3 summarizes the back massage.

Care of Feet and Nails

Feet and nails often need special attention. Assess the appearance of the feet and nails to identify existing problems or clients at risk for foot or nail problems. Table 32-5 lists common foot problems, causes, and treatment. The color and temperature of the skin gives clues to the quality of perfusion (blood flow). Cold feet with a dusky skin color may signal poor circulation. People with diabetes mellitus, older people, and clients with poor circulation are at special risk for foot difficulties, so good foot care and education about self-care

Procedure 32-1
Assisting With the Bath or Shower

Purpose

1. Cleanse the skin, control body odors, and promote self-esteem.
2. Stimulate circulation.
3. Provide an opportunity for assessment of skin and physical mobility.
4. Provide range-of-motion exercises for joints.
5. Promote relaxation and comfort.

Assessment

- Assess client's ability to perform self-care and amount of assistance needed. Evaluate activity tolerance, cognitive function, musculoskeletal function, and level of discomfort to determine type of bath.
  Note: Client should be encouraged to be as independent as possible but should not become excessively fatigued. Pain should not be intensified.
- Assess client preferences for bathing (ie, frequency, time of day, type of skin-care products).
- Review chart to determine what other procedures or therapies the client is receiving to coordinate scheduling and prevent fatigue.
- Identify clients with special considerations for bathing:
  - Older clients: susceptible to dry skin
  - Immobilized clients: pressure areas on dependent and bony parts; need for range-of-motion exercises to joints
  - Clients with altered sensation: risk for burns from hot water
  - Obese or diaphoretic clients: excessive perspiration or moisture on skin surfaces that rub against each other, providing medium for excoriation and bacterial growth
- Review history for precautions regarding movement or positioning.
- Assess client's knowledge and practice of hygiene to determine learning needs.

Equipment

One bath towel
One washcloth
Soap, soap dish, or liquid (nonsoap) cleanser
Personal skin-care products (deodorant, powder, lotions, cologne)
Clean gown or pajamas
Laundry bag

Procedure

1. Prepare bathroom by placing towel or disposable bath mat on floor by tub or shower.
   Rationale: The nurse must maintain cleanliness and safety for the client.
2. Make sure the tub or shower is clean.
3. Don gloves.
4. Accompany or transport client to the bathroom. Some clients may need to use a shower chair for transportation.
   Rationale: Showering or bathing will be tiring. Transportation in a chair will conserve energy.
5. Keep client covered with a bath blanket until water is ready.
   Rationale: Keeping the client warm will prevent chills.

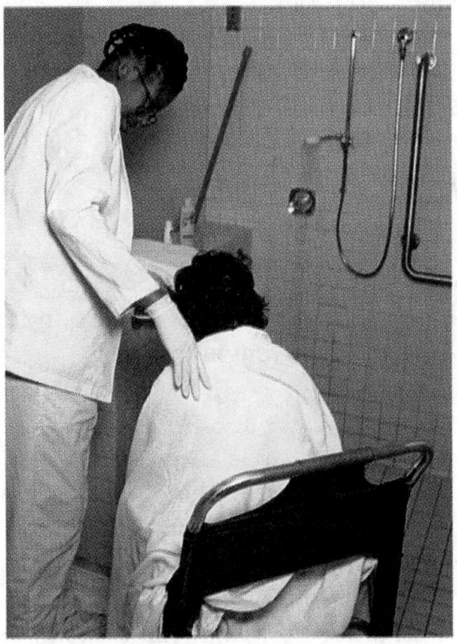

Step 5 • *Wrap client in bath blanket.*

6. Place "occupied" sign on door.
   Rationale: The client needs privacy while bathing. Doors are not usually locked, so nurse can come in to assist client.
7. Fill bathtub halfway with warm water (105°F). Test water or have client test water. If taking shower, turn shower on and adjust temperature.
   Rationale: Testing temperature before entering water prevents burns.
8. Help client into shower or tub, providing necessary assistance.

(continued)

Rationale: Falls can occur in the shower or tub, and the nurse must provide safety for the client.

9. Instruct client in use of safety bars and call bell signal. Client may prefer to sit in shower chair to prevent fatigue.
Rationale: The nurse provides for the client's safety and comfort.
10. If the client is unable to shower independently, stay with the client at all times. (Two nurses may be necessary for some clients.) Use handheld shower to wash client.
Rationale: Hand held shower allows nurse to stay dry.
11. If client is showering or bathing independently, check on client within 15 minutes. Wash any areas he or she could not reach.
Rationale: Prolonged exposure to warm water may cause vasodilation and pooling of blood. This can result in lightheadedness or dizziness.
12. Help client out of tub or shower. Assist with drying.
Note: If client is unsteady, drain water before getting client out of tub to prevent falls.
13. Assist client with dressing and grooming.
14. Help client to room.
15. Return to bathroom to clean tub or shower according to agency policy. Discard soiled linen. Place "unoccupied" sign on door.

Lifespan Considerations

Newborn and Infant

- An infant should not be submerged in water until the umbilical cord has fallen off (around 7–10 days of age) to prevent infection.

Child

- Children younger than 8 years should not be left unattended in a bath to prevent drowning.
- Children often enjoy washing themselves but require supervision to be sure it is done thoroughly.

Adolescent

- Sebaceous glands become active during puberty. Special cleansing agents may be necessary to treat facial acne. Antiperspirants and more frequent baths will help control body odors.

Older Adult

- The older adult is susceptible to dry skin due to reduced sebaceous gland activity, epidermal thinning, and decreased fluid intake. Lotions, bath oil, and decreased use of soap can reduce the drying effects of aging.
- The older adult may have decreased sensation and is at risk for burns from hot water.

Home Care Modifications

- Clients at risk for falling should be instructed to apply lotions and oils after the bath and not put them in bath water. Oils can make the bathtub or shower surfaces more slippery.
- Safety devices, such as tub bars, nonskid tub surfaces, and bathroom carpeting, can be installed to reduce the chance of falls and promote independence.

are essential. Combining teaching with care is a good way to motivate a person with foot problems. The feet of people with peripheral vascular disease must be protected from trauma during foot care, so avoid cutting nails too short and cutting into calluses. Some hospital policies forbid nurses from cutting the toenails of diabetic clients or people with peripheral vascular disease, because healing is slow and the risk of infection following accidental injury is high. These clients often have thick, distorted toenails that are difficult to cut safely, but the nails can be safely filed. Procedure 32-4 outlines nursing care of feet and nails.

Client education concerning care of the feet should include the following:

- Inspect feet daily. You may need a mirror to visualize all areas.
- Avoid habits that will decrease circulation to your feet (smoking, garters, crossing legs).
- Notify your healthcare provider if you notice abnormal sores or drainage, pain, changes in temperature, color, or sensation of the foot.
- Select sturdy, well-fitting footwear with a nonskid sole. Shop for shoes in the afternoon or evening when feet are often larger due to swelling. Break shoes in gradually, carefully observing for signs or irritation or skin breakdown.
- Do not walk barefoot (Ruscin, Cunningham, & Blaylock, 1993).

Hair Care

Shampooing. Shampooing cleans the hair and scalp and helps get rid of excess oil. It promotes circulation to the scalp and provides a relaxing, soothing experience for the client. The nurse can use this opportunity to inspect the hair for dandruff or lice. Shampooing can be done while the client sits in the shower chair, leans

Table 32-5 • Common Foot Problems

Type	*Description*	*Possible Causes*	*Treatment*
Calluses	Flattened thickening of epidermis, often on bottom or side of foot over a bony prominence	Tight shoes or inadequate padding in shoes	Soften by soaking in warm water and abrade with pumice stone.
Corns	Cone-shaped lesion (thickening of epidermis), usually on fourth or fifth toe over a toe joint	Pressure from tight shoes	Softer, better-fitting shoes or foam protective pads. Apply keratolytic agents with salicylic acid to keratinous skin.
Plantar warts	Round or irregular, flattened by pressure, surrounded by cornified epithelium; often painful	Virus, but may be worsened by inadequate circulation or pressure from tight shoes	Remove by curettage, freezing with solid carbon dioxide, or application of salicylic acid.
Bunions (hallax valgus)	Inflammation and thickening of bursa of the great toe joint; enlargement of the joint and displacement of toe	Heredity, degenerative bone and joint disease, and tight shoes or high heels	Surgical intervention may be needed, or symptomatic relief can be achieved by wearing shoes that are wide at the front.
Ringworm, tinea pedis (athlete's foot)	Redness, scaling, and cracking of skin, especially between toes	Fungus, worsened by moist, unventilated environment	Apply antifungal powder or ointment. Change socks daily; wear 100% cotton socks to absorb moisture.
Ingrown nails	Inflammation, swelling, and pain of tissues at edge of nail	Improper trimming of nails, poorly fitting shoes	Prevent by trimming nails straight across and wearing well-fitted shoes. Pain and inflammation are treated with anti-inflammatory agents. Surgical removal of nail may be required.
Foot odor	Excessive foul odor of feet	Possibly from fungal foot infections; exacerbated by hot, moist environment	Decrease excess moisture: use deodorant foot powders, 100% cotton socks, well-ventilated shoes.

back over the sink, leans forward over a pan of water on the bedside table, lies on a stretcher over a sink (if unable to sit), or is in bed with a tray to drain the water. Protect the client from fatigue and chilling during shampooing. Steps in shampooing the hair of a bedridden client are summarized in Procedure 32-5. Dry shampoo is a powder that can be combed or brushed through the hair to remove excess oils and dirt. Cleansing quality is less effective than traditional methods of shampooing, so this treatment is used only when wetting the hair is contraindicated or not feasible.

Brushing and Combing. Combs are usually provided for clients in the hospital, but brushes often must be brought from home. Clients who can brush and comb their hair should be given the equipment and encouraged to do so independently, but clients who cannot comb their own hair need assistance. Brushing hair massages the scalp, stimulating circulation, and facilitates oil distribution along the hair shaft more effectively than combing. Clients with long hair who must spend an extended time in bed need a hairstyle that minimizes matting; combing the hair daily, braiding it, or tying it back helps. If tangles occur, hair is divided into small sections, brushed, and then combed. Tightly curled hair usually requires a wide-toothed comb or a pick and a firm-bristled brush. Combing with the fingers can loosen tangles. A lubricating conditioner or petroleum jelly may be used to soften hair or avoid breaking.

Lice. Infestation with lice is called **pediculosis.** Lice found on the hair of the head, eyebrows, eyelashes, and beard is known as pediculosis capitis; on the body, pediculosis corporis; and in the perineal area, pediculosis pubis.

Head lice and pubic lice attach their eggs, called nits, to hairs with a tenacious substance that makes them

(text continues on page 796)

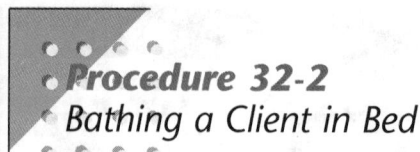

Procedure 32-2
Bathing a Client in Bed

Purpose

Same as Procedure 32-1.

Assessment

Same as Procedure 32-1.

Equipment

Two bath towels
Two washcloths
Bath blanket
Washbasin with warm water (110°–115°F). Test by measuring with bath thermometer or by placing several drops on your inner forearm
Soap, soap dish, or liquid (nonsoap) cleanser
Personal skin-care products (deodorant, powder, lotions, cologne)
Clean gown or pajamas
Bedpan or urinal
Laundry bag
Disposable clean gloves for perineal care

Procedure

1. Close curtains around bed or shut room door.
   Rationale: The client should have privacy for self-dignity.
2. Help client use bedpan, urinal, or commode if needed.
   Rationale: Client will be more comfortable and relaxed after elimination.
3. Close window and doors to decrease drafts.
   Rationale: The nurse provides client comfort and minimizes chilling.
4. Wash your hands.
   Rationale: Handwashing reduces transmission of microorganisms.
5. Raise bed to high position. Lock side rail up on opposite side of bed from your work.
   Rationale: Nurse must prevent back strain while preventing client from falling out of bed.
6. Remove top sheet and bed spread, and place bath blanket on client. Help client move closer to you, and remove gown.
   Rationale: Bath blanket provides for client comfort and warmth. Bringing client closer to you prevents undue muscle strain.
   Note: If top linen is to be reused, place it on back of chair; otherwise, place it in laundry bag.
   Note: If client has an IV line, remove gown from arm, lower IV container, and slide it through gown with tubing. Rehang IV container, and check flow rate.

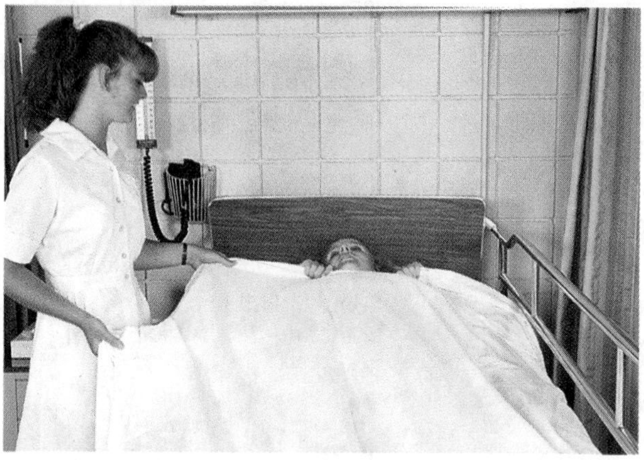

Step 6 • Place bath blanket on client.

7. Lay towel across client's chest.
8. Wet washcloth and fold around your finger to make a mitt.
   a. Fold washcloth in thirds.

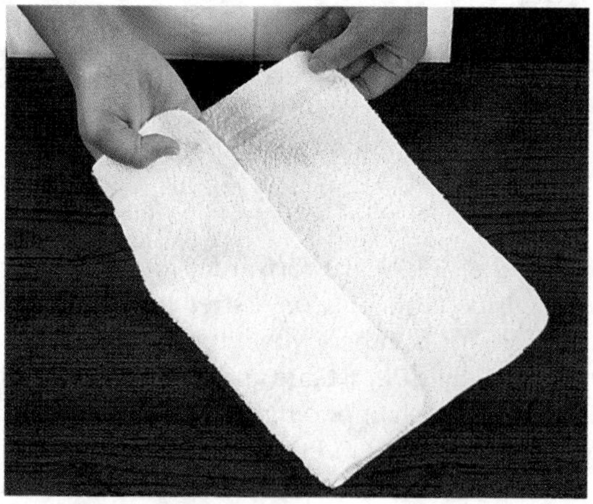

Step 8A • Fold washcloth into thirds.

   b. Straighten washcloth to take out wrinkles.
   c. Fold washcloth over to fit hand.
   d. Tuck loose ends under edge of washcloth on palm.
   Rationale: Mitt retains heat and water better than a loosely held washcloth. Prevents water from dripping on client.
9. Cleanse eyes with water only, wiping from inner to outer canthus. Use separate corner of mitt for each eye.

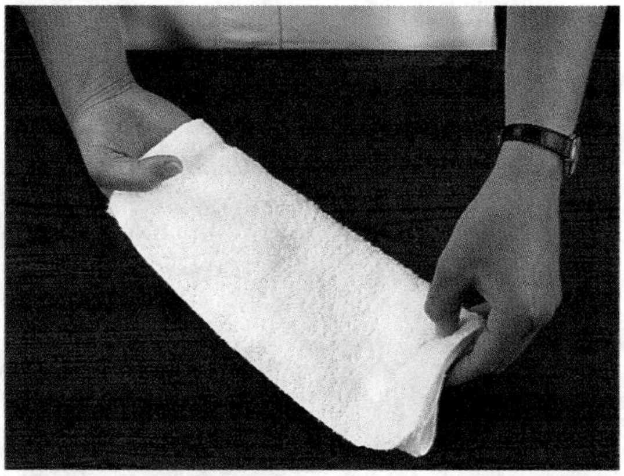

Step 8C • *Fold over to fit hand.*

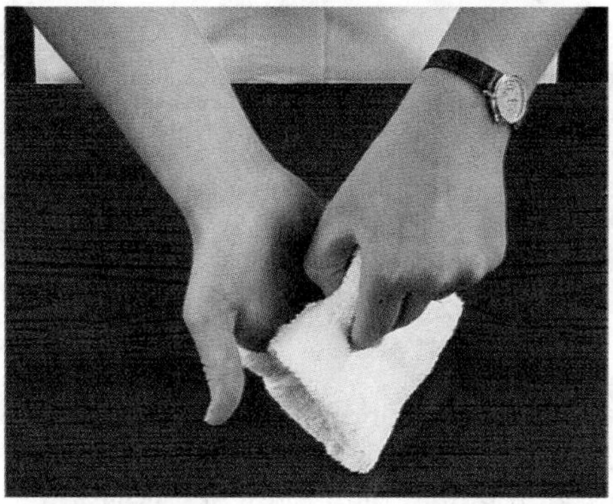

Step 8D • *Tuck end in to make mitt.*

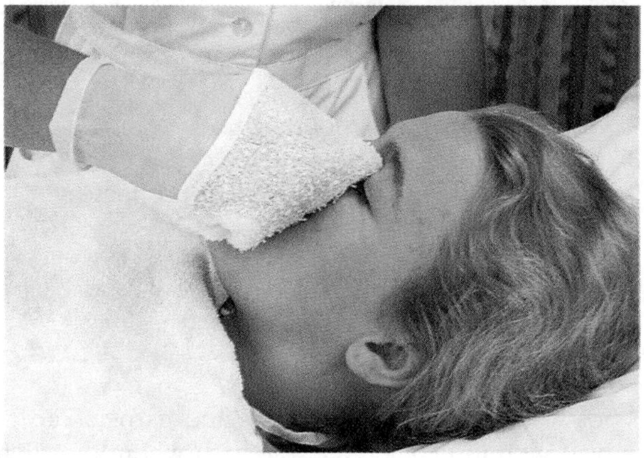

Step 9 • *Wipe each eye with separate corners of cloth.*

Rationale: Washing eye from inner to outer canthus prevents secretions from entering and irritating nasolacrimal ducts. Using separate corners for each eye prevents transfer of microorganisms from one eye to the other.

10. Determine if client would like soap used on face. Wash face, neck, and ears.
    Rationale: Soap can be drying, especially to the face.

    Note: Avoid letting soap bar sit in washbasin, or water will become too soapy for rinse. Liquid nondetergent cleansing agents are available in many institutions to mix directly into bath water. These products are nondrying and need not be rinsed from the skin.
11. Fold bath blanket off arm away from you. Place towel lengthwise under arm. Wash, rinse, and dry the arm using long firm strokes from the fingers toward the axilla. Wash axilla.
    Rationale: Stroking from distal to proximal stimulates circulation and facilitates venous blood return.

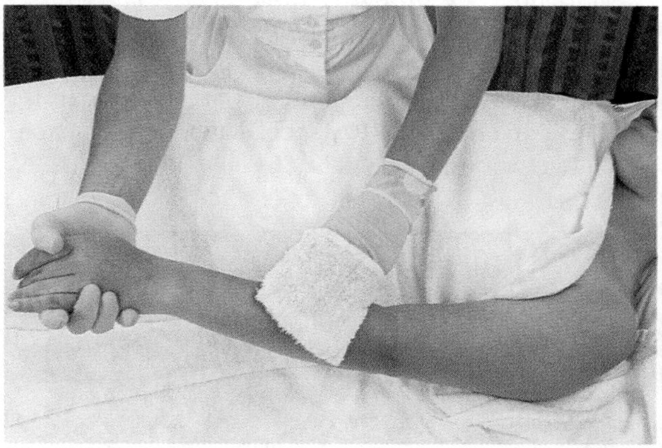

Step 11 • *Wash arm stroking from fingers toward axilla.*

12. (Optional) Place bath towel on bed and put washbasin on it. Immerse client's hand and allow to soak for several minutes. Wash, rinse, and dry hand well. Repeat on other side. Apply lotion.
    Rationale: Soaking softens cuticles and loosens dirt under nails.
13. Repeat for hand and arm nearest you.
14. Apply deodorant or powder according to client's preferences. Avoid excessive use of powder or inhalation of powder.
    Rationale: Hygiene products control excess body moisture and odor. Excessive powder can cause caking, which leads to skin irritation; inhalation can cause respiratory difficulty.
15. Assess temperature of bath water, and change water if necessary.
    Note: Side rails should be up to prevent accidental falls.
16. Place bath towel over chest. Fold bath blanket down to below umbilicus.
    Rationale: The nurse keeps the client warm while preventing unnecessary exposure of body parts.
17. Lift bath towel off chest, and bathe chest and abdomen with mitted hand using long, firm strokes. Give special attention to skin under the breasts

(continued)

and any other skin folds if client is overweight. Rinse and dry well.
Note: A light dusting of bath powder under the breasts or between skin folds absorbs excess moisture and prevents skin maceration and irritation.

18. Help client don a clean gown.
19. Expose leg away from you by folding over bath blanket. Be careful to keep perineum covered.
Rationale: Unnecessary exposure of body parts is prevented.
20. Lift leg, and place bath towel lengthwise under leg. Wash, rinse, and dry leg using long, firm strokes from ankle to thigh.
Rationale: Washing from distal to proximal stimulates circulation and facilitates venous blood return.
21. Wash feet or place in basin of water as for hands. Rinse and dry well. Pay special attention to space between toes.

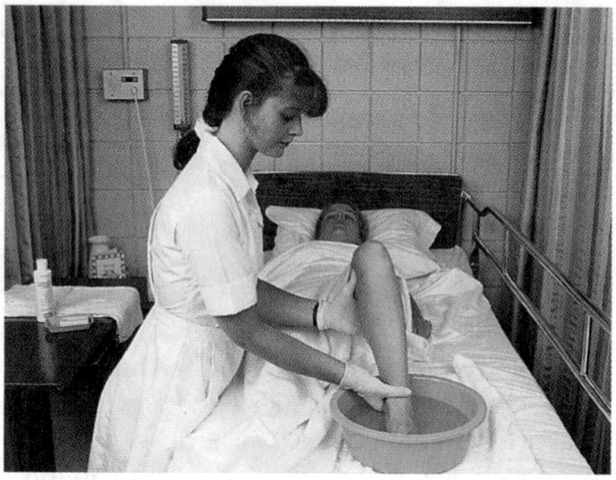

Step 21 • *Place foot in basin of water to soak.*

22. Repeat for other leg and foot.
23. Assess bath water for warmth. Change water if necessary.
24. Assist client to side-lying position. Place bath towel along side of back and buttocks to protect linen. Wash, rinse, and dry back and buttocks. Give a backrub with powder or lotion.
Rationale: Backrub stimulates circulation and promotes comfort.
Note: Wear disposable, clean gloves when cleansing anal area.

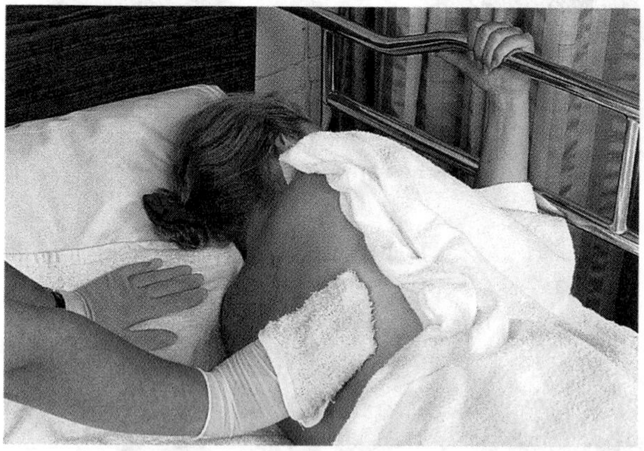

Step 24 • *Assist to side-lying position to wash back and buttocks.*

25. Assist to supine position. Assess if client can wash genitals and perineal area independently. If unable to, drape with bath blanket so that only genitals are exposed. Don disposable, clean gloves; using fresh water and a new cloth, wash, rinse, and dry genitalia and perineum (see text for instructions).
26. Apply powder, lotion, cologne according to client preference.
27. Assist with hair and mouth care.
28. Make bed with clean linen.
29. Clean equipment and return to appropriate storage area.
30. Wash your hands.
31. Chart significant observations.

hard to remove. Nits, which may be visible with a light and magnifying glass, resemble shiny ovals. To the naked eye, they appear similar to dandruff. Lice live on the skin and their bites cause itching. Inflamed bites can be seen along the hairline. Body lice suck blood from the skin and tend to live in the clothing, making them hard to detect. Clues to the presence of body lice are scratching and hemorrhagic lesions on the skin.

The usual treatment for pediculosis is gamma benzene hexachloride (Kwell), which comes in lotion, cream, and shampoo form. Lice can be treated by showering with Kwell. Because of the heavy hair growth of the area, pubic lice are often difficult to remove; the shampoo may be applied and left on for 12 to 24 hours. Linens and clothing used by the client must be washed in hot water. Blankets, furniture, and carpets can be sprayed with insecticide. People with whom the client has had sexual or intimate contact also should be treated.

Dandruff. Dandruff is a chronic, diffuse scaling of the epidermis of the scalp. It is characterized by itching and flaking of whitish scales, which are annoying and embarrassing. Frequent brushing and daily shampooing with a keratolytic shampoo may control the problem, but persistent, severe cases may require medical attention.

Hair Loss. Hair continually grows and renews itself. To promote healthy hair, chemical treatments and ex-

Procedure 32-3
Massaging the Back

Purpose

1. Stimulate circulation to the skin
2. Relieve muscle tension
3. Promote comfort and relaxation

Assessment

- Assess client for muscle fatigue or stiffness, complaints of back discomfort or tension.
- Identify clients with impaired physical mobility who may benefit from back massage.
- Assess skin for localized areas of redness on the back, shoulders, or hips.
- Assess client's desire for back massage.
- Identify conditions that may contraindicate backrub (rib and vertebral fractures, burns, or open wounds).
- Determine any limitations to positioning.

Equipment

Bath blanket
Bath towel (to absorb excess moisture)
Lotion, powder, or alcohol. Lotion is used to lubricate the skin and prevents friction during massage. Powder reduces friction and prevents "sticky" feeling on diaphoretic clients. Powder and lotion are not used together. Alcohol cools the skin but can be drying.

Procedure

1. Help client to side-lying or prone position.
2. Expose back, shoulders, upper arms, and sacral area. Cover remainder of body with bath blanket.
   Rationale: Covering areas not being massaged prevents unnecessary exposure and chilling.
3. Wash hands in warm water. Warm lotion by holding container under running warm water.
   Rationale: Warm hands and lotion prevent startle response and muscle tension from cold lotion and hands.
   Note: Alcohol is applied cold, but warn the client before application.
4. Pour small amount of lotion into palms.
   Rationale: Lubricating palms decreases friction on skin during massage.
5. Begin massage in sacral area with circular motion. Move hands upward to shoulders, massaging over scapulae in smooth, firm strokes. Without removing hands from skin, continue in smooth strokes to upper arms and down sides of back to iliac crest. Continue for 3 to 5 minutes.
   Rationale: Continuous, firm pressure promotes relaxation and stimulates circulation.

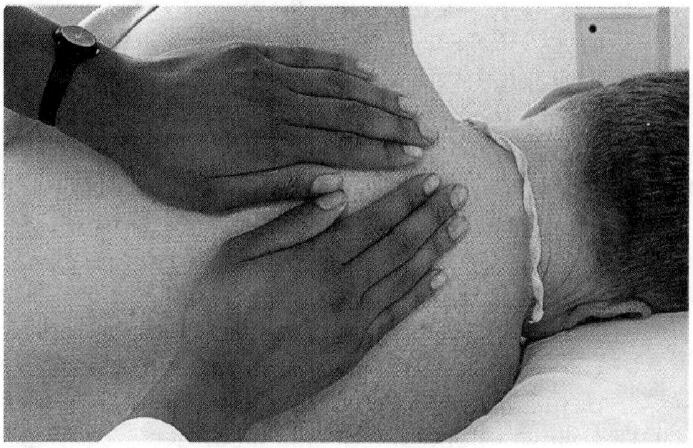

Step 5 • *Move hands upward with firm, circular motion.*

6. While massaging, assess for whitish or reddened areas that do not disappear and broken skin areas. Provide additional massage to reddened areas.
   Rationale: Massage will stimulate circulation to areas at risk for breakdown.
7. If additional stimulation is desired, *petrissage* (kneading) over the shoulders and gluteal area and *tapotement* (tapping) up and down the spine can be done.
8. End massage with long, continuous, stroking movements.
   Rationale: Stroking is the most relaxing of the massage movements.
9. Pat excess lubricant dry with towel. Retie client's gown, and assist to comfortable position.
10. Wash your hands.

cessive heat (drying on the high setting, electric rollers) should be avoided. Cream rinses can be helpful in keeping hair untangled and matt free.

Male-pattern baldness occurs in middle or older age but can occur much earlier in some men. Premature loss of hair can be stressful, impacting self-image and sexual identity. Treatment includes hair pieces, hair transplants, or drugs that stimulate hair growth.

Acute hair loss can occur due to stress, high fever, certain medications, general anesthesia, or childbirth. Most commonly hair loss (**alopecia**) is caused by cancer treatment. Clients need to be warned that hair loss

Procedure 32-4
Performing Foot and Nail Care

Purpose

1. Maintain skin integrity around nails
2. Provide for client's comfort and sense of well-being
3. Maintain foot function
4. Encourage self-care

Assessment

- Note client's gait for limping or unusual position. Unnatural gait can be caused by painful feet or bone and muscle disorders.
- Assess footwear worn by client. Socks should be worn to absorb excess perspiration and avoid fungal infections.
- Identify clients at risk for foot or nail problems:
  - Diabetes is associated with changes in microcirculation to peripheral tissues. The diabetic client is at high risk for infection from breaks in skin integrity and may have decreased sensation to pain as a result of neuropathies.
  - Elderly clients' ability to perform foot and nail care may be impeded by poor vision, obesity, or musculoskeletal conditions that limit their ability to bend and maintain balance.
  - Cerebrovascular accident may alter the client's gait due to foot drop, muscle weakness, or paralysis.
  - Conditions associated with foot and ankle edema (renal failure, congestive heart failure) interfere with blood flow to surrounding tissues and impede proper shoe fit.
- Determine client's ability to perform self-care.
- Inspect nails and skin of fingers, toes, and feet. Assess areas between toes for dryness and cracking.
- Assess client's knowledge of foot and nail care practices.
- Review agency policy for trimming nails. Many agencies require a physician's order to perform nail trimming on high-risk clients.
- Identify clients going to surgery. Nail polish must be removed so nailbeds can be assessed for changes in oxygenation.

Equipment

Waterproof pad
Washcloth, towels
Washbasin, warm water, soap
Lotion
Disposable gloves
Nail clippers, file
Orange stick
Polish remover (if necessary)

Procedure

1. Wash your hands.
2. Help client to chair if possible. Elevate head of bed for bedridden client.
3. Remove colored nail polish if client is scheduled for surgery. Review agency policy to determine if patient may wear clear nail polish.
   Rationale: Colored nail polish prevents observation of the nail beds for changes in color associated with poor oxygenation.
4. Fill washbasin with warm water (100°–104°F). Place waterproof pad under basin. Soak client's hands or feet in basin.
   Rationale: Warm water softens nails, increases local circulation, and reduces inflammation.
   Note: Diabetic clients may have decreased sensation in their extremities. Test water temperature carefully to prevent burns.

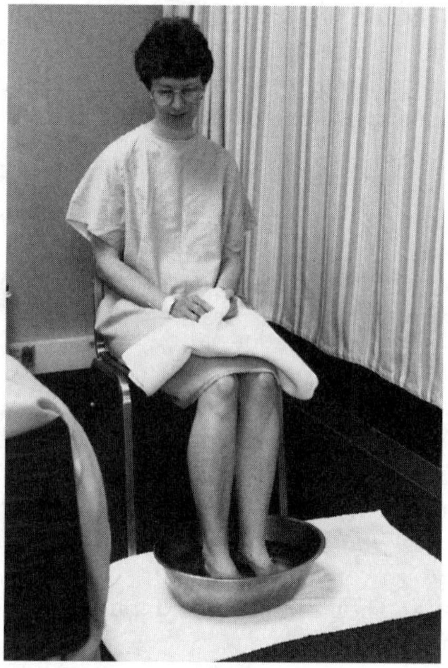

Step 4 • *Soak feet for 10 to 20 minutes.*

5. Place call bell within reach. Allow hands or feet to soak for 10 to 20 minutes.
   Rationale: Softening allows easier removal of dead epithelial cells and reduces possibility of nails cracking during trimming.

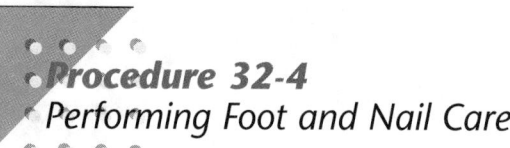

6. Dry the hand or foot that has been soaking. Rewarm water, and allow other extremity to soak while you work on the softened nails.
   Rationale: Soaking the second hand or foot while the nurse works on the first increases efficiency of time.

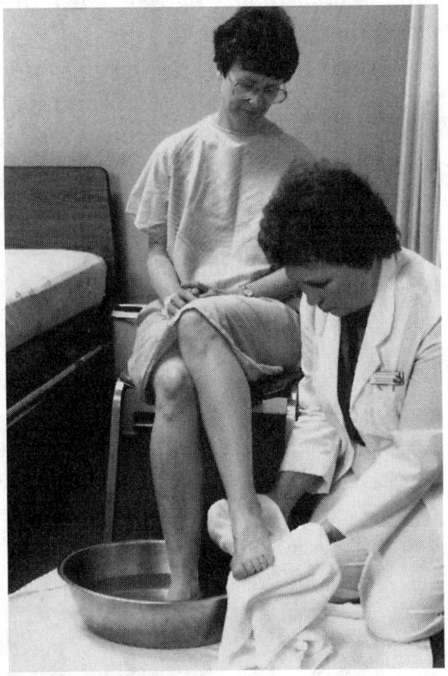

Step 6 • *Dry feet thoroughly.*

7. Gently clean under nails with orange stick.
   Note: If nails are thickened and yellow, client may have fungal infection. Wear disposable gloves to prevent transmission of infection.
8. Beginning with large toe or thumb, clip nail straight across. Shape nail with file. File rather than cut nails of clients with diabetes or circulatory problems.
   Rationale: Trimming straight across prevents splitting of nail and injury to tissues around the nail.
   Note: Clients with severely hypertrophied nails should be referred to a podiatrist or foot clinic for care.
9. Push cuticle back gently with orange stick.
   Rationale: Cuticle care reduces inflamed cuticle and hang nail formation.
10. Repeat procedure with other nails.
11. Rinse foot or hand in warm water.

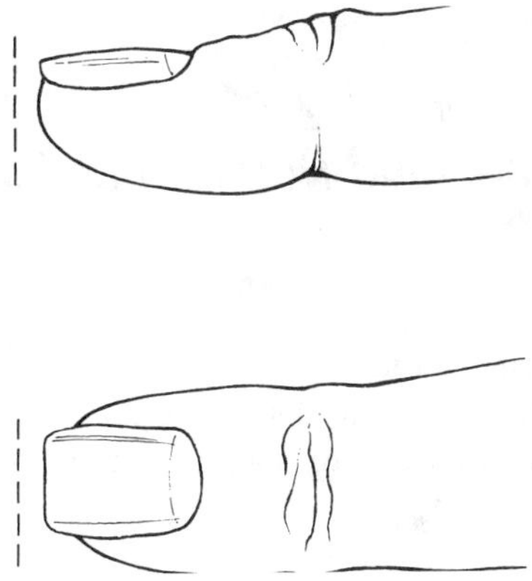

Step 8 • *Cut nails straight across.*

12. Dry thoroughly with towel, especially between digits.
    Rationale: Removing excess moisture inhibits bacterial growth.
13. Apply lotion to hands or feet.
14. Help client to comfortable position.
15. Remove and dispose of equipment.
16. Wash your hands.

Lifespan Considerations

Infant

- Parents must learn to care for nails to prevent the infant from scratching himself or herself. The nails should be cut straight across using blunt scissors. It is easiest to trim the nails when the baby is asleep.

Child

- Nail-biting is often a concern in school-age children. It may be a learned behavior or a symptom of nervous tension. Bad-tasting over-the-counter preparations are available to paint on the nails as a reminder not to bite. Other measures may include positive reinforcement and rewards for "good" days with no nail-biting.

Older Adult

- Elderly clients may have dehydrated epidermal cells and decreased sebaceous gland secretion from normal physiologic effects of aging. This predisposes them to fungal infections and breaks in skin integrity.

may be gradual or sudden and total a few weeks after treatment is started. Following treatment, hair usually regenerates, although it may grow back a different color or texture. Support of the client during this time may include helping to select a hat, wig, or decorative scarf to wear or referral to a community agency, such as the American Cancer Society, which provides support.

Shaving

Shaving may make men feel good about their physical appearance. Most men without beards shave every day, and receiving help with shaving can boost the client's morale. To avoid cuts, soften the beard with warm towels before shaving. Use soap lather or shaving cream,

Procedure 32-5
Shampooing Hair of a Bedridden Client

Purpose

1. Cleanse hair and scalp
2. Promote comfort and self-esteem
3. Apply medication to scalp and hair

Assessment

- Assess condition of hair and scalp.
- Determine agency policy about shampooing hair of bedridden clients. Some agencies require a physician's order.
- Assess activity level of client, and identify positioning restrictions.
- Assess client's preference for hair-care products. Determine whether medicated shampoo has been ordered and is available.

Equipment

Comb and brush
Hair dryer (optional)
Two bath towels, one washcloth
Shampoo (cream rinse is optional)
Water pitcher
Plastic shampoo basin
Washbasin or bucket
Bath blanket
Waterproof pads
Cotton balls (optional)
Hydrogen peroxide (optional, to cleanse matted blood from hair)

Procedure

1. Place waterproof pads under client's head and shoulders, and remove pillow.
Rationale: Bed linen must be kept clean and dry.
2. Raise bed to highest position.
Rationale: This position reduces strain on nurse's back.
3. Remove any pins from hair. Comb and brush hair thoroughly.
Rationale: Tangle removal and distribution of scalp oils through hair result in thorough cleansing.
4. Lay bed to flat position.
5. Place shampooing basin under head. Place bath towel around shoulders and folded washcloth where neck rests on basin.
Rationale: Shoulder padding protects client from becoming wet. Washcloth protects neck from strain and discomfort.
6. Fold bed linens down to waist. Cover upper body with bath blanket.
Rationale: Client should be kept warm and linen protected from water.
7. Place waste basket with plastic bag under spout of shampoo basin on a chair or table at the bedside.
Rationale: Water should run away from face and head into a receptacle.
8. Using water pitcher, wet hair thoroughly with warm water (approximately 110°F). Check temperature by placing small amount of water on your wrist. A bath thermometer may be used.
Rationale: Face and scalp are protected from burns.

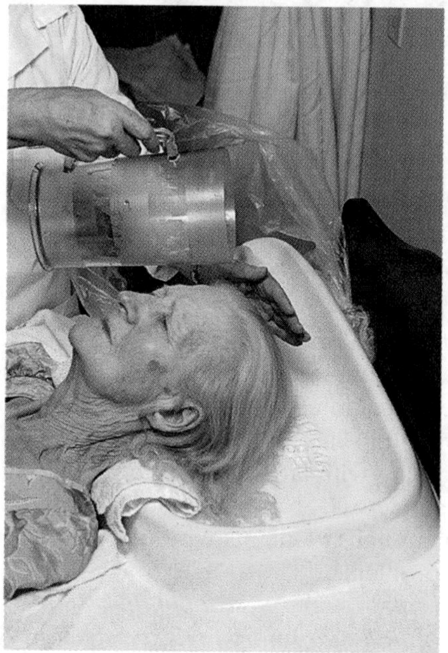

Step 8 • *Run warm water over hair.*

9. Apply small amount of shampoo.
Note: Before shampooing, hydrogen peroxide may be used to dissolve matted blood in hair. Peroxide normally feels bubbly and warm. Reassure client that it will not bleach hair.
10. Massage scalp with fingertips while making shampoo lather. Start at hairline and work toward neck.
Rationale: Massage stimulates circulation to the scalp; systematic lathering ensures thorough cleansing.
11. Rinse hair with warm water. Reapply shampoo, and repeat massage.
12. Rinse hair thoroughly with warm water.
Note: Clean hair "squeaks" when rubbed between fingers.

Rationale: Soap residue in hair may dry and irritate hair and scalp.

13. Apply small amount of conditioner per client request. Rinse well.
    Rationale: Conditioner prevents drying and makes combing easier.
14. Squeeze excess moisture from hair. Wrap bath towel around hair. Rub to dry hair and scalp. Use second towel if necessary.
15. Remove equipment and wet towels from bed. Place dry towel around client's shoulders.
    Rationale: These activities prevent chilling of client.
16. Dry hair with hair dryer. Comb and style.
17. Help client to comfortable position.
18. Dispose of soiled equipment and linen.

Lifespan Considerations

Infant

- Shampooing is usually done during daily bath to prevent seborrhea, a gray, scaly scalp condition (cradle cap).
- Prewarm the room and use warmed towels to prevent chilling infant during bath.

Child

- Pediculosis infestations are common in school-age children. Assess hair carefully for nits (lice eggs).

Adolescent

- Many adolescents shampoo their hair daily. Offering to shampoo their hair may improve their self-esteem and help them feel better than many other nursing interventions.

Older Adult

- Many older adults have decreased subcutaneous tissue and chill quickly. Prewarm towels, and thoroughly dry hair after a shampoo to prevent chilling.
- Older adults may have decreased sensation to heat. Use a hair dryer cautiously on a low heat setting to prevent burning the scalp.

pull the skin taut, and shave in the direction in which the hair grows to decrease irritation (Fig. 32-4). Men with decreased energy and fine motor skills find it easier to use electric shavers, and some agencies provide electric shavers for clients. Clients at risk for excessive bleeding (ie, those with bleeding disorders or taking anticoagulants or large doses of aspirin) should use an electric razor rather than a safety razor to avoid cuts. Some men like to use an aftershave lotion. Men with beards or mustaches may need help trimming them and keeping them clean and free from food particles. Facial hair can be washed during a bath or shower. Mustaches or beards are shaved off only at the client's request.

Shaving underarm and leg hair is an important part of grooming for many women. This is done using basically the same shaving technique as for men.

Oral Care

Brushing the teeth and cleansing and rinsing the mouth are comfort measures. Clients find that having their teeth brushed and mouth cleaned induces feelings of well-being. Rinsing is soothing to the client with a dry mouth. An unclean mouth can harbor bacteria that can multiply and cause other problems. Procedure 32-6 gives guidelines for providing oral care. This procedure also can be used as a teaching tool.

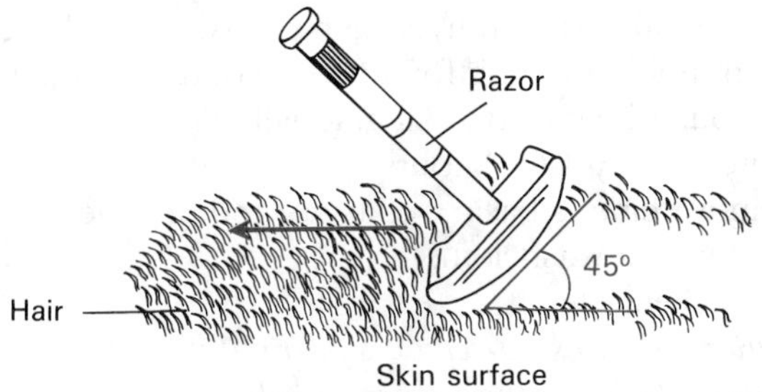

Figure 32-4 • *Shave in the direction of hair growth.*

The nurse or caregiver may need to assist or perform brushing and flossing for clients who are unable to do so. Assisting clients with mouth care gives the nurse an opportunity to teach proper techniques and to stress their importance. By encouraging regular brushing and flossing, the nurse can contribute to the prevention of caries and periodontal disease and help prevent the loss of teeth. Providing oral care also permits the nurse to assess the oral cavity.

Brushing and Flossing. Clients who can brush and floss without help should be encouraged to do so. If the client cannot get out of bed to use the sink, provide the necessary equipment, including a basin for spitting.

A soft-bristled toothbrush with a rounded, even brushing surface and a nonabrasive toothpaste is used for clients with natural teeth. The toothbrush is held at a 45-degree angle to the teeth for the outside of all teeth and the inside of the back teeth. Brushing should begin with the tips angled slightly into the groove around the teeth. In this position, the teeth should be brushed with small rotating motions over two or three teeth at a time. The bristles on the front of the brush are used to clean the inside of the front teeth in a rotating movement. The chewing surfaces can be cleaned

(text continues on page 804)

Procedure 32-6
Providing Oral Care

Purpose

1. Cleanse tooth surfaces to prevent odor and caries
2. Maintain hydrated, intact oral mucosa
3. Promote self-esteem and comfort

Assessment

- Inspect lips, buccal membrane, gums, palate, and tongue for lesions or inflammation.
- Assess for presence of caries or halitosis (bad breath).
- Identify clients at risk for oral hygiene complications:
- Dehydration, NPO status, nasogastric tubes dry the oral mucosa.
- Oral airways accumulate secretions and irritate the mucosa.
- Chemotherapy often results in stomatitis and ulcerations.
- Anticoagulant therapy or clotting disorders predispose the client to gum bleeding.
- Oral surgery or trauma may contraindicate tooth brushing; special rinses may be ordered.
- Determine client's ability to assist with procedure.
- Assess client's risk for aspiration.

Equipment

Toothbrush (sponge-ended swabs may be used for clients at risk for bleeding)
Toothpaste
Cup with water, straw
Emesis basin
Washcloth, towel
Mouthwash (optional)
Dental floss
Disposable gloves (if the nurse provides oral care)

Procedure

1. Wash your hands.
2. Close bedside curtains or room door, and explain procedure to client.
3. Help client to a sitting position. If client cannot sit, help to a side-lying position.
   Rationale: High or semi-Fowler's or side-lying position helps prevent choking and aspiration.
4. Place towel under client's chin.
   Rationale: Bed linens and gown are protected from soiling.
5. Moisten toothbrush with water. Apply small amount of toothpaste.
6. Hand toothbrush to client or don disposable gloves and brush client's teeth as follows:
   a. Hold toothbrush at a 45-degree angle to the gum line.

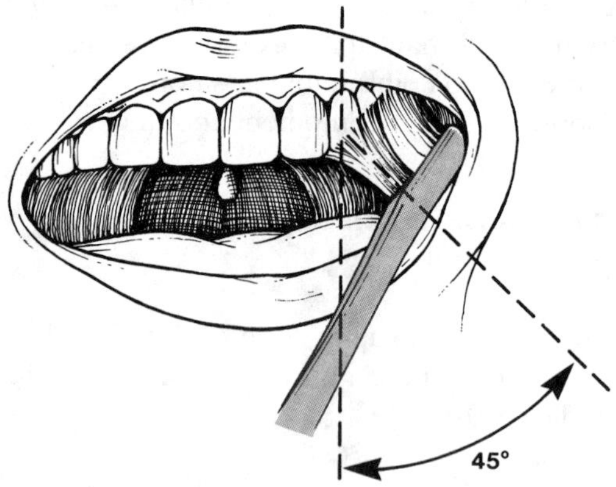

Step 6A • *Brush teeth at a 45-degree angle to the gum line.*

   b. Using short, vibrating motions, brush from the gum line to the crown of each tooth. Repeat until outside and inside of teeth and gums are cleaned.
   Rationale: Angle of toothbrush allows brush to reach all tooth surfaces and to penetrate and cleanse under the gum line, where plaque and tartar accumulate.
   c. Cleanse biting surfaces by brushing with a back-and-forth stroke.
   d. Brush the tongue lightly. Avoid stimulating the gag reflex.
   Rationale: Bacteria accumulate and grow on the tongue surface and must be removed.
   Note: If client is anticoagulated or has a clotting disorder, use a *very* soft toothbrush or a sponge-ended swab to prevent gum bleeding.
7. Have client rinse mouth thoroughly with water and spit into emesis basin.
   Note: If tongue is heavily coated, prepare a mixture of half-strength hydrogen peroxide and have client hold in mouth for a few seconds and then spit out. The coating will gradually dissolve. Repeat every 1 to 2 hours.
8. Remove emesis basin, set aside, and dry client's mouth with washcloth.
9. Floss client's teeth.
   Rationale: Flossing removes particulate matter trapped between the teeth and below the gum line.

a. Cut 10-inch piece of dental floss. Wind ends of floss around middle finger of each hand.

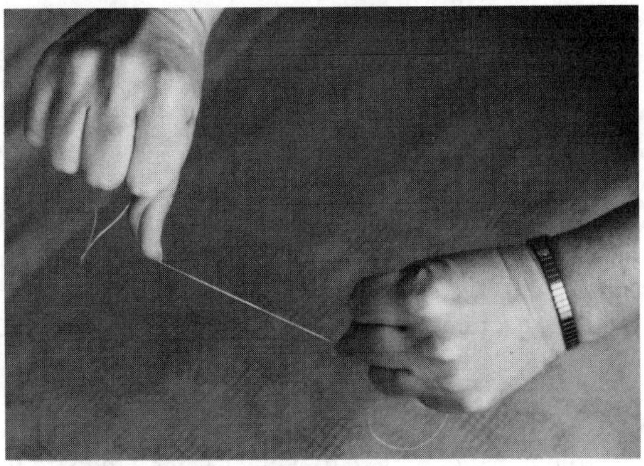

***Step 9A** • Grasp dental floss tightly.*

b. Using index fingers to stretch the floss, move the floss up and down around and between lower teeth. Start at the back lower teeth and work around to the other side.
c. Using thumb and index fingers to stretch the floss, repeat procedure on upper teeth.
d. Have client rinse mouth thoroughly and spit into emesis basin.

10. Remove basin; dry client's mouth.
11. Remove and dispose of supplies. Help client to comfortable position.
12. Wash your hands.

Procedure

Variation for the Unconscious Client

1. Gather equipment.
2. Place client in a side-lying position with head of bed lowered so saliva runs out of mouth by gravity. *Rationale: Side-lying position prevents aspiration.*
3. Place towel or waterproof pad under client's chin.
4. Place emesis basin against client's mouth, or have suction catheter positioned to remove secretions from mouth.
5. Use padded tongue blade to open teeth gently. Leave in place between the back molars. *Never* put your fingers in an unconscious client's mouth. *Rationale: Unconscious clients often respond to oral stimulation by biting down.*
6. Brush teeth and gums as directed previously, using toothbrush or soft sponge-ended swab.
7. Swab or suction to remove pooled secretions. A small bulb syringe or syringe without needle may be used to rinse oral cavity.
8. Apply thin layer of petroleum jelly to lips to prevent drying or cracking.
   Note: Lemon glycerin swabs can be drying to the oral mucosa if used for extended periods.

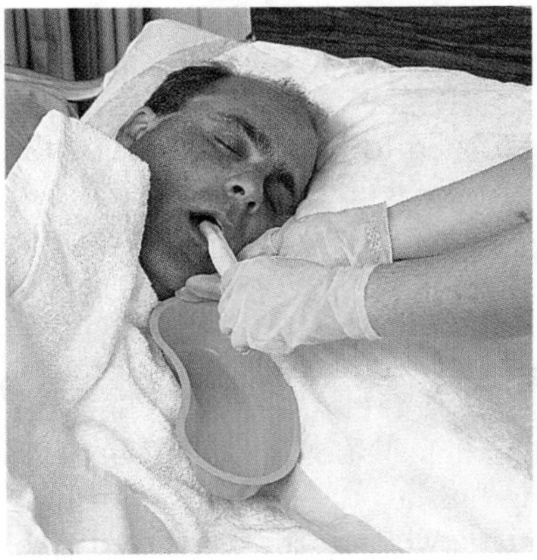

***Step 5** • Using a padded tongue blade, gently open the client's mouth.*

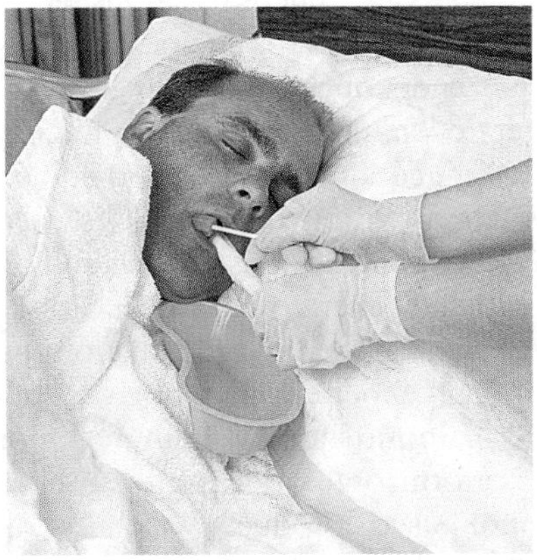

***Step 6** • Using a soft sponge-ended swab, cleanse teeth and mouth.*

Lifespan Considerations

Infant

- A dry gauze or washcloth can be used to remove accumulated secretions from an infant's gums.
- A small, soft-bristled brush is used after first teeth have erupted.

Child

- Children younger than 3 or 4 years may not understand what "rinse" or "spit" means. Do not offer them water to rinse with if they are NPO because they will swallow the rinse.
- Children or teens wearing braces need special attention to remove food particles from the wires.

Older Adult

- Many older adults wear full or partial dentures. Be sure dentures are removed regularly and cleansed. Special denture cleansers are available. The gums or any remaining teeth should be brushed well.

with a brisk back-and-forth motion, taking care not to traumatize the gingival tissue. Brushing of the tongue is important to remove microorganisms and debris. The tongue is brushed toward the throat (with the grain), lightly toward the teeth, and on the sides.

For the client who has difficulty grasping the small handle of an ordinary toothbrush, an electric toothbrush can be used because it has a larger handle that is easier to grasp and requires less manipulation. The handle of a regular toothbrush can be built up with tape, a bicycle handlebar grip, or a split rubber ball.

Flossing finishes the task of removing plaque and debris from between teeth. Unwaxed dental floss is used, avoiding traumatization the gums. The floss should be long enough so that a new section of the floss can be used when it becomes frayed.

Other oral hygiene measures include cleansing and moisturizing the oral mucosa by rinsing with water, saline, dilute mouthwash, or an anesthetic mouthwash. Hydrogen peroxide, once commonly used for oral care, is no longer recommended because nursing research demonstrates mucosal alterations and subjective client complaints when hydrogen peroxide is used (Tombes & Gallucci, 1993). Clients at risk for altered oral mucous membranes include clients who are NPO or dehydrated; undergoing chemotherapy or radiation therapy for cancer treatment; experiencing trauma or surgery to the oral cavity; malnourished or immunosuppressed; or unable to perform oral care. High-risk clients should avoid alcohol-based products, such as commercial mouth washes or lemon glycerine swabs, because these products are drying to tissues. Clients with drainage or lesions in the oral cavity and those who cannot take fluids by mouth may need rinsing and cleansing as often as every 2 hours. Such clients may have dry lips; a water-based lubricant or petroleum jelly can be applied.

Oral Care in the Unconscious Client. Feeding tubes, nasogastric tubes, and constant breathing through the mouth can dry mucous membranes. Because of the risk of aspiration of fluids into the lungs, the unconscious client should be turned on the side during mouth care so that fluids can drain easily. External surfaces of the teeth are brushed in the usual way. To protect fingers, a padded tongue blade is placed between the upper and lower teeth toward the back on one side. Then, using a toothbrush, sponge-tipped applicator, or gauze on a tongue blade, the interior of the teeth and the chewing surfaces are cleaned. To prevent aspiration, small amounts of cleaning solution are used. An oral suction device can be used to remove the fluid safely. See "Variation for the Unconscious Client" in Procedure 32-6.

Denture Care. Determine whether the client wears dentures. If so, encouraging the client to wear them improves eating, talking, and appearance and may boost the client's self-image.

Dentures collect the same debris, plaque, and tartar as natural teeth. If the client cannot care for the dentures, the nurse or caregiver needs to do so, using a brushing technique similar to that for natural teeth. Whenever possible, the client should remove his or her own dentures. If the client is unable, grasp dentures with a gauze pad to prevent slippage. Bottom dentures usually remove easily; upper dentures may need to be gently rocked forward or from side to side to break the vacuum seal created with the upper palate. A soft toothbrush is recommended because hard-bristled brushes can produce grooves in dentures. Soap and water is effective, although a mild commercial cleaning agent can be used. Dentures must be protected from breakage. Keep them in a denture cup while carrying them to the sink, and store them in a covered container if not worn continuously (Fig. 32-5).

The client should rinse the mouth before reinserting the dentures. Gums and tongue should be cleaned with a soft brush when the dentures are out. Massaging the gums with a brush or thumb and forefinger helps to stimulate circulation and toughen the oral mucosa. Dentures should be removed at night so that tissues are exposed to air (Renn, 1989).

Clients, especially those who are older and at greater risk, should be taught the signs and symptoms of oral cancer, emphasizing self-examination. Teach the finger massage technique for stimulation of alveolar mucosa and gingiva to promote healthy tissues. Review and teach denture care.

Eye Care

Some clients need help with eye care, particularly those who have had eye surgery, injury, or infection or unconscious clients who have lost the blink reflex. The nurse assesses eye problems as listed in the accompanying display to individualize care. Observations include noting whether the eyelids are edematous, crusted with secretions, or inflamed with sties and whether the lacrimal ducts are inflamed or tearing excessively. The sclera are examined for discoloration and the conjunctiva for inflammation and degree of redness. Pupil constriction or dilation and response to light and coordination of eye movements also are assessed.

Clients with eye inflammation, draining, or crusting need help cleaning these secretions from the eyes. Eyes should be cleaned with a washcloth or cotton ball soaked with saline or sterile water. Clean from the inside of the eye toward the outside. If infection is not suspected, use a different part of the washcloth for each eye; if infection is present, use a different cloth for each eye. This reduces the potential for spreading infection from one eye to the other.

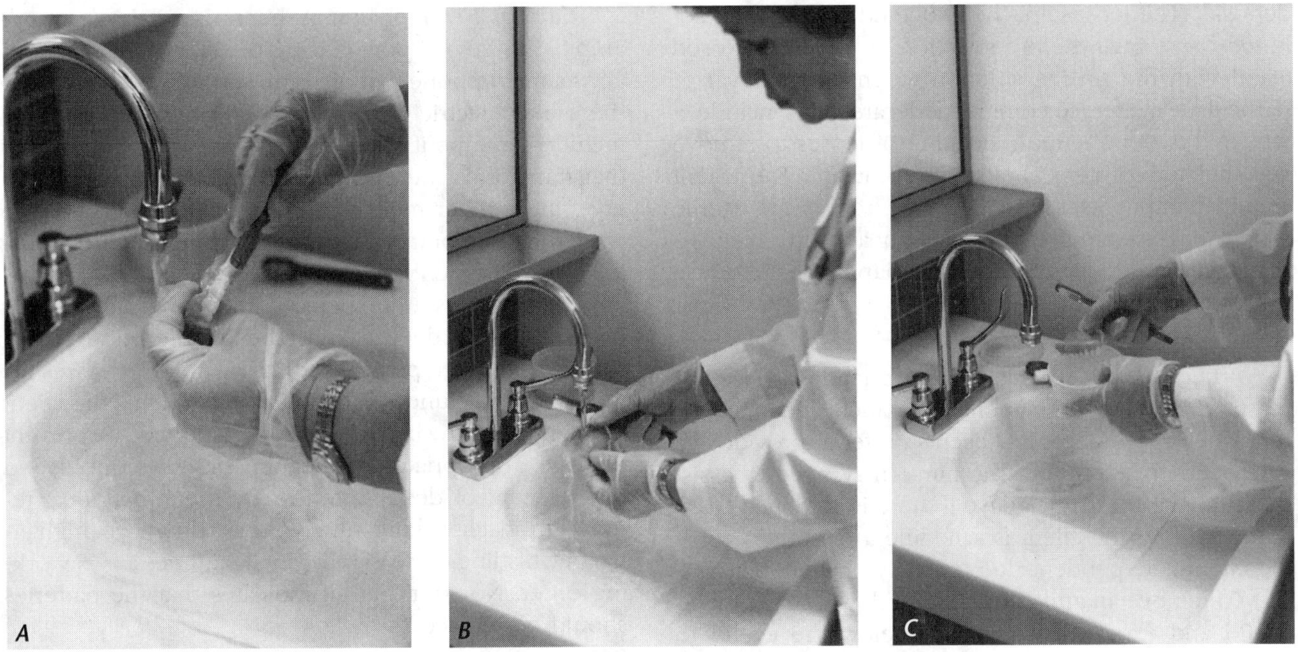

Figure 32-5 *• Denture care. (**A**) The dentures are brushed as though the nurse were brushing natural teeth. (**B**) Dentures are rinsed. (**C**) To prevent damage, dentures should be stored in a plastic container when not in use or when carried to and from the sink.*

Eyeglasses and Contact Lenses. Determine if a visual aid is used; locate the aid, and encourage its use. Safeguarding these aids contributes to the client's independence and safety.

Glasses should be cleaned daily, but clients do not often ask for this kind of help. Glass lenses can be washed under warm water, but plastic ones should be washed with a special cleaning solution. Both can be dried with facial tissue or a lens cloth. Store glasses in a secure place where the client can reach them. When clients are too ill to manage these activities or have other physical limitations to self-care, the nurse must take responsibility for glasses. Their location is noted in the nurses' notes or the Kardex. This allows the nurse on the next shift or the next unit to which the client is transferred to find them.

Contact lenses are a common alternative to glasses. These concave plastic disks cover the pupil and float on the tear layer. Contact lenses may be hard, soft, or gas-permeable hard or soft. Hard lenses are made of rigid plastic that does not absorb air or liquid. Because they restrict oxygen supply to the cornea, their use is limited to 14 hours per day. Some kinds of soft lenses are worn during the day and removed at night, but others can be worn for as long as 14 to 30 days. Disposable contact lenses are a recent innovation that require less care.

Red conjunctiva, excess tearing, and burning pain are symptoms of lens overwear. Secretions and foreign matter (dust, pollen) accumulate under the lenses as they are worn. These substances are irritating to the eye and result in distorted vision and increased risk of infection. Because all contact lenses decrease the flow of oxygen to the cornea to some extent, corneal damage can occur if they are left in place for too long.

Contact lenses must be cleaned and disinfected after removal, using the appropriate method for the type of lens. If the client cannot do so, the nurse must remove and care for the lenses. To care for soft lenses, a cleaning solution is used to loosen and remove film and debris. Rinsing is required after cleaning, using a rinsing and disinfecting solution to remove loosened

Nursing Assessment
Eye Care

- Does the client use eyeglasses or contact lenses or have an artificial eye?
- How does the client rate visual acuity?
- Is the client experiencing eye problems now?
- Are eyelids edematous, crusted with secretions, inflamed with sties?
- What is the appearance of the lacrimal ducts? Are they inflamed, tearing excessively, not tearing at all, or crusted with secretions?
- Are sclera discolored?
- Are conjunctiva inflamed, pale?
- Are pupils dilated, constricted, responsive to light?
- Are eye movements coordinated?

deposits. The lenses are then covered with rinsing solution for storage. Before insertion, each lens is rinsed again with the rinsing solution to ensure removal of particulate matter. Recommended care may include a weekly heat or chemical cleaning of lenses to remove accumulated protein, lipids, and mucin. The client should bring contact lense supplies from home. Sterile saline that is commonly used in healthcare agencies may contain additives and may be inappropriate for use in contact lens care.

Artificial Eyes. Artificial eyes are made of glass or plastic. Some are permanent, but others require daily removal for cleaning. Most clients prefer to provide eye care for themselves, but the nurse may need to assist by removing the artificial eye if there is evidence of inflammation, if the client is scheduled for surgery, or if the client is dependent due to injury or immobility.

To remove an artificial eye, pull down on the lower eyelid and exert slight pressure below the eyelid to overcome the suction holding the eye in place. To ease removal, a small bulb syringe or medicine dropper bulb may be used to create a suction great enough to counteract the suction holding the eye in the socket. The eye can be cleaned with saline and stored in saline or water in a covered, labeled container. The edges of the eye socket are cleaned with saline or tap water and should be inspected for redness, swelling, or drainage. Because of the proximity of the eye to the sinuses and underlying brain tissue, infection in this area is of great concern. To reinsert the eye, pull down on the lower lid and slip the eye into the socket, lifting the upper lid to permit the eye to slide in.

Eye Care in the Unconscious Client. Comatose clients are at risk for corneal ulceration, which can cause blindness. When the blink reflex is lost, eyes may remain open and become dry. To prevent these complications, eyes are kept moist and protected from the air. Liquid tear solution (methylcellulose) or saline can be instilled to prevent drying, or the eyes can be closed and covered with a protective shield.

Ear Care

Healthy ears require little care. Check the external ear for inflamed tissue, drainage, and discomfort. Clean the auricles with a washcloth-covered finger. Excessive cerumen can be removed with the twisted end of a clean washcloth while pulling the auricle down or by irrigation if this method fails. Emphasize the danger of using bobby pins, cotton-tipped applicators, toothpicks, or other sharp objects to remove cerumen. Bobby pins or toothpicks can rupture the tympanic membrane or traumatize the ear canal; cotton-tipped applicators can push the wax further in and block the ear canal.

Care of Hearing Aids. A hearing aid is a sound-amplifying device powered by batteries. The aid contains a microphone that picks up sound waves, changes them into electric signals, and transmits them. It also includes an amplifier for magnifying sound, a receiver that transforms the electric signals back to sound energy, and an ear mold that channels the sound to the tympanic membrane. There are several kinds of hearing aids, as described in the display.

Hearing aids are expensive and significant to their owners. These devices must be handled and stored safely. Note the type of device, how the client cares for it, how well it functions, and what problems the client has with it. Care includes careful handling to prevent damage, appropriate use, cleaning of the ear mold, and replacement of dead batteries. To check batteries, remove from client and turn volume slowly to high. A harsh whistling noise is apparent if batteries are in working order. No sound at all indicates that the batteries should be replaced.

Types of Hearing Aids

- *Behind-the-ear aid,* the most common type, fits over the ear. An ear mold fits into the ear, and the case, containing the microphone, amplifier, receiver, volume control, batteries, and T/M switch, fits behind the ear.
- *In-the-ear aid,* the most compact, has all of the elements located in the ear mold.
- *Eyeglass aid* involves a hearing aid in one or both temples of a pair of eyeglasses. It functions similarly to the behind-the-ear aid, but the components are located in the temples of the glasses.
- *Body-type hearing aid* is used for the most severe hearing losses. The case looks like a pocket-sized transistor radio and can be clipped into a pocket, undergarment, or harness. The case contains the microphone and amplifier and is connected to a receiver, which snaps into an ear mold.

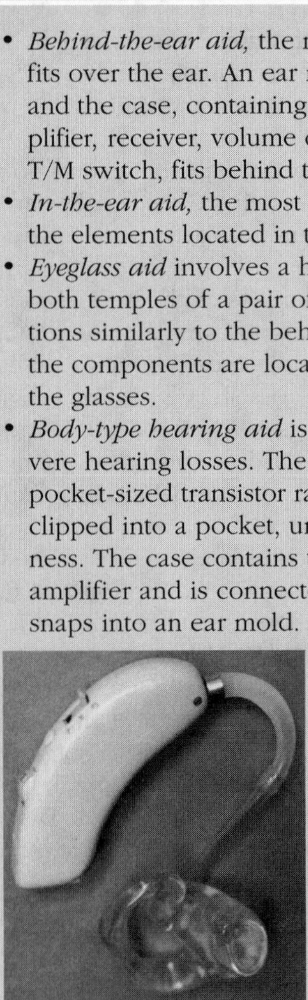

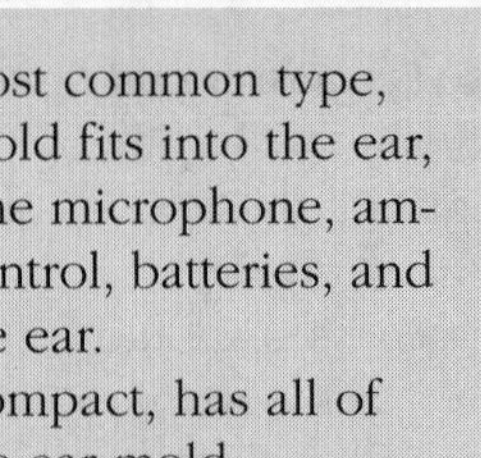

In-the-ear

Behind-the-ear

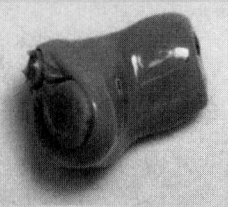

When placing the hearing aid in the ear, turn off the device to protect the ear from sudden loud sound. When the hearing aid is snugly in the ear canal, the volume can be adjusted as needed to promote hearing.

Although the hearing aid amplifies the sound of voices, it also amplifies background sounds. Clients may continue to have difficulty hearing, especially in a noisy setting. To foster optimal hearing, face the client, speak slowly and clearly, and rephrase what is said if the client does not understand. Some hearing-impaired people can lip-read; careful enunciation improves their ability to understand.

Feeding

Clients often have poor appetites because of pain, depression, or medication side effects. The client may find hospital food unfamiliar or unpalatable. The setting may be uncomfortable, noisy, too warm, or too cool, or there may be unpleasant odors or sights. Other frequent causes of decreased food intake are inability to eat without help due to weakness, fatigue, or paralysis. Assess the client's feeding ability and the level of support needed for eating; in this way, assistance can be planned and a teaching program instituted if appropriate.

Often clients are spoon fed in institutional settings even though they are capable of self-feeding if given adequate time (Osborn & Marshall, 1993). Verbal prompts and physical guiding assist the cognitively impaired client to maintain independence and are preferred over spoon feeding.

Because being fed represents a loss of control, the client should be given some role if possible. This is true for people of all ages. Giving the client a choice—for instance, the order in which food is eaten—may relieve some of the helpless feelings. Because the process of helping with eating is time-consuming, the client may feel like a burden. The person feeding the client must avoid reinforcing this belief and should always give the client ample time to chew and swallow. Interventions to meet feeding needs are varied. Examples are listed in the accompanying guidelines. Ensure good body mechanics by positioning the client high enough in bed to match the bed gatch with the client's hips. Raise the head of the bed if the client cannot sit on the side of the bed. A high sitting position is necessary to reduce the danger of choking and aspirating food. See Procedure 37-1 for details on helping a client to eat.

Adequate swallowing is essential for safe eating. Difficulty swallowing (dysphagia) may occur as a result of disease or trauma to cranial nerves. Such damage commonly occurs following a cerebrovascular accident (stroke) or head injury. Diseases such as myasthenia gravis and muscular dystrophy, which cause muscle weakness, also may result in dysphagia. After a stroke or surgical removal of part of the larynx, the client may need to relearn how to initiate swallowing. Consulting a speech therapist or an occupational therapist is important in planning a safe rehabilitation program.

To avoid food aspiration, carefully assess the client's ability to swallow before feeding. Elicit the gag reflex by stroking the inside of the throat with a tongue depressor. This will cause the pharynx to rise and constrict while the tongue retracts (Meehan, 1992). When there is any doubt as to the client's ability to swallow, do not try to feed him or her until obtaining an expert opinion. If a client needs supervision during feeding, this should be indicated on the plan of care. If supervision is delegated to auxiliary personal or family members, the nurse must assess that they understand proper feeding technique and emergency care in case of choking.

Keep verbal cues short and simple while feeding. Multiple verbal cues or conversation during feeding may distract and confuse the client who is cognitively im-

Nursing Care Guidelines
Meeting the Client's Feeding Needs

- Check chart, Kardex, or diet list to determine whether the client has limitations on eating (eg, fasting for laboratory tests or procedures).
- Check each tray for the client's name and the type of diet. Check any questions about the client's chart. Verify the client's name by checking the wristband.
- If pain is a factor limiting food intake or self-feeding ability, time analgesia to permit pain relief at mealtime.
- If fatigue is a problem, schedule a rest period before eating to enhance appetite and increase independence.
- Help the client urinate or defecate prior to meals if needed to enhance mealtime comfort.
- Enhance the setting. Turn on the lights if needed. Provide good ventilation. Remove room odors and disturbing sights, such as soiled dressings.
- Prepare the client for mealtime by finding dentures and eyeglasses, brushing teeth, rinsing mouth, and washing hands.
- Help the client to a comfortable position for eating, usually sitting in high Fowler's position in bed or a chair.
- Clear the overbed table of extraneous items.
- Determine how much help the client needs (ie, uncovering containers, removing food from plastic bags, buttering bread, or cutting meat).
- Plan ahead so that clients who need assistance can be helped while their food is still hot. Food that has cooled can be microwaved.

paired. Use directions like "chew" and "swallow" rather than complete sentences.

Food consistency is important for clients who have difficulty swallowing. Liquids may have to be thickened; dry food, such as crackers and toast, and sticky food, such as peanut butter, should be avoided. Remaining in an upright position following a meal will prevent gastric reflux and possible aspiration.

Blind clients can be oriented to the location of food on a plate by referring to the numbers on a clock. They may be used to developing a mental map of the tray by doing a survey with their fingertips; food can be located by gentle probing with a fork. Knowing what the foods are helps a blind person plan how best to eat them. For example, knowing that peas and mashed potatoes are on the plate enables a blind person to eat the peas more easily by pushing them against the mashed potatoes.

Many eating aids are available. Plates with guards or lips help the client get food onto a utensil. Utensil handles can be padded to make them easier to grasp. Cups with spouts help with drinking. Straws may help clients drink without dribbling.

When feeding infants, the atmosphere should be relaxed and free of interruptions. Parents or other relatives should feed the child if possible. When giving solid food, position the infant to face the feeder at eye level. Finger foods allow the infant to participate in feeding before fine motor skills are developed to enable self-feeding with utensils.

When the meal is finished, assess the food and fluid intake, and record it if indicated. If a calorie count is ordered, record the precise amount of food eaten. Record any pertinent reaction to the meal. Make necessary adjustments in the diet and the plan of care.

Toileting

Clients often require assistance with toileting (ie, walking to the bathroom or being placed on a bedpan). Needing help with these intimate functions may provoke extreme discomfort for some clients; a kind approach helps allay embarrassment. Helping clients to be as independent as possible with toileting is an essential nursing intervention. Most people prize control in this area and benefit greatly from independence in toileting. Even if the only independent self-care a client can manage is to decide when and how elimination will take place, it can help the client feel more in control.

The following measures can help clients manage self-care of elimination. The nurse can teach these methods and help the client determine which ones work best.

Exercise affects micturition by strengthening abdominal and perineal muscles, which enhances voiding and helps to prevent urinary incontinence. For example, Kegel exercises strengthen the muscles of the perineum. These exercises involve contracting the muscles as if trying to stop micturition or by actually practicing stopping the stream of urine while voiding.

Privacy and an opportunity to relax enhances most people's ability to urinate. Worrying about being able to void, especially after surgery or giving birth, may produce tension, so do not pressure clients to void on schedule. The following may help the client urinate:

- Turn on the bathroom water.
- Have the client visualize his or her bathroom at home.
- Warm the bedpan.
- Have the client assume a comfortable position (standing for men).
- Provide analgesia for pain.
- Pour warm water over the perineum.
- Always provide call light within easy reach.

Chapters 41 and 42 give more detail on elimination.

Bedpans. There are two types of bedpans: a *regular bedpan* has a high rim, and a *fracture pan* has a lower rim for clients who cannot raise their buttocks or in whom such movement is contraindicated (Fig. 32-6).

Many clients need help to get on a bedpan. Sitting is the most effective position for passing urine or stool. Some clients can use a bedpan alone if it is left on the bed or covered on a nearby chair; such independence should be encouraged. A trapeze on the bed frame also facilitates moving on and off a bedpan. Procedure 32-7 outlines bedpan use.

Urinal. A man who is on strict bed rest or who is confined to bed due to weakness or disability may use a **urinal,** a metal or plastic receptacle into which the penis can be placed to facilitate urinating without spilling (see Fig. 41-5). The urinal needs to be emptied frequently into a toilet to prevent spilling and odors. Some men cannot void while sitting or lying in bed; sometimes they can be helped to a standing position long enough to void. Incontinent men may be more comfortable if the urinal is left in place. If this is done,

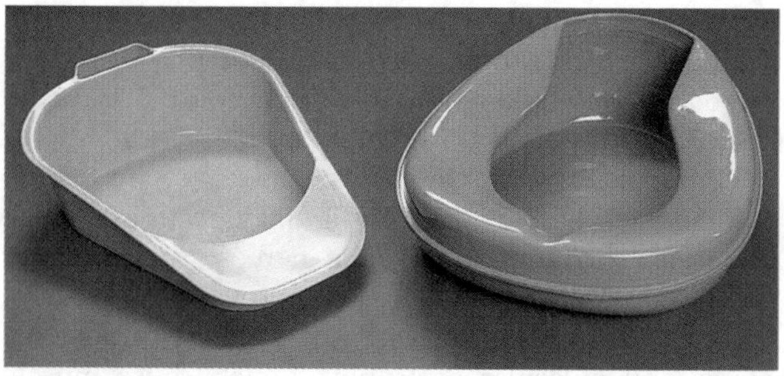

Figure 32-6 **•** *Two types of bedpans.* ***(Left)*** *The fracture bedpan.* ***(Right)*** *Regular bedpan.*

Procedure 32-7
Using a Bedpan

Purpose

1. Provide a means for elimination for clients who are confined to bed or unable to get to the bathroom or bedside commode independently or safely

Assessment

- Assess the client's normal elimination habits and when he or she last voided or defecated.
- Assess level of mobility, positioning restrictions, and degree of assistance required.
- Review orders to determine if urine or fecal specimens are needed.
- Identify medications the client is receiving that would alter the color, consistency, or amount of urine or feces obtained.

Equipment

Clean bedpan or fracture pan (see Fig. 32-6 for two types of bedpans)
Toilet tissue
Washcloth, towel, soap
Air freshener (optional)
Specimen container (if needed)
Cover for bedpan (if toilet for discarding is not in client's room)
Disposable gloves

Procedure

Placing the bedpan

1. Wash your hands. Don clean gloves.
2. Close curtain around bed or shut door.
   Rationale: This provides privacy and reduces embarrassment.
3. Run warm water over rim of pan; dry with towel.
   Rationale: Warming the pan facilitates client relaxation and encourages elimination.
4. Position and lock side rail up on opposite side of bed from which you will work.
   Rationale: Prevents client rolling out of bed when turning on and off bedpan.
5. Raise bed to height appropriate for nurse.
   Rationale: Prevents muscle strain and promotes proper body mechanics.
6. For client who can raise buttocks and assist with procedure:
   a. Fold top linen down on the nurse's side to expose the patient's hips.
   Rationale: The client is minimally exposed to decrease embarrassment and preserve dignity.
   b. Have client flex knees and lift buttocks. Assist client by placing your hand under sacrum, elbow on mattress, and lifting as a lever.
   Rationale: Client's body weight is supported by lower legs and feet. Proper body mechanics by nurse prevent muscle strain.

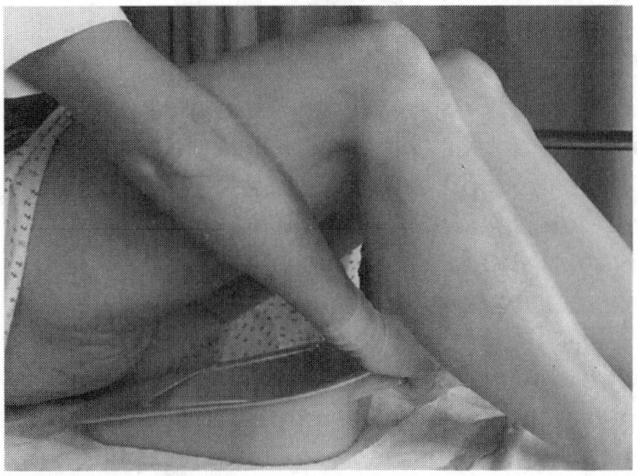

Step 6B • *Lift buttocks to place bedpan.*

   c. Slide rounded smooth rim of regular bedpan under client. If using a fracture pan, slide narrow flat end under buttocks.
   Rationale: Proper placement prevents spillage and shearing trauma of skin in sacral area.
7. For client unable to assist by raising buttocks:
   a. Lower head of bed to flat position.
   b. Fold top bed linens down to expose client minimally.
   c. Help client to roll to side-lying position.
   d. `Place bedpan against buttocks and tucked down against mattress. Hold firmly in place and roll client onto back as bedpan positions under buttocks.

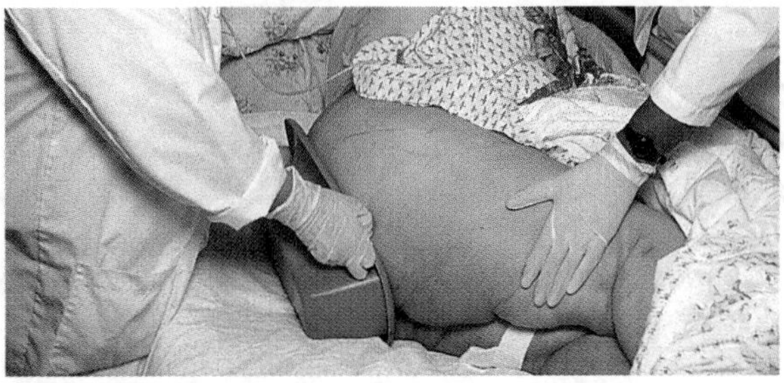

Step 7D • *Placing bedpan from side-lying position.*

(continued)

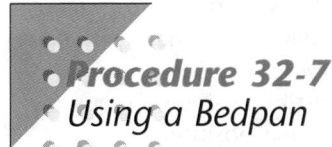

Rationale: Correct placement prevents spillage.

8. Cover client with linen. Place call bell and toilet paper within reach.
   Rationale: Privacy, warmth, independence, and self-dignity are important for the client.
9. Raise head of bed 45 to 80 degrees unless contraindicated.
   Rationale: Sitting position reduces discomfort and strain on lower back and facilitates elimination.
10. Lower bed to lowest position. Place side rails up if indicated.
    Rationale: Client must be kept safe.
11. Wash your hands. Allow client to be alone.

Removing the bedpan

12. Answer call bell promptly.
13. Place soap, wet washcloth, and towel at bedside.
14. Raise bed to appropriate working height for nurse.
    Rationale: Nurse must prevent muscle strain and promote proper body mechanics.
15. Fold back top linens to expose client minimally.
16. Put on disposable clean gloves.
    Rationale: Gloves help prevent contamination of hands with body substances.
17. Assess if client can wipe perineal area. If not, wipe area with several layers of toilet tissue. If specimen is to be measured or collected, dispose of soiled toilet tissue in separate receptacle, not bedpan.
    Note: For female clients, wipe from urethra toward anus to prevent tracking of rectal microorganisms into the urinary meatus. Use as an informal teaching session to reinforce good hygiene practices.
18. For client who can raise buttocks and assist with procedure:
    a. Lower head of bed.
    b. Have client flex knees and lift buttocks. Assist client by placing one hand under sacrum and supporting bedpan with other hand to prevent spillage. Remove bedpan and place on bedside chair.
    c. Offer soap, warm water, washcloth, and towel for client to wash hands or perineal area.
    Rationale: Washing prevents transfer of microorganisms, promotes good hygiene practices, and prevents skin breakdown.
19. For client unable to assist by raising buttocks:
    a. Lower head of bed to flat position.
    b. Fold top linen down to expose client minimally.
    c. Help client to roll off bedpan and onto side. Use one hand to stabilize bedpan during turning to prevent spillage.
    d. Wipe anal area with tissue. Wash perineum with soap and warm water. Pat dry.
    Rationale: This prevents skin breakdown and excoriation.
20. Assist client to comfortable position.
21. Cover bedpan, and remove from bedside. Obtain specimen if required. Empty and clean bedpan and return it to bedside.
    Rationale: Clean pan minimizes spread of offensive odor.
22. Remove and discard gloves. Wash your hands.
    Rationale: Washing reduces spread of microorganisms.
23. Spray air freshener if necessary to control odor, unless contraindicated (client with respiratory conditions, allergies).
    Rationale: Odor is embarrassing to client and visitors. Self-dignity is preserved by minimizing embarrassment.

Lifespan Considerations

Child

- A toilet-trained child is reluctant to use a bedpan, as he or she has been taught not to toilet in bed. Use a potty chair at the bedside if possible.

Older Adult

- It is often difficult for the older adult to use a regular bedpan because of limitation of body movement and arthritis. A fracture pan is less difficult and less painful to use.

the urinal should be plastic, and the scrotum should be padded for protection.

Condom Catheter. A **condom catheter** is a heavy rubber sheath that fits over the penis and is connected to a collection tube and bag. A small bag that can be strapped to the leg may promote self-care for the ambulatory man. Application is outlined and illustrated in Procedure 41-3.

Bedside Commode. As a rule, most clients can progress to the most independent mode of managing elimination that is safe. Many clients on bed rest can tolerate a brief time out of bed to use a bedside **commode,** a portable chair with a toilet seat and a receptacle beneath that can be emptied. In this way, a client who cannot walk to the bathroom can manage toileting independently. A male client could stand to urinate and use the commode for a bowel movement. The nurse

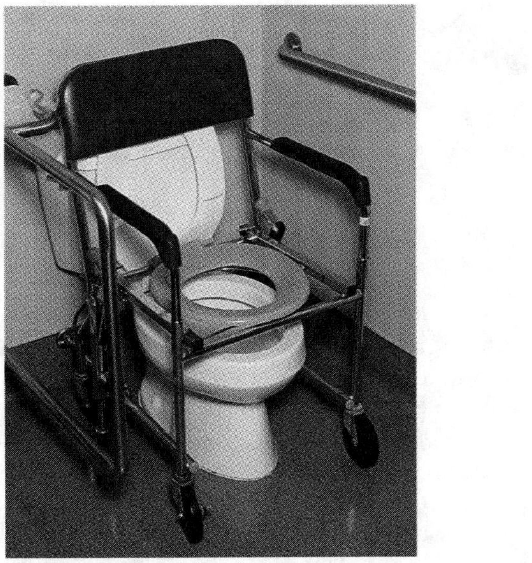

Figure 32-7* • *The commode chair can slide over the toilet when the waste receptacle is removed, allowing clients with mobility problems greater access to the privacy of the bathroom.

may need to provide support for these activities by providing water, a washcloth, and a towel for self-cleaning or by performing the cleaning. A commode chair can often be wheeled into the bathroom and placed over the toilet after the waste receptacle has been removed (Fig. 32-7). This permits the client to use the privacy of the bathroom even if ambulating to the bathroom is not possible.

Dressing

Dressing and undressing consume a great deal of time and energy, which is why chronically and acutely ill people often become fatigued and discouraged. The following interventions are designed to help clients relearn dressing skills:

- Schedule dressing or undressing in conjunction with bathing.
- Encourage the client to use his or her eyeglasses or hearing aid.
- Provide analgesia if needed.
- Organize carefully, and allow ample time.
- Lay clothes out in the order in which they will be needed, and place them within easy reach.
- Choose clothes that are loose and easy to get on and off, with wide sleeves and pant legs and front fasteners. Use Velcro closures when possible. Shoes should have elastic laces or Velcro closures.
- Encourage the client to help select clothes. Suggest street clothes rather than night clothes when appropriate.
- Assess the client's ability to maintain balance.
- Ensure privacy (within the limits of safety).
- If the client has visual deficits, tell him or her when you enter and leave the area.

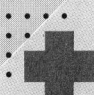

Safety Alert
Self-Care Deficit

- Hold infants and small children firmly, and attend to them when on a high changing table.
- When assisting a person to a bedside commode from bed, lock the bed and the commode firmly before moving to prevent falls.
- To avoid burns, check the water temperature carefully for clients with diminished ability to perceive extremes in temperature.
- Encourage people with balance problems to use handrails in the bathroom.
- Avoid cutting toenails of people with diabetes or other clients with poor circulation to the legs. Filing is usually safe.
- To prevent falls, find sturdy shoes and check the floor for water spills when helping a client ambulate.
- To prevent aspiration of food, sit clients upright in bed or in a chair before meals.
- Raise the side rails on both sides of the bed if you must leave even for a brief time.

- If the client has cognitive deficits, develop a routine to lessen confusion, keep instructions clear and simple, and avoid distractions.
- Teach the use of aids for dressing (eg, long-handled shoehorn, zipper pull, long-handled reacher, buttonhook). Help the client adapt available equipment to meet specific needs.

Care of Unit Environment

The equipment and supplies used by a client while in a healthcare facility are kept in what is called the client's unit.

Overbed tables, which provide a surface for eating and a work space for nurses, have wheels so they can be maneuvered to fit over the bed or over a chair. Some overbed tables have a mirror and storage space for toilet articles.

Small stands are placed at the side of the bed to provide storage space for personal belongings, a basin for bath water, a small curved basin (emesis basin), supplies for oral care, soap, bedpan, urinal, and toilet paper. A towel bar may be attached to the stand. Closet storage for belongings is usually provided as well. A chair, either lightly padded and straight or upholstered, is often provided for the client or visitors.

In many agencies, oxygen and suction outlets are installed on the wall above the bed, and often a sphygmomanometer is mounted on the wall with a blood pressure cuff. The lighting in the unit usually includes diffuse, less intense lighting for general use; a brighter light for client reading; and an intense light for use during procedures and when visualization is needed for diagnostic purposes.

A call light with which the client can summon the nurse is attached to the bed. Often, the call light is part of the sound receiver for the television set and the television channel selector. A television and telephone are commonly available free or for a small fee. Televisions are usually mounted on the wall to facilitate viewing from a Fowler's or flat position. All of this equipment should be explained to the client and family at admission.

Beds. Hospitals beds can be moved to a variety of positions, providing comfort for the client, therapy for some conditions, and proper body mechanics for the nurse. Adjustments in height can usually be made. The high setting permits nurses to perform their tasks without back strain; the low setting permits clients to get in and out of bed easily and safely. Bed position is changed to obtain a specific therapeutic effect. The nurse should be familiar with prescribed bed positions (see display) and how to achieve them. Because bed controls are usually accessible to clients, teaching them how to use the bed enhances independence. Other adjustments that can be made in the beds include the following:

- Elevating the head of the bed to permit eating and other activities
- Simultaneously elevating the head and foot of the bed to prevent sliding toward the foot
- Elevating the foot of the bed when the legs need to be placed above the level of the heart to control swelling
- Tilting the entire bed, with the head of the bed lower than the foot, to enhance circulatory return to the heart

Several kinds of beds are available for clients who cannot turn themselves and are at risk for skin breakdown; these are discussed in Chapter 38.

Mattresses are usually constructed of inner springs. They give good support and are covered with a water- and soil-resistant material to permit cleaning. Foam-rubber mattresses with an eggcrate configuration can be placed on top of the inner spring mattress for clients who must stay in bed for a long time or who find the mattress uncomfortable. Eggcrate mattresses are often not needed with the new types of mattresses that distribute pressure more evenly. Bedboards can be placed under the mattress for added firmness. People with back alignment difficulties may require additional support.

Side rails, a standard part of beds and stretchers, help to prevent accidents caused by clients falling out of bed or getting out of bed by themselves when they are not able to do so safely. They also provide a support for clients to hold while moving in bed and getting up.

Bed Positions

- Flat position: Mattress is completely flat.
- Fowler's position: The lower part of the bed is raised to the following positions:
  - Low Fowler's position: Head of bed is elevated to semisitting position of 15 to 45 degrees. This position also is called semi-Fowler's position.
  - High Fowler's position: Head and trunk are elevated to 80 to 90 degrees. This position also is called simply the Fowler's position.
- Trendelenburg position: The entire bed is tilted with the head downward. This position is not often used because it causes blood pressure to rise and causes hypotension on return to the supine position.
- Reverse Trendelenburg position: Entire bed is tilted with feet downward. Prevents gastric reflux.

Footboards are flat boards of wood or plastic placed at the bottom of the bed at a right angle to the bed. They remove the weight of bedclothes from feet and legs and support the feet to prevent foot drop. Bed cradles also can remove the pressure of bedclothes from the feet and legs. For clients with injured or swollen legs, feet, or toes, removing the pressure of bedclothes may relieve pain and improve circulation.

Poles used for hanging IV containers are located near the bedside in most units. A pole can be inserted into a hole in the bed frame, a free-standing pole can be used, or the containers can be hung from the ceiling.

Bedmaking. A clean, dry, smooth bed enhances the client's feeling of well-being. Linens are changed on the basis of client need and cost, rather than a fixed routine. If the linens are soiled, wet, or stained, they need to be changed. When deciding whether to change linens, however, consider the other needs of the client and the demands of other clients. For instance, if the client is tired and weak, it may be better to pad slightly damp or soiled areas and wait until the client has rested to change the linens. Sometimes straightening and tightening the sheets is adequate. Procedures 32-8 and 32-9 give guidelines regarding making unoccupied and occupied beds.

Asepsis is important in bedmaking. Drainage on used linens may contain microorganisms that can be transmitted through the air when the linens are shaken or through contact with the nurse's hands or clothing. Handle linens carefully without shaking them. Wear gloves during bedmaking if linen soiling is likely. Avoid

Procedure 32-8
Making an Unoccupied Bed

Purpose

1. Provide clean linen and remove sources of skin irritation
2. Promote comfort

Assessment

- Assess client's activity level and ability to get out of bed.
- Determine nursing interventions needed in assisting client out of bed:
  - Vital sign check for orthostatic hypotension
  - Analgesia
  - Position precautions (ie, elevation of body parts)
- Assess client's potential for excessive perspiration, drainage, or incontinence in determining special linen requirements.

Equipment

Bottom sheet
Top sheet
Draw sheet
Blanket
Bedspread (changed only if soiled)
Mattress pad (changed only if soiled)
Pillowcases
Waterproof pads or bath blanket (optional for incontinent or diaphoretic clients)
Linen bag
Bedside table or chair

Procedure

1. Wash your hands.
2. Assemble equipment on bedside table or chair. Do not place on another client's bed.
   Rationale: Prevention of contamination with microorganisms helps maintain a safe environment.
3. Help client to chair at bedside.
4. Raise bed to comfortable working position.
   Rationale: The nurse must promote good body mechanics and reduce muscle strain to back.
5. Loosen linen on one side of bed. Move to other side of bed and loosen all linen.
6. Remove bedspread and blanket, and fold each separately if they are to be reused. Place over back of chair.
   Rationale: Blanket and bedspread are changed only when soiled at most agencies.
7. Remove pillowcases by grasping seamed end with one hand and pulling pillow out with the other. Place pillows on chair. Discard pillowcases in linen bag.
8. Remove each piece of linen separately by rolling into a ball and discarding into linen bag. Be careful to prevent soiled linen from touching your uniform.
   Rationale: Disposing of linen separately minimizes the chance of nurse's uniform being contaminated by soiled linen. Rolling linen into compact unit prevents microorganisms from shaking off during transfer to linen bag.
9. Slide mattress to head of bed if it has slipped to the foot.
10. Wipe mattress with antiseptic solution if grossly soiled. Dry thoroughly.
11. Working from side of bed where linen is stored, spread mattress pad over mattress and smooth out wrinkles.
    Rationale: Wrinkles in linen irritate the skin, can cause pressure areas, and are uncomfortable.
12. Unfold bottom sheet lengthwise on bed with vertical center crease along center of bed. Unfold top layer toward opposite side of mattress. Pull remaining top sheet over head of mattress, leaving bottom edge of sheet even with mattress edge. Smooth bottom sheet with hand.
    Rationale: If a contour sheet is not used, the bottom sheet is tucked in only at the top of the bed so linen can be changed without undoing the top sheet.

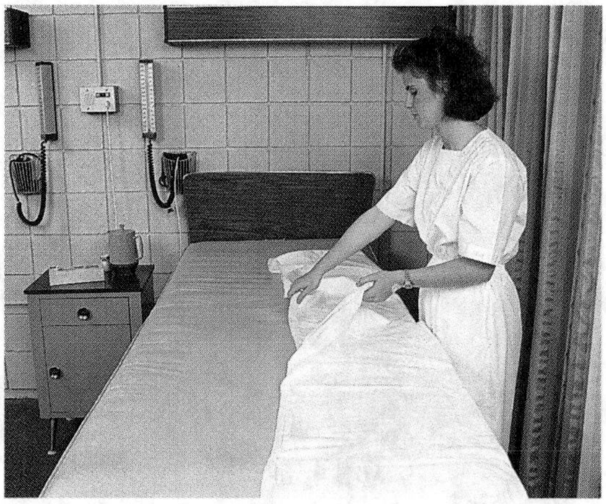

Step 12 • *Center bottom sheet on bed.*

13. Standing near head of bed, tuck the excess sheet under the mattress on your side at the end of the bed.

(continued)

14. Miter the corner on your side:
    a. Grasp side edge of sheet about 18 in down from mattress top.

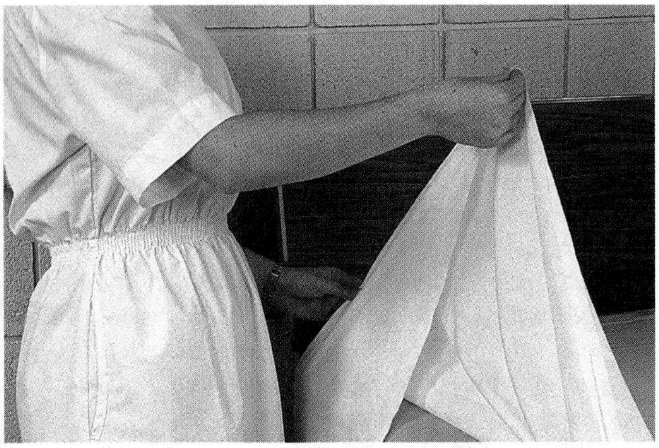

Step 14A • *Pick up selvage edge of sheet.*

    b. Lay sheet on top of mattress to form a triangular, flat fold.

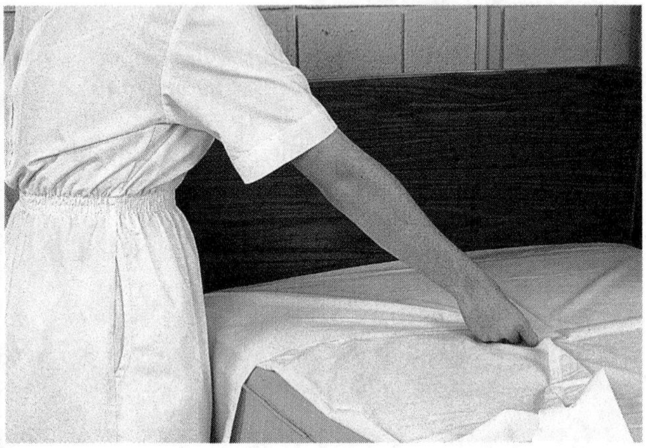

Step 14B • *Lay triangle back on bed.*

    c. Tuck sheet hanging loose below mattress under the mattress without pulling on the triangular fold.

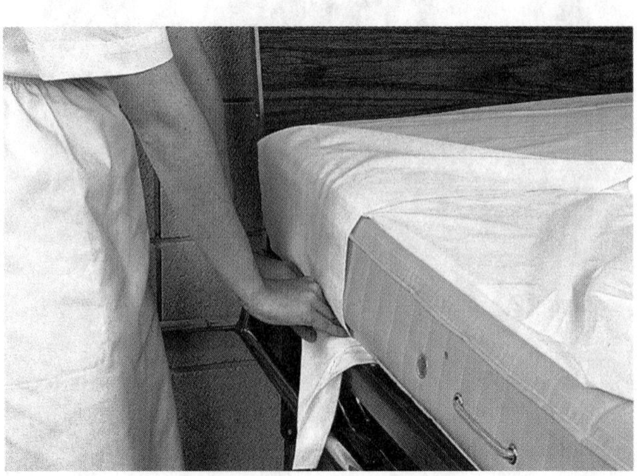

Step 14C • *Tuck hanging part under mattress.*

    d. Pick up top of triangular fold, and place it over side of the mattress.

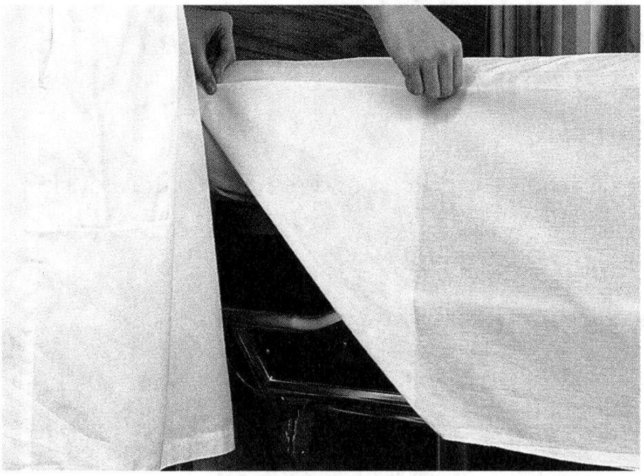

Step 14D • *Drop triangle over side of bed and tuck in.*

    e. Tuck this loose portion of sheet under the mattress.
       Rationale: Mitered corners do not loosen easily when client moves in bed.
       Note: If contour sheet is used, fit elastic edges under corner of mattress.
15. Tuck remaining sheet on that side under the mattress.
16. Lay draw sheet (folded in half) on the bed with the center fold at center of bed. Place top edge of draw sheet about 12 to 15 in from head of bed. Tuck excess draw sheet under mattress.
    Rationale: Draw sheet secures bottom sheet in place to decrease wrinkling.
17. Move to opposite side of bed.
    Rationale: Completing work on one side of bed at a time saves time and decreases energy expenditure.
18. Spread bottom sheet over mattress edge and miter top corner.
19. Tuck excess bottom sheet *tightly* under mattress, pulling gently to smooth out wrinkles.
    Rationale: Taut sheet eliminates wrinkles, which irritate and cause pressure on the skin.
20. Grasp draw sheet, pulling gently. Beginning at middle, tuck draw sheet under mattress firmly. Finish tucking top and bottom.
    Rationale: Tucking middle of draw sheet first prevents wrinkling and poor fit.
21. Return to side of bed where linen is placed.
22. Place top sheet on bed with vertical center fold at center of bed. Unfold sheet with seams facing out and top edge even with top of mattress. Smooth sheet, with excess falling over bottom edge of mattress.
    Rationale: Placing seam side up prevents edges from rubbing and irritating client's skin.
23. Spread blanket and bedspread evenly over bed.
24. Miter the bottom corner, using all three layers of

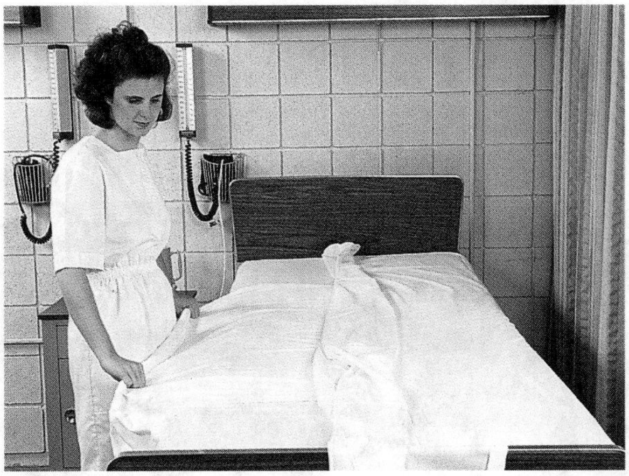

Step 20 • *Tuck draw sheet firmly under mattress.*

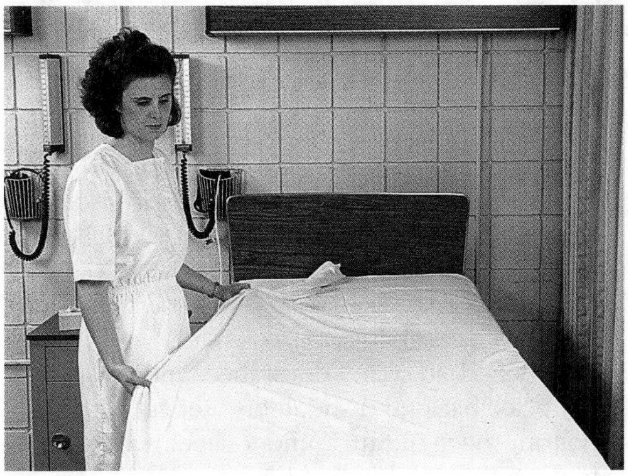

Step 22 • *Center top sheet on bed.*

linen (sheet, blanket, bedspread). Leave sides untucked.

25. Move to opposite side of bed, and miter bottom corner, using all three layers of linen.
    Rationale: Mitering all three layers together saves time and energy. Mitered corners secure top covers but allow easy access in and out of bed by leaving sides free.
26. Standing at bottom of bed, grasp top covers about 10 in from bottom of mattress. Loosen linen slightly by pulling on top covers or forming a pleat.
    Rationale: Additional room for client's feet gives comfort and prevents pressure on toes.
27. Put on clean pillowcases:
    a. Grasp center of pillowcase, with one hand on seamed end.
    b. Gather case, turning it inside out over the hand holding it.
    c. With same hand, grasp middle of one end of pillow.
    d. Pull case over pillow with free hand.
    e. Adjust case so corners fit over pillow.
    Rationale: This method prevents shaking of pillowcase and linen and distributing microorganisms in room.

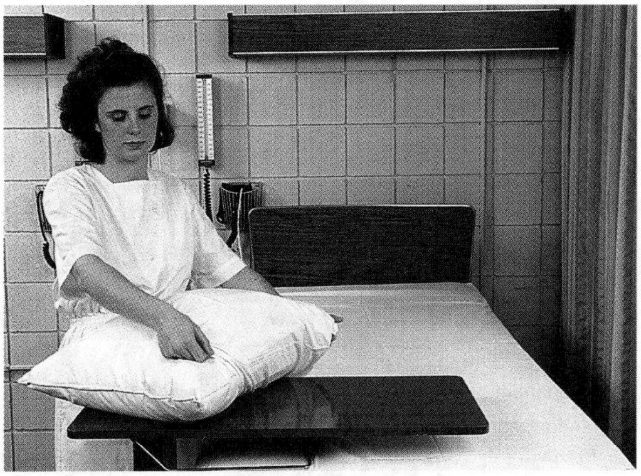

Step 27 • *Replace pillowcase.*

28. Place pillows in center at head of bed.
29. Fold top linen back to one side or fanfolded at bottom of bed.
30. Secure call bell within client's reach, and lower bed.
    Rationale: A call bell within reach helps provide safety for the client.
31. Arrange the bedside table, nightstand, and personal items within easy reach.
32. Discard soiled linen according to agency policy.
33. Wash your hands.

touching your clothing, and wash your hands after handling soiled linens. Soiled linens must be put immediately into a linen bag, not on any surfaces of another client's area. Do not put soiled linens on the floor. If a linen bag is not available, a pillowcase can be slipped over the back of a standard chair to provide a handy receptacle for dirty linens.

To conserve time and energy, pick up all the necessary linens from the linen supply before beginning. One side of the bed is made as completely as possible before moving to the other side. Lowering the head of the bed and raising the bed to a comfortable working height helps prevent back strain.

Community-Based Nursing

Many people who are unable to provide for their own hygiene, feeding, grooming, and toileting independently live in the community. Family and community support are often needed to ensure adequate functioning. Rehabilitation promotes optimal return of function and

Procedure 32-9
Making an Occupied Bed

Purpose

1. Provide clean linen for client who is unable to get out of bed.
2. Promote comfort

Assessment

Same as Procedure 32-8.

Equipment

Same as Procedure 32-8.

Procedure

1. Wash your hands.
2. Assemble equipment on bedside table or chair. Do not place on another client's bed.
   Rationale: Placing linen on clean surface prevents contamination with microorganisms.
3. Close room door or bedside curtains.
   Rationale: The client's privacy must be maintained.
4. Lock side rails up on side of bed opposite from where clean linen is stacked.
   Rationale: Side rails prevent client from rolling out of bed. Also gives client a bar to grasp to assist with turning.
5. Raise bed to comfortable working position. Lower side rail on your side of bed.
   Rationale: Nurse uses good body mechanics to reduce muscle strain on back.
6. Loosen all top linen from foot of bed.
7. Remove bedspread and blanket separately. Without shaking, fold each and place over back of chair if they are to be reused. If they are soiled, hold them away from your uniform, and place in linen bag.
   Rationale: Folding linen enables nurse to discard or handle without contaminating uniform. Shaking linen spreads microorganisms through the air.
8. Leave top sheet on client or cover client with a bath blanket; remove and discard top sheet.
   Rationale: Warmth is provided and unnecessary body exposure is prevented during linen change.
9. Loosen the bottom sheet on your side.
10. Lower head of bed to flat position.
    Note: If client cannot tolerate flat position, lower head of bed as far as client can tolerate.
11. With assistance from another worker, grasp mattress lugs and slide mattress to head of bed if it has slipped down.

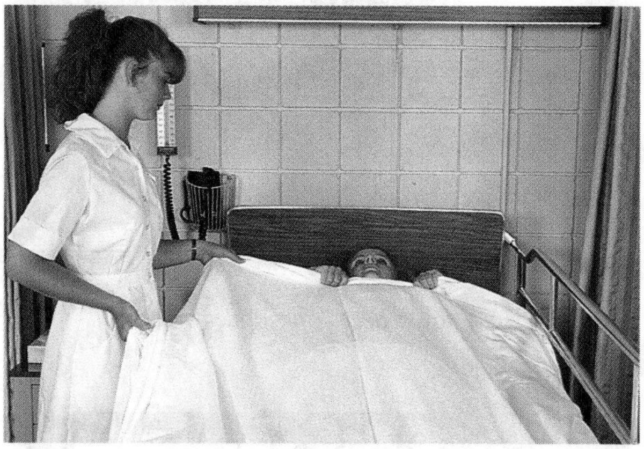

Step 8 • *Cover with bath blanket or leave top sheet in place.*

12. Help client to roll onto side facing away from you. Client may grasp side rail to assist. Additional personnel may be needed to assist with client positioning. Adjust pillow under head.
    Rationale: Side-lying position provides space for placing clean linen on mattress.
13. Tightly fanfold soiled draw sheet and tuck under buttocks, back, and shoulders. Repeat with soiled bottom sheet and tuck under client. Do not fanfold mattress pad unless it is soiled.
    Rationale: Fanfolds under client should be as tight and smooth as possible to provide space for clean linen and enable client to eventually roll back over folds.

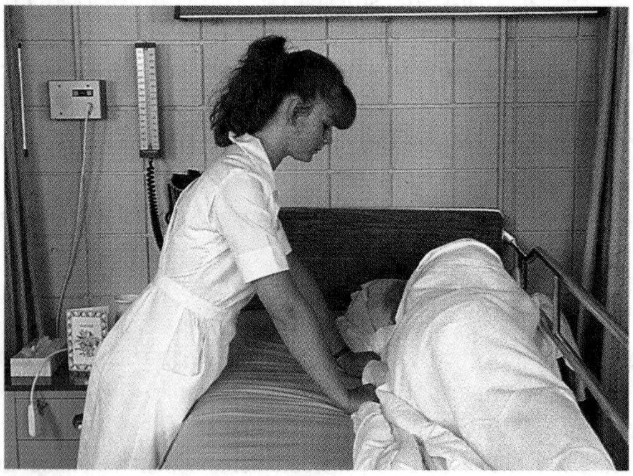

Step 13 • *Fan-fold soiled linens and tuck under client.*

14. Place clean bottom sheet on bed. Unfold lengthwise so bottom edge is even with end of mattress and vertical center crease is at center of bed.

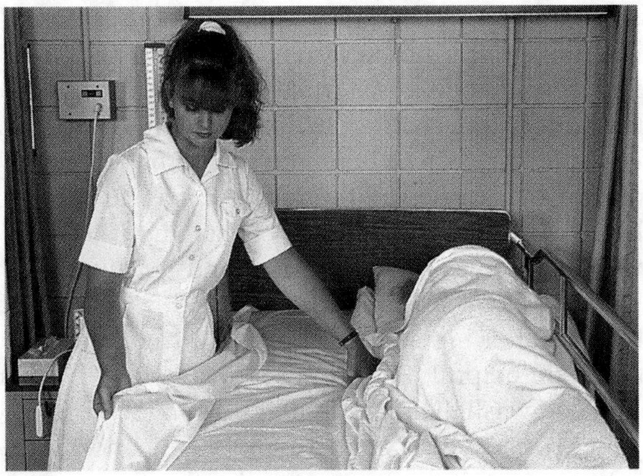

Step 14 *• Unfolding and centering clean linen.*

15. Bring sheet's bottom edge over mattress sides and fanfold top of sheet toward center of mattress and place next to client.
16. Tuck top edge of sheet under mattress. Miter top corner on your side (as in Procedure 32–8). Tuck remaining portion of sheet under mattress.
    Note: If a contour sheet is used, fit elastic edges under corner of mattress.
17. Place draw sheet on bed with center fold at center of bed. Position sheet so it will extend from the client's back to below the buttocks. Fanfold the top edge and place next to client. Tuck excess under mattress.
    Rationale: Draw sheet is used to reposition client and absorb excess perspiration.
18. Lock side rails on your side up and move to other side of bed.
    Rationale: Side rails maintain client's safety.
19. Lower side rail. Help client to roll over folds of linen onto his or her other side. Additional help may be needed if client is unable to move easily.
    Rationale: When second half of bed is exposed, soiled linen can be removed and clean linen replaced.
20. Move pillow under client's head.
21. Remove soiled linen by folding into a square or bundle, with soiled side turned in. Place in linen bag.
    Rationale: These actions reduce transmission of microorganisms and prevent client embarrassment from seeing soiled sheets.
22. Grasp edge of fanfolded bottom sheet and pull from under the client.
23. Tuck top of sheet under top of mattress. Miter top corner.
24. Facing bed, pull bottom sheet tight and tuck excess linen under mattress from top to bottom.
    Rationale: Tucking linen under mattress maintains a tight fit of the sheet and eliminates wrinkles.

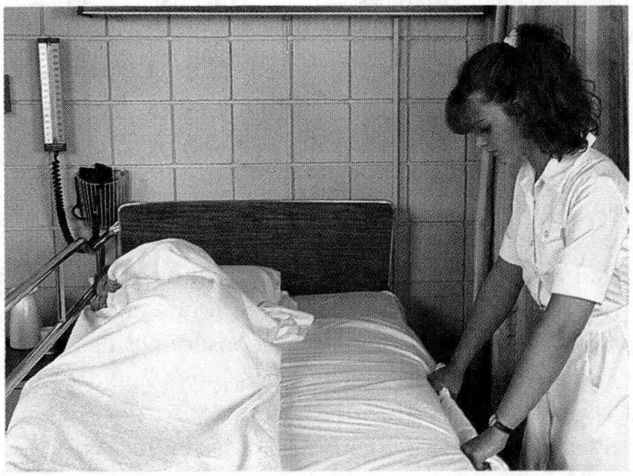

Step 24 *• Smoothly tuck sheets under mattress.*

25. Unfold draw sheet by grasping at center. Tuck excess tightly under mattress. Tuck the middle first, then the top, and finally the bottom.
    Rationale: Tucking the center first prevents the draw sheet from pulling sideways, causing a poor fit and wrinkles.
26. Help client to center of bed.
27. Raise side rail if necessary and move to side of bed where remainder of linen is stored.
28. Place top sheet over client with center crease lengthwise at center of bed with seam side up. Unfold sheet from head to toe.
29. Have client grasp top edge of clean top sheet. Remove bath blanket or soiled top linen by pulling from beneath clean top sheet.
30. Discard in linen bag.
    Rationale: Limiting exposure of body parts gives client dignity.
31. Complete top covers as described in Procedure 32–8.

ability to cope with and remain independent despite limitations.

Before discharge from the acute care facility, the nurse promotes as much independence in self-care activities as possible. An occupational therapist often helps the client develop self-care skills, and the nurse can support this learning on a daily basis. The nurse can help the client anticipate self-care problems at home and plan how to manage them.

Bathing. The home environment should enhance self-care. In the bathtub or shower, hand grips and nonskid mats can protect against falls. For most clients, getting in and out of the tub poses the greatest problem.

Tub seats can be installed so that clients need not lower themselves down into the tub. Hand-held shower appliances also can assist with bathing. The hot-water tank thermostat should be set below 48°C (120°F) to avoid burns during bathing.

For the client who cannot shower or use the bathtub, placing a chair in the bathroom so he or she can wash by the sink may help to conserve energy. Relatives may be available to visit on a weekly basis to supervise or assist with bathing, but often clients are embarrassed to ask relatives or friends to assist with this private, personal activity. If family support is inadequate, home health aides can be used on a routine basis to provide hygiene care for the client at home.

Grooming and Dressing. Independent grooming and dressing also should be assessed and promoted by the nurse before discharge. Many clients do not dress in the hospital and are surprised at how draining this activity can be. Before discharge, clients should be encouraged to practice dressing using energy-conserving measures. The client should sit as much as possible while dressing and should wear clothes that are easy to get on and off. Sweatsuits are often ideal for the client who has difficulty with fine motor skills because they have no buttons or zippers. Slip-on shoes with nonskid soles are easy to put on and help prevent falls. Discuss with the client the psychological benefits of getting dressed, and work out a plan so that he or she can avoid wearing nightclothes during the day.

Hair care provides a morale boost to the homebound client. Hair should be washed before discharge for clients who might have difficulty with this task. Relatives can take the client to a local hairdresser for shampoos and hair care, and some beauticians make house calls. Frequently, a family member or friend can be encouraged to provide such a service. Applying makeup is important to some women, and lack of coordination or energy can make this activity difficult.

Food Preparation and Eating. Buying and preparing food can be exhausting, so provide instructions on easy, nutritious meals. Frozen foods have improved dramatically in recent years and can be nutritious. Relatives can package single-serving meals so they can be reheated. Safety (ie, burn prevention) should be stressed. Meals on Wheels is a community service that provides hot, well-balanced meals for the homebound person for a nominal fee. Few supermarkets deliver groceries, but friends, relatives, or neighborhood young people can shop for the homebound person.

Eating can consume energy. Rest before and after meals should be encouraged. Special utensils can be used by clients with fine motor impairment.

Toileting. Self-care deficit in toileting is an important consideration, and home bathroom facilities should be assessed before discharge. If the bathroom is on a different floor from the bedroom, the client may need a bedside commode or a urinal. If the client is wheelchair-bound, the bathroom doorway must be wide enough for the wheelchair, and the bathroom must be large enough to permit the client to transfer from the wheelchair to the toilet. Some clients find it difficult to lower themselves onto the toilet and get up again. A high-rise toilet seat can be helpful and is indicated for all clients after hip surgery. Hand grips next to the toilet also are helpful. Clients must be able to wipe themselves and wash their hands after toileting. Prepackaged towelettes can be an easy way to wash hands.

Incontinence can be managed with a Foley catheter or disposable diapers. If a catheter is used, a leg bag can be worn under clothes to promote self-image, and a larger collection bag can be used at night. A condom catheter also can be used with the same urine collection system. Disposable diapers for adults are now widely available, although they are more costly than infant diapers. A more streamlined adult incontinence pad (Depends) also is available.

Transfers and Caregiving. Clients with self-care deficits and inadequate support may be unable to manage safely at home and may need to be transferred to an extended care facility or nursing home. When a client is transferred to another healthcare agency, it is important to communicate the level of self-care function to that staff. Transfer forms usually have a place for the nurse to indicate a client's independence in bathing, feeding, grooming, and toileting. Be specific, so optimum independence can be maintained.

A designated caregiver may have to provide much assistance for a client with severe self-care deficit to remain in the community. The role of the nurse expands to include teaching and support for the caregiver. Providing 24-hour care for a client with severe self-care deficits can be emotionally and physically draining. Providing respite care (eg, adult day care) or support groups for the caregiver is important to prevent burnout and improve quality of life for all involved.

Evaluation

Evaluation of self-care deficit is based on the outcome criteria developed from the client goals. Objective and subjective data can be collected from the client to support successful attainment of client-centered goals. Ideally, the client should exhibit increased independence in bathing, grooming, feeding, and toileting. The client should be able to state any limitations and should feel comfortable accepting necessary assistance. The client should demonstrate a positive self-image and satisfaction with accomplishments in self-care despite limitations. The client should be able to use adaptive devices

Nursing Plan of Care
The Client with Self-Care Deficit

Nursing Diagnosis
Bathing/Hygiene Self Care Deficit related to right-sided weakness manifested by impaired ability to wash most body parts

Client Goal
Client will willingly participate in hygiene measures.

Client Outcome Criteria
- During care, client states need for assistance to perform hygiene activities that he or she cannot perform alone.
- After teaching session, client demonstrates bathing face, trunk, and upper extremities, with verbal cuing.
- Before discharge, client verbalizes a realistic plan for bathing at home.

Nursing Intervention	*Scientific Rationale*
1. Assist client to identify self-care deficits in hygiene.	1. Maximum self-participation can occur with improved self-esteem.
2. Encourage client to communicate needs and concerns to nursing staff and significant others.	2. Communication reduces the presence of energy-consuming stressors, such as isolation and worry.
3. Permit and encourage client to accept some dependency and verbalize feelings.	3. A degree of dependence is a necessary part of recovery and rehabilitation for most people.
4. Ensure safety through monitoring and assistance during bathing and hygiene activities.	4. Safety measures reduce the possibility of increased injury due to falls.
5. Schedule hygiene self-care 1 hour after breakfast when client feels rested.	5. Hygiene self-care is a tiring procedure; fatigue can produce confusion.
6. Lay out objects for hygiene care in the order to be used, and place them on client's right side on a chair. Don't hurry client.	6. Nurse gives support and conserves his or her energy. Client can see objects on the right with visual field split.
7. Provide for the greatest amount of privacy possible.	7. Privacy enhances feeling of dignity and self-worth.
8. Assist client to use unaffected hand to wash self, comb hair, and brush teeth within the limits of ability.	8. Activities enhance independence while providing help and support as needed.
9. Evaluate frequently for indications of fatigue by checking pulse and respiratory rate.	9. Ability to sustain concentrated effort may be limited until endurance is developed.
10. Coordinate self-care rehabilitation with occupational and physical therapy and any other involved health professionals.	10. Necessary techniques and assistive devices are used in the most beneficial manner. Represent client in negotiations and making arrangements for care.

to facilitate self-care, and self-care should occur without injury.

Examples of outcome criteria are listed here. Some criteria may be important for more than one goal. Specific outcome criteria must be established for each client.

Goal
Client will actively participate in hygiene measures.

Possible Outcome Criteria
- Client states assistance required to perform hygiene activities during initial interview.
- After teaching session, client uses left hand for bathing face, trunk, and arms, as witnessed by nurse.
- Before discharge, client verbalizes a realistic plan for achieving hygiene measures at home.

- During follow-up home visit, client verbalizes satisfaction with ability to perform self-care.

Goal

Client will safely increase level of independence in eating.

Possible Outcome Criteria

- During next home visit, client demonstrates using a cup with a built-up handle held with both hands to drink thick liquids.
- Before discharge, client verbalizes a plan for managing food preparation at home.

Goal

Client will participate in dressing himself or herself.

Possible Outcome Criteria

- By third week of rehabilitation, client demonstrates ability to put on a loose-fitting dress with Velcro fasteners.
- By fourth week of rehabilitation, client uses a long-handled reacher to put on slip-on shoes.
- Prior to discharge from rehabilitation unit, client expresses a positive approach to solving problems inherent in relearning to dress self.
- Before discharge, client demonstrates dressing using energy conservation techniques.

Goal

Client will manage toileting as independently as possible.

Possible Outcome Criteria

- Within 48 hours, client is able to recognize and communicate the need to go to the toilet.
- Within 5 days, client transfers from bed to wheelchair to toilet or from bed to commode with standby assistance.
- Before discharge, client states plan for managing toileting at home.
- By first home visit, client demonstrates toileting in own bathroom without experiencing fatigue or activity intolerance.

Key Concepts

- Self-care and hygiene are important factors in promoting health.
- With stress or illness, children and adults often regress to a lower developmental level, requiring more assistance with self-care.
- Factors affecting self-care are neuromuscular function, energy level, sensory ability, cognition, motivation, sociocultural factors, environmental resources, and age.
- Sudden alterations in functional ability can occur with injury, acute illness, surgery, altered cognitive states, and pain.
- Chronic illness often poses challenges to independent self-care, because clients must develop coping strategies for functional deficits.
- The nursing assessment provides a specific picture of the self-care deficit to use in planning interventions.
- Although the primary reason for bathing is to enhance cleanliness, warm water and friction enhance circulation, movement provides an opportunity for range of motion, and the experience can be relaxing.
- When providing hygiene care, describe the care measures and obtain permission to proceed. Permission also is needed before cutting hair or shaving facial hair.
- Optimal care of the eyes, ears, and teeth is important in maintaining optimal health. Care must be taken to avoid damage or loss of glasses, contact lenses, hearing aids, or dentures because they are significant to functioning and expensive to replace.
- Identification of inability to self-feed is important to promote nutrition and prevent possible aspiration.
- Providing a clean environment and a smooth, wrinkle-free bed helps promote comfort.

Critical Thinking Challenges

You have added self-care and hygiene to your growing body of knowledge about nursing care. You are prepared to help people with their hygiene and support them in self-care. Now turn back to the situation at the beginning of the chapter, and consider these questions.

1. *Identify factors that might make your client reluctant to participate in morning care.*
2. *Discuss reasons why you as a nurse feel he should participate in morning care.*
3. *Reflect on your feelings when you encounter a client who is dirty and smells bad.*
4. *Identify two or three conclusions you might draw before obtaining more information from the client.*
5. *Predict positive and negative potential consequences of directly approaching this client and "forcing" him to wash.*

References

Doyle, D. L., & Stern, P. N. (1992). Negotiating self-care in rehabilitation nursing. *Rehabilitation Nursing, 17* (6), 319–321, 326.

Jackson, D. B., & Saunders, R. B. (1993). *Child health nursing: A comprehensive approach to the care of children and their families.* Philadelphia: J.B. Lippincott.

Johnston, B. L., Watt, R., & Fletcher, J. (1981). Oxygen consumption and hemodynamic and electrocardiographic responses to bathing in recent postmyocardial infarction clients. *Heart and Lung, 10* (4), 666–671.

Katz, S. (1963). Studies of illness in the aged, the index of ADL's: A standardized measure of biological and psychosocial function. *Journal of the American Medical Society, 185* (12), 914–919.

Katz, S. (1983). Assessing self-maintenance: Activities of daily living, mobility, and instrumental activities of daily living. *Journal of the American Geriatric Society, 31* (12), 721–725.

Meehan, M. (1992). Nursing Dx: Potential for aspiration. *RN, 92* (1), 30–34.

North American Nursing Diagnosis Association (1994). *NANDA nursing diagnoses: Definitions and classifications 1995–1996.* Philadelphia: Author.

Osborn, C. L., & Marshall, M. J. (1993). Self-feeding performance in nursing home residents. *Journal of Gerontological Nursing, 19* (3), 7–14.

Renn, N. (1989). Oral health and hygiene for the elderly: A shared learning experience. *Home Healthcare Nurse, 7* (3), 37–39.

Ruscin, C., Cunningham, G., & Blaylock, A. (1993). Foot protocol for the older client. *Geriatric Nursing, 14* (4), 210–212.

Skewes, S. M. (1994). No more baths! Bag bath a technique that lessens the risk of skin impairment. *RN, 57* (1), 34–35.

Tombes, M. B., & Gallucci, B. (1993). The effects of hydrogen peroxide rinses on the normal oral mucosa. *Nursing Research, 42* (6), 332–337.

Valentine, A. D. (1988). The case for fluoridation. *Midwife, Health Visitor, and Community Nurse, 24* (5), 158, 160.

Bibliography

Easton, K. (1993). Defining the concept of self-care. *Rehabilitation Nursing, 18* (6), 384–387.

Griffin, C. W. (1987). Learning to swallow again. *American Journal of Nursing, 87* (3), 314–317.

Heals, D. (1993). A key to wellbeing: Oral hygiene in patients with advanced cancer. *Professional Nurse, 8* (6), 391–392.

Jopp, M., et al. (1993). Using self care theory to guide nursing management of the older adult after hospitalization. *Rehabilitation Nursing, 18* (2), 91–94.

Kruger, S., et al. (1993). Foot care: Knowledge retention and self care practices. *Diabetic Educator, 18* (6), 487–490.

Miskovich Mehta, S. (1993) The road back to independence: Applying Orem's self-care framework. *Geriatric Nursing, 14* (4), 182–185.

Ney, D. F. (1993). Cerumen impaction, ear hygiene practices, and hearing acuity. *Geriatric Nurse, 14* (2), 70–73.

Wolf, Z. R. (1993). The bath: A nursing ritual. *Journal of Holistic Nursing, 11* (2), 135–148.

Body Mechanics and Mobility

Key Terms	Learning Objectives

Key Terms

Active range of motion
Activity intolerance
Aerobic exercise
Anaerobic exercise
Arthroscopy
Atrophy
Body mechanics
Contracture
Dangling
Deep vein thrombosis
Flaccidity
Foot drop
Gait
Isometric exercise
Isotonic exercise
Mobility
Passive range of motion
Range of motion
Spasticity

Learning Objectives

Upon completion of this chapter, the student will be able to do the following:

- *Explain normal functions of the musculoskeletal system and characteristics of normal movement.*
- *Identify factors that can affect or alter normal mobility, including lifespan considerations.*
- *Describe the impact of immobility on each functional area.*
- *Discuss appropriate subjective and objective data to collect to assess mobility status.*
- *Identify three NANDA nursing diagnoses for the functional area of mobility.*
- *Demonstrate nursing interventions, such as positioning, ambulating, providing range of motion, and using assistive devices.*
- *Plan strategies to avoid musculoskeletal injury during client care.*
- *Develop appropriate community-based nursing interventions for preventing and managing mobility problems.*

33

You are a home health nurse visiting a new client. He is a retired man recently discharged from the hospital after surgical repair of a fractured hip. His wife meets you at the door. She looks tired and anxious. She explains that her husband is reluctant to do anything for himself because it still hurts him to move. He has been sleeping on the sofa bed in the downstairs den and spends the day in the recliner. He uses a urinal rather than walking to the bathroom, which is close by. Getting him to his recliner has been very difficult for the wife, who fears her husband may fall, even with the walker. The wife adds that her husband becomes very upset and yells at her when she encourages him to do more for himself.

In previous chapters, you have learned about the individual, family, and community; communication; client teaching; and home management. All of this infomation is important as you study the situation at the beginning of the chapter. After you study the chapter, you will be able to add body mechanics and mobility to your knowledge base. These are important factors in preventing injury for your clients, your coworkers, and you. When you have finished studying the chapter, consider the Critical Thinking Challenges that conclude the chapter.

Mobility, or the ability to move freely within the environment, is fundamental to normal daily functioning. In a highly mobile society, problems affecting mobility are especially significant. Independence is usually defined by a person's ability to perform activities of daily living (grooming, dressing, and feeding), job-related activities, and role-related activities (as a parent or spouse). Limitations in a person's ability to move normally and spontaneously can affect all of these areas.

Changes in mobility also create more subtle effects, especially in communication. Facial expressions and gestures are significant in nonverbal communication, and talking with someone at eye level promotes equality between those talking. The person who must look up at someone from a chair or bed may feel that he or she is at a psychological disadvantage. Movement also is significant in dispersing negative feelings and tension. Many people find that jogging or participating in athletics helps them to feel healthier and less anxious. Being able to leave uncomfortable or dangerous situations gives most people a feeling of control.

Most people associate mobility with health. When people are confined to bed, they see themselves as sick. Disabilities that affect mobility, such as amputation or a musculoskeletal defect, may impair self-image; the client may see himself or herself as defective or abnormal. Like many aspects of health, mobility can be viewed along a continuum from full mobility to immobility. Full mobility occurs when the person has no physical or psychological factors that limit mobility. Immobility occurs when the person cannot move his or her entire body or a specific body part.

Clients move along this continuum as their abilities change:

- Temporary changes in mobility are often caused by therapeutic treatment, such as traction to repair a fracture.
- Some conditions lead to progressive disability; examples are muscular dystrophy and severe crippling rheumatoid arthritis.
- Permanent changes in mobility occur when physiologic dysfunction that interferes with normal body movement cannot be reversed (ie, spinal cord injuries that result in paralysis or cerebrovascular accidents [strokes] that cause weakness or paralysis on one side of the body).

Rehabilitation is the key to restoring a person with certain disabilities to optimal health, and the nurse plays a significant role in this process.

Normal Mobility

The musculoskeletal system is the supporting framework for the body. It includes the bones and muscles involved in movement and is responsible for the form and shape of the body. The complex activity of movement is coordinated by central and peripheral nerves. Maintaining posture and balance against the force of gravity requires smooth coordination of muscles, joints, and nerves and a stable center of gravity.

Structures of the Musculoskeletal System

The musculoskeletal system consists of bones, muscles, joints, cartilage, connective tissue, and fibrous tendons. Movement is permitted by flexible connections of bones and muscles at the joints.

Bones

Bones are a framework on which muscles, tendons, and ligaments are attached. They facilitate movement, protect vital organs (brain, heart, lungs, liver), store and regulate calcium and phosphate, and form blood cells.

The structure of bones provides for minimum weight and maximum structural strength. Bone tissue is either woven or lamellar. Woven bone is characterized by rapid growth, as in infants, and is generally found where ligaments and tendons insert into the bone of an adult. Lamellar bone is mature with highly organized mineralized plates.

The 206 bones in the body also can be classified by shape: long (arms, legs), short (tarsals, carpals), flat (cranium), and irregular (vertebral). Basic components of the long bones are the diaphysis (shaft) and the epiphyses (ends). Most of the bone is covered by periosteum, which contains nerves and blood vessels. The outer portion of long bones is composed of dense, compact bone with a marrow cavity in the center where the blood-forming cells are located.

Muscles

Skeletal muscles are connected to bones at or across joints and are made up of striated, long muscle fibers usually arranged in a parallel alignment. The formation of the striated fibers allows the muscle to contract (shorten) or extend (lengthen) as required by movement. Contraction occurs when the overlapping striated fibers slide toward each other, thereby shortening and increasing the strength of the muscle.

Muscle contraction requires a complex mechanical, chemical, and electrical interaction. The contraction is initiated when an action potential (electrical charge) moves along the nerve and across the myroneural junction to the muscle. Neurotransmitters, which are chemical substances such as acetylcholine, permit neurologic impulses to be transmitted to the muscle. The transmitting activity occurs when calcium is released into the sarcoplasmic reticulum, which initiates a complex series of biochemical events resulting in muscle contraction. Energy for the work of contraction comes from the metabolism of food, especially fats and carbohydrates.

Muscles are covered by a layer of connective tissue, which joins with tendon fibers at the end of the muscle fiber where the muscle joins the bone. Muscle fibers are innervated by motor neurons originating from the anterior horn of the spinal cord. All muscle fibers connected to a single motor nerve are called a *motor unit.*

During a lifetime, the body has only the number of muscle cells with which it was born; however, the work of the muscle determines the size of the muscle cells. When forceful activity is demanded of the muscle, the muscle hypertrophies (the diameter of the muscle increases), causing an increase in the strength of the muscle. Atrophy, the opposite of hypertrophy, causes the muscle to decrease in strength and size as a result of disuse. Disuse may be related to lack of exercise, aging, enforced rest, or immobilizing devices.

Joints

Joints are the areas where bones meet. The types of joints are fibrous, which do not move (cranial); cartilaginous, which allow minimal movement (costochondral); and synovial, which are movable (joints of the extremities). Synovial joints are lined with synovial tissue, which has a rich blood supply and produces synovial fluid. Synovial fluid lubricates the joint, allowing smooth articulation and easy motion.

Ligaments and tendons connect and support joints. Ligaments stabilize the bones in the joints and are more elastic than tendons. Tendons are specialized tissues. They connect muscle to bone and are surrounded by synovial-like tissues.

Normal Physiologic Function

Carrying out coordinated movement is a complex process. Even with a framework of bones held together by ligaments and covered with soft tissue and skin, normal function cannot occur without coordinated muscle activity and neurologic integration.

Alignment and Posture

Maintaining upright posture requires proper alignment of the bones, muscles, and joints and a stable center of gravity (Fig. 33-1). Alignment is achieved when the joints and muscles are not experiencing extremes in extension or flexion or unusual stress, whether the person is lying down, sitting, or standing.

Upright posture and movement require a balanced *center of gravity,* which is where the weight of the body is centered and where the downward forces of gravity are balanced. The usual line of gravity starts at the top of the head and bisects the shoulders, trunk, weight-bearing joints, and base of support; it runs slightly anterior to the sacrum. In older people, the lumbar spine tends to flatten, and the upper spine and head tend to tilt forward, causing the head to fall forward from the usual line of gravity.

Balance

Maintaining balance is a complex function of counteracting gravity and reflexes to maintain posture. The reticular formation provides the nervous energy for supporting the body against gravity by providing most of the intrinsic excitation required for maintaining tone in the extensor muscles. If a person begins to fall to one side, the extensor muscles on that side stiffen while the extensor muscles on the opposite side relax to prevent the fall.

Equilibrium is provided largely by the vestibular apparatus of the ear, which consists of the cochlear duct, the three semicircular canals, and two large chambers known as the utricle and the saccule. While the cochlear duct is a structure of hearing, the saccule, utricle, and semicircular canals are structures of equilibrium and thus balance. The utricle, saccule, and semicircular canals contain tiny hair cells connected to sensory nerve

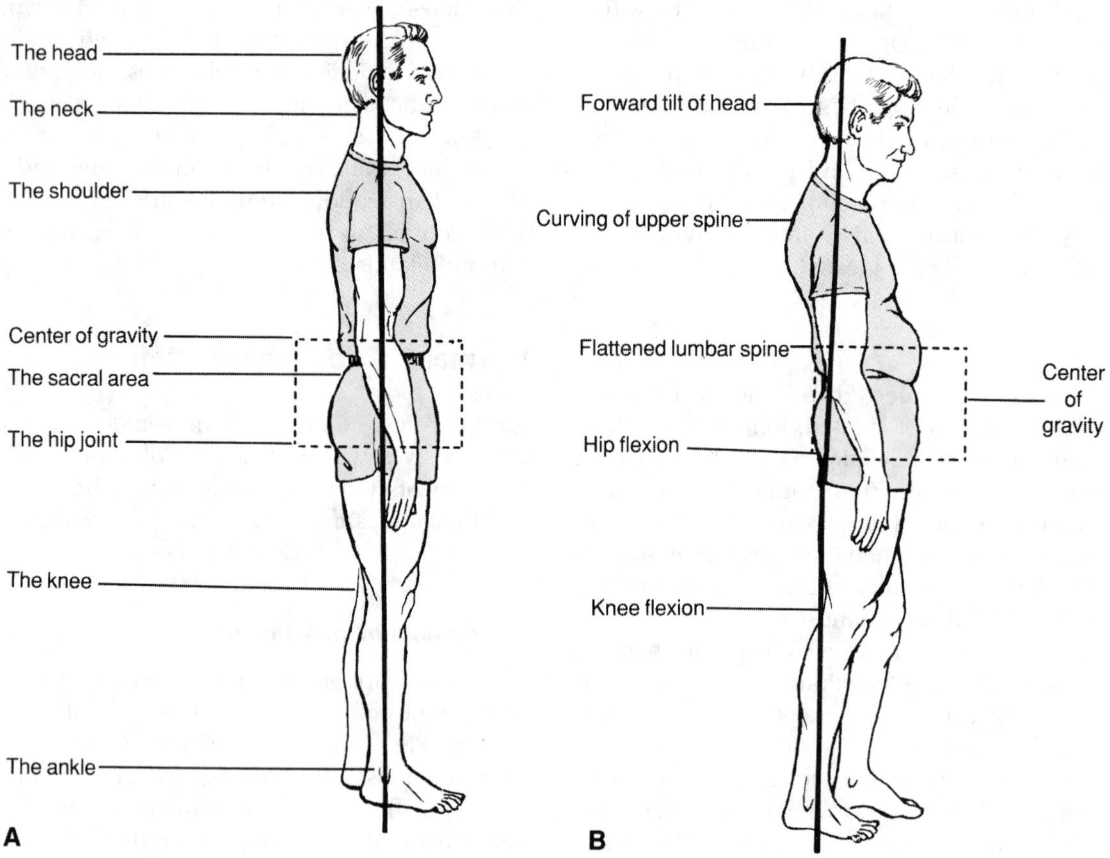

Figure 33-1 • *Vertical gravity line and posture. **(A)** Vertical gravity line and center of gravity. **(B)** Postural changes with age.*

fibers that pass into the vestibular nerve. When the head moves, these hair cells are bent, pulled, or compressed, transmitting signals to the sensory nerves over the appropriate nerve tracts to the area that controls equilibrium and balance.

The saccule and utricle provide information about the position of the head relative to the direction of the force of gravity. The three semicircular canals provide a specialized control of equilibrium by signaling the rate of the change. The superior, posterior, and lateral semicircular canals are arranged at right angles to each other, representing all three dimensions of space. When the head suddenly begins to rotate in any direction, the endolymph, or fluid within the canals, remains stationary while the canals turn. This causes the fluid in the canals to flow in the opposite direction of the rotation of the head. The fluid flow stimulates the hair cells that signal the sensory nerve fibers.

The information from the semicircular canals serves two purposes. The first is to control the muscles that move the eyes so that when the head moves in any direction, the person can keep the eyes fixed on a point of interest. The second purpose is to control the reflex mechanisms for maintaining upright posture and balance (Vander, Sherman, & Luciano, 1994). Vestibular input for equilibrium comes from vision (vestibulo-ocular input) and from skin and joint receptors (vestibulospinal input).

Coordinated Movement

The cerebellum, cerebral cortex, and basal ganglia are responsible for the control of motor functions, such as the mechanisms of alignment, posture, and balance, and for coordinated movement. The cerebellum coordinates the motor activities of movement, the cerebral cortex initiates voluntary motor activity, and the basal ganglia maintain posture. These systems make up the pyramidal and extrapyramidal tracts. The pyramidal tract (the direct corticospinal pathway) initiates transmission of impulses to the spinal cord for voluntary movements. The extrapyramidal tract (the indirect corticospinal pathway) dampens and inhibits impulses to smooth and coordinate skeletal muscle movement.

The cerebellum has a special role in controlling movement: it controls muscles used to maintain steady posture and coordinated, detailed movements. It receives information from the cortex and subcortical centers on what muscles *should* be doing and compares it with information from other neurologic sources about what the muscles *are* doing. Based on that comparison, the cerebellum can initiate impulses to correct the dis-

Procedure 33-1
Using Proper Body Mechanics to Move Clients

Purpose

1. Prevent injury to the nurse's musculoskeletal system
2. Prevent injury to the client during transfer

Assessment

- Evaluate weight of client to be lifted. Arrange for assistance if necessary.
- Assess position and height of client to be lifted.
- Assess knowledge about body alignment and how to maintain it with position changes.

Procedure

1. Plan movement before doing it.
   a. Always lock wheels on bed, stretcher, or wheelchair.
   Rationale: Unexpected movements may offset your balance and result in injury to yourself or client.

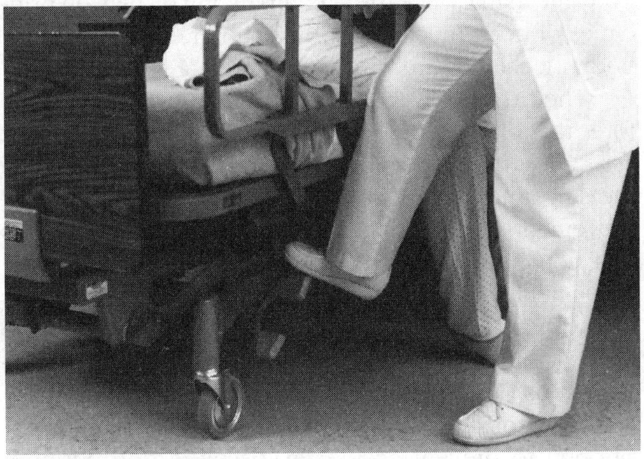

Step 1A • *Lock wheels on bed.*

   b. Allow client to assist during move.
   Rationale: Client participation helps overcome forces resisting the move, encourages client's sense of independence, and provides exercise for client.
   c. Use mechanical aids (ie, lifters, slide boards, body mobilizers) or additional personnel to move heavy clients.
   d. Slide, push, or pull client rather than lifting and carrying when possible.
   Rationale: Your body weight adds power to muscle work. Rocking your own body weight can balance the client's weight when assisting to a standing position.
   e. Tighten abdominal and gluteal muscles before lifting or moving client.
   Rationale: Tightening supports the abdomen and stabilizes the pelvis to provide a firm base of support.
   f. Use smooth, rhythmic, coordinated motions.
   Rationale: Smooth motions use less energy and lead to less muscle strain than jerky motions.
   g. If another person is assisting, plan your movements before beginning.
   Rationale: Prevents uncoordinated movements that may result in muscle strain or injury.
2. Begin all movements with body aligned and balanced.
   a. Face client to be moved, and pivot your body.
   b. Increase base of support by placing both feet flat on floor, knees slightly bent, with one foot slightly in front of the other or one step apart.
   c. Bend knees to lower center of gravity toward client to be moved.
   Rationale: This maintains body balance, reduces risk of falling, and allows larger muscle groups to work together.

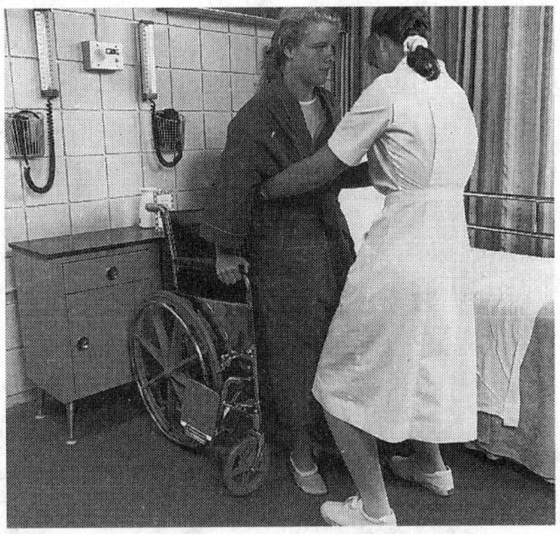

Steps 2B and C • *With feet flat and slightly apart, lower center of gravity.*

3. Elevate adjustable beds to waist level, and lower side rails to prevent stretching.
4. Carry objects close to body, and stand as close as possible to work area.
Rationale: This maintains the workload near the center of gravity to prevent muscle strain and fatigue caused by hyperextension.

Home-Care Modifications

- Teach caregivers the above guidelines for body movements. Redemonstration of learning provides a good opportunity to evaluate technique.

crepancy and ease the motion (Vander, Sherman, & Luciano, 1994). The result is smooth, coordinated movement and developed, fine-motor function, rather than uncoordinated, arrhythmic movements.

Body Mechanics

Body mechanics can be defined as using alignment, posture, and balance in a coordinated effort to perform activities such as lifting, bending, and moving. Proper body mechanics promote safe musculoskeletal function and maintain balance without undue strain on muscles. When nurses use their bodies to perform therapies, assist clients with movement, or move equipment, effective body mechanics are required to prevent injury to the client and nurse. Proper use of body mechanics is explained in Procedure 33-1.

Components of Body Mechanics. Using effective body mechanics means using gravity advantageously in body alignment, posture, balance, and movement. The center of gravity tends to be in the area of the pelvis, slightly anterior to the sacrum. Maintaining a balanced center of gravity during movement is essential for alignment, posture, and balance.

Maintaining balance involves keeping the spine in vertical alignment, the feet positioned for a broad base of support, and the body weight close to the center of gravity. When a person lifts or carries a load, that weight becomes part of the body weight; therefore, that additional weight must be balanced over the center of gravity (Fig. 33-2).

The greater the base of support, the more stability the person has for changing body position while maintaining alignment, posture, and balance. The weight-bearing joints and skeletal muscles of the legs provide a stable base of support, which can be widened by placing the feet farther apart and flexing the hip and knee joints. These activities lower the center of gravity, making it more stable and allowing flexibility in adjusting position to avoid muscle strain. The base of support must be sufficient so that changes in body position do not cause the center of gravity to fall beyond the edge of the base.

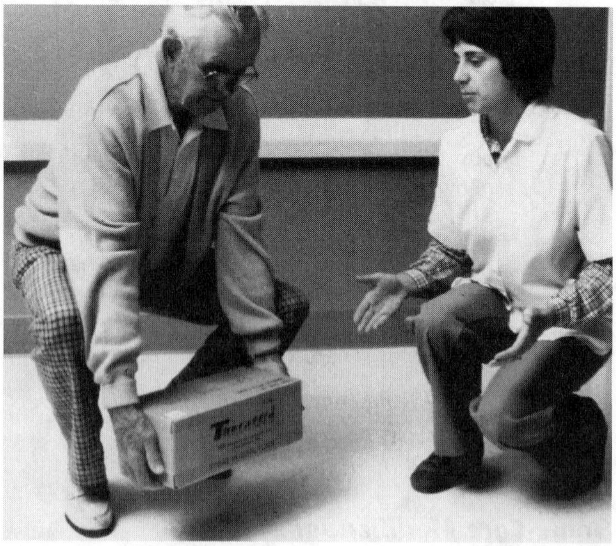

Figure 33-2 • *The nurse instructs a client on proper lifting techniques to prevent back strain and injury. (Courtesy of Overlake Medical Center, Bellevue, WA.)*

Movement is coordinated by opposing voluntary muscle groups and neuromuscular reflexes. The flexor and extensor muscle groups provide the opposing tensions for movement. When the flexors contract to move a joint, the extensors relax; when the flexors relax, the extensors contract. The flexors of the legs are among the largest and strongest muscles in the body and are used for leverage in good body mechanics. The neuromuscular reflexes maintain posture by enabling opposing muscle groups to work together in coordinated movement.

Principles of Body Mechanics. Nurses and clients may fall or incur back injuries as clients are moved from one position or location to another. The more limited the client's mobility, the more the nurse needs to use good body mechanics. See the accompanying display on principles of body mechanics. Some general rules for good body mechanics are presented here.

The first rule is to assess the situation carefully before acting. Planning is crucial. When in doubt, seek assistance before beginning to move a client. Examine the surroundings for potential obstacles to the desired movement (equipment, cords, tubing, or other items that could trip the nurse or hamper the client's free movement). Necessary equipment should be placed out of the way of the nurse and client, usually near the head or foot of the bed. Ventilator tubing, catheters, intravenous (IV) tubing, or wires for cardiac and ventilatory monitoring must be handled by an assistant or positioned to prevent accidental disconnection during a turn or transfer. Using a counting method helps to coordinate the actions of everyone involved in the movement. Counting "one, two, three" with the position change on "three" helps focus everyone's attention and invites active participation of the client.

The second rule is to use the large muscle groups of the legs whenever possible to provide the force for the movement. The back stays straight, the arms maintain a strong grip with elbows slightly flexed, and the hips and knees are bent. Pushing, pulling, or lifting are then accomplished by orienting the torso in the desired direction of movement and straightening the legs. Back injuries that result from moving clients can usually be traced to asymmetric use of muscles. Avoid twisting or moving in a diagonal direction.

The third rule is to perform work at the appropriate height for body position. When helping a client to

Principles of Body Mechanics

Scientific Principles Underlying Body Mechanics

- Less energy is used if all body parts are balanced appropriately.
- The body parts move segmentally and affect balance and function of the musculoskeletal system.
- The greater the base of support, the more stable the body.
- Force can be applied or resisted more effectively when the base of support can be enlarged in the direction of the force.
- Pelvic tilt (contraction of the abdominal and gluteal muscles to stabilize the pelvis) before activity helps protect the lower back from strain and injury.
- Facing the direction of work reduces the chance of injury.
- Less energy is needed to keep an object moving (momentum) than to initiate movement (inertia).
- Moving an object on a level surface requires less effort.
- Reducing friction between the object moved and the surface on which it is moved requires less energy.
- Use of levers reduces energy expenditure.
- Holding an object close to the body requires less energy than holding it farther away.
- Muscle strain can be avoided by using the strong leg muscles when lifting, pushing, and pulling.
- Smooth, continuous movements are easier and safer than sudden, sharp, or uncontrolled movements.
- Using rhythmic movements at a normal speed requires less energy.

Applied Principles of Body Mechanics

- Adjust the height of the work area when possible.
- Assume a starting position that will permit freedom of movement in range, direction, and position.
- Keep body balanced over the base of support with knees relaxed and trunk erect (in relation to the pelvis).
- Bend hips and knees to alter position of body, widening the base of support as needed, for effective leverage and use of energy.
- Face the direction of motion, using the muscles of the lower extremities and shifting body weight for lifting, pushing, and pulling actions.
- Hold objects close to the body when lifting.
- Use rhythmic, smooth, and coordinated motions at a reasonable speed.
- Use elbows, hips, and knees as levers when lifting.
- Use mechanical devices when appropriate.
- Holding the breath during a physical activity is an indication of muscle strain and inefficient use of body mechanics.

move in bed, the bed height should be raised to a level close to the nurse's center of gravity, usually between the hips and waist. Usually, lowering the side rails allows the nurse to move the client as close as possible and avoid awkward positioning involved in reaching over side rails to perform tasks. When moving the client from the bed to a stretcher, the two surfaces should be at the same height so that the client does not need to be lifted.

The fourth rule is to use mechanical lifts or assistance whenever needed to facilitate a move. In many situations, a lift sheet (also called a turn or draw sheet) is helpful. This is a sturdy sheet that is positioned under the client in bed so that it extends from the shoulders to just below the hips. Depending on the client's weight, two or more nurses (distributed on each side of the bed) can use the lift sheet to move the client anywhere on the mattress and then to position the client onto either side. The key to successful use of the lift sheet is coordinating the movement of the lifters.

Moving a client in bed may include turning or repositioning the client relative to the head of the bed. The client should be included in planning for the change and encouraged to assist whenever possible. Overhead trapezes may provide handholds for clients who wish to assist. Putting the bed in the flat, horizontal position minimizes the muscle work needed to reposition the client. If the client cannot assist because of weakness, confusion, or illness, it is better for the client to cross the arms over the chest than to hold onto the nurse's neck or arms. The nurse can then coordinate and carry out the movement without the risk of unpredictable oppositional pulling from the client.

Of the several techniques for transferring a client from the bed to a wheelchair, chair, or commode, the chosen technique depends on the client's ability to assist and cooperate, the nurse's skill, and the number of assistants. The client should wear nonskid footwear and if possible, a transfer belt snugly around the waist. After explaining the sequence of actions to the client, the nurse may use the counting technique to coordinate everyone's efforts. Mechanical lifts are recommended when the client cannot assist or cooperate or when the nurse is uncertain about the safety of the transfer.

Exercise

Exercise that actively requires alignment, posture, balance, and coordinated movement offers many physiologic and psychological benefits. Exercise must be regular and integrated into the person's lifestyle for maximum benefit. Whether a person values and participates in exercise may be influenced by his or her family, culture, job, and health. In recent years, exercise has become more popular as people have taken responsibility for decreasing risk factors and leading a healthier life.

Types of Exercise. Exercise may be classified by the source of energy (aerobic or anaerobic) and by the type of muscle tension (isotonic or isometric).

Aerobic exercise requires oxygen to use the energy provided by the metabolic activities of the skeletal muscles. Vigorous, continuous muscle movement (as in walking, running, cycling, cross-country skiing, aerobic dance, or tennis) may be aerobic exercise if the person's heart rate is high enough to promote cardiovascular conditioning.

Anaerobic exercise occurs when the muscle cannot extract enough oxygen from the blood, and anaerobic pathways are used to provide the additional energy for a short time. This type of exercise is useful in endurance training for athletes.

Isotonic exercise is a dynamic form of exercise in which there is constant muscle tension, muscle contraction, and active movement. Most activities (walking, running, activities of daily living, and range-of-motion exercises) are isotonic.

Isometric exercise is static exercise in which the muscle undergoes tension and contraction but no change in length and no joint movement. Examples of isometric exercise are quadriceps setting to strengthen the quadriceps muscle, maintaining strength in immobilized muscles (casts, traction), and endurance training.

Benefits of Exercise. Exercise provides multiple benefits and affects all physiologic and psychosocial functioning. Exercise strengthens muscles, increases endurance, and promotes joint mobility. Cardiovascular health improves as lung capacity increases, resting pulse rate and blood pressure decrease, and the risk of artherosclosis decreases. Exercise prevents constipation, enhances appetite, and improves sleep quality. Exercise contributes to a feeling of well-being; the activity increases circulating endorphins and promotes the release of tension and stress. Weight loss and improved physical appearance often motivate people to continue exercising regularly. The person who does not exercise regularly is at risk for health problems, just as the immobile client is at risk for problems related to disuse.

In the United States, national health goals listed in *Healthy People 2000* (1991) include physical activity and fitness. Following are two specific goals:

- Increasing to 30% the proportion of people 6 years and older who participate in daily light to moderate physical activity
- Reducing to no more than 15% the proportion of people 6 years and older who engage in no leisure time physical activity

Characteristics of Normal Movement

Full Range of Motion

Range of motion (ROM) is the ability to move all joints through the full extent of intended function. Each joint must be kept actively moving for the joints to maintain mobility, the muscles to maintain strength, and the cardiovascular system to function adequately.

Active ROM means that the person can initiate and perform exercises in which each joint moves through its complete ROM. The healthy person may complete active ROM as a part of everyday activities and exercise.

Joints move through various planes and ROMs, depending on the type of joint. Table 33-1 shows the types of joints and their designated ROMs.

Normal Gait

Walking is the most common form of locomotion. Although most people take the ability to walk for granted, the normal walking **gait,** the style and character of a person's walk, is a coordinated process requiring equilibrium and balanced posture. To walk efficiently, the person must have strong leg muscles (antigravity support), alternate extension and flexion of the legs (stepping ability), have controlled center of gravity for equilibrium, and have neuromuscular ability to initiate forward motion (Vander, Sherman, & Luciano, 1994). The normal walking gait has two phases:

- The stance phase is composed of three events: heel strike, midstance, and push-off.
- The swing phase completes the walking gait with another three events: acceleration, swing through, and deceleration.

Walking is initiated by stepping with a slight forward tilt. The weight of the body is rolled off the ball and toes of one foot and shifted to the heel of the opposite foot and extended leg. In the process, the center of gravity moves from one side to the other and forward at the same time. The body weight is balanced on a narrow base, shifted from one side to the other, and supported alternately on one foot and then the other.

Terms Describing Joint Motion

Adduction	Moving a joint or extremity toward the midline of the body
Abduction	Moving a joint or extremity away from the midline of the body
Rotation, internal	Turning a joint or extremity on its axis toward the body's midline
Rotation, external	Turning a joint or extremity on its axis away from the body's midline
Flexion	Decreasing the angle between two bones
Extension	Straightening a joint
Hyperextension	Moving a joint past normal extension
Supination	Turning the body or a body part to face upward
Pronation	Turning the body or a body part to face downward
Circumduction	Moving a body part in widening circles
Inversion	Turning the feet inward so toes point toward the midline
Eversion	Turning the feet outward so toes are pointing away from the midline
Opposition	Touching the thumb to each finger

Factors Affecting Normal Mobility

Intact Musculoskeletal System

Normal mobility requires adequate muscle strength, bone resiliency and strength, and full ROM of the joints. The integrity of the musculoskeletal system may be affected by anything that interrupts these factors. Muscle strength may be affected by fluid and electrolyte levels, exercise, conditioning, adequate nutrition, or the condition of tendons, ligaments, or soft tissue. Exercise increases muscle tone, mass, and strength and enhances the condition of other musculoskeletal tissues and body organs.

The function of the bones and joints depends on the mineral content of bones, which gives them adequate resilience, and on the flexibility of joints and their tendons and ligaments. Adequate dietary calcium, phosphorus, and vitamin B are essential to maintain bone resilience and an intact skeletal system. Joints must be able to move through their entire ROM so that the body can move freely and maintain mobility.

Nervous System Control

Normal mobility requires the smooth control of movement provided by the nervous system. Motor ability depends on the integrity of the multisynaptic pathways of the afferent and efferent nerves and the central integration provided by the cerebral cortex. Nerve conduction, in turn, needs adequate circulation and an appropriate fluid and electrolyte environment. Balance and stability are the product of equilibrium, which can be affected by some medications, fatigue, or situations that temporarily impair vision and visual input to the vestibular system in the semicircular canals.

Circulation and Oxygenation

The skeletal muscles need adequate amounts of oxygen to function at an optimal level. The lungs must be able to provide oxygen to the hemoglobin while removing carbon dioxide, the by-product of aerobic metabolism in the muscles. The heart must be able to pump adequately to the muscles and to supply other body organs with enough blood to meet the increased demands imposed by exercise. The vasculature must be able to redirect proportionally larger amounts of blood to the muscles, often shunting blood flow away from the gut, during periods of extreme exercise.

Energy

Energy for muscle function is derived from using oxygen and the breakdown products of food to produce muscle contraction. There are two primary types of metabolism: aerobic and anaerobic. In aerobic metabolism, the oxidative processes that produce energy occur in the mitochondria of cells; water and carbon dioxide are the by-products of this process. Aerobic metabolism is the most efficient form of energy production for long-term activity.

In anaerobic metabolism, a process known as glycolysis converts stored glycogen to energy. This process

Table 33-1 • Normal Movement of Body Joints

Location in Body	Type of Joint	Normal Movement
Neck, cervical spine	Pivotal Supine Cervical	Flexion, extension, lateral flexion, rotation

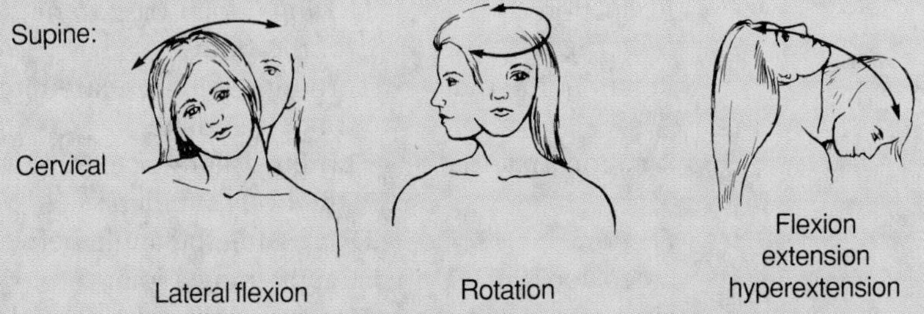

Shoulder	Ball and socket	Flexion, extension, hyperextension, abduction, adduction, internal rotation, external rotation, circumduction

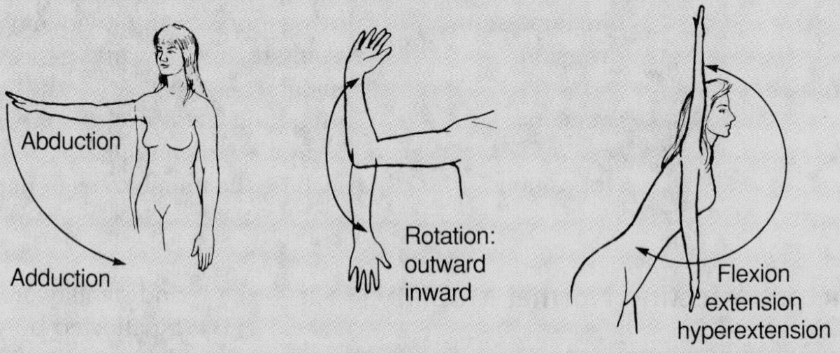

Elbow	Hinge joints	

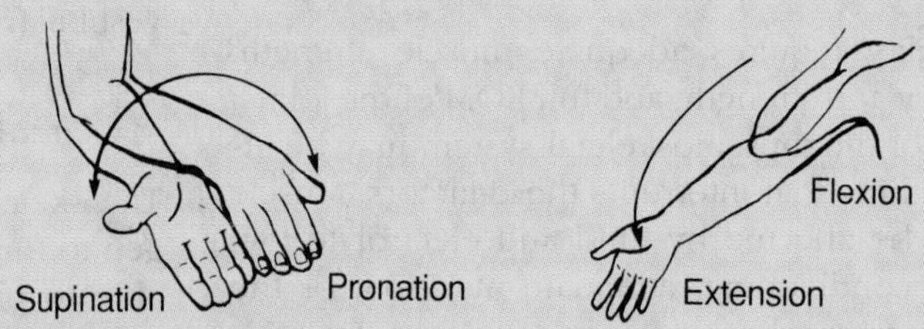

Forearm	Pivotal	Supination, pronation
Wrist	Condyloid	Flexion, extension, hyperextension, adduction, abduction

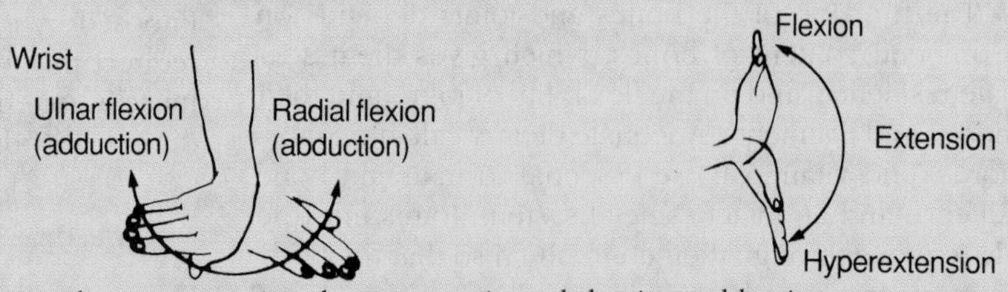

Fingers	Condyloidal hinge	Flexion, extension, hyperextension, abduction, adduction

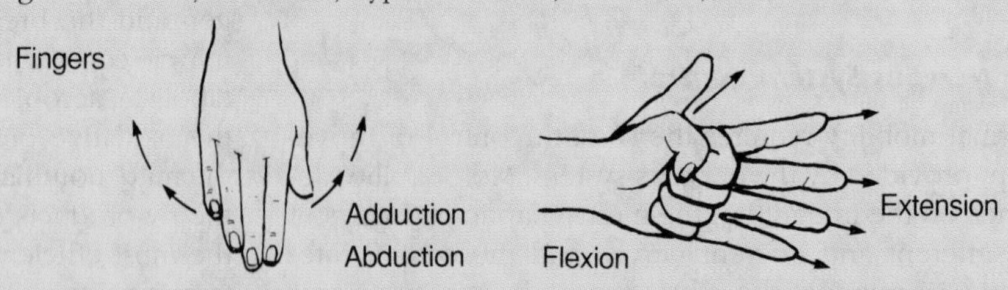

Thumb	Saddle	Flexion, extension, abduction, adduction, apposition

(continued)

Table 33-1 *(Continued)*

<table>
<tr><th>Location in Body</th><th>Type of Joint</th><th>Normal Movement</th></tr>
<tr><td>Hip</td><td>Ball and socket</td><td>Flexion, extension, hyperextension, abduction, adduction, internal rotation, external rotation, circumduction

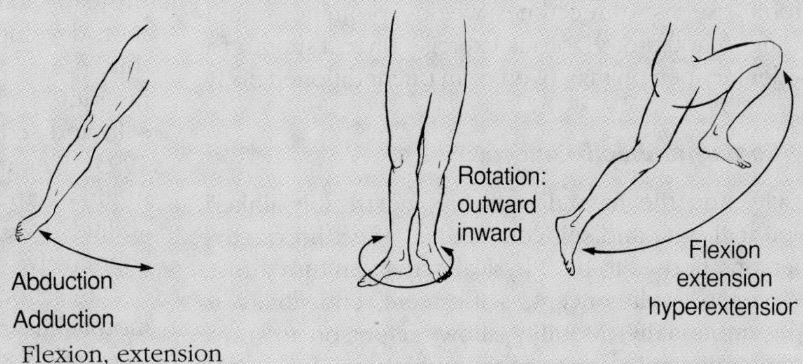

</td></tr>
<tr><td>Knee</td><td>Hinge joint</td><td>Flexion, extension

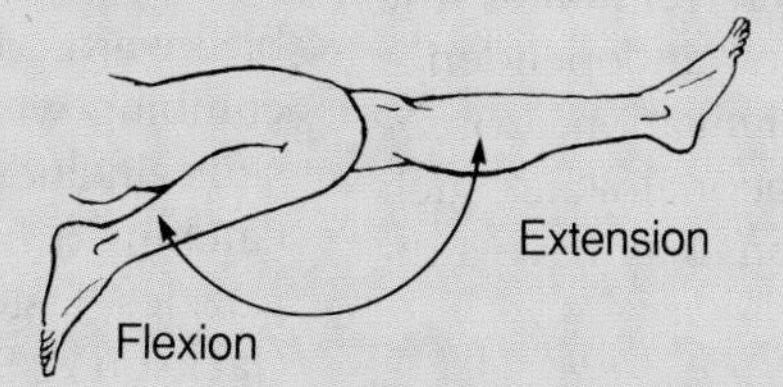

</td></tr>
<tr><td>Ankle</td><td>Hinge joint</td><td>Dorsal flexion, plantar flexion

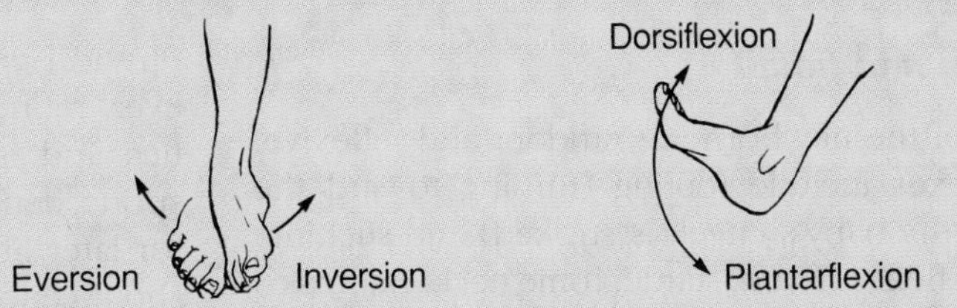

</td></tr>
<tr><td>Foot</td><td>Gliding</td><td>Inversion, eversion</td></tr>
<tr><td>Toes</td><td>Condyloid</td><td>Flexion, extension, abduction, adduction

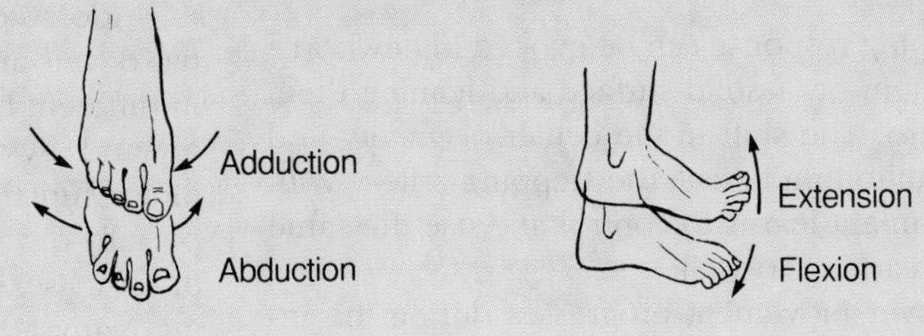

</td></tr>
</table>

provides energy when the oxygen supply is inadequate or delayed; lactic acid is the by-product. The depletion of stored glycogen in the presence of lactic acid produces fatigue in a short time, so this type of metabolism is useful only for short bursts of energy.

Pregnancy

Pregnancy may have an impact on mobility and exercise tolerance. By altering the center of gravity, the expanding uterus affects the pregnant woman's balance. Moderate exercise and toning are usually recommended during pregnancy, but excessive exercise can contribute to heat stress and venous pooling, which can cause hemodynamic changes that affect fetal oxygenation (Yeo, 1994). Swimming is an excellent exercise during pregnancy.

Lifestyle and Habits

The effectiveness of the musculoskeletal system is related to the way in which a person lives. Regular exercise and optimal nutrition are essential to maintain normal mobility and musculoskeletal functioning. If a person has a balanced approach to activity, nutrition, and exercise, mobility will be maintained. The maxim "use it or lose it" is particularly true in regard to the musculoskeletal system: It must be used regularly to maintain function. Regular, ongoing exercise is required for optimal conditioning. About 30 minutes of strenuous aerobic exercise three times weekly promotes conditioning; 6 hours of vigorous exercise once a month for a sedentary person may overtax an unconditioned body.

Coping and Self-Concept

Activity and the mental state are inextricably linked. Emotional state and self-concept can affect how active a person chooses to be. Physical activity in turn affects the person's self-concept, self-esteem, and ability to cope emotionally. Mobility allows a person to move toward enjoyable experiences, which reinforces the activity. The subsequent feeling of independence enhances intellectual and sensory stimulation. Consequently, situations that alter the emotional state, such as fatigue, sadness, grief, or depression, may have a direct effect on mobility.

Lifespan Considerations

Newborn and Infant

Movements of the newborn are random and reflexive. Survival reflexes include rooting (turning toward the breast when the baby's cheek is stroked) and sucking. Subcortical reflexes (Moro, startle, tonic neck, Babinski) subside as higher brain function matures and exerts an inhibitory influence. Protective reflexes (gag, blink, and withdrawal) persist into adulthood (Jackson & Saunders, 1993).

The stepping response can be evoked in newborns by holding them on a solid surface and leaning them slightly forward. The shift in the center of gravity and change in equilibrium initiate the stepping reflex. With maturity, the infant learns to control and use the same reflex when learning to walk.

Control over movement progresses during the infant's first year as the neurologic system matures. Development proceeds from proximal to distal parts and in a head-to-toe fashion; babies progress from being able to control their heads, to rolling over, to crawling, to pulling themselves up to a standing position, to standing, and finally to walking. Each successive task requires increasingly coordinated movement. Refinement of the gross motor skills precedes fine motor skills. The ages at which specific tasks are accomplished vary, but the development always occurs in an orderly progression. Motor activity during the first year characterizes many of the changes that occur in the infant. For this reason, parents often use motor development as a yardstick to evaluate the progress of their infant.

Toddler and Preschooler

The ages from 1 to 5 years are marked by refinement of gross and fine motor skills and by nearly boundless energy. Walking is usually mastered soon after the first birthday. Walking begins with a wide stance and unsteady gait, hence the term **toddler.** Among common developmental tasks mastered in the second and third year of life are coordinated walking, running, jumping, climbing stairs, throwing a ball, feeding oneself, and scribbling with crayons (Jackson & Saunders, 1993). Fine motor skills generally develop more rapidly in girls than in boys. Young children use their physical abilities to explore their environment and to develop cognitively.

Preschoolers continue to increase gross and fine motor skills rapidly. Gross motor activities mastered before school typically include riding a tricycle, walking backward, dancing, skipping, running, jumping, and climbing well (Jackson & Saunders, 1993). Fine motor skills include using crayons to draw or make letters, catching a ball, stringing beads, brushing teeth, doing puzzles, fastening or using zippers, and washing hands (Jackson & Saunders, 1993).

Child and Adolescent

Physical growth slows between 6 and 12 years. However, refinement of gross and fine motor skills continues and is often supported by group activities (eg, sports, dancing, or swimming lessons). Exercise patterns for later life are often determined at this time. Parents should encourage regular physical exercise while avoiding excessive pressure on children to excel. Such expectations can be emotionally and physically damaging for youngsters whose muscles are not fully developed.

Adolescence is a period of rapid physical and sexual development. Because of rapid and varied growth in different body parts, teenagers typically appear gangly and awkward. Consequently, the resulting uneven motor function affects body image, which can be especially distressing for the adolescent. Additionally, the onset of sexual development and growth varies, causing many adolescents to believe that they are not maturing at a normal rate. Most schools require some physical education as a graduation requirement, and many students engage in competitive sports or other school-sponsored physical activities, such as dancing. Physical activities are an acceptable outlet for sexual tension during the adolescent years.

Adult and Older Adult

Between ages 20 and 40 years, relatively few physical changes occur that affect mobility, although late-term pregnancy can limit vigorous physical activity. Adults who have jobs that require repetitive movement (eg, typists, assembly line workers, supermarket checkers,

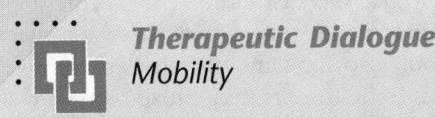

Therapeutic Dialogue
Mobility

Scenes for Thought

Jeannette Frost is an 82-year-old woman who has suffered shoulder problems during the last year and who had a surgical repair of her right shoulder 6 months ago. She comes to the clinic for assessment of her range of motion and pain in the affected shoulder. She drove herself to the clinic.

Effective

Nurse: *Hello Mrs. Frost. I'm Natalie Richmond, the nurse practitioner you'll be seeing today. How are you? (Looking at the chart.)*
Client: *Fine.* She is elegantly dressed, sits quietly, and doesn't smile at you.
Nurse: *(Sits down at the desk and pays attention.) What can I help you with today?*
Client: *I want to see how much more I can do with my arm. I can only raise it this high.* Shows you, using her left arm to help the right. Looks serious.
Nurse: *You're concerned about that arm. (Good eye contact.)*
Client: *Yes. I live alone.*
Nurse: *You live alone, and you're worried you won't be able to manage with your arm the way it is? Am I getting that right? (Using good eye contact.)*
Client: *No, I can manage the way it is. I don't want it to get worse.* Looks more serious. Her eyes are moist.
Nurse: *I can see how concerned you are. I'd like to examine your shoulder and ask you a few questions, then we can talk about the answers to your questions. Does that sound alright with you?*
Client: *Yes, that will be fine.*
(After the assessment, Natalie discusses the swimming and physical therapy that Mrs. Frost is doing and how they're helping to maintain the range of motion she has in her shoulder.)
Nurse: *It seems that the exercises you're doing are keeping your shoulder in the shape it is now. If you stop the exercises, there is a risk that you will lose motion, and it will be harder for you to do your cooking, housework, and entertaining. Otherwise, you're doing a good job. (Pause.) Is there something you want to say?*
Client: *No, I think you answered everything I had on my mind.* Pause. *Could I come back and see you again so you can check to see that the shoulder is still okay?*
Nurse: *Certainly. You can call me, too. Here's my card with my number.*
Client: *Thank you very much.* She smiles.

Less Effective

Nurse: *Hello Mrs. Frost. I'm Nancy Robertson, the nurse practitioner you'll be seeing today. How are you? (Looking at the chart.)*
Client: *Fine.* She is elegantly dressed, sits quietly, and doesn't smile at you.
Nurse: *(Sits down at the desk and pays attention.) What can I help you with today?*
Client: *I want to see how much more I can do with my arm. I can only raise it this high.* Shows you, using her left arm to help the right. Looks serious.
Nurse: *You're concerned about that arm. (Good eye contact.)*
Client: *Yes. I live alone.*
Nurse: *I see that your husband is listed as your emergency contact, but he has a different address. (Looking through the chart then looking at the client questioningly.)*
Client: *Yes. I live by myself.* Looks embarrassed and annoyed.
Nurse: *(Realizing this is not a safe subject.) Well, I can understand you're concerned about doing your housework and cooking and so forth. Let me examine your shoulder and see how much more you might be able to do with your arm. (Assesses range of motion and discusses swimming and physical therapy that Mrs. Frost is already doing and how they're helping to maintain her current functioning.) It seems that this is as good as this shoulder's going to get, Mrs. Frost. But it sounds as though you're doing everything you can to keep it in good shape, so I wouldn't worry if I were you. If it gets any worse, feel free to call me, and we'll go over it again. Okay?*
Client: Getting dressed. *Fine.* No eye contact.
Nurse: *'Bye now.*

Critical Thinking Challenges

Compare and contrast Natalie's and Nancy's actions and assessment styles. • *Analyze how Nancy talked to Mrs. Frost.* • *Recognize the emotions Mrs. Frost exhibited, and infer emotions from her nonverbal behavior.* • *Determine how you might feel working with a client who is reserved and does not show emotions readily.* • *Formulate some helpful skills that could be used when working with Mrs. Frost.*

computer operators) may develop carpal tunnel syndrome, a nerve compression that causes pain and decreases mobility in the hand. As the adult approaches middle age (40–60 years), muscle tone and bone density and mass decrease. Further deterioration in the musculoskeletal system occurs as a person ages. Joints lose elasticity and flexibility. Bone mass decreases, especially in women with osteoporosis, resulting in an increased incidence of fractures. Additionally, altered coordination affects normal gait, and a slowing reaction time delays the overall body response to stressors.

Aging brings postural changes and chronic joint disorders. Flattening of the lumbar spine and changes in the intervertebral disks and vertebral bodies may cause the head and upper spine to tilt forward, shifting the center of gravity. Joint degeneration and bone demineralization also affect balance and gait. As a result, the older person usually has less extension and swing through and more side-to-side sway; weight is transferred from the ball of one foot to the ball of the other foot, leading to a wide-based, short-stepped, shuffling gait.

The older person has more difficulty overcoming inertia and using gravity efficiently. One reason for this is the shift in the center of gravity. In an effort to compensate for the shift, the knees flex slightly for support. The resulting posture is a forward-leaning crouch with a widened base. Chronic health problems or injuries from falls also affect the mobility of older adults.

Altered Mobility

Potential for Altered Mobility

Normal mobility can be altered by congenital problems, conditions that impair the musculoskeletal or neurologic systems, chronic illness that depletes strength and endurance, injury or trauma, affective disorders, and treatments that require restrictive devices or voluntary restriction on movement.

Congenital Problems

Congenital problems can affect normal musculoskeletal or neurologic development. Some, such as congenital hip dysplasia, can be corrected with treatment. Others, such as spina bifida or cerebral palsy, cannot be cured, so the treatment goals are maximal functional mobility and minimal complications.

Neuromuscular Deficits

Any disorder that impairs the ability of the nervous system to control muscular movement and coordination hinders functional mobility. Usually these disorders (for example, muscular dystrophy, Parkinson's disease, and multiple sclerosis) are progressive, slowly eroding and destroying the ability to move normally until the person is confined to bed or a wheelchair.

Impairments of the brain or spinal cord also affect normal movement. Central nervous system control can be disrupted by infectious processes (eg, meningitis), tumors, or cerebrovascular accidents (strokes). Treatment can limit or reverse some damage to the central nervous system, but at times, dysfunction is permanent and severe.

Musculoskeletal Deficits

Any impairment of the musculoskeletal system can affect joint mobility, skeletal strength, and body movement. Demineralization of the bone, as in osteoporosis or multiple myeloma, increases the risk of fractures. Rheumatoid arthritis, degenerative joint disease (osteoarthritis), and gout also limit mobility because movement causes pain. Bone tumors may cause pain as well and may require amputation of an affected limb.

Chronic Health Problems

Chronic illnesses commonly decrease mobility because many chronic disorders limit the supply of oxygen and nutrients needed for muscle contraction and movement. Chronic cardiovascular conditions, such as congestive heart failure or peripheral vascular disease, limit effective blood flow, especially during periods of increased need, such as aerobic exercise. Lung disorders decrease the amount of oxygen delivered to all body tissues, including skeletal muscles. Cancer or other conditions that strain nutritional stores deplete the energy necessary for movement.

Trauma

Trauma usually results in accidental injury to joints, tendons, ligaments, muscles, or bones. The damage may be minor, affecting mobility for only a short (eg, a strain caused by overexerting a muscle or a sprain caused by twisting a joint), or it may be more extensive, involving a dislocated joint, torn tendons, broken bones, or joint replacements. Immobilizing devices are usually used to keep healing body parts in normal alignment.

Severe trauma also can cause extensive damage to the spinal cord or brain. When the spinal cord is severed or severely damaged, paralysis occurs below the level of injury. The term *paraplegia* describes decreased motor and sensory function to the legs. *Quadriplegia* describes paralysis of the arms and the legs.

Affective Disorders

Severe affective disorders can hinder mobility. Depression and catatonic states result in limited mobility, not because of physical impairments but because the person lacks the desire to move. Fear, especially of pain on movement, may cause some people to restrict their movements as well.

Therapeutic Modalities

Sometimes limited movement is the treatment for a medical problem. Restrictive devices, such as casts, braces, and splints, can immobilize certain areas of the body to promote healing. Bed rest is another treatment whereby mobility is restricted for therapeutic benefits. A client may be placed on bed rest for the following reasons:

- To promote healing and tissue repair by decreasing metabolic needs
- To relieve edema (swelling)

- To reduce oxygen requirements of the body
- To decrease pain
- To support a weak, exhausted, or febrile client

Bed rest must be psychologically and physically restful. The definition of bed rest may vary to some extent: Some healthcare providers permit clients on bed rest to use a bedside commode; others insist on strict confinement to bed. No matter what the modality, the more complex the therapy, the more client care will involve collaboration among healthcare specialists. (For a summary of collaborative care, see the example of a critical pathway for a client with a total hip replacement.)

Manifestations of Altered Mobility

The client with altered mobility may have various symptoms of varying intensity. Common manifestations are decreased muscle strength and tone, lack of coordination, altered gait, falls, decreased joint flexibility, pain on movement, and decreased ability to tolerate activity.

Decreased Muscle Strength and Tone

Loss of muscle strength and tone is typical of altered mobility. Normal muscle strength is maintained by frequent contraction of the muscle, which occurs during movement. When movement is limited or abnormal, maximal tension is not applied to muscle groups, which decreases the muscle's ability to contract. This may be accompanied by muscle **atrophy,** a decrease in size, possibly from disuse.

Decreased strength is apparent when the client cannot grasp the nurse's hand strongly or can push only weakly with the legs. Weakness may be so severe that the client's leg muscles cannot support his or her body weight. At other times, decreased strength is less obvious. For example, a client may be able to extend his or her arms in front of the body, but after a few minutes, the arms begin to drift down as the muscles become too fatigued to provide adequate support.

Muscle tone, or the normal resistance to stretch, also decreases with inactivity. Decreased muscle tone is called hypotonicity or **flaccidity.** Decreased tone can cause the muscles to stretch (if they are held in a lengthened position) or contract (if they are held in a shortened position). Neurologic impairment that results in increased muscle tone, often called **spasticity,** also can affect normal movement.

Lack of Coordination

Lack of coordination occurs when neurologic control and regulation of movement are impaired. Usually this is the case when trauma or disease affects the cerebellum, which plays an important role in coordinating voluntary muscle movement. Alcohol and certain drugs, such as barbiturates, also may interfere with normal coordinated movement. Uncoordinated movement appears jerky and uneven and affects the person's ability to move purposefully and efficiently. Many terms are used to describe alterations in coordinated, purposeful movement:

Ataxia is a general term used to describe defective muscle coordination.

A *tremor* is a rhythmic, repetitive movement that can occur at rest or when movement is initiated. A tremor usually interferes with fine motor control, but in Parkinson's disease, it also can interfere with coordinated ambulation.

Chorea is spontaneous, brief, involuntary muscle twitching of the limbs or facial muscles; severe chorea hinders mobility.

Athetosis is movement characterized by slow, irregular, twisting motions.

Dystonia is similar to athetosis but usually involves larger areas of the body.

Altered Gait

Abnormal gait can affect the rhythm, steadiness, or speed of walking.

An ataxic gait is characterized by staggering and unsteadiness.

When walking appears stiff and toes appear to catch and drag, the gait is called spastic.

Walking with feet wide apart in a ducklike fashion is called a waddling gait.

A hemiplegic gait occurs when one leg is paralyzed or neurologically damaged, so the leg is dragged or swung around to propel it forward.

A festinating gait, typified by walking on the toes as if being pushed, is common in Parkinson's disease.

Falls

Clients with mobility limitations are likely to fall from gait changes, weakness, postural hypotension, or diminished coordination. Falls typically result in musculoskeletal trauma, such as fractures, which can further decrease mobility. Sensory and cognitive changes in the older person, combined with medication usage, further increase the risk of falls for this age group. Fear of repeated falls may cause some clients to limit their mobility.

Decreased Joint Flexibility

Decreased joint flexibility typically occurs with altered mobility because decreased movement causes joints to stiffen. This decreases normal ROM, because fibrosis

(text continues on page 845)

Collaborative Care Plan: Critical Pathway (Hospital)

Client Name: ____________________
Case Type: Total Hip Replacement (THR)
DRG: 209
ICD-9: ____________________

Admit Date: ____________
Date Path Initiated: ____________

Expected LOS: 4 days
Actual LOS: ____________
Discharge Date: ____________

Physician: ____________
Case Manager: ____________

Outcome Criteria

	Preop 4–6 wks to 1 wk				Day of Surg/P O Day 1				Post Op Day 2–4			
Client Problems		D	E	N		D	E	N		D	E	N
Knowledge deficit related to pre & po care & sensations, hip precautions, & activity progression.	Client/family verbalizes understanding of pre & po sensations & care; diet & activity progression; hip precautions; equipment needed at home & unusual course of recovery.				Performs C&DB, & incentive spirometer. Performs isometric exercises (ankle pumps, quad & gluteal sets). Demonstrates position & activity restriction (no hip flexion >90°, no crossing legs or internal rotation				States complications to report to MD. Verbalizes understanding of hip precautions, activity & exercise pgm, safety precautions, equipment needed. States S & S of complications & when to notify health provider. Demonstrates ambulation techniques & proper use of walker, crutches, or cane. Verbalizes S & S of bleeding precautions where on anticoagulants.			
Pain related to surgical trauma to tissues, manipulation of hip joint, edema, & muscle spasms.	Verbalizes understanding of pain rating scale (0-10), pain mgt techniques, usage of PCA pump/-epidural analgesia.				Rates pain <4 on scale of 0-10 30 min past IV/IM pain med. Verbalizes understanding of usage of PGA pump				Rates pain <2 on scale 0-10 30 min past po pain med. Transfers & ambulates, performs ADL's with minimal pain. No significant increase in hip pain, calf pain, or chest pain.			
Altered mobility related to pain, weakness, & activity restrictions.	Activity at tol. with assistance devices as needed.				Turn c̄ abduction pillow Transfers from bed to standing position c̄ assist of PT. ______full wt bearing ______partial wt bearing HOB <45° Performs isometric exercises (ankle pumps, quad & glut sets) Follows hip precau-				Demonstrates correct transfer technique s̄ flexing hip >80°. Transfers to reclining chair for meals c̄ full—partial wt bearing Ambulates c̄ assistive devices independently Follows hip precaution Performs isometric exercises. Skin intact. Bowel movement 2-4 days po No evidence of infection or hip dislocation			

	Preop 4–6 wks to 1 wk				Day of Surg/P O Day 1				Post Op Days 2–4			
Client Problems		D	E	N		D	E	N		D	E	N
High risk for neurovascular dysfunction related to trauma to nerves & blood vessels, edema, or incorrect alignment/& positioning	Intact neurovascular (NV) function (6P's) in affected & unaffected extremities →				Intact NV function (6P's): → Absence of polar (coldness) → pallor pulselessness parasthesia paralysis pain in affected extremity				Intact NV function (6P's) No S & S of DVT/PE (no calf, posterior knee pain, swelling, redness, warmth or chest pain)			
High risk for injury related to falls, hip dislocation, and bleeding due to anticoagulants	No injury or falls will occur No hip dislocation (no significant ↑ in pain) No bleeding or blood in stools, urine				→ → → → → →				→ → No bleeding or blood in urine or stools PT/PTT WNL			
Critical Path												
Consult/Referral	Anesthesiologist/surgeon-hip/consult Social services/ Case manager				PT-exercise pgm OT-adaptive aids →				Assess need for Home Health Care (RN or home health aide, VNA services) Arrange for outpt PT services. Follow up visit social service			
Diagnostic Tests	Schedule for pre op labs-CBC, lytes, Chem7, PT/PTT, UA EKG, CXR & Hip or Pelvis X ray T&C 2 u blood Schedule autologous blood donation				Hematocrit Pro Time				→ →			
Assessment	Assess understanding of THR procedure, effect on lifestyle. Assess anxiety/concern related to surgery Neurovascular (NV) assess (6p's) on affected extremity (baseline)				NV (6P's) Assess q 1-2° VS q1° $\times$ 4, then q 4° $\times$ 4 02 sat Assess wound/dsg q 2° Monitor hemovac/constavac q 8° Monitor PCA/epidural-Assess for Sx Hip dislocation Bowel sounds, Guaiac stools if on anticoagulant				NV assess (6P's) q 4hr.VS q 8° DC O_2 sat if >92% Chg dsg-strict asepsis Assess for Sx infection DC hemovac/constavac per order DC PCA/epidural per order Assess Sx dislocation Guaiac stools if on anticoagulant.			

(continued)

Collaborative Care Plan: Critical Pathway (Hospital) *(continued)*

Client Problems	Preop 4–6 wks to 1 wk	D	E	N	Day of Surg/P O Day 1	D	E	N	P O Day 2–6	D	E	N
Treatments	Surgeon visit/ Informed Consent Permit signed Advance Directives Instruct in Hibiclens shower HS Preop				I & O q8, Foley Cath DC PO Day 1/C&DB, incentive spirometer (IS) q 1° TEDS/antiembolism device; remove 30″ q shift IV fluids/PRBC if needed Hip precaution, leg abduction c̄ pillows/brace Isometric exercises O_2 2-4L/NC Reinforce drsg as needed				I & O q 8°, Cath if unable to void C & DB, IS q 2-4° TEDS while up—may be removed HS Heplock IV Hip precaution Isometric exercises DC O_2 if O_2 sat >92% ⟶			
Activity	Up as tolerated c̄ assistive devices if needed				Overhead trapeze Bed rest, turn to unaffected side c̄ abductor pillow Trochanter roll/sandbag to hip Hip precautions, avoid hip flexion >90° Isometric exercises, ankle pumps, quad & glute sets Massage, skin care TED hose				Stand to transfer c̄ PT assist Full wt-bearing Partial wt-bearing High/recliner chair/ raised toilet seat Chair, legs apart, no crossing Up all meals No prolonged sitting or standing; isometric exercises Shower if wound closed Amb. in hall per walker QID No knee gatch on bed			
Diets	Diet as tol NPO p̄ mn and HS prior Surg				Clear liquids–advance as tol IV fluids as needed				Diet as tolerated DC IV's			
Meds	Identify client's routine meds; Teach client about meds, pain mgt (PCA pump) Anticoagulant (Coumadin day before or)				Pain meds—IM/IV/ PCA pump Pain Rating Scale 0-10 Anticoagulants Stool softeners Antibiotics IV				Pain meds PO-DC PCA Admin pain meds prior to exercises, and ambulation Laxative/Stool softeners as needed Suppository if no BM 3 days Comfort measures/-positioning			

Collaborative Care Plan: Critical Pathway (Hospital) *(continued)*

Client Problems	**Preop 4–6 wks to 1 wk**	D	E	N	**Day of Surg/P O Day 1**	D	E	N	**P O Day 2–6**	D	E	N
Teaching	Pre-op class for THR, view video Send PKT home Explain pain mgt (PCA) Coumadin teaching Pathway given to client/family Teach hip precaution				Instruct in correct use of trapeze Review pain rating scale; PCA/epidural Reinforce pre/po care (TCDB, IS, exercises, calf pumps, quads & glute sets Reinforce hip precaution (abduction pillows, no crossing legs, hip flexion >90°, no internal rotation)				Teach bed to chair transfer techniques c̄ walker, crutches, cane Assure client understanding of hip precaution. Reinforce Coumadin teaching Teach equipment/devices & safety precautions Give written DC plan to client/family			
Discharge/Transfer Planning	Assess DC needs & referrals Evaluate potential need for home health/or SNF transfer Assess need for social services				Assess client understanding of DC plan, equipment needs, activity restriction, hip precautions, lifestyle chgs.				Equipment ordered (walker, raised toilet seats, bars in showers) DC meds ordered Home exercise pgm from PT/OT Identify caregiver, community resources Transportation arranged if needed to skilled care facility. Follow up appt 6 wk with MD.			

Shift: D = Day
E = Evening
N = Night

Variance reporting: Write "V" for variance in shift column if outcome not achieved or intervention not performed. Explain the client variance in the progress note.

Initials	Signature	Initials	Signature	Initials	Signature

Collaborative Care Plan: Critical Pathway (Home Health)

Client Name: ____________
Case Type: Ttl Hip Rplcmnt (THR)
DRG: ____________
ICD-9: ____________
Date Path Initiated: ____________
Expected LOS: 2 wks po–2 mo
Actual LOS: ____________
Discharge Date: ____________
Physician: ____________
Case Manager: ____________

Home Health—Outcome Criteria

Client Problems	Post Hospital 2 wks	D	E	N	Post Hospital 6 weeks	D	E	N	Post Hospital 3 months	D	E	N
Knowledge deficit related to post op activity & exercise regime & hip precaution	Client/family will verbalize understanding of exercise pgm, activity progression, hip precautions, safety, medication, diet, and wound care				Client/family will state S & S of complications of hip dislocation (sig. ↑ pain, & loss of sensation) Demonstrates safe transfers, ambulation, & chair activity				Client/family verbalizes understanding of po complications (deep vein thrombosis [DVT], hip dislocation) & when to notify health provider			
Pain & discomfort related to surgical trauma, edema, muscle spasms	Rates pain <2 on scale of 0–10 after po pain med. Performs exercises & ambulation s̄ excessive hip pain (<5)				No pain or pain controlled c̄ po pain med. No significant increase in pain with exercises or ambulation				No pain at rest or with activity No significant increase in pain with exercises or ambulation			
Altered Mobility related to pain, weakness, & activity restriction	Performs isotonic/isometric exercises & ADL c̄ caregiver assistance Adheres to position limits of <80° hip flexion, no internal rotation or adduction Weight bearing ambulation as ordered c̄ assistive devices (walker, crutches) Sits in high (reclining chair) c̄ feet apart; does not cross legs.				Ambulates independently c̄/s̄ assistive devices Performs isotonic & isometric exercises independently Performs ADL's independently Returns to work & ambulates in community (no longer homebound)				Transfers & ambulates safely at home Attains PT outcomes hip flexion >110° c̄ full extension–PT Dcd if outcomes achieved. Performs ADL's/household/work tasks s̄ limitations			
High risk of neurovascular dysfunction related to surgical interruption of nerves & blood vessels, edema, venous stasis or incorrect alignment or position	Neurovascular function intact (6P's)-No pain, paralysis, pallor, polar (cool), pulselessness or paresthesia) in affected extremity				→ No hip dislocation No S&S of DVT or pulmonary embolism				→ → →			
High risk for injury related to falls, hip dislocation, bleeding due to anticoagulants	No injury or falls will occur No hip dislocation (no extreme pain) No bleeding, urine & stools neg for blood Follows hip & safety precaution				→ → → Demonstrates safety in transfers/ambulation				→ → →			

Collaborative Care Plan: Critical Pathway (Home Health) *(continued)*

	Post Hospital 2 wks.				Post Hospital 6 weeks				Post Hospital 3 months			
Client Problems		D	E	N		D	E	N		D	E	N
Critical Path												
Consult/Referral	Home PT visit 2x/wk outpt PT/OT (adaptive aids) Evaluate need for home health aide Home health RN phone call 1-2 wks PO				Home Health visit by RN/case manager for assessment/evaluation of progress. Continue outpt PT services 2-3x/wk Office visit to orthopedic surgeon				Follow-up office visit to orthopedic surgeon 3, 6, 12 mo. Follow-up X rays 2 yrs & 5 yrs Return to family MD Evaluate need for PT services			
Diagnostic Tests	Pro Time 2x/wk for 4–6 wks.				Pro Time 1x wk until Coumadin DC'd or 6 wks.				Possible X-rays hip & pelvis			
Assessment	Safety of home & mobility; hip precautions assessed by PT in home. Neurovascular assessment (6P's); degree of flexion & mobility, status of wound, S & S of complications Assess need for assistive & safety devices.				Home health RN to assess NV (6P's) status in affected extremity (polar (cold) pallor, pain, pulselessness, paresthesia, paralysis) Condition of wound, assess ROM of hip/leg, functional mobility.				Assess NV status of affected extremity, S&S of complication (hip dislocation, DVT) Condition of wound (S&S of infection) & functional mobility			
Treatment	Home PT for 2 wk Implement prescribed exercise pgm all affected joints (isometric – or quad, gluteal sets) & isotonic (or calf pumping). TED hose when OOB for dependent edema Remove staples/steristrips				Outpt PT 2x/wk for 6 wk—3 mo. Continue advancing exercises & ambulation Home health visit by RN to evaluate compliance c̄ exercise pgm, hip precautions, functional mobility, incision, & complications. TED hose for dependent edema—remove at night Assess wound				Home health RN evaluate exercise/activity progression & need for further PT if functional outcome not met, or need for further physician follow-up → →			
Activity	No abduction pillow-Use regular pillow between knees when in bed. Full wt bearing on standard THR. If cementless THR, partial wt bearing & no resistive exercises c̄ assistive device (walker) Sit with high chair, feet together, knees apart Reinforce exercises/strengthening & ROM				Continue pillow between knees when in bed Advance activity & ambulation c̄ or s̄ assistive device (walker if needed) Evaluate & advance exercises for strengthening & ROM				→ Independent ambulation c̄ or s̄ assist devices (if needed for safety) Continue strengthening & ROM exercises			

(continued)

Collaborative Care Plan: Critical Pathway (Home Health) *(continued)*

Client Problems	Post Hosp 2 wks	D	E	N	Post Hospital 6 wks	D	E	N	Post Hospital 3 months	D	E	N
Diet	Diet as tol				⟶	⟶			⟶			
	Adeq. fluids & fiber to prevent constipation				⟶	⟶			⟶			
	Low calorie—avoid obesity				⟶	⟶			⟶			
Meds	Instruct client to take po analgesics prior to exercise & ambulation				PO pain meds PRN & prior to exercises & ambulation.				PO pain meds PRN			
	Assess understanding of meds & side effects											
	Instruct in bowel mgt (LOC, stool softener), Anticoagulants (Coumadin)				Stool softener as needed DC anticoagulant at 6 wks	⟶			⟶			
Teaching	Teach position limits <80 degree hip flexion				Reinforce hip & safety precaution	⟶			⟶			
	No internal rotation or adduction for 6 wks po				Bleeding precaution with Coumadin				Instruct client in need for antibiotics prior to dental work, invasive procedures, or surgery			
	No crossing legs for 3 mo. Reinforce exercises				Reinforce home exercise pgm–gradually increase strengthening & ROM & progress with ambulation				⟶			
	Reinforce safety precautions (handles, grab bars, raised toilet seat, high chair, no throw rugs)											
Discharge/Transfer Planning	Reinforce need for keeping appts c̄ PT/OT.				Evaluate whether PT outcomes met & need to continue to 3 mo.				DC from PT if functional outcomes met			
	Instruct in resources for assistive/adaptive devices				Continue exercises & activity progression				Return to family MD for further followup care.			
	Provide information on community resources (meals on wheels, home health aide)				Reinforce need for continued safety precautions.							

Initials/Signatures:

____

____

____

Shift: D = Day
E = Evening
N = Night

*Variance reporting: Write initials of nurse/health provider in box if outcome met or intervention performed. Write "V" for variance if outcome not met or intervention not performed. Explain client variance in progress notes.

and fixation affect the joint structures. Muscles atrophy when they do not regularly shorten and lengthen during normal muscle contraction. Initially, decreased flexibility and altered ROM occur in affected joints, but if the joints remain immobilized, contractures can occur. A **contracture** is the progressive shortening of a muscle and loss of joint mobility resulting from fibrotic changes in the tissues surrounding the joint.

Pain on Movement

Impaired mobility is often accompanied by pain on movement. Pain can result from physical injury, as in sprains, strains, or torn ligaments, or it may result from degenerative and inflammatory processes. Osteoarthritis (degeneration of the articular surface of weight bearing joints) and rheumatoid arthritis (an inflammatory disorder that affects joints) cause pain on movement, which may cause the client to avoid movement to decrease discomfort.

Incisional pain decreases the willingness of most clients to ambulate during the postoperative period. Pain caused by inadequate blood flow to the extremities (intermittent claudication) also can severely decrease mobility. Cancer, low back pain, and other disorders associated with chronic pain also limit movement.

Activity Intolerance

Decreased ability to tolerate activity often accompanies impaired mobility. **Activity intolerance** is the state in which the person has inadequate physiologic or psychological energy to endure or to complete an activity. A balance must occur between the activity and the client's energy. Symptoms associated with activity intolerance are dyspnea, tachycardia, discomfort, weakness, and fatigue.

Commonly, disorders that affect oxygenation, such as respiratory or cardiac problems, decrease a client's ability to tolerate increases in activity. However, some activity intolerance can be noted in anyone who has been inactive. For example, a 46-year-old man who has been inactive since college will experience activity intolerance if he tries to run 2 miles. Even short periods of immobility can impair activity tolerance.

Impact of Immobility on Function

Immobility affects all areas of function (Table 33-2). Recognizing the possible consequences of immobility allows the nurse to intervene to limit or prevent problems.

Health Perception and Health Management

Immobility often limits the activities and exercise that the client uses to promote health. When mobility decreases, the client is less able to participate in normal activities, including exercise. This decreased activity level can predispose the client to several health problems. Furthermore, impaired mobility or immobility may require the client to learn how to manage such devices as casts, splints, walkers, or canes.

Activity and Exercise

Immobility significantly affects activity and exercise patterns and musculoskeletal, cardiovascular, and respiratory function in several ways.

Muscle Atrophy and Weakness. Immobility decreases muscle strength and mass. In a healthy person who has full freedom of movement, muscles keep their size and strength through frequent muscle contractions. Such contractions occur continually with normal activity and movement. Muscle strength and size are proportional to the conditioning the muscle experiences. In an athlete who vigorously exercises, certain muscles will grow in size and strength, but in a sedentary person who exercises infrequently, the muscles will be smaller and less capable of work.

Reduction in muscle cell size (atrophy) results from the alterations in metabolism that occur during immobility; the body breaks down muscle mass to obtain energy (catabolic metabolism). The resulting changes in strength and mass are substantial and last even after immobility is reversed. Classic experiments by Dietrick et al. (1948) on the effects of immobility on healthy males showed that muscle strength decreased substantially and took 4 to 6 weeks to recover. Leg muscles are affected more by immobilization than other muscles. This is thought to be due to the effects of gravity in maintaining muscle tone. The evidence of atrophy can be seen dramatically when a cast is removed and the limbs are compared.

Endurance (the ability to tolerate exercise) decreases as the muscle atrophies. In many cases, this becomes a vicious cycle. Atrophy experienced by an immobilized client decreases endurance, discouraging the client from engaging in activity and contributing to further atrophy.

Contractures and Joint Pain. In the active, mobile person, movement promotes the formation of new connective tissue that is deposited around joints and muscles. This tissue is loose and pliable and remains so as long as normal body movement occurs. During immobility, stretching of muscles and movement of joints cease, resulting in the deposition of denser, less pliable fibrotic tissue.

Immobility can leave joints fixed and unable to move normally. A **contracture** (progressive shortening of a muscle and loss of joint mobility) results from fibrotic changes that occur when normal mobility is not

Table 33-2 • Comparison of the Effects of Exercise and Immobility on Function

Functional Area	Effects of Exercise	Effects of Immobility
Health perception/ health maintenance	Promotes optimal health and well-being	Increases risk of various health problems
Activity/exercise	Decreases risk of cardiovascular disease Strengthens muscles and increases muscle tone Increases endurance Promotes joint mobility Increases cardiac efficiency Decreases resting pulse rate and blood pressure Improves circulation Increases respiratory rate Increases depth of respirations Improves gas exchange	Causes muscle weakness and atrophy, activity intolerance, contractures Decreases range of motion Increases cardiac workload Causes orthostatic hypotension Increases risk of thrombus formation Decreases lung expansion Promotes retained secretions Impairs gas exchange
Nutritional/metabolic	Increases metabolic rate, appetite, energy Improves skin tone and turgor	Decreases metabolic rate Causes anorexia, negative nitrogen balance, disuse osteoporosis, impaired immunity, skin breakdown, and pressure sore development
Elimination	Increases intestinal tone and motility Increases blood flow to kidneys, promoting optimal excretion of waste products	Decreases intestinal tone and motility Causes constipation, urinary stasis Increases risk of urinary tract infection, renal calculi Decreases bladder tone
Sleep/rest	Improves sleep quality	Decreases sleep quality
Cognitive/perceptual	Increases vitality and well-being	Causes sensory deprivation, confusion, hallucinations, pain and discomfort
Self-perception/ self-concept	Improves appearance, body image, self-concept	Impairs appearance, body image, self-concept
Coping/stress	Reduces stress	Increases stress Produces anxiety, anger, depression, powerlessness
Roles and relationships	Fosters relationships if exercise done in groups	Interferes with roles requiring mobility (eg, going to work, caring for child)
Sexuality	Increases energy available for sexual expression	Can hinder normal sexual expression Immobilizing devices may interfere

maintained. Impaired blood flow to the muscle or joint hastens the formation of contractures. Without appropriate intervention, increasing damage occurs, and a contracture can become irreversible. An irreversible contracture further decreases the person's mobility, because it makes moving the involved muscle difficult or impossible. Contractures also cause disfigurement, which can increase social isolation.

Flexion contractures are most common in immobilized clients. Clients often assume positions of flexion naturally because these positions require less muscle stress and tension to maintain. Also, flexor muscles (those that allow joints to bend) are usually stronger than their extensor counterparts. Common flexor contractures occur at the joints of the elbow, hip, knee, shoulder, wrist, and ankle. **Foot drop** is a contracture in which the foot is fixed in plantar flexion.

Immobility can decrease joint stability as a result of decreased tension exerted by ligaments and muscles secondary to loss of muscle tone. Decreased joint stability is thought to be the cause of aches and pains often experienced by immobilized clients. It also may account for the difficult ambulation and general stiffness that follow inactivity and bed rest.

Increased Cardiac Workload. Cardiac workload is increased in the immobilized client because the heart must work harder when the body is supine than when it is erect. Pooling of blood in the legs usually does not occur in the supine position. With less gravitational pull, blood can be redistributed from the legs to the trunk. This subsequent increase in venous blood returning to the heart means the heart must work harder to circulate the increased volume.

The heart rate also increases in the immobilized client to accommodate the greater amount of blood that must be pumped. Tachycardia (rapid heart rate) in inactive clients is thought to reflect sympathetic nervous system dominance, whereas tachycardia in the active person may reflect parasympathetic dominance (Groer & Shekleton, 1993). An important effect of the increased heart rate in the inactive person is the shorter time between myocardial contractions and therefore the shorter myocardial rest period, which further increase the heart's workload.

Orthostatic Hypotension. *Orthostatic hypotension* is the decreased ability to maintain systemic blood pressure when changing from a supine to an upright position. It is commonly seen after a period of immobility. Position changes do not normally cause systemic blood pressure to drop substantially because arteriolar vasoconstriction prevents large amounts of blood from pooling in the extremities when an upright posture is assumed. Baroreceptors are stimulated when blood flow decreases in the aortic arch and carotid arteries (when, for instance, the person stands up). This in turn triggers increased sympathetic activity, which causes vasoconstriction.

Immobility decreases the effectiveness of this neurovascular reflex. During inactivity, regulatory adjustments are not used and become inactive. Sympathetic stimulation may still occur in response to standing upright, but peripheral vessels do not respond to this stimulation. Therefore, vasoconstriction does not occur, and a drop in blood pressure results.

Another factor that may contribute to orthostatic hypotension is the ineffectiveness of the muscle pump in promoting venous return. This is especially true of muscles atrophied by immobility. As the calf muscles weaken, they are less effective in compressing the veins of the legs and less able to promote venous return. This increases the pooling of blood in the legs and intensifies postural hypotension.

Orthostatic hypotension is not apparent during immobilization, but when the client tries to stand, lightheadedness, dizziness, and increased sympathetic activity (reflected by an elevated pulse rate and diaphoresis) may occur. Loss of consciousness can occur with severe postural hypotension. A postural drop of more than 25 mm Hg in the systolic or 10 mm Hg diastolic blood pressure or an increase of 20 beats/min in pulse rate is considered significant (Skov & Motzer, 1995).

Thrombus Formation and Embolism. A *thrombus* is a blood clot composed of platelets, fibrin, and cellular elements that attaches to the wall of an artery or vein. A thrombus most commonly originates in the large veins of the legs because of the relatively low velocity of blood flow there. This is called *deep vein thrombosis.* When the clot breaks away from the vessel wall and enters circulating blood, it is called an *embolus.* Depending on the size of the original thrombus, the clot can lodge in the circulatory system as the diameter of the vessels decreases. This most commonly occurs when the thrombus enters the pulmonary vasculature, where it interferes with blood flow to the lung (a pulmonary embolus). Large pulmonary emboli can cause immediate death, but small thrombi may produce no clinical symptoms.

Normal hemostatic mechanisms regulate the clotting process so that clots normally do not form in veins and arteries. However, the delicate balance in this system can be altered by factors such as venous stasis (the slowed return or stoppage of circulating blood), hypercoagulability of blood, and trauma or injury to an artery or vein.

Immobility promotes venous stasis. When leg muscles are inactive, venous return to the heart decreases; with time, the gravitational effect of the supine position results in the redistribution of body fluids, with a net decrease in venous return. The numerous bifurcations and valves in veins are thought to promote further stasis. This seems to be even more pronounced in older adults, perhaps explaining in part the increased incidence of thrombus development in an immobilized older client (Groer & Shekleton, 1993). Poor positioning can cause external pressure on blood vessels, which also contributes to inadequate blood flow and promotes the development of thrombi.

Hypercoagulability is not directly caused by immobility, but sometimes immobilized clients become dehydrated, which can increase blood viscosity. Dehydration may partly result from the client's inability to obtain fluids without assistance, and some experts think that elevated serum calcium levels (a common finding in the immobilized client) also affect coagulation.

Decreased Lung Expansion. The immobilized client experiences greater-than-normal resistance to breathing, resulting in underinflation of the lungs and increased work of breathing.

The healthy person keeps the lungs well inflated with practically no effort. In an upright position, the diaphragm can move up and down freely. Airways are cleared of mucous secretions by an efficient mechanism known as the mucociliary escalator. Periodic sighing and coughing helps to keep even the smallest air sacs (alveoli) open and available for gas exchange. Finally, ordinary activity produces enough carbon dioxide to stimulate a smooth, effective pattern of breathing.

The immobile client, however, breathes less deeply than normal and with greater effort. The supine client must overcome two resistances that do not ordinarily work against breathing. First, the diaphragm is prohibited from free movement by the abdominal organs, which shift against it when the client lies down. To achieve full lung expansion, the client's diaphragm must push the organs out of the way with each breath. Second, the client's chest movement is limited by the pressure of the bed against the chest wall. Together these factors result in diminished depth of breathing, which decreases tidal volume. Because the immobilized client's activity level is less than normal, less carbon dioxide is produced. This results in a lower level of stimulation for breathing, causing further reduction of tidal volume.

Decreased depth of breathing can result in the collapse of alveoli, which in turn hinders the exchange of oxygen and carbon dioxide. This condition of alveolar collapse is known as *atelectasis*. In addition to limiting the lungs' ability to exchange gases, atelectasis predisposes the client to pneumonia. The client's ability to cough deeply is often limited; thus, mucus may become trapped in the lung, providing a rich medium for microbial growth.

Retained Secretions. Pulmonary secretions ordinarily perform important protective functions. The mucous layer that blankets the airways ordinarily moves steadily upward. The secretions, which contain inhaled debris, are moved into the throat, where they stimulate a cough. Once this occurs, they are expectorated or swallowed.

Immobility can limit the effectiveness of this protective mechanism by weakening the cough mechanism. With an impaired cough mechanism, clients who produce excessive mucus are at risk for retaining secretions, atelectasis, and pneumonia.

Nutrition and Metabolism

The nutritional and metabolic effects of immobility include decreased metabolic rate, anorexia, negative nitrogen balance, disuse osteoporosis, impaired immunity, and increased potential for development of pressure sores.

Decreased Metabolic Rate. The basal metabolic rate decreases during immobility. The production of many hormones related to metabolic rate, fluid and electrolyte balance, and the stress response is affected by severely restricted activity. The amount and pattern of production of thyroid hormone, adrenocorticotropic hormone, aldosterone, and insulin are all affected. Drug metabolism also is altered. In addition, some studies report a significant weight loss in clients on bed rest despite a lowered metabolic rate (Maloni, et al., 1993). Weight loss is thought to result from loss of muscle mass and diuresis.

Negative Nitrogen Balance. In an active person, a balance exists between protein breakdown and protein synthesis. However, immobility raises the rate of protein breakdown, probably because of muscle atrophy. One way to monitor this process is to measure nitrogen, which is excreted in urine as a waste product of protein breakdown. Elevated urine nitrogen levels occur in most immobilized clients. A negative nitrogen balance results when nitrogen excretion exceeds dietary intake. In such cases, the body lacks adequate nitrogen for protein synthesis, which results in nutritional depletion; this in turn interferes with wound healing and restoration of muscle mass when mobility resumes.

Immobilized clients often have concomitant factors that further deplete nitrogen, such as trauma, burns, surgery, coma, cancer, fever, or infection. Clients with chronic illness or poor nutritional balance before immobilization are at increased risk for negative nitrogen balance.

Anorexia. Anorexia (loss of appetite) is common in immobilized clients. Decreased metabolic rate is accompanied by decreased caloric need. Moreover, if the client is confined to a healthcare facility, the institutional food, eating in a supine position, environmental

Nursing Research
Mobility

Selected Nursing Research Studies

Maloni, J. A., Chance, B., Zhang, C., Cohen, A. W., Betts, D., & Gange, S. J. (1993). Physical and psychosocial effects of antepartum hospital bedrest. *Nursing Research, 42*(4), 197–203.

Mason, D. J., & Redeker, N. (1993). Measurement of activity. *Nursing Research, 42*(2), 87–92.

Neuberger, G. B., Kasal, S., Smith, K. V., Hassanein, R., DeViney, S. (1994). Determinants of exercise and aerobic fitness in outpatients with arthritis. *Nursing Research, 43*(1), 11–24.

Topp, R., & Stevenson, J. S. (1994). The effects of attendance and effort on outcomes among older adults in a long-term exercise program. *Research in Nursing and Health, 17*(1), 15–24.

Whitney, J. D., Stotts, N. A., Goodson, W. H., & Janson-Bjerklie, S. (1993). The effects of activity and bedrest on tissue oxygen tensions, perfusion, and plasma volume. *Nursing Research, 42*(6), 349–355.

Possible Topics for Nursing Inquiry

- What are the risk factors for falls among mobile, noninstitutionalized older people?
- What effect do routine exercise programs have on the development of osteoporosis in postmenopausal women?
- What is the psychological impact of routine exercise on depressed terminal cancer clients?
- What effect does extended immobility have on pain perception?
- What impact does posting specific turning schedules at bedside have on compliance?
- What is the impact of bed exercises on reducing perceptual changes associated with prolonged immobility?

factors, and psychological state can inhibit the appetite. The stress of confinement or adjusting to altered body function may contribute to dyspepsia and gastric stasis, bloating, and distention—all factors that contribute to anorexia. Regardless of the cause, decreased nutritional intake can impair body function and rehabilitation.

Disuse Osteoporosis. In disuse osteoporosis, bone demineralization occurs secondary to immobility. The bone matrix is always in a dynamic state of formation and destruction. Osteoblastic cells are responsible for the proliferation of bone matrix. In contrast, osteoclastic cells destroy bone matrix by absorbing and removing osseous tissue from the bone. Immobility results in an imbalance between osteoblastic and osteoclastic activity, because normal stress and strain imposed on bone through movement are an important part of osteoblastic processes. In the immobilized client, osteoblasts continue to lay down bony matrix, but osteoclasts break down bone faster than osteoblasts can build it. The result is a loss of bony matrix. Disuse osteoporosis results in bones that are more porous, brittle, and susceptible to fractures.

Another significant effect of this process is increased serum calcium that must be excreted from the body. Increasing dietary intake of calcium is helpful in preventing disuse osteoporosis only initially. If renal function is insufficient to excrete excess calcium at an adequate rate, calcium may be deposited into the muscles and joints. This can cause discomfort and interfere with normal musculoskeletal function.

Impaired Immunity. The immune system is weakened during immobility. Catabolism of immunoglobulin G doubles, significantly decreasing the normal concentration of circulating antibodies. Leukocytes are less able to engulf and destroy microorganisms. Lymphatic transport may be decreased as well when skeletal muscles are inactive.

Pressure Sores. Pressure sores form when pressure exerted over an area of skin or subcutaneous tissue exceeds the pressure required for adequate blood flow to the area. This causes cells to die because they are not supplied with oxygen and nutrients and because waste products build up. Pressure is usually concentrated on bony prominences but can occur anywhere that pressure is great. In the supine position, pressure is greatest over the back of the skull and at the elbows, sacrum, ischial tuberosities, and heels. In the sitting position, the greatest pressure is at the ischial tuberosities and the sacrum.

A compensatory mechanism that responds to this inadequate blood flow is reactive hyperemia. When pressure is removed, blood floods the area in an attempt to prevent tissue necrosis. Reactive hyperemia is only effective if it occurs before cellular damage occurs. The critical time varies from one person to another. Usually, the normal person can sense pressure buildup and can change position to reduce discomfort, but this is not always possible for the client with impaired mobility. Clients with neurologic impairment may be incapable of movement or unable to sense the need to change positions.

Healing of pressure sores is difficult and slow, especially in the immobilized client. Pressure sores can prolong immobility and increase the cost and length of confinement. See Chapter 38 for more information about pressure sores.

Elimination

Immobility may alter normal elimination patterns. Common manifestations include constipation, urinary stasis, and increased incidence of urinary tract infections and renal calculi.

Constipation. Even in a healthy person, dietary changes, activity variations, or emotional stress affect normal bowel patterns. The immobilized client faces additional changes. Abdominal and perineal muscles can be weakened by muscle atrophy, making it more difficult for the client to bear down and exert pressure to evacuate stool. As stool descends against the rectum, the stimulus to defecate is felt. In an upright posture, stool descends more quickly into the rectal area, eliciting a strong stimulus. In the supine position, rectal filling is slow, weakening the stimulus for defecation.

The defecation reflex also can be affected if the person postpones defecation after recognizing the stimulus to defecate. This happens frequently in the immobilized client, who may feel embarrassed or may need assistance to use a bedpan. When defecation is delayed, fecal material increases in size and more water is absorbed from the feces, making stool passage even more difficult. Dehydration, common in the immobile client, also can contribute to constipation. The result may be fecal impaction (hard stool contained in the rectum that cannot be removed naturally by defecation). With fecal impaction, the client has a feeling of fullness with a desire to defecate. Often liquid stool seeps around the obstruction formed by the impaction. Fecal impaction can lead to bowel obstruction, so it should be treated promptly with manual removal. Preventive measures should be taken to discourage recurrence.

Urinary Stasis. Normal micturition requires the coordinated interaction of the detrusor muscle of the bladder wall, the perineal muscles, and the internal and external urethral sphincter. As the bladder fills, the person senses the need to void, and the internal urethral sphincter relaxes. Control over external sphincters prevents the elimination of urine until the perineal muscles relax voluntarily.

In the immobilized client, the urge to void may not be heeded. The client may not want to bother the nurse by asking for a bedpan. Some clients try to void when they feel the need but have difficulty relaxing the perineal muscles from the supine position. Delaying micturition causes urine to collect in the bladder. Chronic delay can lead to overstretching of the detrusor muscle, permanent changes in bladder tone, and long-term consequences for normal voiding patterns.

Prostatic enlargement in the older male client also can interfere with bladder emptying, especially in the supine position, which promotes the retention of urine. In the upright position, gravity encourages the continual flow of urine from each renal pelvis into the ureters, and from the ureters to the bladder. When a person is supine, the ureters are above the level of many renal calyces, which means that urine must flow upward against gravity to enter the ureters.

Urinary retention poses significant problems for the immobilized client. One problem, urinary stasis, contributes to urinary tract infections and renal calculi. Bladder distention, another problem, leads to overflow incontinence, which is embarrassing for the client and can contribute to skin breakdown.

Urinary Tract Infection. Stagnant urine makes a good medium for bacterial growth. Bladder distention can cause small tears in the delicate bladder mucosa, which contribute to the incidence of urinary tract infection. When the client experiences distention, catheterization may be necessary to empty the bladder. With any type of catheterization comes the risk of introducing pathogens and infection into the body.

Renal Calculi. Urinary stasis and an increased serum calcium level promote the formation of renal calculi (kidney stones) in the immobilized client. As serum calcium levels rise (the result of calcium loss from the bones), more calcium is excreted. This raises urinary calcium levels. Because calcium can precipitate from solution to form crystals and because stagnant urine encourages the aggregation of crystals, renal calculi pose a significant problem to the immobilized client. Dehydration, common in the immobilized client, also increases the incidence of calculi formation. Additionally, infection caused by some urea-splitting organisms makes the urine more alkaline, which also promotes calculus development. Renal calculi predispose the immobilized client to increased urinary retention, infection, and hydronephrosis, which can contribute to renal damage.

Sleep and Rest

Immobility can interfere with normal sleep patterns. Normal activity, especially physical work, and aerobic exercise produce a sense of fatigue that helps the person fall asleep and obtain restful sleep. The immobilized client may doze frequently during the day, disrupting normal nighttime sleep patterns. The immobilized client must be awakened frequently to be turned, monitored, or given treatment and medications. Such wakings, especially when numerous, impair the quality of sleep. In addition, the immobilized client may sleep in an unfamiliar, noisy environment and may have stressful health concerns that further reduce the amount and quality of sleep.

Cognition and Perception

Because freedom to interact normally with the environment is decreased by immobility, the client has less sensory information available to him or her. This can lead to sensory deprivation, which may prompt the client to provide self-stimulation in the form of visual and auditory hallucinations. Initially this may take the form of simple sensory alterations, such as seeing colors or shapes that are not there or experiencing abnormal sensations, such as itching, heat or cold, and involuntary muscle movement. As deprivation continues, more complex abnormal experiences occur, such as hearing voices or seeing people or events that are not real.

Symptoms include preoccupation with somatic complaints, difficulty with time perception, difficulty with understanding and following directions, crying, and other emotional outbursts. Confusion is common but reversible if normal sensory input returns.

Pain may result from physiologic changes that occur with immobility. Joint stiffness, pneumonia, pressure sores, thrombosis, and emboli can contribute to discomfort for the immobilized client. The perception of pain also may intensify because focusing on discomfort is more common when diversions are limited.

Self-Perception and Self-Concept

Changes in self-perception and self-concept commonly accompany functional motor impairment or immobility. Immobility contributes to a feeling of powerlessness, especially when the client must depend on others. Motor impairment can alter body image, especially if the impairment results from loss of a body part. Self-concept is altered when the client must depend on devices such as crutches, wheelchairs, or walkers. Problems with coordination can cause embarrassment; for example, the client may worry about appearing awkward or even intoxicated. Altered body image can negatively impact self-esteem and lead to a feeling of lowered self-worth.

Coping and Stress Tolerance

Loss of mobility is not something the client chooses or desires. With trauma, the loss occurs suddenly. In some cases, it is permanent, requiring the client to adapt to different functional abilities. Despite supportive social interactions with family and friends, immobilized clients may spend many hours alone and are often bored or lonely. Depression, anger, and anxiety are common.

Different behavior is exhibited by clients who experience stress due to immobility. Some withdraw, limiting social contact even further. Some complain and become more demanding. The client who constantly requests assistance may be responding negatively to the stress of immobility.

Roles and Relationships

Immobility affects role function for many people. For children and adolescents, school and social activities are disrupted (Fig. 33-3) For adults, the ability to work may be impaired and may result in temporary or permanent unemployment with corresponding financial stress. Immobility also disrupts various parental or spousal activities. Normal family life is affected when any family member experiences immobility. Child care may be impossible when a parent is hospitalized or immobilized at home. Arrangements for child care may be difficult to make and stressful for child and parent. Older children may be better able to care for themselves, but they still require emotional support and guidance from parents. Older children may need to assume more responsibility for tasks normally performed by their parents. When a child is immobilized, this may decrease the quantity and quality of time the parents can spend with other children, which may trigger anger and resentment in siblings.

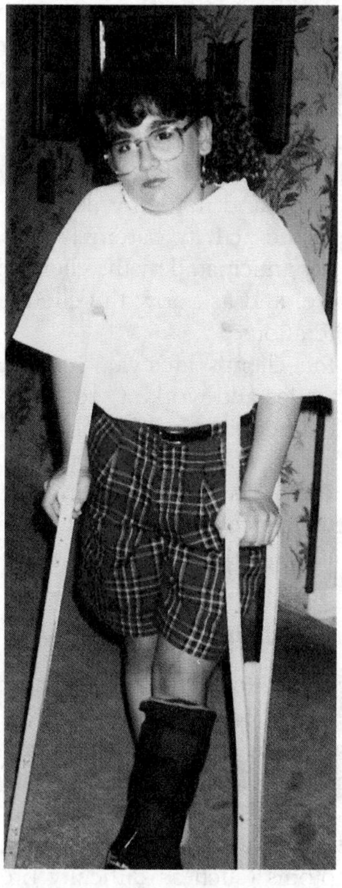

Figure 33-3 • *A broken leg can seem very significant to an adolescent when school and social activities are disrupted.*

Sexuality

Sexual feelings and activities may be affected by mobility limitations. Lack of privacy, depression, fatigue, and physical limitations can contribute to decreased sexual function. Immobility may impede grooming activities that are often important in maintaining sexual identity. For some clients with long-term motor impairments, such as paraplegia, sexual function may be permanently altered, requiring the client to learn new methods of sexual expression.

Impact of Altered Mobility on Activities of Daily Living

Individual Considerations

Impaired mobility can severely restrict the client's ability to perform normal daily activities, either temporarily or permanently. Coordination and muscle strength are necessary for eating, dressing, and grooming. Usually the nurse can show the client ways to function successfully and independently despite physical limitations. This is best accomplished by setting short-term, achievable goals and developing a long-range plan in collaboration with the healthcare team (eg, physician, physical therapist, occupational therapist, psychologist, social worker). For example, ambulatory physical therapy sessions may help the client with mobility problems regain function and independence (Fig. 33-4).

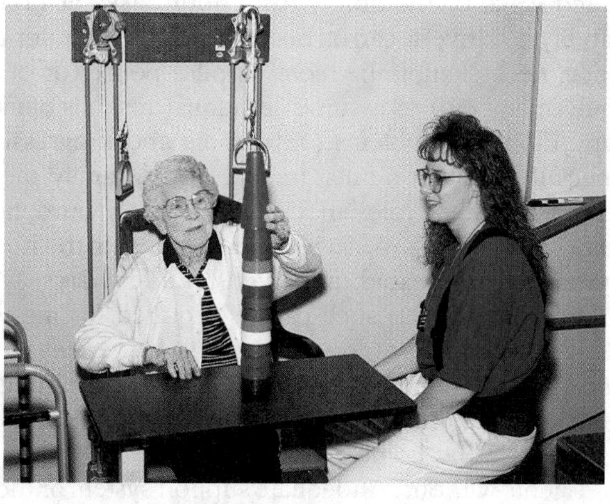

Figure 33-4 • *Outpatient physical therapy sessions can help an older person remain independent as mobility is improved following a cerebral vascular accident (stroke).*

Eating difficulties are most common among clients with arm involvement (often caused by neuromuscular diseases) or hemiparesis or hemiplegia. Special devices can help the client grasp a cup or eating utensils. Many clients who lack the coordination to feed themselves also suffer from difficulty swallowing secondary to neurologic impairment; careful nursing supervision is necessary to prevent aspiration of food.

Dressing is often a problem for clients with problems with fine motor skills. Velcro fasteners can be used in place of buttons or zippers. Sweat pants and other loose-fitting clothes are usually acceptable options for the client who has difficulty dressing.

Because personal hygiene is a private matter for most clients, it is stressful to have to depend on family members or nursing personnel for this care. Clients who can perform some care independently may report it to be physically taxing. Sometimes fatigue and lack of endurance limit the self-care tasks that can be performed.

Gaining access to toilet facilities is difficult for the client who cannot move normally, and bedside commodes may be helpful during hospitalization and at home. For clients with impaired bowel or bladder function related to paralysis, bowel or bladder programs may be implemented to manage possible constipation and urinary incontinence.

Impaired mobility affects other daily activities as well. Performing housework, driving a car, buying groceries, and paying bills may be difficult; social activities may be curtailed, and participation in athletic or exercise programs may be impossible.

Family Considerations

Whether mobility problems are temporary or permanent, family members are usually affected. A spouse who breaks a leg skiing may need to be in a long leg cast for several weeks. This may interfere with job-related tasks or the ability to perform tasks at home. Inability to drive a car or board a bus limits independence, necessitating the more mobile spouse (or other family members) to assume additional responsibilities. Many mobility problems are chronic and progressive, especially in older adults. In such cases, family members in caretaker roles may be excessively burdened. Fulltime, 24-hour care of a bed-ridden client in the home is an exhausting experience even for a few days. With chronic impairment, such care is required for months or years. Adequate support of the primary caregiver, either from other family members, friends, or community agencies, is significant in enabling the immobilized client to remain in the home.

Clients without an adequate support system or those who need special care, for example a quadriplegic client, may need to employ a caregiver or consider seeking care in an intermediate or long-term care facility.

Assessment

To assess the client's mobility, the nurse must collect subjective and objective information from the client. Such data help the nurse understand the client's normal mobility, risk factors for potential alterations in mobility, actual impairments in mobility, and management techniques or devices that the client uses.

Subjective Data

Subjective data are initially collected during the nursing interview when the client enters the healthcare facility; during the initial client contact in the home, community, or elsewhere; and at routine intervals as necessary to update information.

Functional Pattern Identification

The nurse must determine the client's normal activity pattern. The client should describe his or her ability to move normally and perform activities of daily living. A rating scale may be useful for documenting the client's independence, partial independence, or complete dependence in various activities involving mobility, such as ambulation, toileting, dressing, bathing, and household chores. Ask the client to describe any recent change in mobility or activity level. Determine the client's normal patterns of exercise and leisure activities. If the client actively engages in aerobic exercise, determine the frequency and appropriateness of the activity.

Assess the client's satisfaction with his or her current activity level, and note any desire on the client's part to change the activity pattern. Explore any alterations in activity anticipated by the client after discharge or in the future, and ask how the client plans to deal with these alterations.

Discuss the client's lifestyle. Some people enjoy sedentary activities and work at sedentary jobs. Others work at jobs that require vigorous physical exertion and take part in sports and physical activities during their leisure time. People who grew up in a family that valued quiet activities commonly carry the pattern of inactivity into adulthood.

Risk Pattern Identification

Interviewing the client also can help the nurse identify risk factors that can contribute to impaired mobility. For example, inadequate aerobic activity may increase the risks for chronic disease and deconditioning. Determine whether the client feels weak or fatigued after routine exercise and activity. Ask the client to describe any distressing symptoms (such as difficulty breathing, pain, or increased heart rate) with activity; document the degree of exercise and the degree of stress. Ask the client how long the symptoms have occurred and how long they persist after the activity ends. Evaluate the client's risk for falls. Factors that increase this risk include decreased mobility, altered cognition, the use of alcohol or drugs that impair balance, postural hypotension, and a cluttered environment.

Document current or chronic health problems that may limit mobility or decrease activity tolerance. Common and notable medical conditions are respiratory disease, cardiac disease, anemia, peripheral vascular disease, arthritis, cerebrovascular accidents, multiple sclerosis, Parkinson's disease, brain tumors, head injuries, fractures, spinal cord injuries, and amputations. Evaluate the impact of medical conditions on mobility.

Dysfunction Identification

Document any inability of the client to move normally and easily. Encourage the client to explain any problems with mobility or activity tolerance and any adaptations used to promote optimal functioning at home. If the client reports any limitation in mobility, determine the extent of the problem, when it first occurred, and whether the client knows the cause.

Ask the client whether the mobility problem has been improving or worsening and how it affects his or her functional abilities in other areas. Document what the client can do independently so that independence within his or her capabilities can be encouraged.

Ask the client whether he or she uses devices to assist with ambulation (eg, prostheses, canes, walkers, crutches). If surgery is planned and if assistive devices will be used afterward, the client may be asked to demonstrate skills previously learned.

Perform a comprehensive functional health assessment to determine the impact of decreased mobility on all functional health areas. Note any complications resulting from limited mobility (eg, pressure ulcers or renal calculi). To guide the assessment, review Table 33-2, which describes the effects of immobility on functional health patterns.

Discuss how impaired mobility has affected the client's roles and relationships, self-concept, self-esteem, and body image. Identify family and community support services and evaluate past and present coping strategies.

Objective Data

In addition to collecting subjective information, the nurse uses physical examination and diagnostic test results to help evaluate the client's mobility.

Physical Assessment

Physical examination findings contribute information about alignment; balance; coordination; gait; joint structure and function; muscle mass, tone, and strength; and activity tolerance. For the most part, the nurse uses the technique of inspection to visualize these qualities. When mobility appears normal, more extensive assessment techniques are usually unnecessary, but if mobility is impaired, a more detailed assessment may be indicated.

Alignment. Assessing alignment is the first step in determining mobility. First, determine the center of gravity. Proper alignment should be maintained while sitting and standing. When alignment is normal, an imaginary line can be drawn through the earlobe, shoulder, hip, femoral trochanter, knee, and front of the ankle. Symmetry of organs and bones should be noted. Normal spinal alignment is characterized by concave curvature of the cervical spine, convex curvature of the thoracic spine, and concave curvature of the lumbar spine. Extreme curvature of the spine may be abnormal. *Scoliosis,* a lateral deviation of the thoracic spine, can be detected by watching the client bend at the waist from a standing position. *Lordosis,* an abnormal concavity of the lumbar spine, and *kyphosis,* an exaggerated curvature of the thoracic spine, are less common spinal deviations.

Balance. Assess balance by asking the client to sit or stand with eyes closed. Observe his or her ability to maintain a normal erect posture through postural adjustments. Swaying to one side indicates an inability to maintain balance through normal physiologic mechanisms.

Coordination. Watching the client perform normal activities, including ambulation, allows the nurse to evaluate the coordination of movement. Look for fluid, well-controlled movement. The client should be able to initiate the desired movement quickly without hesitation. Fine motor skills can be assessed by asking the client to perform a simple skill, such as unbuttoning a shirt or signing papers.

Gait. Watch the client walk to evaluate his or her gait. Normal gait should be rhythmic and even; the stride should be symmetric with full extension. The head should remain erect, and the knees and feet should point forward. Arms should swing alternately with leg movements. The full weight of the body should be easily supported. Observing the client's shoes to detect patterns of wear also can provide the nurse with information about gait.

Joint Structure and Function. Observation and palpation can detect redness, swelling, or warmth around the joint. Listen for a crunching or grating sound (crepitus), which can occur when bones rub against one another during movement because of inadequate protection or lubrication in the joint. Observe the client's facial expression and nonverbal signs of discomfort during movement. If observation discloses stiffness or guarding during certain body movements, evaluate joint mobility by moving the involved joint through its full ROM (see Table 33-1). When doing this, note the amount of resistance encountered and whether the client complains of discomfort.

Muscle Mass, Tone, and Strength. Normal muscle mass, tone, and strength can vary greatly from one person to another. Athletes may have bulging, well-defined muscles and great strength and endurance. Older adults may have weak, small muscles with little tone. Increased strength and tone are usually found on the person's dominant side.

Assess muscle strength by evaluating the client's ability to perform activities of self-care, such as feeding, dressing, toileting, and grooming. Strength and coordination can be estimated by observing the ease with which the client carries out these tasks. Evaluate the strength of specific muscle groups by asking the client to grip your hand or to use certain muscle groups to push against resistance.

Muscle size in the arms and legs is determined by observation and by comparing measurements. A decrease in circumference in the affected limb usually reflects muscle atrophy from immobility. Atrophy indicates a loss of muscle tone, which decreases endurance.

Postural Blood Pressure. To help determine if a client can safely ambulate, measure postural blood pressure (see Chap. 22 for instructions). A drop in blood pressure when the client changes from a supine to a sitting position suggests a risk for impaired ambulation. Complaints of dizziness, lightheadedness, diaphoresis, and tachycardia may accompany orthostatic hypotension and are indications that fainting may occur if ambulation continues.

Risk for Falls. Determine whether independent ambulation is safe. Some healthcare facilities list risk factors contributing to falls and ask the nurse to calculate a score to determine clients at greatest risk (for more information, see Chap. 29). Risk factors include the following:

- Advanced age (especially older than 70 years)
- Visual impairment
- History of falls
- History of dizziness, postural hypotension, or syncope
- Cognitive impairments, such as confusion
- Use of drugs or alcohol that can impair balance, coordination, or cognitive abilities
- Incontinence

Activity Tolerance. In assessing activity tolerance, observe the client before, during, and after activity to detect abnormal responses. The most common parameters measured are the pulse rate and the respiratory rate. Normally, both increase during activity. Resting vital signs should be within a normal range before activity starts. If activity begins when the client is experiencing hypotension, tachycardia, or tachypnea (rapid, irregular breathing), he or she has little energy in reserve to meet the body's increased need for oxygen during exercise.

When activity resumes after bed rest or the level of prescribed activity increases, observe the client carefully for signs of distress, such as dyspnea, diaphoresis, or dizziness. In high-risk clients, such as those with cardiac or respiratory conditions, the nurse may be directed to monitor pulse or respiratory rate during activity and to discontinue the activity if values are outside the prescribed range. After activity, pulse and respiratory rates should return to preactivity baseline values within 3 minutes.

Diagnostic Tests and Procedures

Common diagnostic tests used to evaluate musculoskeletal function are radiographic studies and direct visualization of joints. Laboratory values, such as hemoglobin and hematocrit, may be helpful when assessing activity tolerance.

Radiographic Studies. X-rays are useful in differentiating traumatic injuries, such as sprains, dislocations, and fractures. X-rays also help assess the demineralization of bone that occurs in osteoporosis. Radiographic studies using injected, radiopaque dye can help evaluate problems with the spine or joints. Defects are revealed by an abnormal pattern of dye distribution in the body part. *Arthrograms* permit visualization of joints and are often used to diagnose tears in ligaments or cartilage. *Myelograms* rely on radiopaque dye to highlight the spinal column to detect ruptured vertebral disks or other structural defects.

Arthroscopy. **Arthroscopy** is the examination of a joint with a fiberoptic instrument to diagnose abnormalities. Minor corrective surgery also can be performed to remove torn cartilage or repair torn ligaments.

Hematologic Studies. Hemoglobin and hematocrit values can be used to evaluate the client's reserve for activity. Clients with low hemoglobin values have difficulty transporting adequate oxygen to body tissues. Activity expectations may need to be modified for clients with hemoglobin values of less than 10 g/dL. Low hematocrit values often reflect blood loss or inadequate volume replacement. When clients have low hematocrit values, they are likely to experience postural hypotension and activity intolerance.

Nursing Diagnoses

North American Nursing Diagnosis Association (NANDA) diagnoses that relate to mobility are Impaired Physical Mobility, Activity Intolerance, and Risk for Disuse Syndrome.

Diagnostic Statement: Impaired Physical Mobility

Definition

Impaired physical mobility is a state in which the individual experiences a limitation of ability for independent physical movement (NANDA, 1994).

Defining Characteristics

Defining characteristics include inability to move within the physical environment purposefully, including bed mobility, transfer, and ambulation; reluctance to attempt movement; limited ROM; decreased muscle strength, control, or mass; imposed restrictions of movement, including mechanical, medical protocol; impaired coordination (NANDA, 1994).

Related Factors

Related factors include intolerance to activity or decreased strength and endurance, pain or discomfort, perceptual/cognitive impairment, neuromuscular impairment, musculoskeletal impairment, and depression or severe anxiety (NANDA, 1994).

Diagnostic Statement: Activity Intolerance

Definition

Activity intolerance is a state in which an individual has insufficient physiologic or psychological energy to endure or complete required or desired daily activities (NANDA, 1994).

Defining Characteristics

Defining characteristics include verbal report of fatigue or weakness (critical), abnormal heart rate or blood pressure response to activity, exertional discomfort or dyspnea, electrocardiographic changes reflecting arrhythmias or ischemia (NANDA, 1994).

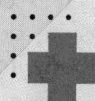

> **Safety Alert**
> *Body Mechanics and Mobility*
>
> - When transferring a client to a wheelchair, make sure the wheels are locked to avoid chair movement and possible falls.
> - To avoid injury to the caregiver when a client starts to fall, gently guide the person to the floor, rather than attempting to hold the client up.
> - Take postural blood pressures before getting clients up to decrease the chance of falling due to postural hypotension.
> - Use ambulation belts when transferring or ambulating clients who are likely to fall.
> - Obtain needed help when transferring or ambulating clients; working independently can risk injury to the client and the caregiver.
> - When performing ROM, discontinue movement if the client complains of pain. Damage could occur if stiff areas are overextended.
> - When turning and positioning clients, always keep side rails up if a staff member is not there to prevent falls.
> - Make sure all clients who need assistance with mobility have their call lights at all times. Instruct them to call for the nurse if they need to ambulate.
> - Keep rooms free of clutter, and provide adequate lighting to prevent falls.
> - Logroll any client following spinal injury or spinal surgery to prevent additional spinal trauma.

Related Factors

Related factors include bed rest or immobility, generalized weakness, sedentary lifestyle, and imbalance between oxygen supply and demand (NANDA, 1994).

Diagnostic Statement: Risk for Disuse Syndrome

Definition

Risk for disuse syndrome is a state in which an individual is at risk for deterioration of body systems as the result of prescribed or unavoidable musculoskeletal inactivity (NANDA, 1994).

Defining Characteristics

Presence of risk factors, such as paralysis, mechanical immobilization, prescribed immobilization, severe pain, altered level of consciousness (NANDA, 1994). Complications from immobility can include pressure ulcers, constipation, stasis of pulmonary secretions, thrombosis, urinary tract infection or retention, decreased strength and endurance, orthostatic hypotension, decreased range of joint motion, disorientation, body image disturbance, and powerlessness.

Risk Factors

See under "Defining Characteristics."

Related Nursing Diagnoses

Lack of normal movement affects all areas of function. The client with a nursing diagnosis of Impaired Physical Activity or Activity Intolerance is usually at risk for many other problems. Self-Care Deficits in Bathing/Hygiene, Feeding, Dressing/Grooming, Toileting are common because these tasks require normal movement and coordination. The disruption of various body systems can result in Impaired Skin Integrity, Risk for Infection, Urinary Retention, Constipation, Altered Nutrition: Less Than Body Requirements, Impaired Gas Exchange, or Ineffective Airway Clearance. Risk for Injury is greater because the risk for falls increases with impaired mobility. Sensory/Perceptual Alterations can occur, and Pain may increase. Sexual Dysfunction may be an appropriate diagnosis if spontaneous, normal movement is limited, resulting in a negative change in sexual expression.

Because mobility directly relates to a person's sense of independence, decreased mobility affects personal feelings. Body Image Disturbance, Self Esteem Disturbance, Anxiety, and Powerlessness can occur when normal movement is impaired. Altered Role Performance results because some of the responsibilities as a spouse, parent, or employee may require normal movement. Social Isolation and Impaired Verbal Communication can occur when the client withdraws from social interaction. Ineffective Family Coping or Individual Coping often results from the stress imposed by altered mobility or the need to adjust to permanent disability.

Outcome Identification and Planning

After nursing diagnoses and related factors have been identified, the nurse, client, and family plan interventions and expected outcomes. The accompanying display summarizes some of the interventions that are used in problems with mobility. The next section also discusses interventions.

General goals for clients with impaired mobility might include the following:

Client will increase endurance and tolerance for physical activity.

Client will actively participate in prescribed therapies to promote optimal healing and restoration of mobility.

Planning

Examples of Nursing Interventions Used in Common Altered Mobility Problems

Mobility Assistance

- Turning and positioning
- Transferring
- Assisting with ambulation
- Teaching (preventing falls, ambulation and transfers, using ambulation aids)

Preventing Complications From Immobility

- Range-of-motion exercises
- Leg exercises
- Deep breathing and coughing
- Adequate hydration
- Skin care
- Bowel program

Client will comply with measures to prevent potential complications of immobility.

Client will maintain optimal function despite mobility restrictions.

Implementation

Nursing Interventions to Promote Health and Function

Physical Fitness Promotion

In the United States, machines have reduced the need for physical labor, leading many into sedentary lifestyles. This decrease in activity has been implicated in the rising incidence of many diseases. However, physical fitness has recently become more fashionable, spurring many people to walk, jog, or participate in exercise programs. Health clubs are available in most communities, and even some employers are incorporating gymnasiums into the workplace for after-hour use. Nonetheless, a relatively small percentage of the population is physically fit.

The nurse is frequently in a position to promote physical fitness. By stressing the importance of exercise for physical and emotional health, the nurse can help prevent mobility problems. Physical fitness teaching opportunities occur in many areas of nursing. For example, the school nurse can help young people develop good exercise habits. Physical education should be part of the curriculum in all grades. The school nurse should work with physical education teachers and coaches to promote well-balanced programs. The nurse in clinical practice can teach clients about the value of exercise when they make routine visits to private physicians and clinics. Nurses are often part of the team for weight-reduction programs. Nurses can be role models by remaining physically fit.

Exercise Programs. Exercise programs must be performed regularly to be effective. For example, aerobic exercise is most beneficial when performed at least three times a week for at least 30 minutes of accelerated heart rate. Exercise tolerance should be increased gradually to avoid excessive stress on muscles and joints. Pain during exercise is a signal to stop. People may drop out of an exercise program because of pain and soreness if they begin too aggressively.

Exercise programs are part of the rehabilitation process for many clients. Group exercise activities are often planned for clients in extended-care facilities. After a heart attack or cardiac surgery, a specific exercise program is recommended. Exercise is used after a stroke to strengthen affected muscles. Many diabetic clients follow an exercise program to obtain better control over blood glucose levels. The client who has undergone orthopedic surgery is encouraged to exercise certain muscles and joints. In many healthcare facilities, the physical therapy staff is usually responsible for supervising exercise programs, but the nurse can encourage and reinforce the prescribed therapies.

Injury Prevention

Injuries from accidents commonly cause impaired mobility, but many accidents can be prevented (see Chap. 29). The nurse can play a significant role in accident prevention:

- Promote automobile safety, and instruct clients to wear seat belts and use proper restraint devices for young children.
- Teach about drug and alcohol counseling.
- Help clients provide a safe environment for themselves and their families.
- Provide instruction about accident prevention in the workplace.

Nursing Care Guidelines
Moving Clients

- Assess client's abilities and limitations.
- Medicate client to provide optimal pain relief.
- Organize environment, and request needed help to ensure safety.
- Explain what you are going to do and how you expect the client to help.
- Permit client to do as much as capabilities allow.
- Consider safety precautions (eg, lock wheels, use transfer belt).
- Use good body mechanics.
- Keep movements smooth and rhythmic.
- Prevent trauma (eg, friction against skin, pulling joints, grabbing muscles).
- Check client for proper body alignment and comfort, and provide client with call bell before leaving.

Nursing Interventions for Altered Mobility

Positioning

Therapeutic positioning is used to prevent complications when mobility is limited. The client may be placed in specific positions to facilitate diagnostic tests or surgical intervention. Common positioning postures include prone (face down), supine (lying on back), high Fowler's (head of the bed elevated 80–90 degrees), semi-Fowler's (head of the bed elevated 30–45 degrees), dorsal recumbent (supine with legs flexed in an elevated position), knee-chest position, Trendelenburg (supine with head lower than feet), lateral or side-lying position, and Sims' (semiprone between a prone and side-lying position). These positions are illustrated in Figure 33-5. Positions most commonly used for the immobile client include supine, Fowler's, semi-Fowler's, prone, side-lying, and Sims'.

Regardless of the specific position, general principles of body mechanics should be used in any position change. Proper body alignment must be maintained, and all body parts must be supported. Pressure, especially over body prominences, should be avoided by adequately padding these areas. Such positioning aids as pillows, splints, footboards, and foam rubber or sheepskin protectors are helpful (Table 33-3). Various organizational skills are required for turning and positioning clients. Among them are the following:

- Think through the task before beginning.
- Ensure that all needed equipment is within easy reach.
- Decide whether help from other staff members will be needed, and ensure that they are in the room before beginning the position change. If there is a possibility that help may be needed, always request it.
- Explain to the client exactly what will happen before beginning the position change.
- Enlist the client's assistance whenever possible, giving instructions and encouragement as necessary.
- When the position change has been completed, ask if the client is comfortable. Reposition as necessary.
- Tell the client how long he or she will remain in the position. Provide a call device within easy reach.

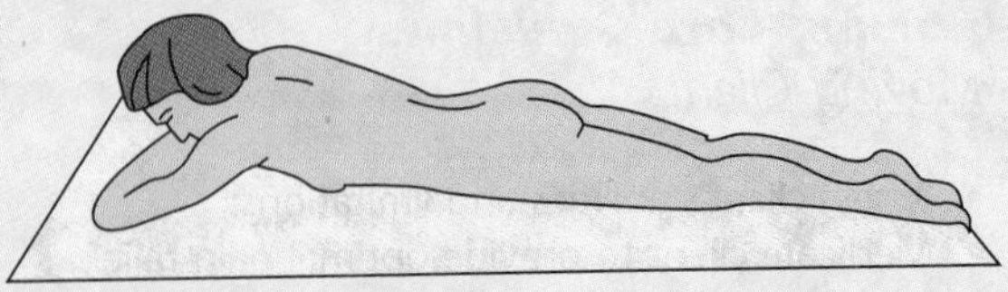

Prone: The client lies face down. Arms may cushion the head or may be flexed. An alternative position for an immobilized client, the prone position is contraindicated after abdominal surgery and in clients with respiratory or spinal problems.

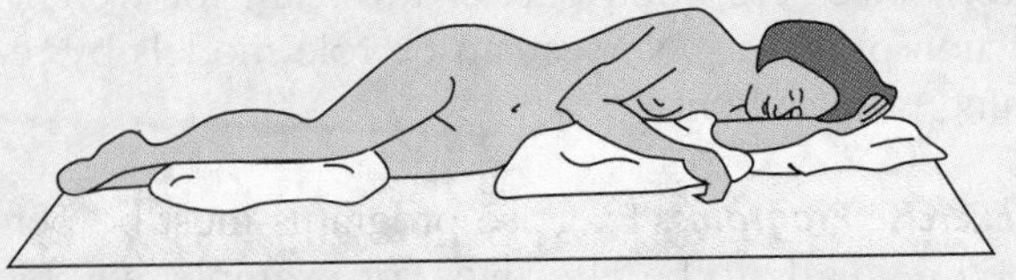

Side-lying: The client lies on the side with weight on hip and shoulder. Pillows support and stabilize uppermost leg, arm, head, and back. A choice position for clients with pressure on bony prominences of the back and sacral pressure sores, side-lying is not used after hip replacement and other orthopedic surgery.

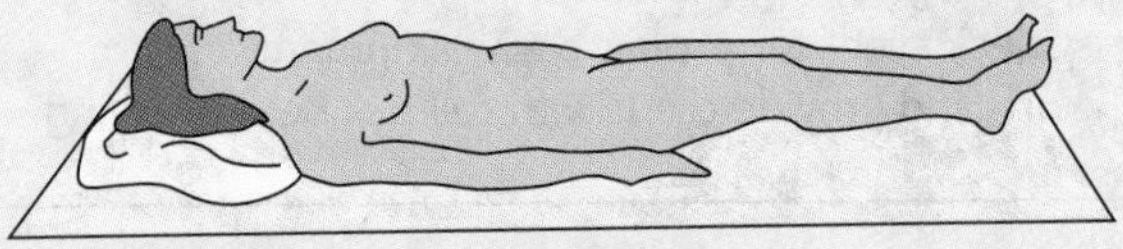

Supine: The client lies flat on back. Pillows may be used under the head, knees and calves to raise heels off the mattress. An alternative position for a client on bedrest, the prone position is used after spine surgery and some spinal anesthesia. It is not used for clients with dyspnea or at risk for aspiration.

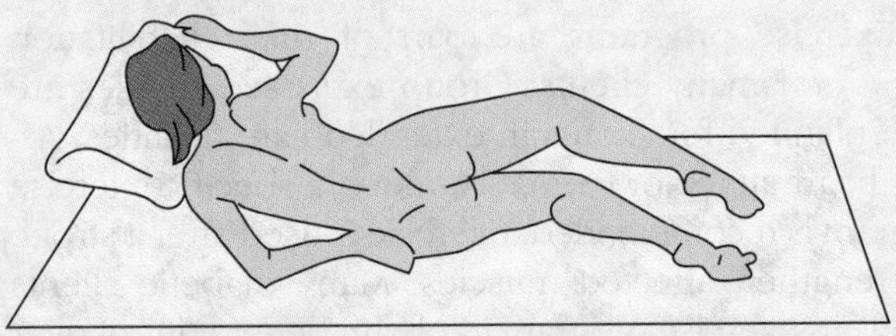

Sims': In this semiprone position the client lies on the side with weight distributed toward the anterior ileum, humerus, and clavicle. Pillows support the flexed arms and legs. The position is contraindicated by many spine or orthopedic conditions.

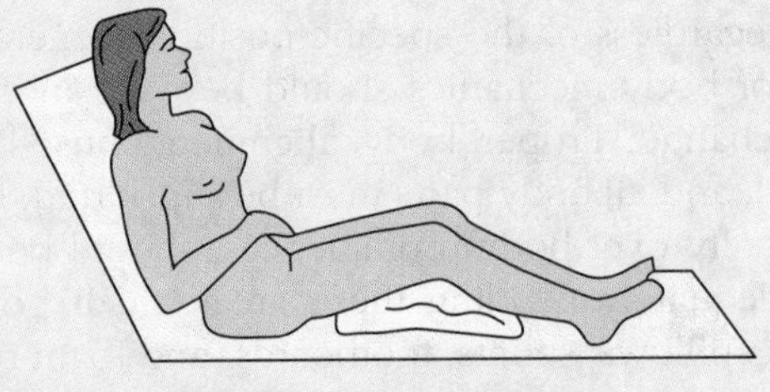

Fowler's: This sitting position raises the client's head 80°–90°. Pillows can be used under the head and arms and a footboard may also be used. The position improves cardiac output, promotes ventilation and eases eating, talking, and watching TV. It is not used after spine or brain surgery.

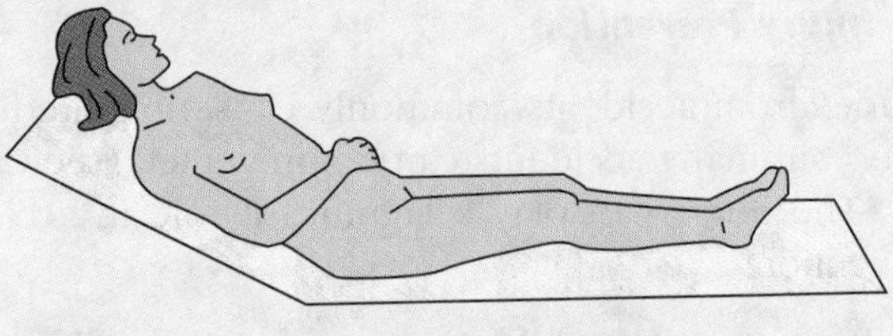

Semi–Fowler's: In this semi–sitting position the client's head is elevated 30°–45°. This position has the same advantages and contraindications as Fowler's position.

(continued)

Figure 33-5* • *Common client positions. Among selected body positions, the prone, supine, Fowler's, semi-Fowler's, side-lying, and Sims' positions are typically chosen for clients in health-care facilities; whereas the dorsal recumbent, lithotomy, knee-chest, and Trendelenburg positions are typically used during certain tests and surgical procedures.

- Document position changes and the client's tolerance of specific positions in the chart.

Proper positioning, outlined in Procedure 33-2, is important in preventing complications. A client with partial mobility can usually be taught positioning techniques to use with or without the nurse's assistance, but immobile clients rely on the nursing staff or caregiver to reposition them. Helping promote functional mobility is an important independent responsibility of the nurse, who works within mobility restrictions ordered by the healthcare provider or physical therapist. Unless contraindicated, clients should be moved to a chair twice a day (see the accompanying display for guidelines on moving clients).

Turning Schedules. According to most reports in the nursing literature, immobile clients should be turned and repositioned every 2 hours, but there is little research to show that this schedule is therapeutic for all

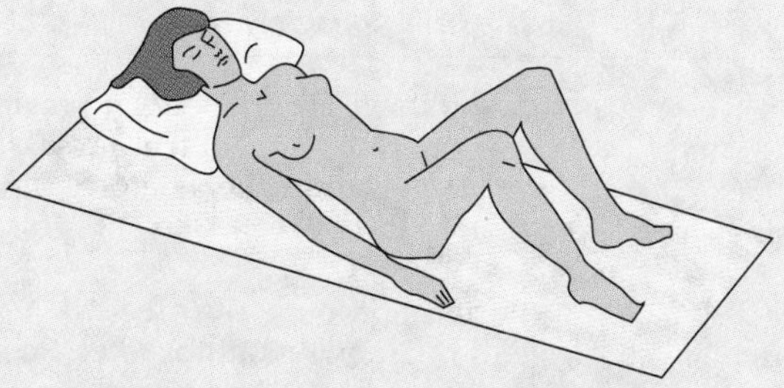

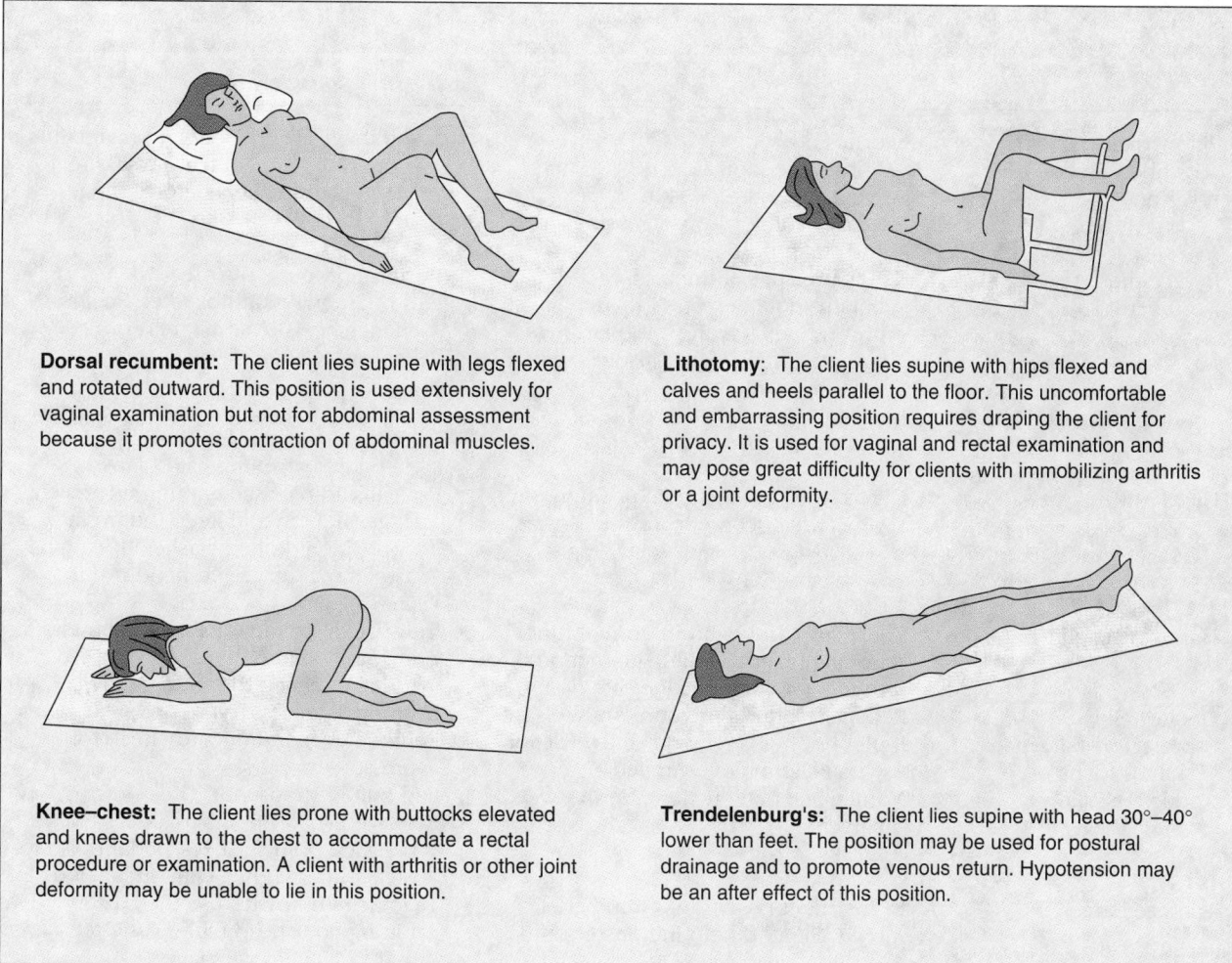

Dorsal recumbent: The client lies supine with legs flexed and rotated outward. This position is used extensively for vaginal examination but not for abdominal assessment because it promotes contraction of abdominal muscles.

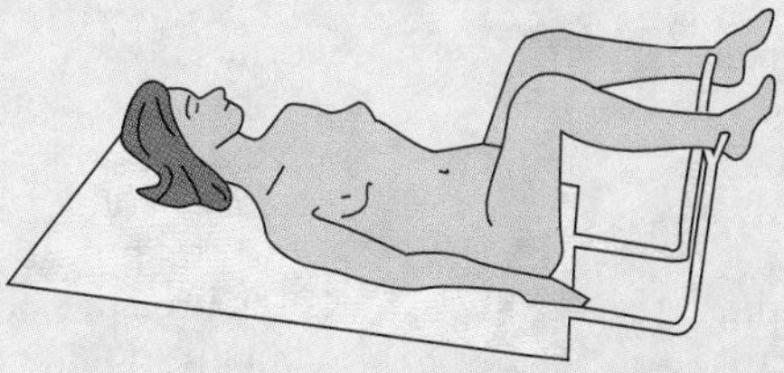

Lithotomy: The client lies supine with hips flexed and calves and heels parallel to the floor. This uncomfortable and embarrassing position requires draping the client for privacy. It is used for vaginal and rectal examination and may pose great difficulty for clients with immobilizing arthritis or a joint deformity.

Knee–chest: The client lies prone with buttocks elevated and knees drawn to the chest to accommodate a rectal procedure or examination. A client with arthritis or other joint deformity may be unable to lie in this position.

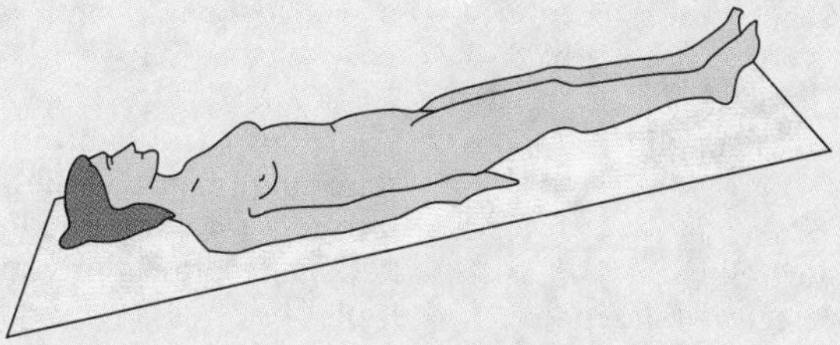

Trendelenburg's: The client lies supine with head 30°–40° lower than feet. The position may be used for postural drainage and to promote venous return. Hypotension may be an after effect of this position.

Figure 33-5 • *(continued)*

clients. More frequent turning may be needed. Significant factors include the amount of adipose tissue, skeletal structure, underlying pathophysiology, comfort level, skin condition, and level of mobility. Assessing for skin condition and signs of pressure is important in determining the turning schedule. Decreased capillary refill and blanched or reddened areas indicate the need for more frequent turning.

Turning schedules should be incorporated in the plan of care and posted at the bedside whether the client is receiving care in the home, a long-term care facility, or a hospital. This helps ensure consistency of care between different shifts and different caregivers. In extended-care facilities, where many clients require frequent position changes, a specific rotation pattern may be developed to ensure that various positions are used in an orderly fashion.

Logrolling. Logrolling (as described in Procedure 33-2) is a technique used for clients who have had surgery or an injury involving the back or spine. To prevent further trauma and injury, the body must be moved as a unit so that the spinal column does not bend or twist. Instruct the client to keep his or her body as stiff as possible and to avoid any sudden moves during the procedure. A draw sheet can be helpful in logrolling clients smoothly, especially if they are obese. When turning a client, pillows are placed between the legs. Leave the pillows in place if the client remains in the side-lying position.

Managing Clients with Hip Fractures. When turning clients who have had hip fractures or hip surgery, take special care to prevent adduction of the affected hip and leg. Dislocation of the hip can result from movement of the leg toward or past the midline of the body (adduction). To avoid this, abductor pillows should be used. If unavailable, regular pillows should be placed between the legs, and an additional staff member should support the affected leg so that it will not fall, even momentarily, during the move.

Joint Mobility Maintenance

Each joint's mobility is maintained by normal body movements that exercise the joint through its full ROM. Almost all daily activities are full of intricate movements that exercise each joint fully, but when mobility is altered,

Table 33-3 • Positioning Aids

Aid	Purpose	Nursing Considerations
Pillow (feather, foam, or fiber-filled); various sizes	Elevates body part Supports client on side Prevents pressure on skin Increases comfort by decreasing stress and strain on body parts	Use pillows small enough to maintain proper body alignment. Assess for allergies to feathers before using.
Bed cradle	Keeps pressure of linen off feet	Position properly over feet.
Footboard	Maintains dorsiflexion of the feet, preventing foot drop. If board has antirotation blocks, it also can prevent hip rotation.	Pad board with bath blanket. Position client's heels over mattress or use heel protectors.
Trochanter roll	Prevents external rotation of legs when in a supine position	Trochanter roll should be placed from client's iliac crest to mid-thigh. Can be made by rolling bath blanket.
Hand roll	Keeps hand in functional position; prevents finger contractures	Roll should be large enough to prevent finger flexion and keep thumb in opposition. Rolled washcloth may be used if manufactured hand roll is unavailable.
Hand-wrist splint	Keeps arm and hand in normal functioning position (slight adduction of thumb and dorsiflexion of wrist)	Individually made for each client: Pad inside of splint. Remove every 4 hours to check for pressure areas.
Heel or elbow protectors (sheepskin or foam)	Reduces mattress pressure on heels or elbows; helps remove elbow friction when client moves in bed	Launder as necessary. Remove every 4 hours to check for pressure areas.
Abduction pillow	Maintains hip abduction after hip surgery	Pad pillow straps. Remove every 4 hours to assess for pressure points. Check pedal pulse to detect interference with circulation.
Trapeze bar	Helps client raise trunk from bed Allows client to help in transfers and position changes Allows client to strengthen upper arms through exercise	Teach client how to use the bar. Avoid hitting your head when you are assisting client with care.
Side rail	Helps weak client turn independently Protects client from falling out of bed	Keep in raised position to aid client mobility and ensure client safety.
Turn sheet	Helps reposition client; can be secured to side rail to support client in side-lying position	Position from midthorax to below hips. Roll sheet close to client to obtain better support when moving client. Can be made from bath blankets if manufactured models are unavailable.

joints stiffen. If the immobility and stiffness continue, the joint becomes fixed (a contracture), and movement becomes difficult or impossible. The aim of nursing interventions is to maintain joint mobility and prevent contractures.

Types of ROM. A client who can perform ROM unassisted is said to have **active ROM.** A client who needs the nurse's assistance to perform ROM is said to have **passive ROM.** Assistive ROM indicates that the client can participate in ROM exercises with assistance. For example, after a stroke, the client may have weakness on one side of the body. With direction, the client may use the strong muscles on the unaffected side to exercise the weaker muscles on the affected side.

General Principles of ROM Exercises. ROM exercises should be initiated as soon as possible, because changes in affected joints can occur after only 3 days of impaired mobility (Loeper, 1992). Allow the client to participate as fully as he or she can. Perform ROM exercises in a systematic order at a designated time each day (usually during morning care). For high-risk clients, ROM exercises may be indicated more often. In some facilities, physical therapists help immobile clients perform ROM exercises at the bedside.

ROM exercises should be done smoothly and gently. Stop if the client complains of pain or if resistance is encountered. Support the joint distal to the one being exercised. A healthcare provider's order and specific instructions should be obtained to perform ROM

Procedure 33-2
Positioning a Client in Bed

Purpose

1. Maintain skin integrity and prevent deformities of the musculoskeletal system
2. Maintain proper body alignment
3. Provide comfort
4. Maintain optimal position for ventilation and lung expansion

Assessment

- Assess client's body alignment and comfort level in current position.
- Review chart for conditions that influence ability to move or to be positioned (ie, fractures, paralysis, spinal injury).
- Assess for tubes, IV lines, incisions, or equipment that may alter the positioning procedure.
- Assess client's level of consciousness and ability to understand and follow directions.
- Assess client's ability to assist with positioning.
- Assess client's weight and your strength. Determine if additional assistance is needed.

Equipment

Pillows
Draw sheet or turning sheet
Side rails

Procedure

Moving a Client Up in Bed (One Nurse)

1. Explain procedure and rationale to client.
Rationale: Explanation reduces anxiety and increases cooperation.
2. Lower head of bed to flat position, and raise level of bed to comfortable working height.
Rationale: This decreases gravitational pull of upper body and promotes good body mechanics by decreasing back strain.
3. Remove all pillows from under client. Leave one at head of bed.
Rationale: Pillows prevent accidental head injury against top of bed frame.
4. Instruct client to bend legs, put feet flat on bed, and place arm nearest you under your arm and around your shoulder.
Rationale: Client will be able to assist by pushing legs against bed.
5. Place your feet in broad stance with one foot in front of the other. Flex your knees and thighs.
Rationale: Lowering center of gravity ensures using large muscle groups of legs.
6. Place one arm under client's shoulders and one arm under thighs.
Rationale: The heaviest parts of client's body are supported.
7. Rock back and forth on front and back legs to count of three. On third count, have client push with feet as you lift and pull the client up in bed.
Rationale: Rocking motion develops momentum, which promotes smooth lifting with minimal exertion by the nurse.
8. Elevate head of bed, and place pillows under head. Raise side rails, and lower bed to lowest level.
Rationale: Provides for client comfort and safety.

Procedure

Moving Helpless Client Up in Bed (Two Nurses)

1. Explain procedure and rationale to client.
Rationale: Explanation reduces anxiety.
2. Lower head of bed to flat position, and raise level of bed to comfortable working height.
Rationale: This minimizes back strain.
3. Remove all pillows from under client. Leave one at head of bed.
Rationale: Pillow prevents accidental head injury against top of bed frame.
4. One nurse stands on each side of bed with legs positioned for wide base of support and one foot slightly in front of the other.
5. Each nurse rolls up and grasps edges of turn sheet close to client's shoulders and buttocks.
Rationale: Turn sheet is used to distribute client's weight and prevent shearing injury to skin by reducing friction during move.

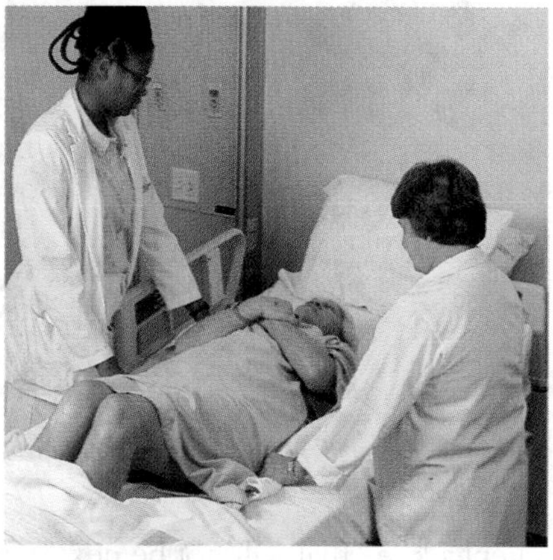

Step 5 • *Grasp turn sheet near client's shoulders and buttocks.*

(continued)

6. Flex knees and hips. Tighten abdominal and gluteal muscles.
   Rationale: Using large muscle groups of legs and tightening muscles during transfer prevents back injury.
7. Rock back and forth on front and back legs to count of three. On third count, both nurses shift weight to front leg as they simultaneously lift client toward head of bed.
   Rationale: Rocking motion develops momentum, which provides a smooth lift of client with minimal exertion by nurses.
8. Elevate head of bed, and place pillows under client's head. Adjust other positioning pillows as necessary. Put up side rails and lower bed to lowest level.
   Rationale: This provides for client comfort and safety.

Procedure

Positioning Client in Side-Lying Position

1. Lower head of bed as flat as client can tolerate.
   Rationale: Client turns easier from flat position.
2. Elevate and lock side rail on side client will face when turned.
   Rationale: This prevents accidental injury from falling out of bed during turn.
3. Place arm that client will turn toward away from his or her body. Fold other arm across chest.
   Rationale: This facilitates turning by preventing client from rolling onto bottom arm.

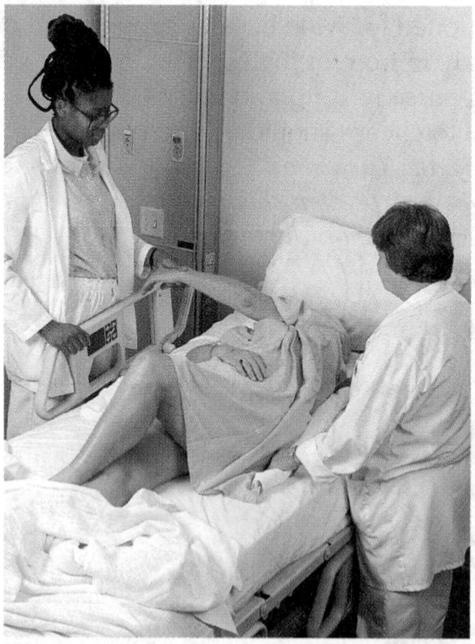

Step 3 • *Have client reach toward side rail with opposite arm.*

4. Flex client's knee that will not be next to mattress after turn. Have client reach toward side rail with opposite arm.
   Rationale: Client assists with position change.
5. Assume a broad stance with knees slightly flexed.
   Rationale: This stance increases balance, lowers center of gravity, and encourages use of large muscle groups during movement.
6. Using draw sheet, gently pull client over on side.
   Rationale: You can evenly support heaviest part of client during turn.
7. Align client properly, and place pillows behind back and under head.
   Rationale: The client is supported in a side-lying position.

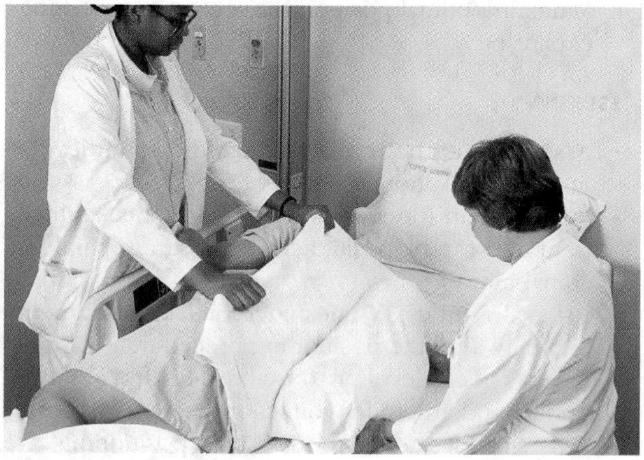

Steps 6 and 7 • *Using draw sheet pull client onto side, placing pillow behind back.*

8. Pull shoulder blade forward and out from under client. Support client's upper arm with pillow.
   Rationale: Joints are protected from weight and strain. Ventilation also may improve because chest can expand more fully.
9. Place pillow lengthwise between client's legs from thighs to foot.
   Rationale: This keeps leg aligned and prevents pressure on bony prominences.

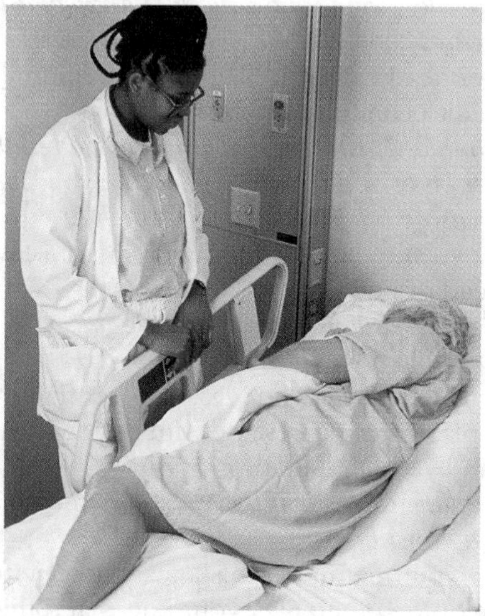

Steps 8 and 9 • *Support arm and legs with pillows.*

Procedure

Logrolling

1. Obtain assistance. Two or three nurses are usually required.
2. All nurses stand on same side of bed, with feet apart, one foot slightly ahead of the other. Flex knees and hips.
   Rationale: This stance increases balance and stability and ensures use of large muscle groups when turning client.
3. Use one pillow to support client's head during and after turn.
   Rationale: Pillow maintains alignment of cervical spine.
4. Place pillows between client's legs.
   Rationale: Pillows support the uppermost leg and prevent adduction during turn.
5. Instruct client to fold arms over chest and keep body stiff.
   Rationale: Spine is kept in alignment during turn.
6. Reach across client and support head, thorax, trunk, and legs. On count of three, roll client in one coordinated movement to lateral position.
   Rationale: Alignment of whole body is maintained during turn.
7. Support client in alignment with pillows as described in "Side-lying position."
   Note: Clients with suspected or known spinal injuries should wear cervical collars to prevent injury to the spinal cord whenever turning or moving in bed.

Home-Care Modifications

- Teach caregivers principles of body alignment, and explain the types of assistive devices used to support and maintain the body in alignment.
- Teach caregivers about devices used to protect bony prominences and prevent pressure sores (ie, sheepskins, foam mattresses, heel and elbow protectors).

for clients with acute arthritis, fractures, torn ligaments, joint dislocation, or acute myocardial infarction. Procedure 33-3 details ROM technique.

Automatic ROM Equipment. Mechanical devices, such as continuous passive range-of-motion machines, have been developed to provide continuous ROM to a specific joint. Such devices are most commonly used after orthopedic surgery, usually of the knee, when such exercise promotes joint mobility and permits rapid rehabilitation. The equipment extends the joint to a prescribed angle for a prescribed period, continuously cycling according to parameters set by the healthcare provider.

Ambulation

Early ambulation significantly reduces complications of immobility. Walking exercises almost all body muscles and promotes joint flexibility. Most surgical clients are permitted and encouraged to get out of bed and walk on their first postoperative day. Early ambulation significantly reduces the formation of venous clots and atelectasis, thereby decreasing respiratory and circulatory complications after surgery. Even a short period of immobility decreases a client's exercise tolerance, so assistance is usually required when the client resumes walking. Musculoskeletal or neurologic alterations typically require temporary or permanent assistance with ambulation (see Procedure 33-4).

Dangling the Legs. **Dangling** is a preliminary step to ambulation, especially for clients who may be unable to ambulate initially. The activity involves sitting on the side of the bed and dangling the legs. Often this occurs on the evening of surgery or when weight bearing is not permitted. Dangling helps to prevent postural hypotension when it precedes the client's first ambulatory steps.

When assisting the client to dangle his or her legs, raise the head of the bed slowly as high as the client can tolerate. This not only decreases the distance the client needs to move but also uses the bed to help the client into a sitting position. To further assist the client to an upright position, have the client move as close to the edge of the bed as possible. Face the client, and establish a broad base of support, flexing your hips, knees, and ankles. Moving the client to a sitting position occurs in one smooth movement, supporting the client under the knees and around the shoulders (Fig. 33-6). The nurse should tighten the gluteal and abdominal muscles to avoid back strain or injury.

Some clients can independently reach a sitting position. The easiest way to accomplish this is to have the client roll onto his or her side, grasp the mattress with the lower arm, and use the other hand to push up while swinging the legs over the side of the mattress (Fig. 33-7). After achieving this position, the client can maintain it by placing the hands palm down on the mattress for balance.

Assisting the Client With Ambulation. Assisting the client to ambulate safely begins by thoroughly assessing his or her muscle strength and coordination. First, assist the client to a sitting position on the side of the bed. If the client complains of dizziness, is diaphoretic, or has orthostatic hypotension (confirmed by blood pressure measurement), postpone ambulation. If dangling is well tolerated, ambulation can proceed.

Procedure 33-3
Providing Range-of-Motion Exercises

Purpose

1. Maintain joint mobility
2. Improve or maintain muscle strength
3. Prevent muscle atrophy and contractures

Assessment

- Review medical history to determine specific limitations to joint mobility.
- Assess client's level of consciousness and physical ability to assist or independently perform range-of-motion (ROM) exercises.
- Assess for redness, tenderness, pain, swelling, or deformities around joints.

Equipment

No special equipment is required except a bed.

Procedure

1. Explain procedure and purpose to client.
   Rationale: Explanation reduces anxiety and encourages cooperation.
2. Position client on back with head of bed as flat as possible. Elevate bed to comfortable working height.
   Rationale: Adjusting bed promotes proper body mechanics to prevent muscle strain for nurse.
3. Stand on side of bed of joints to be exercised. Uncover only the limb to be exercised.
   Rationale: This provides warmth and privacy.
4. Perform exercises slowly and gently, providing support by holding areas proximal and distal to the joint.
   Rationale: This prevents discomfort and muscle spasms from jerky movements.
5. Repeat each exercise five times.
   Note: Discontinue or decrease ROM if client complains of discomfort or muscle spasm.
6. Neck:
   a. Move chin to chest.
   b. Bend head toward back.
   c. Tilt head toward each shoulder.
   d. Rotate head in circular motion.
   e. Return head to erect position.
7. Shoulder:
   a. Raise client's arm from side to above head.
   b. Abduct and rotate shoulder by raising arm above head with palm up.
   c. Adduct shoulder by moving arm across body as far as possible.

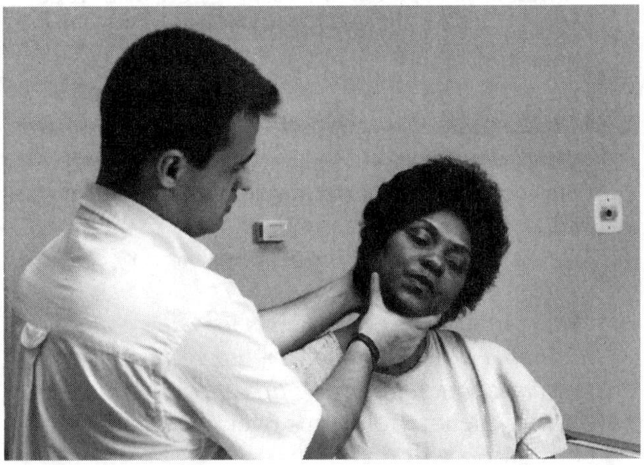

Step 6C • *Rotate client's head.*

   d. Rotate shoulder internally and externally by flexing elbow and moving forearm so that palm touches mattress; then reverse the motion so that back of client's hand touches mattress.
   e. Move shoulder in a full circle.
8. Elbow:
   a. Bend elbow so that forearm moves toward shoulder.

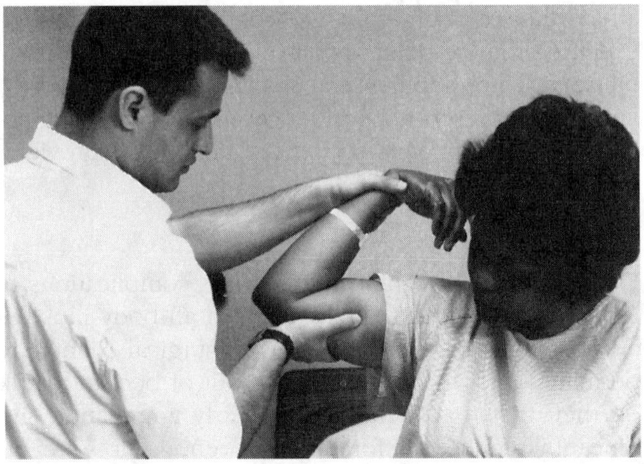

Step 8A • *Bend elbow so that forearm moves toward shoulder.*

   b. Hyperextend elbow as far as possible.
9. Wrist and hand:
   a. Move hand toward inner aspect of forearm.
   b. Bend dorsal surface of hand backward.
   c. Abduct wrist by bending toward thumb.
   d. Adduct wrist by bending toward fifth finger.
   e. Make a fist; extend the fingers.
   f. Spread fingers apart, then together.
   g. Move thumb across hand to base of fifth finger.

10. Hip and knee:
    a. Lift leg and bend knee toward chest.
    b. Abduct and adduct leg, moving leg laterally away from body and returning to medial position.
    c. Internally and externally rotate hip by turning leg inward, then outward.
    d. Take special care to support joints of larger limbs.
11. Ankle and foot:
    a. Dorsiflex foot by moving it so toes point upward.
    b. Plantarflex by moving foot so toes point downward.
    c. Curl toes down, then extend.
    d. Spread toes apart, then bring together.
    e. Invert by turning sole of foot medially.
    f. Evert by turning sole of foot laterally.
12. Move to other side of bed and repeat exercises.
13. Reposition client comfortably.
14. Document ROM.

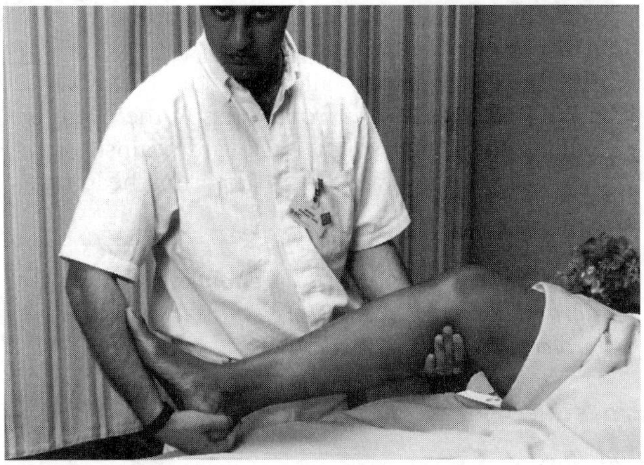

Step 11A • *Flex foot so that toes point upward.*

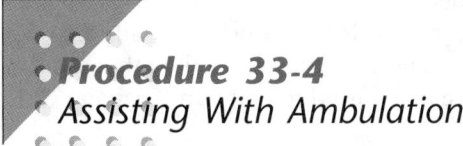

Procedure 33-4
Assisting With Ambulation

Purpose

1. Promote safe ambulation free of falls or injury
2. Increase muscle strength and joint mobility
3. Prevent complications of immobility
4. Promote self-esteem and independence

Assessment

- Review chart for conditions that impair ambulation (arthritis, fractures, paralysis) and for healthcare provider's orders for ambulation or ambulating aids (walkers, canes, crutches).
- Assess comfort level. Medicate as ordered with analgesics. Plan ambulation for time when analgesics have peak action.
- Assess range of motion and muscle strength. Determine if extra assistance is required.
- Obtain baseline vital signs. Obtain orthostatic vital signs if client has been on prolonged bed rest or is at risk for orthostatic hypotension for other reasons.

Equipment

Ambulation aid (crutches, cane, walker) if required
Transfer belt (optional), clothing, or robe
Well-fitting shoes or slippers with nonskid soles

Procedure

1. Explain procedure and purpose of ambulation to client. Decide together how far and where to walk.
   Rationale: Explanation reduces anxiety and facilitates cooperation.
2. Place bed in lowest position.
3. Assist client to sitting position on side of bed. Assess for dizziness or faintness. Obtain orthostatic vital signs if complaints are present. Allow client to remain in this position until he or she feels secure.
   Rationale: This minimizes orthostatic hypotension and resulting falls or injury.
4. Help client with clothing and footwear.

(continued)

Procedure

One Nurse

1. Wrap transfer belt around client's waist (optional according to previous assessment).
   Rationale: Transfer belt provides a firm hold for the nurse and prevents injury to the client.

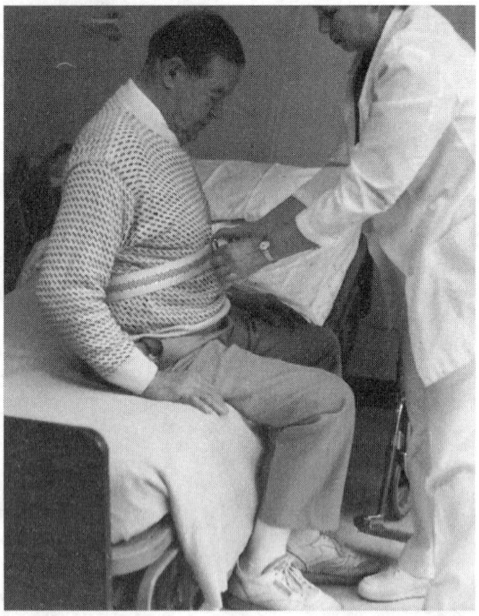

Step 1 • Place transfer belt snugly around waist.

2. Assist client to standing position, and assess client's balance. Return to bed or transfer to chair if very weak or unsteady.

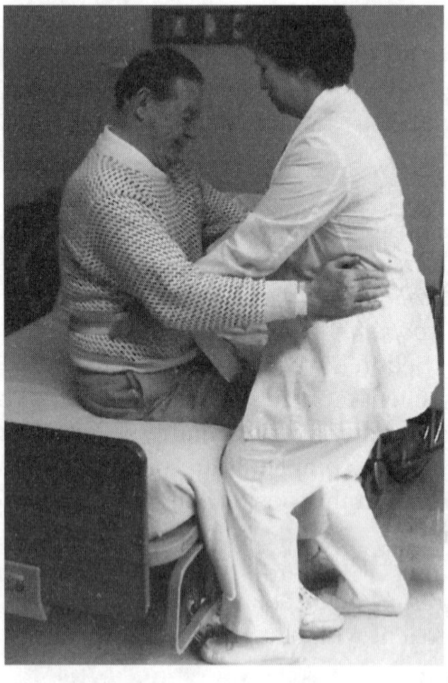

Step 2 • Assist client to standing position, using a wide base of support and with knees flexed.

3. Position yourself behind client while supporting him or her by waist or transfer belt.
   Rationale: Client can stand erect and does not lean to one side for support from nurse.
4. Take several steps forward with client. Assess strength and balance.
5. Encourage client to use good posture and to look ahead, not down at feet.
   Rationale: Promote good balance.
6. Ambulate for planned distance or time.
7. If client becomes weak or dizzy, return to bed or assist to chair.
8. If the client begins to fall, place your feet wide apart with one foot in front. Support the client by pulling his or her weight backward against your body. Lower gently to floor, protecting head (see Fig. 33–7).
   Rationale: Nurse's foot position widens and stabilizes the base of support and enables nurse to support client's weight with large muscle groups. This protects nurse from back strain.

Procedure

Two Nurses

1. Assist client to sitting position as described.
2. Assist client to standing position with one nurse on each side.
3. Each nurse grasps client's upper arm with the nearest hand and the elbow with the other hand. One nurse may be used to carry and manage equipment.
   Rationale: Support is provided during ambulation to prevent falls.
   Note: May use a transfer belt around client's waist. Each nurse should grasp belt with near hand and elbow with the other hand.
4. Walk with client using slow, even steps. Assess strength and balance.
   Rationale: This promotes stability of client.

Procedure

Using a Walker

1. Assist client to sitting and standing position.
2. Have client grasp walker handles.
3. Client moves walker ahead 6 to 8 in, placing all four feet of walker on floor.
4. Client moves forward to walker.
5. Nurse should walk close behind and slightly to side of client.
   Rationale: If client begins to fall, nurse can support him or her and prevent injury.
6. Repeat above sequence until walk is complete.

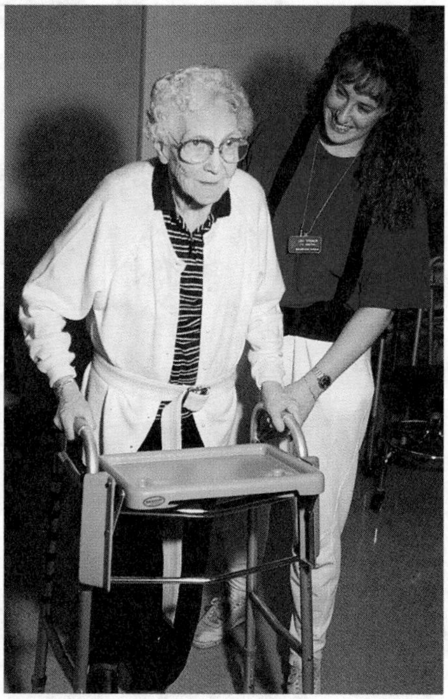

Step 5 • *The nurse should walk behind and to the side of the client.*

Home-Care Modifications

- To provide safety and prevent falls at home, throw rugs and small pieces of furniture should be removed so client will not trip on them.
- Client should always wear shoes with nonskid soles.
- The bathroom is a common place for falls and injury. Placing a large rug with a skid-resistant backing on the floor can prevent falls from slipping on wet floors.

Have the client wear shoes or slippers with nonskid soles, and clear the path of obstacles that might cause the client to trip. Many hallways have railings the client can grip. A weak or unstable client may prefer to push a chair or wheelchair to provide extra support and balance. Encourage the client to look straight ahead to promote balance and prevent dizziness.

All equipment (IV tubing, indwelling catheter, drains) must be secured to a pole. The nurse assisting the client should not carry equipment so that his or her hands are free in case the client falls. Watch IV lines carefully. Commonly, the change in position decreases the distance between the bottle and the infusion site, thereby decreasing gravitational force and affecting the flow rate. This usually causes blood to flow up the IV tubing. Unless corrected by readjusting the flow rate, blood may clot at the infusion site, and the IV will have to be restarted. Encourage the client to keep the arm in which the IV is infusing at the side rather than using it to push the IV pole. Nasogastric suction can usually be discontinued while the client is ambulating and reconnected on return to the room.

While the client is walking, assess for steadiness of gait, diaphoresis, and complaints of fatigue. Pulse and respiratory rate should be monitored before and after ambulation to determine cardiorespiratory response to exercise.

Transfer Belts. Transfer belts (sometimes called safety belts or ambulation belts) should be used if the client is weak or has problems with coordination. The transfer belt is a canvas belt that can be applied around the waist and tightened over clothing (see the example in Procedure 33-4). The nurse grips the transfer belt as the client walks so that he or she can provide aid if the client begins to fall. If the client becomes dizzy or starts to fall, slowly and gently lower the client to the floor, and call for help (Fig. 33-8). If the client is at high risk for falls, two nurses may be required to assist with ambulation.

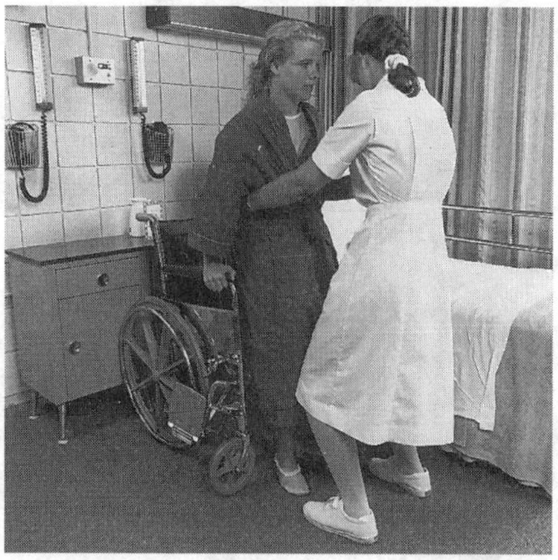

Figure 33-6 • *The nurse assists the client to the side of the bed in one smooth movement. The nurse supports the client under the knees and around the shoulder and swings the client into a sitting position.*

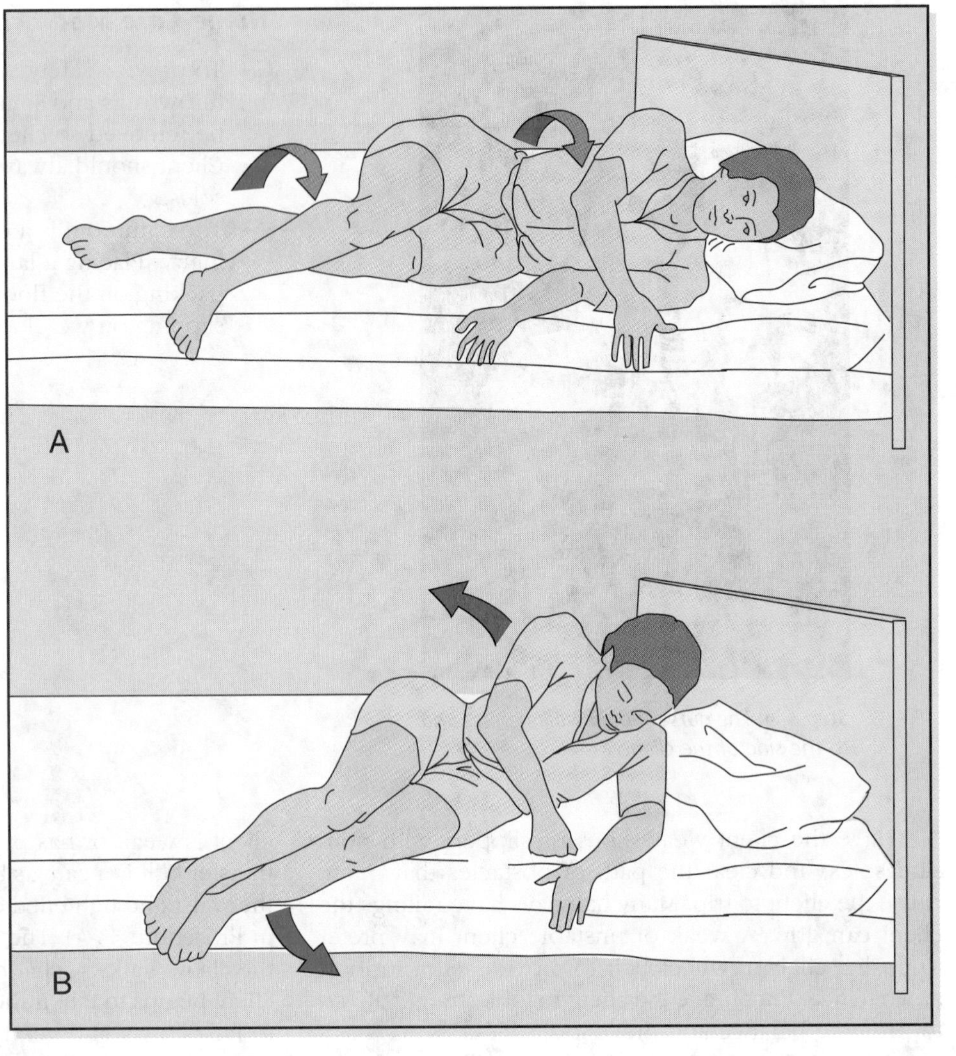

Figure 33-7 • *Many clients can reach a sitting position independently when taught the proper method.* ***(A)*** *The client rolls over onto his or her side.* ***(B)*** *The client grasps the mattress with the lower arm and uses the other hand to push up while swinging the legs over the side of the bed.*

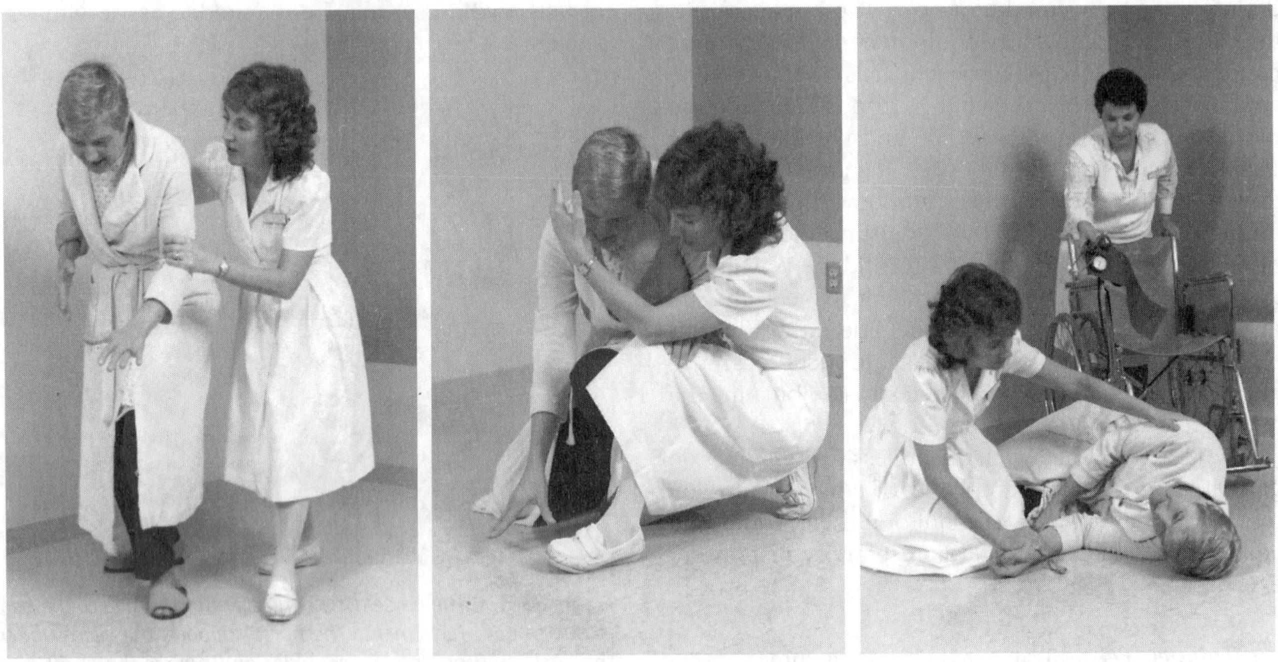

Figure 33-8 • *Ensure safety during a fall by supporting and gently lowering the client to the ground, then calling for help. Do not try to hold the client up, because this can result in injury to you.*

Mechanical Aids. Mechanical devices can help the client with certain limitations to ambulate safely. During ambulation, walkers, canes, quad canes, and crutches help bear a portion of the client's weight, promote stability, and maintain balance. The physical therapist is usually responsible for instructing the client how to use these devices initially, but usually the client requires additional instruction or supervision.

Canes are useful for clients who can bear weight but need support for balance or who have decreased strength in one leg. The cane acts as an additional "leg," providing the client with three points of support during ambulation. The client holds the cane in the hand opposite the weak or injured leg, then moves the affected or weak foot forward with the cane as the weight of the body remains on the stronger extremity (Fig. 33-9). When climbing stairs, the strongest leg advances up the stair first, followed by the cane and the weaker leg. This process is reversed when descending stairs: The cane and the weaker leg are followed by the stronger leg. Instruct the client to look straight ahead rather than at the feet while walking.

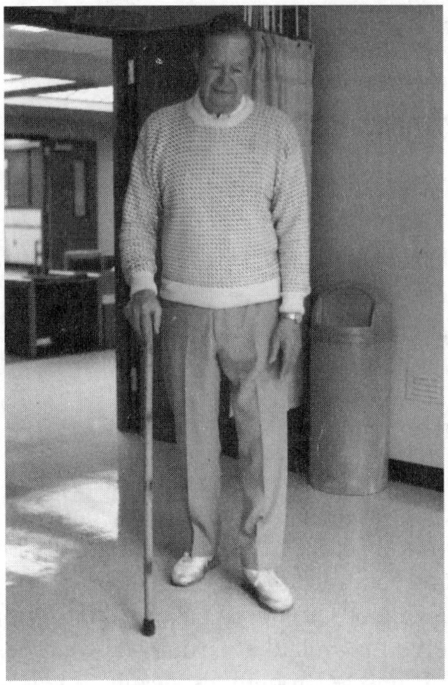

Figure 33-9 • *Using a cane to ambulate.*

Canes are made of wood or metal and should be about waist high. A variety of canes are available, ranging from a simple straight-leg cane to a three-or four-pronged cane (often called a quad cane).

Walkers are lightweight, tubular metal structures that provide more support than canes. Four rubber-tipped legs give walkers a wide base of support. The client grips the walker, picks it up, and moves it forward. The client may use a two-point or three-point gait when ambulating with the walker. Clear hallways of obstructions. Some walkers have wheels and a seat so that clients who tire can sit and rest or propel themselves by pushing with their feet.

Crutches allow the client to walk without weight bearing on the legs. Crutches may be indicated when the client has a sprain, fracture, or nonwalking cast. Underarm crutches usually serve these short-term purposes. The client must use the arms, not the shoulders, to support the body weight. Using the shoulders can cause skin breakdown at the axilla and nerve damage to the brachial plexus. Underarm crutches must be fitted correctly. About 2 in should remain between the axilla and the top of the crutch when the crutch is placed 2 in in front of and 6 in to the side of the foot.

Crutches also may be used for additional support that weak or paralyzed legs cannot provide for walking. For long-term use, Lofstrand crutches, which have metal bands encircling the forearms, are used. The client on crutches may use several gaits (see Procedure 33-5):

When the client can bear partial weight on both feet, the *four-point gait* may be used. The right crutch is placed forward, followed by the left foot, then the left crutch is moved forward, followed by the right foot.

When the client can bear weight on only one foot, the *three-point gait* is used. Here, both crutches and the weaker leg move forward first, followed by the stronger leg.

The *two-point gait* requires at least partial weight-bearing on each foot, as each crutch moves at the same time as the opposing leg.

The *swing-through gait* is often used by paraplegics, who move both crutches forward, then swing the body beyond the crutches to propel themselves forward.

To function independently, the client on crutches must learn how to rise from a sitting position and climb and descend stairs. This instruction is usually done by a physical therapist. The client also should be taught to inspect the rubber tips of crutches for wear. Prompt replacement of worn tips can prevent falls.

Muscle Strengthening to Facilitate Ambulation. Certain muscle groups may need strengthening before some clients can walk. Immobility weakens muscles, which may lead to muscle atrophy. Clients on bed rest should be taught to contract their quadriceps, gluteal, and abdominal muscles regularly, because these muscles are important for ambulation. Clients who will use crutches or walkers need to strengthen their arm muscles as well, because increased arm strength will be necessary to support their body weight. *Setting* is a term used to refer to isometric strengthening of muscles. The client concentrates on one muscle at a time, contracting it for 10 seconds and then permitting it to relax completely. This is repeated a prescribed number of times.

Procedure 33-5
Helping Clients With Crutchwalking

Purpose

1. Increase client's level of activity after musculoskeletal injury.
2. Assist client to walk safely with crutches using the least amount of energy.

Assessment

- Review medical history to determine reason for needing crutches and whether client is to bear weight on one leg only or can partially bear weight on affected side.
- Assess client's ability to balance himself or herself.
- Observe for unilateral or unusual weakness.
- Assess muscle strength, especially in legs and arms.
- Determine if client has experience with crutchwalking.
- Determine appropriate size crutch.

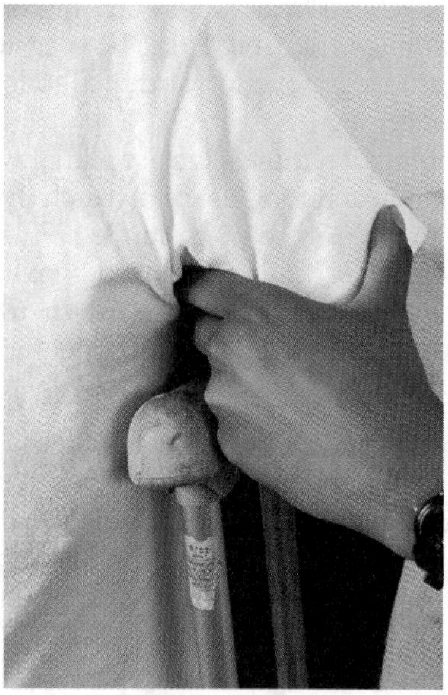

Assessment: Measuring crutches for proper fit.

Equipment

Crutches with suction tips, hand grips, and axillary pads
Shoes with nonskid soles

Procedure

Four-Point Gait

1. Client stands erect, face forward in tripod position. Client places crutch tips 6 in in front of feet and 6 in to side of each foot.

   Rationale: This is the position used to start crutchwalking. It provides a wide base of support so stability and balance are increased.

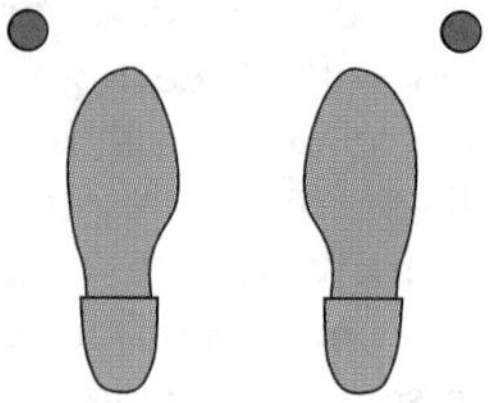

Step 1 • *To assume beginning tripod position, place crutch tips 6 inches ahead and to the side of each foot.*

2. Client moves right crutch forward 6 in.

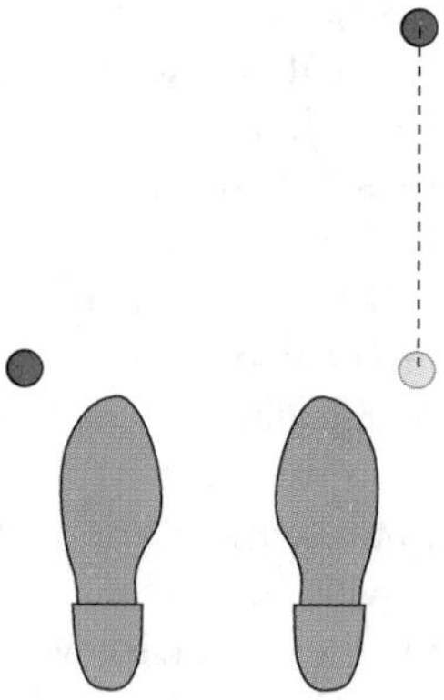

Step 2 • *Move right crutch forward.*

3. Client moves left foot forward to level of right crutch.

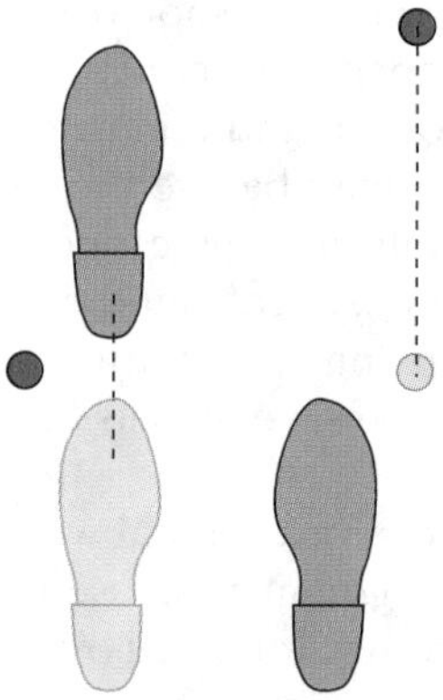

Step 3 • *Move left foot forward.*

4. Client moves left crutch forward 4 to 6 in.

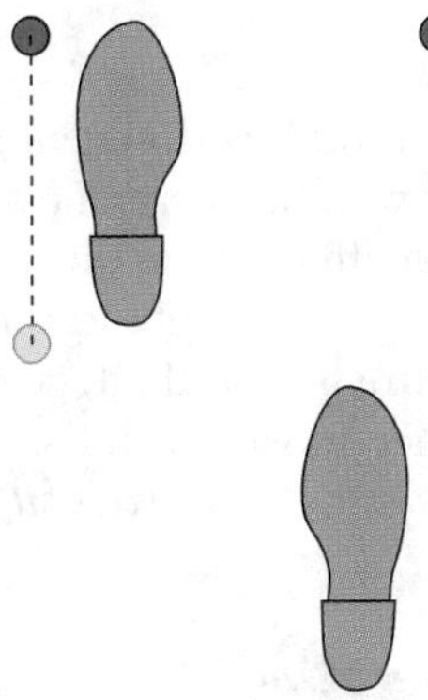

Step 4 *• Move left crutch forward.*

5. Client moves right foot forward to level of left crutch.

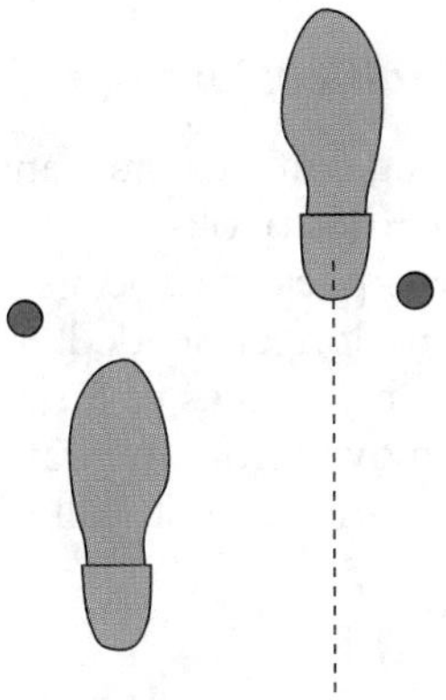

Step 5 *• Move right foot forward.*

6. Repeat sequence.
   Rationale: This gait is the safest and most stable because three points are always on the ground. The crutch and foot positions mimic arm and foot positions during regular walking. The client must be able to bear weight partially on the affected side to perform this gait.

Procedure

Three-Point Gait

1. Beginning in tripod position, client moves both crutches and affected leg forward.

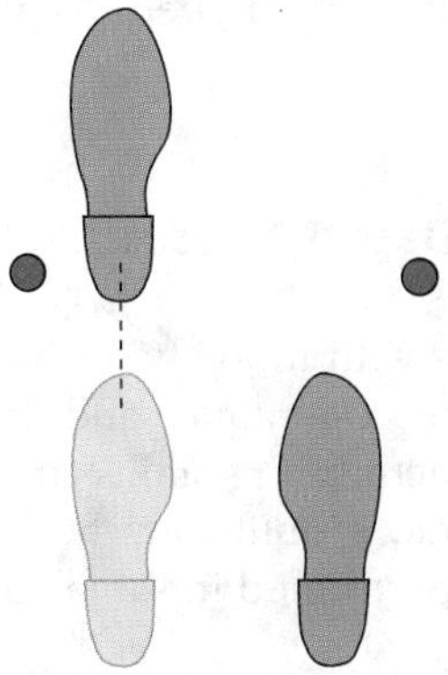

Step 1 *• Move both crutches and the affected leg.*

2. Client moves stronger leg forward.

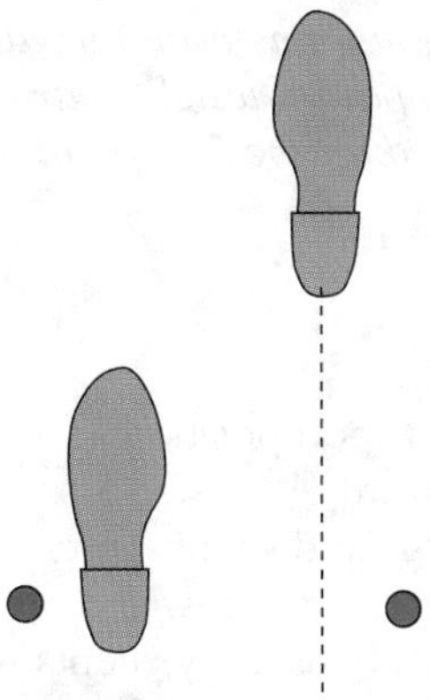

Step 2 *• Move stronger leg forward.*

3. Repeat sequence.
   Note: Client must bear his or her entire weight on the stronger leg to perform this gait.

Procedure

Two-Point Gait

1. Beginning in tripod position, client moves left crutch and right foot forward.

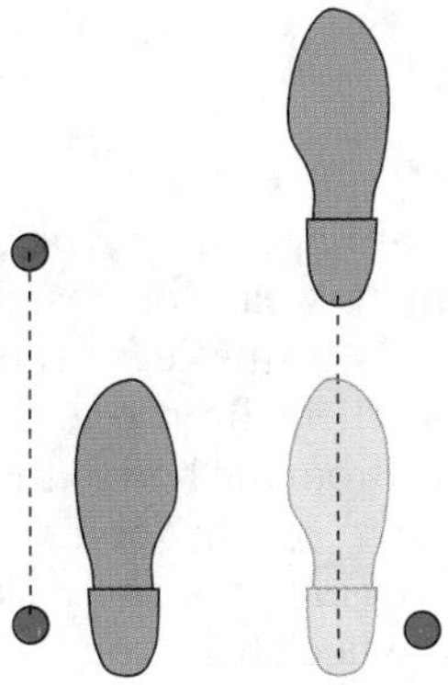

Step 1 *• Move left crutch and right leg forward.*

2. Client moves right crutch and left foot forward.

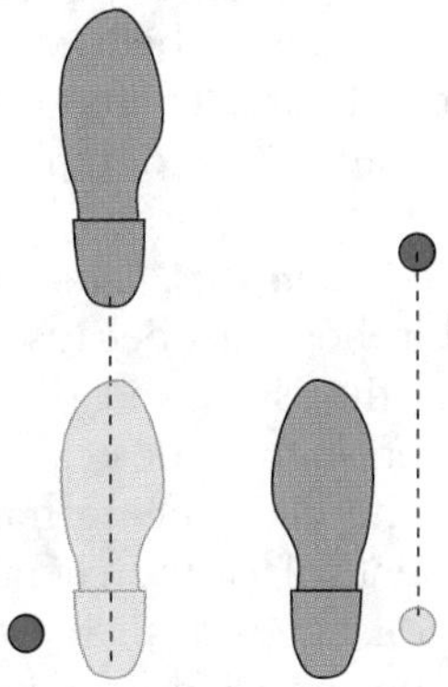

Step 2 *• Move right crutch and left leg forward.*

(continued)

3. Repeat sequence.
   Rationale: Crutch and foot movement is similar to arm and leg movement in normal walking. This gait requires partial weight bearing on both feet and is faster than the four-point gait.

Procedure

Swing-To Gait

1. Client forms tripod position and moves both crutches forward.
2. Client lifts legs and swings to crutches, supporting body weight on crutches.
   Note: Frequently used by clients with paralysis of legs and hips or those wearing weight-supporting braces on their legs.

Procedure

Swing-Through Gait

1. Client forms tripod position and moves both crutches forward.
2. Client lifts legs and swings through and ahead of crutches, supporting weight on crutches.
   Note: Similar to swing-to gait but requires much more strength and coordination.

Procedure

Climbing Stairs

1. Beginning in tripod position facing stairs, client transfers body weight to crutches.
2. Client places unaffected leg on stair.
3. Client transfers body weight to unaffected leg.
4. Client moves crutches and affected leg to stair.
5. Repeat sequence to top of stairs.
   Rationale: The crutches always support the affected leg.

Lifespan Consideration

- Older clients may not have the strength or balance necessary to feel comfortable or safe using crutches. A walker may be preferable.

Home Care Modifications

- The client using crutches must anticipate problems. If he or she carries books to school or a briefcase to work, a backpack may be a solution until crutches are no longer needed.
- Throw rugs, small pieces of furniture, and toys should be removed from the traffic pattern to provide for safety and ease of walking with crutches.

Transfers

Assisted transfers are necessary when the client is unconscious, extremely weak, or has decreased muscle strength or paralysis in the legs. Transfers usually involve moving the client from one flat surface to another, for example, from the bed to the stretcher or vice versa (see Procedure 33-6). Another transfer involves moving the client from the bed to a sitting position, either in a chair or wheelchair (see Procedure 33-7).

Safety is important during transfers. Doing an assessment to identify client abilities and limitations permits the nurse to individualize the transfer technique and plan for extra help as needed. Proper body mechanics will help to prevent injury to the client and nurse. Equipment (transfer belts, transfer boards or sleds, roller boards, hydraulic lifts) can make transfers easier and safer. Table 33-4 describes common aids.

Two- or Three-Person Lifts. Lifts or carries by staff are seldom used in hospitals because they are usually uncomfortable for the client and pose safety risks for the nurse. However, such carries can be used in emergencies or when the client being transferred is light. When lifting a client, place the client's arms over the chest and have colleagues available to lift each body area. When moving the client to another flat surface, one nurse grasps the client under the head and shoulders, one under the hips, and a third under the thighs and legs. If the client is being lifted to a chair, one nurse holds the client under the arms around the chest, and the second supports the hips and legs. Synchronize the lift by counting to three. Using proper body mechanics is essential to prevent injury to the lifters.

Hydraulic Lifts. A hydraulic lift is a mechanical device that permits a client to be transferred from the bed to a chair (Fig. 33-10). It is used when transferring a client may pose a safety risk to the client or the nurse. The lift has a canvas or fabric sling that fits under the client and hooks into a metal frame. Before using any hydraulic device, read the manufacturer's guidelines for proper operation. The client may become frightened when lifted away from the bed, so provide verbal support.

Community-Based Nursing

Most individuals with mobility problems manage independently in the community and at home. Acute injuries, such as fractures or sprains, are often treated with immobilizing braces until they heal. Most orthopedic surgery is now performed in same-day surgery centers,

(text continues on page 876)

Procedure 33-6
Transferring a Client to a Stretcher

Purpose

Transfer a client without injuring nurse or client

Assessment

- Review medical history for conditions that influence or contraindicate ability to move (ie, fractures, paralysis, spinal injury, generalized muscle weakness, cardiac or respiratory disease that limits exertion).
- Assess client's range of motion and muscle strength.
- Assess cognitive function or ability to understand and follow directions.
- Assess comfort level. Medicate as ordered with analgesics.
- Assess client's weight and your strength. Determine if assistance is needed.

Equipment

Stretcher
Transfer sled

Procedure

1. Explain procedure and purpose to client.
   Rationale: Explanation reduces anxiety and increases cooperation.
2. Place stretcher parallel to bed.
3. Raise bed to same level as stretcher. Lower side rails. Lock wheels on bed.
4. One or two nurses stand on side of bed without stretcher. Two nurses stand on side of bed with stretcher.
5. Loosen draw sheet on both sides of bed.
   Rationale: Draw sheet assists in transferring client.
6. Nurses on side without stretcher help client to roll toward them onto his or her side. They may use draw sheet to pull client onto side or use logrolling technique.
7. Nurses on stretcher side of bed slide transfer sled under draw sheet and under client's buttocks and back.
8. Roll client onto transfer sled into supine position. Place client's arms across his or her chest.
   Rationale: This prevents injury to arms during transfer.

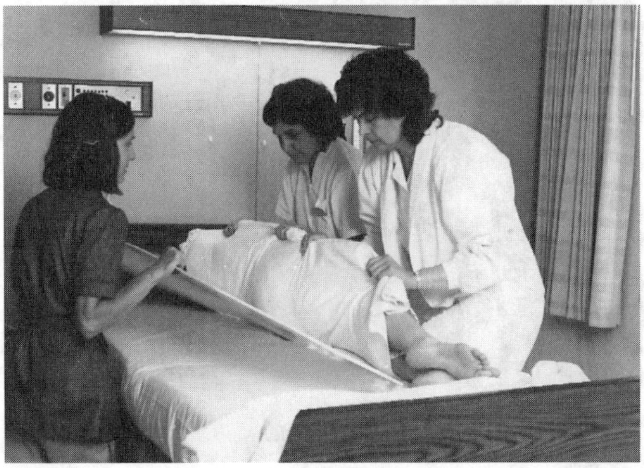

Step 7 • *Slide transfer sled under client's buttocks and back.*

9. Move stretcher parallel to bed, and lock wheels.
   Rationale: This prevents unexpected movements of stretcher during transfer.
10. Nurses on stretcher side of bed assume a broad stance.
    Rationale: A broad stance provides a stable base of support.
11. Warp end of draw sheet over curved end of transfer sled and slide client onto stretcher on count of three.
    Rationale: This provides smooth motion for transfer.

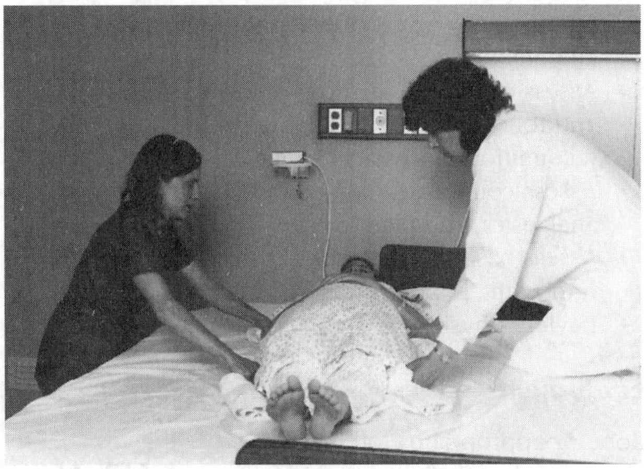

Step 11 • *Smoothly slide client onto stretcher.*

12. Roll client slightly up onto side, and pull transfer sled out from under him or her.

(continued)

13. Lock side rails up on bed side of stretcher and move stretcher away from bed.
    Rationale: This provides for client's safety.

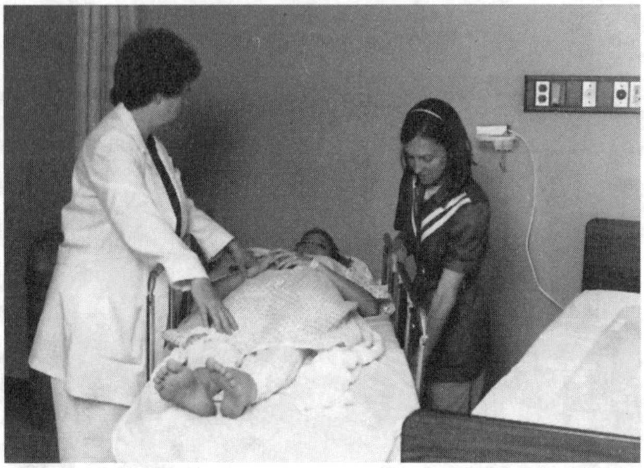

Step 13 • *Lock side rails on stretcher.*

14. Place cover over client and lock safety belts across client's chest and waist. Adjust head of stretcher according to client limitations.
    Rationale: Comfort, warmth, and safety are provided.

Lifespan Considerations

Infants and Children

- Infants can be safely moved by one person.
- Children may be moved by one or two people.

Adults

- Depending on level of musculoskeletal function, adults may be able to slide onto a stretcher with minimal assistance.

Procedure 33-7
Transferring a Client to a Wheelchair

Purpose

1. Prevent complications of immobility
2. Increase independence and promote self-esteem
3. Prevent muscle strain to nurse

Assessment

- Assess musculoskeletal function: Joint mobility; paresis or paralysis of extremities; fractures, amputations.
- Assess cognitive function: Ability to understand and follow directions; short-term memory and recognition of physical limitations to movement.
- Assess comfort level. Medicate as ordered with analgesics, and plan transfer when pain is relieved.
- Assess baseline vital signs. Assess for history of orthostatic hypotension.
- Review physician's orders for activity level.

Equipment

Robe or appropriate clothing
Slippers or shoes with nonskid soles, transfer belt, wheelchair, restraints (optional as needed)

Procedure

1. Explain procedure to client.
   Rationale: Explanation reduces anxiety and gains client's cooperation.
2. Position wheelchair at 45-degree angle or parallel to bed. Remove footrests and lock brakes.
   Rationale: This facilitates a smooth, safe transfer.

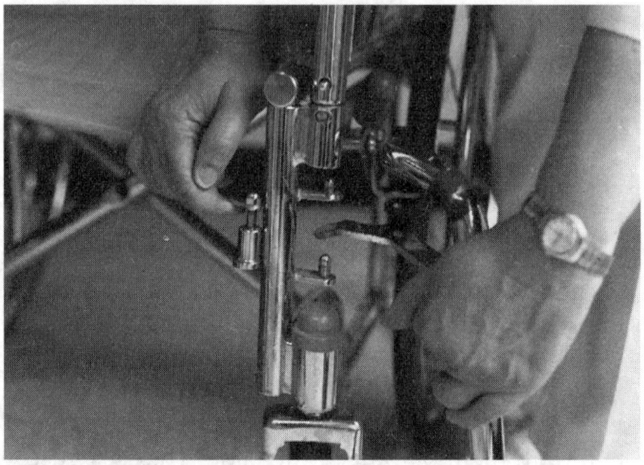

Step 2 • *Remove footrests from wheelchair to facilitate transfer.*

3. Assist client to side-lying position, facing the side of bed he or she will sit on.
4. Lock bed brakes; lower bed to lowest level, and raise head of bed as far as client can tolerate.
   Rationale: Amount of energy needed to move to a sitting position is decreased.

5. Lower side rail, and stand near client's hips with foot near head of bed in front of and apart from other foot.
   Rationale: Nurse's center of gravity is placed near client's greatest weight.
6. Place one arm under client's shoulders and one arm over client's thighs.
7. Swing client's legs over side of bed. At the same time, pivot on your back leg to lift client's trunk and shoulders.
   Rationale: Gravity lowers client's legs over bed while nurse transfers weight in the direction of motion.
8. Stand in front of client, and assess for balance and dizziness.
   Rationale: Prevents falls or injuries from orthostatic hypotension.
9. Help client to don robe and nonskid footwear.
   Rationale: Nonskid soles reduce risk of falling.
10. Apply transfer belt if necessary.
    Rationale: Risk of falling during transfer is reduced.

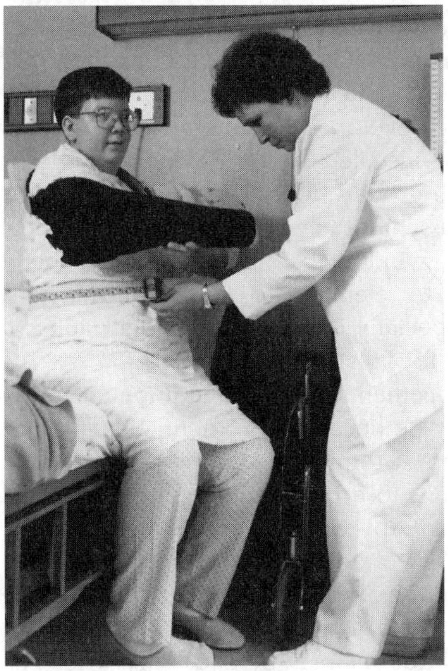

Step 10 • *Fasten transfer belt.*

11. Spread your feet apart and flex your hips and knees.
    Rationale: Center of gravity is lowered and base of support is broadened to provide stability and smooth movement using large muscle groups of legs.
12. Put your hands around client's waist or grasp back of transfer belt.
    Rationale: Balance and support are provided.
13. Have client slide buttocks to edge of bed until feet touch floor.
14. Rock back and forth until client stands on the count of three.
    Rationale: Rocking motion prevents muscle strain by giving client's weight momentum and requiring less energy to lift.

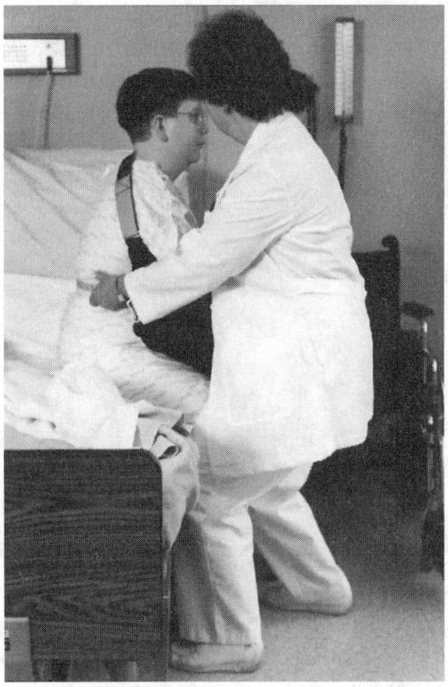

Step 14 • *On the count of three, assist client to a standing position.*

15. Brace your front knee against client's weak knee as client stands.
    Rationale: Weak knee is prevented from buckling and client is prevented from falling.
16. Pivot on back foot until client feels wheelchair against back of legs; keep your knee against the client's knee.
    Rationale: Proper position is ensured before sitting.
17. Instruct client to place hands on chair armrests for support. Flex your knees and hips as you assist client into chair.

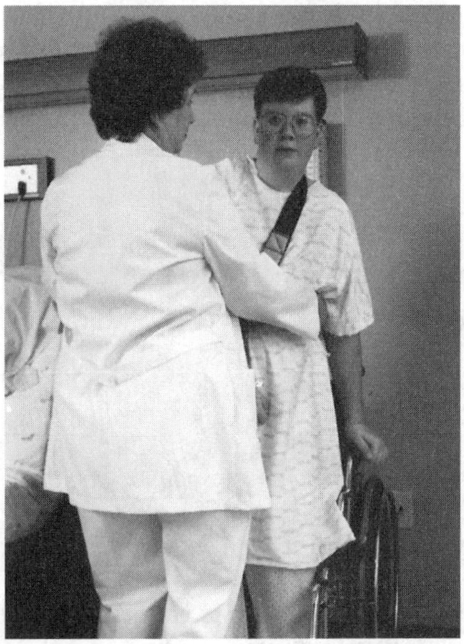

Step 17 • *Pivot into wheelchair; have client grasp arm rests.*

(continued)

Rationale: Good body mechanics prevents back injury by supporting weight with large muscle groups.

18. Assess client's alignment in chair, and secure with restraints as necessary. Provide call light.
Rationale: This promotes comfort and provides for safety.

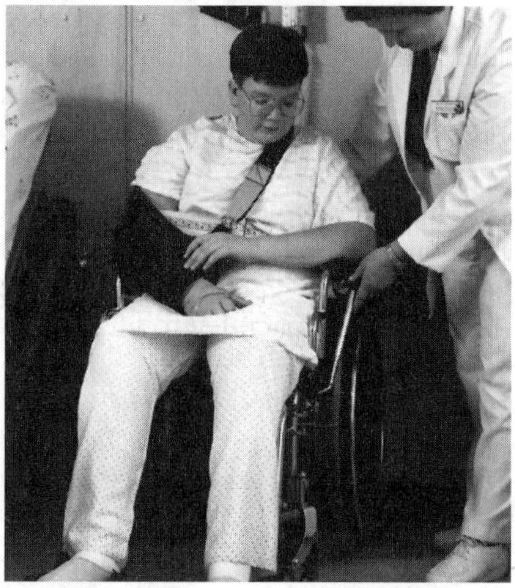

Step 18 • *Assess client's alignment and comfort.*

allowing the client to be discharged a few hours after the surgery. With adequate support, even chronic neuromuscular problems, for example, from cerebrovascular accident, Parkinson's disease, or multiple sclerosis, can be managed at home.

Client teaching aims at helping the client learn to use special equipment and to live with motor limitations. The client and family should learn about transfer techniques, ambulation techniques, and special equipment. The physical therapist may do much of this instruction, with reinforcement from the nursing staff. Written instructions help reinforce initial learning and are useful for reference at home.

In some situations, the nurse may assess the client's home, expecially for safety. Ask about the physical layout of the house, including the number of stairs, the location of bedrooms and bathrooms in relation to living areas, and the ability to accommodate special equipment in the house (eg, whether a wheelchair can fit through doorways). If disabilities are permanent, reconstruction may be necessary; for example, ramps can be built to permit easy wheelchair access.

Stress the importance of safety to the client returning home with impaired motor function. Clutter and area rugs should be removed to prevent falls. Plans should be developed for emergencies. Smoke detectors should be installed, and the person's bedroom should be on the ground floor. The local fire department can provide a symbol to place in the handicapped person's bedroom window. Arrangements may be made for someone to telephone or check on the person daily; this is especially important for older adults who are at high risk for falls.

Arrangements for special equipment and home services may be necessary. Sometimes equipment can be rented, or customized equipment may be made. Written referrals to home health agencies for nursing care, physical therapy, or other support services may be made as well. Telephoning such personnel to relay preliminary information promotes communication before discharge.

Modifications may be necessary when care continues in the home setting. When possible, the home situation should be simulated. For example, if a hospital bed will not be available at home, practice transfers in a highbed position using a transfer sled or board. The client should discuss how he or she will manage such activities as bathing and cooking.

Often much family support is necessary for the client to manage at home. Family members should feel knowledgeable and comfortable in assuming this responsibility and should schedule time for respite from such responsibilities as well. This will allow them to recover their strength and enthusiasm. The nurse can give relatives a telephone number of support groups to contact if problems arise.

Great strides have been made in recent years to accommodate people with disabilities. Public buildings

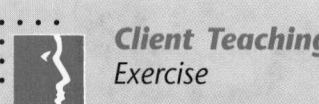

Client Teaching
Exercise

Instruct the client as follows:

- *Establish a regular exercise routine with aerobic activities that are enjoyable.*
- *Start an exercise program gradually, and obtain medical clearance as needed.*
- *Practice deep breathing to decrease the potential for respiratory complications when immobilized.*
- *Drink adequate fluids during periods of immobility to prevent urinary stasis and constipation.*
- *Perform leg exercises every hour while in bed to promote circulation and prevent thrombus formation.*

Table 33-4 • Transfer Equipment

Device	Purpose	Nursing Considerations
Transfer sled (also called transfer board)	Smooth, flat surface placed under a supine client to ease the transfer to another flat surface	Use only when transfer surfaces are at the same height. Avoid pinching client's skin when positioning board.
Roller board	Also assists with transfers from one flat surface to another; consists of metal frame covered with longitudinal rollers encased in a fabric covering	Board is placed in the gap between the bed and the stretcher. Draw sheet is used to slide client across.
Transfer belt	Used for support during transfers or ambulation, especially for clients who are weak or dizzy or have poor balance	Fasten belt snugly over clothing. Use whenever ambulation may be unsteady.
Hydraulic lift	Used to transfer immobile clients from bed to chair or bathtub. Lift has a canvas sling that fits under client and hooks into metal frame. Client can then be elevated and transferred using the hydraulic mechanism.	Reassure clients that they will not fall.

now have wheelchair access, and special facilities can be found in some public restrooms. Some buses and vans are equipped to handle wheelchairs. Barrier-free, equal accessibility to public buildings is a right that is guaranteed to all individuals under federal law.

Evaluation

Measuring outcome criteria helps determine whether the client has achieved mobility goals. Outcome criteria must be individualized for each client, but the outcome criteria listed here may be appropriate.

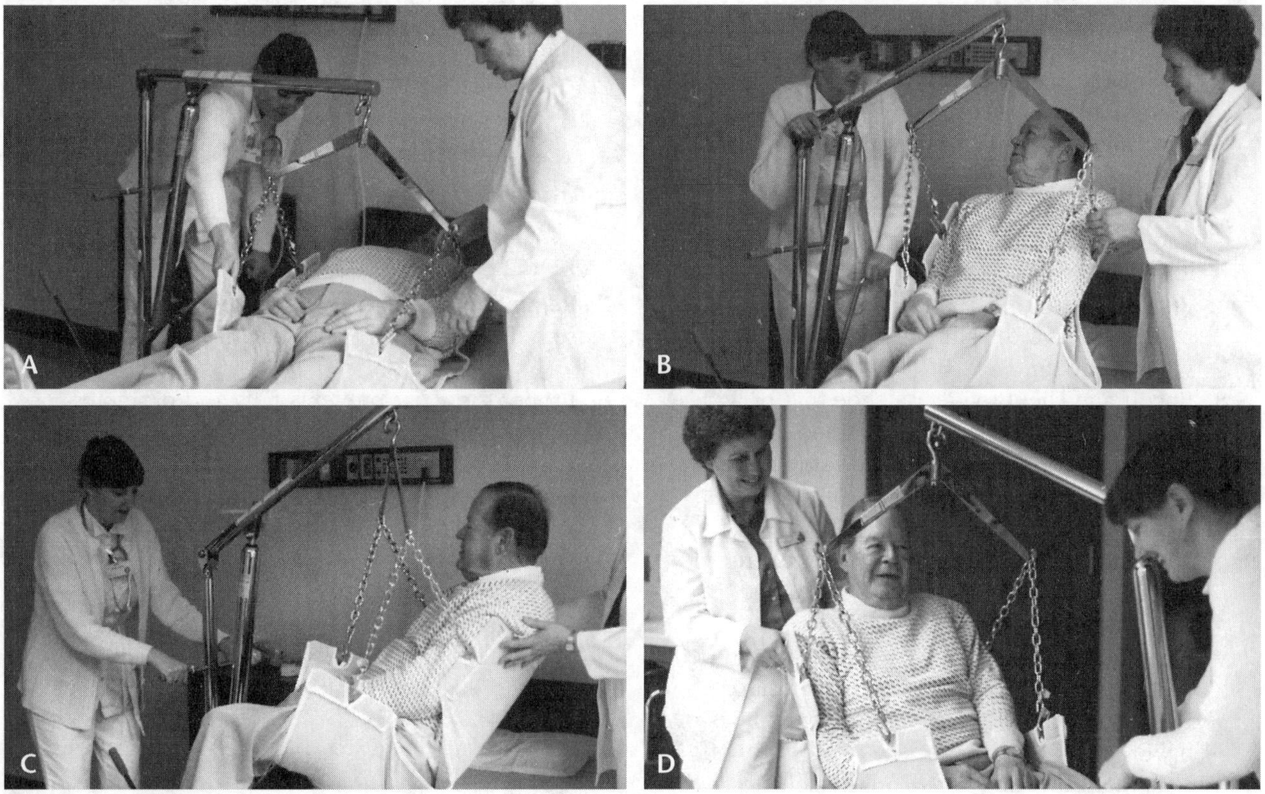

Figure 33-10 *• Using a hydraulic lift.* ***(A)*** *Attach fabric sling to frame.* ***(B)*** *Engage hydraulic system to raise client from bed.* ***(C)*** *Move client to chair.* ***(D)*** *Lower client to chair. Sling remains in place and is reattached to frame when client is moved back into bed.*

Nursing Plan of Care
The Client With Impaired Physical Mobility

Nursing Diagnosis

Impaired Physical Mobility related to right-leg above-the-knee amputation, as manifested by inability to move purposefully within the environment.

Client Goal

The client will move within the environment to perform ADLs.

Client Outcome Criteria

- Client's hip maintains its flexibility throughout recovery and rehabilitation.
- Client maintains balance and support by standing on left leg (with help of crutches or walker) 1 week after surgery.
- Client demonstrates safe transfer technique (in and out of bed, commode, wheelchair) by 1 week after surgery.

Nursing Intervention	*Scientific Rationale*
1. Keep stump flat and unrotated; do not place pillows under stump.	1. Keeping stump flat prevents contracture.
2. Encourage active ROM exercises every 8 hours.	2. Improves joint flexibility.
3. Provide a program of frequent position changes that includes having client lie prone for 1/2-hour intervals every 8 hours.	3. Frequent position changes enhance mobility and prevent contractures.
4. Avoid long periods of sitting in bed or in a chair.	4. Sitting up flexes the stump and can cause contractures.
5. Take postural blood pressure measurements before client gets up.	5. This will detect orthostatic hypotension and prevent falls.
6. Encourage client's active participation in physical therapy. • Discuss value of increasing muscle strength in the remaining leg. • Note time when physical therapy is scheduled and ensure that client has eaten and is medicated (if needed) by that time.	6. Encouraging physical therapy sessions should motivate client.
7. Remind client to use abdominal and gluteal muscles to avoid leaning to right side of body when standing.	7. Reminding client which muscles to use while standing promotes better balance.
8. Encourage client to wear a shoe that provides good support and has a nonskid sole.	8. Proper footwear prevents falls and promotes ambulation.
9. Instruct client to perform good foot care daily.	9. Foot care is essential because injury to remaining foot will greatly reduce mobility and independence.
10. Show client how to use trapeze for exercise and in preparation for transfer. • Attach trapeze above bed. • Demonstrate use of trapeze to maneuver in bed and to transfer from bed to sitting position. • Encourage strength in the upper extremities by having client pull on trapeze to lift body off bed, then lowering himself or herself slowly.	10. Demonstrating use of equipment increases client compliance with self-transfers. Using trapeze for exercise should strengthen upper extremity muscles.

(continued)

Nursing Plan of Care
The Client With Impaired Physical Mobility (Continued)

11. When client is in wheelchair, encourage him or her to lift body by pushing down on the arms of the wheelchair.	11. Muscle strength is increased in upper extremities. This prevents prolonged pressure and development of pressure sores.
12. Develop a program of isometric exercises, and have client perform 10 repetitions three times a day. For example: Lie on back, squeeze cushion between legs. Lie on back, spread legs apart against belt buckled around thighs. Lie on stomach, lift stump toward ceiling. Lie on back, raise stump, then lower stump and hip, pushing down toward bed.	12. Isometric exercise should maintain muscle tone in right stump and left leg; spelling out exercises reinforces client's understanding of them.
13. Teach transfer from bed to chair using stand-pivot technique.	13. A client with good strength in remaining leg should be able to transfer safely to chair using this technique.
Use transfer belt.	Enables you to grip client better during transfer
Client should wear shoe with nonskid sole.	Decreases chance of slipping during transfer
Verbally guide client through procedure.	Provides cuing for movement necessary during transfer
Praise successful efforts.	Psychological support and praise increase client motivation and reinforce client's effort.

Goal

Client will exhibit increased endurance and tolerance for physical activity.

Possible Outcome Criteria

- Within 24 hours, client states importance of gradually increasing activity or exercise.
- Client increases amount of exercise or degree of activity daily according to preset parameters.
- With activity or exercise, client discontinues activity if adverse symptoms (eg, dyspnea, tachycardia, pain, vertigo) are experienced.

Goal

Client will actively participate in prescribed therapies to promote optimal healing and restored mobility.

Possible Outcome Criteria

- Client assists with turning by using trapeze and pushing with legs as instructed during repositioning.
- Client increases ambulation for a longer period each day.
- Client demonstrates use of crutches or walker before discharge.
- Client demonstrates safe transfer technique before discharge.

Goal

Client will comply with measures to prevent potential complications of immobility.

Possible Outcome Criteria

- Client practices leg exercises every hour to prevent possible thrombus formation during activity restriction.
- Client practices deep breathing and coughing every hour to minimize pooling of secretions.
- Client increases fluid intake to eight glasses of water per day to prevent urinary tract infection and renal calculi.
- Client performs ROM exercises daily as instructed to maintain joint flexibility.

Key Concepts

- The normal functions of the musculoskeletal system are proper body alignment, posture, balance, and coordinated movement.
- Proper body mechanics use alignment, balance, and coordinated movement to perform activities such as lifting, bending, and moving in a safe and efficient manner.
- ROM is the ability to move a joint through the full extent of its normal movement. Active ROM is

when a client can independently move the joint; passive ROM is when another person must do this for the client.

- Normal walking gait consists of the stance phase and the swing phase. It requires coordinated effort, balance, and equilibrium.
- Normal mobility requires an intact musculoskeletal system, nervous system control, adequate circulation and oxygenation, adequate energy, appropriate lifestyle values, and a suitable emotional state.
- Symptoms of altered mobility are decreased muscle strength or tone, lack of coordination, altered gait, decreased joint flexibility, pain on movement, and decreased activity tolerance.
- Immobility affects all functional health areas and can contribute to many serious complications.
- Nursing assessment includes subjective data collection to determine normal mobility, risk factors for altered mobility, and any current impairments to mobility. Objective data provide information about body alignment, balance, coordination, gait, joint flexibility, muscle tone and strength, and blood pressure affected by positional changes.
- NANDA nursing diagnoses in the functional area of mobility are Impaired Physical Mobility, Activity Intolerance, and Risk for Disuse Syndrome.
- Nursing interventions to assist the client with mobility problems include turning and positioning, providing ROM exercises, transferring, assisting with ambulation, and teaching how to use ambulation aids.
- Client goals concerning mobility should focus on promoting optimal mobility, increasing endurance and tolerance to exercise, preventing complications from immobility, and adapting to mobility restrictions.

Critical Thinking Challenges

Now reread the clinical situation involving the older client recovering from a hip fracture and his wife at the beginning of this chapter. Apply the knowledge you have gained to this situation and your client's plan of care. Consider the following.

1. *Prioritize your assessment in this situation.*
2. *Describe how you will assess your client's mobility status.*
3. *From the information provided, consider possible nursing diagnoses. Prioritize them, and give rationales for your choices.*
4. *Propose ways in which collaboration with other healthcare professionals would be beneficial.*
5. *Plan ways to help ensure your client's safety.*

References

Dietrick, J., et al. (1948). Effects of immobilization upon various metabolic and physiologic functions of normal men. *American Journal of Medicine, 4*(1), 3–36.

Jackson, D. B., Saunders, R. B. (1993). *Child Health Nursing: A Comprehensive Approach to the Care of Children and their Families.* Philadelphia: J.B. Lippincott.

Groer, M., & Shekleton, M. (1993). *Basic pathophysiology: A holistic approach* (4th ed.). St. Louis: C.V. Mosby.

(1991). *Healthy People 2000* Washington, DC: U.S. Department of Health and Human Services (PHS #91-50213).

Loeper, J. M. (1992). *Positioning.* In Bulechek, G. M., McCloskey (eds.) *Nursing Interventions,* 2nd ed. Philadelphia: W. B. Saunders.

Maloni, J. A., Chance, B., Zhang, C., Cohen, A. W., Betts, D., & Gange, S. J. (1993). Physical and psychosocial effects of antepartum hospital bedrest. *Nursing Research, 42*(4), 197–203.

North American Nursing Diagnosis Association (1994). *Nursing diagnoses: Definitions and classification 1995–1996.* (Author).

Skov, P., Motzer, S. U. (1995). History taking and physical examination. In Woods, S. L., Sivarajan, E. S., Halpenny, C. J., and Motzer, S. U. (eds) *Cardiac nursing* (3rd ed.). Philadelphia: J.B. Lippincott.

Vander, A. J., Sherman, J. H., & Luciano, D. S. (1994). *Human physiology: The mechanisms of body function.* New York: McGraw-Hill.

Yeo, S. (1994). Exercise guidelines for pregnant women. *Image,* 26(4), 265–269.

Bibliography

Galarneau, L. (1993). An interdisciplinary approach to mobility and safety education for caregivers and stroke patients. *Rehabilitation Nursing,18*(6), 395–399.

Holm, K., et al. (1989). Immobility and bone loss in the aging adult. *Critical Care Nursing Quarterly, 12*(1), 46–51.

Lake, F. R., et al. (1990). Upper-limb and lower-limb exercise training in clients with chronic airflow obstruction. *Chest, 97,* 1077–1082.

Langemo, D. K., et al. (1990). Explicating the relationship of health measures and self-esteem to exercise practices in adults. *Health Education,21*(4), 7–11.

Mason, D. J., & Redeker, N. (1993). Measurement of activity. *Nursing Research, 42*(2), 87–92.

Miers, L. J., et al. (1990). The cardiovascular response to exercise in the patient with congestive heart failure. *Journal of Cardiovascular Nursing, 4*(3), 47–58.

Naso, F., et al. (1990). Endurance training in the elderly nursing home patient. *Archives of Physical Medicine and Rehabilitation, 71,* 241–243.

Neuberger, G. B., Kasal, S., Smith, K. V., Hassanein, R., DeViney, S. (1994) Determinants of exercise and aerobic fitness in outpatients with arthritis. *Nursing Research, 43*(1), 11–24.

Olson, E. V. The hazards of immobility. *American Journal of Nursing, 67,* 780–785.

Olson, E. V., et al. (1990). The hazards of immobility. *American Journal of Nursing, 90*(3), 43-48.

Topp, R., & Stevenson, J. S. (1994). The effects of attendance and effort on outcomes among older adults in a long-term exercise program. *Research in Nursing and Health, 17*(1), 15–24.

Volderi, C., et al. (1990). The relationship of age, sex, gender and exercise practices to measures of health, life-style, and self-esteem. *Applied Nursing Research, 3*(1), 20–26.

Whitney, J. D., Stotts, N. A., Goodson, W. H., & Janson-Bjerklie, S. (1993). The effects of activity and bedrest on tissue oxygen tension, perfusion, and plasma volume. *Nursing Research, 42*(6), 349–355.

Oxygenation: Respiratory Function

Key Terms	Learning Objectives
Alveoli *Apnea* *Atelectasis* *Bronchioles* *Bronchospasm* *Diffusion* *Dyspnea* *Hyperventilation* *Hypoventilation* *Hypoxemia* *Hypoxia* *Oxygen saturation* *Pulse oximetry* *Respiration* *Tracheostomy* *Ventilation*	*Upon completion of this chapter, the student will be able to do the following:* • *Identify factors that can interfere with effective oxygenation of body tissues.* • *Describe common manifestations of altered respiratory function.* • *Contrast changes in respiratory function and problems over the lifespan.* • *Describe important elements in the respiratory assessment.* • *List appropriate nursing diagnoses and outcomes for the client with altered respiratory function.* • *Describe nursing measures to ensure a patent airway.* • *Discuss safe administration of oxygen using different modes of delivery.* • *Describe the impact of respiratory dysfunction on activities of daily living.* • *Identify home-care considerations for the respiratory client.*

34

You are a nurse working in an intermediate care facility. Your facility has served primarily geriatric clients in the past. Recently, the facility has begun to care for stable, ventilator-dependent clients. Although staff respiratory therapists regularly monitor them, the arrival of these clients has caused considerable anxiety among the nursing staff. You have volunteered to serve on a committee to address concerns of the nursing staff.

In this chapter you will add information about gas exchange and respiratory function to your growing knowledge base of nursing care. You will see how this chapter relates to previous chapters, such as Medication Administration, Safety, Home Management and Care, and Self-Care and Hygiene. When you have completed the chapter, Critical Thinking Challenges at the end of the chapter will help you work through the situation above.

The function of the respiratory system is gas exchange. This replenishes the body's supply of oxygen and eliminates the waste gas carbon dioxide from the blood.

An important nursing responsibility is assessment of respiratory function. The nurse gathers information from the client, listens to breath sounds with a stethoscope, interprets laboratory tests, and makes important observations to determine the effectiveness of the client's breathing. Assessment also allows the nurse to identify risk factors that could cause respiratory dysfunction.

The nurse is responsible for promoting normal respiratory function regardless of the practice area in which she or he works. The school nurse may conduct classes on the hazards of smoking, the perioperative nurse will instruct the preoperative client in deep-breathing techniques, and the community nurse may screen for and teach about tuberculosis prevention.

The nurse also helps improve breathing in the client with altered respiratory function. From positioning of the debilitated client to managing sophisticated life-supporting ventilator systems, the nurse plays a vital role in assisting the client with respiratory disease.

Normal Respiratory Function

Understanding normal respiratory function allows the nurse to appreciate better the problems of dysfunction. This chapter discusses the processes of breathing and gas exchange, and their relation to health.

Structure of the Respiratory System

Breathing delivers air to the lungs, where gas exchange occurs. Before air reaches the lungs, it passes through a series of structures and tubes collectively called the airways (Fig. 34-1).

The upper airway consists of the mouth, nose, and pharynx. The mouth and nose are the normal entry portals for air. They are connected by the nasopharynx, which funnels incoming air into the lower portions of the pharynx. Below the pharynx lies the larynx, or voice box. This cartilaginous structure (commonly called the Adam's apple) marks the transition from the upper to the lower airway.

The lower airway consists of the trachea, or windpipe, and its many branches. The average adult trachea is 10 to 12 cm long and 2 to 2.5 cm in diameter. It branches into left and right mainstem bronchi. These become smaller tubes, first giving rise to lobar bronchi, then segmental bronchi. The airways continue to branch in tree-like fashion, generating 23 successively smaller (and increasingly numerous) sets of tubes.

The smallest of these tubes are the **bronchioles**, which connect the larger conducting airways with the lung parenchyma. This gas-exchanging portion of the lung is made up of millions of tiny air sacs, or **alveoli**. These thin-walled epithelial structures are in contact with a lush capillary network. Oxygen reaching the alveoli crosses the epithelium into the blood, where it is transported to the heart and from there to body tissues.

The tracheobronchial tree and the lungs occupy the thoracic cavity. Inflation and deflation of the lungs depends on complex, coordinated neuromuscular activity. The lungs move only passively: they stretch and recoil in response to muscular movement. The diaphragm (which separates the chest from the abdominal cavity) and the intercostal muscles (which lie between the ribs) are the primary muscles of breathing. These muscles respond to impulses from the central nervous system, which uses information obtained from specialized nerve centers located in the aorta and carotid arteries.

Normal Function of the Respiratory System

Breathing accomplishes two vital tasks: it makes oxygen (O_2) available to the blood, and it allows carbon dioxide (CO_2) to be removed from the blood. Oxygen is carried by the blood through arteries to all cells and tissues, where it is used for metabolism and growth. Oxygen is essential for life: without it, cells die. Carbon dioxide is a waste product of metabolism that continuously enters the blood from the cells. Carbon dioxide is carried through the veins to the heart, and from there to the lungs, where it is excreted. Regulation of carbon dioxide by breathing is also essential because carbon dioxide greatly affects the acid-base balance of the blood.

The respiratory system's function is to ensure that breathing takes place in an efficient and effective manner. When the respiratory system functions properly, breathing is practically effortless; however, chronic and

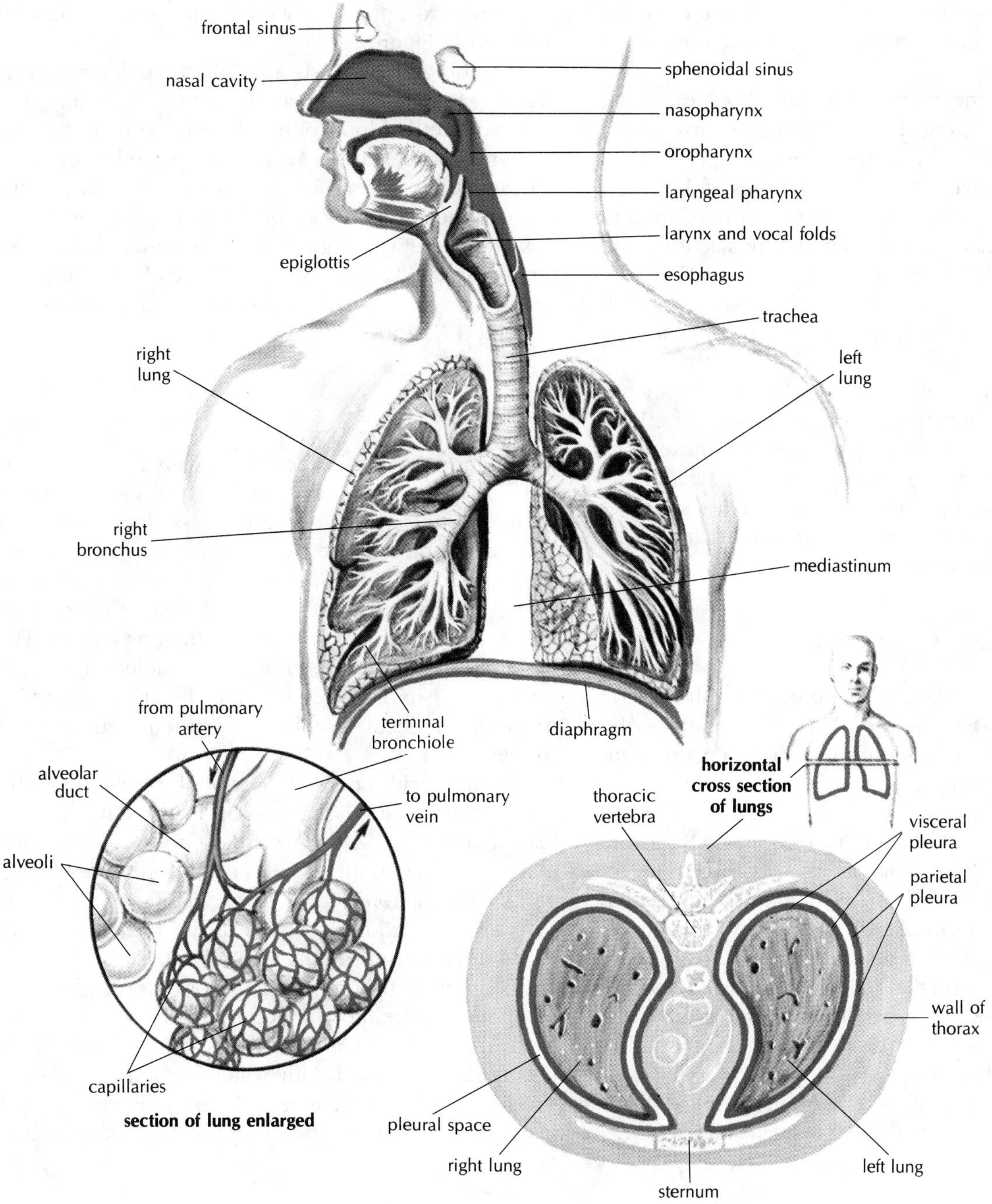

Figure 34-1 • *Respiratory system.*

acute respiratory diseases can greatly affect the breathing process. They can cause severe physical discomfort and emotional stress, and may be life-threatening or fatal.

Distribution of Air in the Lungs

Breathing, or **ventilation**, is the physical process of moving air into and out of the lungs. Ventilation allows air to enter the respiratory system so that gas exchange can take place. The mechanical process of ventilation is the result of volume and pressure changes in the chest cavity, or thorax.

During inspiration, the diaphragm and external intercostal muscles contract. Their contraction enlarges the volume of the thorax, and decreases intrathoracic pressure. The expanding chest wall pulls the lungs outward. As the lungs expand, pressure within the airways drops. As airway pressure falls below atmospheric pressure, air rushes into the lungs.

During exhalation, the process reverses. The diaphragm and intercostal muscles relax, causing the thorax to return to its smaller resting size. Pressure in the chest increases, thus allowing air to flow out of the lungs.

Ordinarily, little effort is required to draw air through the conducting airways. The larger airways are held open by cartilage and are large enough for air to flow freely. The smallest conducting tubes of the lower airway, the bronchioles, are made primarily of smooth muscle. They remain open by smooth muscle tone and usually provide little resistance to breathing. Because there are millions of bronchioles, they have a collectively large diameter; thus, pulling air through these tiny tubes is easy.

After air finally passes through 20 or more branches of airways, it reaches the respiratory units of the lung parenchyma. Each alveolus that makes up these units is in contact with dozens of capillary channels of the pulmonary circulation. The hundreds of millions of alveoli in the lung parenchyma thus provide an amazingly large surface area for gas exchange.

Gas Diffusion

Oxygen and carbon dioxide move between the alveoli and the blood by **diffusion**. This is the process by which molecules move from an area of greater concentration or pressure to a lower one.

Breathing continually replenishes the lungs' oxygen supply, so the partial pressure of oxygen (PO_2) in the alveoli is relatively high. Simultaneously, breathing removes carbon dioxide from the lungs, so the partial pressure of carbon dioxide (PCO_2) is low in the alveoli. Blood that returns to the lungs via the pulmonary circulation is the blood that has been used by the body's tissues, so it is low in oxygen and rich in carbon dioxide. Oxygen diffuses from the alveoli into the blood because PO_2 is higher in the alveoli than it is in the capillary blood. For similar reasons, carbon dioxide diffuses from the blood into the alveolar space. The exchange of gases across the alveolar-capillary membrane is illustrated in Figure 34-2.

The blood that passes through the pulmonary capillaries enters the systemic circulation as freshly oxygenated arterial blood. When it reaches the tissues the exchange process once again takes place but in opposite directions. Metabolic processes in the tissues use oxygen and produce carbon dioxide, so tissue PO_2 is low and its PCO_2 is high. Thus, when arterial blood enters tissue capillaries, oxygen diffuses from the blood to the tissues and carbon dioxide from the tissues to the blood (Barnes, 1994).

Gas Transport

As oxygen crosses the alveolar-capillary membrane into the blood, it is transported to the tissues in two forms. Small amounts of oxygen are physically dissolved in plasma, but most of the oxygen being carried to the tissues is attached to hemoglobin molecules on red blood cells. Hemoglobin has the unique ability to carry oxygen in its molecular form, rather than as an ion. This is significant because tissues require molecular oxygen for metabolism. Each red blood cell contains many hemoglobin molecules and can carry large amounts of oxygen.

In the healthy person, hemoglobin acts somewhat like a magnet, attracting oxygen in the lungs and releasing it to the tissues in response to their need. Normal blood flow to the tissues is therefore necessary for tissue oxygenation to take place.

Carbon dioxide is carried in the blood in several forms. It is transported in a dissolved state, but it also can combine with some amino acids to form carbamino compounds. The most important transport mechanism for carbon dioxide is in its dissociated form. When chemically combined with water, carbon dioxide dissociates into bicarbonate ions. These ions form the primary component of the bicarbonate buffer system,

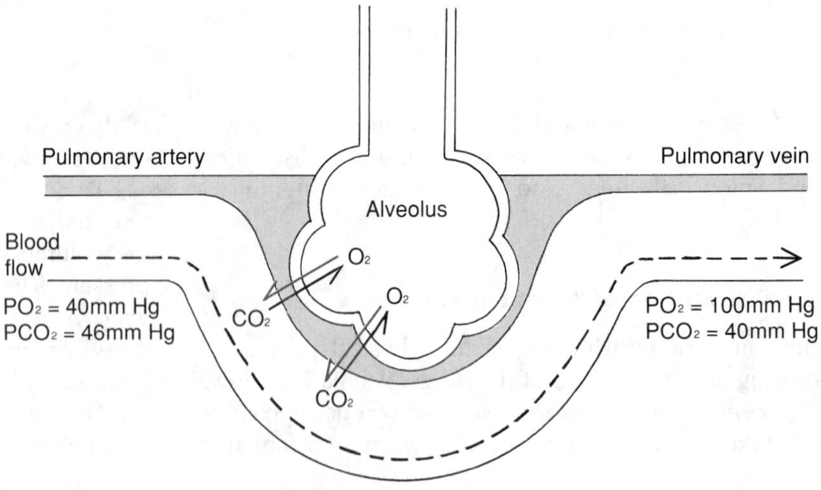

Figure 34-2 • *Gas exchange in the pulmonary capillary.*

which plays a major role in acid-base balance within the body.

Control of Ventilation

The process of ventilation is regulated through neural pathways, which are influenced by many factors. Specialized neurons in the brain stem, known collectively as the respiratory centers, generate regular impulses. These impulses are transmitted to the respiratory muscles, causing them to contract and relax rhythmically.

Many neural pathways provide input to the respiratory centers. Stretch receptors in the lung and chest wall limit how far the lungs can expand. These receptors increase the efficiency of breathing by limiting the work the respiratory muscles must do. Peripheral sensory neurons, notably pain and cold receptors, can also provide input to these centers. Finally, although regular rhythmic breathing is primarily an involuntary function, voluntary thought can be a strong influence.

Perhaps the most important influence on the respiratory centers comes from the peripheral and central chemoreceptors. Specialized neural tissue in the aortic arch and carotid arteries (peripheral receptors) and the medulla (central receptors) are sensitive to the blood's chemical content. All of these receptors are sensitive to circulating blood levels of carbon dioxide and hydrogen ions. The peripheral receptors are also stimulated by decreases in the partial pressure of oxygen in arterial blood (PaO_2). These chemoreceptors are linked by neural pathways with the respiratory centers. Information from these specialized tissues greatly influences our pattern of breathing.

Of all the stimuli affecting the chemoreceptors, carbon dioxide plays the primary role in determining the frequency and depth of ventilation. If carbon dioxide levels in the blood increase, the chemoreceptors are stimulated and we breathe more deeply and rapidly. The opposite is also true: our breathing decreases when carbon dioxide levels decrease. Normal breathing is usually regular and smooth because carbon dioxide levels remain fairly constant. If the blood level of carbon dioxide rises or falls appreciably, it ordinarily soon returns to normal by alterations in breathing patterns. The chemoreceptors also increase ventilation if arterial blood pH or PaO_2 falls substantially, but in general the degree of response to these conditions is less than when alterations in the partial pressure of carbon dioxide in arterial blood ($PaCO_2$) occur.

Defenses of the Respiratory System

A major function of the upper airway is to warm and humidify inspired air. The generous blood flow of the nasal cavity warms inspired air, and its mucosal lining imparts humidity. This moisture and warmth is necessary to maintain the fluid character of the mucus in the lower respiratory tract.

The upper airway also cleans the air we breathe. The nose is a highly effective filter for foreign particles. Dust and irritants are trapped in the hairs lining the nostrils or in the mucus layer of the nasal passages. Incoming air is further purified by the tonsils and adenoids, which are protective lymphoid tissues in the pharynx.

The upper airway protects the lower airway from infection and from injury due to aspiration. The epiglottis acts as a trapdoor, preventing large particles of food or foreign matter from being accidentally aspirated into the lower airway. Below this structure, the vocal cords, false cords, and aryepiglottic folds act as secondary protection against aspiration.

The conducting tubes of the lower airway further filter and clean incoming air. Lining these airways is an epithelial layer containing millions of ciliated cells and mucus-producing glands. This mucous membrane produces a "mucus blanket" that efficiently traps bacteria and microscopic foreign particles. The ciliated cells provide motion to the mucus blanket, allowing it to carry trapped matter upward and out of the respiratory tract. This "mucociliary elevator" protects the airways by constantly sweeping potentially harmful material out of the lungs. At the alveolar level, specialized scavenger cells called macrophages help decrease the risk of infection by eating bacteria and any minute particles that may have bypassed the mucus blanket.

The lungs and airways are also protected by the sneeze and cough reflexes. Irritants trapped in the nose stimulate sneezing. This helps to expel the trapped material from the nasal passages, thereby decreasing the irritation and helping to prevent infection.

The most important lung defense is a strong and effective cough (Shapiro, et al., 1995). Coughing clears the lower airways much like sneezing helps cleanse the nose. A forceful expulsion of air from the lungs can remove large amounts of germ-laden mucus. This action is vital for keeping the lungs free of infection. Coughing also helps to prevent mucus plugs from forming in airways and to remove plugs that have already formed. In this way, airways are kept open so all areas are available for gas exchange.

Normal Breathing Pattern

Although normal breathing varies depending on age, in general it is smooth, even, and regular. A description of a person's breathing pattern must include information about the rate and depth of breathing, its rhythm, and the effort required to take each breath.

Normal or "quiet" breathing of a person at rest occurs at a rate of 12 to 20 breaths per minute in the older child and adult (Table 34-1). The rate does not

Table 34-1 • Respiratory Rates Through the Lifespan

Age Group	Breathing Rate (breaths/minute)
Newborn	30–60
1–5 years	20–30
6–10 years	18–26
10–adult	12–20
Older adult (60 years and older)	16–25

vary significantly from one minute to the next unless the person's activity level changes. Usually an awake person breathes slightly faster than one who is asleep.

The rhythm of the healthy adult's breathing is steady. All breaths are evenly spaced, with an equal interval between each breath. Exhaling normally takes twice as long as inhaling.

Normally, each breath is about the same size. Despite an occasional sigh or yawn, the chest of a person who is breathing quietly will be seen to rise and fall the same amount from breath to breath. People who use their diaphragms effectively to breathe make their abdomens rise and fall. The average adult moves about a half a liter of air per breath.

Normal breathing is nearly effortless. Little muscular work is required to move air through the lungs. Because of this, quiet breathing is almost unnoticeable; ordinarily no sounds are associated with it.

Factors Affecting Respiration

Respiration, or the exchange of oxygen for carbon dioxide, is highly complex and depends on many factors. Specific physiologic conditions, level of general health, lifestyle, and environment all affect the process.

Body Position

An upright posture allows for the greatest ease of lung expansion. The diaphragm can move up and down most readily when the abdominal organs are not pressed against it. Standing or sitting erect allows gravity to pull the organs down; thus, the diaphragm must push against less resistance. Breathing requires more effort when lying down, because the abdominal contents push against the diaphragm (Barnes, 1994).

Activity and Exercise

Strenuous exercise increases oxygen demand by the body and increases carbon dioxide production. For these reasons, the rate and depth of ventilation increases during exercise. This helps to provide more oxygen to the tissues and to get rid of the extra waste gas. The cells of the well-conditioned person who exercises strenuously and regularly use oxygen more efficiently than those of the sedentary person. Thus, an athlete normally breathes more slowly and deeply while at rest than someone who is less fit.

Age

The aging process changes all organ systems, including the lungs. They become naturally stiffer with age, and the work needed to stretch them increases. Older people, even those without lung disease, usually breathe more shallowly and slightly faster than the young adult.

Pregnancy

During the last trimester of pregnancy, the fetus and amniotic sac grow large enough to displace the diaphragm upward. The mother then breathes faster and more shallowly, even to the point of hyperventilation. During the last few weeks of pregnancy, breathing can become uncomfortable.

Body Weight

An obese person may experience the same restriction and discomfort in breathing as the pregnant woman. The extra work required to carry extra body weight increases oxygen demands. At the same time, the chest is restricted in its movements (especially in the supine position), so breathing is more difficult.

Environment

All humans are exposed to the same concentration of oxygen: the atmosphere contains about 21% oxygen. Although the concentration of oxygen does not change appreciably, its partial pressure decreases steadily as altitude increases. The partial pressure of oxygen in the atmosphere at 10,000 feet above sea level is only about two-thirds of its partial pressure at sea level. This lower oxygen pressure at higher elevations means that less oxygen is available to the lungs for gas diffusion. Therefore, less oxygen can enter the blood, and tissues receive less oxygen. Thus, even healthy people are likely to experience shortness of breath and activity intolerance at higher elevations.

People's reactions to weather conditions are highly personalized. Some tolerate heat and humidity well; others may complain of difficulty breathing under these conditions. The same is true for cold or dry climates or for sudden changes in weather. People who move to different climates may experience slight changes in breathing patterns until they become acclimated to their new surroundings.

Lifespan Considerations

Like the heart, the lungs perform a lifetime of continual work; however, the structure and function of the respiratory system do undergo normal changes during life.

Newborn and Infant

In the uterus, the fetus's lungs grow rapidly. Branches of airways sprout during the first weeks of pregnancy, and alveoli continue to develop throughout pregnancy. Until the 24th or 25th week of pregnancy, the fetus's lungs do not have enough properly functioning alveoli to make breathing effective (Koff, et al., 1993). It takes another 10 weeks or more for fully functional lungs to develop in the fetus. Surfactant, which decreases surface tension and permits alveolar expansion, is not produced in sufficient quantities until late in gestation. For this reason, infants born prematurely may require ventilatory support. Surfactant replacement therapy is now being used for respiratory distress in the premature infant, and is being used experimentally in adults with adult respiratory distress syndrome (Sinski & Corbo, 1994).

The newborn's first breath requires tremendous physical effort. At birth, the lung is collapsed and the alveoli are filled with amniotic fluid. Although the birth process helps squeeze some of this fluid out of the lungs, it takes several breaths before the alveoli are fully opened.

The newborn breathes rapidly (30 to 60 breaths per minute), and in general larger neonates breathe more slowly than smaller ones (Koff, et al., 1993). The newborn's breathing pattern is characterized by occasional pauses of several seconds between breaths. This periodic breathing is normal during the first 3 months of life, but frequent or prolonged periods of **apnea** (cessation of breathing of 20 seconds or longer) are abnormal.

Toddler and Preschooler

As the child leaves infancy, the breathing pattern evens out considerably. The respiratory rate of the young child continues to decline. By the child's third year the rate should decrease to around 20 to 30 breaths per minute, and the rhythm is smooth and regular. During this period, the child must be protected from aspirating foreign objects, which can obstruct his or her small air passages. Providing safe toys and avoiding hard candy or small, hard pieces of food are important to ensure normal respiratory function in this age group.

Child and Adolescent

As the school-age child grows, the rate of breathing steadily slows, until the adult rate of around 12 to 20 breaths per minute is reached. During this period, generally good respiratory health is the rule.

During adolescence, more than 90% of all smokers begin their habit, and thus initiate the gradual decline in their lung function. One of the most valuable (and most difficult) functions of the nurse is to educate adolescents about the health risks of smoking.

Adult and Older Adult

Structural and functional changes occur in the respiratory system in the later decades of life. The thoracic wall becomes more rigid and the lungs become less able to stretch. There is no significant decrease in total lung capacity, but ventilation of non–gas-exchange areas of the lungs increases. The protective functions of the lung are impaired: there is decreased ciliary activity, and the cough is less propulsive and effective in airway clearance. Finally, gas exchange is affected: normal PaO_2 decreases by 10% to 15% (Shapiro, et al., 1995). These respiratory changes contribute to the activity intolerance and increased incidence of respiratory infections in older adults.

Altered Respiratory Function

Many factors can alter normal respiratory function. Smoking, lack of exercise, poor nutrition, drugs and alcohol, exposure to hazardous fumes or pollutants, cardiopulmonary disorders, developmental abnormalities, restrictive lung movement, airway obstruction, and emotional distress can cause or contribute to illness in general and breathing problems in particular. Conversely, a healthy cardiopulmonary system, clean air, exercise, proper nutrition, and avoiding smoking promote healthy lungs.

Potential for Altered Function

All parts of the respiratory system must be in good working order for effective respiration. Narrowed airways, or lungs that are stiff and difficult to expand increase the work of breathing. This in turn makes breathing an inefficient, oxygen-consuming activity. Weakened respiratory muscles or dysfunctional pathways between nerves and muscles can also prevent proper ventilation. If an insufficient amount of air enters the lungs with each breath, blood oxygen levels (as indicated by PaO_2) will decrease, resulting in **hypoxemia**, an abnormally low amount of oxygen in the blood.

Nursing Research
Respiration

Selected Nursing Research Studies

Ackerman, M. H. (1993). The effect of saline lavage prior to suctioning. *American Journal of Critical Care, 2(4),* 326–330.

Glass, C., Grap, M. J., Corley, M. C., & Wallace, D. (1993). Nurses' ability to achieve hyperinflation and hyperoxygenation with a manual resuscitation bag during endotracheal suctioning. *Heart & Lung, 22,* 158–165.

Hill, M., Harrell, J., & McCormick, L. (1992). Predictors of smokeless tobacco use by adolescents. *Research in Nursing and Health, 15,* 359–368.

Narsavage, G., & Weaver, T. (1994). Physiological status, coping, and hardiness as predictors of outcomes in chronic pulmonary obstructive disease. *Nursing Research, 43(2), 90–94.*

Possible Topics for Nursing Inquiry

- Does suctioning using in-line systems decrease the risk of infection?
- What factors contribute to depression among clients with COPD?
- How does wearing oxygen supply devices outside the hospital affect the client's self-image?
- After initial instruction, how many clients can effectively use the metered-dose inhaler?
- What are effective nursing measures to prevent nasal irritation when receiving oxygen via cannula?

The lungs must have an adequate number of functional alveoli. The respiratory epithelium must be intact and unscarred, so that oxygen and carbon dioxide can pass readily through it. The gas exchange units must also have properly functioning pulmonary capillaries. Enough blood must be flowing through these capillaries so that gas exchange can take place.

Increased Work of Breathing

All bodily functions that require muscle movement involve a certain amount of work. For the healthy person, breathing is practically effortless: the work involved is minimal. It normally becomes noticeable only during strenuous exercise. This is because normal lung tissue is stretchy, and because the airways are open to allow air to flow through them. Thus, a breath requires little energy to expand the lungs.

In altered respiratory function, the amount of work needed for breathing becomes significant because the amount of oxygen needed for respiratory muscles increases. Although these muscles ordinarily use less than 5% of the oxygen available in the blood, under extreme conditions (when the work of breathing is very high) they may use up to 50% of all the oxygen available to the body tissues (Shapiro, et al., 1995). Because blood oxygen supply is limited, increased work of breathing can deprive other tissues of needed oxygen. The client who experiences increased work of breathing is at risk for oxygen deprivation and exhaustion.

There are two general causes of increased work of breathing: restricted lung expansion and airway obstruction.

Restricted Lung Movement. Certain conditions and diseases may cause the lung to stiffen, or may restrict expansion of the chest. This can alter normal respiration in three ways:

Stiffer lungs (or lungs that are not allowed to expand fully) tend to shrivel, and their alveoli collapse. This condition is called **atelectasis**. The amount of space available for gas exchange in the lungs decreases.

Some diseases cause lung tissue to swell and thicken. Oxygen has greater difficulty in passing through thickened alveolar walls.

Because stiff lungs require more work to expand, the respiratory muscles must consume a disproportionate amount of oxygen.

In all three cases, less oxygen is available to the blood for the tissues.

Actual stiffening of the lung tissues can result from acute or chronic lung injuries. Smoke inhalation, pulmonary fibrosis, respiratory distress syndrome (of the adult or infant), and infections such as pneumonia are examples of disorders that make lung tissues swell and stiffen. These types of problems are classified as restrictive lung disorders.

Not all restrictive problems are caused by lung injuries or lung diseases, however. A client can have perfectly healthy lungs, but if other factors prevent the lungs from expanding completely, the same problems with oxygenation occur. Pain from a surgical incision is a common example of this. The discomfort of stretching the wound's stitches often forces the client to breathe shallowly; this is why atelectasis is common in postsurgical clients. Other factors that can restrict breathing include severe obesity, chest or abdominal binders, abdominal distention by gas or fluid, medications or anesthesia, rib injuries, musculoskeletal chest deformities, and severe weakness or neuromuscular disorders.

Airway Obstruction. Any process that reduces the diameter of either the upper or lower conducting airways causes increased airway resistance. Breathing then requires more effort because air must be drawn through a narrower passageway.

Airways become obstructed in several ways. Lumens become plugged by foreign material, mucus, or abnormal growths. Children who aspirate small objects experience airway obstruction. The client who is dehydrated or who has chronic bronchitis, cystic fibrosis, or asthma may experience airway obstruction from excessive mucus production. Clients with lung cancer may experience difficulty breathing as tumors obstruct large bronchi.

Airway resistance can also be increased by inflammation caused by chemical or physical irritants. Inflammation makes airways swollen and edematous. As the walls of the airways thicken, lumen size decreases. Asthma, bronchitis, and bronchiolitis are examples of conditions in which small airways become inflamed and narrowed. Croup and epiglottitis, most common in young children, obstruct upper airways by swelling the tissues of the throat.

Finally, altered bronchial smooth muscle tone also causes airway obstruction. Normal smooth muscle tone maintains the patency of the smallest airways, the bronchioles. Allergy or injury may cause the smooth muscle to become hyperreactive to stimuli. This greatly increases smooth muscle tone, which narrows airway lumens and makes breathing difficult. Airway hyperreactivity, or **bronchospasm**, is a common problem for clients with asthma and chronic obstructive pulmonary disease (COPD). By contrast, clients with emphysema experience breathing problems because of abnormally low bronchial smooth muscle tone. Years of damage to the bronchiole walls make them floppy and unable to remain open during exhalation. Air becomes trapped in the alveoli, leaving little space for fresh air and making full inspiration difficult (Jess, 1992).

Lifestyle and Habits

In addition to pathologic problems, a person's daily activities and habits can also alter normal breathing patterns.

Smoking. The most important lifestyle choice that can affect respiration is smoking. Smokers are far more likely than nonsmokers to acquire emphysema, chronic bronchitis, and lung cancer, as well as heart and cardiovascular disease. By producing more mucus and by slowing the mucociliary escalator, smoking inhibits mucus removal and can cause airway blockage. This promotes bacterial colonization and infection. Regardless of whether clinically identifiable lung disease is present, smokers usually breathe more rapidly than nonsmokers.

Drugs and Alcohol. Barbiturates, narcotics, and some sedatives (whether legal or illegal) can depress the central nervous system, with a resulting decrease in respiration. Alcohol in large doses can achieve the same effect, but it usually leads to respiratory problems of a different nature. In the chronic alcohol abuser, insufficient nutritional intake results in the body's inability to manufacture hemoglobin and plasma proteins. A decrease in hemoglobin reduces the blood's oxygen-carrying ability; a deficiency of plasma proteins can alter fluid balance and cause fluid to leak into the lungs. Of more immediate concern in the intoxicated person is the danger of vomiting and aspirating stomach contents into the lungs. Alcohol depresses the reflexes that protect the airways, so if vomiting occurs, stomach contents can easily slip into the trachea, choking the victim. If the victim is revived, aspiration is likely to cause pneumonia.

Nutrition. Without proper diet, plasma proteins and hemoglobin cannot effectively be made by the body. This occurs not only in the alcohol abuser but in people who are malnourished from poverty or from eating disorders. In addition, sufficient caloric and protein intake is required for respiratory muscle strength. People with diminished muscle strength work harder at breathing with even slight activity. Adequate fluid intake is necessary to keep secretions thin and easy to expectorate so that airways remain patent.

Adequate nutrition is also essential for maintaining a competent immune system. Alcohol abusers and malnourished people are at greater risk for contracting pneumonia and other respiratory infections than are well-nourished people.

Stress. The stress of illness can increase oxygen demand and cause increased breathing. In addition, anxiety often causes an increase in the breathing rate. In extreme cases of anxiety, the victim hyperventilates and may complain of asthma-like symptoms.

Environment

The places where we live and work can greatly affect our breathing status. As noted earlier, altitude and climate can affect breathing in people with healthy lungs. People with lung disease feel the adverse effects of high elevation or oppressive weather far more acutely than healthy people. Clients with lung disease often need oxygen when traveling in airplanes because commercial airliners are not pressurized to sea-level conditions. Some asthmatics breathe more easily in warm, dry climates; others may find a damp climate more soothing. People with COPD often find it more difficult to breathe when the weather is hot and humid because humidity contributes to air viscosity. People with COPD or asthma experience more exacerbations of their disease during changes in the weather. Some clients with lung disease benefit from moving to a climate more agreeable to them; others find no difference in their breathing.

Air Pollution. Industrialized urban areas may have elevated levels of air pollutants. Substances emitted by cars and factories, such as hydrocarbons and oxidants, interfere with oxygenation by directly damaging the lung. Carbon monoxide inhibits the attachment of oxygen onto hemoglobin. Because they are respiratory irritants, pollutants cause increased mucus production and may contribute to bronchitis and asthma. Workers in industrial plants or in certain occupations may be exposed to strong concentrations of specific pollutants and harmful dust. These workers may be prone to development of breathing problems. Air pollution in the home is also of concern. The role of second-hand smoke (smoke from someone else's cigarette) continues to attract the attention of researchers for its effects on breathing.

Pollens and Allergens. Specific substances that cause allergic responses can affect respiration, sometimes severely. The body's attempt to rid itself of substances it perceives as harmful results in the release of chemical mediators that cause an inflammatory response. Substances that trigger such a response are called *allergens.* Pollens, dust, foods, or almost any substance can be an allergen. The allergic response precipitates a series of events that leads to tissue damage.

Hay fever is the result of allergies confined to the nose and upper airways. Its dripping nose, itchy eyes, and swollen mucous membranes are annoying and uncomfortable but not life-threatening. When allergic responses take place in the lungs, breathing difficulties are far more severe. Small airways become edematous, mucus production is increased, and inflammatory chemical mediators cause bronchospasm. These are the hallmarks of common allergic asthma. If it is severe and uncontrolled, allergic asthma can be fatal.

Manifestations of Altered Respiratory Function

Cough, sputum production, shortness of breath, and chest pain are basic symptoms of respiratory disease (Wilkins, et al., 1990).

Cough

A cough is usually a reflexive response to irritation in the airways. Smoke is certainly an irritant, and coughing is the natural response to smoke. There is no such thing as a "normal" cough. Any cough, regardless of how obvious its origin, is most often an indication that the lungs or airways are being subjected to some form of irritation. A cough's primary function is to help clear offending substances from the airways. A cough also serves as a warning signal: it should alert the cougher to the fact that the airways are being assaulted by possibly harmful stimuli, and that steps should be taken to prevent further irritation.

Coughs can be triggered by a seemingly endless list of chemical or physical substances, or by physical conditions such as hot, dry air. Anything that enters the airway that does not normally belong there can provoke a cough. A cough that accompanies a disease may come from mediators released from inflamed tissues. These mediators, such as histamine, irritate the airways and can trigger a cough.

Not all coughs originate from lung problems. The client with borderline heart failure, for example, often has a chronic cough. Some people may cough for no apparent reason, as a nervous habit.

Because coughs are so prevalent, their value as a diagnostic sign is limited. Many people live with a cough, expressing concern only when it changes in severity or frequency. By contrast, some people may have a serious lung disease but a minimal cough.

Sputum Production

As with a cough, sputum production may be one of the natural consequences of irritation, but it is never really normal. In general, respiratory mucus, or sputum, is another protective feature of the airways. However, it is normally produced in such small amounts that a cough from a healthy person is dry and nonproductive. Raising mucus with a deep cough indicates that the lungs are attempting to clear away irritants. Although the lungs may seem to be the obvious source of expectorated sputum, sometimes coughed-up secretions originate in the nose or throat. It is necessary to determine whether the client raises the secretions with a genuine deep cough, or if he or she snorts or "hawks" them out. When a cough is productive, it is important to establish the source of the sputum and to assess its color, volume, consistency, and any other noteworthy characteristics.

Especially frightening can be the coughing up of blood, or hemoptysis. Blood-filled secretions that originate in the lungs may indicate a serious condition, such as lung cancer or tuberculosis. Often, however, bloody secretions originate in the nose. Drainage from the nose or mouth can drip backward into the throat, staining the mucus of the lower airways. These sources of bleeding should be ruled out before the lungs are assumed to be hemorrhaging.

Shortness of Breath

Everyone must move a certain amount of air into and out of the lungs every minute to meet the body's metabolic demands. When we cannot breathe sufficiently to meet these requirements, we experience the discomfort of breathlessness. This difficulty in catching the breath is known as **dyspnea**. The various levels of dyspnea are outlined in the display.

Levels of Dyspnea

Level I:	Client can walk 1 mile at own pace before experiencing shortness of breath.
Level II:	Client becomes short of breath after walking 100 yards on level ground or climbing a flight of stairs.
Level III:	Client becomes short of breath while talking or performing activities of daily living.
Level IV:	Client is short of breath during periods of no activity.
Orthopnea:	Client is short of breath lying down.

The most common cause of dyspnea is the increased work of breathing that occurs with lung disease. Clients with asthma or emphysema work harder to breathe because their airways are narrower than normal. Clients with pneumonia must work harder at breathing because their lungs do not stretch as readily as normal, and because atelectasis prevents full gas exchange. Very weak clients, or people with neuromuscular diseases such as polio or myasthenia gravis, may experience dyspnea because of weakened respiratory muscles.

Along with increased work of breathing, other causes of dyspnea may need to be assessed. High levels of carbon dioxide or low levels of oxygen in the blood may directly cause breathlessness (DesJardins, 1993). People with chronic congestive heart failure often experience shortness of breath because of excess fluid in the lungs and low blood oxygen levels. People who become dyspneic during anxiety attacks often have no heart or lung disease.

Shortness of breath is a subjective symptom of lung problems. Some clients with severe lung disease appear to breathe with great difficulty, yet at such times they may report that their breathing is fine. Others may complain of severe dyspnea even when objective data (such as blood gas values or pulmonary function tests) indicate no apparent problem.

Chest Pain

Chest pain can be associated with a wide variety of conditions. Although many common causes of chest pain are nonrespiratory, there are several breathing problems that can lead to it. Diseases characterized by inflammation or infection often cause pain. Inflammatory mediators such as histamine may directly stimulate nerve endings, some of which may be exposed and made hypersensitive by the disease process. This occurs in the airways of the client with bronchitis, who complains of a burning sensation with each cough. Acute bronchitis can make the simple act of breathing painful, because the flow of cooler air across sensitized nerves can cause them to react violently. Mediators may also be responsible for edema formation, which can further contribute to pain as swollen tissues exert pressure on nerves. Clients with pneumonia often experience pain with deep breathing, because each breath increases pressure on pain receptors that are already compressed and irritated by swollen, inflamed lung tissue.

Sometimes chest pain may be the result of cracked ribs or pulled muscles. Clients with severe coughs may actually separate ribs from the cartilage that holds them together. Prolonged or harsh coughing can make the chest muscles sore.

Other Signs of Respiratory Dysfunction

The secondary signs that may appear in a client with lung disease are less common than the four primary signs, but they are nonetheless important indicators of respiratory problems.

Abnormal Breath Sounds. The breath sounds heard through a stethoscope can change as a result of lung changes. Crackles, wheezes, and pleural friction rub are examples of abnormal breath sounds. These are described further in the section on Assessment.

Accessory Muscle Use. Healthy people use the muscles of the neck and upper chest to help "catch their breath" during vigorous exercise. The client with breathing problems uses them to counter episodes of dyspnea. Accessory muscle use is often evident by a forward-leaning posture. The nurse can readily observe the client raising the shoulders with each breath, and straining the muscles of the neck in an effort to maximize chest expansion. Often clients with chronic breathing problems use accessory muscles habitually, even at rest.

Cyanosis. Cyanosis is a bluish discoloration of the skin caused by a decreased amount of oxygen in the blood. Hemoglobin, the major carrier of oxygen in the blood, is bright red when saturated with oxygen. When not carrying oxygen, it becomes deep blue. Central cyanosis, seen in the mucous membranes of the eyes and mouth, must never be ignored because it indicates the presence of serious oxygenation problems (Carpenter, 1993). It should be distinguished from peripheral cyanosis, an example of which is blue fingertips on a cold day. Such problems are relatively benign, and are indicative only of local vasoconstriction.

Clubbing. Clubbing is an unusual phenomenon seen in many clients with lung or heart disease. For reasons that are unclear, the tips of the fingers and toes become rounded and enlarged. It is thought that long-term tissue hypoxia causes an alteration of local blood flow in the digits, which in turn affects the tissue growth (Wilkins, et al., 1990). Clubbing occurs in lung cancer and in lung diseases such as lung abscess.

Impact of Respiratory Dysfunction on Activities of Daily Living

Individual Considerations

Debilitation caused by lung disease can range from mild to severe. The client has less and less tolerance for activity as the disease progresses. The client's ability to perform common, day-to-day activities may be impaired because of breathlessness or oxygen dependence. Some clients become dyspneic with simple tasks such as shaving, cooking, or talking. The client with advanced symptoms may be unable to perform these and other activities because of breathlessness.

Meals can pose a problem for the homebound client. Unless help is available, preparing meals can be exhausting work. Eating is an energy-expending activity. Many people with advanced lung disease cannot eat three large meals daily without feeling severely dyspneic. Many clients will prefer to avoid dyspnea by avoiding eating, but this leads to a vicious cycle: the client has insufficient energy to eat, yet without eating both weight loss and energy loss will continue. This can contribute to feelings of depression and hopelessness.

Some respiratory clients solve this dilemma by modifying the usual routine of three square meals a day. Instead, they eat several smaller but nutritionally balanced meals. This helps conserve oxygen and prevents the excessive buildup of pressure against the diaphragm caused by larger meals. This regimen provides needed nutrition without causing the breathlessness brought on by a full stomach.

Dressing is also tiring for some respiratory clients. Some may prefer to remain in their bedclothes all day. Whenever dressing is physically possible, the client should be encouraged to dress daily. This is important for self-esteem and helps keep clients from thinking of themselves as invalids. Garments should be loose-fitting and easy to slip into. Dressing should be done slowly, while sitting down.

Getting into and out of a bathtub can exhaust the breathless client, so showering may be preferred. The client with a laryngectomy or permanent tracheostomy tube can shower but should take care to avoid flooding the stoma with water. A washcloth held over the tube prevents this. A shower also imparts humidity to the mucous lining of the airways.

Toilet concerns of the respiratory client are important to consider. Constipation can cause abdominal distention, thereby limiting diaphragm movement. Extra straining can also tire the client and cause shortness of breath. Prescribed stool softeners and good hydration can help to prevent constipation.

Mobility within the home can be a problem for the client with extreme dyspnea. Use of prescribed oxygen during periods of daily in-home activity is helpful in building up tolerance to exertion. Use of stairs can be especially difficult and may necessitate moving sleeping areas to the main floor of the house. Frequent rest during periods of activity is needed.

Mobility outside the home can also present special problems for the client with poor respiratory function. Public transport may be available but may be several blocks from the client's home. Thus, the client may have to rely on taxis or a private car. If the client uses oxygen and wants to fly, advance arrangements must be made with the airline. The client who is a marginal candidate for oxygen therapy may find a greater need for it on an airplane or at a high elevation.

Respiratory clients are often less communicative than other clients. This may be because of depression and feelings of isolation. However, some are less talkative because the act of speaking can cause shortness of breath. It is difficult to inhale while speaking, so the dyspneic client typically speaks in short, terse sentences. This may make respiratory clients appear crabby and unpleasant, but in fact they may be merely attempting to conserve their energy.

Family Considerations

Respiratory dysfunction can impact the entire family, especially if the dysfunction is severe or chronic. The client with chronic respiratory disease is susceptible to infection, so infected family members or young children should limit exposure to minimize infection risk. When the client expectorates large quantities of sputum, it can be unpleasant for family members and may limit inviting friends to visit. Listening to or staying with a loved one in respiratory distress can cause much anxiety. Family members should know emergency CPR to deal with a respiratory arrest until emergency medical help can arrive.

Caregiver burden depends on the degree of respiratory dysfunction. End-stage respiratory disease or chronic conditions can involve 24-hour care of a ventilator- or oxygen-dependent family member. Premature infants or children with cystic fibrosis often require continual ventilatory support for many years. In such situations, the parent also may grieve over the loss of the opportunity to raise a "normal" child. In end-stage respiratory disease, the person may be bedridden due to inability to supply oxygen for even minimal demands.

Assessment

The basis for appropriate nursing interventions is a thorough respiratory assessment. Information from the assessment enables the nurse to identify potential or actual nursing diagnoses and to individualize nursing care.

If relevant data are missed or go unreported by the nurse, the respiratory client's condition may worsen or may even become life-threatening.

Although it is essential to gather facts from the client, the person who is severely short of breath may be unable to respond fully to a battery of questions. The hypoxic client may respond with confused answers, and forcing the dyspneic client to speak can worsen shortness of breath. The nurse must be sensitive to the client's ability to answer questions, and may need to defer some questions until a more opportune time.

Subjective Data

Relevant subjective information to be gathered by the nurse includes data to help identify the client's functional breathing pattern. The nurse must also identify factors that show the client to be at risk for respiratory dysfunction. Finally, the nurse must be alert to the presence of breathing problems in the client.

Functional Pattern Identification

Unlike eating, sleeping, or elimination patterns, normal breathing is usually nondescript. Unless a person has experienced previous breathing problems, he or she is likely to have taken no notice of the normal breathing pattern. Few people can provide specific information about how often or how deeply they breathe. The nurse may generally assume that the client with no previous history of lung disorders breathes normally.

The normal breathing pattern of the person with chronic respiratory problems may differ greatly from that of the healthy person, however. For example, the client with chronic asthma may ordinarily breathe with a slight wheeze. Although this would be considered uncomfortable and abnormal by most people, the asthmatic client may have grown to tolerate it. Indeed, because asthmatics know from past experience how difficult breathing can be, they may regard the slight wheeze as normal, and consider only a severe wheeze as abnormal.

Similarly, the client with COPD may grow to accept as normal shortness of breath after walking two city blocks. Only if exercise tolerance decreases below this standard might the client begin to consider that something is wrong.

These examples show that the nurse must take care in eliciting information about normal breathing patterns. Clients who indicate that their breathing is ordinarily fine or unremarkable may have adjusted to a baseline breathing pattern that is abnormal for most people. The nurse can identify the normal functional breathing pattern by asking relevant questions about cough, dyspnea, sputum production, and discomfort associated with breathing. Although these symptoms are normally assessed with regard to the client's complaints, they also may give some insight into the normal breathing pattern.

The nurse should establish whether a cough is ordinarily present, for example, and if so, at what times of the day it usually occurs. The client may deny being usually short of breath unless the nurse can specify degrees of dyspnea to which he or she can relate. The nurse can ask how far the client can walk before needing to rest ("A mile; a city block; a flight of stairs; 20 feet?"). The client can be asked how much sputum he or she usually coughs up ("A teaspoon; a tablespoon; a half cup?") and about its color. Many other questions are listed in the accompanying display. Family members and people close to the client may be helpful in providing supportive information.

Nursing Assessment

Initial Respiratory Assessment Questions

- Describe your cough.
- Does the cough produce sputum? If so, how much?
- Does the cough occur at any particular time of day, or under any particular circumstances? Is it constant, or intermittent?
- What is the color and consistency of the sputum? Is it thick or thin? Is it difficult to raise? Is there any odor or bad taste to the sputum? Has there been any blood in the sputum?
- When do you become short of breath? How much activity can you tolerate before you become dyspneic? How severe is the dyspnea?
- Do you have pain associated with breathing? Where is the pain located? How can it be described? Is it continuous, does it occur only on inspiration, or during coughing, or at other noticeable times?

Risk Identification

Causes of the client's breathing problem may be rooted in long-term habits, occupational exposure, or past illnesses. The nursing history must include information about the risk factors that can lead to respiratory dysfunction.

Information about smoking habits is most important for providing insight into the client's condition. The duration and extent of cigarette smoking is sometimes expressed in terms of "pack-years": 1 pack-year is equal to smoking one pack of cigarettes a day for a year. A person who has smoked two packs a day for 40 years would thus be said to have an 80 pack-year smoking history. Chronic bronchitis, emphysema, and lung cancer are directly related to smoking and are more likely to occur in clients with long histories of heavy smoking.

Other lifestyle factors can also affect lung health. The client who has lived in poverty and is malnourished, for example, is more at risk for infections such as tuberculosis. This and other respiratory infections are also more common in alcohol abusers. These people are likely to have problems fighting infection because of self-neglect and the lowered effectiveness of their immune systems.

Work history often provides relevant information. Many occupations involve exposure to fumes or dust such as silicon and asbestos, which are toxic to lung tissue. Agricultural workers are exposed to organic dusts such as molds that can cause infections and asthma-like symptoms.

Family and personal history are also essential to a thorough evaluation. Cystic fibrosis is genetically transmitted, as is α_1-antitrypsin deficiency, which causes emphysema that develops in early adulthood. The client with asthma often recalls a childhood with allergies and eczema. A history of dental problems may explain a client's bronchiectasis or lung abscess.

Dysfunction Identification

The nurse should determine whether the client has come to the hospital with a completely new breathing problem, or whether help is being sought because of a change in a chronic respiratory condition. Acute breathing problems are frightening, so people with no history of previous respiratory difficulties usually seek medical help quickly when they find they are having trouble breathing. Some clients with chronic lung disease will also seek early help for breathing changes. But, because many chronic clients are taught by their physicians to recognize and treat certain changes in breathing status, some may wait longer than others before seeking medical and nursing help. Sometimes infection worsens their already poor breathing sufficiently to motivate them to seek extra care. A full description of the symptoms that have led the client to seek care can help clarify the cause of the immediate breathing problem.

When gathering information about the onset and duration of recent breathing problem, the nurse should determine whether the problem is continuous or intermittent. If the problem seems to be continuous, perhaps some new exposure has triggered a hypersensitivity reaction, such as new carpeting or a new pet. The client may have contracted an infection that has progressed or has remained subacute. If the problem comes and goes, the nurse should ask whether the client can identify the circumstances that bring on the difficulty. Perhaps the client's breathing worsens at certain times of the day, or when the client engages in certain activities.

The nurse should also assess cough, dyspnea, sputum production, and discomfort or pain. Relevant questions are listed in the accompanying display.

Breathing problems are accompanied by a variety of emotions. Acute episodes of dyspnea bring anxiety and fear. Panic occurs when the client feels severely dyspneic. The discomfort caused by difficult breathing can make the client worry that breathing may stop altogether. Some clients become verbal and express their panic in words, but others become quiet and withdrawn. The nurse must recognize that either response may accompany breathlessness. With either response, the client needs reassurance that the breathing complaint is being taken seriously.

Clients with chronic respiratory problems may experience self-consciousness and embarrassment because of their dysfunction. Because breathlessness may interfere with the ability to communicate, the chronic respiratory client may feel isolated and appear aloof. This can contribute to frustration and irritability, and may end in depression caused by continued illness and loss of independence.

The nurse can assess these feelings by asking appropriate questions and by observing the client. Observations made by the client's family and friends and other members of the healthcare team are invaluable in helping the nurse determine how the client is adjusting to the illness.

Decreased self-sufficiency can cause stress in the client's support system. The spouse, family, or significant others may need to assume a greater role in the client's care. The nurse must assess the understanding and abilities of the client and those who will assist the client at home.

Objective Data

In addition to the subjective information obtained through the nursing history, objective, measurable data must be gathered. This information includes observations made by the nurse, information gained by hands-on examination of the chest, and laboratory data.

Physical Assessment

The primary techniques used in physical assessment are inspection, palpation, percussion, and auscultation. Sputum is visually examined.

Inspection. An essential observation is the rate and pattern of respiration. The respiratory rate is significant because a steady amount of air must enter and leave the lungs every minute to ensure proper blood levels of oxygen and carbon dioxide. Excessively slow breathing can cause hypoxemia and hypercapnia, or abnormally high carbon dioxide in the blood. Conversely, breathing too fast causes excessive elimination of carbon dioxide, which causes dizziness and possibly respiratory alkalosis. Rapid breathing by the severely debilitated client may lead to exhaustion and even respiratory arrest.

Breathing pattern is also important to assess. Normal respirations should be smooth and regular. Except in the newborn, uneven or irregular breathing can indicate airway obstruction, or it can signal neurologic or muscle problems. As noted earlier, infants breathe rapidly and often have regular brief periods of apnea between groups of breaths. This is abnormal only when the apnea periods are frequent or last more than 10 or 15 seconds (Koff, et al., 1993). Assessment of breathing rate and pattern is described in Chapter 22.

The nurse should also take note of the client's breathing effort by noting obvious use of shoulder or neck muscles. The client with COPD often sits in a forward-leaning position, using the accessory muscles to help enlarge the chest cavity and make room for more air. This indicates shortness of breath, and may be seen in clients without COPD as well. Other obvious signs of dyspnea should be noted, such as gasping, audible wheezing, or panting respirations. In the infant, flaring of the nostrils and retractions of the ribs during inspiration are notable signs of air hunger and extraordinary work of breathing.

In addition to describing the breathing pattern, the nurse should observe the client's color. Cyanosis around the lips and under the tongue indicates serious hypoxemia.

Finally, the nurse inspects the chest to detect obvious chest deformities, wounds, or masses. The overall shape of the chest is important but less obvious. In COPD, the client's chest becomes hyperinflated over time because of an inability to exhale fully. This increases the anterior-posterior chest diameter, resulting in a barrel-shaped appearance.

Palpation. The hands are used to assess abnormalities such as swelling or tenderness. Palpation is also used to determine the extent and pattern of thoracic expansion and to note the position of the trachea. Abnormal chest wall vibrations transmitted through inflamed or fluid-filled lung tissues may be detected by palpation.

Percussion. Tapping on different areas of the chest with the fingertips produces characteristic sounds. Percussion is used to detect fluid-filled or consolidated portions of the lung. A keen ear and experience with pulmonary assessment are needed to interpret correctly the various alterations in pitch, intensity, duration, and quality of percussion notes.

Auscultation. Listening to breath sounds with a stethoscope provides vital information for evaluating the client's respiratory status. Normal breath sounds, classified as bronchial, bronchovesicular, and vesicular, are described in Chapter 21.

The most important reason for listening to the chest is to determine whether air is moving through all areas of the lung. When auscultating with a sensitive stethoscope, the nurse should be able to hear air moving in all lung fields. Breath sounds should be equally loud on both sides of the chest.

Absent or distant-sounding breath sounds in any area of the lung can indicate airway obstruction, or can mean that fluid or air has accumulated in the pleural space. A "quiet chest" in an asthmatic who is experiencing severe shortness of breath is a grave sign of poor ventilation and impending respiratory failure.

The quality of breath sounds can also be assessed by auscultation. Normal breathing should make soft rustling sounds, like a breeze blowing gently through leaves on trees. Only inspiratory sounds should be noticeable; expiration should be quiet.

The nurse must also become familiar with abnormal breath sounds. These have been described in a variety of terms through the years. Official nomenclature (as developed by the American Thoracic Society) is presented here, but the nurse should be aware that alternative terminology is commonly used (Pierson & Kacmarek, 1992). Abnormal breath sounds are summarized in Figure 21-11.

Crackles (also called rales) are *discontinuous* sounds heard on inspiration and indicate the presence of fluid in the lungs. These sounds are often heard in clients with obstructive diseases or pneumonia. When they are coarse and loud and occur with severe dyspnea, crackles may be a telling sign of congestive heart failure and pulmonary edema.

Wheezes are *continuous* sounds created by air passing through narrowed airways. They are differentiated by pitch and sound quality. High-pitched, musical sounds are caused by air traveling through bronchospastic or edematous airways. Expiratory wheezes are commonly heard in the client with asthma and COPD. Coughing does not usually make this type of wheeze disappear. In many cases, bronchodilators and corticosteroids are required to open the client's airways and ease breathing. Inspiratory wheezes can be heard when the upper airways are swollen and edematous. The most severe type of inspiratory wheeze is called stridor, heard most commonly in children with croup or epiglottitis. If upper airway obstruction becomes too severe, an artificial airway (such as an endotracheal tube or a tracheostomy) must be used to ensure an open passage for breathing.

A coarse wheeze is a low-pitched, rumbling sound that indicates the presence of sputum in the airways. These sounds, often called gurgles or rhonchi, are common in clients with chronic bronchitis, cystic fibrosis, or in any disorder in which an excess of mucous secretions are produced. Often gurgles clear with a strong cough. If the client has a weak cough and cannot clear the secretions, coarse gurgles can indicate the need for airway suctioning.

A *pleural friction rub* produces a dry, rubbing or grating sound that is caused by inflammation of pleural surfaces as they rub against the chest wall. A pleural friction rub can be heard best on inspiration but is also present during expiration and does not disappear with a cough. This abnormal breath sound is loudest over the lower lateral anterior surface of the lung.

Sputum Assessment

If the client is coughing up sputum, it should be inspected. Normal respiratory secretions are clear or white. Normal sputum has no odor and is of medium consistency. Sputum that is thick and sticky is usually difficult to expectorate. It may indicate that the client is poorly hydrated. Sputum produced by clients with asthma is stringy, like thickened egg white. Life-threatening pulmonary edema produces frothy, pinkish secretions.

Sputum that is yellow or greenish or has a putrid or musty odor usually indicates infection. When infection is suspected, a sputum sample should be collected in a sterile container and sent to the laboratory for examination.

Blood-streaked mucus indicates airway inflammation, and although it can be alarming, it usually is not serious. It commonly occurs during harsh coughing episodes in clients with bronchitis. Frankly red, bloody mucus (**hemoptysis**) is a sign of continual bleeding somewhere in the airways, and it must be thoroughly investigated.

Diagnostic Tests and Procedures

The most commonly used tests for assessing respiratory status are chest x-ray, pulmonary function tests, sputum culture, and analysis of arterial blood gases. More specialized tests include bronchoscopy, lung scans, pulmonary angiography, skin testing for allergies in asthma, and skin tests for tuberculosis.

Chest X-ray. The chest x-ray is widely used to identify pathologic changes in the lung and chest that may explain the client's breathing problems. From a chest x-ray the radiologist can detect abnormal fluid or air in the pleural space. The x-ray can also show whether portions of the lungs are consolidated (as in pneumonia) or underinflated (as in atelectasis). Tumors are sometimes first detected by routine x-rays. The chest x-ray is also used to determine the position of catheters and tubes and to monitor a client's response to therapy. Lung scans and angiography are specialized radiographic techniques used to study blood flow and ventilation in the lung.

Pulmonary Function Tests. Specialized breathing tests measure lung size and airway patency. Spirometry produces graphic representations of lung volumes and flows. These graphs are essential in determining the severity of a client's restrictive or obstructive lung disease. Common measurements include tidal volume, vital capacity, and forced expiratory volume in 1 second (FEV-1). More highly specialized pulmonary function tests can provide additional information on lung characteristics.

Sputum Culture. The client who has a productive cough, is febrile, and may otherwise show signs of infection should have a sample of sputum evaluated by the laboratory. A Gram stain can be performed quickly to determine whether an infection is present. Sputum is cultured to identify the specific agent causing the infection. A sensitivity test done at the same time will indicate the best antibiotic to use against the causative agent, but 2 to 3 days are needed for results.

Arterial Blood Gas Monitoring. Blood levels of oxygen, carbon dioxide, and pH are the most reliable indicators of gas exchange. Arterial blood sampling provides the most complete and accurate picture of the client's gas exchange status. PaO_2 is one of the best indicators of how much oxygen is available to tissues. When the PaO_2 is lower than normal, tissues may experience **hypoxia**. This is dangerous to all tissues and organs, but can be especially damaging to the heart and the brain, where it can result in a myocardial infarction or a cerebrovascular accident. Although PaO_2 normally declines with age, an abnormally low PaO_2 always indicates gas exchange problems (Shapiro, 1994). PaO_2 decreases in direct proportion to severity of lung impairment (see the accompanying display).

In addition to oxygenation, arterial blood sampling also indicates how effective the lungs are at removing carbon dioxide. Regulation of this metabolic waste product by the lungs is essential for normal acid-base balance of the blood. This affects many functions, including the drive to breathe, affinity of hemoglobin for

Levels of Hypoxemia

Mild:	PaO_2 of 60–80 mm Hg
Moderate:	PaO_2 of 40–60 mm Hg
Severe:	PaO_2 of less than 40 mm Hg

Note: PaO_2 naturally declines with age. For every year over 60, subtract 1 mm Hg from the normal range. For example, a man of 70 would be expected to have a PaO_2 of 70–90 mm Hg.

Also, the newborn infant is normally hypoxemic during the first 12–24 hours of life. A PaO_2 of 80–100 mm Hg is achieved after this time.

Table 34-2* • *Normal Arterial Blood Gas Values

PaO_2:	80–100 mm Hg
$PaCO_2$:	35–45 mm Hg
pH:	7.35–7.45
HCO_3^-:	22–26 mEq/L
Base excess:	± 2

oxygen, and cardiac function. The $PaCO_2$ stays nearly constant in the person with healthy lungs. A $PaCO_2$ lower than 35 mm Hg indicates **hyperventilation**, or breathing in excess of metabolic needs. Healthy people are able to hyperventilate voluntarily. Hyperventilation is common during an asthma attack, and occurs in some clients with head injuries. It may also occur involuntarily during extreme anxiety.

A $PaCO_2$ above 45 mm Hg indicates **hypoventilation**. This means the person's breathing is insufficient to clear carbon dioxide adequately from the blood. Hypoventilation is caused by severe airway obstruction, and is a serious problem for clients with advanced COPD. It is also caused by respiratory failure in clients whose respiratory drive has been diminished by narcotics, barbiturates, or trauma.

Arterial blood sampling also indicates the blood's acidity or alkalinity. The pH is a measure of the acid-base balance of the blood. Biochemical processes essential to all cellular life require a close balance of the blood's acids and bases. Normally, arterial blood pH ranges from 7.35 to 7.45. Arterial pH below 7.35 is described as acidosis, whereas pH above 7.45 indicates alkalosis (Table 34-2). A more detailed discussion of acid-base balance is presented in Chapter 36.

Pulse Oximetry. Pulse oximetry offers a noninvasive means for approximating oxygenation, whereas arterial blood sampling provides precise information about blood gases. The pulse oximeter uses infrared light to determine the percentage of hemoglobin that has combined with oxygen. A sensor attached to the client's finger or earlobe allows assessment of heart rate and oxygen saturation, either intermittently or continuously. Oximetry is a convenient and painless alternative to needle sticks, it is simple to use, and provides immediate data. These advantages make it invaluable as a tool for determining the need for oxygen therapy and for assessing its effectiveness.

The oximeter registers arterial oxygen saturation (SaO_2). An SaO_2 greater than 95% is considered normal, whereas values lower than 93% usually indicate the need for oxygen therapy and further assessment.

Several factors affect the accuracy and proper interpretation of oximetry. The client must have adequate peripheral blood flow for the oximeter to detect a pulse. Conditions such as room lighting, client motion, cigarette smoking, or dark polish on the client's fingernails can affect sensor accuracy. Carbon monoxide poisoning results in false high readings, and edema at the sensor site produces false low readings (Ehrhardt & Daleiden, 1994). Most important, interpretation of SaO_2 depends on the operator's understanding of hemoglobin and its unique properties. Because of the manner in which hemoglobin combines with oxygen, relatively slight changes in SaO_2 may actually reflect large changes in blood oxygenation. Experience and clinical judgment help the skilled practitioner relate oximetry readings to client condition. Refer to Procedure 34-1 for guidance in using pulse oximetry.

Bronchoscopy. Bronchoscopy allows the physician to visualize the airways directly. A flexible fiberoptic tube connected to a viewing screen is inserted through the client's nose. The scope is directed into the trachea and bronchi by a hand-held control. The bronchoscope can be used to collect sterile sputum specimens or tissue samples for laboratory examination, or to withdraw large sputum plugs or aspirated objects that have obstructed the airways.

Skin Tests. One type of skin test is performed to identify client allergies to specific substances. By determining possible sources of airway hypersensitivity in asthmatic clients, allergists can help these people avoid the offending substances. These tests also help the allergist devise serums for desensitizing the client. Another type of skin test is used to establish whether a client has been exposed to tuberculosis. The purified protein derivative test is a vital screening tool that helps identify those people who may be carrying this disease.

Nursing Diagnoses

Client assessment data can substantiate a potential or actual nursing diagnosis. Nursing diagnoses included in this category are Ineffective Breathing Pattern, Ineffective Airway Clearance, and Impaired Gas Exchange. In 1992, NANDA added Inability to Sustain Spontaneous Ventilation and Dysfunctional Ventilatory Weaning Response, but because these are nursing diagnoses encountered in critical care units, they will not be developed in depth here (NANDA, 1994).

Diagnostic Statement: Ineffective Breathing Pattern

Definition

Ineffective Breathing Pattern is the state in which an individual's inhalation and/or exhalation pattern does not enable adequate pulmonary inflation or emptying (NANDA, 1994).

Procedure 34-1
Monitoring With Pulse Oximetry

Purpose

1. Monitor arterial oxygen saturation (SaO_2) noninvasively.
2. Make an early detection of clinical hypoxemia.
3. Assess tolerance to tapering of oxygen therapy.

Assessment

- Identify clients at risk for hypoxemia (ie, respiratory and cardiac disease) who would benefit from pulse oximetry.
- Identify if client would benefit from continuous versus intermittent oximetry monitoring.
- Assess client's baseline respiratory status to include vital signs, skin and nailbed color, breath sounds, shortness of breath, alterations in breathing patterns, current oxygen supplementation, presence of arrhythmias, and tissue perfusion of extremities.
- Review laboratory hemoglobin values to identify anemic clients whose oxygen content in the blood may be low although their SaO_2 is within normal levels.
- Observe client's height, weight, and size, and note any allergies to adhesive to choose appropriate sensor.

Equipment

Pulse oximeter
Nail polish remover, if needed

Procedure

1. Select appropriate type of sensor. A wide variety of sensors are available in sizes for neonates, infants, children, and adults. In addition, there are clip-on, adhesive, or disposable sensors. To select the appropriate sensor, consider the client's weight, level of activity, whether infection control is a concern, allergies, and the anticipated duration of monitoring.
Rationale: Proper sensor will increase accuracy of reading.
2. Explain purpose of procedure to client and family.
Rationale: Understanding the procedure increases compliance and prevents anxiety.
3. Instruct client to breath normally.
Rationale: Consistent breathing prevents large fluctuations in minute ventilation and inaccurate reflections of SaO_2 levels.
4. Select appropriate site to place sensor.
Note: Avoid using lower extremities that have compromised circulation, or extremities receiving infusions or other invasive monitoring.
If client has poor tissue perfusion due to peripheral vascular disease, or is receiving vasoconstrictor medications, a nasal sensor or forehead sensor may be considered.
Rationale: Decreased circulation can falsely alter the SaO_2 measurements from the pulse oximeter.
5. Remove fingernail polish or acrylic nail from digit to be used.
Rationale: Polish and artificial nails can interfere with accurate measurements.
6. Attach sensor probe and connect it to the pulse oximeter. Make sure the photosensors are accurately aligned.
Rationale: Proper alignment is essential for accurate SaO_2 measurement.

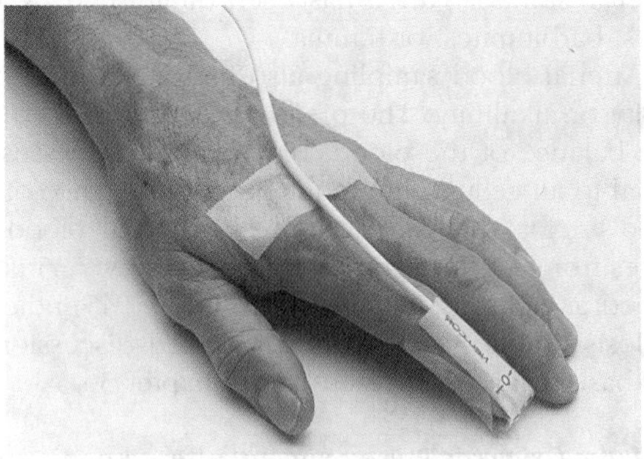

***Step 6** • Attach sensor probe.*

7. Watch for pulse sensing bar on face of oximeter to fluctuate with each pulsation and reflect pulse strength. Double-check machine pulsations with client's radial or apical pulse.
Rationale: A weak signal or missed pulsations will not produce an accurate measurement.
8. If continuous pulse oximetry is desired, set the alarm limits on the monitor to reflect the high and low oxygen saturation **and** pulse rates. Ensure that the alarms are audible before leaving client.
Rationale: Client safety is ensured and staff attention will be immediate to low critical oxygen saturation values.
Note: Inspect the sensor site every 4 hours for tissue irritation or pressure from the sensor.
9. Read saturation on monitor and document as appropriate with all relevant information on client's chart. Report SaO_2 less than 93% to physician.

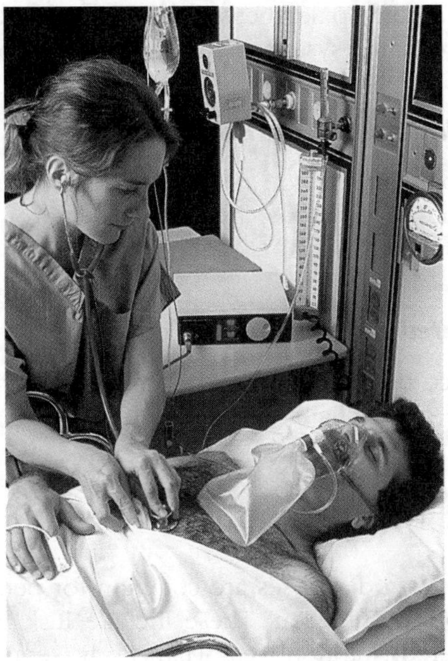

Step 7 • Compare apical pulse with pulsations detected by oximeter.

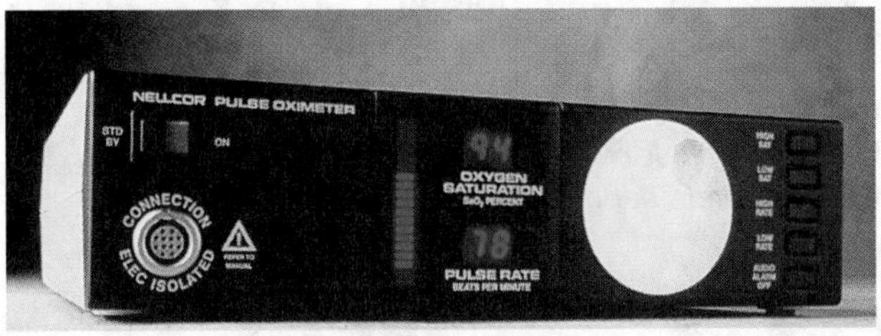

Step 9 • Read oxygen saturation from monitor.

Rationale: Documentation provides healthcare team with baseline information and response to therapy. SaO2 of less than 93% indicates need for increased oxygen.

Lifespan Considerations

Use a sensor that is appropriate for the client's weight and size.

Infants and Children

- May express fear of being burned or hurt by the light on the sensor.
- Show the sensor to them and let them touch it or place it on Mom or Dad's finger before placing it on the child.

Older Adults

- Clients who have peripheral vascular disease or who smoke cigarettes or use nicotine gum may have reduced tissue perfusion. This can make monitoring difficult and interfere with the accuracy of the readings.

Home-Care Considerations

- Because they are portable, pulse oximeters may be used in home care to monitor oxygen therapy.

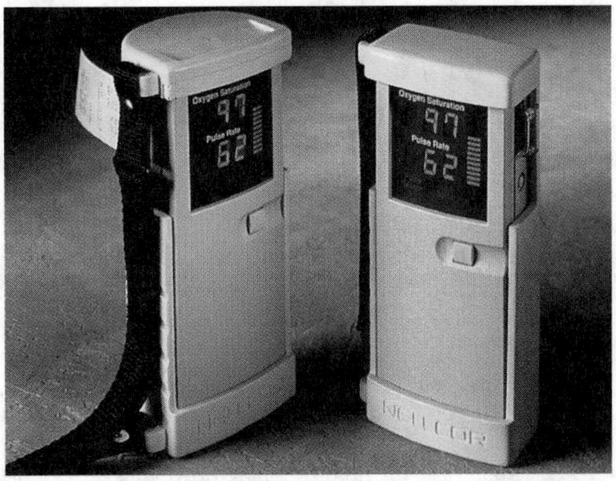

Portable oximeters are convenient for monitoring oxygen saturation in the home.

All photos in this Procedure are courtesy of Nellcor Incorporated, Pleasanton, California.

Defining Characteristics

Dyspnea, shortness of breath, tachypnea, fremitus, abnormal arterial blood gas values, cyanosis, cough, nasal flaring, respiratory depth changes, assumption of three-point position, pursed-lip breathing or prolonged expiratory phase, increased anteroposterior diameter, use of accessory muscles, altered chest excursion (NANDA, 1994).

Related Factors

Many factors, such as neuromuscular impairment, pain, musculoskeletal impairment, perceptual or cognitive impairment, anxiety, decreased energy, and fatigue can contribute to Ineffective Breathing Pattern (NANDA, 1994).

Diagnostic Statement: Ineffective Airway Clearance

Definition

Ineffective Airway Clearance is the state in which an individual is unable to clear secretions or obstructions from the respiratory tract to maintain airway patency (NANDA, 1994).

Defining Characteristics

Abnormal breath sounds (rales [crackles], rhonchi [wheezes]); changes in rate or depth of respiration; tachypnea; effective or ineffective cough, with or without sputum; cyanosis; dyspnea (NANDA, 1994).

Related Factors

Related factors for Ineffective Airway Clearance include decreased energy and fatigue, tracheobronchial infection, obstruction, secretion, perceptual or cognitive impairment, and trauma (NANDA, 1994).

Diagnostic Statement: Impaired Gas Exchange

Definition

Impaired Gas Exchange is the state in which an individual experiences a decreased passage of oxygen and/or carbon dioxide between the alveoli of the lungs and the vascular system (NANDA, 1994).

Defining Characteristics

Confusion, somnolence, restlessness, irritability, inability to move secretions, hypercapnia and/or hypoxia (NANDA, 1994).

Related Factor

Imbalance of ventilation and perfusion contributes to impaired gas exchange (NANDA, 1994).

Related Nursing Diagnoses

Other nursing diagnoses are common for people with respiratory dysfunction. These include Risk for Infection, Altered Nutrition: Less Than Body Requirements,

---

Therapeutic Dialogue
Respiratory Care

Scenes for Thought

Marvin Ottaway is a 60-year-old man in the hospital for stabilization of his pneumonia. He's sitting up in bed with the O_2 nasal prongs lying on his chest, somewhat short of breath but smiling when he sees you at the door.

Effective

Client: *Hello, Nancy, it's good to see you again today! I haven't seen you for a week!* Smiling broadly, breathing rapidly.
Nurse: *Hello, Mr. Ottaway. (Speaking slowly and clearly.) My name is Barbara, actually, and this is the second time I've met you. Who is Nancy?*
Client: Looking confused and somewhat alarmed. *But . . . you're Nancy, my sister-in-law!*
Nurse: *(Standing quietly by the bed with hand on his arm. Gently replaces the O_2 prongs.) I'm Barbara, your nurse, Mr. Ottaway. Tell me a little about Nancy.*
Client: Still breathing somewhat quickly but beginning to warm to the subject. *Oh, she's lovely; been married to my brother for 30 years, and always treats me like one of the family. You know, Sunday dinner, Christmas at their place with all the kids. I miss her. She hasn't been to see me lately.* Looks worried.
Nurse: *You really like her, don't you? (Still standing next to the bed.)*
Client: Looks at Barbara with sudden recognition. *Oh, now, I remember you. I'm sorry, sometimes my mind isn't clear. I can't remember things like I used to.* Looks embarrassed.
Nurse: *No need to apologize. Sometimes the lack of oxygen from the pneumonia can play tricks with your memory. It's important to keep the oxygen in place so you can get the benefit.*
Client: *Okay, I'll try to remember.*
Nurse: *Would it be okay if I reminded you?*
Client: *Sure! That'd be great!* Smiling broadly.

Less Effective

Client: *Hello, Nancy, it's good to see you again today! I haven't seen you for a week!* Smiling broadly, breathing rapidly.
Nurse: *Hello, Mr. Ottaway. (Speaking slowly and clearly.) My name is Betsy, actually, and this is the second time I've met you. Who is Nancy?*
Client: Looking confused and somewhat alarmed. *But . . . you're Nancy, my sister-in-law!*
Nurse: *(Gently replaces the O_2 prongs.) I'm Betsy, your nurse, Mr. Ottaway. You really need to keep this oxygen on, you know. If you don't have enough oxygen you're going to get confused. That's why you think I'm Nancy. (Smiling, speaking in a gentle tone.)*
Client: *But you are! I'd know my own kin! Why are you telling me you're not?!* Becoming agitated and frightened.
Nurse: *Quiet down, now. The oxygen will start to work soon, then you'll recognize me. (Still speaking quietly, putting hand on his arm.)*
Client: *No, I want Nancy! What have you done with her?!* Becomes more agitated. Finally calms down after oxygen and a mild sedative have been administered.

Critical Thinking Challenge

- *Explain the relationship between oxygen deprivation, confusion, and anxiety.*
- *Compare and contrast how the two nurses presented reality.*
- *Identify dialogue that caused Mr. Ottaway's anxiety level to increase or decrease.*

Pain, and Sleep Pattern Disturbance. Breathing difficulties and respiratory disease also affect the client's ability to carry out activities of daily living. Possible nursing diagnoses related to this include Risk for Activity Intolerance or Self-Care Deficit. Anxiety, Self-Esteem Disturbance, and Ineffective Individual or Family Coping are examples of possible psychosocial nursing diagnoses. Knowledge Deficit regarding treatment plan, and Impaired Adjustment are also potential nursing diagnoses for many clients with respiratory dysfunction.

Outcome Identification and Planning

After nursing diagnoses and related factors have been established, the nurse and client identify outcomes. The following general areas should be included in the formulation of client goals and outcomes:

Client will demonstrate knowledge regarding prevention of respiratory dysfunction.
Client's tissues will have adequate oxygenation.
Client will mobilize pulmonary secretions.
Client will effectively cope with changes in self-concept and lifestyle.

Client outcomes differ substantially depending on the prognosis. For the client with an acute respiratory problem, the goal will be to recover without any residual respiratory complications. Goals for the chronic respiratory client will focus on the client's ability to live within limitations imposed by the disease, and to accept changes in lifestyle and self-concept. For the terminal respiratory client, goals should be to maintain adequate comfort and to accept impending death.

Interventions are aimed at restoring, maintaining, and promoting respiratory health. Examples of nursing interventions often used in respiratory dysfunction are listed in the display and discussed in the following section.

Planning

Examples of Nursing Intervention Used in Respiratory Dysfunction

Airway maintenance

- Positioning
- Hydration
- Humidification (eg, nebulizers or humidifiers)
- Coughing
- Increased mobility
- Chest physiotherapy
- Postural drainage
- Suctioning
- Airway care

Inadequate gas exchange

- Positioning for optimum lung expansion
- Deep breathing
- Pursed-lip breathing
- Incentive spirometry
- Oxygen administration (via cannula, mask, Venturi mask, rebreathing mask)
- Bronchodilator therapy
- Ventilators

Ineffective breathing pattern

- Verbal cues regarding respiratory rate or depth
- Judicious use of pain medication
- Anxiety management

Implementation

The nurse plays a central role in educating clients with respiratory dysfunction, as well as preventing and treating this problem.

Nursing Interventions to Promote Health and Respiratory Function

The nurse can become involved in hospital or community activities that promote healthy lungs. The nurse is a credible teacher who can provide clients in the hospital, in the community, in schools, and at community-sponsored health fairs with facts about the dangers of smoking. Industrial nurses promote respiratory health by teaching workers how to avoid harmful exposures, and to recognize early symptoms of respiratory problems. In many areas, organizations such as the American Lung Association focus on pulmonary health promotion. They sponsor "Better Breather" clubs for those with chronic breathing problems, and are active in supporting clean air legislation.

The nurse uses a number of therapies to promote respiratory function. Adequate hydration, deep breathing, coughing, use of the incentive spirometer, positioning, and ambulation all assist in promoting optimal lung function and preventing pneumonia or atelectasis.

Hydration

All physiologic functions and systems depend on proper hydration. Inadequate moisture in the airways makes respiratory mucus thick and difficult to cough up. Sticky, tenacious sputum that coats the respiratory tract increases work of breathing for any client, and makes breathing especially difficult for those with chronic lung disease. Mucus that is hard to expectorate promotes infection because the bacteria it traps have time to multiply. Dried, sticky mucus also causes excessive coughing, which worsens pain in postoperative or trauma clients. Unnecessary coughing also can deprive clients of sleep and may lead to dyspnea. Finally, mucus plugs in the airways can lead to atelectasis and decreased oxygenation.

The nurse can help maintain the mobility of mucus by encouraging fluids in all clients who are at risk for dried secretions. Unless the client is severely restricted in the amount of fluid allowed, water and juices should be taken frequently to keep the sputum thinned. In some clients milk products may tend to thicken secretions, so they should be avoided. For clients who are weak or need assistance in obtaining fluids, the nurse should offer fluids regularly. Clients whose oral intake is restricted may require additional aerosol therapy to ensure secretion mobility.

Positioning and Ambulation

Changing positions and movement in general helps to shift respiratory mucus in the airways. This is beneficial because the mucus moves into portions of the airways where it may generate a cough, making expectoration easier. This keeps mucus from pooling and decreases the risk of bacterial colonization and infection.

Mucus tends to pool in the airways of people with limited mobility. Bedridden clients, clients experiencing pain, and clients with limited exercise tolerance (because of heart or lung disease) often retain secretions. The client with an artificial airway, such as a tracheostomy, and the client whose cough is otherwise impaired are also prone to mucus pooling.

To assist these clients in the removal of secretions, the nurse should see that they change position often. Whenever possible, the client with unilateral lung problems should be positioned with the good lung down to promote optimal matching of ventilation and perfusion (Yeaw, 1992). Moving the client from one side to another or assisting with ambulation when possible assists the natural clearance mechanisms of the lung.

Ambulation is difficult for some respiratory clients because of dyspnea with exertion. Whenever possible, the nurse should help promote exercise tolerance by encouraging independence. Additional benefits of increased exercise tolerance include decreased oxygen consumption and extra strength for effective coughing. Portable oxygen may be needed during periods of ambulation (Burton, et al., 1991).

Deep Breathing

Shallow breathing or an ineffective cough can lead to mucus plugging, atelectasis, hypoxemia, and pneumonia (Shapiro, et al., 1995). Taking deep breaths helps to expand alveoli and promote an effective cough, which decreases the risk of atelectasis.

Deep breathing is essential for the prevention of pulmonary complications in the at-risk client. Pain, lung disease, muscle weakness, or neurologic impairment can hinder a client's ability to breathe deeply. A major task of the nurse is to coach and encourage the client in deep-breathing techniques. The technique is explained in Procedure 34-2.

Deep breathing is useful for all clients, especially the postoperative client. There are no contraindications to deep breathing: anyone can do it at any time. Deep breathing may cause discomfort for the client with an abdominal incision or broken ribs, but it is only beneficial. A deep breath can open alveoli that have collapsed as a result of shallow breathing. It also stimulates the specialized cells of the alveoli that are responsible for surfactant production (DesJardins, 1993). A deep breath also strengthens the cough and aids in the movement of mucus in the airways. The nurse should instruct the client to deep-breathe by inhaling slowly through the nose, then holding the breath for 2 or 3 seconds at the peak of inspiration. This allows the air to distribute throughout the airways. The client can then exhale passively through the mouth.

Incentive Spirometry

An incentive spirometer is a simple device designed to encourage deep breathing. Its simplicity, minimal cost, and effectiveness have made incentive spirometry a commonly prescribed therapy.

The incentive spirometer motivates the client to breathe deeply by offering the incentive of being able to measure progress. Models of incentive spirometers vary greatly, but all provide the client some observable indicator of how deep a breath has been taken. Some models use a bellows-like device that deflates as the client inspires, others use ping-pong balls that float. Regardless of the device used, the client is visually motivated to take increasingly deeper breaths. The client and nurse set realistic goals for each breathing session, and the client works independently toward achieving each goal. Incentive spirometry motivates the client to take responsibility for the success or failure of deep-breathing therapy. Properly performed, it provides all the benefits of deep breathing. A reasonable schedule for this therapy is 8 to 10 breaths hourly during waking hours (Scanlan, Spearman, & Sheldon, 1995). Care should be taken to perform the exercises slowly, to avoid hyperventilation. Procedure 34-3 explains the procedure.

Coughing

Retained secretions cause increased work of breathing and may contribute to atelectasis and hypoxemia. No single measure controls respiratory secretions more effectively than a strong cough. A cough is a sudden, explosive exhalation that pushes secretions upward. To

Procedure 34-2
Teaching Coughing and Deep-Breathing Exercises

Purpose

1. Facilitate respiratory functioning by increasing lung expansion and oxygenation.
2. Encourage expectoration of mucus and secretions that accumulate in the airways after general anesthesia and immobility.

Assessment

- Assess client's risk factors for development of respiratory complications (ie, general anesthesia, history of pulmonary disease or smoking, chest wall trauma, cold or respiratory infection within past week).
- Assess quality, rate, depth of respiration.
- Auscultate breath sounds.
- Inspect placement of incision and evaluate whether it interferes with chest expansion.
- Evaluate client's physical ability to cooperate and perform pulmonary exercises:
  - Level of consciousness
  - Language or communication barriers
  - Ability to assume Fowler's position
  - Expression of pain (medicate as ordered)

Equipment

Pillows for positioning and to split incision

Procedure

Deep Breathing

1. Assist client to Fowler's or sitting position.
   Rationale: Upright position allows increased diaphragmatic excursion secondary to downward shift of internal organs from gravity.
2. Have client place hands palm down, with middle fingers touching, along lower border of rib cage.
   Rationale: This position allows client to feel movement of diaphragm indicating a deep breath.
3. Ask client to inhale slowly through the nose, feeling middle fingers separate. Hold breath for 2 or 3 seconds.
   Rationale: Inhaling through nose allows air to be filtered, warmed, and humidified. Holding breath allows lungs to expand fully.
4. Have client exhale slowly through mouth. Repeat three to five times.
   Rationale: Slow expulsion of air frequently initiates the coughing reflex, which facilitates expectoration of mucus.

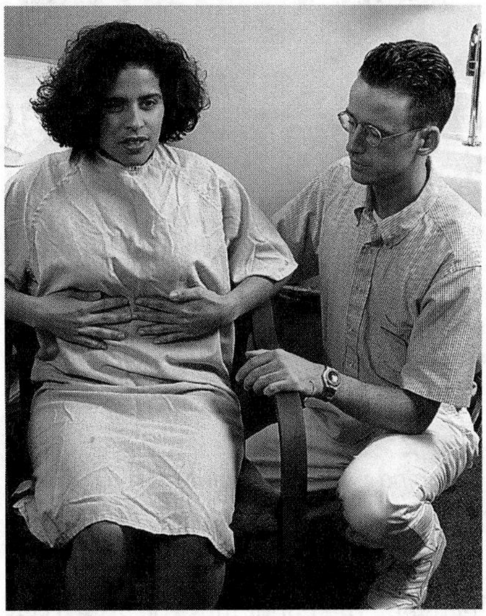

***Step 2** • Hands placed along lower rib cage allow client to feel diaphragm movement.*

Procedure

Controlled Coughing

1. If voluntary coughing does not occur, have client take a deep breath, hold for 3 seconds, and cough deeply two or three times. Nurse should stand to the client's side to ensure the cough is not directed at him or her.
   Note: Client must cough deeply, not just clear the throat.
   Rationale: Several consecutive coughs are more effective than one single cough at moving mucus up the respiratory tree.
2. If the client has an abdominal or chest incision that will be painful during coughing, instruct the client to hold a pillow firmly over the incision (splinting) when coughing.
   Rationale: Coughing uses abdominal and accessory respiratory muscles, which may have been cut during surgery. Splinting supports the incision and surrounding tissues and reduces pain during coughing.
3. Instruct, reinforce, and supervise deep-breathing and coughing exercises every 2 to 3 hours postoperatively.

(continued)

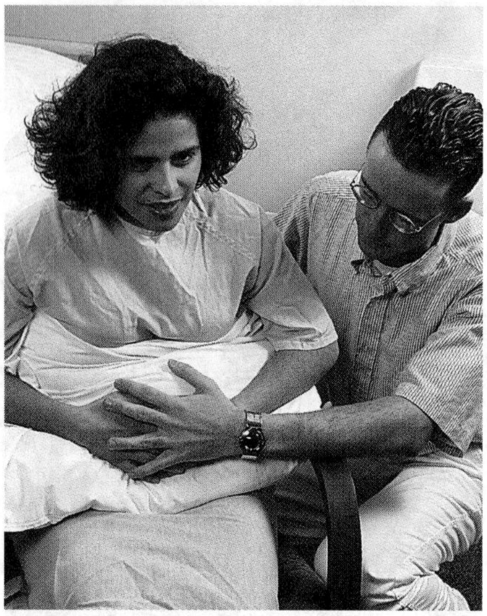

Step 2 • Splinting with a pillow during coughing promotes comfort.

Rationale: Performing these exercises every 2 to 3 hours will facilitate pulmonary ventilation and promote airway clearance without overtiring the client.

4. Document procedure.

Lifespan Considerations

Infants and Children

- Infants cannot cooperate with coughing and deep-breathing exercises, but crying is thought to hyperinflate the lungs.
- Young children learn through games and imitation. A preoperative game of "Simon Says" is one way to teach them lung exercises: "Simon Says" is one way to teach them lung exercises: "Simon says touch your nose," "Simon says stick out your tongue," "Simon says take a deep breath," "Simon says cough."

cough effectively, the client must be able to take a deep breath and generate rapid airflow (see Procedure 34-2).

For many clients, producing a strong cough is difficult or impossible. The client experiencing postoperative or trauma pain may be unable or unwilling to take the deep breath needed to cough. Clients with COPD are often unable to exhale quickly enough to generate an effective cough. Some clients are simply too weak to cough, and others may not understand how to produce an effective cough. Finally, a client with a tracheostomy or endotracheal tube cannot cough with optimal efficiency because the glottis cannot close.

The nurse must be an effective coach to elicit a proper cough. Many clients need encouragement and assistance, and all clients should be told clearly the rationale for coughing. Different types of coughs should be used by different clients.

Deep Cough. The postoperative client who does not have lung disease should be encouraged to cough deeply. This will not only help to mobilize secretions but will help to open collapsed alveoli. The client should inspire as deeply as possible, and hold the breath a second or so while closing the glottis. The air is then released as the client suddenly opens the glottis.

The deep cough can cause pain around the incisional area in clients who have had abdominal or thoracic surgery. To help control the pain, the client can support the incisional area with a pillow, using it as a splint to immobilize the wound. In clients with severe incisional discomfort, it is helpful to schedule coughing sessions after pain medications have been administered.

Stacked Cough. Some clients find it painful to cough despite premedication. For them, a stacked cough may be less uncomfortable and almost as effective. Stacked coughing is the release of several short blasts of air instead of one deep cough. This type of cough prevents excessive stretching of sutures and also minimizes the airway collapse that may come with deep coughing.

Low-Flow (Huff) Cough. A third type of cough is called low-flow or "huff" coughing. This method of clearing the airways is most effective for clients with COPD. The airways of these clients tend to collapse with rapid exhalation, so slowing their airflow actually is more facilitative for expelling secretions. The client is instructed to inhale deeply. Instead of closing the glottis and generating high pressure, the client then says "huff" three or four times while exhaling.

Quad Cough. Clients with neuromuscular disease, or those who are quadriplegic, often need direct assistance to generate an effective cough to prevent respiratory dysfunction. The client takes a deep breath, or the nurse provides a deep breath with a manual resuscitation bag. The deep breath is then held for a moment. With hands placed just below the client's rib cage, the nurse assists the client by quickly pushing in and upward, much like performing the Heimlich maneuver. The resultant rush of air acts as a cough by helping to dislodge mucus from the airways.

Nursing Interventions for Altered Respiratory Function

Aerosol therapy, oxygen administration, positive pressure therapies, chest physiotherapy, management of artificial airways, and suctioning may be necessary inter-

Procedure 34-3
Promoting Breathing With the Incentive Spirometer

Purpose

1. Improve pulmonary ventilation and oxygenation.
2. Loosen respiratory secretions.
3. Prevent or treat atelectasis by expanding collapsed alveoli.

Assessment

- Identify clients at risk for atelectasis.
- Complete respiratory assessment (ie, history of smoking, breath sounds, respiratory rate and rhythm, sputum production).
- Review physician's orders for incentive spirometry.

Equipment

Incentive spirometer (flow-oriented or volume-oriented)
Note: Type of incentive spirometer is usually determined by equipment available through respiratory therapy.
Mouthpiece (if not already connected to spirometer)
Nose clip (optional)

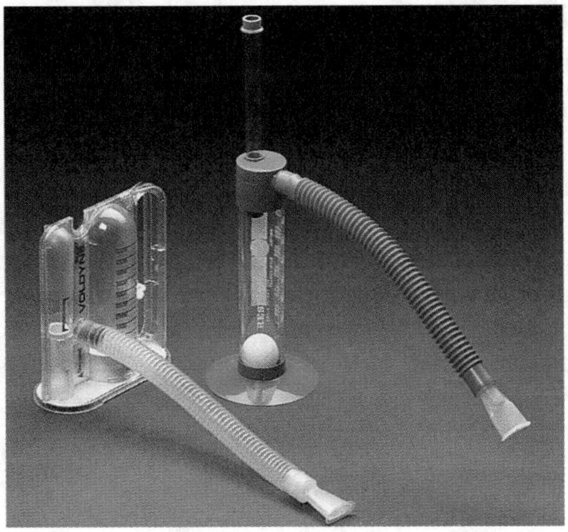

Procedure

1. Wash your hands.
   Rationale: Handwashing reduces transfer of microorganisms.
2. Assist client to high Fowler's or sitting position.
   Rationale: This position facilitates optimal lung expansion.
3. Instruct client in procedure:
   a. Seal lips tightly around mouthpiece.
   Rationale: A sealed mouthpiece prevents leakage of air around mouthpiece.
   b. Inhale slowly and deeply through mouth. Hold breath for 2 or 3 seconds.
   Rationale: Holding the breath maintains maximal inflation of alveoli.
   Note: Client can see his or her progress by watching the balls elevate or lights go on, depending on type of equipment used.

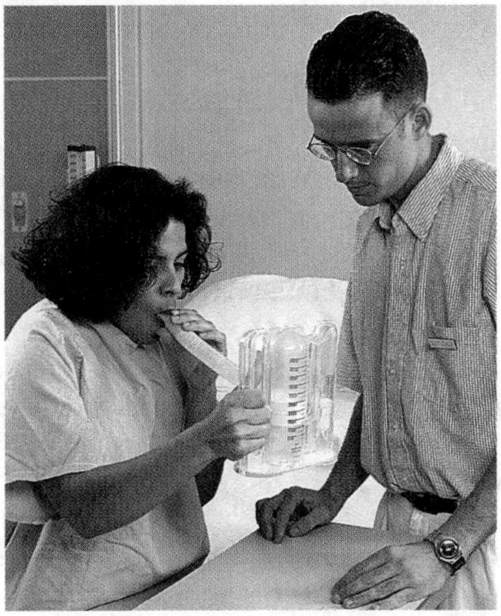

Step 3B • *Inhale slowly and deeply through the mouth, holding breath for 2–3 seconds.*

   c. Exhale slowly around mouthpiece.
   d. Breathe normally for several breaths.
4. Repeat procedure 5 to 10 times every 1 to 2 hours, per physician's orders.
5. Wash your hands.

Lifespan Considerations

- Clients who are too young to follow directions, are cognitively impaired or malnourished, or lack necessary motor skills are likely to be unsuccessful at using incentive spirometry.

ventions to help promote optimal oxygenation for the client with respiratory dysfunction.

Aerosol Therapy

An aerosol is a suspension of microscopic liquid droplets in air or oxygen. Aerosol therapy may be given for any of the following reasons:

- To add moisture to oxygen delivery systems
- To hydrate thick sputum and prevent mucus plugging
- To administer various drugs to the airways

Thick, dried sputum is difficult to raise, even with the most powerful cough. Despite adequate hydration, a client's sputum may dry out. When this happens, aerosol therapy is beneficial. A large-volume nebulizer or an ultrasonic nebulizer will deliver a moist fog continuously to the airways. The mucus blanket is loosened as it absorbs the water, which facilitates its removal. The watery mist also soothes inflamed airways. Heating the water in the nebulizer increases the amount of moisture delivered.

The nurse must check the reservoir frequently to ensure it is filled with sterile water. It must be screwed together tightly to ensure full delivery of the prescribed level of oxygen. The large-bore tubing must be drained often to prevent buildup of condensation. Temperature of the mist should be monitored to prevent burning the client. Finally, because aerosols loosen dried secretions, the nurse must help the client remove them by coughing or suctioning.

Aerosol Medications. A variety of drugs are administered by aerosol. Bronchodilators reverse bronchospasm most quickly when administered directly to the lungs. Although they are commonly used and highly effective, these agents are powerful medications that may have serious side effects. All clients receiving bronchodilators should be closely monitored for signs of increased heart rate, nervous agitation, and restlessness. These medications are packaged in a wide variety of dosages, so the nurse should carefully check the ordered dose against the available unit-dose packages. Inhaled corticosteroids are used to fight lung inflammation. For clients with asthma and chronic lung disease, aerosol steroids offer a safe alternative to oral steroids with their long-term negative systemic effects. Other types of medications delivered by aerosol include cromolyn sodium (Intal; Fisons Corporation, Bedford, MA) or nedocromil, which are used to prevent asthma attacks. Antibiotics may also be delivered by aerosol to clients with cystic fibrosis, to counter stubborn lung infections. Table 34-3 lists common respiratory medications.

Aerosolized medications are usually administered by two main delivery systems. To optimize aerosol effectiveness, the nurse must become familiar with the proper use of these delivery devices.

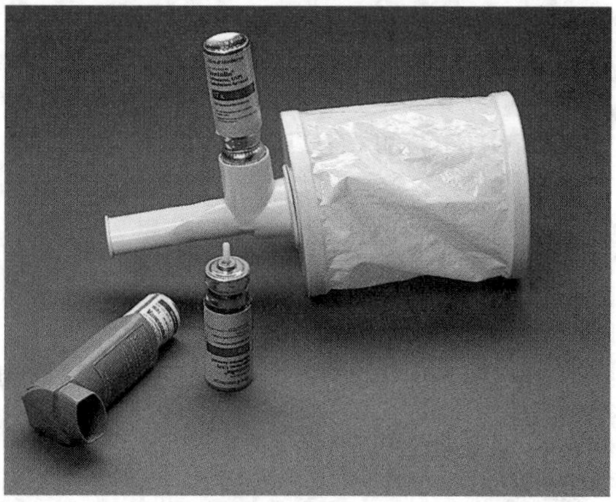

Figure 34-3 • *Metered-dose inhaler (MDI) and MDI with spacer.*

Metered-Dose Inhalers. Gas-powered, cartridge-type nebulizers called metered-dose inhalers (MDIs) provide the client with a premeasured dose of aerosolized medication. Squeezing the gas cartridge discharges a single puff of medication that the client inhales deeply into the lungs. Usually, two puffs provide a single dose. MDIs are ordinarily self-administered by the client, but the nurse is often responsible for providing instruction in their use. These devices are portable, compact, and highly convenient to use. For many people they are simple to operate, but coordination of inspiration with inhaler activation poses difficulty for some. An aerosol chamber (or "spacer") that attaches to the MDI helps to minimize this problem and improves the MDI's efficiency. Figure 34-3 shows an MDI and an MDI with a spacer.

Because MDIs are used to deliver practically any type of respiratory medication, clients may use several MDIs in their medication regimen. A complete understanding of each medication's actions and dosing schedule is essential for optimal management of respiratory symptoms.

Hand-Held Nebulizers. Small-volume nebulizers (Fig. 34-4) offer an alternative to clients who are unable to

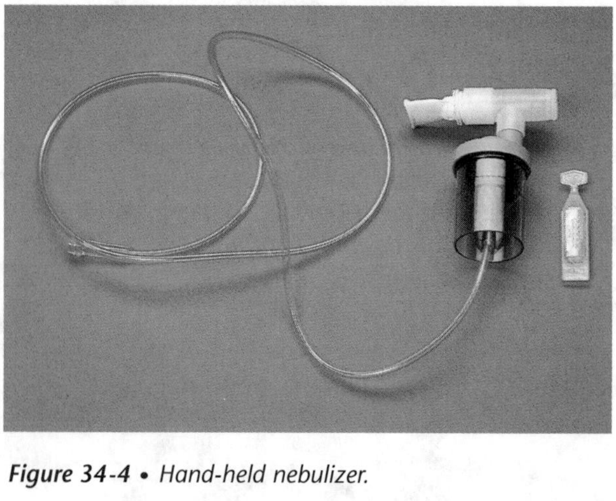

Figure 34-4 • *Hand-held nebulizer.*

Table 34-3 • Common Medications for Patients with Respiratory Conditions

Agent	How Provided	Clinical Notes
Bronchodilators		
Isoetharine (Bronkosol) Metaproterenol (Alupent) Terbutaline (Brethine, Bricanyl) Albuterol (Ventolin, Proventil) Ipratropium (Atrovent)	MDI, unit-dose packs, solution for administration via hand-held nebulizer or IPPB; some solutions for injection	1. Used to treat wheezing from asthma, COPD 2. May cause nervousness and tremors 3. May cause tachycardia; note heart rate before and after treatment 4. Aerosol chamber (or "spacer") improves dispersal of medication
Theophylline (Theo-Dur, Slo-bid), aminophylline, many others	Oral via tabs and liquids; injectable intravenous solution is aminophylline	1. Same as 1–3 above 2. Side effects include nausea, headache, agitation 3. Toxic effects may include cardiac arrhythmias and seizures 4. Blood levels should be monitored, kept at 10–20 μg/dL 5. Wide variety of available preparations; use extra caution in administration
Anti-inflammatory agents		
Beclomethasone (Beclovent, Vanceril) Flunisolide (AeroBid) Triamcinolone (Azmacort)	MDI	1. These agents are locally acting steroids; they decrease inflammation in asthma and COPD 2. These agents are not effective in acute dyspnea attacks 3. Patient should rinse mouth after use
Antiasthmatic agent		
Cromolyn sodium (Intal) Nedocromil	MDI; solution for administration via hand-held nebulizer; powdered for administration via Spinhaler	1. Maintenance drug used to decrease frequency and intensity of asthma attacks 2. NOT to be used during acute asthma attack 3. May require several weeks for noticeable effects 4. Few side effects (cough, dry mouth)

MDI, metered dose inhaler; IPPB, intermittent positive pressure breathing; COPD, chronic obstructive pulmonary disease.

operate MDIs. Instead of providing a full dose of medication in one or two breaths, the hand-held nebulizer delivers a steady stream of aerosolized medicine that is breathed over the course of several minutes. This eliminates the problem of trying to coordinate inspiration with cartridge activation. These devices are operated by means of a compressor, or by oxygen at 4 to 5 liters per minute.

The client inhales deeply and holds each breath for a moment. This allows for more effective deposition of the aerosol into distant portions of the airways. The client continues breathing slowly in this manner until the nebulizer is empty.

Oxygen Therapy

Some clients need oxygen therapy to maintain adequate arterial blood oxygen levels. Lung disease, cardiovascular problems, blood disorders such as anemia, and high metabolic demands of healing tissues can limit the body's oxygen supply. These clients may require supplemental oxygen to maintain an acceptable PaO_2.

Oxygen therapy is used primarily to reverse hypoxemia. This action can help to accomplish three fundamental goals (Shapiro, et al., 1995):

- Improved tissue oxygenation
- Decreased work of breathing in dyspneic clients

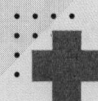

Safety Alert
Respiratory Care

- Do not smoke or use heat-generating devices nearby when oxygen is in use. Oxygen accelerates combustion and a fire may result.
- Handle oxygen cylinders with care. Damage to the tank or its valve can result in an explosion.
- Closely monitor oxygen administration and be sure the prescribed concentration or liter flow rate is not exceeded. Hypoventilation, oxygen toxicity, and eye damage may occur in selected clients who are given too much oxygen.
- When suctioning a client, hyperinflate and preoxygenate with 100% oxygen before each attempt. This will help prevent atelectasis and hypoxemia.
- Limit each suctioning attempt to 15 seconds to minimize the risk of trauma and hypoxemia.
- Monitor clients receiving theophylline preparations closely for tonic effects such as nausea, tachycardia, and nervous agitation. This bronchodilator can cause cardiac arrhythmias and seizures in excessive doses.

- Decreased work of the heart in clients with cardiac disease

First, increasing the amount of oxygen available to the client's lungs increases the amount of oxygen available to the blood. This makes more oxygen available for the vital organs.

Second, the hypoxemic client must often work harder at breathing to maintain adequate blood oxygen levels. As a result, the respiratory muscles use a disproportionate amount of oxygen just to maintain the process of breathing. By replacing the oxygen used by the overworked muscles, the client can expend less effort breathing.

Third, hypoxemia normally causes the heart to beat faster. This is a compensatory mechanism: by increasing the amount of blood flow to tissues, the heart can make up for a decreased amount of oxygen in the blood. By reversing the hypoxemia that causes this increased heart rate, myocardial work can be decreased.

General Principles of Oxygen Administration. For the average client with lung disease, oxygen therapy helps eliminate dyspnea and so improves comfort. For the critically ill client, meticulous oxygen therapy can be life-saving.

Oxygen is prescribed either in terms of flow or concentration, depending upon client needs and the capabilities of the delivery device used. Oxygen flow is expressed in liters per minute. Concentration is expressed as a percentage, or as fraction of inspired oxygen. A general rule for safe oxygen therapy is to use the lowest oxygen concentration or flow possible to achieve an acceptable blood oxygen level.

When oxygen is administered, the client's response should be assessed regularly to determine the need for continuation or adjustment of therapy. The client's color, alertness, heart rate, and breathing effort are general indicators of the effectiveness of oxygen therapy. Arterial blood gas monitoring and pulse oximetry provide more specific information concerning client response to oxygen therapy. For most clients, the aim of oxygen therapy should be to maintain the PaO_2 above 60 mm Hg, or the SaO_2 above 90%. It is rarely necessary to exceed a PaO_2 of 90 mm Hg, or an SaO_2 greater than 97%. Most often, oxygen is used continuously for as short a time as possible, until the client can maintain satisfactory blood oxygenation without it. Most clients require relatively low concentrations of oxygen to correct hypoxemia. See Procedure 34-4 for a general guide to administering oxygen.

Selection of Oxygen Systems. A variety of equipment is available to provide oxygen in a wide range of flows and concentrations. Many of these are pictured in Figure 34-5. The nurse should be familiar with the proper operation and capabilities of several oxygen devices.

The client's oxygenation status determines which oxygen delivery device is most appropriate. Although comfort is also a factor, the best oxygen device for each client is the one that is capable of providing his or her oxygen needs. If only a small amount of additional oxygen is needed to maintain adequate oxygenation, a cannula or low-concentration Venturi-type mask can be used. If the client requires a moderate amount of oxygen, a simple mask is suitable. When a high concentration of oxygen is needed, a reservoir-type mask or more sophisticated system is required. Table 34-4 compares and contrasts a variety of commonly used oxygen delivery systems. Refer to Procedure 34-4, which outlines guidelines for administering oxygen via cannula or mask.

Transtracheal catheters, implanted surgically, are becoming more common. These catheters (12 Fr or smaller) are inserted through the client's neck into the trachea. They are attached to a portable "walker" oxygen system. A significant advantage of this oxygen delivery device is that less oxygen is wasted because the oxygen from the catheter enters the lung directly. The client is managed well on less oxygen.

Safety Considerations. Because oxygen is a drug, a prescription is required for its use. The fact that it is so commonly and sometimes casually prescribed may give the impression that oxygen is harmless. Although oxygen is generally safe when used properly, certain precautions must be observed. As with all drugs, there is the potential for causing harm with misuse.

(text continues on page 913)

Procedure 34-4
Administering Oxygen by Nasal Cannula or Mask

Purpose

Deliver low to moderate levels of oxygen to relieve hypoxia.

Assessment

- Assess respiratory status (ie, breath sounds, respiratory rate and depth, presence of sputum, arterial blood gases if available, past medical history). *Note:* For clients with chronic obstructive pulmonary disease (COPD), hypoxemia is often the stimulus to breathe because they chronically have high blood levels of carbon dioxide. If additional oxygen is needed, a low-flow system is essential to maintain slight hypoxemia so breathing is stimulated.
- Assess for clinical signs and symptoms of hypoxia: anxiety, decreased level of consciousness, inability to concentrate, fatigue, dizziness, cardiac arrhythmias, pallor or cyanosis, dyspnea.
- Review chart for physician's order for oxygen to include method of delivery, flow rate, duration of therapy.

Equipment

Appropriate oxygen delivery system:
- Nasal cannula and tubing (O_2 concentrations: 22%–44%)
- Simple oxygen mask (O_2 concentrations: 40%–60%)
- Partial rebreather, mask–low-flow system (O_2 concentrations: 50%–70%)
  - Reservoir bag allows client to rebreathe a portion of exhaled air.
  - Bag must not totally deflate during inspiration, or O_2 flow rate should be increased.
- Nonrebreather mask
  - Delivers the highest O_2 concentrations possible without mechanical ventilation (80%–90%).
  - One-way valve prevents room air or exhaled air from being inspired.
- Venturi mask
  - Delivers O_2 concentrations accurate within 1% (24%–50%).
  - Frequently used with clients with COPD.

Oxygen source
Flow meter
"No smoking" sign
Humidifier and distilled water (optional)

Procedure

1. Wash your hands.
   Rationale: Handwashing reduces transmission of microorganisms.
2. Explain procedure to client. Explain that oxygen will ease dyspnea or discomfort and inform client concerning safety precautions associated with oxygen use. If the client is using the cannula, encourage him or her to breathe through the nose.
3. Assist client to semi- or high-Fowler's position, if tolerated.
   Rationale: These positions facilitate optimal lung expansion.
4. Inset flow meter into wall outlet. Attach oxygen tubing to nozzle on flow meter. If using a high O_2 flow, attach humidifier.
   Rationale: Oxygen in high concentrations can be drying to the mucosa.

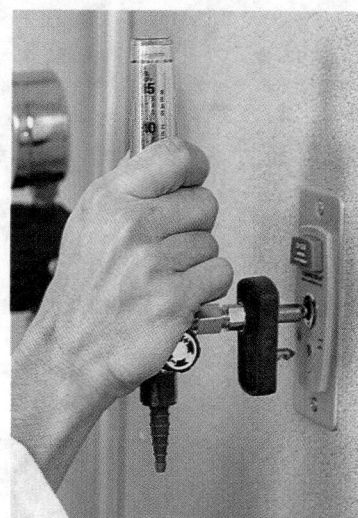

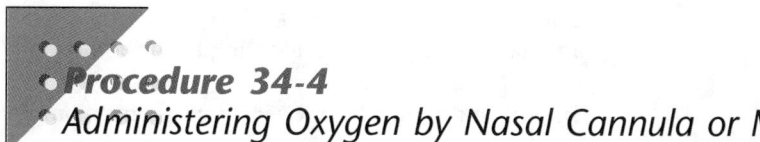

***Step 4** • Insert flow meter into wall outlet.*

5. Turn on the oxygen at the prescribed rate. Check that oxygen is flowing through tubing.
6. Cannula.
   a. Place cannula prongs into nares.
   b. Wrap tubing over and behind ears.
   c. Adjust plastic slide under chin until cannula fits snugly.

   Note: The cannula permits some freedom of movement and does not interfere with the client's ability to eat or talk.

(continued)

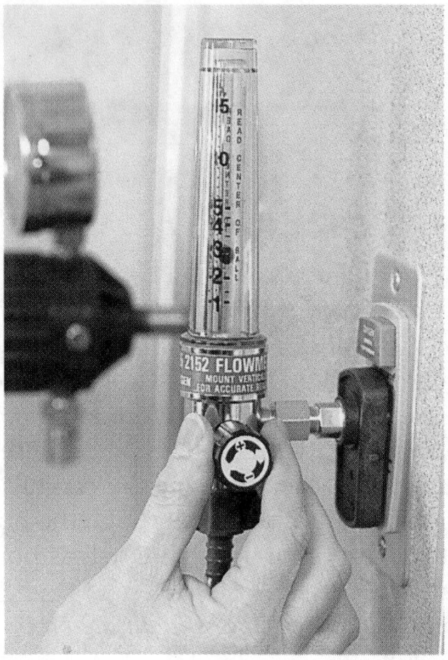

Step 5 • *Turn on oxygen at prescribed rate.*

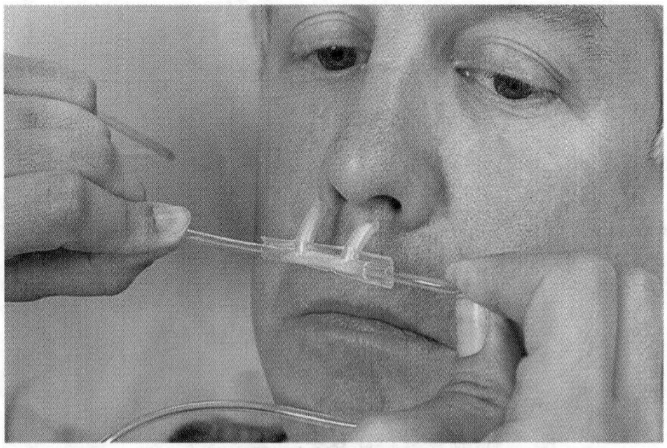

Step 6A • *Place cannula prongs into nares.*

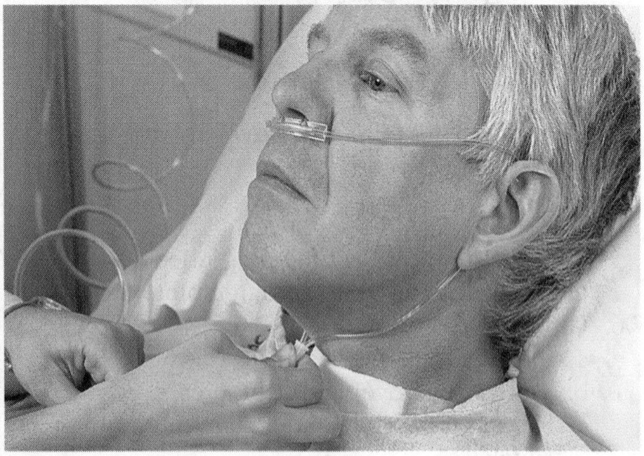

Step 6C • *Adjust plastic slide under chin until cannula fits snugly.*

7. Mask.
   a. Place mask on face, applying from the nose and over the chin.
   b. Adjust the metal rim over the nose and contour the mask to the face.
   Rationale: When the mask fits the face properly, little oxygen escapes.
   c. Adjust elastic band around head so mask fits snugly.
   Rationale: Client is more likely to comply with therapy if equipment fits comfortably.

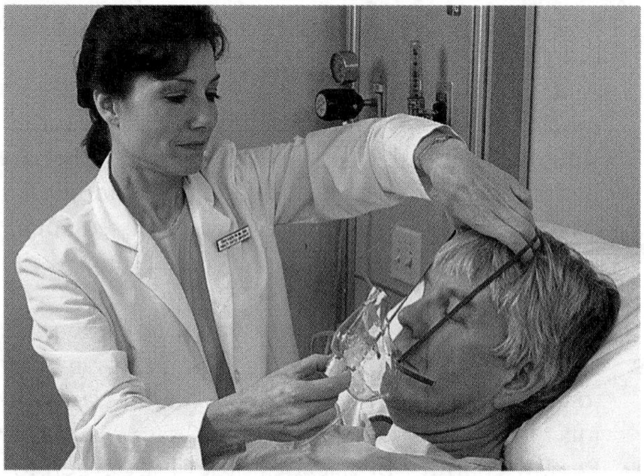

Step 7 • *Apply oxygen mask over mouth and nose.*

8. Assess for proper functioning of equipment and observe client's initial response to therapy.
   Rationale: Assessment of vital signs, color, breathing pattern, and orientation helps the nurse evaluate effectiveness of therapy and detect clinical evidence of hypoxia.
9. Monitor continuous therapy by assessing for pressure areas on the skin and nares every 2 hours and rechecking flow rate every 4 to 8 hours.
10. Document procedure and observations.

Lifespan Considerations

Infants and Children

- Isolettes (incubators) and tents are used for administering oxygen and humidity to infants and newborns. It is difficult to maintain high concentrations of oxygen in an isolette or tent, but it is nonintrusive and nonirritating.
- Plan nursing care so tent or isolette is entered as little as possible to prevent oxygen levels from dropping.
- Children frightened by the oxygen tent may feel more secure with their favorite toy or blanket.

Home-Care Modifications

- In-home oxygen supply is delivered by cylinders, liquid oxygen, or oxygen concentrators. Portable oxygen systems are available to increase independence and social activities.
- Equipment vendor and home-care nurse should instruct client on how to use oxygen equipment and how often the equipment must be filled.
- The client should be informed about using an oxygen vendor whose services include

  Trained personnel to instruct the client in use and maintenance of the equipment.
  24-hour emergency service.
  Monthly follow-up visits for equipment maintenance and client instruction.
  Vendor insurance billing.
- Needing oxygen at home can be a psychological trauma for the client. Clients should be encouraged to share their fears and concerns. A local support group of other clients using home oxygen may help clients to discuss their feelings.

When oxygen therapy is begun, the nurse should inform the client of the importance of wearing the oxygen device. A "no smoking" sign must be posted in the client's room, and the warning strictly enforced. Although oxygen is not flammable, it greatly accelerates combustion and could cause a fire from a small spark.

The flow of oxygen should be checked often to ensure that the prescribed amount is being delivered. If a humidifier or nebulizer is used (to minimize the drying effect of oxygen on the airways), the nurse must ensure that the reservoir is filled with water and is attached properly. A leak in the delivery system can prevent the client from receiving the full amount of oxygen, so all connections must be tight.

Oxygen therapy has the potential for causing serious health consequences in some clients. Relatively low oxygen concentrations can damage the retina of the eye in newborns, resulting in blindness. For this reason, all newborns receiving oxygen therapy must be meticulously monitored.

High concentrations of oxygen are toxic to lung tissue. Severely ill clients who require intense oxygen therapy for extended periods of time may suffer lung dam-

(text continues on page 915)

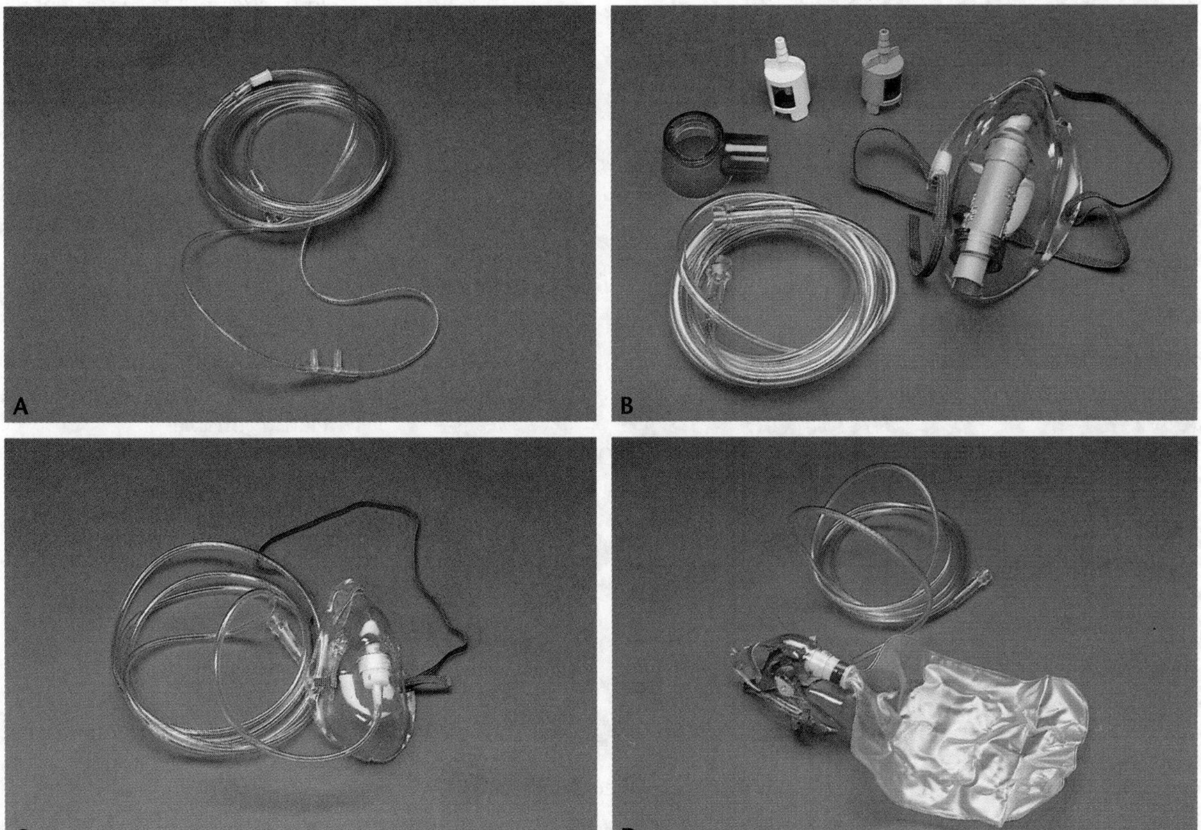

Figure 34-5 • *Common oxygen delivery devices. (**A**) Cannula. (**B**) Venturi mask. (**C**) Simple oxygen mask. (**D**) Reservoir mask.*

Table 34-4 • Oxygen Therapy Equipment

Device	Oxygen Capability	Nursing Considerations
Cannula (nasal prongs)	22%–44% when operated at 1–6 L/min	1. Most commonly used oxygen device because of convenience and client comfort 2. Delivered oxygen concentration can vary with client breathing pattern. "Rule of Four" used to estimate concentration: for each L/min of O_2, concentration increases by 4% (eg, 1 L/min provides 22%, 2 L/min provides 26%) 3. Limit maximum O_2 flow to 6 L/min to minimize drying of nasal mucosa; use humidifier prn 4. Nasal passages must be patent for client to receive O_2; mouth breathing does not appreciably diminish delivered O_2 5. Delivered O_2 concentration can vary, depending on client's breathing pattern. Relatively consistent O_2 delivery with quiet, steady breathing
Transtracheal catheter	0.5–2 L/min	1. Device is surgically implanted in trachea of O_2-dependent client as alternative to cannula 2. Advantages: efficient use of O_2 (no waste, because all O_2 is delivered directly to lungs); practically invisible so client feels less self-conscious 3. suitable only for clients who can care for device
Venturi mask	24%–50% when operated at 3–8 L/min as specified by manufacturer	1. Provides precise and consistent O_2 concentration 2. Essential to adjust mask according to specifications to ensure accurate O_2 delivery 3. Noisy; like all masks may cause claustrophobia
Simple mask	40%–60% when operated at 6–10 L/min	1. Most common midrange O_2 delivery device 2. Minimum of 5 L/min O_2 required to prevent client from rebreathing exhaled carbon dioxide 3. As with cannula, actual delivered O_2 concentration varies with breathing pattern 4. Not suitable for client with COPD because of potential for excessive oxygenation
Reservoir mask	up to 90% + when operated at 10–15 L/min	1. Used for critically ill client 2. Use sufficient flow to keep O_2 reservoir inflated

(continued)

Table 34-4 • *(Continued)*

Device	Oxygen Capability	Nursing Considerations
Large volume pneumatic nebulizer	21%–100% when operated at 12–15 L/min	1. Used to deliver O_2 with continuous aerosol therapy; required by many clients with artificial airways (eg, tracheostomies) 2. Temperature must be monitored and tubing must be drained frequently
Incubator	22%–40% +	1. Enclosure used for environmental control for newborn infants 2. Extremely imprecise O_2 delivery: accuracy varies each time unit is opened
Oxyhood	22%–90% + when operated at 7–12 L/min	1. Precise O_2 delivery for newborns and small infants 2. Minimum O_2 flow of 7 L/min flushes infant's exhaled carbon dioxide 3. Oxygen must be prewarmed and humidified to prevent infant heat loss 4. Frequent analysis needed to prevent excessive oxygenation
Oxygen tent	21%–30% +	1. Primarily used by small child unable to wear mask or cannula 2. Mainly used as "mist tent" to deliver high humidity to children with croup 3. Extremely inefficient O_2 delivery system; O_2 delivery fluctuates because leaks are common

COPD, chronic obstructive pulmonary disease.

age as a result. Although this is not a serious concern for the average client who uses a nasal cannula, oxygen toxicity poses a danger for the client who needs intensive respiratory care.

Oxygen can cause hypoventilation in some clients with advanced COPD. Some of these clients breathe primarily as a response to hypoxemia. If they receive too much oxygen, their PaO_2 rises excessively and their drive to breathe decreases. This causes hypoventilation, which can lead to respiratory arrest. Although this is relatively uncommon, it is difficult to predict which clients may be affected by this problem, so all clients with COPD must be considered at risk. For this reason, clients with COPD must be maintained only with low concentrations of oxygen. If a client with COPD requires higher concentrations of oxygen to achieve minimally acceptable blood gases, the client should be observed carefully in an intensive care setting.

Finally, a client may become psychologically dependent on oxygen. This can be expensive, and at the least poses an unneeded fire hazard.

Assisted Ventilation

When clients are unable spontaneously to breathe deeply or have difficulty maintaining optimal respirations, they may benefit from positive pressure breathing or ventilation with a manual resuscitation bag.

Positive Pressure Breathing. Intermittent positive pressure breathing (IPPB) or bilevel positive airway pressure (BiPAP) therapy uses a mechanical ventilator to assist inspiration. The client's inspiratory effort triggers the ventilator, which pushes air into the lungs. The positive pressure helps prevent and treat atelectasis by helping to open underinflated alveoli. Continuous positive airway pressure (PAP) uses oxygen under constant pressure to accomplish this objective.

To optimize its benefits, positive pressure therapy should be administered by experienced personnel. The nurse or respiratory care practitioner (RCP) must assess each client's breathing needs and individualize the treatment accordingly. The ventilator is adjusted to provide the best breathing pattern for each client. The nurse or RCP allows for rest periods at appropriate times and assesses the client continuously for adverse effects.

Positive pressure breathing is not usually ordered unless other, more simple hyperinflation therapies, such as deep breathing and incentive spirometry, have been ineffective. The equipment is expensive, and specially trained personnel are needed to provide and monitor therapy. Complications can be serious; these include hyperventilation, spread of infection, air swallowing with resultant gastric distention, danger of causing or worsening a pneumothorax, and the possibility of increasing air trapping in clients with obstructive diseases.

Manual Resuscitation Bag and Mask. When the client is unable to sustain adequate ventilation, a manual resuscitation bag and mask can be used until recovery occurs or an airway can be inserted and mechanical ventilation begun or death pronounced. A manual resuscitation bag is basic emergency equipment. This bag can also be used to hyperinflate lungs just before suctioning, and can be adapted to attach to a tracheostomy or endotracheal tube if the face mask is removed. (A resuscitation bag is pictured in Procedure 34-6.)

To deliver effective ventilation, the client's chin should be tilted back and the jaw pulled forward to open the airway. The mask is held tightly over the client's mouth and nose, maintaining a good seal with one hand as the other hand is used to compress the bag, delivering air into the lungs. The bag is self-inflating, and a one-way valve allows exhaled air to escape. A normal rate of inflations for an adult is 16 to 20 breaths per minute. The tidal volume delivered, as well as the amount of oxygen, can vary depending on the rate and technique used in compressing the bag (Glass, et al., 1993).

Ventilators

Ventilators are mechanical devices used to provide artificial breathing for clients who cannot breathe effectively. Until recently, these machines were used only in the intensive care unit. Now, ventilator clients increasingly are cared for on general medical-surgical and rehabilitation units. Intermediate care facilities that deal exclusively with ventilator-dependent clients are becoming common, and the use of ventilators in the home is growing steadily.

Positive-pressure ventilators deliver oxygen under pressure to clients who cannot breathe effectively. These machines range from simple pressure-limited devices to microprocessor-driven, volume-limited ventilators. Their use ranges from full ventilatory support to simply assisting the client who is too weak to maintain effective ventilation for long periods.

Ventilators require frequent monitoring by specially trained personnel. The person who is caring for a ventilator client must become familiar with the ventilator's alarm system. The ventilator's alarms indicate changes in the client's condition or possible machine malfunction.

More information on negative-pressure ventilators follows in the Community-Based Nursing section of this chapter. For additional information on intensive ventilator care, consult texts on respiratory therapy or critical care nursing.

Chest Physiotherapy

This treatment is commonly prescribed to help clear the airways of excessive bronchial secretions. It is based on the premise that mucus can be knocked or shaken from the walls of the airways and helped to drain from the lungs. Chest physiotherapy is a mainstay of treatment for many clients with cystic fibrosis, COPD, and pneumonia.

The primary techniques of this method of secretion mobilization are percussion, vibration, and postural drainage. Any of these physiotherapy techniques can be used alone, but they are most effective when used together. The client's ability to tolerate these procedures may limit the vigor with which they are applied, so positioning and clapping techniques may need to be modified.

Percussion. Percussion produces a wave of energy that is transmitted through the chest wall to the mucus-coated bronchial tubes. The chest is struck rhythmically with cupped hands over the area where secretions are located. Care must be taken to avoid striking over the spine or kidneys, on female breasts, or on incisions or broken ribs. Pneumatic or electrical chest percussors are effective substitutes for manual percussion.

Vibration. Vibration works in much the same manner as percussion. In this technique, the nurse's hands are used like a gentle jackhammer. They are placed on the client's chest and are rapidly and vigorously vibrated during the client's exhalation. This technique may help dislodge secretions and stimulate a cough.

Postural Drainage. Postural drainage uses gravity to assist in the movement of secretions. The client is placed in various positions to facilitate the flow of mucus from different segments of the lung (Fig. 34-6). Placing a mucus-filled segment of the lung higher than the rest of the lung allows the mucus in that segment to flow more readily downward toward larger airways. The mucus is then more easily removed by coughing or suctioning.

Not all postural drainage positions are well tolerated by all clients. The Trendelenburg (head-down) position can increase shortness of breath in the client with COPD because the abdominal organs limit diaphragm movement. Lying head-down can increase intracranial pressure and should be used cautiously for clients with head injuries. It can also be very stressful for clients with cardiac problems. The nurse or therapist who ad-

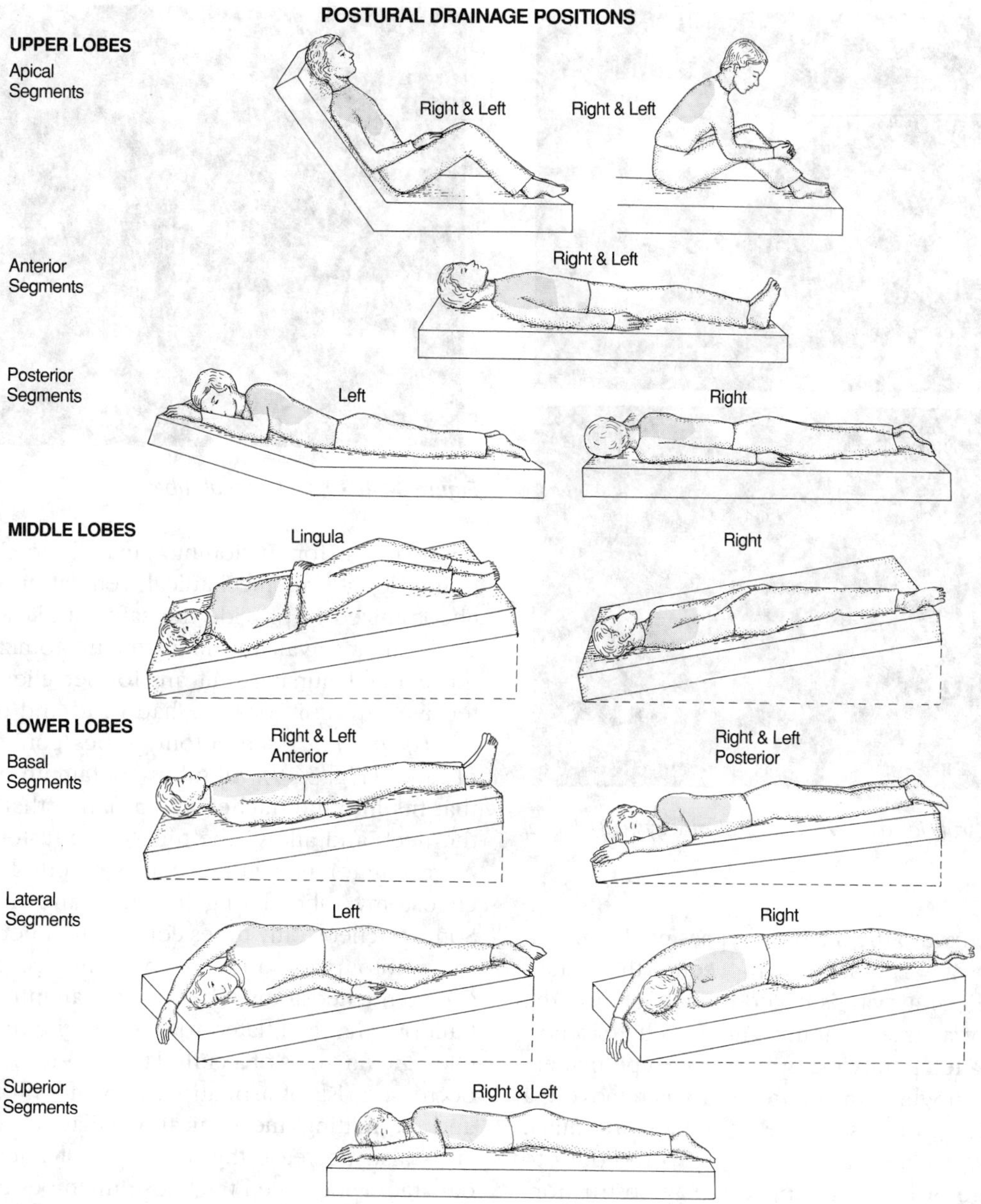

Figure 34-6 • *Various postural drainage positions are used to mobilize secretions from specific lobes and segments of the lung.*

ministers postural drainage may need to modify the treatment for clients who cannot tolerate the prescribed positions.

Artificial Airways

An artificial airway is a device that is inserted through the mouth, nose, or throat to provide direct assess to the lungs. Oropharyngeal airways, nasopharyngeal airways ("nasal trumpets"), endotracheal tubes, and tracheostomy tubes are examples of artificial airways.

Oral or Nasal Pharyngeal Airways. These airways are used to bypass upper airway obstructions or to facilitate secretion removal (Fig. 34-7). Oropharyngeal airways (see Fig. 34-7A) are simple to insert but are poorly tolerated by all but the comatose client. The noncomatose client is likely to gag on an oropharyngeal airway, so a nasal trumpet (see Fig. 34-7B) is preferable. These airways should be well lubricated with water-soluble gel before they are inserted.

Endotracheal Tubes. An endotracheal tube is a plastic tube inserted through the nose or mouth into the trachea (Fig. 34-8). These airways are used to ventilate a client during surgery or when mechanical ventilation is necessary.

Tracheostomy. The **tracheostomy** is an artificial airway consisting of a plastic tube surgically implanted just

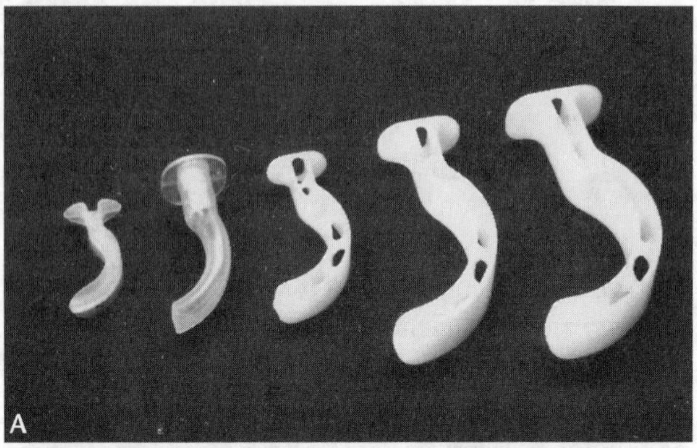

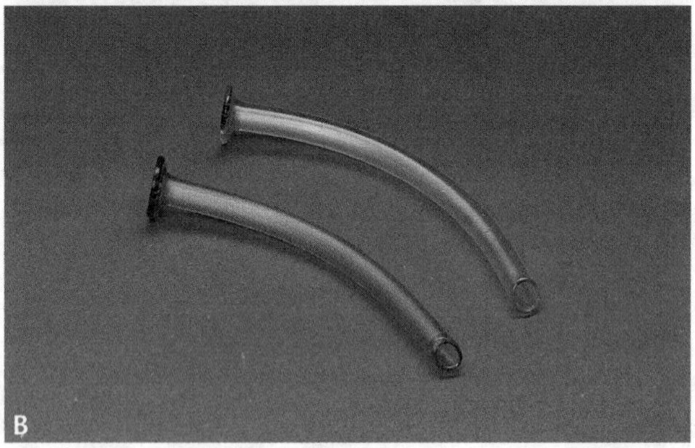

Figure 34-7 • *Artificial airways. **(A)** Oral airways. **(B)** Nasal trumpets.*

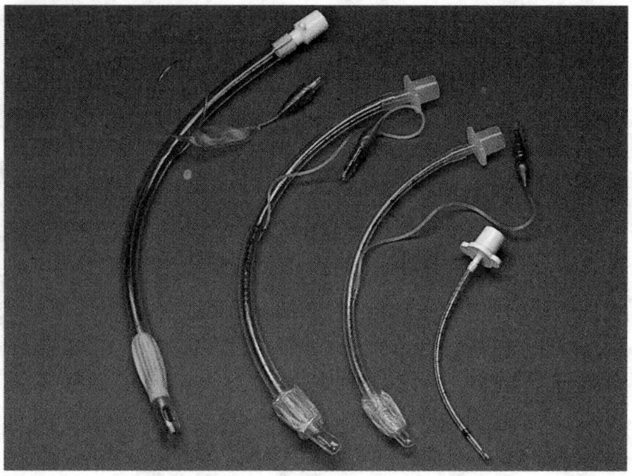

Figure 34-8 • *Endotracheal tubes.*

below the larynx into the trachea, bypassing the mouth and upper airway. The surgical procedure that establishes the artificial airway is called a tracheotomy; the resultant airway is a tracheostomy. This procedure is most often done as a temporary measure. Unlike a permanent laryngectomy, in which the entire larynx is removed, a tracheotomy leaves the structure of the airway intact.

Indications. A client may require this procedure to bypass a severe or recurrent upper airway obstruction. The client who regularly aspirates food or stomach contents may need a tracheostomy to protect the airway. A few clients may need this type of airway to help with secretion control because a tracheostomy provides ready access for suctioning. Finally, the client who requires long-term mechanical ventilation may be tracheotomized to provide the safest and most stable artificial airway available. Many tracheotomized clients on the general nursing unit are former clients of the intensive care unit, or have had head and neck surgery.

Equipment. Tracheostomy tubes come in a variety of types (Fig. 34-9). All tubes contain an outer cannula that fits into the trachea and a flange that rests against the neck and allows the tube to be fastened in place. An obturator is a guide that is inserted into the tracheostomy tube during insertion and then removed. Some tracheostomy tubes contain an inner cannula that locks into place and can be removed for cleaning. Cuffed tracheostomy tubes contain an inflatable cuff (or balloon) that is inflated to stabilize the tube in the trachea. Advantages of a cuffed tracheostomy tube include decreased risk of aspiration, prevention of air leakage, and permitting mechanical ventilation. Low-pressure cuffs also decrease the incidence of tracheal mucosal damage. Fenestrated tracheostomy tubes are tubes that have holes in the outer cannula. When the client is being ventilated, the inner cannula remains in place, but when weaning is attempted the inner cannula can be removed and the cuff deflated, allowing the client

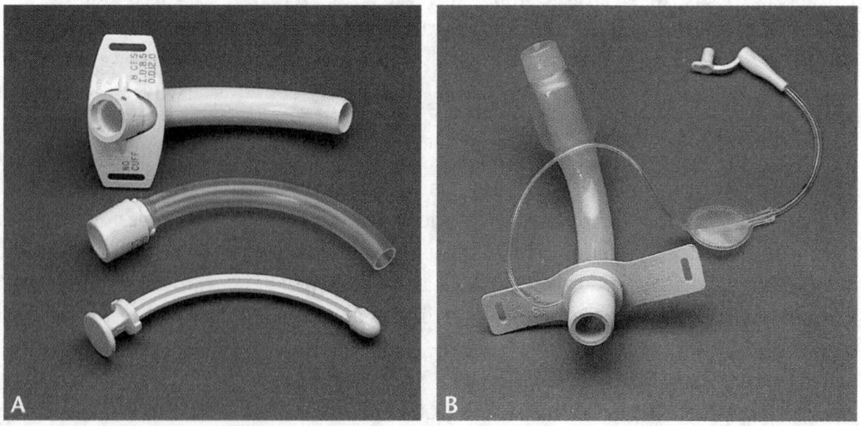

Figure 34-9 • *Tracheostomy tubes. **(A)** Uncuffed tube with inner cannula and obturator. **(B)** Cuffed tube.*

to breathe around the tube and through the fenestration. Another advantage of the fenestrated tube is that speaking is possible when the tracheostomy is plugged because the hole permits exhaled air to flow over the vocal cords. It is essential that the tube never be plugged if the cuff is inflated because this could cause suffocation and possible death (Weilitz & Dettenmeier, 1994).

Risks. Risks of a tracheostomy are numerous. Immediately after surgery, bleeding of the incision is common. Dressings must be changed frequently during this period. The nurse must also assess the extent of blood loss and be prepared to call the surgeon if bleeding is excessive.

Fastidious care of the stoma is necessary to keep it free of infection. Because the tracheostomy bypasses the defenses of the upper airway, the client is at risk for pneumonia. Thus, during the postoperative hospitalization period, sterile technique should be used when cleaning the tracheostomy site and when suctioning the client.

Clients who are tracheotomized often have marginal breathing ability. It is this type of client who must be protected most diligently against plugging of the tube. Dried secretions can completely occlude the tube, creating a respiratory emergency. For this reason, tracheostomy clients must be well hydrated, and the air they breathe must be completely humidified by a nebulizer or high-output humidifier.

A tracheostomy also poses communication problems. Because the vocal cords are above the level of the tracheostomy tube, the client cannot speak. A tablet and pencil can save both the client and the nurse a great deal of frustration. Specialized tracheostomy tubes, such as the Olympic Trach-Talk (Olympic Medical, Seattle, WA) can be attached to a standard tracheostomy tube, making speech possible. Tracheostomy buttons are used temporarily to plug the tracheostomy so that the client's ability to breathe through the natural airway can be assessed. When these are in place, the client can once again speak.

Such devices are more effective for some clients than for others. They are appropriate for use only by the client with strong spontaneous respirations. The nurse must scrupulously follow the directions for each of these specialized devices. Improperly applied, they are unlikely to work, and they may cause complete airway blockage.

Body image is a potential problem for these clients. The tracheotomized client may feel embarrassed or inadequate because of the stoma. The client may perceive the stoma as ugly and disfiguring, and may be embarrassed by its messy, bubbling secretions. Feelings of failure and depression may result from the inability to perform such a basic life function as breathing without assistance. The client is also likely to feel fear and anxiety about the inability to speak.

The nurse can be supportive and help to allay these fears. When the tracheostomy is temporary, the nurse can reassure the client that the ability to communicate will return and the incision will heal completely. This will help the client better to accept the temporary disfigurement.

Tracheostomy Care. Tracheostomy care is necessary to decrease infection risk and to ensure that crusted secretions do not plug the tube. Dried mucus must be removed from the inner cannula of the tube and from around the incision site. Stoma dressings must also be changed regularly. Commercially made tracheostomy dressings are available, or gauze may be folded to size. Dressings should not be cut with scissors because threads from the gauze can cause an inflammatory reaction at the stoma. If the client has large amounts of secretions, tracheostomy dressings should be changed as often as necessary. If the tracheostomy produces few secretions, the dressing may need changing only once or twice a day. Well established dry tracheostomies may require no dressing. Great care must be taken while changing the security ties that hold the tracheostomy tube in place because an unsecured tube can easily be coughed out. Tracheostomy care often is best performed by pairs of nurses, to minimize the danger of accidental extubation. Detailed instructions on tracheostomy care are given in Procedure 34-5.

Suctioning

In clients who cannot cough effectively to expectorate mucus, atelectasis and pneumonia may develop. Excessive mucus can even cause asphyxiation from choking. To prevent this, the nurse may have to suction the airways.

To suction the airways, the nurse inserts a catheter through the nose, mouth, or tracheal tube. The catheter is attached to a portable or wall unit suction device, which provides the suction pressure for secretion removal. Effective suctioning can clear the oral cavity and nasopharyngeal areas of secretions. Secretions deep in the trachea are more difficult to remove, but the suctioning procedure is similar regardless of where the secretions are found. Procedure 34-6 gives complete instructions on secretion removal by suctioning.

Some clients produce excessive amounts of oral secretions. These clients can use a "tonsil tip" (Yankauer) suction tube to evacuate excess saliva and thick mucus from the back of the throat. This suction catheter is also attached to wall or portable suction.

Potential Hazards of Suctioning. Clients with deep bronchial secretions may require deep endobronchial suctioning. Properly performed, suctioning can greatly improve airflow in the lungs and thus promote oxygenation. However, the procedure carries several risks. Because oxygen is withdrawn along with mucus from the airways, suctioning can cause temporary hypoxia.

(text continues on page 923)

Procedure 34-5
Providing Tracheostomy Care

Purpose

1. Maintain airway patency by removing encrusted mucous secretions.
2. Prevent infections of the tracheal site.
3. Promote cleanliness and prevent skin breakdown at stoma site.

Assessment

- Assess for excess peristomal secretions, excess intratracheal secretions, or soiled tracheostomy dressing and ties.
- Assess respiratory status: breath sounds, respiratory rate, skin color, labored breathing, flared nares or sternal retractions, arterial blood gases.
- Identify factors that influence tracheostomy care:
  Inadequate nutritional status predisposes client to infection, poor healing, and weak cough reflex.
  Respiratory infection: pulmonary secretions increase in amount. Note color, amount, and odor. Fluid status: inadequate hydration increases tenaciousness of secretions. Client may have difficulty coughing thick secretions up.
  Humidity: tracheostomy collars deliver humidified air to prevent dry, cracked membranes and thickened secretions.
- Identify type of tracheostomy tube used and if inner cannula is present.
- Assess client's ability to understand and perform independent tracheostomy care.

Equipment

Sterile tracheostomy care kit containing:
- Two basins
- Small brush or pipe cleaners
- 4″ × 4″ gauze
- Commercially available tracheostomy dressing
- Twill tape or tracheostomy ties

Hydrogen peroxide
Normal saline
Sterile gloves
Scissors
Tracheostomy suction supplies

Procedure

1. Wash your hands and don gloves.
   Rationale: Handwashing and gloves reduce transmission of microorganisms.
2. Explain procedure to client. Place in semi- to high-Fowler's position.
3. Suction tracheostomy tube. Before discarding gloves, remove soiled tracheostomy dressing, and discard with catheter inside glove.
   Note: Follow Procedure 34–6, Suctioning Secretions from Airways, but insert catheter through tracheostomy tube and advance about 10 to 12 cm in an adult.
   Rationale: Removing secretion maintains a patent airway while doing tracheostomy cleaning.
4. Replace oxygen or humidification source and encourage client to deep-breathe as you prepare sterile supplies.
5. Open sterile tracheostomy kit. Don sterile gloves. Pour normal saline into one basin, hydrogen peroxide into the second. Open several sterile cotton-tipped applicators and one sterile precut tracheostomy dressing and place on sterile field. If kit does not contain twill tape, cut two 15″ ties and set aside.
   Rationale: Preparing equipment allows for smooth, organized performance of tracheostomy care.

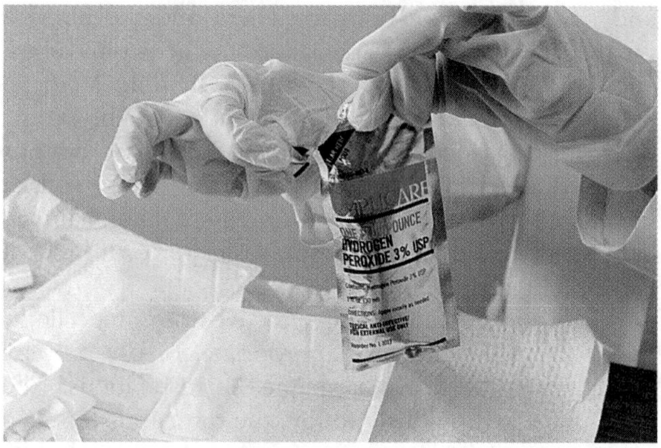

Step 5 • *Pour sterile hydrogen peroxide into basin.*

6. Remove oxygen or humidity source.
   Note: For tracheostomy tube with inner cannula, complete Steps 8 to 25. For tracheostomy tube without inner cannula or plugged with a button, complete Steps 13 to 25.
7. Unlock inner cannula by turning counterclockwise. Remove inner cannula.
8. Place inner cannula in basin with hydrogen peroxide.
   Rationale: Hydrogen peroxide loosens and removes secretions from inner cannula.

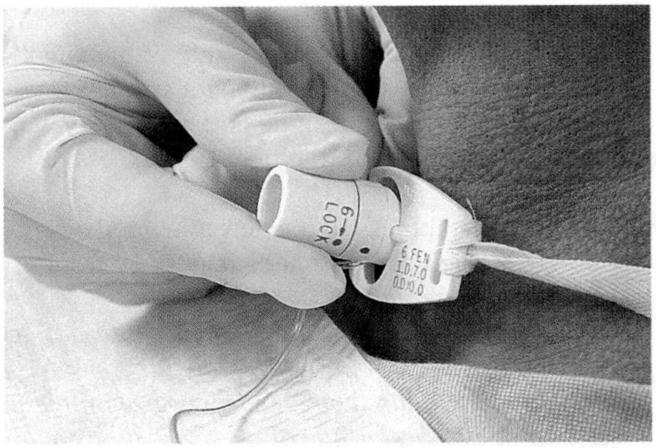

Step 7 • *Unlock inner cannula by turning counterclockwise.*

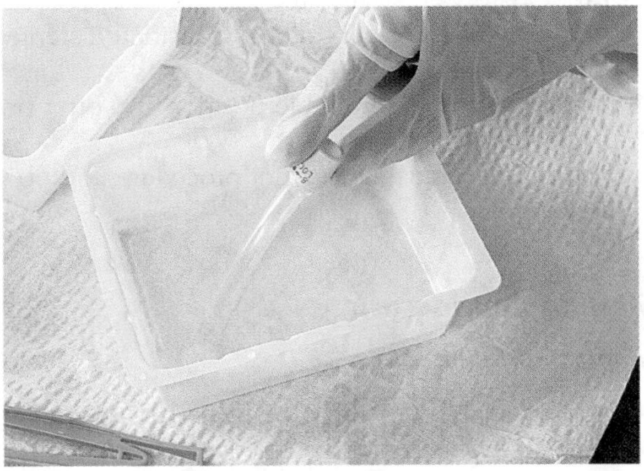

Step 8 • *Place inner cannula into basin with hydrogen peroxide.*

9. Replace oxygen source over or near outer cannula.
   Rationale: Constant supply of oxygen must be maintained to prevent respiratory or cardiac distress.
   Note: Not all clients require a constant oxygen supply during tracheostomy care.
10. Clean lumen and sides of inner cannula using pipe cleaners or sterile brush.

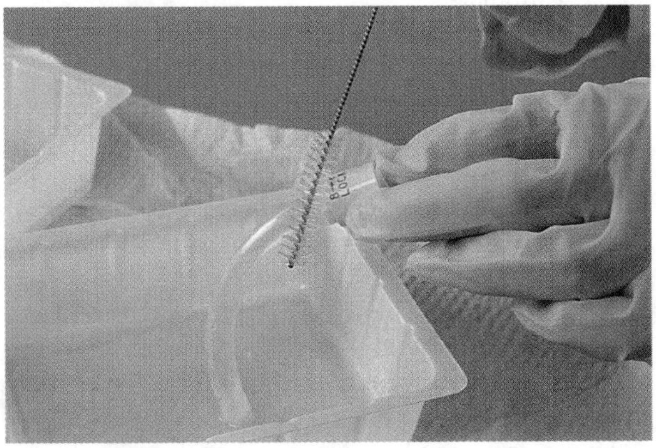

Step 10 • *Clean inner cannula with brush.*

   Rationale: Mechanical force and friction are needed to remove thick or dried secretions.
11. Rinse inner cannula thoroughly by agitating in normal saline for several seconds.
   Rationale: Rinsing and agitation remove secretions and water from cannula and provide lubrication to each insertion.
12. Remove oxygen source and replace inner cannula into outer cannula. "Lock" by turning clockwise until the two blue dots align. Replace oxygen or humidity source.
   Rationale: Oxygen is reestablished to a secured inner cannula.

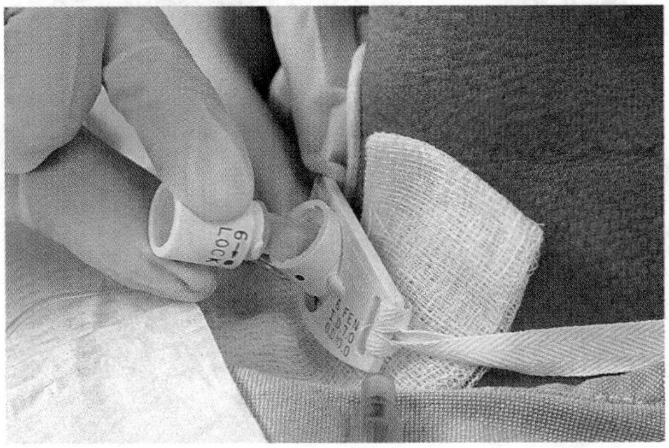

Step 12 • *Replace inner cannula, then lock into place.*

13. Clean stoma under faceplate with circular motion using hydrogen peroxide-soaked cotton applicators. Clean dried secretions from all exposed outer cannula surfaces.

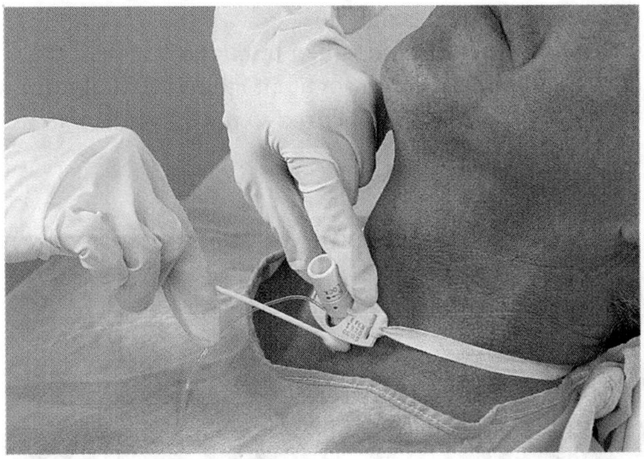

Step 13 • *Clean secretions from tracheostomy site with cotton applicator.*

14. Remove foaming secretions using normal saline-soaked cotton-tipped applicators.

(continued)

Rationale: Hydrogen peroxide can be irritating to the skin.

15. Pat moist surfaces dry with 4″ × 4″ gauze.
    Rationale: Moist surfaces support growth of microorganisms and skin excoriation.
16. Place dry, sterile, precut tracheostomy dressing around tracheostomy stoma and under faceplate. Do not use cut 4″ × 4″ gauze.
    Rationale: Frayed cotton fibers could be aspirated into the trachea.

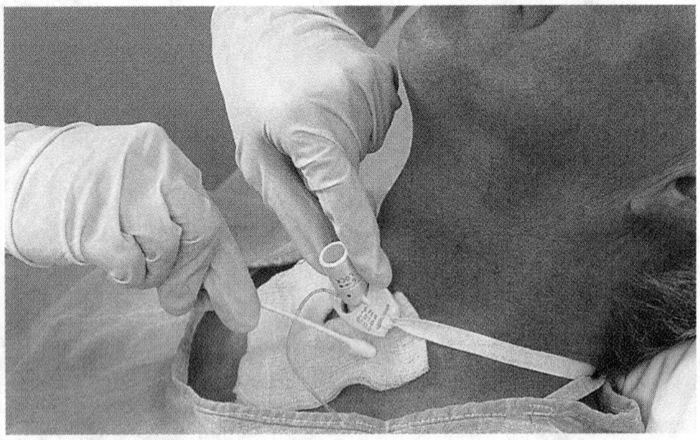

Step 16 • *Replace new precut tracheostomy dressing.*

17. If tracheostomy ties are to be changed, have an assistant don a sterile glove and hold the tracheostomy tube in place.
    Rationale: This action prevents accidental displacement of the tracheostomy tube if the client moves or coughs when the ties are not secure.
18. Cut a ½″ slit approximately 1″ from one end of both clean tracheostomy ties. This is easily done by folding back on itself 1″ of the tie and cutting a small slit in the middle.
19. Remove and discard soiled tracheostomy ties.
20. Thread end of tie through cut slit in tie. Pull tight.
    Rationale: The tie is secured to the faceplate without using knots.

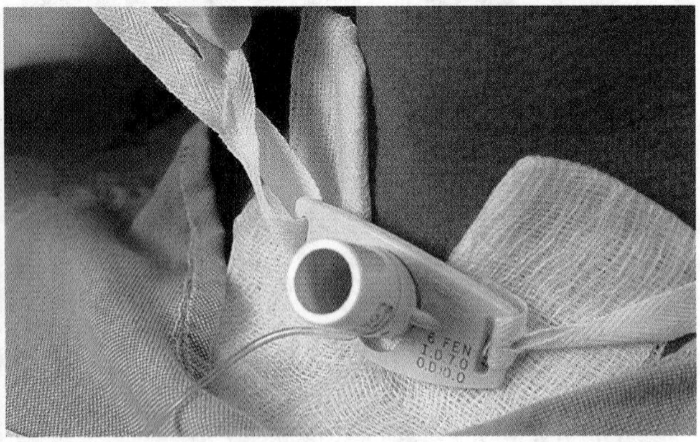

Step 20 • *Thread end of tie through cut slit in tie. Pull tight.*

21. Repeat Step 19 with the second tie.
22. Bring both ties together at one side of the client's neck. Assess that ties are only tight enough to allow one finger between tie and neck. Use two square knots to secure the ties. Trim excess tie length.
    Note: Assess tautness of tracheostomy ties frequently in clients whose neck may swell from trauma or surgery.
    Rationale: Ties must be taut enough to prevent accidental dislodging of tracheostomy tube, but loose enough not to cause choking or pressure on the jugular veins. Ties at side of neck are more comfortable for the client.
23. Remove gloves and discard disposable equipment. Label, date, and store reusable supplies.
    Note: Opened normal saline is considered sterile for 24 hours.
24. Assist client to comfortable position and offer oral hygiene.
25. Wash your hands. Document procedure and observations.

Lifespan Considerations

Infants and Children

- Additional assistants may be necessary during tracheostomy care to prevent active children from dislodging or expelling their tracheostomy tubes.
- Parents may be encouraged to participate with the procedure in an effort to comfort the child and promote client teaching.

Home-Care Modifications

- The client or caregiver must be taught:
    That handwashing is the most important step before touching the tracheostomy.
    The function of each part of the tracheostomy tube.
    To remove, change, and replace the inner cannula.
    It is recommended that the inner cannula be cleaned two or three times a day.
    To clean the tracheostomy stoma.
    To suction tracheal secretions.
    To assess for symptoms of infection (ie, increased temperature, increased amount of secretions, change in color or odor of secretions).
- A vaporizer may be used in the home to replace moisture into the air.
- The client may wear a scarf or 4″ × 4″ over the tracheostomy if the air is dusty.
- Home care may be a clean rather than sterile procedure:

Plain single-use paper cups may be used for soaking the inner cannula.
Tap water may be used to rinse secretions from the inner cannula.
Gloves need not be worn, but thorough handwashing is imperative.

- A list of needed supplies and equipment and the names of medical supply houses is useful.
- Names and telephone numbers of healthcare professionals who are available for emergencies or advice 24 hours a day should be readily available.

Many studies over the last decade have demonstrated the significance of hyperinflation and hyperoxygenation before each suctioning attempt to minimize hypoxemia and atelectasis (Mancinelli-Van Atta & Beck, 1992).

Suction should be applied intermittently to help minimize damage to the delicate mucosal lining of the trachea by the catheter. Ten to 15 seconds is the recommended time limit for each suction attempt (Bolecheck & McCloskey, 1992). Only as much suction as necessary to remove secretions should be used. Usually the suction regulator should be set between 80 and 120 mm Hg for larger children and adults, and 60 to 80 mm Hg for infants.

Saline lavage, a practice commonly used to loosen thick secretions, can cause a significant (although temporary) drop in oxygenation, so this procedure must be used only with selected clients, and only with caution (Ackerman, 1993). In some clients it is used to stimulate a strong cough.

In addition to causing hypoxia, suctioning can cause cardiac arrhythmias, hypotension, and atelectasis. Because suctioning can stimulate a gag reflex, vomiting (with the potential for aspiration) is possible. Suctioning can greatly relieve the dyspnea that accompanies excessive secretions, but for nearly all clients it is frightening and unpleasant. The nurse should be prepared to offer a great deal of reassurance.

Emergency Airway Measures

Airway obstruction is a medical emergency requiring immediate attention. Because airway obstruction hinders breathing, the airway must be cleared to prevent suffocation and cardiorespiratory arrest. The most common cause of airway obstruction is the tongue, which can fall back into the airway and interfere with ventilation and gas exchange. The neurologically impaired client, such as the comatose client or one with a cerebral vascular accident, is most at risk for this problem. Because the airway is only partially occluded, the person is able to breathe with effort. The partial obstruction is identified by loud snoring sounds as the client inspires. The obstruction is relieved by positioning the client on either side. If this is undesirable or impractical, an oral or nasal airway may be needed.

The choking victim who has aspirated foreign matter into the airway (such as food) is in grave danger. The nurse must quickly assess the situation and be ready to initiate steps to open the airway. On discovering the choking victim, the nurse must quickly determine the relative extent of airway obstruction. If the choking victim is coughing loudly and gasping for breath, the airway is only partially obstructed. In this case the victim should be allowed to cough, with no assistance from the nurse. The cough will be more effective than any interventions the nurse can take. The nurse should not slap the victim's back because this may lodge the obstructing material even more deeply in the airway.

If high-pitched inspiratory stridor is heard, the airway is near-totally obstructed. At best, the victim can produce only a very weak cough. If the victim cannot cough at all and makes no sounds, the airway is totally obstructed. In either case, treatment is the same. The nurse who discovers the choking victim should stay with the victim while calling for help. The person arriving first to help will be ready to alert the cardiopulmonary resuscitation team, if necessary, and to offer other support. The nurse must then take immediate action to clear the obstruction by using the Heimlich maneuver.

Heimlich Maneuver. The Heimlich maneuver is recommended by the American Heart Association (AHA) for the treatment of foreign body obstruction in adults and children (AHA, 1993). In this procedure, abdominal thrusts are used to generate high pressures that can dislodge an aspirated obstruction. After establishing that the choking victim cannot cough or speak, the nurse must act quickly. The nurse stands behind the victim, and wraps his or her arms around the victim's waist. With one fist against the abdomen and the other grasping the opposite wrist, the nurse squeezes rapidly and tightly, using an upward thrusting motion. This must be repeated until the obstruction is successfully dislodged, or until the victim loses consciousness. Managing an obstructed airway is outlined in Procedure 34-7.

If unconsciousness occurs, the victim is laid in a supine position. The nurse should sweep the victim's mouth with the fingers in an attempt to pull out any obstruction. If no obstruction is evident, the nurse must try to ventilate the victim with a manual resuscitator or with mouth-to-mouth breathing. This is followed by abdominal thrusts, and the sequence is repeated until it is successful.

The Heimlich maneuver or any abdominal thrust technique is not recommended for pregnant women or

(text continues on page 926)

Procedure 34-6
Suctioning Secretions From the Airways

Purpose

1. Remove excess mucous secretions to maintain patent airway.
2. Collect sputum or secretions for diagnostic testing.

Assessment

- Assess respiratory system:
  Note rate, depth, rhythm of respirations.
  Note noisy, wet, or gurgling respirations.
  Auscultate breath sounds.
- Assess client's ability to cough. Note amount and character of sputum.
- Assess vital signs. Compare to baseline vital signs. Note an elevation in temperature.
- Assess level of consciousness and ability to protect airway (ie, presence of cough reflex). Note any drainage from mouth.

Equipment

Portable or wall suction apparatus with tubing and reservoir
Sterile suction kit containing:
  Appropriate-sized catheter: infants, 5 to 8 Fr; children, 8 to 10 Fr; adults, 12 to 18 Fr
  Pair of gloves
  Container for saline to flush and lubricate catheter
Sterile saline (may be provided in kit)
Water-resistant disposal bag
Facial tissues
Towel (optional)

Procedure

1. Wash your hands.
   Rationale: Handwashing prevents transmission of microorganisms.
2. Explain procedure and purpose to client.
   Rationale: Explanations reduce anxiety and encourage cooperation with procedure.
3. a. Position the conscious client with an intact gag reflex in a semi-Fowler's position.
   Rationale: The semi-Fowler's position helps prevent aspiration of secretions.
   b. Position the unconscious client in a side-lying position facing you.
   Rationale: A side-lying position facilitates drainage of secretions by gravity and prevents aspiration.
4. Turn suction device on and adjust pressure: infants and children, 50 to 75 mm Hg; adults, 100 to 120 mm Hg.
   Rationale: Excessive negative pressure traumatizes mucosa and can induce hypoxia.
5. Open and prepare sterile suction catheter kit.
   a. Unfold sterile cup, touching only the outside. Place on bedside table.

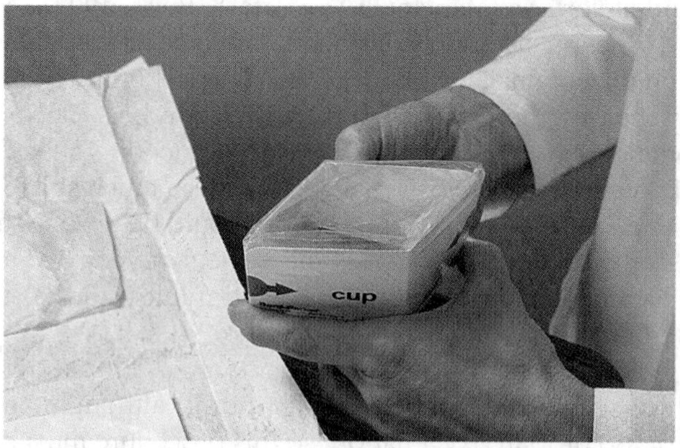

Step 5A • *Open and prepare sterile suction catheter kit.*

   b. Pour sterile saline into cup.

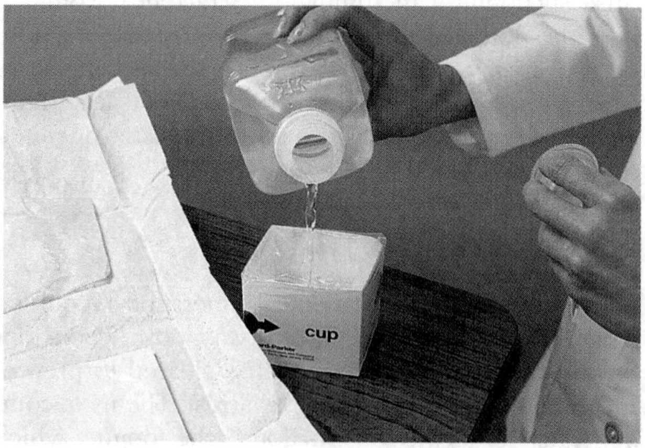

Step 5B • *Pour sterile saline into cup.*

6. Preoxygenate client with 100% oxygen. Hyperinflate with manual resuscitation bag.
   Rationale: Preoxygenation helps prevent hypoxia; hyperinflation decreases atelectasis caused by suctioning.
7. Don sterile gloves. If kit provides only one glove, place on dominant hand.
   Rationale: Dominant hand will remain sterile. A clean disposable glove may be used on nondominant hand to protect yourself from mucous membrane and sputum exposure.

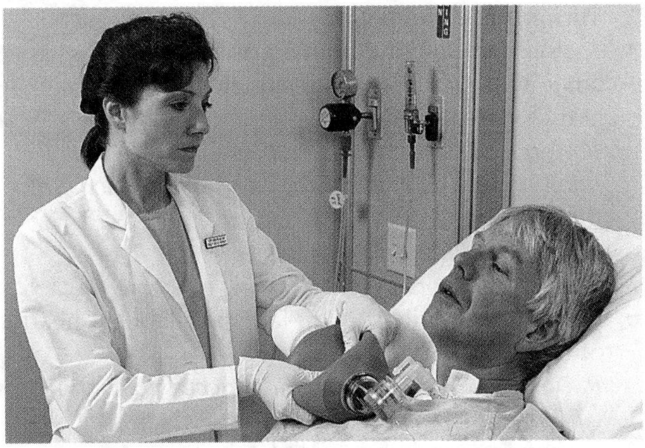

Step 6 • *Preoxygenate and hyperinflate prior to suctioning.*

8. Pick up catheter with dominant hand. Pick up connecting tubing with nondominant hand. Attach catheter to tubing without contaminating sterile hand.

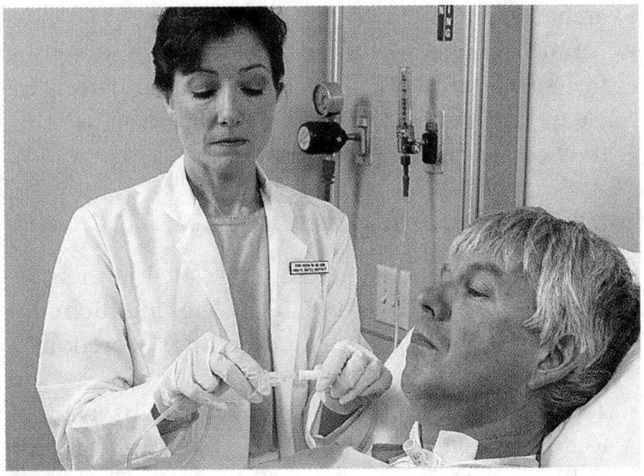

Step 8 • *Attach catheter to suction tubing.*

9. Place catheter end into cup of saline. Test functioning of equipment by applying thumb from nondominant hand over open port to create suction. Return catheter to sterile field.
   Rationale: Lubrication makes catheter insertion easier and ensures proper functioning of suction equipment.
10. Insert catheter into trachea through nostril, nasal trumpet, or artificial airway during inspiration.
    Rationale: Inspiration opens epiglottis and facilitates catheter movement into trachea.
11. Advance catheter until resistance is felt. Retract catheter 1 cm before applying suction.
    Rationale: Retracting catheter slightly prevents mucosal damage.
    Note: Client usually will cough when catheter enters trachea.
12. Apply suction by placing thumb of nondominant hand over open port. Rotate the catheter with

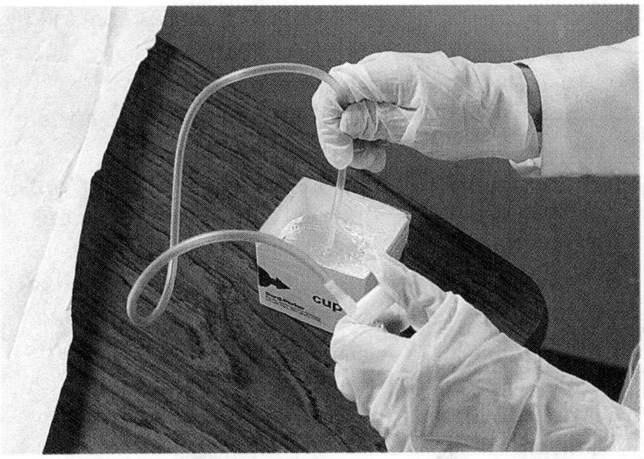

Step 9 • *Flush saline through catheter.*

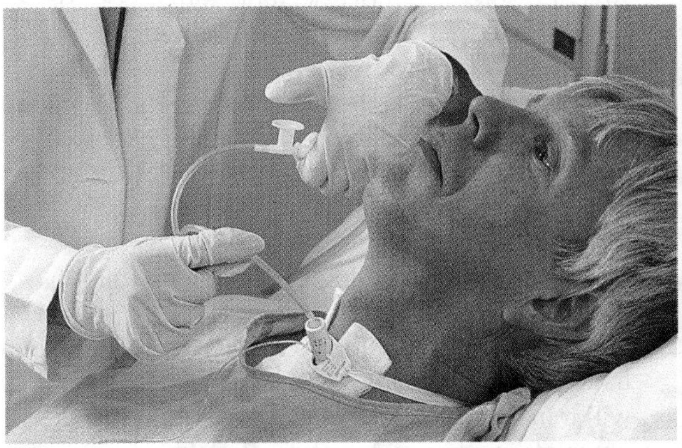

Step 10 • *Insert catheter into trachea without applying suction.*

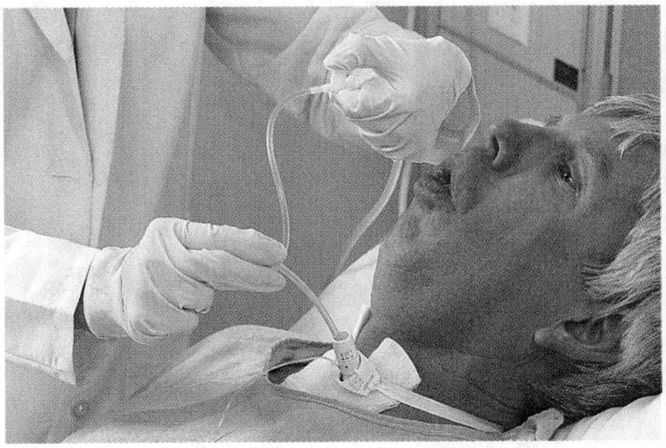

Step 12 • *Apply suction as you withdraw the catheter.*

your dominant hand as you withdraw the catheter. This should take 5 to 10 seconds.
Rationale: Rotation of catheter prevents trauma to mucous membrane from prolonged suctioning of one area. Limiting the suction time to 10 seconds or less prevents hypoxia.

13. Hyperoxygenate and hyperinflate using manual resuscitation bag for a full minute between subsequent suction passes. Encourage deep breathing.

(continued)

Rationale: Prolonged suctioning can induce hypoxia.

14. Rinse catheter thoroughly with saline.
    Rationale: Rinsing clears secretions from catheter.
15. Repeat Steps 10 to 14 until airway is clear.
16. Without applying suction, insert the catheter gently along one side of the mouth. Advance to the oropharynx.
    Rationale: Oropharynx is suctioned after trachea because the mouth is not as clean as the trachea. Directing the catheter along the side of the mouth prevents stimulation of the gag reflex.
17. Apply suction for 5 to 10 seconds as you rotate and withdraw catheter.
    Rationale: Rotation of the catheter prevents trauma to the mucous membrane.
    Note: Be sure to remove secretions that pool beneath the tongue and in the vestibule of the mouth.
18. Allow 1 to 2 minutes between passes for the client to ventilate. Encourage deep breathing. Replace oxygen if applicable.
19. Repeat Steps 16 and 17 as necessary to clear oropharynx.
20. Rinse catheter and tubing by suctioning saline through.
21. Remove gloves by holding catheter with dominant hand and pulling glove off inside-out. Catheter will remain coiled inside the glove. Pull other glove off inside-out. Dispose of in trash receptacle.
    Rationale: Client secretions are contained inside gloves to reduce transmission of microorganisms.

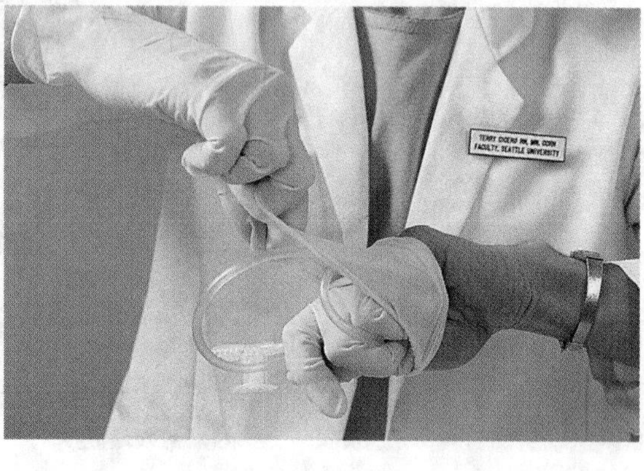

***Step 21** • Remove glove, pulling it over catheter in other hand.*

22. Turn off suction device.
23. Assist client to comfortable position. Offer assistance with oral and nasal hygiene. Replace oxygen device if used.
    Rationale: Accumulated respiratory secretions irritate the mucous membranes and are unpleasant for the client.
24. Dispose of disposable supplies.
25. Wash your hands.
26. Ensure that sterile suction kit is available at head of bed.
    Rationale: Provides immediate access to suction equipment when needed.
27. Document procedure and observations.

Lifespan Considerations

Infants and Children

- Infants and young children have airways that are easily occluded by a small amount of secretions. The nasal airway is smaller in diameter, the epiglottis is higher, and the tongue is proportionately larger.
- A bulb syringe is often used to aspirate secretions from an infant's nasal and oral cavities. This is a clean rather than a sterile procedure because the trachea is not entered.

Home-Care Modifications

- Clients may need to be taught to suction their secretions if they have difficulty coughing them up. Maintaining adequate hydration thins secretions and facilitates their removal.
- The type and number of microorganisms available to contaminate the respiratory system are different at home than in the acute care setting. The client or caregiver may be taught to use plain paper cups for suctioning, not a sterile basin. The cups should be kept in a sealable package. A clean cup is removed from the bottom of the package for each suctioning effort. The package should be resealed between uses.
- Suction catheters can be clean, not sterile. They should be washed in soapy water, rinsed well, and soaked in a vinegar-and-water solution.
- To decrease expenses, saline solution can be made by boiling water and adding salt.

for infants. For these choking victims, chest thrusts should be used instead.

Dyspnea Management

Causes of Dyspnea. Most dyspnea is caused by exertion. The range of activity required to precipitate dyspnea varies widely from one person to another. Some clients with lung disease live relatively unrestricted lifestyles and experience dyspnea infrequently. For others, dyspnea is almost constant, brought on by the simplest activities of daily living.

Anxiety and emotional distress are also common causes of dyspnea. Regardless of its initial source, anx-

Procedure 34-7
Managing an Obstructed Airway (Heimlich Maneuver)

Purpose

Remove a foreign body from obstructing the airway to prevent anoxia and cardiopulmonary arrest.

Assessment

- Identify disorders that put clients at greater risk for airway obstruction:
  - Cerebral vascular accident with hemiparesis
  - Neuromuscular disorders
  - Seizure disorders
  - Tumors of neck or esophagus
  - Decreased level of consciousness
  - Heavy narcotic or sedative use
  - Alcohol intoxication
  - Diminished or absent cough and gag reflex
- Assess clients for signs and symptoms of airway obstruction.
  - Symptoms *not needing* immediate intervention:
    - Ability to speak
    - Ability to breathe in and out
    - Ability to cough
    - Stable vital signs
    - *Note:* Stay with the client and allow him or her to cough to clear airway.
  - Symptoms *needing* immediate intervention:
    - Universal distress signal for complete airway obstruction
    - Irregular, slow, shallow breathing
    - Apnea
    - High-pitched wheezing
    - Inability to cough forcibly or at all
    - Inability to speak
    - Vomitus in mouth or on face
    - Loose, free-floating dentures
    - Cyanosis
    - Abnormal pulse (irregular, rapid, or slow)
- Determines which variation of the Heimlich maneuver (chest thrusts, finger sweep) to use.

Equipment

No equipment is mandatory; suction equipment and emergency cart are useful if in hospital setting.

Procedure

Conscious Adult (Heimlich Maneuver)

1. The client will be standing or sitting.
2. Stand behind the client.
3. Wrap your arms around client's waist.
4. Make a fist with one hand. Place thumb side of fist against client's abdomen, above the navel but below the xiphoid process.

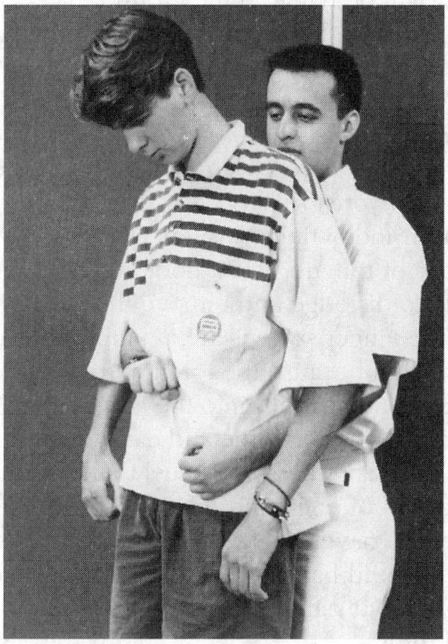

Step 4* • *Place thumb side of fist against client's abdomen below xiphoid process.

5. Grasp fist with other hand.

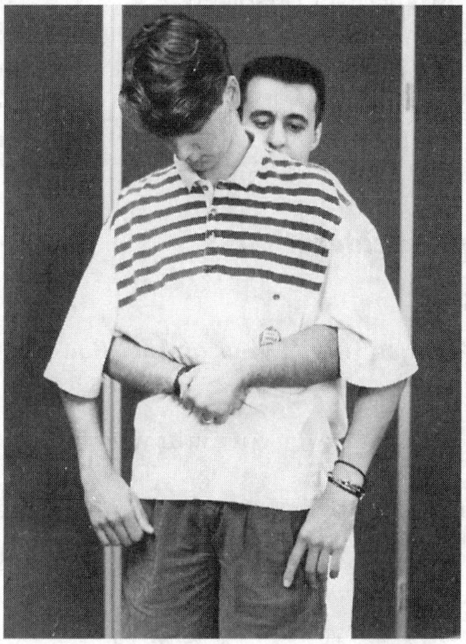

Step 5* • *Grasp fist with other hand and press with quick upward thrust.

6. Press fist into abdomen with a quick upward thrust. *Rationale: A quick upward thrust increases intratho-*

(continued)

racic pressure and creates an artificial cough, which forces air and foreign objects out of the airway.

7. Repeat distinct separate thrusts until foreign body is expelled or client becomes unconscious.

Procedure

Unconscious Client (Heimlich Maneuver, Abdominal Thrust)

1. Client will be lying on the ground.
2. Turn client on back and call for help.
3. Finger sweep.
   a. Use tongue–jaw lift to open mouth.
   Rationale: Tongue–jaw lift draws tongue way from back of throat to relieve obstruction or visualize foreign body.
   b. Insert index finger inside cheek and sweep to base of tongue. Use a hooking motion if possible to dislodge and remove the foreign body.
   Note: Finger sweeps are avoided in infants and children because the foreign body can easily be pushed further into the airway. Remove only if clearly visible and easily reached.
4. Straddle client's thighs or kneel to the side of thighs.
5. Place heel of one hand on epigastric area, midline above the navel but below the xiphoid process.
6. Place second hand on top of first hand.
7. Press heel of hand into abdomen with a quick upward thrust.
   Rationale: A quick upward thrust increases intrathoracic pressure and creates an artificial cough to force air and foreign body out of airway.
   Note: Be careful to thrust in the midline to prevent injury to the liver or spleen.
8. Repeat abdominal thrusts 6 to 10 times.
9. If airway is still obstructed, attempt to ventilate using mouth-to-mouth respiration and head tilt–chin lift.
10. Repeat Steps 5 to 8 until successful.

Lifespan Considerations

Procedure

Infants Younger Than 1 Year of Age (Back Blows and Chest Thrusts)

1. Straddle infant over your arm with head lower than trunk.
2. Support head by holding jaw firmly in your hand.
3. Rest your forearm on your thigh and deliver four back blows with the heel of your hand between the infant's scapula.
4. Place free hand on infant's back and support neck while turning to supine position.
5. Place two fingers over sternum in same location as for external chest compression (one fingerwidth below nipple line).
6. Administer four chest thrusts.
7. Repeat Steps 1 to 6 until airway is not obstructed.

Procedure

Children Older Than 1 Year of Age

1. Perform Heimlich maneuver with child standing, sitting, or lying as for adult, but more gently.
2. Rescuer may need to kneel behind child or have child stand on a table.
3. Prevent foreign body airway obstruction in infants and children by teaching parents or caregivers to:
   a. Restrict children from walking, running, or playing with food or foreign objects in their mouths.
   b. Keep small objects (ie, marbles, beads, beans, thumb tacks) away from children younger than 3 years of age.
   c. Avoid feeding popcorn and peanuts to children younger than 3 years of age, and cut other foods into small pieces.
4. Parents and caregivers should be instructed in the management of foreign body airway obstruction.

Procedure

Pregnant Women or Very Obese Adults (Chest Thrusts)

1. Stand behind client.
2. Bring your arms under client's armpits and around chest.
3. Make a fist and place thumb side against *middle* of sternum.
4. Grasp fist with other hand and deliver a quick backward thrust.
5. Repeat thrusts until airway is cleared.
6. Chest thrusts may be performed with client supine and hands positioned with heel over lower half of sternum (as for cardiac compression). Administer separate downward thrusts until airway is clear.

iety that causes dyspnea is in turn made worse by dyspnea. This creates a vicious cycle.

Finally, dyspnea not caused by exertion or anxiety may be the result of organic problems. Infection, pulmonary embolism, bronchospasm, or changes in the client's underlying condition may all trigger difficulty breathing.

Assisting the Dyspneic Client. Effective treatment of dyspnea addresses both its physical and psychological components. Common interventions used to manage dyspnea include anxiety control, activity modification, and comfort measures that modify the client's breathing pattern.

Regardless of its specific cause, dyspnea can be extremely frightening, both for the client who is experiencing it and for the nurse who must treat it. To help the client, the nurse must remain calm while offering reassurance. Speaking calmly, slowly, and offering one simple direction at a time help minimize the client's anxiety. Listening empathetically and helping the client relax are sometimes all that is needed to relieve their dyspnea. When uncontrolled anxiety is the primary cause of a client's dyspnea, the physician may prescribe mild antianxiety medication.

Comfort measures include the use of positioning. Usually the client is most comfortable sitting upright because this allows the diaphragm to move freely. If oxygen is ordered, the nurse should see that it is operating as prescribed. The nurse should also focus the client's efforts on slowing the breathing rate. The client should breathe through the nose if possible, using the diaphragm for inspiration. The nurse can assist in this by gently pushing down on the client's shoulders, which discourages the inefficient use of accessory muscles. Usually, with gentle encouragement and reassurance, the breathing rate will gradually decrease and the dyspnea will pass. Whenever dyspnea occurs, the nurse must try to establish its immediate cause and its severity. Comfort measures are always appropriate, as is oxygen when a standing order is available. Many institutions have policies allowing nurses to begin oxygen therapy for the dyspneic client while a physician's order is being sought. When oxygen and comfort measures do not decrease dyspnea within a short period of time, or when dyspnea appears suddenly and without warning, the physician should be notified.

Pursed-Lip Breathing. Pursed-lip breathing helps clients with obstructive lung diseases such as COPD or asthma release trapped air from hyperinflated lungs.

To perform pursed-lip breathing, the client takes a deep breath and holds it for a moment, then exhales slowly through lips that are held almost closed. By pushing the air against the small orifice made by the pursed lips, pressure builds backward through the airways. This back-pressure effect prevents airway collapse by pushing them open throughout exhalation. This allows more air to escape during exhalation and helps prevent air trapping.

Hyperventilation Management

The client who hyperventilates exhibits rapid breathing and symptoms such as dizziness and tingling sensations; arterial blood gases indicate a $PaCO_2$ below 35 mm Hg. The client may or may not experience subjective feelings of dyspnea. Nursing efforts should be directed at decreasing client anxiety and getting the client to breathe at a slower rate.

If simple encouragement cannot accomplish this, a paper bag may be used as a rebreathing device. The client breathes in and out of the bag for several breaths. By rebreathing the exhaled carbon dioxide from the bag, the client's $PaCO_2$ can gradually return to normal. This will naturally slow the rate of breathing, and the dizziness and tingling sensations should disappear. As with dyspnea, a complete assessment of hyperventilation is needed, and referral to the physician may be required.

Hypoventilation Management

Hypoventilation occurs when a client's breathing cannot meet metabolic requirements. It is identified definitively by blood gases that show a $PaCO_2$ far above the client's normal range. The hypoventilating client is often groggy and breathing slowly. This may be caused by pharmacologic depression of the respiratory centers of the brain or by severe lung disease.

If the client is heavily sedated or has received a large dose of anesthesia or pain medication, the nurse must encourage him or her to breathe more deeply. The client must be watched closely and told to take deep breaths frequently. Gradually the effect of the medication will diminish, and breathing will return to normal. Until it does, the nurse must observe the client closely and continually encourage breathing.

Airway obstruction caused by severe lung disease can also lead to hypoventilation. For such clients the nurse must assess the need for secretion removal and bronchodilators. By actively helping the client to cough, or by suctioning the airways or administering a bronchodilator, the nurse can help the client open the airways. This will allow for greater breathing efficiency and better gas exchange. Positive pressure breathing with BiPAP or IPPB will also help the client breathe more deeply and decrease $PaCO_2$.

If hypoventilation cannot be reversed by these measures, more aggressive therapy (such as intubation and mechanical ventilation) may be needed. Because all cases of hypoventilation are serious, the physician should always be notified.

Community-Based Nursing

Most respiratory clients are managed in the community, except for periods of acute respiratory dysfunction or exacerbation of a chronic respiratory condition. Home respiratory therapy can include hand-held aerosol treatments, chest physiotherapy, oxygen, or ventilator care. How much and what kind of home therapy the client receives depends on many factors, including the client's

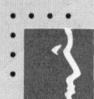

Client Teaching
Respiratory Function

Instruct the client as follows:

- *Learn to breathe correctly. Using the diaphragm helps the client with chronic lung disease to increase breathing efficiency. Breathe with your abdomen: push out with inspiration, and exhale by pulling your abdomen in.*
- *Use pursed-lip breathing to exhale more fully. To do this, almost close your lips, forming a small circle, and exhale slowly against the lips, as if you are whistling.*
- *If you are taking prescribed medications for your breathing, do not use over-the-counter medications without your healthcare provider's advice. Undesirable interactions can occur.*
- *Use bronchodilators according to the prescribed schedule. Exceeding the prescribed dose can cause serious side effects, such as heart irregularities and seizures.*
- *To help keep secretions thin and easy to cough up, drink at least six glasses of water each day (unless contraindicated).*
- *Notify your healthcare provider if your breathing becomes more difficult, your sputum increases in amount or changes color, or you have an elevated temperature. These signs may indicate respiratory infection.*
- *When using oxygen at home, instruct friends and family members not to smoke. Keep oxygen away from open flames and space heaters.*

age, ability to learn procedures, family support, degree of impairment, and motivation. The nurse is often the one to assess these characteristics for the purpose of making recommendations to the physician. Often, the nurse is also responsible for making home-care arrangements and for much of the teaching involved.

Infection Control

Pieces of equipment normally considered disposable after 2 or 3 days in the hospital, such as cannulas or small-volume nebulizers, are likely to be used for much longer in the home. Hospital procedures performed under sterile conditions, such as tracheostomy care and suctioning, may be done using clean technique at home. Because these differences in procedure can foster germ growth, one of the most important aspects of home nursing care of the respiratory client is infection control. Although cost considerations and limited facilities make sterilization difficult, infection control at home can be practically as effective as it is in the hospital.

The nurse must ensure that the client clearly understands the importance of infection control, because potentially lethal pneumonia may result from respiratory infection. The client must be taught effective cleaning of all equipment. To assess compliance, the nurse should secure an order for periodic culturing of equipment. The client should also have yearly influenza vaccinations and should avoid crowds during flu season. The client with COPD should be encouraged to discuss pneumonia immunization with the physician.

The client must learn the signs of impending respiratory infection. Increased sputum production, change of sputum color to yellow or green, fever, and increasing difficulty in raising sputum often signal the onset of infection. If the client has a standing order for antibiotics, it is appropriate to begin taking the medication when these signs appear. If relief is not obtained within a day or two, the physician should be contacted. Appreciable amounts of blood in the sputum, a severe increase in shortness of breath, or any other severe symptoms should be referred immediately to the physician.

Medications

Home use of respiratory medications can be simplified by prepackaged unit-dose medications, but these are more expensive than stock bottles of medications. If the client can learn to measure dosages, stock bottles may be more cost-effective. The client should be taught to recognize side effects of medications and to understand why they are dangerous. The dangers of taking medications more frequently than ordered should also be stressed. If the medications provide no relief, the client should be taught to call the physician.

Home Oxygen Systems

The respiratory equipment used by clients at home also differs from hospital equipment. At home the client can receive oxygen from high-pressure cylinders, liquid gas systems, or electrically powered concentrators. Compressed oxygen from high-pressure tanks is best for the client who only occasionally requires supplemental oxygen. Liquid oxygen systems allow the client to leave home. Portable "walkers" can be filled from a stationary unit at home. The walkers are small enough to be carried or wheeled in a small cart, yet they hold up to several hours' worth of oxygen (Fig. 34-10). A concentrator is a device that chemically separates oxygen from room air. It is an excellent choice for the client who requires continuous oxygen in low concentrations.

Home ventilators are also quite different from those found in the intensive care unit. Choices range from wrap-around pulmonary-aid belts, which assist clients whose breathing is weak, to negative-pressure chest shells and positive-pressure portable ventilators that provide full ventilatory support.

The companies that rent these items or supply the oxygen should be well established and reliable. They

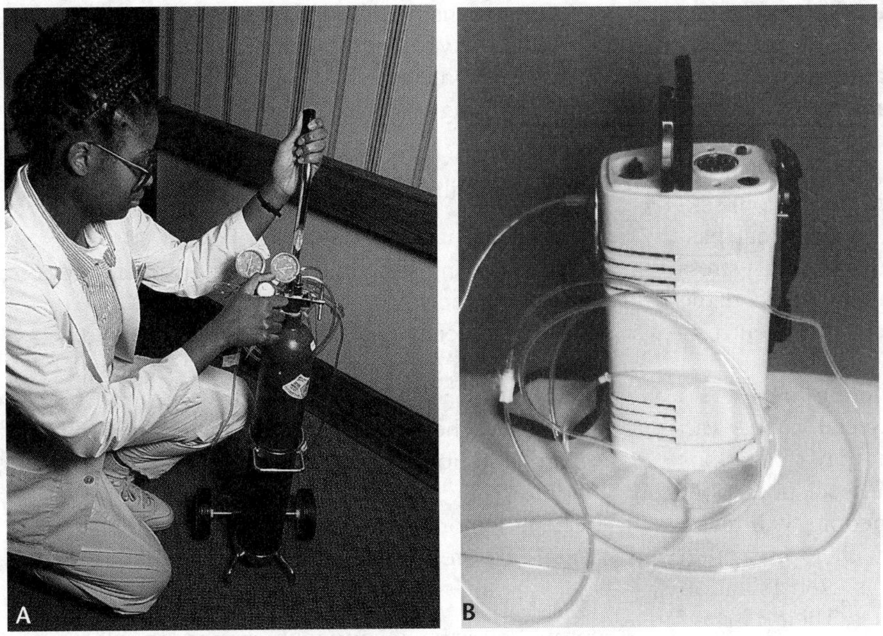

Figure 34-10 • *Portable oxygen. **(A)** E cylinder used as back up emergency oxygen supply or for short period of ambulation. **(B)** Portable oxygen walker—fill with liquid oxygen for longer period of ambulation.*

should be able to provide service 24 hours every day. The client should have the telephone numbers of the suppliers and must be able to get service whenever necessary. Reputable suppliers often hire respiratory therapists to visit the client routinely at home and to assess respiratory status and equipment function. Coordination between these services and community health nursing services should be arranged.

Energy Conservation

Activities of daily living can be seriously affected by respiratory dysfunction, but with slight modifications they can be performed by most clients. Energy conservation and the motivation to be independent are keys to success.

The nurse should base suggestions for modifying activities of daily living on a thorough assessment of the extent to which each activity has been affected by respiratory dysfunction. For instance:

If meal preparation is a problem, the nurse may be able to provide a referral to a "Meals on Wheels" program.

Sponge baths may be a practical alternative to tub bathing if mobility is impaired.

An elevated toilet seat may help decrease the work needed to rise from the toilet.

It is neither practical nor desirable for the client to avoid activity, but modifications may be necessary to prevent activity from causing dyspnea. This may mean the client may require assistance either in performing activities or in approaching them more efficiently. The nurse can help the client establish an activity schedule that allows for more time than the healthy person would require. Energy-saving measures such as sitting while performing basic tasks helps to eliminate one source of breathlessness. Unsupported arm activities, such as combing hair or reaching for items on an upper shelf, increase dyspnea and may need to be modified (Breslin, 1992). Activities may be spaced between rest periods to prevent overexertion.

Clients must take care not to exceed their physical abilities, but they should be encouraged to work gradually toward increasing exercise tolerance. Helping the client to set realistic goals is of utmost importance. Conversely, goals should provide enough challenge to allow the client to feel the endeavor is worthwhile. The nurse must recognize the value of small accomplishments and offer praise and encouragement because progress at building endurance is often slow.

Fostering Self-Esteem

Like most of us, the person with lung disease wants to be an independent, contributing member of society, feeling self-reliant and not burdensome to others. The ability to get around independently and to do meaningful work can help foster these feelings. These activities are also essential to avoid the debilitating effects of depression.

Work is often a source of satisfaction and self-esteem. The diagnosis of pulmonary disease does not mean the person is automatically unable to work. If the client derives satisfaction from a job, it is important for him or her to continue working as long as possible. Frequent illness can make it difficult for the severely dyspneic client to hold a demanding job. Although it is not always feasible for the client's employer to offer schedule flexibility, this option should be explored.

Respiratory disease can severely inhibit both sexual desire and sexual performance. Chronic fatigue, shortness of breath, and embarrassment caused by excessive mucus or dyspnea are often reasons the client with respiratory problems loses sexual function. Sexual difficulties may be common among respiratory clients, but they can be surmounted. Prescribed bronchodilators should be used before beginning sexual relations. This will help the client avoid dyspnea throughout sexual activity. The nurse can inform the client that passive positions save energy. Finally, the nurse must stress the importance of open communication between the client and his or her partner, and help the client recognize that adjustments will be necessary.

The nurse can help further by offering suggestions for activities outside of the home. Social outlets can help the client to cope with the day-to-day frustrations of lung disease. The American Lung Association sponsors classes and support groups for people with respiratory disease. Nurses, physicians, or therapists often are guest speakers at such gatherings. Rehabilitation programs offer more structured activities. Their purpose is to increase the client's ability to function with lung disease. Such programs may provide breathing retraining, exercise, and diet and occupational counseling.

Evaluation

The nurse works with the client to develop goals. Outcome criteria are specific observable indicators that can measure goal attainment. For each general goal, outcome criteria are suggested, but it is important to individualize outcome criteria depending on the client's current breathing status.

Goal

Client will demonstrate knowledge regarding prevention of respiratory dysfunction.

Possible Outcome Criteria

- After teaching session, client demonstrates deep-breathing and coughing techniques.
- After teaching session, client discusses the physiologic effects of smoking.
- Client joins and regularly attends meetings of a stop-smoking program for 6 months.

Goal

Client will demonstrate knowledge regarding optimal management of respiratory dysfunction.

Possible Outcome Criteria

- After teaching session, client lists signs of respiratory infection and knows when to call the physician.
- After teaching session, for any medication administered for respiratory problems, client describes the name of the drug, dose to be taken, action of the medication, side effects of the medication, and any special considerations for administration.
- Before discharge, client demonstrates the safe use of home oxygen equipment.
- After teaching session, client demonstrates pursed-lip breathing.

Goal

Client will mobilize pulmonary secretions.

Possible Outcome Criteria

- After teaching session, client demonstrates proper coughing technique.
- Client drinks at least six glasses of water a day, as indicated in daily log.
- Caregiver or parent demonstrates proper techniques of chest physiotherapy, including percussion, vibration, and postural drainage, by the next home visit.
- Client demonstrates correct self-suctioning technique before discharge.

Goal

Client will effectively cope with changes in self-concept and lifestyle.

Possible Outcome Criteria

- Within 6 months of diagnosis, client verbalizes how the respiratory condition has caused changes in lifestyle.
- Within a week of diagnosis, client identifies support people to provide emotional strength.
- By end of teaching session, client lists community agencies and services that he or she plans to use.
- Before discharge, client demonstrates oxygen-conserving measures such as sitting while dressing and planning rest periods.
- Before discharge, client verbalizes sexual positions requiring less oxygen expenditure.

Key Concepts

- The primary functions of breathing are the delivery of oxygen to the blood, the removal of carbon dioxide from the blood, and maintenance of acid-base balance.
- Breathing is normally almost effortless, but the work required for breathing increases tremendously when the airways are obstructed by inflammation, bronchospasm, or excessive mucous secretions.
- Deep breathing and coughing are two of the most important measures for preventing pulmonary complications, such as atelectasis and pneumonia.
- Adequate hydration is essential to keep respiratory secretions moist and easily coughed up from the respiratory tract.

Nursing Plan of Care
The Client With Ineffective Airway Clearance

Nursing Diagnosis

Ineffective Airway Clearance related to tracheobronchial infection, as manifested by weak cough, adventitious breath sounds, and copious green sputum production.

Client Goal

Client will mobilize pulmonary secretions.

Client Outcome Criteria

- After teaching session, client demonstrates proper coughing techniques.
- Client drinks at least six glasses of water per day while in hospital.
- Client demonstrates correct self-suctioning technique before discharge.

Nursing Intervention	*Scientific Rationale*
1. Provide and teach the client the importance of adequate hydration. Encourage fluids (2,000–3,000 mL per 24 hours). Monitor intake and output. Avoid milk and milk products. Ultrasonic nebulizer treatment.	1. Adequate hydration thins secretions, which prevents mucus from plugging airways. Evaluate hydration status of client. Milk products tend to thicken secretions. Moisten and aid mobility of respiratory secretions.
2. Position and encourage to cough to promote mobilization of secretions. Deep breathing every 2 hours. Huff coughing. Assume sitting position if possible.	2. Open alveoli and prevent further atelectasis. Prevent airway collapse. Permit deep inspiration and forceful abdominal contractions necessary for coughing.
3. Administer analgesic before cough session if pain limits coughing effectiveness.	3. If client fears pain, he or she hesitates to breathe deeply and cough effectively.
4. Provide or teach client tracheal suctioning if he or she is unable to remove secretions with effective coughing. Hyperoxygenate with 100% O_2 before and after suctioning procedure. Suction for no longer than 15 seconds per suctioning attempt. Provide opportunities for client to practice and demonstrate suctioning technique if self-suctioning is necessary.	4. A weak, nonproductive cough causes secretions to be retained in airways and interfere with gas exchange. Hypoxemia, which can occur during the suctioning procedure, is prevented. Longer periods of suction can contribute to tissue trauma and hypoxemia. Suctioning is a complex motor skill that requires practice for skill acquisition and comfort.
5. Provide or teach postural chest physiotherapy as ordered. Have client or family members demonstrate when comfortable with skill mastery.	5. Secretions drain from major airways using the force of gravity.

- Clients with COPD must not receive too much oxygen because it can cause hypoventilation. They normally require only 2 to 3 liters per minute through a nasal cannula, or 28% through a Venturi mask.
- Smoking is the single most important factor affecting pulmonary health.
- Common manifestations of respiratory dysfunction are cough, dyspnea, chest pain, and sputum production.
- Major nursing interventions for the respiratory client are measures to promote airway patency, improve the distribution of air in the lungs, and promote oxygenation.

- Airway maintenance interventions include hydration, aerosol therapy, positioning, coughing, chest physiotherapy, suctioning, and management of artificial airways.
- Hyperinflation techniques, such as deep breathing, incentive spirometry, and intermittent positive pressure breathing or BiPAP, help prevent atelectasis and promote a strong cough.
- Oxygen therapy raises the amount of oxygen in the lungs, thereby making more oxygen available to the blood and tissues.
- Dyspnea, excessive mucous secretions, dried secretions, hyperventilation, and hypoventilation are common nursing problems of the respiratory client.
- Home care must be individualized for the respiratory client. Ability to perform activities of daily living and manage home procedures must be considered carefully before discharge.

Critical Thinking Challenges

Gas exchange, respiratory function, and nursing care related to oxygenation are now part of your knowledge base. You should be able to see how this chapter relates to issues of safety, home management, and self-care. Now turn back to the situation at the beginning of this chapter, and think about how you can effectively represent your fellow nurses on the committee. The following will guide your thinking.

1. *Identify the nurses' concerns about the clients and about themselves that may contribute to feelings of anxiety.*
2. *Compare and contrast special needs of these ventilator-dependent clients with those of the average geriatric client.*
3. *Describe how nursing personnel may collaborate with respiratory care personnel to optimize care for these clients.*
4. *Identify and plan strategies that may make the nursing staff feel more comfortable caring for the new clients.*

References

Ackerman, M. H. (1993). The effect of saline lavage prior to suctioning. *Am J Crit Care, 2,* 326–330.

American Heart Association (AHA). (1993). *Basic life support heart saver guide: A student handbook for cardiopulmonary resuscitation and first aid for choking.* Dallas, TX: Author.

Barnes, T. A. (1994) *Core textbook of respiratory care practice.* (2nd ed.) St. Louis: C. V. Mosby.

Breslin, E. H. (1992). Dyspnea-limited response in chronic obstructive pulmonary disease: Reduced unsupported arm activities. *Rehabilitation Nursing, 17* (1), 12–20.

Bolecheck, G., & McCloskey, J. A. (1992). *Nursing interventions essential nursing treatments* (2nd ed.). Philadelphia: W. B. Saunders.

Burton, G., Hodgkin, J., & Ward, J. (1991). *Respiratory care* (3rd ed.). Philadelphia: J. B. Lippincott.

Carpenter, K. (1993). A comprehensive review of cyanosis. *Critical Care Nurse, 13* (4), 66–72.

DesJardins, T. (1993). *Cardiopulmonary anatomy and physiology: Essentials for respiratory care.* (2nd ed.) Albany, NY: Delmar Publishers.

Ehrhardt, B., & Daleiden, J. (1994). Pulse oximeters: Follow these tips to ensure accurate readings. *Nursing94, 24* (8), 32V–32X.

Glass, C., Grap, M. J., Corley, M. C., & Wallace, D. (1993). Nurses' ability to achieve hyperinflation and hyperoxygenation with a manual resuscitation bag during endotracheal suctioning. *Heart Lung, 22,* 158–165.

Jess, L. W. (1992). Chronic bronchitis and emphysema: Airing the differences. *Nursing92, 22* (3), 34–42.

Koff, P. B., Eitzman, D., & Neu, J. (1993). *Neonatal and pediatric respiratory care* (2nd ed.) St. Louis: C. V. Mosby.

Mancinelli-Van Atta, J., & Beck, S. (1992). Preventing hypoxemia and hemodynamic compromise related to endotracheal suctioning. *Am J Crit Care, 1,* 62–79.

North American Nursing Diagnosis Association (NANDA). (1994). *Nursing diagnoses: Definitions and classification 1995-1996.* Philadelphia: Author.

Pierson, D., & Kacmarek, R. (1992). *Foundations of respiratory care.* New York: Churchill-Livingstone.

Scanlan, C. L., Spearman, C. B., & Sheldon, R. L., (1995). *Egan's fundamentals of respiratory care* (6th ed.) St. Louis: C. V. Mosby.

Shapiro, B., Harrison, R., Kacmarek, R., & Cane, R. (1995). *Clinical application of respiratory care* (5th ed.). Chicago: Year Book Medical Publishers.

Shapiro, B., Peruzzi, W. T., & Templin, R. (1994). *Clinical application of blood gases* (5th ed.) St. Louis: Mosby YearBook.

Sinski, A., & Corbo, J. (1994). Surfactant replacement in adults and children with ARDS: An effective therapy? *Critical Care Nurse, 14* (6), 54–59.

Weilitz, P., & Dettenmeier, P. (1994). Test your knowledge of tracheostomy tubes. *Am J Nurs, 94* (2), 46–50.

Wilkins, R. L., Sheldon, R. L., & Krider, S. J. (1990). *Clinical assessment in respiratory care* (2nd ed.). St. Louis: C. V. Mosby.

Yeaw, E. M. (1992). How position affects oxygenation: Good lung down? *Am J Nurs, 92* (3), 26–29.

Bibliography

Ahrens, T. (1993). Changing perspectives in the assessment of oxygenation. *Critical Care Nurse, 13* (4), 78–83.

Boutotte, J. (1993). T.B.: The second time around. *Nursing93, 23* (5), 42–49.

Boutotte, J. (1994). What to do if you've been exposed to TB. *Nursing94, 24* (6), 26.

Carroll, P. (1992). Nursing the thoracotomy patient. *RN, 55* (6), 34–42.

Dantzker, J., MacIntyre, N., & Bakow, E. (1994). *Comprehensive respiratory care.* Philadelphia: W. B. Saunders.

Davies, B. L., MacLeod, J. P., & Ogilvie, H. M. (1990). The efficacy of incentive spirometers in post-operative protocols for low-risk patients. *Canadian Journal of Nursing Research, 22*(4), 19–36.

Della Bella, L. A. (1992). Steroidphobia and the pulmonary patient. *Am J Nurs, 92* (2), 26–29.

Fiorentini, A. (1992). Potential hazards of tracheobronchial suctioning. *Intensive and Critical Care Nursing, 8,* 217–226.

Gift, A. G. (1991). Psychologic and physiologic aspects of acute dyspnea in asthmatics. *Nurs Res, 40* (4), 196–199.

Grossbach, I. (1993). Case studies in pulse oximetry monitoring. *Critical Care Nurse, 13* (4), 63–65.

Handerhan, B. (1991). Recognizing pulmonary embolism. *Nursing91, 21* (2), 107–110.

Hill, M., Harrell, J., & McCormick, L. (1992). Predictors of smokeless tobacco use by adolescents. *Res Nurs Health, 15,* 359–368.

Leffert, C. C., & Luecke, L. (1993). Assessing and treating pulmonary edema. *Nursing93, 23* (7), 54.

Litwack, K., Saleh, D., & Schultz, P. (1991). Postoperative pulmonary complications. *Critical Care Nursing Clinics of North America, 3,* 77–82.

McIntosh, D., Baun, M., & Rogge, J. (1993). Effects of lung hyperinflation and presence of positive end-expiratory pressure on arterial and tissue oxygenation during endotracheal suctioning. *Am J Crit Care, 2,* 317–325.

Miller, P., (1992). Using pulse oximetry to make clinical nursing decisions. *Orthopedic Nursing, 11* (4), 39–42.

Narsavage, G. L., & Weaver, T. E. (1994). Physiologic status, coping, and hardiness as predictors of outcomes in chronic obstructive pulmonary disease. *Nurs Res, 43* (2), 90–94.

Pfister, S. (1993). Management of a transtracheal oxygen catheter in a mechanically ventilated patient. *Critical Care Nurse, 13* (4), 52–58.

Tampinco-Golos, I. C. (1993). Thoracotomy. *Nursing93, 23* (8), 63–64.

Tasota, F. J., & Wesmiller, S. W. (1994). Understanding A.B.G.s. *Nursing94, 24* (5), 34–45.

West, A. L., (1992). The patient with bronchospasm: Assessment, triage, and teaching adjuncts. *Journal of Emergency Nursing, 18,* 511–517.

White, K. (1993). Using continuous SvO2 to assess oxygen supply/demand balance in the critically ill patient. *AACN Clinical Issues in Critical Care Nursing, 4* (1), 134–147.

Oxygenation: Cardiac Function and Tissue Perfusion

Key Terms

Angina
Aneurysm
Arrhythmia
Arteriosclerosis
Contractility
Diastole
Infarction
Ischemia
Myocardium
Perfusion
Sequential compression devices
Stenosis
Systole
Thrombus
Transient ischemic attack

Learning Objectives

Upon completion of this chapter, the student will be able to do the following:

- *Discuss factors that contribute to normal cardiac output and tissue perfusion.*
- *Describe the consequences of altered cardiovascular function and their causes.*
- *Understand how altered cardiovascular function can impact normal activities.*
- *Discuss cardiovascular changes that occur during the lifespan.*
- *Perform a basic nursing assessment of cardiovascular function.*
- *Identify common procedures and diagnostic tests used in the evaluation of the cardiovascular client.*
- *State relevant nursing diagnoses for the client with cardiovascular dysfunction.*
- *Discuss several nursing measures directed at promoting and restoring cardiovascular function.*

35

A 59-year-old trial lawyer comes in for his yearly physical, accompanied by his wife. His history reveals a positive family history for cardiac disease, and his father died at age 60 of a massive myocardial infarction (MI). He has been under stress lately at work (a very important trial) and at home (his 24-year-old daughter has returned home with two young children after a recent divorce). He used to play golf twice a week but recently has not had time. Physical examination reveals BP of 178/94, pulse 94, and respirations 14. When you tell your client his vital signs, he states, "Now don't you start yelling at me about my blood pressure. I'm as healthy as they come, and I am not about to go on any crazy vegetarian diet."

In previous chapters, you studied about health maintenance and client teaching. These chapters relate to your care of this client during his physical. This chapter adds information about cardiovascular function to your knowledge base. It helps you understand risk factors for this client. When you have completed the chapter, you will be better able to reply to this man and plan for his care by studying the Critical Thinking Challenges at the end of the chapter.

Throughout a person's life, the heart and blood vessels work together as the main components of the cardiovascular system. The primary function of this system is to transport oxygen and nutrients to the tissues and to deliver the end-products of tissue metabolism to appropriate organs for their excretion.

The proper function of every organ and tissue depends on the efficiency and effectiveness of the cardiovascular system. A healthy heart is essential to provide an adequate flow of blood into the blood vessels. The blood vessels distribute the blood and precisely regulate the amount of blood available to every tissue of the body. The fact that this takes place 24 hours a day for 70 or more years attests to the remarkable durability of this system.

This chapter focuses on the vital role played by the cardiovascular system in the maintenance of overall health. Dynamics of normal circulation are discussed, and the role of the nurse in supporting cardiovascular health is examined.

Normal Cardiovascular Function

Structure of the Cardiovascular System

The Heart

The heart is a hollow, muscular organ that acts as a powerful pump. Its job is to circulate blood throughout the body. Because blood contains the nutrients and oxygen that are essential for life, the heart is responsible for providing all tissues with a constant supply of fresh, life-sustaining nutrition.

Heart Tissues. The heart consists of three layers. The innermost layer of the heart, the endocardium, is made of endothelial cells and connective tissue. The thick muscular middle layer is called the **myocardium.** The outer layer of the heart, or epicardium, is a thin-walled sac that surrounds the heart and attaches it to the diaphragm and sternal wall of the thorax.

The bulk of the heart is muscle. Similar to both striated (skeletal) and smooth muscle, cardiac muscle is unique because of its automaticity. The heart is capable of beating without external neural stimuli. Its rhythmicity is created by its own automatic electrical conduction system that generates and conducts electrical impulses.

Heart Structure. The heart is a hollow organ, with dividing walls that form four chambers. It is divided into left and right halves by a strong muscular wall, or septum. These halves are further divided crosswise by a "fibrous skeleton" of connective tissue. The upper chambers are called the atria, and the lower chambers are called the ventricles.

The muscle on the left side of the heart is much thicker than the muscle on the right. The left side of the heart must generate higher pressures than the right to pump blood to all tissues of the body; the right side of the heart serves only the low-resistance pulmonary system of the lungs.

Valves. Valves separate the atria from the ventricles. Attached to rings of connective tissue, the valves are fibrous structures that open and close in response to pressure differences between chambers. Each of these atrioventricular (AV) valves appears as flaps or leaflets that fold together to form a tight seal between chambers. The tricuspid valve separates the right atrium from the right ventricle; the mitral valve separates the left atrium and left ventricle.

Valves also separate the ventricles from the large blood vessels they fill. These valves are called semilunar valves, because of the half-moon shape of their leaflets.

Coronary Circulation. The coronary circulation provides the heart tissue with oxygenated blood. A pair of main coronary arteries, each with multiple branches, delivers fresh blood to all layers of the heart. One artery serves the right side of the heart; the other serves the left.

The Blood Vessels

The heart empties its contents into an interconnected network of arteries, capillaries, and veins. These are collectively called blood vessels. These vessels range in size from microscopic to over an inch in diameter. Arteries convey blood away from the heart; veins carry blood from the tissues back to the heart. They are linked together by smaller vessels called capillaries.

Arteries. Arteries are relatively thick-walled, muscular vessels. This gives them strength and elasticity, which allows them to withstand the high pressure of blood being constantly forced into them by the heart. The smallest arteries, called arterioles, connect to the capillaries and regulate the flow of blood into them.

Capillaries. These near-microscopic vessels run through all the body's tissues. Capillaries in the skin, muscles, and other tissues of the body are narrow channels with few branches; those in the lungs are multichanneled. The thin endothelial walls of all capillaries are permeable, which allows for the exchange of nutrients and waste products between the blood and tissues.

Veins. After blood has passed through capillaries, it drains into the veins. Veins are less muscular than arteries, and therefore more distensible. Because of their distensibility, veins can stretch to accommodate relatively large volumes of blood. At their junction with capillaries, veins are small. These empty into successively larger veins, finally ending in the superior and inferior vena cavae. Together these vessels return deoxygenated blood from the systemic circulation to the right atrium of the heart.

The Cardiovascular System

The heart and blood vessels comprise the cardiovascular system. It is a closed circuit, with all of its many branches beginning and ending at the heart. This system has two major portions: the pulmonary circulation and the systemic circulation. The pulmonary circulation carries blood through the gas exchange portion of the lungs, where carbon dioxide is released, and oxygen is absorbed. The systemic circulation then transports oxygenated blood and nutrients to all body tissues.

Normal Function of the Heart and Blood Vessels

The normal heartbeat is a repetitive cycle of rhythmic contraction and relaxation. With each contraction, during the period called **systole,** blood is ejected from the atria into the ventricles and from the ventricles into the arteries. Between contractions, in the period called **diastole,** the heart muscle relaxes, and its chambers fill with blood. Throughout the cycle, blood continually flows past the body's tissues, exchanging vital nutrients for their wastes.

The cardiac cycle begins with the generation of a small electrical impulse within the heart. This impulse is translated into mechanical activity, which results in muscle contraction and pumping motion.

Heart

The effectiveness of the heart as a pump depends on several factors. Three of the most important factors are its ability to generate and conduct electrical impulses, its ability to fill and empty properly, and the strength with which it can contract.

Impulse Conduction. Whereas contraction and relaxation of most muscles are controlled by the nervous system, the heart has its own inherent, automatic ability to control its activity (Fig. 35-1). Impulses that stimulate contraction normally originate in specialized cells (sinoatrial [SA] node) near the top of the right atrium. In the SA node, small but significant chemical changes regularly occur. Concentrations of ions, such as potassium, sodium, and calcium, inside and surrounding the SA node fluctuate suddenly and rapidly. This rapid ionic fluctuation causes a change in the electric potential of the cells, known as depolarization. This generates a small electrical impulse. Because the SA node establishes impulses that determine the rate at which the heart beats, it is often called the pacemaker of the heart. As this wave of depolarization travels through the heart, it leads to muscle contraction. After the impulse has passed over the cells, their ionic concentrations return to previous levels (repolarization), and the muscle relaxes.

From the SA node, the electrical impulse travels over the surface of the atria. This causes smooth and uniform atrial contraction. When the impulse reaches the lower portion of the atria, it is delayed briefly before it continues into the ventricles. This delay is important because it allows time for the atria to contract fully. Thus, the atria can empty their contents into the ventricles before the lower chambers contract.

Leaving the atria, the impulse is channeled through the AV node, the bundle of His, and into its right and left branches. It finally enters the many Purkinje fibers that extend throughout the ventricular muscle. As the impulse spreads, the ventricular myocardial cells contract. This entire sequence of electrical events takes less than 1 second. It occurs 60 to 100 times during each minute of life.

Blood Flow Through the Heart. The electrical impulse generates an orderly, sequential contraction. The coordinated contraction of all muscle fibers is essential for maximum cardiac pumping power. Proper valve function is another essential element for effective pumping.

The valves act as doorways between the atria and ventricles and between the ventricles and their major arteries. They allow blood to flow in one direction only, maximizing efficiency and preventing the backflow of blood (Fig. 35-2). This unidirectional action of the valves allows the heart chambers to develop high pumping pressures. This is necessary to ensure that blood is ejected with sufficient force to reach the furthest tissues of the body.

Between heartbeats, the heart is at rest. During this time, the atria fill passively, receiving blood from the vena cavae (on the right side of the heart) and the pulmonary veins (on the left). When the atrial muscle cells contract, pressure builds within the atrial chambers. The pressure forces the AV valves to open, and the blood is pushed into the ventricle below each atrium.

As the ventricles fill, the spreading electrical impulse causes a similar mechanical action in the ventricles. The

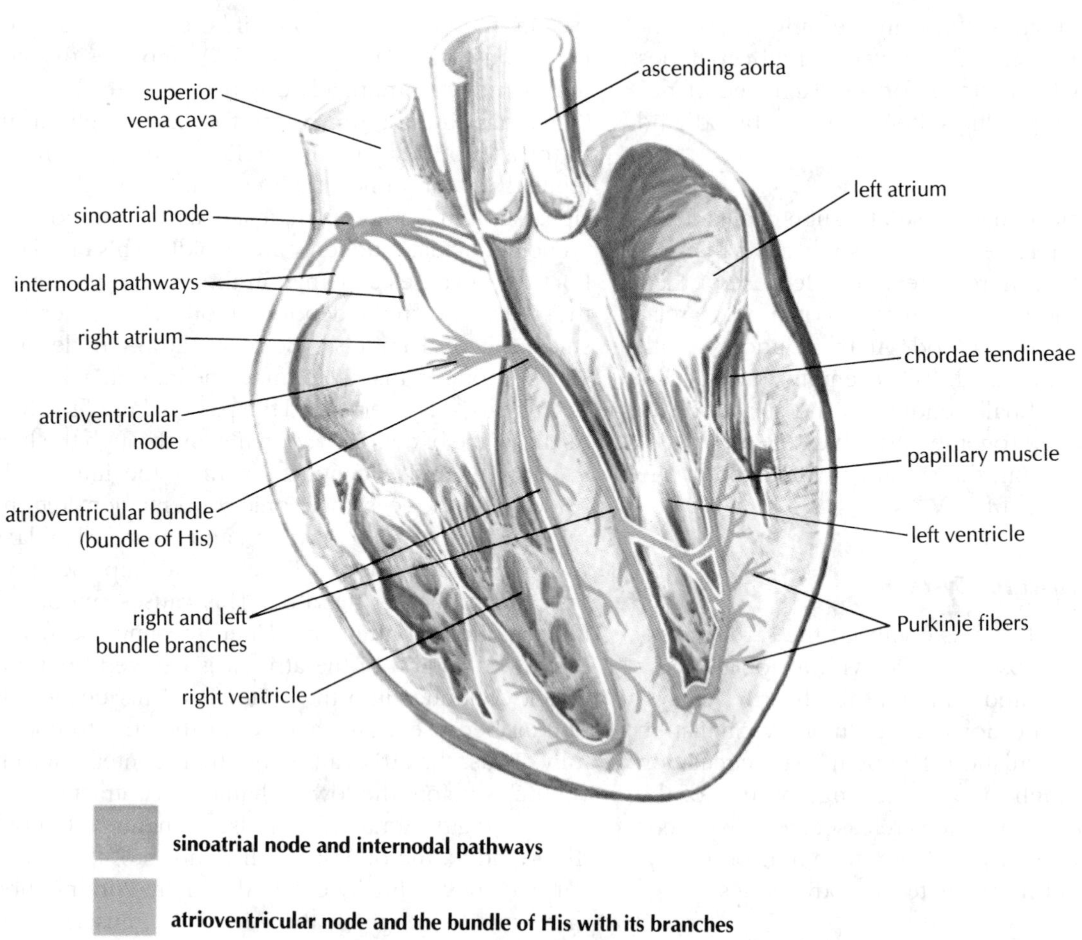

Figure 35-1 • *The conduction system of the heart. The sinoatrial node generates the electric impulse that begins the heartbeat. The excitation wave travels throughout the muscle of each atrium, causing it to contract. The atrioventricular node is stimulated, but the slower conduction through this node allows time for the aorta to contract and complete the filling of the ventricles. The excitation wave travels rapidly through the bundle of His and then throughout the ventricular walls by means of the bundle branches and Purkinje fibers. The entire musculature of the ventricles contracts almost at once.*

ventricular muscle cells begin to contract, squeezing the volume of blood inside the chamber. The rising pressure within the ventricles forces the AV valves to close. As the pressure in each ventricle rises, the valves to the pulmonary artery and the aorta are eventually forced open. The blood from the right ventricle is ejected into the pulmonary circulation for gas exchange, and the blood from the left ventricle enters the systemic circulation.

Cardiac Output. The amount of blood pumped by the heart each minute is referred to as cardiac output. In the normal resting adult, cardiac output is approximately 5 to 6 L/min. The healthy person is able to increase cardiac output to several times this amount in response to changing metabolic demands.

Cardiac output is a function of two factors, heart rate and stroke volume. Heart rate is simply the number of times the heart beats each minute. Stroke volume refers to the amount of blood ejected by the heart with each beat. An increase or decrease in either of these factors may change cardiac output.

Heart rate is primarily determined by the heart's pacemaker, the SA node. This tissue receives information constantly from the autonomic nervous system. The parasympathetic branch of this system slows heart rate; the sympathetic branch increases it. Increased metabolic activity (such as vigorous exercise) produces cardiac-stimulating metabolites; it also stimulates the sympathetic nervous system. Thus, cardiac output increases under these conditions to meet the extra demands of the tissues.

Stroke volume depends on three factors. First, the amount of blood that enters the heart determines how much can be pumped out. Healthy heart muscle is usually able to stretch to accommodate the volume of blood returning to it. Second, stroke volume also depends on the natural strength of the heart muscle, or its **contractility.** Like any muscle, the healthy, well-exercised

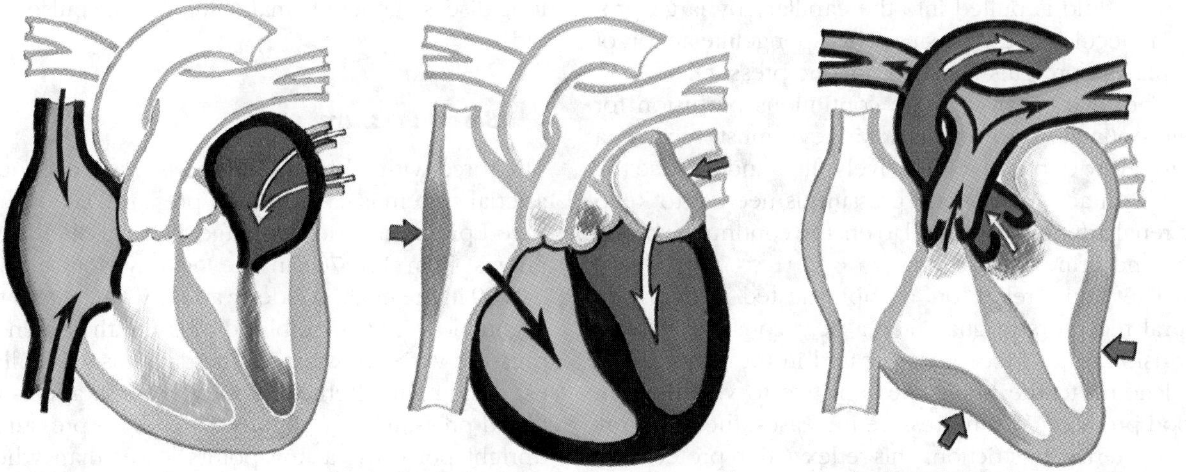

Diastole
Atria fill with blood which begins to flow into ventricles as soon as their walls relax.

Atrial Systole
Contraction of atria pumps blood into the ventricles

Ventricular Systole
Contraction of ventricles pumps blood into aorta and pulmonary arteries.

Figure 35-2 • *Pumping cycle of the heart.*

heart is a stronger and more efficient heart, so it is able to eject a larger volume of blood with each beat. Finally, stroke volume depends on the resistance to blood flow offered by the circulatory system.

Blood Vessels

Arteries, capillaries, and veins are dynamic structures that are essential for adequate distribution and perfusion of blood to body tissues.

Distribution of Blood Flow. As the heart ejects blood, the thick, muscular walls of the arteries stretch slightly, then rebound. The relative stiffness and elasticity of the arteries allow the blood to maintain its forceful forward momentum. This is important to maintain blood pressure and ensure that the blood has enough force to reach the tissues.

The smallest arteries are called arterioles. They are the primary regulators of blood flow, and they play a key role in the moment-to-moment regulation of blood pressure. These tiny vessels are able to increase or decrease their caliber to meet local tissue needs. For example, a jogger's active leg muscles require more oxygen and nutrients than do the digestive tract organs. Metabolites from the working leg muscles, rapid depletion of the local muscle oxygen supply, and the autonomic nervous system cause the arterioles serving the leg muscles to dilate. By opening wider, the vessels allow more blood to flow into the legs to meet the tissue needs. At the same time, arterioles within the digestive tract may actually constrict, limiting the amount of blood entering it. In this manner, the body is able to direct blood flow to where it is needed most.

By the time blood enters the capillaries, its pressure and velocity have decreased greatly. The slower flow rate of blood through the capillaries is necessary to allow sufficient time for tissues to extract oxygen and nutrients. The slow flow also allows the tissues adequate time to deposit their wastes into the blood so they can be removed.

The veins collect blood from all the capillaries. Blood flows slowly in the veins; the initial force of the heartbeat is greatly diminished by the time the blood has passed through the capillaries. In addition, venous blood must overcome gravity in the upright person. Backward flow of the venous blood would be a problem were it not for one-way valves in the veins. Skeletal muscles, particularly those of the legs, squeeze the veins, pushing blood forward and opening the valves. As the muscles relax, the valves of the veins snap shut, preventing backflow.

Tissue Perfusion. To maintain life, all living cells of the body must have a constant supply of oxygen and nutrients. The flow of blood through the tissues of the body is called tissue **perfusion.**

Individual cells and tissues receive oxygen, glucose, and various ions through the walls of capillaries. Their thin endothelial walls are permeable to most small molecules. In the arterial end of the capillary, the forward force of the blood helps to push fluid and soluble particles out of the vessel. This fluid surrounds the cells, and nutrients are exchanged for wastes. Oxygen and other molecules enter the cells primarily by diffusion, moving from an area where they are highly concentrated (the fluid) to an area of lower concentration (the cell). Metabolites such as carbon dioxide diffuse from the cell into the fluid, also in response to a concentration difference.

At the venous end of the capillary, tissue pressure forces some of the fluid back into the vessel. The remaining fluid is pulled into the capillary by large protein molecules in the plasma. This spongelike action of the plasma proteins is called oncotic pressure.

The vital organs require continuous perfusion for their optimal function. The kidneys must receive a steady flow of blood to effectively filter and cleanse the blood. An adequate blood pressure is needed to keep the renal arteries patent and to ensure continuous blood flow and urine production.

The brain relies on a sophisticated network of neural receptors to guarantee a near constant level of perfusion. These receptors, located in the major arteries leading to the brain, are sensitive to variations in blood pressure. When pressure increases, the receptors cause arterial constriction. This reflex action protects the brain's delicate capillaries from possible injury caused by a sudden rise in pressure. If blood pressure drops, the arteries dilate, thus ensuring a consistent flow of blood through the brain despite a possible momentary decrease elsewhere.

The coronary arteries that nourish the heart tissue are perfused primarily during the resting portion of the cardiac cycle (diastole). Adequate coronary perfusion depends, to a great extent, on adequate cardiac output. Within the normal range of heart rate, there is usually sufficient time for the coronary arteries to fill completely.

Characteristics of Normal Cardiovascular Function

Heart rate, blood pressure, skin temperature, and skin color all help to identify normal cardiovascular function.

Heart Rate

In the healthy adult, the heart beats rhythmically, with an equal time interval between each beat. Also, every beat is normally the same strength or intensity as all other beats. The normal heart rate in the adult is around 70 beats/min, although this value can vary greatly from one person to another. Resting heart rate in the person who exercises regularly is usually lower than in the person who does not. For this reason, the range for normal heart rate is from 60 (or lower) to 100 beats/min.

Exertion normally increases heart rate. The heart beats faster to meet the additional metabolic demands of hard-working muscles. It continues to do so for a short while after the exertion has stopped. The level and duration of heart rate increase depend on the level of exertion and the conditioning of the person. The well-conditioned person experiences a smaller and shorter increase in heart rate with exertion than the person who does not exercise regularly.

In general, heart rate is highest in the newborn, and it decreases steadily through early and middle adulthood. The person who is free of cardiovascular and lung disease generally maintains a stable pulse well into old age.

Blood Pressure

The force with which the blood is pushed through the arterial system is called blood pressure. Like heart rate, blood pressure varies with age. Normal blood pressure ranges from 120/70 (in the healthy young adult) to 140/89 in the healthy elderly adult. Women tend to have slightly lower average blood pressure than men. Blood pressure varies throughout the day; it is generally highest during late afternoon. Body position affects normal blood pressure only slightly. The blood pressure of an upright person is a few points lower than when it is measured in the same person who is lying down. Finally, physical exertion causes minimal changes in diastolic blood pressure, but systolic pressure can rise by as much as 60 to 80 mm Hg (Rowell, 1986).

Skin Temperature and Color

Skin temperature is a rough indicator of cardiovascular function. The person with good circulatory status is warm, with a fairly uniform skin temperature over all parts of the body. Cool ambient temperatures may cause local constriction of blood vessels in exposed skin, such as the hands, face, or ears. Under such conditions, these areas are cool to the touch. Warm outside temperatures do not raise skin temperature appreciably, however, because the sweating mechanism helps to cool the body. Skin temperature increases somewhat with strenuous exercise. In this situation, blood vessels dilate to release excess body heat.

Skin color also reflects circulatory status. It can roughly indicate the level of blood oxygenation and adequacy of local blood flow. Because skin color varies so greatly among individuals, it is difficult to apply general norms. Regardless of external skin color, however, the mucous membranes of all people are generally deep pink. These areas include the inner linings of the lips and mouth and the inner lining of the eyelids.

Factors Affecting Normal Cardiovascular Function

Heart rate, blood pressure, and the other indicators of cardiovascular function can vary from one person to another. They also can fluctuate normally within the same person. Several factors are responsible for this variance.

Age

The rapid metabolic rate of the newborn demands tremendous blood flow to developing tissues. Thus, the heart rate is considerably faster in the infant than in the older child, whose growth rate has slowed. The heart rate of the adult whose bodily growth has almost stopped is slower still. Only in old age, when the vascular system has narrowed and stiffened somewhat, does the heart rate again increase slightly.

This loss of elasticity of the blood vessels also is responsible for an increased blood pressure in the elderly (Craven, 1995). The heart must pump the blood with greater force to move it through the narrowed network of vessels. In turn, the additional effort required of the heart forces it to beat faster to meet its own metabolic demands.

Activity and Exercise

Increased metabolic requirements of exercising muscles force the heart to beat faster. The contraction and relaxation of muscles against veins increase return of blood to the heart; consequently, cardiac output increases. The increase in metabolism raises the temperature of the muscle. Increased muscle temperature, in turn, causes vascular dilation, which increases local blood flow. Locally acting vasoactive mediators and the muscles' rapid depletion of their oxygen supply also may cause local vasodilation.

Exercise may protect the cardiovascular system. In addition to promoting weight reduction, regular vigorous exercise helps to control serum levels of cholesterol, a major factor in the onset of atherosclerosis (Newton & Sivarajan-Froelicher, 1995).

Gender

Heart rate and blood pressure vary slightly between the sexes. The average man has a slower pulse but higher blood pressure than the average postpubescent woman. In women, blood pressure may increase slightly after menopause, probably as a result of hormonal changes.

Body Position

Because blood is a fluid, it is affected by gravity. It tends to pool in the lower, gravity-dependent areas of the body. In the standing person, blood must overcome gravity to reach the heart. The heart must work slightly harder to force blood through the system because venous blood must be forced upward.

In contrast, in the supine person the blood vessels are on the same level as the heart. In this case, gravity promotes venous return to the heart. For this reason stroke volume is generally greater when a person is lying down than when the same person is standing. In the healthy person, the supine position usually causes a drop in systolic blood pressure with a slight rise in diastolic blood pressure.

As the client changes from a supine to sitting position, a normal postural response includes an increased heart rate of 5 to 20 beats/min, a drop in systolic blood pressure less than 10 mm Hg, and an increase in diastolic pressure of about 5 mm Hg (Skov & Underhill Motzer, 1995).

Coping and Stress Tolerance

The autonomic nervous system causes momentary increases in blood pressure and heart rate when fear, pain, or anxiety is experienced. Stimulation of the adrenal gland to release epinephrine can prolong this effect. When these emotions are extreme, the opposite can occur, with a resultant drop in blood pressure.

Much has been written about personality types and their predisposition toward heart disease (Haynes, Feinleib, & Kannel, 1980; Jenkins, 1982; Rosenman, 1974; Rosenman, et al., 1970). For many years, the hard-striving, competitive, highly assertive person with the "type A" personality was believed to suffer an appreciably higher incidence of heart attacks than the easy-going, relaxed, more cooperatively oriented "type B" person. Recent studies have raised questions about the validity of this belief and suggest one personality component, hostility, may more directly correlate with increased cardiac risk (Newton & Sivarajan-Froelicher, 1995).

Lifestyle and Habits

Smoking increases heart rate, blood pressure, and peripheral vascular resistance. Many over-the-counter and prescription medications, including those for noncardiovascular problems, can affect heart rate, blood pressure, or local blood flow. Drinkers of caffeinated coffee and cola usually have higher heart rates and blood pressures than those who drink decaffeinated beverages. Excessive alcohol intake has been associated with hypertension and increased cardiovascular risk, so prudent alcohol consumption of less than one ounce per day is recommended (National High Blood Pressure Education Program, 1993).

Lifespan Considerations

Although the functions of cardiac output and tissue perfusion remain unchanged throughout life, age-related changes in hemodynamics do occur.

Newborn and Infant

The newborn's heart rate is normally 130 to 160 beats/min. Its rhythm is commonly irregular. A heart rate of less than 100 in a newborn is cause for alarm. As the infant matures, the heart rate becomes more rhythmic and slower, but it can easily increase during activity or when the infant cries.

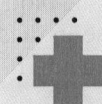

> **Safety Alert**
> *Cardiac Clients*
>
> - Never ignore chest pain; unrelieved chest pain should be reported to medical personnel immediately.
> - Teach all cardiovascular clients to avoid Valsalva's maneuver (exhaling against a closed glottis) because this can significantly increase blood pressure and decrease venous return. Teach clients to blow out slowly when pulling up in bed or attempting to have a bowel movement.
> - Teach cardiovascular clients to avoid isometric exercises, which tend to cause changes in blood pressure and heart rate.
> - Teach clients receiving diuretics or antihypertensive medications to change position slowly to avoid orthostatic hypotension and to prevent potential falls.
> - Do not palpate both carotid pulses at the same time because this can interfere with blood supply to the brain. When obtaining the carotid pulse, avoid rubbing the area because this can stimulate parasympathetic discharge and cause severe bradycardia.

Blood pressure is lowest during the newborn period. The newborn's systolic pressure is low, usually in the mid-40s. By 1 month of age, average systolic pressure is 80 to 90 mm Hg, with diastolic pressure ranging from the mid-40s to 60 mm Hg. By 1 year of age, the average blood pressure is around 96/65 mm Hg.

Toddler and Preschooler

The heart rate slows somewhat as the infant becomes a toddler. Steady activity, however, is likely to keep it high throughout the daytime hours. By the end of this period, the heart rate has decreased to a resting rate of around 100 beats/min.

Blood pressure varies slightly within this age group but generally remains within the 95 to 100/65 mm Hg range.

Child and Adolescent

As the heart increases in size, its rate continues to decline. Blood pressure changes are gradual and slight during this period. At any age during this time, boys generally have slightly higher blood pressure and lower heart rate than girls. By the age of 17 years, heart rate and blood pressure have stabilized at the adult values of 60 to 80 and 120/70, respectively.

Adult and Older Adult

By the time the person reaches adulthood, age-related changes have already occurred within the cardiovascular system. As maturing continues, these changes may lead to decreased activity tolerance and decreased endurance. Along with natural "wear and tear," diet, stress, smoking, and several other lifestyle factors may have contributed to the processes of calcification, fatty degeneration, and diminished elasticity of the blood vessels. This is likely to account for the gradual and expected rise in blood pressure as the adult grows older. Because of the added work this places on the heart, the heart rate is often slightly higher in the older adult.

Diseases leading to problems with tissue perfusion are uncommon in early adulthood. Peripheral vascular disease and its resultant perfusion problems increase in frequency with age. Disorders such as diabetes mellitus, chronic hypertension, kidney disease, or problems with lipid metabolism cause peripheral vascular disease in the elderly (Craven, 1995).

Although coronary heart disease (CHD) is not considered part of the normal aging process, it has traditionally affected older adults. There is growing evidence that lifestyle changes have led to lower death rates from CHD during the last several decades, with the greatest reduction in deaths occurring among younger middle-aged adults. This finding implies that CHD development is indirectly related to age, insofar as duration of exposure to CHD risk factors is longer in the elderly (Gillum, Folsom, & Blackburnz, 1984; Pell & Fayerweather, 1985; Newton & Sivarajan-Froelicher, 1995).

Altered Cardiovascular Function

For years, cardiovascular disease has ranked as America's number one cause of death and debilitation. Worldwide, its incidence has grown steadily as modernization has spread. It is a contributing factor in untold numbers of cases of debilitating and disabling conditions.

Because of the complexity of the cardiovascular system, the potential for altered function is great. A host of factors can adversely affect cardiovascular function. Lifestyle choices, such as nutritional status, exercise, and smoking, along with trauma and pathologic conditions, can contribute greatly to problems of the heart and blood vessels.

Potential for Altered Cardiovascular Function

Tissue oxygenation requires that all portions of the cardiovascular system work properly. Alterations in the conduction system, improper opening or closing of the valves, or damage to cardiac muscle fibers can diminish the effective pumping ability of the heart. Changes in the blood vessels and in the blood can create the potential for altered function.

Decreased Pumping Ability of the Heart

Conduction problems, valve dysfunction, or muscle damage can decrease the ability to pump blood effectively, resulting in congestive heart failure (CHF). An example of a Critical Pathway for a client with CHF summarizes collaborative care.

Conduction Problems. Proper function of the conduction system ensures the orderly contraction of myocardial muscle fibers. This results in a coordinated, concerted pumping action, with all muscle fibers operating as a unit. If the conduction system is damaged or malfunctions, the electrical impulses it generates do not spread sequentially through the muscle. Thus, the fibers that normally contract together may do so out of sequence or may contract independently of each other. This discordant fiber contraction affects the inherent rhythm of the heart and may impair its ability to pump effectively.

An **arrhythmia** is an abnormality in heart rhythm, commonly caused by disturbances in the conduction system. Arrhythmias are diagnosed by electrocardiography (ECG). Arrhythmias range from minor, clinically insignificant abnormalities to life-threatening conditions. Arrhythmias may be caused by damage to the heart muscle, diminished coronary blood flow, decreased blood oxygen levels, medications, alterations in serum electrolytes (such as potassium or calcium), stress (from exercise, fever, or emotional stress), or overstretching of the heart muscle.

Valve Dysfunction. The four valves of the heart must be able to open fully and close tightly to guarantee forward blood flow. Any of the heart's valves may be damaged by inflammation, infection, or trauma, or they may be congenitally malformed. The most common cause of acquired valve damage is rheumatic fever. Generally, valve damage results in **stenosis** (narrowing). This condition can limit stroke volume and force the heart to work much harder than normal to maintain an adequate cardiac output. With time, the heart becomes less able to maintain normal cardiac output, and heart failure occurs.

Muscle Damage. To maintain normal rhythm, the heart requires a constant supply of oxygen and nutrients. If blood flow decreases through the coronary arteries, the active muscle becomes hypoxic. Unless blood flow is restored, portions of the heart muscle can die. This is called an MI, or heart attack. The person who survives a heart attack may have areas where the damaged heart muscle tissue is replaced by scar tissue.

A second cause of cardiac muscle damage or weakening is severe overwork of the heart. The normal heart responds to extra work by enlarging. Eventually, excessive demands stretch the heart to its limits. It finally weakens and fails. Increased vascular resistance (often caused by **arteriosclerosis,** or hardening of the arteries), excessive blood volume, and alterations in blood viscosity are common contributing factors in the development of heart failure.

Finally, the heart muscle can be damaged by infection, inflammatory or infiltrating metabolic disease, nutritional deficiencies, trauma, and drug abuse (Laurent-Bopp, 1995).

Altered Blood Flow

Conditions that affect the arteries and veins can alter tissue perfusion and cardiac output.

Arterial Dysfunction. Conditions that affect the structure of the arteries disrupt their normal function. Arteries can become occluded, or they can dilate abnormally because of **aneurysms** (weakened areas of arterial walls).

Atherosclerosis is by far the most common cause of arterial occlusion. This condition is characterized by fatty deterioration of the arterial smooth muscle walls. With time, the lumen of the arteries narrows as the arterial walls absorb increasing amounts of circulating fat particles, or lipids. Affected vessels also become stiff and fibrinous and eventually may close completely. The resultant change in the walls of the vessel is called *plaque* formation (Fig. 35-3). This degenerative process occurs gradually, over a period of years. It is more common in susceptible people and is associated with a wide range of lifestyle factors. High blood pressure, high serum lipid levels, and cigarette smoking are the most important of these (Newton & Sivarajan-Froelicher, 1995). Atherosclerosis is the primary cause of peripheral vascular disease and CHD. It is the most common disorder of the cardiovascular system. It seriously compounds the problems of hypertension and is the most important factor in the majority of strokes and heart attacks.

Other important causes of arterial occlusion include infection, inflammation, or trauma to the arteries. Arteries also can have increased smooth muscle tone as a result of increased sympathetic nervous system stimulation. Finally, arteries can be occluded by edema (swollen tissues) and thrombi (blood clots).

Capillary Dysfunction. As passive structures, capillaries are mainly affected by the arteries, veins, and sur-

(text continues on page 948)

Collaborative Care Plan: Critical Pathway: Congestive Heart Failure (CHF)

Client Name:____________
Case Type: ____________
DRG:____________
ICD-9:____________

Admit Date:____________
Date Path Initiated:____________

Expected LOS:____________
Actual LOS:____________
Discharge Date:____________

Physician:____________
Case Manager:____________

Outcome Criteria

	Day 1				Day 2				Day 3–6			
Client Problems	CCU/MICU	D	E	N	Telemetry	D	E	N	Telemetry/Floor	D	E	N
Decreased cardiac output related to ↓myocardial contractility, altered conduction, & valve defects	No life-threatening dysrhythmias HR < 120 – regular skin pink, warm, dry Cap. refill < 3 sec. Palpable peripheral pulses Bil SBP > 100 UO > 30 cc/hr				NSR–no ectopy Serum K 3.5–5 HR 60–100 reg Skin pink, warm, dry Cap. refill < 3 sec. Palp. periph. pulses SBP > 100 < 140 DBP > 50 < 90				NSR Serum K 3.5–5 HR 60–100 reg. Skin pink, warm, dry Cap. refill < 3 sec. Palp. periph. pulses SBP > 90 < 140 DBP > 50 < 90 UO > 30 cc/hr.			
Altered gas exchange related to pulmonary congestion, V/Q mismatching, ↓diffusion	02 Sat > 90% Minimal crackles in lung bases Resp < 24 unlabored PO2 > 60 Dyspnea on exertion				02 Sat > 95% Decreased crackles heard in lungs R < 20 unlabored P02 > 80mm Hg No dyspnea on exertion				02 Sat > 95% HR < 20 over baseline on amb. Lungs clear Chest x-ray clear R < 20 unlabored No dyspnea			
Activity intolerance related to imbalance between oxygen supply–demand, dyspnea, fatigue	Turns in bed, feeds self; performs self toilet measures No dyspnea or fatigue				Tolerates commode or sits in chair TID without dyspnea, chest pain, fatigue Participates in ADL's without discomfort or fatigue				Performs ADL's without fatigue, dyspnea, or chest pain. Ambulates with QID SBP +/– 10 mmHg over baseline HR < 20 BPM over baseline			
Fluid volume excess related to pulmonary congestion, venous pooling	Resp < 24 unlabored Lung sounds clear without crackles & diminished in bases No dependent edema Wt. loss 1 lb/day until baseline				Resp 12–20 unlabored Lungs clear No edema No JVD Wt. loss 1 lb/day until baseline				Resp 12-20 unlabored Lungs clear No edema No JVD No wt. gain			
Anxiety RT dyspnea, fear of death, & hospitalization	Verbalizes fears & concerns related to hospitalization & diagnosis, fear of death				Relaxed non-verbals & posture Identifies source of anxiety & possible coping mechanisms				Identifies appropriate coping mechanisms & sources of social support			
INTERVENTIONS												
Consult/Referral	Cardiologist Pulmonologist Social Service				Assess need for dietary consult & RT				Assess need for Home Health Care Social Service referral			
Diagnostic Tests	Chest x-ray EKG Lytes, Chem Profile CBC, cardiac enzymes, BUN/Cr UA ABG's				Chest x-ray EKG Lytes BUN/Cr Possible Echo				Lytes BUN/Cr			

(continued)

Critical Pathways *(continued)*

	Day 1				Day 2				Day 3–6			
INTERVENTIONS	CCU/MICU	D	E	N	Telemetry	D	E	N	Telemetry/Floor	D	E	N
Assessment	VS q 15" until stable then q hr; Cardiac monitor; Assess heart sounds S_3/S_4 Lungs (crackles) Edema, JVD Daily wt I&O q hr-Foley cath Art line/Swan Ganz cath				VS q 4hr Focus on heart sounds (S_3 or S_4) & lungs (crackles or wheezes) Edema, JVD Daily wt. I&O q 8 hr – DC Foley DC Monitor/Art line/Swan Ganz cath				VS q 8 hr Assess heart & lung sounds q 8 hr, crackles, wheezes Edema, JVD Daily wt I&O q 8 hr			
Treatments	Insert IV – #18 – 20G Incentive Spirometer (IS) per q 2 hr O_2 4 L/NC or intubation/ventilator O_2 saturation (pulse oximetry) SVN q 4/hr				Saline Lock IV when adequate PO IS q 2–4hr O_2 2L/NC PRN O_2 Sat SVN q 4/hr				DC Saline Lock IS q 4 DC O_2 when O_2 sats > 92%			
Activity	Bed rest c̄ BSC HOB ↑45–90 Conserve energy Balance rest c̄ activity				BRP ⟶ chair X 3 OOB as tol Assist c̄ all ADL's				Ambulate in hall X 3 → up ad lib Self ADL's Shower daily			
Diet	Clear liquids as tol.				Low Na, low cholesterol cardiac soft				Low Na, low cholesterol cardiac diet as tol.			
Meds	Diuretic IV Anti-anxiety Rx Assess need for nitrates (NTG drip, patch) or KCl replacement Morphine SO4 Inotropes (Dobutamine, Dopamine) Digoxin				Diuretics PO Evaluate need for preload & after load reducers – DC NTG → drip Nitropaste Ace Inhibitors. Stool softener/LOC KCl replacement				Diuretics PO Digoxin PO NTG paste Stool softeners – KCl replacement Discharge prescription written			
Teaching	Explain CCU environment, routines, procedures Teach pain rating scale & mgt tech. Involve family in all teaching Give critical path to pt/family				Teach CHF disease process, trt. regimen. Give CHF teaching pkt Instruct pt in need for freq rest periods & conservation of energy Begin medication teaching				Reinforce CHF teaching & answer questions. Review medications & importance of smoking cessation. Activity progression Diet teaching, esp NAS Daily record wt, edema Teach importance of weight control			
Discharge/Transfer Planning	Assess home care situation, physical arrangements, social support, care giver. If stable, transfer to telemetry Case manager visit				Assess DC needs of pt Contact social worker, Home health if needed				Review DC orders/meds c̄ pt/family. Arrange follow up appt & when to contact MD Cardiac rehab, smoking clinic nutrition referral if needed Emerg phone #'s			

Initials/Signatures:

D=Day
E=Evening
N=Nite

Write "V" for variance in the box if expected outcome not met or staff intervention not performed. Client variances must be explained in t' e progress note.

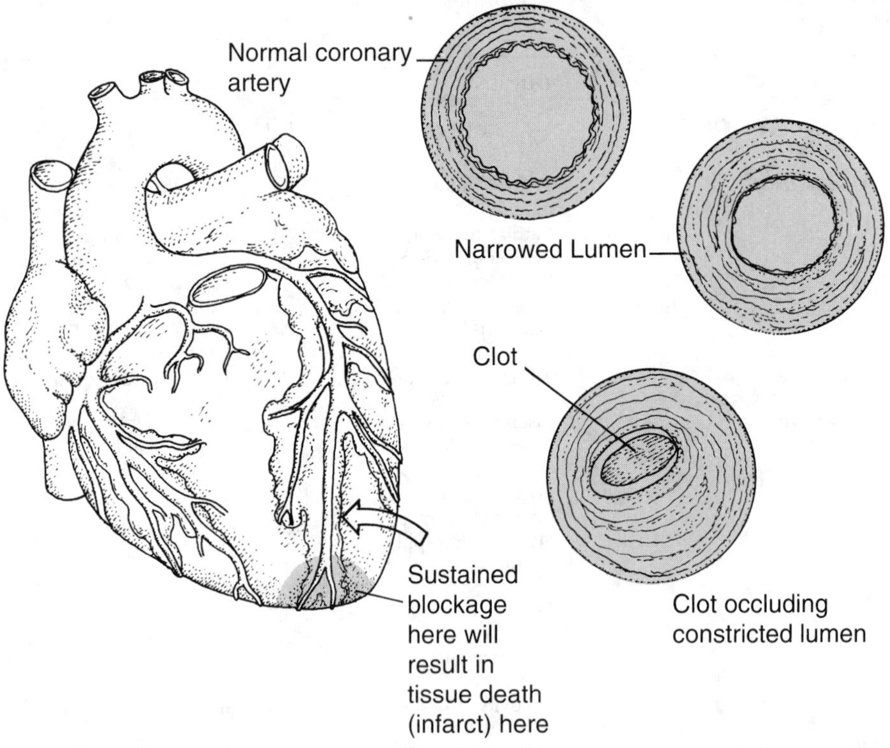

Figure 35-3 • *Atherosclerotic plaque: a buildup of fat, cholesterol, fibrin, cellular waste products, and calcium on the endothelial lining of an artery.*

rounding tissues. Capillaries can become occluded by pressure from surrounding tissue. This can happen when tissues are swollen by edema, bruising, or tumors.

Capillaries can become leaky and can cause or contribute to tissue edema. Increased blood pressure or venous congestion can excessively stretch the walls of the capillaries, allowing fluid to leak out into interstitial tissues as edema. Toxins, trauma, and inflammation can increase capillary permeability, thereby promoting fluid leakage. Finally, capillaries can leak if plasma proteins are deficient, because these substances are responsible for exerting the osmotic pressure that retains fluid in the blood vessels.

Venous Pooling. Decreased venous blood flow can aggravate hypertension and cause ischemia. Unless blood is kept moving steadily through the veins, tissue edema or clot formation may occur. Causes of venous pooling include right heart failure and ineffective venous valves.

If the right side of the heart is weakened by disease or the pulmonary vasculature is highly resistant, the heart may be unable to pump effectively. Blood collects in the vena cavae faster than the heart can pump it into the pulmonary system. Blood flow slows as the larger and then the smaller veins become engorged with pooled blood.

Venous valve incompetency can be caused by trauma or vein inflammation (phlebitis). More often, however, gravity and muscle inactivity are responsible for valve dysfunction and venous pooling. In the upright person, gravity hinders venous return, thereby promoting the gradual collection of blood in the veins of the lower leg. A person who must stand or sit for long periods (or who is immobile, such as a client confined to bed) does not have the benefit of regular muscle compression against the veins. As more blood collects in the leg veins, the veins can become dilated and distorted varicosities develop (VanEtta, 1995). The valves become so overstretched that their edges cannot approximate, so blood moves backward and forward through the incompetent valves.

An additional effect of venous pooling is increased myocardial work. Because stroke volume depends on how much blood enters the heart, venous pooling limits venous return. To maintain normal output, the heart must beat faster. This added work is compounded by the fact that increased venous pressure causes increased vascular resistance. Thus, the heart must increase its efforts to push against the pooled blood.

Altered Blood Composition

The blood carries essential nutrients to the cells, but it can do this effectively only if the composition of the blood is normal and if blood volume is sufficient to fill the cardiovascular system. Alterations in the red blood cells or plasma or changes in circulating blood volume or consistency can affect cardiovascular function.

Altered Red Blood Cells. The red blood cells are responsible for delivering oxygen, which is carried on the hemoglobin portion of the cell. An insufficient number of red blood cells (as in anemia) or damage to the hemoglobin molecules results in tissue hypoxia. Hypoxia affects all tissues, but the brain and heart are particularly sensitive to oxygen deprivation.

Altered Plasma Composition. The liquid portion of the blood carries glucose, electrolytes, and trace minerals and nutrients to the cells. Changes in the normal levels of any of these substances or in pH can cause alterations in cardiovascular function. For example, slight changes in serum potassium levels can cause serious arrhythmias. Increased sodium intake can cause an increase in blood volume, which increases cardiac work. An acidotic blood pH can decrease the ability of hemoglobin to carry oxygen.

Altered Blood Volume. To function optimally, the cardiovascular system must contain a relatively constant blood volume. Dehydration or hemorrhage causes a decrease in circulating volume. Because tissue perfusion depends on a sufficient volume of circulating blood, any decrease in volume can lead to tissue hypoxia. This occurs in the condition commonly called shock.

Excessive blood volume can occur in individuals with congestive heart failure, kidney failure, and mismanagement of intravenous (IV) fluid therapy. Excess blood volume causes increased blood pressure. The heart must work harder than normal to pump the additional blood through the vascular system. The additional blood volume and pressure also overload capillaries, causing edema. In the peripheral tissues, overloading causes swelling and decreased perfusion. If fluid overload occurs in the lung, pulmonary edema fills the air sacs and causes asphyxiation and possibly death.

Altered Blood Viscosity. The thickness (or viscosity) of the blood is generally consistent. Thinner, less viscous blood flows more quickly than normal blood through the vessels. Increased blood flow increases venous return to the heart. This usually forces the heart to pump faster to empty itself.

The opposite condition, called polycythemia, results in thicker, more viscous blood. Polycythemic blood flows more slowly through the vessels. To pump this thicker blood through the system, the heart must work harder than usual.

Cardiovascular Risk Factors

Many factors contribute to the development of cardiovascular problems. Adequate knowledge of these risk factors and the impact they have on cardiovascular health can encourage lifestyle changes that help to prevent cardiovascular dysfunction. See the accompanying display of controllable, uncontrollable, and contributory risk factors for cardiovascular disease. Healthy People 2000, which encourages national health promotion and disease prevention, has targeted reduction of CHD deaths to no more than 100 per 100,000 people (reduced from 135 per 100,000 in 1987; Healthy People 2000, 1991). Guidelines for decreasing specific cardiovascular risk factors, such as smoking, physical fitness, and dietary fat, are included along with specific goals for high-risk groups.

Coronary Heart Disease Risk Factors

Controllable Risk Factors

Cigarette smoking
High blood pressure
Hyperlipoproteinemia (high blood lipids; results from excessive intake of cholesterol and saturated fats)
Sedentary lifestyle
Stress
Obesity

Uncontrollable Risk Factors

Gender—risk increases for all men; risk increases for women after menopause
Family history of heart disease
Age—risk increases with age
Diabetes mellitus

Contributing Factors

Lack of exercise
Oral contraceptives
Excessive alcohol intake

Smoking. Smoking has been called the most important modifiable risk factor for cardiovascular disease and has caused more deaths due to cardiovascular disease than lung cancer or chronic obstructive pulmonary disease (Newton & Sivarajan-Froelicher, 1995). Smoking increases the heart rate, increases blood pressure, constricts arterioles, and may cause irregular cardiac rhythm. It enhances the process of atherosclerosis and is the major cause of peripheral vascular disease. Smoking also limits the oxygen-carrying capacity of the blood by displacing oxygen with carbon monoxide.

Nutrition. The relationship between dietary factors and cardiovascular problems is complex, but a diet high in saturated fats and cholesterol is strongly associated with atherosclerotic lesions. Cholesterol is the primary component of the plaque (fatty lesion) that gradually occludes arteries. This leads to peripheral vascular disease and hypertension, which greatly increase the chance of MI from coronary artery disease or stroke from cerebral vascular disease.

The role of salt in foods has received close scrutiny. Because sodium is hydrophilic, a diet high in salt can increase blood volume and cardiac work. This can seriously aggravate chronic hypertension or congestive heart failure. Convenience foods and preserved foods often contain a large amount of sodium. Increased sodium intake in sodium-sensitive individuals can increase the incidence of hypertension (Sollek, 1995). Studies concerning the role of potassium, magnesium, and calcium intake on cardiovascular health are being conducted.

Body Size and Body Fat. Being overweight places excessive demands on the cardiovascular system. The extra adipose tissue must be supplied with blood to meet its metabolic requirements. The extra cells are served by miles of blood vessels. To perform the additional work of pumping blood to these tissues, the heart may become enlarged. Blood pressure increases, but perfusion may decrease. Obesity also has been shown to correlate positively with cardiovascular disease. Recent studies have shown that central distribution of excess weight (around the midsection) poses greater risk than more peripheral distribution (thighs) (Newton & Sivarajan-Froelicher, 1995).

Exercise. A sedentary lifestyle leads to an increased risk for cardiovascular disease (Newton & Sivarajan-Froelicher, 1995). Just as regular exercise strengthens leg and arm muscles, it also makes the heart stronger and improves its pumping efficiency. Increased blood circulation also helps prevent the formation of thrombi and atherosclerotic plaques by decreasing platelet stickiness and serum cholesterol. Thus, a well-conditioned person has a lower risk of heart or circulatory problems than a person who does not exercise regularly.

Cardiovascular problems may be related to the client's job. Occupations that require the worker to stand or sit for long periods promote venous pooling and predispose the person to varicose veins and possible hypercoagulation problems. A sudden change from a sedentary occupation to a physically demanding job may aggravate cardiovascular problems.

Medical and Family History. Some cardiovascular problems may result from current or previous medical conditions. Diabetes mellitus is often accompanied by serious circulatory changes. Rheumatic fever can be responsible for damage to the heart valves. In addition to rheumatic fever, recent systemic infections, particularly those that have gone untreated or have responded poorly to antibiotic therapy, may increase the client's risk for endocarditis.

Trauma also can be responsible for cardiovascular problems. Severe trauma may cause direct damage to vascular beds. Vessel trauma coupled with edema can result in diminished blood flow to the injured area. Recent long bone fractures can cause emboli. High blood pressure is an important risk factor for stroke, MI, and dissection (bursting) of aneurysms.

Although it is clear that many cardiovascular problems have no hereditary basis, genetics may play a role in certain disorders. For example, some clients may report that an unusually high number of close relatives have suffered strokes or heart attacks. Hypertension also is more prevalent in some families than in others. Thus, a positive family history for cardiovascular disease must be considered carefully.

Medications and Drug Use. Prescription or over-the-counter drugs may affect cardiac output or blood pressure. Asthma preparations and some cold remedies may substantially increase heart rate and blood pressure. Diuretics (prescribed or so-called natural diuretics from health stores) can decrease blood volume and alter electrolyte balance. This can cause potentially dangerous changes in heart rhythm. Birth control pills significantly enhance the process of blood clot formation and increase the risk of embolism.

The use of illicit drugs can have serious cardiovascular complications. IV use of any drug provides an entry for bacteria into the bloodstream and puts the user at high risk for bacterial endocarditis. Impurities in the injected drug can cause cardiac inflammation and may form the nucleus of an embolism. Repeated IV injections can result in phlebitis and eventual destruction of the vessel.

Cocaine use has been increasingly associated with sudden cardiac arrest, because it increases oxygen demand and reduces supply (Jensen, 1995). Overdoses of opiates (such as heroin or morphine) can cause severe hypotension. They also may induce pulmonary edema.

Stress. Stress is often mentioned as a cause of high blood pressure, angina, and MI. Its precise role in the development or progression of these disorders has not been established, but its association with cardiovascular disease is well known. People with preexisting cardiac problems who encounter extraordinary or protracted periods of business, family, or personal stress may be at added risk for exacerbations of these problems.

Manifestations of Altered Cardiovascular Function

Cardiovascular function is altered in many ways and has a wide range of manifestations. Vital signs are typically affected. When cardiovascular changes cause tissue ischemia, common indicators of inadequate tissue perfusion include pain and changes in the skin and sensorium. Edema and **thrombus** (clot) formation are manifestations and causes of alterations in blood flow.

Nursing Research
Cardiovascular Health

Selected Nursing Research Studies

Fleury, J. (1992). The application of motivational theory to cardiovascular risk reduction. *Image Journal of Nursing Scholarship, 24*(3), 229–238.

Hahn, W., Brooks, J. A., & Hartsough, D. (1993). Self-disclosure and coping styles in men with cardiovascular reactivity. *Research in Nursing & Health, 16*(4), 275–82.

Hawthorne, M. (1994). Gender differences in recovery after coronary artery surgery. *Image Journal of Nursing Scholarship 26* (1), 75–80.

Puntillo, K., & Weiss, S. (1994). Pain: Its mediators and associated morbidity in critically ill cardiovascular surgical patients. *Nursing Research, 43*(1), 31–37.

Possible Topics for Nursing Inquiry

- To what extent do antiembolism stockings affect heart rate and blood pressure?
- Does upper body extremity effort cause increased incidence of angina compared with similar energy output from lower extremities?
- How do diets low in vegetables and fruit affect the cardiovascular health of children?
- What effect does the use of clinical simulation have on decreasing a new graduate's anxiety regarding code management?

Finally, organ dysfunction and possible failure are manifestations of altered cardiovascular status.

Changes in Vital Signs

Changes in cardiovascular status are reflected by changes in blood pressure, pulse character and rate, and respiratory rate.

Blood Pressure. Blood pressure may fluctuate with changes in cardiac output and tissue perfusion. Decreased circulating volume or increased venous pooling may be indicated by orthostatic hypotension. This condition is present when blood pressure drops more than 25 mm Hg systolically or 10 mm Hg diastolically after assumption of an upright position (Skov & Underhill Motzer, 1995). Abnormally low blood pressure (below 100/60 mm Hg), accompanied by other indicators of diminished oxygenation, is a serious sign of decreased cardiac output.

High blood pressure, formerly called hypertension, is undoubtedly the most common manifestation of altered blood flow, affecting 30% of the adult population (Joint National Committee, 1993). It is the most common risk factor for cardiovascular disease in developed and developing countries (Sollek, 1995). A complex phenomenon, high blood pressure contributes to the morbidity and mortality of millions of people annually.

High blood pressure is nearly always caused by narrowing of the arteries. To maintain a normal, constant cardiac output, the heart must work harder to force blood through the narrowed vessels. High blood pressure also promotes atherosclerosis, which further increases blood pressure. Researchers have postulated that primary high blood pressure is caused by an increased level of circulating vasoactive substances or by increased sympathetic nervous system activity. Increased blood pressure may be caused by changes in sodium excretion or in arterial smooth muscle contractility caused by changes in calcium absorption (Sollek, 1995).

High blood pressure can affect anyone, but it occurs most often in those with a positive family history, men, and the elderly. Urban dwellers, particularly African-Americans, are most susceptible. Important modifiable risk factors include smoking, sodium intake, high serum lipids, weight control, and stress. High blood pressure is unique in that it is a manifestation of cardiovascular dysfunction and in turn, a cause of further dysfunction, causing severe tissue and organ damage.

Pulse Character. Diminished or absent pulses may indicate inadequate blood flow to an area. Although the pulse normally becomes fainter as the distance from the heart increases, absence of pulse may indicate vessel occlusion, especially when differences occur bilaterally. Complete vessel occlusion is most often associated with other signs, such as skin changes and pain. In some people, the most distal peripheral pulses (the dorsalis pedis and posterior tibial) may not be palpable but may be confirmed with the use of a Doppler instrument (Gehing, 1992).

Pulse Rate. The heart rate increases in response to increased oxygen demand. It decreases at rest when oxygen demands are low. A heart rate of 100 beats/min at rest may indicate problems with cardiac output if known contributing factors (such as fever, pain, medications, or anxiety) are absent. An increase in heart rate greater than 20 beats/min during mild activity (such as walking or moving to the commode) may indicate that decreased cardiac output is contributing to activity intolerance. Conversely, heart rate that does not increase with exercise may indicate the heart is unable to adjust to changing oxygen demands (Richie & Sivarajan-Froelicher, 1995). Heart rate should return to baseline within 3 minutes after exercise.

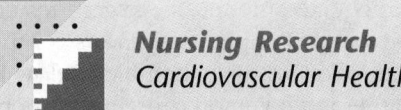

Respiration. Respiratory rate and effort often increase in the person with cardiovascular dysfunction. Decreased cardiac output or diminished tissue blood flow limits the amount of oxygen available to the tissues. As activity increases and tissues demand more oxygen, respiration increases to supplement blood oxygenation. Shortness of breath can occur in the person with heart or circulatory problems with even slight activity, because the cardiovascular system is unable to meet the added oxygen demand. In extreme cases, the person may experience shortness of breath at rest or when lying down. Finally, a hacking cough is a common manifestation of heart failure.

Ischemia

Decreased tissue perfusion causes tissue hypoxia because less oxygen is available for metabolism. The tissue also experiences starvation because less blood flow brings fewer nutrients and abnormalities due to the build-up of waste products. This condition of inadequate perfusion, along with its consequences, is called **ischemia.** Subnormal tissue perfusion causes suboptimal tissue function. Although ischemia is better tolerated by some tissues than others, it is never desirable. The manifestations of ischemia include pain, changes in skin and sensorium, and organ dysfunction.

Pain. Pain occurs commonly with ischemia when tissues are deprived of oxygen. The exact mechanism by which this occurs is not fully understood, but it has been hypothesized that peripheral nerve endings may be stimulated by pressure caused by cellular edema, or the nerves may release chemical pain mediators as a response to their own hypoxia (Jensen, 1995). Reversal of hypoxia by restoring blood flow eliminates the pain if the tissue is still viable. Pain that is not lessened by rest or by measures to improve blood flow and oxygenation may signal tissue infarction.

Angina is chest pain associated with decreased coronary blood flow. **Intermittent claudication** is limb pain caused by poor blood flow.

Changes in Skin Color, Temperature, and Character. Alterations in cardiac output and tissue perfusion can become apparent by changes in the skin.

Skin color varies widely, so changes in color may not be evident in all people. In light-skinned people, however, sudden constriction of peripheral blood vessels (caused by fear, low cardiac output, or trauma) causes blanching of the skin. Clients experiencing these circumstances appear "ashen." Chronically decreased tissue perfusion or anemia causes pallor. Rubor is a bluish-red skin coloration caused by hyperemia, or increased blood flow. Temporary increases in skin perfusion cause flushing, as is evident during fever or times of embarrassment. Cyanosis occurs when hemoglobin is not carrying an adequate amount of oxygen, resulting in a bluish appearance. Peripheral cyanosis (of the fingers, toes, and ear lobes) occurs when blood flow is restricted. Cold weather is a common cause of transient peripheral cyanosis and usually is not clinically significant. In contrast, central cyanosis is a serious sign of decreased oxygenation. It appears around the lips and tissues of the oral cavity.

Skin temperature rises with increased blood flow to the skin; vascular constriction or poor perfusion cools the skin. If the sympathetic nervous system has caused the constriction (eg, in shock), sweat glands may become activated, and the client will feel clammy to the touch.

Skin character changes occur with alterations in perfusion. Chronically poor perfusion may result in loss of hair in the affected area, thickened nails, and shiny, dry skin indicative of inadequate tissue nutrition. Some people with chronic heart disease also have clubbed fingers and toes.

Poor perfusion causes tissue malnutrition. This leaves the cells weak, edematous, and unable to withstand normal wear and tear. Skin lesions, dermatitis, and ulcerations can develop readily in clients with compromised skin perfusion. Chronically limited arterial flow to an area can cause skin breakdown, with possible tissue necrosis and gangrene.

Changes in Sensorium. The brain is extremely sensitive to any alterations in normal blood flow. When cerebral blood supply diminishes even slightly, changes in sensorium occur. Most commonly, the client is restless and anxious. Confusion, fatigue, listlessness, and slurred speech may occur with a prolonged decrease in cerebral blood flow, as in shock. Chronic brain ischemia limits cognitive function.

When the blood supply to the brain is acutely diminished or completely interrupted, dizziness and loss of consciousness may occur. This occurs when the vessels to the brain are blocked or when cardiac output is abnormally low. A **transient ischemic attack (TIA)** is a temporary decrease in blood flow to the brain, with brief disturbances in speech, vision, and mobility; confusion; and numbness felt on one half of the body. TIAs are important warning signs of possibly impending strokes.

Complete lack of blood flow to specific areas of the brain causes tissue infarction, resulting in a cerebrovascular accident ("stroke").

Edema

An excess of fluid collected in the interstitium is called edema. Often it is the result of venous pooling caused by heart failure or incompetent venous valves. The capillaries become engorged, stretching the epithelium and eventually allowing fluid to leak from the overstretched vessel. This extravascular fluid collects in the surrounding tissue.

The resultant edema can cause pain by compressing local nerves. More importantly, swollen tissues compress capillaries and smaller arteries, limiting blood flow and causing ischemia.

Thrombus Formation

A thrombus is a solid mass or clot, which can develop in veins and steadily increase in size until it occupies the entire lumen of the vein. This halts blood flow because the clot becomes a barrier to incoming arterial blood. Wherever a clot blocks a vessel, ischemia, infarction, and tissue necrosis can occur.

An embolus occurs when a thrombus breaks loose and travels in the circulation. If the embolus lodges in the pulmonary artery, it is called a pulmonary embolism. Pulmonary emboli disrupt blood flow to the affected portion of the lung, disrupt gas exchange, and if large enough, can cause death.

Thrombi can form in any blood vessel, but they are particularly likely to form in the deep veins of the legs. The surgical client, the immobile client, and those with added risk for clot formation are the most susceptible to thrombus formation. Inappropriate blood clot formation is another potential consequence of venous pooling. Polycythemia, infection, malignancy, pregnancy, and oral contraceptives greatly increase the risk of clot formation (Knowlton-Moravec, 1995).

Organ Dysfunction and Failure

The vital organs require consistent, normal cardiac output and perfusion for optimal function. High blood pressure or ischemia can have serious consequences for the brain, the kidneys, or other vital organs. The greater the impairment of perfusion, the greater the possibility of permanent damage and possible organ failure.

Impact of Cardiovascular Dysfunction on Activities of Daily Living

Because oxygen is necessary for all activities, impaired cardiovascular function can limit the ability to perform normal activities. Frequently, the client will depend on family or friends to assist with many functions that he or she can no longer perform.

Individual Considerations

The functional range of activities for the client with cardiovascular problems varies widely. Some clients are severely disabled by their disease; others may experience little change in their activity levels. The ability to perform activities of daily living (ADLs) is determined by the extent to which the disease has affected oxygen delivery to tissues. Because all activity increases tissue oxygen demands, severe ischemia greatly limits activity. Conversely, minor alterations in blood flow or cardiac output have less effect on ADLs.

Frequently, after an acute cardiovascular episode, such as an MI or stroke, ability to perform normal ADLs may be severely restricted. The hospitalized cardiac client is often restricted from any form of activity for 1 to 2 days after an uncomplicated MI. Activity is slowly increased and individualized to ensure balance between oxygen demand and oxygen supply. The client may continue to experience fatigue after discharge. The time needed to return to work, normal social interaction, and normal sexual activity varies but is ordinarily within 6 to 8 weeks of discharge.

The client with impaired circulation, especially with severe peripheral vascular disease, may limit activity due to pain. Time needed for walking from place to place must include adequate time for rest. Clients who have limited perfusion of their hands experience a decrease in strength, and simple tasks, such as opening jars and using eating utensils, may become more difficult.

The client who has had a stroke can initially have great difficulty accomplishing ADLs. As the condition improves, the ability to perform ADLs varies greatly, depending on the extent of brain damage caused by the stroke.

Family Considerations

Cardiovascular dysfunction or disability impacts the entire family. Adequate support of the spouse or caregiver is important during this time (Levin, 1993). Any client who has limited activity tolerance probably needs help with normal tasks that require extensive movement or effort. Frequently, this changes role relationships; a family member may need to assume the role of caregiver or even breadwinner if the client is no longer able to work. Many cardiovascular problems are chronic and progressive, so the burden of care continually increases. Family members need to be taught cardiopulmonary resuscitation (CPR) and what to do in emergency situations. The threat of a sudden cardiac emergency can cause much anxiety among family members, which can contribute to social isolation if the family is afraid to leave the person alone. In some communities, service groups are available to help with shopping, meal preparation, housekeeping, or transportation.

Assessment

To formulate accurate nursing diagnoses and establish appropriate interventions, the nurse must assess the client's cardiovascular status. This includes gathering subjective data, most of which come from the health history. Objective data may include information gained through a physical examination of the client and from laboratory and diagnostic tests.

The extent and timeliness of this assessment vary depending on the immediate condition of the client. All clients must be assessed thoroughly and methodically, but this is easier in clients with stable or chronic cardiovascular conditions. Acutely ill clients who are experiencing severe chest pain or other acute symptoms must be assessed rapidly and on a moment-to-moment basis. In such cases, intervention is begun immediately, and evaluation is ongoing. Only after the client is stabilized can a thorough assessment be conducted. The method of assessment described here focuses on the client with stable cardiovascular problems.

Subjective Data

The nursing history helps the nurse identify patterns of normal cardiovascular function. To use the nursing history to its fullest, the nurse must be aware of factors that may place the client at risk for cardiovascular problems. The nurse also must be able to use information from the nursing history (and objective data sources) to identify basic patterns of cardiovascular dysfunction so that appropriate intervention can be initiated.

Functional Pattern Identification

Like breathing, normal cardiovascular function is taken for granted; as a continuous process, the regularity of the system becomes virtually unnoticeable. The nurse can gain information about the client's normal functional pattern by assessing activity tolerance. The ability to perform a normal range of daily activities and to tolerate a reasonable level of physical exertion strongly indicates good cardiovascular health. Most people experience no chest pain or other remarkable discomfort while at rest or while engaged in moderate activity. Practically everyone is aware that strenuous work or exercise causes the heart to beat faster and more forcefully. Because this is recognized as normal, few people would call these changes "pain" or "discomfort." Consequently, complaints of chest pain with activity always warrant a full investigation.

The nurse assesses activity tolerance by first determining whether the client experiences pain, discomfort, or any other symptom during physical activity. The majority of people who report no pain or activity restriction are usually free of significant cardiovascular disease. People with cardiovascular problems often experience discomfort, pain, or other symptoms at a lower level of activity than the healthy person. This usually leads to self-imposed restriction of activities as the person adjusts to the condition.

Risk Identification

Many factors contribute to the development of cardiovascular problems. Direct observations and the nursing history can be instrumental in identifying those factors. The nurse should question the client concerning past cardiovascular conditions, such as a previous MI, stroke, or circulatory difficulties. The nurse also must determine any functional deficits that resulted from these conditions and the management program the client is using. Increased risk can be assessed by asking the client if any close family members have had cardiovascular problems.

The nurse should determine the extent of the client's smoking. The number of packs of cigarettes smoked daily and the number of years smoked (pack-per-year history) are important measures of the client's total exposure to smoking.

Dietary intake of saturated fats, cholesterol, and sodium should be assessed. Clients can be asked directly about cooking habits and dietary patterns, but many people are unaware of the fat, cholesterol, and sodium content of specific foods. It may help to ask the client to describe a normal day's intake and ask for an estimate of specific high-risk foods (eg, "how many eggs do you eat per week?"). Despite an increased emphasis on health, much of the prepackaged supermarket food and food sold in "fast food" restaurants contain an extremely high percentage of fat and sodium. Because many people regularly eat these convenience foods, the nurse should investigate the client's eating habits with this in mind.

Activity and exercise patterns should be assessed to determine increased risk for cardiovascular dysfunction. Questions such as, "How often do you exercise each week, and what type of activities do you enjoy?" may be helpful. Assess how much of the client's work day is comprised of sedentary activity.

Information concerning any medications the client is taking must be obtained. Many medications have side effects that can have an impact on cardiovascular function. If the medication is specifically for a cardiovascular condition, the nurse should assess the length of time the medication has been taken, the dose, the client's knowledge of the medication, and any side effects the client may have experienced. The use or abuse of recreational drugs, especially IV drugs or cocaine, should be determined.

Dysfunction Identification

Finding out why the client has sought medical care is the first step in determining the nature of the client's health complaint. The client should be allowed to explain in his or her own words without interruption. After the initial explanation, the nurse should seek specific clarification concerning the problem.

Nursing Assessment

Initial Questions for the Client Experiencing Chest Pain

- When did the pain start?
- What were you doing when it began?
- Does anything you do make it go away?
- Does the pain increase with deep breathing or movement?
- Does the pain go anywhere else (eg, to the arms, neck, or back)?
- Do you feel any other unusual symptoms (eg, shortness of breath, nausea, dizziness, fear)?
- What is the nature of the pain? Is it pressure, stabbing, dull, crushing, sharp, constant?

Pain is the most common reason people with cardiovascular dysfunction seek medical and nursing aid. The nurse should determine the specific nature of the pain: its location, its intensity, and the circumstances that cause it. See the display listing questions to ask the client who is experiencing chest pain.

Activity restriction is an important subjective measure of cardiovascular dysfunction. The nurse must establish the level of activity associated with the onset of pain or discomfort. Some relevant questions to determine activity restriction include, "do the symptoms occur only during strenuous exercise, such as running or playing basketball?" "Do they occur when walking at a normal pace? If so, how far can you walk before the symptoms begin?" "Does quiet household activity bring on the symptoms?" "Do you experience the symptoms during periods of rest?" "Do any other circumstances, such as weather or emotional stress, tend to cause or exaggerate the problem?" "Do the symptoms appear at particular times of the day?"

Other subjective complaints may occur with cardiovascular problems. A nocturnal cough or dyspnea, dizziness, "blackouts," swelling of hands or ankles, and changes in skin color or sensation are significant. The nurse must gather as much specific information concerning these symptoms as possible. This information forms the basis for physical examination and further diagnostic investigation.

Objective Data

Physical Assessment

Physical examination of the client is helpful to assess cardiovascular status and detect actual or potential alterations in cardiovascular function.

Inspection. Observing the client's general behavior and appearance yields significant information about tissue perfusion and cardiac output. Because the brain is extremely sensitive to any decrease in blood flow, assessment of sensorium and level of consciousness provides clues about cerebral perfusion. Decreased cardiac output, vascular disease, or both can change cognitive and perceptual function.

Sensorium is often the first indicator of perfusion to be assessed because it is readily apparent in the nurse's first interactions with the client. People with normal cerebral perfusion usually speak in a normal cadence, answer questions quickly and appropriately, and are oriented to person, place, and time. They are able to follow directions. The nurse should note slowness of speech or other overt difficulties with speaking. Inappropriate responses to questions or statements, confusion, apathy, decreased understanding, disorientation, restlessness, or anxiety are all possible signs of decreased cerebral perfusion. Level of consciousness is indicated by client arousability. The well-perfused client is easily aroused; one who requires much stimulation to respond may have diminished cerebral blood flow.

Appearance of the client also provides information about circulatory status. Because skin color can roughly indicate blood flow adequacy, the person should be examined for central and peripheral cyanosis. In light-skinned clients, pallor or blanched skin is evidence of possible ischemia or anemia. Localized skin discolorations, such as bruises, redness, or mottling, also should be noted. The presence of dependent edema (in the hands, sacrum, or ankles) indicates possible circulatory problems. Neck veins should be relatively flat; engorgement of these veins implies inefficient right heart pumping.

The legs and arms should be inspected for changes in hair distribution, shiny skin, ulcerations, edema, and venous distention. Any varicosities should be noted. Toenails and fingernails should be smooth; ridged, thickened, hornlike nails indicate decreased peripheral perfusion. Digits are normally round in shape, but exaggeratedly rounded, "clubbed" fingertips are associated with oxygenation problems, from lung or cardiovascular disease.

Palpation. The well-perfused client is warm and dry to the touch. Although cool extremities are normal in many people, chronically cold fingers and toes often indicate poor circulation.

Capillary refill time also reflects peripheral tissue perfusion and cardiac output. This is determined by pressing a nailbed until it blanches (Fig. 35-4). Pressure is released, and the time it takes for the nail to return to its original color is noted. This "capillary refill time" is ordinarily less than 3 seconds. A longer refill time indicates narrowing of the blood vessel serving the digit, decreased circulating blood volume, or otherwise decreased cardiac output.

Edema also is palpated and its extent noted (Fig. 35-5). Edema has traditionally been described in terms

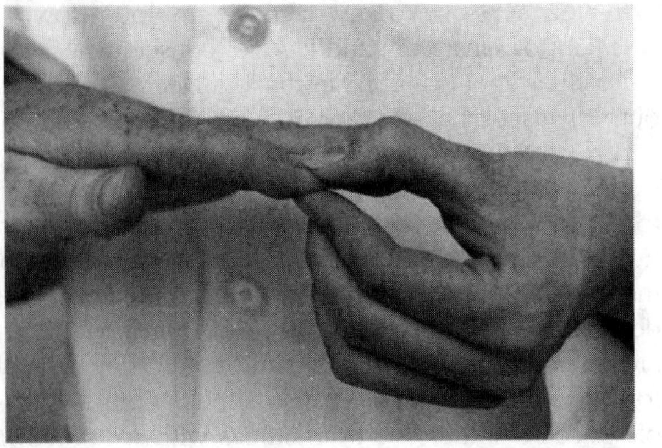

Figure 35-4 *• Test for capillary refill time. Pressure is applied to nail bed and then released. Time for nail to regain color is noted.*

of a scale ranging from zero (no edema present) to four (severe, pitting edema). This scale offers a subjective but moderately useful means for indicating the amount of edema present.

More accurate means of measuring edema include serial measurements of affected extremities or abdominal girth (for ascites). Daily weight assessment also can indicate the extent of edema present. A weight gain of 10 lb (indicative of 5 L of extracellular fluid volume) precedes visible edema in most clients (Skov & Underhill Motzer, 1995).

Homan's sign is assessed by experienced practitioners to determine the possibility of deep vein phlebitis. This test is performed by bending the client's foot upward toward the leg (dorsiflexion). When performed properly, pain or tenderness in the calf suggests vein inflammation.

Pulse is palpated for quality and rate. Regularity of rhythm, pulse intensity, and the number of beats per minute are noted. Peripheral circulation is assessed, with the nurse checking femoral, popliteal (behind the knee), and dorsalis pedis (ankle) pulses for equal intensity in both legs. If an irregular pulse is detected, the apical and radial pulses should be assessed simultaneously to detect the presence of a pulse deficit (refer to Procedure 22-3).

Auscultation. A stethoscope is used to determine blood pressure, count the apical pulse, and identify normal and abnormal heart sounds.

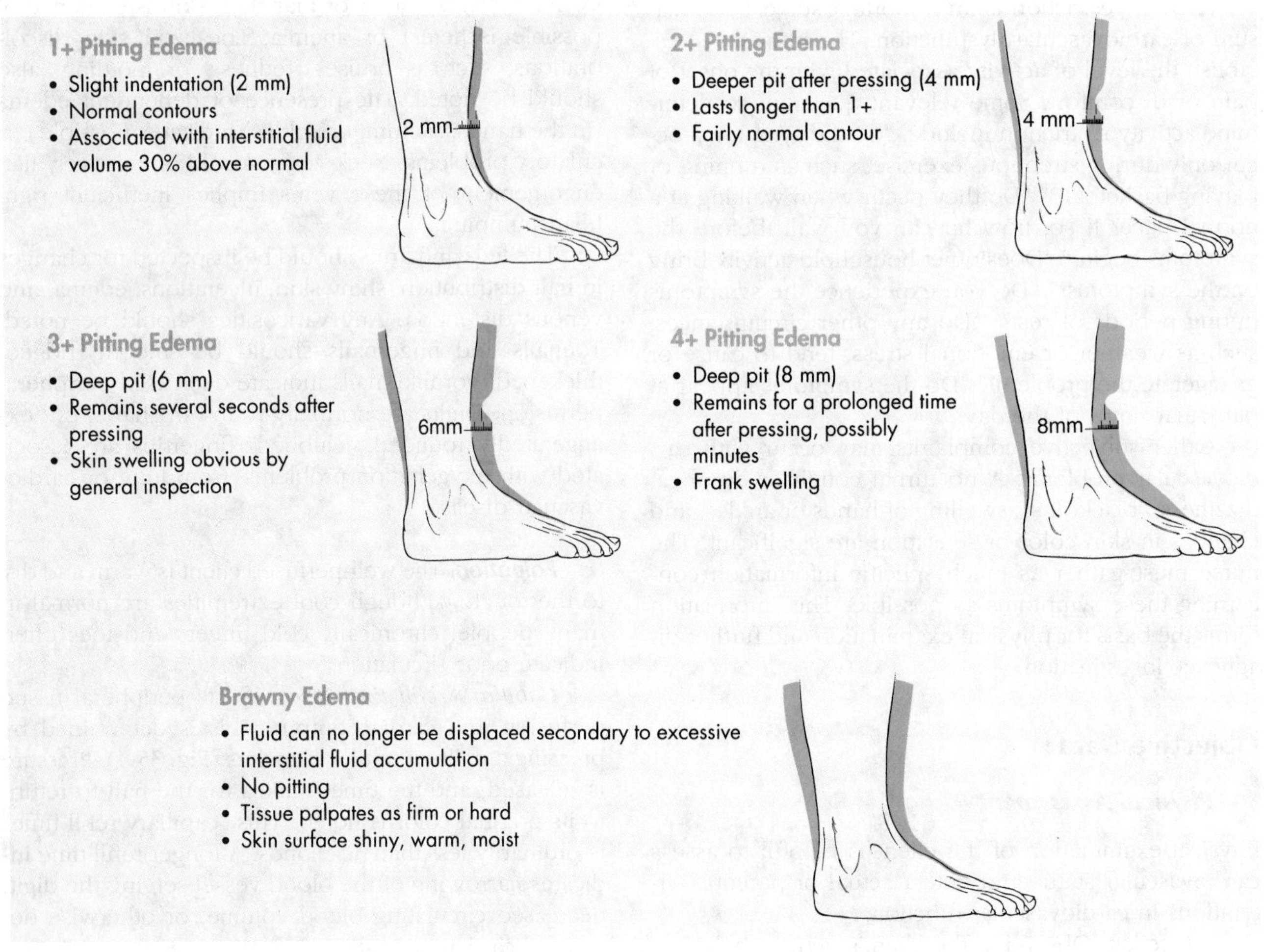
1+ Pitting Edema
• Slight indentation (2 mm)
• Normal contours
• Associated with interstitial fluid volume 30% above normal
2 mm
2+ Pitting Edema
• Deeper pit after pressing (4 mm)
• Lasts longer than 1+
• Fairly normal contour
4 mm
3+ Pitting Edema
• Deep pit (6 mm)
• Remains several seconds after pressing
• Skin swelling obvious by general inspection
6mm
4+ Pitting Edema
• Deep pit (8 mm)
• Remains for a prolonged time after pressing, possibly minutes
• Frank swelling
8mm
Brawny Edema
• Fluid can no longer be displaced secondary to excessive interstitial fluid accumulation
• No pitting
• Tissue palpates as firm or hard
• Skin surface shiny, warm, moist

Figure 35-5 *• Edema can be graded by gently pressing the edematous area with the fingers for up to 5 seconds.*

Blood pressure is assessed to establish the presence of hypotension, high blood pressure, and positional differences. (For a detailed discussion of pulse and blood pressure assessment, see Chap. 22.)

Apical pulse is determined by auscultation to establish its rate and character. This is a simple yet essential measurement for the complete assessment of the client who has a pulse that is difficult to palpate or a heart rate that is irregular. It also is necessary to auscultate the apical pulse when administering certain medications, notably cardiac glycosides, such as digoxin.

Normal heart sounds, murmurs, or other adventitious sounds also are audible by stethoscope. Normal heart sounds, S_1 and S_2, are the "lub" and "dub" that are normally heard as the heart valves close. Abnormal heart sounds, such as murmurs, gallops, or clicks, and normal heart sounds are discussed in Chapter 21. Interpretation of these sounds takes a considerable amount of practice and a strong understanding of their underlying physiology.

Diagnostic Tests and Procedures

The most common tests and procedures are described briefly here. For a more detailed discussion of diagnostic tests and procedures, consult Chapter 22 or a text on cardiovascular nursing. Table 35-1 lists selected tests and diagnostic procedures used to assess cardiovascular function.

Laboratory Studies. Several laboratory tests yield useful information concerning cardiovascular function. These tests range from basic blood assessment to highly sophisticated assays.

The complete blood count (CBC) provides information on white blood cells, platelets, and sedimentation rate. In addition, the CBC determines the number of red blood cells, hemoglobin, and hematocrit. These latter measures are important indicators of the oxygen-carrying capability of the blood.

Cardiac enzymes are proteins that are liberated from cells when tissue damage occurs. Serum levels of creatine kinase (CK), CK-MB, and lactic dehydrogenase are measured to confirm a suspected MI.

Kidney function studies can indicate problems with perfusion. Blood urea nitrogen and creatinine may be elevated in clients with hypoperfusion of the kidneys.

Deviations from normal levels of *serum electrolytes* can adversely affect cardiovascular function. Arrhythmias result from potassium imbalances. Sodium increases lead to extra fluid volume and increased cardiac work. Levels of these electrolytes are affected by diuretics and other drugs that affect cardiac function. They also are altered by changes in kidney function, acid-base status, and fluid balance.

Blood lipids include cholesterol and triglycerides. Lipids, linked to proteins known as lipoproteins, also are measured. Elevated blood levels of low-density lipoproteins are strongly associated with peripheral vascular disease and coronary artery disease. Conversely, high-density lipoproteins have been associated with a reduced risk for cardiovascular diseases. Although this test does not confirm or rule out the presence of cardiovascular disease, it is a useful screening tool for identifying those who are at risk (Goe, 1995).

Diagnostic Procedures. A variety of invasive and noninvasive procedures have been devised to study the

Table 35-1 • Selected Tests and Procedures Used to Assess Cardiovascular Function

Test/Procedure	Purpose
Complete blood count	Yields information on platelets, presence or absence of infection, oxygen-carrying capacity; to diagnose anemias, nutritional deficiencies, and selected metabolic disorders
Blood chemistry tests	Determine serum electrolytes, lipids; also creatinine and BUN to assess kidney function
Serum enzymes	Rule out or confirm myocardial infarction (MI)
EKG	Identify arrhythmias, determine types and extent of heart damage from MI
Stress EKG (treadmill)	Identify cardiac abnormalities not evident on resting EKG
Echocardiography	Measure heart size and thickness; observe valve function; measure cardiac output
Heart catheterization	Measure pressure within heart chambers to determine heart strength, valve competency, cardiac output, and fluid volume status
Angiography	Outlines blood flow through vessels to identify blockages, aneurysms

cardiovascular system. Some are simple and require relatively basic skills and equipment. Others can be conducted only in the most technologically advanced facilities.

Diagnostic procedures yield information about cardiac function or blood flow. Tests relating to the heart include those that measure its electrical conductivity (such as electrocardiography and exercise testing) and those that measure its size and mechanical ability (such as echocardiography and cardiac catheterization). Angiography and hemodynamic monitoring provide precise information concerning blood flow.

Electrocardiography (ECG) records electrical impulse conduction of the heart in the resting client. Electrodes are placed on specific areas of the client's limbs and chest. The electrodes are connected to a highly sensitive voltmeter, which controls a delicate pen. As the electrodes detect electrical impulses, the pen scribes a tracing on a moving strip of paper. The various deflections of the ECG tracing correspond to the individual events of the cardiac conduction cycle (Fig. 35-6).

Electrodes are placed on several areas of the limbs and chest to provide several "views" of cardiac impulses. Many views (called "leads") are needed to differentiate among the various conditions that can affect the heart, because abnormalities may not appear in all leads. Single-lead ECGs are useful for continuous monitoring of a client, but the standard 12-lead ECG is needed for a thorough evaluation of the heart's electrical conductivity. When properly interpreted, the ECG can detect myocardial damage, cardiac ischemia, alterations from normal heart rhythm, changes in heart position or size, or problems within the conduction system.

Exercise testing can assess a person's response to cardiovascular stress. In some people, problems of cardiac ischemia may not be detectable with a conventional resting ECG because these problems may occur only during periods of activity.

The test involves the use of a treadmill, a "moving sidewalk" with adjustable speed and slope. The client begins walking at a normal pace on the treadmill. The ECG and blood pressure are monitored continually while the speed and slope of the treadmill are gradually increased. The test usually lasts about 15 minutes, unless it is terminated because of ECG or blood pressure changes or by the client's fatigue, pain, or shortness of breath. Exercise testing allows practitioners to determine with some precision the degree of the person's functional ability.

Echocardiography uses ultrasonic waves to diagnose structural defects of the heart. This technique evolved from the use of marine sonar equipment, in which sound is bounced off structures, forming identifiable patterns. A penlike probe sends high-frequency sound waves through the chest wall. The waves produce "echoes" as they bounce off the heart, and the echo pattern is recorded. Using these patterns, cardiologists can obtain an accurate view of the heart without performing potentially dangerous invasive procedures, such as catheterization. Myocardial muscle thickness and motion, structure and motion of the valves, the size of the chambers, and the presence of fluid around the heart can be detected with echocardiography.

Catheterization of the heart and large vessels is used to determine precise information concerning valve function and cardiac muscle strength. Various types of catheters can be inserted through a vein or artery and directed (under fluoroscopy) into the chambers of the heart. The catheter is able to measure the pressure generated within each of the chambers and to establish how efficiently the heart is pumping.

Some types of cardiac catheters also can measure cardiac output and pressures within the pulmonary vascular system. Because they furnish information about vascular pressures, indwelling catheters are valuable tools in fluid and blood pressure management. Pulmonary artery and central venous pressure catheters are used for this purpose.

Arterial catheters allow the nurse to monitor arterial blood pressure closely and to draw blood for evaluation of oxygenation and acid-base status. Arterial and other indwelling vascular catheters, are used only where constant monitoring is possible, usually in an intensive care setting.

Blood flow studies determine the patency and shape of blood vessels and the direction and volume of blood flow through them. The simplest and least expensive test of this type is Doppler examination. Doppler instruments enhance the turbulent sounds made by blood as it circulates through the heart or vessels. Using ultrasound technology, the Doppler instrument produces a graphic representation of the course of blood flow.

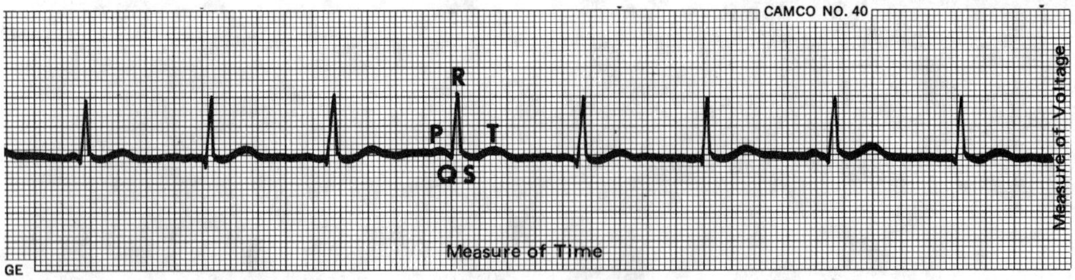

Figure 35-6 • *An electrocardiogram provides valuable information about the heart's ability to conduct impulses.*

Angiography uses a radiopaque dye to outline blood vessels and to confirm or rule out vessel blockage. This technique also is used to detect aneurysms. Radionuclide examinations use radioactive substances to detect MI and decreased myocardial blood flow.

The chest x-ray can establish the size and shape of the heart and aorta and detect pulmonary congestion or edema. It is used to confirm correct placement of indwelling heart catheters and pacemakers.

Nursing Diagnoses

Appropriate nursing diagnoses concerning the client's response to altered cardiovascular function are based on accurate interpretation of assessment data. The two primary North American Nursing Diagnosis Association (NANDA) nursing diagnoses that specifically address problems of cardiovascular function are Altered Tissue Perfusion and Decreased Cardiac Output. Activity Intolerance also is a significant problem for many clients with cardiovascular dysfunction, although Activity Intolerance is not exclusively a cardiovascular problem.

Diagnostic Statement: Altered Tissue Perfusion (Renal, Cerebral, Cardiopulmonary, Gastrointestinal, Peripheral)*

Definition

Altered tissue perfusion is the state in which an individual experiences a decrease in nutrition and oxygenation at the cellular level due to a deficit in capillary blood supply (NANDA, 1994).

* The cerebral, renal, and gastrointestinal subcomponents require further work.

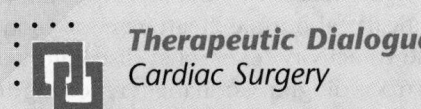

Therapeutic Dialogue
Cardiac Surgery

Scenes for Thought

Jean Norman is a 77-year-old woman with snowy curls and a stately air. She's lying in her bed in the ICU with tubes and beeping monitors around her. She turns to you as you approach with an extra blanket; one of your colleagues had told you Ms. Norman had requested one.

Effective

Client: *Thank you for the blanket, dear. I'm so cold here.* She speaks softly and weakly.
Nurse: *How are you feeling otherwise, Ms. Norman? (Arranging the blanket over her.)*
Client: *Very tired and sore. I guess a bypass operation takes a lot out of you.* She smiles weakly. *But I'm sure it will turn out fine.* She doesn't maintain eye contact.
Nurse: *I wonder if you have some doubts about that. (Standing at the bedside, looking at her.)*
Client: Looks at you in surprise. *Why, what do you mean, dear?*
Nurse: *I was just wondering if you might be a little more worried than you let on. You seem to be the kind of person that doesn't want to trouble others with your worries. Is that so?*
Client: Her eyes fill with tears, and she looks toward the hallway where her husband is sitting. *Yes. I'm really worried about my heart and the scar on my chest and if I'll ever be able to be as active as I was.* Crying.
Nurse: *(Holding her hand, standing quietly by the bed.)*
Client: *I know I'm being silly. People go through this operation all the time.* Drying her eyes.
Nurse: *It's usual for people to be worried. I'm glad you decided to share that worry with me. Would you like to talk a little more about it? Maybe I can help.*
Client: *Do you think so? You don't think I'm being neurotic about this?*
Nurse: *I'm not sure what you mean by neurotic, but I know that you seem fearful, and sometimes talking about fears helps them become more manageable.*
Client: *That's true.* She begins to talk about her fear of becoming an invalid and not being able to golf with her husband.

Less Effective

Client: *Thank you for the blanket, dear. I'm so cold here.* She speaks softly and weakly.
Nurse: *How are you feeling otherwise, Ms. Norman? (Arranging the blanket over her.)*
Client: *Very tired and sore. I guess a bypass operation takes a lot out of you.* She smiles weakly. *But I'm sure it will turn out fine.* She doesn't maintain eye contact.
Nurse: *You seem to be doing just great—look at your blood pressure, temperature, and EKG! I don't think I've seen too many people recover from surgery this fast, honestly. Are you in much pain right now? (Standing quietly by the bed and holding her hand.)*
Client: *A little. If you have some time perhaps you could get me something?* Still smiling.
Nurse: *Right away, Ms. Norman. You only have to let me know. (Smiling and giving her hand a warm squeeze.)*
Client: *Thank you, dear. I appreciate it.* Squeezing back.

Critical Thinking Challenge

• Both nurses cared for Ms. Norman's needs. Compare and contrast the dialogues and detect what made the second dialogue less effective. • Explain the relationship between fear and pain. • Relate fear and recovery, giving reasons for your decisions. • Evaluate the wisdom of a person who has recovered from bypass surgery going golfing.

Defining Characteristics

Table 35-2 lists defining characteristics with the chances that the characteristics will be present in the diagnoses, as outlined by NANDA. NANDA does note that additional work and development are necessary for the subcomponents involving cerebral, renal, and gastrointestinal blood flow.

Related Factors

Related factors include interruption of arterial blood flow, interruption of venous blood flow, exchange problems, hypovolemia, and hypervolemia (NANDA, 1994).

Diagnostic Statement: Decreased Cardiac Output

Definition

Decreased cardiac output is a state in which the blood pumped by an individual's heart is sufficiently reduced so that it is inadequate to meet the needs of the body's tissues (NANDA, 1994).

Defining Characteristics

Defining characteristics include variations in blood pressure readings, arrhythmias; fatigue; jugular vein distention; color changes in skin and mucous membranes; oliguria; decreased peripheral pulses; cold, clammy skin; rales; dyspnea, orthopnea; restlessness; change in mental status; shortness of breath; syncope; vertigo; edema; cough; frothy sputum; gallop heart rhythm; and weakness (NANDA, 1994).

Related Factors

NANDA has not yet developed related factors.

Diagnostic Statement: Activity Intolerance

Definition

Decreased activity intolerance is a state in which an individual has insufficient physiologic or psychological energy to endure or complete required or desired daily activities (NANDA, 1994).

Defining Characteristics

Defining characteristics include verbal report of fatigue or weakness (critical), abnormal heart rate or blood pressure response to activity, exertional discomfort or dyspnea, and electrocardiographic changes reflecting arrhythmias or ischemia (NANDA, 1994).

Related Factors

Related factors include bedrest or immobility, generalized weakness, sedentary lifestyle, and imbalance between oxygen supply and demand (NANDA, 1994).

Table 35-2 • Defining Characteristics for Altered Tissue Perfusion

	Chances That Characteristics Will Be Present In Given Diagnosis	Estimated Sensitivities and Specificities; Chances That Characteristic Cannot Be Explained By Any Other Diagnosis
Skin temperature, cold extremities	High	Low
Skin color		
Dependent blue or purple	Moderate	Low
Pale on elevation; color does not return on lowering of leg*	High	High
Diminished arterial pulsations*	High	High
Skin quality: shining	High	Low
Lack of lanugo	High	Moderate
Round scars covered with atrophied skin		
Gangrene	Low	High
Slow-growing, dry, brittle nails	High	Moderate
Claudication	Moderate	High
Blood pressure changes in extremities		
Bruits	Moderate	Moderate
Slow healing of lesions	High	Low

*Highly specific and sensitive for diagnosis.

Adapted from North American Nursing Diagnosis Association (1990). *Taxonomy I revised 1990, with official nursing diagnosis.* St. Louis, MO: Author.

Related Nursing Diagnoses

Other nursing diagnoses are common for people with cardiovascular dysfunction. These include Fluid Volume Excess; Risk for Infection; Altered Nutrition: Less than body requirements; Pain; and Sleep Pattern Disturbance. Circulatory problems and heart disease also affect the client's ability to carry out ADLs. Possible nursing diagnoses related to this include Fatigue or Self-Care Deficit. Anxiety, Ineffective Individual Coping, and Ineffective Family Coping are examples of possible psychosocial nursing diagnoses. Knowledge Deficit is common as clients often must learn about new medications, diet, or management strategies to cope with cardiovascular dysfunction.

Outcome Identification and Planning

Outcomes are individualized based on the client's health status. In general, the following are appropriate goals for the cardiovascular client:

- Client will demonstrate adequate knowledge concerning cardiovascular dysfunction, prevention, or care.
- Client will maintain adequate cardiac output.
- Client will demonstrate adequate tissue perfusion with adequate oxygenation of body tissue.
- Client will cope effectively with resulting changes in self-concept and lifestyle.

Specific outcomes for the healthy person focus on prevention of cardiovascular problems by increased awareness of risk factors associated with cardiovascular dysfunction. Outcomes pertinent to the client admitted with an acute problem focus on recovery from the cardiovascular problem without residual complications. Realistic outcomes for the chronic cardiovascular client focus on helping the client to live within limitations imposed by the disease and to improve acceptance of changes in lifestyle and self-concept. Outcomes for the terminal cardiovascular client should revolve around the maintenance of adequate comfort and acceptance of impending death.

Examples of nursing interventions commonly used in planning for clients with cardiovascular problems are summarized in the accompanying display.

Planning

Examples of Nursing Interventions Used for Cardiac Problems

Activity Intolerance

- Monitor pulse, respiratory rate, and subjective feelings during activity.
- Space activities.
- Permit rest periods before activity.
- Limit activity 1 hour after meals.
- Teach energy conservation measures.

Edema

- Instruct client to avoid constricting garments.
- Instruct client to elevate edematous area.
- Instruct client to avoid dependent positioning.
- Teach client about fluid- or sodium-restricted diet.
- Apply antiembolism stockings.

Pain (due to inadequate oxygen supply)

- Instruct client to stop activity when pain occurs.
- Administer nitroglycerin or vasodilators as ordered.
- Pace activities within client's limits.
- Instruct client to avoid cold temperature and smoking.
- Instruct client to report unrelieved pain to appropriate healthcare professional.

Implementation

Nursing Interventions to Promote Health and Function

Risk Factor Modification

The primary prevention of cardiovascular disease starts with an understanding of its causes. The nurse can be instrumental in promoting cardiovascular health by instructing people and groups on the dangers posed by the many risk factors associated with cardiovascular disease. Teaching is provided in the areas of smoking cessation, nutrition, and activity. Presenting information concerning risk factors in a nonsensational, objective manner can help consumers choose appropriate behavior modification measures.

The nurse can help clients who are seeking to modify their risk for cardiovascular disease by being knowledgeable about (and taking part in) local support groups and classes that focus on this goal. The recent proliferation of self-help programs, fitness clubs, and aggressively advertised diets has provided the consumer with many choices. The nurse should be able to offer guidance in program selection and help the client identify (and avoid) programs that promise overly simplistic or unrealistic means to cardiovascular health.

The client may need to be made aware of appropriate supervised physical activity programs. If the client has a known medical problem or is older than 35 years, the nurse should recommend a complete physical examination before the client starts an exercise regimen.Various classes or support groups may be available to help the client alter unhealthful lifestyle habits.

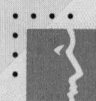

Client Teaching
Cardiovascular Conditions

Instruct the client as follows:

- *Restrict fat, cholesterol, and sodium in your diet to promote cardiovascular health.*
- *If you have chronic angina, take nitroglycerin before activities requiring exertion.*
- *If you take digoxin, monitor your pulse and notify your doctor if the pulse rate falls below 60 (unless instructed otherwise), or you are experiencing irregularities of rhythm, nausea, weakness, or visual changes; these symptoms may indicate digoxin toxicity.*
- *If you have poor peripheral circulation, examine your feet daily for redness or signs of skin breakdown. Poor circulation decreases sensation and increases the time it takes for sores to heal.*
- *Do not cross your legs or wear constricting clothing because impaired circulation can occur.*
- *If you experience ischemia (angina or intermittent claudication), alternate periods of activity with periods of rest to lessen pain.*
- *Apply antiembolism stockings before getting out of bed in the morning to prevent dependent edema and to make application easier.*

Diet management, smoking cessation, and stress management programs are often sponsored by the hospital or other local agencies. Nurses may be instrumental in developing and implementing such programs in the private workplace. The goal of these programs is the promotion of cardiovascular health.

Prevention of Venous Stasis

Venous stasis in the client with limited mobility may result in edema and embolization. The nurse helps to reduce the risk of dangerous clot formation by taking measures to improve the return of blood to the heart. Leg exercises, antiembolic stockings, sequential compression devices, and avoidance of constriction help to prevent venous stasis.

Leg Exercises. Leg exercises improve circulation and prevent venous stasis. Leg exercises are commonly taught to preoperative clients to prevent postoperative circulatory complications. These simple exercises are helpful for any client with impaired mobility, especially those on bed rest.

Leg exercises alternately contract and relax the quadriceps and gastrocnemius muscles of the lower extremity. Contraction of these muscles helps promote the flow of blood back to the heart. Three separate leg movements can be encouraged (Fig. 35-7). First, have the client perform *calf-pumping* exercises, which involve alternate dorsiflexion and plantar flexion of the feet. Second, have the client bend one knee, sliding the foot up as far as possible along the mattress and back again. This process should be repeated with the other leg. Finally, have the client alternately raise and lower each straight leg off the mattress as far as comfort allows.

Leg exercises should begin as soon as the client returns from surgery or whenever the client is immobile. Exercises should be performed at least once every 1 to 2 hours while the client is awake. If the client is not able to perform leg exercises independently because of decreased strength or neurologic impairment, the nurse must assist with passive leg exercises, encouraging as much client participation as possible.

Antiembolism Stockings. Immobility deprives the bedridden client of the circulatory benefit of muscular contraction against the veins. Venous engorgement can be offset in these clients by the use of antiembolic stockings. Antiembolism stockings are made of strong elastic material. They are not the same as support hose, because they provide varying degrees of compression at different areas of the leg (Bright & Georgi, 1994). When correctly fitted and applied, they exert external pressure against the vein wall, decreasing pooling in the extremities. The stockings promote venous return in much the same manner as the leg muscles, using continuous instead of intermittent pressure.

To do their job effectively, antiembolism stockings must fit properly. Stockings that are too large for the client cannot provide sufficient vein compression; stockings that are too tight can shut off blood flow to the legs. Guidelines for proper measurement and size selection of antiembolism stockings are available from the manufacturer and should be followed instead of estimating stocking size by the height or weight. Wrinkles or poorly made seams can lead to pressure sores on the skin. Instructions on application of antiembolism stockings are given in Procedure 35-1.

The nurse must inspect the client's legs and feet regularly to ensure that circulation is not impeded by the stockings. Antiembolism stockings are usually removed for 30 minutes once every 8 hours. When in place, the toes should remain warm, and there should be no obvious constriction or excoriation caused by the stockings. The stockings should be applied in the morning, before the client has gotten out of bed. This allows them to be fitted while the client's legs are least edematous.

Pneumatic Compression Devices. Intermittent compression devices improve venous return by alternating pressure exerted against the extremity by inflating and deflating plastic sleeves that are wrapped around the leg. The pneumatic compression device consists of an air

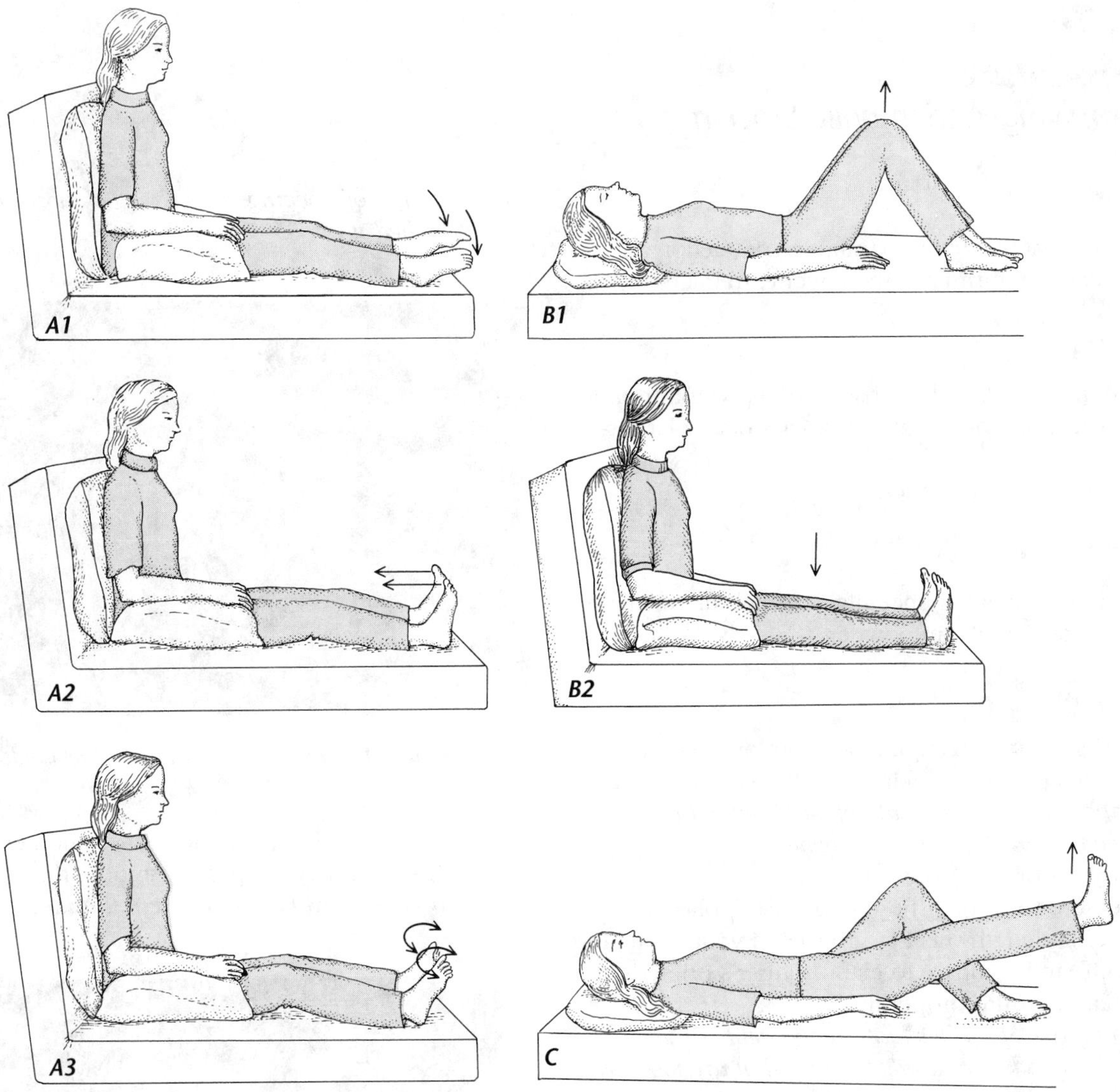

Figure 35-7 • *Leg exercises to improve circulation.* ***(A)*** *Calf pumping exercises: dorsiflexion and plantarflexion. (1) Point toes of both feet toward the foot of the bed; relax. (2) Pull toes toward the chin; relax. (3) Make circles with both ankles, one direction and then the other; repeat three times; relax.* ***(B)*** *Knee flexion and extension (1) With knees flexed and feet flat on the bed, (2) slide feet forward as far as possible and (1) back to flexed position.* ***(C)*** *Raising and lowering leg. Raise and lower each straight leg alternatively while the other leg is flexed. Raise as far as comfort allows without straining.*

pump, extremity sleeves, and connecting tubing. Pneumatic compression devices are of two types: intermittent or sequential. Sequential compression devices (SCD) sequentially compress various chambers within the extremity sleeve to promote venous return. A complete cycle can take 75 seconds to 5 minutes. Each of these devices is attached to an air pump that alternates inflation and deflation of the sleeve. Frequently, SCDs are ordered for the immobilized client or the surgical client while on bed rest. Antiembolic hose are often worn underneath the plastic sleeves to decrease irritation from the plastic and provide extra support. When the client gets up to ambulate, the devices are removed, and once ambulation has resumed sequential compression devices are usually discontinued. Pneumatic compression devices should not be used in clients with arterial occlusive disease, severe edema, cellulitis, or infection of the extremity. Refer to Procedure 35-2 for application of sequential compression devices.

Avoiding Constriction. Immobilized and inactive clients must be warned against venous constriction. Any article of clothing that exerts excessive pressure on the calves or thighs may constrict the veins. This diminishes venous return and promotes the formation of clots and varicosities. The use of garters or the practice of wearing stockings knotted above the knee should be dis-

text continues on pg. 965

Procedure 35-1
Applying Antiembolic Stockings

Purpose

1. Supplement the action of muscle contraction and aid venous return from the lower extremities

Assessment

- Identify clients at high risk for deep vein thrombosis (eg, long-term bed rest or cardiovascular disease).
- Obtain physician order.

Equipment

Stockings (available in knee-high or thigh-high lengths)
Baby powder or talcum powder

Procedure

1. Position client in supine position for one-half hour before applying stockings.
   Rationale: Veins should not be distended with blood when stockings are applied.
2. Provide for client privacy.
3. Measure for proper fit prior to first application. Measure length (heel to groin) and width (calf and thigh) and compare to manufacturer's printed material to ensure proper fit.
   Rationale: Stockings that are too tight can lead to venous occlusion, and stockings that are too loose will not promote venous return.

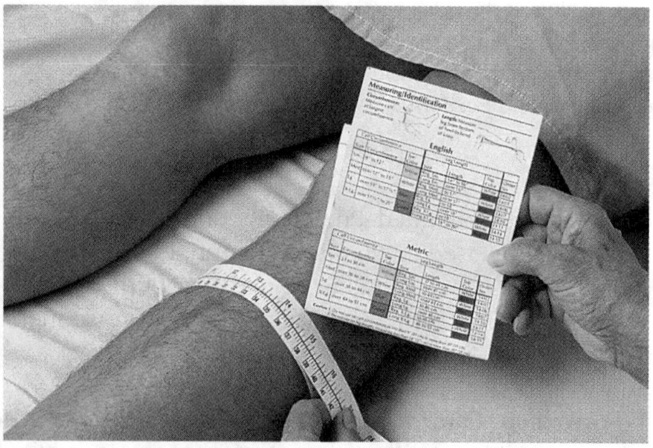

Step 3 • *Measure to ensure proper fit.*

4. Turn stocking inside out, tucking foot inside.
   Rationale: Inside out method allows for easier application of stocking, because stocking is not bunched up.

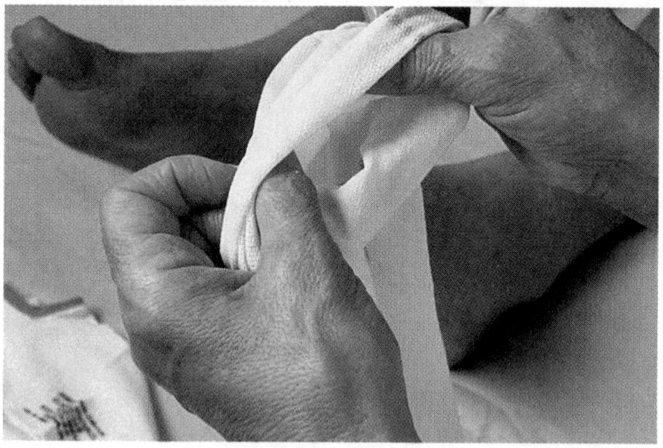

Step 4 • *Turn stocking inside out, tucking heel inside.*

5. Ease foot section over client's toe and heel, adjusting as necessary for proper smooth fit.
   Rationale: Wrinkles impede circulation.

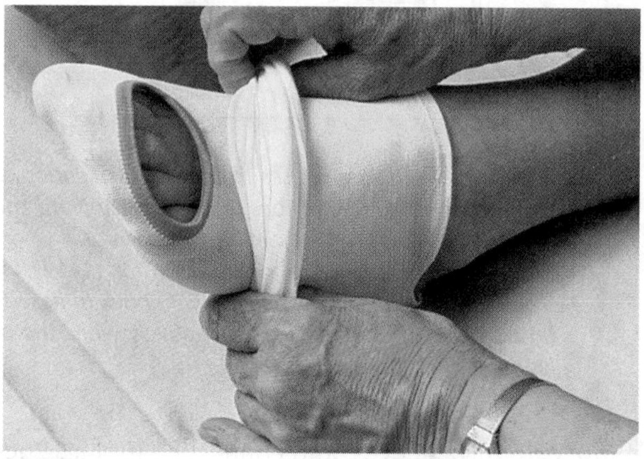

Step 5 • *Ease foot section over toe and heel.*

6. Gently pull the stocking over the leg, removing all wrinkles.
   Rationale: Irregularities in fit may cause pressure areas.
   Hint: Baby powder or talc lightly sprinkled over the foot and leg may make stocking application easier.
7. Assess toes for circulation and warmth. Check area at the top of the stocking for binding.

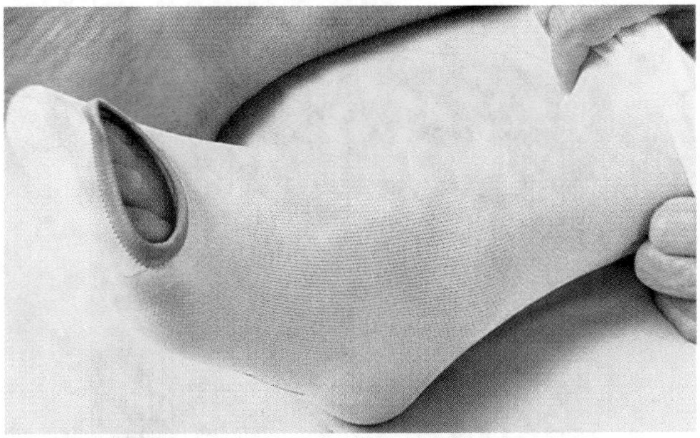

Step 6* • *Pull stocking over the rest of leg.

Rationale: Constriction and rolling down of stockings during wear is a result of poor fit and can impede circulation and cause thrombosis.

8. Antiembolic stockings should be removed at least twice daily.
Rationale: Permits skin to be washed and assessed for edema or irritation.

Lifespan Considerations

Children

- Antiembolic stockings are infrequently used in children.

Special Considerations

The Obese Client

- Proper fitting of antiembolic stockings is difficult with the obese client, requiring special attention for areas of constriction and binding.
- Elastic (Ace) bandages may be an alternative to provide antiembolic protection in clients from whom correct fit is impossible with standard stocking sizes.

Home-Care Modifications

- Clients need to be instructed to remove stockings regularly for skin inspection and cleansing.
- Be sure clients understand that commercial support stockings *are not* a substitute for medical antiembolic stockings.

couraged. Socks with tight elastic bands around the tops and short-legged pants with tight elastic or belted bottoms should be avoided.

In addition to garments, orthopedic casts made of plaster or other materials can tighten and restrict blood flow. Warm fingers or toes indicate sufficient blood flow, but cool extremities, numbness or tingling, and limited capillary refill may indicate a need for altering the cast or recasting.

The nurse should point out that crossing the legs creates pressure points against veins and should be avoided. Clients who must sit for extended periods (such as at work) should be careful not to create venous constriction by sitting too far back in chairs. The back of the calves should not rest against the edge of the chair because this compresses the veins. These people also should be taught to flex their leg muscles periodically and to stand and walk frequently to encourage venous return.

Nursing Interventions for Altered Cardiovascular Function

Quality of life for the client with cardiovascular function often depends on teaching and support provided by the healthcare provider. Important areas for instruction include medication management, edema reduction, pain management, and energy conservation. The nurse also must be skilled at providing CPR in an emergency.

Client Teaching

The client with cardiovascular disorders should be taught to recognize warning signs of decreased cardiac output or decreased perfusion. Signs and symptoms that indicate the need for medical help are listed in the display. The nurse should be certain the client is aware of the importance of infection prevention. The client also should be instructed in how to promote blood flow and reduce edema, promote skin integrity, and avoid fatigue.

The cardiovascular client often must take numerous medications. The quality of the nurse's teaching can help promote client compliance with the medication regimen. Cardiovascular drugs are complex and may be confusing to the client. Therefore, it is beneficial to include the client's spouse or significant other in discussions concerning medications. The nurse should explain clearly the reasons for taking prescribed medications and provide written information. Telling the client that the drug is for his or her heart is inadequate because the client may have several prescribed heart medications. Simple yet accurate descriptions of each medication's action help the client appreciate and remember the importance of complying with the medication regimen. The nurse also should stress the importance of taking medications as ordered. The client must be warned against missing doses or stopping a medication without consulting the physician. The nurse must be certain the client understands how and when to take medications, whether any foods or other substances should be

Client Teaching
Indications for Seeking Medical Advice

Instruct the client as follows:

Call Your Doctor When You Experience

- *Unusual insomnia or extreme, prolonged fatigue after physical exercise*
- *Angina pain that does not subside with rest or after three nitroglycerin tablets taken 5 minutes apart (for clients who have documented chronic angina)*
- *Sudden confusion or incoordination*
- *Unusual fatigue*
- *Prolonged depression*

Call An Ambulance (911, If Available) When You Experience

- *New, sustained pressure or pain in the chest, arms, neck, or jaw (if this is not a normal occurrence)*
- *Rapid, irregular, or unusually slow heart beat (if this is abnormal)*
- *Dizziness or fainting*
- *Severe pain and loss of normal color in an extremity (which is not due to exposure to cold)*

avoided (to prevent interactions), and what side effects to expect. The client also should be taught to recognize signs of overdose or toxicity and when to contact the physician.

Reasons for other medical therapies should be explained thoroughly. The client's usual lifestyle and culture should be taken into consideration when schedules for treatments and medications are planned. Flexibility should be allowed when possible.

Edema Reduction

Peripheral edema can impede blood flow to the tissues. It is unsightly and often uncomfortable or painful for the client. Control of edema is an important nursing priority (Fig. 35-8).

Elevation of Limbs. One of the simplest measures for reducing edema is to elevate affected limbs. This allows gravity to assist venous return to the heart and helps to decrease venous pressure, reducing the leakage of fluid from vessels and promoting its reabsorption. Vessels can reopen, and perfusion is improved.

Venous constriction should be avoided when elevating edematous limbs. The legs should be fully supported when elevated, and there must be no pressure points. The leg should not be lifted so high that a con-

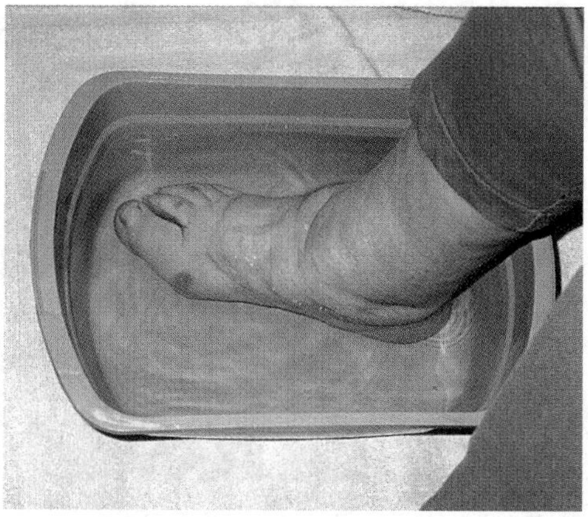

Figure 35-8 • Foot care is very important for the client with edema or peripheral vascular disease. Note the edema and reddened areas that could easily break down.

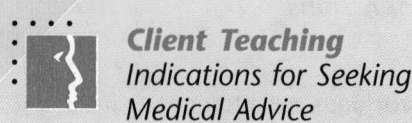

striction occurs at the groin. The knee gatch on the hospital bed should not be used because this restricts venous flow behind the knee.

Diet Teaching. The client with fluid retention problems usually benefits from a low-sodium diet. Because sodium molecules attract water, limiting salt intake helps to control edema. The nurse can help the client develop an awareness of the importance of salt and sodium restriction.

Limited use of table salt is a logical first step in a sodium-restricted diet, but the client also must understand "hidden" sodium content. The client should learn to look for sodium content on the labels of beverages, health products, over-the-counter medicines (especially antacids), and in foods. The client should avoid highly processed convenience foods. Vinegar, spices, and herbs can be used as a replacement for salt in cooking. Finally, the client should be encouraged to discuss possible salt substitutes with the physician.

Fluid Restriction. Clients who have fluid volume excess must restrict fluid intake until balance is restored. Intake and output are monitored carefully to assess fluid status. An intake of more than 2 L (2,000 mL) greater than output suggests fluid retention. The client also should be weighed daily, preferably at the same time and ideally before breakfast. Weight should not vary by more than 1 kg (2 lb) per day.

Positioning

Body position affects cardiac work and tissue perfusion. The heart works harder in the supine position than in the upright position. Lying flat promotes venous return. Because all vessels are at the same level of the heart, gravity's effect on the blood is minimized. Blood can flow more freely into the vena cavae. The increased volume of blood entering the atria increases stroke volume.

For the client with compromised cardiac status, such as the client with an MI or heart failure, lying supine can be uncomfortable and can increase the work of the heart. A semi-Fowler's position for these clients reduces their cardiac work by limiting venous return.

Conversely, the client who is in shock should not be placed in the semi-Fowler's position. Without sufficient blood to fill the vascular space, the shock victim requires improved cardiac output. Recommended positioning for a hypotensive client is with legs elevated 20 to 30 degrees to improve venous return and blood perfusion to vital organs (Bulechek & McCloskey, 1992). Research has not shown the Trendelenburg (head down) position to improve mean arterial blood pressure significantly. During this period, the hypotensive client also must receive specific treatment for the cause of the shock to ensure restoration of perfusion to all vital organs.

On a smaller scale, positioning can be used to improve perfusion to selected underperfused areas. Arterial flow is enhanced by gravity. Allowing ischemic hands or feet to hang in dependent positions may improve perfusion; however, this is contraindicated in the edematous client.

Pain Management

Some cardiovascular clients experience infrequent, relatively slight pain; others have constant debilitating pain. Helping these clients to manage their pain is an essential nursing skill.

Chest Pain. Complaints of chest pain must never be ignored. It has many causes, but unless proven otherwise, chest pain in the cardiac client must be assumed to be a serious sign of cardiac hypoxia. Although the client may want to attribute some chest pains to anxiety or excitement, these are unlikely causes. People with normal coronary arteries do not experience chest pain with anxiety or excitement.

When acute chest pain is evident, the client should stop all activity and rest. The client should sit comfortably; lying flat inhibits full chest expansion and limits gas exchange in the lung, so this position should be avoided. Oxygen should be started as ordered.

Sublingual nitroglycerin should be administered if it has been ordered for chest pain. Blood pressure should be assessed 5 minutes after this medication has been given, because nitroglycerin is a vasodilator, and blood pressure may fall. If the pain is not relieved after two repeat doses of nitroglycerin, the physician should be notified, or the family should call 911 or emergency services.

The client should rest after an episode of pain. The nurse should document the duration, activity during onset, and vital signs during the episode and should report this information to the physician.

Clients with chronic angina can be helped primarily by assistance with activity management. They should be taught to monitor their pulse rates and to pace activities to prevent increases of greater than 20 beats/min above the baseline rate. Activities should be done on an empty stomach whenever possible to avoid acute angina. Because blood is diverted to the gut after eating, less oxygen is available to the muscles, including the heart. For this reason, the nurse should not schedule procedures or activities, such as bathing or walking, right after meals. If sublingual nitroglycerin is ordered, the client should take a dose before performing an activity that has previously produced pain.

Claudication and Peripheral Ischemic Pain. These categories of pain from peripheral vascular disorders are not life-threatening, but the discomfort they produce can be crippling. Pain may be precipitated by cold surroundings, cigarette smoking, or activities that exceed individual tolerance. Nursing measures to prevent such pain are directed at enhancing oxygen delivery to tissues by improving blood flow or by decreasing oxygen demand.

Heat helps relieve peripheral vascular pain. Warm, moist heat applied to the extremities promotes vasodilation, thereby improving circulation to the tissues. This is accomplished through the use of warm compresses or by soaking the hands or feet in a basin of warm water. A warm pad may be wrapped around a limb.

Chronically impaired perfusion of extremities can cause impaired perception of the sensation of heat. For this reason, the client with vascular disease is prone to burns. The nurse must exercise great care to avoid excessively hot soaks or compresses. Their temperature should not exceed 95° to 100°F (35°–38°C). When a heating pad is used, it should be covered with a towel or pillowcase and not allowed to come into direct contact with the skin.

Increased Activity

Gradual rehabilitation of the hospitalized client following an acute episode (MI, CVA) can begin with simple in-bed activity. Examples of nonstrenuous exercises include rotation and dorsiflexion of the ankles and working the feet against a footboard. Self-care activities, such as shaving, washing, eating, or brushing the teeth, should be encouraged. These activities help prevent deconditioning by maintaining joint mobility and preserving some muscle tone. They also may help to maintain the client's spirits by forcing the realization that the condition has not rendered him or her helpless.

Activity can be increased daily on the basis of the client's tolerance or by exercise prescription. As the

Procedure 35-2
Applying Sequential Compression Device (SCD)

Purpose

1. Promote venous return from legs to decrease the risk of deep vein thrombosis and pulmonary embolism in clients with reduced mobility

Assessment

- Identify clients at increased risk for development of deep vein thrombosis.
- Assess skin integrity and identify any existing leg condition that would be exacerbated by use of the plastic sleeve or compression device. Clinical examples in which use of SCE is contraindicated are
  - -Dermatitis, cellulitis
  - -Postoperative vein ligation
  - -Gangrene
  - -Recent skin graft
  - -Massive edema of legs
  - -Extreme deformity of legs
  - -Suspected or existing deep vein thrombus
- Verify physician order

Equipment

Antiembolism stockings
Measuring tape
Compression sleeves
Inflation unit

Procedure

1. Measure leg to ensure proper sleeve sizing.
   Note: Knee length—one size fits all; thigh length—measure length of leg from ankle to the popliteal fossa.
   Measure circumference of thigh at the gluteal fold.

Extra small	Circumference 22 in	Length 16 in
Regular	Circumference 29 in	Length 16 in
Extra Large	Circumference 35 in	Length 16 in

   Rationale: Proper sleeve size ensures proper fit and function of the sleeve.
2. Apply antiembolism stockings. Ensure that there are no wrinkles or folds (see Procedure 35-1).
   Note: Stockinette or ace wraps are recommended options if unable to fit client with antiembolism stockings.
   Rationale: Wearing stockings decreases the risk of skin irritation and diaphoresis under the plastic sleeves.
3. Place client in supine position.
   Rationale: Proper positioning helps secure plastic sleeve.
4. Place a plastic sleeve under each leg so the opening is at the knee, and solid portion is in the popliteal region behind the knee.
   Note: If only one sleeve is required, leave the other sleeve in package and connect to control unit.
   Rationale: Unit will not reach proper pressure if single sleeve is left to inflate in unconfined area.

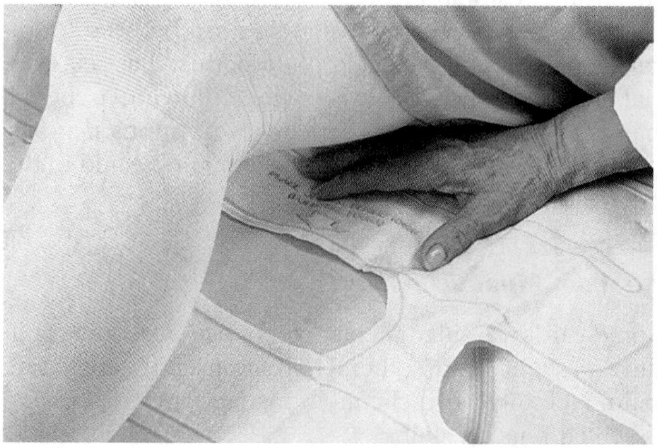

Step 4 • Place plastic sleeve under leg.

5. Fold outer section of the sleeve over the inner portion, and secure with Velcro tabs. Check sleeve fit. Two fingers should fit between the sleeve and leg.
   Rationale: Proper fit prevents irritation to the leg and allows unit to reach adequate inflation pressure.

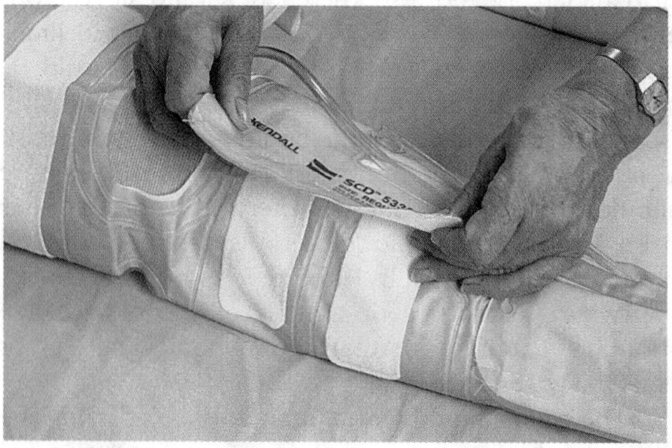

Step 5 • Secure plastic sleeve around leg.

6. Connect tubing to control unit. The premarked arrows on the tubing from the sleeve and from the controller must be aligned to make adequate connection. Turn machine on.
   Rationale: Control unit performs a system self-check.

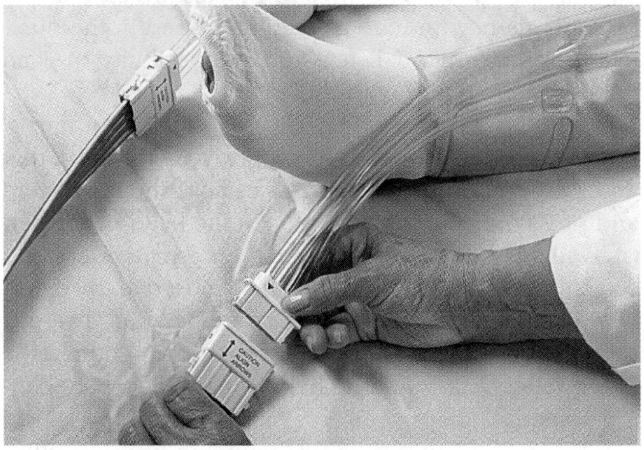

Step 6 • *Connect tubing to control unit.*

7. Adjust control unit settings as necessary. Unit control is preset with sleeve cooling in "off" position and audible alarm in "on" position. Sleeve cooling should be in "on" position at all times except during surgery. Ankle pressure should be set at 35–55 mm Hg.
   Rationale: Plastic sleeves can become warm and uncomfortable if cooling is in "off" position. Skin and stocking under sleeve can become wet with diaphoresis which increases risk for impaired skin integrity. Cooling may be turned "off" during surgery to preserve client warmth.
8. Recheck control unit settings whenever unit has been turned off.
   Rationale: The unit will convert to preset mode.

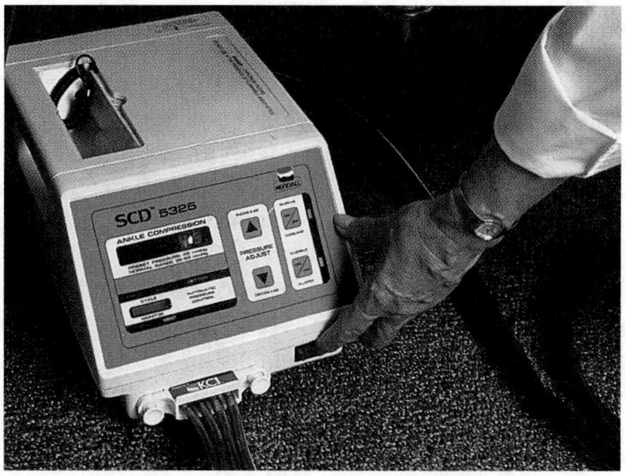

Step 7 • *Turn on control unit.*

9. Respond to and promptly correct all "fault" indicator alarms.
   Note: The control unit will sense and indicate four pressure "fault" conditions.
   1. Pressure failed to drop to zero during the ventilation cycle.
   2. The ankle pressure failed to reach 20 mm Hg for five consecutive cycles.
   3. The ankle pressure exceeded 90 mm Hg.
   4. Internal diagnostics error has occurred.

   Rationale: Adequate functioning of unit is imperative to prevent complications
10. Document time and date of application. If SCD is applied to only one leg, document reason.
11. Assess and document skin integrity every 8 h.
    Rationale: Frequent assessment of skin integrity is necessary to prevent and provide early intervention in case of skin irritation.
12. Remove sleeves and notify physician if client experiences tingling, numbness, or leg pain.
    Rationale: These findings may indicate nerve compression.

client progresses to ambulation, accurate assessment is essential to prevent the client from attempting to do more than he or she is ready to do. The nurse must observe the client closely for subjective signs of pain. The cardiac client should be monitored by telemetry, which records the electrocardiogram while the client is walking. Changes in blood pressure, mentation, or color, or complaints of lightheadedness or weakness are indications that the exercise is too strenuous. The client should sit and rest immediately. Breathlessness or increased heart rate lasting for more than 10 minutes after exercise indicates a need to go slower in the rehabilitation effort. Nocturnal insomnia or daytime fatigue also may mean that the previous day's exercise has been too strenuous.

Energy Conservation

Closely related to pain management and activity intolerance is energy conservation. Pain can occur when the client exceeds normal activity tolerance. Effective conservation of energy can promote activity tolerance and thus can help prevent pain.

Repeated movement of the upper arms should be avoided by newly diagnosed clients with MI. This movement increases the metabolic demands of the arm muscles. The heart is forced to pump harder for the blood to overcome gravity.

The client should be warned against using Valsalva's maneuver, which occurs during grunting. Air in the chest pushes against a closed glottis, raising intrathoracic pressure. This can suddenly increase blood pressure while simultaneously hindering venous return. Activities involving lifting or pushing heavy objects and straining during bowel movements often involve the Valsalva maneuver. The client with an acute MI should be instructed to avoid the stress this places on the heart by consciously maintaining a steady breathing pattern or exhaling slowly during such activities.

The most important energy conservation measure for the cardiovascular client is rest. Regular rest periods should be provided. The client should rest undisturbed for 1 hour after meals. Rest should be encouraged before and after activities such as bathing or when lengthy treatments are scheduled.

Activities should be spaced to avoid fatigue. Periods of work should alternate with rest or lighter activity. During activities, the client should sit whenever possible to avoid cardiovascular strain. When activities or tasks require gathering several materials, good planning is essential to eliminate unnecessary and inefficient wasted effort. The client should immediately stop any activity that produces fatigue, breathlessness, pressure, or pain.

Cardiopulmonary Resuscitation

Cardiac arrest is the most serious emergency that can occur. When a client's heart stops, acute hypoxia begins to destroy all tissues. Unless oxygenation is restored quickly, the victim will die. CPR is a means of artificially supporting circulation and oxygenation until the victim's heart begins beating on its own.

CPR is a systematic approach to life support that has been revised and refined over the years. In 1992, the National Conference on Cardiopulmonary Resuscitation and Emergency Cardiac Care recommended some changes in protocols. Basic CPR is outlined in Procedure 35-3.

Most agencies require practically all personnel to be trained in basic cardiac life support (BCLS). The ability to maintain a cardiac arrest victim's breathing and circulation with basic CPR skills is essential to the success of all resuscitation efforts. The Red Cross and other agencies offer classes for BCLS certification. These courses can be completed in 1 day, often through the employing agency.

Advanced cardiac life support (ACLS) requires extensive training and rigorous testing. People certified in ACLS are trained in ECG interpretation and advanced airway management. They are qualified to administer cardioactive drugs or electrical shock (defibrillation) as needed.

Hospital resuscitation is often referred to as a "code" (eg, cardiac arrests may be announced as "code 199" or "code blue"). The "code" team consists of physicians, nurses, pharmacists, and respiratory therapists. All members of the code team should be certified in ACLS.

The nurse may be the first person to discover a cardiac arrest victim. Knowing what to do before and after help arrives increases the chances for the victim's survival. Along with the techniques of CPR, the nurse must be proficient in handling many duties at the scene of a cardiac arrest. The following discussion focuses on some of the important nursing aspects of hospital CPR efforts. Specific cardiac arrest protocols are established by each agency and are usually published in the nursing procedure manual. It is the responsibility of each nurse to be familiar with these protocols.

Initial Management. After quickly establishing that an arrest has occurred, the nurse must shout for help and press the emergency button at the head of the bed (if available). At the same time, the hospital telephone operator must be alerted. The nurse must dial the emergency number and announce to the operator, "There is a cardiac arrest on (floor or wing), room (number)." The operator can summon help using the hospital paging system.

The nurse's first calls for help should bring other nurses to the room. They bring the emergency supplies ("crash cart"), while the first nurse begins preparations for CPR. Whether or not assistance comes immediately, *the discovering nurse must stay with the victim* and continue to call for help until it arrives.

If the client has been sitting upright, the bed must be lowered to a flat position. The overbed table should be moved away from the bed for easy access to the client. The nurse should remove the pillow from under the client's head. If the bed is elevated to stretcher level, it should be lowered. All of these adjustments must be made as quickly as possible, and CPR must be initiated immediately. Other nurses can move the furniture from around the bed to make room for the crash cart, defibrillator, and ECG machine.

The Code Team. Management of a cardiac arrest usually requires no fewer than four people. The first team member is responsible for establishing and managing the client's airway. This is often a nurse anesthetist, anesthesiologist, or respiratory therapist. The second performs chest compressions to maintain circulation. The third team member establishes IV lines and administers medications. The fourth member maintains an accurate record of medications and interventions and can help by retrieving needed supplies. Team members may switch roles during the resuscitation effort and take turns at compressions, because this is especially fatiguing.

After Resuscitation Begins. Once the code team has taken charge, the nurse who discovered the person should remain with the team to provide essential information. The circumstances under which the person

(text continues on page 975)

Procedure 35-3
Administering Cardiopulmonary Resuscitation (CPR)*

Purpose

1. Restore cardiopulmonary functioning
2. Prevent irreversible brain damage from anoxia

Assessment

- Determine that the client is unconscious. Shake the client and shout at him or her to confirm unconsciousness rather than being asleep, intoxicated, or hearing impaired.
- Assess for presence of respirations.
- Assess carotid artery for pulse.
  Note: Presence of pulse *and* respiration contraindicates initiation of CPR.

Equipment

A hard surface: Client may be placed on floor, ground, or backboard.
No additional equipment is necessary, but in the hospital setting, an emergency (crash) cart with defibrillator and cardiac monitoring should be brought to the bedside by additional personnel. A crash cart usually contains

Airway equipment
Suction equipment
Intravenous equipment
Laboratory tubes and syringes
Prepackaged medications for advanced life support

Procedure

One Rescuer—Adult Client

1. Verbally ask, "Are you okay?" Assess to determine responsiveness. Shake gently.
   Rationale: Need for resuscitation must be determined.
2. Call for help.
   Rationale: The majority of adults with sudden cardiac arrest are in ventricular fibrillation. Recent studies confirm that survival is linked to early access to defibrillation from emergency medical systems.
3. Turn client onto back while supporting head and neck. Place a cardiac board under the back or place client on the floor.
   Rationale: A firm surface is needed for adequate compression of the heart between the sternum.
4. Open the airway.
   a. Use a head tilt/chin lift maneuver.
   Rationale: Moving the jaw forward lifts the tongue away from the back of the throat and opens the airway.

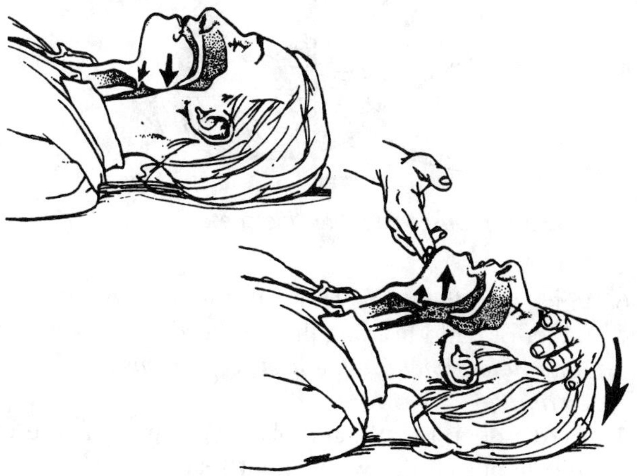

Step 4A • *Open the airway. Relieve airway obstruction by head tilt/chin lift maneuver.*

   b. Use the modified jaw thrust if a neck injury is suspected.
   Rationale: Jaw thrust maneuver can be accomplished without extending the neck and exacerbating a potential neck injury.

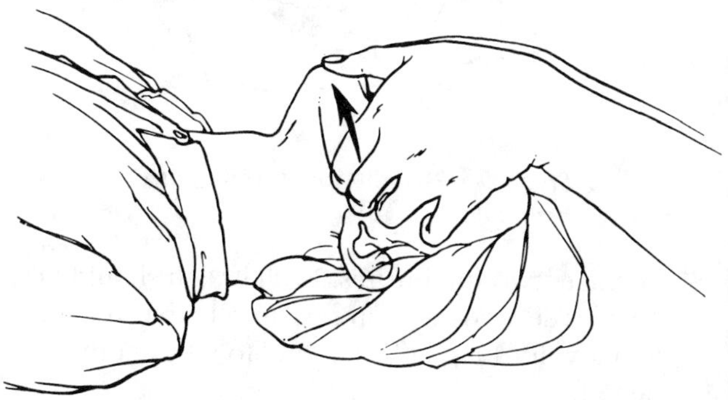

Step 4B • *Open the airway using jaw thrust maneuver.*

(continued)

5. Place your ear over client's mouth, and observe the chest for rising with respiration. *Listen, look,* and *feel* for breathing for 3 to 5 seconds.

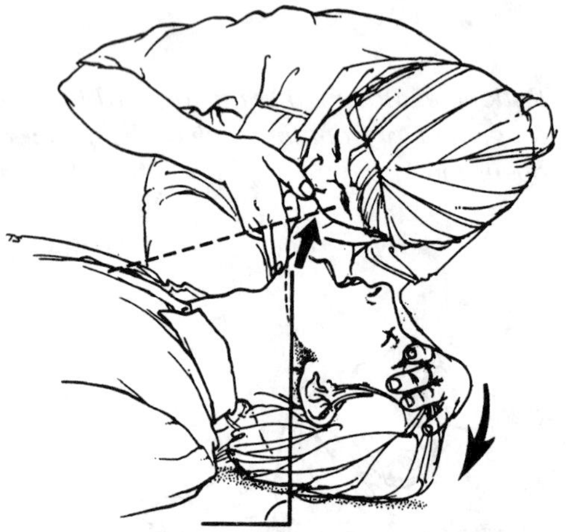

Step 5 • *Observe for breathlessness.*

6. Pinch the client's nostrils with thumb and index finger of hand holding the forehead.
   Rationale: Pinching the nostrils prevents air from escaping.
7. Take a deep breath, and place your mouth around the client's mouth with a tight seal.
   Note: If client wears dentures, they should remain in place to enable an airtight seal.
   Rationale: Tight seal is required for effective ventilation.

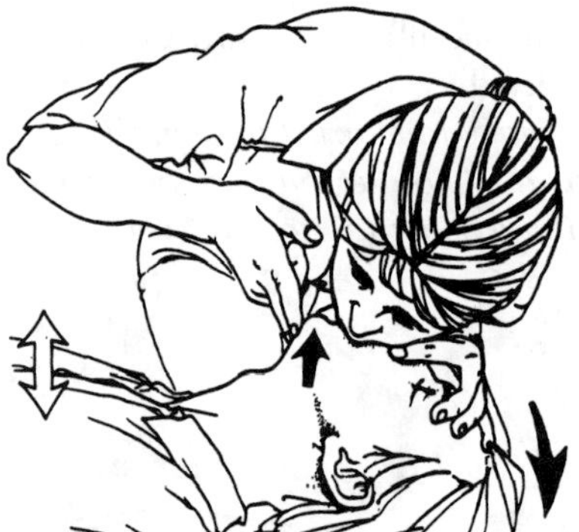

Step 7 • *Perform mouth-to-mouth breathing.*

8. Ventilate two full breaths. Each breath should take 1.5 to 2 seconds to deliver. Pause between breaths to allow for lung deflation and to take another deep breath.
   Rationale: Slow ventilations and complete exhalation between breaths decrease gastric distention, regurgitation, and aspiration.
9. Assess for carotid pulse for 5 to 10 seconds on the side next to which you are kneeling. Maintain head tilt with the other hand.
   Rationale: The carotid is the most accessible, reliable, and easily learned location for checking the pulse in adults and children. The pulse area should be pressed gently to avoid compressing the artery. Serious medical complications may occur if chest compressions are performed on a person who has a pulse.
   a. Locate the larynx.

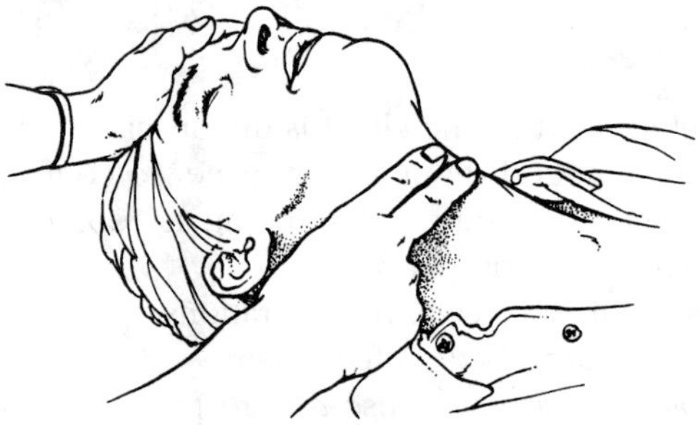

Step 9A • *Locate the larynx.*

   b. Slide the fingers into the groove between the trachea and muscles at side of neck to feel carotid pulse.

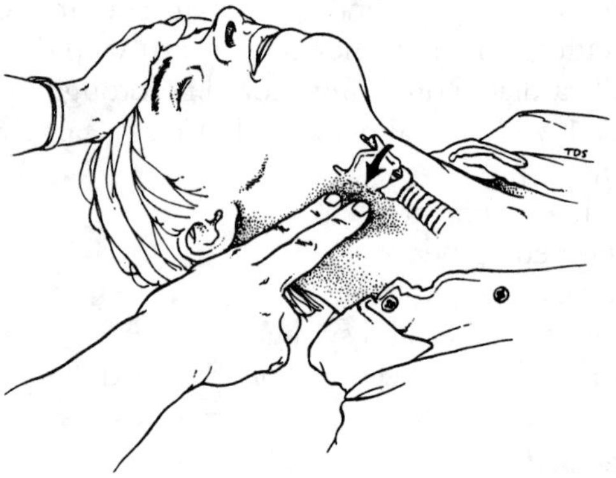

Step 9B • *Slide the fingers to the groove to feel the carotid pulse.*

10. *If client is pulseless,* start chest compressions.
11. With hand nearest client's legs, place middle and index fingers on lower ridge or near ribs, and move fingers up along ribs to the costal-sternal notch (in center of lower chest).
12. Place middle finger on this notch and the index finger next to the middle finger on the lower end of the notch.
13. Place heel of other hand along the lower half of the sternum, next to the index finger.
    Rationale: Careful attention to hand placement during cardiac compression prevents fractured ribs and organ trauma.
14. Remove first hand from the notch and place heel of that hand parallel over the hand on the chest. Interlock fingers, keeping them off client's chest.

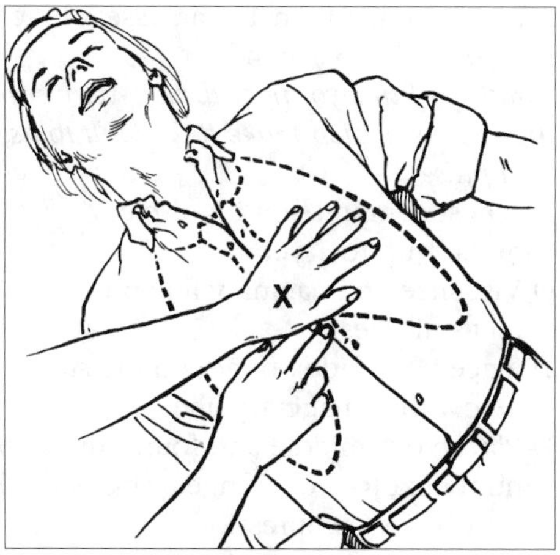

Steps 12 & 13 • *Find correct position for external chest compression.*

Rationale: This prevents trauma from pressure on the ribs.

15. Keeping your hands on sternum, extend your arms, locking the elbows, with your shoulders directly over the client's chest.
Rationale: Weight of your upper body and strength of both arms are needed for adequate cardiac compression. Placing your shoulders over client's chest provides additional muscle power and prevents hands from slipping off sternum and breaking ribs.
16. Press down on chest, depressing sternum 1.5 to 2 in. *Rationale: Compresses the heart between sternum and vertebrae to pump blood out of heart.*

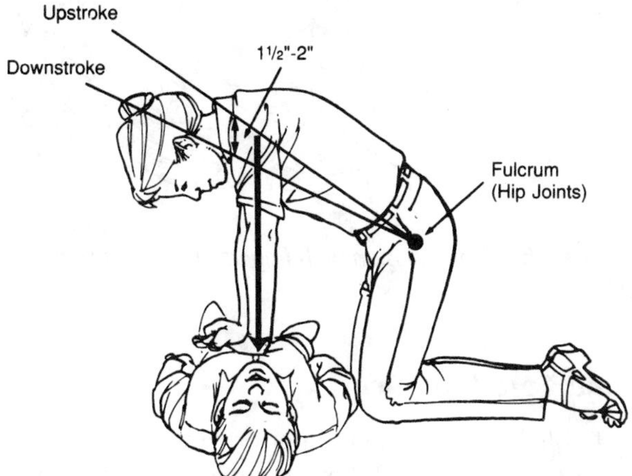

Step 16 • *Keeping shoulders over person's chest, depress sternum 1.5 to 2 inches.*

17. Completely release compression while maintaining your hand position. Repeat in a smooth rhythm 80 to 100 times/min.
Note: Saying the mnemonic "one and two and . . . fifteen" may help maintain the rhythm.
Rationale: Pressure on the sternum must be released between compressions to allow the heart to fill with blood. Leave your hands in position on the chest to prevent internal injury from malposition of the hands.
18. Ventilate with 2 full breaths after every 15 chest compressions.
19. Repeat 4 cycles of 15 chest compressions and 2 ventilations.
20. Reassess for carotid pulse. If client is pulseless, continue CPR. Reassess for carotid pulse every few minutes.
Note: Never interrupt CPR for longer than 7 seconds.
Rationale: Stopping CPR can result in cerebral anoxia and brain damage.

Procedure

Two Rescuers—Adult Client

1. When second rescuer arrives, the first rescuer stops CPR after completing two ventilations and assesses for a carotid pulse for 5 seconds.
2. The second rescuer moves into the chest compression position
3. If pulselessness continues, the first rescuer states "no pulse" and delivers one ventilation.
4. The second rescuer begins chest compression while counting out loud, "one and two and three and four and five and." The compression rate is 80 to 100/min.
5. The first rescuer gives one full ventilation after every five chest compressions. The first rescuer also assesses carotid pulse during chest compressions to evaluate effectiveness.

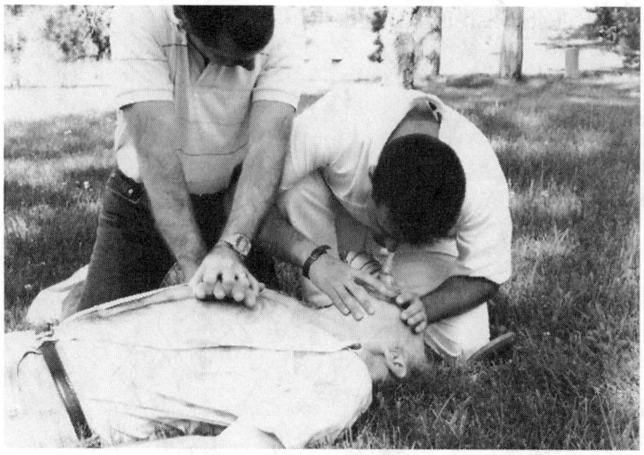

Steps 4 & 5 • *Two rescuers synchronize chest compression and ventilation.*

6. If second rescuer wishes to change positions, he or she states, "Change, one and two and three and four and five and."

(continued)

7. The first rescuer delivers the ventilation then moves into the chest compression position.
8. The second rescuer moves to the ventilator position and assesses for a carotid pulse for 5 seconds. If pulseless, resume CPR.
   Note: Do not interrupt CPR for more than 7 seconds.

Procedure

One Rescuer CPR—Infant and Child

1. Assess unresponsiveness.
2. Call for help.
3. Place child on hard surface. Provide basic life support for 1 full minute before activating emergency medical system.
   Rationale: Airway obstruction and respiratory arrest are the most common causes of collapse in children. Early support is essential and should be attempted first.
4. Open the airway using head tilt/chin lift. Avoid overextension of head in infants.
   Rationale: Overextension of the head is thought to collapse the trachea in infants, causing an airway obstruction.
5. Place your ear over child's mouth, and observe chest for rise.
   Listen, look, and *feel* for breathing.
   Note: If airway obstruction from food or foreign object is suspected, perform Heimlich maneuver.
6. If breathlessness is determined, seal mouth and nose and ventilate twice (1 to 1.5 seconds for each breath). Observe for chest rise.
   Note: Infants and small children may require the rescuer to place mouth over the mouth and nose to establish an airtight seal.

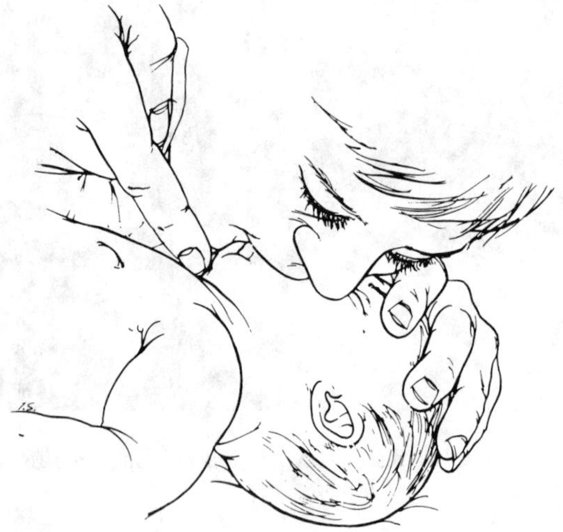

Step 6 • *Seal mouth and nose to ventilate.*

7. Assess pulselessness by palpating for carotid artery on near side in children older than 1 year. In infants younger than 1 year, assess brachial or femoral pulse for 5 seconds.
   Rationale: Infants younger than 1 year have short, chubby necks, which make it difficult to assess the carotid pulse.
8. Begin chest compression if pulseless.
   a. For infant up to 1 year:
      1) Visualize an imaginary line between the infant's nipples.
      2) Place your index finger on the sternum just below this imaginary line.
      3) Place your middle and fourth finger on sternum next to index finger. This is the location for cardiac compression.
   b. For child 1 to 8 years of age:
      1) Placement of hand on sternum is the same as for adult CPR. Use heel of one hand to compress sternum 1 to 1½ inches 80 to 100 times/min.
      2) Continue chest compressions, and ventilate at the rate of one breath to five compressions.
      3) Continue CPR as for an adult.

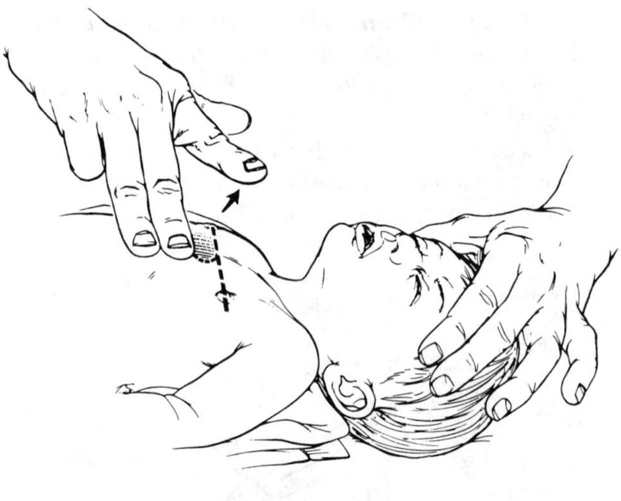

Step 8 • *Chest compression with fingers on infant up to 1 year old.*

Home-Care Modifications

- Public education in the performance of CPR must be emphasized. CPR is a complex skill, and efforts to decrease the complexity for lay people must be addressed.
  Emphasis should be placed on teaching one-rescuer CPR because two-rescuer CPR is rarely used by lay rescuers.
  Courses should be developed to allow people to concentrate on an area of basic life support that most closely applies to their life situation. For example, families of clients with heart disease

may learn one-rescuer CPR of adults, while parents may learn only infant/child resuscitation and Heimlich maneuvers.

- Nonphysicians who initiate CPR should continue resuscitation efforts until:
  Spontaneous circulation and ventilation are effectively restored.
  Another competent person is available to continue CPR.
  A physician or physician-directed team assumes responsibility.
  The rescuer is physically exhausted and unable to continue CPR.

*All art is from Emergency Cardiac Care Committee and Subcommittees: AHA guidelines for cardiopulmonary resuscitation and emergency cardiac care. *JAMA, 268*: 2193, 1992. Copyright 1992, American Medical Association.

was found, the client's prearrest status, primary diagnoses, recent medications, and recent laboratory data are relevant. The nurse also may be needed to assist with procedures. The person in charge assigns specific duties to members of the code team. Those who are not actively participating in the resuscitation efforts should leave the room.

Consideration of privacy is important. If the room is shared by another client, the roommate should be moved elsewhere if possible. If this is not practical, the curtain should be drawn, and a nurse should stay with the second client. This client may be anxious; his or her questions should be answered honestly.

Finally, one of the most difficult tasks for the nurse is in dealing with the sorrow and fears of the victim's loved ones. These people need support during and after the resuscitation. The nurse provides honest information but should not speculate on the client's condition. Questions concerning the client's immediate condition should be answered only by those who are absolutely certain of it.

Community-Based Nursing

The majority of clients with cardiovascular dysfunction are managed in the community. Hospital stays for acute episodes, such as MI or open heart surgery, have decreased dramatically in length during the last decade. Many other less acute problems are diagnosed in ambulatory settings and are completely managed at home.

Community-based care is often focused on prevention, especially among high-risk individuals. On routine examination, if a client is found to be overweight, sedentary, to smoke, or have high cholesterol levels, lifestyle modification education is appropriate. Often detection of elevated cholesterol or hypertension is a significant motivating factor for making necessary changes. Follow-up is important for these clients (Fig. 35-9).

Medication Management

Cardiovascular dysfunction is frequently managed with medications. Often multiple medications may be necessary, and regimens are complex and difficult to follow. Side effects can be unpleasant and potentially serious, at times making compliance difficult. Table 35-3 provides some drug classes that are commonly used to treat cardiovascular problems. The nurse discharging the client from an acute care agency or who works in a clinic or physician's office should explain drug effects, side effects, and special considerations to the client. If the client is unable to remember or could become confused, the family or caregiver also should be involved. Many cardiovascular medications (eg, antihypertensive agents, nitrates) can cause postural hypotension, resulting in a fall or injury. Clients should be cautioned to get out of bed slowly and avoid hot baths, which could increase vasodilation and syncope.

Cardiac Rehabilitation

For many clients, cardiovascular problems need not permanently prevent them from enjoying a normal lifestyle. The purpose of rehabilitation is to help the cardiovascular client restore or improve lost function. This goal depends on physical endurance, which is improved by graded physical activity. Thus, although rest is an essential part of the management of cardiovascular problems, activity also must play a part.

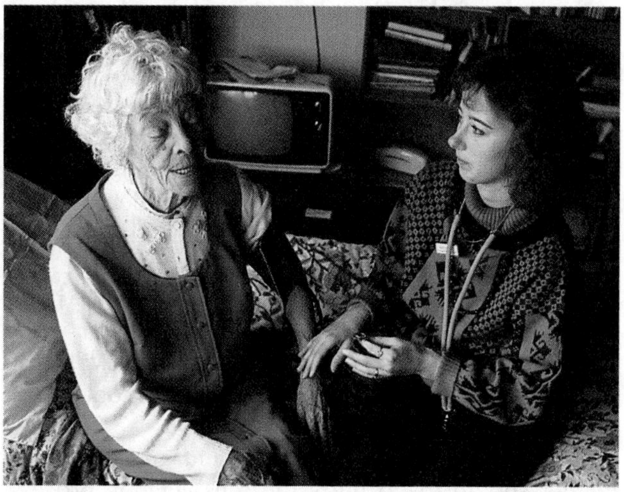

Figure 35-9 • *Monitoring blood pressure in the home may be necessary for some elderly clients. (Courtesy of Seattle University School of Nursing and Yesler Terrace.)*

Table 35-3 • Medications Affecting Cardiac Function and Tissue Perfusion

Medication	Example	Drug Action	Side Effects
Cardiac glycoside	Digoxin	Increases cardiac contractility; decreases heart rate	Bradycardia, arrhythmias
Antihypertensive agents			
Beta-adrenergic blockers	Inderal	Decreases blood pressure	Low blood pressure, dizziness, syncope
Calcium channel blockers	Nifedipine		
Vasodilators	Apresoline		
ACE inhibitors	Captopril		
Vasopressor	Norepinephrine	Increases blood pressure	High blood pressure
Antiarrhythmic	Quinidine sulfate	Regulates heart rhythm	Hypotension, dizziness
Nitrates	Nitroglycerine	Relieves angina via peripheral vasodilation	Hypotension, headache
Antilipid agents	Lovastatin	Decreases cholesterol levels, reducing atherosclerosis risk	Nausea, bowel changes
Diuretics	Lasix	Reduces edema and fluid volume by increasing urinary output	Electrolyte imbalance (hypokalemia), volume depletion
Anticoagulants	Heparin	Decreases potential for clot formation	Bleeding

Promotion of activity tolerance starts after the medical problem has been identified and treated. Next, a functional assessment of the client is conducted. Only after the client's physical, mental, and emotional readiness for rehabilitative measures has been thoroughly assessed can appropriate measures be implemented.

Exercise should be part of a continuing rehabilitation program after the client's discharge from the hospital. A program of gradual progressive exercise is prescribed by the physician. The nurse should teach the client about safe exercise practices at home. Warm-up exercises prevent sudden demands on the heart; cooling down exercises help prevent pooling of blood in the legs. Exercise should not be performed in extremes of weather, nor should it be performed within 1 hour of meals. Isometric exercises should be avoided because they involve Valsalva's maneuver.

The client also should be instructed to recognize untoward symptoms of overexertion, such as palpitations or fluttering in the chest, racing pulse, pain, and pressure. The nurse should instruct the client how to take the pulse using the carotid or radial sites. The client should stop activity if the pulse rate exceeds the specific target zone prescribed by the physician. If the pulse lowers with activity, if it becomes irregular, or if the heart rate does not return to its resting level within 10 minutes after exercise, the client should contact the physician.

Patience is essential for the client and the nurse; neither should try to hurry the rehabilitation process. Exercise must be graduated, with more strenuous activities being added to the regimen only as client tolerance allows. The client must be warned against the following belief: "If this much exercise is good, twice as much will cure me in half the time." Exercise can provide several valuable physiologic and psychological benefits to the client with cardiovascular disease, but it is not a cure all. Exercise is one facet of a multipronged approach to regaining health. Adherence to prescribed medical therapies, reduction of stress, and modification of lifestyle risk factors are vital parts of any successful rehabilitation program.

Sexual Activity

A common area of concern for the client with cardiovascular dysfunction is the possible impact such limitations will have on sexual function. Following cardiac surgery or an MI, sexual activity may be limited until recovery permits more strenuous activity. Another common concern is the fear that another serious cardiac episode may occur during sexual activity. This can create much stress for the client and the sexual partner. The nurse can instruct the client to use positions that require less energy expenditure (eg, side lying), take nitroglycerin prior to sexual activity, avoid sexual activity following a large meal or after heavy consumption of alcohol, and stop and rest if any chest pain occurs.

Emergency Situations

The client and family members need to be knowledgeable concerning emergency situations. Nitroglycerin should always be available so that it can be quickly administered if chest pain occurs. Nitroglycerin should be refilled whenever it has passed the expiration date to ensure potency in case an emergency occurs. If after three doses, each administered 5 minutes apart, the chest pain persists, 911 or emergency community services should be notified. The client should not attempt to drive to the hospital. All family members should complete BCLS and be able to administer CPR.

Evaluation

Clients with cardiovascular dysfunction show widely variable rates of progress. For this reason, specific goals for these clients must be individualized. Together, the nurse and client can establish realistic goals with appropriate outcome criteria for measuring goal attainment.

General goals for all clients with cardiovascular dysfunction include the following:

Goal

Client will demonstrate adequate knowledge concerning cardiovascular dysfunction prevention or care.

Possible Outcome Criteria

The following should occur by the end of the teaching session:

- Client demonstrates an understanding of cardiovascular risk factors by reciting those that apply to him or her and discussing their physiologic effects.
- Client describes a specific plan and timetable for modifying his or her cardiovascular risk factors.
- Client states the following for any medication administered for cardiovascular problems: name of the drug, dose to be taken, action of the medication, side effects of the medication, and any special considerations for administration.
- Client describes the rationale(s) for prescribed therapies.
- Client lists and describes signs or symptoms that warrant calling the physician.

Goal

Client will demonstrate adequate tissue perfusion with adequate oxygenation of body tissue.

Possible Outcome Criteria

The following will occur within 48 hours of initiation of nursing interventions:

- Client reports absence of severe ischemic pain and improvement in comfort.
- Client demonstrates improved color and temperature of extremities.
- Client demonstrates improved activity tolerance by experiencing decreasing pain with ambulation.

Goal

Client will effectively cope with changes in self-concept and lifestyle.

Possible Outcome Criteria

The following will occur by the second home visit:

- Client verbalizes how his or her cardiovascular condition has caused life changes.
- Client identifies support people from whom emotional strength can be derived.
- Client demonstrates energy conservation measures, evidenced by sitting while dressing and planning rest periods.
- Client discusses realistic plans concerning return to work and other normal activities.

Key Concepts

- Good cardiovascular function depends on a healthy heart to pump blood, an adequate blood volume, and healthy blood vessels to distribute blood to tissues.
- Tissue perfusion, or the flow of blood through the tissues of the body, is essential for cell viability. Tissue perfusion depends on adequate functioning of the cardiovascular system to supply body tissues with oxygen and to remove waste products.
- Normal cardiovascular function usually produces a pulse rate between 60 and 100 beats/min, a blood pressure between 100/60 and 150/85, and an absence of pain on exertion.
- Normal cardiovascular function is affected by age, gender, exercise, body position, temperature, stress, smoking, and the ingestion of drugs or alcohol.
- Age-related changes in hemodynamics occur throughout a person's life.
- Altered cardiovascular function can occur when the heart is less effective as a pump (eg, arrhythmias, muscle damage, valve dysfunction), when the blood vessels are not able to deliver blood adequately to the tissues (atherosclerosis, vein problems, clots, or emboli), or when abnormalities occur within the blood (anemia, low blood volume).
- Modifiable cardiovascular risk factors include smoking, high cholesterol, obesity, lack of exercise, hypertension, stress, and abuse of IV drugs.
- Manifestations of altered cardiovascular function include changes in vital signs, ischemic pain, changes in the color or temperature of the skin, changes in sensorium, edema, organ system failure.
- Cardiovascular dysfunction can have a great impact on a person's ability to perform ADLs and may necessitate lifestyle changes.

Nursing Plan of Care
The Client With Activity Intolerance

Nursing Diagnosis

Activity Intolerance related to an imbalance between oxygen supply and demand manifested by verbal reports of fatigue or weakness; abnormal heart rate or blood pressure response to activity; exertional discomfort or dyspnea.

Client Goal

Client will balance activity with physical limitations.

Client Outcome Criteria

- Client's heart rate has regular rhythm and remains between 60 and 100 beats/min at rest. (Values may require adjustment for clients with chronic cardiovascular or pulmonary problems.)
- Client's heart rate rises in proportion to level of activity and does not exceed prescribed maximum limits.
- Client's blood pressure remains within normal limits for the person's age group; fluctuations with position are minimal.

Nursing Intervention	Scientific Rationale
1. Limit activity 1 h after meals.	1. Blood flow is directed to digestive tract to aid digestion; increases workload on the heart.
2. Plan heavy activities (eg, morning hygiene, ambulation) to alternate with rest period of 1 to 2 h.	2. Careful scheduling allows for uninterrupted rest period. Spacing activity conserves energy and avoids activity intolerance.
3. Offer prescribed nitroglycerine before activity or when pain develops with activity.	3. Nitrates vasodilate, decreasing venous return and decreasing cardiac workload.
4. Monitor pulse, blood pressure, and respiratory rate before, during, and after activity.	4. Sudden changes in vital signs indicate activity intolerance and provide a parameter for scheduling activity.
5. Gradually increase activity within physician's activity order.	5. Gradual increase in activity level helps client build endurance and better tolerate increased activity.

Client Goal

Client will effectively cope with necessary lifestyle and activity changes.

Client Outcome Criteria

- Client demonstrates energy-conserving measures, as evidenced by sitting while dressing and planning rest periods during hospital stay.
- Client discusses realistic plans concerning return to work and other normal activities by end of hospital stay.

Nursing Intervention	Scientific Rationale
1. With client, establish a plan for day's activity schedule.	1. Offering opportunity to plan activity periods increases client's feeling of control.
2. Educate client regarding signs of activity tolerance (eg, shortness of breath, increased heart rate)	2. Knowledge of symptoms of activity intolerance helps client identify activity tolerance and manage own activity level.
3. Encourage goal-setting for future activity periods (ie, "Next time, what would you hope to be able to do for yourself?").	3. The goal-directed client is in greater control of situation. Communicates confidence that progress will occur.
4. Explore with the client inventive ideas to conserve energy (eg, doing tasks from a chair rather than standing; sitting in shower).	4. Conservation of energy increases energy available for other, more important activities and increases independence.

- The nurse is instrumental is promoting optimum cardiovascular health by teaching risk modification for the general public.
- Nursing measures that can help maximize cardiovascular health and prevent complications include risk factor modification, prevention of venous stasis, client teaching, edema reduction, positioning, pain management, increased activity, and energy conservation.
- Cardiac arrest is a medical emergency for which CPR must be quickly and effectively performed to prevent morbidity and mortality.

Critical Thinking Challenges

Now that cardiovascular function, health maintenance, and client teaching are part of your knowledge base, you should be better able to plan care for the lawyer having his yearly physical. Turn to the situation at the beginning of the chapter, and consider the following.

1. *Evaluate risk factors that could negatively impact your client's cardiovascular health.*
2. *Analyze his readiness to learn, listing factors that could affect his readiness level.*
3. *Prioritize teaching plans to improve your client's cardiovascular health.*
4. *Plan two possible approaches to encourage compliance with necessary lifestyle changes.*
5. *Reflect on how you as a nurse feel when a client is reluctant to make positive lifestyle changes.*

References

Boulechek, G., & McCloskey, J. A. (1992). *Nursing interventions essential nursing treatments* (2nd ed.). Philadelphia: W.B. Saunders.

Bright, L. D., & Georgi, S. (1994). How to protect your patient from DVT. *American Journal of Nursing, 94* (12), 28–32.

Craven, R. F. (1995). Physiologic adaptations to exercise and immobility. In S. Woods, E. Sivarajan-Froelicher, J. Halpenny, & S. Underhill (Eds.), *Cardiac nursing* (3rd ed) (pp. 180–184). Philadelphia: J.B. Lippincott.

Gehing, P. (1992). Perfecting the art: Vascular assessment. *RN, 55* (1) 40–48.

Gillum, R. F., Folsom, A. R., & Blackburnz, H. (1984). Decline in coronary heart disease mortality. *American Journal of Medicine, 76* (6), 1055–1065.

Goe, M. R. (1995). Laboratory tests using blood. In S. Woods, E. Sivarajan-Froelicher, J. Halpenny, & S. Underhill (Eds.), *Cardiac nursing* (3rd ed) (pp. 259–278). Philadelphia: J.B. Lippincott.

Haynes, S. G., Feinleib, M., & Kannel, W. B. (1980). The relationship of psychosocial factors to coronary heart disease in the Framingham Study III. Eight-year incidence of coronary heart disease. *American Journal of Epidemiology, III* (1), 37–58.

Healthy People 2000: *National health promotion and disease prevention objectives.* U.S. Department of Health and Human Services, Public Health Service, DHHS Publication #(PHS) 91–50213.

Jenkins, C. (1982). Psychosocial risk factors for coronary heart disease. *Acta Medica Scandinavica (Suppl), 660,* 123–136.

Jensen, S. (1995). Pathophysiology of myocardial ischemia and infarction. In S. Woods, E. Sivarajan-Froelicher, J. Halpenny, & S. Underhill (Eds.), *Cardiac nursing* (3rd ed) (pp. 212–225). Philadelphia: J.B. Lippincott.

Joint National Committee on Detection, Evaluation, and Treatment of High Blood Pressure-Fifth Report (1993). NIH Publication #93–1088. Washington, DC: National Institutes of Health.

Knowlton-Moravec, C. (1995). Hematopoiesis, coagulation, and bleeding. In S. Woods, E. Sivarajan-Froelicher, J. Halpenny, & S. Underhill (Eds.), *Cardiac nursing* (3rd ed) (pp. 101–120). Philadelphia: J.B. Lippincott.

Laurent-Bopp, D. (1995). Heart failure. In S. Woods, E. Sivarajan-Froelicher, J. Halpenny, & S. Underhill (Eds.), *Cardiac nursing* (3rd ed) (pp. 555–571). Philadelphia: J.B. Lippincott.

Levin, R. (1993). Caring for the cardiac spouse. *American Journal of Nursing, 93* (11), 50–53.

National High Blood Pressure Education Program: *Guidelines for educating nurses in high blood pressure control (1993).* National Heart, Lung and Blood Institute. NIH Publication. Washington DC, U.S. Department of Health, Education, and Welfare.

North American Nursing Diagnosis Association (1994). *Nursing diagnosis: Definition and classifications 1995–1996.* Philadelphia, PA.

Newton, K., & Sivarajan-Froelicher, E. (1995). Coronary heart disease risk factors. In S. Woods, E. Sivarajan-Froelicher, J. Halpenny, & S. Underhill (Eds.), *Cardiac nursing* (3rd ed) (pp. 200–211). Philadelphia: J.B. Lippincott.

Pell, S., & Fayerweather, W. E. (1985). Trends in the incidence of myocardial infarction and in associated mortality and morbidity in a large employed population, 1957–1983. *New England Journal of Medicine, 312* (16), 1005–1011.

Richie, D., & Sivarajan-Froelicher, E. (1995). Exercise and activity. In S. Woods, E. Sivarajan-Froelicher, J. Halpenny, & S. Underhill (Eds.), *Cardiac nursing* (3rd ed) (pp. 708–724). Philadelphia: J.B. Lippincott.

Rosenman, R. H. (1974). The role of behavior patterns and neurogenic factors in the pathogenesis of coronary heart disease. In R. S. Eliot (Ed.), *Stress and the heart* (pp. 123–141). Mt. Kisco: Futura.

Rosenman, R. H., Friedman, M., Strauss, R., et al. (1970). Coronary heart disease in the Western Collaborative Study Group: A follow-up experience of 4–1/2 years. *Journal of Chronic Diseases, 23,* 173–190.

Rowell, L. B. (1986). *Human circulation regulation during physical stress.* New York: Oxford University Press.

Skov, P., & Underhill Motzer, S. (1995). History taking and physical examination. In S. Woods, E. Sivarajan-Froelicher, J. Halpenny, & S. Underhill (Eds.), *Cardiac nursing* (3rd ed) (pp. 226–258). Philadelphia: J.B. Lippincott.

Sollek, M. V. (1995). High blood pressure. In S. Woods, E. Sivarajan-Froelicher, J. Halpenny, & S. Underhill (eds.), *Cardiac Nursing* (3rd ed.) (pp. 751–797). Philadelphia: J. B. Lippincott.

VanEtta, D. (1995). Peripheral vascular disease. In S. Woods, E. Sivarajan-Froelicher, J. Halpenny, & S. Underhill (Eds.), *Cardiac nursing* (3rd ed) (pp. 831–841). Philadelphia: J.B. Lippincott.

Bibliography

American Heart Association (1993). Basic life support heart saver guide—a student handbook for cardiopulmonary resuscitation and first aid for choking. Dallas, TX.

American Medical Association. (1992). Pediatric basic life support. *JAMA, 268,* 2256, 2257.

Bates, B. (1995). *A guide to physical examination* (6th ed.). Philadelphia: J.B. Lippincott.

Boose Fabius, D. (1994). Solving the mystery of heart murmurs. *Nursing 94, 24* (7), 39–44.

Carpenito, L. J. (1993). *Nursing diagnosis: Application to nursing practice* (5th ed.). Philadelphia: J.B. Lippincott.

Conn, V., Taylor, S., & Casey, B. (1992) Cardiac rehabilitation program participation and outcomes after myocardial infarction. *Rehabilitation Nursing, 17* (2), 58–62.

Daumer, R., & Miller, S. P. (1992). Effects of cardiac rehabilitation on psychosocial functioning and life satisfaction of coronary artery disease clients. *Rehabilitation Nursing, 17* (2), 69–74.

Fleury, J. (1992). The application of motivational theory to cardiovascular risk reduction. *Image Journal of Nursing Scholarship, 24* (3), 229–238.

Hahn, W., Brooks, J. A., & Hartsough, D. (1993). Self-disclosure and coping styles in men with cardiovascular reactivity. *Research in Nursing and Health, 16* (4), 275–782.

Hawthorne, M. (1994). Gender differences in recovery after coronary artery surgery. *Image Journal of Nursing Scholarship, 26* (1), 75–80.

Nash, C., & Jensen, P. (1994). When your surgical patient has hypertension. *American Journal of Nursing, 94* (12), 38–44.

Puntillo, K., & Weiss, S. (1994). Pain: Its mediators and associated morbidity in critically ill cardiovascular surgical patients. *Nursing Research, 43* (1), 31–37.

Rigotti, N. A., Thomas, G. S., & Leaf, A. (1983). Exercise and coronary heart disease. *Annual Review of Medicine, 34,* 391–412.

Sollek, M. V., & Lee, K. A. (1995). High blood pressure. In S. Woods, E. Sivarajan-Froelicher, J. Halpenny, & S. Underhill (Eds.), *Cardiac nursing* (3rd ed) Philadelphia: J.B. Lippincott.

Nutrition and Metabolism

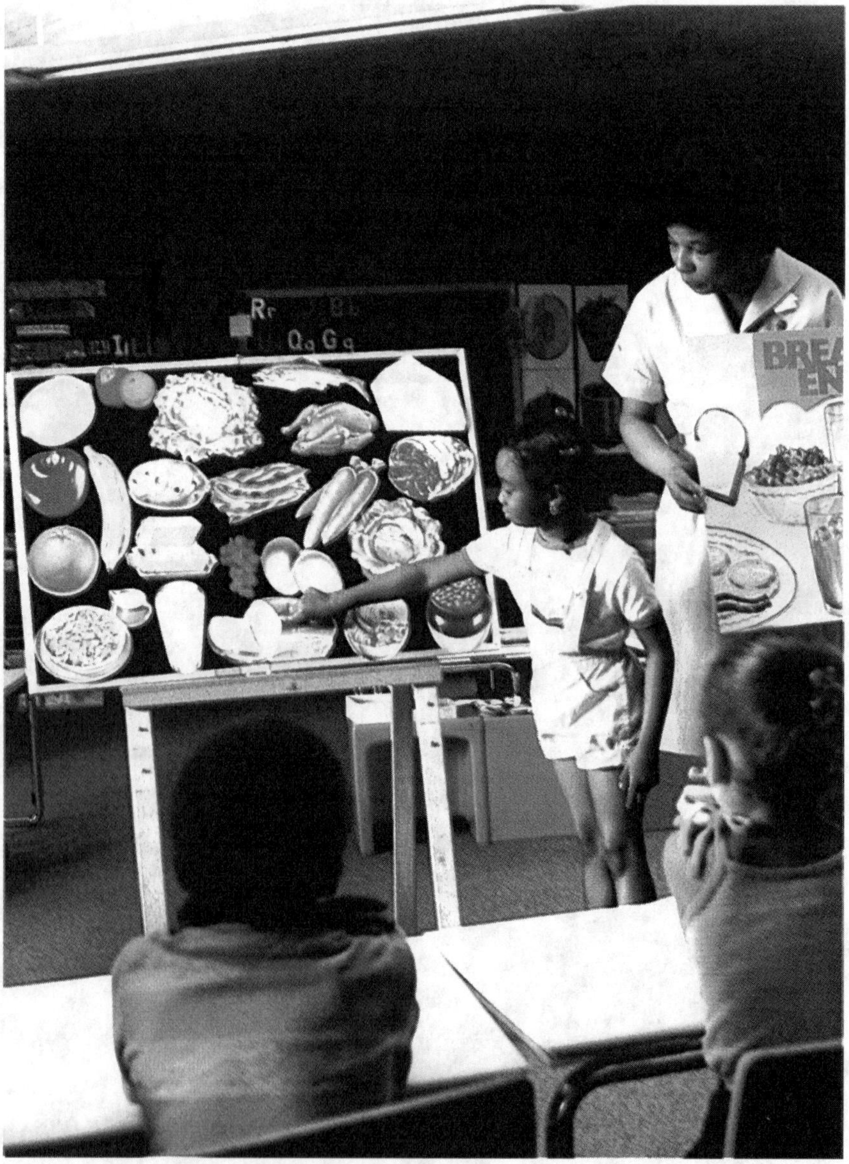

UNIT IX

Assessing for nutritional and metabolic needs and intervening to meet those needs encompass a wide range of nursing activities. Using the nursing process as a framework, Unit IX explores the many facets of nutrition and metabolism. These areas of human function include not only the intake and use of food and fluids but also such indicators of nutritional and metabolic status as skin and tissue integrity, immune system function, and body tempature regulation.

The first two chapters in this unit discuss the concepts and nursing care associated with acid–base and fluid and electrolyte balance and the intake of food and fluids. Maintaining a chemical balance within the body and meeting adequate nutritional needs require accurate assessments and nursing diagnoses that result in effective nursing interventions. Every client encounter reveals a client need for nursing care because these areas of function require the nurse to emphasize health promotion as well as health restoration or support. The next three chapters in this unit explore concepts and nursing care pertinent to situations that indicate the status of nutritional and metabolic function: skin integrity and wound healing, the body's defenses against infection, and thermoregulation.

This unit discusses concepts, principles, and nursing care issues relevant for every client. In addition to emphasizing nursing interventions to promote health and function, each chapter features assessments and holistic interventions for high-risk situations as well as nursing needs for clients with altered function.

Fluid, Electrolyte, and Acid–Base Balance

Key Terms	Learning Objectives

Key Terms

Acid
Active transport
Anion
Base (or alkali)
Buffer
Cation
Diffusion
Electrolyte
Extracellular fluid
Filtration
Hyperosmolar
Hypertonic
Interstitial fluid
Intracellular fluid
Intravascular fluid
Ion
Osmolality
Osmolarity
Osmosis
Osmotic pressure

Learning Objectives

Upon completion of this chapter, the student will be able to do the following:

- *Describe physiologic factors that affect fluid, electrolyte, and acid–base homeostasis.*
- *Describe common alterations in fluid, electrolyte, and acid–base balance.*
- *Recognize the impact of age on fluid and electrolyte status.*
- *Describe assessment parameters for the client with potential or actual fluid and electrolyte imbalance.*
- *Identify appropriate nursing diagnoses for clients with fluid imbalance.*
- *Implement appropriate client teaching to prevent or manage fluid and electrolyte imbalance.*

36

You are a student nurse working on a medical unit, and one of your assigned clients has a diagnosis of pneumonia. In shift change report, you are told that she has had diarrhea for the last 4 days accompanied by a 10-lb weight loss. She has been experiencing fever and chills, and she had no urine output during the *last shift. The laboratory called with the following results: serum Na^+, 128 mEq/L; serum K^+, 4.1 mEq/L; blood urea nitrogen, 28 mg/dL; and blood glucose, 326 mg/dL.*

In previous chapters, you studied phases of the nursing process and learned how to apply them to clinical situations. In this chapter, you will add information about fluid, electrolytes, and acid–base balance to your growing knowledge base. Fluid and electrolytes affect body homeostasis every minute, and illness affects fluid and electrolyte balance. After you have studied this chapter, turn to the Critical Thinking Challenges at the end of the chapter to help sharpen your thinking skills.

Health and normal body functioning depend on fluid, electrolyte, and acid–base balance. Vascular fluid is essential for the maintenance of adequate blood volume, blood pressure, and cardiovascular system functioning. Interstitial fluid surrounding the cells of the body is important in the transportation of oxygen, nutrients, hormones, and other essential chemicals from the blood to the cell cytoplasm. Both vascular and interstitual fluids also are important for waste removal. Intracellular fluid is critical for maintaining cell size and function. Optimal cell function depends on the volume and composition of body fluids being maintained within a narrow, normal range.

The balance of fluids, electrolytes, acids, and bases within the body is carefully regulated and depends on physiologic control mechanisms. Simple activities of daily life, such as vigorous exercise, skipping meals, or sunbathing, could upset the precise balance of fluids, electrolytes, acids, and bases if the body were not capable of making adjustments. Healthy adults and children compensate for such physiologic challenges; for example, on a hot summer day, most people will increase their fluid intake due to thirst, and their urine volume will decrease. At the same time, changes in the rate of respirations and urine composition are important in regulating acid–base balance.

Symptoms, such as vomiting and diarrhea, or therapies, such as surgery, can temporarily disrupt fluid, electrolyte, and acid–base homeostasis despite general good health. For example, sustained vomiting or diarrhea may require intervention by a healthcare professional to institute fluid replacement therapy. Chronic diseases, such as heart failure, kidney impairment, or liver dysfunction, seriously disrupt the body's ability to maintain fluid, electrolyte, and acid–base balance. People with such medical problems are in constant danger of excesses or deficits, which can be life-threatening.

The nurse plays a vital role in promoting normal fluid, electrolyte, and acid–base balance and in preventing life-threatening imbalances. Client teaching regarding the importance of adequate food, fluid, and electrolyte intake and the management of common problems, such as fever, vomiting, and diarrhea, can prevent imbalances. Nursing assessment of fluid, electrolyte, and acid–base balance is essential in early detection of imbalances so that appropriate interventions can begin promptly. Interventions such as promoting the appropiate fluid intake, assisting with eating, monitoring intravenous infusions, and administering medications can all help to maintain fluid, electrolyte, and acid–base balance.

Normal Fluid and Electrolyte Balance

Body fluid is composed primarily of water, which contains chemical compounds called electrolytes. Two aspects of body fluid are monitored and controlled by the body:

- Volume of fluid in the extracellular space
- Water concentration (osmolarity) of body fluid

Individuals can experience an excess or deficit of either or both of these aspects of body fluid. As background, it is important to review the location and characteristics of fluids in the body.

Fluid Compartments

From 45% to 80% of body weight is fluid; the variation depends on body fat, gender, and age, as illustrated in Table 36-1. Because fat contains proportionately less fluid than muscle, obese individuals contain relatively less fluid than lean individuals. Women, who have more adipose tissue than men, also have a lower fluid content. Fluid accounts for 46% to 52% of the body weight in adult women and 52% to 60% of the body weight in

Table 36-1 • Variations in Total Body Fluid According to Age and Sex

Age	Total Body Fluid (% Body Weight)
Premature infant	85%
Newborn (full-term)	70%–80%
12 months	64%
Puberty to 39	Male: 60% Female: 52%
40–60	Male: 55% Female: 47%
Older than 60	Male: 52% Female: 46%

From Metheny, N. (1992). *Fluid and electrolyte balance: Nursing considerations* (p. 5) (2nd ed.). Philadelphia: J.B. Lippincott.

Table 36-2 • Normal Serum Electrolyte Values

Electrolyte	Serum Value
Cations	
Sodium (Na^+)	135–145 mEq/L
Potassium (K^+)	3.5–5.0 mEq/L
Calcium (Ca^{++})	4.3–5.3 mEq/L (8.5–10.5 mg/dL)
Magnesium (Mg^{++})	1.5–2.5 mEq/L (1.8–3.0 mg/dL)
Anions	
Chloride (Cl^-)	95–108 mEq/L
Bicarbonate (HCO_3^-)	22–26 mEq/L
Phosphorus (PO_4^-)	1.7–2.6 mEq/L (2.5–4.5 mg/dL)

Normal value ranges may vary slightly from laboratory to laboratory.

adult men. Infants have a greater proportion of body fluid than adults.

The fluids in the two major body fluid compartments (intracellular and extracellular) vary in electrolyte composition and location. The primary electrolytes of the **intracellular fluid** (which is located within body cells) are potassium, phosphate, and sulfate. The primary electrolytes of the **extracellular fluid** (ECF, consists of all the fluid outside the cells) are sodium, chloride, and bicarbonate. The concentrations of the primary extracellular electrolytes are listed in Table 36-2. The ECF is further divided into the *intravascular fluid*, which consists of the fluid inside the blood and lymphatic vessels, and *interstitial fluid*, which is the fluid between the cells. Adults have about two-thirds of their total fluid within the intracellular compartment and one-third in the extracellular compartment (Fig. 36-1). In contrast, newborns have more extracellular than intracellular fluid. By 3 months of age, infants have equal amounts of intracellular fluid and ECF, and by 1 year, they approach the same distribution as adults (Metheny, 1992). The maintenance of the proportional distribution of ECF between the vascular and interstitial spaces depends on three factors:

- Protein content of the blood (serum proteins, predominantly albumin and globulin)
- Integrity of the vascular endothelium (the layer of cells lining blood vessels)
- Hydrostatic pressure inside the blood vessels

The protein content of the blood and vascular endothelium function to keep fluids within the blood vessels, while the hydrostatic pressure tends to force fluid out of the vessels. In healthy individuals, these forces are equally balanced.

Extracellular Fluid Volume

The most important regulated aspect of body fluid balance is the volume of ECF. The body monitors ECF volume with stretch receptors known as pressure or barore-

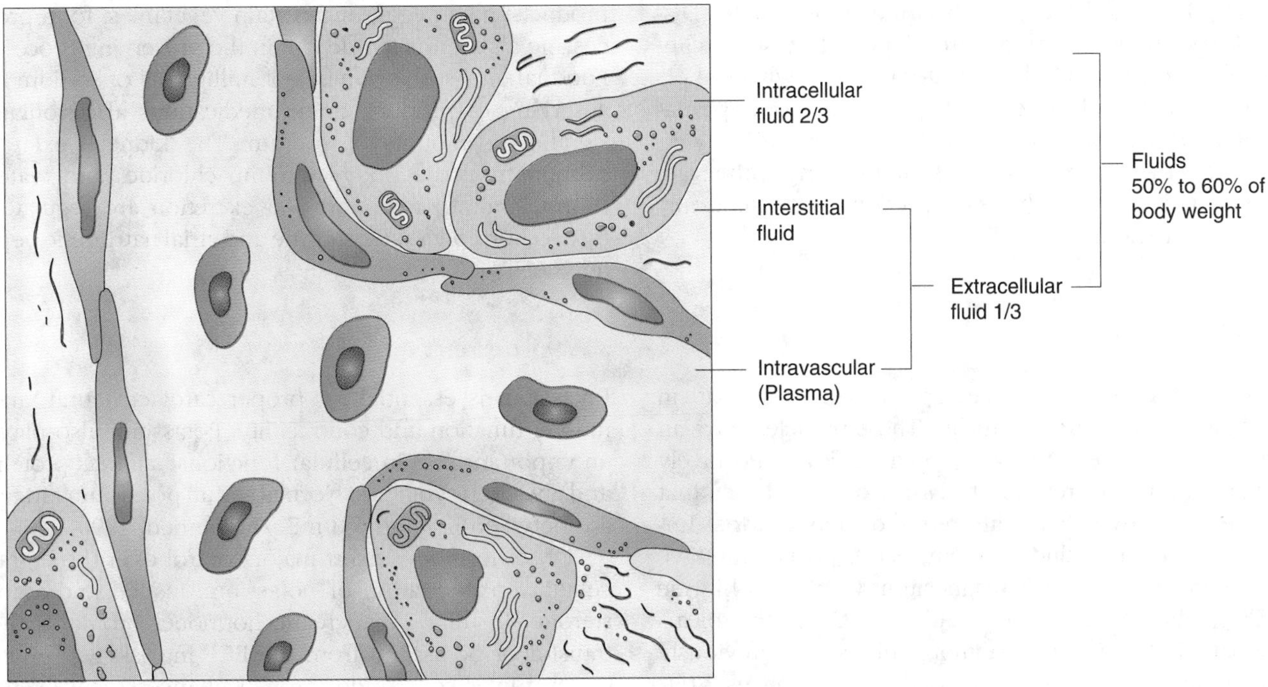

Figure 36-1 • Fluid compartments, showing intracellular fluid and extracellular fluid (which contains intravascular and interstitial fluid). Total body fluid is 50% to 60% of body weight.

ceptors located in major arteries and veins. The renin-angiotensin-aldosterone hormone system then regulates extracellular volume by adjusting fluid intake and the urinary excretion of sodium, chloride, and water to maintain the extracellular volume within normal limits. Extracellular volume is the most protected aspect of body fluid balance because without an adequate extracellular volume, blood pressure cannot be maintained. Prolonged periods of very low blood pressure are known as shock, a lethal condition (see Chap. 35).

Water Concentration (Osmolarity) of Body Fluid

The second aspect of body fluid that is regulated is osmolarity. **Osmolarity** refers to the proportion of dissolved particles (solute) in a volume of fluid.

The normal range for osmolarity is between 275 and 290 mOsm/L. (see following section on osmotic pressure; Rose, 1994). Hypothalamic cells, known as osmoreceptors, monitor changes in body fluid osmolarity and respond by varying the secretion of antidiuretic hormone (ADH) from the posterior pituitary. When body osmolarity falls due to an excess of water in relation to solute, ADH secretion is inhibited; when osmolarity increases due to a decrease in water in relation to solute, ADH secretion is increased. ADH regulates the concentration of the urine by influencing water reabsorption in the distal tubule and collecting duct of the nephron. When body osmolarity is increased, ADH is secreted, the urine becomes more concentrated, water is retained, and plasma osmolarity decreases. Conversely, when osmolarity is decreased, ADH secretion is inhibited, and the urine becomes more dilute. Disorders of body osmolarity are identified by some clinicians as disorders of body water balance, while others refer to these imbalances as hyponatremia or hypernatremia because an excess or deficit of water directly influences the concentration of sodium; along with its accompanying anions, this is the predominant osmotically active particle in the ECF.

Electrolytes

Electrolytes are chemical compounds that dissociate in solution into separate particles. These particles carry an electrical charge and are known as **ions.** Positively charged ions are referred to as **cations,** and ions that have a negative charge are referred to as **anions**. Important cations include sodium (Na^+), potassium (K^+), calcium (Ca^{++}), and magnesium (Mg^{++}). Chloride (Cl^-), phosphate (HPO_4^-), sulfate (SO_4^-), and bicarbonate (HCO_3^-) are common anions. As previously mentioned, the concentration of these electrolytes is different in the intracellular and ECF compartments. The most common electrolytes in the ECF are sodium, chloride, and bicarbonate, whereas potassium, phosphate, and sulfate are found in greatest concentration in the intracellular fluid.

Electrolytes are measured in terms of their combining power, or the ability of cations to combine with anions, rather than by their absolute weight in solution. The milliequivalent is the measure of this chemical activity. The amount of electrolytes in a solution is most commonly expressed in terms of milliequivalents per liter (mEq/L). For example, 1 mEq of Mg^{++} will combine with 2 mEq of Cl^-.

Electrolyte balance refers to maintaining the concentration of each electrolyte in the serum within normal limits. Electrolyte imbalance refers to an increase or decrease of the concentration of ions within the serum. Because the concentration of cellular electrolytes is not commonly available, the healthcare worker relies on changes in the serum levels to reflect body electrolyte imbalance. Normal serum electrolyte ranges for the adult are given in Table 36-2. Normal values vary somewhat between laboratories. Trends in electrolyte concentration over time should be monitored whenever possible rather than making a diagnosis based on a single laboratory value.

Sodium

Sodium is the most abundant cation in the ECF. Normal serum sodium levels are between 135 and 145 mEq/L. Changes in the serum sodium level reflect changes in body water balance or osmolarity and therefore *do not* reflect sodium intake and output directly. Sodium is found in table salt (sodium chloride), dairy products, meat, eggs, and certain vegetables; food processing also tends to add salt in the preserving process. Food labels list the number of milligrams of sodium in a serving of product. Some medications also contain significant amounts of sodium. The kidneys excrete sodium from the body. Sodium, chloride, and water (normal saline) retention and excretion are regulated by two hormones, aldosterone and atrial natriuretic peptide (ANP).

Potassium

Potassium is essential for proper cardiac, neural, and muscle function and contractility. Potassium also plays an important role in cellular functions, such as protein and glycogen synthesis. Normal serum potassium ranges are between 3.5 and 5.0 mEq/L (Tannen, 1990).

Two hormones exert major control over the extracellular concentration of potassium: insulin and aldosterone. Insulin, a pancreatic hormone, promotes the transfer of potassium from the ECF into skeletal muscle and liver cells. Aldosterone enhances renal excretion of potassium. An increase in serum potassium stimulates the release of insulin and aldosterone to lower the concentration of the ion. Conversely, a decrease in serum potassium inhibits the release of aldosterone and insulin to reduce excretion of the ion.

The body needs a minimum 30 mEq/d of potassium, and a typical Western diet contains 50 to 100 mEq/d (Tannen, 1990). The kidneys play the major role in the maintenance of potassium balance, varying excretion with daily intake. Potassium also is excreted from the body in the stool and in perspiration.

Calcium

Normal serum calcium levels are between 8.5 and 10.5 mg/dL (Pak, 1990). Approximately 99% of the calcium within the body is located within the bones and teeth. The remainder is located in the serum. Calcium is present in the blood primarily in two states: ionized and bound to protein. Approximately 50% is ionized, with the remainder bound to proteins, mainly albumin. The level of ionized calcium is most important for physiologic function. Because a large portion of the calcium is bound to albumin, it is important to look at the serum albumin levels when evaluating laboratory data. If serum albumin levels are decreased, which may happen with liver disease or cachexia, the level of ionized calcium may or may not also be decreased. The laboratory can then be asked to measure the ionized calcium level, which is normally 2.0 to 2.5 mEq/L (Pak, 1990).

Calcium is indispensable for healthy functioning. The cell membrane structure depends on calcium, because it promotes cell to cell adhesion. Calcium also is important in wound healing, synaptic transmission in nervous tissue, membrane excitability, muscle contractility, and providing the structure for teeth and bones. Calcium is essential for blood clotting and is critical in metabolic reactions involved in energy production (glycolysis).

There are many good dietary sources for calcium. Dairy products, such as milk, cheese, and yogurt, are excellent sources. Sardines, whole grains, and leafy, green vegetables also contribute calcium. Food labels indicate the percent of the daily value of calcium contained in a serving.

Magnesium

The normal serum magnesium level is 1.4 to 2.0 mEq/L (1.7–2.4 mg/dL; Cronin, 1990). Seventy percent of magnesium is in the bones, and 30% is in the soft tissue and body fluids. Like potassium, magnesium is primarily an intracellular ion, with only 1% in ECF. Magnesium is important in regulating neuromuscular function and cardiac activity. Alterations in magnesium are often paralleled by changes in potassium, and the signs and symptoms of a deficit of either ion are similar. In addition, a magnesium deficiency is often accompanied by hypocalcemia (Cronin, 1990). Good dietary sources of magnesium include green, leafy vegetables; legumes; citrus fruit; peanut butter; and chocolate. The kidney regulates magnesium levels by reabsorbing the ion when serum levels are low and excreting it when serum levels are high.

Fluid and Electrolyte Distribution

The membranes of individual cells, the vascular capillary walls, and the lymphatic capillary walls are semipermeable membranes that separate fluid compartments. Movement between compartments is constant and necessary for cell viability. Water and some electrolytes move easily across these semipermeable membranes, but larger molecules, such as proteins, are less able to move across capillary walls. The mechanisms by which fluid movement occurs include osmosis and filtration. Electrolytes and other dissolved particles move by means of diffusion, filtration, and active transport. These mechanisms respond to fluid pressures, which include hydrostatic pressure and oncotic pressure.

Processes of Fluid and Electrolyte Movement

Diffusion. **Diffusion** is the process of molecules moving from an area of higher concentration to an area of lower concentration. Molecules are in constant motion; if a highly concentrated substance is placed in one side of a container of fluid, the molecules will bounce off each other until they are equally distributed in the solution.

Diffusion is an important process in maintaining electrochemical neutrality. Electrochemical neutrality, a state in which the numbers of anions and cations are balanced within each fluid compartment, is the normal condition within compartments. If any compartment contains an excess of cations, then an identical number of anions must diffuse into the compartment so that the charge is balanced. The same is true if an excess of anions is present: A sufficient number of cations will diffuse into the compartment to balance the electrical charge and ensure electrochemical neutrality.

Osmosis. **Osmosis** refers to the movement of a fluid through a semipermeable membrane. A semipermeable membrane allows some substances to travel through but not others. Osmosis can occur if a semipermeable membrane separating two fluid compartments is permeable to water, and if one compartment contains a greater concentration of a dissolved substance (hyperosmolar) than the other compartment (hypo-osmolar). Water passes through the membrane to the area of greater concentration of the dissolved substance. The net effect of osmosis is to equalize solution concentrations on both sides of the membrane. The principle to

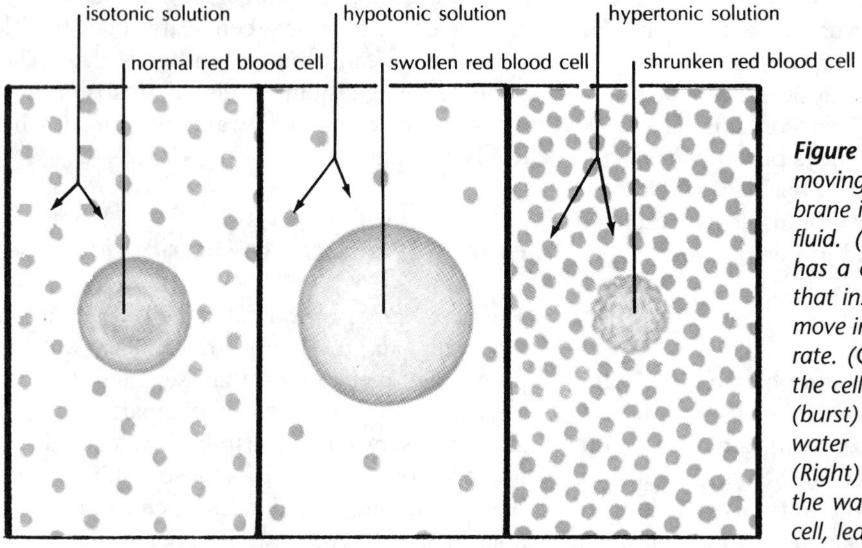

Figure 36-2 *• Osmosis. Water molecules moving through a red blood cell membrane in three different concentrations of fluid. (Left) The normal saline solution has a concentration nearly the same as that inside the cell, and water molecules move into and out of the cell at the same rate. (Center) The dilute solution causes the cell to swell and eventually hemolyze (burst) because of the large number of water molecules moving into the cell. (Right) The concentrated solution causes the water molecules to move out of the cell, leaving it shrunken.*

remember is given a semipermeable membrane, water always moves in the direction of greater concentration of dissolved particles (Fig. 36-2). Capillary vessel walls and cell walls are semipermeable membranes.

Active Transport. **Active transport** is the process by which ions and other molecules move across membranes from an area of lesser concentration to an area of greater concentration. Energy is required to move ions against a concentration gradient. Enzymes, such as sodium potassium ATPase, are involved in active transport. A specific carrier molecule binds with each ion transported against the concentration gradient. The carrier and the combined ion move through the semipermeable membrane and then separate. Active transport can be inhibited by decreasing the temperature of the cell, decreasing the supply of glucose and nutrients available to the cell, and exposing the cell to medications or toxins.

The process of active transport can be illustrated by the functioning of the sodium–potassium pump in the body. A high concentration of sodium ions is present in ECF (135–145 mEq/L), whereas a low concentration of sodium is present in the intracellular fluid (10 mEq/L). Sodium ions diffuse across the cell membrane into the cell down this concentration gradient. If left unchecked, intracellular sodium would continue to rise, extracellular sodium would continue to fall, and cell function would be disrupted. The sodium–potassium pump prevents sodium from accumulating inside the cell by actively transporting sodium out. The difference in concentration of sodium and potassium in intracellular and extracellular compartments is essential for the initiation of action potentials, nerve impulse propagation, and muscle contraction.

Filtration. **Filtration** involves the transfer of water and dissolved substances through a permeable membrane from a region of high pressure to a region of low pressure. Hydrostatic pressure, or the pressure exerted by fluid against the walls of its container, promotes the flow of fluid out of the capillaries (Fig. 36-3). Filtration

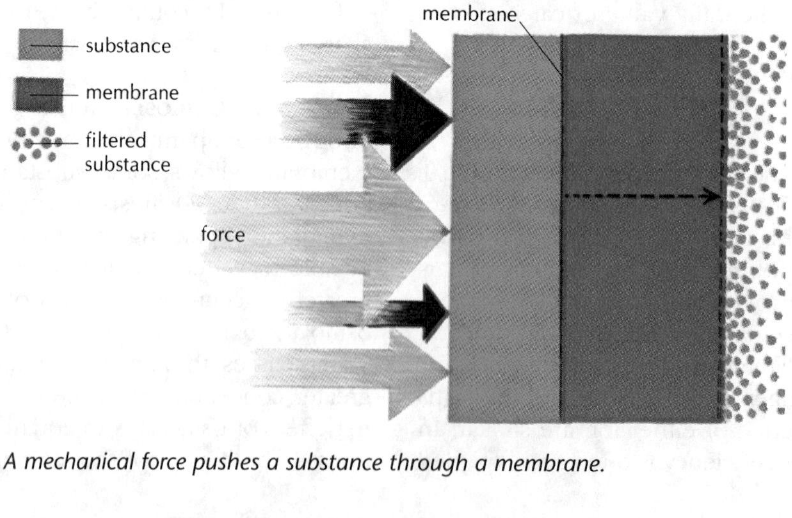

Figure 36-3 *• Filtration. A mechanical force pushes a substance through a membrane.*

occurs within the glomerular capillaries of the kidney and in tissue capillaries.

Pressures Affecting Fluid and Electrolyte Movement

Pressure differences are important in determining fluid movement between and within the intracellular fluid and ECF compartments. The most important pressures involved in fluid movement are osmotic pressure and hydrostatic pressure.

Osmotic Pressure. **Osmotic pressure,** the force of attraction for water by undissolved particles, helps to keep fluid within blood vessels and opposes net flow outward. Osmotic pressure depends on the osmolarity of the solution. Osmolarity refers to the proportion of dissolved particles (solute) in a volume of fluid. **Osmolality** refers to the concentration of dissolved substances on the basis of weight to weight rather than weight to volume. Osmolarity is expressed in milliosmols per liter (mOsm/L), whereas osmolality is expressed in milliosmols per kilogram (mOsm/kg). Because body fluids are very dilute, these terms are often used interchangeably.

The normal osmolality of blood plasma is approximately 275 to 290 mOsm/kg (Rose, 1994). Plasma proteins contribute to the osmotic pressure because they are hydrophilic, which means they attract water. Another term for the osmotic pressure that is produced by plasma proteins is colloid oncotic pressure.

Fluids can differ in osmolarity depending on the concentration of their solutes (see Fig. 26-1). The major extracellular substances that contribute to the movement of water between the ECF and cell cytoplasm are sodium, chloride, and glucose. A solution that has the same osmotic pressure or osmolarity as blood plasma is called iso-osmotic or isotonic. When an isotonic solution enters the circulation, there is no net movement of water across the membrane, so cells retain their normal size. Normal saline (0.9%) is an isotonic solution. A hypo-osmotic or hypotonic solution has a concentration of solute that is less than blood plasma. When a hypotonic solution (such as water) surrounds cells, water will cross the membrane into the cells, causing them to swell. The opposite is true for a hyperosmotic or hypertonic solution. In a hypertonic solution, the concentration of solute is greater than blood plasma. When a hypertonic solution such as 3% sodium chloride (hypertonic saline) is infused, water will leave cells, causing the cells to decrease in size.

Hydrostatic Pressure. Hydrostatic pressure promotes filtration of fluid from an area of higher pressure to an area of lower pressure, such as from the blood vessels into the interstitial fluid compartment. Factors that affect hydrostatic pressure include the arterial blood pressure, the force with which the heart pumps blood, the rate of blood flow, and venous pressure.

Filtration Pressure. Hydrostatic pressure minus osmotic pressure equals the filtration pressure. To illustrate what happens as blood circulates through the capillary bed, the filtration pressure needs to be examined (Fig. 36-4). In the arteriole, the net hydrostatic pressure of the blood is about 32 mm Hg, and the osmotic pressure is 22 mm Hg. The filtration pressure of the arteriole is the difference between them, or +10 mm Hg. Be-

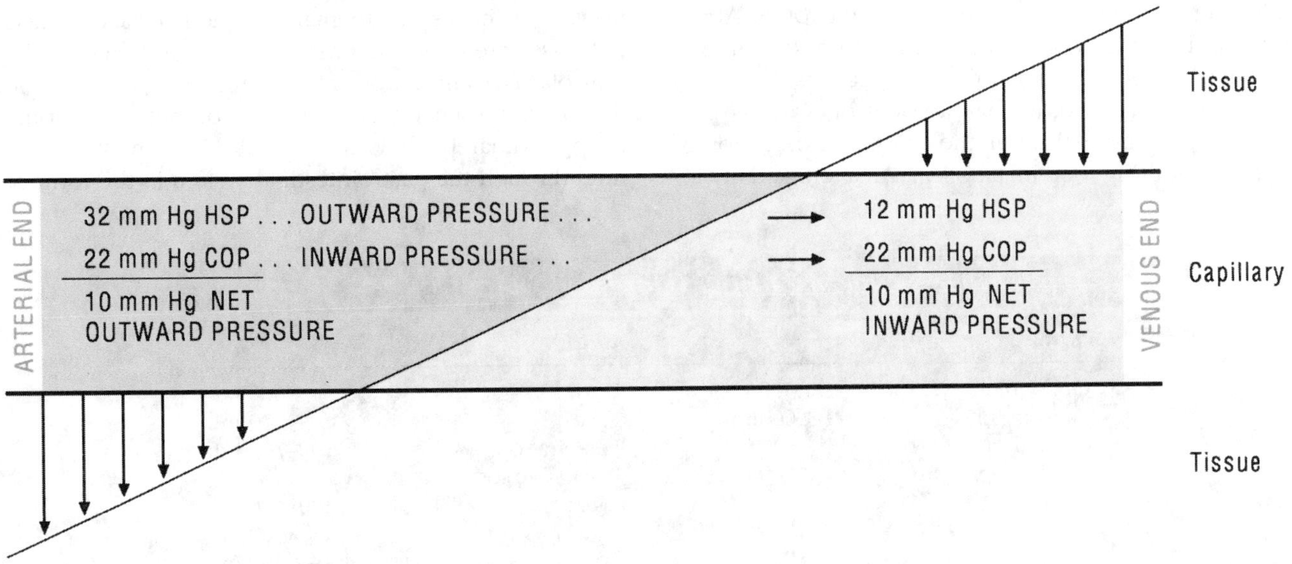

Figure 36-4 • Filtration pressure in a capillary. In the arterial end of a capillary, fluid is pushed out into the tissues; in the venous end, fluid is absorbed back into the circulation.

cause this is a positive pressure, fluid filters out of the vessel into the interstitial fluid. However, in the venule, hydrostatic pressure is 12 mm Hg, while the osmotic pressure remains 22 mm Hg. The filtration pressure is the difference, which is −10 mm Hg. Because this is a negative pressure, fluid will filter from the interstitial fluid back into the venous capillaries and venules.

This process of fluid leaking out of the arterioles, only to be reabsorbed in the venules, is continuous. It also is the manner by which the body is able to transport oxygen and other nutrients to the cells and remove waste products. In the healthy person, this process is balanced so that almost all filtered fluid is returned to the vascular space. The lymphatic vessels return excess fluid to the circulation through the thoracic duct and at the same time carry cells and proteins from the periphery through the lymph nodes. If the hydrostatic pressure is greatly increased or the osmotic pressure is greatly reduced, some of the filtered fluid remains in the interstitial space, and this accumulation is called edema. Blockage of lymph drainage also can produce edema.

Factors Affecting Fluid and Electrolyte Balance

In the healthy person, homeostasis demands a balanced fluid and electrolyte status. Normally, fluids and electrolytes lost from the body are replenished through adequate intake. Hormonal controls and kidney function regulate this process; Table 36-3 gives a summary of typical intake and output for a 24-hour period. Hormones also influence the movement of electrolytes in and out of cells.

Fluid Intake

Water enters the body through the oral route. About two-thirds of ingested water is in the form of drinking water or other beverages; the remainder is contained in other foods. Also, a small amount of water is produced by the body through the process of oxidation of hydrogen during food metabolism. An average daily intake for an adult is 1,300 mL of water (about six glasses). An additional 1,000 mL of water is obtained from foods, especially fruits and vegetables, which are about 80% to 90% water. About 300 mL of water is obtained through food oxidation (Metheny, 1992).

The thirst mechanism helps to regulate fluid intake. The thirst center is located in the hypothalamus and is stimulated by an increase in plasma osmolarity or a decrease in blood volume. Psychological factors or a dry mouth also may stimulate thirst. Adequate intake of fluids will satisfy thirst if blood volume is restored and osmolarity returns to normal. The level of serum osmolarity at which individuals begin to experience thirst has been shown to be decreased in pregnancy and elevated in the older adults (Sterns & Spital, 1990).

Food Intake

In addition to food providing approximately one-third of the body's fluid needs, food provides the body with electrolytes. Calcium is abundant in dairy products. Sodium is found in salt, processed meat and food, bread products, and dairy products. Bananas, melons, oranges, apricots, broccoli, raisins, and dates are all good sources of potassium. A well-balanced diet contains all the necessary electrolytes.

Fluid and Electrolyte Output

Water and electrolytes can be lost from the body in four ways: through the kidneys as urine, through the skin as perspiration, through the lungs as insensible water loss, and through the gastrointestinal tract in stool or vomit.

The kidney is the main organ regulating fluid balance. Glomerular filtration and tubular reabsorption permit the kidneys to conserve or excrete water and electrolytes as necessary to maintain homeostasis. These processes are controlled through the hormonal regulation of ADH and aldosterone, which are discussed in the following section. Normal urine output for 24 hours is approximately 1,500 mL if intake is normal. Loss of fluid through the gastrointestinal system in the form of

Table 36-3 • Typical 24-Hour Intake and Output

Intake		*Output*	
Oral Fluids	1,300 mL	Urine	1,500 mL
Fluid in food	1,000 mL	Feces	200 mL
Oxidation of food	300 mL	Perspiration	100–200 mL
Total	2,600 mL	Insensible loss	
		Skin	300–400 mL
		Respiration	300 mL
		Total	2,400–2,600 mL

Therapeutic Dialogue
Edema in Pregnancy

Scenes for Thought

Eileen Watkins is 35 years old and happily pregnant for the second time. Her first child, Katie, is 4 years old. Eileen and Katie are in the clinic for Eileen's 6-month checkup.

Effective

Nurse: *Hello ladies. How are you both today?*
Client: *Hi, Sarah. We're doing just fine, right Katie?* Hugs the little girl.
Nurse: *Let me get some weight and blood pressure readings on you, Eileen. (Does so, and Katie gets her weight read, too.) You know, I think your blood pressure is a little high this month, Eileen. Have you noticed anything different with you?*
Client: Looks worried. *What do you mean different?*
Nurse: *Have you had headaches, feet swelling, feeling extra tired? (Good eye contact.)*
Client: Looks down at her feet. *A little, right around the ankles and over the instep.* Looks up at you. *Is there a problem?* Katie looks over at her mother's face.
Nurse: *(Reaching down to assess the edema—2+ pitting over the ankle.) Nothing unusual for most pregnant women. If I remember, you had some swelling when you were pregnant with Katie, right?*
Client: *Yes, but not this early; it was in the 8th month, I think.*
Nurse: *(Checking the chart.) That's right. This seems to worry you. (Good eye contact.)*
Client: *Yes. I guess I thought everything was going to be the same as last time—easy, no problems.* Smiles at Katie, a little sadly.
Nurse: *Is there something particular worrying you about this?*
Client: *I didn't tell you last time; my mother lost three babies after her blood pressure got really high and her legs swelled up. I remember that it happened when I was about 10 years old, and it really scared me. I was so glad when my pregnancy was so easy.*
Nurse: *I understand your worry. You're scared that you'll swell up like your mom and have the same problems.* Client nods; she looks scared. Katie is keeping a close eye on her mom. *Well, let's work on this together. There are a number of ways I can think of to take care of this.*
Client: *You mean putting my feet up and staying off the chips? I do that already. What else should I do?* Sounds a little frustrated.
Nurse: *First, let's chat a little more. I want to find out about your daily routine and then talk about some salt hidden in foods that might not be so obvious. Before all that, I just want to say that we can work on this together. Even Katie can help. (Puts hand over Eileen's.)*
Client: *Okay. I'm listening.* Takes a breath and settles in.

Less Effective

Nurse: *Hello ladies. How are you both today?*
Client: *Hi, Cindy. We're doing just fine, right Katie?* Hugs the little girl.
Nurse: *Let me get some weight and blood pressure readings on you , Eileen. (Does so, and Katie gets her weight read, too.) You know, I think your blood pressure is a little high this month, Eileen. Have you noticed anything different with you?*
Client: Looks worried. *What do you mean different?*
Nurse: *Have you had headaches, feet swelling, feeling extra tired? (Good eye contact.)*
Client: Looks down at her feet. *A little, right around the ankles and over the instep.* Looks up at you. *Is there a problem?* Katie looks over at her mother's face.
Nurse: *(Reaching down to assess the edema—2+ pitting over the ankle.) Nothing unusual for most pregnant women. If I remember, you had some swelling when you were pregnant with Katie, right?*
Client: *Yes, but not this early; it was in the 8th month, I think.*
Nurse: *Yes, it's a little earlier than last time, Eileen, but you're 4 years older, you're working harder now with Katie and your job to take care of, and besides, it's summertime! Edema is always worse in the summer. (Pats Eileen's hand.) Don't worry, Eileen. You're fine. Let me give you some information on salt in your food that might be hidden in stuff like biscuit mix. This is a really good pamphlet . . . (Continues to talk about hidden sodium and resting throughout the day in a reassuring tone.)*
Client: Listening carefully and anxiously, holding Katie close.

Critical Thinking Challenge

- *Relate anxiety to the ability to hear and learn.* • *Detect what Cindy did to deal with Eileen's anxiety about the pedal edema.* • *Analyze how you could tell one was more effective than the other by looking at body language.* • *Determine what emotions you would assess on Eileen's next checkup.* • *Describe how you would assess for them if you were Sarah and then if you were Cindy.*

feces is usually minimal (approximately 200 mL; Metheny, 1987).

Loss of fluid through the skin in the form of perspiration accounts for an average daily loss of 100 to 200 mL of fluid. In addition to perspiration, insensible fluid loss through the skin amounts to about 300 to 400 mL/d. Insensible water loss occurs when water molecules move from an area of higher concentration (the body) to an area of lower concentration (the atmosphere). This differs from perspiration, during which sweat glands actively expel water through the skin.

The final route for fluid loss is through the lungs during respiration. Exhalation not only contains carbon dioxide, but also water vapor. The loss of water through respiration is approximately 300 mL/d (Metheny, 1992). As body temperature increases with fever, the amount of fluid lost as perspiration, insensible water loss, and from the lungs with respiration increases proportionally.

Hormonal Control

Three hormones, aldosterone, ANP, and ADH, regulate fluid balance in the body. They work by adjusting the urine output and concentration to maintain fluid and electrolyte balance. ECF volume is regulated by the renin-angiotensin-aldosterone system and ANP, while body water balance or osmolarity is controlled by ADH. Parathyroid hormone (PTH) is involved in the regulation of body calcium and phosphate balance, while insulin influences the distribution of potassium between the intracellular fluid and ECF.

Renin-Angiotensin-Aldosterone System. The renin-angiotensin-aldosterone system regulates ECF volume. Renin release is stimulated by decreased arterial blood pressure, decreased renal blood flow, increased renal sympathetic nerve activity, or a low-salt diet. Renin, an enzyme secreted by juxtoglomerular cells in the kidney, splits angiotensinogen into angiotensin I. Angiotensinogen is produced by the liver and circulates in the blood. Converting enzyme in the lungs and other vascular beds converts angiotensin I into angiotensin II. Angiotensin II stimulates aldosterone secretion and is a potent vasoconstrictor.

Aldosterone, which is produced by the adrenal cortex, regulates sodium reabsorption in the distal tubules and collecting ducts of the kidney. Because chloride and water passively accompany the reabsorbed sodium, the result of aldosterone action on the kidney is the reabsorption of saline, a 0.9% solution of sodium chloride, which is ECF.

Atrial Natriuretic Peptide. ANP has recently been found to be produced by the cardiac atria in response to changes in ECF volume. When atrial pressure is increased, ANP is released by the atrial myocytes and acts on the nephron to increase sodium excretion. Release of ANP is inhibited by low atrial pressures.

Antidiuretic Hormone. ADH is produced in the supraoptic and paraventricular nuclei of the hypothalamus. From these nuclei, ADH passes down axons into the posterior lobe of the pituitary, where it is stored. When plasma osmolarity increases and activates the hypothalamic osmoreceptors, ADH is released into the systemic circulation. ADH maintains the osmolarity of the blood within normal limits by adjusting the amount of water excreted in the urine. The hormone acts on the distal tubules and collecting tubules in the kidney, making them more permeable to water. This permeability increase promotes water reabsorption and serves to conserve water in the body. In the presence of an increased ADH, the urine becomes more concentrated. Conversely, if plasma osmolarity is decreased due to an excess of water in relation to solute, ADH release is inhibited, resulting in a decrease in the water permeability of the distal tubules and collecting duct. When water permeability is decreased, the urine is more dilute, water is lost from the body, and plasma osmolarity increases.

Under typical circumstances, ADH release is controlled by changes in plasma osmolarity. However, when arterial blood pressure is markedly diminished, such as with heart failure and shock, ADH is released regardless of plasma osmolarity in response to input from the vascular baroreceptors (Abraham, 1994).

Parathyroid Hormone. PTH, along with vitamin D and calcitonin, helps to regulate the calcium and phosphate balance in the body. The presence of PTH causes serum calcium levels to increase by increasing gut and renal reabsorption of calcium and releasing calcium from bone. Usually, there is a reciprocal relationship between calcium and phosphorus levels. PTH increases serum calcium levels but decreases serum phosphate levels, and conversely, decreased secretion of PTH will lower serum calcium levels and increase serum phosphate concentration.

Lifespan Considerations

Age is a significant factor in fluid and electrolyte balance. The very young and older adults are more likely to experience fluid or electrolyte imbalances. An understanding of age-related differences is important so that a nurse can participate in the prevention, identification, and management of fluid and electrolyte problems.

Newborn and Infant

Infants have a proportionally larger percentage of weight (70%–80%) as water than adults (60%). Preterm infants have an even greater amount of body water, up to 90% (Metheny, 1992). A greater amount of the water is within the extracellular compartment in the infant as compared with the adult. The infant also has a greater surface area in relation to weight than the adult. Hence, a proportionally larger volume of fluid can be lost through the skin. Fluid requirements vary according to age, as do normal urine outputs. Generally the infant has greater fluid requirements and greater fluid losses. The kidneys of the infant are immature, lacking the ability to concentrate urine fully (Blackburn, 1994; Robillard, Segar, Smith, & Jose, 1992). Metabolic rate is high in the infant, as is the respiratory rate, both of which contribute to increased insensible loss of fluid.

Fluid loss can occur very rapidly in this age group. Parents need to be taught how potentially serious vomiting or diarrhea can be for the infant and the importance of contacting their healthcare provider and appropriate fluid replacement if these symptoms occur (MMWR, 1994).

Toddler and Preschooler

Approximately 62% of the toddler's weight is water. Fluid requirements vary but are generally 1,000 to 1,200 mL for a 24-hour period. Urine output increases from approximately 500 to 700 mL/d at 2 years to 600 to 850 mL/d at 5 years. Water loss through the skin, respiration, urine, and stools is proportionally greater for the young child than for the adult.

Child and Adolescent

The ratio of total body water to total body weight decreases throughout childhood and adolescence. By the time the child is 12 years old, the percentage of body water to body weight is approximately the same as in the adult. Children in this age group often drink soda or sugared beverages to supply their fluid needs. Water and other more nutritious fluids, such as milk and fruit juices, should be encouraged. Children and adolescents need to be cautioned against the potential dangers of excessive exercise without adequate fluid replacement, especially in hot weather, because muscle damage (rhabdomyolysis) and fluid and electrolyte imbalances can occur (Tannen, 1990). Balanced dietary intake is important to promote normal electrolyte balance. Dietary intake may be erratic in the adolescent. Fad diets or purging to lose weight, which have become increasingly frequent among adolescent girls, can cause severe fluid and electrolyte imbalances.

Adult and Older Adult

Water accounts for 46% to 52% of the body weight in adult women and 52% to 60% of the body weight in adult men. The lower water content in women is due to greater amounts of adipose tissue. In middle age, there tends to be an increase in adipose tissue, thus accounting for a continual decrease in total body fluids after the age of 40. After 25 years, there is a decline in the number of nephrons in the kidney. By the time an individual is 85 years old, there are 30% to 40% fewer functioning nephrons. Consequently, the kidney has less ability to concentrate urine and conserve body fluids (Faull, Holmes, & Baylis, 1993). When adults older than 65 years were compared with younger adults (mean age 22 years), the plasma osmolarity at which the older group experienced thirst was increased, which means they have an increased risk of developing a water deficit (Mack, et al., 1994).

Adults most often develop fluid and electrolyte imbalances after an acute illness or elective surgery. Older adults commonly experience alterations in fluid and electrolyte status secondary to chronic diseases, such as renal failure or heart failure. Diuretics, commonly given to treat high blood pressure and heart failure, can cause hypernatremia or hypokalemia. Excessive use of laxatives can reduce gastrointestinal absorption of potassium, promoting hypokalemia and fluid loss. Some older people may restrict their fluid intake to prevent urinating in the middle of the night or while they are away from home. Although calcium levels are often normal in older adults, calcium leaves the bones of the body, predisposing the person to osteoporosis and consequently, fractures when falls occur.

Normal Acid–Base Balance

For cells to operate with maximum efficiency, they need oxygen, nutrients, electrolytes, a controlled temperature, and an otherwise predictably stable environment. An important component of cellular environment is the hydrogen ion concentration (H^+), which is regulated within extremely narrow limits. The maintenance of this narrow concentration range is called acid–base balance. Such vital functions as nerve conduction, hormonal activity, and cardiac rhythm depend on a stable acid–base environment. Because significant deviations from normal blood H^+ may be life-threatening, nurses need a thorough understanding of the processes of acid–base balance.

Acids, Bases, and pH

Any substance that can donate free H^+ ions to a solution is called an **acid**. By contrast, any substance that can decrease H^+ concentration in a solution is a **base** (also called an *alkali*).

An example of a *strong* acid is hydrochloric acid (HCl), which is found in the stomach. When HCl enters into solution, it breaks down (or dissociates) almost completely into hydrogen and chloride ions. A small amount of a strong acid in water can generate a large number of free H^+ ions.

Sodium hydroxide (lye) is one example of a strong base. In solution, it binds with some of the H^+ provided by water, greatly reducing the number of free H^+ ions. Weak acids and bases differ from strong acids and bases; they only partially dissociate in solution, thus causing much smaller changes in H^+. Solutions that contain more acid than base are described as acidic, whereas solutions containing relatively more base are termed basic (or alkaline).

The number of H^+ ions in any solution is indicated indirectly by means of the pH scale (Fig. 36-5). This scale (actually the negative log of the hydrogen ion concentration) describes the degree of acidity or alkalinity of solutions. The pH scale ranges from 1 to 14, with 7 representing a neutral solution that is neither acidic nor alkaline. A solution with a pH between 1 and 7 is acidic. Weak acids have a pH only slightly below 7, whereas the strongest acids have pH values closer to 1. Similarly, bases have pH values above 7, with higher pH values indicating increasingly strong bases.

Acids and Bases in the Blood

The body's ECF has an average pH of between 7.37 and 7.43 (Rose, 1994). This very narrow pH range is maintained by buffers that limit pH changes in the body fluids and by elimination of acids from the body through the lungs (carbon dioxide) and kidneys.

A very important acid in the body is carbonic acid. The waste substance carbon dioxide is produced each moment by cells as they use oxygen to metabolize glucose. By itself, carbon dioxide could be considered a neutral compound, but as it enters the blood, it combines chemically with water to form carbonic acid. This weak, unstable acid partially dissociates to H^+ and HCO_3^- (bicarbonate) ions:

$$H_2O + CO_2 \rightarrow H_2CO_3 \rightarrow H^+ + HCO_3^-$$

Carbonic acid and bicarbonate ion together form what is known as a buffer pair (a weak acid and its accompanying conjugate base). Although there are several other buffer systems in the body, the bicarbonate-carbonic acid buffer system is the most important for two reasons. First, because all the buffer systems are in equilibrium, changes in the bicarbonate-carbonic acid system reflect changes in all the other systems. Second, the body regulates the carbon dioxide level by changes in the respiration rate (ventilation), and it regulates the bicarbonate level by adjusting the amount of bicarbonate lost in the urine or the amount regenerated by the kidneys.

Factors Affecting Acid–Base Balance

The balance between blood acids and bases is extremely closely regulated. Compared with the electrolytes, which are present in the plasma in millimolar (10^{-3} molar) concentrations, the concentration of H^+ in the blood is normally 1 million times smaller; that is, H^+ is present in nanomolar (10^{-9} molar) amounts. Death usually results if blood pH falls below 6.8 or increases above 7.8 (Rose, 1994). Because metabolism continually produces acids and bases, maintenance of the pH within its incredibly narrow limits depends on two processes; buffering and compensation. Buffers allow acids or bases to be transported from where they are produced to where they are excreted, while the compensatory processes either excrete acids and bases or retain acids or bases to compensate for losses.

Buffers are substances that help prevent large changes in pH by absorbing or releasing H^+ ions. Thus, when the blood has an excess of acid, successful buffering prevents a large drop in pH despite the influx of extra H^+ ions into the blood. In such cases, buffers combine with the additional H^+ ions released by the acid, minimizing the potentially damaging effect of extra free H^+ ions in the blood. Similarly, a deficit of blood acid or excess of base can result in a serious increase in pH. Successful buffering will cause extra H^+ ions to be released into the blood.

The body relies on several buffer mechanisms. The plasma proteins, such as albumin and globins, along

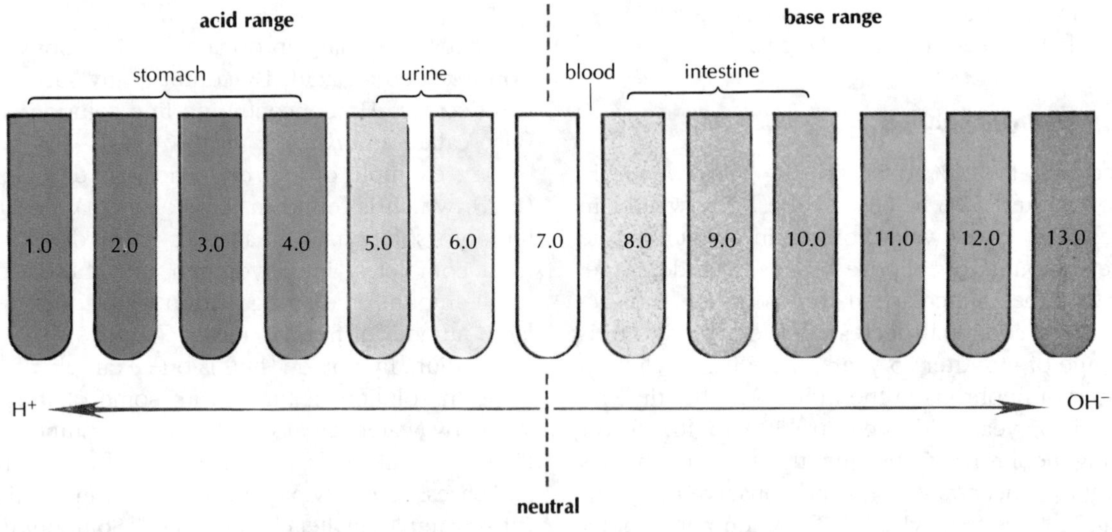

Figure 36-5 • The pH scale measures degree of acidity or alkalinity.

with hemoglobin in the red blood cell, have limited capacities for regulating H^+ ion concentration. Compounds such as phosphate and ammonia assist in the removal of H^+ ions to the urine and thus play a part in acid–base balance. Bone also participates in buffering.

The respiratory and renal systems are involved in normal excretion of acid and base from the body and compensation for any imbalances. Moment-to-moment maintenance of acid–base status is handled by the lungs, because they can react almost instantly to minute changes in blood pH. The kidneys are responsible for regulating gradual or long-term changes in acid–base balance. They are slower than the lungs to react to changes, taking hours to days to respond. Failure or impairment of either system can lead to life-threatening illness; therefore, preservation of optimal lung and renal function should be a goal for nurses caring for any client at risk for acid–base imbalance.

Respiratory Compensation

The lungs are directly responsible for controlling the amount of carbon dioxide in the blood. Carbon dioxide diffuses into the blood from the tissues and is carried primarily as carbonic acid, bicarbonate, and hydrogen ions. When the blood reaches the lungs, these substances recombine into carbon dioxide, which rapidly diffuses into the lung and is exhaled. The lungs normally maintain carbon dioxide levels in the arterial blood ($PaCO_2$) between 36 and 44 mm Hg (Rose, 1994).

When large amounts of carbon dioxide are being produced by the tissues, the lungs respond with an increase in the rate and depth of ventilation, which increases the rate at which this acid is excreted and prevents any significant change in pH. The respiratory system reacts in an opposite manner if carbon dioxide production decreases. Because breathing also is needed to supply oxygen to the blood and to regulate carbon dioxide, people are able to decrease ventilation only to a limited extent.

Renal Compensation

The kidneys play a major role in the regulation of acid–base status. By manipulating the rate of excretion or retention of H^+ and HCO_3^- ions, they greatly influence the maintenance of the normal base-to-acid balance.

Gradual increases in the blood acids are buffered in two ways by the kidneys. They will increase excretion of H^+ ions into the urine and return HCO_3^- ions to the blood. Additional serum bicarbonate is thus made available to absorb more free H^+ ions, and normal pH can be reestablished.

The kidneys balance a gradual loss of blood acid (or excess of blood base) by increasing retention of H^+ ions and increasing the excretion of HCO_3^- ions into the urine. Thus, any rise in pH is prevented as the relative concentration of bases and acids is kept in the correct ratio.

The response of the kidneys to acid–base imbalance is generally long-lasting; however, it can take as long as 2 days before the kidneys' response is complete. For this reason, the kidneys are less effective than the lungs in handling sudden changes in acid–base status. Table 36-4 gives normal values for arterial blood gases.

Altered Fluid, Electrolyte, and Acid–Base Balance

Altered States of Fluid, Electrolyte, or Acid–Base Balance

Disruptions in homeostasis can affect fluid balance, electrolyte balance, or acid–base balance. Fluid imbalances include ECF volume excess or deficit and water excess or deficit. Electrolyte imbalances include excesses or deficits of potassium, calcium, or magnesium. Acid–base imbalances encompass the problems of res-

Table 36-4 • Normal Arterial Blood Gas Values

Abbreviation	Normal Range	Definition
pH	7.37–7.43	Reflects the hydrogen ion concentration of arterial blood Acidosis: < 7.37 Alkalosis: > 7.43
$PaCO_2$	35–45 mm Hg	Reflects partial pressure of carbon dioxide in arterial blood Hypocapnia: low partial pressure of carbon dioxide in arterial blood, < 35 mm Hg Hypercapnia: high partial pressure of carbon dioxide in arterial blood, > 45 mm Hg
PaO_2	80–100 mm Hg	Partial pressure of O_2 in arterial blood
HCO_3^-	22–26 mEq/L	Amount of bicarbonate in arterial blood

piratory acidosis, respiratory alkalosis, metabolic acidosis, and metabolic alkalosis.

Frequently, more than one imbalance occurs at a time. For simplicity, each imbalance is discussed separately. Refer to a medical-surgical nursing text for more information on complex problems of fluid and electrolyte imbalance.

Fluid Imbalances

A state of fluid imbalance can occur if there is too much or too little fluid in any of the fluid compartments. There are two major categories of fluid balance problems: ECF volume balance problems and water or osmolar balance problems. For each category, there can be either a deficit or excess. A client may present with any of eight possible combinations of fluid balance problems: an ECF volume excess or deficit or a water excess or deficit or a combination of an ECF and a water balance problem. To simplify and organize your assessment and intervention decisions, first assess ECF volume and then water balance.

Extracellular Fluid Volume Deficit. ECF volume deficit involves the loss of ECF containing equal proportions of solute, primarily sodium, chloride and bicarbonate, and water (normal saline). This loss of isotonic fluid causes a decrease in the volume of the ECF compartment. There are two subdivisions of the ECF: the vascular volume, which is the fluid inside blood and lymph vessels, and the interstitial volume, which is the fluid between the cells. Other common terms that are used for ECF volume deficit include hypovolemia, saline deficit, and isotonic dehydration. ECF volume deficit can occur because of inadequate intake or abnormal losses, such as vomiting or diarrhea.

A special type of ECF volume balance problem known as "third spacing" occurs when fluid leaves the vascular volume and is trapped within the interstitial fluid in a given area of the body (Metheny, 1992). A "third space" is any area where fluid accumulates and is physiologically unavailable to return to its appropriate compartment. For example, collection of fluid in the peritoneal cavity is known as ascites. There is no actual "third space," and the retained fluid is within the interstitial space; however, this terminology is relatively common.

Symptoms of an ECF volume deficit include orthostatic or postural changes in pulse rate and blood pressure (an increase in pulse rate and sometimes a decrease in blood pressure when the individual changes from the lying to standing position); weak, rapid pulse; weight loss (except in third spacing); dry mucous membranes; thirst; poor skin turgor; decreased urine output; and slow-filling peripheral veins. Serum sodium values do *not* change noticeably because the fluid that is lost has the same concentration of electrolytes as the serum. Treatment of ECF volume deficit includes either oral or intravenous replacement of sodium, chloride, and water in the same concentrations that are found in body fluid (normal saline). The client must be protected from injury that could occur secondary to postural hypotension.

Extracellular Fluid Volume Excess. ECF volume excess involves an increase of ECF composed of a 0.9% solution of sodium, chloride, and water (normal saline). Increases in ECF volume often occur with cardiac failure, renal failure, or liver disease. When excess fluid cannot be eliminated, hydrostatic pressure forces some of it into the interstitial space, where it is observable as edema. A significant increase in ECF volume has to occur before edema is visible.

Rapid weight gain (greater than 0.5 kg/d) is the most significant symptom indicating ECF volume excess. A weight gain of 1 kg reflects retention of 1 L of saline. Other symptoms may include increased blood pressure, bounding pulse, and fullness of neck veins. Although one might predict that urine output would be increased when there is an ECF volume excess, it is often decreased because of the underlying cause, such as heart or renal failure. Excess extracellular volume can leak into the lungs, causing pulmonary edema, which is indicated by dyspnea, orthopnea (difficulty breathing when supine), and abnormal breath sounds (rales). As with ECF volume deficit, serum sodium values will be within normal limits unless the client also has a water balance problem.

Medical management of ECF volume excess involves restriction of sodium and saline intake (low-sodium diet) and administration of diuretics. The underlying pathology is identified and treated.

Water or Osmolar Balance. Water or osmolar balance problems occur when water intake is increased or decreased markedly or when water is retained or excreted excessively. To determine whether there is a water balance problem, the serum osmolarity must either be measured or estimated. Because osmolarity is the number of dissolved particles in solution, body fluid osmolarity can be estimated by counting the number of particles per unit volume of body fluid. This seemingly impossible task is simplified by the fact that the most abundant extracellular particle that is osmotically active is the sodium ion and its accompanying anion, either chloride and bicarbonate. The only other molecule that makes a contribution to serum osmolarity that influences the distribution of body fluid is glucose. (Other molecules, such as urea, also contribute to serum osmolality, but because they move easily across cell membranes, they have no net effect on body fluid volume distribution.) Use the following formula to estimate serum osmolarity:

$$\text{estimated serum osmolarity} = (\text{serum sodium} \times 2) + \left(\frac{\text{serum glucose}}{100} \times 5.6\right)$$

Therefore if a client had a serum sodium of 135 mEq/L and a glucose level of 90 mg/dL, his or her estimated serum osmolarity would be:

$$\begin{aligned}\text{estimated serum osmolarity} &= (135 \times 2) + (90/100 \times 5.6)\\ &= 270 + (0.90 \times 5.6)\\ &= 270 + (5.04)\\ &= 275 \text{ mOsm/L}\end{aligned}$$

Because water moves freely across almost all cell membranes, the serum osmolarity indicates intracellular osmolarity except for relatively brief periods when changes in one fluid compartment have not yet had time to equilibrate with the other.

Water moves down its concentration gradient from areas of higher concentration to areas of lower concentration. For example, if a client is given a hyperosmotic intravenous solution, such as 2× normal saline, the osmolarity of the ECF will increase, and water will move from the cells into the ECF until the osmolarity of both compartments is the same. Conversely, if a client takes in too much water, the osmolarity of the ECF will decrease, and water will move from the ECF into the cells. When clients get an intravenous infusion of dextrose 5% in water, which initially has an osmolarity close to blood, the glucose is subsequently metabolized and actively transported into cells, leaving the water behind in the ECF. This water then distributes one-third into the ECF and two-thirds into the intracellular fluid; this results in a decreased osmolarity of all the body fluids.

Water Deficit or Hyperosmolarity. A water deficit or serum hyperosmolarity occurs when there is a decrease in water intake, an increase in water loss in the urine, or an excess intake of solute. The estimated serum osmolarity will be >295 mOsm/L, depending on the glucose level, and the serum sodium may be greater than 145 mEq/L. As serum osmolarity increases, water is drawn from the intracellular compartment, causing cellular shrinking. As fluid is pulled from the cells of the brain, confusion, agitation, convulsions, coma, and death may result. Other symptoms include decreased urine output with an increase in urine concentration, thirst, and dry mucous membranes (Takamata, Mack, Gillen, & Nadel, 1994). Other terms used for water deficit include hypernatremia, hypertonic dehydration, and hypertonicity.

Water Excess or Hypo-osmolarity. A water excess or serum hypo-osmolarity occurs when there is an increase in water intake, abnormal secretion of ADH, or decreased urinary output of water. The estimated serum osmolarity will be < 275 mOsm/L, depending on the glucose level, and the serum sodium will be less than 135 mEq/L. As serum osmolarity decreases, water diffuses down its concentration gradient into cells, with the major impact on the cells of the central nervous system resulting in lethargy, irritability, confusion, personality changes, seizures, coma, and death. Additional signs and symptoms include anorexia, nausea, vomiting, weakness, and cramps. Other terms used for water excess include hypotonic disorder, hyponatremia, and hypotonicity.

Electrolyte Imbalance

Electrolyte balance is significant for maintaining normal physiologic function. Too much or too little potassium, calcium, or magnesium in the blood can cause serious disruptions in homeostasis and, when severe, can be life-threatening.

Potassium Imbalance. An excess of serum potassium (above 5.0 mEq/L) is known as hyperkalemia, and a deficit of serum potassium (below 3.5 mEq/L) is known as hypokalemia.

Hyperkalemia. Hyperkalemia most often accompanies kidney failure, because renal impairment prevents the proper excretion of excess potassium. Hyperkalemia also has been associated with cellular damage, which results in potassium being released into the ECF; with insulin deficiency, which decreases the amount of potassium moving into the cell; and with adrenal deficiency, which is due to decreased production of aldosterone. Rapid infusion of potassium intravenously can cause hyperkalemia.

An increase in the serum potassium concentration leads to an increased responsiveness of the cell membranes to stimuli, which can be seen in changes in skeletal, smooth, and cardiac muscle. Anxiety, irritability, gastrointestinal hyperactivity (diarrhea and intestinal cramping), characteristic electrocardiogram changes, and cardiac arrhythmias (irregular heart rate or rhythm) may be present. If serum potassium is elevated (above 8 mEq/L), responsiveness of the cell membranes to stimuli is decreased. Symptoms similar to those of hypokalemia then appear.

Medical treatment for hyperkalemia depends on how elevated it is. Treatment of very high levels includes intravenous calcium gluconate to oppose potassium's effect on the membrane potential of excitable cells, followed by an infusion of insulin and glucose to move potassium into the cell. Potassium can then be removed from the body by dialysis or the administration of ion exchange resins. Moderate elevations of potassium may be treated with diuretics and potassium exchange resins. The underlying cause for the hyperkalemia should be detected and treated.

Hypokalemia. Hypokalemia occurs with abnormal loss of potassium, inadequate replacement, or movement into cells (which may occur when insulin is given).

A reduction in serum potassium concentration leads to a decreased responsiveness of cellular membranes to stimuli. The resulting lack of responsiveness to stimuli leads to characteristic skeletal muscle, smooth muscle, renal, and cardiac manifestations. Symptoms usually appear when serum potassium is below 3 mEq/L. Muscle weakness and fatigue are common. Muscle weakness begins in the lower extremities and moves up the trunk to the upper extremities. In severe cases of hypokalemia, the respiratory muscles are affected. A decreased responsiveness of the smooth muscle in the gastrointestinal area can produce abdominal distention, nausea, vomiting, constipation, and paralytic ileus. Because the effectiveness of ADH depends on an adequate serum level of potassium, increased urination (polyuria) and thirst (polydipsia) frequently accompany hypokalemia. Arrhythmias and characteristic electrocardiogram changes occur in the presence of hypokalemia. Low serum potassium levels may suppress insulin release, thus elevating blood glucose level.

Hypokalemia is corrected by increasing the intake of potassium by encouraging potassium-rich foods in the diet, administering oral potassium supplements, using potassium-sparing diuretics, or administering potassium intravenously if the potassium is very low. The underlying cause for potassium loss should be identified and preventive teaching implemented if indicated.

Calcium Imbalance. Hypercalcemia is an elevated serum calcium level and occurs when serum calcium concentration rises above 10.5 mg/dL. Hypocalcemia refers to a low serum calcium level and occurs when the serum calcium concentration falls below 8.5 mg/dL.

Hypercalcemia. Hypercalcemia occurs with excessive intake of vitamin D, excessive intake of milk or alkaline "antacids," hyperparathyroidism, immobilization, and reduced renal function. The presence of several types of cancer also can cause hypercalcemia by a variety of mechanisms.

Hypercalcemia causes decreased neuromuscular excitability, which can result in various symptoms, such as muscle weakness, lack of coordination, confusion, lethargy, and impaired memory. Gastrointestinal problems, such as nausea, vomiting, and constipation, pruritus, kidney stones, and bone pain can occur in the person with high serum calcium levels.

Hypocalcemia. Hypocalcemia is associated with para-thyroid deficiency, vitamin D deficiency, and renal disease. Some malignancies, pancreatitis, various treatments (such as massive blood transfusion), and the abuse of laxatives or enemas can decrease serum calcium levels.

A reduction in calcium in the serum can cause spontaneous discharge of sensory and motor fibers of the peripheral nervous system. The following symptoms are produced in the client as the serum calcium falls. Mild hypocalcemia begins with paresthesia, which is a tingling in the hands, fingers, feet, or around the mouth. Tetany is manifested by grimacing, muscle twitching, cramping, hyperactive reflexes, and severe flexion of the wrist and ankle joints. If untreated, laryngospasm, seizures, and cardiac arrest can cause death.

Oral calcium supplements should be given in mild cases of hypocalcemia. In more severe cases, intravenous calcium must be given slowly. Rapid intravenous replacement of calcium can result in cardiac arrhythmias. Seizure precautions may be necessary.

Magnesium Imbalance. Hypermagnesemia is defined as a serum concentration of magnesium greater than 2.0 mEq/L, and hypomagnesemia is a serum concentration of magnesium less than 1.4 mEq/L.

Hypermagnesemia. Hypermagnesemia can occur in renal failure, diabetic ketoacidosis, or when magnesium sulfate is given in therapy (Metheny, 1992). It also can occur with the use of magnesium-based laxatives. High serum magnesium levels depress muscular irritability, which can cause hypotension, weakness, depressed reflexes, paralysis, bradycardia, respiratory failure, and cardiac arrest.

Hypomagnesemia. Hypomagnesemia can be due to impaired intake, impaired intestinal absorption, and excessive urinary excretion secondary to diuretics and chronic alcoholism. Hypomagnesemia causes neuromuscular irritability, which can be seen in tremors, cramps, difficulty swallowing, and cardiovascular changes.

Acid–Base Imbalance

An arterial pH between 7.37 and 7.44 is necessary for efficient cellular metabolism. Because the pH scale is actually the negative log of the hydrogen ion concentration, a person is acidotic when the arterial pH is less than 7.37 and alkalotic when the pH is greater than 7.44. Acidosis and alkalosis can be categorized as either respiratory or metabolic, depending on the primary cause and either acute or chronic depending on the underlying cause. Disturbances in acid–base balance can severely alter blood oxygen transport, neurologic function, and cardiac rhythmicity.

Acidosis. Respiratory acidosis is present when low pH is caused by hypoventilation. Metabolic acidosis occurs either when excess acid is ingested or created (diabetic ketoacidosis) or when the kidneys are unable to retain enough bicarbonate ion to buffer free hydrogen ions in the blood.

Respiratory Acidosis. Respiratory acidosis is indicated by a low pH accompanied by an elevated arterial level of carbon dioxide ($PaCO_2$ greater than 44 mm Hg.) The lungs normally maintain blood concentrations of carbon dioxide between 36 and 44 mm Hg (Rose, 1994). When breathing ability is compromised by lung diseases such as asthma or emphysema or by depressed neural or muscular function (such as with narcotic overdose, head trauma, or polio), carbon dioxide accumulates in the blood. As this acid increases, free hydrogen ion concentration is increased, causing pH to drop. With time, the kidneys compensate for this build-up of acid by increasing the excretion of H^+ ion into the urine and the return of HCO_3^- to the blood. In this way, normal pH can be reestablished.

Metabolic Acidosis. Metabolic acidosis is characterized by a low pH and a decreased plasma HCO_3^- level (below 22 mEq/L). It can occur with loss of bicarbonate from severe diarrhea, or with acid accumulation (such as ketoacids, caused by diabetes, or lactic acids, caused by oxygen deprivation).

The respiratory system compensates for metabolic acidosis by increasing ventilation, thus increasing the rate of carbonic acid excretion resulting in a fall in $PaCO_2$. This respiratory compensation occurs relatively rapidly but cannot alone return the acid–base balance to within normal limits. Renal compensation with the excretion of H^+ ion and retention of HCO_3^- takes hours to occur and can, in conjunction with respiratory compensation, return the pH to within normal limits if the kidneys are not the cause of the metabolic acidosis.

Alkalosis. Respiratory alkalosis is caused by hyperventilation. Metabolic alkalosis occurs when there is excessive loss of body acids or with unusual intake of alkaline substances.

Respiratory Alkalosis. Respiratory alkalosis is present when a high pH is accompanied by decreased blood carbon dioxide levels (below 36 mm Hg). Hyperventilation (caused most commonly by anxiety and asthma) increases carbon dioxide (carbonic acid) excretion, leading to a relative excess of blood base and an increase in pH. To compensate, the kidneys increase the excretion of HCO_3^- into the urine, and pH returns toward normal. Intervention may be required to reduce the hyperventilation.

Metabolic Alkalosis. Metabolic alkalosis is often caused by vomiting or vigorous nasogastric suction. In addition, endocrine disorders or ingesting large amounts of antacids can bring about metabolic alkalosis. The loss of stomach acid or an excessive amount of base in the stomach will cause H^+ shifts in the blood, and pH will increase.

Compensation for this disorder includes a decrease in ventilation, which allows blood carbon dioxide to rise. The kidneys respond to metabolic alkalosis by retaining acid and excreting HCO_3^-. Renal compensation for metabolic alkalosis is impaired if the individual has an ECF volume deficit or hypokalemia (Rose, 1994).

Nursing Research
Fluid and Electrolyte Balance

Selected Nursing Research Studies

Treas, L. S., & Latinis-Bridges, B. (1991). Efficacy of heparin in peripheral venous infusions in neonates. *Journal of Obstetrical and Gynecological Nursing, 21,* 214–219.

Wright, A., Hecker, J., & McDonald, G. (1995). Effects of low-dose heparin on failure of intravenous infusions in children. *Heart & Lung, 24,* 79–82.

Cosgray, R., Davidhizar, R., Giger, J. N., & Kreisl, R. (1993). A program for water-intoxicated patients at a state hospital. *Clinical Nurse Specialist, 7,* 55–61.

Gerber, A. M., James, S. A., Ammerman, A. S., Keenan, N. L., et al. (1991). Socioeconomic status and electrolyte intake in black adults: The Pitt County Study. *American Journal of Public Health, 81,* 1608–1612.

Burge, R. I. (1993). Dehydration symptoms of palliative care cancer patients. *Journal of Pain and Symptom Management, 8,* 454–464.

Possible Topics for Nursing Inquiry

- Does the education of new parents about the fluid needs of neonates and how to mange diarrhea decrease the incidence of hospitalization for fluid replacement?
- What is the most effective way to teach clients about the prevention of fluid balance problems?
- What is the impact of client education about fluid and diet treatment plans on subsequent morbidity, number of hospitalizations, and cost of care?
- What are the most effective interventions for managing the sensation of thirst for clients who must restrict their fluid intake?
- What is the most effective method of increasing fluid intake for older clients with decreased thirst?

Potential for Altered Fluid, Electrolyte, and Acid–Base Balance

Many factors can increase the risk for fluid, electrolyte, or acid–base imbalance, including inadequate oral intake, excessive loss of fluid or electrolytes, stress, chronic illness, and surgery.

Inadequate Oral Intake

Many factors can affect the ability to achieve adequate fluid intake. Fluids and food have to be readily accessible. Older adults may be unable to get out to shop for or prepare a well-balanced diet, thus decreasing their intake of needed electrolytes and fluid. People in bed may be too weak to reach for and drink fluids and too fatigued to consume entire meals. Infants have to rely on others to meet their fluid and nutrient needs.

Psychological factors, such as depression or confusion, also may contribute to decreased oral intake. Some people may purposely limit oral intake to lose weight or decrease the number of times they must void. Often, lack of knowledge regarding the consequences of these actions contributes to such behavior.

Physiologic factors such as nausea can limit oral intake. In addition, the ability to swallow may be impaired after a stroke, or the discomfort of a sore throat may limit swallowing.

Excessive Loss

Fluid and electrolyte problems can occur when an individual experiences abnormal loss of fluid or electrolytes.

Vomiting, diarrhea, diaphoresis, or increased urine output secondary to the administration of diuretics may cause such a loss.

Vomiting depletes the body of fluid and electrolytes. As hydrochloric acid is lost from the stomach, hydrogen, sodium, and chloride ions are depleted, leading to a metabolic alkalosis and ECF volume deficit. Gastric fluid also is high in potassium and loss may contribute to hypokalemia. Vomiting compounds fluid and electrolyte problems because the ability to maintain adequate intake is reduced.

Diarrhea depletes the body of fluid and electrolytes. Intestinal secretions contain bicarbonate; thus, diarrhea may cause metabolic acidosis. Intestinal contents are rich in sodium, chloride, water, and potassium, and diarrhea can contribute to an ECF volume deficit and hypokalemia. The development and promotion of oral rehydration fluids, which replace the fluid and electrolytes lost in diarrhea, has significantly reduced worldwide death rates from diarrheal disease, particularly among infants (Avery & Snyder, 1990).

Diaphoresis, or excessive sweating, can increase the loss of fluid and electrolytes. Sweat is a hypotonic fluid containing sodium, potassium, and chloride. Diaphoresis can occur with increased physical activity, fever, or exposure to elevated environmental temperatures.

Diuretics are prescribed to increase the excretion of sodium, chloride, and water in clients with high blood pressure or with chronic heart, renal, or liver problems. At times, the medications may remove too much ECF from the body, resulting in a deficit. Many diuretics (eg, thiazides) also promote the excretion of potassium from the body, increasing the risk for potassium depletion.

Stress

Stress caused by many factors, such as physical trauma, anxiety, and pain, can affect fluid and electrolyte balance. When stress occurs, aldosterone production is increased, causing ECF retention. Stress also increases ADH production, resulting in decreased renal excretion of water.

Chronic Illness

Many chronic medical problems adversely affect a person's ability to maintain normal fluid, electrolyte, and acid–base homeostasis. Chronic renal problems, heart problems, and respiratory problems are commonly accompanied by imbalances. Other problems, such as liver disorders, cancer, and diabetes mellitus, also result in fluid and electrolyte imbalances.

Renal Failure. As kidney function decreases due to loss of nephrons, there may be an abnormal accumulation of sodium, chloride, potassium, and fluid in the body, resulting in ECF volume and water excesses. The kidneys are less able to regulate electrolyte excretion, so abnormal levels may occur. Hyperkalemia and hypocalcemia are common. Because normally more acid wastes are produced than alkaline wastes, metabolic acidosis occurs when the kidneys fail.

Cardiac Failure. As the heart fails to pump effectively and circulate blood, blood pressure falls; the secretion of aldosterone and ADH is stimulated, often resulting in ECF volume and water excesses. This fluid collects in the lungs, increasing the risk of pulmonary edema, and the rest of the body, where it is apparent as pitting or dependent edema. Fluid volume excess is complicated by the fact that as the heart pumps less effectively, decreased blood reaches and perfuses the kidneys, thus increasing fluid retention.

Respiratory Failure. Chronic respiratory problems affect acid–base balance. Progressive destruction of alveoli limits the lungs' functional ability to excrete carbon dioxide (carbonic acid). The pH of the blood falls, and chronic respiratory acidosis occurs.

Surgery

Many preoperative and postoperative factors influence the surgical client's fluid and electrolyte status. Preoperatively, the client may be kept *non per os* (NPO, nothing by mouth) and may receive enemas. During surgery, increased insensible water loss occurs as the internal body structures are exposed to air and blood is lost; the amount depends on the type of surgery. Potassium levels frequently fall after surgery due to cellular trauma and inadequate intake. As cells are destroyed, potassium is released from inside the cell, which will cause a temporary increase in serum potassium. As this potassium is excreted in the urine, serum potassium can become reduced, and supplemental potassium may be necessary. Frequently, the postoperative client is NPO or on a restricted diet for a period. Drainage from nasogastric tubes or surgical drains increases the potential for loss of fluids and electrolytes (Norris, 1993). Emotional stress, pain, nausea, and vomiting are common postoperatively and can contribute to fluid and electrolyte imbalance.

Pregnancy

Physiologic changes occur during pregnancy that can alter fluid, electrolyte, and acid–base status. Fluid retention and edema occur frequently, although the exact mechanism underlying this is not completely understood (Paller & Ferris, 1990). Aldosterone production increases during pregnancy. There is an overall increase in blood volume and total body fluid volume. Acid–base balance is altered. Hyperventilation is caused by higher progesterone levels and may result in alkalosis as the $PaCO_2$ decreases.

Manifestations of Fluid, Electrolyte, or Acid–Base Imbalances

Although each specific fluid, electrolyte, or acid–base imbalance has specific symptoms, general groups of symptoms frequently accompany states of imbalance: a significant difference between intake and output plus changes in mental status, vital signs, tissue turgor, and muscle tone. The degree of the imbalance, the suddenness with which it occurs, and the client's age will determine the symptom severity. When evaluating manifestations, it is important to see if all data support the same conclusion. Suspect a fluid, electrolyte, or acid–base imbalance for any client who presents the following signs or symptoms.

Imbalance of Intake and Output and Body Weight

Intake and output should be approximately equal for a 24-hour period. When output is significantly greater or less than intake, the nurse should suspect a fluid balance problem after making certain that the intake and output record is accurate, because mistakes are common. Comparison of daily body weights is a good way to confirm apparent discrepancies in intake and output. Normally, urine output is around 1,500 mL/24-hour period, but a wide range of individual variation is normal, depending on many factors. A decrease in urine volume and increase in body weight will indicate an ECF volume deficit; an increase in urine volume and decrease in weight indicate an ECF volume excess.

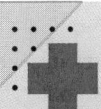

> ***Safety Alert***
> *Fluid and Electrolyte Balance*
>
> - Carefully monitor infants when they are losing or being given fluids. They are at increased risk for fluid and electrolyte balance problems because of their immature kidneys and increased body surface area in relation to their body size.
> - Advise new parents to call their healthcare provider if they are unsure if a particular food or fluid is safe for their infant.
> - Monitor postural heart rate and blood pressures when getting clients with an extracellular fluid volume deficit out of bed. Have them take several minutes to get up, going in slow steps from lying to sitting to standing. Be sure someone is present when they are getting up.
> - Teach family members how to assist the client if the individual is receiving care at home.
> - If there is an unexplained change in a client's level of consciousness, be sure to estimate serum osmolarity or request that a blood sample be sent to the laboratory for analysis if current results are not available. Water excess or deficit can cause changes in a client's level of consciousness.
> - Monitor clients receiving intravenous potassium carefully and be sure the infusion rate does not exceed 10 to 20 mEq/h unless there is extreme hypokalemia. Clients with renal failure are at risk for hyperkalemia and need careful monitoring. Rapid changes can be serious and even fatal.

When evaluating trends in intake, output, and weight, consider at least the last 48 hours or longer for some chronic health problems. Look for a pattern of imbalance between intake and output or increases or decreases in weight.

Changes in Mental Status

Subtle changes in a person's ability to understand and relate to his or her environment are some of the earliest indications of a fluid or electrolyte imbalance. Level of consciousness (LOC) is the state of awareness and arousal of an individual. Changes in LOC can occur with changes in serum osmolarity (water balance). At first, changes are minor and may not be picked up unless the nurse knows the client well. The client may simply feel fatigued, restless, or apprehensive. Confusion can occur as the imbalances become more severe. Changes in LOC can vary from excessive excitability to lethargy. Lethargy can progress to coma and eventually death. The abruptness of the onset of the imbalance will increase the severity of symptoms.

Changes in Vital Signs

Many fluid, electrolyte, or acid–base imbalances are accompanied by a change in the client's vital signs. Observe for changes from baseline vital signs.

Respiratory Rate and Depth. Deep, labored respirations may occur to compensate for metabolic acidosis, whereas shallow respirations may be present in alkalosis. In ECF volume excess, fluid can accumulate in the lungs, decrease oxygenation, and be accompanied by dyspnea. Lung auscultation can detect rales, a subtle sign of fluid excess, prior to frank dyspnea.

Heart Rate and Rhythm. The quality of the pulse depends in part on the vascular volume. With ECF volume excess, the pulse may be strong, full, and bounding, while with ECF volume deficit, the pulse is usually weak, thready, and rapid. Irregular heart rhythms are common in potassium, calcium, and magnesium imbalances.

Postural Pulse Rate and Blood Pressure. An increase in pulse rate and perhaps a decrease in blood pressure will occur in ECF volume deficit. To assess for an ECF volume deficit, determine the effect that position change has on pulse rate and blood pressure. The blood pressure and pulse are first measured in the supine position and then with the client standing (postural vital signs). Because clients who have a marked ECF volume deficit may become faint or dizzy when they stand, have help available and be vigilant to prevent client injury when taking postural vital signs. An increase in pulse rate of more than 20 beats/min is a more sensitive indicator of ECF volume deficit than decreases in blood pressure. A drop of greater than 15 mm Hg in systolic pressure or a 10 mm Hg drop in diastolic pressure with an increase in pulse rate frequently means the client is volume depleted (Woods, Sivarajan-Froelicher, Halpenny, & Motzer, 1995). Postural pulse and blood pressure readings are a useful assessment tool for the nurse to use routinely for all clients at risk for volume depletion (eg, postoperatively). Increased blood pressure may sometimes occur with ECF volume excess.

Abnormal Tissue Hydration

When ECF volume or water imbalances occur, tissues can retain excess fluid, appearing edematous (turgid) or lose fluid, appearing dry and shriveled. Tissue hydration can be noted in the mouth, where the mucous membranes and tongue can appear dry with ridges due to lack of moisture. Tissue turgor, or the ability of the skin to return to normal position immediately after being pinched, is affected by fluid imbalance (Fig. 36-6). Poor tissue turgor occurs in ECF volume deficit or when elasticity is lost from the skin during normal aging.

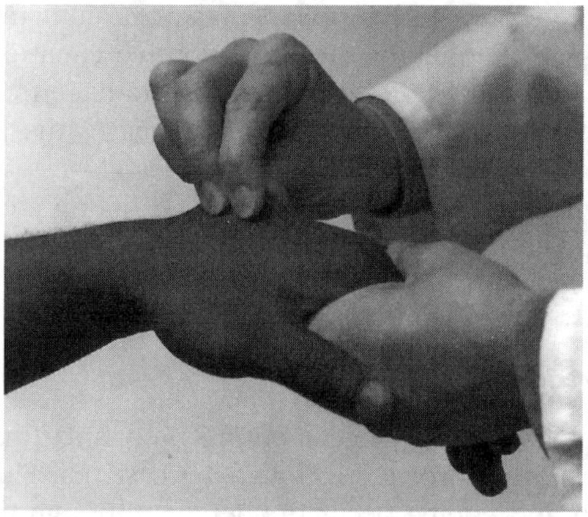

Figure 36-6 • *Normally the skin is elastic and returns to its original shape rapidly when pinched, as in this photo. When there is fluid loss, however, the skin is not elastic and does not return to its normal shape as rapidly.*

Edema, or the presence of fluid in the interstitial space, is not observable in most clients until 2.5 to 3.0 L of fluid has been retained (Rose, 1994). Edema is most noticeable in dependent areas of the body (eg, the legs when walking, the back and sacral area when supine in bed). When edema is severe, an indentation can be left when a finger is pressed into the edematous tissue; this is known as pitting edema.

Abnormal Muscle Tone or Sensation

Changes in muscle tone and muscle irritability frequently accompany imbalances. Increased or decreased neuromuscular excitability manifests as increasing irritability, muscle weakness, twitching, or cramping. Changes in gastrointestinal neuromuscular tone result in anorexia, nausea, constipation, and vomiting. Clients with electrolyte imbalance may experience tingling and other paresthesias. The nurse also should observe clients for seizure activity, which can occur in severe imbalances.

Impact of Fluid, Electrolyte, or Acid–Base Imbalance on Activities of Daily Living

Individual Considerations

The ability of the client with a fluid, electrolyte, or acid–base imbalance to perform common activities of daily living may be impaired. Because the client may tire easily, activities may need to be limited, with frequent rest periods during energy-consuming activities. If a client assumes an upright posture and experiences any "light-headedness" or dizziness, it is important to teach him or her to change positions slowly, perhaps going from lying to sitting before standing up if in bed.

The individual also should wait until dizziness subsides before ambulating. The client's ability to perform activities of daily living safely may be limited.

Family Considerations

Families can be instrumental in assisting the client to avoid fluid and electrolyte imbalances by assisting him or her in this basic activity of daily living. With some clients (especially older people), the client may not feel thirsty and would benefit from having family members remind them to drink adequate fluids. Confusion also may occur, so the nurse or family caregiver needs to make sure that safety precautions are implemented, including orienting the client to person, place, and time; keeping the side rails up; and assisting the client with activities of daily living that cannot be safely done independently. If mobility becomes a problem, stand-by assistance may be necessary to ensure safety. Aids such as ambulation belts, walkers, and canes can assist the client to ambulate more safely, thus supporting activities of daily living.

Assessment

Gathering data concerning the fluid and electrolyte status of an individual is important to determine potential problems and actual disturbances. Subjective and objective data are obtained in the nursing assessment through the nursing history, physical assessment, and through evaluating information obtained from laboratory and diagnostic tests.

Subjective Data

The collection of subjective information helps the nurse identify the normal pattern of fluid and electrolyte status for the client, any risk factors that may predispose the client to fluid and electrolyte imbalance, and any actual dysfunctions that are present.

Functional Pattern Identification

The nurse usually begins the assessment of a client's fluid and electrolyte status by obtaining or reviewing his or her history. In this process, the nurse gains an understanding of normal fluid status for the person and any factors that may predispose the person to imbalance. The client should be questioned regarding normal functional patterns of intake and output and any recent changes that have occurred. Special diet restrictions, such as sodium restriction or the use of salt substitutes should be noted. Reported increased thirst or a decreased fluid intake also are significant. The amount and pattern of urine output also should be assessed, along with any changes.

Risk Identification

The collection of subjective data also can help the nurse identify risk factors that could contribute to dysfunction. The nurse should elicit information concerning recent acute illness. Vomiting or diarrhea is especially important to document, as is the presence of a fever or diaphoresis. Document the severity and duration of these problems.

Certain chronic diseases also predispose a person to fluid and electrolyte imbalance. The client should be questioned about the presence of the renal failure, congestive heart failure, respiratory dysfunction, diabetes mellitus, diabetes insipidus, Addison's disease, Cushing's disease, or thyroid disease. If any of these are present, the client should be questioned regarding his or her individualized management plan and any complications that have occurred.

The client should be questioned regarding the any prescription or nonprescription medications he or she is taking. Various medications, such as insulin, diuretics, steroids, laxatives, and antacids, can contribute to fluid and electrolyte disturbances. The use of vitamin and mineral supplements also should be noted.

Finally, assess spiritual or sociocultural factors that may affect fluid and electrolyte balance. Religious beliefs, such as refusal to receive blood products, could increase the potential for fluid deficit problems if a client hemorrhages after surgery. A fixed income or the lack of transportation could prevent a person from getting medicine or food to comply with medical treatment.

Dysfunction Identification

The nurse can use the subjective data he or she collects to help identify actual fluid and electrolyte problems. Actual fluid and electrolyte imbalances are most likely to cause altered cognitive functioning or imbalances of intake and output and weight. The client can provide information regarding significant differences from their normal patterns of intake or output. It is important to validate subjective data with objective information gained through the physical assessment and the evaluation of laboratory test results before an actual diagnosis is made.

Objective Data

In addition to gathering subjective data, the nurse also collects objective data concerning the client's fluid and electrolyte status through physical assessment of the client and reviewing laboratory test results.

Physical Assessment

Objective data are obtained from all functional health patterns. Physical assessment data can be collected by assessing intake and output, body weight, vital signs, skin for turgor and hydration, edema, and fullness of neck and hand veins. More invasive assessment techniques include monitoring central venous pressure and pulmonary artery pressure (PAP).

Monitoring Intake and Output. Monitoring intake and output helps evaluate fluid and electrolyte status. The physician may order intake and output assessment (I & O) on a client after surgery or when evaluation of medical problems, such as congestive heart failure, is necessary. Often the nurse decides when it is important to monitor a client's intake and output. Guidelines that the nurse can use include when fluid intake or urinary output is less than normal; when abnormal losses are occurring, such as from a surgical drain or vomiting; when intravenous therapy is being administered; when the client has medical problems that affect fluid or electrolyte status; and when the client is not physiologically stable, such as after surgery or trauma.

Intake measurements include oral and parenteral fluids. Oral fluids include any liquids ingested or any foods that will become liquid at room temperature. Jello, sherbet, popsicles, and ice cream are types of solid foods that should be included in intake and output. Pureed food is not considered fluid intake. Other oral intake includes feedings delivered through any tube that enters the body (eg, a nasogastric tube going into the stomach through the nose, a jejunostomy tube entering the jejunum through the abdomen, or a gastrostomy tube entering the stomach through the abdomen). Parenteral intake includes any intravenous fluids, intravenous medications, and blood products administered.

Output measurements include urine, liquid stool, vomit, drainage from a wound or operative site (eg, chest tube, Hemovac drain), and drainage from a nasogastric tube. Diaphoresis or drainage on a dressing cannot be precisely measured, but if they are excessive, their presence can be noted without an exact value for output. If greater precision is required, dressings or wet bedding can be weighed to estimate fluid loss.

Intake and output are recorded on a graphic sheet, which is individualized for each agency. Most forms permit the nurse to list the intake and output and obtain subtotals for each shift and a total for the entire 24-hour period (Fig. 36-7). Some agencies also have worksheets that can be posted on the client's door or on the bathroom door to alert all staff that the client needs intake and output recorded. When clients are having their intake and output recorded, teach them and their families about their procedure so they can assist with accurate recording. The cubic centimeter (cc) or milliliter (mL) is the standard of measurement, rather than household measures, such as cups or ounces. One cubic centimeter is equal to 1 mL, and there is approximately 30 mL in a fluid ounce.

Intake measurements are often obtained by knowing the standard measurements of containers. Often what is normal for the agency will be printed on the intake and output sheet as a handy reference for the nurse. For example, when a milk carton contains 240 mL and the client drinks half of the milk, 120 mL is recorded. All intake must be included. Sips of water taken during the day can add up to significant intake, as can oral medications, such as antacids, that are given frequently. Ice chips should be recorded as approximately half their volume.

Urine output is measured every time the client voids. Toilet paper should be kept separate from the urine to obtain an accurate measurement. If the client voids in a bedpan or a commode, the urine is transferred into a calibrated container so that a measurement can be obtained. If the client is able to get up to the toilet, a measuring device (sometimes called a hat) is placed between the toilet seat and the toilet to collect the urine (Fig. 36-8). If a voiding cannot be measured, it is usually indicated on the intake and output record (eg, 320 mL plus incontinent × 1). If a client has a Foley catheter, the collection bag is usually emptied, and the urine is measured at the end of each shift unless the bag becomes full sooner. Other drainage also is usually emptied and measured at the end of each shift.

In addition to measuring and recording intake and output, the nurse evaluates patterns and values that are outside the normal range. Intake and output should be roughly equal, as seen in Table 36-3. For an adult, the urinary output is usually 40 to 80 mL/h, or approximately 1,500 mL/d. Typically, the intake of fluid is 1,300 mL/d. The reason there is a difference in intake and output is that water also is ingested in food. When a person has significant other losses (eg, vomiting, diarrhea), it also may affect urinary output. Urine values less than 30 mL/h indicate renal failure or marked ECF volume deficit. If large discrepancies occur between intake and output, it is important to ascertain the accuracy of the data collected. Because many people may be responsible for recording intake and output, some intake or output could have inadvertently not been recorded.

Body Weight. Assessing weight provides data concerning fluid balance. Rapid changes in weight indicate body fluid changes. Each kilogram of weight lost or gained equals approximately 1 L of fluid. A rapid loss of 2% of total body weight indicates a mild fluid deficit, whereas a rapid loss of 8% or more indicates a severe fluid deficit (Metheny, 1992).

Daily weights are often ordered for clients who are at risk for ECF volume problems. Weights should be measured at the same time of day (preferably in the morning before breakfast), with the client wearing the same clothing, using the same scale to ensure accuracy.

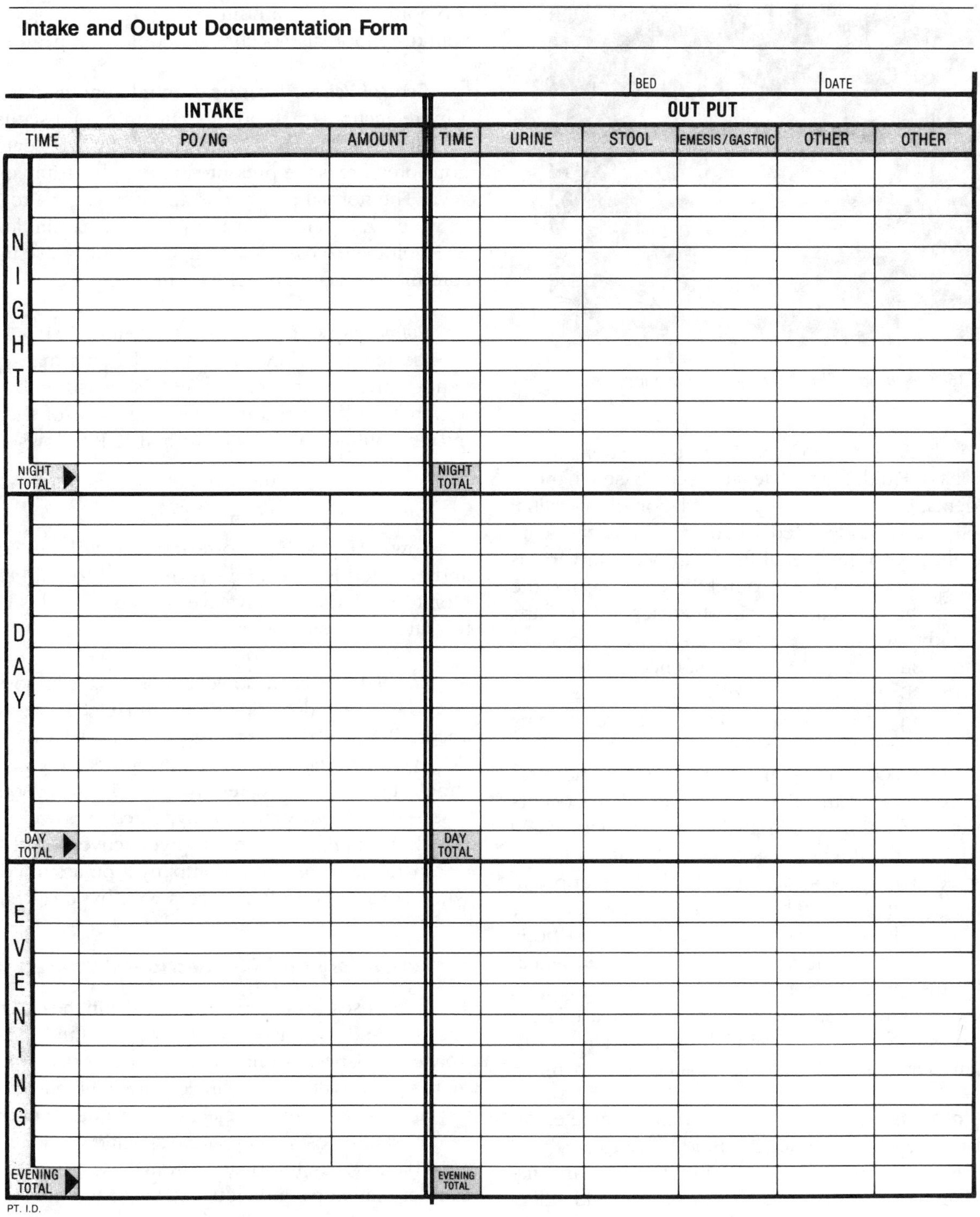
Intake and Output Documentation Form
BED
DATE
INTAKE
OUT PUT
TIME
PO/NG
AMOUNT
TIME
URINE
STOOL
EMESIS/GASTRIC
OTHER
OTHER
NIGHT
NIGHT TOTAL
NIGHT TOTAL
DAY
DAY TOTAL
DAY TOTAL
EVENING
EVENING TOTAL
EVENING TOTAL
PT. I.D.

Figure 36-7 • *Example of an input/output form.*

If a client is too ill or weak to stand to be weighed, a bed scale weight can be obtained. A bed scale is a portable scale on wheels onto which the client can be transferred and weighed.

The data from intake and output and daily weight are used together to evaluate for fluid imbalance. A decreasing output in conjunction with an increasing weight indicates ECF volume retention. A sudden weight loss with low urine output may indicate ECF volume deficit.

Integumentary Assessment. Changes in the skin and mucous membranes can indicate fluid imbalance. The general appearance of the skin is important to note. Flushed, dry skin may signal a fluid volume deficit. Lack of tearing or perspiration also is important to note. Vari-

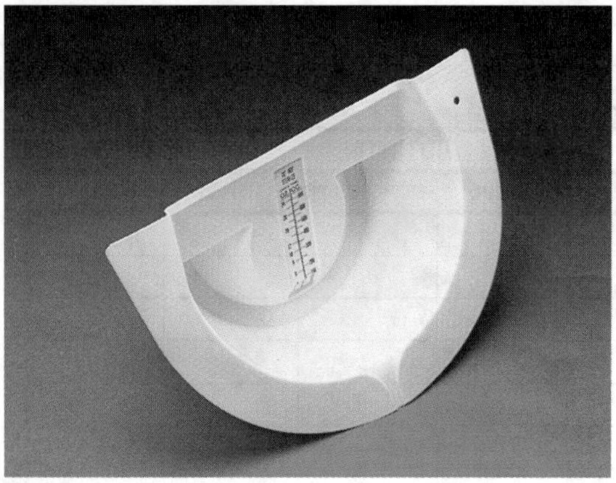

Figure 36-8 • *Urinary "hat" for measuring urine.*

ations in hydration are discussed in the section "Manifestations of Fluid, Electrolyte, and Acid–Base Balance."

Edema, or the excessive accumulation of interstitial fluid, also can be detected when examining the skin. This collection of interstitial fluid can occur in various parts of the body, such as around the eyes, around the sacrum, in the extremities, or in other dependent parts of the body. Edema is best assessed by pressing a finger into tissue over a bony prominence, such as the lower tibia. Edema is measured by the use of + signs, ranging from + to ++++. One + indicates edema that is just perceptible (2 mm); ++ and +++ indicate moderate edema (4–6 mm); and ++++ indicates severe edema (8 mm or more). Pitting edema occurs when an indentation remains in the skin (often for 15–30 seconds) after a finger presses into edematous tissue. Pitting edema is not apparent until there is approximately a 10% increase in body weight. Edema also may be evaluated by measuring the circumference of body parts (eg, leg or abdomen). If the circumference is measured at the same location with the same technique, an increase in circumference would indicate increased fluid in the interstitial space. Accumulation of fluid in the abdominal cavity (ascites) is often evaluated in this manner.

Vital Signs. Vital signs are important parameters to monitor and detect potential fluid, electrolyte, and acid–base imbalances. Variations in vital signs are discussed in the section, "Manifestations of Fluid, Electrolyte, and Acid–Base Balance."

Neck Veins. Distention of neck veins accompanies ECF volume overload. The jugular veins are visible in the neck. Changes in jugular vein distention can indicate alterations in ECF volume. To assess jugular vein distention, place the client in a sitting position with the head elevated to 30 to 45 degrees. The neck should be straight in alignment with the body. With the client in this position, the distention within the jugular vein should not extend more than 2 cm above the sternal angle (angle of Louis). An increase in ECF volume may be indicated by distention of the neck veins from the top portion of the sternum to the angle of the jaw. Neck vein distention also occurs in people with heart failure.

Central Venous Pressure. Central venous pressure is a more accurate method of evaluating fluid status than visually inspecting neck vein distention. The central venous pressure is the pressure in the right atrium or vena cava. The normal pressure is approximately 4 to 11 cm of water. An increase in the pressure may indicate an ECF volume excess or heart failure. A decrease in pressure may indicate an ECF volume deficit.

Pulmonary Artery Pressure. Evaluating PAP is a more precise method of evaluating fluid status than central venous pressure monitoring. PAP is measured by using a catheter placed through the right side of the heart into the pulmonary artery. Normal PAP follows:

$$\frac{20 \text{ to } 30 \text{ mm Hg}}{8 \text{ to } 15 \text{ mm Hg}}$$

Low PAP readings correspond to volume deficits, and elevated PAP readings correspond to fluid excess. Monitoring PAP is an invasive procedure and is limited to critical care situations.

Bowel Assessment. Bowel elimination is important to consider when detecting fluid and electrolyte imbalances. Because diarrhea predisposes an individual to ECF volume and electrolyte disorders, any diarrhea should be evaluated carefully. Bowel tones should be assessed and hypoactive or hyperactive bowel sounds noted. Abdominal distention, hypoactive bowel tones, or a paralytic ileus can accompany a potassium deficit, while constipation often occurs with hypercalcemia.

Laboratory and Diagnostic Tests

The nurse uses laboratory data to assist in the early identification and continuous monitoring of fluid and electrolyte imbalances. Trends revealed in laboratory data are more significant than any single value. The nurse should be familiar with serum electrolyte values, hematocrit, serum or urine osmolality, urine-specific gravity, and arterial blood gases. Information from these laboratory tests can help the nurse individualize his or her plan of care.

Serum Electrolytes. Monitoring serum electrolyte values permits the nurse to evaluate trends and assess whether electrolyte imbalances are developing, improving, or getting worse. Electrolytes are usually obtained and evaluated in groups rather than singularly. Two standardized groupings are common. A profile including serum calcium, carbon dioxide, chloride, phosphate, magnesium, potassium, and sodium may be ordered to help screen electrolyte abnormalities. A more comprehensive profile that also includes other blood components, such as glucose, blood urea nitrogen, creatinine, and protein (total, albumin globulin ratio), can be helpful when evaluating the total fluid and electrolyte status. Normal reference values for each blood chemistry are found in Appendix B. Because venous blood samples are used to measure the quantity of electrolytes, serum electrolyte values reflect amounts within ECF.

Serum Osmolality. Serum osmolality can be obtained with a venous blood sample. Normal osmolality is 275 to 290 mOsm/kg. Serum osmolality is decreased in water excess and elevated in water deficit.

The nurse may double the serum sodium to obtain a rough approximation of serum osmolarity. If necessary, the nurse is able to estimate more accurately serum osmolarity by using the following formula: 2× plasma sodium concentration + (blood glucose ÷ 100 × 5.6). Although urea contributes to the absolute value of the serum osmolarity, it is not used in the calculation because it crosses cell membranes easily and does not influence water distribution.

Urine Osmolality. Urine osmolality measures the solute concentration of the urine. Increasing the amount of nitrogenous wastes, such as urea, creatinine, and uric acid, will elevate the urinary osmolarity. The circulating amount of ADH will affect urine osmolality. Normal urine osmolality ranges from 50 to 1,200 mOsm/kg. The more concentrated the urine, the greater the urine osmolality. Comparison of plasma and urine osmolarity can be informative. If the kidneys are functioning normally, urine osmolarity should be elevated when plasma osmolarity is elevated and decreased when plasma osmolarity is decreased. That is, the kidneys should be retaining water when plasma osmolarity is increased and losing water when the blood is hypo-osmotic. If the urine concentration is not what one would predict from the plasma osmolarity, then the client may have a renal problem.

Specific Gravity. Specific gravity measures the weight of a substance compared with an equal part of water. The specific gravity of water is 1.000. With normal fluid intake, urine-specific gravity is usually 1.010 to 1.020. A higher specific gravity is obtained when the urine is concentrated, whereas a lower specific gravity is obtained when the urine is dilute. The urine-specific gravity and osmolarity are correlated.

Hematocrit. Hematocrit measures the percentage of whole blood that is composed of red blood cells. Because the hematocrit evaluates the relationship between red blood cells and plasma, an increase or decrease in either red blood cells or plasma will affect the hematocrit. Loss of red blood cells, as in hemorrhage, will lower hematocrit, whereas conditions that increase red blood cell production, such as polycythemia, will increase hematocrit. Alterations in ECF volume also can alter hematocrit. ECF volume deficit may increase hematocrit, whereas ECF volume excess will decrease hematocrit.

Arterial Blood Gases. Arterial blood gases include the pH, partial pressure of carbon dioxide ($PaCO_2$), partial pressure of oxygen (PaO_2), bicarbonate (HCO_3^-), and oxygen saturation of hemoglobin (O_2 sat). These blood gases are used to evaluate acid–base balance and pulmonary function. A pH below 7.37 indicates acidosis, whereas a pH greater than 7.44 indicates alkalosis. Normal ranges for other blood gas values are given in Table 36-4.

Nursing Diagnoses

Using information gathered in the assessment, the nurse is able to identify actual or potential fluid and electrolyte problems. Two nursing diagnoses related to fluid disturbances have been accepted by the North American Nursing Diagnosis Association (NANDA): Fluid Volume Deficit and Fluid Volume Excess, which can be actual or potential nursing diagnoses. To make them more useable, these diagnoses have been expanded here to ECF Volume Excess or Deficit and Water Excess or Deficit. These fluid imbalances also can be actual or potential, and a client can present with both an ECF volume and a water balance problem. These diagnoses are more useful than those offered by NANDA because they reflect the way the body monitors and regulates body fluid balance and the diagnoses indicate how the problem should be managed.

Diagnostic Statement: Fluid Volume Deficit

Definition

ECF volume deficit is the state in which an individual experiences a deficit of vascular and interstitial fluid volume (ECF).

Defining Characteristics

Clients with an ECF volume deficit may have the following signs and symptoms: decreased urine output, increased urine concentration, sudden weight loss, decreased venous filling, increased hematocrit, decreased PAP, decreased central venous pressure, increased pulse rate and hypotension (especially on standing), thirst, decreased skin turgor, decreased pulse volume or pressure, changes in mental state, increased body temperature, dry skin, and dry mucous membranes.

Related Factors

Related factors include individuals with prolonged or marked loss of body fluids, hypoaldosteronism, and a prolonged decrease in intake of fluids or food. Those who use diuretics also have an increased probability of experiencing ECF volume deficit.

Diagnostic Statement: Fluid Volume Excess

Definition

Fluid volume excess is the state in which an individual experiences an excess of vascular and interstitial fluid volume (ECF).

Defining Characteristics

The signs and symptoms of ECF volume excess include edema, effusions, weight gain, shortness of breath, orthopnea, fluid intake greater than output, S/3 heart sound, pulmonary congestion on chest x-ray, abnormal breath sounds and rales (crackles), change in respiratory pattern, change in mental status, decreased hematocrit, increased central venous pressure and PAP, jugular vein distention, oliguria, decreased specific gravity of the urine, and azotemia.

Related Factors

Factors that predipose to ECF volume excess include hyperaldosteronism, excess fluid intake, excess sodium intake, renal failure, heart failure, and liver failure.

Diagnostic Statement: Water Excess

Definition

Water excess or serum hypo-osmolarity is the state in which the individual has an excess of body water in relation to solute. It can result from an increase in water or a decrease in solute and is present when estimated serum osmolarity is <275 mOsm/L.

Defining Characteristics

The signs and symptoms of water excess include estimated or measured serum osmolarity <275 mOsm/L, confusion, headache, cramps, delirium, personality changes, convulsions, coma, anorexia or nausea or vomiting, weight gain, and a low specific gravity of the urine.

Related Factors

Related factors include cardiac, hepatic, or renal failure; excess water intake (oral or intravenous); and the syndrome of inappropriate ADH secretion.

Diagnostic Statement: Water Deficit

Definition

Water deficit or serum hyperosmolarity is the state in which the individual has a deficit of body water in relation to solute. It can result from a decrease in water or an increase in solute and is present when estimated serum osmolarity is >290 mOsm/L.

Defining Characteristics

The signs and symptoms of a water deficit include measured or estimated serum osmolarity >290 mOsm/L, increased specific gravity of the urine, lethargy, disorientation, delusions, irritability, convulsions, coma, thirst, oliguria or anuria, tachycardia, and sometimes fever.

Related Factors

Inadequate water intake, particularly in the very young, very old, and those physically or mentally incapable of independently getting water can contribute to the development of a water deficit. In addition, excess intake or production of solute, such as may occur with diabetes mellitus or overdoses, and excess water loss may be contributing factors.

Related Nursing Diagnoses

Many other nursing diagnoses can be present in clients with fluid and electrolyte imbalances. Related nursing diagnoses can be actual or potential, and early identification permits the nurse to intervene successfully. Self-Care Deficit or Activity Intolerance can occur if fatigue, weakness, or muscular irritability is present. Risk for Injury can occur if electrolyte or fluid imbalances cause postural hypotension, loss of consciousness, or impaired cognition. Impaired Skin Integrity is frequently associated with edema, and Constipation or Diarrhea is often associated with fluid or electrolyte imbalances. Knowledge Deficit or Noncompliance can occur when new treatment regimens are instituted without adequate client teaching.

Outcome Identification and Planning

After nursing diagnoses and related factors are identified, the nurse and the client or family plan outcomes and interventions. In many situations, planning may be done with family or support people rather than the client. Examples of some interventions that can be used in planning are listed in the accompanying display and discussed in the next section of this chapter.

The nurse and client or client's family work together to set realistic, individualized goals. Goals of nursing intervention for a client with altered fluid, electrolyte, acid–base balances focus on prevention, early recognition of the alteration, intervention in contributing factors, and provision of therapies to restore normal function. Goals must be individualized based on the client's history, areas of risk, evidence of altered function, and

Planning

Examples of Nursing Interventions Used for Common Fluid and Electrolyte Problems

Extracellular Fluid Volume Excess

- Administer diuretics as ordered.
- Limit intake of foods and fluids containing sodium.
- Weigh daily.

Extracellular Fluid Volume Deficit

- Encourage the oral intake of salty fluids, such as chicken broth, bouillon, or sugar-salt solutions.
- Administer intravenous fluids, such as normal saline or lactated Ringer's solution as ordered by the healthcare provider.

Water Excess

- Limit oral or intravenous (dextrose 5% in water) water intake.
- Explain why intake is being limited, and provide oral care.

Water Deficit

- Encourage oral intake of fluids, such as fruit juices, sodas, and tea.
- Administer intravenous fluids, such as dextrose 5% in water as ordered by the healthcare provider.

related objective data. Examples of client goals for the client with altered fluid and electrolyte balance follow:

The client will reestablish normal ECF volume, water, and electrolyte balance.

The client will demonstrate knowledge regarding how to promote future ECF volume, water, and electrolyte balance.

The client will have an absence of complications from ECF volume, water, or electrolyte imbalance.

The nurse and client together can determine specific outcome criteria to individualize the plan of care. Short-term goals (ie, the client will increase fluid intake to 2,000 mL/24 hours) may be easy to reach within a short period of time. Other goals may involve changes in long-established dietary patterns, which may take much longer.

Implementation

Nursing intervention is important in preventing and promoting adequate fluid and electrolyte balance and in treating imbalances as they occur. Client teaching, assisting with fluid and dietary intake, and monitoring and managing intravenous infusion of fluids or blood are all important nursing interventions to promote optimal fluid and electrolyte balance.

Nursing Interventions to Promote Health and Function

Teaching people in the community or those seeking assistance within the healthcare system is an important nursing role to prevent fluid and electrolyte problems from occurring. Nurses can help people understand how fluid and electrolyte imbalances occur and how they can be prevented. The type of fluid replacement that people use should be matched to the type of fluid that is being lost. If there is a deficit of ECF volume, consuming mildly salty solutions, such as chicken broth, is appropriate. Some "sports drinks" contain electrolytes; however, they are relatively costly. One liter of boiled or clean water containing 1/2 teaspoon of salt and 8 teaspoons of sugar is an inexpensive substitute (Avery & Snyder, 1990). Fruit juices (except tomato juice), sodas, and other sugar drinks can be considered as water.

Teaching can occur in a variety of settings and for all age groups. A few teaching elements are listed in the accompanying display. The nurse who interacts with new parents should stress fluid needs of the newborn; how quickly serious problems can develop if the infant develops vomiting, diarrhea, or a fever; and symptoms that warrant contacting a physician (MMWR, 1994). Follow-up teaching can occur as the child grows, explaining normal fluid requirements and dietary patterns. When the child is ill, the nurse can explain measures to help the parents adequately replace the fluid that is lost. Balanced electrolyte solutions are available commercially. Ice pops and other frozen treats may be helpful in encouraging fluid intake in the reluctant child.

The school nurse can reinforce teaching in health classes. Often school-age children are involved in sports activities. Encouraging adequate fluid intake before, during, and after strenuous exercise is important, particularly in hot weather. The dangers of fad diets and eating disorders should be discussed, especially among adolescents.

Nurses who work in industry should be aware of working conditions that could affect fluid and electrolyte balance. When employees must work in hot, humid environments performing strenuous exercise, periodic breaks should be scheduled so that adequate fluid replacement is possible. The nurse may be influential in supporting policies and legislation to ensure such practices.

Health teaching is especially important among older adults. Classes can be offered in senior citizen centers or community agencies to reinforce good diet and fluid

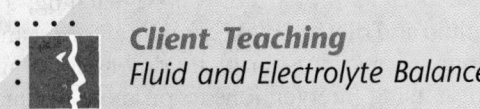

Client Teaching
Fluid and Electrolyte Balance

Instruct the client as follows:

- *Drink at least six glasses of water daily unless advised otherwise.*
- *When you have increased loss of body fluids, make an inexpensive replacement fluid by adding 1/2 teaspoon of salt and 8 teaspoons of sugar to 1 L of clean or boiled water (Avery & Snyder, 1990).*
- *If you exercise vigorously or are in a warmer than usual climate, replenish fluid and electrolyte loss with the fluid described above or with commercial replacement solutions.*
- *Diarrhea and vomiting that are severe or last for more than 24 hours in an infant should be reported to the healthcare provider. Infants are especially susceptible to rapid and serious problems with fluid balance.*
- *Do not give supplemental water to healthy infants until they are old enough to begin eating solid food. Newborns' kidneys are unable to handle large volumes of water, and symptomatic water excess has been reported to two 2-month-old infants fed excess bottled water (MMWR, 1994).*
- *If you are on a special diet to increase or decrease the intake of an electrolyte, ask for a list of recommended foods and those that are discouraged.*

requirements. Often older individuals take medications, such as diuretics, that can affect fluid and electrolyte balance. Teaching is important to ensure client compliance and help prevent any problems that can occur with treatment. Clients can be taught to detect signs of fluid and electrolyte imbalance, such as rapid weight gain or loss, swelling, changes in normal urine output, muscle weakness, or abnormal skin sensation; they also can be given guidelines for when to notify a physician.

Nursing Interventions for Altered Fluid and Electrolyte Status

Planned nursing interventions are important for promoting optimum fluid and electrolyte balance (Cullen, 1992). The nurse must individualize his or her approach for specific clients, considering their current condition.

Oral Fluids

Depending on the client's current status, oral fluids may need to be regulated. The nurse may determine the nursing assessment and nursing diagnosis. If the nurse has identified a potential or actual ECF volume or water deficit, he or she will want to institute a plan to increase oral intake of mildly salty fluids or water; if the nursing diagnosis is potential or actual ECF volume or water excess, the nurse will want to curtail oral intake of salt and salty fluids or water. The physician also may order that fluids be restricted or encouraged.

Increasing Oral Fluids. "Force fluids" or "push fluids" are general terms indicating that increased fluid intake is required. Individual goals should be set for each client, depending on the current fluid status. To enhance compliance, explain why the increased fluid intake is desirable, and involve the client in setting goals for fluid intake. Client teaching and goal setting may include the family if the client is unable or reluctant to drink fluids independently. Encourage the family members to offer sips of fluid frequently during their visits, and teach them how to record on the intake and output sheet.

Ensure that fluids are placed and kept within the client's reach. Determine what temperature of water is preferred, and change the water pitcher as often as needed to maintain that temperature. If the client is unable to drink independently, offer fluids and encouragement for drinking during every client interaction. Some clients may verbally refuse fluids, but when the straw or glass is placed in their mouth and encouragement is given, they may decide to drink. Providing fluids that the client especially likes may increase fluid intake. It is important to consider any dietary restrictions when providing clients with additional fluids. For example, a diabetic client should have sugar-free soft drinks, and a client on a potassium-restricted diet should not be offered fluids high in potassium, such as orange juice. Encourage foods that have a high fluid content, such as custards, soups, and ice creams.

When a specific fluid order is given (eg, increase fluids to 2,000 mL/24 hours), plan how much should be consumed in each shift. The largest volume is usually consumed during the daytime and early evening. Large amounts taken close to bedtime may necessitate getting up to the bathroom during the night, consequently interrupting sleep.

Adequate fluid replacement also is necessary for clients who are receiving tube feedings. These clients may need additional water to prevent water deficit. They often cannot independently drink when they are thirsty or even notify the nurse of their thirst. For this reason, assess carefully the fluid needs of clients receiving tube feedings, and administer water as needed.

Restricting Oral Fluids. Oral fluids may need to be restricted when ECF volume or water excess is present or when certain medical conditions occur, such as congestive heart failure or renal failure. Assisting the client to comply with limited fluid intake despite thirst can be a challenge.

The physician's orders for fluid restriction will include the number of milliliters of fluid to be taken per 24 hours. Most fluid restrictions include all fluids ingested. When a free water restriction is ordered, only free water is restricted, because other fluids, such as tomato juice or milk, which contain at least 150 MEq/L of sodium, would not contribute further to a water excess (Sterns & Spital, 1990).

The nurse and client plan how best to allocate the allotted fluid during a 24-hour period. Some clients prefer to drink fluids with their meals, whereas others prefer to save fluids for between meals. Most fluids are designated for day and evening shifts, with about 100 mL left over for nights in case the client has to take medication or wants a drink. Ice chips may be helpful for people on fluid restriction. Ice melts to one half its volume and should be noted as such on the intake and output record. Water pitchers may be removed from the room and water offered in small cups to avoid the temptation of drinking too much at one time. Diversional activities also may help the client focus less on the thirst he or she is experiencing.

To minimize thirst for clients on fluid restrictions, avoid salty or very sweet fluids. Gum and hard candy may temporarily relieve thirst by drawing fluid into the oral cavity because the sugar content increases oral tonicity. Fifteen to 30 minutes later, oral membranes may be even drier than before. To avoid this rebound effect, try to encourage sugar-free candy and gum. Dry foods, such as crackers and bread, also may increase the client's feeling of thirst. Thirst may be decreased by allowing the client to rinse his or her mouth frequently. A sip of water is taken, swished around the oral cavity, and then spit out before it is swallowed. Mouth washes containing alcohol should be avoided because they have a drying effect. Frequent oral care is necessary for anyone on a fluid restriction. Lips can be moistened with a water-soluble gel to prevent drying and cracking.

Electrolyte Replacement

From the nursing assessment, the nurse can identify clients at risk for electrolyte deficit or excess. The nurse can help to promote optimum electrolyte balance by teaching the client about foods that should be restricted or encouraged and administering oral or intravenous electrolyte supplements.

Diet Teaching. Once the nurse has identified the potential for an electrolyte imbalance, a diet teaching plan can be individualized. The client should be provided with a list of foods high or low in the identified electrolyte and given some guidelines for the amount to be consumed each day (Table 36-5). For example, for the client who has recently been ordered a thiazide (potassium-depleting) diuretic, the nurse may indicate that it is important to eat at least one banana or one other potassium-rich food each day.

Electrolyte Supplements. When normal dietary intake is not sufficient, electrolyte supplements can be administered orally or intravenously. The intravenous administration is usually reserved for severe electrolyte imbalances or when the client is unable to take anything orally. Liquid oral potassium supplements taste unpleasant and should be mixed with juice to promote compliance. Intravenous preparations of potassium must be administered carefully because concentrated infusion can damage the veins or cause rebound hyperkalemia, which is potentially lethal.

Table 36-5 • Selected Dietary Sources for Electrolytes

Electrolyte	Dietary Source
Sodium (Na^+)	Salt (sodium chloride), monosodium glutamate (MSG), soy sauce, dairy products (milk, cheese), processed food (luncheon meats, bacon), snack foods (peanuts, chips, pretzels), bouillon, canned or packaged soup, pickles, olives, sauerkraut, tomato juice
Potassium (K^+)	Fruits (banana, cantaloupe, apricots, peaches, dates, raisins), vegetables (avocado, navy beans, potatoes, squash, carrots, cauliflower), orange juice, tomato juice
Calcium (Ca^{++})	Dairy products (milk, cheese, yogurt, ice cream), dark green vegetables (broccoli, spinach, greens), sardines, salmon, oysters, tofu
Magnesium (MG^{++})	Nuts and peanut butter, egg yolk, milk, whole grain cereals, bananas, citrus fruit, dark green vegetables, legumes, seafood, chocolate

Intravenous Therapy

Intravenous therapy is frequently used with clients to prevent or treat fluid and electrolyte imbalances. In the hospital, the nurse is responsible for initiating, monitoring, and discontinuing the intravenous infusion. The type and amount of intravenous fluid and electrolyte replacement are ordered by the physician. Fluid therapy also is provided in the home, and family members or visiting nurses assist with monitoring the therapy (see Chap. 26).

Community-Based Nursing

Many clients continue treatment for fluid and electrolyte imbalances in the home. Fluid and electrolyte imbalances may necessitate dietary changes. Certain restrictions may be enforced, or certain foods may need to be encouraged. Lists of such foods should be given to the client and a plan worked out as to who will do the shopping and prepare the meals. These tasks may prove tiring for those who are weak from fluid or electrolyte imbalances.

Clients with fluid and electrolyte imbalances may have various medications prescribed. The medication, purpose, dosage, frequency, precautions, and potential side effects and complications should be emphasized. If the client has a prescription for a medication (eg, diuretics), it is important to explain the manifestations of the potential electrolyte imbalance and methods of circumventing the problem. For example, for the client taking diuretics that enhance excretion of potassium, the importance of potassium replacement by taking ordered supplements or making necessary dietary changes (eg, eating bananas, dried apricots, and other fruits daily) must be emphasized.

Because fluid and electrolyte imbalances may cause poor coordination, weakness, confusion, and altered gait, the nurse should emphasize the need for a safe home environment. Such teaching may include assistance with ambulation or suggestions for safety features in the home (installing night lights and hand railings next to the tub or toilet and removing throw rugs).

Explaining to the client the symptoms that need to be relayed to the physician is an important part of client teaching. For example, some physicians may want to be informed if the client gains more than 5 lb or has vomiting or diarrhea that lasts for more than 1 day. All client teaching is beneficial for preventing future occurrences of fluid and electrolyte imbalances.

Evaluation

The nurse uses specific outcome criteria to measure the attainment of client goals. If outcome criteria have not been achieved, the nurse can revise his or her plan of care or set more realistic goals. The process of evaluation and revision of care is dynamic and continual.

Outcome criteria should be individualized for the client. Possible outcome criteria are given as a guide.

Goal

The client will reestablish normal fluid and electrolyte balance.

Possible Outcome Criteria

- The client maintains equal intake and output within 300 mL/24 hours.
- By discharge, the client demonstrates weight within 2 kg of baseline weight (give specific amount of weight to be lost or gained).
- The client does not experience sudden changes in weight (increasing or decreasing more than 1 kg/d).
- By discharge, the client reestablishes electrolyte values within normal limits.
- The client experiences a decrease in postural pulse and blood pressure changes.
- By discharge, the client verbalizes that he or she does not have excessive thirst.
- By discharge, the client does not have edema.
- By discharge, the client does not have concentrated urine.

Goal

The client will demonstrate knowledge regarding how to promote fluid and electrolyte balance.

Possible Outcome Criteria

- By the conclusion of the teaching session, the client verbalizes the importance of drinking eight glasses of water per day.
- By the conclusion of the teaching session, the client lists foods that are high in sodium and verbalizes needed modifications in diet.
- The client maintains a daily record of weight for the next month.
- The client notifies the physician of any significant weight gain.
- By the conclusion of the teaching session, the client verbalizes a plan to cope with temporary problems of diarrhea or vomiting.
- By the conclusion of the teaching session, the client lists foods high in potassium.

Goal

The client will have an absence of complications from fluid or electrolyte imbalance.

Possible Outcome Criteria

- The client stands and walks without falling.
- The skin remains intact despite edema until edema is reduced.

Nursing Plan of Care
The Client with Fluid Volume Deficit

Nursing Diagnosis

Fluid Volume Deficit related to inadequate oral intake as manifested by concentrated urine, change in urine output, dry mucous membranes, postural hypotension, and change in serum sodium.

Client Goal

Client will reestablish normal fluid and electrolyte balance.

Client Outcome Criteria

- Client maintains equal intake and output within ± 300 mL/24 h.

Nursing Intervention	*Scientific Rationale*
1. Monitor intake and output.	1. Observation of trends in intake and output provides essential data regarding client's fluid and electrolyte status and guides interventions. Intake should approximately equal output, but observing for trends and significant increases or decrease is more important than specific numbers.
2. Monitor serum electrolytes, serum osmolality, specific gravity, and hematocrit.	2. Monitoring provides essential data regarding client status and guides interventions. (Common abnormal laboratory values in fluid volume deficit include increased Hct, increased serum sodium, increased serum osmolality, increased specific gravity.)
3. Increase oral fluid intake to at least 2,000 mL/24 h or as ordered by physician.	3. Increased intake of fluids (and high fluid-content foods) helps correct fluid volume deficit and maintain adequate hydration.
4. Monitor IV fluid therapy as prescribed.	4. Fluids must be provided when adequate intake cannot be obtained by oral intake alone. Monitoring ensures infusion at prescribed rate and allows early detection of complications.
5. Assess fluid preferences.	5. Client is more likely to increase fluid intake with fluids that are appealing.
6. Ensure optimal access to preferred fluids, and assist as needed.	6. Availability and assistance are necessary to ensure increased fluid intake.
7. Give positive reinforcement or verbal cuing as necessary.	7. Reinforcement helps to increase compliance for clients who may be forgetful or disinterested.

Client Goal

Client will demonstrate knowledge regarding how to promote fluid and electrolyte balance

Client Outcome Criteria

- Client verbalizes the importance of drinking eight glasses of water per day by the end of the teaching session.
- Client lists foods that are high in sodium and verbalizes needed modifications in diet by discharge.
- Client maintains a daily record of weight for next month.
- Client verbalizes a plan to cope with temporary problems of diarrhea or vomiting by discharge.

(continued)

Nursing Plan of Care
The Client with Fluid Volume Deficit *(continued)*

Nursing Intervention	*Scientific Rationale*
1. Assess reason for inadequate fluid intake before admission.	1. There are many possible reasons for inadequate intake (eg, increased need secondary to diarrhea, depression, desire to decrease voidings, and inability to access and prepare food). It is important to understand the reason to individualize plan for care and prevention.
2. Teach client or family about the significance (eg, rehospitalization, potential for confusion and injury) and prevention (eg, daily fluid requirement, method for recording intake) of fluid volume deficit.	2. Increased knowledge leads to increased compliance and more successful outcomes.
3. Provide a list of symptoms of or conditions that increase risk for fluid volume deficit (eg, diarrhea) that require contact with a physician.	3. This may result in earlier treatment. Written material may be cited in the future to help ensure compliance.

Evaluation is important to ensure that the goals of promoting optimum fluid and electrolyte balance, preventing complications of fluid and electrolyte imbalance, and increasing the client's knowledge to prevent fluid and electrolyte imbalance are achieved. Modification of the plan of care or more realistic outcome criteria may be necessary if the goals have not been attained.

Key Concepts

- Homeostasis of body fluids, electrolytes, and pH is necessary for cellular function and the maintenance of health. Homeostasis is maintained by processes such as diffusion, osmosis, active transport, and filtration that facilitate fluid or electrolyte movement.
- Intracellular fluid refers to the fluid within the cells of the body, whereas ECF refers to the intravascular fluid and the interstitial fluid.
- Cations are positively charged electrolytes (sodium, potassium, calcium, and magnesium), and anions are negatively charged electrolytes (chloride, phosphate, sulfate, and bicarbonate). Balance between anions and cations is a dynamic process necessary to maintain neutrality.
- States of altered fluid balance include ECF volume excess or deficit and water excess or deficit.
- States of electrolyte imbalance include hyperkalemia, hypokalemia, hypercalcemia, hypocalcemia, hypermagnesemia, and hypomagnesemia.
- States of altered acid–base balance include respiratory acidosis, metabolic acidosis, respiratory alkalosis, and metabolic alkalosis.
- Inadequate intake; excessive loss through vomiting, diarrhea, diaphoresis, or diuretics; stress; chronic illness, such as renal failure, cardiac failure, or respiratory failure; surgery; or pregnancy can increase the potential for altered fluid, electrolyte, and acid–base balance.
- Alterations in normal fluid, electrolyte, or acid–base balance are manifested by imbalances in intake and output, changes in mental status, changes in vital signs, abnormal states of tissue hydration, or abnormal neuromuscular status.
- Intake and output, weight, edema, tissue turgor, neck vein and hand vein engorgement, and vital signs are all important objective data to collect to identify actual problems in fluid and electrolyte status.
- Laboratory data, such as serum electrolytes, serum osmolality, urine-specific gravity, and arterial blood gases, also provide important information for identifying potential disruption in fluid and electrolyte status.
- Important nursing interventions include preventive health teaching; regulating oral fluids; assisting

with electrolyte replacement; initiating, regulating, and monitoring intravenous therapy; and monitoring blood transfusions.

Critical Thinking Challenges

Now that you have studied fluid, electrolyte, and acid–base balance, you should be able to understand laboratory results and other signs and subjective and objective data related to your client at the beginning of the chapter. Review the situation, and consider the following.

1. *Summarize the information you have about this client's ECF volume, water balance, and electrolyte balance.*
2. *Based on this information, make a tentative nursing diagnosis for each of the following: ECF volume status, water balance, and electrolyte balance. Describe what additional data you need to confirm or correct your nursing diagnoses.*
3. *Propose types of oral fluids you would offer this client to drink, and give your reasons.*
4. *Discuss your safety concerns for this client, and outline how you would plan her care to ensure safety.*
5. *Plan what teaching you would do today and before the client is discharged.*

References

Abraham, W. T., & Schrier, R. W. (1994). Body fluid volume regulation in health and disease. *Advances in Internal Medicine, 39*, 23–47.

Blackburn, S. T. (1994). Renal function in the neonate. *Journal of Perinatal and Neonatal Nursing, 8*(1), 37–47.

Avery, M. E., & Snyder, J. D. (1990). Oral therapy for acute diarrhea. The underused simple solution. *New England Journal of Medicine, 323*, 891–894.

Cronin, R. E. (1990). Magnesium disorders. In J. P. Kokko & R. L. Tannen (Eds.), *Fluid and electrolytes* (pp. 631–645) (2nd ed.). Philadelphia: W.B. Saunders.

Cullen, L. (1992) Interventions related to fluid and electrolyte balance. *Nursing Clinics of North America, 27*(2), 569–597.

Faull, C. M., Holmes, C., & Baylis, P. H. (1993). Water balance in elderly people: Is there a deficiency of vasopressin? *Age and Ageing, 22*(2), 114–120.

Mack, G. W., Weseman, C. A., Langhans, G. W., Scherzer, H., Gillen, C. M., & Nadel, E. R. (1994). Body fluid balance in dehydrated healthy older men: Thirst and renal osmoregulation. *Journal of Applied Physiology, 76*(4), 1615–1623.

Metheny, N. M. (1992). *Fluid and electrolyte balance: Nursing considerations* (2nd ed.). Philadelphia: J.B. Lippincott.

Norris, S. O. (1993). Managing low cardiac output states: Maintaining volume after cardiac surgery. *AACN Clinical Issues in Critical Care Nursing, 4*(2), 309–319.

Pak, C. Y. C. (1990). Calcium disorders: Hypercalcemia and hypocalcemia. In Kokko, J. P., & Tannen, R. L. (eds). *Fluid and electrolytes.* (2nd ed.) Philadelphia: W. B. Saunders, 596–630.

Paller, M. S., & Ferris, T. F. (1990) Fluid and electrolyte disorders of pregnancy. In J. P. Kokko & R. L. Tannen (Eds.), *Fluid and electrolytes* (pp. 906–921) (2nd ed.). Philadelphia: W.B. Saunders.

Robillard, J. E., Segar, J. L., Smith, F. G., & Jose, P. A. (1992). Regulation of sodium metabolism and extracellular fluid volume during development. *Clinics in Perinatology, 19*(1), 15–31.

Rose, B. (1994). *Clinical physiology of acid–base and electrolyte disorders* (4th ed.). New York: McGraw Hill.

Sterns, R. H., & Spital, A. (1990). Disorders of water balance. In J. P. Kokko & R. L. Tannen (Eds.), *Fluid and electrolytes* (pp. 139–194) (2nd ed.). Philadelphia: W.B. Saunders.

Takamata, A., Mack, G. W., Gillen, C. M., & Nadel, E. R. (1994). Sodium appetite, thirst, and body fluid regulation in humans during rehydration without sodium replacement. *American Journal of Physiology, 266* (5 Part 2), R1493–R1502.

Tannen, R. L. (1990). Potassium disorders. In J. P. Kokko & R. L. Tannen (Eds.), *Fluid and electrolytes* (pp. 195–300) (2nd ed.). Philadelphia: W.B. Saunders.

Woods, S., Sivarajan-Froelicher, E., Halpenny, J., & Motzer, S. U. (1995). *Cardiac nursing* (3rd ed.). Philadelphia: J.B. Lippincott.

Bibliography

Brown, R. G. (1993). Disorders of water and sodium balance. *Postgraduate Medicine, 93*(4), 227–244.

Duggan, C., Santosham, M., Glass, R. I. (1992). The management of acute diarrhea in children: oral rehydration, maintenance, and nutritional therapy. *Morbidity and Mortality Weekly Report, 41(RR-16)*, 1–20.

Kositzke, J. A. (1990). A question of balance-dehydration in the elderly. *Journal of Gerontological Nursing,* 16(5), 4–11.

MMWR (2 Feb 1994). Hyponatremic seizures among infants fed with commercial bottled drinking water—Wisconsin, 1993. *Morbidity and Mortality Weekly Reports, 43*(35), 641–643.

Ozuna, L. A., & Adkins, A. T. (1993). Development of a vital-sign/fluid-balance flow sheet. *Oncology Nursing Forum, 20*(1), 113–115.

Phillips, P. A., Johnston, C. I., & Gray, L. (1993). Disturbed fluid and electrolyte homeostasis following dehydration in elderly people. *Age and Ageing, 22*(1), S26–S33.

Porth, C. M., & Erickson, M. (1992). Physiology of thirst and drinking: Implication for nursing practice. *Heart and Lung, 21*(3), 273–282.

Walpert, N. (1990). An orderly look at calcium metabolism disorders. *Nursing 90, 20*(7), 60–64.

Nutrition

Key Terms	Learning Objectives

Key Terms

Absorption
Anorexia
Basal metabolism
Calorie (kilocalorie)
Carbohydrates
Complete proteins
Digestion
Disaccharides
Fats
Fiber
Glycogenesis
Incomplete protein
Metabolism
Monosaccharides
Nutrients
Partially complete proteins
Polysaccharides
Proteins
Vitamins

Learning Objectives

Upon completion of this chapter, the student will be able to do the following:

- *Identify essential nutrients, and give examples of good dietary sources for each.*
- *Describe normal digestion, absorption, and metabolism of carbohydrates, fats, and proteins.*
- *List factors that can affect normal dietary patterns.*
- *Discuss nutritional considerations across the lifespan.*
- *Describe manifestations of altered nutrition.*
- *Describe nursing interventions to promote optimal nutrition and health.*
- *Discuss nursing responsibilities for interventions used to treat altered nutritional states.*

37

You are a high school nurse. Several teachers have expressed concern about observed weight loss in a particular female student, so you bring her to your office. You observe that her body weight is significantly lower than what would be ideal. She is fairly pleasant and appears to be cooperative. She reports that her intake is adequate and normal. You must decide how to address this issue.

In previous chapters, you discovered the importance of holistic nursing and individual responsibility in health maintenance. In this chapter, you will expand your knowledge base about nutritional requirements and meeting nutritional needs. After you read the chapter, you should be able to combine holistic nursing and health maintenance to concepts and facts about nutritional needs. Information related to nutrition will help you provide nursing care for the high school student's situation. Critical Thinking Challenges at the end of the chapter will help you consider nutritional concerns.

As part of a holistic approach to good health, a nutritionally adequate diet is vital for promoting normal growth and development and preventing deficiency states. Optimal nutrition is essential to maintain health and prevent disease. An adequate diet is necessary to maintain bodily functions, promote healing, maintain healthy tissues, maintain body temperature, and build resistance to infection.

Nutrients are biochemical substances obtained from ingested food and fluids. Carbohydrates, proteins, and fats are nutrients that supply the body with energy. Vitamins, minerals, and water are not sources of energy but are important in regulating body processes.

The body cannot synthesize essential nutrients in adequate amounts; therefore, they must be provided through the diet. Dietary intake of nonessential nutrients is not required, because these nutrients can be synthesized in adequate amounts by the body or are not required for body functioning.

Nurses are in key positions to access, monitor, and promote good nutrition. In a variety of settings (eg, health fairs, classes in schools and community centers, and interactions with families during health screening), they can teach principles of normal nutrition. Nurses also screen for altered nutritional states to detect obesity, malnutrition, and anorexia. Nutritional assessment also is important for all preoperative clients. Nurses teach clients how to adapt to dietary restrictions when special diets are necessary. Nurses also are responsible for monitoring nutritional therapies, such as enteral tube feedings or total parenteral nutrition (TPN), which may be necessary to maintain optimal nutrition in clients with significant impairments.

Normal Nutritional Function

The body uses nutrients to build and maintain body tissues, furnish energy, and regulate body processes (Eschleman, 1991). Cell make up is constantly changing. Nutrients are needed to supply building materials, for example, calcium for teeth and bones or fat for padding and support of vital organs. Each cell requires energy to fulfill its task, such as health maintenance or walking. Chemicals in the form of nutrients act and react to regulate body processes, which can be as basic as breathing or as circumstantial as wound healing. Water, which makes up one-half to two-thirds of adult weight, is an important regulator in body processes.

In a complex series of processes, the body breaks down the ingested nutrients into a form that can be absorbed and used. **Metabolism** is the process by which energy from nutrients can be used by the cells or stored for later use. Anabolic processes build up substances and body tissues; catabolic processes break down substances or body stores. These reserves are used when the person is not eating, as in a serious illness, or when there is an increased need for nutrients, as in pregnancy.

Energy obtained from food is measured in the form of a large calorie or kilocalories (abbreviated calories or cal or kcal) or in Canada, kilojoules (KJ). The large **calorie** is the amount of heat required to raise one kilogram of water 1°C.

Structure of the Digestive System

The digestive system consists of the organs of the gastrointestinal (GI) tract, through which food enters, travels, and exits the body (mouth, pharynx, esophagus, stomach, small intestine, large intestine), and accessory organs that play a role in the process of digestion (tongue, salivary glands, teeth, liver, pancreas, and gallbladder).

The mouth is lined with mucous membrane. The tongue is composed of skeletal muscle and is covered with mucous membrane. The papillae, which are the elevations on the tongue, contain the taste buds. The salivary glands are sublingual (the interior part of the mouth under the tongue), submandibular (the posterior part of the floor of the mouth), and parotid (near the temporomandibular joint). The salivary glands secrete saliva, which contains the salivary enzymes involved in mastication. Mastication includes chewing, reducing the size of food particles, and mixing the food with saliva.

The pharynx extends from the base of the skull to the esophagus and is composed of muscle lined with

Nursing Research
Nutrition

Selected Nursing Research Studies

Grant, L. P., Wanger, L. I., & Neill, K. M. (1994). Fiber-fortified feedings in immobile patients. *Clinical Nursing Research, 3*(2), 166–172.

Heitkemper, M. M., Bond, E. F., Shaver, J. F., & Georgers, J. M. (1990). Menstrual cycle factors related to increased gastric contractile response to tube feeding. *Journal of Parenteral and Enteral Nutrition, 14*(6), 634–639.

Johnson, A. A., Knight, E. M., Edwards, C. H., Oyemode, U. J., Cole, O. J., Westney, O. E., Westney, L. S., Laryea, H., & Jones, S. (1994). Selected lifestyle practices in urban African American women. *Journal of Nutrition, 124*(6Suppl.), 963S–972S.

Little, R. E., Lambert, M. D., & Worthington-Roberts, B. (1990). Drinking and smoking at 3 months postpartum by lactation history. *Paediatric and Perinatal Epidemiology, 4*(3), 290–302.

Springer, N. S., Bogue, E. L., Arnold, M., Yankou, D., & Oakley, D. (1994). Nutrition locus of control and dietary behaviors of pregnant women. *Applied Nursing Research, 7*(1), 28–31.

Possible Topics for Nursing Inquiry

- What is the effect of prompted cueing on nutritional intake in nursing home clients?
- What is the relationship of preoperative albumin levels on postoperative wound healing and incidence of wound infection?
- How does nurse follow-up teaching affect compliance with a low-sodium diet?
- What is the impact of continuous versus intermittent tube feedings on the sensation of hunger and desire to eat?
- What are the nutritional risk factors for low-birth-weight infants during the first year of life?

mucous membrane. Food and air pass through this organ before reaching the appropriate outlet (the epiglottis for food and the bronchi for air). The epiglottis closes off the airway during swallowing. The esophagus extends from the pharynx to the stomach and transports food from the mouth to the stomach. It is a long, collapsible tube composed of muscular walls lined with mucous membrane.

The stomach lies in the upper portion of the abdominal cavity. It is connected to the esophagus at the upper end and to the duodenum at the lower end. The stomach varies in size according to body size, sex, and distention. The stomach is lined with mucous membrane and has a muscle layer and an outer fibroserous layer.

The small intestine lies in the abdominal cavity and measures about an inch in diameter and 20 ft in length. It has a mucous lining, two muscle layers, and an outer visceral peritoneal layer.

The small intestine consists of the duodenum, the jejunum, and the ileum.

The large intestine, located at the lower end of the GI tract, is about 2 to 3 in in diameter and 6 ft long. It has a mucous lining, a muscle layer, and an outer visceral peritoneal layer. The large intestine consists of the cecum, the colon (ascending, transverse, descending, and sigmoid), and the rectum (see Fig. 42-2).

The accessory organs of digestion are located outside the GI system, but their secretions are conveyed there by ducts. The liver, the largest gland in the body, lies in the right upper quadrant of the abdominal cavity. Bile produced in the liver is transported through the hepatic duct and the cystic duct to the gallbladder, where it is stored and concentrated. The common bile duct transports bile to the duodenum, where it participates in digestion. The pancreas is located behind the stomach and lies in the curvature of the duodenum. Pancreatic enzymes are transported to the duodenum through the pancreatic ducts.

Normal Function of Nutrients

Nutrients, or food containing elements for normal body functioning, are divided into six categories: carbohydrates, proteins, fats, vitamins, minerals, and water. Energy is provided by the metabolism of carbohydrates, fat, and protein. Water is essential to maintain normal fluid balance and promote normal digestion, absorption, and metabolism of food. Vitamins and minerals are organic and inorganic compounds important for normal body processes.

Carbohydrates

Carbohydrates are simple sugars (**monosaccharides** and **disaccharides**) and complex sugars (**polysaccharides**). They are composed of carbon, hydrogen, and oxygen. The polysaccharides are hydrolyzed into simple sugars during digestion by acid hydrolysis and digestive enzymes. Sugars, syrups, molasses, honey, fruit, and milk are excellent sources of simple carbohydrates. Complex carbohydrates are contained in bread, cereal, potatoes, rice, pasta, crackers, flour products, and legumes.

The main function of carbohydrates is to provide energy. Each gram of oxidized carbohydrate yields about 4 kcal. Carbohydrates also are important in oxidizing fats in normal fat metabolism; promoting desirable bacterial growth in the GI tract, which is vital to the synthesis of B-complex vitamins; producing the carbon component in the synthesis of nonessential amino acids; and producing other essential body acids and compounds.

Polysaccharides not digested in the GI tract are one of the main components of dietary fiber. Dietary **fiber** is a minimal source of energy but plays an essential role in stimulating peristalsis and maintaining normal bowel elimination. Another characteristic of carbohydrates is their protein-sparing action. Protein sparing is when the body uses carbohydrates rather than protein as a source of energy, thus sparing protein for the vital function of tissue building.

The circulation of blood supplies glucose to the cells as a source of energy and for the production of vital substances. The blood glucose level is maintained within relatively narrow limits (about 80–110 mg/dL). In the fasting state, the blood glucose level is about 60 to 80 mg/dL, but shortly after a meal, the level can rise to 140 to 160 mg/dL (Patrick, et al., 1991). *Hyperglycemia*, in which the blood glucose level is higher than normal due to inadequate production or use of insulin, occurs in diabetes mellitus. *Hypoglycemia*, in which the blood glucose level is lower than normal, can be symptomatic of liver or pancreatic abnormalities.

Protein

Proteins are vital to growth, development, and the normal functioning of nearly all body systems. They are major constituents of most living cells and body fluids, including bones, skin, teeth, muscle, hair, blood, and serum. **Proteins** are organic compounds composed of polymers of amino acids connected by peptide bonds. They contain carbon, hydrogen, oxygen, and nitrogen. Depending on the specific amino acids of which they are composed, proteins also may contain phosphorus, iron, sulfur, or copper. These proteins are synthesized by the body for specific functions, including hemoglobin for carrying oxygen to tissues, insulin for blood glucose regulations, and albumin for regulating osmotic pressure in the blood. These functions generally cannot be performed by another body protein.

The main functions of proteins include growth, regulation of body functions and processes, replacement of cellular proteins, and energy. Protein catabolism supplies 4 kcal/g. Protein also plays an important role in regulatory functions and in the body's immune system. Catalytic enzymes derived from proteins function in the regulation of digestion, absorption, metabolism, and catabolism.

Dietary proteins can be classified as complete, partially complete, or incomplete. **Complete proteins** contain sufficient amounts of the essential amino acids to maintain body tissues and promote body growth. Essential amino acids must be supplied by the diet because they cannot be synthesized by the body at a rate sufficient to meet the body's needs. Nonessential amino acids can be synthesized by the body from available sources. An adequate diet contains a good supply of essential and nonessential amino acids. Good sources of complete proteins are meat, fish, poultry, milk, cheese, and eggs.

Partially complete proteins contain sufficient amounts of amino acids to maintain life but do not promote growth. **Incomplete proteins** do not contain sufficient amounts of all essential amino acids to maintain life, build tissue, or promote growth. By themselves, incomplete proteins are not compatible with maintaining life. Sources of incomplete protein are dried peas and beans, peanut butter, seeds, fruits and vegetables, bread, cereal, rice, and pasta.

A person's protein requirement depends on his or her state of health, age, body weight, state of nutrition, stress level, activity level, and other factors. One measure of the protein requirement is a person's state of nitrogen balance. Nitrogen equilibrium, the normal state for a healthy adult, exists when the amount of nitrogen taken in equals the amount of nitrogen excreted. A state of *positive nitrogen balance* exists when the intake of nitrogen is greater than the amount excreted. This situation exists when new tissues are being synthesized, as in recovery from illness, athletic training, pregnancy, and childhood growth. A *negative nitrogen balance* exists when the excretion of nitrogen exceeds the intake. This is an undesirable condition that may exist when a disease is causing excessive tissue breakdown or when the diet is inadequate in protein, calories, or both.

Fat

Fats, also called lipids, include neutral fats, oils, fatty acids, cholesterol, and phospholipids. **Fats** are organic substances composed of carbon, hydrogen, and oxygen. They are a significant component of the American diet.

Fat is a component of all body cells and makes up approximately 20% of the body weight of healthy, nonobese people. Fat performs many important functions in the human body, including cellular transport, insulation, protection of vital organs in the form of padding, provision of energy, energy storage of adipose tissue, vitamin absorption, and transport of fat-soluble vitamins (eg, vitamins A, D, E, and K).

The energy value of fats is significant, supplying 9 kcal/g of oxidized fat. This is more than twice as much energy per gram than is provided from oxidation of an equal amount of protein or carbohydrate. Fats also have a significant satiety value: They give us a feeling of fullness because they remain in the stomach longer than carbohydrates or protein.

Fats are classified as saturated or unsaturated, based on chemical differences. Saturated fats have two hydrogen atoms attached to each of the carbon atoms in the carbon atom chain. An unsaturated fat has a single hydrogen atom missing from each of two side-by-side carbon atoms; thus, a double bond will be formed between the two carbon atoms. This difference is significant in terms of the physical characteristics of the fats, including such factors as melting point, hardness, and the ability to form an emulsion.

Most sources of fats contain a combination of saturated and unsaturated fatty acids. Sources of animal fats, especially beef and lamb, generally contain a higher percentage of saturated fatty acids and are harder than vegetable sources of fatty acids. Coconut oil, palm oil, and palm kernel oil also are highly saturated. Chicken fat contains a significantly higher percentage of unsaturated fatty acids and is measurably softer than beef or lamb fat. Fish and vegetable sources are classified as unsaturated, because they contain a higher percentage of unsaturated fatty acids and are generally softer than animal fats.

Vitamins

Vitamins are organic compounds that are essential to the body in small quantities for growth, development, maintenance, and reproduction (Table 37-1). They do not supply energy but they assist in the use of energy nutrients. Most vitamins (except vitamins D and K) cannot be synthesized by the body and must therefore be supplied by the diet. Recommended dietary allowances (RDAs) specify the intake of vitamins needed to supply normal daily requirements. Vitamins are present in small quantities in food. In varying degrees, they can be destroyed by exposure to light, air, heat and during food preparation. Because of this, fresh foods are usually the best source of vitamins. Some foods, such as fortified milk or cereals, have extra vitamins added.

Vitamins are classified as fat soluble or water soluble. Fat-soluble vitamins (A, D, E, K) are absorbed with fat into the circulation. A deficiency of fat-soluble vitamins can occur when fat digestion or absorption is altered. Excess fat-soluble vitamins are stored in the liver or adipose tissue; thus, excessive intake of vitamins A and D can cause toxicity.

The water-soluble vitamins are vitamin C and the B-complex vitamins. Water-soluble vitamins are not stored in the body, although some body tissues can hold limited amounts. Adequate daily intake of water-soluble vitamins is recommended to prevent deficiencies. When the intake of water-soluble vitamins exceeds the amount absorbed by the tissues, the excess is excreted in the urine.

Fat-Soluble Vitamins

Vitamin A. Vitamin A is important in the following:

- Maintenance of normal vision, especially in dim light
- Maintenance of healthy epithelium
- Promotion of normal skeletal and tooth development
- Promotion of normal cellular proliferation

The effects of a vitamin A deficiency are significant, and in many countries, vitamin A deficiency is the most prevalent vitamin deficiency.

Signs of Vitamin A Deficiency. Signs of vitamin A deficiency follow:

- Night or total blindness
- Epithelial changes, such as keratinization (progressive degeneration of the cells that may lead to infections in the eyes, ears, or nasal passages)
- Follicular hyperkeratosis (skin changes leading to rough, dry, and scaly skin)
- Dryness of the eyes (xerophthalmia)
- Inadequate tooth and bone development

The RDA of vitamin A for adult men is 1,000 RE (or 5,000 IU [international units]) and for adult women, 800 RE (or 4,000 IU); more is needed for pregnant or lactating women (National Research Council, 1989). Vitamin A is stored in the liver, and excessive intake can be toxic. Sources of vitamin A are listed in Table 37-1.

Vitamin D. Vitamin D is synthesized in the skin (by ultraviolet light activity), in the liver, and in the kidney. Vitamin D is important in the following:

- Intestinal absorption of calcium
- Mobilization of calcium and phosphorus from bone
- Renal reabsorption of calcium

These effects increase the blood levels of calcium and phosphorus, allowing for normal mineralization of bone and cartilage and maintenance of calcium extracellular fluid for normal muscle contraction.

A deficiency in vitamin D intake is significant because it leads to an inadequate absorption of calcium and phosphorus and to a deficiency of mineralization in bones and teeth. The bones become soft and cannot bear weight, resulting in skeletal deformities. Signs of vitamin D deficiency follow:

- Rickets in children
- Poor dental health
- Tetany (low serum calcium resulting in muscle twitching and convulsions)
- Osteomalacia (soft bones and a tendency toward spontaneous fractures secondary to vitamin D and calcium deficiency)

The RDA of vitamin D for adults is 5 μg and 10 μg for pregnant or lactating women (National Research

text continues on page 1027

Table 37-1 • Summary of Vitamins

Vitamin and RDA	Functions	Deficiency Signs and Symptoms	Food Sources
Fat-Soluble Vitamins			
Vitamin A Vitamin precursor: carotene Vitamin: retinol Adult RDA Men: 1,000 μg RE* Women: 800 μG RE	Formation of visual purple, which enables the eye to adapt to dim light; normal growth and development of bones and teeth; formation and maintenance of skin and mucous membranes	Night blindness; bone growth ceases and bone shape changes; skin becomes dry, scaly, rough, and cracked; eyes become dry, decreased saliva secretion → difficulty chewing, swallowing → anorexia; decreased mucous secretion of the stomach and intestines → impaired digestion and absorption → diarrhea, increased excretion of nutrients; susceptible to respiratory, urinary tract, and vaginal infections	Preformed retinol: liver, fish liver oils, whole + fortified milk and dairy products; fortified margarine, and fortified breakfast cereals. Carotenes: dark green and yellow vegetables (eg, sweet potatoes, winter squash, carrots, broccoli, spinach, "greens," peaches, apricots, and canteloupe)
Vitamin D Vitamin precursors: ergosterol, 7-dehydrocholesterol Vitamins: D_2 (ergocholecalciferorl), D_3 (cholecalciferol) Adult RDA 19–24-year-olds: 10 μG After age 24: 5 μG	Maintenance of levels of calcium and phosphorus for normal bone mineralization	Rickets; osteomalacia (in adults)	Fortified milk, margarine, and breakfast cereals; small amounts in butter, egg yolk, liver, salmon, sardines, and tuna fish
Vitamin E Tocopherol Adult RDA Men: 10 mg α-TE Women: 8 mg α-TE	Protection of vitamin A and PUFA from being destroyed; protection of cell membranes	Increased RBC hemolysis; in infants, causes anemia, edema, and skin lesions	Vegetable oils, wheat germ, leafy vegetables, soybeans, corn, peanuts, pecans, walnuts, margarine, and salad dressings made with vegetable oils
Vitamin K Vitamin K_1 (phylloquinone) Vitamin K_2 (menaquinone) Adult RDA Men: 80 micrograms Women: 65 micrograms	Essential for the formation of five proteins necessary for normal blood clotting	Delayed blood clotting → hemorrhage; hemorrhagic disease of the newborn	Green leafy vegetables, cabbage, cauliflower, spinach, cheese, egg yolk, and liver.

Vitamin and RDA	Functions	Deficiency Signs and Symptoms	Food Sources
Water-Soluble Vitamins			
Vitamin C (Ascorbic Acid) Adult RDA Men and women: 60 mg	Antioxidant; collagen formation: enhancement of intestinal absorption of iron; conversion of folate to its active form; metabolism of certain amino acids	Bleeding gums; pinpoint hemorrhages under skin; scurvy	Guava, broccoli, brussels sprouts, green peppers, strawberries, "greens," citrus fruits, potatoes, tomatoes, and cabbage
Thiamine (Vitamin B_2) Adult RDA Men: 1.2–1.5 mg Women: 1.0–1.1 mg	Energy metabolism, especially the metabolism of CHO; normal nervous system functioning	Beriberi; fatigue; muscle weakness and wasting; anorexia; edema, enlarged heart	Pork, liver, organ meats, whole and enriched grains, nuts, legumes, potatoes, eggs, and milk
Riboflavin (Vitamin B_2) Adult RDA Men: 1.4–1.7 mg Women: 1.2–1.3 mg	CHO, protein, and fat metabolism	Dermatitis; cheilosis; glossitis, photophobia; reddening of the cornea	Milk and dairy products, organ meats, eggs, enriched grains, and green leafy vegetables
Niacin {Vitamin B_2) Adult RDA Men: 15–19 mg NE Women: 13–15 mg NE	CHO, protein, and fat metabolism	Pellagra: (4 Ds) Dermatitis, diarrhea, dementia, death, if untreated	Kidney, liver, poultry, lean meat, fish, yeast peanut butter, enriched and whole grains, dried peas and beans, and nuts

(continued)

Table 37-1 *(continued)*

Vitamin and RDA	Functions	Deficiency Signs and Symptoms	Food Sources
Water-Soluble Vitamins			
Vitamin B_6 (Pyridoxine) Adult RDA Men: 2.0 mg Women: 1.6 mg	Amino acid metabolism; blood formation; maintenance of nervous tissue; conversion of tryptophan to niacin	Dermatitis, cheilosis, glossitis, abnormal brain wave pattern, convulsions, and anemia	Chicken, fish, peanuts, oats, yeast, wheat germ, pork, organ meats, egg yolk, whole grain cereals, corn, potatoes, and bananas
Folacin (Folic acid) Adult RDA Men: 200 μg Women: 180: μg	Amino acid metabolism; DNA and RNA synthesis; proliferation of cells; blood formation	Glossitis, diarrhea, macrocytic anemia	Green leafy vegetables, asparagus, broccoli, liver, organ meats, milk, eggs, yeast, wheat germ, and kidney beans
Vitamin B_{12}(Cobalamin) Adult RDA Men and women: 2 μg	RNA and DNA synthesis blood formation maintenance of nervous tissue; CHO, protein, and fat metabolism; folate metabolism	GI changes; macrocytic anemia → pallor, dyspnea, weakness, fatigue, and palpitations; neurologic	Liver kidney, fresh shrimp and oysters, meats, milk, eggs, and cheese
Pantothenic Acid Adult RDA Men and women: safe and adequate intake 4–7 mg	CHO, protein, and fat metabolism	Not observed in humans	Animal tissues, whole grain cereals, legumes, milk, vegetables, fruit
Biotin Adult RDA Men and women: safe and adequate intake 30–100 μg	Fat and CHO metabolism; glycogen formation	Observed only under experimental conditions	Liver, organ meats, egg yolk, milk, and yeast. synthesized by GI flora.

Source: Dudek, S. G. (1993). *Nutrition handbook for nursing practice* (2nd ed.). Philadelphia: J.B. Lippincott.

Council, 1989). Sources of vitamin D are listed in Table 37-1. Excessive amounts can be toxic.

Vitamin E. The physiologic effects of vitamin E are not well understood. The major function is thought to be its role as an antioxidant, in which it assists in maintaining the integrity of cellular membranes and protecting vitamin A from oxidation.

Vitamin E deficiency is rare, but signs of severe deficiency are increased hemolysis of red blood cells, poor reflexes and impaired neuromuscular functioning, and anemia.

The RDA of vitamin E for adult men is 10 mg α-TE and for adult women, 8 mg α-TE (more for pregnant or lactating women; National Research Council, 1989). Sources are listed in Table 37-1. Vitamin E is not stored in the body to any appreciable extent, and toxicity is rare.

Vitamin K. An adequate intake of vitamin K is necessary for the formation of prothrombin and other clotting factors. The major physiologic effect of vitamin K appears to be its role in blood coagulation.

Vitamin K deficiencies are manifested in two ways: an increased tendency to hemorrhage (prolonged clotting time) and hemorrhage disease of the newborn. This disease of the newborn is most common in premature or anoxic neonates.

RDAs for vitamin K were set for the first time in 1989 (Dudek, 1995). The RDA for adult men is 80 µg/d and for adult women, 65 µg/d. Approximately half of the body's requirement of vitamin K is synthesized by bacteria in the lower intestinal tract. Sources are listed in Table 37-1. Vitamin K is not stored in the body to an appreciable extent. Large amounts are not usually toxic except in the newborn.

Water-Soluble Vitamins

B-Complex Vitamins. Each B-complex vitamin has its own function and RDA.

Vitamin B_1 (thiamine) functions in carbohydrate metabolism, and adequate thiamine intake will result in healthy nerve functioning and normal appetite and digestion. Deficiency symptoms are poor appetite, apathy and mental depression, fatigue, constipation, edema, cardiac failure, and neuritis. The disease associated with inadequate thiamine intake is beriberi. Acute beriberi adversely affects the cardiac, nervous, and GI systems. Death can result from cardiac failure. The RDA of thiamine is 1.5 mg for men and 1.1 mg for women, with additional amounts recommended for pregnant or lactating women (National Research Council, 1989). Sources are listed in Table 37-1.

Vitamin B_2 (riboflavin) functions in protein and carbohydrate metabolism and contributes to healthy skin and normal vision. Deficiency symptoms are cheilosis (cracking and fissures at the corners of the mouth), dermatitis, and increased vascularization of the cornea and other vision irregularities. The RDA of riboflavin is 1.7 mg for men and 1.3 mg for women, with additional amounts recommended for pregnant or lactating women (National Research Council, 1989). Sources are listed in Table 37-1.

Vitamin B_3 (niacin) is involved in glycogen metabolism, tissue regeneration, and fat synthesis. The niacin deficiency disease is pellagra; its symptoms are fatigue, headache, loss of appetite and weight loss, abdominal pain, diarrhea, dermatitis, and neurologic deterioration. The RDA of niacin is 19 mg for men and 15 mg for women, with additional amounts recommended for pregnant or lactating women (National Research Council, 1989). Sources are listed in Table 37-1.

Vitamin B_{12} (cyanocobalamin) functions in the formation of mature red blood cells and in the synthesis of DNA and RNA. It requires intrinsic factor for absorption. A vitamin B_{12} deficiency leads to pernicious anemia, other forms of anemia, and neurologic deterioration. The RDA of vitamin B_{12} is 2 μg for adults, with additional amounts recommended for pregnant or lactating women. This vitamin is found only in animal foods (meats, fish, poultry, milk, and eggs).

Other important B vitamins are vitamin B_6, pantothenic acid, folic acid, and biotin. Deficiencies are rare.

Vitamin C. Vitamin C is important in the following:

- Protection against infection
- Adequate wound healing
- Collagen formation
- Iron absorption
- Metabolism of several important amino acids

Vitamin C is an antioxidant and thus protects vitamins A and E from excessive oxidation. Signs of vitamin C deficiency follow:

- Inadequate formation of collagen (poor wound healing), increased susceptibility to infection, retardation of growth and development, joint pain, anemia
- Scurvy (now rare, but formerly common among sailors whose diets lacked fresh fruits and vegetables, particularly citrus fruits)

The RDA for vitamin C is 60 mg for adults and 70 to 90 mg for pregnant or lactating women (National Research Council, 1989). Sources of vitamin C are listed in Table 37-1. Little vitamin C is stored in the body, so a daily supply is needed. Although megadoses (30–100 times the recommended allowances) of vitamin C have not been proven toxic, excessive doses are not advised due to the possibility of kidney stone formation and GI disturbances.

Minerals

Minerals are inorganic substances found in nearly all body tissues and fluids. When plant or animal tissue is

Table 37-2 • Summary of Several Minerals

Mineral and RDA	Functions	Deficiency Signs and Symptoms	Food Sources
Calcium 18–24 y: 1,200 mg 25 y and older: 800 mg	Bone and teeth formation and maintenance; blood clotting; nerve transmission; muscle function; cell membrane permeability	Stunted growth; rickets, osteomalacia; osteoporosis (porous bones); tetany (low serum calcium)	Milk and dairy products; green leafy vegetables; whole grains; nuts and legumes; seafood
Phosphorus 18–24 y: 1,200 mg 25 y and older: 800 mg	Bone and teeth formation and maintenance; acid–base balance; energy metabolism; cell membrane structure; hormone and coenzyme regulation	Stunted growth; rickets (due to excessive excretion rather than dietary deficiency)	Meat; poultry; fish; eggs; legumes; milk and dairy products; soft drinks
Magnesium Men: 350 mg Women: 280 mg	Bone formation; smooth muscle relaxation; protein synthesis; CHO metabolism	Alcoholism or renal disease: tremors leading to convulsive seizures	Green leafy vegetables; nuts; legumes; whole grains; seafood
Iron Men: 10 mg Women: 15 mg	Oxygen transport through hemoglobin and myoglobin; constituent of enzyme systems	Depletion of iron stores, anemia (microcytic, hypochromic), pallor, decreased work capacity	Liver; lean meat; dried beans; fortified cereals
Iodine 150 μg	Constituent of thyroid hormones that regulate BMR	Goiter (not a problem in the United States)	Iodized salt; seafood; milk; eggs; bread
Zinc Men: 15 mg Women: 12 mg	Tissue growth, development, and healing; sexual maturation and reproduction; constituent of many enzymes in energy and nucleic acid metabolism	Impaired growth, sexual maturation, and immune system functioning; skin lesions; acrodermatitis enteropathica; decreased sense of taste and smell	meat; oysters; seafood; milk; egg yolks; legumes; whole grains

Adapted from Dudek, S. G. (1993). *Nutrition handbook for nursing practice* (2nd ed.). Philadelphia: J.B. Lippincott.

burned, what remains is ash or mineral matter. Minerals help build body tissues and regulate metabolism. There are more than 25 known minerals in the adult body, but the most notable are described here and in Table 37-2.

Calcium. Nearly all the calcium in the body is found in the bones and teeth. The bones provide the framework for the body and are a storage area for calcium to keep the plasma concentration of calcium relatively constant. Calcium also is important in the following:

- Conversion of prothrombin to thrombin and other steps of the coagulation process
- Nerve impulse transmission by participating in the formation of acetylcholine
- Regulation of materials in and out of cells
- Contraction and relaxation of muscles, most notably the heart muscle

Calcium is absorbed mainly from the duodenum by active transport. Calcium also is passively diffused across the intestinal mucosa from the jejunum and the ileum. The amount of calcium absorbed is mainly determined by the body's need. About 30% to 40% of the calcium in the diet is absorbed in the healthy adult. Growing children and adolescents and pregnant and lactating women absorb a greater percentage of their dietary calcium because of the increased need. Some of the ingested calcium forms insoluble salts, which cannot be absorbed.

Absorption of calcium is assisted by adequate amounts of vitamin D, parathyroid hormone, ascorbic acid, lactose, several other amino acids, and physical activity. Calcium absorption can be decreased by inadequate amounts of vitamin D, insufficient exposure to sunlight, decreased amounts of ascorbic acid, decreased physical activity, and emotional stress. Other factors, such as a high consumption of dietary fiber and excessive phosphorus intake, impair the absorption of calcium. These factors are still being researched.

The effects of calcium deficiency can be profound. *Rickets*, a disease of infants and children caused by inadequate calcium and vitamin D, involves the inadequate deposition of calcium and phosphorus in the bone. Symptoms include soft bones, enlarged joints, enlarged skull secondary to delayed closure of the cranial fontanels, bowed legs, and spinal and chest deformities. *Osteomalacia*, the adult form of rickets, results from an inadequate intake of calcium, phosphorus, and vitamin D. The mineral content of the bone is reduced, but the bone stays the same size.

Osteoporosis involves a reduction in bone mass. It is mainly seen in women older than 50 years who have had a chronically insufficient intake of calcium. Other factors contributing to the development of osteoporosis may include decreased estrogens, heredity, smoking, race, and decreased physical activity. Symptoms vary in severity and may include reduced bone mass, leading to poor posture; increased fragility of bones, leading to an increase in bone fractures; and delayed healing of fractured bones. Malabsorption syndromes can lead to problems in calcium absorption, and osteoporosis can develop. Low dietary intake of calcium also has been associated with hypertension; research is continuing (Shils, Olson, & Shike, 1994).

The RDA for calcium is 800 mg for adults, with additional amounts recommended for adolescents, young women, and pregnant or lactating women (National Research Council, 1989). Sources are listed in Table 37-2.

Iron. Most of the iron in the body is found in hemoglobin, the red-pigmented iron-containing protein. Hemoglobin carries oxygen from the lungs to the tissues and helps transport carbon dioxide to the lungs. Iron also is found in the body's myoglobin, an iron–protein deficiency compound in the muscle that is an oxygen storage system for the muscles.

Iron deficiencies may manifest themselves in iron-deficiency anemia. This form of anemia is not uncommon, especially in infants and menstruating women. In anemia, circulating hemoglobin is reduced, and the blood cannot provide for the oxygen needs of the tissues. Iron-deficiency anemia may result from a diet chronically deficient in iron. Other factors that may lead to iron-deficiency anemia are blood loss, chronic disease, pregnancy and lactation, diarrhea, and other nutritional deficiencies (protein and calorie). Symptoms of iron-deficiency anemia are excessive fatigue, lethargy, and poor resistance to infection. Because obtaining sufficient iron to combat anemia by dietary measures alone is impractical, recommended treatment includes taking iron salts (ferrous sulfate or gluconate) along with a well-balanced diet.

The RDA of iron for adult men is 10 mg and for adult women, 15 mg, with additional amounts recommended for pregnant or lactating women (National Research Council, 1989). Good sources of iron are listed in Table 37-2.

Sodium. Sodium is found primarily in the extracellular fluid in the body and helps maintain the body's fluid and acid–base balance. RDAs for sodium intake have not been set. The average diet contains more sodium than the body requires, and sodium deficiencies (except in rare circumstances) have not been identified. Many people would benefit from eating less sodium, and sodium restriction is important for people with heart disease, hypertension, edema, renal disorders, liver disease, congestive heart failure, and toxemias of pregnancy. Only 10% of sodium intake is from natural sources, including salt, salt compounds, milk, meat, poultry, fish, and eggs, while 75% of sodium comes from processed foods.

Potassium. Potassium is found primarily in the intracellular fluid of the body and functions in fluid balance, protein synthesis, and regulation of muscle contraction. RDAs have not been set, and deficiencies have not been identified, except in cases of severe vomiting and diarrhea and diabetic acidosis. Potassium restriction is indicated for clients with renal impairment and renal failure. Potassium is present in many foods, including protein-rich foods, bread, cereal, fruits, and vegetables.

Iodine. Although considered a trace element, iodine is an important mineral. The primary location of iodine in the body is the thyroid gland. Iodine is a component of the thyroid hormones, thyroxine and triiodothyronine. These hormones help regulate energy metabolism, nervous and muscle cell functioning, and mental and physical growth.

A chronic deficiency of iodine can lead to endemic goiter. The major initial symptom is an enlarged thyroid gland. This condition is especially significant in pregnant women because it can lead to physical and mental retardation in the fetus. In its severe form, this condition in the infant is known as *cretinism.* Cretinism is rare in the United States but remains a problem in certain areas of Central and South America, Africa, and Asia. Characteristics of cretinism are muscle flabbiness, weakness, dry skin, thick lips, skeletal retardation, and severe mental retardation. Thyroid hormone given early to infants can be of some value, but certain physical and mental deficiencies are irreversible. Everyone, especially pregnant women, should eat a diet sufficient in iodine.

The RDA of iodine for adult men and women is 150 µg, with additional amounts recommended for pregnant or lactating women (National Research Council, 1989).

Fluorine. Fluorine is found primarily in the bones and teeth. It maintains bone structure and reduces tooth decay by strengthening tooth enamel. There is no RDA, but the estimated safe intake level is 1.5 to 4.0 mg/d for adults (National Research Council, 1989). Flouride is found in the diet, the water, and the soil in generally safe and adequate amounts. Many areas in the United States have added fluoride, a fluorine compound, to the water in amounts equivalent to the normal soil concentration (1 part fluoride per 1 million parts water or soil).

Water

Water is necessary to maintain normal cell function. Water is obtained by drinking fluid and eating foods with a high water content (fresh fruits and vegetables) and by the oxidation of food. Thirst signals the need for water and encourages a person to drink. Fluid balance is covered in Chapter 36.

Normal Function of the Digestive System

The digestive system performs the vital function of converting food into substances that can be absorbed and used by the cells of the body. This conversion involves the processes of digestion, absorption, metabolism, and excretion.

Digestion

Digestion is the process by which foods are broken down to be used by the body for growth, development, healing, and prevention of disease. Digestion includes the mechanical and chemical processes necessary to convert the food into a physically absorbable state.

Mechanical Process. The mechanical process of digestion consists of the following events:

1. Mastication takes place in the mouth. Food particles are reduced in size and mixed with enzymes in saliva.
2. Deglutition (swallowing) begins in the mouth and continues in the pharynx and the esophagus.
3. Churning movements and peristalsis move the ingested material through the stomach and into the duodenum.
4. In the small intestine, the ingested material is further churned and mixed with digestive enzymes. It comes in contact with the intestinal mucosa to allow for absorption.
5. Peristalsis moves the ingested material into the large intestine.
6. Further churning, peristalsis, and absorption help move the ingested mass along the full length of the large intestine, where it is stored until it is evacuated from the body.

Chemical Process. The chemical processes of digestion change the composition of ingested material. Most carbohydrates and all fats and proteins must be chemically reduced for absorption.

Carbohydrate digestion involves the hydrolysis of polysaccharides (with the exception of cellulose and other fibers) into disaccharides by the amylase enzymes found in saliva and pancreatic juices. Hydrolysis is a chemical process between a compound and water that results in the division of the compound into simpler components. A polysaccharide is a carbohydrate compound containing three or more saccharide groups; a disaccharide contains two saccharide groups; a monosaccharide contains only one saccharide group. Disaccharides are further hydrolyzed into monosaccharides by the enzymes sucrase, maltase, and lactase secreted by the intestines.

Fat digestion is accomplished by emulsification of fats, which is facilitated by bile. Emulsification involves breaking down fats into smaller fat droplets and dispersing these droplets into solution. The pancreatic enzyme lipase hydrolyzes the small fat droplets into fatty acids and glycerol.

Protein digestion involves the hydrolysis of the larger protein compounds into amino acids. This is done by the protease enzymes, which include pepsin from the gastric fluid, trypsin and other proteases from the gastric fluid, trypsin and other proteases from the pancreatic fluid, and peptidases from the intestinal fluid.

Absorption

Absorption is the process by which the digested protein, fats, carbohydrates, vitamins, minerals, and water are actively and passively transported through the intestinal mucosa into the blood or lymphatic circulation. The proteins, such as amino acids, and the digested carbohydrates and simple sugars, in the form of monosaccharides, are absorbed into the bloodstream through the intestinal capillaries. The fats, in the form of glycerol and fatty acids, are absorbed into the lymphatic system through the lymphatic capillaries in the intestinal villi. Some finely emulsified neutral fats are absorbed undigested into the capillaries.

Metabolism

After the undigested food is digested and absorbed, it is ready to be metabolized. *Metabolism* is the complex chemical process that occurs in the cells to allow for energy use and for cellular growth and repair. Metabolism involves catabolic and anabolic processes: catabolic processes break down complex substances into simpler substances (eg, tissue breakdown), and anabolic processes convert simple substances into more complex ones (eg, tissue repair).

Carbohydrate Metabolism. Short-term glucose excesses are changed into glycogen in the presence of insulin by the liver cells. This is an anabolic process called **glycogenesis.** Glycogen is stored in the liver and skeletal muscles until needed and is then converted back into glucose by a catabolic process called glycogenolysis.

Longer term storage of glucose in the presence of insulin takes the form of fat deposits (adipose tissue). When the amount of glucose entering the cells is not enough to meet cellular demands, gluconeogenesis (the formation of glucose from protein and fat in the liver) occurs. This catabolic process yields 4.1 kcal of energy per gram of oxidized carbohydrate (Linder, 1991).

Fat Metabolism. Fats are converted to adipose tissue and stored in the body's fat deposits. Stored fat deposits make up the body's largest reserve energy source. The catabolism of fats involves the hydrolysis of fat into glycerol and fatty acids. The fatty acids are then converted by a series of chemical reactions known as ketogenesis into ketone bodies. In the tissue cells, ketones are converted the citric acid cycle into energy, carbon dioxide, and water. Glycerol is converted by gluconeogenesis into glucose. Fats are a more concentrated source of energy than carbohydrates, yielding 9 kcal of energy per gram of catabolized fat.

Protein Metabolism. Protein anabolism builds tissues, produces antibodies, replaces blood cells, and repairs tissues. Temporary excesses of protein are stored in the liver and in skeletal muscle. Protein catabolism involves the hydrolysis of cellular proteins into amino acids in the tissue cell. It also involves the deamination process of amino acids, in which an amino group is split off from an amino acid to form ammonia and keto acid. This process takes place in the liver cell to form glucose and urea.

Excretion

The excretory organs (kidneys, sweat glands, skin, lungs, and intestines) remove waste products from the body. Water, toxins, salts, and nitrogen wastes are excreted through the kidneys, skin, and sweat glands. Carbon dioxide and water are excreted through the lungs. Digestive and metabolic wastes are excreted through the intestines and rectum.

Characteristics of Normal Nutrition

Normal nutrition involves a balanced intake of food to meet the energy requirements necessary for organ function, body movement, and work. Adequate food intake also provides raw materials for the production of enzymes and the production of cells necessary for growth, replacement of tissues, and tissue repair. See the display for the characteristics of a well-nourished person.

Ideal Body Weight

Normal nutritional intake usually results in body weight appropriate for a person's height and frame. Ideal body weight (IBW) is the estimated weight optimal for body functioning and health. Ranges for IBW according to height and body frame are listed in standardized tables (see Appendix D). Sometimes such information can be misleading, because it does not always reflect accurately the amount of body fat present. For example, a

Characteristics of a Well-Nourished Person

- Normal weight and height for age, body build, and developmental stage
- Adequate appetite
- Active, alert, and able to maintain adequate attention span
- Firm, healthy skin and mucous membranes
- Erect posture, with straight arms and legs
- Well-developed muscles without excess body fat
- Normal schedule of tooth eruption and healthy teeth and gums
- Normal urinary and bowel elimination patterns
- Normal sleep patterns
- Normal hemoglobin, hematocrit, and serum protein levels
- Absence of diet-related abnormalities

body builder may be heavier than the IBW listed but may have a less than average amount of body fat.

A rule of thumb for estimating IBW is that a 5-ft woman should weigh about 106 lb; 5 lb should be added for each additional inch. The IBW for a 5-ft man is 105 lb, to which 6 lb should be added for each additional inch.

Physical Status

Normal nutrition is apparent in the normal appearance of many parts of the body. The client's general appearance should reflect alertness and responsiveness. The skin should have normal tone and good turgor. The mouth, gums, and lips should appear moist, pink, and free from lesions. Hair and nails should appear healthy. Bones should hold the body erect, and muscles should maintain good tone. Normal reflexes should be apparent. The abdomen should appear flat and undistended.

Normal Laboratory Values

Laboratory values are usually within normal ranges in healthy people. Normal hematocrit and hemoglobin values suggest adequate iron stores if hydration status is normal. Plasma protein values, such as serum albumin, reflect normal adequate protein intake.

Normal Nutrition Pattern

At one time, healthcare personnel were concerned about individuals with nutrient deficiencies, and guidelines were written to help prevent these deficiencies. Current concerns, however, are related to avoiding excesses for possible prevention of chronic diet-related diseases. A discussion of normal nutrition and other nutritional advice for healthy eating follows. Because no single food supplies all essential nutrients, individuals are encouraged to eat a variety of foods.

The Food Guide Pyramid

The food guide pyramid, as recommended by the U.S. Department of Agriculture (USDA, 1992), provides a general guide for planning nutritious, appetizing meals. The pyramid emphasizes food from five major food groups; bread, cereal, rice, and pasta; vegetables; fruits; meat, poultry, dry beans, eggs, and nuts; milk, yogurt, and cheese. Fats, sugars, and alcohol are included in a sixth group. Guidelines suggest an appropriate daily number of servings from each group (Fig. 37-1).

Bread, Cereal, Rice, and Pasta Group. Bread, cereal, rice, and pasta are important food sources in many countries. Rice, wheat, and corn are worldwide dietary staples. This group includes whole grains, breads, cereals, rice, noodles, pasta, and products made with enriched flour and cereal. Six to 11 daily servings are recommended; one serving is about half a cup of a cooked product (pasta, rice, or cereal), one slice of bread, or one ounce of uncooked cereal (USDA, 1992).

Breads and cereals are good sources of thiamine, iron, niacin, and riboflavin. Many breads and cereals are enriched, especially those processed and sold in the United States. Enrichment with vitamins and minerals adds to their nutritive value. Whole grains also are excellent sources of zinc, copper, B vitamins, vitamin E, and fiber. These foods are a good source of carbohydrates, calories, and incomplete proteins, and are low in fat.

Vegetable Group. The vegetable group includes cooked and uncooked parts of plants. Three to five servings of vegetables are recommended daily (USDA, 1992). One serving is roughly equal to one cup of raw leafy vegetables or half a cup of a cooked vegetable.

Vegetables provide vitamins A and C, folate, and minerals, such as iron and magnesium. Because they are low in fat and provide fiber, they are excellent for human nutrition. Nutritional plans can be colorful, using dark green leafy vegetables (such as spinach and romaine lettuce) and deep yellow vegetables (such as carrots and sweet potatoes). Legumes and other vegetables should be included.

Fruit Group. Fruit and fruit juices make up the fruit group. The food guide suggests two to four servings of fruit a day (USDA, 1992). A medium apple, banana, or orange counts as a serving. A serving also includes half a cup of chopped, cooked, or canned fruit or three-fourths of a cup of fruit juice.

In addition to being important sources of vitamins A and C and potassium, fruits are low in fat and sodium. As a group, these foods have a high water content and are generally low in calories and protein. They are free from cholesterol.

Fresh whole fruit is the best source because of their high fiber content. Juice has no fiber content. Heavy syrups and sweetened drinks should be avoided.

Meat, Poultry, Fish, Dry Beans, Eggs, and Nuts Group. Two to three servings from this group are recommended daily (USDA, 1992). A serving is 2 to 3 oz of the edible part of meat, fish, or poultry. Included in this group are eggs, dry beans or peas, lentils, soybeans, nuts, and peanut butter. One ounce of meat is roughly equal to one egg, half a cup of dry beans or peas, or 2 tablespoons of peanut butter.

The meat group is an excellent source of protein and is a good source of B vitamins and minerals (iron and zinc). Other foods in the group similarly provide protein and most vitamins and minerals. Some shellfish

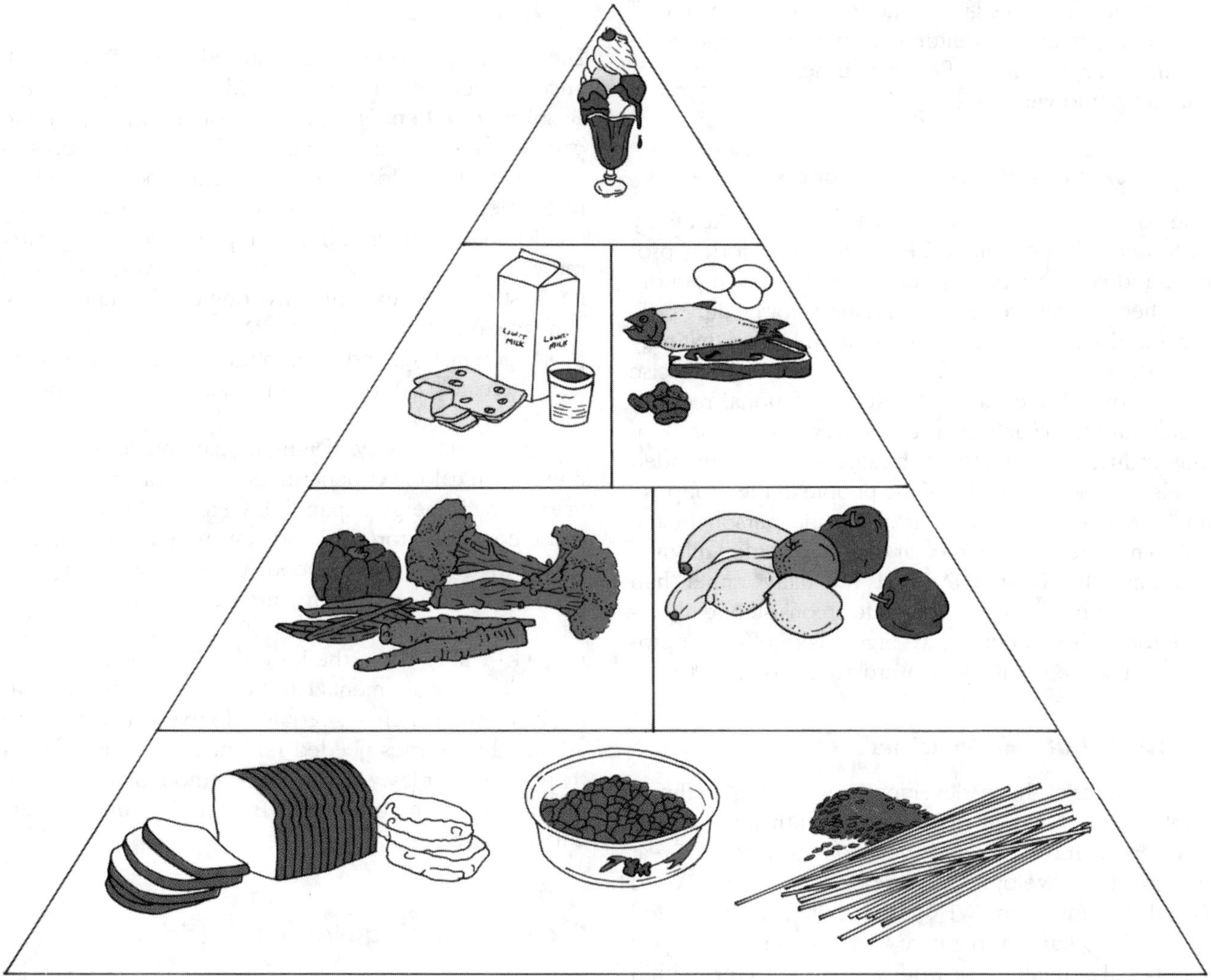

Figure 37-1 • *The Food Guide Pyramid: A Guide to Daily Food Choices. USDA, April 1992.*

are a good source of calcium, and saltwater fish are a good source of iodine. This group can contain a large amount of fat, depending on the cut of the meat, the type of meat, and the method of processing and preparation. Animal food can contain a significantly larger amount of cholesterol and saturated fat, but fish is generally lower in cholesterol and saturated fat. Egg yolks in particular contain a large amount of cholesterol.

Milk, Yogurt, and Cheese Group. The milk group is an important source of nutrition for all people but is especially important for infants, children, and pregnant or lactating women. The recommended number of daily servings depends on the person's physiologic needs, age, and developmental level. Children younger than 12 years need two or three servings; adolescents need four servings; adults need two or three servings; pregnant women need three or four servings; lactating women need four servings. One serving equals a cup (8 oz) of milk or yogurt, about 1.5 oz of natural cheese, or about 2 oz of processed cheese.

Milk is an excellent source of calcium, phosphorus, and riboflavin. It also is fairly rich in sodium, potassium, magnesium, vitamin A, thiamine, vitamin B_6, vitamin B_{12}, niacin, and vitamin D. Milk is an excellent source of protein, but it has little iron. The fat content of milk depends on the type of product. In recent years, many people have started drinking low-fat milk and eating low-fat cheese to decrease their fat intake.

The nutritional characteristics of cheese are similar to those of milk, depending on the type of cheese. One noteworthy difference (which could be important for people with a deficiency) is that cheese contains only a trace amount of lactose.

Fats, Oils, and Sweets Group. The foods in this group (for example, sugar, jelly, jam, shortening, butter, margarine, salad dressings, soft drinks, and alcoholic beverages) add flavor, variety, and interest to meals. There is no recommended number of daily servings. Most people should use them sparingly. The intake of sugar and fats, especially saturated fats, should be minimized. Foods in this group add to the energy value of diets but generally add little nutritive value. One noteworthy exception is fortified margarine, a fair source of vitamin A and vitamin E.

Recommended Dietary Allowances

The Food and Nutrition Board of the National Academy of Sciences has developed RDAs for kilocalories, protein, and certain vitamins and minerals (see Appendix D). These values are recommendations for healthy people and do not take into consideration factors that may significantly increase metabolic demands (eg, exercise or hypermetabolic states). Because nutritional requirements vary with age, sex, pregnancy, and lactation, separate values are given for each category. Recommended levels include about 98% of the people in the group, so an RDA may be more than a specific person in the group may need at a particular time. A common mistake is to think the "D" in RDA stands for "daily" rather than "dietary," which would necessitate a consistent daily intake for each nutrient. An average intake of each nutrient for 1 week is sufficient (Wardlaw & Insel, 1990).

World Nutrient Guidelines

Many countries have developed nutrition guidelines. Canada's Department of National Health and Welfare developed recommended nutritional intakes. Great Britain also developed a nutrition guide. The World Health Organization (WHO), together with the United Nations Food and Agriculture Organization, developed nutritional guidelines for worldwide use. Factors within each country and the opinions of scientists vary, explaining the slight differences in recommendations.

Nutrient Density

The concept of *nutrient density* can be used to evaluate the nutritional quality of foods. Foods that provide more nutrient value than kilocalories are nutrient dense. Foods with low nutrient density (eg, sugar or alcohol) provide energy but often lack essential nutrients. Foods that are nutrient dense are preferred to promote optimal nutrition.

Dietary Guidelines for Americans

Because many Americans overeat and lead sedentary lives, the number of people with cardiovascular problems, diabetes, and cancer has risen significantly. To reverse this trend, dietary guidelines were established in 1980 by the USDA and U.S. Department of Health and Human Services. They were revised in 1985 and 1990. The most current revision is 1995. These guidelines are outlined in the Client Teaching display later in this chapter.

Energy Balance

Dietary patterns should be adjusted to maintain a balance between caloric intake and energy expenditure. **Basal metabolism** is the amount of energy required to carry out involuntary activities at rest (such as breathing, circulating blood, or maintaining body temperature). Men usually have a higher basal metabolic rate (BMR) than women due to a proportionally greater muscle mass. Other factors, such as growth, infection, fever, stress, and extreme environmental temperatures, can increase BMR. Decreased BMR can be due to aging, prolonged fasting, and sleeping. Increased physical exercise creates caloric demands above basal requirements.

To maintain body weight, dietary intake of calories must equal caloric expenditures. When caloric intake is greater than energy expanded, weight gain occurs, because energy is stored in body fat. When caloric intake is less than energy expended, weight loss occurs, because body stores of energy are depleted. For an average person, a daily deficit of 500 calories (3,500 calories/wk) will result in the loss of 1 lb a week.

Caloric requirements can be calculated by estimating how much energy is required for basal activities and adding the calories needed for voluntary muscular activity. The display shows one method of calculating kilocalorie energy output for BMR and voluntary muscular activity.

Factors Affecting Normal Nutrition

Normal diets vary widely among people. Some of the factors affecting a person's nutritional status are discussed here.

Physiologic Factors

Healthy body functioning promotes digestion and absorption of food. Healthy teeth and gums or well-fitting dentures are important for chewing, which is necessary to break up food particles to facilitate digestion. The GI system must function well for optimal use of ingested nutrients. Hormone production of insulin and pancreatic digestive enzymes also is important for food use.

Physical factors can affect a person's ability to buy, transport, cook, and eat food. Physical mobility and energy are necessary for shopping, cooking, and eating. When a person cannot complete such tasks due to physical limitations, assistance may be necessary to ensure adequate nutrition.

Lifestyle and Habits

Eating patterns are highly individualized and greatly determined by personal preference. Food preferences and

Calculating Energy Requirements

Shortcut for Estimating Energy Output: Basal Metabolism

Use the factor 1.0 kcalorie per kilogram of body weight per hour for men or 0.9 for women. The following is an example for a 150-lb man.

1. Change pounds to kilograms:

$$\frac{150 \text{ lb}}{2.2 \text{ lb}} \times 1.0 \text{ kg} = 68 \text{ kg}$$

2. Multiply weight in kilograms by the BMR factor:

$$68 \text{ kg} \times 1 \text{ kcal/kg/h} = 68 \text{ kcal/h}$$

3. Multiply the kcalories used in 1 h by the hours in a day:

$$68 \text{ kcal/h} \times 24 \text{ h/d} = 1{,}632 \text{ kcal/d}.$$

Energy for BMR equals 1,632 kcal/d.

Shortcut for Estimating Energy Output: Voluntary Muscular Activity

The figures we use are crude approximations based on the amount of muscular work a person typically performs in a day. To select the one appropriate for you, remember to think in terms of the amount of *muscular* work performed. Don't confuse being *busy* with being *active*.

- For sedentary (mostly sitting) activity (a typist), add 50% of the BMS.
- For light activity (a teacher), add 60%.
- For heavy work (a roofer), add 100% or more.

If the man we used in the previous example were a typist, we would estimate the energy he needed for physical activities by multiplying his BMR kcalories per day by 50%.

1,632 kcal/d × 50% = 816 kcal/d. His energy need for activities equals 816 kcalories per day.

Reprinted by permission from pp. 90, 91 of *Nutritional and diet therapy: Principles and practice* (2nd ed.), by Cataldo, C., Nyenhuis, J., & Whitney, E.;

eating habits are often set during childhood and may be handed down from one generation to the next. Some families are adventurous and love trying new recipes; other families derive security from having certain meals prepared in exactly the same way repeatedly. If a child is raised in a family that eats throughout the day, rather than having three distinct meals, this pattern will seem normal and will probably influence his or her eating patterns throughout life. The amount and type of food eaten also are determined by early experience. If a child is given large servings and rewarded with desserts, overeating may become a problem later in life. The atmosphere created at mealtime also subtly affects our feelings about food and eating.

Peer pressure and sex-role stereotypes can affect eating patterns. Adolescents survive for years on hamburgers, french fries, pizza, and soda (Fig. 37-2*A*). A man may be less likely to order a salad for lunch than a woman (Fig. 37-2*B*); likewise a woman may feel less comfortable eating a big steak sandwich.

Food fads also can affect dietary patterns. Some foods can be linked with beliefs about health that are not grounded in scientific fact.

A professional person who works long hours and is single may not have enough time to shop for and cook food. A family with two working parents may eat out for the same reason. Although they have time to cook and shop, some single older adults may have limited motivation to cook and eat meals alone. People who lead active lives with strenuous physical exertion may need more frequent meals and more calories to meet their minimal nutritional requirements. On the other hand, sedentary people who spend hours in front of the television may gain weight from decreased physical activity and increased snacking.

Culture and Beliefs

Culture plays a significant role in the type of food eaten and feelings about diet and nutrition. Staple products may vary among different cultural groups; for example, Asians may eat rice with most meals, and Italians may prefer pasta. Spices and methods of cooking also vary from culture to culture.

Some religions dictate when or if certain foods can be eaten and how food is to be prepared. An example of this is the Jewish dietary law, which restricts (among other things) eating dairy and meat products at the same time. Most religions have special foods that are traditional for specific religious observances.

Economic Resources

An adequate diet may be related to a person's finances. Money is needed to buy and transport food and to obtain and maintain the equipment needed to cook and store food safely. The lower a person's economic level, the less likely it is that his or her diet is nutritionally ad-

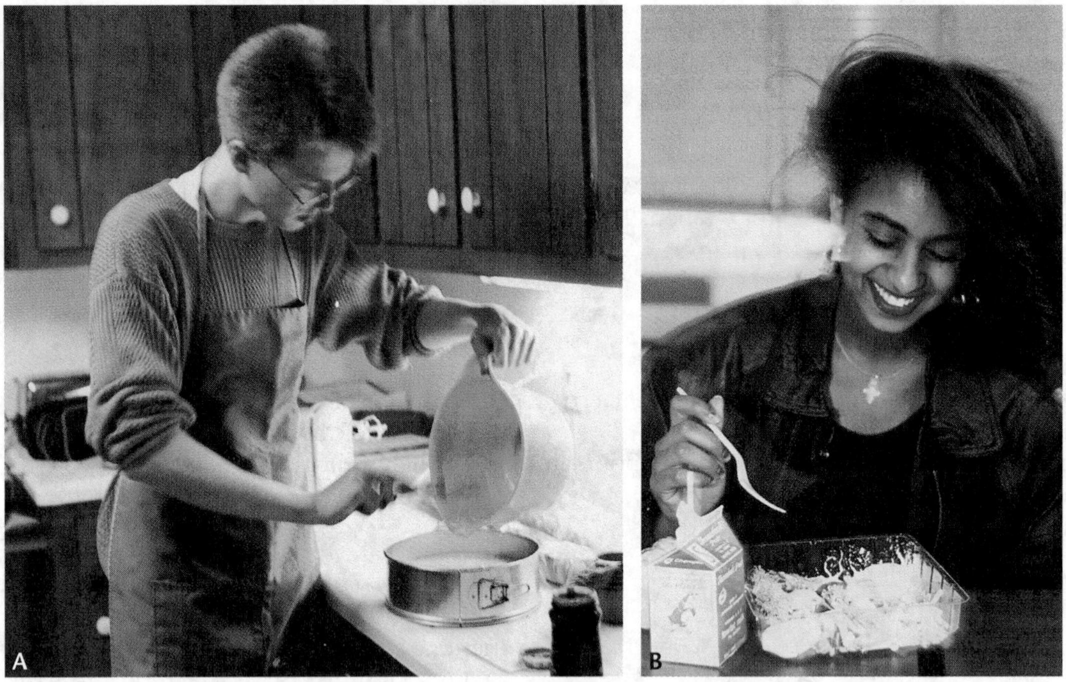

Figure 37-2 • *One of the factors in nutrition is lifestyle. (A), Preparing food at home encourages nutritionally balanced meals. (From Jackson, D.B., & Saunders, R.B. (1993).* Child health nursing: A comprehensive approach to the Care of children and their families. *Philadelphia, J.B. Lippincott.) (B), Women may tend to eat salads more than men. (USDA photo.)*

equate. Low-income areas often have fewer grocery stores, with less selection and often higher prices. People with low incomes may not have available transportation to shop outside their neighborhoods. Affluent people can stock up when items are on sale, stretching their food budget; poor people cannot do so.

Low-income families often must sacrifice their food budget to leave enough money for other bills. The result may be less expensive meals that are low in protein and high in starch. Sources of protein, such as meat and dairy products, are usually expensive and require refrigeration.

Gender

Nutritional requirements vary slightly between men and women. Men usually need more calories and protein to maintain a larger muscle mass. Women have proportionally more adipose tissue and need fewer calories to maintain body weight. To prevent anemia, woman need more dietary iron to offset losses from menstruation.

Pregnancy and Lactation

The pregnant woman's diet should include a substantial increase in calories, protein, calcium, folic acid, and iron. Often a prenatal multivitamin and mineral supplement is prescribed. The pregnant woman should gain weight throughout her pregnancy as prescribed and monitored by her healthcare professional. Pregnant women at particular risk for nutritional deficiencies are adolescents, underweight women, obese women, women with chronic nutritional problems, women who smoke or ingest alcohol or drugs, low-income women, and women with chronic illnesses, such as diabetes or anemia.

The lactating woman also has special needs. Minor deficiencies in the lactating woman's diet are more likely to influence her nutritional state than the nutritional quality of her milk. Major deficiencies in the woman's diet may result in a decrease in the nutritional quality and quantity of her milk. Lactating women need to increase their intake of calcium, protein, fluid, and calories. These increases are important because the quality and quantity of breast milk produced directly affects the adequacy of the breast-feeding infant's diet (Worthington-Roberts & Williams, 1993).

Lifespan Considerations

Although people vary widely in their nutritional needs throughout the lifespan, people have certain characteristics in common at different ages.

Newborn and infant

Adequate nutrition during infancy is important because the infant's growth and development are more rapid during the first year of life than at any other time. Birth weight usually doubles within the first 4 to 6 months and triples by 12 months. The newborn needs more calories per pound of body weight because the BMR is so high. The infant's growth and development also are influenced by genetic characteristics and the quality of prenatal nutrition and care.

Milk is the food of choice for the newborn. If the infant is breast-fed, it should begin as soon after birth as possible. For the first 3 days after birth, the mother's breasts produce colostrum, a thin, watery fluid. Breast milk, which contains about 20 calories/oz, is produced after the third day. Weight gain may be less rapid in the breast-fed infant. Feedings are usually frequent (eg, every 2–3 hours) because breast milk is easily digested. Breast milk gives the infant immunity against some bacteria and viruses, decreases the production of bacteria in the intestine, decreases the incidence of allergies, and provides a well-balanced, ideal source of nutrition. The breast-feeding mother should avoid taking drugs, because small amounts can be transferred to the breast milk and ingested by the infant.

Formula is a safe and nutritious substitute for mothers who prefer not to breast-feed or cannot do so. Iron-fortified commercial formulas should be used until at least 6 months of age. Most formulas are modified cow's milk, which has been heat-treated to aid digestion. Soy formulas and predigested formulas also are available.

Food (juices, fruits, vegetables, and iron-fortified cereal) is gradually added to the infant's diet to provide additional nutrition and to begin to accustom the infant to food of different textures, flavors, and consistencies. The age at which these foods are introduced varies according to the infant's need, the practices of the health-care provider, and the influence of the infant's culture and environment. Cereal, fruits and vegetables, and egg yolk are added at about 4 to 6 months. When teeth begin to erupt at about 6 months, crackers and teething biscuits are often added. New foods should be introduced one at a time so that the offending food can be identified if allergies develop. In the second half of the first year, motor development has improved so that the infant can begin to sit up, eat finger foods, and drink from a cup.

Toddler and Preschooler

Adequate nutritional intake is important between the ages of 1 and 5 years because this is a period of physical growth and development. Variations between toddlers necessitate some differences in their diets. During this period, the growth rate begins to decline, and the appetite decreases as less food is needed to meet normal metabolic demands. The child's appetite may be erratic. Teeth continue to erupt into the second and sometimes the third year. Muscle mass and bone density increase. This requires adequate protein, calcium, and phosphorus in the diet. Energy levels remain high, requiring adequate caloric intake.

Independence in feeding greatly increases during this period as the child increases coordination and ability to use eating utensils. Many children can feed themselves by age 2. Mental abilities and language development are increasing, so the child is better able to communicate food likes and dislikes. Values and attitudes about eating develop during this period. It is important not to use food to punish, reward, bribe, or convey love. Some children may become picky eaters, especially when not eating gains them attention from their parents.

Maintaining adequate dietary habits for toddlers and preschoolers is important because good habits are established at an early age. The most common dietary deficiency in this age group is iron deficiency, which leads to iron-deficiency anemia. A diet that includes iron-rich foods is indicated, and iron supplements may be necessary. Vitamins A and C also may be deficient in the diets of toddlers and preschoolers, so they must eat foods rich in these vitamins. Active children in this age group benefit from nutritious between-meal snacks.

Child and Adolescent

Children's growth rates vary greatly. The digestive system matures, and permanent teeth erupt. Children can eat larger meals less frequently, requiring fewer calories per unit of body weight. Adolescence is a period of rapid growth and sexual maturation.

A diet that includes adequate carbohydrates and the recommended allowances of protein, vitamins, and minerals for the individual age group, physical status, and developmental level is necessary for optimal health. Nutritional deficiencies that are most common during childhood and adolescence are iron, calcium, vitamin A, and vitamin C (Pipes & Trahms, 1993). Adequate amounts of these vitamins and minerals must be included in the diet. Health problems that respond well to nutritional intervention during this age include dental caries, anemia, and obesity.

School lunch programs play an important role in providing nutritionally balanced, low-cost meals (Fig. 37-3). Some schools also have a breakfast program and a snack program. These programs usually are available free or at a reduced cost for needy children. In addition to providing a substantial part of the daily nutrition needs for children, these programs make a valuable contribution in terms of nutrition education and developing good nutrition habits.

Social pressure and emotional stress can have adverse effects on the young person's efforts to maintain a nutritionally adequate diet. Peers may dictate dietary choices. Fewer meals may be eaten at home; fast food, soda, and candy are often favorites. Smoking, drinking, and substance abuse also can affect nutritional status.

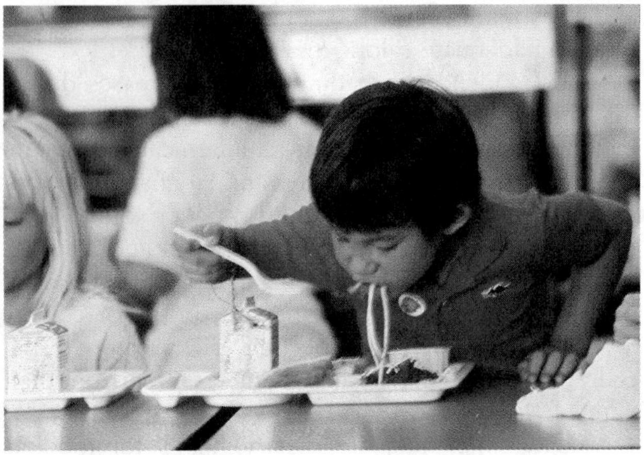

Figure 37-3 • *Children can receive well-balanced meals through a school lunch program. (USDA photo.)*

The child or adolescent may experience an unbalanced pattern of activity or rest. Increased participation in sports requires additional caloric intake. Weight gain is common during the preadolescent period as the body prepares for rapid growth. If the child leads a sedentary life and eats a high-calorie diet, weight gain can be excessive and can contribute to obesity. On the other hand, weight consciousness, especially among adolescent girls, can lead to fad diets, anorexia nervosa, and bulimia.

Adult and Older Adult

Growth stops and metabolism declines during adulthood, so fewer calories are required. Weight gain is common, especially if physical activity is limited. Calcium deficiency and osteoporosis can be a concern for adults, especially postmenopausal women. Adults should maintain a calcium intake of 800 to 1,200 mg/d throughout adulthood. Adequate intake of calcium is especially important before age 30, when peak bone mass is being attained (Robinson & Weigley, 1984). Among adult Americans, nutritional excesses are more common than deficiencies.

Inadequate nutritional intake during this time may be due to increased daily demands that decrease the time and energy available for buying, cooking, and eating food. Dietary patterns can be affected when both parents in a family work. Some adults lack adequate resources or knowledge about good nutrition. Pregnancy and lactation, as discussed previously, greatly alter nutritional requirements.

Physiologic changes that have a major impact on nutrition occur in later years. Metabolic rate continues to decline. Even though the need for calories decreases, the need for iron and vitamins remains high. A woman's need for iron, however, decreases after menopause. The diets of many elderly people are deficient in calories; calcium; vitamins A, C, D, and B-complex; folate; thiamine; and riboflavin (Shils, et al., 1994). Adequate fiber intake is necessary to prevent constipation, a common problem in older adults. The senses of taste and smell diminish, which can affect enjoyment of eating and cause decreased intake of food. Digestion is affected by a change in the contents of bile and pancreatic secretions, decreased peristalsis, and decreased blood flow to the GI tract. Periodontal disease and ill-fitting dentures can make chewing difficult and painful.

For older adults, socioeconomic factors can contribute to inadequate nutrition (Fig. 37-4). Transportation for shopping and carrying groceries can be problems for the older person with impaired mobility. Older adults may have trouble using cooking appliances because of failing eyesight and arthritis or because of the complexity of modern appliances. Selecting economical, nutritious foods can be difficult for the older shopper because of the wide variety of products available.

Social isolation also can hinder nutrition. Those who have lost friends and live far from relatives may become lonely and depressed, making it more difficult to cook and eat.

Several community resources have been developed to help older adults continue living at home by combating the problems mentioned previously. Programs for home-delivered meals, such as Meals on Wheels, provide nutritious, low-cost meals for older people. This program is able to remain low in cost partly because of a volunteer staff. Food stamps and food banks are useful to older adults. Another excellent resource for older adults is a local senior center, which can provide meals, health screening and medication assistance, transportation assistance, dietary counseling, recreational activities, and assistance and referral for economic and legal problems.

Altered Nutritional Function

The body constantly undergoes renewal. If proper nutrition is not provided, body tissues will not be adequately maintained, energy will not be adequate for activities, and normal body processes will suffer.

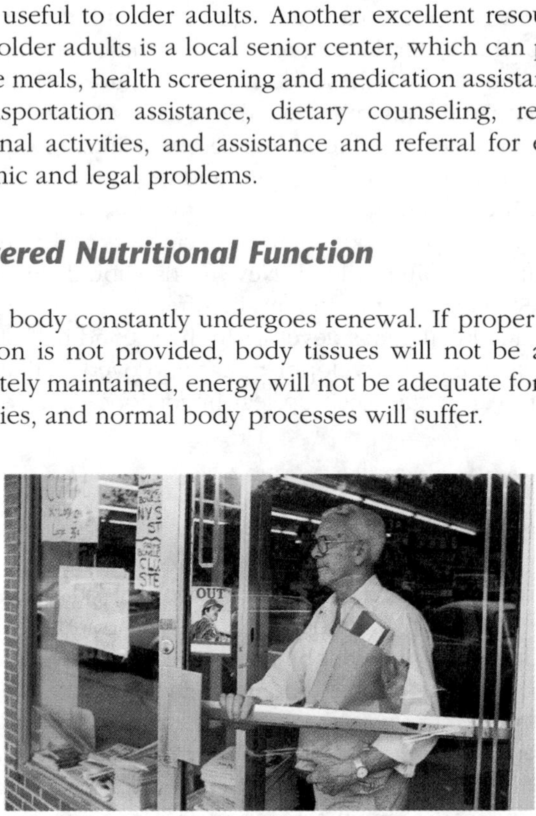

Figure 37-4 • *Learning proper food selection and preparation and ability to shop are significant to the individual's health.*

Potential for Altered Nutrition

Inadequate intake of essential nutrients can impair nutritional status. Problems associated with excessive intake have emerged only recently and are limited primarily to developed countries in which food is plentiful and lifestyles are more sedentary.

Despite adequate intake, some people experience altered nutritional status because of inadequate digestion and absorption of nutrients. Medical conditions causing inflammation or obstruction of the GI tract decrease nutrient absorption. Inadequate production of hormones or enzymes can affect digestion and absorption. A person who cannot use ingested nutrients may decrease his or her food intake due to anorexia, nausea, bloating, or vomiting.

Inadequate Intake of Nutrients

Inability to Acquire and Prepare Food. People who are unable to purchase, transport, and prepare food will often suffer from inadequate intake unless other people or agencies can be found to fulfill this need. In third world countries, starvation is common due to drought and famine. Starvation or malnutrition also can occur in developed nations when people lack the resources to obtain adequate food. A confused or disoriented person may not remember to eat or may be unable to organize the complex tasks of buying and cooking food independently.

Inadequate Knowledge. Some people may not eat a balanced diet because they lack information about nutrition. A person is likely to eat only what tastes good or is convenient if he or she does not know or care that such an eating pattern can be unhealthy. The consequences of poor nutrition are not immediately observable, so the motivation to change bad eating patterns may not be strong.

Swallowing Impairment. People who have difficulty swallowing may be unable to ingest enough nutrients to meet daily requirements. Swallowing impairment can occur when the gag reflex is absent due to neurologic dysfunction (such as a cerebrovascular accident) or muscle weakness. Obstruction of the oropharyngeal cavity secondary to a tumor or edema also can impair swallowing.

Discomfort During or After Eating. When a person experiences discomfort during or after eating, he or she may decrease food intake. A sore throat, a tonsillectomy, a mouth lesion, or ill-fitting dentures may be causes.

Anorexia. **Anorexia**, or loss of appetite, can occur for a variety of reasons. Depression, GI dysfunction, infectious, illnesses, malignancies, and the side effects of many medications can cause anorexia and the resultant decrease in food intake.

Nausea and Vomiting. Nausea and vomiting interfere with normal food intake. They may be due to motion sickness, viral or bacterial infections of the GI tract, gallbladder disease, general anesthesia, disruption of inner ear function, side effects of various medications, and pregnancy. Some people may feel nauseated or vomit from unpleasant smells or sights.

Excess Intake of Nutrients

Calories. Caloric intake in excess of daily energy requirements results in storage of energy in the form of increased adipose tissue. As the percentage of stored fat increases, a person becomes overweight or obese. Excess weight increases the stress on body organs and predisposes the person to chronic health problems, such as diabetes mellitus and hypertension. Excessive caloric intake does not ensure an adequate intake of essential nutrients: The obese person may be malnourished due to a lack of essential vitamins or nutrients.

Fats. Americans have a higher percentage of fat in their diets than do people in many other countries; studies have shown that fat makes up about 40% of the calories in the American diet (Shils, et al., 1994). An excess intake of fat has been related to obesity, an increased risk of coronary artery disease (especially increased intake of saturated fats), and several forms of cancer, including breast, colon, and uterine cancer. Dietary modifications can lower fat and cholesterol intake.

Inability to Use Ingested Nutrients

Inflammation of the Gastrointestinal Tract. Inflammation of the lining of the GI tract causes discomfort and interferes with the absorption of nutrients.

Esophagitis, an inflammation of the esophagus, can be caused by burns, poisons, infections, or chronic vomiting. This causes discomfort and impairs swallowing.

Gastritis is characterized by inflammation of the mucosal layer of the stomach, which can proceed to ulceration if untreated. Mucosal cells of the stomach can atrophy and become unable to absorb vitamin B_{12}, leading to pernicious anemia (Shils, et al., 1994).

Cholecystitis is an inflammation of the gallbladder, usually caused by the presence of gallstones. The presence of inflammation and stones causes pain after the ingestion of a meal high in fat, because the gallbladder spasms as it attempts to release bile to assist with fat digestion.

Inflammatory bowel disease (eg, Crohn's disease, or ulcerative colitis) greatly affects absorption of nutri-

Therapeutic Dialogue
Loss of Appetite

Scenes for Thought

Mrs. Kwai Wu is an 82-year-old woman admitted to your unit weighing 40 kg. She is 150 cm tall, and her worried family has reported that she eats only rice and tea twice a day since 2 weeks ago. Her husband died suddenly 2 months ago. Her laboratory values indicate that she is dehydrated and anemic. She is weak but oriented to time, place, and person. She objects to the need for hospitalization.

Effective

Nurse: *Good morning, Mrs. Wu. I'm your nurse, Carl Bonnette. How do you feel, today?*
Client: *Alright, I guess.* Looks at nurse and then away.
Nurse: *I was wondering if we could talk a little about your not eating. Would you be willing to do that? (Giving choice.)*
Client: *My family has been talking to me about that for 2 weeks. I'm tired of all the nagging.* Continues to look away. Sad expression on face.
Nurse: *They're concerned about you, and so am I. We're all afraid you're going to get sicker and sicker because you aren't eating enough. I'm afraid you might die. (Presenting reality).*
Client: *That might happen. I don't really mind that. I'm old and my family doesn't need me around anymore.* Looks sad; makes eye contact with nurse.
Nurse: *I wonder what your feelings about eating have to do with the death of your husband? (Exploring.)*
Client: *It's so much trouble to cook for just me. I didn't feel like it.* Continues to look sad.
Nurse: *One of the other reasons that people stop eating is because of feeling sad and lonely. Are you having any of those feelings? (Exploring.)*
Client: *I suppose so, but isn't that normal? I miss my husband.* A tear rolls down her face.
Nurse: *I can see you do. (Sits quietly, uses therapeutic silence.) Nurse continues to sit with client, and they talk more about Mrs. Wu's feelings of loneliness and how she'll cope with her new status of widowhood.*

Less Effective

Nurse: *Hello, Mrs. Wu. I'm Jonathan Hopkins, your nurse for today. I have your breakfast tray here. Shall I put it over here where you can reach it? (Offering choice.)*
Client: *If you want to.* Looks at nurse, then looks away.
Nurse: *I notice you haven't eaten anything but some juice since yesterday. Does the food not appeal to you? (Exploring.)*
Client: No. *It isn't what I'm used to.* Looks sad.
Nurse: *I can understand that. I'd like to ask the dietitian to come up and talk to you so you can help her arrange for the kind of foods you're used to. Would that be okay? (Offering choices.)*
Client: *Fine.* Turns her head away and looks disinterested.
Nurse: *Good! I'm sure she can come up with something that will increase your appetite, so you can eat and get strong again. I'll be back in a little while with your medication.*
Client: Turns to wall, and pulls up covers. Closes eyes.

Critical Thinking Challenges

Associate loss of appetite with depression on a physiologic level. • Identify questions that this scenario raises in your mind about the Chinese culture and death. • Discuss what success you think the dietitian will have in helping Mrs. Wu find something she'd like to eat. Give your reasons. • Identify the clues Jonathan ignored that Carl noticed.

ents and water from the intestine. The intestinal inflammation greatly increases the movement of nutrients through the GI tract, resulting in severe diarrhea. Treatment frequently requires resection of large inflamed areas of the intestine, permanently altering absorption in the area.

Obstruction of the Gastrointestinal Tract. Any obstruction caused by scar tissue, benign or cancerous growths, or structural abnormalities can alter normal nutritional status. Esophageal obstruction can severely limit intake or restrict oral intake to fluids. A hiatal hernia is a protrusion of the stomach upward into the mediastinal cavity, causing esophageal reflux, or the backflow of stomach contents into the esophagus, resulting in heartburn. Intestinal obstruction usually necessitates withholding all oral intake until the obstruction has resolved or has been surgically corrected.

Malabsorption of Nutrients. Malabsorption syndromes can be caused by the inability to tolerate certain foods. An allergic reaction to gluten, which is found in wheat, rye, oats, and barley, can affect absorption. Gluten causes mucosal villi to atrophy, decreasing their absorptive abilities. Lactose intolerance occurs when there is a deficiency of lactase, a digestive enzyme that breaks down the sugar commonly found in milk.

A decrease in pancreatic enzyme production occurs in some pancreatic disorders, resulting in altered digestion of fats and protein. In cystic fibrosis, an inherited disorder, excessive mucus plugs pancreatic ducts, leading to altered protein and fat digestion.

Malabsorption also can occur secondary to surgical intervention. Gastric or intestinal resection removes large areas of the GI tract normally involved in absorption of nutrients. Decreased blood flow to the GI tract can decrease the rate of nutrient absorption.

Diabetes Mellitus. Diabetes mellitus is a chronic condition in which insufficient amounts of insulin are produced or the body cannot effectively use circulating insulin. Insulin is a hormone essential for proper metabolism of fats and carbohydrates. When adequate insulin is unavailable, the transfer of glucose into the cell is impaired, and the glucose level of the blood rises. Thus, the available energy source cannot be used by the body.

Increased Metabolic Demand

Certain conditions increase the body's nutritional requirements, potentially contributing to altered nutritional status:

- Periods of rapid growth (infancy, adolescence, or pregnancy)
- Conditions that increase the BMR (fever, exercise, or hyperthyroidism)
- Stress (from emotional distress, fear, surgery, or illness)
- Cancer (greatly increases the metabolic rate, which can result in rapid weight loss despite normal food intake)

Surgery

Surgery greatly increases the risk for nutritional deficits. Studies by Shirreff (1990) note weight and serum albumin losses for all clients studied after surgery. Increased metabolic demands due to the stress of surgery and wound healing, along with inadequate postoperative intake, compound nutritional deficits. Many surgical clients are nutritionally depleted at the time of the operation due to chronic illness or GI problems.

Cancer and Cancer Treatment

Cancer greatly increases metabolic demands of the body, and cancer cells compete with normal cells for nutrients. Cancer clients often experience anorexia, nausea, vomiting, and depression, all of which can decrease food consumption. Radiation or chemotherapy also can alter normal nutrition because loss of appetite, nausea, and vomiting are commonly associated with such treatments. Mouth lesions (known as stomatitis) often occur with cancer therapy, causing pain and difficulty with chewing. Chemotherapy and radiation cause fatigue, decreasing the amount of energy available for cooking and eating.

Alcohol and Drug Abuse

Excessive, chronic ingestion of alcohol can impair nutrition. Normal eating may be greatly affected when excessive alcohol intake occurs, impairing the necessary intake of calories and nutrients. Money normally spent on food may be used to buy alcohol. Deficiency of B vitamins (thiamine, folate, niacin, and B_6) is common because these are necessary to metabolize alcohol. Alcohol's toxic effect on the intestinal mucosa can impair the normal absorption of nutrients. Chronic alcohol use also can cause irreversible changes to the cells of the liver, affecting the liver's role in metabolic pathways.

Drug abuse also can affect nutrition. Addiction to heroin or cocaine can decrease the user's desire for food, because preoccupation with buying drugs disrupts normal daily routines. Other drugs, such as amphetamines and barbiturates, can cause an increase or decrease in food intake.

Psychological State

A person's psychological state can affect his or her desire to eat. Anxiety causes some people to increase their food intake; others eat less when they feel anxious. Depression often decreases the person's appetite and depletes the energy available for cooking and eating. Some people may willingly alter eating patterns to help achieve weight loss. Rather than changing eating patterns, rapid weight loss is often obtained through crash diets. **Anorexia nervosa** is an eating disorder in which the person refuses to eat due to a fear of becoming overweight, even in the presence of normal or less than ideal body weight.

Manifestations of Altered Nutrition

Indications of altered nutrition are overweight, obesity, underweight, recent significant weight loss or gain, decreased energy levels, altered bowel patterns, and altered appearance of the skin, hair, teeth, and mucous membranes (Table 37-3). If the client's weight varies significantly from IBW, a nutrition problem is likely.

Overweight

A person is said to be overweight if his or her body weight exceeds IBW by 1% to 20%. The National Center for Health Statistics estimates that more than 20 million American adults (or 31%–35% of the adult population) are overweight (Shils, et al., 1994). A person gains weight when he or she takes in more calories than the body needs.

Obesity

A person is obese if he or she is more than 20% over IBW. Morbid obesity is obesity that can interfere with normal functioning, such as mobility or breathing.

Table 37-3 • Signs of Poor Nutrition and Possible Nutrient Deficiency

Signs	Possible Lacking Nutrient
Hair: thin, coarse, lacking luster, breaks easily	Protein
Skin: excessive bruising, bleeding	Vitamin K
Skin: pressure sores, poor wound healing	Vitamin C and protein
Gums: swollen, bleeding	Vitamin C
Muscles: wasting	Protein
Lack of growth	Protein, calories
Skeletal: poor posture, painful joints, bowed legs, increase in bone fractures	Calcium, vitamin D, vitamin C, protein
Mental: confusion, motor weakness	Thiamine: niacin, B complex

Excess calories do not ensure adequate nutritional intake, so the obese client may be undernourished in many important nutrients.

Underweight

A person is said to be underweight if he or she is 10% less than IBW. This occurs when caloric intake is insufficient to meet the body's nutritional requirements.

Recent Significant Weight Gain or Loss

Minor fluctuations in weight occur on a day-to-day basis due to fluid losses and gains, but changing weight patterns over weeks or months may indicate altered nutrition. A significant weight gain (5% in 1 month or 10% in 6 months) can occur when a person eats more than the body needs for energy expenditure. This can happen when a person becomes less active or when the intake of food is increased due to stress or boredom. Significant weight loss, especially when intake has remained constant, can indicate hypermetabolic states, such as cancer or hyperthyroidism, or an inability to use ingested nutrients.

Decreased Energy

Nutrition provides the body with energy to perform normal cellular processes and carry out normal movement and activities. When nutritional deficits occur, adequate energy may be unavailable. Fatigue or activity intolerance are common manifestations of altered nutrition. The client may complain of feeling tired or weak.

Altered Bowel Patterns

Inadequate dietary intake may affect bowel function and regularity. Constipation can occur when fiber or fluid intake is inadequate. Diarrhea can occur when large quantities of fresh fruits are eaten. With food intolerance (eg, lactase deficiency) or malabsorption syndrome, GI distress occurs. When a client's bowel regularity changes, nutritional deficits must be ruled out as a causative factor.

Altered Skin, Teeth, Hair, and Mucous Membranes

Skin, nails, hair, and mucous membranes are rapidly growing tissues that continuously require adequate nutrition for growth. Protein is especially important in this process. Vitamin deficiencies are often manifested by altered development and growth of skin, teeth, hair, and mucous membranes. When protein is lacking, hair may become thin, lack luster, and break easily. Skin heals slowly and may appear thin and fragile when nutrition is inadequate. Mucous membranes may develop sores and bleed easily. Teeth and gums are more prone to disease.

Impact of Dysfunction on Activities of Daily Living

Individual Considerations

Altered nutrition may marginally or seriously affect activities of daily living (ADLs). Poor dietary habits can affect a person's ability to work or a child's performance in school. Poor nutrition reduces a person's energy to carry out ADLs and affects normal growth and development. Ingesting alcohol impairs the person's intellectual and physical performance.

Increased susceptibility to common illnesses and chronic diseases is often a consequence of inadequate nutrition. For example, the person who has a long history of high fat intake may have chronic cardiovascular disease that will affect all aspects of ADLs. If a man who has depended on his wife for meal preparation loses her, this may contribute to poor nutrition because he has not developed the skills for shopping and meal preparation.

Family Considerations

Any illness, dietary deficiency, or other problem not prevented by healthy nutrition disrupts a family's usual level of functioning. Lack of transportation and low income limit the family's ability to obtain food for adequate nutrition. Some low-income families may need to use available money for housing or heat, reducing the amount of money available for adequate nutrition.

If the person who is the primary food preparer is unable to fix meals, the nutrition of the entire family may decline as they resort to "fast foods" and foods that are high in calories and low in nutrition. If the nursing mother has poor nutrition, the infant who depends on her for nutrition also will become poorly nourished. Because so much family socialization centers around food and meals, disruption of those socialization opportunities may have an effect on the socialization ADLs.

Assessment

Subjective Data

In a nutritional assessment, the nurse determines the person's nutritional health. Information is collected by interviewing the client about normal dietary patterns and preferences, risk factors that may contribute to nutritional alterations, and actual nutritional deficits.

Functional Pattern Identification

The nurse asks questions to determine the client's normal eating patterns and food preferences. The client is asked to describe his or her appetite as good, fair, or poor and whether eating is usually a pleasant experience.

Asking the client to describe food and fluid intake on a typical day gives the nurse a sense of what is normal for the client. Two surveying methods can be used, the 24-hour recall or the food diary. The 24-hour recall asks the person to recall and record the type, quality, and method of preparation of all food eaten within a 24-hour period. In the food diary, the person keeps a log of the amount, time, and manner of preparation for all food consumed within a specific period of time. This time period can vary but is often 3 days to 1 week; this permits the evaluation to be affected less by "one time only" dietary indiscretions. Both surveying methods are subject to recall and recording errors.

The client is asked about food likes and dislikes, normal timing of meals, and routine snacks. Does the client follow a special diet for any reason, have food allergies, or limit the intake of certain foods? Cultural or religious dietary concerns are discussed. For some clients, it may be important to inquire how stress affects eating patterns. Some people under stress limit their food intake, but others increase the amount and frequency of food consumption.

Who in the family is responsible for shopping and cooking, or are such responsibilities shared by more than one family member? The nurse should determine whether the client uses prepackaged, prepared food and how many times per week the client eats out.

Risk Identification

The nutritional assessment helps to identify clients at risk for nutritional deficits. The client's knowledge and values related to nutrition are determined by asking questions such as, "Do you feel your diet helps promote health?" and "What (if any) changes in your diet do you feel might be beneficial?" If the client is on a specific diet, asking which foods are important to include or avoid can help assess the client's understanding of the dietary restrictions. Who prescribed the diet? Was it a neighbor or a nutritionist?

The nurse identifies the presence of anorexia, chewing problems, sore mouth, dysphagia, nausea and vomiting, and when present, how long food intake has been affected. Chronic or acute health problems affecting the GI tract (eg, ulcers, gallbladder disease, inflammatory bowel disease) are noted. Chronic health conditions (eg, diabetes mellitus, cancer, renal disease, heart disease, lung disease) are documented, and their effect on appetite and food intake is assessed. Any condition that impairs swallowing (eg, a neurologic impairment) and its specific deficits are noted.

Assessing socioeconomic factors helps to determine possible nutritional deficits. Does the client have money and transportation to buy nutritious food? Are safe storage and adequate cooking facilities available? Does the client or caretaker have the energy to shop for and prepare meals?

Intake of over-the-counter drugs, excessive alcohol, and illicit drugs, such as cocaine and heroin, is documented. The use of vitamin and mineral supplements and prescription medications, such as insulin, antacids, chemotherapeutic agents, and steroids, should be noted, and any impact on nutrition should be assessed.

Dysfunction Identification

Nutrition can be impaired if the client cannot buy and prepare food, is unwilling or unable to eat, has excessive intake, or cannot use ingested nutrients. Such dysfunctions are often determined by asking questions.

Nutritional alterations can be identified if the client's weight is significantly greater or less than IBW.

Reports of significant recent weight loss without altered diet indicate an inability to meet normal nutritional requirements. A dietary intake that supplies significantly less than the RDA also helps to identify a deficit. Signs and symptoms, such as fatigue, muscle wasting, and obesity, show nutritional dysfunction.

Objective Data

Objective data are gathered by general observation, anthropometric measurements, calorie counts, mouth examination, and swallowing evaluation. Laboratory and diagnostic tests can provide data to evaluate nutritional status and the functional ability of the GI system.

Physical Assessment

General Observations. General observation provides important information on nutritional status. An adequately nourished person should appear robust, vital, and energetic and should have erect posture. Skin, hair, and nails should appear healthy. Compare the display on characteristics of a well-nourished person with Table 37-3.

Anthropometric Measurements. Anthropometric measurements include height and weight, skinfold measurements, and arm circumference measurements (Fig. 37-5). Skinfold and arm circumference measurements are reserved for nutritional screening.

Height and weight are measured and compared with a table of standard measurements grouped by age, sex, and body frame. Small, medium, or large body frame can be estimated by measuring wrist circumference. Ask what the person thinks his or her IBW is; this may vary from standardized tables.

Skinfold measurements are used to help determine fat stores in the body. The triceps skinfold and the subscapular skinfold are most commonly used. Using a caliper, the fold of skin, which includes the subcutaneous tissue but not the underlying muscle, is measured. Measurements are compared with a table of standards grouped by age and sex to detect excess fat.

Mid-arm circumference measurements are taken of the upper arm to provide information about the muscle mass. Because muscles are the major protein stores, measuring arm circumference helps evaluate protein status. Again, measurements are compared to a table of standards.

Calorie Count. When inadequate intake is suspected, calories can be counted. The nurse records the percentage eaten of each food served. This information is used by the dietitian to calculate the calories and to evaluate whether the caloric intake is adequate for the client's needs.

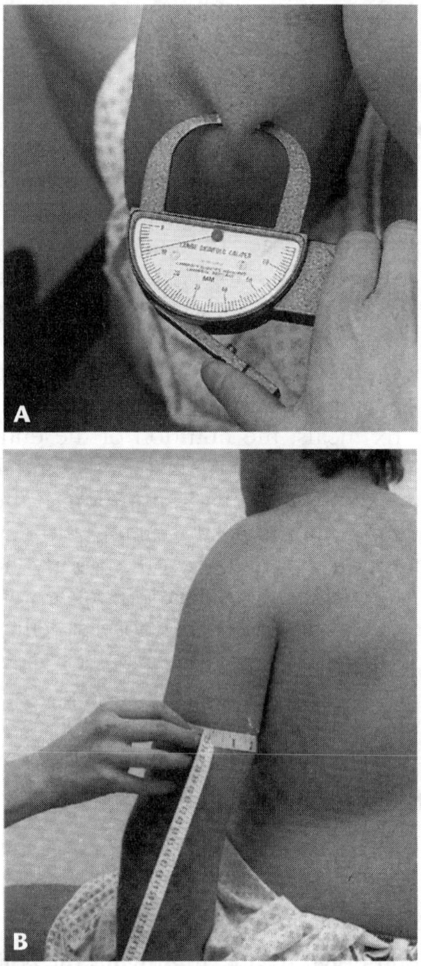

*Figure 37-5 • Anthropometric measurements. **(A)** Calipers are used to measure triceps skin fold. **(B)** A tape measure is used to measure the upper arm. Values are compared with standards to detect increased body fat.*

Mouth Inspection. The nurse observes the condition of the teeth, gums, and mucous membranes. Mucous membranes should be moist and adequate saliva present. Caries, excessive plaque, and gingivitis are noted. If the client uses dentures, proper fit and condition are evaluated. Lesions of the oral cavity (canker sores, stomatitis, *Candida* infections) should be detected and treated promptly, because discomfort associated with such lesions can alter food intake.

Swallowing Evaluation. A swallowing evaluation is necessary when potential difficulty in swallowing is suspected. Often the client is referred to a speech therapist for a swallowing evaluation, but the nurse may need to evaluate swallowing abilities to determine whether feeding is safe. A swallowing evaluation includes assessment of motor function of the facial, oral, and tongue muscles; cough reflex; swallowing reflex; and gag reflex (DiIorio & Price, 1990).

Motor function is assessed by observing the face, jaw, and tongue for symmetry and strength during normal movements. Asking the client to cough will permit evaluation of the briskness and strength of the cough reflex, which is necessary to clear aspirated food from the airway. Ability to swallow is evaluated by placing the index finger and thumb on the client's laryngeal protuberance and asking the client to swallow. As the client with an intact swallowing reflex swallows, the nurse will feel the larynx elevate.

Finally, the gag reflex is evaluated by stroking the client's right or left pharyngeal wall with a tongue blade.

Diagnostic Tests and Procedures

Biochemical data can be used to confirm a diagnosis, help determine the necessary dietary modification, or help identify specific nutritional deficiencies before clinical signs appear. Evaluating blood and urine is most useful when analyzing a client's nutritional state. The most common laboratory data used are hemoglobin, serum albumin, serum transferrin, and total lymphocyte count. Anergy testing can be done to identify severe nutritional deficits.

Hemoglobin. A hemoglobin count measures the blood's oxygen- and iron-carrying capacity. A decreased hemoglobin value indicates decreased iron intake or decreased iron reserves, which often are present in anemia.

Serum Albumin. Serum albumin accounts for more than half of the body's total serum protein. Serum albumin values reflect protein intake or absorption. Values of less than 3.5 g/dL may indicate nutritional deficits. A low albumin level also can be related to overhydration and may not necessarily indicate malnutrition.

Serum Transferrin. Transferrin, a blood protein that binds with iron and is important in its transport, is considered a sensitive indicator of protein deficiency. Transferrin, which is synthesized in the liver, increases when iron stores are low and decreases when iron stores are high. Changes in protein intake or visceral protein stores are more rapidly reflected in serum transferrin levels than in serum albumin levels.

Creatinine Excretion. The rate of creatinine formation is proportional to total muscle mass. Creatinine is released during skeletal muscle metabolism and is excreted from the body through the kidneys. Creatinine excretion is usually measured by collecting and measuring creatinine in all voided urine during a 24-hour period. As muscles atrophy during malnutrition, creatinine excretion decreases.

Immunocompetence Testing. Immunity is affected by nutritional status. In severe nutritional depletion, the client may be unable to mount an immune response (anergy). Commonly this is seen as the lymphocyte count decreases with protein depletion. Skin testing also may be performed to evaluate the impact of nutritional deficits on immune function. Antigen skin tests (eg, tuberculosis, *Candida,* mumps) can be used to evaluate the client's response to antigens to which he or she has already been sensitized. If no skin response is observed after 48 hours, anergy is present (Curtas, Chapman, & Megurd, 1989). Anergy indicates the need for aggressive nutritional support.

Nursing Diagnoses

By assessing the client, the nurse can identify strengths, nutritional risk factors, and altered nutritional states. Four accepted North American Nursing Diagnosis Association (NANDA) nursing diagnoses have been identified for the area of nutrition: Altered Nutrition: Less than body requirements; Altered Nutrition: More than body requirements; Altered Nutrition: Potential for more than body requirements; and Impaired Swallowing.

Diagnostic Statement: Altered Nutrition: Less Than Body Requirements

Definition

Altered Nutrition: Less than body requirements is the state in which in an individual's intake of nutrients is insufficient to meet metabolic needs (NANDA, 1994).

Defining Characteristics

One of the following defining characteristics or clinical cues that point to this nursing diagnosis must be present:

- Loss of weight with adequate food intake
- Loss of weight due to food intake less than recommended

Note: Body weight of 20% or more less than ideal may be critical in consequence to body functioning.

Related Factors

These conditions may result from inability to ingest or digest food, inability to absorb nutrients, or increased body requirements. Many etiologies or contributing factors may be associated with these changes in health status. Biologic factors that result in weight loss may include a painful, inflamed buccal cavity, weakness in the muscles required for swallowing, or abdominal pain with pathology, such as cramping, diarrhea, or steatorrhea. Psychological factors include lack of interest or aversion to eating, immediate sensation of satiety after ingestion of food, or perceived inability to digest food. Economic factors include reported or evidence of lack of food. Lack of information, misinformation, or misconceptions about nutrition also may be related to weight loss. Some conditions, such as cancer, thermal injuries, and sepsis, result in increased body requirements.

Diagnostic Statement: Altered Nutrition: More Than Body Requirements

Definition

Altered Nutrition: More than body requirements is the state in which an individual's intake of nutrients exceeds metabolic needs (NANDA, 1994).

Defining Characteristics

This nursing diagnosis is implicated when one of the following characteristics is present:

- Body weight 10% to 20% more than ideal for height and frame
- Triceps skinfold greater than 15 mm in men, 25 mm in women

Related Factors

Excessive intake in relation to metabolic need results in weight gain. Related factors may include sedentary activity, which decreases metabolic rate. Hypothyroidism also may decrease metabolic rate. Excessive intake may be related to a reported or observed dysfunctional eating pattern. Some eating patterns that may contribute to weight gain include pairing food with other activities; concentrating food intake at the end of the day; eating in responese to external cues, such as time of day or social situation; or eating in response to internal cues other than hunger, such as emotional distress.

Diagnostic Statement: Altered Nutrition: Potential for More Than Body Requirements

Definition

Altered Nutrition: Potential for more than body requirements occurs when an individual is at risk of experiencing an intake of nutrients that exceeds metabolic needs (NANDA, 1994).

Defining Characteristics

The major characteristics or clinical cues that point to this nursing diagnosis include at least one of the following:

- Obesity in one or both parents
- Rapid transition across growth percentiles in infants or children
- Reported or observed dysfunctional eating pattern

Related Factors

Contributing factors may include reported use of solid food before 5 months of age, use of food to comfort or reward, pairing food with other activities, concentrating intake at the end of the day, or eating in response to external or internal cues other than hunger. All of these behaviors may result in excessive intake in relation to metabolic need.

Diagnostic Statement: Impaired Swallowing

Definition

Impaired Swallowing occurs when an individual has decreased ability to voluntarily pass fluids or solids from the mouth to the stomach (NANDA, 1994).

Defining Characteristics

- Major: observed evidence of difficulty swallowing (eg, stasis of food in oral cavity, coughing or choking)
- Minor: evidence of aspiration (NANDA, 1994)

Related Factors

Related factors include neuromuscular impairment (eg, decreased or absent gag reflex, decreased strength or excursion of muscles involved in mastication, perceptual impairment, facial paralysis), mechanical obstruction (eg, edema, tracheostomy tube, tumor), fatigue, limited awareness, and reddened, irritated oropharyngeal cavity (NANDA, 1994).

Related Nursing Diagnoses

Altered nutritional status affects many functional areas and can contribute to many other nursing problems. Alterations in normal elimination patterns (Diarrhea, Constipation) can occur due to nutritional deficits or the inability to use ingested nutrients. Decreased nutritional status greatly increases the risk for infection and delays wound healing. Skin breakdown (Impaired Skin Integrity, Impaired Tissue Integrity) also is more common in the poorly nourished person. Fluid status alterations (Fluid Volume Deficit) can occur in severe malnutrition. Altered nutritional status often results in fatigue, because the energy supply to the cells of the body is inadequate. When this occurs or when morbid obesity is present, the client may develop Activity

Intolerance or Self-Care Deficit. If these conditions are extreme, such limitations can affect the person's ability to manage independently in the home setting (Impaired Home Maintenance Management).

Knowledge Deficit often occurs in clients who are placed on new diets (eg, diabetic or heart clients) or new nutritional therapies (eg, hyperalimentation or tube feedings). Noncompliance with diet orders or dietary restrictions can occur. Altered nutritional status frequently affects appearance as body weight is gained or lost. Extreme alterations in body weight can lead to Body Image Disturbance, Self-Esteem Disturbance, and Social Isolation.

Outcome Identification and Planning

After the nursing diagnoses and related factors are identified, client goals and nursing interventions are planned. Client goals for nutrition include ensuring adequate nutritional intake and understanding and complying with dietary modifications. Common goals in nutrition include the following:

Client will use a nutritionally sound dietary intake to meet body requirements and promote health.

Client will maintain dietary intake adequate to meet energy expenditures of the body.

Client will demonstrate adequate knowledge to adhere to dietary prescription or therapies to promote health.

The client's cooperation is needed to plan and set goals because the client is responsible for his or her own nutrition, unless someone else does the meal planning for the client.

Planning will revolve around the client's motivation and abilities. If the client is not able to shop and prepare food, a support person must be included in the planning. Most nursing interventions for healthy nutritional balance are educational. Examples of nursing interventions commonly used in planning for nutritional education and support are listed in the accompanying display and are discussed in the next section of this chapter.

Planning

Examples of Nursing Interventions Used in Common Nutritional Problems

Less Nutrition Than Body Requires

- Encourage and cue verbally to eat.
- Provide high-protein and high-caloric snacks, (ie, small, frequent "meals").
- Give dietary supplements (ie, liquids), because they are easy to consume and leave the stomach quickly.
- Use enteral tube feedings.
- Use peripheral parenteral nutrition or total parenteral nutrition.

More Nutrition Than Body Requires

- Explain low-calorie diets and low-fat diets.
- Identify and encourage healthy eating habits and patterns.
- Give encouragement and positive reinforcement.
- Refer for behavior modification techniques.
- Encourage increased activity and regular exercise.
- Refer to support groups and appropriate agencies for weight reduction.

Impaired Swallowing

- Provide rest period before meals.
- Position client upright in chair or high-Fowler's position in bed with neck slightly flexed.
- Thicken liquids.
- Provide small bites, and check for pocketing of food.
- Provide simple, short verbal cues to "chew," "swallow," and so forth.
- Keep stimuli to a minimum to prevent distractions.
- Provide enough time, and appear unrushed.
- Initiate appropriate referrals as needed.
- Provide nutrient-dense foods to help limit volume of food needed.

Implementation

Nursing Interventions to Promote Health and Function

In collaboration with the healthcare team, the nurse is responsible for promoting optimal nutrition through health teaching. Nutritional counseling can occur in the community or hospital. Promoting optimal nutrition by providing assistance and creating an atmosphere that encourages eating also is an important nursing role.

Client Teaching

Nurses are active in promoting good nutrition in a variety of settings. Examples are health fairs, schools, prenatal classes, health screening visits, and at home. The goal of such education is to encourage good nutrition by increasing the person's understanding of the importance of a healthy diet (see display).The nurse in these settings can refer people at risk to appropriate private and community resources.

Some hospitalized clients are receptive to nutrition teaching. Statements can be directed toward actions the client can take immediately (eg, "While your incision is healing, it's important to eat enough protein"). Informal diet instruction can occur when helping clients make

Client Teaching
Dietary Guidelines for Americans

Instruct the client as follows:

- Eat a variety of foods. *Eat a variety of foods daily, choosing different foods from each group, including fruits, vegetables; whole grain and enriched breads, cereals, and other products made from grains; milk, cheese, yogurt, and other products made from milk; meats, poultry, fish, eggs, and dry beans and peas.*
- Balance the food you eat with physical activity; maintain or improve your weight. *To help control overeating, eat slowly, take smaller portions, and avoid "seconds." To lose weight, eat a variety of foods that are low in calories and high in nutrients. Eat more fruits, vegetables, and whole grains prepared without added fats or sugar; eat less fat and fatty foods; eat less sugar and sweets; drink little or no alcoholic beverages; increase your physical activity.*
- Choose a diet with plenty of vegetables, fruits, and grain products. *Choose three or more servings of various vegetables, two or more servings of various fruits, and six or more servings of grain products. Increase fiber intake by eating more of a variety of foods that are natural sources of fiber.*
- Choose a diet low in fat, saturated fat, and cholesterol. *Choose lean meat, fish, poultry, and dry beans and peas as protein sources; use skim or low-fat milk and milk products; moderate your use of egg yolks and organ meats; use fats and oils sparingly, especially those high in saturated fat, such as butter, cream, lard, heavily hydrogenated fats (some margarines), shortenings, and foods containing palm and coconut oils; choose liquid vegetable oils most often because they are lower in saturated fat; trim fat off meats; remove skin from poultry; have meatless meals occasionally; broil, bake, or boil rather than fry; read labels carefully to determine amount and type of fat in foods.*
- Choose a diet moderate in sugars. *Use sugars sparingly if your calorie needs are low. Avoid excessive snacking, and brush and floss your teeth regularly.*
- Use salt and sodium only in moderation, if at all, in cooking and at the table. *Choose foods lower in sodium instead of high-sodium foods. Use salted snacks, such as chips, crackers, pretzels, and nuts, sparingly. Read food labels carefully to determine the amounts of sodium. Use lower-sodium products, when available, to replace those that have higher sodium content.*
- If you drink alcoholic beverages, do so in moderation. *Women should drink no more than one drink a day; men should not drink more than two drinks a day. Alcohol should not be consumed by women who are pregnant or trying to conceive; individuals who plan to drive or engage in other activities that require attention or skill; individuals using medicines, even over-the-counter kinds; individuals who cannot keep their drinking moderate; and children and adolescents.*

Report of the Dietary Guidelines Advisory Committee on the Dietary Guidelines for Americans, 1995, to the Secretary of Health and Human Services and the Secretary of Agriculture.

menu selections. The nurse can praise food choices, emphasizing the importance each food plays in staying healthy. Gentle encouragement can be given to improve diet selections (eg, "Have you tried 1% milk rather than 2% milk? Many people don't notice the difference, and it's a good way to reduce the fat intake in your diet").

Clients often question the nurse about nutrition or ask for suggestions for altering diets. For example, an overweight client may ask the nurse's opinion of a new diet recommended by a friend. The nurse must provide the person with accurate factual information, encouragement, praise, and referral to appropriate resources.

Optimal Intake Promotion

Illness often affects eating, and the nurse plays a role in encouraging optimal nutrition for clients. The room should be clean, well ventilated, free from strong odors, and facilitate enjoyment of food. The atmosphere should be relaxing. Interruptions, such as treatments and procedures, should be avoided during mealtime. Oral care before eating promotes comfort. Medications to control nausea and pain should be timed so that optimal relief is achieved at mealtimes.

Food should be served in an appetizing manner and at the right temperature. Microwave ovens can be used to rewarm cooled food. Food preferences should be considered, and the food should be arranged attractively. Small servings are preferable because they do not overwhelm the client. Family members should be encouraged to bring favorite foods from home, as long as such food is permitted on the client's diet.

Pleasant company can improve the incentive for eating for some clients, but conversation should not distract the client. Staff or relatives can provide verbal cues and encouragement during eating for the confused or reluctant client.

It is preferable to get clients out of bed and sitting in a chair for meals. This position facilitates chewing and swallowing and prevents reflux of stomach contents. Some clients may need assistance in cutting food, opening packages, or eating. Procedure 37-1 suggests methods for assisting clients with feeding.

Procedure 37-1
Assisting an Adult With Feeding

Purpose

1. Maintain nutritional status.
2. Provide a time for socialization.

Assessment

- Assess client's physical and emotional ability to feed self (ie, motor function, coordination, level of consciousness, vision, interest, depression),
- Assess eating habits and food preferences. Cultural and religious beliefs may eliminate certain food from the diet.
- Review history for food allergies.
- Assess ability of GI tract to absorb and digest oral nutrition (ie, presence of bowel sounds, regular bowel movements, history of GI disorders, Crohn's disease, duodenal ulcers, pancreatitis, cholecystitis, ulcerative colitis).
- Review physician's orders for type of diet.

Equipment

Personal hygiene supplies for client to wash hands
Glasses, if necessary
Special devices (splints, prostheses, spoons, cups)
Meal tray
Oral hygiene equipment

Procedure

1. Prepare client's environment for meal:
   a. Remove urinals, bedpans, dressings, trash.
   b. Ventilate or aerate room for unpleasant odors.
   c. Clean overbed table.
   Rationale: Clean, uncluttered environment enhances appetite.
2. Prepare client for meal:
   a. Help client urinate or defecate.
   b. Help client wash face and hands.
   c. Assist with oral hygiene
   d. Help client apply dentures, glasses, or special appliances.
   e. Assist to upright position in bed or chair.
   Rationale: Comfort and optimal physical condition stimulate appetite and help client ingest meal.
3. Wash your hands before touching meal tray.
   Rationale: Clean hands help prevent transfer of microorganisms.
4. Check client's tray against diet order.
   Rationale: Diets are prepared for specific clients.
5. Place tray on overbed table and move in front of client.
6. Prepare tray. Open cartons, remove lids, season food, cut food into bite-size pieces.
   Rationale: Clients with impaired physical or cognitive function may be unable to prepare food for eating.
7. Place a napkin or towel under client's chin, and cover clothing.
8. If client can feed self, the nurse may leave at this point. Return after 10 to 15 minutes to determine if client is tolerating diet.
   Rationale: Self-care enhances feelings of independence and positive self-esteem.
   Note: Do not leave clients with overly hot liquids or food unless they are fully independent with feeding.
   Rationale: Decreased sensation or lack of motor coordination could result in burns from hot foods or liquid.

9.A. If client can sit in a chair but needs help to eat, sit in chair facing client.

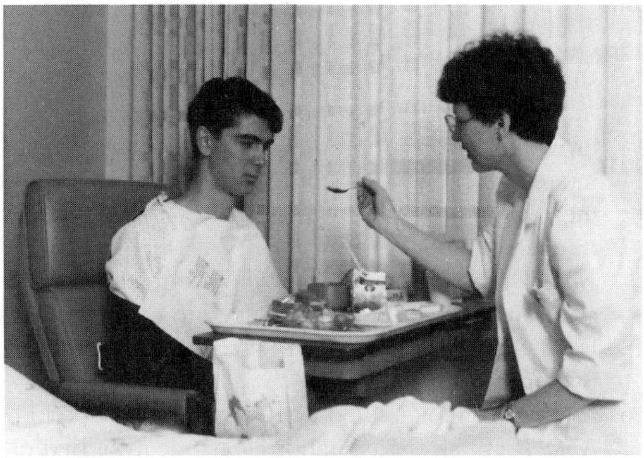

Step 9A The nurse assists the client in a chair.

(continued)

9.B. If client must remain in bed, nurse may stand to feed client.
Rationale: An unhurried social impression should be conveyed to client

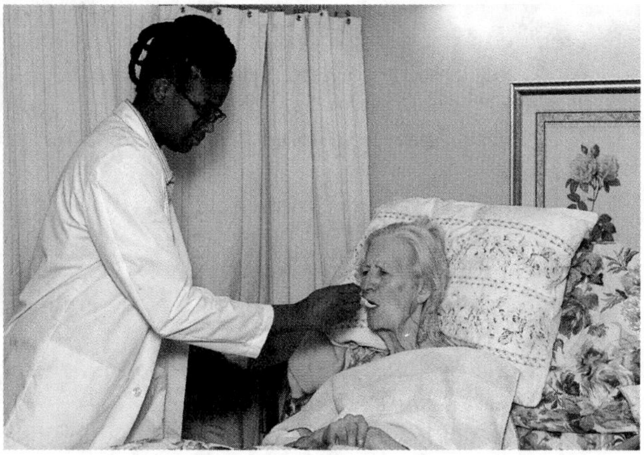

Step 9B The nurse assists the client in bed.

10. Allow client to choose the order he or she would like to eat. If client is visually impaired, identify the food on the tray.
11. Warn client if food is hot or cold.
12. Allow enough time between bites for adequate chewing and swallowing.
Rationale: Allowing sufficient time to eat helps digestion.
13. Offer liquids as requested or between bites. Use a straw or special drinking cup if available.
Rationale: Liquids assist in swallowing.
14. Provide conversation during meal. Choose topic of interest to client. Reorient to current events, or use meal as an opportunity to educate on nutrition or discharge plans.
Note: Do not talk to clients who are relearning swallowing techniques; they need to concentrate.
15. Help client wash hands and face and perform oral hygiene after meal.
16. Assist to comfortable position, and allow rest period.
Note: If at risk for aspiration, leave head of bed elevated for 30 minutes after eating.
17. Record fluids and amount of meal consumed, if ordered.
Rationale: Documentation allows for monitoring of fluids and nutritional status.
18. Remove and dispose of tray.
19. Wash your hands.

Lifespan Considerations

Infant

- Infants do not usually need food other than breast milk or formula until 4 to 6 months of age. Strained or blended foods may be introduced at that time.
- Infant cereal is recommended as first solid because of its iron content.
- At 6 months of age, infants are interested in self-feeding with a spoon or teething crackers.

Toddler

- Toddlers are often independent and insist on feeding themselves.
- Appropriate "finger foods" include meatballs, hard-boiled eggs, cooked carrots, peas, fruit slices (without skins), cheese pieces, dry cereal, crackers.

Preschool

- This is a period of slow growth, so a decrease in appetite can be expected.
- Using foods in color games and allowing the child to help with food preparation (stirring gelatin and pudding, peeling oranges, washing vegetables) stimulate the child's interest and teach good eating habits.

Adolescent

- Ages 10 to 11 (girls) and 12 to 13 (boys) are a period of rapid growth. Larger consumption of nutrients and calories is needed.
- Girls beginning menstruation need increased iron in their diets.

Older Adult

- Elderly patients may have diminished appetites from loss of taste and smell and decreased number of taste buds.
- Many older adults wear dentures. Poorly fitting dentures can impair their ability and desire to eat properly
- Fewer calories are usually needed in this age group because of decreased activity and slowing metabolism.

Home Care Modifications

- Loneliness and poverty may decrease a client's ability or interest in eating balanced meals at home.
- Federal programs, such as food stamps and supplemental security income, can increase the food-buying power for clients at home.
- In 1972, a federally funded nutrition program for the elderly was instituted that provides low-cost, nutritious meals served in community settings. These programs also provide socialization for lonely elderly.

Nursing Interventions for Altered Function

Nursing responsibility for the client with altered nutrition includes providing special diets and nutritional supplements and monitoring nutritional therapies, such as TPN and tube feedings. Client teaching is important in each of these therapies.

Withholding Food

The term *NPO*, or nothing by mouth (Latin, *non per os*), is used when clients cannot ingest food or fluids orally. Withholding food may be indicated in the following situations:

- To rest the GI tract to promote healing
- To clear the GI tract of contents before surgery or diagnostic procedures
- To prevent aspiration during surgery or in high-risk clients
- To give normal intestinal motility time to return during the postoperative period
- To treat severe vomiting or diarrhea
- To treat medical problems, such as bowel obstruction or acute inflammation of the GI tract

Well-nourished clients can tolerate lack of food for a few days, but fluids must be provided to prevent fluid and electrolyte disturbances. Some clients find it difficult to be unable to eat. The following nursing measures can promote comfort during this period:

- Provide frequent oral hygiene.
- Give ice chips, hard candy, and gum or mouth rinses if permitted.
- Avoid exposure to people eating or advertisements for food.

If the NPO period is longer than a few days, alternate forms of nutritional support may be necessary.

> ***Safety Alert***
> *Feeding Clients*
>
> - Keep hot liquids away from toddlers or confused clients who may accidentally spill them.
> - When ability to swallow is questionable, never give oral food or fluids until a complete evaluation is done.
> - Sit clients upright when eating to minimize the chance of accidental aspiration.
> - Use caution when using microwave ovens to reheat food. Burns can result from steam when containers are opened or if portions of the food become very hot.
> - Always check proper tube placement before beginning tube feedings to prevent accidental aspiration of feedings.
> - Dilute infant formulas or tube feedings according to manufacturer's specifications to avoid administering highly osmotic solutions, which could cause significant fluid and electrolyte imbalances.
> - Be familiar with the Heimlich maneuver, and use it to dislodge aspirated food particles if the client cannot independently clear airway.

Special Diets

Dietary intake must often be altered to promote healing and restore health. Objectives of dietary treatment may be to increase or decrease weight, allow an organ to rest, remedy nutritional deficits, promote healing, and provide nutrients the body can metabolize.

When a client can eat any food, the diet called general, regular, or house. A regular diet is well balanced and supplies the metabolic requirements of a sedentary person (about 2,000 calories/d). Menus allow the client to select from a wide variety of choices, but all offerings are nutritionally planned to supply recommended daily allowances. Special requests or preferences (such as vegetarian or kosher diets) and food allergies should be reported to the dietary department when the client is admitted.

It may be necessary to modify the diet's texture, consistency, calories, or other nutrients if the client has had surgery or has a medical condition that requires an altered diet (Fig. 37-6). Modifications of consistency are clear liquid, full liquid, soft, and mechanical soft.

Clear Liquid. This diet includes only liquids that lack residue, such as juices without pulp (eg, apple, cranberry), tea, gelatin, soda pop, and clear broth. It is used as a first diet postoperatively, before some diagnostic tests, and after an acute episode of vomiting or diarrhea.

Full Liquid. A full liquid diet includes all fluids and foods that become liquid at room temperature (ice cream, sherbet). This diet may be ordered postoperatively after a clear liquid diet has been well tolerated or for clients who cannot chew food adequately.

Soft. Soft diets include soft foods and those with reduced fiber content, which require less energy for digestion. Soft diets are appropriate for the person who has difficulty chewing or who has no teeth. *Mechanical soft* diets are further chopped or pureed. Soft diets also may be used for the postopertive client as the diet progresses from full liquid.

Diet as Tolerated. Diet as tolerated is ordered when the client's ability to tolerate certain foods may change, such as during the postoperative period or after GI dis-

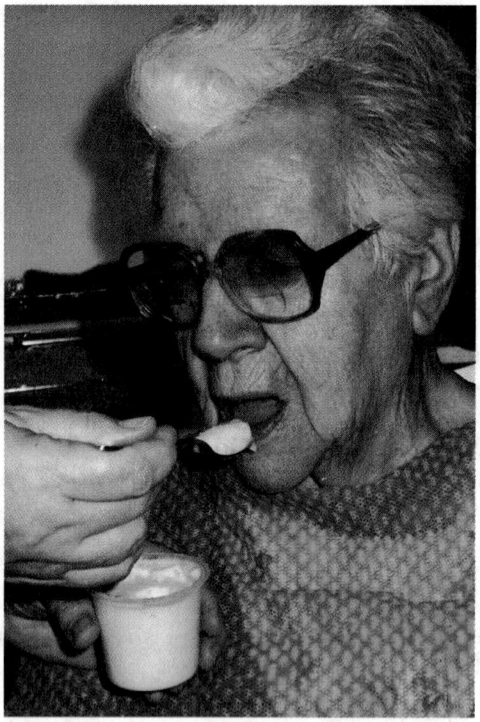

Figure 37-6 • Special diets are planned for some clients.

tress. The nurse orders the diet based on the client's appetite and ability to eat. For example, on the first postoperative day, a client may be given a clear liquid diet. If no nausea occurs, normal intestinal motility has returned, and the client feels like eating, the diet may be advanced to a regular diet.

Restrictive Diets. Diets may be ordered to fulfill a special requirement in a client with chronic disease or altered metabolism. For example, a client with cardiac problems may need to limit sodium and cholesterol, an obese client may need calorie restriction, and a diabetic client may follow a prescribed American Diabetes Association diet. Examples of such dietary modifications for different diseases are given in Table 37-4. Such dietary restrictions must be considered, because any food or fluid given must fit the restrictions.

When a client is placed on a restrictive diet, teaching must promote necessary dietary changes. The dietician may do initial diet teaching, and the nurse reinforces such teaching. Written materials are available to assist in client teaching. Changes in long-established eating patterns are difficult for many clients, and goals must be realistic and individualized for each client.

Nutritional Supplements

Nutritional supplements may be added to the prescribed diet to provide necessary nutrients, especially during periods of increased metabolic demand. Supplements can take the form of protein-rich formulas or vitamins and minerals. Protein supplements, such as Ensure, can be requested by the nurse and ordered by the physician. These supplements are typically milkshake-type drinks given between meals three or four times a day to increase calorie and protein intake. Malnourished clients or clients with excessive metabolic demand from trauma, fever, infection, surgery, or cancer benefit from such therapy.

Enteral Tube Feedings

Enteral nutrition is the direct delivery of nutrients into the GI system. Tube feedings are nutritionally balanced commercial formulas that are given through a tube directly into the esophagus, stomach, jejunum, or duodenum. Access to the GI system can be achieved by inserting a tube through the nose into the stomach or intestine.

Table 37-4 • Dietary Modifications for Diseases

Disease	Modification
Renal disease	Restrict intake of sodium, potassium, protein, and possibly fluids.
Liver disease (cirrhosis)	Restrict intake of sodium; increase intake of protein, unless hepatic coma is pending; then protein is virtually eliminated.
Congestive heart failure	Restrict intake of sodium and calories.
Coronary artery disease	Restrict intake of sodium, calories, and fats (saturated fats and cholesterol).
Burns	Increase intake of calories, protein, vitamin C, and the B-complex vitamins.
Respiratory (emphysema)	A soft, high-calorie, high-protein diet is recommended.
Tuberculosis	Increase intake of protein, calories, calcium, and vitamin A.
Hypertension	Restrict sodium intake; lose weight, if appropriate.

If long-term tube feedings are likely, a surgical procedure is performed to create an opening directly into the stomach or intestines through which feedings can be directly administered. A *gastrostomy* is an opening into the stomach. A newer procedure for gastrostomy placement involves endoscopic percutaneous insertion of a mushroom catheter into the stomach (Fig. 37-7). Known as *percutaneous endoscopic gastrostomy,* this procedure is safer and less expensive because it does not require a general anesthetic and can often be done on an ambulatory basis (Starkey, et al., 1988). Because GI motility is not decreased by surgery or anesthesia in this procedure, feedings can start immediately. An opening into the jejunum (*jejunostomy*) is often used when aspiration has been a problem (Eisenberg, 1989). A *gastrostomy/jejunostomy* tube can be inserted if decompression is necessary along with feeding. A double-lumen tube allows feeding to enter the jejunum while a second lumen drains the stomach (Eisenberg, 1989).

Indications. Tube feedings provide nutrition to clients who cannot swallow or who have an esophageal obstruction. Obstruction can occur secondary to edema from head or neck surgery or trauma (eg, swallowing caustic substances or inhaling smoke). Tube feedings also are indicated when the client's decreased level of consciousness prevents safe eating. Tube feedings can be used as adjunctive therapy for clients who can eat but who cannot consume adequate nutrients to meet the nutritional demands of the body (eg, cancer clients). Premature infants who have an inadequate sucking reflex or lack of strength to feed also can be fed through gavage. Tube feedings are appropriate only when the client can absorb nutrients from the GI tract (Fig. 37-8).

Types of Tubes. The type of tube used to deliver enteral feedings depends on where and how the feeding is delivered. A nasogastric tube, such as a Levin tube, can be used for short-term tube feedings. Because such tubes are relatively rigid and have a large diameter compared with the nasal passage, discomfort and mucosal breakdown are common with prolonged therapy. More flexible, small-bore tubes have been developed when long-term feeding is indicated, but a surgical opening of the GI tract is undesirable. These tubes vary in size from 6 to 12 French and are composed of polyurethane, silicon, or polyvinyl chloride. Most have weighted distal tips and are placed using a stylet. The tubes are radiopaque so that tube placement can be confirmed by x-ray. Nasogastric tubes are attached to the nose with tape.

Tubes that are surgically placed in the stomach or intestines are usually larger in diameter and made of plastic or rubber. Initially, they are sutured in place to prevent leakage and avoid dislodgement. Aseptic care of the incision is important until healing has occurred. The tube can be clamped off between feedings. When the incision has healed, the tube can be removed and reinserted when feeding is required.

Enteral Formulas. Enteral feedings consist of nutritionally balanced formulas. Many brands are available commercially; they vary in relative proportions of nutrients and calories, osmolality, and ease of digestibility and absorption. Most formulas can be stored unrefrigerated until opened, but then should be refrigerated to limit microbial growth.

Continuous Versus Intermittent Feedings. Enteral feedings may be given on an intermittent or continuous basis, as summarized in Procedure 37-2. The physician orders the rate of infusion and the formula to be used. Continuous feedings are permitted to flow in at the prescribed rate using gravitational drip method, or they are

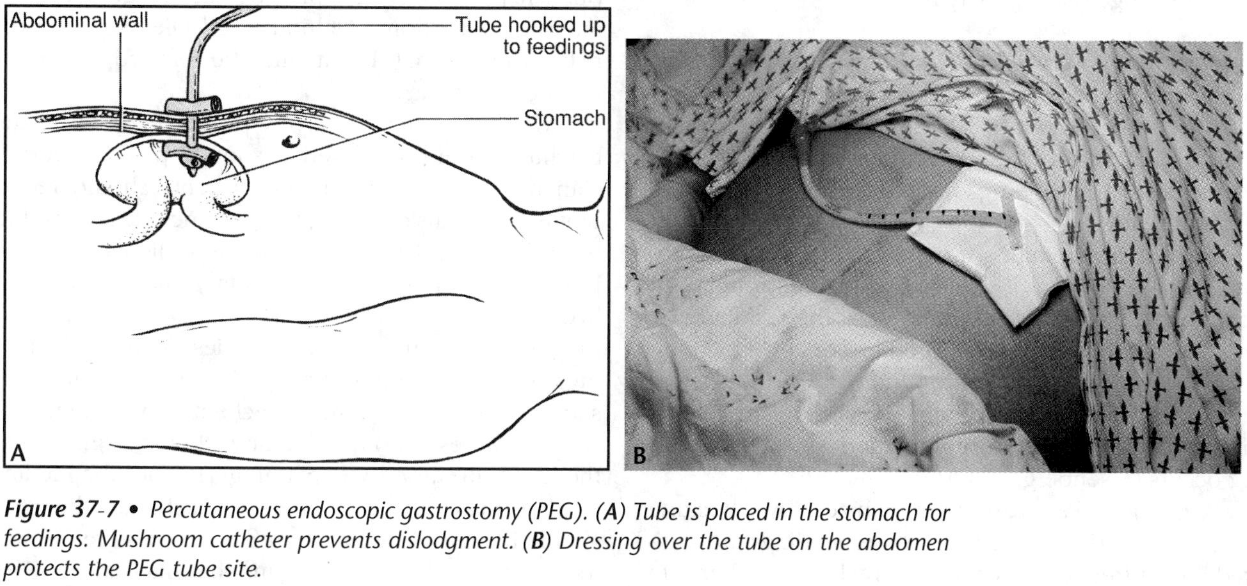

Figure 37-7 • *Percutaneous endoscopic gastrostomy (PEG). **(A)** Tube is placed in the stomach for feedings. Mushroom catheter prevents dislodgment. **(B)** Dressing over the tube on the abdomen protects the PEG tube site.*

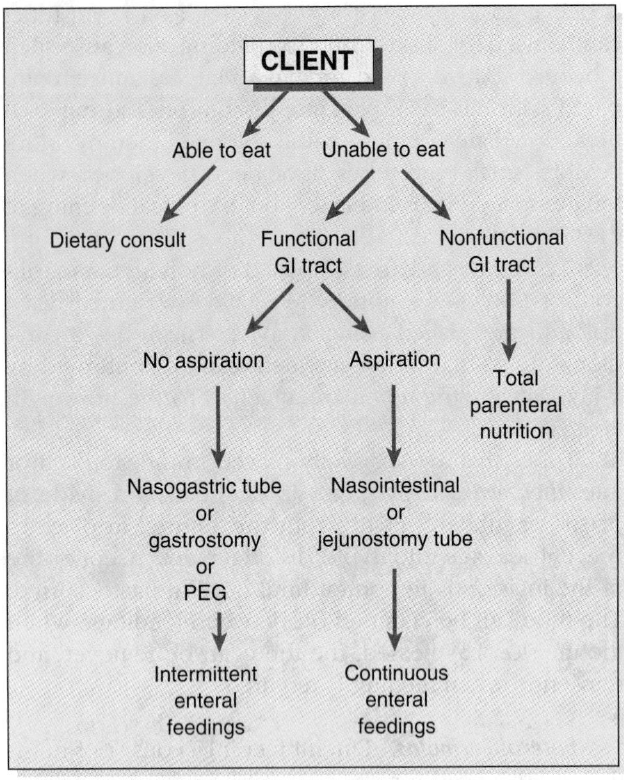

Figure 37-8 • *Indications for selection of different types of nutritional support. (Modified from Eisenberg, P. (1989). Enteral nutrition: Indications, formulas, and delivery techniques.* Nursing Clinics of North America, *24(2): 326.)*

monitored by an infusion pump. For the client who is eating, feedings may be ordered to infuse continuously during the night and are discontinued a few hours before breakfast to stimulate the appetite.

Intermittent feedings are given at specific intervals, usually corresponding to mealtimes. Intermittent feedings should be given slowly over a 15-minute period using a syringe or by gravity flow.

Hazards and Complications. Nursing responsibilities for the client receiving tube feedings include prevention and assessment of complications, such as nausea, vomiting, aspiration, fluid and electrolyte imbalance, diarrhea, intestinal cramping, occlusion of the tube, and hyperglycemia.

Nausea and vomiting usually occur when the feeding is administered at a rate faster than the formula can be absorbed. To assess for this, check the residual volume left in the stomach after feedings or at periodic intervals if tube feedings are continuous. If residuals are greater than 100 mL, the feeding should be stopped or the rate decreased, because aspiration is likely if vomiting occurs (Eisenberg, 1989).

Aspiration also can be minimized by checking proper placement of the tube before feedings are initiated and at frequent intervals and by keeping clients in Fowler's position at all times when feedings are infusing and for 30 minutes after an intermittent feeding. Blue food coloring can be added to the formula of clients at risk for aspiration. If blue-tinged respiratory secretions are produced, aspiration has probably occurred.

Diarrhea, intestinal cramping, and fluid loss are related to the high osmolality of the formulas used. Diluting the concentration by adding water or giving the client adequate free water may present severe osmotic fluid shifts. Slow administration of room-temperature feedings helps limit GI intolerance.

Feeding tubes, especially those with small-bore lumens, clog easily. Tube occlusion, even for a short period of time, must be avoided. Clogging can be prevented by frequent flushing of the tube with water, especially after giving medications.

Hyperglycemia may occur in clients who cannot produce enough insulin to deal with the carbohydrate load in the formula. For diabetic clients and any high-risk person, blood glucose monitoring permits careful regulation of increased insulin need.

Community-Based Nursing

Nutrition is an important consideration in independent management at home. The nurse should assess whether the client can buy, prepare, and eat food; often clients need assistance with shopping or cooking. Family and friends may be available to help for a short time. The nursing plan of care should reflect the client's needs and support from others, if necessary. Nurses can enlist the help of others to provide services for the client.

Clients with chronic health problems pose greater nutritional challenges. Many local and national agencies, such as the American Cancer Society, American Heart Association, and American Diabetes Association, publish pamphlets that provide dietary guidance and realistic suggestions. Malnourished clients or those at risk for nutritional deficits may be referred to community health agencies.

When new restrictive diets are ordered for clients, teaching should be started as soon as possible. A dietician may begin the teaching. Clients should receive written materials outlining foods to include and exclude from the diet. The nurse can help clients determine how best to incorporate the dietary changes into their lives.

Nutritional support technologies, such as tube feedings or TPN, are often managed at home. In many instances, the nurse teaches the client how to administer such therapies at home. Teaching should begin early in the hospitalization by explaining TPN or tube feedings as they are performed. Before discharge, the client should be able to demonstrate necessary administration techniques and solve problems that may occur. When

Procedure 37-2
Administering Nutrition Via Nasogastric or Gastrostomy Tube

Purpose

1. Provide enteral nutrition for clients who cannot swallow or who have an esophageal obstruction.
2. Provide nutrition to comatose or semiconscious clients.
3. Provide additional nutrients for clients who cannot orally consume total caloric requirements.

Assessment

- Assess client's nutritional status and identify need for tube feedings:
  - Impaired swallowing
  - Decreased level of consciousness
  - Head, neck, or facial surgery or trauma
  - Extraordinary caloric requirements
  - Review chart for food allergies and physician's order as to type, amount, rate, route, and frequency of feeding.
- Assess client's GI system:
  - Observe and palpate for distention, tenderness.
  - Auscultate bowel sounds.
  - Determine time of last bowel movement.
  - Assess for presence of existing feeding tube.

Equipment

Formula
Blue food coloring (optional)
Disposable gavage bag and tubing
60-cc catheter tip irrigation syringe
Infusion pump (optional)
Water
Measuring container

Procedure

1. Wash your hands.
2. Close room door or curtains around bed.
   Rationale: Privacy decreases embarrassment.
3. Explain procedure to client.
4. Help client to high-Fowler's position by elevating head of bed at least 60 degrees or assisting to a chair. If high-Fowler's position is contraindicated, help client to a right side-lying position with head slightly elevated.
   Rationale: Positions prevent aspiration of formula into lungs and facilitate flow of feeding into intestine.
5. Confirm placement of tube in stomach:
   a. Attach 60-mL irrigation syringe to tube and inject 10 mL of air while auscultating over epigastrium.

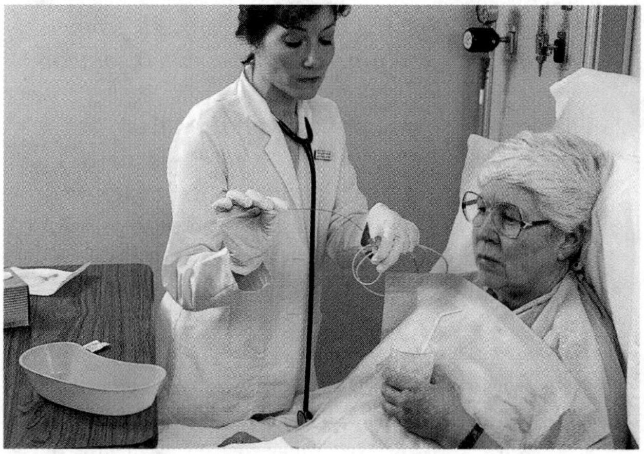

Step 4 The client is in a high-Fowler's position.

   Rationale: Air can be heard entering stomach.
   Note: Auscultation of air is not always a reliable index of tube placement when a small-bore feeding tube is used.
   b. Aspirate all stomach contents, and measure for residual.
   Rationale: Presence of gastric fluid confirms tube placement in the stomach. Gastric residuals are checked to evaluate if gastric emptying is adequate.
   c. If 100 mL or more than half of the last feeding is aspirated, contact the physician before proceeding with tube feeding. The feeding is usually held.
   d. Reinstill the aspirated gastric contents through the tube and into the stomach.
   Rationale: Gastric content is rich in electrolytes. Electrolyte imbalance could occur if residuals are discarded.
6. Prepare correct amount and strength of formula. Formula should be room temperature. Add several drops of food coloring (optional).
   Rationale: Strength and amount of formula are gradually increased to prevent diarrhea and gastric intolerance. Formula should be at room temperature because it will not be warmed or cooled by the oral and esophageal mucosa as occurs in normal swallowing. Cold formula can cause abdominal cramping and discomfort; hot formula can burn the stomach. Food coloring is frequently used when tube-feeding clients are at risk for aspiration. If formula is aspirated, nasotracheal suction reveals bluish secretions. Check agency policy.

Procedure

Bolus of Intermittent Feeding

1. Remove plunger from irrigation syringe. Clamp gastric tubing and attach syringe. If using gavage bag, attach tubing to gastric tube.
   Rationale: Clamping tubing prevents air from entering stomach and prevents stomach contents from leaking out.
2. Fill syringe or gavage bag with formula.
3. Allow feeding to flow in slowly (10–15 min). If using syringe, raise or lower syringe to adjust flow rate by gravity. Refill syringe as needed without disconnecting, avoiding air spaces in tubing. If gavage bag is used, hang bag on IV pole, and adjust flow rate with clamp on tubing.
   Rationale: Feedings given too rapidly cause nausea, vomiting, flatus, and abdominal cramps.
4. Clamp tubing just as feeding is completing. Rinse tube with 30 to 60 mL tap water. Do not allow air to enter tubing.
   Rationale: Clamping tubing prevents air from entering stomach to reduce bloating or cramps. Rinsing with water clears the gastric tube to prevent blockage and bacterial growth.
5. Clamp gastric tube, and disconnect from syringe or gavage bag.
6. Have client remain in high-Fowler's or elevated side-lying position for 30 to 60 minutes after feeding.

Procedure

Continuous Feeding

1. Connect gavage tubing to gastric tube.
2. Hang gavage bag on IV pole
3. Pour in desired amount of formula.
   Note: Usually hang amount of formula to infuse in 3 hours. Check agency policy.

4a. Connect tubing to infusion pump.

4b. Set rate.
   Rationale: If feeding is infused too rapidly, vomiting and cramps may result.

5. Clients on continuous feedings should have gastric residuals checked every 4 to 6 hours, according to agency policy. Then flush tubing with 30 to 60 mL of water.
   Rationale: This assesses for adequate absorption of feeding and verifies correct placement of tube.
6. Have client remain in high-Fowler's or in slightly elevated right side-lying position.
7. Wash any reusable equipment with soap and water. Change equipment every 24 hours or according to agency policy.
   Rationale: Clean equipment prevents inadvertent administration of spoiled or contaminated feeding.
8. Wash hands.
9. Document appropriately.

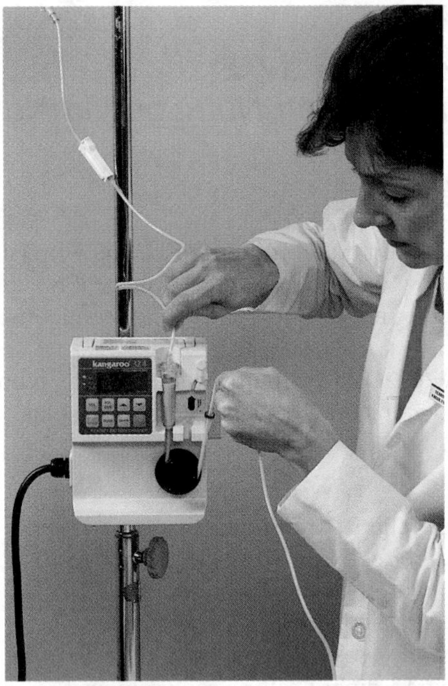

Step 4A Gavage tubing is placed in infusion pump.

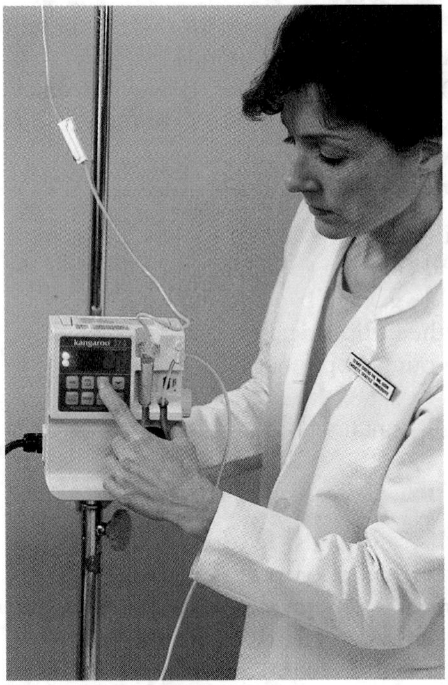

Step 4B The infusion rate is set.

Lifespan Considerations

Infants and Children

- Intermittent feeding and reinsertion of nasogastric feeding tube at each feeding are recommended in children. There is significant risk of stomach perforation, nasal airway obstruction, and ulceration and irritation of the mucous membrane if a feeding tube is left in continuously.

Home Care Modifications

- Clients are encouraged to participate in the preparation and procedure of tube feeding if possible to increase their feelings of independence and self-esteem.
- Client or caregiver must be educated in correct techniques and rationales as stated above.
- Feedings can be provided from commercially prepared formulas or home-blended foods. Formulas may be thinned with juice, milk, or water.
- Caregiver must be taught proper storage of extra formula:
  - Commercially prepared formulas should be sealed and stored in refrigerator once the can is open. Use within 24 hours.
  - Home-blended feedings should be tightly sealed, dated, and refrigerated. Use within 24 hours after preparation.
- Tube-fed clients may feel isolated or may have altered self-esteem and body image from the loss of sensory and social stimulation associated with eating. Feedings can be scheduled with family mealtimes.
- If medically permitted, the client can consume some favorite foods orally. If swallowing is contraindicated, it may be possible for the client to chew and taste a few favorite foods, then spit them out.
- Follow-up and consultation with a home health nurse often allows clients and caregivers to arrange creative solutions to problems or concerns that arise.

possible, family members or caregivers should be included in teaching sessions. Arrangements for equipment and supplies should be made before discharge, and the client should be provided with the name of the vendor.

Governmental programs have been developed for people who need dietary enhancement and nutrition education. Nurses are actively involved in providing education and care through such programs. Community-based programs include the following:

- Senior center services
- Home-delivered meals
- Food stamps
- Missions and shelters
- Women, Infants, and Children (WIC), a nutrition and healthcare program for pregnant women, new mothers, infants, and children
- Child-care centers
- School lunch programs
- The M&I Program (maternal and infant nutritional supplementation and healthcare)

In addition to providing food for groups at risk, many of these services also provide nutrition education and counseling. The Nutrition Education and Training program has been developed to help public schools incorporate nutrition education in their curricula.

Community resources also include the nutritional services of public health nurses, nutritionists, home health caregivers, and welfare agency workers. These people provide education, assistance with meal planning and food buying, consultation, nutrition referrals, and research.

International agencies promote health and nutritional adequacy on a worldwide level. These programs include the United Nations Food and Agriculture Organization, WHO, and the United Nations Children's Fund.

Evaluation

Nursing interventions related to nutrition are helpful if the nurse and client agree that progress has been made toward the identified outcomes. Progress is easily measured by outcome criteria established in the planning phase. The following are general goals identified previously in this chapter with outcome criteria for clients, although goals and outcome criteria are always individualized.

Goal

Client will use nutritionally sound dietary intake to meet body requirements and promote health.

Possible Outcome Criteria

- Within 24 hours, client describes a diet that provides his or her RDAs as indicated by age, sex, and physiologic state.
- Within 3 days, client verbalizes use of proper daily food selection from the food guide pyramid.
- Client uses healthful diet by limiting the intake of saturated fats, refined sugar, and sodium, as witnessed by the nurse at five meals during the next 5 days.
- By discharge, client's skin and nails demonstrate absence of clinical signs of nutrition deficiency or excess.
- During hospitalization, client's blood glucose, albumin, and so forth remain within normal limits as shown in laboratory tests.

Nursing Plan of Care
The Client With Altered Nutrition

Nursing Diagnosis

Altered nutrition: Less than body requirements, as manifested by being underweight, having a low hematocrit, and having an inadequate intake of calcium, iron, protein, vitamin A, and vitamin C.

Client Goal

Client will construct a diet that meets the RDA standards, is psychologically satisfying, can be readily understood, and is relatively easy to prepare or obtain.

Client Outcome Criteria

- Client obtains correct, useful information in which he or she expresses confidence.
- Client describes the basic function of nutrients.
- Client uses a diet that contains adequate amounts of all nutrients to meet the RDA standards.
- Client reports satisfaction with the diet and an increased energy level.
- Client increases weight within the normal range for height, age, and sex.

Nursing Intervention	*Scientific Rationale*
1. Assess client laboratory values (hematocrit, hemoglobin, serum albumin) and physical parameters (height, weight, skin-fold measurements).	1. To detect deviations from baseline and deviations from normal standards so that measures can be taken to correct deficiencies
2. Assess the client's ability to obtain food.	2. To detect possible problems to minimize or prevent financial or physical limitations from contributing to an inadequate diet
3. Assess the client's motivational level and ability to learn and follow the new diet prescription.	3. To detect potential problems to prevent motivational or learning difficulties from interfering with obtaining a nutritionally adequate diet
4. Instruct the client in the new diet prescription, and assess understanding (increased intake of protein, calcium, iron, vitamins A and C, and calories).	4. To provide an improved intake of nutrients, especially those that had been determined to be low
5. Provide the client with written information on the basic functions of the major nutrients; discuss this information with the client, and assess understanding.	5. To provide the client with basic information for personal use; written format assists the client in retaining the information
6. Answer client's questions; discuss areas of concern; provide the client with additional reference material as necessary.	6. To assist the client toward increased knowledge; to relieve uncertainties; to improve knowledge of self-care activities
7. Assess the client family history of diabetes and the client's predisposing characteristics toward the possible development of diabetes.	7. To establish a baseline of information so that potential problems can be prevented or detected early and treated promptly.

Goal

Client will maintain dietary intake adequate to meet energy expenditures of body.

Possible Outcome Criteria

- Within 24 hours, client describes dietary changes necessary to meet adequate caloric intake when demand is increased (eg, pregnancy, lactation, adolescence, trauma, or surgery).
- Client works toward maintaining ideal body weight by exercising daily during next week.
- For 1 month, client uses nutritional supplements (eg, protein supplement, vitamins) during periods of increased demand.

Goal

Client will demonstrate adequate knowledge to adhere to dietary prescription or therapies to promote health.

Possible Outcome Criteria

- After teaching session, client lists foods to avoid on special diet (eg, low sodium, low fat).
- Before discharge, client describes how to alter lifestyle (eating in restaurants, preparing food) to comply with dietary restrictions.
- Before discharge, client discusses realistic use of family and community support groups to ensure adequate nutrition after discharge.
- Before discharge, client or caregiver demonstrates how to administer hyperalimentation or tube feedings.
- After conclusions are reached, the nurse and client can decide whether to readjust previous goals, establish new goals, or terminate goals.

Key Concepts

- Adequate nutritional intake is important to maintain body functions, promote healing, maintain healthy tissues, maintain body temperature, and build resistance to infection.
- Essential nutrients are carbohydrates, protein, fat, vitamins, minerals, and water.
- Complex physiologic processes, including digestion, absorption, and metabolism, permit the body to break down food so that the body can use it as energy.
- Great variations exist in dietary intake among people, but guidelines can be useful when evaluating adequate intake.
- Manifestations of altered nutrition include body weight that is above or below ideal, a recent significant weight gain or loss, decreased energy, altered bowel patterns, and altered skin, teeth, hair, or mucous membranes.
- Nutritional needs vary across the lifespan.
- The health assessment includes collecting subjective data on normal eating patterns, risk factors for nutritional deficits, and identification of altered nutrition.
- Anthropometric measurements (height and weight, skinfold measurements, and arm circumference), calorie counts, and swallowing evaluation can provide objective data to help assess a client's nutritional state.
- NANDA nursing diagnoses in the functional area of nutrition are Altered Nutrition: Less than body requirements; Altered Nutrition: More than body requirements; and Impaired Swallowing.
- Nursing interventions to promote optimal nutrition include client teaching and measures to encourage eating.
- Therapeutic diets are used to promote health, manage disease, or encourage healing.
- A variety of community programs are useful for client referral for nutritional needs.

Critical Thinking Challenges

Now that you have added the many facets of nutrition to your knowledge base, turn back to the situation at the beginning of the chapter.

1. *Describe your immediate impressions, and identify the knowledge and values that led you to these impressions.*
2. *Contrast and compare your assessments for possible biologic and psychological factors related to weight loss.*
3. *Identify and discuss what ethical or legal issues you as a nurse must consider.*
4. *Select other healthcare professionals who might be helpful in this situation, and explain how you think they could collaborate with you.*

References

Curtas, S., Chapman, G., & Megurd, M. (1989). Evaluation of nutritional status. *Nursing Clinics of North America, 24,* 301–311.

DiIorio, C., & Price, M. E. (1990). Swallowing: An assessment and practice guide. *American Journal of Nursing, 90*(7), 38–46.

Dudek, S. G. (1995). *Nutrition Handbook for Nursing Practice.* (2nd ed.). Philadelphia: J.B. Lippincott.

Eisenberg, P. (1989). Enteral nutrition: Indications, formulas, and delivery techniques. *Nursing Clinics of North America, 24,* 315–337.

Eschleman, M. M. (1991). Introductory *Nutrition and Diet Therapy.* (2nd ed.). Philadelphia: J. B. Lippincott.

Linder, M. C. (1991). *Nutritional biochemistry and metabolism.* New York: Elsevier.

National Research Council. (1989). *Food & Nutrition Board Recommended Dietary Allowances.* (10th ed.). Washington, DC: National Academy Press.

North American Nursing Diagnosis Association (1991). *Taxonomy I revised 1991, with official nursing diagnoses.* St. Louis, MO: Author.

North American Nursing Diagnosis Association (1994). *Nursing diagnoses: Definitions and classification 1995–1996.* Philadelphia: Author.

Patrick, M., Woods, S., Craven, R., et al. (1991). *Medical-surgical nursing: A pathophysiological approach* (2nd ed.). Philadelphia: J.B. Lippincott.

Pipes, P. L., & Trahms, P. L. (1993). *Nutrition in infancy and childhood* (5th ed.). St. Louis: C.V. Mosby.

Robinson, C. H., Weigley, E. S., & Mueller, D. H. (1993). Basic Nutrition and Diet Therapy. (7th ed.). New York: MacMillan.

Shils, M. E., Olson, J. A., & Shike, M. (1994). *Modern nutrition in health and disease.* Philadelphia: Lea & Febiger.

Shirreff, A. (1990). Preoperative nutritional assessment. *Nursing Times, 86*(8), 69–72.

Starkey, J. F., et al. (1988). Taking care of Percutaneous endoscopic gastronomy (PEG). *American Journal of Nursing, 88*(1), 42–45.

U.S. Department of Agriculture and US Department of Health and Human Services (1990). *Nutrition and your health: Dietary guidelines for Americans* (3rd ed.). Home and Garden Bulletin No. 232.

U.S. Department of Agriculture (1992). *USDA's food guide pyramid.* Home and Garden Bulletin No. 249.

Wardlaw, G., & Insel, P. (1990). *Perspectives in nutrition.* St. Louis: Mosby-Yearbook, Inc.

Worthington-Roberts, B. S., & Williams, S. R. (1993). *Nutrition in pregnancy and lactation* (5th ed.). St. Louis: Mosby-Yearbook, Inc.

Bibliography

Anastasi, J. K., & Lee, V. S. (1994). HIV wasting. How to stop the cycle. *American Journal of Nursing, 94*(6), 18–24.

Burns, C. M. (1994). Toward healthy people 2000: The role of the nurse practitioner and health promotion. *Journal of the American Academy of Nurse Practitioners, 6*(1), 29–35.

Cheney, C. L., Weiss, N. S., Fisher, L. D., Sanders, J. E., Davis, S., & Worthington-Roberts, B. (1991) Oral protein intake and the risk of graft-versus-host disease after allogeneic marrow transplantation. *Bone Marrow Transplantation, 8*(3), 203–210.

Cope, K. A. (1994). Nutritional status: a basic "vital sign." *Home Healthcare Nurse, 12*(2), 29–34.

Fain, J. A. (1994). Assessing nutrition education in patients with weak literacy skills. *Nurse Practitioner Forum, 5*(1), 52–55.

Hall, G. R. (1994). Chronic dementia: Challenges in feeding a patient. *Journal of Gerontological Nursing, 20*(4), 21–30.

Karkeck, J. M. (1993). Nutrition support for the elderly. *Nutrition in Clinical Practice, 8*(5), 211–219.

Keithley, J. K., & Eisenberg, P. (1993). The significance of enteral nutrition in the intensive care unit patient. *Critical Care Nursing Clinics of North America, 5*(1), 23–29.

Keithley, J. K., & Kohn, C. L. (1990). Managing nutritional problems in people with AIDS. *Oncology Nursing Forum, 17*(1), 23–27.

Killen, J. D., Hayward, C., Wilson, D. M., Taylor, C. B., Hammer, L. D., Litt, I., Simonds, B., & Haydel, F. (1994). Factors associated with eating disorder symptoms in a community sample of 6th and 7th grade girls. *International Journal of Eating Disorders, 15*(4), 357–367.

Kim, I., Williamson, D. F., Byers, T., & Koplan, J. P. (1993). Vitamin and mineral supplement use and mortality in a U.S. cohort. *American Journal of Public Health, 83*(4), 546–550.

Lewis, C. M. (1986). *Nutrition and nutritional therapy in nursing.* Norwalk, CT: Appleton-Century-Crofts.

Margetts, B. M., & Jackson, A. A. (1993) Interactions between people's diet and their smoking habits: the dietary and nutritional survey of British adults. *British Medical Journal, 307*(6,916), 1381–1384.

Melkus, G. D. (1994). Obesity: Assessment and intervention in a primary care practice. *Nurse Practitioner Forum, 5*(1), 28–33.

Merrill, A. (1994). Home care of a malnourished AIDS client. *Home Healthcare Nurse, 12*(2), 39–42.

Merrill, A. (1994). Nutrition intervention for the HIV positive client. *Home Healthcare Nurse, 12*(2), 35–38.

Mion, L. C., McDowell, J. A., & Heaney, L. K. (1994). Nutrition assessment of the elderly in the ambulatory care setting. *Nurse Practitioner Forum, 5*(1), 46–51.

Monaghan, D. (1994). Let us ensure a healthier nation. Community nutrition and dietetics. *Professional Nurse, 9*(7), 482, 484–485.

Mow'e, M., Bohmer, T., & Kindt, E. (1994). Reduced nutritional status in an elderly population (> 70 yr.) is probable before disease and possibly contributes to development of disease. *American Journal of Clinical Nutrition, 59* (2), 317–324.

Schreiner, B., & Brondum, L. A. (1994). Nutrition in pediatric primary care: Assessment and common problems. *Nurse Practitioner Forum, 5*(1), 13–23.

Shuster, M. H., & Mancino, J. M. (1994). Ensuring successful home tube feeding in the geriatric population. *Geriatric Nursing, 15*(2)67–81.

Weigley, E. S. (1994). Nutrition in nursing education and beginning practice. *Journal of American Dietetic Association, 94*(6), 654–656.

Wells, L. (1994). At the front line of care. The importance of nutrition in wound management. *Professional Nurse, 9*(8), 525–530.

Winson, G. (1994). Gastrointestinal problems in patients with AIDS. *Nursing Times, 90*(25), 36–39.

Worthington, P., & Wagner, B. (1989). Total parenteral nutrition: Advances in nutritional support. *Nursing Clinics of North America, 24,* 355–369.

Skin Integrity and Wound Healing

Key Terms

Abrasion
Approximated
Débridement
Dehiscence
Dermis
Desquamation
Epidermis
Eschar
Evisceration
Fistula
Laceration
Macerated
Pruritus
Purulent
Sanguinous
Serosanguinous
Serous
Subcutaneous tissue

Learning Objectives

Upon completion of this chapter, the student will be able to do the following:

- *Discuss factors that affect normal integumentary function.*
- *Identify manifestations of altered integumentary function*
- *Describe normal wound healing and factors that affect it.*
- *List categories of support surfaces used in pressure ulcer prevention.*
- *Discuss nursing assessment of skin integrity and wound healing.*
- *Discuss nursing interventions to prevent pressure ulcers or altered skin integrity.*
- *Explain scientific principles in the application of heat and cold to promote wound healing.*
- *Describe categories of wound dressings and their indications.*

38

You are a home health nurse. You make visits twice a week to a client with a stage 3 pressure ulcer on his heel. The client is recovering from a cerebrovascular accident and receives daily visits from a physical therapist for exercise and mobility. The client's wife is actively involved in his care. You are planning today's care.

You have been building a knowledge base of clinical nursing care as you have studied previous chapters. In this chapter, you learn about the importance of good skin care. You will help your client learn preventive care, and you will learn how to give first aid and care for wounds. When you have finished this chapter, you should be able to work through the Critical Thinking Challenges at the end of the chapter.

Skin, also called integument, is the external covering of the body and is the body's largest organ. It helps protect the body and has sensory and regulatory functions. Disruptions in normal skin integrity can interfere with important skin functions.

A *wound* is a break in skin integrity. Accidental wounds can occur when the skin is exposed to extremes in temperature or pH, caustic chemicals, excessive pressure, moisture, friction, trauma, or radiation. An *incision* is a type of wound created intentionally as a part of surgical treatment. Regardless of the cause of the wound, the body responds to any injury with a complex restorative process called *wound healing.*

The nurse has a significant role in preventing impaired skin integrity and promoting optimal healing when disruptions in the skin or underlying structures occur. The nurse teaches clients how to avoid accidental injury, provides first-aid measures for traumatic skin injuries, manages wound care for lesions or surgical incisions, and prevents pressure ulcers in clients at risk.

Normal Integumentary Function

The nutritional-metabolic health pattern provides the framework for normal and abnormal skin function. The body's nutritional-metabolic function is preserved by the skin and its interrelationships with nutrition, fluid balance, and thermoregulation (Cox, et al., 1989).

Structure of the Skin

The skin, a vital organ, is part of the integumentary system. Various skin appendages are included in this system.

Skin Layers

The skin has two major tissue layers: epidermis and dermis (Fig. 38-1).

The **epidermis** is the outer layer of skin. It is avascular and relies on the dermis for its nutrition. The epidermis specializes to form the hair, nails, and glandular structures. The epidermis is composed of layers of stratified squamous epithelial cells. The thin, outermost layer of the epidermis (the stratum corneum or horny layer) is continously shed in a process called **desquamation**. The major cell of the epidermis, the keratinocyte, produces keratin, the primary material in the shed layer of cells. Basal layers of the epidermis contain melanocytes, which produce *melanin,* the brown substance that colors the skin.

The **dermis** underlies the epidermis and is the thickest skin layer. It is composed of tough connective tissue and is well vascularized. The major cell of the dermis, the fibroblast, produces the proteins collagen and elastin. Lymphatic vessels and nerve tissues also

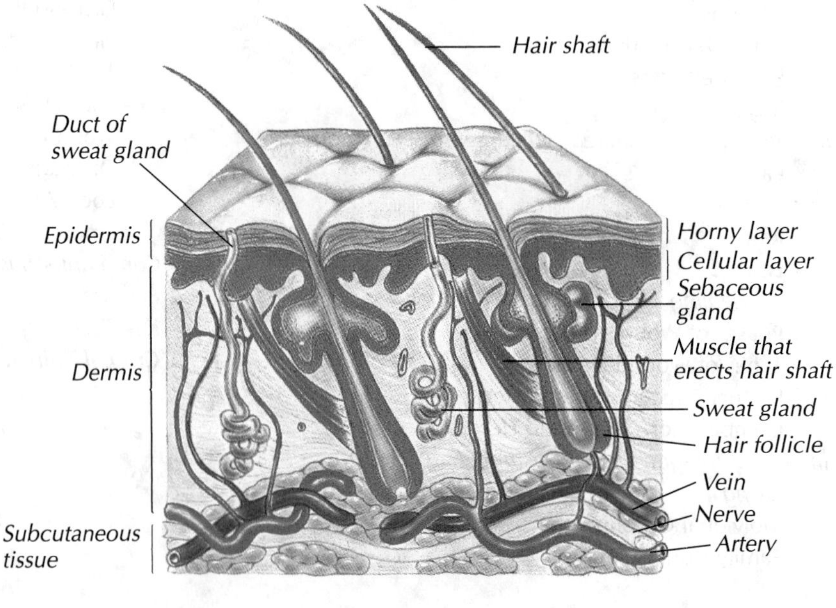

Figure 38-1 • *Cross-section of skin and underlying structures. (From Bates, B. (1995). A guide to physical examination and history taking, 6th ed. Philadelphia, J. B. Lippincott.)*

are found in the dermis. This dermal matrix supports and nourishes the constantly changing epidermis.

Subcutaneous tissue underlies the skin. It consists primarily of fat and connective tissues that support the skin.

Skin Appendages

The skin appendages (hair, nails, eccrine sweat glands, apocrine sweat glands, and sebaceous glands) are formed by invagination of the epidermis into the underlying dermis. Hair consists of keratinous fibers and grows on the entire skin surface, except palms and soles. Nails are formed by rapidly dividing epidermal cells in the nailbed. Hair and nails have no nerve endings or blood supply. The eccrine and apocrine glands are sweat glands; eccrine glands, which are widely distributed throughout the skin, help transport sweat to the outer skin surface, and apocrine sweat glands are found primarily in the axilla and the genital area. The apocrine duct empties into the hair follicle. Sweat produced by apocrine glands contributes to a characteristic body odor when the secretions are decomposed by bacteria. Sebaceous glands secrete sebum, which lubricates the outer layer of the skin. These glands are found in the greatest concentration over the head and upper chest.

Normal Physiologic Function

The skin has many functions: protection, thermoregulation, sensation, metabolism, and communication.

Protection

Intact skin protects the body from physical and chemical injury. Infection is less likely when intact skin provides a barrier to microorganisms. The cells that provide protection are Langerhans' and the keratinocytes in the epidermis and the macrophages and mast cells beneath the epidermis basal layer. Melanin provides protection from the sun's ultraviolet rays. Sebum, secreted by sebaceous glands, gives the skin an acidic pH, which retards the growth of microorganisms. Additionally, microorganisms that inhibit the growth of pathogens are present on the skin. These resident skin flora include *Staphylococcus, Streptococcus,* yeast, and others (Wysocki, 1992).

Thermoregulation

Through dilation and constriction of the blood vessels in the dermis, the skin helps to regulate the temperature of the body and adjust to external changes of temperature. Vasoconstriction produces shivering, which helps the body maintain its temperature in cool environments. Sweating cools the body through evaporation of fluid and dissipation of heat. Large volumes of fluid can be lost through profuse sweating during exercise or warm external temperatures.

Sensation

The skin contains networks of nerves that are sensitive to pain, itch, vibration, heat, and cold. These nerve endings are contained within the dermis, and some extend into the epidermis. The fine hair on body surfaces also provides sensation because of the sensory nerves that surround the hair follicles.

Metabolism

From the sun's ultraviolet rays, the skin synthesizes vitamin D, which is necessary for efficient absorption of calcium and phosphorus.

Communication

The skin provides a means of communication through facial expression and physical appearance. Facial skin and underlying muscles can produce expressions, such as frowning, blinking, winking, and other forms of nonverbal messages. The skin plays an important role in providing some aspects of body appearance and attractiveness. The skin, hair, and nails are often decorated and provide a basis for cultural sex differences.

Characteristics of Normal Skin

Characteristics of normal skin include color, temperature, moisture, texture, thickness, turgor, and odor.

Color

Normal skin tones vary among races, depending on the production and accumulation of melanin in the skin. The greater the accumulation of melanin, the darker the skin tone. In races with darker skins, melanocytes produce more melanin when the skin is exposed to sunlight; skin tones can range fron tan to dark brown or black. The skin color of lighter-pigmented races also varies, ranging from ivory to pink. Areas of hyperpigmentation, such as freckles, normally occur in light-skinned people. Some races have yellow or olive undertones to their skin color. In all people, sun-exposed areas, such as the face or arms, can be darker.

Temperature

Skin is normally warm, but peripheral areas, such as the feet or hands, may be cool if vasoconstriction in the skin has occurred.

Moisture

Normally the skin is dry to the touch, but moisture can accumulate in folds of the skin. Moisture can be felt on the skin if the person is in a warm climate or has recently exercised. Anxiety can increase the moisture normally detected in the axilla or palms of the hands.

Texture and Thickness

The texture of unexposed skin is smooth, but areas exposed to friction (such as the soles of the feet or the palms of the hands) may become rough and hypertrophied. Sun exposure, aging, and smoking also can make skin less smooth. Skin thickness varies depending on the body location. The skin on the soles of the feet may be a 1/4-in thick, but the skin covering the eyelids may be only 1/50-in thick.

Normal skin has good elasticity and rapidly returns to its normal shape when pinched between the thumb and forefinger. As a person ages, skin turgor normally decreases. Skin turgor also can be affected by other factors, such as loss of fluid.

Odor

Skin is usually free from odor, but a pungent aroma is normal with perspiration, especially in the axilla and groin.

Nursing Research
Skin Care and Wound Healing

Selected Nursing Research Studies

Barnes, D., & Payton, R. G. (1993). Clinical application of the Braden Scale in the acute-care setting. *Dermatology Nursing, 5*(5), 386–388.

Bostrum, J., & Kenneth, H. (1992). Staff nurse knowledge and perceptions about prevention of pressure sores. *Dermatology Nursing, 4*(5), 365–368.

Kemp, M. G., Kpanke, D., Tordecilla, L., et al. (1993). The role of support surfaces and patient attributes in preventing pressure ulcers in elderly patients. *Research in Nursing and Health, 16,* 89–96.

Possible Topics for Nursing Research

- What is the effect on wound healing of listening to music during dressing changes?
- What is the effect of dry versus moist cold therapies for pruritus relief?
- What is the incidence of pressure-ulcer development in immobile clients with hemoglobin values less than 9 g/100 mL?
- How effective are various tape-removal techniques on preventing tissue damage?
- What nursing interventions can increase sunscreen use by adolescents?

Factors Affecting Normal Integumentary Function

Normal skin viability depends on blood flow, nutrient supply, personal hygiene, habits, and the integrity of the epidermis. Age-related changes and photoaging due to chronic overexposure to the sun also can affect normal integumentary status.

Circulation

Adequate blood flow to the skin is necessary for healthy, viable tissues. Adequate skin perfusion requires four factors:

- The heart must be able to pump adequately.
- The volume of circulating blood must be sufficient.
- Arteries and veins must be patent and functioning well.
- Local capillary pressure must be higher than external pressure.

Alterations in any of these factors can lead to skin that has abnormal color, texture, thickness, moisture, and temperature or becomes ulcerated.

Nutrition

A well-balanced diet promotes healthy skin. With a deficiency of protein or calories, hair becomes dull and dry and may fall out, and skin becomes dry and flaky. Adequate intake of vitamins A, B_6, C, and K; niacin; and riboflavin is important to prevent abnormal skin changes. Adequate intake of iron, copper, and zinc is important to prevent abnormal pigmentation and changes in nails and hair.

Lifestyle and Habits

Lack of cleanliness can hinder skin health, because washing removes debris, bacteria, and sweat from the skin and keeps pores open and unclogged. Hygiene practices vary widely among people and cultures. Repeated exposure to ultraviolet radiation in the form of sunlight or artificial tanning lights produces characteristic changes, including wrinkling, altered texture, and laxity of the skin.

Knowledge

The client's understanding of skin care and hygiene is an important factor in maintaining skin integrity. The need for cleaning the body is the first step. Skin care is especially important in the heat and direct sunlight of the summer and the cold, chapping winds of the winter. Ill clients should know the importance of frequent repositioning in bed or chair. Parents should be taught how to care for their newborn's skin. Cognitive changes could affect safety when using items such as heating pads, stoves, hot pans, frozen items, and hot and cold water.

Condition of the Epidermis

To maintain its protective function against invading microorganisms, the epidermis should be free from any breaks. The natural moisture of skin should be maintained, because abnormal drying can cause microscopic cracks in the skin.

Lifespan Considerations

Skin changes during the lifespan, with the greatest variations occurring in the very young and in the older adult.

Newborn and Infant

The neonate's skin is thinner and more sensitive than that of the older infant. Superficial blood vessels are so prominent that they give the newborn's skin a characteristic red color. Only the sebaceous glands are active during early infancy. Milia are sebaceous retention cysts that can be seen as white, opalescent spots around the chin and nose. They appear during the first few weeks of life and disappear spontaneously. Fine hair called lanugo covers the newborn's body. It also is lost during the first weeks of life and replaced by hair of a different color and texture. Infants characteristically have long, thin fingernails and toenails that often scratch their delicate skin.

The infant's skin is susceptible to blistering, chafing, and rashes related to friction or irritation. Exposure to a warm, humid environment can lead to prickly heat, and frequent bathing can cause dryness, leading to other skin problems. Exposure to cold environmental temperatures may produce hypothermia because infants have a decreased ability to thermoregulate. Contact dermatitis and bacterial infections can occur from exposure to soiled diapers.

Other common skin disorders of infancy are diaper rash and eczema. Diaper rash can be avoided by keeping the infant clean and dry and by avoiding rubber pants, disposable diapers, or detergents to which the baby is sensitive. Eczema may be an allergic response to foods, soaps, or other stimuli, so new foods should be introduced one at a time into the infant's diet.

During the first year of life, the proportion of subcutaneous fat increases. Raw areas called *intertrigo* may develop in obese youngsters as skin rubs against skin. The proportion of subcutaneous fat decreases in the second year of life, and intertrigo is less common.

Toddler and Preschooler

After the first year of life, the normal child shows little changes in the skin until puberty. As motor skills develop, children are more prone to accidents, which can cause lacerations or abrasions. Falls increase as the child learns new skills (walking, running, jumping) but does not yet have adequate motor coordination. Despite the risk of injury, children must have the freedom to develop their skills. Children often spend an extensive amount of time outdoors. Sunscreen should be applied to protect the skin from sun damage.

Toddlers and preschoolers also are susceptible to burns. Hot liquids should be kept out of their reach, and they should be kept away from heaters, barbecue grills, stoves, and fires. Electric outlets should be capped with protective covers to prevent accidental electrical burns.

Today, more children attend day-care centers or nursery schools, increasing the risk of contracting communicable diseases. The poor hygiene practices of most young children compound the problem of disease transmission in this age group. The importance of handwashing must be taught at an early age.

Child and Adolescent

The skin remains stable until adolescence. Skin integrity is most affected by communicable illness in this age group. Impetigo and head lice can occur, which can be embarrassing for the child and family and can require absence from school. Older children are more aware of their bodies and are concerned when rashes or scars affect their appearance. The nurse can identify rashes in children and institute measures to avoid the spread of infectious diseases that impair skin integrity. The nurse also can provide emotional support for parents and children, so the child is better able to cope with the stress and discomfort of skin disruptions.

During adolescence, pubic, axillary, and other body hair appears. The most common skin disorder of adolescence is acne vulgaris. As the sebaceous glands enlarge at puberty, the production of sebum increases. Acne lesions result from plugging of pilosebaceous glands. Lesions form primarily on the face and neck and to a lesser extent, on the back, chest, and shoulders. Because adolescence is a time when physical appearance is important to self-concept, severe acne can be emotionally disturbing to the adolescent.

Adolescents engage in many leisure activities that involve sun exposure (eg, swimming, outdoor sports, sunbathing). Because excessive sun exposure has been linked to skin cancer, they should be taught to protect their skin by using effective sunscreen products.

Adult and Older Adult

Skin changes are part of the normal aging process. As skin ages, it generally becomes thinner because dermal and subcutaneous mass is lost. Because sebaceous and sweat glands are less active, dry skin is more common as a person ages. Wrinkling and poor skin turgor result from the loss of elastic fibers and collagen changes in the dermal connective tissue. Because circulation to the skin is reduced, healing is slower. Skin breakdown occurs more easily, and tissue repair takes longer. There is less hair and nail growth. The nails may become thicker and brittle, and hair may lose pigment and turn gray. *Pruritus* (itching) commonly occurs in older adults, due mainly to dry, scaling skin.

There is a marked increase in the size and number of benign skin growths in older adults, which can affect the person's appearance and self-concept. *Skin tags* are loose flaps of skin that occur mainly around the neck, eyelids, and axillary areas. *Keratoses* are horny growths that are slow-growing proliferations of the keratinizing cells of the epidermis. *Senile lentigines,* also called age or liver spots, are pigmentation changes that occur on sun-exposed areas. Although many skin changes are benign, older people should have regular skin examinations because the incidence of malignant skin problems increases with age.

Altered Integumentary Function

Potential for Altered Integumentary Function

Allergies, infections, growth disorders, accidental and surgical wounds, burns, and pressure ulcers can significantly impair skin integrity. Any impairment in skin integrity is likely to threaten normal skin function.

Allergic Reactions

Allergic reactions and skin inflammation are responses to injury mediated by histamine release. The reactions may be caused by external or internal irritants. The irritants may be chemical (shampoo, skin creams, detergents, cosmetics, clothing, plants such as poison ivy or poison oak) or mechanical (for example, rubbing against an irritant, such as wool). Berries, shellfish, chocolate, sulfur, and penicillin may cause skin reactions. *Dermatitis* is an inflammation of the skin. Dermatitis most often produces epidermal and dermal damage or irritation and can be accompanied by pain, itching, redness, and blisters. Chronic dermatitis produces changes in the epidermis, including thickening, scaling, and increased pigmentation.

Infections

Skin infections can be bacterial, viral, or fungal. Streptococcal and staphylococcal organisms are responsible for most bacterial infections. Impetigo, which usually is caused by beta-hemolytic streptococci, is the most common bacterial skin infection. Herpesvirus infection is the most common viral cause of skin disruption. Common locations are the lips, face, mouth, and genitals. Many communicable childhood illnesses of viral origin cause rashes. Pruritus often accompanies these rashes and may lead to secondary infection.

Fungal infections can infect nonhairy skin (tinea corporis), scalp (tinea capitis), genital region (tinea cruris or "jock itch"), nails (tinea unguis), and most commonly, the feet (tinea pedis or "athlete's foot"). Candidal (formerly called monilial) fungal infections often occur when normal body flora is disrupted secondary to antibiotic therapy or immunosuppression.

Abnormal Growth Rate Disorders

When the skin is produced at an abnormal rate by malignant or nonmalignant processes, normal integrity can be disrupted.

Psoriasis is a nonmalignant, chronic disorder that greatly increases the rate of skin production; the normal epidermal turnover rate of 14 to 20 days is accelerated to 3 to 4 days. The elbows, knees, scalp, and soles of the feet are common sites for psoriasis. Periods of remission are followed by exacerbations, which can be triggered by stress, infection, or environmental factors.

Benign or malignant *neoplasms* also can affect skin integrity. Most benign neoplasms result from viral infections or normal aging, but most malignant lesions result from prolonged exposure to ultraviolet radiation.

Wounds

Any trauma to the skin, such as a wound, creates a risk for altered skin function. Wounds can be divided into broad categories of accidental and surgical (Table 38-1).

Accidental. Common accidental wounds are abrasions, lacerations, and puncture wounds. An **abrasion** is caused when skin rubs against a hard surface. Friction scrapes away the epithelial layer of skin, exposing the epidermal or dermal layer. Falls onto hands, elbows, or knees cause most abrasions. A **laceration** is an open wound or cut. Most lacerations affect only the upper layers of skin and subcutaneous tissue underneath, but permanent damage may occur if there is injury to in-

Table 38-1 • Types of Wounds

Wound	Description
Broad Categories	
Accidental	Unintentional injury, such as knife, gunshot, burn; jagged edges; bleeding; unsterile
Surgical	Planned therapy, such as surgical incision, needle introduction; clean edges; controlled bleeding; controlled surgical asepsis
Skin Integrity	
Open	Break in skin or mucous membranes; may bleed with tissue damage; infection risk
Closed	No break in skin integrity, but soft tissue damage present; may have internal injury and bleeding
Descriptors	
Abrasion	Wound involving friction of skin; superficial; dermatologic procedure for scar-tissue removal
Puncture	Intentional or unintentional penetrating trauma; made by sharp instrument that penetrates skin and underlying tissue
Laceration	Ragged wound edges with torn tissues; object may be contaminated; infection risk
Contusion	Closed wound; bleeding in underlying tissues caused by blunt blow; bruise
Classifications of Surgical Wounds	
Clean	Closed surgical wound that did not enter gastrointestinal, respiratory, or genitourinary systems; low infection risk
Clean/contaminated	Wound entering gastrointestinal, respiratory, or genitourinary systems; infection risk
Contaminated	Open, traumatic wound; surgical wound with break in asepsis; high infection risk
Infected	Wound site with pathogens present; signs of infection

ternal structures, such as muscles, tendons, blood vessels, or nerves. Accidents involving automobiles, machinery, or knives may result in lacerations. A puncture wound is made when tissue is penetrated by a sharp, pointed instrument. Damage to underlying structures or gross contamination with debris and pathogens may result. Nails, pins, tacks, and other sharp objects are common causes.

Surgical. Surgical wounds vary from simple and superficial (such as a thyroidectomy incision) to deep and contaminated (such as an abdominal incision done for septic peritonitis). They may be divided into several categories (see Table 38-1).

The severity of the wound determines the time for healing, the degree of pain, the probability of wound complications, and the presence of any tubes, drains, or suction devices.

Ostomies are surgical openings in the abdominal wall that allow part of an organ to open onto the skin. Many medical conditions, such as cancer of the intestine or urinary bladder or an inflammatory bowel disease, may require an ostomy. Because the skin surrounding the opening (stoma) may be continuously exposed to feces, urine, or intestinal secretions, skin irritation may develop if appropriately fitted ostomy pouches and products are not used.

Stasis Dermatitis

Stasis dermatitis is caused by impaired venous return secondary to venous disease or structural alterations in the legs. Pooling of blood leads to edema, vasodilation, and plasma extravasation, all of which result in dermatitis by increasing the distance between the blood vessels and the skin they nourish (Torrence, Hovanec, Bartunek, & Brodell, 1993). A stasis ulcer is illustrated in Figure 38-2.

Pressure Ulcers

Pressure ulcers, sometimes called decubitus ulcers or bed sores, result when capillary blood flow to the skin is impeded. These ulcers occur primarily as the result of unequal distribution of pressure over bony prominences. Because of decreased blood flow, the supply of nutrients and oxygen to the skin and underlying tissues

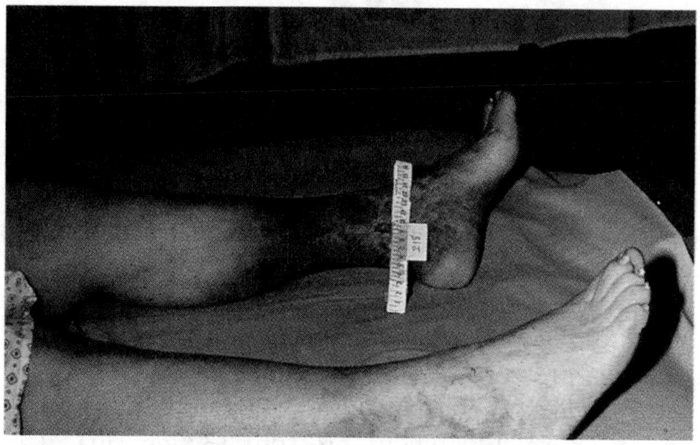

Figure 38-2 • Stasis ulcer on lower leg.

Ulcer Staging by Development

Stage I Ulcer

Nonblanchable erythema of the skin over a bony prominence or area of pressure. Usually stage I ulcers are reversible if pressure is relieved.

Stage II Ulcer

The ulcer is superficial and presents as an abrasion, shallow crater, or blister. This partial-thickness skin loss involves the epidermis or dermis. The ulcer is usually painful. Assessment of stage I pressure ulcers may be difficult in dark-skinned individuals.

Stage III Ulcer

Full-thickness skin loss involving damage or loss of subcutaneous tissue that may extend down to, but not through, underlying fascia. The ulcer presents clinically as a deep crater with or without undermining of adjacent tissue. Stage III ulcers can require months to heal.

Stage IV Ulcer

Full-thickness skin loss with extensive destruction, tissue necrosis, or damage to muscle, bone, or supporting structures (for example, tendons or joint capsule); may have undermining or sinus tracts. Months or years can elapse before a stage IV ulcer heals.

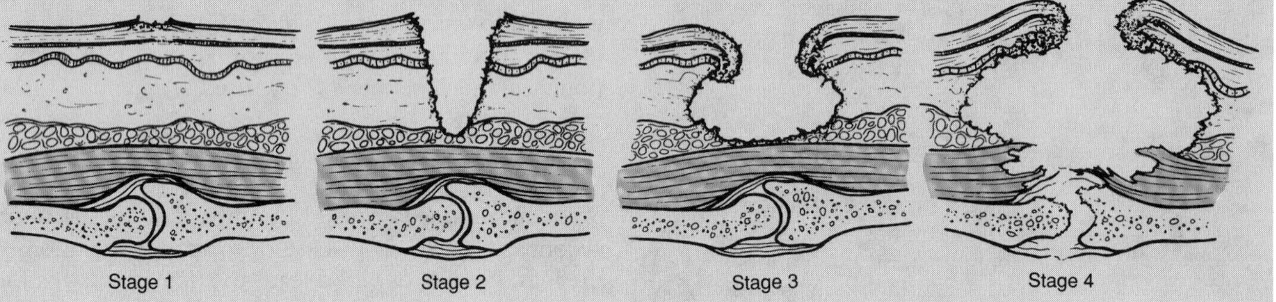

is impaired. This causes cells to die and decompose and an ulcer to form.

Ulcers may be superficial, involving the epidermis and dermis, or deep, involving underlying tissue layers; they are classified according to their stage of development. These are described and illustated in the accompanying display. Infection and sepis may occur because of the destruction of the skin's protective cover and because of the proximity of the blood vessels, which may pick up large numbers of contaminants from the wound. Ulcers may develop a dark black crust, called **eschar**. When eschar is present, accurate staging of the pressure ulcer is not possible until the wound has been débrided.

Risk Factors. Factors causing ulcer formation include increased pressure and decreased tissue tolerance. Pressure can be increased by decreased mobility, decreased activity, and decreased sensory/perceptual ability. Extrinsic factors that decrease tissue tolerance and increase the likelihood of pressure ulcer development are moisture, friction, and shearing force. Other contributing factors are malnutrition, age or low arteriolar pressure. Often the relationship between risk factors ultimately causes a pressure ulcer to develop.

Pressure. When unevenly distributed, pressure can exceed normal capillary pressure (32 mm Hg). The greater the pressure and the longer the duration, the more likely it is that a pressure ulcer will develop. Any rigid object (such as a bed or chair) puts pressure on the skin. When the client is sitting or lying, gravity increases the pressure over bony prominences. Normally, a person unconsciously shifts his or her body weight to prevent the occlusion of capillaries due to increased pressure. Everyone has had the experience of numbness or prickly sensation in an area of the body to which blood flow was impeded due to pressure. However, people who cannot sense increased pressure or who cannot independently reposition themselves (eg, paraplegic or comatose clients) are at risk for the development of pressure ulcers.

Mental Status. Altered mental status can occur when clients are confused, comatose, or on medications that alter normal cognitive processes. When this occurs, clients are less aware of pressure build-up and may not reposition themselves as needed to prevent ulceration. Altered mental status may contribute to incontinence and inadequate self-care, which can increase the potential for ulcer formation.

Moisture. Moisture can predispose skin to breakdown. Skin that is continually bathed in moisture softens, increasing its susceptibility to trauma and infection. Skin continually exposed to moisture becomes **macerated.** Macerated tissue is lighter in appearance than healthy tissue and is damaged more easily. Incontinence often causes the client to lie in urine or feces. Di-

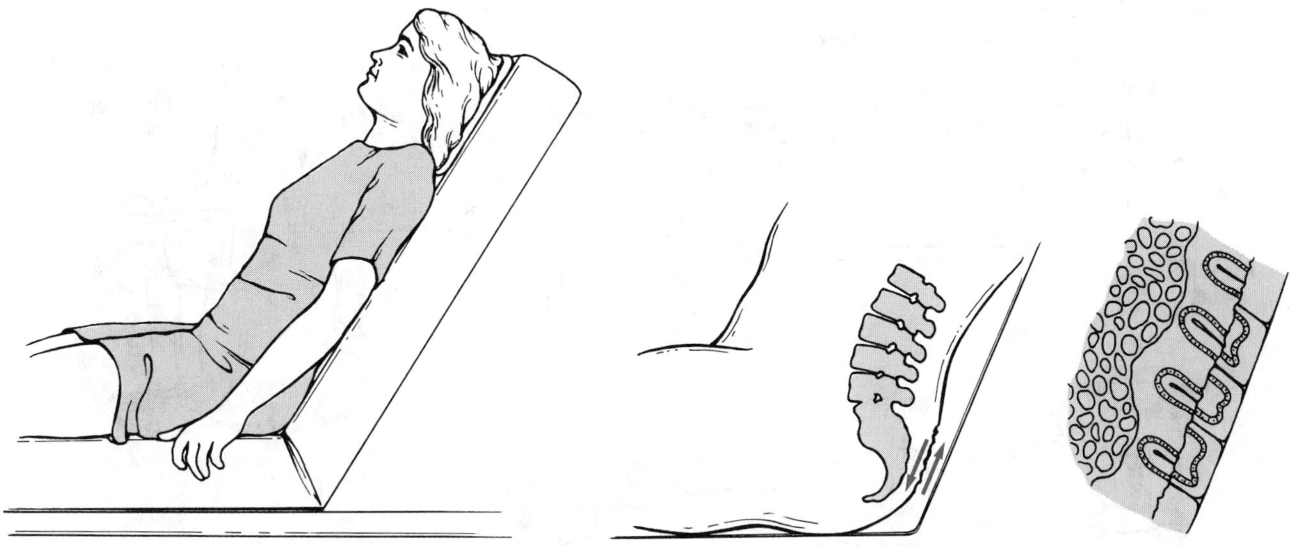

Figure 38-3 • *Shearing force contributes to pressure ulcer development when opposing forces cause capillaries to stretch and tear as the client slides down in bed.*

aphoresis or inadequate drying after hygiene, especially in skin folds, can increase moisture and encourage the growth of yeast, leading to rashes.

Friction. Friction occurs when two surfaces rub together. When skin rubs against a firm surface, such as wrinkled bedding, small abrasions can occur, increasing the possibilty of ulcer formation. Adequate lubrication of the skin and care when handling, moving, and washing clients limits the negative effect of friction.

Shearing Force. Shearing force occurs when tissue layers move on each other, causing blood vessels to stretch as they pass through subcutaneous tissue (Fig. 38-3). Most commonly this occurs when the client slides down in bed or is pulled up in bed. The client's skin remains relatively immobile because friction anchors it to the sheets, but deeper structures, such as fascia, move with the client, as they are attached to the bone. In the process, capillaries in the underlying tissue are stretched and often torn, increasing the risk of ulcer formation.

Nutrition and Metabolism. Altered nutritional status increases the risk of pressure ulcer development. In nutritionally depleted clients, capillaries become more fragile, and as they break, blood flow to the skin can be impaired. Severely malnourished clients experience weight loss, decreased subcutaneous tissue, and decreased muscle mass. This limits the amount of padding between skin and underlying bone, aggravating the effects of pressure over bony prominences.

Common Locations. Pressure ulcers most commonly develop over bony prominences, where body weight is distributed over a small area with inadequate padding (Fig. 38-4). The majority of pressure ulcers develop in the pelvis. When supine, the greatest points of pressure are the back of the skull, the elbows, the sacrum and coccyx, and the heels. When sitting, the greatest points of pressure are the ischial tuberosities and the sacrum.

Burns

A burn involves damage to tissue as the result of exposure to excessive heat, electricity, caustic chemicals, or radiation. Burns range from minor injuries, such as simple sunburn, to major insults that cause significant life disruptions. The degree of damage depends on the type of burn, its extent and depth, and the client's preburn state of health.

Partial-thickness burns may be superficial or moderate to deep. A superficial partial-thickness burn (first degree; epidermal) is pinkish or red with no blistering; a mild sunburn is a good example. Moderate to deep partial-thickness burns (second degree; dermal or deep dermal) may be pink, red, pale ivory, or light yellow-brown. They are usually moist with blisters. Exposure to steam may cause this type of burn.

A full-thickness burn (third degree) may vary from brown or black to cherry red or pearly white. Thrombosed vessels and blisters or bullae may be present. The full-thickness burn appears dry and leathery. Sometimes when fascia, muscle, or bone is extensively damaged, the injury is called a fourth-degree burn.

Thermal burns, the most common type, are caused by contact with a variety of heat sources, including flames, hot liquids, hot surfaces, and steam. Chemical burns are caused by contact with noxious substances. The amount of tissue damaged as a result of chemical injury depends on the concentration of the chemical and the length of exposure. The severity of an electrical burn depends on the type and voltage of the current, the pathway the current takes through the body, and the duration of contact. Radiation burns occur when a

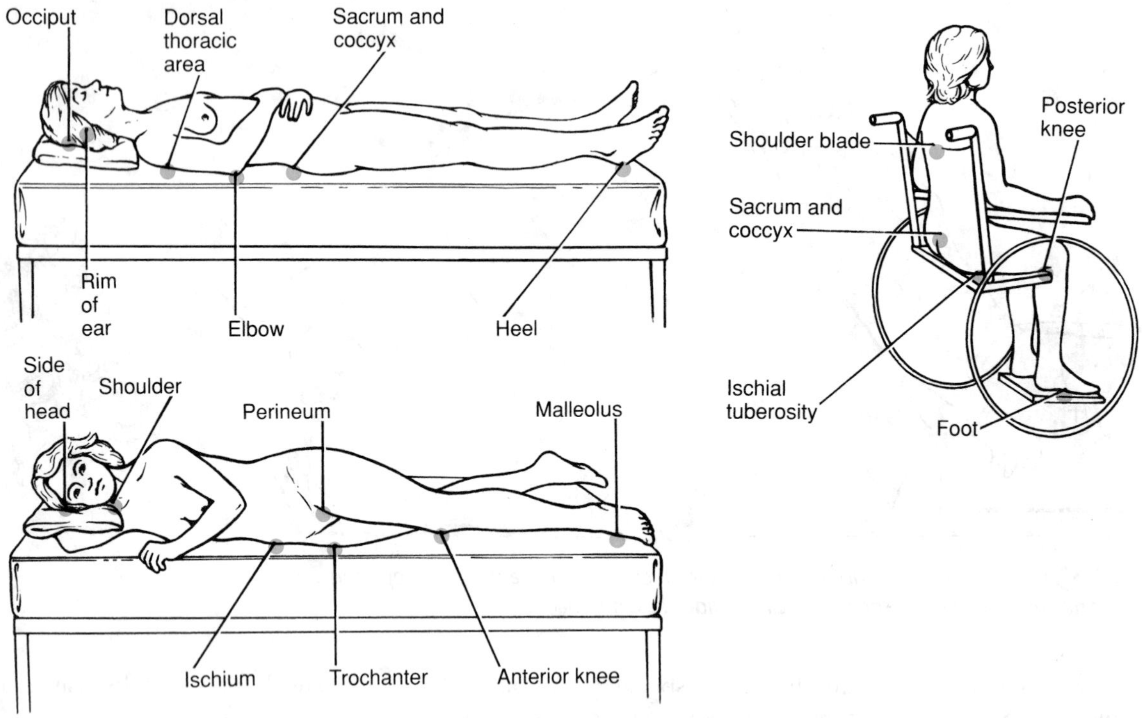

Figure 38-4 • *Common locations for pressure ulcers when supine and sitting.*

person is accidentally exposed to radiation or when radiation is used as a form of therapy. If intense enough, radiation can kill cells through ionization.

Manifestations of Altered Integumentary Function

Disruption in normal skin integrity can manifest as rashes, lesions, open wounds, pain, or pruritus; often more than one of these symptoms may occur. Any break in the epidermal layer of the skin signifies that skin integrity is altered. Often the disruption to the epidermis is evident but may be smaller and less obvious; microscopic breaks in the skin may manifest as redness due to inflammation.

Pain

When the nerves within the skin are stimulated, pain may be felt. Alterations to the normal integrity of the skin can increase the quantity of impulses propagated along these nerves. Destruction of the epidermis and dermis creates exquisite pain, but it is not uncommon for clients to report less pain over time or with pressure ulcers involving deeper tissues.

Pruritus

Pruritus, or itching, is a common symptom associated with many skin and systemic problems. The majority of diseases that cause itching are inflammatory or allergic. Pruritus is often the cause of secondary lesions, because scratching breaks skin surfaces. Common causes of pruritus include the following:

- Infestation by mites or lice
- Inflammatory reactions due to irritants or allergens
- Skin diseases of rapid cell proliferation, such as psoriasis
- Sunburn
- Overdrying of the skin
- Liver or renal disease

The itching sensation arises from a particular pattern of sensory impulses as the result of multifiber stimulation either directly or by release of chemical mediations. Prostaglandins, lymphokines, and opioid peptides are some of the chemical mediators involved in the sensation of itching (Hägermark, 1992).

Rash

Many conditions, such as excessive heat, communicable disease, allergy, or emotional distress, can cause a *rash*, a general term used for a temporary skin eruption. A rash is described according to its characteristics and distribution on the body's surface. A macular rash is level with the skin surface; a papular rash involves solid elevations above the skin surface. A generalized rash covers most areas of the body; a localized rash is limited to specific areas. Pruritus may accompany a rash.

Lesions

A *lesion* involves the loss of structure or function of normal tissue. Lesions may vary in size from a fraction of a millimeter to many centimeters in diameter. Lesions also are described by their characteristics and distribution.

Various terms are used to describe different lesions, as shown in Table 38-2. A *wheal*, which normally occurs from insect bites or allergic skin reactions, is an elevated, irregularly shaped area of cutaneous edema. *Urticaria,* more commonly called hives, is a linear wheal that forms in response to capillary dilatation and passive transudation of plasma. Vesicles, bullae, and pustules are superficial elevations of skin formed by fluid. A *vesicle* is less than 1 cm in diameter and is filled with serous fluid. A *bulla* is a vesicle greater than 1 cm in diameter. A *pustule* is filled with pus rather than serous fluid. *Eczema,* which is a symptom rather than a disease, is an acute or chronic inflammatory condition in which erythema, papules, vesicles, scales, crusts, or scabs appear alone or together. It is a severe form of atopic dermatitis.

Lesions also can be classified by shape, arrangement, and distribution. Primary lesions arise in previously normal skin, and secondary lesions may develop from primary lesions. Examples of secondary lesions include scales, crusts, and fissures. In the acute form of dermatitis, vesicles develop, burst, and ooze, and crusts form.

Wound Healing

When the skin is wounded, a type of healing by replacement occurs. The nature of this healing process is similar for wounds of similar depth, but the time frame for healing depends on the location of the wound, its extent, the regenerative capacity of the injured cells, and the client's overall health.

Phases of Wound Healing

Wounded skin is repaired by regeneration or connective tissue repair. The type of healing that occurs depends on the depth of the injury to the skin.

Inflammation is the first phase of healing in partial and full-thickness wounds. Injury to tissue prompts the responses of hemostasis, edema, and attraction of leukocytes to the wound bed. The inflammation phase lasts approximately 3 days.

Regeneration follows the inflammatory phase in the healing of partial-thickness wounds. Epidermal cells reproduce and migrate across the surface of the partial-thickness wound, which is called re-epithelialization. When epithelial cells have covered the base of the wound, cells continue to replicate, increasing the number of layers of cells in the epidermis to assimilate the thickness of healthy epidermis.

In full-thickness wound healing, *proliferation* occurs after inflammation. Granulation tissue is produced, filling the wound with connective tissue. Granulation tissue consists of a matrix of collagen embedded with macrophages, fibroblasts, and capillary buds. Open wounds (other than primarily closed) undergo contracture during this phase of healing. Contraction can be identified by its effect of pulling the wound inward, leading to a decrease in depth and dimension of the wound. The proliferative phase lasts from day 4 postinjury to about day 21 in a normally healing full-thickness wound.

Maturation is the final stage of full-thickness wound healing. It begins about 3 weeks after the injury and may last up to 2 years. The number of fibroblasts decreases, collagen synthesis stabilizes, and collagen fibrils become increasingly organized, resulting in greater tensile strength of the wound. The tissue generally reaches maximum strength in 10 to 12 weeks, but even after complete healing, only 70% to 80% of the original strength can be expected.

Types of Wound Healing

Wounds heal differently depending on whether tissue loss has occured. The major types of wound healing are classified as primary, secondary, and tertiary intention (Fig. 38-5).

Healing by Primary Intention. Wounds with minimal tissue loss, such as clean surgical incisions or shallow sutured wounds, heal by *primary intention.* The edges of the primary wound are **approximated** or lightly pulled together. Granulation tissue is not visible, and scarring is generally minimal. Infection risk is lower when a clean, surgical wound heals by primary intention.

Healing by Secondary Intention. Wounds with tissue loss, such as deep lacerations, burns, and pressure ulcers, have edges that do not readily approximate. They heal by *secondary intention:* The open wound gradually fills with soft pinkish-red buds that bleed easily **(granulation tissue)**. Eventually, epithelial cells grow over these granulations, completing the cycle. Scarring is more prevalent, and because the wound is open for a longer time, it becomes colonized with microorganisms that may lead to infection.

Healing by Tertiary Intention. Healing by tertiary intention occurs when there is a delay between injury and wound closure. This type of healing also is referred to as a delayed primary closure. This may happen when a deep wound is not sutured immediately or is

(text continues on page 1076)

Table 38-2 • Basic Types of Skin Lesions With Examples

Primary Lesions (May Arise From Previously Normal Skin)

Circumscribed, Flat, Nonpalpable Changes in Skin Color

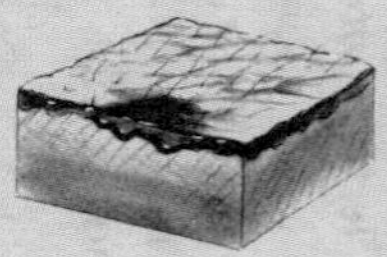

Macule—Small spot. Examples: freckle, petechia

Patch—Larger than macule. Example: vitiligo

Palpable Elevated Solid Masses

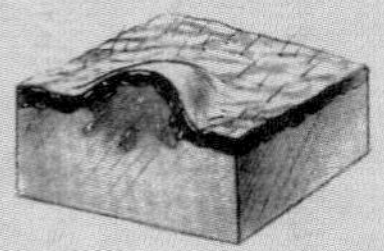

Papule—Up to 0.5 cm. Example: an elevated nevus

Plaque—A flat, elevated surface larger than 0.5 cm, often formed by the coalescence of papules

Nodule—larger than 0.5 cm; often deeper and firmer than a papule

Tumor—A large nodule

Wheal—A somewhat irregular, relatively transient, superficial area of localized skin edema. Examples: mosquito bite, hive

Circumscribed Superficial Elevations of the Skin Formed by Free Fluid in a Cavity Within the Skin Layers

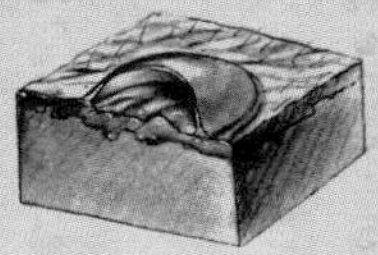

Vesicle—Up to 0.5 cm; filled with serous fluid. Example: herpes simplex

Bulla—Greater than 0.5 cm; filled with serous fluid. Example: second-degree burn

Pustule—Filled with pus. Examples: acne, impetigo

Secondary Lesions (Result From Changes in Primary Lesions)

Loss of Skin Surface

Erosion—Loss of the superficial epidermis; surface is moist but does not bleed. Example: moist area after the rupture of a vesicle, as in chickenpox

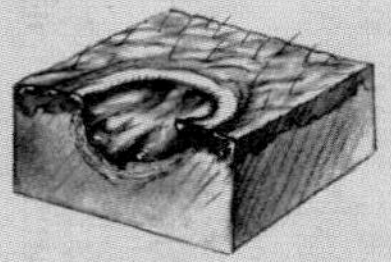

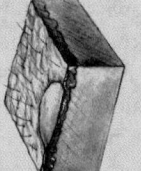

Ulcer—A deeper loss of skin surface; may bleed and scar. Examples: stasis ulcer of venous insufficiency, syphilitic chancre

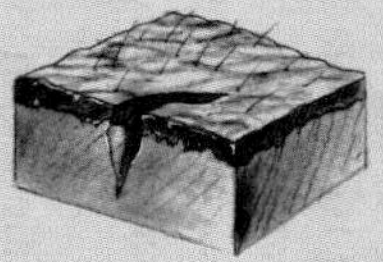

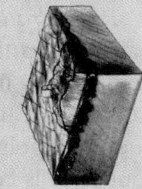

Fissure—A linear crack in the skin. Example: athlete's foot

Material on the Skin

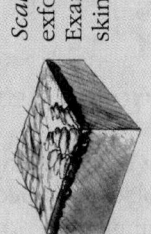

Crust—The dried residue of serum, pus, or blood. Example: impetigo

Scale—A thin flake of exfoliated epidermis. Examples: dandruff, dry skin, psoriasis

Miscellaneous Lesions

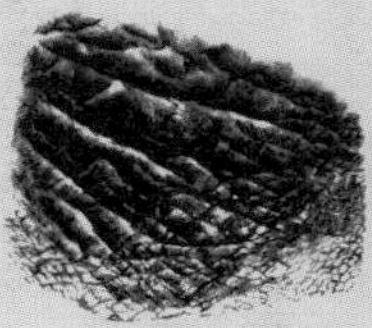

Lichenification—Thickening and roughening of the skin with increased visibility of the normal skin furrows. Example: atopic dermatitis

Atrophy—Thinning of the skin with loss of the normal skin furrows; the skin looks shinier and more translucent than normal. Example: arterial insufficiency

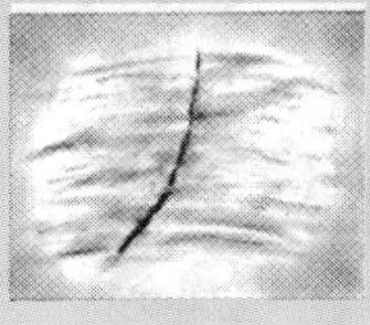

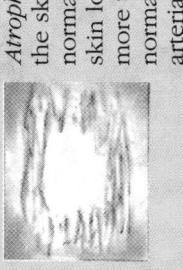

Excoriation—An abrasion or scratch mark. It may be linear, as illustrated, or rounded, as in a scratched insect bite.

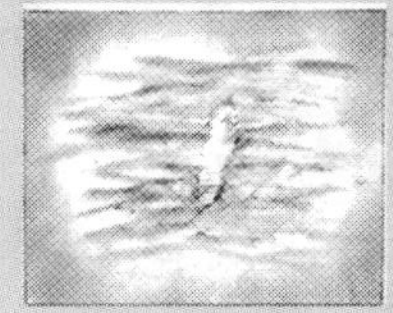

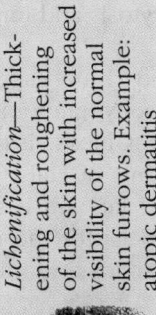

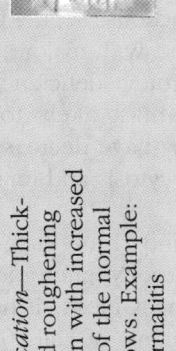

Scar—Replacement of destroyed tissue by fibrous tissue. May be thick and pink (hypertrophic) or thin and white (atrophic), but does not extend beyond the injured area

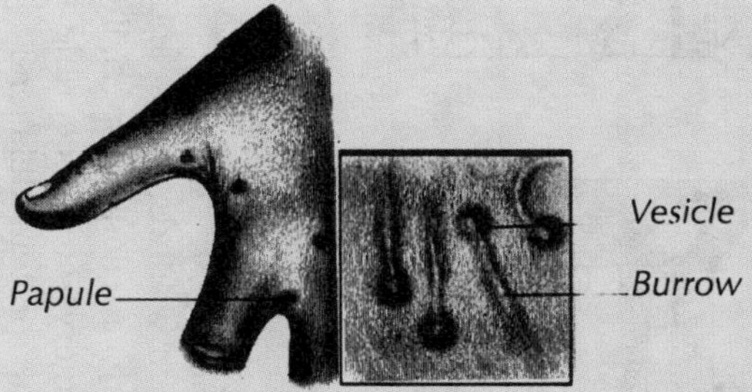

Burrow of Scabies—A person with scabies has intense itching. Skin lesions include small papules, pustules, lichenified areas, and excoriations. With a magnifying lens, look for the *burrow* of the mite that causes it. A burrow is a minute, slightly raised tunnel in the epidermis and is commonly found on the finger webs and on the sides of the fingers. It looks like a short (5–15 mm), linear or curved, gray line and may end in a tiny vesicle.

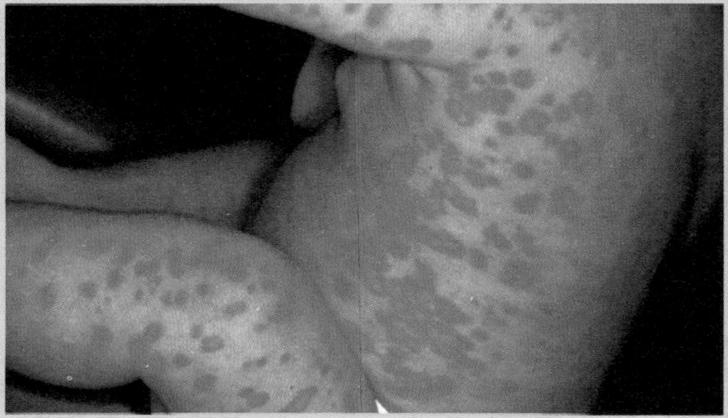

Wheals (urticaria) in a drug eruption in an infant.

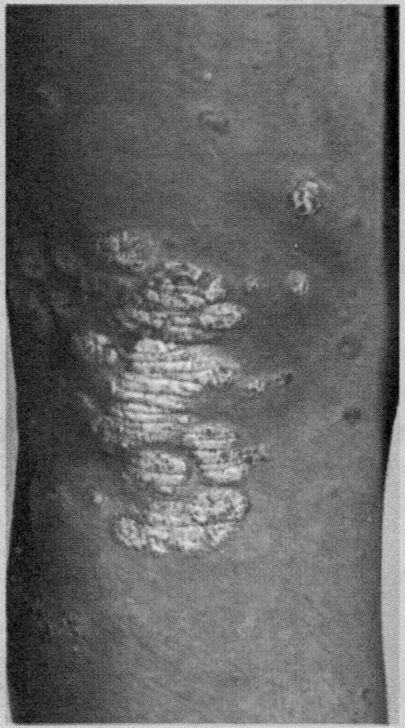

Plaques with scales on the front of a knee (in psoriasis)

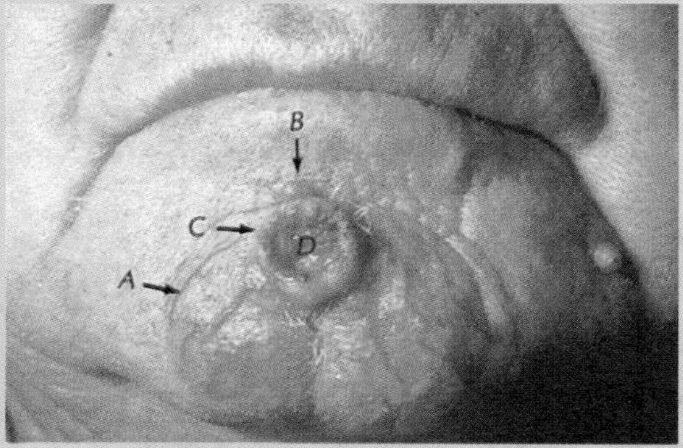

(A) Telangiectasia, (B) nodule, (C) tumor, (D) ulcer (in squamous cell carcinoma)

Source: Bates, B. (1995). *A guide to physical examination and history taking* (6th ed.). Philadelphia: J.B. Lippincott. Source of colored photos: Sauer, G. C. (1991). *Manual of skin diseases* (5th ed). Philadelphia: J. B. Lippincott.

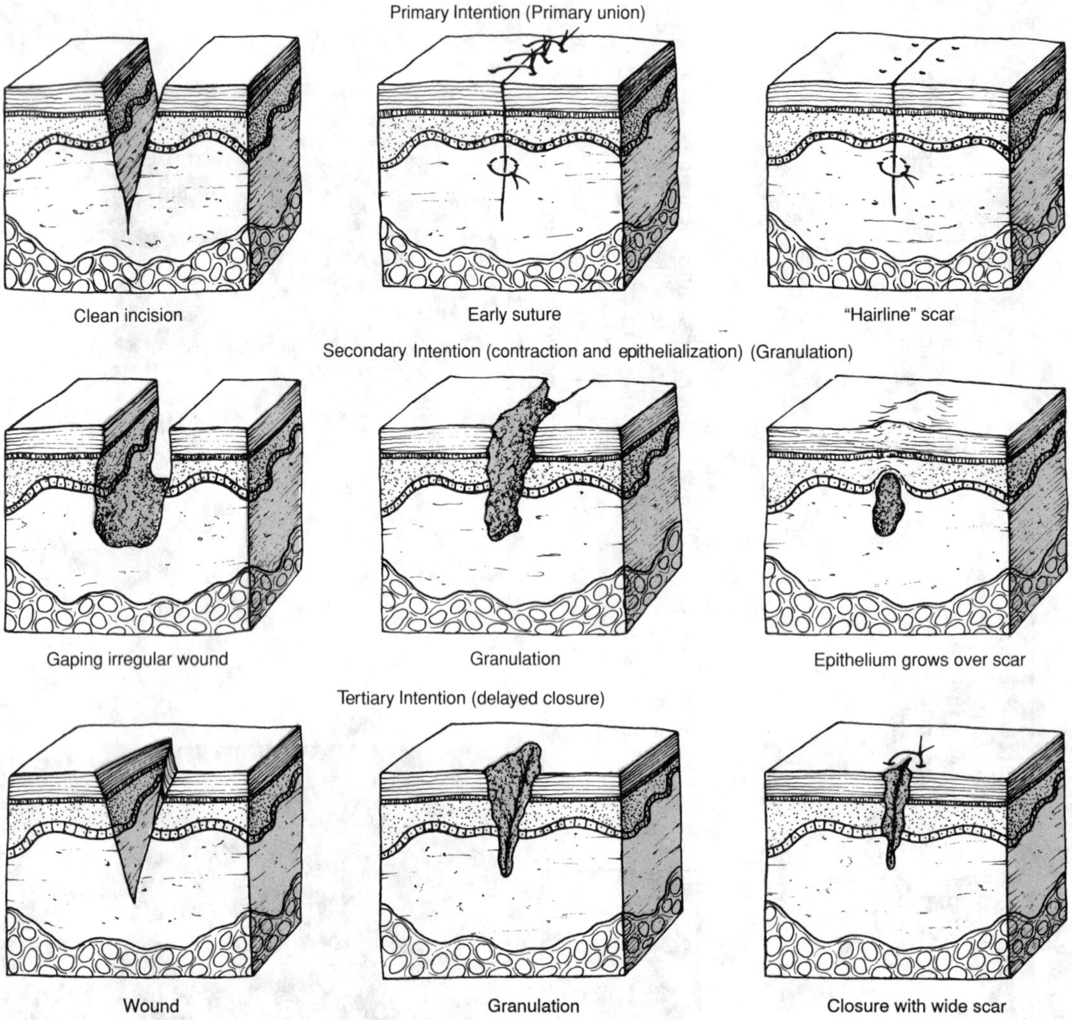

Figure 38-5 • Wound healing by primary, secondary, and tertiary methods.

purposely left open until there is no sign of infection. When a wound heals by tertiary intention, a deeper and wider scar is common.

Factors Affecting Wound Healing

Many variables promote or inhibit wound healing. Systemic factors, such as nutrition, circulation, oxygenation, and immune cellular function, affect wound healing. Individual factors, including age, obesity, smoking history, and drug therapy, also can affect the rate of wound healing. Finally, local factors, such as the nature of the injury, the presence of infection, and the local wound environment, play a part in enhancing or retarding the wound healing process. The type of dressing used to cover a wound affects the local wound environment.

Systemic Factors

Nutrition. Sound nutrition is essential for optimal wound healing. Nutritional deficiencies retard wound healing by inhibiting collagen synthesis. Nutritional requirements increase with stresses, such as surgery, large open wounds, burns, and infections. Septic, burn, and surgical clients (especially those with major abdominal surgery) are susceptible to protein deficiency. Clients with protein deficiencies are most likely to develop wound infections because they have decreased leukocytic functions (such as phagocytosis and immunogenesis).

Protein and vitamins A and C are especially important in healing wounds. Carbohydrates and fats also play key roles in wound healing. Glucose is needed for the increased energy requirements of cells (especially leukocytes and fibroblasts), and fats are essential because they are the building blocks for the cell membranes being formed. Many vitamins and minerals are important in wound healing:

- Vitamin A promotes epithelialization and enhances collagen synthesis and cross-linking.
- Vitamin B complex is a cofactor of enzyme systems.
- Vitamin C (ascorbic acid) is essential for collagen production; with decreased amounts of vitamin C, the tensile strength of the wound decreases.

Ascorbic acid also enhances capillary formation and decreases capillary fragility. It provides a defense to infection by playing a role in the immune response.
- Vitamin K is essential in the synthesis of prothrombin, which is important in coagulation.
- Minerals such as iron, zinc, and copper are involved in collagen synthesis.

Circulation and Oxygenation. Circulation to the involved wound and oxygenation of the tissues greatly influence wound healing. Wound healing slows whenever there is reduced local blood flow, which is why venous stasis ulcers and pressure ulcers are so notoriously hard to heal. Decreased arterial oxygen tension alters both collagen synthesis and formation of epithelial cells (Whitney, 1989). When hemoglobin levels are reduced by more than 15%, such as in severe anemia, oxygenation is reduced, and tissue repair is altered. Anemia may combine with preexisting states, such as diabetes or arteriosclerosis, to impair blood flow further and retard wound healing.

Immune Cellular Function. Drugs and therapies can affect immune cellular function and therefore wound healing. Immunosuppressive drugs, such as corticosteroids, which may be given to prevent organ rejection in transplant clients, also depress the natural defenses against infection and mask inflammatory response. Immunosuppressive agents also usually suppress protein synthesis, wound contraction, and epithelialization (Silane & Oot-Giromini, 1990).

Cancer clients are often at risk for delayed wound healing and infection. Some clients have deficient or defective circulating antibodies. Chemotherapy and radiation treatments often retard wound repair. Chemotherapeutic agents, such as 5-fluorouracil, inhibit fibroblast replication and collagen synthesis, whereas vincristine suppresses antibody production. Radiation therapy negatively affects fibroblastic activity.

Individual Factors

Age. Changes that are part of the normal aging process can hinder wound healing. Circulation slows slightly, compromising oxygen delivery to the wound. Changes occur in clotting process, and the inflammatory response and phagocytosis are impaired, increasing the risk of infection. Fibroblastic activity and collagen synthesis decrease with age, so cell growth, differentiation, reconstruction are slower. Because the scar tissue produced is less pliable, there is a greater risk that the body part will have a functional problem. Impaired healing may result from associated factors, such as poor nutrition, which is more common in the older population, rather than as a direct result of the aging process.

Obesity. Wound healing may be retarded in obese clients. Because adipose tissue is relatively avascular, it provides only a weak defense against microbial invasion and impairs delivery of nutrients to the wound. Obese clients are at increased risk for complications and are often advised to lose weight before elective surgery. In general, surgery on an obese person takes longer, and suturing adipose tissue can be difficult. The potential for wound dehiscence and infection also is greater in the obese client.

Smoking. Physiologic changes occur in smokers that hinder wound healing. Functional hemoglobin levels decrease, impairing oxygen release to the tissues. Long-time smokers have an increased number of platelets, and the platelets are more adhesive. This hypercoagulability leads to the formation of thrombi, which may block small vessels. Oxygen delivery to the tissues may ultimately be compromised, which delays wound healing.

Medications. Many drugs, in addition to those that directly affect the immune response, affect wound healing. Oral anticoagulants, given to decrease potential thrombus formation, increase the potential for bleeding into the wound. Even over-the-counter drugs, such as aspirin and nonsteroidal anti-inflammatory drugs, decrease platelet aggregation and prolong bleeding time. Antibiotics may be prescribed preoperatively for certain operations that carry a high risk for postoperative infection. The prophylaxis is generally given for only a short time, because when antibiotics are used for a long time, the risk of infection can increase, and wound healing can be delayed.

Stress. Physical and emotional stress triggers the release of catecholamines; they cause blood vessels to constrict, decreasing blood flow to the wound. Stress can be caused by trauma, pain, and acute or chronic illness.

Local Factors

Nature of the Injury. Usually, a surgical incision made using strict aseptic technique heals faster than, for instance, a deep wound embedded with gravel from a bicycle accident. The deeper the wound and the more extensive the tissue loss, the longer the wound will take to heal. Even the shape of the wound has an effect: the greater the irregularity, the more prolonged the wound healing process. If trauma has caused hematomas (blood clots) to form, this also can impede healing.

Presence of Infection. Infection hampers wound healing. When debris is not fully débrided or cleansed from a wound, infection is common. Infection may be introduced by inadequate handwashing and poor dressing-change techniques. Infection may result from a surgical procedure, especially when a contaminated area, such as the gastrointestinal or genitourinary tract, is the operative site.

Local Wound Environment. Many factors in the local wound environment affect healing. The pH should be between 7.0 and 7.6; it can be altered by drainage, which may need to be contained or siphoned away for proper healing.

Bacterial growth must be controlled, because infection slows the healing process. The elimination of all microorganisms is not required nor desirable because the normal flora help to regulate some of the events occurring in wound healing. Excess debris and drainage can slow the healing process, yet a moist surface is essential to the activity of the cells (platelets, leukocytes, fibroblasts, and epithelial) at work to heal the wound.

Tension or stress on the wound is a factor in healing. Undue stress can be caused by improper handling of the wound during surgery or any activity that puts tension on the wound during the early postoperative period (eg, applying a dressing or binder incorrectly, stress during movement). Vomiting, coughing without splinting, and abdominal distention can cause tension on an abdominal incision, potentially interfering with wound healing.

Complications of Wound Healing

Inadequate or delayed wound healing can cause complications: hemorrhage, hematoma formation, infection, dehiscence, evisceration, and fistula formation. Such complications can lead to increased mortality and morbidity and at best, delay recovery.

Hemorrhage. After the intial trauma, bleeding is expected, but within several minutes, hemostasis occurs as part of the first phase of wound healing. However, when large blood vessels are severed or the client has poor clotting ability, bleeding may continue. Hemorrhage may occur later in the postoperative period if a suture slips, a clot dislodges, erosion through a blood vessel occurs, or abnormal stress or trauma is applied to the wounded area.

Hemorrhage may occur internally or externally. External bleeding is obvious: bloody drainage, more than normally expected, is visible from the wound. Dressings may become saturated with blood, and blood may even pool under the client. Internal bleeding is less observable and may be indicated by swelling of the affected area, an abnormal amount of bloody drainage from a catheter or drain, an increase in pain, or abnormal vital signs.

Hematomas. A **hematoma**, a localized collection of blood, appears as a swelling or mass underneath the skin surface and often has a bluish color. Small hematomas are readily absorbed into the systemic circulation as debris from the wound, but larger hematomas may take weeks to reabsorb, creating dead space and dead cells that inhibit healing. A large hematoma near a major artery or vein is especially dangerous, because local pressure exerted by the hematoma can disrupt blood flow. Large hematomas may require evacuation or surgical removal to promote optimal wound healing.

Infection. A break in skin integrity, whether due to a surgical incision or accidental trauma, gives microorganisms a portal for entry into the body. Bacterial contamination of the wound can result in infection if the client's defenses are inadequate. The incidence of wound infection depends on the following:

- Local factors: contamination, degree of closure, presence of foreign bodies
- Treatment factors: surgical technique, environmental conditions
- Host factors: client's age, nutritional status, chronic health problems
- Virulence of the organism

Symptoms of an infected wound are purulent drainage, an inflamed incisional area, fever, and an elevated white blood cell count. Wound infections greatly increase the cost of medical care and can substantially lengthen recovery time. See Chapter 39 for detailed information on wound infection.

Dehiscence. **Dehiscence** is a total or partial disruption in wound edges (Fig. 38-6). Wound separation is synonomous with dehiscence but is most commonly used to describe surgical incisions in which the skin has separated, but underlying subcutaneous tissue has not parted. As wound edges separate, an increase in drainage usually occurs. Dehiscence most commonly occurs before collagen formation is complete in high-risk clients (3–14 days after injury). Obesity, poor nutritional status, and increased stress on the incisional area through abdominal distention or trauma increase the risk of dehiscence. Clients often report feeling that their incision has "given way" after activities, such as coughing or vomiting, that increase the pressure on the incision. Dehiscence also may occur when sutures or staples are removed before the wound is healed adequately.

Evisceration. **Evisceration** is the protusion of viscera through an abdominal wound opening (see Fig. 38-6). Evisceration can follow dehiscence if the opening extends deeply enough to allow the abdominal fascia to separate and internal organs to protrude. Evisceration often occurs when dehiscence occurs suddenly. When evisceration occurs, reassure the client, cover the area with sterile saline dressings, and notify the surgeon immediately. Do not try to push viscera back into the abdomen. The client usually must return to surgery for wound closure and receive antibiotics, because infection is more likely when dehiscence and evisceration have occurred.

Fistula. A **fistula** is an abnormal tubelike passageway that forms between two organs or from one organ to the outside of the body. Fistula tracts can be the result of poor wound healing after tissue injury from surgery. Fistulas also may result from illness, such as

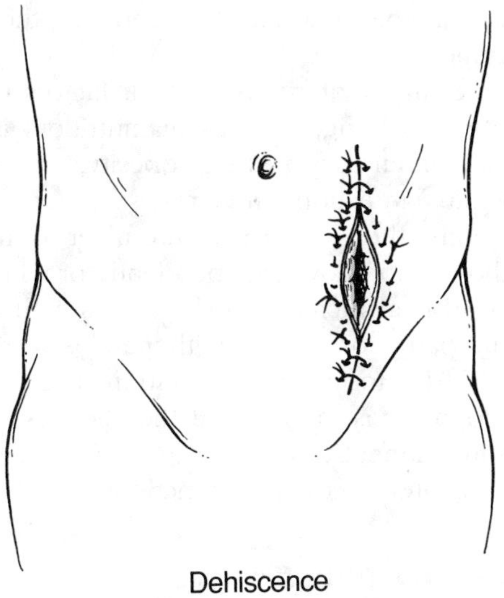

Dehiscence

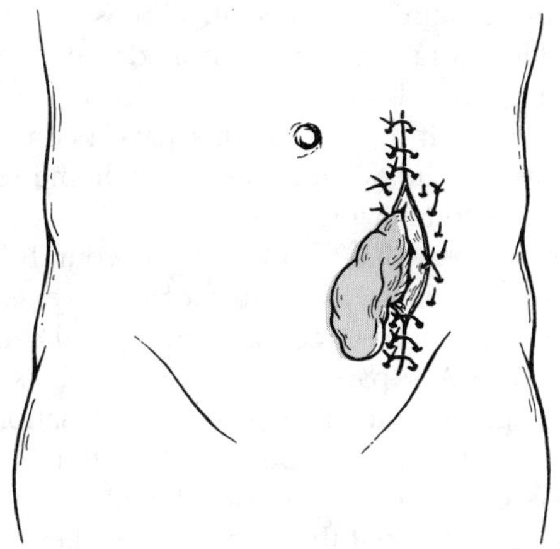

Evisceration

Figure 38-6 • *Dehiscence is the disruption of wound edges; evisceration is the protrusion of viscera through that wound opening.*

inflammatory bowel disease. Normal wound healing promotes tissue layer closure, thus preventing abnormal communication between organs of the body. The name of the fistula designates the site of the abnormal communication; for example, a rectovaginal fistula is an abnormal opening between the rectum and the vagina that permits feces to enter the vagina.

When a fistula opens onto the outside skin surface, drainage (especially gastric or intestinal) may contribute to skin breakdown. Fistulas may be managed conservatively with good nutrition and bowel rest, or they may require surgical closure.

Impact of Integumentary Dysfunction on Activities of Daily Living

Altered skin integrity can change a client's ability to perform activities of daily living (ADLs). Some skin conditions restrict the client to home because of treatment demands, discomfort, or limitations on their ability to return to work with open lesions or wounds.

Individual Considerations

Systemic reponses to skin alterations, such as fever and malaise, may lower the client's activity tolerance. Nutritional needs are higher during healing, and the client may feel unable to prepare the meals necessary to provide adequate calories and nutrients. Clients who have activity restrictions due to wound and skin problems may be unable to spend time on their feet to cook, groom, and perform other ADLs. This may lead to social isolation, altering the client's ability and motivation to perform ADLs.

Adults who are experiencing impaired skin integrity often manage their own care, if supplied with adequate information. Clients with coexisting diseases or disabilities and those with wounds requiring complex management plans often require assistance with care by a healthcare professional or trained family member. Clients with wounds in difficult-to-reach areas require help with the use of topical products, such as ointments or dressings. An older woman with lower extremity ulcers, for example, might require assistance to secure a dressing and apply a compression stocking to her leg.

Family Considerations

Wound management can be a financial burden if it is not covered by medical insurance. Obtaining special equipment and supplies often becomes the responsibility of the family if the client's mobility level prevents them from leaving the home. Clients often rely on family members for transportation to medical follow-up appointments and wound therapies, such as whirlpool. These demands impact the family member's schedule and occupational demands.

Family members may be asked to learn how to provide wound care. The ability and willingness of family members to provide this care depends on cultural factors, prior relationships between client and family, and general health of the family member. When working with older clients, the nurse must inquire about the health of the client's spouse before assuming any care can be delegated to him or her.

Assessment

A systematic assessment of skin integrity and wound healing is essential. It provides data to identify potential or actual problems and allows the nurse to develop an individualized plan of care. Subjective and objective data are collected during the first encounter with the client, and assessment is ongoing to detect changes in skin integrity, wound healing status, and the potential for further skin problems.

Subjective Data

Interviewing the client allows the nurse to gather data about the client's normal skin status, the history of skin problems, and the presence of risk factors that can increase the potential for altered skin integrity or wound healing. Subjective data also provide detailed information on the development of actual skin or wound problems and their prior management.

Functional Pattern Identification

When interviewing the client, the nurse should ask what the client's skin, hair, and nails are normally like. Reports of excessively dry or oily skin should be noted. Questions about normal skin-care practices and individual preferences help the nurse to individualize care. The nurse should assess what self-care activities the client can independently perform. If the client has been unable to care for his or her hair or nails, arrangements for such care can be made.

If the client manages a chronic skin or wound condition, the nurse should document specific management techniques. For the ostomy client, the nurse documents the usual care required to keep the skin around the stoma free from irritation and breakdown. For the client with an acute wound, the nurse gathers information about normal wound-management practices. In all skin impairments, the effect of the problem on ADLs is evaluated.

Risk Identification

The interview helps the nurse identify clients at risk for problems with skin integrity or delayed wound healing.

Obtain an allergy history, with a description of the allergic response (including dermatologic symptoms) and identification of the allergen. For clients with a positive allergy history, note specific foods, medications, or products (eg, soaps or tape) on the client's record. When a client reports numerous allergies, avoid new products that may cause an allergic response.

Obtain a history of past skin conditions. Ask what factors triggered the problem, whether the condition was seasonal or aggravated by stress, and how the client handled the problem (eg, home remedies, over-the-counter preparations). Question the client about a family history of skin problems, because some dermatologic problems (eg, eczema, psoriasis) commonly run in families.

Document any recent exposure to factors that can cause skin trauma, rash, or lesions. Note any contact with family members or others with infectious illnesses (eg, measles, chickenpox, scabies, lice). Travel to foreign countries or activities such as hiking or camping can expose the client to parasites or poisonous plants. Exposure to caustic chemicals, excessive heat, or radiation also may be important in identifying the risk for skin alterations.

Prior to any surgery, assess risk factors that may delay wound healing, such as malnutrition, impaired circulation, immunosuppression, obesity, smoking, diabetes mellitus, infection, and stress.

Determine the risk for pressure ulcer formation. A client who cannot move independently or who will be immobilized is at increased risk. Clients with diabetes with neuropathy or clients with paralysis are at increased risk due to impaired sensation. The risk for ulcer development is increased if the client is malnourished, is incontinent of urine or feces, is obese or very thin, or has altered cognitive functioning.

Dysfunction Identification

Ask the client if any skin problems (rash, sores, or breaks in the skin) are present. If present, ask about the problem, duration, what it looked like when it first appeared, if and how it spread, and any associated symptoms. Ask if any treatments have been used, including medical advice and therapies, home remedies, and over-the-counter preparations.

If an accident has resulted in a wound, burn, or other injury, evaluate the nature of the events leading to the trauma. Note any contamination of the area with dirt or debris. Ask parents about their child's injuries, and if they give vague or suspicious explanations, a follow-up evaluation should be done to determine if child abuse has occurred. For all accidental wounds, even minor ones, ask about the status of the client's tetanus immunization, and update it if necessary.

Interview questions also can help assess the impact a skin condition or wound has on ADLs. Such conditions can affect self-concept, causing the client to withdraw from social interaction. Watching the client's nonverbal cues helps the nurse assess the psychological impact of the skin impairment.

Objective Data

Objective information obtained during the physical examination can identify actual problems in skin integrity or wound healing. Inspection and palpation help the nurse to collect objective data about skin integrity and wound status. Laboratory and diagnostic tests may confirm a diagnosis of cancer or the presence of infection.

Physical Examination

Inspection of the Skin. A general inspection of the skin is followed by a more detailed examination of any abnormalities noted. Examine the skin for color, vascularity, turgor and mobility, texture, and the presence or absence of lesions. A good source of light is essential. Compare for symmetry in contralateral areas throughout the examination.

Skin color varies from one person to another, from one part of the body to another, and according to race. Some pigment variations are normal. Pigment changes also normally occur during pregnancy. Other changes in skin color may be evidence of systemic disease. Cyanosis (bluish discoloration) in nailbeds may be due to vasoconstriction, although cyanosis in the mouth or conjunctiva may indicate hypoxemia secondary to heart or lung dysfunction. The yellow hue of jaundice may indicate liver or biliary disease.

Skin texture refers to the palpable and visible surface structure, its fineness or coarseness, and whether it is scaly, crusted, or macerated. Skin may appear thick and tough or thin and friable. Note the presence of any edema and presence of absence or peripheral pulses when assessing clients with ulcers or wounds of the extremities.

When any skin abnormality is present, note its shape, pattern, distribution, and color. Note whether the abnormality is localized or generalized and whether distribution is symmetric. Lesions can occur in clusters, circles, or lines, or their placement may be irregular. Measure the size of the lesion so that changes in size can be detected.

Examine the client's hair and nails. Inspect the hair for distribution, quantity, and quality. Absence of hair growth on lower extremities can indicate decreased peripheral circulation. Thinning and brittle nails may be caused by nutritional deficits or impaired circulation. Nail clubbing (see Fig. 21-7), a change in the angle of the fingernail and nail base, is associated with chronic respiratory and cardiac dysfunction. Capillary refill time is illustrated in Figure 35-5.

Pressure Ulcer Risk Assessment. Structured assessment tools are available to assist in the prediction of clients who require pressure ulcer prevention. The two risk assessment tools that have been tested extensively are the Braden Scale and the Norton Scale. These scales provide a numeric score to rate the individual client's level of risk (Panel for the Prediction and Prevention of Pressure Ulcers in Adults, 1992).

Inspection of the Wound. Inspection permits the nurse to evaluate wound healing and detect possible wound complications. Appraise the general appearance of the wound, type and amount of drainage, functioning of drainage systems, amount and characteristics of incisional pain, and signs of wound complications, such as infection.

General Appearance. Note the size and shape of the wound, and compare it with previous measurements. Size is usually estimated in centimeters. When wound healing is watched carefully, size and shape may be measured weekly with concentric circle overlays, tracings, or photographic measures (Etris, Pribble, & LaBrecque, 1994).

Clean surgical incisions are usually closed with sutures, staples, or clips so the skin edges are well approximated to promote healing. Initially the incision may appear slightly swollen or red due to normal inflammation. Usually within 1 week of surgery, the wound edges heal together, and swelling subsides. When staples have been in for a prolonged period, they may rise and show signs of inflammation where they enter the skin.

When wound edges are not well approximated and healing does not occur by primary intention, it occurs by granulation. Intially the area appears red, as capillary beds proliferate from connective tissue that will eventually develop. As healing occurs, epithelium grows over these capillary beds, and the wound decreases in size. This shrinkage in wound size can be observed and measured.

Drainage Systems. Drainage devices are placed in the wound when the surgeon anticipates a large amount of fluid accumulation, which inhibits wound healing. Closed drainage systems consist of a drain attached to a portable or external suction source. Open drainage systems, such as a Penrose drain, drain directly from the wound and are associated with a higher rate of wound infection.

A *Penrose drain* is a hollow, flat, rubber tube placed directly into the incision or into a stab wound in the incisional area (see Fig. 38-16). It allows fluid to drain through capillary action into absorbent dressings. Penrose drains may be advanced or shortened to drain different areas.

A *Hemovac* is placed into vascular areas where bloody drainage is expected after surgery. Suction is maintained by compressing a springlike device (see Procedure 38-4, Step 7). When inspecting a Hemovac drain, expect bloody drainage, and ensure that the Hemovac remains in the compressed state. Suction can be interrupted if leaks are present in the system or if the Hemovac has filled with drainage.

A *Jackson-Pratt* or grenade drain permits drainage to collect in a bulblike device, which can be compressed to create gentle suction (see Fig. 38-14). Suction is lost when the bulb is expanded from too much drainage or a leak in the system.

Inspect the drainage system to ensure patency and function. Drains may or may not be sutured in place, so take care not to inadvertently remove them during inspection.

Wound Drainage. The type and amount of drainage varies depending on the type, location, and depth of the wound. Note the amount, color, consistency, and odor of any drainage. Terms commonly used to describe wound drainage follow:

- **Serous** drainage is clear, watery, and plasmalike.
- **Sanguinous** drainage is bloody, as from a fresh wound.

- **Serosanguinous** drainage is pale and thin and contains plasma and red cells.
- **Purulent** drainage contains white cells and microorganisms and occurs when infection is present. It is thick and opaque and can vary from pale yellow to green or tan, depending on the offending organism.

In closed systems, the amount of drainage can be accurately monitored by measuring what is emptied from the drain collector. The greatest amount of drainage is expected in the early postoperative period. The amount tapers off as edema subsides and fluid is removed from the site. Most surgeons remove drains when drainage is minimal. An unexpected increase in drainage can precede wound complications, such as dehiscence. A change in the character of drainage also is important to observe and report, especially if there is a sudden increase in bloody drainage or if drainage become purulent.

Assessing the amount of drainage is more difficult when a closed drainage system is not used. The nurse can help to quantify the amount of drainage by noting the number of dressings that were saturated and the number of times the dressing required changing. When the dressing is not being changed (as in a fresh postoperative wound), drainage is sometimes circled on the dressing and marked with a date and time.

Inspection for Infection. Observe for symptoms that may indicate infection in the wound, such as pain, redness, swelling, induration, and purulent drainage. Systemic signs include fever and an elevated white blood count. Wound infection can occur at any time, but often such infections do not become apparent until late in the postoperative period or after débridement procedures. See Chapter 39 for a detailed discussion of wound infections.

Palpation. Palpation can be used along with inspection to gather objective data about wound status of skin. Use gloves when palpating skin surfaces to avoid exposure to infectious agents. Palpation is helpful in assessing raised sufaces of the skin and the skin texture and temperature. When wound infection is suspected, gently palpate the incisional area to detect swelling or induration.

Diagnostic Tests and Procedures

Laboratory and diagnostic tests may be performed to confirm the cause of a skin or wound abnormality. Most commonly, a culture and sensitivity is done to identify infectious organisms that can cause a skin lesion or infect a wound. See Chapter 35 for more information on wound cultures. A biopsy is sometimes performed to rule out malignant causes of skin abnormalities.

Nursing Diagnoses

Impaired Skin Integrity and Impaired Tissue Integrity are North American Nursing Diagnosis Association (NANDA) diagnoses used to identify problems with skin breakdown and healing. Impaired Skin Integrity is used to identify potential or actual problems that involve only the epidermal or dermal layer. Impaired Tissue Integrity is used when the damage involves more than the dermis; often connective tissue, muscles, and nerves are involved.

Diagnostic Statement: Impaired Skin Integrity

Definition

Impaired Skin Integrity is the state in which an individual's skin is adversely altered (NANDA 1994).

Defining Characteristics

Of the defining characteristics or clinical cues that point to this diagnosis, disruption of epidermal or dermal tissue must be present (NANDA, 1994).

Minor characteristics that may be present but are not required for this diagnosis include the following:

- Denuded skin (patchy loss of epidermis)
- Erythema (redness)
- Lesions or pruritus (itch)

Related Factors

Enviromental factors may cause or contribute to Impaired Skin Integrity. These may include hyperthermia or hypothermia, which damage the skin, causing burns or frostbite; chemical substances, radiation, or mechanical factors, such as shear or friction, which destroy the epidermis; and physical immobility or immobilization leading to pressure ulcers or excessive moisture leading to macerated skin.

Somatic factors contributing to Impaired Skin Integrity may include those that lower the tissue tolerance to pressure, such as emaciation, decreased skin turgor, altered metabolic states, and altered circulation.

Diagnostic Statement: Impaired Tissue Integrity

Definition

Impaired Tissue Integrity is the state in which an individual experiences damage to mucous membrane, corneal, integumentary, or subcutaneous tissue (NANDA, 1994).

Defining Characteristics

Of the defining characteristics or clinical cues that point to this diagnosis, damaged or destroyed tissue (cornea, mucous membrane, integumentary, or subcutaneous) must be present.

The etiologic or contributing factors that may have contributed to Impaired Tissue Integrity are similiar to those listed under Impaired Skin Integrity (see above).

Related Nursing Diagnosis

Client problems that led to the injury to skin or tissue may be listed as nursing diagnoses. For example, a client with the diagnosis of Impaired Physical Mobility can develop Impaired Skin Integrity. Clients with diagnoses of Altered Nutrition: Less than Body Requirements, Sensory/Perceptual Alterations, Bowel Incontinence, Stress, Reflex, Urge, Functional or Total Incontinence also may develop the need for the diagnoses of Impaired Skin Integrity or Impaired Tissue Integrity.

The inability of the client to meet the physiologic requirements for wound healing may be summarized in the nursing diagnosis. Nutrition or fluid intake may be inadequate. Any break in the skin produces Risk for Infection and Pain. The client with skin and tissue injury effects may have the diagnosis Risk for Infection and in the case of extensive burns, Ineffective Thermoregulation or Fluid Volume Deficit. Body Image Disturbance, and Self Esteem Disturbance commonly accompany skin impairments. When severe, this can cause Anxiety, Ineffective Individual Coping, or Social Isolation.

Outcome Identification and Planning

Planning for nursing interventions to promote skin integrity is based on the data gathered in the assessment and the resulting nursing diagnoses and outcome identification. They fall into the general categories of promoting skin integrity and providing an environment for optimal healing. Examples of nursing interventions commonly used in achieving these categories are listed in the accompanying display and are discussed in the following section.

Client-centered goals for skin and tissue integrity involve preventing damage and promoting optimal healing of damaged tissues.

- The client's skin will remain intact without areas of local inflammation.
- The client's wounds will demonstrate evidence of healing.
- The client will demonstrate increased knowledge of skin care.
- The client or family will comply with the treatment plan to promote wound healing and skin integrity.

These goals must be individualized to reflect the needs of the person at risk. At that point, goals are supported by specific nursing interventions.

Planning

Examples of Nursing Interventions Used in Common Skin Problems

- Keep skin clean and dry, changing client's position frequently to relieve pressure areas.
- Maintain adequate hydration to skin through adequate fluid intake by the client.
- Provide adequate nutrition for client to ensure optimally well-nourished skin cells.
- Observe for redness, heat, swelling, pain, or change in function in skin areas.
- Teach effective application of heat or cold as therapies for decreasing inflammation, improving healing, and reducing pain.
- Apply dressings to wounds appropriately for the purpose to be achieved for that particular wound.
- Assist client in determining appropriate mattress or cushions for avoiding pressure areas.

Implementation

Nursing interventions are aimed at promoting optimal skin integrity, preventing skin or tissue damage, and treating impaired skin to promote optimal wound healing, prevent infection, and produce optimal skin function.

Nursing Interventions to Promote Health and Integumentary Function

Nursing care plays an important role in preventing skin alterations. Optimal skin integrity is maintained by promoting adequate oxygen, nutrients, water, and waste removal for the skin and mucous membranes.

Skin Care

There are several basic principles of skin care (see the display). One of the most important involves maintaining intact skin because it is the body's first line of de-

Principles of Skin Care

- Intact skin is the body's first line of defense against trauma and infection.
- Breakdown of the skin's integrity must be prevented.
- Skin must be adequately hydrated.
- The body's cells must be adequately nourished.
- Adequate circulation is needed to maintain cells.
- Skin hygiene is necessary.
- Skin sensitivity varies among people and according to their health status.

fense against trauma and infections. Measures to prevent irritation or injury are imperative. Skin breakdown can be prevented by avoiding mechanical irritation from rubbing or friction. Remove tape carefully, and pat skin dry to avoid traumatizing delicate skin. To minimize chemical irritation, use mild soap, plain water, or products containing emollients. Very young, older, emaciated, or obese clients may have particularly sensitive skin that is more prone to chemical irritation.

Maintaining adequate hydration of the skin also contributes to healthy skin function. Because very dry skin is susceptible to breakdown, avoid drying agents, such as alcohol, and use lotions or creams with lanolin. Clients with dry skin should be bathed only once or twice a week. However, skin that is exposed to excessive moisture for prolonged periods can lead to bacterial growth and irritation. Clients who are incontinent of urine or stool or who perspire excessively need prompt, thorough, frequent washing and drying. Areas where skin lies in folds (eg, under the breasts, in the gluteal folds) can collect moisture and need special attention. A gauze pad or a light dusting of powder may help prevent moisture build-up in skin folds.

Adequate nutrition is essential for normal skin integrity. Adequately nourished cells can better resist injury and disease, so a diet with appropriate vitamins, minerals, and protein is essential. A client who has poor absorption of nutrients, excessive losses of protein, or inadequate food and fluid intake may need additional nutritional support (high-protein supplements, total parenteral nutrition) to prevent skin breakdown and ensure healing.

Adequate circulation also is needed to maintain cell life. Inadequate blood flow to the skin results in ischemia and tissue breakdown. Keeping clients warm prevents vasoconstriction. Treating underlying cardiac or circulatory problems helps ensure adequate blood flow to the skin. Clients with impaired venous circulation from the legs and feet require leg elevation and compression to heal venous ulcers (McColloch, Marler, Neal, & Phifer, 1994). Getting adequate exercise and avoiding constrictive clothing can help ensure optimal blood flow. Frequent turning and repositioning can avoid localized obstruction of blood flow due to increased pressure.

Client Teaching

Hygiene teaching is important to maintain skin integrity. Because clients with impaired sensation from neuropathies or paralysis are less able to sense injury to the skin, they should be taught to inspect skin surfaces (especially the feet) routinely for signs of breakdown. When wearing new shoes, they should avoid blisters and irritation. Prevention strategies can decrease the incidence of amputation in people with diabetes (Kaufman, 1994). Because temperature discrimination also is affected, hot-water heaters should be turned down to avoid accidental burns.

Hygiene teaching is important for the parents of a newborn. Teaching should include how to prevent skin trauma (for example, clipping fingernails short and putting mittens on the child when scratching is anticipated). Reassure parents about normal skin changes or congenital lesions of the skin. Parental bonding with the infant can be hindered if the parents view the infant as deformed or scarred.

Education about trauma prevention is important. Many automobile accidents (which can lead to skin and tissue injury) can be avoided by careful driving, adhering to speed limits, using seat belts, and driving cars with air bags. Bicycle injuries can be prevented or limited by observing safety rules and wearing helmets.

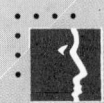

Client Teaching
Protection of Skin

Instruct the client as follows:

- *If you have decreased skin sensations, inspect your skin carefully and take actions to prevent skin injury resulting from trauma or burns.*
- *Reduce your risk of skin cancer by avoiding overexposure to the sun and using effective sunscreen products.*
- *Report any change in size, shape or color of moles and other lesions to your healthcare provider.*
- *Reduce skin irritation by regular applications of lotion and moisturizers, especially if you are an older adult.*
- *Install smoke detectors and learn to use fire extinguishers, and routinely practice what to do if fire breaks out.*
- *Keep dry any areas that hold moisture (eg, under the breasts, between fat folds, between the legs) to prevent maceration of skin.*

Smoke detectors should be installed to prevent serious burns. See Chapter 29 for more information on safety.

Protection from the Sun

All clients should be taught the importance of limiting exposure to ultraviolet radiation (sunlight and artificial tanning lights). The use of clothing, wide-brimmed hats, and sunglasses to protect frequently exposed areas is often the most practical. For fair- to light-skinned individuals, sunscreen with a minimum sun protection factor of 15 should be used daily. The sun should be avoided for infants younger than 6 months, because sunscreen is not recommended. The use of tanning machines for cosmetic purposes should be discouraged.

Pressure Ulcer Prevention

Most pressure ulcers can be prevented and many stage one ulcers can disappear with pressure relief. Prevention is less costly than treatment financially and in its impact to the individual. Once a client is determined to be at risk and the factors that produce that risk are determined, nursing measures are implemented. A synopsis of the interventions for prevention of pressure ulcers is provided (see display). Structured pressure ulcer prevention programs within inpatient facilities have demonstrated success in decreasing the incidence of nosocomial pressure ulcers (Murray & Blaylock, 1994).

Risk for pressure ulcers can be decreased by using a pressure-reducing support surface (pad, mattress, or product that distributes pressure more evenly across the body surface) on the bed or chair used by the individual at risk. A variety of such beds, mattresses, and cushions are available. Most manufacturers conduct research on the pressure-reducing effect of their product; however, more research is needed to compare the effect of products when used with at-risk clients, rather than with healthy, young volunteers.

Support surfaces may be purchased, rented, or leased for client use. The primary goal for any of these products is to prevent and manage pressure-related skin breakdown. Choosing a particular support surface for a client requires consideration of the product efficacy, desired effect, anticipated duration of treatment, client preferences, cost, upkeep, and impact on client mobility.

The support surfaces used for pressure ulcer care and prevention can be broadly catorgorized as static and dynamic overlays, mattress replacements, and specialty beds, which include low air loss beds and air fluidized beds. Kinetic therapy beds and obese beds may

Pressure Ulcer Prediction and Prevention

Risk Prediction

- Identify clients at risk, and specific factors placing them at risk.

Skin Care

- Maintain and improve tissue tolerance to pressure to prevent injury. Inspect pressure points once a day; document all findings.
- Cleanse skin regularly and whenever soiled, using a mild cleansing agent and warm, not hot, water.
- Minimize factors that dry the skin. Treat dry skin with moisturizers.
- Do not massage bony prominences.
- Minimize exposure of skin to incontinence, perspiration, or wound drainage.
- Protect skin from friction and shear.
- Provide adequate calories and nutrients.
- Maintain or improve mobility, activity level, and range of motion.

Pressure Reduction for At-Risk Clients

- Reposition every 2 hours.
- Use pillows to keep bony prominences from rubbing against each other.
- Keep heels from pressing on the bed if the client is completely immobile.
- When the client is on his or her side, avoid positioning directly on the trochanter.
- Limit the time the head of the bed is elevated.
- Lift, do not drag, clients to move them up in bed. Use overbed trapeze.
- Place clients on a pressure-reducing device when in bed.
- Avoid prolonged sitting. Reposition or shift the client's weight every hour.
- For chair-bound clients, place a pressure-reducing device on the chair that maintains good postural alignment, balance, and stability.
- Use a written plan regarding the use of positioning devices and repositioning schedules.

Education

- Provide structured education about pressure ulcer prevention to healthcare providers, clients, and family or caregivers.

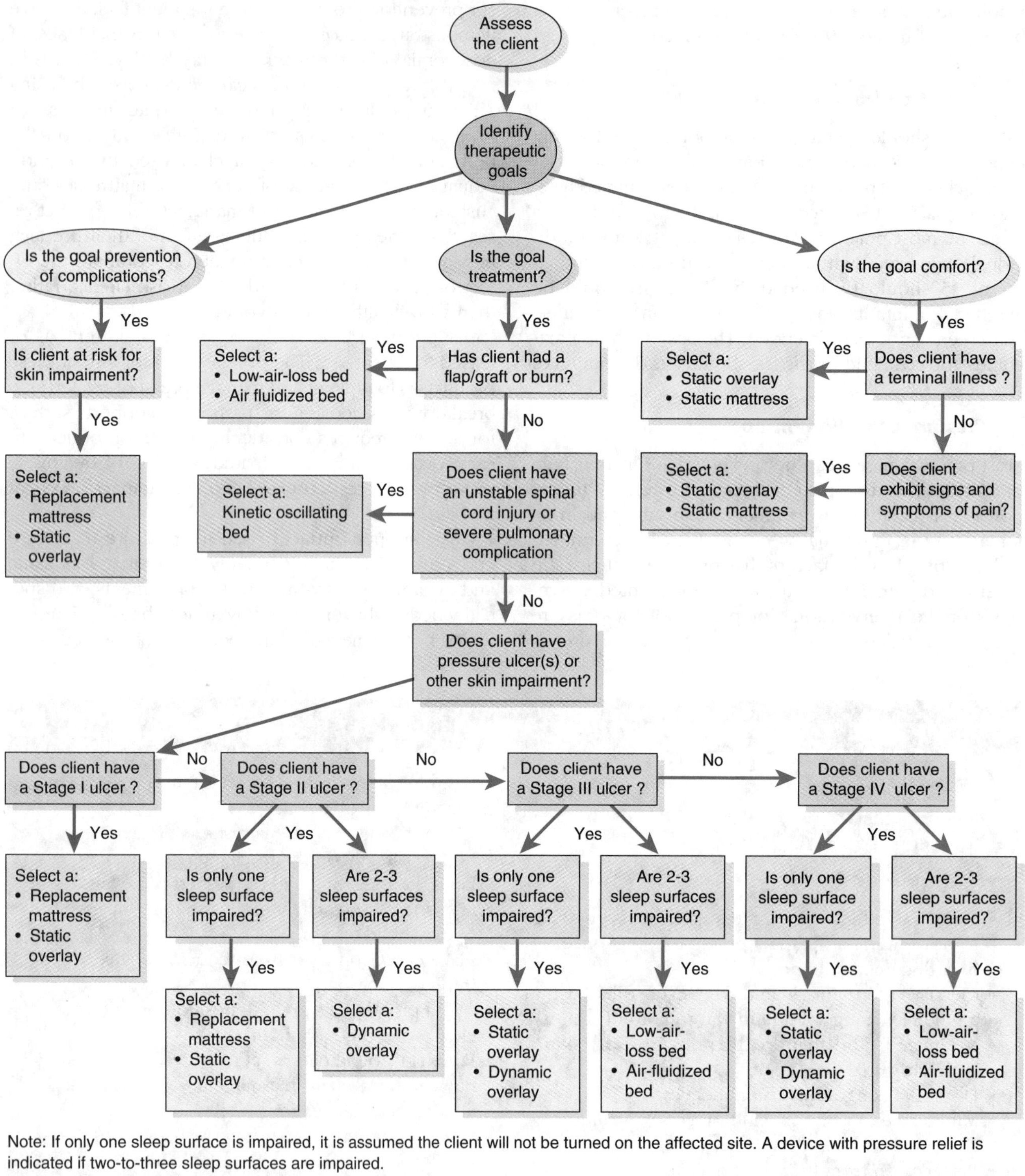

Figure 38-7 • *Support surface algorithm (Thomason, S., Hawley, G. G., & Wurzel, J. (1993). Modified and reprinted with permission of the author.)*

reduce pressure; however, their purposes are primarily to promote respiratory function (kinetic beds) and to provide a sleep surface for clients who weigh more than 300 lb (obese bed).

Given the wide variety of available support surfaces, it can be difficult to decide which product will best meet the needs of individual clients. To narrow and standardize the selection of support surfaces, many inpatient facilities create algorithms or guidelines. One such algorithm is displayed in Figure 38-7.

Mattress Overlays. An overlay is a product placed on top of the existing bed mattress. Overlays can be made of foam or filled with air, gel, or water. Eggcrate

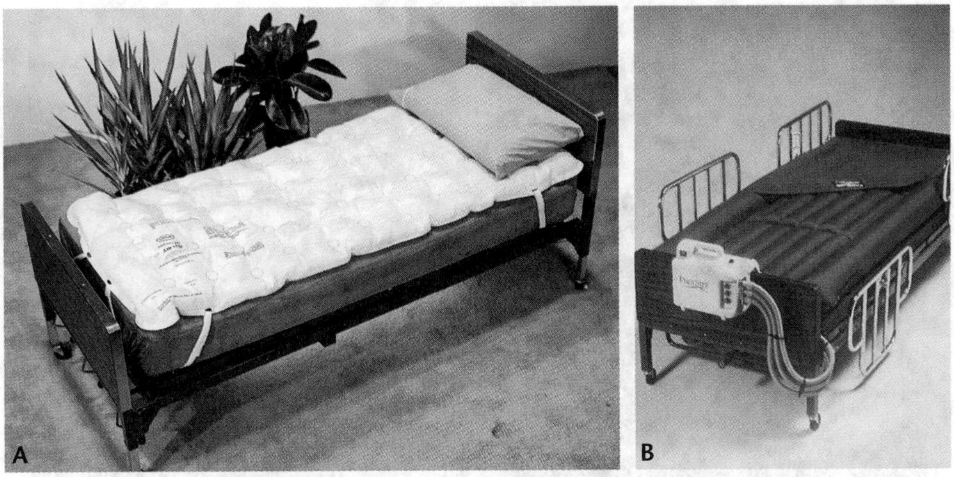

*Figure 38-8 • Examples of air-filled overlay mattresses. **(A)** Static air flotation mattress with corner straps gives 17 to 25 mm Hg interface pressure relief. (Photo courtesy of Lotus Health Care Products, Naugatuck, CT.) **(B)** Dynamic air-filled overlay mattress. This particular mattress has elevated sides for futher protection. The control section at the foot of the bed has three individually controlled air-flow sections. There is a built-in adjustable heater also and convenient CPR switch. (Photo of First Step ® Plus courtesy of KCI Therapeutic Services, San Antonio TX.)*

foam, a loose, convoluted overlay, provides little pressure reduction unless the base of the foam is at least 4 in high. It is most appropriately used as a comfort measure. Foam overlays with greater density and thickness provide pressure reduction when used with normal weight clients. Air-filled overlays also reduce pressure when the product is correctly inflated. Air-filled overlays may be static (like an air mattress) or dynamic (attached to a motorized air blower or pump). Examples are given in Figure 38-8.

Replacement Mattresses. Replacement mattresses are used on a standard bed frame after removing the original mattress. Replacement mattresses reduce some pressure because of their design, which includes layers of dense foam or foam and gel combinations within a lightweight, bacteriostatic cover. There is little independent research on the pressure-reducing effects and durability of these products because they are relatively new to the market of support surfaces.

Specialty Beds. Specialty beds for use in pressure ulcer care include low airloss beds and air-fluidized beds (Fig. 38-9). Low airloss beds consist of multiple air-filled, horizontally positioned cushions within a traditional electrical bed frame. The cushion in the seat area contains a higher amount of air to support the increased weight required in this area when the head of the bed is elevated. Air-fluidized beds use a high flow rate of air to blow fine particles of silicone within a protective cover. The resulting support surface behaves like a liquid and feels similar to a waterbed. When the airflow is turned off, the beads settle to the bottom of the bed and become a firm hard surface, holding the client in position until the airflow is resumed.

Nursing Interventions for Altered Integumentary Function

Wound care is planned by the members of the health-care team, and nursing interventions are significant for promoting optimal wound healing and skin integrity. Nursing interventions to encourage independence, reinforce client accomplishments, and teach the client and family to achieve optimal self-care are important. Depending on the type of wound, the nurse may want to protect the area to promote optimum regeneration of tissue, cleanse the area to treat or prevent infection, or débride the area to remove debris that impairs wound healing. Heat and cold also can be used as therapeutic modalities to promote healing and provide pain relief.

Pruritus Relief

Pruritus often accompanies skin problems. Nursing management is aimed at relieving the situations that cause pruritus, decreasing the associated discomfort, and preventing additional trauma to the skin.

Pruritus is often caused by excessive drying of the skin, especially in older clients. Lotions and moisturizing creams should be applied regularly to promote rehydration of dried areas. Bathing should be limited; if soap is used, it should be thoroughly rinsed from the skin, and specific brands that increase irritation should not be used. Oil may be added to the bath water, but

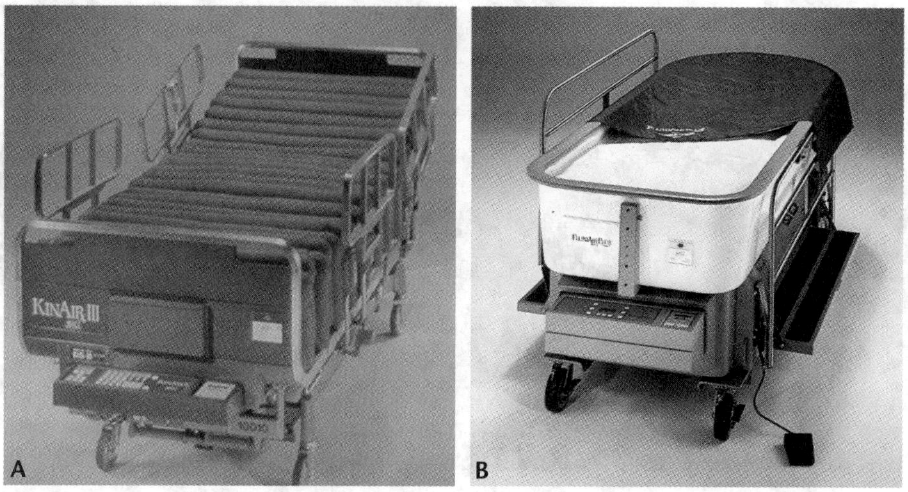

Figure 38-9* • *Examples of specialty beds.* (A) *KinAir ® III is an air-flotation, low air-loss support surface that provides pressure relief. At the foot of the bed there is a microprocessor computer control panel that precisely controls air flow and temperature. A built-in digital scale and heater are included. The bed also has a CPR quick-release lever.* (B) *Air-fluidized bead therapy is provided by FluidAir ® & FluidAir Plus ®. This system supports the client on fluidized silicon-coated microspheres. It has a computerized control panel, digital scale, and quick release for CPR. Steps are built in the side. Fluidization levels can be adjusted for client comfort. A dual-model cooling system allows a cooler temperature when the client needs it. (Photos courtesy of KCI Therapeutic Services, San Antonio TX.)

care should be taken because oil makes the bathtub slippery and may contribute to falls. Using tepid, not hot, water and gently patting the skin dry also decrease skin irritation.

Explaining the importance of not scratching may increase compliance for adults, but cautions rarely work for young children. Keeping children's fingernails cut short and having them wear cotton gloves may decrease skin trauma. Diversional activities also may help focus a child's attention away from unpleasant sensations.

Cool baths and moist, cool compresses promote vasoconstriction and provide relief. Baking soda or oatmeal baths are soothing. The physician may order medications to be used as needed. Antihistamines and sedatives, although commonly used, have systemic side effects. Topical medications, such as corticosteroids or antibiotics, can decrease inflammation or treat infection. A paste made from baking soda and water also can be applied to decrease itching.

First Aid for Minor Wounds

Basic principles in caring for minor accidental wounds are to promote hemostasis, cleanse the wound, and protect it from further injury.

Bleeding can be controlled by putting direct pressure on the wound or by elevating the affected part. Initial bleeding may help remove dirt and contaminants from the wound.

Cleansing the wound removes potential sources of infection. Try to remove foreign materials, such as dirt or cinders, unless the wound is extensive or the client complains of excessive pain. For most minor wounds, running water as an irrigating solution and mild soap as a cleansing agent are recommended.

After bleeding has subsided and the area has been cleansed, the wound is protected with a sterile or clean dressing. Small cuts may be left open to the air. Extensive wounds may require a bulky dressing applied with pressure to minimize movement.

The wound should be assessed for potential complications; any client with a wound that requires more extensive treatment should be referred to the appropriate healthcare agency. Signs of infection usually take up to 24 hours to develop. Exudate, fever, or severe redness and swelling indicate that the wound needs medical attention. When excessive bleeding occurs, sutures are usually necessary to ensure healing by primary intention.

First Aid for Minor Burns

The type of burn dictates the appropriate first-aid measures. In all cases, it is important to halt the burning process and prevent further damage.

In thermal burns, the heat source must first be removed. If someone is on fire, immediate action should be to "stop, drop, and roll." After the heat source has been removed, the burned area should be flushed with copious amounts of cool water. If done quickly, this action halts the burning process by speeding heat dissipation, and it relieves pain. The client's clothing and jewelry in the affected area should be removed, because clothing and metal can retain heat. If clothing sticks to the burned area, cut around it rather than pulling, which may traumatize underlying burned tissues. Ointments and home remedies should be avoided because they can complicate burn healing.

Treatment of chemical burns is similar to that of thermal burns. The first step is to remove the client's clothing and flush the burned area with water, which dilutes the chemical and halts the burning process. If a large area has been exposed, placing the client in a shower may be the easiest way to flush the burned area. Brush powdered chemicals off the area before irrigating. Avoid splashing any of the irritant, because even dilute exposure to some chemicals can result in burns or irritation of mucous membranes. Some chemicals (eg, alkali powders) may react with water to produce heat, so industrial nurses should be knowledgeable about the chemicals used in their workplaces.

Before treating an electrical burn, the victim must be freed from the electrical source. If the person is still in contact with the electrical current, it must be turned off at its source. If you must separate the victim from energized currents, make sure you are well grounded, and use nonconductive equipment, such as a lineman's glove, polydacron rope, or dry wood. After removing the victim from the current, if the injury site or clothing are smoldering, douse them with water to dissipate the heat. Cardiopulmonary resuscitation may be necessary, because ventricular fibrillation or cardiac arrest often occurs with electrical burns. After stabilizing a victim of an electrical burn, contact the power company and describe any malfunction or problem that led to the burn. The company will conduct a safety inspection of the electrical system.

Treatment of Denuded Skin

Denuded skin can occur from many causes. When it occurs on the buttocks or perineal area, it is often the result of urinary or fecal incontinence. The most important factor leading to skin healing in these cases is resolution of the underlying problem. The reasons for incontinence must be investigated and treated. A urinary catheter may be needed temporarily to allow the surface of the skin to re-epithelialize. Options for protecting skin from incontinent stool include adult briefs and protective ointments, rectal pouches, and rectal tubes. There are advantages and disadvantages associated with each of the options (Bosley, 1994). While the skin is protected, measures must be taken to resolve the underlying cause of the incontinence.

Topical Wound Therapy

A dressing is a protective covering placed on a wound. Dressings may be used for any of the following reasons:

- Absorb drainage
- Prevent contamination
- Prevent mechanical injury to the wound
- Help maintain pressure so that excessive bleeding is avoided
- Immobilize the wound so that further trauma does not occur
- Provide comfort for the client

The type of dressing used depends on the type of wound, location, status, and personal preference.

Types of Dressings. A large variety of dressings are available for topical wound therapy (Hess, 1994). These dressings can be broadly grouped into categories, based on their characteristics and indications (Table 38-3). Of all the products listed, gauze dressings have been used in wound care the longest. They are versatile and easy to use. Because they do not keep the surface of open wounds moist, they are often moistened with saline before packing into large cavities.

Polyurethane film, polyurethane foam, and hydrocolloid dressing are often selected for topical therapy of partial-thickness wounds and stage I and II pressure ulcers. These dressings provide protection for wounds and provide a moist wound environment. They can be left in place up to 1 week unless the wound requires more frequent visualization or the amount of drainage overwhelms the capacity of the dressing.

Hydrogels are used to encouraged granulation within full-thickness wounds and to provide comfort in tender, partial-thickness wounds. Alginate products, the newest of the listed dressings, are known for their capacity for absorption. Alginate is indicated in deep, heavily draining, open wounds.

Some of the newest products being placed on wounds are ointments and lotions containing platelet-derived growth factors. These products are being evaluated for their effect on stimulating and hastening healing in chronic wounds (Turner, 1990).

Methods of Securing Dressings. Tape, Montgomery straps, gauzes, ace wraps, stretch nets, or binders can hold a dressing in place. *Tape* is the most commonly used securing device. Adhesive tape is not often used on the skin; it holds securely, but removal can be painful. If adhesive tape must be used, hair should be clipped before application, and an adhesive remover solution used when the tape is gently pulled from the skin. Nonallergenic paper or plastic tape is preferred for dressings that adhere to the skin.

Older people and others with fragile skin require paper tape or nonadhesive products to secure dressings without tape. Microfoam tape is a pliable, foam-like tape used for compression or pressure dressing.

Montgomery straps or ties, used when dressings require frequent changing, are commercially prepared

Table 38-3* • *Types of Dressings, Characteristics, and Indications

Category	*Characteristics*	*Indications*
Alginate dressings 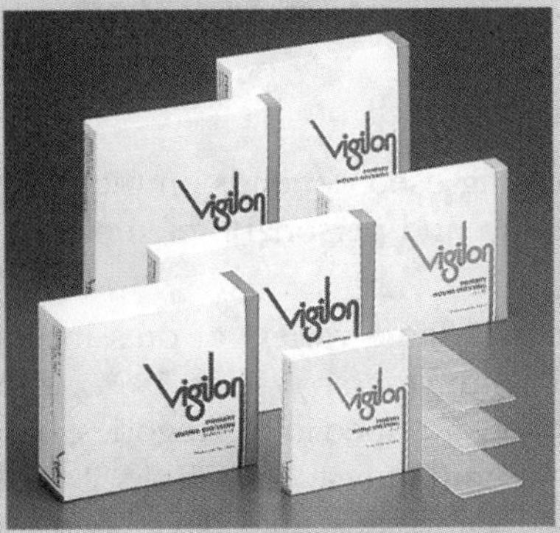	• Highly absorbent product designed to be placed inside the wound • Require a cover dressing • Available in sheet form or as packing strips	• Deep, noninfected, heavily draining wounds
	Kaltostat ® Fortex, a high-capacity alginate dressing effective for use on draining wounds. (Courtesy of ConvaTec, a Bristol-Myers Squibb Company, Princeton, NJ.)	
Gauzes	• Woven cotton material available in many sizes and thicknesses • Nonocclusive, allowing environmental oxygen to reach the wound surface • Highly absorbent • May be moistened with sterile saline to create a moist packing for larger wounds	• Newly created surgical incisions or wounds requiring pressure for hemostasis • Packing of deep wounds • Cover dressing over hydrogels and other primary dressings
Hydrocolloid wafer dressing 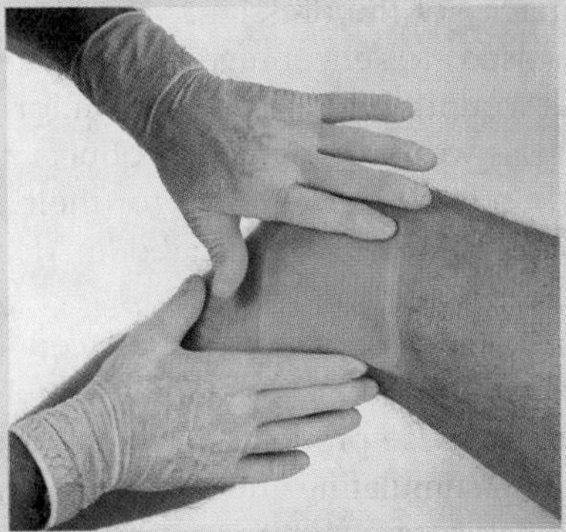	• Adhesive-backed pad, often tan in color, made of hydroactive materials • Pad absorbs excess exudate into its matrix, maintaining a moist wound surface • Most are occlusive, keeping environmental oxygen from reaching the wound • Moderate absorptive properties	• Partial-thickness wounds • Pressure ulcers • Venous leg ulcers
	Replicare ™, a hydrocolloid wafer with bacteria-proof, water-proof exterior that becomes transparent when saturated, signalling dressing change is needed. (Courtesy of Smith Nephew, Largo, FL.)	
Hydrogels 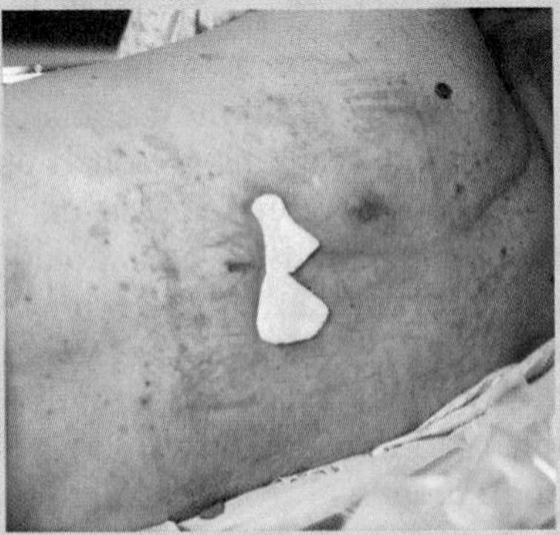	• Hydrophylic polymer product with a high percentage of water within their matrix • Available in transparent sheet-like wafer or as tube gel • Provide moderate absorption of drainage and a moist wound environment • Sheetlike wafer provides cooling sensation on the skin	• Partial-thickness wound • Pressure ulcers, stage II-IV (with a cover dressing, such as gauze) • Minor burns • Skin graft donor sites
	Bard ® Vigilon ®, an inert continuous hydrogel sheet. (Courtesy of C.R. Bard, Inc., Murray Hill, NJ.)	

(Continued)

Table 38-3 • Types of Dressings, Characteristics, and Indications (continued)

Category	Characteristics	Indications
Polyurethane foam	• Pads of compressed foam (vary in thickness according to brand, which sometimes have an adhesive backing) • Mild to moderate absorptive capacity, depending on thickness • Provide a moist wound surface	
Transparent adhesive dressings	• Clear, polyurethane film with adhesive backing • Different brands allow varying levels of moisture vapor to evaporate through the dressing. • Maintains a most wound surface • Multiple sizes and shapes • No absorptive properties	• Partial-thickness wounds • May be used instead of tape to secure a gauze pad or other type of absorbent dressing in place • Wounds with minimal exudate • Protective cover for areas exposed to friction (sacrum and heels in bed-bound clients, for example)

strips of nonallergenic tape (Fig. 38-10). Ties are inserted through the holes at one end. Montgomery straps help prevent skin breakdown because they eliminate the need to remove tape with every dressing change.

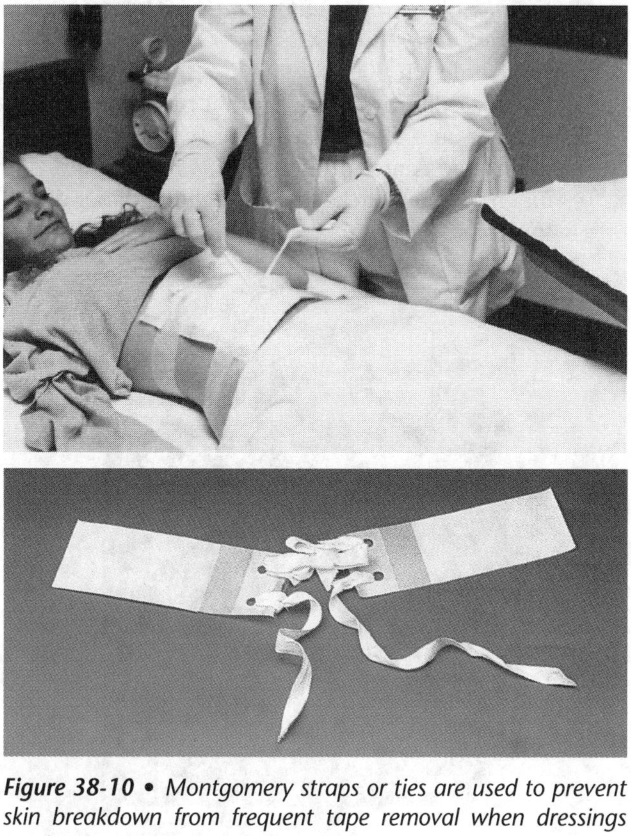

Figure 38-10 • Montgomery straps or ties are used to prevent skin breakdown from frequent tape removal when dressings need to be changed often.

Changing the Montgomery straps is required only when they become loose or soiled.

Bandages, binders, and *stretch nets* can be used to hold gauze dressings in place. They are discussed and illustrated later in this chapter.

Dressing Changes. The type of dressing used and the frequency of dressing changes are determined by wound status, type of dressing, amount of drainage, and frequency of wound assessment required. Sometimes the physician may order the type of dressing and the frequency of dressing changes, but other times the nurse determines what type of dressing will best promote healing. Hydrocolloid dressings, for example, may be left in place for 1 week on clean, partial-thickness wounds. Procedures for changing a dry sterile dressing and applying wet-to-dry dressings are given in Procedures 38-1 and 38-2.

Packing. Sterile packing can be inserted into an infected wound or an open wound that has the potential for infection. Packing prevents the wound from closing prematurely, which could lead to microorganism growth and abscess formation. Packing is commercially prepared in long, thin strips. Usually plain or saline moistened gauze packing is used, but gauze impregnated with iodophor, petrolatum, or povidone-iodine also is available. A sterile cotton applicator is used to insert packing into the wound until it is loosely filled.

Packing also may be used after surgery on areas of the body that are hard to suture (eg, vagina, nasal septum) to apply pressure and prevent blood loss from

(text continues on page 1094)

Procedure 38-1
Changing a Dry Sterile Dressing

Purpose
1. Protect wound from trauma and external contamination
2. Provide opportunity to assess the wound
3. Provide a dry environment for wound healing

Assessment

- Assess location and degree of pain. Medicate if necessary.
- Assess for presence of generalized symptoms of infection (ie, elevated temperature, leukocytosis, diaphoresis).
- Assess dressing for drainage. Observe bed clothes and linen for drainage.
- Review medical history, and identify factors that may contribute to delayed wound healing (ie, poor nutritional status, age, obesity, immunosuppressive therapy, disorders such as anemia or diabetes mellitus).
- Assess client's ability to cooperate during procedure. Arrange for assistance if necessary to ensure client's safety during procedure.
- Note client allergies to tape or dressing materials.

Equipment

Clean gloves, sterile gloves
sterile, prepackaged dressing(s)
Sterile towel
Sterile cup
Clean, flat work surface
Tape (micropore or paper)
Montgomery straps (optional)
Disposable suture-removal set for scissors and forceps (optional)
Cleansing solution as ordered, applicator
Plastic bag

Procedure

1. Close client's door or close curtains around bed. Explain procedure to client.
2. Position client comfortably. Expose only wound area.
   Rationale: The client should be kept safe and comfortable.
3. Wash your hands.
   Rationale: Handwashing helps prevent spread of microorganisms.
4. Make a cuff on top of plastic bag and place within easy reach of dressing table.
   Rationale: Cuff allows contaminated dressing to be easily contained without contaminating outside of bag.
5. Put on clean disposable gloves.
   Rationale: Gloves protect nurse from becoming contaminated by wound drainage.
6. Remove dressing from wound, and discard into plastic bag.
   Note: If dressing adheres to wound, pour a small amount of sterile saline on the wound to loosen the dressing and prevent disruption of healing tissue.

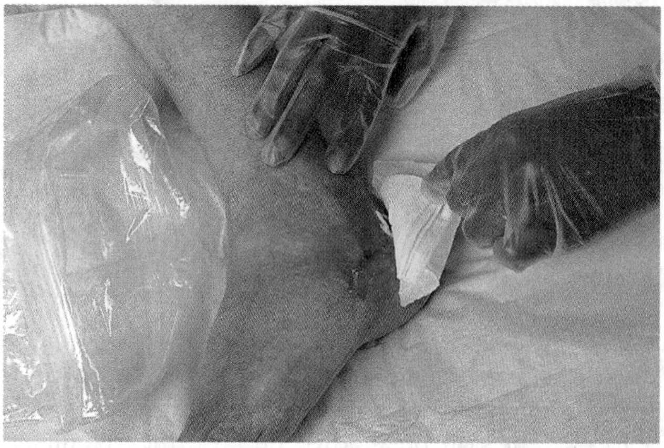

Step 6 • Remove soiled dressing.

7. Dispose of gloves. Wash your hands.
   Rationale: Gloves are contaminated. Handwashing helps prevent spread of microorganisms.
8. Set up sterile supplies.
   a. Open sterile towel, and hold it by the edges.
   b. Place it on a clean, flat surface without contaminating the center of the towel.
   c. Open dressing package(s) by peeling paper down to expose dressing. Let it fall onto the sterile field.

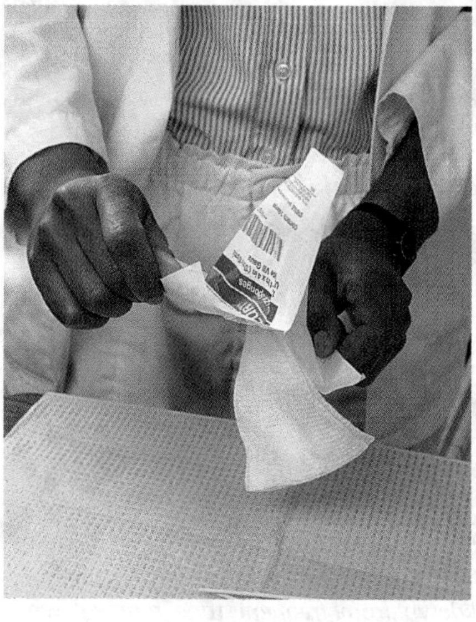

***Step 8C** • Open sterile dressings and let fall onto sterile field.*

d. Open cleansing solution container, and pour solution into sterile cup.

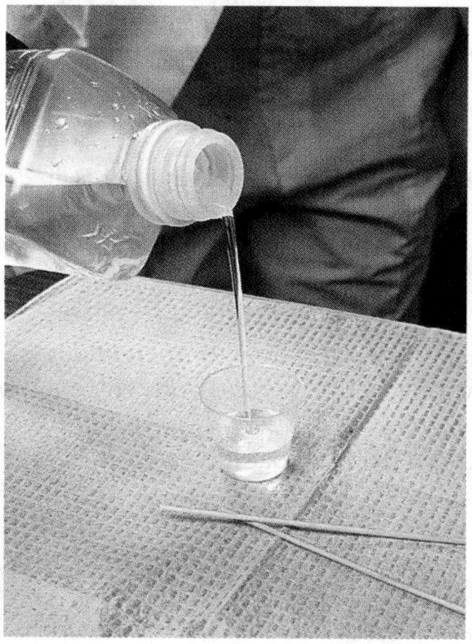

***Step 8D** • Pour container of cleansing solution.*

e. Open applicator packages. Set materials at the side of the sterile field.
Rationale: Setting up sterile supplies after removing and discarding the soiled dressing allows the nurse to assess what dressing material is needed and to make changes if necessary without charging the client for unneeded supplies.
Optional: Instead of using the sterile towel as a sterile field, the nurse may open the dressing packages and suture set carefully, allowing the inside of the packaging material to serve as the sterile field.

9. Don sterile gloves. Grasp applicators at nonabsorbent end and dip them into the cleansing solution.

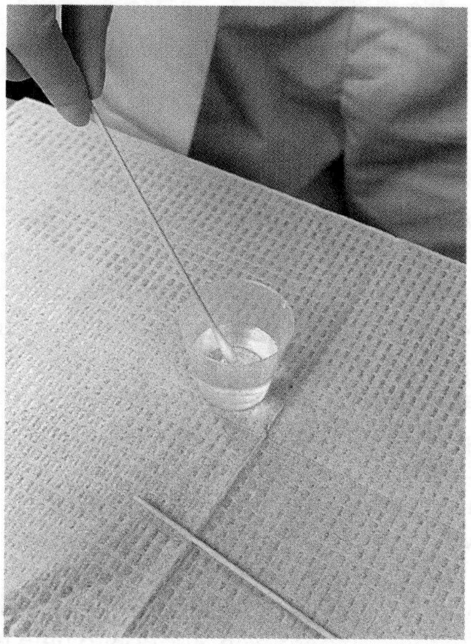

***Step 9** • Dip cotton tip applicators into cleansing solution.*

10. Clean drainage from the center of the wound outward. Use each applicator once and discard it. Do not place it back into the cleansing solution.
Rationale: Cleansing from the wound out prevents introduction of microorganisms into the wound. Using applicators only once prevents the transfer of microbes into the cleansing solution container.

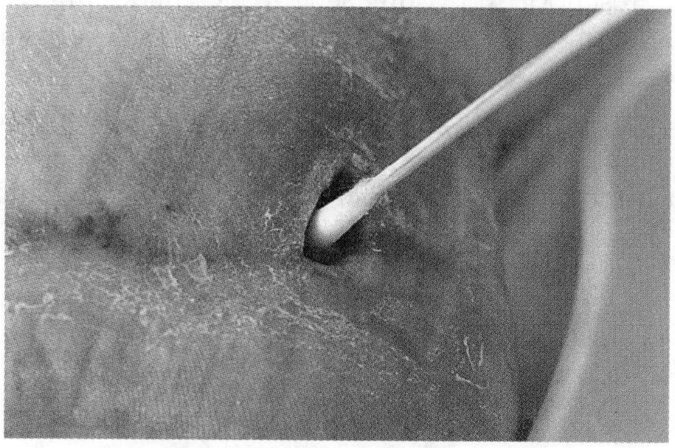

***Step 10** • Clean wound from the least contaminated area to most contaminated area.*

11. Dry the wound with gauze held by forceps.
Rationale: Microorganisms grow well in dark, moist environments.
12. Inspect the incision for bleeding, inflammation, drainage, and healing. Note any areas of dehiscence (opening or gaping of wound edges).
Rationale: Inadequate healing or complications must be noted and treated immediately.
13. Apply sterile dressings one at a time over the wound.
Rationale: Careful application of dressings prevents introduction of microorganisms into the wound.

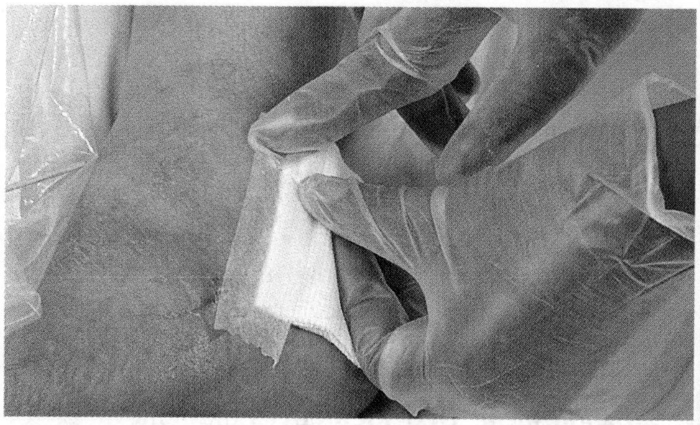

***Step 13** • Apply sterile dressing over the wound.*

14. Wash your hands.
Rationale: Handwashing helps prevent spread of microorganisms.
15. Document procedure and observations.

(continued)

Lifespan Considerations

Children

- Young children need to be reminded not to touch the incision when their dressing is removed. An assistant may be needed to prevent the child from moving and contaminating the wound or the sterile field.
- Preschool and young school-age children may feel that the part of their body covered by a dressing is not there. It reassures them to see the body part. Allow them to see their incision if they are interested.
- If the child is not toilet trained and the dressing becomes wet with urine or feces, change the dressing. Consider using wide plastic tape over the dressing to keep it dry.

Older Adult

- As skin ages, it loses its elasticity and becomes more sensitive. Adhesive tape may tear the skin. Paper tape or Montgomery straps are more protective.

Home Care Modifications

- When a client needs to change dressings at home, instruct him or her:
- That handwashing before and after the dressing change is the most important aspect of maintaining asepsis. For some dressing, gloving is not required.
- Where to buy and how to open and use dressings.
- How to clean the wound and which antiseptic to use.
- Signs of infection that indicate the need to call the nurse or physician.

small capillaries. When packing has been inserted during surgery, this should be noted on the client's record so that it is not accidentally removed when the dressing is changed. Pressure packing is usually left in place for 2 or 3 days and then removed by the surgeon or by the nurse with a physician's order so that it does not become a reservoir for the growth of microorganisms.

Wound Cleansing and Disinfection. The purpose of wound cleansing is to remove debris, contaminants, and excess exudate. Wound cleansers should not contain agents that are harmful to the cells involved in wound healing. This is especially important in the care of chronic wounds, such as pressure ulcers. Sterile normal saline (0.9% NaCl) is the cleansing solution of choice for chronic wounds. Many commercial wound cleansers are available, with varying levels of toxicity to cells (Wright, 1993). Commercial wound cleansers contain agents such as surfactant, which may facilitate the removal of wound debris. Procedure 38-3 describes how to irrigate a wound.

Intact skin is prepared for surgical incisions or invasive procedures using a process called skin preparation. Skin preparation often involves the use of antiseptic solutions, such as iodine or chlorhexidine, to scrub the surface of the skin. This decreases the possibility of infection from breaking the intact skin barrier and is an appropriate use of disinfectants.

Débridement. **Débridement** is the removal of foreign material or dead tissue from a wound to discourage the growth of microorganisms and to promote wound healing. There are four main types of débridement: mechanical, surgical, enzymatic, and autolytic (Rodeheaver, 1994). Surgical débridement refers to the use of sharp instruments to débride the wound, and it can be done in surgery or at the bedside. Physicians and other providers who specialize in wound care (eg, enterostomal therapy nurse, physical therapist) perform sharp débridement. Mechanical débridement is most commonly done with the use of a wet-to-dry dressing. Saline-moistened gauze is gently packed into the wound, covered with a lightweight gauze, and allowed to dry before removal. The dry dressing, when removed, pulls out the debris that has adhered to its surface. Enzymatic débridement refers to the process of chemical products being placed within the wound to help break down the necrotic debris. Autolytic débridement is a process of removing debris and necrotic tissue using the body's own fluids and cells. Autolytic débridement occurs when an occlusive dressing is applied over a wound and left in place while wound exudate and body fluids build up. The wound fluid softens the eschar, making it easier to remove and in some cases, totally dissolves debris so that it can be irrigated from the wound during a subsequent dressing change.

Wound Support

Supporting the wound area and preventing stress and tension on the incision help promote healing.

Butterflies and Steristrips. Butterflies and Steristrips can be applied to wounds to approximate wound edges and promote healing. A butterfly is a type of adhesive strip shaped like a butterfly. One edge is adhered to the skin and is pulled until wound approximation is achieved; then the other adhesive side is adhered to the skin. On small wounds, a butterfly may eliminate the need for sutures. Steristrips are commercially prepared adhesive strips used for the same purpose. They come in different widths. Tincture of benzoin may be applied to the skin before application to help them stick longer.

Procedure 38-2
Applying Wet-to-Dry Dressings

Purpose

1. Débride the wound
2. Promote healing
3. Protect the wound from contamination and mechanical trauma

Assessment

- Review the physician's orders for type and strength of solution to be used and frequency of dressing changes.
- Assess location and size of wound to determine needed dressing supplies.
- Assess client's level of comfort. Give analgesics as needed before wound care.
- Review nursing notes for previous wound description and for presence of generalized symptoms of infection (ie, elevated temperature, leukocytosis).

Equipment

Clean disposable gloves
Sterile gloves
Sterile dressing instrument set (forceps, scissors)
Sterile thin-mesh gauze dressing
Sterile gauze dressings
Extra sterile gauze dressings or ABD pads
Sterile basin
Prescribed sterile solution
Sterile saline
Tape or ties
Waterproof disposal bag
Sterile cotton-tipped applicators (optional)
Sterile drape (optional for sterile field)

Procedure

1. Prepare client and remove dressing according to Steps 1–5 of Procedure 38-1.
   Note: Forceps may be used to remove a soiled dressing. If dressing adheres to underlying tissues, do not moisten it. Gently remove the dressing while assessing client's discomfort level.
   Rationale: Dressing removal is intended to débride exudate and necrotic tissue from the wound. Moistening the dressing impairs the débridement process.
2. Observe dressings for amount and characteristics of drainage. Note odor and color.
   Rationale: Assessment of dressings reveals any wound infection.
3. Observe wound for eschar (thick layer of dead cells and dried plasma), granulation tissue (reddish capillary loops that bleed easily), or epithelial skin buds.
   Rationale: Wound must be assessed for healing.
4. Prepare sterile supplies. Open sterile instruments, sterile basin, solution, and dressings.
5. Place fine-mesh gauze into basin, and pour the ordered solution over mesh to saturate.
   Rationale: Gauze touching the wound surface must be thoroughly moistened to increase its absorptive ability.
   Note: If the wound is very large, warm the ordered solution to body temperature to prevent excessive loss of body heat.
6. Don sterile gloves.
   Rationale: Gloves prevent contamination of wound or supplies and protect nurse from contamination from body fluids.
7. Cleanse wound with antiseptic solution as prescribed or with normal saline, moving from least to most contaminated areas.
   Rationale: When cleaning debris from wound, steps are taken to prevent spread of contamination.
8. Squeeze excess fluid from gauze dressing.
   a. Gently pack moistened gauze into the wound.

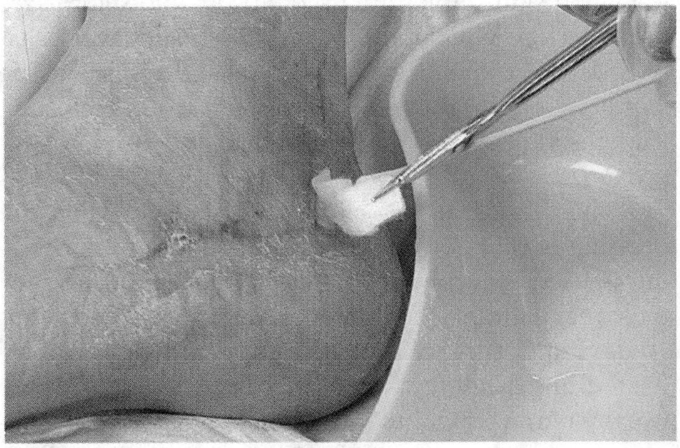

Step 8A • *Gently press gauze into wound.*

   b. If wound is deep, use forceps or cotton-tipped applicators to press gauze into all wound surfaces.

(continued)

Rationale: Moist gauze absorbs drainage and adheres to necrotic debris as it dries.

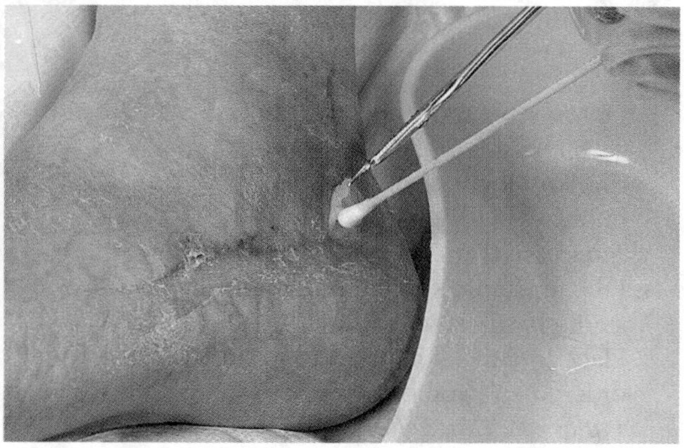

Step 8B Press gauze into all wound surfaces.

9. Apply several dry, sterile 4 × 4's over the wet gauze.
   Rationale: Extra pads help absorb excess moisture from under dressings.
10. Place ABD pad over dry 4 × 4's.
   Rationale: The wound is protected from contamination.
11. Dispose of sterile gloves.
12. Secure dressings with tape, Kerlix gauze (for circumferential dressings), or Montgomery ties.
13. Assist client to a comfortable position.
14. Wash your hands.
15. Document procedure and observations.

Lifespan Considerations and Home Care Modifications

See Procedure 38-1.

Sutures, Staples, and Clips. Support is provided in a surgical incision by using sutures, surgical staples, or surgical clips to hold the incision together until healing occurs. The type of material used for wound closure affects wound healing.

A suture, the material used to sew an incision together, can be absorbable (eg, catgut or chromic) or nonabsorbable (eg, nylon, silk, or polypropylene). The type of suture used depends on the size and location of the wound, how strong the suture material needs to be, the desired cosmetic effect, and the surgeons's preference. Generally, the least amount of suture and the smallest size of suture results in optimal wound closure.

Skin staples are made of stainless steel and are minimally reactive to the body as a foreign substance. Often when skin staples are used, absorbable sutures are used to close viscera and underlying tissue layers. Staples decrease the risk of infection and reduce tissue handling because they allow faster wound closure. Larger stainless-steel clips also may be used to approximate wound edges.

Sutures, staples, or clips are inspected when the dressing is changed or routinely if a transparent dressing is used. The physician determines how long they must remain in place. Sutures are usually removed 7 to 10 days after surgery if wound edges are well approximated and healing appears normal. Skin staples are usually removed in 5 to 7 days, but larger retention sutures may remain in place for a longer time. Sometimes the physician orders the removal of every other staple or suture to ensure that adequate healing has occurred and to avoid dehiscence. Most surgical clients also have absorbable sutures in place holding deeper layers of tissue or fascia together.

Staples are removed with a staple remover (Fig. 38-11). It is inserted under each staple, and the handle is

(text continues on page 1098)

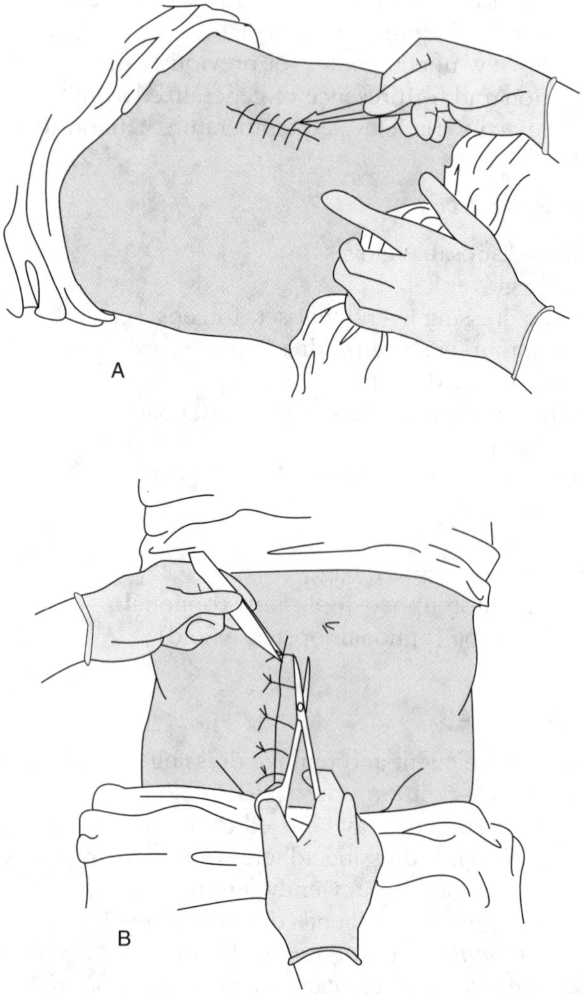

Figure 38-11 • ***(A)*** *Staples are removed by inserting a staple remover under each staple and compressing the handle, causing the staple to bend in the middle.* ***(B)*** *To remove a suture, cut close to the skin and use forceps to pull through, taking care to avoid pulling the visible part of the suture through underlying tissue.*

Procedure 38-3 Irrigating a Wound

Purpose

1. Cleanse the wound by removing debris and exudate
2. Occasionally, instill medication into the wound
3. Promote wound healing

Assessment

- Review physician's orders for type and strength of solution to be used for irrigation.
- Assess location and size of wound to determine needed dressing supplies.
- Assess client's comfort level. Give analgesics as needed before wound care.
- Assess for symptoms of anxiety.
- Review chart for presence of generalized symptoms of infection (ie, elevated temperature, leukocytosis).

Equipment

Sterile dressing instrument set and dressing materials, as in Procedure 38-2
Sterile gloves
Sterile basin
Mask, goggles, and gown may be indicated to protect nurse's eyes, mouth, and clothes from splatter
Clean basin to collect contaminated irrigating solution
Prescribed irrigating solution warmed to body temperature
Sterile irrigating solution
Sterile Robinson catheter (optional for deep wounds)
Waterproof disposal bag
Waterproof underpad
35-cc syringe and 19-gauge needle

Procedure

1. Close door or curtains around bed. Explain procedure to client.
2. Position client comfortably to allow irrigating solution to flow by gravity across the wound and into a collection basin.
   Rationale: Solution must flow from least contaminated to most contaminated area. Gravity directs the flow.
3. Expose only the wound area. Place waterproof pad under client.
   Rationale: Linen is protected from spill of irrigating solution.
4. Wash your hands.
   Rationale: Handwashing helps prevent transfer of microorganisms.
5. Don mask, goggles, and gown if needed.
   Rationale: Nurse's mucous membranes and clothing must be protected from accidental splashing of wound irrigation.
6. Remove dressing and inspect wound. See steps 1 to 4 of Procedure 38-2.
7. Pour warmed irrigating solution into sterile basin.
   Rationale: Warmed solution is more comfortable for client.
8. Open irrigating syringe, and place into basin with solution.
9. Place second basin at distal end of wound.
   Rationale: Basin will catch contaminated irrigating solution.
10. Don sterile gloves.
    Rationale: Wearing gloves maintains surgical asepsis.
11. Fill irrigating syringe with solution. Holding syringe tip about 1 in above the wound; gently flush all areas of the wound. Continue flushing until solution draining into basin is clear.
    Rationale: Holding syringe tip above tissue prevents trauma to granulation tissue. Irrigating until clear ensures that all debris and exudate are removed.

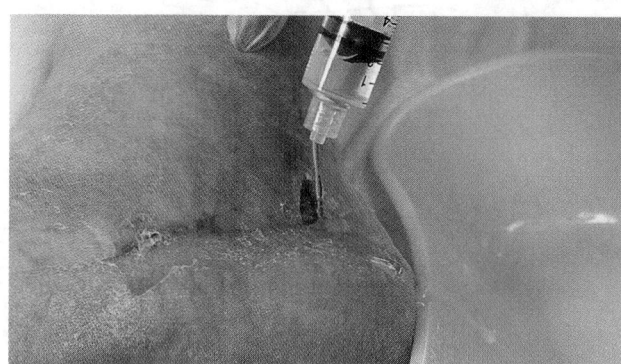

Step 11 • *Flush the wound with irrigating solution.*

12. If the wound is deep, attach a Robinson catheter to filled syringe with irrigating solution. Gently insert catheter into wound and flush until returning solution is clear.
    Rationale: Catheter introduces solution deeper into wound.
    Note: When refilling irrigation syringe with solution, disconnect catheter, fill syringe, and reconnect catheter. This prevents contaminating the basin of solution with microorganisms from the catheter.

(continued)

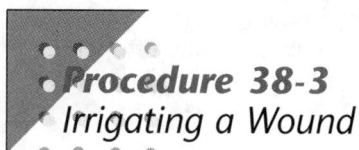

13. Dry surrounding skin thoroughly.
    Rationale: Excess moisture on skin promotes growth of microorganisms and skin breakdown.
14. Apply sterile dressing.
    Rationale: Sterile dressing provides protective barrier over wound.
15. Remove and discard gloves.
16. Secure dressing with tape or Montgomery straps.
17. Assist client to a comfortable position.
18. Dispose of equipment.
    Note: Retain remaining bottle of sterile solution for future irrigations. Mark date and time of opening on bottle for reference. Dispose according to agency policy.
19. Wash your hands.
20. Document procedure and observations.

Lifespan Considerations and Home Care Modifications

Refer to Procedure 38-1.

compressed. The pressure causes the staple to bend in the middle, and the edges pop out of the skin. The client may experience minor discomfort as the staples are removed. Steristrips are usually applied after the staples are removed to support the wound until healing is more complete.

Sutures are removed with a forceps and scissors. The suture is cut close to the skin, and the forceps is used to remove the suture (see Fig. 38-11*B*). Care must be taken to avoid pulling the visible portion of the suture through underlying tissue, because this can contaminate the incisional area and contribute to an infection. Sutures may be intermittent or continuous, and the nurse must discern the suturing technique before removing the sutures. As with staples, Steristrips are often applied after suture removal.

Ace Wraps and Bandages. Ace wraps are bandages used to support an area and often to secure a dressing (Fig. 38-12). Incorrectly applied, Ace wraps and gauze

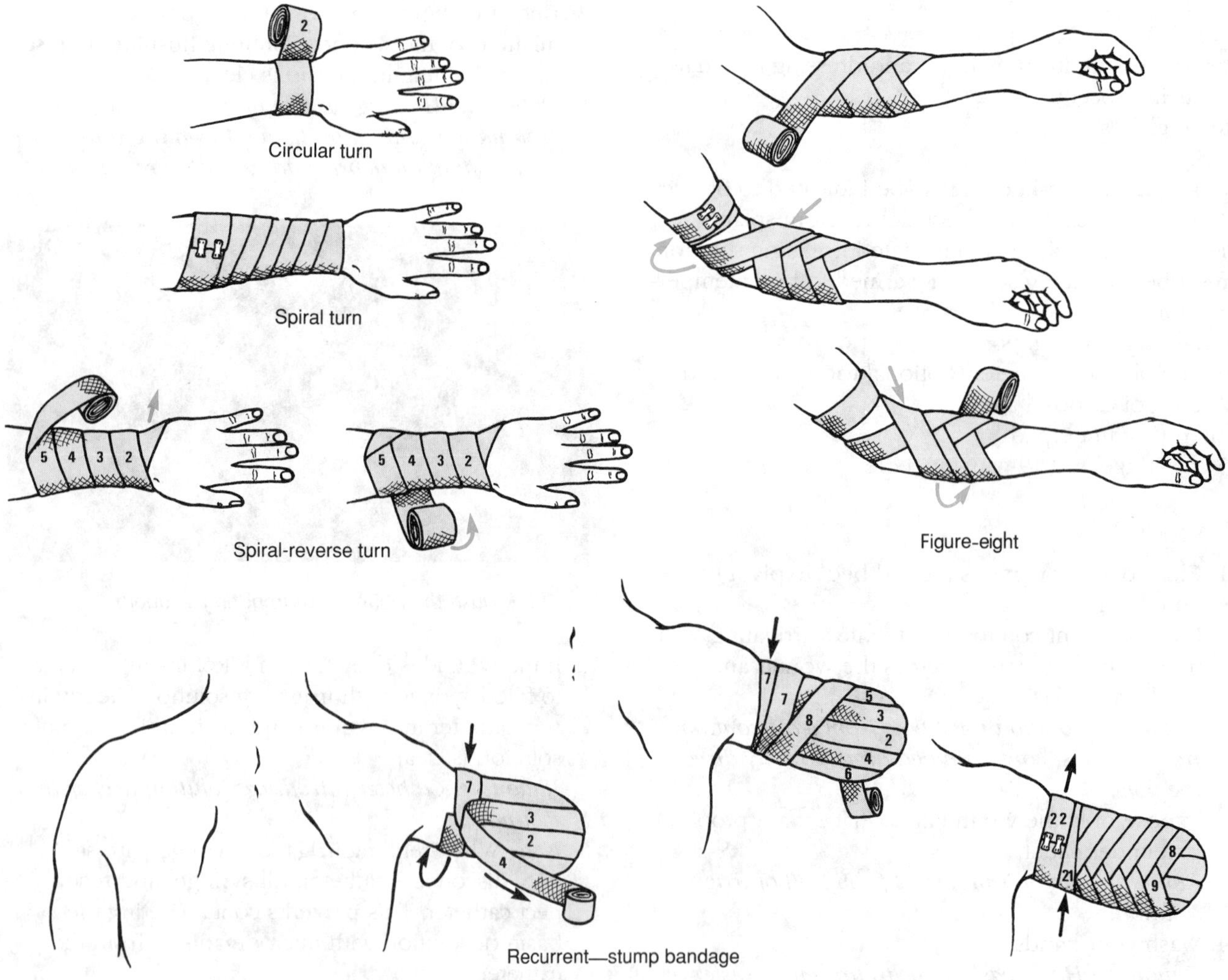

Figure 38-12 *• Techniques for bandage application.*

wraps can lead to edema and impaired circulation. Pressure, when applied circumferentially to an extremity, should be more snug at the distal end of the extremity to facilitate venous return.

Circular turns anchor bandages in place by overlapping the previous bandage turn completely.

Spiral turns are used to cover cylindric body parts, such as the wrist or arm, ascending the body part by overlapping the previous turn by one-half or two-thirds the width of the bandage.

Spiral reverse turns, useful when bandaging the leg, thigh, or forearm, require a twist that reverses the bandaging direction halfway through each turn.

Figure-8 turns consist of overlapping, alternating ascending and descending oblique turns that resemble a figure 8. This technique is especially useful when bandaging a joint.

Recurrent or stump bandaging is used for the head, digits, or amputated limbs. The bandage is anchored with a few circular turns, then turned back over itself, repeating until the distal end of the body part is covered. Once the end is covered, the bandage is anchored by using figure-eight and circular turns.

Frequent assessment of body parts distal from the bandage site (eg, fingers, toes) is important to detect impaired circulation promptly. Cyanosis, paller, coolness, numbness, tingling, swelling, or absent or diminished pulses are signs that circulation may be decreased. Many bandages are routinely removed so that the area can be inspected and areas of pressure avoided. If a bandage was applied by a physician or during surgery, the nurse may need an order before removing or adjusting it.

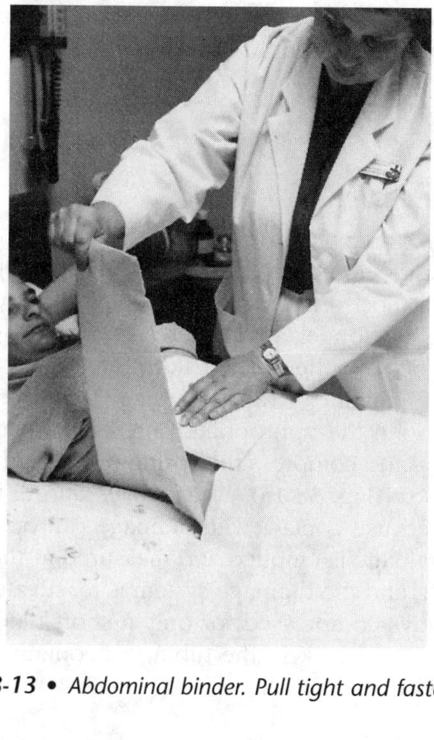

Figure 38-13 • Abdominal binder. Pull tight and fasten Velcro.

Binders. **Binders** are used to support a specific body part or to hold dressings in place. The use of Velcro in binders has increased their ease of application and comfort. Velcro fasteners permit individualized adjustments and securely fasten the binder in place, while permitting quick and easy release. Binders come in different shapes and sizes depending on the area for use. The binders most commonly used for support are abdominal binders and slings.

An *abdominal binder* is used to support the torso, especially after abdominal surgery (Fig. 38-13). It is usually a straight piece of elastic fabric, 15 to 20 cm wide and long enough to go around the torso.

A *sling* is used to support the arm, usually after trauma or injury. Commercially manufactured slings use Velcro for fastening and adjustments. If a commercial sling is unavailable, a triangular piece of cloth can be placed under the bent arm and folded as necessary to create a proper support. The sling is tied to the side of the neck so that the knot does not press against the cervical vertebrae.

Drainage Management

A large amount of wound drainage can inhibit wound healing and impair skin integrity around the wound. Nurses promote optimal wound healing by ensuring that drainage systems function properly and by advancing or removing drains as ordered by the physician. Nurses also protect skin from irritation by changing dressings frequently when caustic drainage is present.

Drains must be patent to remove drainage from the wound effectively. Clients should be prevented from lying on drainage systems because this can kink or compress the drain, thereby obstructing drainage flow. Some drains are sutured in place, but others are not, so care must be taken not to remove a drain accidentally. When the client ambulates, the drainage container is pinned to the client's clothing; this avoids placing excessive tension on the drainage system and incisional area, especially when the system is full of drainage. Preventing tension on the drainage system also decreases client discomfort.

Closed Drainage Systems. Appropriate suction permits drainage to be evacuated from the wound. If the drain is attached to external suction, check that the prescribed amount of suction is registered on the suction source. When the attachment tube is disconnected, suction should be apparent.

When closed drainage systems (such as Hemovac or Jackson-Pratt; Fig. 38-14) are used, suction is usually maintained by compression of a spring or bulb. Steps in maintaining portable wound suction are outlined in

Procedure 38-4
Maintaing a Portable (Hemovac) Wound Suction

Purpose

1. Facilitate healing by removing drainage from the incisional area where granulating tissue is forming

Assessment

- Assess client for generalized signs of infection (ie, elevated temperature).
- Assess drainage for amount, color, clarity, and odor.
- Assess the client for inflammation for discomfort around the drain.

Equipment

Clean disposable gloves
Calibrated drainage receptacle

Procedure

1. Explain procedure, assist client to a comfortable position; pull curtains or close door.
2. Wash your hands. Don clean disposable gloves.
   Rationale: Handwashing and gloves help prevent transfer of microorganisms.
3. Expose Hemovac tubing and container while keeping client draped.
   Rationale: Privacy and warmth are provided for the client.
4. Examine tubing and container for patency and suction seal.
   Note: If the system's seal is broken, the Hemovac reservoir will be expanded and not compressed.
5. Open the drainage plug (it is labeled).
6. Pour drainage into a calibrated receptacle without contaminating the drainage spout.
   Rationale: Transfer of microorganisms to the wound is prevented by this action.
   Rationale: A closed drainage system is established.
7. Reestablish suction by placing reservoir on a firm, flat surface. With drainage plug open, compress the unit and reinsert drainage plug.

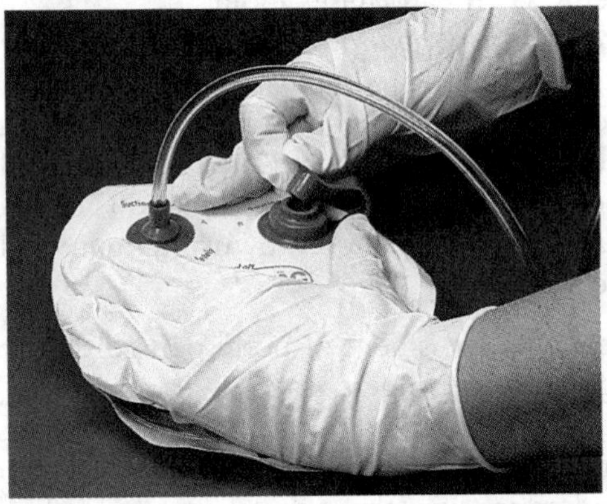

Step 7 • *Compress the reservoir and close the drainage plug.*

8. Remove and discard gloves.
9. Return client to a comfortable position.
10. Measure drainage and record amount, color, and any other pertinent information.

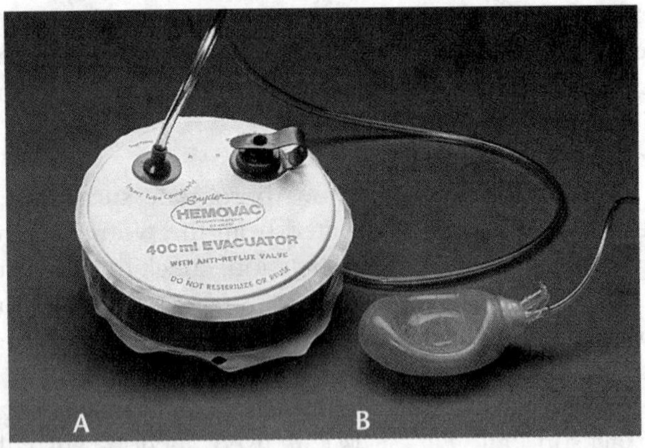

Figure 38-14 • *Closed drainage systems. **(A)** Hemovac. **(B)** Jackson-Pratt or grenade.*

Procedure 38-4. Specific instructions accompany drainage systems and should be consulted before handling.

When most drainage systems expand fully, gentle suction is no longer available to assist drainage flow. This can occur if there is a leak in the system or if the collection container is full of drainage. To reactivate the suction, open the appropriate port, empty drainage if necessary, and compress the spring or bulb while closing the port (Fig. 38-15). Wear gloves during this procedure because contact with drainage can occur. Routinely, drainage is emptied and measured at the end of each shift, and the drainage system is reactivated. If the system stays compressed for only a short time, it usually indicates a leak in the tubing or container, which may need replacement.

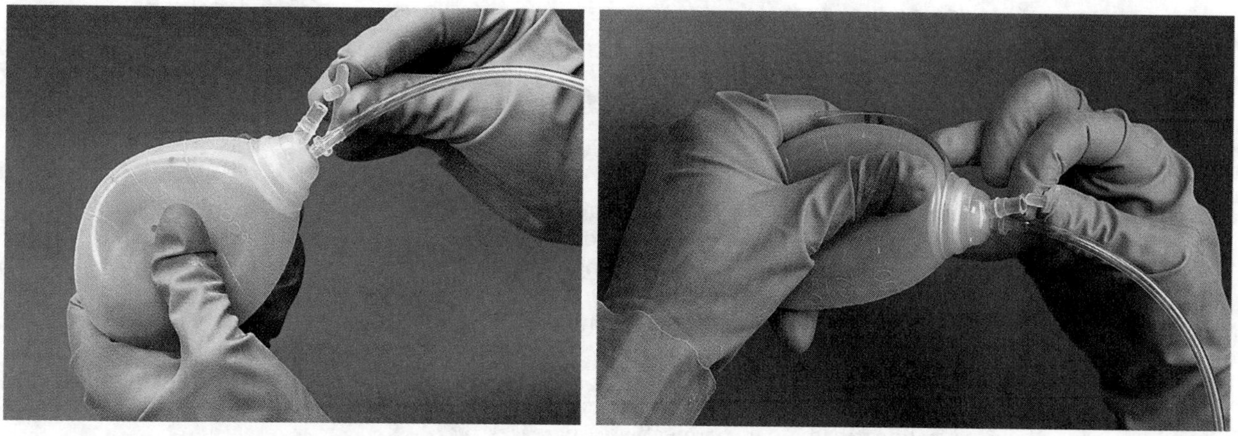

Figure 38-15 • Recharging a Jackson-Pratt drainage system. Also see Procedure 38-4, Step 7.

Advancing and Removing Drains. Drains are advanced or removed when little drainage is being discharged. Advancing a drain means pulling in a small amount, rather than removing it entirely. Advancing a drain allows evacuation of drainage from different areas of a wound without the need for more than one drainage tube.

To advance or shorten a drain, any sutures holding the drain in place must first be removed. When shortening a Penrose drain, a sterile safety pin is attached to the end of the drain (Fig. 38-16). This helps to prevent inadvertent loss of the drain back to the wound. Any excess part of the drain is cut off with scissors. Advancing some drains can cause the client discomfort. This can be minimized by asking the client to breathe deeply as the drain is pulled and by premedicating the client. After drain advancement or removal, increased drainage can be expected for a short time.

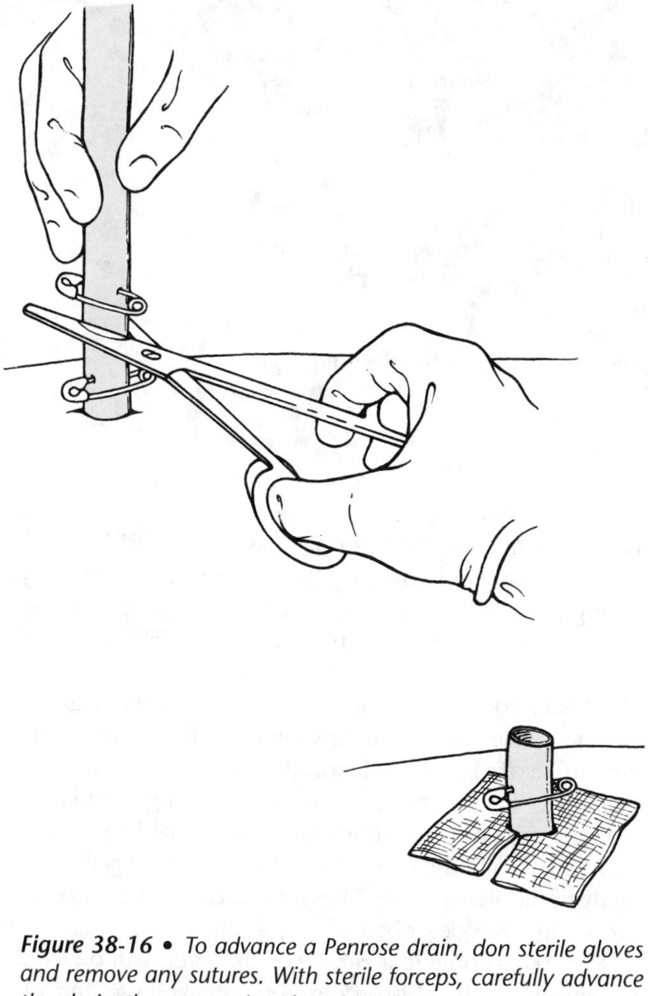

***Figure 38-16** • To advance a Penrose drain, don sterile gloves and remove any sutures. With sterile forceps, carefully advance the drain the appropriate length and attach a second sterile safety pin to prevent inadvertent loss back into the wound. Cut between the pins. Place a gauze square around the drain to absorb drainage and protect skin integrity.*

Local Application of Heat and Cold

Heat and cold are used in a variety of therapeutic interventions to promote healing (Table 38-4).

Cold therapies are usually used early in wound management to control hemorrhage, edema, and pain. Cold is used to control local bleeding because it causes vasoconstriction, which decreases blood flow to the area. Cold helps control swelling by reducing the permeability of capillary walls and the escape of extracellular fluids.

Heat therapies are used to increase blood flow, resolve inflammation, improve healing of soft tissues, and relieve muscular pain and stiffness. Local heat causes vasodilation, increasing the supply of oxygen, nutrients, leukocytes, and antibodies to the tissues. The increased blood flow also promotes removal of metabolic wastes and dissipation of heat. Heat increases the local cellular metabolic processes, which in turn increases the demand for more oxygen. As a result of this activity, soft tissues heal. The inflammatory process also is accelerated when heat is applied because heat reduces the viscosity of blood. This allows leukocytes and antibodies to reach the infected area more quickly. Heat allows pus to consolidate in infected areas. Heat also promotes muscular relaxation and relieves muscle tension, spasms, and joint stiffness. A disadvantage of local heat

Table 38-4 • Uses for Heat and Cold

Effect	Physiologic Mechanism	Selected Uses
Heat Application		
Promotes healing and suppuration (consolidation of pus)	Vasodilation leads to increased blood flow, thus increasing oxygen and nutrients to the area and promoting removal of waste products	Surgical wounds, infected wounds, hemorrhoids, episiotomies
Decreases inflammation by accelerating inflammatory process	Increases capillary wall permeability, increases leukocyte and antibody flow to area, promotes action of phagocytes	Phlebitis, IV infiltration
Decreases musculoskeletal discomfort	Increases sensory nerve conduction, promotes muscle relaxation, decreases viscosity of synovial fluid	Low back pain, menstrual cramps, contractures, arthritis, muscle spasms
Cold Application		
Controls bleeding	Vasoconstriction decreases blood flow, which in turn decreases metabolic tissue demands and the supply of oxygen and nutrients	Fractures, trauma, superficial lacerations, puncture wounds
Decreases edema	Decreases capillary permeablility; causes vasoconstriction	Sprains, muscle strains, sports injuries
Relieves pain	Decreases nerve conduction velocity; induces numbness or paresthesia	Arthritis, trauma, musculoskeletal injuries

is that increased capillary permeability can increase edema formation.

Safety Considerations. Client safety is an important consideration when using heat or cold, because they can damage tissues or alter thermoregulation. Table 38-5 lists precautions for the safe use of heat or cold.

The duration of application is important. Maximum vasodilation or vasoconstriction usually occurs in 30 minutes, and prolonged application may result in burns or freezing. Very young or older clients have a decreased ability to tolerate heat and cold and are more likely to suffer adverse effects. Impaired circulation, impaired sensation, or impaired cognitive abilities also increase the incidence of injury. Body areas where heat or cold therapy is used can be more or less sensitive, depending on the sensitivity or thickness of skin. Impaired skin integrity increases the chance that heat or cold application could damage tissues. Extensive exposure to heat or cold can have systemic and local effects. Unexpected adverse effects can occur, especially in high-risk clients, such as the very young or older adults. Refer to Chapter 40 for more details.

Cold Packs and Ice Bags. Cold packs and ice bags are used to deliver local dry cold. Commercial cold packs contain an alcohol-based solution that is released inside the bag when it is squeezed or kneaded, creating a cold temperature. The outer covering is soft and pliable, so it can be molded to fit the contours of the body and applied directly to the skin surface. These packs cannot be refrozen. Procedure 38-5 describes how to apply a cold pack.

Ice bags come in a variety of sizes and can be used to control localized bleeding, reduce swelling, and reduce pain. Some ice bags are made of rubber and have screw-on caps for filling. Before applying a rubber bag, a cloth cover should be applied over the rubber surface to avoid irritating the skin and to maintain med-

Table 38-5 • Precautions for the Safe Use of Heat and Cold

Assessment Factor	Rationale
Acute sudden pain that may indicate abscessed tooth or appendicitis	Application of heat may cause rupture, with systemic spread of infection.
Broken skin or deep open wounds	Subcutaneous and visceral tissues are more sensitive to temperature extremes. Fewer pain and temperature receptors are available to warn of possible tissue damage.
Circulatory impairment (peripheral vascular disease, diabetes)	Cold application vasoconstricts, thus decreasing circulation to the already compromised area. Heat is not dissipated well from the area, making tissue damage more likely.
Sensory deficits (cerebrovascular accident, paraplegia, quadriplegia)	Alterations in nerve conduction limit the sensation of temperature or pain, thus increasing the likelihood of tissue damage.
Mental status impairment (confusion, decreased level of consciousness)	Decreased reliability of reporting pain and altered sensation increases the possibility of tissue damage.
Age extremes	Very young children have immature thermoregulation, cannot communicate pain or discomfort specifically, and cannot alter their environment. Elderly have reduced sensation to pain and often have another impairment (eg, circulatory, sensory) that compounds the risk. Heat should not be applied to the abdomen of a pregnant woman because fetal growth could be affected.
Metallic implants (pacemakers, total joint replacements)	Metal is a good conductor of heat, thus increasing the potential for burns because the implant cannot be readily removed

ical asepsis. When using cold therapy with children, it is often helpful to use a plastic glove with a "face" marked on it as a way of decreasing fear.

Cold Compresses. Cold compresses are used to relieve swelling and inflammation. Gauze pads are moistened with chilled saline or water and applied to the appropriate area. If applied to an open wound, asepsis must be maintained. Compresses easily conform to the contour of the intended area and can soften exudate. Because cold compresses quickly warm to the temperature of the client's skin, they need to be changed frequently. If left on the wound for a prolonged period, maceration can occur.

Warm Compresses. Warm compresses are generally applied to open wounds to improve circulation and promote suppuration. If an open wound is involved, surgical asepsis principles must be followed, but medical asepsis is sufficient if the compress is applied to intact skin. Compresses mold easily to body contours. Commercially packaged sterile compresses are available, which must be heated under an infrared lamp before opening and application. If commercially prepared compresses are unavailable, solution can be warmed and applied to gauze pads. Avoid using temperatures that might cause burns.

The heat of a warm compress dissipates quickly, but heat can be retained longer by applying a layer of plastic over the compress. If a constant warm temperature is desired, the nurse can apply a heating mechanism over the compress (eg, an aquathermia pad), but because moisture conducts heat, the temperature of the heating mechanism must be low.

Warm Soaks. Warm soaks involve immersing a body part in a warm liquid (usually water) to promote relaxation, improve circulation, or soften wound exudate. They also can be used to apply a medicated solution. Warm soaks usually take about 20 minutes, and the solution may need to be changed because cooling may occur.

Sitz Baths. A sitz bath provides moist heat to the pelvic and perineal area. A sitz bath is used after rectal or perineal surgery or after vaginal delivery to decrease inflammation and discomfort. The client sits in a special tub or in a basin that fits onto the toilet seat, so the legs and feet remain out of the water. Using a bathtub does not serve the same purpose, because immersing the entire body in warm water nullifies the effect of local heat applied to the pelvic area. The client's feet and upper torso should remain covered to prevent chilling. The sitz bath is filled with warm water (105°–

Procedure 38-5
Applying a Cold Pack

Purpose

1. Promote capillary vasoconstriction to prevent or decrease edema of traumatized tissue, to control bleeding, or to reduce pain

Assessment

- Identify the purpose for cold therapy.
- Examine the condition of the affected skin or injury.
- Assess sensitivity of affected area to temperature and touch to determine if client has impaired sensation to cold.
- Determine baseline level of pain.
- Obtain baseline vital signs, and assess client's ability to tolerate cold therapy (see Lifespan Considerations).
- Review physician's order for frequency and duration of therapy.
- Assess client's understanding of procedure.

Equipment

Ice bag, collar, and ice or commercially prepared ice pack
Pillowcase or bath towel

Procedure

1. Prepare ice pack. Fill bag or collar two-thirds full with crushed ice. Expel excess air from bag and secure cap. Commercial pack must be squeezed or kneaded.
   Rationale: Excess air in ice bag acts as insulation and interferes with cold conduction. Squeezing commercial pack releases alcohol-based solution to activate cold.
2. Place towel or pillowcase over cold pack.
   Rationale: Direct contact of ice pack to skin can cause destruction of skin cells from intense vasoconstriction.
   Note: Some commercial packs have an outer insulating wrap and can be applied directly to skin.
3. Close bed curtains or room door.
4. Assist client to a comfortable position, and expose only area to be treated.
   Rationale: Client privacy and comfort are maintained.
5. Apply prepared ice pack to area to be treated. Secure with tape or ties if necessary. Cover client.
6. Monitor condition of skin after 5 minutes.
   Rationale: Skin should be slightly pale and cool to touch. Cold therapy is too intense if skin surface is blue or mottled.
7. Remove pad after 30 minutes, and observe condition of treated skin.
   Rationale: Maximum effect of cold therapy is achieved in 30 to 60 minutes. After 60 minutes, a secondary vasodilation will occur. Wait 1 hour before reapplying.
8. Assist client to a comfortable position, and dispose of ice or commercial pack.
   Rationale: Plastic ice collars and bags are reusable if not soiled. Commercial ice packs cannot be frozen for reuse.

Lifespan Considerations

Infants

- Infants lose body heat readily. Ice packs are generally contraindicated because of the potential for loss of core body heat. Cold therapy may be used cautiously on limited areas (ie, an extremity).

Toddlers and Children

- Increased cooperation and compliance can be achieved if the child thinks of the ice pack as a friendly object. A plastic glove or ice bag with a face marked on it changes it from a treatment to a friend.

Older Adults

- Clients with atherosclerosis may have decreased blood supply to a body part. If cold is applied to an area with decreased circulation, treatment-induced vasoconstriction may cause tissue damage.
- Clients with cardiovascular or pulmonary disease are at risk for fluid overload if cold is applied on a large area or extremity. Cold-induced vasoconstriction shifts blood into the central circulation and may cause heart failure or pulmonary edema. Be alert to the client's overall circulatory status before applying cold.

Home-Care Modifications

- Ice packs are frequently ordered for home use. Assess the client's or significant other's knowledge of the procedure and safety measures. Educate as necessary.

110°F or 40°–43°C). A plastic bag with attached tubing is filled with warm water and inserted into the portable sitz bath, where it slowly replenishes warm water during the procedure. Sitz baths usually last for about 20 minutes. Because heat is being applied to a large area of the body, vasodilation can occur, causing the client to feel lightheaded and faint. If this occurs, the nurse should assess the client for a rapid pulse, pale facial color, or complaints of nausea. If these signs and symptoms are present, the sitz bath should be discontinued.

Paraffin Baths. Paraffin baths, a mixture of heated paraffin wax and mineral oil, are used for arthritic clients with painful joints. The treatment is usually given by a physical therapist.

Hot Packs. Dry local heat can be applied with hot-water bottles or K-packs. Hot-water bottles are similar to ice bags, but they are filled two-thirds full with hot water (125°F or 52°C for a normal adult, 110°F or 43°C for a young child or debilitated adult). Make sure the temperature of the water will not burn the client. Place a cloth covering over the rubber container to avoid irritation to the skin. The water should remain warm for 20 to 45 minutes, depending on its initial temperature. Hot-water bottles are used infrequently in hospitals and long-term care facilities but are common in the home setting. Electric heating pads also are common in the home setting.

K-packs or commercial hot packs are disposable, commercially prepared packages that produce specified amounts of heat when squeezed or kneaded. They cannot be reused.

Heating Pads. A thermostat controls the amount of heat the unit delivers. When a heating pad is used, the client should be advised not to lie on the unit or operate it near moisture, because this increases the chance of a burn. A heating pad should not be applied to the skin for longer than 20 to 30 minutes at any one time.

Aquathermia Pads. An aquathermia (water flow) pad is a popular heat-producing device used for treating muscle spasms and mild inflammation. This unit consists of a waterproof pad through which water circulates; the temperature of the circulating water can be controlled. The unit is filled two-thirds full of water and should be checked periodically for evaporation. If significant evaporation occurs, the unit must be refilled. The waterproof pad should not be in direct contact with the client's skin. It is usually covered with a pillowcase or towel. The pad is positioned over the intended area and left there for 20 to 30 minutes. The client should not lie on the pad, because pressure prevents normal distribution of the circulating water.

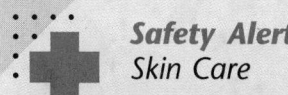

Heat Lamps. Heat lamps are used to increase circulation and provide comfort to small areas, such as episiotomy incisions. The area to be treated must be free of moisture, which could conduct heat. The heat lamp is placed an appropriate distance away from the treatment area (at least 45 cm), and low-wattage bulbs (40-60 watts) are used. The treatment lasts about 20 minutes. During treatment, the client's skin should be assessed periodically to ensure that no burn occurs. Heat lamps are contraindicated in pressure ulcer care.

> ***Safety Alert***
> *Skin Care*
>
> - Monitor clients with decreased sensation to skin surfaces closely when using heating pads or hot water. Thermal burns may result from impaired temperature perception.
> - Never use the high setting on heating pads or other heating units. During use, inspect the skin frequently for signs of thermal damage.
> - Move and position the immobile client carefully to prevent injury to the skin as a result of shearing force.
> - Monitor postoperative wounds carefully, and prevent undue stress to the wound by supporting the wound during coughing or vomiting.
> - Monitor toddlers and preschoolers around hot liquids, cigarettes, heaters, barbecue grills, and stoves to prevent thermal burns.

Emotional Support

Skin conditions may cause low self-esteem and altered body image, especially if the face or other highly visible area is disfigured. The client may choose isolation over appearing in public. Getting the client to express feelings about perceived or actual disfigurement is the first step in facing the problem. The nurse, with the client, can identify appropriate diversional activities. Support people can help the client work through the isolation. Referrals to appropriate community resources can be made to help avoid isolation.

Community-Based Care

Skin disorders and wounds require regular care and assessment for complications. Some clients can obtain their care at home, while others require temporary hospitalization or home care. Regardless of where the care is provided, the following principles apply:

- The environment should be clean.
- Wound care supplies must be accessible and available.

Therapeutic Dialogue
Skin Cancer

Scenes for Thought

Mrs. Cook is a 72-year-old woman who has a busy and active life in the retirement community where she lives. You are the community health nurse who makes frequent visits to the retirement community. Today Mrs. Cook wants to see you "about a rash."

Effective

Nurse: *Hi there, Mrs. Cook. How are you?*
Client: *Hi, Rhonda. I'm so glad to see you, I was worried you wouldn't be here today.* Looks concerned and a little scared.
Nurse: *Here I am. What can I help you with?*
Client: *I'm worried about this mole I have on the back of my neck. It gets rubbed by my collars, and yesterday I found blood on the collar in the same place as the mole. Could you look at it?* Shows you. There is a small amount of dried blood on the mole.
Nurse: *How long have you had the mole?*
Client: *Years and years. I never noticed anything about it until now, though.* Continues to look worried.
Nurse: *What worries you about this, Mrs. Cook?*
Client: *Cancer. My husband had a lot of these removed, and both my parents had skin cancer. Could it be cancer?* Her body stiffens as she waits for the answer.
Nurse: *It could be, but it may not be either. The dermatologist needs to see it and will possibly remove it in the office. Then it'll be sent to the pathologist for examination of the cells. You should know if it's cancer or not within a week. What do you think?*
Client: *I think I'd better make the dermatology appointment today. I want to know as soon as possible. Thanks, Rhonda.*

Less Effective

Nurse: *Hi, Mrs. Cook. What can I do for you today?*
Client: *I need to show you this mole. It's been bleeding when it rubs up against my collars.* Looks worried.
Nurse: *(Looks at the mole carefully) I don't see any problem right now, Mrs. Cook, but I think you need to be seen by the dermatologist. Shall I make the appointment for you? (Looks up the physician's number in the card file.)*
Client: *No, no I'll do it myself. I'll use the one that removed my husband's skin cancer.* Still looks worried.
Nurse: *That sounds like a good plan. At least the physician will be familiar to you. Is there anything else?*
Client: *No, that's okay. Have a good week.* Leaves office with mouth set, hurries to phone.

Critical Thinking Challenge

• Analyze what the first nurse did that the second nurse didn't do. • Detect what clue the second nurse missed and what difference it made. • In both instances Mrs. Cook called a dermatologist and will be seen, evaluated, and helped. Compare and contrast the nursing care supplied by each nurse. • Infer how Mrs. Cook will seek care in the future from either nurse.

- The client should receive adequate calories and nutrients to facilitate healing.
- The person providing wound or skin care should demonstrate the ability to perform the procedures and should know what symptoms to report to the healthcare provider.

All immobile clients and their caregivers require information about prevention of pressure ulcers: Frequent turning and proper positioning, hygiene, and nutrition. Topical wound care products and methods of use must be described and demonstrated. The use of pressure-reducing support surfaces should be encouraged. Clients often require nursing assistance to select an appropriate support surface for their use.

Clients who need dressing changes must demonstrate the ability to perform wound care or receive assistance from a caregiver or healthcare worker in that process. Clients and involved family members should be taught how to detect infection and how to monitor the client's temperature. Instructions (written and verbal) that include information on where to buy supplies should be provided. Clients who are unable to afford the needed products should receive assistance in making the treatment plan workable, which may include referral for assistance with healthcare expenses. Family members' acceptance of the skin impairment and their willingness to assist with care boosts the client's self-esteem.

Wound and skin problems can take an extended time to resolve. Instruct clients about the frequency of required follow-up medical appointments and symptoms of complications or recurrence. As indicated, teach about the etiology of the disorder, control or risk factors, and the importance of maintaining healthy skin function.

Evaluation

The evaluation of client-centered goals determines whether the outcome criteria have been met. Outcome criteria should be individualized for each client and revised as necessary. Below are client goals and possible outcome criteria concerning the prevention of tissue damage and promotion of optimal wound healing.

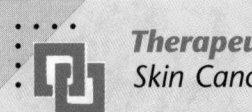

Nursing Plan of Care
The Client With Impaired Skin Integrity

Nursing Diagnosis

Impaired Skin Integrity related to pressure, friction, and immobility manifested by 3 cm stage II sacral pressure ulcer

Client Goal

Client/family will comply with regimen to prevent and treat pressure ulcers.

Client Outcome Criteria

- Client discusses pressure ulcers in his or her own words.
- Client describes five contributing factors to pressure ulcer development.
- Client inspects skin daily.
- Before discharge, client demonstrates interventions to relieve pressure effectively.

Nursing Intervention	*Scientific Rationale*
1. Teach the client and family what pressure ulcers are; use photos.	1. Knowledge is important in developing values to maintain preventive health practices
2. Discuss factors that can increase incidence of pressure ulcer formation.	2. Specific knowledge allows client to develop specific interventions that help prevent pressure ulcers.
3. Teach the client or family to inspect all pressure points daily and to use a mirror for hard to visualize areas.	3. Daily inspection helps to detect any evidence of skin abnormality promptly.
4. Elicit client preference for equipment (eg, support surfaces), skin treatment, turning schedules.	4. Active involvement of client in individualizing prevention plan helps ensure compliance.

Client Goal

Client's skin will demonstrate evidence of healing of existing wounds.

Client Outcome Criteria

- Client demonstrates increased granulation tissues in healing wound.
- Client demonstrates absence of redness, swelling, and purulent drainage.

Nursing Intervention	*Scientific Rationale*
1. Reposition q2h, increasing frequency of positioning if redness or blanching does not disappear.	1. Repositioning relieves pressure, which can include capillary blood flow leading to tissue damage and ulcer formation.
2. Do not allow client to lie on healing pressure ulcer. Turn right to left, left to right, and right to prone.	2. Delicate healing tissues are more susceptible to trauma and impaired blood flow; pressure delays healing.
3. Use pillows to position and support pressure points.	3. Padding decreases pressure and friction, which can increase pressure sore development.
4. Get up in chair at least 30 minutes twice a day	4. Different body positions and movement improve overall circulation and relieve pressure from ulcer area.
5. Communicate turning schedule on wall at client's bedside.	5. Communication of specific times and positions helps promote compliance with turning schedule.
6. Avoid high-Fowler or semi-Fowler position while in bed.	6. These positions increase shearing force, which impairs circulation as client slides down in bed.

(continued)

Nursing Plan of Care
The Client With Impaired Skin Integrity *(continued)*

Nursing Intervention	Scientific Rationale
7. Use turning sheet when moving client up in bed.	7. This action decreases shearing force and friction from bed when moving client.
8. Apply pressure-reducing or pressure-relieving overlay.	8. Special mattress overlays decrease the chance of occlusion of capillary blood flow, which can increase pressure sore development and delay healing.
9. Keep skin clean and dry, especially after episodes of incontinence.	9. Moisture promotes maceration of tissues and delays healing.
10. Apply hydrocolloid dressing to pressure ulcer; change every 7 days unless barrier is broken. Inspect each shift.	10. Hydrocolloid dressing protects ulcer to promote healing and prevent infection.
11. Encourage protein and vitamin-rich diet; assess dietary intake, and assist with menu choices.	11. Adequate nutrition is necessary for wound healing.

Goal

Client's skin will remain intact without areas of local inflammation.

Possible Outcome Criteria

- Client develops no skin lesions or pressure ulcers.
- Client develops no redness or abrasions of the skin.
- Client has intact skin without excessive drying or flaking.

Client's skin will show evidence of healing of existing wounds.

Possible Outcome Criteria

- Within 24 hours, wound edges are well approximated.
- Within 48 hours, healing wound has increased granulation tissue.
- By discharge, wound has no redness, swelling, or purulent drainage.

Goal

Client will identify principles of preventive skin care.

Possible Outcome Criteria

- After teaching session, client verbalizes interventions that can prevent pressure ulcer formation.
- Client identifies causes of mechanical or chemical tissue destruction.
- Client demonstrates routine skin care to prevent excessive drying or abrasions.
- Client discusses effective use of heat or cold therapies to prevent skin injury.

Goal

Client or family will comply with treatment plan to promote wound healing and skin integrity.

Possible Outcome Criteria

- After teaching session, client states important measures to promote skin integrity and wound healing.
- Client maintains adequate nutritional intake.
- By discharge, client or family demonstrate wound care and dressing change.
- Client discusses signs of wound infection and when to contact a healthcare provider.
- Client or family demonstrates proper use of special equipment needed to promote skin integrity.

Key Concepts

- The health of skin depends on adequate blood flow, adequate nutrition, intact epidermis, and proper hygiene.
- The skin's normal physiologic functions are protection, thermoregulation, sensation, metabolism, and communication.
- The very young and the very old are most susceptible to skin disruption.
- Potential for alterations in skin function include allergic reactions, infections, abnormal growth rate, wounds, pressure ulcers, and burns.
- Altered skin integrity may be manifested by pruritus, rash, lesions, pain, and inadequate wound healing.
- Understanding the types of wound healing (primary, secondary, or tertiary intention) is vital for proper wound assessment and management.

- Depth of injury affects choice of topical treatment.
- Hemorrhage, infection, dehiscence, evisceration, and fistula formation are potential complications of wounds.
- Factors affecting wound healing include oxygenation and nutrient supply, immune cellular function, age, obesity, smoking, drug intake, stress, nature of the injury, wound infection, and environment.
- In the nursing assessment, data are collected about normal skin status, risk for skin impairment, and identification of altered skin integrity.
- Planned nursing interventions are important to prevent pressure ulcer development and trauma to skin.
- Gauzes, transparent film, polyurethane foam, hydrocolloids, hydrogels, and alginates are categories of dressings used in topical care.
- Wound support can be provided by sutures, staples, clips, Steristrips, bandages, and binders.
- Effective management of drainage systems (ensuring patency, reactivating and advancing drains) promotes optimal wound healing.
- Local application of heat and cold can decrease inflammation, improve healing, and reduce pain.
- Home care is important for long-range promotion and maintenance of skin integrity.

Critical Thinking Challenges

Now that you have added skin care and wound healing to your knowledge base, turn to the situation at the beginning of the chapter, and plan care for your client using the following as your guide.

1. *Describe assessments you will make today and on subsequent visits.*
2. *Summarize factors that could affect the rate of wound healing in this client.*
3. *Outline teaching you will provide to help prevent further occurrence of pressure ulcers.*
4. *List the primary nursing diagnoses that will guide your care and other related nursing diagnoses that might apply in this situation.*
5. *Plan collaboration with the client, family, and other healthcare providers.*

References

Bosley, C. (1994). Three methods of stool management for patients with diarrhea. *Ostomy/Wound Management, 40* (1), 52–57.

Cox, H. C., Hinz, M. D., Lubro, M. A., et al. (1989). *Clinical applications of nursing diagnosis.* Baltimore: Williams & Wilkins.

Etris, M. B., Pribble, J., & LaBrecque, J. (1994). Evaluation of two wound measumement methods in a multi-center, controlled study. *Ostomy/Wound Management, 40* (7), 44–48.

Hägermark, O. (1992). Peripheral and central mediators of itch. *Skin Pharmacology, 5,* 1–8.

Hess, C. T. (1994). Wound care products: A directory. *Ostomy/Wound Management, 40* (3), 70–72, 74, 76–78, 80, 82–84, 86, 88–90, 92, 94.

Kaufman, M. W. (1994). Preventing diabetic foot ulcers. *MEDSURG Nursing, 3* (3), 204–210.

McCulloch, J. M., Marler, K. C., Neal, M. B., & Phifer, T. J. (1994). Intermittent pneumatic compression improves venous ulcer healing. *Advances in Wound Care, 7* (4), 22–24, 26.

Murray, M., & Blaylock, B. (1994). Maintaining effective pressure ulcer prevention programs. *MEDSURG Nursing, 3* (2), 85–93.

North American Nursing Diagnosis Association (1994). *NANDA nursing diagnoses: Definitions and classification 1995–1996.* Philadelphia: Author.

Panel for the Prediction and Prevention of Pressure Ulcers in Adults. (1992). *Pressure ulcers in adults: Prediction and prevention.* Clinical Practice Guideline, Number 3. AHCPR Publication No. 92–0047. Rockville, MD: Agency for Health Care Policy and Research, Public Health Service. U.S. Department of Health and Human Services.

Rodeheaver, G., Barastani, M. M., Brabec, M. E., Byrd, H. J., Salzberg, C. A., Scherer, P., & Vogelpohl, T. S. (1994). Wound healing and wound management: Focus on debridement. *Advances in Wound Care, 7*(1), 22–24, 26–29, 32–39.

Silane, M., & Oot-Giromini, B. (1990). Systemic and other factors that affect wound healing. In W. Eaglstein, C. Baxter, P. Mertz, et al. (Eds.), *New directions in wound healing.* Princeton, NJ: E.R. Squibb & Sons.

Torrence, B. P., Hovanec, R., Bartunek, C. & Brodell, R. T. (1993). Stasis dermatitis: Practical pearls for the dermatologic nurse. *Dermatology Nursing, 5* (3), 186–193.

Turner, T. D. (1990). The development of wound management products. In D. Krasner (Ed.), *Chronic wound care: A clinical source book for health care professionals.* King of Prussia, PA: Health Management Publications.

Whitney, J. D. (1989). Physiologic effects of tissue oxygenation on wound healing. *Heart and Lung, 18,* 466–474.

Wright Jr., R. W. (1993). Fibroblast cytotoxicity and blood cell integrity following exposure to dermal wound cleansers. *Ostomy/Wound Management, 36* (7), 33–36, 38, 40.

Wysocki, A. B. (1992). Skin. In R. A. Bryant (Ed.), *Acute and chronic wounds, nursing management.* St. Louis: Mosby Year Book.

Bibliography

Boyle, D. M. (1994). The older patient with cancer: Teaching/learning considerations for ostomy, wound, and continence management. *Progressions—Developments in Ostomy, Wound, and Continence Management, 6* (1), 11–21.

Braden, B. J., & Bergstrom, N. (1987). A conceptual schema for the study of etiology of pressure sores. *Rehabilitation Nursing, 12* (1), 8–12.

Bryant, R. A. (1992). *Acute and chronic wounds.* St. Louis: Mosby Year Book.

Goldstein, B. G., & Goldstein, A. D. (1992). *Practical dermatology.* St. Louis: Mosby Year Book.

Jester, J., & Weaver, V. (1990). A report of clinical investigation of various tissue support surfaces used for the prevention, early intervention and management of pressure ulcers. *Ostomy/Wound Management, 36* (1), 39–45.

Kemp, M. G. (1994). Critiquing clinical research on support surfaces. *Ostomy/Wound Management, 40* (2), 18–22, 24, 25.

Kim, M. J. (1993). *Pocket guide to nursing diagnoses* (5th ed.). St. Louis: Mosby Year Book.

Krasner, D. (1990). *Chronic wound care: A clinical source book for healthcare professionals.* King of Prussia, PA: Health Management Publications.

Nicol, N. H., & Fenske, N. A. (1993). Photodamage: Cause, clinical manifestation, and prevention. *Dermatology Nursing, 5* (4), 263–277.

Proehl, J. A. (1993). *Adult emergency nursing procedures.* Boston: Jones and Bartlett Publishers.

Thomason, S., Hawley, G. G., & Wurzel, J. (1993). Speciality support surfaces: A cost containment perspective. *Decubitus, 6* (6), 32–34, 36–38, 40.

Weaver, V., & Jester, J. (1994). A clinical tool: Updated readings on tissue interface pressures. *Ostomy/Wound Management, 40* (5), 34–43.

The Body's Defenses Against Infection

Key Terms

Agranulocytes
Antibody
Antigen
Colonization
Culture and sensitivity
Granulocytes
Incidence
Interferon
Leukocytosis
Neutropenic
Normal flora
Nosocomial infection
Opportunistic
Pathogens
Purulent
Symbiotic
Virulence

Learning Objectives

Upon completion of this chapter, the student will be able to do the following:

- *Name the major components of the immune system and some natural barriers to infection.*
- *Identify clients at risk for infectious diseases.*
- *Name four common nosocomial infections.*
- *Recognize common manifestations of infection.*
- *Identify common laboratory and diagnostic tests used to identify or confirm an infectious process.*
- *Describe major consequences of an infectious process.*
- *Identify the components of infection treatment.*
- *Describe nursing measures that strengthen defense mechanisms against infection.*

39

You are a nurse doing tuberculosis surveillance for the Public Health Department. Your new client is a 31-year-old man who had a positive purified protein derivative (PPD) test last week when he was admitted to the hospital after a brawl in a local bar. Your client left the hospital AMA (against medical advice) before a definitive diagnosis of tuberculosis could be made. When you find your client, he is drinking in the same bar. After you introduce yourself, he swears at you, telling you to go away, he is not sick, and he does not need any nurse nosing into his affairs.

So far you have developed a broad base of nursing care techniques founded on solid professional concepts. In previous chapters, you studied asepsis and wound healing. In this chapter, you will learn more about normal and abnormal resistance in the body's defense system. As you read this chapter you will learn about caring for people with potential for infection, and how to protect yourself and others who come in contact with infected clients. The Critical Thinking Challenges at the end of the chapter will help you apply this body of knowledge to the client who may have tuberculosis.

Infectious diseases have changed history by wiping out large numbers of people, stopping industrial growth, causing migrations, and altering social structures. Infection continues to make a significant impact. Sexually transmitted diseases such as herpes, gonorrhea, and AIDS have spread rapidly in the past two decades because of changing sexual practices and now have enormous social consequences. Tuberculosis, once thought of as a communicable disease that was well controlled, is increasing dramatically, and in some instances proving to be drug resistant. More infectious organisms are developing resistance to antibiotics, posing a very serious challenge to healthcare providers.

Infections consume billions of dollars in healthcare costs and are a major cause of absenteeism from work and school. They are a common cause of death in Third World countries, and cause significant morbidity and mortality in the developed world.

For infection to occur, an uninterrupted chain of conditions must be present allowing microorganisms to grow, reproduce, be passed from place to place, and to enter a susceptible host. This "chain of infection" is described in detail in Chapter 25 and illustrated in Figure 25-1. When the chain of infection remains intact, people must rely on their bodily defenses to fight disease-causing microorganisms.

Normal Resistance to Infection

Humans are bathed in a sea of microorganisms called **normal flora**. Their presence in or on the body is normal and is usually **symbiotic**, meaning that there is no harm to either organism. These organisms live on the skin, in the nasopharynx, in the gastrointestinal tract, and on other body surfaces.

Infection is the result of an interaction between an agent that can alter the normal functioning of the body and a host that provides an environment for the agent's replication and growth. Microorganisms that can cause disease are called **pathogens**.

Characteristics of Normal Resistance to Infection

The body's defenses against infection can be divided into two major groups:

Nonspecific natural barriers include the skin and the mucous membranes covering the gastrointestinal, respiratory, and urinary tracts.

Specific acquired defenses occur in response to a particular organism and are mobilized to fight that specific invader.

The types of human defenses against infection are outlined in Table 39-1.

Nonspecific Natural Defenses

A person's general health (including nutritional status, lifestyle, and stress level) is an important factor in determining his or her resistance, along with age, sex, and place of residence.

Cultural Factors. A population's exposure to an infectious agent over generations can lead to increased resistance to that microorganism. For instance, measles was carried by European explorers to the New World, causing the deaths of millions of inhabitants of the Americas. Today, Africans and African-Americans who have the genetic disease of sickle cell anemia do not contract malaria, presumably because the shape of the cell makes it difficult for the parasite to enter. Because malaria kills more than a million people a year, this is an important form of immunity, but it carries its own consequences as a disease. Many ethnic groups have developed cultural habits that act as a barrier to the spread of infection, and scientists are sorting out the differences between customs and genes. The same is true of religious rituals and practices.

Mechanical and Chemical Barriers. Intact skin and mucous membranes that cover body cavities are the most important barriers to infection. Infection is rare if these barriers remain intact. The physical barriers of the skin and mucous membranes are aided by their chemical composition, and some barriers also have specialized cells. Normal flora that grows on healthy tissues uses the local nutrients. Lack of nutrients and oxygen can inhibit the colonization and growth of pathogens. Mechanical forces, such as tears, saliva, and urine, wash bacteria from surfaces as they flow through ducts and tracts. Peristalsis increases the mechanical cleansing of organ walls. **Interferon** is a nonspecific chemical inhibitor secreted by body cells in response to invasion by viruses.

White Blood Cells. Leukocytes, another name for white blood cells (WBCs), and the inflammatory response make up the second line of defense to microbial invasion. Many leukocytes functions as *phagocytes*, ingesting and thus destroying microbes. There are two categories of WBCs:

- **Granulocytes** are polymorphonuclear cells that contain granules of digestive enzymes. Specific types of granulocytes include neutrophils, eosinophils, and basophils.
- **Agranulocytes** are mononuclear cells that lack digestive enzymes. Monocytes and lymphocytes are examples of agranulocytes.

Table 39-2 lists the actions of various white cells. Appendix B also includes a table of differential WBC counts.

Table 39-1 • Human Defenses Against Infection

Defense	Examples
Nonspecific Natural Defenses	
Individual factors	Heredity Good hygiene practices Good nutritional status Immunization history
Anatomic barriers	Skin Mucous membranes
Mechanical removal of micro-organisms	Gastrointestinal motility Ciliary action in the respiratory tract Cleansing effect of the flow of urine Expulsive effect of coughing and sneezing Lavaging effects of tears and saliva Shedding of uterine lining in menstruation Flow of organ secretions through ducts (eg, bile)
Chemical factors*	Acidity of gastric secretion Acidity of vaginal secretions Acidity of fatty acids of the skin Lysozyme enzymes in tears, nasal secretions, urine, and saliva Hormones secreted by the adrenal cortex and pancreas Indigenous microflora (competition)
Local tissue factors	Tissue surface receptor (occupancy) Inflammation
White blood cell function	Fever Phagocytosis
Acquired Specific Resistance†	Immune response Cellular immunity (T lymphocytes elaborate killer cells and helper cells) Humoral immunity (B lymphocytes produce antibodies to specific microorganisms) Memory of the organisms produces lasting immunity

*Factors that retard growth and provide less favorable media for growth.
†Resistance may be acquired naturally if the person has had the infectious disease or has been immunized.

Inflammatory Response. Inflammation is a nonspecific response to tissue injury that may be caused by microbial invasion or mechanical, chemical, or heat injury. The purpose of inflammation is to limit the extent of the injury. Blood vessels dilate and plasma flows out of the capillaries into the irritated tissue. WBCs migrate into the area; neutrophils are usually first, followed by the clean-up crew of monocytes. The area then begins to show the four signs of inflammation:

- ***Redness*** from blood accumulation in the dilated capillaries
- ***Warmth*** from the heat of the blood
- ***Swelling*** from the accumulation of fluid
- ***Pain*** from pressure or injury to the local nerves.

The area is red, warm, swollen, and tender. It is inflamed but not necessarily infected. The inflammatory response is discussed further in Chapter 38.

Inflammation and phagocytosis work together to contain microorganisms. If they are successful, a collection of dead leukocytes, digested bacteria, dead tissue cells, and plasma may form into the material called ***pus***.

Fever. Elevated body temperature also aids in the battle against infection. The hypothalamus raises the body's thermostat in response to pyrogens, and cell metabolism increases. Pyrogens are released by some phagocytic cells (granulocytes, monocytes, and macrophages) after being stimulated by microorganisms or endotoxins (Wertz, 1991).

Research has shown that fever (defined as a body temperature above 101°F or 38.2°C) helps combat infection by interrupting viral replication and slowing the rate of bacterial growth. Fever is also reported to increase the mobility of leukocytes and to enhance

Table 39-2 • White Blood Cell Functions in Infection

Cells	Action
Neutrophils	Phagocytes. They ingest and break down foreign particles, particularly bacteria and parasites. They are also an important link in the generation of fever to combat the proliferation of microorganisms.
Eosinophils	Allergic reaction. They increase in response to allergic and parasitic conditions when there is an antibody–antibody response.
Basophils	Unknown. They contain heparin and histamine in their granules, which may be important in preventing blood clotting during an inflammatory response.
T lymphocytes	Synthesis of immunoglobins. Effective in destroying bacteria, viruses, and cancer cells, they recognize antigens and stimulate B lymphocytes and macrophages. Three types have been identified: helper cells, which stimulate other leukocytes; killer T cells, which recognize and destroy virus-infected cells; and suppressor cells, which tell the other cells to stop fighting after the antigenic substance is cleared. They produce cellular immunity.
B lymphocytes	Synthesis of antibodies. Important in the immune response, they are stimulated by the T cells to divide and produce the plasma cells, which then produce specific antibodies to the antigen. The memory of the antigen is carried on memory cells that produce lasting immunity to the specific microorganism. They produce humoral immunity.
Macrophages	Scavenger cells. They dispose of cellular debris. Their numbers increase in the late stage of acute infections and during chronic infections. Levels also rise in response to viral, bacterial, and parasitic infections. They are considered important in activating the lymphocytes and are found in the reticuloendothelial system.

their ability to phagocytize microorganisms. Also, the effects of endotoxins are shortened with elevated temperatures.

Fever is thought to have a beneficial effect on the outcome of an infection if other body systems are not compromised. If fever is too high or is prolonged, however, the client may become severely debilitated or suffer convulsions.

Specific Acquired Defenses: Immunity

Another important defense against infection is the specific response of acquired defenses that develop immunity. **Antigens** are foreign particles, such as microbes, that enter the host, but they may be a person's own cells in some autoimmune diseases. The specific response to an antigen takes place at two sites: in the blood (humoral immunity) and in the cells of the lymphatic system (cellular immunity).

The immune system response is stimulated when antigens enter the lymphatic and circulatory systems. The antigens are phagocytized by macrophages, monocytes, or neutrophils, and the microbe is digested. Portions of the microbe are antigenic determinants, particles that stay with the phagocyte and are carried to the lymphoid tissue in the lymph nodes or the spleen. The phagocyte, usually a macrophage, presents this processed antigen to the lymphocytes, which then work to produce immunity.

There are two types of lymphocytes: T lymphocytes and B lymphocytes. Both originate from stem cells in the bone marrow that differentiate to become the lymphopoietic cells. Some of them pass through the thymus gland in the chest and are modified to form the thymus-dependent lymphocytes or T lymphocytes (also known as T cells). The others are modified by unknown mechanisms and become B lymphocytes. There are several subgroups of lymphocytic cells, and much research is being done on their functions. Table 39-2 lists lymphocyte functions.

The immune system, if properly functioning, can produce resistance to recurrence of a disease. Immunity to a specific pathogen usually follows an active infection, which may or may not be symptomatic. Other forms of immunity can be produced to prevent a specific disease from occurring.

The immune system conveys lasting resistance to infection by forming a "memory" of the antigen within the body. T lymphocytes and B lymphocytes, the building blocks of the immune system, accumulate in lymph nodes along lymphatic vessels and are exposed to all antigens except those that enter the bloodstream directly. These lymphocytes are heavily concentrated in the tonsils and spleen, which are important tissues in children and young adults.

Cellular Immunity. Cellular immunity, principally consisting of T-lymphocyte activity, is stimulated by fungi, protozoa, some viruses, and bacteria. After the T lymphocytes are stimulated, they enter the circulation from the lymphoid tissues and seek the site of the microbe. At the site, the lymphocytes produce proteins called lymphokines that draw more phagocytes to the area, keep them there to fight the invader, and increase their killing power. Lymphokines disappear after the antigen has been eliminated, but some of the T cells remain in the tissues and keep a memory of the antigen. Memory T lymphocytes are reactivated rapidly if the same antigen reappears.

Humoral Immunity. Humoral immunity takes place in the bloodstream. B lymphocytes produce humoral immunity by producing antibodies that convey specific resistance to many bacterial and viral infections. B lymphocytes are stimulated by the antigenic determinants contained within the macrophages, and produce plasma cells. The plasma cells then produce antibodies that are released into the bloodstream from the lymphoid tissue. Antibodies, also called immunoglobulins, circulate in the bloodstream and interact there with the antigens they encounter; this gives rise to the term humoral, or blood, immunity.

Antibodies are formed in response to substances found in bacterial cell walls, toxins, microbial enzymes, viruses, and other individual allergens. They can make the bacteria more susceptible to phagocytosis or help in bacterial cell lysis. Antibodies formed in response to a virus neutralize the virus, act as antitoxins, or cause the microbes to clump together or precipitate. Others simply make it easier for microbes to be ingested by phagocytes. Memory B lymphocytes remain in lymphoid tissue, where they can become reactivated if the pathogen reappears.

The complement system, a series of proteins found in the bloodstream, also aids in the antigen-antibody reaction. The complement system enhances phagocytosis of microbes, helps in lysis of bacterial cell walls, and encourages the inflammatory response.

Active Immunity. Active immunity is produced when the immune system is stimulated, either naturally or artificially, to produce antibodies. Natural immunity follows the course of an infection: the client experiences a disease and produces a good response to the antigen. Active immunity can also be produced by vaccination (the injection of weakened or killed organisms into a person, stimulating antibody production and producing an artificially acquired active immunity).

Passive Immunity. Passive immunity does not involve the host's immune response; rather, immunity is transferred to the recipient. This can be done in two ways. Antibodies can pass from the mother via the placenta to the fetus, or through breast milk to the newborn. Also, antibodies from a person or animal that has had the disease can be taken from the blood and given to a person for temporary passive protection. Passive immunity, which provides only temporary protection, is given in the form of immune globulins when there is not enough time for the person to acquire active immunization or when a vaccine does not exist for the disease.

Factors Affecting Normal Resistance to Infection

A person's ability to resist infection is affected by his or her intact skin or mucous membranes, hygiene, nutrition, environment, and immunization status.

Intact Skin and Mucous Membranes

Intact epithelial surfaces of the skin and mucous membranes stop microbial invasion. Epithelial surfaces include the skin; the linings of the oral, anal, vaginal, gastrointestinal, respiratory, and urinary tracts; the conjunctiva; and the lining of the external ear. Few pathogens can penetrate these intact anatomic boundaries.

Secretions and mechanical functions help to remove organisms that are deposited and colonized on these surfaces. For organisms to invade tissues, they must first attach to the surface, and this attachment is impeded by the local pH, mobility of the surface, flow of mucus, beating of cilia, washing of the surface by fluids, and renewal of surface cells by desquamation.

Personal Hygiene

Routine personal grooming fosters normal host defenses against infection. Normal cleansing of the skin is important in removing transient microorganisms and decreasing colonization. Handwashing is the most significant way to decrease the spread of microorganisms. Hygiene also helps to lubricate skin surfaces and to maintain an intact epidermis. Routine oral care removes debris and plaque, which attract microorganisms to the mouth. Routine washing of clothes and accessories also decreases the number of microorganisms on the body.

Nutrition

Adequate nutrition is essential for normal host defense against infection. The body's ability to synthesize antibodies, which are proteins, becomes ineffective if protein stores are depleted. Adequate energy, supplied by the breakdown of ingested food, is necessary to mount an effective attack against invading organisms.

Environment

Environmental factors influencing resistance to infection include sanitation, climate, and population density. Adequate treatment of water and waste products is essential to prevent the spread of infection. Government agencies supervise and control the treatment of human waste. Communities ensure that garbage is collected and sewage is chemically treated before it enters the water system. Adequate sanitation reduces the number of microorganisms.

Warm, moist climates provide a good environment for the growth of organisms or vectors (eg, mosquitoes or ticks) that can transmit disease. Cold temperatures increase the amount of time most people spend indoors, which is why the incidence of colds and viruses rises during the winter. Densely populated areas increase the transmission of infection. Avoiding overcrowding, both in the community and in each household, can decrease the risk of infection.

Immunization

Vaccines are made of inactivated viruses or bacterial cells that cannot multiply in the body or weakened (attenuated) organisms that multiply slowly in the body but do not cause symptoms. Some vaccines produce lifelong immunity, but others require periodic booster doses to maintain immunity.

Nursing Research
Infection

Selected Nursing Research Studies

Bertone, S., et al. (1994). Quantitative skin cultures at potential catheter sites in neonates. *Infection Control and Hospital Epidemiology, 15,* 315–318.

Boyce, J. (1992). Methicillin-resistant *Staphylococcus aureus* in hospitals and long term care facilities: Microbiology, epidemiology, and preventative measures. *Infection Control and Hospital Epidemiology, 13,* 725–737.

Cardo, D., et al. (1993). Validation of surgical wound surveillance. *Infection Control and Hospital Epidemiology, 14,* 211–215.

Fanning, C., et al. (1991). Urinary tract infections: A survey. *Canadian Journal of Infection Control, 6(3),* 68–69.

Graham, S., et al. (1993). Frequency of changing enteral alimentation bags and tubing, and adverse patient outcomes in a long term care facility. *Canadian Journal of Infection Control, 8* (2), 41–43.

Possible Topics for Nursing Inquiry

- How reliable is fever as a symptom of infection in clients older than 65 years of age?
- How successful in reducing the incidence of infection is a teaching program encouraging preschool workers to provide proper hygiene after preschoolers' toileting?
- What is the incidence of nonvaccinated children in community shelters for the homeless?
- What is the incidence of bacteremia when alcohol versus Betadine is used to clean intravenous ports before injection?
- How successful are current blood bank standards in preventing HIV-contaminated blood from reaching the public?

Lifespan Considerations

The ability to defend against infection can be affected by age-related factors. The very young and the very old have high rates of infection because their defense mechanisms against infections are less effective.

Newborn and Infant

The immune system does not become fully operational until about 6 months of age. Before then, the infant's resistance to infection comes from the antibodies passed via the placenta and breast milk. Neonates have difficulty localizing infections (preventing the spread of organisms from the site of contact). Their phagocytes have difficulty trapping microbes, and they do not produce enough antibodies. Viral diseases such as chickenpox or herpes simplex, acquired from the birth canal or from infected siblings, can cause severe disseminated disease.

Neonates have immature thermoregulatory mechanisms and do not become febrile. Instead, they manifest infections more subtly: they become lethargic or restless, or stop feeding. After 2 to 4 months of age, infants begin producing antibodies, and by 6 months their lymphocytes are fully operational if they have had adequate nutrition (Alcamo, 1991; Donowitz, 1992).

Toddler and Preschooler

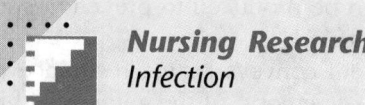

Preschool children need supervision to prevent infections. They are exposed to many pathogens as they increase their mobility, and they have poor personal hygiene. Toddlers often play in dirt, they are incontinent of urine and feces, and they put things in their mouths. Although they are developing mature immune systems, they may not have been exposed to pathogens to give them immunity. By age 3 to 4 years, the immune system has matured to a level similar to that of adults in producing antibodies. Childhood vaccinations are timed to take advantage of this developing immunocompetence.

Children are continually exposed to bacterial and viral illness. When viral diseases occur in children, they are often milder than in adults. Children may develop lifelong immunity from some of these viral infections, but diseases caused by bacteria, such as ***Salmonella*** and ***Shigella***, do not produce immunity and may recur frequently.

The most common infections in early childhood are respiratory tract infections. Because children's eustachian tubes are shorter and straighter than those of adults, middle ear infections (otitis media) are common as bacteria pass to the ear canal from the nasopharynx. Children may suffer many colds each year, but by age 5 or 6 years their immune system and body defenses have matured to a level where the infections are more localized. The common communicable diseases are transmitted as children play with others.

Preventing infections in early childhood requires

- Good hygienic care of the child and his or her food
- Adequate vaccinations
- Early infection treatment to prevent spread or preventable complications
- Isolation from infected people

Child and Adolescent

Communicable diseases are most prevalent as children enter school and organized play activities, and they are most common during the winter, when children stay indoors. Children are also exposed to skin diseases such as impetigo (from staphylococcal infections), roundworm infestations, and lice (from sharing combs, clothes, and sports equipment). There is a high incidence of streptococcal infections in children aged 6 to 12 years, resulting in pharyngitis, tonsillitis, and scarlet fever.

Accidents are common in this age group, resulting in abrasions, lacerations, and fractures. Although most accidents from play and sports are relatively minor, they carry an infection risk.

Sexually transmitted diseases such as infectious mononucleosis, chlamydia, herpes simplex, syphilis, gonorrhea, and AIDS are on the rise in adolescents. Young adults who contract them run an increased risk of serious consequences; for example, pelvic inflammatory disease in young women is a major cause of ectopic pregnancy and infertility, and inflammation and infection of the urethra and testes can lead to sterility in men. The immune system should be fully mature by adolescence but may be compromised by malnutrition or acquired deficiencies (Farley, 1991; Halverson & Graham, 1991).

Adult and Older Adult

Immunity to many diseases is established by adulthood. Adults have fewer respiratory tract infections but more chronic lung diseases, which can increase infection risk. Sexually transmitted diseases continue to be a major problem in this age group, depending on the person's lifestyle. Accidents, both industrial and recreational, have infectious complications. Many deaths from motor vehicle accidents are caused by infections that can cause organ failure.

Infections in a pregnant woman can be transmitted across the placenta to the fetus. A minor or subclinical infection can be passed to the fetus, who may suffer either minor consequences, major congenital anomalies, or death.

As people age, the effects of their lifestyles begin to affect their ability to resist infection. The thymus begins to shrink in late adolescence and continues to diminish into middle age, leading to a decline in cell-mediated and humoral immunity. Cardiovascular disease, cancer, diabetes, obesity or malnutrition, alcoholism, anxiety, depression, and stress have all been shown to decrease defense mechanisms against infection. The medications and treatments used to combat these diseases may also decrease immune system function. Adults with chronic diseases require more frequent hospitalization, putting them at risk for **nosocomial infections** (infections acquired while receiving healthcare).

With the increase in air travel and the development of global economic ties, people are traveling more and living in foreign countries where they may be exposed to infectious diseases that are not endogenous to their native area. They may then take these infectious organisms home, contributing to the spread of infection. Because they have their initial exposure as adults, the symptoms and complications of the disease may be severe (Wertz, 1991).

The skin of older people becomes thinner and drier. It loses elasticity and fat and receives less circulation, leading to an increased susceptibility to injury and infection. Bedridden clients are more susceptible to the development of infected decubitus ulcers.

There are changes in other defense mechanisms with aging. The pH of body secretions changes, peristalsis slows, and the endogenous flora changes with age and medications. The cough and gag reflexes of older clients may be impaired after a stroke or from medications that cloud their thinking. Loose-fitting dentures and impaired swallowing mechanisms may lead to aspiration, which can contribute to respiratory infection.

Older adults may have problems with urinary retention, which leads to bacterial growth in stagnant urine and decreased cleansing of the urethra by a brisk stream of urine. Incapacitated adults may be incontinent of urine and feces, causing excoriation of the skin in the perineal and sacral regions and further contributing to infections. If they are confused or agitated, older clients may carry microorganisms from these areas to their nose or mouth if they are not given adequate help with hygiene.

The immune systems of older adults may be impaired. WBC counts do not always rise in response to infections, and phagocytosis is ineffective. There is a decreased inflammatory response, and body temperature may not be elevated in response to an infection. The ability to wall off and limit the spread of infection is decreased. There is a decreased cellular immune response, and old infections such as tuberculosis may be reactivated. Both nonspecific and specific responses to microbial invasion are diminished (Smith, et al., 1992).

As a cause of death in older adults, infections are exceeded only by cancer and myocardial infarction; urinary tract and respiratory tract infections are the most common and the most lethal. Infections use up energy necessary for other body processes. Older people have twice the incidence of influenza as young adults, and the mortality rate is higher. They are also vulnerable to postoperative infections, particularly when the chest or abdomen is the operative site.

Increasing numbers of older adults in the United States live in nursing homes. They are at increased risk for infection for a variety of reasons: their chronic diseases may predispose them to infection, they may be housed in crowded rooms with other infected clients, they may have invasive devices such as Foley catheters, and they may be unable to take adequate nutrition by mouth. The inability to care for their own hygienic needs, coupled with the inadequate staffing in many long-term care facilities, increases infection risk. Additional exposure to infection may come from visitors with active respiratory infections or caregivers who fail to wash their hands before and after care.

Altered Resistance to Infection

Potential for Infection

Infection transmission can occur because of the virulence of the infectious agent or because of alterations in normal host defense mechanisms. Often, the combination of many factors leads to an infection.

Presence of Infectious Agents

The type and number of microorganisms and their virulence, pathogenicity, and invasiveness determine whether an infection occurs. **Virulence** means the vigor with which the organism grows and multiplies, ***pathogenicity*** is its ability to cause harm, and ***invasiveness*** involves its ability to penetrate tissues. Large numbers of organisms that are virulent, pathogenic, and invasive are most likely to cause infection.

The **incidence** of infection can be represented by this equation:

$$\text{Incidence of infection} = \frac{\text{Bacteria} \times \text{Virulence}}{\text{Host Defenses}}$$

In the past, only a few organisms were thought to be pathogenic, but that idea is changing as we recognize that almost any microorganism can cause disease, given the right conditions for entry and growth in the body. Even normal flora can cause disease under the right circumstances. Such organisms are **opportunistic**: although normally not considered pathogens, they can take advantage of being in the right place at the right time and cause infection.

Bacteria, viruses, fungi, and parasites are pathogenic organisms. Common infectious diseases caused by bacteria and viruses are listed in Table 39-3.

Bacteria. The group of organisms called bacteria contains thousands of species, but only a few hundred of them cause human disease. They are what most people think of when they say "germs." Gram-positive bacteria such as staphylococci are commonly found in wound infections and food poisoning; streptococci contribute to skin, wound, and respiratory infections. Gram-negative rods, which comprise much of the normal flora of the bowel, are often associated with hospital-acquired infections started by self-contamination of the client. They are also the most common cause of urinary tract infections (UTIs).

Anaerobes, or organisms requiring reduced oxygen tension for growth, are often associated with serious infections. They are often seen in infections in which a mixture of organisms are present (polymicrobial infections) and are part of the normal flora of the mouth, intestines, and female genital tract.

Toxins liberated by bacteria include exotoxins and endotoxins. Exotoxins of gram-positive bacteria are diffusible and cause tissue injury. Exotoxins are liberated by bacteria that cause tetanus, diphtheria, botulism, cholera, and staphylococcal food poisoning. Gram-negative bacteria usually contain toxic substances in their cell wall; these are released on cell lysis and are called endotoxins. Endotoxins are particularly potent poisons when they gain access to the bloodstream.

Viruses. The replication process of viruses is unique. A virus invades a living cell many times its size, uses the cell's metabolism, and produces copies of itself

(text continues on page 1125)

Table 39-3 • Common Infectious Diseases

Infection	Agent	Transmission	Symptoms	Possible Complications	Prevention
General Infections					
Common cold	Rhinovirus	Respiratory droplet	Sneezing, nasal and sinus stuffiness, nasopharyngeal irritation, watery eyes, chills, malaise.	Pneumonia, otitis media	Avoid direct contact with infected individuals. Keep body defenses strong through good nutrition, exercise.
Influenza	Virus	Respiratory droplet	Cold-like symptoms, fever, body stiffness and discomfort; gastrointestinal symptoms of vomiting and diarrhea with some strains of flu	Pneumonia	Avoid direct contact. Keep body defenses strong. Flu virus vaccines are available.
Childhood Infections					
Measles (rubeola)	Virus	Respiratory droplet or secretions or direct contact	Fever, malaise, anorexia, photophobia, coryza, cough, Koplik spots on lateral surface of the mouth followed a few days later by a red rash	Encephalitis	Measles vaccine is available. Avoid contact with infected individuals if not immunized. Wear a mask if contact with an infected person is necessary.
German measles (rubella)	Virus	Respiratory droplet or body secretions (urine, blood, feces). Can cross placenta to fetus during pregnancy.	Malaise, headache, swollen lymph glands, anorexia, low-grade fever, and runny nose followed by maculopapular rash	Severe retardation and birth defects if contracted in utero	Obtain rubella vaccine. Avoid contact with infected people if not immuned. Wear mask if contact with infected person is necessary.
Mumps	Virus	Respiratory droplet or contact with saliva	Malaise, muscle aches, headache, anorexia, swollen and tender parotid glands, fever	Encephalitis, arthritis, deafness, sterility in adult men	Obtain mumps vaccine. Avoid contact with infected people if not immunized. Mask may help decrease infection.
Chickenpox	Varicella-zoster virus	Respiratory droplet, contact with lesions before they have scabbed over	Fever, malaise, anorexia, rash characterized by macules, papules, and vesicles that crust over; pruritus secondary to rash	Secondary skin infections due to scratching	Vaccine is available. Isolate infected person until lesions are scabbed over or disappear.
Scarlet fever	Streptococcal bacteria	Respiratory droplet or direct contact	Sore throat, bright red tongue, high fever, nausea, vomiting, rash	Rheumatic fever glomerulonephritis, renal failure	Avoid direct contact with infected people. Isolate the patient until 24 hours after antibiotic treatment.

(continued)

Table 39-3 *(Continued)*

Infection	Agent	Transmission	Symptoms	Possible Complications	Prevention
Pertussis (whooping cough)	Gram-negative bacillus ***(Bordetella pertussis)***	Respiratory droplet	Cold symptoms that progress to a severe cough that includes a "whoop" as the glottis closes during deep inspiration. Vomiting, epistaxis, and hemorrhaging can occur from severe coughing bouts.		Pertussis vaccine is available. Isolate the patient from nonimmune people and use a mask during acute infectious stage.
Neurologic Infections					
Encephalitis	Enterovirus, arbovirus, or as a sequela of measles, rubella, chickenpox, or influenza	Respiratory droplet or direct contact with gastrointestinal secretions	Fever, vomiting, aching head, neck, and back muscles, drowsiness, convulsions, paralysis, coma	Brain damage	Vaccinations are available for measles, rubella, chickenpox, and influenza.
Meningitis	Gram-negative bacteria or virus	Respiratory droplet, spread to meninges through the bloodstream	Fever, anorexia, intense headache, intolerance to light and sound, delirium, convulsions, coma	Shock, respiratory distress, brain damage	
Polio	Virus	Ingestion of contaminated food and water	Nausea, vomiting, cramps, paralysis of arms, legs and body; if nerve supply is affected, impaired swallowing and breathing	Permanent paralysis	Salk or oral Sabin vaccination is available. Take enteric precautions for infected clients.
Sexually Transmitted Diseases					
Syphilis	Spirochete ***Treponema pallidum***	Sexual contact, mother to fetus via placenta, blood transfusion if donor is in early stage of disease and undiagnosed	Primary stage: genital lesion, enlarged lymph nodes Secondary stage (6 weeks later): lesions of skin and mucous membrane, with generalized symptoms of headache and fever	Tertiary stage: central nervous system and cardiovascular damage, paralysis, psychosis	Public should be educated on safe sex practices. Screen blood donors. Do serologic testing before and during pregnancy. Avoid contact with body secretions from infected clients.
Gonorrhea	Gonococcus ***Neisseria gonorrhoeae***	Sexual contact; mother to fetus during delivery	Yellow mucopurulent discharge of the genital area, painful or frequent urination, pain in the genital area; may be asymptomatic	Sterility, cystitis, arthritis, endocarditis	Public should be educated on safe sex practices. Mother should be tested before delivery. Newborn's eyes should be treated with silver nitrate. All contacts should be treated with antibiotics.
Genital herpes	Virus Herpes simplex type 2	Sexual contact; mother to fetus during vaginal delivery	Genital soreness, pruritus, and erythema. Vesicles appear that usually last for about 10 days, during which time transmission of virus is likely		Public should be educated on safe sex practices. Sexual contact should be avoided when lesions are present. Infected mothers should have a cesarean delivery.

Chlamydia	Bacteria *Chlamydia trachomatis*	Sexual contact; mother to fetus during vaginal delivery	Mucopurulent genital discharge, genital pain, dysuria	Sterility	Public should be educated on safe sex practices. Sexual contact should be avoided when lesions are present. Infected mothers should have a cesarean delivery.
Acquired immunodeficiency syndrome (AIDS)	Human immunodeficiency virus (HIV)	Sexual contact; exposure to blood or blood products; mother to fetus	Active phase: rash, cough, malaise, night sweats, lymphadenopathy Asymptomatic phase: no symptoms but test is positive for HIV antigens AIDS-related complex (ARC): lymphadenopathy, diarrhea, oral candidiasis, weight loss, fatigue, skin rash, recurrent infections, fever AIDS: rare infections such as ***Pneumocystis carinii*** pneumonia or rare cancers such as Kaposi's sarcoma or B-cell lymphomas	Neurologic impairment	Public should be educated on safe sex practices, especially high-risk groups. Blood or blood products used for transfusion should be carefully screened. Intravenous drug abusers should not share needles. Universal precautions should be used consistently in all health-care settings. Institute measures to avoid needlesticks among health-care workers.
Blood-Borne Infections					
AIDS (see above)					
Hepatitis A	Hepatitis A virus (HAV)	Contaminated water or food or fecal–oral contamination	Malaise, anorexia, nausea, vomiting, fever, headache, abdominal pain, jaundice, enlarged liver	Hepatic damage or failure, encephalopathy	Public should be educated on good sanitation and personal hygiene, especially after using the toilet and before handling food. Food handlers and day-care workers should be educated and monitored. Enteric precautions should be taken with all infected individuals. Immune globulin may be given to travelers visiting endemic areas.
Hepatitis B	Hepatitis B virus (HBV)	Transfusion with infected blood or blood products (less common with other body fluid contact), punctures with HBV-contaminated sharps, mother to fetus in utero	Malaise, anorexia, nausea, vomiting, fever, headache, abdominal pain, jaundice, enlarged liver	Hepatic damage or failure, encephalopathy	Hepatitis B vaccine is recommended for high-risk individuals who often come in contact with blood. If exposed, immune globulin may be given. Screen blood donors. Avoid needlesticks. Use universal precautions.

(continued)

Table 39-3 *(Continued)*

Infection	Agent	Transmission	Symptoms	Possible Complications	Prevention
Food- or Water-Borne					
Typhoid fever	Bacteria ***Salmonella typhi***	Contaminated water or food, contact with urine or feces of a carrier	Headache, weakness, fever, rash, abdominal tenderness, diarrhea, decreased level of consciousness (stupor, delirium, coma)	Intestinal hemorrhage or perforation	Water sanitation and waste disposal should be regulated and flies should be controlled. Vaccinations should be given in regions with contaminated water supply. Good handwashing after using the toilet should be encouraged. Use enteric precautions for infected clients. Milk and dairy products should be pasteurized.
Salmonella	Bacteria (various species of *Salmonella*)	Contaminated food, especially inadequate refrigeration or sanitation; improperly cooked meat	Vomiting, diarrhea, abdominal cramps, fever	Dehydration, shock due to fluid volume deficit	Food, especially eggs and poultry, should be properly handled, refrigerated, and cooked.
Shigella	Bacteria ***Shigella***	Contaminated water or food; crowded environments such as jails or institutions	Vomiting, diarrhea, abdominal cramps, fever	Dehydration, possibly leading to shock	Food should be properly stored and prepared.
Accident-Related					
Tetanus (lockjaw)	Bacteria ***Clostridium tetani***	Puncture wound from needle, nail, dog bite, or gunshot wound	Increased neuromuscular tone and irritability, twitching, convulsions	Respiratory arrest and death	Keep immunization current; after accident, booster dose or tetanus may be given to stimulate recall. If prolonged time has elapsed since booster, combination of antitoxins (tetanus immune globin) and tetanus and diphtheria toxoids is given.

while either destroying the cell or changing the cell's genetic makeup. Viruses cause AIDS, chickenpox, colds, cold sores, encephalitis, hepatitis, herpes, influenza, measles, mononucleosis, mumps, polio, rabies, shingles, pneumonia, and many other diseases. They have been associated with some cancers and leukemias and with many autoimmune diseases, including multiple sclerosis, rheumatoid arthritis, and diabetes.

Fungi. Only a few fungal infections cause disease in humans, but fungi can be deadly if they disseminate through the body tissues. Unicellular fungi, called yeasts, that cause disease in humans are often normal flora of the skin and mucous membranes. They do not injure the host until defenses are lowered (eg, ***Candida*** in the mouth of infants [thrush], or in cancer or AIDS clients). Antibiotic use, which can destroy normal bacterial flora, also contributes to fungal infections. Infestations of yeast by inhalation of spores can cause coccidioidomycosis or histoplasmosis lung infections. The most common yeast infections affect the skin, hair, and nails, such as athlete's foot, ringworm, and groin itch.

Parasites. Parasites that infect humans are either protozoa, helminths, or arthropods. Parasitic infections are associated with poor socioeconomic conditions with inadequate sanitation measures for water and sewage. When public health measures do not control these organisms, disease is prevalent.

Protozoal infections are common in underdeveloped countries and probably cause more suffering worldwide than any other group of diseases. Trichomoniasis, a sexually transmitted disease, is the one common protozoal disease in the United States and causes 2.5 million infections annually (Alcamo, 1992). Other diseases include African sleeping sickness, malaria, and giardiasis. Pneumocystosis, a disease of the alveolar sacs, is increasing in frequency in immunosuppressed cancer clients and in clients with AIDS.

Helminths are flatworms and roundworms. Some invade the tissues; others live in the gastrointestinal tract or blood. When infected pork is insufficiently cooked, trichinae pass to human muscles, causing trichinosis. Pinworms are found worldwide and are one of the most common parasites in humans. Roundworms are also passed among humans, and are common. Flatworms are best known from reports of intestinal tapeworms. Another form, flukes, may enter the human bloodstream.

Arthropods include mites, ticks, fleas, lice, and fly larvae. The arthropods cause a skin irritation from the toxins they introduce when they bite humans. The dermatitis they cause is often further complicated by bacterial superinfections. They also serve as vectors for some protozoal infections and for dreaded bacterial infections such as bubonic plague (Alcamo, 1991).

Type of Infection

Colonization is the introduction of microorganisms onto a body surface where they grow and multiply but do not invade the body or cause an immune response or symptoms (Wertz, 1991). The host, if ill or in a vulnerable state, may become ill and get an infection. There is a difference between being infected and becoming ill. Illness results when the agent gains the upper hand and there is a change from the normal state of health. When an obvious complex of symptoms occurs, the infection is called a clinical disease. When the body successfully resists being overwhelmed by the infection, it is called subclinical. There may be few symptoms, and the host may be unaware of the exposure, but antigens form that can be recovered from the person's blood.

Infection is described as primary when it occurs in an otherwise healthy person or secondary when it develops in a weakened client.

Local Versus Systemic. An infection may be localized to a single area of the body, or it may disseminate to deeper organs. When it spreads to other body systems, the infection is called ***systemic***. If bacteria spread through the bloodstream, the term ***bacteremia*** is used. Another term, ***septicemia***, is often used as a synonym, but it more accurately refers to the presence of microorganisms (or their toxic products) in the bloodstream that are disrupting normal body functions. Streptococcal or staphylococcal blood infections were formerly called "blood poisoning."

Acute Versus Chronic. An infection may be acute or chronic depending on the severity and duration of symptoms. An acute infection usually develops rapidly, causes symptoms, comes to a climax, and then fades fairly quickly. A chronic infection, on the other hand, can linger: symptoms usually develop more slowly, and convalescence may take months. An acute infection can become chronic when the body cannot rid itself of the organism.

Nosocomial Infections

Nosocomial infections are infections associated with healthcare delivery. Nosocomial infections can occur during a physician visit if poor aseptic practices are used, during a home visit if the nurse has not washed his or her hands after care of the previous client, or in the ambulatory surgery center if strict surgical asepsis is not observed (Fig. 39-1). Nosocomial infections occur frequently in nursing homes, jails, and other residential facilities where high-risk individuals are cared for by auxiliary staff who may be overworked and poorly trained.

Statistics related to nosocomial infections are monitored for hospitals. About 5% to 6% of all hospitalized

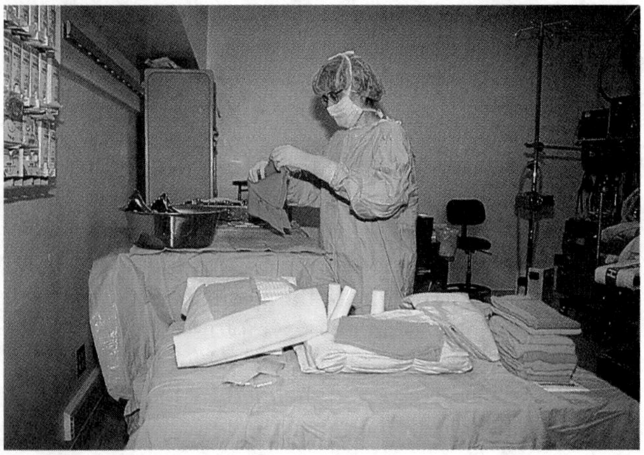

Figure 39-1 • Strict surgical asepsis is needed in the operating room to prevent infection.

clients acquire a nosocomial infection. Most of these infections involve the urinary tract, surgical or traumatic wounds, the respiratory tract, or bacteremias in association with intravascular lines. The rate of such infections in nonhospitalized clients is not as well documented, but probably also significant.

Risk for Urinary Tract Infections. The incidence of UTIs in clients is directly related to instrumentation. The most common causes of UTIs are continuous indwelling Foley catheters and diagnostic or therapeutic procedures that traumatize the urethral mucosa or introduce organisms into the bladder.

Catheter-associated infections result from a lack of strict aseptic technique during catheter insertion, a break in the closed drainage system, an ascending infection by organisms from the perineum of a client with fecal incontinence, and direct contamination from a caregiver's hands. The accompanying display lists factors contributing to the incidence of UTI. See Chapter 41 for detailed information on preventing and treating UTIs.

Risk for Wound Infections. Contributing to the significant problem of wound infections are

- More complicated, longer surgical procedures
- The increase in the number of older clients with chronic diseases who are having surgery
- New surgical procedures in which foreign materials (such as heart valves, joints, vessels, or orthopedic hardware) are implanted
- The increase in the number of organ transplant recipients who require immunosuppressive agents
- The increased use of diagnostic or treatment modalities that expose clients to bacteria or suppress their normal host resistance.

Three factors contribute to the incidence of wound infection: local tissue, treatment, and the host factors (see the display). The longer the client is in an acute-care agency, the more likely the probability of wound infection (Parent, 1992). Today's trends of earlier hospital discharges and treatment in ambulatory surgical centers have reduced wound infection rates.

Risk for Respiratory Infections. Most hospital-acquired respiratory infections are caused by gram-negative organisms that often are the antibiotic-resistant flora of the institution. These are often polymicrobial infections.

Many factors can predispose the client to respiratory tract infections, including factors that

- Increase secretion production
- Decrease chest wall movement
- Inhibit secretion clearance
- Depress the respiratory drive
- Increase the risk of microbial colonization.

Refer to the display for factors that predispose the client to respiratory infections.

Smoking, atelectasis, chronic lung disease, obesity, alcoholism, and malnutrition contribute to the development of respiratory infections. Compromised host defenses lead to increased rates of infection and increased morbidity and mortality. See Chapter 34 for specific information on preventing and treating respiratory infections.

Risk for Bacteremias. Bacteremias are caused by microorganisms that enter the bloodstream from infected wounds or contaminated devices. The most common causes of bacteremias are contaminated intravascular catheters and monitoring devices. When microorganisms enter and proliferate in the bloodstream, serious infections can occur, including cellulitis, septicemia, endocarditis, and distal infections in the lung, liver, and spleen (Messner, et al., 1994).

Risk for Bone and Joint Infections. Bone infection, or osteomyelitis, is a serious type of infection that is difficult to treat. Healthy bone has an excellent blood supply, but because of its rigid structure, once pus forms inside the periosteum, increased pressure develops that can occlude the bone's blood supply. This produces areas of infected, devitalized bone. Ligaments and tendons have poor blood supplies and do not resist infection well. Joints contain avascular cartilage and menisci, and because of the inadequate blood supply, antibiotics cannot reach the infecting organism in bactericidal concentrations.

Bone and joint infections are associated with orthopedic injury or surgery, peripheral vascular disease, decubitus ulcers, infected puncture wounds, or long-term use of intravenous therapy that causes bacteremia.

Factors Predisposing to Infections

Factors Predisposing to Urinary Tract Infection

Factors Increasing Contamination of Urethral Area

- Fecal incontinence
- Atrophic changes (senile vaginitis)
- Environment

Factors Facilitating Urethral Ascent of Organisms

- Catheterization
- Surgery
- Sexual intercourse
- Pelvic relaxation with aging
- Urethral incompetence (incontinence)
- Diapering incontinent clients

Factors Reducing Flow of Urine

- Outflow obstruction (urethral stricture, prostatic hypertrophy, fecal impaction)
- Neurogenic bladder
- Inadequate fluid intake (dehydration)

Factors Promoting Bacterial Colonization

- Foreign body (tumor, calculi)
- Aging (epithelial cell changes, reduced mucus production, waning immunity)

Factors Predisposing to Wound Infection

Local Factors

- Degree of contamination of the wound
- Virulence of contaminating organisms
- Adequacy of local blood supply
- Amount of necrotic or injured tissue in the wound
- Degree of closure of the wound
- Presence of dead spaces, hematomas, and seromas
- Presence and type of foreign bodies
- Location of the wound
- Mechanism of injury

Treatment Factors

- Length of stay in an acute-care facility
- Time, type, and thoroughness of treatment
- Duration of operative procedure(s)
- Timeliness and appropriateness of antibiotic administration
- Appropriate surgical closure
- Surgical technique
- Appropriateness of wound dressing
- Nutritional support
- Adequacy of oxygenation and tissue perfusion
- Use of invasive devices for monitoring, drainage, and fluid or nutritional support
- Adequate treatment of coexisting infections

Host Factors

- Age
- General immunologic competence
- Chronic health problems
- Preoperative nutritional status
- Obesity
- Remote infections
- Extent of injury (multiple wounds or extensive surgery)

Factors Predisposing to Respiratory Infection

Factors Increasing Secretion Production

- Smoking
- Intubation
- Chemical irritation (air pollution, allergies, inhalation anesthetics, aspiration of gastric contents, impaired cough or swallowing mechanisms)

Factors Decreasing Chest Wall Movement

- Pain (chest or abdominal injuries or incisions)
- Obesity
- Abdominal distention
- Tight casts or bandages
- Age
- Skeletal deformities (traumatic or congenital [eg, scoliosis])

Factors Inhibiting Secretion Clearance

- Weak cough
- Dry, tenacious secretions
- Dehydration
- Chronic lung disease
- Decreased diaphragmatic movement (neurologic deficits, paralysis, muscle weakness)

Factors Depressing the Respiratory Center (Hypoventilation)

- Sedatives
- Narcotics
- Altered levels of consciousness (resulting from trauma or cerebrovascular events)
- Acid–base imbalance

Factors Increasing Risk of Microbial Colonization

- Extended hospital stay
- Residence in long-term care facility
- Enotracheal intubation
- Tracheostomy
- Superinfection after long-term use of antibiotics
- Malnutrition
- Primary or acquired immune deficiency
- Contaminated respiratory equipment
- Steroids
- Immunosuppressive therapy
- Poor personal hygiene practices

Compromised Host

A few infections occur as a direct result of the virulence of the infectious agent or its by-products, but most infections occur as a result of decreased host defenses. Before an infectious process becomes a disease, there must be a breakdown or impairment of the physical and chemical barriers to bacterial colonization, the inflammatory and febrile response, and the response of the WBCs, including those involved in immunity. Unfortunately, this occurs frequently in a person's life.

Decreased resistance to infection may be the result of age, preexisting diseases, medical therapy, malnutrition, or stress. The body's anatomic barriers may be broken by many conditions. The accompanying display lists many host factors that can alter resistance to infection.

Factors That Alter Resistance to Infection

Conditions of Client

- Diabetes mellitus
- Advanced malignancy
- Obesity
- Malnutrition or nutritional deficiencies
- Uremia
- Burns
- Trauma
- Leukemia
- Premature birth
- Advanced age
- Drug and alcohol abuse
- Chronic pulmonary disease
- Cardiovascular disease
- Peripheral vascular disease
- Obstructive stones in gallbladder and ureteral ducts
- Immune deficiency diseases
- Immobility
- Cigarette smoking

Therapeutic Procedures

- Intravascular lines
- Indwelling urinary catheters
- Extensive surgical procedures
- Implantation of prosthetic devices
- Hyperalimentation
- Endotracheal and tracheostomy tubes
- Feeding tubes
- Radiation

Medications

- Steroids
- Cancer therapy
- Inappropriate or prolonged use of antibiotics
- Antimetabolites

Breaks in Skin and Mucous Membranes. Breaks in skin and mucous membranes predispose a person to infection. Both natural and therapeutic processes can alter intact epithelial surfaces. Skin in infants and older adults is thin and more easily broken or penetrated by microorganisms. Some medications, such as steroids, cause thinning of the skin and increase the potential for breakdown.

Surgical intervention and many diagnostic procedures break normal skin integrity, greatly increasing the possibility of infection. Therapeutic procedures invade every epithelial surface. Nasogastric tubes, urinary catheters, suction catheters, and rectal thermometers can cause surface abrasions and obstruct the natural flow of cleansing fluids.

Invasive Devices. Any invasive device that enters the body provides a portal of entry for microorganisms, thus increasing the chance for infection. Invasive devices are often used to treat illnesses. Tubes through the skin and body orifices provide microorganisms with direct access to internal organs and the bloodstream. Intravascular lines are inserted to give medications and fluids or to serve as monitoring devices. Urinary catheters or tubes placed in the gastrointestinal tract for decompression or feeding also increase infection risk. Surgical drains placed postoperatively to promote adequate wound drainage provide an access route for microorganisms into the wound.

Stasis of Body Fluids. Stagnant secretions in the body provide a warm, moist environment that fosters bacterial growth. Normal defense mechanisms prevent stasis of body fluids, but these can be altered. Tubes inserted into the trachea or drugs that cause sedation may bypass or suppress the normal cough and sneezing clearance of respiratory secretions. Smokers inhibit normal nasopharyngeal ciliary action by inhaling toxic chemicals in cigarette smoke. Tumors or other obstructions in ducts of exocrine glands obstruct the flow of normal secretions, providing a medium rich for microbial growth. Decreased fluid intake, immobility, and urinary tract obstruction foster urinary stasis, increasing the risk of urinary tract infection.

Inadequate Nutrition. Malnutrition depresses almost every normal defensive response to infection. Neutrophil and microphage function is defective, blood levels of complement are low, and both cellular and humoral immune reactions are diminished. When infection occurs, cellular metabolism increases as the body tries to fight it. Because increased metabolism requires increased calories and protein, inadequate protein stores decrease the body's ability to manufacture antibodies and WBCs. A vicious cycle occurs, with increased nutritional needs and decreased body reserves. Residents of Third World countries experience this cycle of malnutrition and infection many times during their lives. Malnutrition may also occur if the client cannot eat because of anorexia or indwelling tubes in the gastrointestinal tract.

Stress. Stress increases greatly when a client is ill or hospitalized. Surgery or trauma are emotionally and physically stressful. Physical or emotional stress causes the body to release cortisol, which can increase the risk of infection. Cortisol increases the level of serum glucose, a good medium for bacterial growth. The metabolic rate is increased, depleting energy stores necessary for tissue healing and the production of antibodies. Extreme continuous stress causes exhaustion, which limits a person's ability to resist infection.

Humoral Immune Dysfunction. The immune system's ability to finish the killing process by producing memory cells and antibodies can be impaired in several ways. Immunodeficiency may be congenital or acquired. Diseases affecting immunocompetence include AIDS, alcoholism, the presence of preexisting infection, burns, cancer, the absence or removal of the spleen in children, bone marrow depression from radiation or chemotherapy, chemical poisoning, and malnutrition.

Coexisting Medical Problems. Cancer, especially if it affects bone marrow production of leukocytes, increases the risk of infection. Cancers such as leukemia may accelerate the rate of leukocyte production, but the cells are immature and ineffective in fighting infection. Treatment of many forms of cancer by chemotherapy or radiation may cause bone marrow suppression, affecting the body's ability to resist infection.

Some diseases affect the factors that attract neutrophils and wandering macrophages to the site of infection. This attraction, called chemotaxis, is decreased in diabetes mellitus, cirrhosis, and uremia. Clients with burns have impaired neutrophils that do not ingest and destroy microorganisms efficiently. Because neutrophils release mediators of inflammation, impairment of their number and effectiveness has a profound effect on host defenses.

Medical problems that affect the circulation of blood and nutrients can impair host defenses. Cardiovascular conditions, such as peripheral vascular disease and congestive heart failure, can limit the body's ability to supply leukocytes and antibodies to the site of an infection, thus decreasing the infection-fighting potential.

Inflammatory disorders can also increase the risk of infection. The inflammatory response normally helps destroy and contain microbes to prevent systemic infection. However, inflammation can be destructive if it causes loss of vascular control and if the tissue exudate is extensive enough to provide a medium for microbial growth.

Drug Therapy. Drug therapy can cause defects in the host's response to infection. Steroids, chemotherapy, antimetabolites, and the inappropriate or prolonged use of antibiotics can increase the risk of infection. Opportunistic infection (sometimes referred to as superinfection) can occur with antibiotic therapy. If the course of antibiotic administration is prolonged or if an incorrect antibiotic is chosen, bacterial growth may be stimulated as normal flora in the gut, mouth, and skin is destroyed. These opportunistic organisms can take advantage of the alteration in the normal flora, leading to serious infections in the host.

Manifestations of Infection

The way an infection becomes apparent varies depending on the infectious agent, the host, and the organ system involved. Nonspecific symptoms may precede overt clinical signs. Common manifestations of infection are listed in the accompanying display.

Nonspecific Symptoms

The human body has a variety of internal sensors that signal when something is wrong. Often this inner sense is the first warning of an impending infection. These early warnings include malaise (a general sense of feeling not completely well), listlessness, inability to concentrate, uneasiness, light-headedness, weakness, muscle or joint discomfort, headache, and anorexia. As the person becomes more ill, the symptoms change from subjective, vague complaints to objective findings.

Fever

Fever is a common manifestation of infection and should be considered a sign of infection until other causes are ruled out. Fever is the response of the thermoregulatory center in the hypothalamus to circulating pyrogens. These pyrogens are released when phagocytic cells (granulocytes, monocytes, and macrophages) are stimulated by microorganisms or endotoxins (Wertz, 1991). Very young children tend to produce high fevers (up to 105°F or 40°C) in the presence of infection, but older people may not show a fever or may produce only a low-grade fever when infection is present.

During the first postoperative day, an elevated temperature is most likely caused by the physiologic stress of surgery or atelectasis. Pneumonia is most likely to

Common Manifestions of Infection

Wound Infection

- Redness, swelling, pain
- Localized heat
- Fever
- Purulent or malodorous drainage
- Bruising around incision or induration of area around wound

Urinary Tract Infection

- Urgency and increased frequency of urination
- Burning with urination (dysuria)
- Cloudy, bloody, or malodorous urine (pyuria, hematuria)
- Fever
- Flank pain

Respiratory Disease

- Nasal congestion or discharge
- Productive cough
- Fever, increased pulse and respiratory rate
- Sore throat
- Painful breathing (pleuritic chest pain)
- Difficulty in breathing (dyspnea)

Gastroenteritis

- Severe abdominal cramping and nausea after eating
- More than usual number of stools and/or loose, watery, or bloody stools

cause a fever during the second to fifth postoperative day, urinary tract infection on the second to eighth postoperative day, and wound infection from the third to eleventh postoperative day. Deep operative infection or infected prosthetic devices may be detected when fever develops weeks or months after surgery.

Increased Pulse and Respiratory Rate

Infection increases the body's metabolic rate, which increases the heart rate. The pulse may become bounding. The rate and depth of respiration also increase as the body tries to get rid of excess waste products produced during increased metabolism.

Inflammatory Symptoms

Infection stimulates the inflammatory response to promote leukocyte migration to the area. The inflammatory response is discussed in detail in Chapter 38. As inflammation occurs, the area appears red, swollen, and warm.

Pain

Most infections cause discomfort. Pain can occur when inflammation causes swelling within an enclosed area, or when normal function is impeded. Examples of pain caused by infection include the following:

- Pleuritic pain when breathing, with a respiratory infection
- Burning on voiding, with a urinary tract infection
- Pain on swallowing, with a streptococcal throat infection.

Purulent Drainage

As WBCs migrate to the infection, **purulent** (containing pus) drainage may be observed. Because of the increased numbers of WBCs, body fluids such as urine or sputum may become cloudy or whitish-yellow. Purulent drainage is usually thicker than normal and often foul-smelling.

Enlarged Lymph Nodes

During an infection, the lymph nodes that drain an infected area may become enlarged and easily palpable ("swollen glands"). As the swelling increases, the nodes may also become tender. During inflammation, the lymphatic capillaries dilate as excess interstitial fluid, proteins, and invading microorganisms enter the lymphatic system. The swelling shows that lymphocytes and macrophages in the lymph node are fighting the infection and trying to limit its spread.

Rash

A rash may accompany many conditions. It often occurs with primary infections of the skin (eg, impetigo) but may accompany some generalized infectious diseases. The diagnosis of many communicable childhood diseases is made on the specific characteristics of the rash. Many rashes cause pruritus, and scratching may disrupt the skin's integrity, which can result in secondary skin infections.

Gastrointestinal Symptoms

Acute gastrointestinal inflammation can be caused by viruses, bacteria, and toxins produced by certain bacteria and parasites. Anorexia, nausea, and vomiting often occur when the stomach lining is inflamed; diarrhea is more common when the small or large intestine is inflamed.

"Traveler's diarrhea" may occur when tourists drink water and eat uncooked food that contains endemic bacteria or parasites. Travelers have little previous exposure to these microorganisms, so they have limited antibodies to fight the infectious agent.

Impact of Infection on Activities of Daily Living

Individual Considerations

Depending on the severity and duration of the infection, the client's normal daily activities may be affected. The client may experience pain or other physical discomfort, may be separated from his or her peers, and may be disfigured or have a long-term disability. The community suffers from loss of the client's economic contribution and inability to participate in church, political, or charitable activities.

An infection saps the energy needed for normal daily activities. The infected client may not have enough energy for normal grooming. If the infection is located in a joint or requires bed rest, mobility is affected. Pain and the need for antibiotics during the night can disrupt normal sleep patterns. The appetite may be affected, or vomiting and diarrhea may accompany infection or antibiotic therapy.

Because of infection, infants may fail to meet nutritional needs for growth and development. Toddlers may experience delays in developmental task attainment, such as walking or talking, and may suffer separation anxiety if they require hospitalization. School-age children miss the opportunity to participate in school projects and may fall behind in schoolwork. Adolescents and young adults may miss social or athletic events.

Family Considerations

Infection risk increases for all family members whenever one family member is infected, especially if transmission occurs via the airborne route. When one family member is ill, it is especially important for hygienic practices (eg, handwashing, not sharing eating utensils) to be followed. Separation of high-risk family members (eg, newborn or immunocompromised family members) may be necessary. Infectious illness can also pose financial hardship for the family.

Parents may find it necessary to stay home from work or pay for someone to watch the sick child (if such a person can be found). Wage-earners may lose their salary if they do not have sick time as an employee benefit, and may be forced to pay for medical care if they do not have medical insurance.

Routines may need to be shifted so others in the family can take on the responsibilities of the ill person. Sexual and social relations can be hindered because of fatigue. The family's food intake may be affected if the infected person is the one who buys and prepares food. If infection is acute and of short duration, the impact on the family is usually minimal and easily handled. If infections are severe or prolonged, significant impact on the family can occur.

Assessment

The nursing assessment includes gathering data from the nursing history, physical examination, and laboratory and diagnostic tests. As part of the nursing history, the nurse should observe for signs of infection and should ask about the client's infection risk factors, paying careful attention to cues given by the client or caregiver. The nurse collects information from the client and secondary sources such as the family, employee health-care providers, and friends or coworkers. Diagnostic studies and laboratory data are also important sources of information to identify or rule out infection.

Subjective Data

Subjective data is collected from the client to help the nurse determine normal patterns, the risk for infection, and a history of specific infections.

Functional Pattern Identification

The nurse is interested in the client's normal defense system against illness. The nurse should ask the client or caregiver about measures normally taken to avoid illness, including questions about the client's usual pattern of rest and exercise, nutrition, use of vitamins and folk remedies, and understanding of germ exposure. The nurse should obtain a history of immunizations and determine whether they are complete and current. A description of the client's usual experience of illness, including childhood diseases, allows the nurse to determine if the pattern is normal.

Examples of information are given in the accompanying display.

Risk Identification

The nurse should closely screen the client for infection risk and should document any recent exposure to infectious illness. Sometimes this means asking questions such as, "Has anyone in your immediate family recently been infected with (specify disease)?" School records and community documentation of infectious disease outbreaks should be considered in evaluating each client for risk. Questions about the client's general health (such as normal sleep and exercise patterns, nutritional history, use of drugs, cigarettes, or alcohol, and sexual practices) should be included. Any chronic health conditions, such as heart disease, lung disease, or diabetes, and their treatment should be explored. It is important to determine whether the client has been treated with chemotherapy or radiation because such treatment often increases the risk of infection by suppressing the immune system. A medication history should also be taken, focusing on immunosuppressive drugs such as

Nursing Assessment
Health Interview Information

- Immunization history, history of exposure to communicable diseases, and any recent acute infections.
- Chronic diseases that have been complicated by infections and the usual method of treatment. Ask about the signs and symptoms the client has experienced and the medications the client has used.
- Medications or medical therapy the client is receiving (eg, antibiotics, steroids, immunosuppression drugs, chemotherapy, or radiation therapy).
- Client's usual diet and its nutritional adequacy.
- Client's patterns of sleep, exercise, and recreation to determine health beliefs and lifestyle factors that may contribute to the risk of infection.
- History of nausea, vomiting, diarrhea, anorexia, general malaise, muscle aches, or headaches.

steroids and the current or previous use of antibiotics (see the Nursing Assessment display).

Dysfunctional Identification

Manifestations of common infections were listed in a previous display. If an infection was one of the reasons the client sought medical assistance, the nurse's questions should elicit more specific information:

- How long has the infection been present?
- What symptoms first occurred?
- Was the occurrence of the infection associated with any change in routine?
- How does the infection affect the client's ability to perform activities of daily living?

If an infection was not one of the reasons the client sought advice, but the client displays symptoms of infection, further questioning is indicated:

- Is there any pain, redness, swelling, or abnormal drainage? When did it start? How long has it lasted? What is its intensity?
- Has the client suffered nausea, vomiting, diarrhea, malaise, or general aches and pains (symptoms that accompany many viral infections)?

Information about the client's present level of functioning in each of the health patterns should be obtained when infection is present. The nursing history (as opposed to the medical history) focuses on how the infection has affected the client's ability to function normally and to carry out usual activities and routines.

Objective Data

Physical Assessment

The nurse performs a physical assessment to provide more information on the presence of infection and how it has affected the client's functional ability.

General Inspection. The nurse gets a general impression of the client when they first meet. The nurse can see whether the client is comfortable or in obvious pain. Signs of fatigue can be detected in the client's posture and in how he or she moves. Abnormal skin color and the presence of rashes or lesions are often apparent, and swelling and signs of inflammation can also be detected.

Vital Signs. Vital signs are monitored frequently to detect the presence of infection or to monitor its progress. The accuracy of such assessment is important in determining the presence of infection. In a client with an infection, the nurse often finds an elevated temperature (often above 101°F), an elevated pulse rate, and an increased respiratory rate.

When evaluating the significance of vital signs that differ from baseline values, the nurse must consider other factors that could be responsible. It is helpful to look at the pattern of changes in vital signs. A consistently elevated and rising temperature is significant. Often the physician obtains cultures and begins to look for the source of a possible infection when the temperature rises above 101°F. Some people, however, such as older adults and immunosuppressed clients, may not show a fever when infection is present.

Auscultation of Breath Sounds. Auscultating breath sounds can help detect respiratory infections. Pneumonia can alter normal breath sounds, producing rales, rhonchi, and wheezes. Atelectasis, which can predispose a client to respiratory infection, is noted by diminished breath sounds.

Auscultation of Bowel Sounds. Auscultating bowel sounds can help detect increased intestinal peristalsis. Increased peristalsis often accompanies microbial irritation of the gut, which can cause diarrhea.

Palpation of Lymph Nodes. Lymph nodes can enlarge and become tender because of localized and systemic infection. Gentle palpation using the tips of the middle three fingers can detect any enlargement in lymph nodes. Normally, cervical lymph nodes are less than 1 cm in diameter and are soft and mobile. The nurse should note any tenderness during palpation.

Diagnostic Tests and Procedures

Because clinical signs sometimes provide insufficient evidence to identify a pathogen, diagnostic procedures are used to detect and identify the source of an infection. Laboratory analysis and culturing of body fluids and x-rays and other imaging methods are used to locate the source of infection. Antibiotic sensitivities and therapeutic drug monitoring are used to identify optimal drug therapy. Common studies included in an initial infection workup are

- Complete blood count, including hemoglobin, hematocrit, and WBC count
- Urinalysis
- Erythrocyte sedimentation rate (ESR or sed rate).

When infection is strongly suspected, the physician may also order a series of WBC counts with differentials and body fluid cultures and sensitivities.

White Blood Cell Count. The number of WBCs, or leukocytes, rises in response to infection, tissue necrosis, stress, and neoplastic changes in bone marrow. A rise in circulating WBCs to above the normal adult range of 5,000 to 10,000 cells/mm^3 is called **leukocytosis**. Infectious processes may be discovered by examining the WBCs and differentiating the cell types. By examining the types of WBCs, a diagnosis can be confirmed and progress can be followed. The cells are counted and the cell types are reported as a percentage of the total number (see Appendix B).

Neutrophils normally compose about 50% to 70% of all WBCs. Their numbers increase during infection. When the infection is severe or prolonged, the body cannot manufacture neutrophils quickly enough, causing the release of immature granulocytes (also called bands) into the blood. This increase in the number of immature cells is called a leftward shift in the granulocytic differential count. This shift is considered a strong indication of bacterial infection. The greater the leftward shift, the more worrisome the infection appears. When the proportion of neutrophils increases, the client's resistance is good and the body is considered to be fighting the infection well.

Very low neutrophil counts, often associated with cancer or chemotherapy, greatly increase infection risk. When the neutrophils fall below 500/mm^3 the client is **neutropenic**, and neutropenic precautions are instituted to prevent possible lethal infections (Gawlikowski, 1992). Common signs of infection are often mediated by neutrophils, so when counts are very low symptoms of infection may be absent.

Some clients, such as those who are malnourished, older, immunosuppressed, or on steroids, cannot produce more WBCs in response to an infection. In these cases, the absence of an increase in total WBCs or a lack of clarity on the differential does not rule out infection.

To obtain a WBC and differential, a specimen of 5 to 10 mL of blood is sent to the laboratory in a vacuum tube with a solution to prevent clotting. Results from the laboratory are reported in both absolute numbers and the relative percentage of subtypes of WBCs. Abnormal results should be reported to the physician.

Urinalysis. The urine is routinely examined to check for kidney and endocrine function and to identify the presence of UTI. Urinalysis provides information about the color, pH, specific gravity, and presence of protein, glucose, and ketones in the urine. Microscopic examinations search for casts, red blood cells and WBCs, epithelial cells, and bacteria. Changes in color, concentration, or odor of the urine may indicate an infectious process. Alkaline urine (pH above 8) may indicate bacteriuria. High levels of glucose and protein may indicate systemic infection or UTI. Erythrocytes or WBCs or their cellular casts may also indicate infection, but may be caused by noninfectious inflammatory conditions. Large numbers of white cells usually indicate a UTI. A clean-catch or midstream urine specimen is requested if more than four WBCs are found or if bacteria are seen on the slide made from the urine sample. See Chapter 41 for more information on collecting urine samples. Abnormal results should be reported to the physician so that treatment can be started.

Erythrocyte Sedimentation Rate. The ESR measures the rate at which red blood cells settle in unclotted blood in millimeters per hour. The result is elevated both in acute noninfectious inflammatory conditions and in infectious processes. Collagen disease, tissue necrosis, malignancies, and stress can also increase the rate of sedimentation. This test is most commonly used to provide a crude estimate of a disease process and of the response to therapy. Because it is affected by drugs and other factors, all medications the client is taking should be brought to the laboratory's attention.

Culture and Sensitivity. Cultures are obtained from body fluids to isolate the source of unknown fevers and to identify the microorganism causing the signs of clinical infection. Culture specimens are obtained from blood, sputum, stool, throat or wound exudate, and urine, as well as spinal, joint, pleural, and other body cavity fluids. Most specimens are obtained using sterile swabs with a solid or liquid medium, a sterile container with a lid, or a sterile syringe with a sterile bottle of medium to receive the specimen.

Specimens are sent to the laboratory for Gram stain and culture and sensitivity results. Properly prepared Gram stains provide information as soon as the slide smears are prepared and give broad classifications of the microorganisms. This information may be used to order antibiotic therapy while waiting for specific culture results. Results of Gram stains can be obtained from the laboratory in less than 30 minutes; it usually takes 24 to 36 hours to grow good cultures and 48 hours to obtain growth and sensitivity results.

Sensitivity testing of microorganisms to antibiotics is a benefit of obtaining good culture specimens. After microorganisms are grown in culture media, different concentrations of antibiotics are added to a known quantity of the inoculum to test their ability to inhibit growth or to kill the organism. The laboratory reports the names of the organisms present and whether they are sensitive or resistant to specific antibiotics. The drugs are then tested for their range of effectiveness against the pathogen.

The accuracy of laboratory analysis for all cultures is only as good as the specimen provided. Factors affecting the results of the analysis include

- Contamination of the specimen
- Delay in sending the specimen (which increases the growth of contaminating organisms and causes deterioration of the constituents to be examined)
- Use of inappropriate containers and culture media
- Failure to identify the source of the specimen
- Failure to tell the laboratory about current client medications (eg, antibiotics) that may affect the analysis.

The nurse can elicit the client's cooperation by explaining why the specimen is being obtained. Specimens should be taken before starting antibiotics that could alter the results. They should be labeled with the time, date, and site of collection and should be delivered immediately to the laboratory. When cultures are being obtained, aseptic technique should be used and gloves should be worn by the caregiver to avoid potential transmission of pathogens (see Procedure 39-1, Obtaining a Wound Culture).

Many healthcare agencies allow nurses to culture suspect exudates from tubes or wounds as a matter of policy. Because the cost of processing a specimen is often not covered by insurance without a physician's order, however, a written order should be obtained to decrease the financial burden on the client.

Blood Culture. Blood cultures are ordered when there is a high degree of suspicion that an infectious process is occurring. Blood cultures are usually obtained from two separate venipuncture sites. Because indwelling intravascular lines may be contaminated with surface pathogens or seeded by microorganisms that are localized to the catheter tip, blood is not usually drawn for culture from previously inserted lines. The ideal specimen is drawn just before or during the rise in temperature because the pathogens are usually circulating in high concentrations at that time.

Obtaining a blood culture requires a set of culture bottles, a sterile syringe, two sterile needles, skin preparation equipment, and a tourniquet. The skin is cleaned according to the institution's procedure; usually a combination preparation of povidone-iodine (Betadine; Purdue Frederick, Norwalk, CT) and alcohol is recommended. The tops of the culture bottles are cleaned and allowed to dry. Gloves are worn while the sterile needle and syringe are used to aspirate blood. The needle is then usually changed before inoculating the culture media into special vacuum bottles. After ensuring hemostasis at the puncture site, the nurse removes the gloves and washes his or her hands before transporting the specimen to the laboratory.

Sputum Culture. Sputum cultures are obtained in a fever workup when the client has a productive cough. Because infections may be located in either the upper or lower respiratory tract, a good culture specimen should contain little saliva; saliva and postnasal drip secretions contaminate the specimen. Sputum ideally should be obtained in the morning, before the client eats. It should be collected in a sterile container with a lid and should be transported to the laboratory as soon as it is obtained (unless it is a 24-hour specimen, which usually is placed in a special fixative).

Occasionally a client cannot cooperate with sputum specimen collection, or a specimen must be obtained from a client who is endotracheally intubated. A specimen is then obtained by suctioning with a sterile suction catheter via the nasotracheal or endotracheal route. The physician may also elect to insert a small catheter through a needle into the trachea and aspirate secretions transtracheally. Specimens can also be obtained through bronchoscopy. Again, specimens should be transported immediately to the laboratory.

Throat Culture. Throat cultures are obtained with a sterile cotton swab that is touched to the back of the throat as the client says "aaahh." This should be done as quickly as possible because it may trigger the gag reflex. Maintaining sterility, the swab is placed into a culture medium and transported to the laboratory.

Wound Culture. Wound cultures are taken when signs of local inflammation or purulent discharge from the wound are noted. Suitable culture media or kits are obtained from the hospital supply service. Fresh exudate should be used for culture specimens. After removing the dressing, any crusted drainage should be gently wiped away with sterile gauze before swabbing the area. The specimen should be obtained from deep in the wound, if possible; swabs from the skin are usually of no value.

Body Cavity and Fluid Culture. Body cavity and fluid cultures are obtained using aseptic technique when there is an indication of inflammation in the area. Spinal taps, joint aspirations, and pleural cavities are commonly cultured for microorganisms based on clinical observations and a high index of suspicion for an infectious process. Special kits are available from the hospital supply service, and sterile technique is always used. The nurse assists the physician in obtaining these specimens by ordering supplies, positioning and draping the client, and ensuring rapid transport of the specimens to the laboratory.

Stool Culture. Stool cultures may be ordered to rule out infectious causation of diarrhea. Cultures are usu-

Procedure 39-1
Obtaining a Wound Culture

Purpose

1. Identify organisms colonized within a wound so that antibiotics sensitive to the microorganisms can be prescribed, as needed.

Assessment

- Conduct frequent surveillance of surgical incisions and other wounds for signs of inflammation and infection (ie, redness, swelling, warmth, drainage).
- Monitor vital signs for evidence of infection (ie, increased temperature, pulse).
- Identify and document amount, color, and odor of any drainage from wounds.
- Assess client for level of discomfort associated with dressing changes and premedicate if necessary with analgesics.
- Ensure early identification of factors that contribute to potential development of wound infections.

Equipment

Sterile culture swab (anaerobic or aerobic) and transport container
Disposable, clean gloves
Sterile dressing and tape
Name label and completed laboratory requisition

Procedure

1. Wash hands and apply disposable gloves.
   Rationale: Washing and gloves protect hands from contact with drainage and prevent transfer of microorganisms.
2. Remove soiled dressing. Observe drainage for amount, odor, and color.
   Rationale: The wound is assessed for signs of infection.
3. Clear and remove exudate from around wound with antiseptic swab.
   Rationale: Old drainage and microorganisms from wound could interfere with accurate culture and sensitivity report.

Procedure

Obtaining Aerobic Culture

1. Steps 1 to 3 above.
2. Using sterile swab from culture tube, insert swab deep into area of active drainage. Rotate swab to absorb as much drainage as possible.
   Rationale: Adequate sample is necessary for culture of organism.

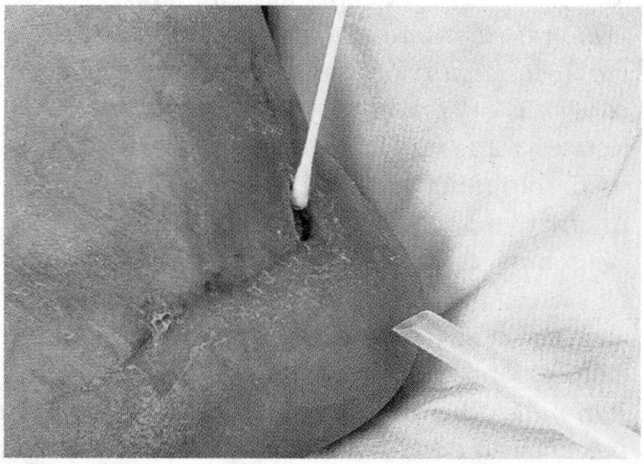

Step 2 • *Insert culture swab into wound to obtain sample.*

3. Insert swab into culture tube, taking care not to touch the top or outside of the tube.
   Rationale: The outside of the culture tube must remain free of pathogenic microorganisms to prevent possible spread of infection to others.
4. Crush ampule of medium and close container securely.
   Rationale: Culture medium keeps bacteria alive until analysis is complete. It is essential not to introduce other microorganisms.

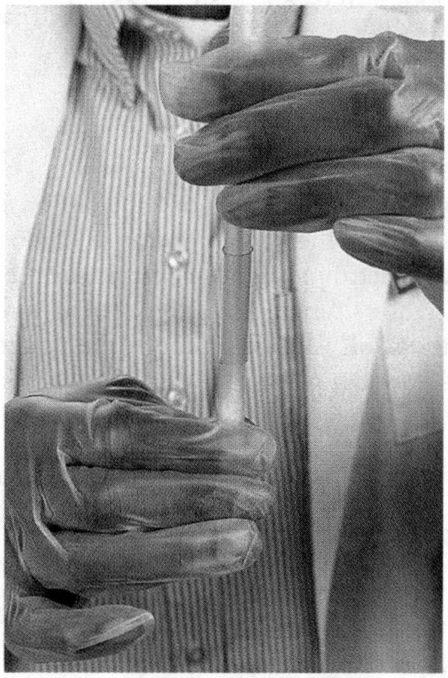

Step 4 • *Crush ampule of medium.*

5. Continue with Step 4 below.

(continued)

Procedure

Obtaining Anaerobic Culture

1. Steps 1 to 3 at beginning of procedure.
2. Using sterile swab from special anaerobic culture tube, insert swab deeply into draining body cavity.
Rationale: Drainage sample is taken from deep cavity to identify organisms that may grow where oxygen is not present.

3a. Rotate swab gently and remove. Quickly place swab into inner tube of collection container.

3b. Alternative method: insert tip of syringe with needle removed into wound and aspirate 1 to 5 mL of exudate. Attach 21-gauge needle to syringe, expel all air, and inject exudate into inner tube of the culture container.
Rationale: The inner tube of the culture container has either a carbon dioxide or nitrogen environment to prevent potential contaminating organisms from growing until the laboratory analysis is complete.
Note: Drainage is sampled from only one drainage site per culture swab. If a specimen is required from another site, repeat the above steps to identify accurately microbes present at each drainage site.

4. Label each culture tube and send specimens with appropriate laboratory requisition immediately to the laboratory.
Rationale: Bacteria grow rapidly within culture media of specimen tubes. Cultures should be prepared quickly for accurate results.
Note: Some agencies require that specimens be transported in clean plastic bags to further to prevent transfer of microorganisms.
5. Clean and apply sterile dressings to the wound, as ordered.
Rationale: Cleansing and sterile dressing protect the wound from environmental contamination; dressing contains further drainage to prevent spread of infection.
6. Remove and discard gloves. Wash hands.
Rationale: Risk of transmission of microorganisms must be reduced.
7. Assist client to comfortable position.
8. Document all relevant information on the client's chart. Include the location the specimen was taken from, and the date and time. Record the appearance of the wound, and the color, odor, amount, and consistency of the drainage. Record how the client tolerated the procedure and any discomfort that was experienced.

Lifespan Considerations

Infants and Children

- Perform procedures that are uncomfortable or potentially fear-inducing in areas other than the child's room, so the child continues to regard his or her room as a safe place.

Home-Care Considerations

- Teach client the signs and symptoms of infection and what to report to his or her healthcare provider.
- When cultures are obtained from the client at his or her home, transport the specimens as quickly as possible to the closest laboratory for analysis.

ally necessary to examine the stool for leukocytes and to identify enteric pathogens of bacterial or fungal origin. Parasites, another common cause of diarrhea, lay eggs in the gastrointestinal tract that can be detected on examination. When a client is being screened for parasitic infection, stool specimens are collected daily for 3 days. Moving organisms can easily be detected in fresh specimens.

Stool specimens should be collected in a sterile bedpan and transferred to a sterile container with a sterile tongue blade. On the laboratory form, the nurse should identify the test required, the organism being screened, and note if the client has been out of the country or backpacking in remote areas. Stool specimens can be affected by urine, toilet paper, soap, disinfectants, antibiotics, antacids, barium, laxatives, enemas, and cool temperatures.

Serology Tests. Serology tests are sometimes done as part of a fever workup. Early in the course of the infection, an acute-phase blood specimen is collected. If the cause of the infection is not determined by the third week, a convalescent-phase specimen is obtained, and both specimens are examined simultaneously for a change in antibody titer. The laboratory needs to know the clinical signs and symptoms of the client and the client's immunization history. By comparing antigen-antibody reactions of the two specimens, a diagnosis can be made.

Therapeutic Drug Monitoring. Drug monitoring is used to determine the concentration of a drug in blood. Blood levels of antibiotics are tested to avoid possible toxic effects such as renal damage (nephrotoxicity) and eighth cranial nerve damage (ototoxicity). The timing of specimen collection is of critical importance in drug monitoring. For the laboratory and physician to interpret the plasma drug level, they must know when the last dose of antibiotic was given and when the specimen was obtained. The highest level of drug concentration (peak level) should occur shortly after the drug is given, and the lowest level (trough level) should occur just before a dose is due to be administered. The goal of therapy is to keep the peaks from being too high and the troughs from being too low. Specimens must be labeled as to whether they are being analyzed as a peak or trough specimen. Depending on the test results, the amount of the antibiotic and the frequency of dosing may be adjusted to match the client's rate of metabolism and drug clearance.

Diagnostic Imaging. Rapid advances are being made in the ability to visualize internal organs and to evaluate them for infection. After these tests, the nurse must monitor vital signs, and when contrast material is used, observe for any signs of allergic reaction.

Chest x-rays are used to diagnose pneumonia, lung abscesses, and tuberculosis. Endoscopic procedures are used to visualize the respiratory and gastrointestinal tract and to obtain specimens for microbiologic testing. Computed axial tomography (CT or CAT) is used to obtain multidimensional images of the body, which are interpreted by computer to construct images of internal structures. By visualizing the differences in densities of organs, and organ deformity, the study can help locate abscesses or other areas of infection. The study can be done with contrast media, which enhances visualization of normal versus abnormal tissue.

Magnetic resonance imaging is expected to be used with increasing frequency to detect infection of the nervous system. The procedure uses opaque contrast materials, injected intravenously, that have affinities for concentrations of WBCs in abscesses or other areas of infection.

Nursing Diagnoses

Risk for Infection is the only North American Nursing Diagnosis Association (NANDA)-accepted nursing diagnosis related to infection. If an infection is actually present in a person, the problem is collaborative, necessitating intervention from nurses, physicians, pharmacists, and other members of the healthcare team. Nurses can independently develop individualized plans to help prevent infection for clients at risk.

Diagnostic Statement: Risk for Infection

Definition

Risk for Infection is the state in which an individual is at increased risk for being invaded by pathogenic organisms (NANDA, 1994).

Risk Factors

Risk factors for infection include

- Inadequate primary defenses (broken skin, traumatized tissue, decrease in ciliary action, stasis of body fluids, change in pH secretions, altered peristalsis)
- Inadequate secondary defenses (decreased hemoglobin, leukopenia, suppressed inflammatory response) and immunosuppression
- Inadequate acquired immunity, tissue destruction, increased environmental exposure, chronic disease, invasive procedures, malnutrition, pharmaceutical agents, trauma, rupture of amniotic membranes, insufficient knowledge to avoid exposure to pathogens (NANDA, 1994).

Related Nursing Diagnoses

Other nursing diagnoses are common in people with infections. Knowledge Deficit may occur because inadequate knowledge of hygiene or infection control measures can contribute to increased incidence of infection. Many infected people are discharged to home with new treatments and protocols to master.

Pain is another common nursing diagnosis associated with infection. The inflammation that accompanies infection causes discomfort, and discomfort also occurs secondary to the fever that accompanies many infections. Sleep Pattern Disturbance can occur if discomfort is great.

Depending on the infection's location, the function of various body systems can be affected. Impaired Physical Mobility can occur if the infection is in an extremity or bed rest is needed to treat the infection. Altered Urinary Elimination can occur with a urinary tract infection. Bowel Incontinence can occur if the infection results in diarrhea or if the client experiences diarrhea as a side effect of antibiotic therapy. Impaired Gas Exchange is common with lung infections.

Impaired Skin Integrity can occur secondary to the rashes that accompany many infections or because of impaired healing of surgical incisions in the presence of an infection.

Nursing diagnoses also involve psychosocial aspects of functioning. Self-Esteem Disturbance can result when a person assumes the sick role or adjusts to a changing body image. Anxiety and Ineffective Individual Coping can occur when clients and their families are faced with severe infection. Altered Role Performance may be a consequence when an infection limits a person's ability to work, go to school, or carry out normal family responsibilities. Sexual Dysfunction can occur because of lowered energy reserves or as a direct consequence of a sexually transmitted disease.

Outcome Identification and Planning

After the identification of nursing diagnoses, the nurse and client make plans for care. Client goals and outcome criteria are developed that focus on preventing the occurrence of infections and minimizing potential

Planning

Examples of Nursing Interventions Used in Infection Prevention and Control

- Teach your client and other household cohabitants about methods of preventing infection
- Participate in infection prevention in the healthcare agency in which you work
- Observe Centers for Disease Control and Prevention guidelines
- Participate in immunization programs
- Promote host defenses and client comfort
- Promote personal hygiene
- Support adequate rest and relaxation
- Promote adequate nutrition and fluid intake
- Promote ambulation and position changes
- Support pulmonary toilet
- Provide comfort measures
- Observe neutrogenic precautions
- Monitor use of antibiotics
- Prevent further spread of infection
- Collaborate with other community agencies (city, state or province, national, international) in education, monitoring, and treatment of infections

complications. Examples of client goals related to infection include

Client or caregiver will demonstrate adequate knowledge to recognize and report signs of infection.
Client or caregiver will use good health practices to prevent occurrence and spread of infection.
Client will participate in planning of treatment regimens to prevent infection and minimize complications.

Planning for nursing interventions is directed at the following:

- Controlling the spread of infection
- Providing education to modify risk behaviors
- Supporting normal defense mechanisms and behaviors that prevent infection
- Reducing or eliminating the adverse effects of infection on functional abilities
- Detecting behaviors that increase the potential for infection
- Participating in community planning and activities for infection prevention

Examples of nursing interventions are listed in the accompanying display and discussed in the next section of this chapter.

Implementation

The perception of health and health management is influenced by the client's developmental level, cultural and religious beliefs, social interactions, and biologic framework (Gordon, 1994). Nursing interventions and therapeutic regimens that fail to consider this interaction of biology, behavior, and beliefs fail to achieve their highest goals.

Nursing Interventions to Promote Health and Function

Nurses collaborate with many other disciplines and public agencies to teach preventive health practices, monitor the incidence of infection, and manage infection.

Client Teaching

Protection from infection starts with people and their household cohabitants. People protect themselves and their families by using good hygiene practices, maintaining household cleanliness, eating a well-balanced diet, and exercising regularly. They enhance their protection by getting recommended vaccinations against communicable diseases associated with childhood or with foreign travel. Some factors in client teaching are listed in the accompanying display.

Immunization Programs

Nurses participate in establishing programs for people and groups to receive immunizations. They help to identify outbreaks of infectious disease in the community, give vaccinations, establish record-keeping mechanisms, and counsel people about precautions and pos-

Client Teaching

Infection Prevention

Instruct the client as follows:

- *Wash your hands after toileting and before eating.*
- *Eat a well-balanced diet to help prevent and combat infection.*
- *Keep immunizations up to date; communicable diseases can be serious or fatal*
- *Ask all family members to participate in infection prevention*
- *Learn the common signs of infection (redness, warmth, swelling, fever, increased or abnormal discharge, pain) and know when it is necessary to notify a healthcare professional.*
- *Learn how to monitor your body temperature accurately to detect infection early.*
- *Properly dispose of contaminated articles or secretions (eg, tissues, dressings) to prevent the spread of microorganisms.*
- *Finish the complete prescription for antibiotics even if the symptoms of infection have subsided.*

sible complications of immunization. Nurses work in clinics, schools, and industry to teach about immunizations.

Immunizations may be given by injection, oral solutions, or nasal sprays. To avoid multiple injections, they are given in combination with each other (when the compounds are stable and there is minimal danger of overwhelming the immune system). Booster injections of some vaccines are given throughout the lifespan to stimulate the memory cells of the immune system. Table 39-4 provides guidelines for immunizations for healthy infants and children.

Because of frequent changes, new immunization guidelines must be obtained yearly. This information is available from the Advisory Committee on Immunization Practices of the U.S. Public Health Service and from the Committee on Infectious Diseases of the American Academy of Pediatrics. Similar committees exist in Canada and the World Health Organization.

Immunization records should be maintained by parents during childhood and given to the children as they leave home. Physicians need to record this information and make clients aware of any unusual reaction when they occur. Commonly, excellent vaccination records are kept through the first years of school, but then the parent or child neglects to update the record. This information may be needed if questions arise about whether immunizations are current (especially tetanus, after an accidental injury).

Contraindications to vaccinations include immunodeficiency states, allergy to eggs, or previous allergic reactions. Live vaccines should not be given during pregnancy, during acute debilitating disease, or during periods of severe malnutrition.

Immunization for High-Risk Groups

In addition to routine childhood immunizations, certain individuals who are at increased risk need additional immunization. All healthcare workers and people exposed to blood and body fluids should receive immunizations

Table 39-4 • Recommended Childhood Immunization Schedule, United States

	Age									
Vaccine	*Birth*	*2 mos*	*4 mos*	*6 mos*	*12[5] mos*	*15 mos*	*18 mos*	*4–6 yrs*	*11–12 yrs*	*14–16 yrs*
Hepatitis B[1]	HB-1									
		HB-2		HB-3						
Diphtheria, Tetanus, Pertussis[2]		DTP	DTP	DTP	DTP or DTaP at 15 + m			DTP or DTaP	Td	
H. influenzae type b[3]		HIb	HIb	HIb	HIb					
Polio		OPV	OPV	OPV				OPV		
Measles, Mumps, Rubella[4]					MMR			MMR or	MMR	

Vaccines are listed under the routinely recommended ages. Shaded bars indicate range of acceptable ages for vaccination.

[1]Infants born to hepatitis B antigen (HB_1Ag)-negative mothers should receive the second dose of hepatitis B vaccine between 1 and 4 months of age, provided at least 1 month has elapsed since receipt of the first dose. The third dose is recommended between 6 and 18 months of age.

Infants born to hepatitis B surface antigen (HBsAg)-positive mothers should receive immunoprophylaxis for hepatitis B with 0.5 ml hepatitis B immune globulin (HBIG) within 12 hours of birth, and 0.5 ml of either Merck Sharpe & Dohme vaccine (Recombivax HB) or of SmithKline Beecham vaccine (Engerix-B) at a separate site. In these infants, the second dose of vaccine is recommended at 1 month of age and the third dose at 6 months of age. All pregnant women should be screened for HBsAg in an early prenatal visit.

[2]The fourth dose of DTP may be administered as early as 12 months of age, provided at least 6 months have elapsed since DTP3. Combined DTP–(*Haemophilus influenza* type b) products may be used when these two vaccines are to be administered simultaneously. DTaP (diphtheria and tetanus toxoids and acellular pertussis vaccine) is licensed for use for the fourth and/or fifth dose of DTP vaccine in children 15 months of age or older, and may be preferred for these doses in children in this age group. Td (diphtheria and tetanus toxoids for people $\geq$ 7 years of age) is recommended at 11 to 12 years of age, provided at least 5 years have elapsed since the last dose of DTP or DT.

[3]Three Hib conjugate vaccines are available for use in infants: HbOC [HibTITER] (Lederle Praxis); PRP-T [ActHIb; OmniHIB] (Pasteur Merieux, distributed by SmithKline Beecham; Connaught); and PRP-OMP [PedvaxHIB] (Merck Sharp & Dohme). Children who have received PRP-OMP at 2 and 4 months of age do not require a dose at 6 months of age. After the primary infant Hib conjugate vaccine series is completed, any licensed Hib conjugate vaccine may be used as a booster dose at age 12 to 15 months.

[4]The second dose of MMR vaccine should be administered EITHER at 4 to 6 years of age OR at 11 to 12 years of age, depending on state school requirements.

[5]Vaccines recommended in the second year of life (12–15 months of age) may be given at either one or two visits.

Approved by the Advisory Committee on Immunization Practices (ACIP), the American Academy of Pediatrics (AAP), and the American Academy of Family Physicians (AAFP), January, 1995. Vaccines for hepatitis A and chickenpox are being added to the recommendations.

Table 39-5 • Adult Immunizations for High-Risk Groups

Vaccine	High-Risk Groups
Diptheria–tetanus	All adults who have not been immunized during last 10 years, especially after puncture wounds or trauma
Measles–mumps–rubella (MMR)	Adults who have never had the disease or been immunized, especially woman of childbearing age All healthcare workers Adults who were born before 1956 and were immunized before 12 months
Pneumococcal infections	Elderly older than 65 years of age Residents of institutions (eg, prisons, nursing homes) Adults with chronic medical problems, especially respiratory or cardiovascular disease
Influenza	Healthcare workers Elderly, especially those in nursing homes Adults with chronic health problems, especially diabetes, respiratory, and cardiovascular disease
Hepatitis B	All healthcare workers Intravenous drug users Hemodialysis clients Hemophiliac clients Immigrants from countries with endemic disease Sexually active people with multiple partners

for hepatitis B virus. Older adults, the chronically ill, or people with respiratory dysfunction should get annual influenza shots and pneumococcal vaccines. Table 39-5 provides a more complete list of adults at risk and specific immunizations that are recommended. Additional vaccinations may be required when a person travels to a foreign country, where different diseases are endemic.

Nursing Interventions for Altered Function

When an infection becomes established, nursing measures are directed toward helping the client combat the illness and preventing the spread of the infection to others. Because nothing is more important in controlling infection than maintaining the natural barriers to infection, nurses devote a great deal of time to supporting these defenses. Enhancing host defenses is both preventive and supportive therapy.

Personal Hygiene

Decreasing the number of microorganisms present on body surfaces can help prevent and fight infection. Handwashing is the most significant measure to decrease the transient growth of microorganisms. Clients should be encouraged to wash their hands after using the toilet, before eating, and after contact with articles likely to be contaminated. Regular bathing, shampooing, and general grooming are important in keeping body surfaces clean. In some instances, such as before a surgical procedure, antimicrobial soap may be used to impede microbial growth further.

Daily brushing and flossing of teeth remove microorganisms that collect in the oral cavity. Regular dental check-ups are important so that plaque and tartar, which provide good foci for bacterial growth, can be removed from the teeth.

Special eye care must be given to clients who have an impaired blink reflex or cannot produce tears. Regular cleansing of the eye and the instillation of artificial tears help prevent eye infections.

Protection of Skin and Mucous Membranes

Intact skin and mucous membranes provide a physical barrier against the invasion of possible pathogens. Adequate hydration and lubricants or creams can prevent

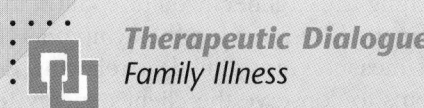

Therapeutic Dialogue
Family Illness

Scenes for Thought

The community health nurse is responsible for visiting 20 families per week. Today she will see the Holden family, which consists of Ann, aged 38, John, aged 39, Maureen, aged 11, and John, Jr., aged 9 years. As she drives up to the small, neat house, she notices that the family car is in the driveway, an unusual occurrence because John is usually at work when the nurse comes to see the family.

Effective

Nurse: *(Knocking on the door.) Ann, it's Evelyn Mason.*
Client: *Hello, Evelyn, come on in.* She looks tired and pale, you notice.
Nurse: *(Settling in on the couch with Ann beside her.) How are things?*
Nurse: *Not wonderful. We're all sick with the stomach flu, and John and I have been up most of the night either with the kids or being sick ourselves. It's just miserable.*
Nurse: *I noticed the car outside and wondered about John being home. What can I help you with while I'm here? (Sitting quietly and attentively.)*
Client: *Well, I know you usually come to check on Maureen's diabetes, and I don't want to trouble you with the rest of it.*
Nurse: *It's no trouble. Maureen's health and the family's health are connected. I'll be happy to do what I can for you.*
Client: Looks relieved. *Well, could you maybe check us all over before you go, just to make sure it is the stomach flu and not something else? And then, I need some advice about what to feed us all. We're all thirsty but some things don't really agree with me, and John, Jr. won't drink juices. I'm not sure what to do.*
Nurse: *Sure, no problem. Shall I start with you since you're right here? (Continues to sit with her without moving.)*
Client: *I'd rather you start with Maureen. You know, these things hit her harder than the rest of us.* Somewhat anxious face.
Nurse: *Okay. Let's go see her.*

Less Effective

Nurse: *(Knocking on the door.) Ann, it's Rosie Connors.*
Client: *Hello, Rosie, come on in.* She looks tired and pale, you notice.
Nurse: *(Settling in on the couch with Ann beside her.) How are things?*
Client: *Not wonderful. We're all sick with the stomach flu, and John and I have been up most of the night either with the kids or being sick ourselves. It's just miserable.*
Nurse: *I know how that is! Especially when everyone gets it at once. No wonder you look tired. I'll bet a good night's sleep would feel just great! (Smiling warmly and sympathetically.)*
Client: *That's the truth.* Smiling wearily. *I suppose you need to see Maureen now. I know you're busy.*
Nurse: *Okay. How's she doing, by the way? (Goes with Ann to see Maureen, chatting as they go.)*

Critical Thinking Challenge

• Detect what the first nurse did differently from the second nurse. • Infer how likely Ann is to ask the first nurse questions about the family's health in the future. • Compare this with Ann's inclinations in the future to ask the second nurse questions about the family's health. • Analyze at what point the second nurse could have picked up cues from Ann that indicated she might like some help.

excessive drying. A water-soluble lubricant can be applied to the nares or lips to prevent cracking. Avoiding trauma that could impair skin integrity is important. Harsh chemicals and excessive heat or friction can abrade skin and should be avoided.

For bedridden clients, establishing regular turning schedules and massaging bony prominences decrease the chance of skin breakdown and possible infection. Specialized equipment such as kinetic beds or special mattresses may be used for high-risk clients.

Rest and Relaxation

Adequate rest and freedom from stress are important in fighting and preventing infection. Sleep disturbances can occur when clients must be awakened at night for antibiotic therapy. If this is necessary, other activities (such as vital signs and dressing changes) should be scheduled to coincide with antibiotic administration. The environment should be kept quiet and comfortable to induce sleep. Naps during the day may be indicated. Activities that promote relaxation and reduce stress should be encouraged.

Nutrition and Hydration

Clients with infections require high-calorie, high-protein diets with adequate vitamins to promote healing and to manufacture the components of the immune system. Fever increases the metabolic needs of body tissues. Loss of nutrients from vomiting, diarrhea, and wound drainage often necessitates supplemental feedings, such as between-meal snacks. Hyperalimentation may be necessary if the client cannot consume adequate nutrition orally. Providing frequent, small meals that the client likes and can manage increases the chances of meeting nutritional goals. Giving oral hygiene before and after meals enhances client enjoyment and decreases the chances for opportunistic infection of the mouth. As always, it is important to avoid any food with questionable methods of preparation or refrigeration.

Infection often causes large fluid losses from sweating, vomiting, diarrhea, or excessive wound drainage. Adequate hydration is important to prevent drying and cracking of the skin and mucous membranes. The nurse should encourage adequate fluid intake to preserve intravascular volume and to maintain adequate urinary output. Decreased urine volume increases urinary stasis and the risk of UTI. If the client cannot drink, intravenous fluid administration may be necessary.

Ambulation and Positioning

Regular periods of aerobic exercise should be encouraged, if possible. If mobility is limited, the nurse should encourage as much activity as the client can tolerate without excessive fatigue. Ambulation promotes circulation, facilitates chest wall excursion, promotes digestion, and decreases stasis of bodily fluids.

When ambulation is impossible, clients may require assistance with turning and positioning. Clients should be assisted in turning every 2 hours while awake and every 2 to 4 hours while sleeping. Ambulation resumes as soon as the client's condition permits. Extremities may need to be elevated to facilitate drainage when infection is present.

Pulmonary Toilet

Encouraging clients to cough, deep-breathe, blow their nose, and move promotes clearance of respiratory secretions, which may become infected if allowed to pool in the lower respiratory tract. Retained secretions prevent adequate gas exchange at the alveolar level and reduce the amount of oxygen available to the tissues to combat infection, heal injured tissues, and meet metabolic needs. Secondary infections are commonly associated with impaired respiratory tract function.

Clients should be taught to cover their mouths when they cough or sneeze to prevent droplet transmission of microorganisms. When blowing the nose, one nostril should always remain open to prevent secretions from becoming forced into the ear canal. Youngsters should be taught not to pick their noses because infected organisms can easily be transmitted to other parts of the body and other people. Everyone should be taught to dispose properly of tissues and respiratory secretions. See Chapter 34 for detailed information on pulmonary hygiene and care.

Comfort Measures

Manifestations of infection such as aches and pains, feelings of lethargy or malaise, fever, chills, nausea and vomiting, and itching cause generalized discomfort that is most often managed by relieving the symptoms. In general, comfort measures are aimed at relieving debilitating symptoms to conserve the client's energy for healing and fighting infection.

Aches and pains are treated with mild analgesics or narcotics, based on their impact on rest, sleep, and ambulation. Feelings of malaise may be relieved with warm broth, a cool cloth to the head, warm blankets, and rest. Fevers may be treated, if prolonged or excessive, with tepid sponge baths, antipyretics, or cooling blankets. Shaking chills can be relieved by warm blankets and warm fluids, but may require intravenous meperidine if prolonged. Nausea and vomiting may be relieved by removing objects with objectionable odors from the client's room, offering carbonated beverages, providing a darkened, quiet room, or in more severe cases by withholding oral intake and giving antiemetics. Itching may be treated with moist, cool cloths, calamine lotion, pastes made from baking soda, or prescribed antihistamines (eg, diphenhydramine).

Neutropenic Precautions

Neutropenia is present when the absolute neutrophil count (ANC) falls below 1,000 cells/mm^3. Serious bacterial infection is almost certain if the ANC falls below 500 cells/mm^3 (Carter, 1993). When neutrophils fall lower than 200 cells/mm^3, the inflammatory response is absent even in the presence of infection (Carter, 1993). When neutropenic precautions are indicated, the client is placed in a private room and visitors are limited, especially children or people with any signs of infection. Handwashing is essential for all who enter the room, and the door may be kept closed to limit airborne exposure. The client should wear a mask whenever it is necessary to leave the hospital room. Care is taken to prevent any breaks in mucous membranes: oral care is gentle and flossing is avoided; razors with blades are not used; rectal temperature are not taken; injections are avoided whenever possible (Gawlikowski, 1992). Sources of pathogens in the environment, such as stagnant water, fresh flowers, or potted plants are removed. Low microbial diets, which avoid fresh vegetables and fruits, or undercooked or raw meat, are indicated (Flyge, 1993).

Clients who are neutropenic after chemotherapy experience a predictable drop in neutrophils, which at its lowest point is referred to as nadir. Nurses can estimate when nadir will be experienced based on the specific chemotherapeutic drug administered. It is important to teach clients that this is the time they will be most susceptible to infection, so preventive measures are essential. Crowds or other likely sources of infection exposure must be avoided. Granulocyte colony–stimulating factors have been developed using DNA technology. These factors are administered to stimulate the production of neutrophils, thus decreasing the degree and duration of neutropenia (Flyge, 1993).

Antimicrobial Therapy

Antimicrobial agents are used to combat the growth and replication of microorganisms. Giving these drugs and monitoring therapy is a collaborative function of nurses, physicians, pharmacists, and laboratory technicians.

Antibiotics should be given based on the presumed antibiotic sensitivity of the infecting species. A culture and sensitivity is obtained to determine appropriate antibiotic therapy. Antibiotics should not be used routinely in all infections. Several species of organisms have mutated over the years since antibiotics were introduced, and now are resistant to all but a few toxic drugs.

One must remember what antibiotics can and cannot do. They do not cure the client: at best, they slow the growth of or kill the organism, which is necessary for recovery from infection. They control the size of the microbial population with which the client's immune system must contend. Antibiotics "buy time" during which the client's own immune system can be mobilized. Eliminating the microbes may prevent further injury, but a return to normality depends on the body's healing capacity (Alcamo, 1991).

Antibiotics as a group have a wide range of safety, but they can produce severe allergic reactions and toxic effects. Clients should be asked about allergies and the drugs they currently use so that incompatibilities can be detected. Renal and hepatic failure, interactions with other drugs, the client's underlying disease, and extremes of age predispose the client to adverse reactions. Both the very young and the very old have impaired renal clearance of drugs, and their dosage should be adjusted accordingly. Monitoring blood levels of antibiotics is one method of ensuring safety and optimal effectiveness.

Antibiotics may eradicate the endogenous flora of the skin and mucous membranes of the mouth, gastrointestinal tract, and vaginal tract. This flora normally protects the host's mucous membranes, and when it is eliminated, opportunistic organisms may invade the tissues. **Superinfection** is a secondary infection that often occurs when normal flora is destroyed by antibodies, immunosuppression, or cancer treatment. These infections are more common when antimicrobials are given in large doses, when several antimicrobials are given concurrently, or when broad-spectrum antibiotics are used. Often such infection appears 4 to 5 days after antimicrobial therapy is begun. Superinfections commonly are fungal infections of the mouth or vagina.

Prevention of Infection Spread

Nurses perform interventions that prevent the spread of infection to others. Aseptic practice (handwashing; cleaning, disinfecting and sterilization; use of barriers; isolation systems; and surgical asepsis) are discussed in Chapter 25.

Handwashing and sterile technique are two significant factors in preventing the occurrence and transmission of infection in healthcare settings (Fig. 39-2). Although experts say that proper handwashing can reduce nosocomial infection rates by 50%, several studies have demonstrated that it is the least common infection control measure used in hospitals (Larson, 1992; Meengs, et al., 1994). See Chapter 25 for specific information on handwashing.

Examples of sterile techniques (surgical asepsis) include inserting intravenous or urinary catheters, giving injections, irrigating drainage devices, and changing dressings on open surgical wounds.

Often the nurse is the first person to identify symptoms indicating infection and to institute precautions for the transmission of infection. Various isolation systems are discussed in Chapter 25.

Clients and their families should be instructed about proper methods for disposal of body secretions such as sputum, feces, urine, and wound drainage. The nurse should provide the client with tissues to cover the nose and mouth while coughing and sneezing, and disposal bags should be within convenient reach. Full bags should be emptied and replaced. Diapers should be rinsed in the toilet.

> ***Safety Alert***
> *Infection Prevention*
>
> - Wash your hands! The most common cause of transmission of microorganisms is contact with unwashed hands.
> - Adhere strictly to aseptic technique when indicated.
> - Institute preventive measures to ensure that skin and mucous membranes remain intact. Disruptions in the epithelial layer greatly increase the risk of infection.
> - Avoid any contact with body fluids with bare hands. Use gloves.
> - Change gloves between patients.
> - Report any exposures (eg, needlestick injury) promptly so treatment can be initiated.

Community-Based Nursing

Nurses can work at different levels to plan, implement, and evaluate health practices. Preventing the spread of microorganisms must take place at four levels: the person and family or household cohabitants, the community, the nation, and the world.

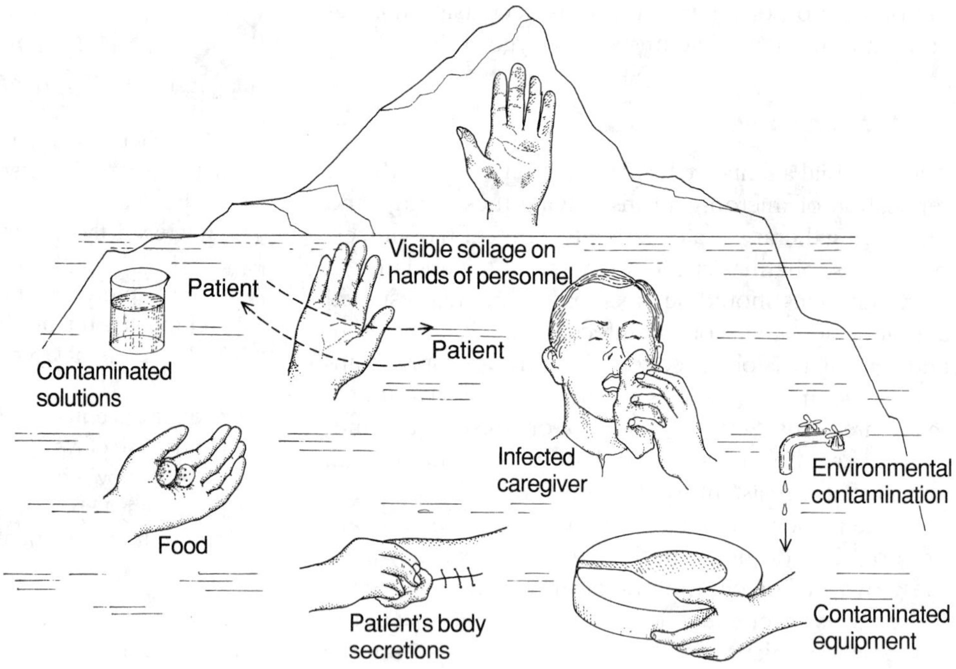

Figure 39-2 • *Contamination iceberg. Visible soilage on the hands of personnel is only the tip of the iceberg. The risk for carrying infection is greater, but many times it is hidden.*

Home-Care Management

Home-care management may be as simple as caring for a person with influenza or as complex as managing home care for a person with terminal cancer recovering from extensive surgery. Many clients are discharged to home from acute-care facilities with indwelling devices that increase the risk for infection. Whether the care is short or long term, avoiding infectious complications and supporting the family is important in maintaining functional abilities.

There is a trend toward keeping all but the most seriously ill clients at home for the delivery of healthcare. Hospitalization, once thought to protect the client who was severely immunosuppressed, is now controversial. Once hospitalized, these clients are more likely to be infected with virulent, sometimes drug-resistant, organisms.

The caregiver must be taught how to evaluate vital signs, give medications, and observe for signs of toxicity. Basic aseptic practices should be taught to the client and family members. The importance of handwashing and proper disposal of contaminated supplies is stressed. The caregiver may require instruction in basic hygiene measures such as bathing, toileting, and oral care. Instruction in sterile technique is necessary for managing intravenous devices and medications.

The caregiver should be taught to wear rubber gloves when caring for the client with a known infection. Lightweight rubber gloves, the kind commonly used for dishwashing and household cleaning, are suitable for the home care of clients with diarrhea or wound infections. These gloves can be washed with mild soap and water and reused after drying. They must be kept separate from those used in food preparation or dishwashing.

Community Infection Control Programs

Community regulations controlling quality of drinking water, food served in public places, and the disposal of sewage and solid waste are important aspects of community-based infection control. Many communities and states have passed laws forbidding unimmunized children from attending school. Some bar children with active infections from the classroom. Community or regional health authorities gather statistics on the incidence of infectious diseases in their communities. They decide which diseases pose a hazard to the community's well-being and must be reported to their agency.

Some countries have public health agencies that gather statistics from the regional reports and compile them for yearly comparisons. They govern the quality of air, water, food, and wastes that cross state, regional, or international boundaries, and set standards for reduction of pollutants and microorganisms. They bar people with designated acute infections from immigrating into the country, and prohibit the return of native citizens without proof of immunizations against diseases endemic in the areas to which they have traveled.

Several international health organizations gather statistics from national groups and have formed commissions for the education of healthcare providers. These organizations establish priorities for infection control and make recommendations about immunizations for international travel. International commissions also provide supplies and personnel for some immunization programs.

Evaluation

The success of a program to avoid or contain infection requires cooperation between the client and the healthcare team. Excellent communication is required and high levels of trust must be established. People must assume responsibility for their own behavior and healthcare practices, and the healthcare system must educate the public and scrutinize its own infection prevention practices. Healthcare workers must be diligent in practicing infection control.

The optimal outcome of efforts to control infection (which is not always attainable) is freedom from the signs and symptoms of infection. Some outcome criteria for goals involving infection include

Goal
Client will demonstrate adequate knowledge to recognize and report signs of infection.

Possible Outcome Criteria

- Client or caregiver lists four signs of infection after teaching session.

Nursing Plan of Care
The Client at Risk for Infection

Nursing Diagnosis
Risk for infection related to delayed wound healing, immunosuppressive treatment for cancer of the bowel, and age manifested by insufficient knowledge of wound healing and infection.

Client Goal
Client/family will demonstrate knowledge about methods of preventing and detecting infection.

Client Outcome Criteria

- Client/family member describes methods to avoid infection after teaching session.
- Client/family member verbalizes signs and symptoms of infection after teaching session.
- Client/family member demonstrates acceptable technique in applying a dressing by next visit.
- Client/family member describes food and fluid that will meet nutritional needs by next visit.

Nursing Intervention	Scientific Rationale
1. Begin instruction of wound care as early in the course of recovery as possible. Include family member.	1. This prepares client and involves family in wound management before discharge.
2. Review principles of good handwashing before wound care.	2. Handwashing is the single most important mechanism in stopping the transmission of pathogenic organisms.
3. Demonstrate the technique for dressing change (see Procedure 34-1). Allow time for practice and a return demonstration.	3. Technical skills are better acquired if they are observed and practiced.
4. Demonstrate removal of old dressing, including how to discard in moisture-proof bag.	4. Proper waste disposal is important in preventing the spread of microorganisms.
5. Review the causes of wound contamination.	5. Better understanding aids client compliance.
6. Discuss activities that may cause trauma to the wound and how to avoid them.	6. Trauma can prevent wound healing and increase the chance of infection.
7. Review signs and symptoms of infection, encouraging client and family to ask questions.	7. Early detection and treatment of infection decreases incidence of serious complications.
8. Instruct client in the importance of well-balanced diet high in protein calories. Discuss sources of vitamin C and vitamin supplements.	8. Wound healing requires protein and calories for building new cells. The immune system depends on protein and calories to produce antibodies.
9. Provide the client with written instruction concerning how to change the dressing and when to call the physician.	9. Instructions given in the hospital may be forgotten when at home. Written instructions provide a handy reference.

- Before discharge, client or caregiver verbalizes indications that would require contacting a healthcare professional.
- After teaching session, client or caregiver demonstrates accurate monitoring of body temperature.

Goal

Client will use good health practices to prevent the occurrence and spread of infection.

Possible Outcome Criteria

- Client or caregiver demonstrates good handwashing technique after the teaching session.
- Before discharge, client or caregiver verbalizes proper methods of infection control to be used at home.
- By discharge, client verbalizes selected strategies to minimize the risk of infection.

Goal

Client will comply with treatment regimens to help cure infection and prevent possible complications.

Possible Outcome Criteria

- Client keeps the next three appointments with healthcare providers.
- Client uses recommended aseptic practices for dressing changes or invasive devices, as evidenced by a return demonstration at the next home visit.
- Client takes prescribed medications to treat or prevent infections, as reported to the nurse at the next appointment.

Key Concepts

- Microorganisms are everywhere but usually do not cause harm.
- The body has an elaborate system of barriers to invasion by microorganisms.
- Infections are responsible for more visits to healthcare facilities than any other reason.
- Infection requires an uninterrupted chain of events; infection cannot occur if any link in the chain is broken.
- Although a few infections are caused by the microorganism's ability to cause disease almost every time it comes in contact with a human, most infections are caused by a breakdown of host defenses.
- Host defenses are specific and nonspecific.
- The four signs of inflammation are redness, warmth, swelling, and tenderness.
- Fever is an important mechanism in fighting infection, but it consumes a great deal of metabolic energy.
- T lymphocytes and B lymphocytes form memory cells that can be reactivated on reexposure to an antigen. This is the basis of lasting immunity.
- Production of cellular immunity and antibodies takes 2 to 4 weeks after the first exposure to an organism.
- Immunizations are given to children and adults to prevent some infectious diseases.
- Because communicable childhood diseases may have severe complications, all children should be immunized.
- Very young and very old people have decreased resistance to infection. Both nonspecific and specific barriers to infection are affected.
- A communicable disease is caused by an agent that is easily transmitted among hosts.
- The inflammatory response helps control the spread of infection, but if it goes on too long it can harm the client.
- The most common hospital infections are urinary tract infections, wound infections, respiratory tract infections, and bacteremias from intravascular line insertion.
- A compromised host is a person whose natural barriers to infection have been decreased by medical therapy, a chronic condition, or an inadequate immune system.
- A culture and sensitivity is necessary to identify the specific organism causing an infection and possible antibiotics useful for treatment.
- Preventing infection is an individual, community, national, and international responsibility.
- Increasing numbers of clients are being treated at home for chronic conditions or rehabilitation, and many of them have several risk factors for infection. Nurses must assume the responsibility for teaching these clients or their caregivers how to avoid infection.

Critical Thinking Challenges

Now that you have increased your knowledge base concerning infection and infection control, look again at the situation at the beginning of the chapter and work through the following challenges.

1. *Analyze how you feel personally after this verbal attack.*
2. *Propose possible factors contributing to your client's reluctance to talk to a nurse from the public health department.*

3. *Prioritize what is most important for your client at the present time, and explain how you can help your client achieve these goals.*
4. *Knowing that drug-resistant strains of tuberculosis have recently developed, weigh the rights of this client to refuse treatment with the rights of the general public to live in a safe environment.*

References

Alcamo, I. E. (1991). *Fundamentals of microbiology* (3rd ed.). Reading, MA: Addison-Wesley.

Carter, L. (1993). Influence of nutrition and stress on people at risk for neutropenia: Nursing implications. *Oncology Nursing Forum, 20,* 1241–1250.

Donowitz, L. G. (1992). Infection in the newborn. In R. P. Wenzel (Ed.), *Prevention and control of nosocomial infections* (2nd ed.). Baltimore: Williams & Wilkins.

Farley, M. P. (1991). Multiple trauma. In M. Patrick, S. L. Woods, R. Craven, et al. (Eds.), *Medical-surgical nursing: Pathophysiological concepts* (2nd ed.) (pp. 1576–1601). Philadelphia: J. B. Lippincott.

Flyge, H. (1993). Meeting the challenge of neutropenia. *Nursing 93, 23* (7), 61–64.

Gawlikowski, J. (1992). White cells at war. *Am J Nurs, 92* (3), 45–51.

Gordon, M. (1994). *Nursing diagnosis: Process and application* (3rd ed.). St. Louis: Mosby.

Halverson, S. G., & Graham, S. K. (1991). Infections and inflammatory disorders affecting reproductive function. In M. Patrick, S. L. Woods, R. Craven, et al. (Eds.), *Medical-surgical nursing: Pathophysiological concepts* (pp. 1499–1523). Philadelphia: J. B. Lippincott.

Larson, E. (1992). Skin cleansing. In R. P. Wenzel (Ed.), *Prevention and control of nosocomial infections* (2nd ed.). Baltimore: Williams & Wilkins.

Meengs, M., Giles, B., Chisholm, C., Cordell, W., & Nelson, D. (1994). Handwashing frequency in an emergency room department. *Journal of Emergency Nursing, 20* (3), 183–188.

Messner, R., & Zink, K. (1992) Nosocomial pneumonia: Combating a hospital menace. *RN, 55(6)* 48–53.

North American Nursing Diagnosis Association (NANDA). (1994). *Nursing diagnoses: Definitions and classification 1995–1996.* Philadelphia.

Parent, P. (1992). Infection control: Management strategies for adult patients in the critical care environment. *Critical Care Nursing Quarterly, 15* (3), 1–9.

Smith, P., Roccaforte, J., & Daly, P. (1992). Infection and the immune response in the elderly. *Ann Epidemiol, 2,* 813–822.

Wertz, M. J. (1991). Infection. In M. Patrick, S. L. Woods, R. Craven, et al. (Eds.), *Medical-surgical nursing: Pathophysiological concepts.* Philadelphia: J. B. Lippincott.

Bibliography

Avalos-Block, S. (1994). Getting a rise out of tuberculosis with the P.P.D. skin test. *Nursing 94, 24* (8), 51–53.

Bertone, S., et al. (1994). Quantitative skin cultures at potential catheter sites in neonates. *Infection Control and Hospital Epidemiology, 15* (5), 315–318.

Cardo, D., et al. (1993). Validation of surgical wound surveillance. *Infection Control and Hospital Epidemiology, 14* (4), 211–215.

Daugherty, J., Hutton, M., & Simone, P. (1993). Prevention and control of tuberculosis in the 1990's. *Nurs Clin North Am,* 28, 599–611.

Fanning, C., et al. (1991). Urinary tract infections: A survey. *Canadian Journal of Infection Control, 6* (3), 68–69.

Graham, S., et al. (1993). Frequency of changing enteral alimentation bags and tubing, and adverse patient outcomes in a long term care facility. *Canadian Journal of Infection Control, 8* (2), 41–43.

Messner, R. L., et al. (1994). Preventing peripheral IV infection. *CINA Journal, 10* (1), 9–12.

Morita, M. (1993). Methicillin-resistant *Staphylococcus aureus:* Past, present and future. *Nurs Clin North Am, 28,* 625–637.

Shovein, J., & Young, M. (1992). MRSA: Pandora's box for hospitals. *Am J Nurs, 92* (2), 48–49.

Wujcik, D. (1993). Infection control in oncology patients. *Nurs Clin North Am, 28,* 639–650.

Thermoregulation

Key Terms	*Learning Objectives*
Antipyretic *Basal body temperature* *Basal metabolic rate* *Core temperature* *Febrile* *Fever* *Hyperthermia* *Hyperpyrexia* *Hypothermia* *Insensible evaporation* *Metabolism* *Set point* *Surface temperature*	*Upon completion of this chapter, the student will be able to do the following:* • *Explain how the body increases or decreases heat production to regulate body temperature.* • *Describe the effects of various factors on the body's thermoregulation.* • *Outline lifespan considerations for temperature regulation.* • *Describe manifestations of altered body temperature.* • *Discuss appropriate assessment parameters concerning thermoregulation.* • *List four NANDA nursing diagnoses concerning potential or actual altered body temperature.* • *Discuss the importance of client teaching in prevention and treatment of altered thermoregulation.* • *Perform appropriate nursing interventions for fever management*

40

An elderly widow, who lives in the Northeast, slipped and fractured her hip 3 weeks ago. After surgery to repair her hip and a short stay on a rehabilitation unit to improve her mobility, she was sent home with a visiting nurse referral. As you enter the home on the first visit, you see your client sitting in a recliner chair with a sweater on and a shawl over her shoulders. It is still winter, and the house appears cool. You notice a draft when you pass by a window. Your client states she is doing OK with her walker but is reluctant to move much because she does not want to fall again. You ask her how she is eating, and she tells you she is not very hungry, usually having cereal and fruit for breakfast and a sandwich later in the day. She says her neighbor comes in every so often to bring her a warm meal. She complains of some pain, but verbalizes concern that she will not be able to fill another prescription until her social security check arrives. Your client's three children live out of state.

This situation is common. As you read through this chapter, you will learn about many factors that might contribute to a problem with temperature regulation. Use this information, along with your knowledge base of the nursing process, lifespan development, mobility, and home management, to individualize a plan of care for your client. At the end of this chapter, the Critical Thinking Challenges will provoke critical thinking about your client's situation.

A person's body temperature is a sensitive indicator of physiologic changes occurring in the body. These changes can be the result of a disease process, a traumatic injury, or a therapeutic intervention. Monitoring the client's temperature is one of the common routine procedures performed on any person within the health-care system.

The nurse is often the person to screen clients using temperature monitoring, identifying deviations in temperature and reporting significant findings to the physician so that appropriate therapy can be instituted. Although the skill itself is readily learned, the physiology underlying thermoregulation is complex. For nurses to provide competent care for clients with normal or abnormal temperature states, the nurse must possess a sound understanding of the physiologic processes involved in temperature regulation.

Normal Thermoregulation

Core temperature, or the temperature of the interior body tissues, remains almost constant (within −0.6°C [1°F]) in a healthy state. In contrast, a person's **surface temperature,** or the temperature of the skin and tissue immediately underlying the skin, rises and falls according to the temperature of the surrounding environment (Guyton, 1991). Core temperature is the product of the precise balance between heat production and heat loss. Figure 40-1 illustrates behavioral and physiologic factors involved in the production and loss of heat from the body.

Heat Production

Heat is continually produced in the body as a byproduct of the chemical reactions taking place in all body cells. This collective process is known as **metabolism.** The rate of heat production is directly determined by

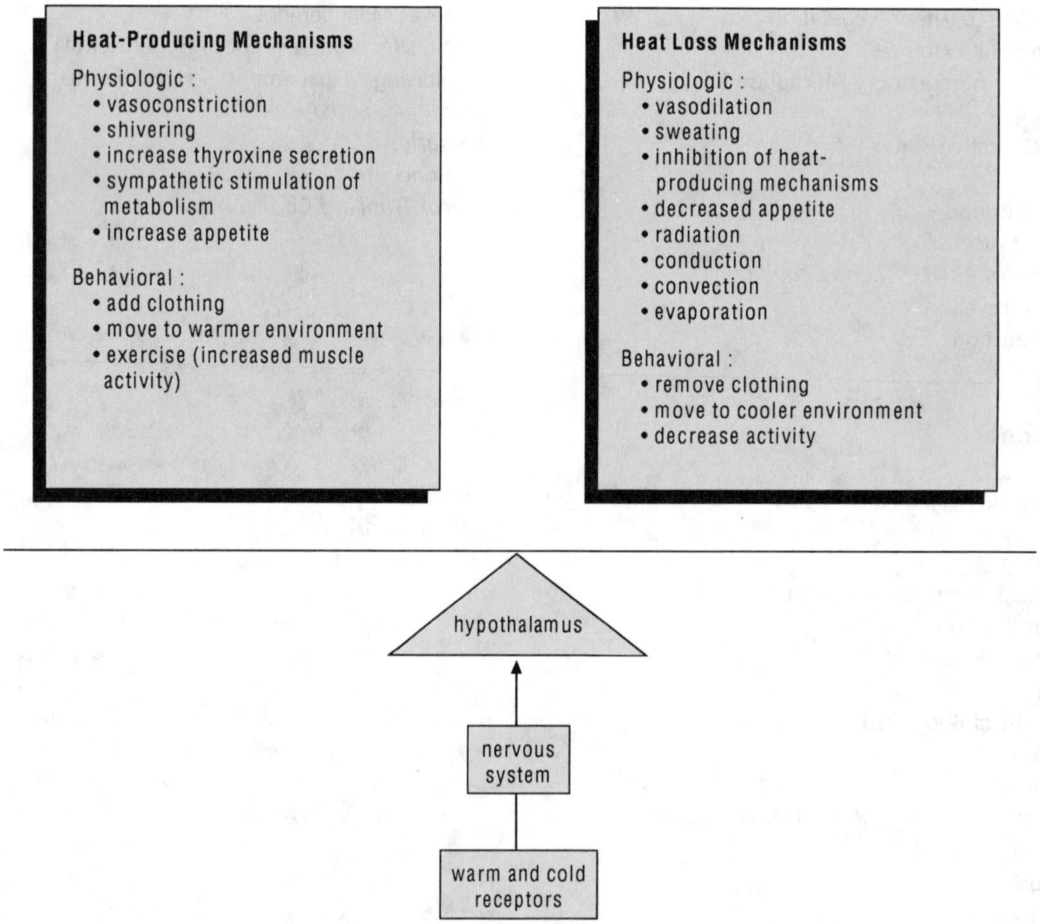

Figure 40-1 • *Body temperature is the balance between heat production and heat loss.*

a person's metabolic rate. Factors such as level of activity, age, hormones, psychological well-being, nutritional status, body temperature, and environmental temperature can increase or decrease the metabolic rate and consequently alter the amount of heat produced. In a resting state, most of the body heat is produced in the body core, which includes the trunk, viscera, and brain. During exercise, most of the heat is produced in the musculature. The process of thermoregulation maintains a fairly constant core temperature regardless of where the heat is being produced.

Basal Metabolic Rate

The **basal metabolic rate** (BMR) is the amount of energy used by the body during absolute rest in an awake state. To measure the BMR, the person is placed in basal conditions, as outlined in the display. The rate of oxygen used by the body is then measured with a metabolator. Metabolic rate can then be calculated in terms of kilocalories per square meter of body surface (kcal/m^2).

The BMR varies with age and sex. A young child has a metabolic rate almost twice that of an adult because of the growth process that occurs in children (Guyton, 1991). The BMR decreases rapidly from birth to about 20 years and then declines more gradually.

Temperature, both external and internal, affects the BMR. People living in a tropical climate will probably have a lower BMR than people living in a temperate zone, and their BMRs will be more closely related to their body weight than to their surface area.

Nursing Care Guidelines
Basal Conditions for Measuring BMR

- No food consumption for 12 hours because digestion of food increases the metabolic rate.
- A restful night of sleep because rest reduces the activities of the sympathetic nervous system and other metabolic excitants to their minimum level.
- No strenuous exercise after waking; rest in a reclining position for 30 minutes before the test. This is most important because of the profound effect exercise has on metabolism.
- A comfortable position and little psychological stimulation to reduce the degree of sympathetic activity.
- Environmental temperature between 20°C to 26.6°C (68°–80°F). Temperatures lower than this range increase sympathetic nervous activity, and higher temperatures cause discomfort and sweating.

From Guyton, A. C. (1991). *Textbook of medical physiology* (8th ed.). Philadelphia: W.B. Saunders.

Exercise or Muscle Activity

Exercise or muscle activity has profound effects on a person's metabolic rate, particularly if the person participates in some form of strenuous activity. Maximal muscle exercise can increase the body's overall heat production significantly, approaching 40°C (104°F) following exercise, such as running a marathon.

Thyroid Hormones

The thyroid hormones thyroxine and triiodothyronine also have a profound effect on the rate of body metabolism. These hormones increase the metabolic rate in most cells of the body, except those in the brain, testes, spleen, and retina. To maintain a normal BMR, the precise amount of thyroid hormone must be released at the appropriate time. This controlling function is regulated by the thyroid-stimulating hormone, which is secreted by the anterior pituitary gland.

People who have excessive levels of thyroid hormones (hyperthyroidism) have a higher metabolic rate and a temperature chronically elevated by as much as 0.5°C (1°F). The converse is true for people with low thyroid hormone levels (hypothyroidism) (Ganong, 1993).

Sympathetic Nervous System

Stimulation of the sympathetic nervous system, with the release of norepinephrine and epinephrine, increases the metabolic process within many cells. In the newborn, the sympathetic stimulation of the mitochondria in a certain type of fat tissue called brown adipose tissue (BAT), increases the metabolic rate of the BAT, resulting in an increased rate of heat production. This marked increase in metabolism and subsequent heat production is referred to as nonshivering thermogenesis (Bliss-Holtz, 1993). The magnitude of the effect of BAT thermogenesis in adults is questionable, and it is being investigated by numerous researchers.

Heat Loss

Just as heat is continuously being produced by the body, it also is continuously being lost. Heat is lost from the body by four processes: radiation, conduction, convection, and evaporation. Figure 40-2 depicts heat loss by each of these four processes. An understanding of these processes enables the nurse to control the amount of heat lost from the body.

Radiation

All objects that are not at absolute zero temperature radiate heat in the form of infrared heat rays. Heat loss in this manner is based on the principle that objects facing each other are always radiating heat toward one

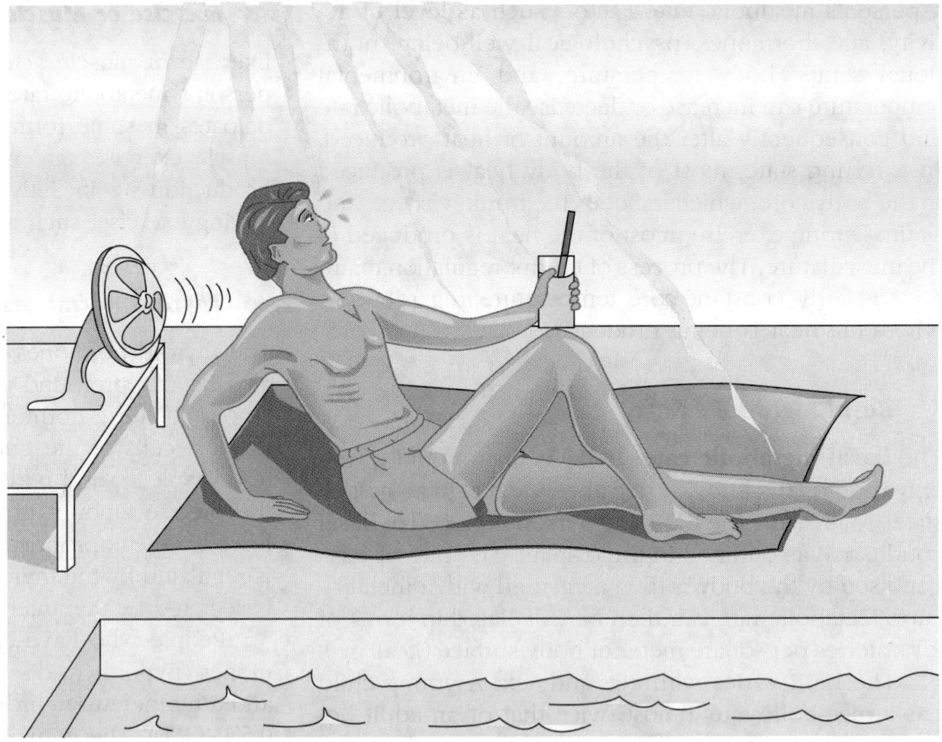

Figure 40-2 • Heat loss from the body can occur by four processes: radiation, conduction, convection, and evaporation. While this man sunbathes, the heat is transferred from the sun by radiation; the fan increases heat loss by convection; the ice water increases heat loss by conduction; and sweating increases heat loss by evaporation.

another. If the temperature of the body is greater than the environment, then a greater quantity of heat is radiated to the environment than to the body, and vice versa. A nude person in a room of normal temperature loses about 60% of his or her total body heat through radiation (Guyton, 1991). The nurse must consider heat lost by radiation when implementing procedures that expose the client's skin surface to the environmental temperature (eg, preparing the client for a surgical procedure in the cool operating room, adjusting the room temperature to compensate for heat loss during a bath, caring for a neonate in an isolette).

The amount of heat lost by radiation can be reduced by covering the body with closely woven fabrics. Dark clothing absorbs more solar rays than light-colored fabrics. The same is true for dark skin tones compared with light ones.

Conduction

Conduction of heat is the transfer of heat from one object to another through direct contact. When a person grasps an empty metal container, heat will be conducted readily from the hand to the container, but within a few minutes, the temperature of the container equals that of the hand; thereafter the container actually acts as an insulator to prevent further heat loss from the hand. The body only loses minute amounts of heat through conduction to other objects.

The body does lose considerable amounts of heat to the air through conduction, however. If the air immediately adjacent to the skin is cooler, then the heat from the body will warm the air. Once the air next to the skin equals the temperature of the skin, there is no further loss of heat from the skin surface. Wearing several layers of clothing allows layers of warmed air to be created, thus insulating the body and helping to keep it warm. If the clothing becomes wet, its effectiveness as an insulator is lost because the conductivity of water increases the rate of heat transmission as much as 20-fold or more (Guyton, 1991).

The body also loses heat to water by conduction. Because water can absorb more heat than air can, the body cannot form a zone of insulation to reduce heat loss. The rate of heat loss from the skin can be high when it is immersed in water that is cooler than body temperature. Water used to bathe clients should be slightly above body temperature, unless the client has an elevated temperature, a condition called **febrile.** For febrile clients, the water should be warm but below body temperature, so the water will absorb heat from the client.

Heat also is conducted from the internal organs of the body to the surface of the skin by the flow of blood. The skin and subcutaneous tissues, particularly the fat, insulate the body. Fat conducts heat only one-third as readily as other tissues. Women tend to have a thicker layer of subcutaneous fat than men. This insulating property of the skin and subcutaneous tissues plays an important role in maintaining a consistent core temperature.

A person can gain heat from the environment if it is warmer than their skin surface. This is not a source of heat production and normally has little effect on the thermoregulation process; however, it can be a threat to the person if the temperature is extremely hot, and the body is not able keep the core temperature within a normal range.

Convection

For heat to be lost from the body by convection, it must be conducted from the body to the air and then carried away by air currents. Normally, a warm layer of air exists adjacent to the skin surface. As the air becomes heated, it rises and passes into the cooler air mass. If the skin surface is in contact with air currents, the process of convection is increased. If during this process the temperature of the skin surface is cooled to equal the temperature of the air, then the rate of heat loss cannot increase. Instead, the rate at which heat can be conducted from the core of the body to the skin is the factor that then determines the rapidity of heat loss.

Heat loss by convection can be increased by opening windows or by forcing the exchange of air by placing a fan in a room. Activity, such as walking or running, also increases the amount of heat lost by convection.

Evaporation

Evaporation causes heat loss as water is transformed to a gas. Water is continuously lost through evaporation from the skin and lungs at a rate of about 600 mL/d (Guyton, 1991). This is referred to as **insensible evaporation,** and it cannot be controlled for purposes of temperature regulation because it results from continual diffusion of water molecules through the skin and respiratory tract mucosa, regardless of body temperature. Diaphoresis (sweating) is a process by which the body can increase the amount of heat that is normally lost through evaporation. Normally, diaphoresis occurs in states, such as fever or strenuous exercise, when heat loss is required to maintain body temperature.

When the temperature of the surroundings becomes greater than the temperature of the skin surface, the only means by which the body can rid itself of heat is evaporation. In a very hot, humid environment, evaporation of water from the body is reduced because the surrounding air is already saturated. This can pose a potential health risk for some people, such as the elderly.

Normal Pattern of Body Temperature

The normal oral temperature of a healthy adult is considered to be 37°C (98.6°F); however, this is an average value. Each person has a unique circadian thermal rhythm that may be slightly higher or lower than 37°C. Table 40-1 outlines the normal temperature ranges for people throughout the lifespan.

Table 40-1 • Normal Temperature Ranges

Age	*Site*	*Degrees Celsius*	*Degrees Fahrenheit*
Newborn	Axilla	35.5–37.5	96–99.5
6 months	Axilla	37.5	99.5
5 years	Oral	37	98.6
13 years	Oral	36.6	97.8
Adult	Oral	37	98.6
> 70 years	Oral	36	96.9

The body has several repetitious patterns, one of which is the circadian thermal rhythm, which occurs in a 24-hour cycle. Studies have identified 5 PM to 7 PM (1700-1900 hours) as the peak of the daily cycle, when body temperature is likely to be elevated (Holtzclaw, 1992). Body temperature is lowest in the early morning.

Normal monthly fluctuations in body temperature occur in women because of hormonal factors. Progesterone, a female hormone secreted by the ovaries, is believed to have a thermogenic effect that causes the core temperature of many women to be elevated by 0.6°C (1°F) in the last half of their menstrual cycle (Shaver, 1991). This rise in temperature occurs at ovulation. By measuring oral body temperature every morning before rising (basal conditions), a woman can determine when ovulation has occurred. This early morning body temperature measurement is known as the **basal body temperature** and provides the basis for the rhythm method of birth control.

Various parts of the body normally have different temperature readings. The rectal temperature is considered to be the most representative of core body temperature, because this site varies least with environmental changes. Oral temperature is considered to be 0.6°C (1°F) lower than the rectal temperature (Guyton, 1991), and it is affected by many factors, including the ingestion of hot or cold fluids, smoking, and mouth breathing (Holtzclaw, 1992). The reason for the higher rectal temperature is that the mouth is constantly being cooled by evaporation. The axillary temperature is considered to be 0.6°C (1°F) lower than the oral temperature. Variations in temperature readings can occur within a particular site. For example, the posterior sublingual pocket of the mouth has been found to be significantly higher than the area under the front of the tongue (Erickson, 1980).

Factors Affecting Normal Body Temperature

Body temperature is determined by the delicate balance that occurs between heat production and heat loss, as shown in Figure 40-1. Normal body temperature depends mainly on physiologic processes and, to a lesser extent, on behavioral responses.

Physiologic Processes

The integrated functioning of many body systems is required to maintain the body temperature within a normal range. The hypothalamus, nervous system, circulatory system, shivering mechanism, and sweat glands interdependently play a significant role in thermoregulation. The skin plays an important role for systemic and local temperature regulation.

Hypothalamus. The hypothalamus, often considered the body's thermostat, is able to maintain the internal temperature of the body within half a degree of the normal average range (Guyton, 1991). The preoptic area, located in the most anterior portion of the hypothalamus, contains thermosensitive neurons that directly respond to the temperature of the blood. When these neurons detect that the temperature of the blood is too warm, signals radiate to the "heat-loss center" located in the anterior portion of the hypothalamus. This anterior center is composed mainly of parasympathetic nerves that, when stimulated automatically, initiate mechanisms to decrease body heat. If cold is detected, signals are sent to the "heat-promoting center" located in the posterior portion of the hypothalamus. This center operates mainly through the sympathetic nervous system, which stimulates mechanisms to produce body heat.

Nervous System. The nervous system is the communicating mechanism to assist the hypothalamus to maintain body temperature within the critical temperature level, which is referred to as **set point**. Mechanisms controlling heat loss and heat gain are coordinated by the nervous system to return the body continually to this set point for optimal functioning. The heat center in the preoptic area of the hypothalamus is mainly responsible for detecting heat, but the detection of cold relies mainly on the cold receptors of the skin. To a lesser extent, the cold receptors in the spinal cord and abdominal organs also serve this purpose (Guyton, 1991). Temperature sensors receive information about the temperature of the internal or external environment and transmit this information to the hypothalamus along neural pathways. Once the signals have been reached by the heat-sensitive neurons in the hypothalamus, messages are then sent to initiate heat-producing or heat-reducing mechanisms.

Circulatory System. The circulatory system functions as a transportation mechanism responsible for carrying heat from the body core, where heat is produced, to the body surface. Once heat arrives at the body surface, it can be transferred to the air through radiation, conduction, convection, and evaporation. When the hypothalamus sends out messages to cool the core temperature, the blood vessels dilate, increasing the blood flow to the skin surfaces. Conversely, vasoconstriction occurs when the body needs to conserve heat. The degree of vasoconstriction is controlled by the sympathetic nervous system. In the most exposed parts of the body, such as the hands, feet, and ears, the blood is supplied directly from the arterioles to the veins. This allows for tremendous variation in the rate of blood flow. In such areas, the rate of blood flow can be almost zero, or it can increase to 30% of the cardiac output (Guyton, 1991).

Skin. The skin plays a major role in thermoregulation. The skin contains mainly cold (and some warmth) receptors, which send signals to the hypothalamus. When the skin is chilled over the entire body, immediate reflex effects are initiated to increase the body temperature. First, a strong reflex causes shivering, which produces heat. Concurrently, vasoconstriction of the blood vessels occurs, and the sweating process is inhibited. When only a portion of the body is affected by a temperature change (eg, when a person places one hand in warm water), local skin reflexes occur. These reactions are caused by the local effects of temperature changes directly on the blood vessels and sweat glands and by local cord reflexes conducted from the skin receptors to the spinal cord and back to the same skin area. The intensity of such a reaction is monitored by the hypothalamus to prevent excessive heat exchange from locally cooled or heated areas of the body (Guyton, 1991).

The skin also contains numerous blood vessels that transport heat from the core of the body to the skin surface, where heat loss mechanisms disperse the heat to the air. In addition, the skin acts as an insulator. Fat tissues within the subcutaneous layer of the skin help to keep heat inside the body.

Shivering Mechanism. The shivering mechanism is an involuntary motor activity that increases body temperature through increased heat production. Shivering is controlled by a center located in the posterior hypothalamus. This center is extremely sensitive and becomes activated when the body temperature falls a fraction of a degree below the set point. When stimulated, nonrhythmic impulses are transmitted, which increase the tone of the skeletal muscles. Once the muscle tone reaches a critical level, shivering results. To help maintain normal body temperature, heat production can rise as high as four to five times normal during maximum shivering.

Sweat Glands. Sweat glands located beneath the dermal layer of the skin secrete a watery solution containing high concentrations of sodium and chloride. This secretion passes through tiny ducts onto the skin surface. Once on the surface of the skin, it evaporates, thus cooling the surface of the skin. As the skin cools, the blood flowing near the surface of the skin also is cooled. The anterior hypothalamus initiates the sweating process through impulses transmitted in the autonomic pathways to the spinal cord and then through the sympathetic outflow to the skin everywhere on the body.

Behavioral Responses

Humans can help regulate body temperature through behavioral responses. A person must be alert and physically able to manipulate the environment successfully to use behavioral responses to assist with temperature control. To increase body temperature, a person can put on more clothes, raise the temperature of the room, or increase physical activity. To decrease body temperature, a person can remove clothing, increase convection currents by sitting near a fan or breeze, or move to a cooler environment.

Lifespan Considerations

The very young and the elderly are at high risk when any deviation from normal body temperature occurs. Understanding the developmental considerations in thermoregulatory mechanisms will help the nurse prevent and treat altered temperature states.

Newborn and Infant

The premature neonate is neurologically underdeveloped, with limited capability for thermoregulation. Low birth weight significantly decreases the amount of body fat available to act as insulation. Premature newborns have temperature receptors on their face in the trigeminal area. The premature newborn is placed in an incubator so that the temperature of the environment can be carefully regulated.

All newborns are at risk for alterations in temperature regulation because of a number of factors. A large surface area compared to weight creates problems in maintaining the heat infants produce. When body temperature decreases, the newborn produces heat by nonshivering thermogenesis through the oxidation of brown fat. This increases the metabolic rate and can cause hypoglycemia, elevated serum bilirubin, and metabolic acidosis (Bliss-Holtz, 1993). Newborns and infants are unable to make behavioral adjustments in their environment or clearly communicate discomfort by means other than crying. During the first year of life, the immune system is immature, so infants are prime candidates for infection, which in turn produces fever.

The infant depends totally on parents or other caregivers to assist with temperature regulation by maintaining a constant, comfortable environmental temperature. Parents frequently must be taught not to overdress a newborn. Many parents also must be taught how to take an axillary temperature for their newborn.

Toddler and Preschooler

As the child enters the second year of life, thermoregulation is more stable, although not fully mature. Weight gain during the first year has added fat to help insulate the body from heat loss.

A common neurologic disorder associated with fever that affects a small portion of young children is febrile convulsions. Most febrile convulsions occur after 6 months of age, with increasing frequency until 36 months. They are unusual after 6 years of age (Jackson & Saunders, 1993). The cause of the convulsions is unknown, but they occur during a temperature rise rather than after prolonged elevation. Convulsions can be frightening for parents. The nurse frequently assumes the role of teacher, helping parents become knowledgeable on how to treat fever or convulsions in their young children.

Child and Adolescent

As children grow and develop, their sweat glands and shivering mechanism become more functional. By the time the child reaches puberty, these two temperature-regulating mechanisms are fully functional.

Childhood illnesses continue to cause fever in the school-age child and adolescent. Adolescents begin to take part in many activities, such as hiking and sledding, that may expose them to extremes in environmental temperature (Fig 40-3). Sports that require excessive exertion in warm temperatures (eg, running laps in football practice) should be done with caution. If youngsters participate in skiing or hiking, they should be informed on how to dress properly to avoid exposure. Swimming lessons should include information on

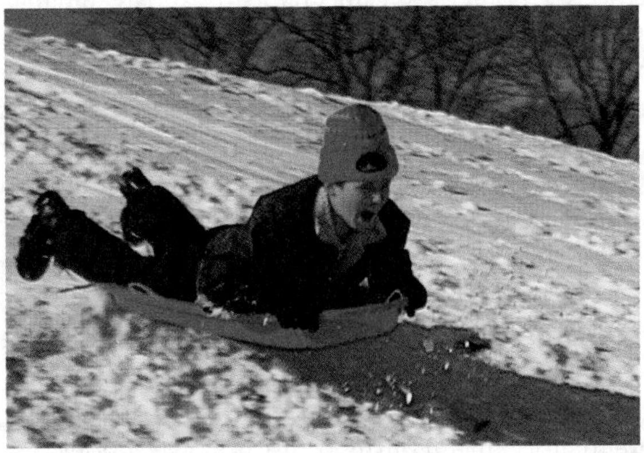

***Figure 40-3** • Bitter cold temperatures increase the risk of hypothermia as a young person enjoys sledding.*

how to protect oneself from hypothermia if accidental exposure to cold water is possible.

Adult and Older Adult

The thermoregulating system of the adult is fully operational to maintain core body temperature. Unless adults are exposed to some form of trauma (eg, head injury, accidental hypothermia) or disease process (eg, skin disorders that disrupt the ability to sweat, tumors involving the hypothalamus, breakdown in the immune system) that impedes the functioning of their regulatory system, their bodies can cope with minor deviations in body temperature.

The normal temperature range decreases as people reach old age. This implies that the elderly have less heat to lose. Also, their BMR has decreased, they are less active, and they can be poorly nourished, which can decrease fat stores that act as insulators. The elderly are particularly sensitive to extremes in the environmental temperature because of the decreased functioning of their thermoregulatory system. The older population has been found to have an increased body temperature threshold before sweating begins and a decreased sweating rate (Yurick, Spier, Robb, & Ebert, 1989). The elderly also may live in poorly ventilated apartments and have inadequate resources for heating or cooling their homes. Cognitive changes may make the older person less mentally capable of making appropriate behavioral responses, especially if drugs such as hypnotics or alcohol are used. The elderly have a much higher mortality rate associated with abnormal temperature states than infants. Perhaps this higher mortality rate occurs because the elderly are not given the same degree of protection and nurturing as infants.

Altered Thermoregulation

Despite finely tuned physiologic mechanisms for temperature control, situations can occur that overwhelm the body's homeostatic mechanisms and result in abnormal body temperature. Abnormal body temperature can be slight, such as low-grade fever, or life-threatening, as in severe cases of hypothermia or hyperthermia. Knowledge of factors that can alter normal body temperature is important for the nurse in preventing and treating alterations in thermoregulation.

Potential for Altered Thermoregulation

Extremes in environmental temperature, altered thermoregulatory mechanisms, infection, strenuous exercise, and stress can cause deviations from normal body temperature.

Environmental Extremes

The person's environment may influence the temperature of the body. Exposure to very warm temperatures for an extended time can lead to hyperthermia. **Hyperthermia** is a state in which the body temperature increases without a change in the set point. Humans are capable of surviving extremes of environmental temperature, provided precautions are taken to avoid injury. The extremes of heat a person can safely tolerate depend on the moisture content of the air. If the air is dry and there are air currents present to allow evaporation, a person may tolerate a temperature of 65.5°C (150°F) for several hours; however, if moisture is present in the air and the environmental temperature is high, the process of evaporation is impeded, and the person can only tolerate a temperature of 34.4°C (94°F). If a person has existing health problems (such as heart disease) or is required to do physical work, even moderately elevated temperatures may be difficult to tolerate.

A period of acclimatization occurs when a person is suddenly exposed to very warm temperatures. At first, physical work is difficult, and the person may actually feel weak and ill. After a few days, sweat mechanisms become more effective in cooling the body. As acclimatization occurs, sweat composition changes to contain less sodium (Guyton, 1991); this decreases the likelihood that fluid and electrolyte imbalances will occur.

Exposure to temperatures that are well below freezing present local and systemic problems, because such extremely low temperatures can result in freezing of the skin's surface and lowering the body's core temperature. When the core temperature of the body falls below 33°C (92°F), the ability of the hypothalamus to regulate body temperature is impaired.

Altered Thermoregulatory Mechanisms

Any condition that interferes with normal mechanisms of thermoregulation can contribute to altered body temperature.

Nervous System Impairment. Tumors or trauma to the brain or spinal cord interfere with nervous system control over temperature regulation. If the spinal cord is severed in the neck above the sympathetic outflow from the cord, as in the quadriplegic client, the hypothalamus can no longer control the degree of vasoconstriction or sweating anywhere in the body. Local temperature reflexes originating in the skin, spinal cord, and intra-abdominal receptors can still function, but their effectiveness is limited. A person with this sort of disability must rely on behavioral responses or environmental control for temperature regulation.

Malignant Hyperthermia. Malignant hyperthermia is an inherited condition in which normal thermoregulatory mechanisms can be disrupted by the administration of certain anesthetic agents. Following the administration of halothane, succinylcholine, or lidocaine, the regulatory mechanisms of the hypothalamus are suppressed. The client may experience tachycardia, arrhythmias, muscle rigidity (especially of the jaw), and extremely elevated body temperature. Temperature of the body increases rapidly due to a hypermetabolic state (Donnelly, 1994). The client's body temperature may reach 44°C (111°F). Excessive body temperature can cause irreversible cell injury, especially to brain cells. Survival depends on early recognition of the symptoms of malignant hyperthermia and immediate treatment to lower body temperature. Because this is an inherited problem, all people undergoing surgery should be questioned concerning any family member experiencing adverse reactions to anesthetic agents. Survival rates have increased dramatically in the last decade due mainly to early recognition and treatment (Kaus & Rockoff, 1994).

Circulatory Impairment. Circulatory problems can impede normal temperature regulation. Clients with peripheral vascular disease or neuropathy (decreased blood flow to the nerves) are not able to constrict or dilate blood vessels to control heat loss from the body. Treatment with medications, such as antihypertensive agents, also can interfere with vasoconstriction as a regulatory mechanism.

Skin Impairment. Damage to large areas of skin can impede the body's ability to regulate body temperature. Severe burns can cause a hypermetabolic state that increases body temperature. In severely burned clients, above-normal body temperature is often present for a few weeks until the core temperature can be readjusted. Damage to the microcirculation of the skin decreases the client's ability to retain body heat. For this reason, the environment of the client with severe burns must be controlled to prevent significant drops in body temperature.

Endogenous Pyrogens. Infection caused by bacteria, viruses, fungi, and other microbes elevates normal body temperature. These agents cause the host to produce specific proteins called endogenous pyrogens (EP). EPs are released from immunologically active phagocytic cells. Some tumor cells also are capable of producing EPs (Holtzclaw, 1992).

EPs are transported to the brain, where they alter the firing rate of the temperature-sensitive neurons located in the preoptic area of the hypothalamus. As a result, the set point is increased, causing the thermoregulatory center to sense the existence of a lower-than-desired temperature (Fig. 40-4). This causes the thermoregulatory center to initiate heat-conserving and heat-producing mechanisms, such as shivering, until the core temperature reaches the new set point (Guyton, 1991).

It usually takes the body several hours to reach the higher set point. During this period, the person experiences chills and feels cold, even though the body temperature may be elevated. The skin surface feels cold, and the person shivers. Once the higher temperature is reached, the person feels neither hot nor cold.

When the factor causing the release of EP is removed and the level of circulating EP falls, the hypothalamic thermostat is set at a lower, often normal rate. This triggers the hypothalamus to initiate heat-loss

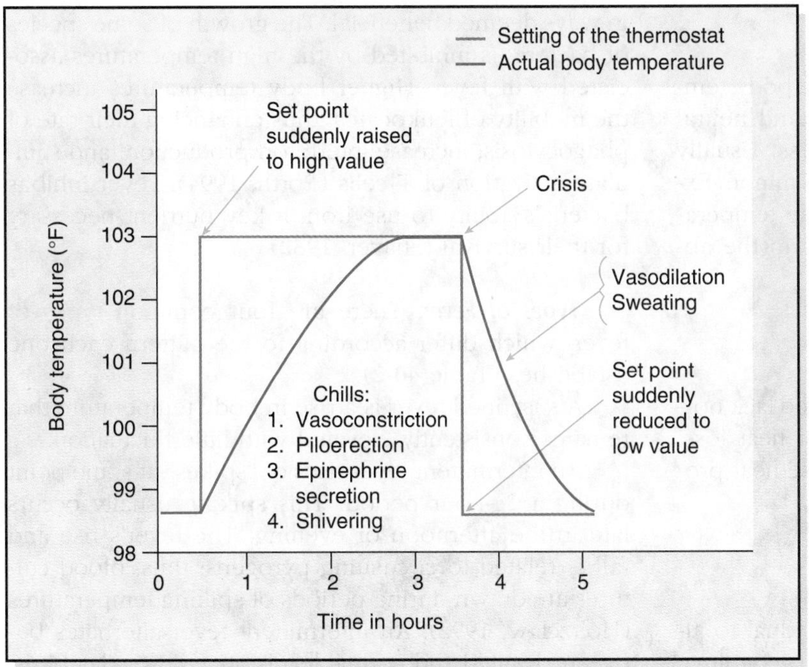

Figure 40-4 • *Effects of changing the set point of the hypothalamic temperature control. (From Guyton, A. C. (1991).* Textbook of medical physiology, *ed. 8. Philadelphia, Saunders.)*

mechanisms. When this happens, the person will experience intense sweating and sudden development of hot skin because of vasodilation. This sudden change is known as the "crisis" and often heralds the return to normal body temperature.

Exercise

An increase in muscle activity increases metabolic rate and heat production. Exercise causes the body temperature to vary according to the strenuousness of the activity. Very strenuous exercise, such as long-distance running, can raise the rectal temperature to 40°C (104°F) in healthy people (Guyton, 1991). If the person is already febrile, then exercise can cause the temperature to rise even higher.

Conversely, inactivity can decrease normal heat production. A paralyzed person who is in a very cool environment cannot use body movement to increase body temperature effectively. This increases the likelihood that hypothermia can occur.

Altered Cognitive States

To use behavioral responses to alter body temperature, a person must be cognitively alert and able to interpret environmental stimuli. The confused client may be unaware that the ambient temperature of his or her surroundings is abnormal and therefore may not dress appropriately or regulate environmental temperature.

Medications and drugs that impair cognitive states also can affect temperature regulation. Narcotics, sedatives, and alcohol decrease levels of consciousness and sensation, thus decreasing the recognition of (and behavioral responses to) abnormal temperature.

Stress

Physical and emotional stress can cause the body temperature to rise because of the hormonal and neural stimulation concurrent with a state of stress. Usually such fluctuations in body temperature are minor. Extreme stress of surgery can cause low-grade temperatures for the first 24 hours postoperatively in the absence of infection.

Altered Nutrition

People who are severely nutritionally depleted lack normal body fat to act as an insulator against heat loss. Lack of appetite and inability to eat decrease heat produced through the metabolism of food.

Drugs and Alcohol

Drugs and alcohol can predispose an individual to altered thermoregulation. Any drug that impairs cognitive ability can impact thermoregulation. For example, the client who is drunk may not be aware or able to seek shelter as outside temperatures drop. Peripheral heat dissipation is impaired by drugs that decrease sweating (eg, drugs with anticholinergic effects). A hypersensitivity reaction to drugs can cause fever. The fever resolves when the drug is stopped. Neuroleptic malignant syndrome can occur in 1% of individuals when neuroleptic medications are administered. In addition to high tempertures, the client may experience tachycardia, labile blood pressure changes, dyspnea, brain damage, and in approximately 30% of cases, death (Porth, 1994).

Manifestations of Altered Thermoregulation

Alterations causing above-normal body temperature are evidenced by fever, heat cramps, heat exhaustion, and heatstroke. Below-normal body temperature can be seen in hypothermia or frostbite.

Pyrexia or Fever

Pyrexia, or **fever,** can be defined as a regulated state in which the body's core temperature rises above the normal level for that person during rest. A low-grade fever is a temperature slightly elevated to approximately 37.1°C to 38.2°C (98.8°–100.6°F). A temperature elevation above 38.2°C is considered a high-grade fever, and temperature elevations above 40.5°C (104.9°F) are referred to as **hyperpyrexia**.

Fever is an adaptive state if it is kept within acceptable limits. Although the adaptive value of fever is not fully understood, research has provided evidence of some body mechanisms that are influenced by fever in ways deemed beneficial. The growth of some species of bacteria is inhibited by the high temperatures associated with fever. Higher body temperatures increase the mobility of leukocytes, thus enhancing their rate of phagocytosis; increase interferon production; and stimulate activation of T cells (Porth, 1994). Fever inhibits bacteria's ability to use iron, a key nutrient necessary for their survival (Shaver, 1982).

Types of Fever. There are four common types of fever, which differ according to the pattern each one establishes (Table 40-2).

A sustained fever is a rise in body temperature that remains consistently elevated with little fluctuation.

An intermittent fever rises or "spikes" at some point during a 24-hour period. This spiking usually occurs late in the afternoon or evening. The fever's rise and fall is related to circulating pyrogens; thus, blood cultures are drawn during periods of spiking temperatures (Holtzclaw, 1992). An intermittent fever alternates between elevated and normal levels on a day-to-day basis.

Table 40-2 • Differences in Types of Fevers

Type of Fever	*Fever Pattern*
Sustained fever	Rise in temperature above normal that remains consistently high with little fluctuation
Intermittent fever	Rises or spikes at some point during 24-hour period; usually late afternoon or evening
Remittent fever	Rise in temperature that is always elevated, but amount of elevation fluctuates
Relapsing fever	Elevated temperature lasting for several days, alternating with several days of normal temperature

A remittent fever occurs when the temperature is always elevated, but the amount of elevation may fluctuate. This could occur when a client has a temperature of 38°C to 38.5°C for most of the day that rises to 40°C in the late afternoon.

A relapsing fever is characterized by an elevated temperature lasting several days, alternating with several days of normal temperature.

Phases of Febrile Episodes. A febrile episode has three distinct phases—the chill phase, the fever phase, and the flush phase or crisis. Each phase exhibits unique symptoms.

During the chill phase, the body's heat-producing mechanisms are attempting to increase the core body temperature. The client will experience a feeling of being cold and may shiver. The appearance of goose flesh, which is caused by the contraction of the arrector pili muscles in an attempt to trap air around body hairs, may be evident. The client's skin will appear pale and cool due to vasoconstriction.

The fever phase occurs when the fever has reached the new, higher set point. The client's skin feels warm to the touch and appears flushed because of vasodilation. During this phase of the fever, the client feels neither hot nor cold. The client may experience thirst if fluid volume deficit has occurred. The client may complain of general malaise, weakness, and aching muscles, which are due to the increased rate of protein catabolism. In addition, the client may be either drowsy or restless. An unchecked fever can cause the client to become delirious and suffer from convulsions because of the irritation to nerve cells in the brain.

The flush or crisis phase is the third phase in a febrile episode. During this phase, the client experiences profuse diaphoresis, decreased shivering, and possible fluid volume deficit. The client's skin will appear flushed and warm to the touch because of vasodilation.

Heat Exhaustion

Heat exhaustion (or heat prostration) occurs from exercising in the heat. Exercising in warm temperatures results in the loss of large amounts of fluid through sweating, especially if fluid is not replaced. Body temperature may be slightly elevated or even below normal, but the loss of fluids causes significant circulatory problems. The client will experience tachycardia, dyspnea, and hypotension. The skin will be pale and feel cold and clammy. To treat heat exhaustion, the person should lie in a dorsal recumbent position and drink salty fluids. To prevent further episodes, people can ingest sodium (salt tablets) before exercise and drink balanced electrolyte solutions during exercise.

Heat Cramps

Heat cramps are painful, intermittent spasms of the skeletal muscles brought about by vigorous exercise and profuse sweating, which disturb the body's sodium balance. When people experience these cramps, they should cease their activity and replace depleted sodium with sodium tablets or fluids high in sodium content (eg, tomato juice).

Heatstroke

Heatstroke occurs when the body temperature rises beyond a critical temperature to a higher range of 41.1°C to 42.2°C (106°–108°F; Guyton, 1991). This rise in body temperature is precipitated by exposure to high environmental temperatures and the inability to rid the body of heat at an acceptable rate. Consequently, as the hypothalamus becomes excessively heated, its heat-regulating ability becomes depressed, and sweating diminishes. Thus, a high body temperature will perpetuate itself unless checked by external temperature-reducing interventions.

The person experiences dizziness, abdominal distress, and delirium, which will lead to unconsciousness if the temperature is not reduced. These symptoms are probably the result of circulatory shock brought on by the excessive loss of fluid and electrolytes. Hyperpyrexia, an excessively high body temperature, can cause damage to the body tissues, particularly to the brain cells.

Elderly people, particularly those who are in the lower socioeconomic group, are more prone to heatstroke during environmental heat waves. This can be attributed to poor ventilation and preexisting health problems, such as poor nutrition and respiratory and cardiac diseases. Also, the sweat mechanism is less efficient in the elderly, limiting their ability to safely cope with high environmental temperatures.

Hypothermia

Hypothermia is a state in which the core body temperature is lower than normal for a person. This condition can be artificially induced for therapeutic reasons, or it can result from unintentional exposure to extremely cold environmental temperatures.

When the core temperature of the body falls below 33°C (92°F), thermoregulation is impaired. A vicious cycle begins: Low body temperature causes the metabolic rate to decrease, which decreases the amount of heat produced by the body. Insufficient heat is available to return the body temperature to a normal range, which in turn slows the metabolic rate even more. If this cycle continues uninterrupted, death will occur when the core temperature reaches about 24°C (75°F) (Guyton, 1991).

Induced (Artificial) Hypothermia. Induced, or artificial, hypothermia is the deliberate lowering of the core temperature to a range of 30°C to 32°C (86°–89.6°F) (Rafalowski, 1987). This hypothermic state is induced by administering drugs that depress the hypothalamic thermostat or by encasing the client in a cooling blanket, which gradually decreases the core temperature. A person can remain in this state of suspended animation for days or several weeks without damage to body tissues (Guyton, 1991).

Induced hypothermia is used during cardiac surgery to decrease the metabolic rate, thus preserving the function of vital organs. It also reduces blood loss, due to the vasoconstrictive effect of the hypothermia. It may be used as a treatment for clients who are hyperpyrexic, when the core temperature is above 40°C (104°F). Hypothermia also is induced to prevent or reduce intracranial pressure in neurosurgical clients.

Accidental Hypothermia. Accidental hypothermia occurs when a person is unintentionally exposed to a cold environment that causes the core temperature to be reduced below an acceptable normal temperature. The severity of hypothermia depends on the age and health status of the person and the length of time he or she is exposed to the cold environment.

Hypothermia causes body functions to be depressed and impairs the function of the hypothalamus. Consequently, heat-producing mechanisms are diminished, so the person becomes even colder. When a person feels cold, he or she becomes drowsy, which reduces the body's ability to produce heat through muscle activity. Eventually the person becomes comatose and dies.

Factors that impact cognition and thermoregulation can greatly increase the incidence and severity of hypothermia. Excessive alcohol intake, the use of drugs (especially phenothiazines or barbiturates), trauma or cerebral vascular accident that inhibits movement all increase the risk for hypothermia (Pezzella, 1994). The homeless are especially vulnerable to hypothermia.

Frostbite

Frostbite occurs when the skin is exposed to extremely cold temperatures, freezing its surface. The most susceptible areas of the body to frostbite are the digits of the hands and feet, the earlobes, and the tip of the nose. Careless application of ice packs also can result in freezing the skin surface. If the frozen area is bathed immediately in warm water, not exceeding 43.3°C (110°F), it can be thawed without permanent damage. Otherwise, prolonged freezing impairs the circulatory network in the affected area, resulting in permanent tissue damage. Gangrene can develop in the damaged tissue, and amputation of the frostbitten area may be necessary.

Impact of Altered Temperature on Activities of Daily Living

Individual Considerations

Altered temperature states have differing effects on how well a person can perform normal daily activities. The warmer environment causes the person to be lethargic and have less energy to perform normal daily activities. Appetite tends to decrease, with a consequent decrease in the amount of food eaten. At the same time, thirst increases, increasing normal fluid intake. For people with preexisting health problems, such as a cardiac condition, a respiratory condition, or obesity, increased environmental temperatures prove more taxing. Daily activities, especially those involving physical exertion, will be uncomfortable and will place them at risk for developing conditions associated with hyperthermia.

People living in warm environmental temperatures must dress with light-weight, loose-fitting clothing to allow air currents to circulate close to their skin and promote cooling. Bathing is usually more frequent to promote comfort and prevent body odor. For people unable to take care of their own hygiene needs, this can prove difficult.

Cold environmental temperatures pose different problems. People are at risk for developing hypothermia if they do not take appropriate measures when exposed to cold environmental conditions. People living in these environments must wear several layers of densely woven fabrics to trap layers of air, providing insulation from cold outdoor temperatures. They must either stay indoors more or protect their skin surfaces from freezing when they venture outdoors. Outdoor physical exercise may be limited in periods of extreme cold.

Economic burdens may be great for those living in extreme environmental climates. Monthly heating or air-conditioning bills may severely stress the person's finances, especially if that person is living on a fixed income. Some jobs may be dangerous when temperatures are extremely hot or extremely cold. The welder who must work in a shop that is not air-conditioned may be at risk for heatstroke. Likewise, the ski instructor who must work when extremely cold conditions persist may develop hypothermia or frostbite. Sometimes work is canceled when weather conditions prove dangerous, thus economically affecting the worker.

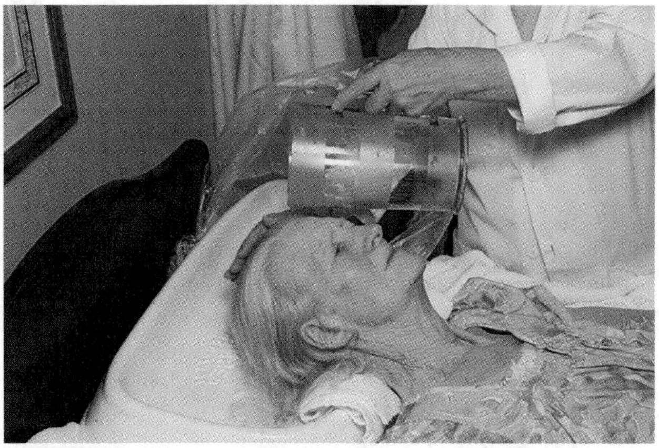

Figure 40-5 • *As you look at this older person, identify possible risk factors for altered thermoregulation.*

Family Considerations

Family and friends may need to care for a person during a febrile illness. Usually such an illness is of short duration and poses minimal hardships on the family. If a child experiences a febrile illness, a parent may have to take off from work. In some instances, this can pose a financial hardship.

When multigenerations live within the same residence, a comfortable environmental temperature may vary for different individuals. For an elderly person to maintain normal temperature, the thermostat may have to be set at 75°F, which younger people may find uncomfortably warm. During summer months, air conditioning may be required, which could pose a financial burden to the family.

Assessment

When collecting information about a client's temperature status, the nurse is gathering data for screening, to determine if a problem exists, or for monitoring an existing problem. Objective and subjective data are important to elicit from the client.

Subjective Data

Interviewing the client helps the nurse to understand the client's normal body temperature range, isolate any risk factors that may predispose the client to alterations in body temperature, and identify actual altered temperature states (Fig. 40-5).

Functional Pattern Identification

When questioned about normal body temperature, some clients may be able to tell the nurse their normal temperature range. More likely, the client will describe his or her temperature as normal or elevated. If a temperature elevation has been present, people often monitor their temperature and can provide the specific temperature measurements they have obtained.

Clients also can provide information about whether they generally feel cold or warm, the temperature at which they keep their thermostat set, and how many blankets they use at night. This information about what is normal for the client will help the nurse adjust the environment to promote comfort whenever possible.

Risk Identification

The client history helps elicit information identifying risk factors the client may have for abnormal temperature states. Any past occurrence of hyperthermia or hypothermia should be documented. Metabolic problems, such as cancer or endocrine imbalances, can alter metabolic rate and should be noted. A systems review should detect problems in circulation, neurologic status, and skin integrity, because all can affect normal thermoregulatory mechanisms. Chronic illnesses, such as cardiac problems, respiratory disease, or obesity, should be considered risk factors for altered temperature status. The medication history should be assessed for the use of drugs that affect vascular tone or level of consciousness, because these drugs increase the risk for altered temperature status.

Risk identification also should include environmental and situational data. The type of home in which the client lives and the adequacy of heating and air conditioning should be ascertained. Information concerning the client's employment or leisure activities should be explored, especially noting if these activities take place outdoors in climates with temperature extremes, or if they involve strenuous physical exertion.

If the client is scheduled for a surgical procedure that involves the administration of anesthetic agents, the nurse should inquire if there is a history of malignant hyperthermia in the family. If the client reports that any family member had difficulty or died suddenly during surgery or in the immediate postoperative period, the anesthesiologist should be notified.

Dysfunction Identification

If the nurse obtains a temperature reading outside the range of normal or if the client verbalizes having an abnormal body temperature, additional information should be collected to help determine the cause of the temperature abnormality. If the temperature is elevated, the nurse should seek information to determine how long the client has been aware of the elevated temperature, whether the client has experienced any chills or diaphoresis, and whether the client feels hot or cold. Questions can be directed to understand better whether the fever has established any pattern (intermittent, remittent, relapsing), what the client thinks is the cause of the fever, and how the client has been treating the fever. The nurse also should consider other factors that can cause elevated temperature, such as strenuous activity, ingestion of hot liquids, ovulation, degree of hydration, environmental temperature, and anxiety.

If the temperature is lower than normal for the client's age, the nurse may suspect the client is suffering from hypothermia. The nurse will need to validate this hypothesis by determining the client's mentation, feelings of warmth or cold, nutritional status, previous activity level, socioeconomic class, and medications taken. The nurse should inquire as to what the client thinks caused the hypothermia. In addition, the nurse should consider other factors that may cause low body temperature, such as a low environmental temperature, ingestion of cold liquids before measuring the temperature, or other factors that could have caused an inaccurate reading.

Objective Data

Objective data collection should include accurate measurement of body temperature and observation of physical signs and symptoms that may indicate temperature abnormality or fluctuation.

Assessment of Body Temperature

Measuring the body temperature is a way of assessing the function of the thermoregulatory system. This is accomplished by measuring the core body temperature at various locations of the body. The temperature varies throughout the body, and no single value is "the" body temperature. The most common site for measuring the temperature is the oral cavity, specifically the posterior sublingual pocket located at the base of the tongue. For specific information on how to determine body temperature accurately at various body sites, refer to Chapter 22.

One study recommends that the optimal time to measure body temperature to screen for fever is once a day at 6 PM (1800 hours). This recommendation is based on the influence of the circadian thermal rhythm on a person's body temperature (Samples, VanCott, Long, King, & Kersenbrock, 1985).

Other vital signs should be monitored along with temperature to evaluate whether changes in other vital signs correspond appropriately with the diagnosed alteration of body temperature.

Inspection

Areas of the body should be inspected for signs of alterations in body temperature. The skin should be observed for color, temperature, moisture, and the presence of piloerection (goose flesh) or shivering. The nurse should note whether color and temperature changes are localized or occur over most of the body. General observations should include the client's level of consciousness, body weight, and the state of nutrition and hydration.

Nursing Diagnoses

Subjective and objective data assist the nurse in identifying actual and potential problems of altered body temperature. The North American Nursing Diagnosis Asso-

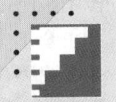

Nursing Research
Thermoregulation

Selected Nursing Research Studies

Bliss-Holtz, J. (1993). Determination of thermoregulatory status in full-term infants. *Nursing Research 42*(4), 204–207.

Caruso, C. C., Hadley, B. J., Shukla, R., Frame, P., & Khoury, J. (1992). Cooling effects and comfort of four cooling blanket temperatures in humans with fever. *Nursing Research, 41(2), 68–72.*

Fulbrook, P. (1993). Core temperature measurement: A comparison of rectal, axillary, and pulmonary artery blood temperature. *Intensive and Critical Care Nursing, 9(4), 217–224.*

Possible Topics for Nursing Inquiry

- How effective are tepid sponge baths in reducing core body temperature?
- Are normal circadian thermal patterns influenced by dietary intake?
- What is the effect of a routine exercise program on core body temperature in people older than 65 years?
- What is the effect on body temperature of giving cool versus warm fluids to a client with a fever?

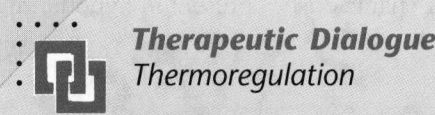

Therapeutic Dialogue
Thermoregulation

Scenes for Thought

Your client, Carmen Morales, aged 35, is in your clinic for her periodic check-up for hypertension and nutrition. She is the chief financial officer of a growing computer supply firm.

Effective

Nurse: *Hello, Carmen. How are you doing? (Sitting down at the desk with the chart.)*
Client: *Just fine, Teri, how are you?* Looks a little tense and fidgety, you notice.
Nurse: *I'm fine, thanks for asking. (Taking blood pressure.) Hmm, the pressure is a little high this month. Anything going on that might contribute to that?*
Client: *You mean besides the expansion at work and the kids having colds and my husband being in Denver all week?* Laughs. *No, nothing I can think of!*
Nurse: *Sounds like there's a lot going on.*
Client: *And my grandmother.* Sighs.
Nurse: *Your grandmother? What's happening with her?*
Client: *She's driving us all bats! She is constantly complaining about how cold it is in the house and keeps turning up the heat; so we're all sweating and she's comfortable. Meanwhile, the heating bills are going up.* Sighs again. *Maybe the kids got their colds from all the heat?* Looks at you questioningly.
Nurse: *Colds are caused by viruses, not temperature changes. What do you think is happening with your grandmother?*
Client: *I have no idea. She seems very healthy. She does all my cooking and laundry, God bless her. What do you think?*
Nurse: *I think it's because of her age. You know, people have lower temperatures as they get older, and they feel colder than younger people do. So they always have to wear sweaters and turn up the heat, even in the summer.*
Client: *Yes, I've noticed that about her.* Pauses thoughtfully. *I guess I should talk with her a little and try to work out something so we can all function together.*
Nurse: *Let me know how it works out. I'd like to assess your salt and fluid intake, okay?*
Client: *Sure. I have to get back to work soon, too. Let's do it.*

Less Effective

Nurse: *Hello, Carmen. How are you doing? (Sitting down at the desk with the chart.)*
Client: *Just fine, Toni, how are you?* Looks a little tense and fidgety, you notice.
Nurse: *I'm fine, thanks for asking. (Taking blood pressure.) Hmm, the pressure is a little high this month. Anything going on that might contribute to that?*
Client: *You mean besides the expansion at work and the kids having colds and my husband being in Denver all week?* Laughs. *No, nothing I can think of!*
Nurse: *Sounds like there's a lot going on. (Writing in the chart and reading past entries.)*
Client: *And my grandmother.* Sighs.
Nurse: *She's adding to the stress, too? You're really having a tough time lately. I'll bet your eating habits are suffering a bit, yes? Let's go over your nutrition and see what's up.*
Client: *Okay.*

Critical Thinking Challenges

• Identify some clues that Toni wasn't truly listening to Carmen • Appraise what part knowledge deficit plays in Carmen's response to her grandmother's behavior • Deduce some false assumptions Carmen might have made about her grandmother's behavior

ciation (NANDA) has identified four accepted nursing diagnoses involving temperature alteration: Risk for Altered Body Temperature, Hypothermia, Hyperthermia, and Ineffective Thermoregulation.

Diagnostic Statement: Risk for Altered Body Temperature

Definition

Risk for altered body temperature is the state in which an individual is at risk for failure to maintain body temperature within a normal range (NANDA, 1994).

Defining Characteristics

The following are defining characteristics: presence of risk factors, such as extremes of age and weight; exposure to cold, cool, warm, or hot environments; dehydration; inactivity or vigorous activity; medications causing vasoconstriction or vasodilation; altered metabolic rate; sedation; inappropriate clothing for environmental temperature; illness or trauma affecting temperature regulation (NANDA, 1994).

Related Factors

Related factors are the same as risk factors.

Diagnostic Statement: Hypothermia

Definition

Hypothermia is the state in which an individual's body temperature is reduced below normal range (NANDA, 1994).

Defining Characteristics

Major characteristics are reduction in body temperature below normal range, shivering (mild), cool skin, and pallor (NANDA, 1994).

Minor characteristics are slow capillary refill, tachycardia, cyanotic nailbeds, hypertension, and piloerection (NANDA, 1994).

Related Factors

Related factors include exposure to cool or cold environments, illness or trauma, damage to hypothalamus, inability or decreased ability to shiver, malnutrition, inadequate clothing, consumption of alcohol, medications causing vasodilation, evaporation from skin in cool environment, decreased metabolic rate, inactivity, and aging (NANDA, 1994).

Diagnostic Statement: Hyperthermia

Definition

Hyperthermia is a state in which an individual's body temperature is elevated above his or her normal range (NANDA, 1994).

Defining Characteristics

The major characteristic is an increase in body temperature above normal range (NANDA, 1994).

Minor characteristics include flushed skin that is warm to the touch, increased respiratory rate, tachycardia, seizures, or convulsions (NANDA, 1994).

Related Factors

Related factors include exposure to hot environment, vigorous activity, medications or anesthesia, inappropriate clothing, increased metabolic rate, illness or trauma, dehydration, inability or decreased ability to perspire (NANDA, 1994).

Diagnostic Statement: Ineffective Thermoregulation

Definition

Ineffective thermoregulation is the state in which an individual's temperature fluctuates between hypothermia and hyperthermia (NANDA, 1994).

Defining Characteristics

Defining characteristics include fluctuations in body temperature above or below the normal range. See also major and minor characteristics present in hypothermia and hyperthermia (NANDA, 1994).

Related Factors

Related factors include trauma or illness, immaturity, aging, and fluctuating environmental temperature (NANDA, 1990).

Related Nursing Diagnoses

People with altered body temperature are at risk for other problems. Those with hyperthermia may experience Fluid Volume Deficit, Activity Intolerance, Risk for Injury, and Altered Nutrition: Less than body requirements. Hypothermia may cause Pain, Altered Tissue Perfusion, and Impaired Skin Integrity.

Outcome Identification and Planning

Client outcomes are individualized for each client who is at risk for developing, or who has, actual problems in maintaining normal body temperature. Goals should focus around the following:

Client will maintain body temperature within normal range.
Client will identify factors that can precipitate alterations in body temperature.
Client will verbalize strategies to prevent and treat deviations from normal body temperature.

Planning for nursing interventions focuses on preventing problems of thermoregulation, educating the client to manage and prevent problems, and assisting in regulating temperatures when alterations have occurred. Examples of some nursing interventions for altered states of theromoregulation are listed in the accompanying display and discussed in the following section.

Implementation

Nursing Interventions to Promote Health

Client Teaching

The nurse's position is ideal for teaching people how to avoid potential problems with thermoregulation and what to do if such problems occur. Teaching can occur in many settings and in social interactions with the general public.

The nurse can be a credible teacher for the parents of a newborn. Instruction about thermoregulation is imperative for parents of the premature infant. Explanations should include a discussion of the immaturity of

Planning
Examples of Nursing Interventions for Altered Thermoregulation

Hypothermia

- Increase environmental temperature.
- Apply layers of clothing or blankets.
- Keep clothing dry.
- Increase physical activity.
- Increase intake of food and warm fluids.

Hyperthermia

- Decrease environmental temperature.
- Increase air movement (eg, fans).
- Remove clothing.
- Sponge skin with cool water.
- Replenish fluids.
- Decrease physical activity.

the infant's ability to regulate temperature. The nurse should instruct the parents to protect the newborn from temperature extremes (eg, to avoid chilling during the bath, to avoid overdressing the infant). The nurse also should explain how to monitor axillary temperature and when to contact the physician regarding a fever.

The public should have a good knowledge of hypothermia and hyperthermia. Proper dress for different weather conditions is important. Keeping the head covered to prevent excessive loss of heat is important, because 40% of body heat can be lost through the head.

Client Teaching
Thermoregulation

Instruct the client as follows:

- *To obtain your oral temperature properly, place the thermometer in the posterior sublingual pocket, which is right under the tongue. Smoking, drinking, chewing gum, and exercise can affect accuracy of the temperature reading obtained.*
- *Wear light-weight, loosely woven fabrics that are light in color to keep cool in hot weather. Drink extra fluid when weather is very hot.*
- *To prevent hypothermia, dress in several layers of clothing (wool is an especially good insulator), making sure to keep your head warm and all clothing dry.*
- *If you are elderly, you are less able to tolerate extremes in temperature.*
- *If you are elderly, you are less likely to have a fever during an infectious episode and may normally run subnormal temperatures.*

When weather conditions are extreme, ways to cope with severe hot or cold weather should be emphasized. This is especially important for the elderly or those with chronic illnesses, such as respiratory or cardiac disease. Community resources to help people pay for high heating or cooling bills or to install insulation to make their homes more energy efficient may be available for those on a fixed income. The nurse can refer people to such community services.

The nurse can speak to community groups, such as the Boy Scouts or Girl Scouts, to explain the effects of temperature extremes and how to avoid thermoregulation problems. Health classes, which are frequently taught by the school nurse, also offer an excellent opportunity to instruct youngsters on such problems. Senior citizen centers welcome instruction on how problems of thermoregulation can be avoided in the elderly.

People indulging in strenuous exercise, especially in hot weather, should be taught to replenish fluids and recognize signs of hyperthermia. The school nurse is an excellent authority for seeing that athletic events and practices are conducted safely so that children are not exposed to heatstroke. The industrial nurse monitors working conditions so that employees are not exposed to unhealthy working conditions.

Nursing Interventions for Altered Thermoregulation

The nurse treats clients with altered body temperature in a variety of clinical settings. The nurse uses interventions for fever management, hyperthermia, and hypothermia to help clients regain normal body temperature when an imbalance has occurred.

Fever Management

The management of a fever varies according to the phase of the fever and the signs or symptoms the client is experiencing (see the display).

Management During Chill Phase. Nursing interventions during the chill phase focus on client comfort. Blankets or extra clothing can be provided to help the client feel warmer. The client should be given adequate nourishment and fluids to meet the body's needs due to increased metabolic rate. The client with a preexisting respiratory or cardiovascular problem may require activity restriction or supplemental oxygen to meet the demands of the increased metabolic rate. The nurse should monitor the client's vital signs frequently to detect any deviations from the normal range and determine the effect of the fever on other body systems.

Management During Fever Phase. Once the fever has reached the new higher set point, nursing interventions

Nursing Care Guidelines
Care of the Febrile Person

During the Chill Phase

Client can experience feeling cold; shivering, paleness of skin; skin cool to touch; appearance of "goose-flesh"; increase in body temperature.

Nursing Interventions

- Apply extra blankets.
- Increase fluid intake.
- Restrict activity.
- Supply supplement oxygen if client has preexisting cardiac or respiratory problem.

During Fever Phase

Client can experience feeling neither hot nor cold; dry oral mucosa; thirst; possible dehydration; general malaise, weakness, aching muscles; drowsiness or restlessness; possible convulsions; possibility of becoming comatose.

Nursing Interventions

- Cover with light, warm clothing to avoid chilling client.
- Encourage fluids (cool).
- Restrict iron from diet if necessary.
- Promote rest.
- Apply lubricant to dried lips and nasal muscosa.
- Use tepid sponging if temperature becomes very high.
- Increase air circulation to encourage cooling.
- Implement safety precautions to protect client if restless or delirious, or if convulsions occur.

Flush Phase

Client can experience profuse sweating; decreased shivering; possible dehydration; flushed skin; skin warm to touch.

Nursing Interventions

- Use tepid sponging; avoid chilling client.
- Encourage oral fluids (cool).
- Restrict activity.
- Cover with light clothing or bed linens.

will continue to focus on client comfort and adequate client hydration. The client should be covered with adequate clothing to prevent shivering. Frequently, mouth care is important, because lips and mucous membranes may become dry. Cool oral fluid should be encouraged, preferably fluids high in protein to cope with the increased rate of metabolism. Food or fluids high in iron should be avoided, because bacteria need good iron supplies to survive (Shaver, 1982). The client should be encouraged to rest.

If the temperature approaches 40°C (104°F), the client may be given a tepid sponge bath to promote cooling by evaporation and conduction. To promote further heat loss, the temperature of the environment can be cooled and the circulation of the air increased using fans.

If the client becomes restless, delirious, or convulses, client safety becomes an additional concern for the nurse. Padded siderails may be indicated to prevent the client from falling out of bed or becoming injured if the siderail is struck. The client should be monitored closely if convulsions are anticipated, and safety precautions should be instituted to prevent injury.

Management During Flush Phase. Nursing interventions during the flush phase continue to focus on client comfort and hydration. The client should be covered with a minimal amount of light clothing to prevent conservation of heat. Cool, tepid sponging and increased air circulation assist the client's cooling mechanisms to reduce the core temperature. The diaphoretic client's clothing and bed linens must be changed frequently to prevent skin breakdown and provide client comfort. The nurse should assist the client to maintain adequate hydration by encouraging cool liquids. Physical activity should be limited to prevent heat production.

Antipyretics. Drugs such as aspirin, acetaminophen, and aminopyrine are called **antipyretics** because they lower the setting of the hypothalamic thermostat so that the temperature of the body falls. Antipyretics may be used to reduce the temperature when the fever becomes a threat to the client's well-being. Aminopyrine, which decreases the normal body temperature, may be used by physicians to induce a hypothermic condition.

Antipyretics should be used judiciously in children and the elderly because of their body size and metabolic function. The use of antipyretics has been questioned in routine fever treatment, because higher body temperatures may help support body defenses to fight infection, but most authorities agree that antipyretics are advisable for fever above 40°C (Holtzclaw, 1992).

Aspirin is effective in lowering an elevated temperature but will not reduce the temperature to a lower than normal range or reduce body temperature that has been elevated by vigorous exercise. Aspirin promotes heat loss by dilating blood vessels and fostering diaphoresis but does not affect heat production in the body. Often, people take aspirin mainly to reduce the aches and discomforts associated with fever. Aspirin should not be given to children with flulike illnesses because it has been associated with Reye's syndrome, a potentially fatal condition involving liver damage and encephalopathy (Reeves-Swift, 1990).

When a nurse administers an antipyretic to a febrile client, the client's temperature should be taken immediately before the medication is given and approximately 1 hour later to determine if the medication has had the desired effect.

Tepid Baths. Tepid baths or sponging is administered to febrile clients when their temperature reaches a seriously elevated level. These may be administered to the client when his or her temperature is consistently high, not during the chill phase of a fever. Tepid water is used to avoid the chilling effects of cool water. This procedure may be either soothing or uncomfortable for the client, depending on the client's skin temperature. Tepid baths or sponging are intended to replace artificially the body's sweating mechanism by cooling the surface of the skin, thereby cooling the blood being delivered to the body core. Also, this procedure promotes cooling by the process of evaporation. The nurse must be cautious to avoid chilling the client, which will trigger the shivering mechanism. Before administering a tepid sponge bath, the nurse should measure the client's temperature, and it should be measured 30 minutes after the procedure to determine the effectiveness of the intervention.

A study by Neuman (1985) suggests that sponging febrile children should be abandoned as a method of reducing elevated body temperature caused by an infectious process. Research has demonstrated that the administration of antipyretics without sponging is just as effective as combining the two procedures (Neuman, 1985). Alcohol sponging is not recommended because rapid evaporation increases the risk of shivering, and the fumes can be noxious.

Hypothermia Blankets. These special blankets can be used to reduce the temperature of the hyperpyrexic client. The blanket consists of rubber or vinyl coils through which distilled water or alcohol is pumped. The temperature of the fluid can be programmed by a control device similar to a thermostat. When cooling is desired, the blanket is usually set slightly lower than normal body temperature (eg, 35°C or 96°F). A rectal probe is inserted into the client to monitor core body temperature constantly so that excessive cooling does not occur. During use of the hypothermia blanket, medication may be necessary to block the shivering mechanism.

Management of Hyperthermia

Many conditions other than fever that involve sustained elevation of core body temperature above the normal range require therapeutic intervention. Based on a sound understanding of thermoregulation, the nurse should focus care on decreasing heat production and increasing heat loss from the body. The environment should be cool and the circulation of air increased by the use of fans. Fluid intake should be encouraged, and physical activity should be limited.

When a client experiences heatstroke, immediate measures must be instituted to prevent cellular damage and possible mortality. Application of ice packs to the head, axilla, and groin, where there are abundant blood vessels close to the skin surface, assists in quickly lowering core body temperature. Spraying or sponging the affected person with water establishes an artificial sweating mechanism and allows heat loss by means of evaporation. If conscious, the person should be encouraged to take oral fluids. Transfer to a medical facility where the client can be closely monitored is often necessary for anyone suffering from heatstroke. A hypothermia blanket, medications, and intravenous fluids may be needed to stabilize the client.

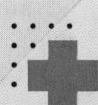

Safety Alert
Thermoregulation

- Protect infants from extremes in temperature, and avoid chilling during bathing.
- Do not permit children younger than 2 years in a hot tub.
- Monitor the temperature using rectal probe when a hypothermia blanket is used so that core body temperature will not drop too low.
- After hypothermia, rewarm the client slowly to prevent massive vasodilation and possible shock.
- Do not administer aspirin to children with flulike illness, because its administration has been linked with potentially lethal Reye's syndrome.
- Provide prompt treatment for heatstroke; it is a medical emergency that must be promptly treated to prevent cellular damage.

Management of Hypothermia

When treating hypothermia, the nurse should use measures to promote heat production and limit heat loss from the body. The environment should be warm, with layers of clothing applied to trap air between layers to act as insulation. In severe cases of hypothermia, more aggressive rewarming by immersion into warm fluids or using external heat sources may be necessary. Warming should occur gradually to prevent massive vasodilation, which can lead to shock. In severe cases, extracorporeal rewarming through hemodialysis or use of the cardiopulmonary bypass may be needed (Walhout, 1992).

If frostbite is present, the affected area should be bathed in water not exceeding 43.3°C (110°F) to prevent permanent damage (Guyton, 1991). The area should not be rubbed or bumped, because frozen skin can be easily damaged.

Community-Based Care

People of all ages need to know how to prevent hyperthermic conditions, such as heat cramps and heatstroke, and hypothermic conditions, such as hypothermia and frostbite. Nurses share information on how to treat these conditions at home and when to seek professional help.

Fevers are commonly treated in the home. The nurse needs to provide information concerning the different stages of fever and the appropriate care during each phase. Information about caregiving should include aspects related to nutrition, fluid balance, activity, heat reduction techniques, and nonprescription medications. Teaching may be required as to how to measure temperature at various body sites with equipment purchased at the local drug store. Information is given regarding when to seek professional advice.

The elderly need to know that the aging process creates changes in their perception of temperature and their ability to cope with environmental changes. Changes in lifestyle and control of the environment should be discussed to prevent alterations in body temperature.

Community health nurses often assess the home environment. Some clients may need to be counseled regarding home heating and cooling. Air-conditioning units may be important for people with chronic health problems who live in hot areas. Heating systems should be safe and efficient. Houses should be well insulated to promote comfort and decrease the cost of heating or cooling. Furnace filters should be changed frequently to prevent excessive dust in the environment. Space heaters should be used with caution and positioned away from flammable items. Kerosene heaters should be well vented to prevent carbon monoxide poisoning. Community agencies are available to assess individual heating systems and in some cases to help financially with the high cost of heating or cooling for those who cannot afford to pay.

Evaluation

Evaluation is an ongoing part of the nursing process. As a nurse completes an intervention, the client must be reassessed to determine if the intervention was effective. This reassessment or evaluation process is accomplished by comparing the actual client outcomes with the outcome criteria established for each client goal.

Client goals and outcome criteria need to be individualized for each client with potential or actual problems with thermoregulation. Examples of appropriate goals and outcome criteria for selected clients follow:

Goal

Client will maintain body temperature within normal range.

Possible Outcome Criteria

- Client maintains body temperature within 1 degree of normal body temperature.
- Client does not complain of feeling uncomfortably cold or warm.

Goal

Client will identify factors that can precipitate altered body temperature.

Possible Outcome Criteria

By the end of the teaching session, the following will occur:

- Client verbalizes three risk factors for developing hypothermia.
- Client verbalizes three risk factors for developing hyperthermia.
- Client identifies factors within his or her lifestyle that could contribute to altered body temperature.

Goal

Client will verbalize strategies to prevent and treat deviations from normal body temperature.

Possible Outcome Criteria

By the end of home visit, the following will occur:

- Client describes three ways to alter the environment to prevent altered body temperature.
- Client discusses how to monitor temperature and how to manage fever at home.
- Client identifies when a healthcare provider should be consulted in the occurrence of altered body temperature.

Key Concepts

- Heat is continuously being produced in the body as a by-product of the chemical reactions taking place in all body cells.
- Body temperature is the delicate balance between heat produced and heat lost.
- Heat production in the body is influenced by the person's BMR, the thyroid hormone level, stimulation of the sympathetic nervous system, and the level of muscle activity.

Nursing Plan of Care
The Client With Ineffective Thermoregulation

Nursing Diagnosis

Ineffective Thermoregulation related to the aging process, as evidenced by low body temperature

Client Goal

Client will maintain body temperature within normal range.

Client Outcome Criteria

- Client maintains body temperature within ± 1° of normal body temperature for next 48 hours.
- Client expresses comfort related to heat or cold for next 48 hours.

Nursing Intervention	*Scientific Rationale*
1. Monitor oral temperature daily at 6 PM.	1. Temperature should be assessed using the same site to ensure consistency. The oral site is accurate and easy to use. 6 PM is when the temperature is highest because of the circadian thermal rhythm, and taking the measurement at the same time also ensures consistency.
2. Encourage client to walk for 20 minutes daily.	2. Exercise increases the metabolic rate, which produces heat.
3. Increase temperature of the environment (room).	3. A warmer environment helps prevent heat lost to the environment by radiation and conduction.
4. Encourage client to wear layers of tightly woven clothing.	4. Layers of clothing trap the air between the layers and provide insulation, thus reducing heat loss.

Client Goal

Client will identify factors that can precipitate altered body temperature.

Client Outcome Criteria

- By end of teaching session, client verbalizes three risk factors for developing hypothermia.
- At next appointment, client identifies factors within his or her lifestyle that could contribute to altered body temperature.

Nursing Intervention	*Scientific Rationale*
1. Encourage client to eat a well-balanced diet.	1. Eating properly prevents loss of fat. Fat is needed to help insulate the body and reduce heat loss.
2. Teach the client about interventions to prevent hypothermia (eg, layering clothing, immediately removing wet clothing, increasing activity).	2. If the client understands the ways to prevent hypothermia, he or she is more likely to comply.

- Heat is lost from the body by means of radiation, conduction, convection, and evaporation.
- The hypothalamus, nervous system, circulatory system, shivering mechanism, and sweat glands interdependently play significant roles in the thermoregulation of the entire body.
- When assessing body temperature, the nurse must consider the effects that age, hormones, exercise, and stress have on the person's thermoregulating mechanism.
- A person's core temperature fluctuates according to his or her circadian thermal rhythm. In addition, a woman's menstrual cycle influences her core temperature.
- Death generally occurs when the core body temperature reaches 44°C to 45°C (112°–114°F) or when the core temperature drops below 24°C (75°F).
- Three common types of fevers are intermittent, remittent, and relapsing fevers.

- The nurse should be able to recognize the early symptoms of malignant hyperthermia, heat cramps, heat exhaustion, and heatstroke and implement appropriate independent and collaborative interventions.

Critical Thinking Challenges

Return to the situation at the beginning of this chapter, and apply your new knowledge about thermoregulation to consider the following questions.

1. *Outline factors that might contribute to altered thermoregulation for this client.*
2. *Prioritize assessment data, and plan your process for deciding with the client what is most important in her plan of care.*
3. *Identify appropriate community agencies or supports that might be helpful at this time.*
4. *Describe your own feelings when visiting a client whose basic needs of food and shelter are being met only minimally.*

References

Bliss-Holtz, J. (1993). Determination of thermoregulatory state in full-term infants. *Nursing Research, 42*(4), 204–207.

Donnelly, A. (1994). Malignant hyperthermia: Epidemiology, pathophysiology, and treatment. *AORN, 59*(2), 393–408.

Erickson, R. (1980). Oral temperature differences in relation to thermometer and technique. *Nursing Research, 29,* 157–164.

Ganong, W. F. (1993). *Review of medical physiology* (16th ed.). Los Altos, CA: Lange Medical Publications.

Guyton, A. C. (1991). *Textbook of medical physiology* (7th ed.). Philadelphia: W.B. Saunders.

Holtzclaw, B. J. (1992). The febrile response in critical care: State of the science. *Heart and Lung, 21*(5), 482–501.

Jackson, D. B., & Saunders, R. B. (1993). *Child health nursing: A comprehensive approach to the care of children and their families.* Philadelphia: J.B. Lippincott.

Kaus, S. J., & Rockhoff, M. A. (1994). Malignant hyperthermia. *Pediatric Clinics of North America, 41*(1), 221–237.

North American Nursing Diagnosis Association (1994). *NANDA nursing diagnoses: Definitions and classifications* (1995–1996). Philadelphia: Author.

Neuman, J. (1985). Evaluation of sponging to reduce body temperature in febrile children. *Canadian Medical Association Journal, 132,* 641–642.

Pezzella, D. (1994). Responding to the hypothermic patient. *Nursing 94, 24*(2), 50–51.

Porth, C. M. (1994). *Pathophysiology: Concepts of altered health status* (4th ed.). Philadelphia: J.B. Lippincott.

Rafalowski, M. M. (1987). Relationship of core temperature at time of blanket removal to subsequent core temperatures in clients immediately after coronary artery bypass. *Heart and Lung, 16,* 9–13.

Reeves-Swift, R. (1990). Rational management of a child's acute fever. *American Journal of Maternal Child Nursing, 15*(2), 82–85.

Samples, J. F., VanCott, M. L., Long, C., King, I. M., & Kersenbrock, A. (1985). Circadian rhythms: Basis for screening fever. *Nursing Research, 34,* 377–379.

Shaver, J. (1982). The basic mechanisms of fever: Considerations for therapy. *Nurse Practitioner, 10,* 15–19.

Shaver, J. (1991). Assessment of reproductive function. In M. L. Patrick, et al. (Eds.), *Medical–surgical nursing: Pathophysiological concepts* (2nd ed.) (pp. 1904–1913). Philadelphia: J.B. Lippincott.

Walhout, M. F. (1992). Treatment for hypothermia. *RN, 55*(4), 50–55.

Yurick, A. G., Spier, B. E., Robb, S. S., & Ebert, N. J. (1989). *The aged person and the nursing process* (3rd ed.). Norwalk, CT: Appleton-Century-Crofts.

Bibliography

Carpenito, L. J. (1995). *Nursing diagnoses: Application to clinical practice* (6th ed.). Philadelphia: J.B. Lippincott.

Caruso, C. C., Hadley, B. J., Shukla, R., Frame, P., & Khoury, J. (1992). Cooling effects and comfort of four cooling blanket temperatures in humans with fever. *Nursing Research, 41*(2), 68–72.

Giuffre, M., Heidenreich, T., & Pruitt, L. (1994). Rewarming cardiac surgery patients: Radiant heat versus forced warm air. *Nursing Research, 43*(3), 174–178.

Morgan, S. P. (1990). A comparison of three methods of managing fever in the neurological client. *Journal of Neuroscience Nursing, 22*(1), 19–24.

Mravinac, C. M., Dracup, K., & Clochesy, J. M. (1989). Urinary bladder and rectal temperature monitoring during clinical hypothermia. *Nursing Research, 38,* 73–76.

Elimination

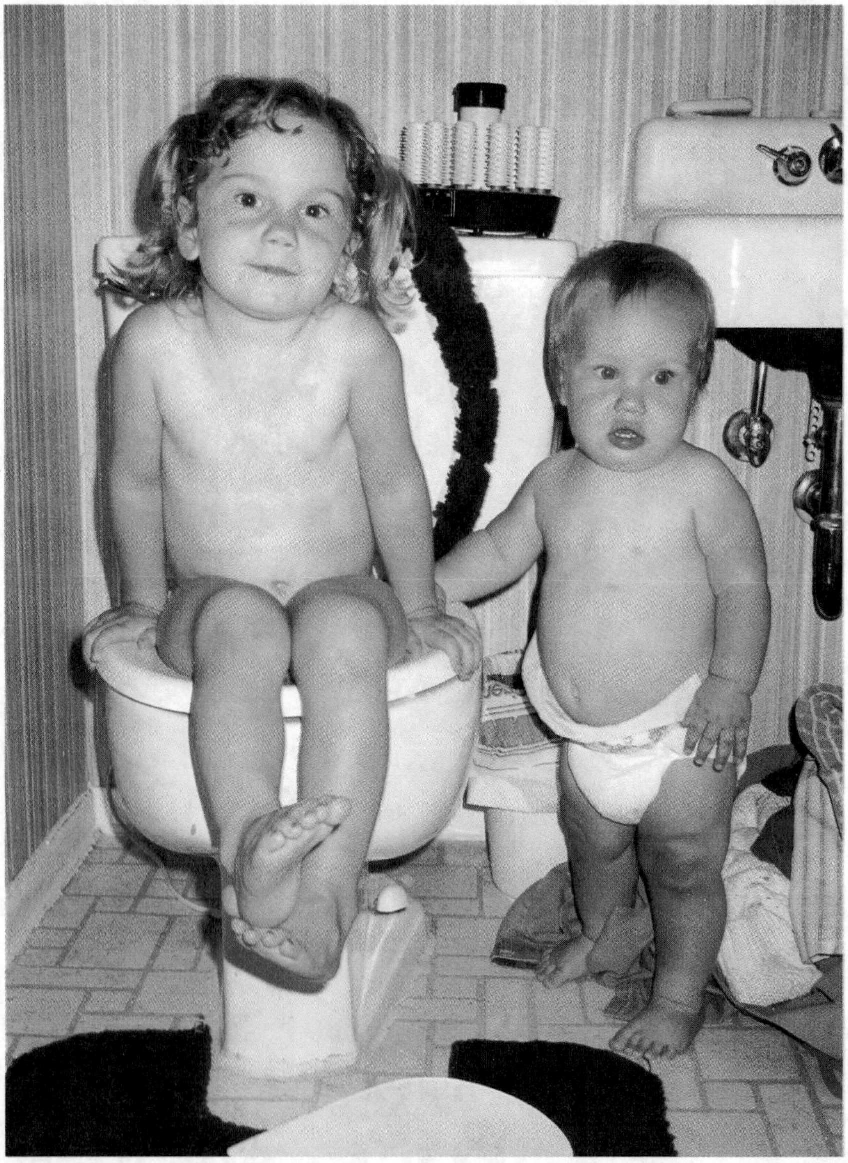

UNIT X

Elimination of body wastes is a universal human function. It is also an area of concern for most clients in a healthcare facility and in the home, where self-care becomes the focus. Unit X explores the functions of urinary and bowel elimination.

Each chapter considers the concepts and principles related to normal function. The nursing process serves as a framework to present the knowledge base necessary to assess function and either plan to promote heath and function or to intervene for altered function. The assessment discussion focuses on uncovering the normal pattern of elimination for each client, as well as the use of any devices, such as laxatives, to control elimination problems. Each chapter emphasizes client teaching to promote normal elimination and considers all forms of elimination, including those that require devices, such as ostomy bags.

Elimination is a concern for every client regardless of the problem for which they need nursing care. Unit X is applicable to every client the nurse encounters.

Urinary Elimination

Key Terms

Anuria
Continuous bladder irrigation
Detrusor muscle
Diuresis
Dysuria
Enuresis
Hematuria
Indwelling catheters
Intermittent catheterization
Micturition
Oliguria
Peritoneal dialysis
Polyuria
Postvoid residual
Pyuria
Renal dialysis
Urinary incontinence
Urinary retention

Learning Objectives

Upon completion of this chapter, the student will be able to do the following:

- *Describe the normal structure and function of the urinary system.*
- *Outline the process of micturition.*
- *List and describe alterations in normal voiding patterns.*
- *Describe factors that can alter normal urinary function.*
- *Recognize age-related differences in urinary elimination.*
- *Discuss nursing assessment of urinary function.*
- *Identify nursing diagnoses related to urinary elimination.*
- *Describe nursing interventions to promote normal urinary elimination.*
- *Discuss interventions for altered urinary function.*
- *Develop appropriate collaborative and community-based nursing interventions to manage voiding problems.*

41

You are a nurse working with John, an 18-year-old who has been recovering for 2 weeks after a motor vehicle accident on the night of his senior prom. John has been in traction and has had a Foley catheter in place for 2 weeks, draining large amounts of urine. Yesterday you noted John's urine was cloudy and he had a temperature of 37.8°C. When you report these findings to the physician, he discontinues John's catheter and orders a urine sample for culture and sensitivity. You enter the room to remove his catheter, and he says, "It's about time I had some attention to my penis. It has been feeling quite neglected during this hospital stay."

This chapter on urinary elimination will discuss alterations in urinary function that will help you to analyze this situation and plan appropriate individualized care for John. As you read the chapter, you also should reflect on how comfortable you feel asking questions concerning elimination or performing procedures involving the perineal area. Critical Thinking Challenges about John's situation are provided at the end of this chapter.

The elimination of fluid waste is an essential function of the human body. Failure of the urinary system to function properly can result in serious, possibly life-threatening conditions. Less serious urinary dysfunction, although not life-threatening, can be embarrassing and debilitating for the person.

The nurse is instrumental in promoting optimal urinary function and preventing urinary complications for all clients. The nurse individualizes teaching and specific interventions to help clients of all ages deal with problems of incontinence, urinary retention, and prevention of urinary tract infection (UTI). An understanding of the anatomy and physiology of the urinary system, and of the factors that can affect normal and abnormal functioning of urinary elimination, is important for the nurse in individualizing client care.

Normal Urinary Function

Structures of the Urinary Tract

Structures within the urinary tract include the kidneys, where the urine is formed; the ureters, which connect the kidneys with the bladder; the bladder, which stores urine; and the urethra, which permits the urine to exit from the body (Fig. 41-1).

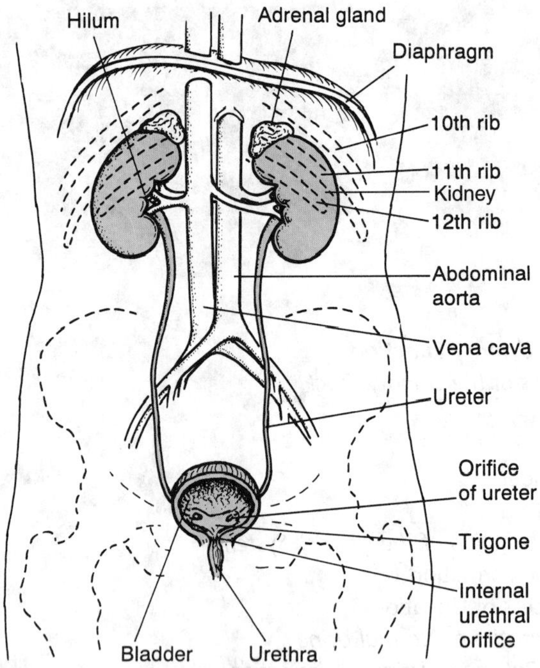

Figure 41-1 • *Anatomic structures of the urinary tract.*

Kidneys

The two kidneys are located on the posterior abdominal wall, in front of and on either side of the vertebral column. They lie approximately between the 12th thoracic and 3rd lumbar vertebrae. Each kidney is enclosed by a fibrous capsule and supported by a mass of adipose tissue.

The functional unit of the kidney is called a nephron (Fig. 41-2). Each kidney has over 1,000,000 nephrons, and each nephron is capable of forming urine. The nephron consists of the glomerulus, Bowman's capsule, proximal convoluted tubules, loop of Henle, the distal tubule, and the collecting duct. The glomerulus is a network of blood vessels, surrounded by Bowman's capsule, where the formation of urine begins. The tubules, loop of Henle, and collecting ducts are passageways that permit the urine to flow to the bladder. More important, they selectively reabsorb or secrete substances from the urine so that fluid and electrolyte balance is maintained.

Ureters

The ureters are narrow (1.25 cm), smooth muscle tubes that serve as passageways for urine to flow from the kidneys to the bladder. Peristaltic movement in the ureters propels the urine toward the bladder. The frequency of the peristaltic movement ranges from once every 10 seconds to once every 2 to 3 minutes (Guyton, 1995). A flap of mucous membrane, which acts as a valve, covers the juncture between the ureters and the bladder. Under normal conditions, this prevents reflux of urine up through the ureter into the kidney.

Bladder

The bladder is the storage compartment for urine. It is a hollow, smooth muscle that lies behind the sym-

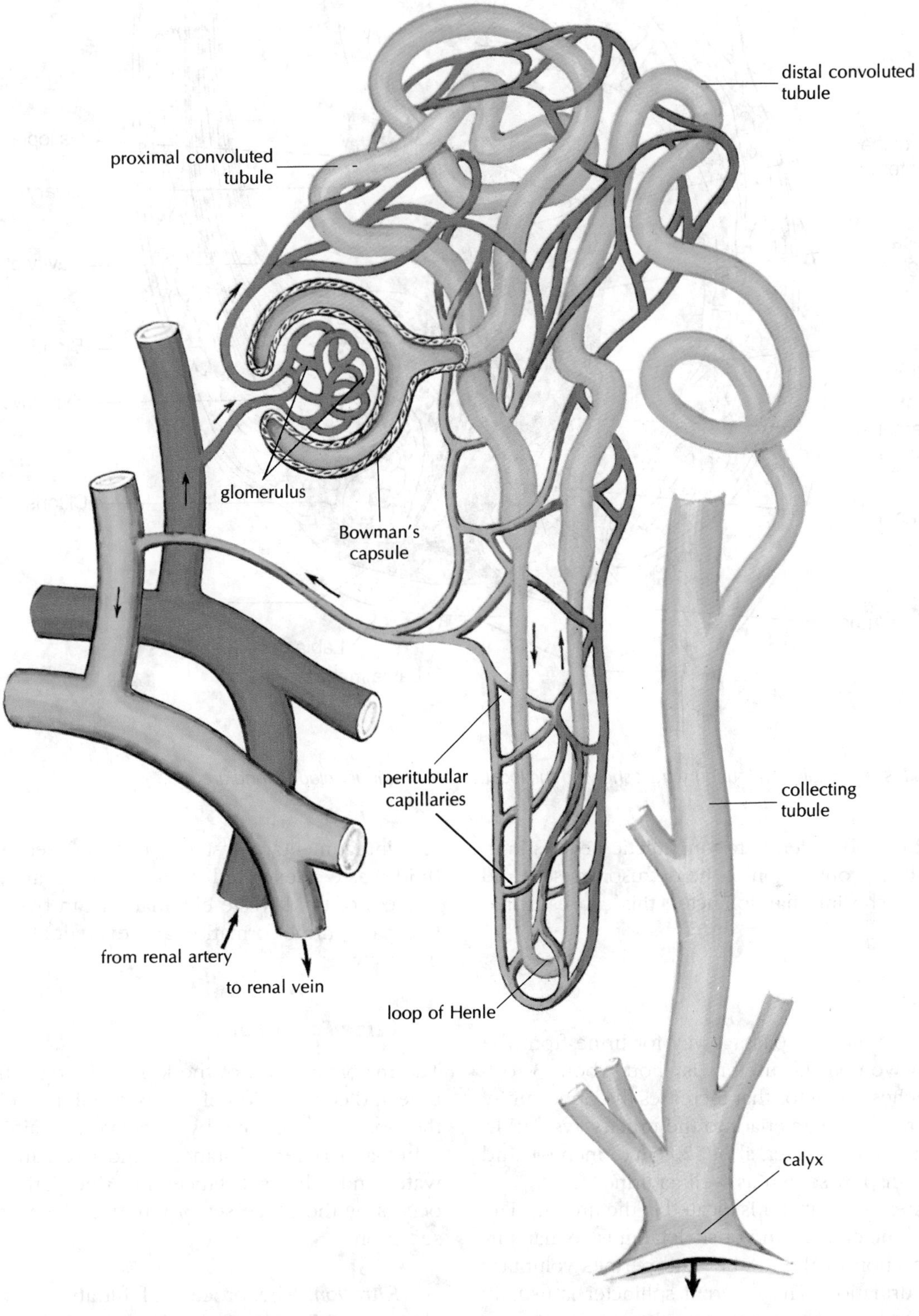

Figure 41-2 • *The nephron: the functional unit of the kidney.*

physis pubis when empty. In the woman, the bladder is located in front of the uterus and the vagina, as illustrated in Figure 41-3. In the man, the bladder is located in front of the rectum and above the prostate gland (see Fig. 52-1).

The body of the bladder is composed of three layers of smooth muscle. The inner and outer layers are longitudinal, whereas the middle layer is circular. Collectively, these three layers are called the **detrusor** muscle. The bladder is hollow when empty but is capable of expansion to hold a considerable amount of urine.

The lower portion of the bladder, approximately 2 to 3 cm long, is called the bladder neck or internal urinary sphincter. Autonomic nervous innervation affects smooth muscle control of the internal sphincter. Sympathetic impulses cause the sphincter to contract, keeping

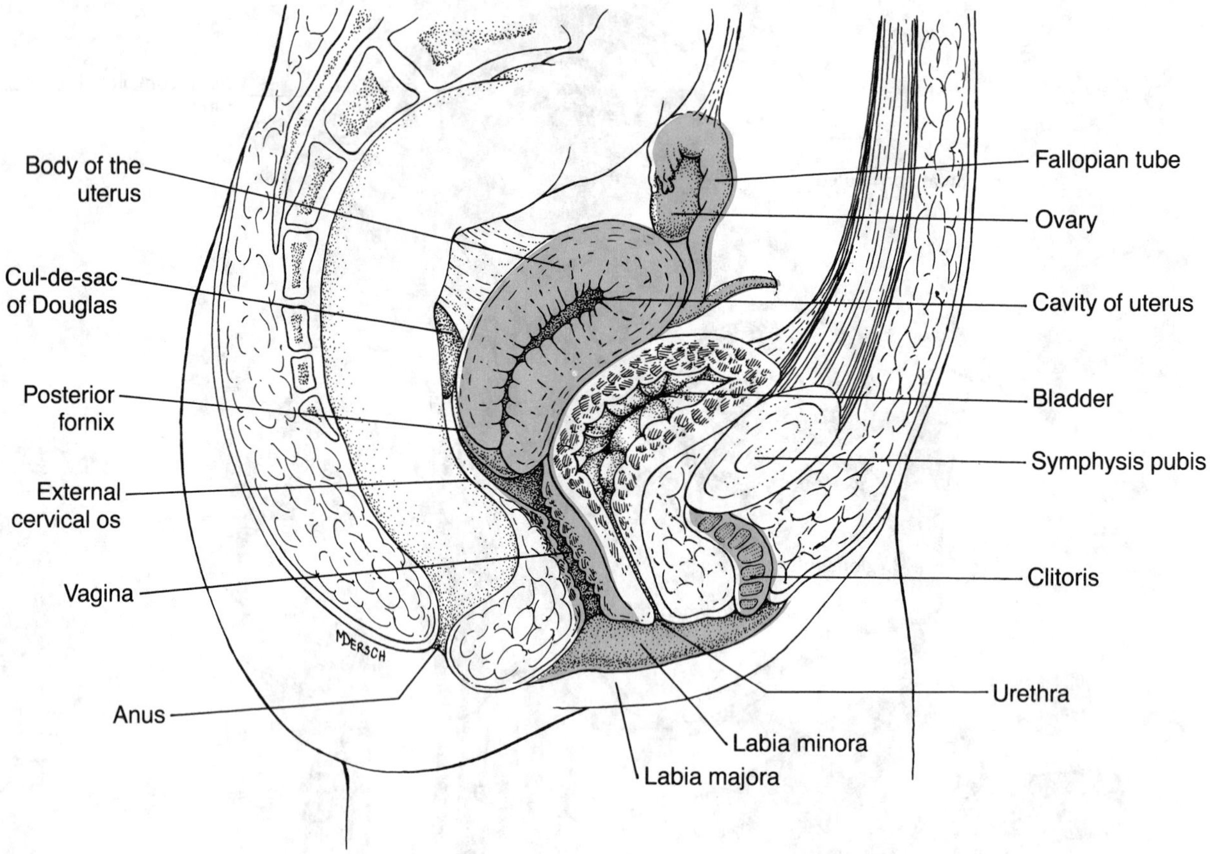

Figure 41-3 • *Female genitourinary tract showing the location of the urinary bladder and urethra.*

the urine in the bladder. Parasympathetic nerve stimulation results in contraction of the detrusor muscle and relaxation of the internal sphincter; this causes urination to occur.

Urethra

The urethra is the exit passageway for urine from the bladder. In women the urethra is short, about 3 to 5 cm (1–2 inches), a factor that increases the opportunity for the entrance of bacteria into the urinary system. In men, the urethra is longer, about 20 cm (8 inches), and serves to transport semen as well as urine.

The external sphincter is located in the urethra. The external sphincter is a band of skeletal muscle that surrounds a section of the urethra and permits voluntary control of urination. The external sphincter is usually contracted to keep the urethra closed and prevent constant emptying of urine from the bladder. When the external sphincter relaxes, urine can flow out from the bladder.

Normal Function of the Urinary System

The elimination of fluid waste from the body is the function of the urinary system. Small amounts of fluid waste are excreted by the gastrointestinal, respiratory, and integumentary systems, but the great majority of fluid waste is excreted through the renal system. The process of fluid waste elimination can be divided into two parts, urine formation and excretion of urine from the body.

Urine Formation

The major function of the kidney is regulation of volume and composition of the extracellular fluid (ECF) of the body. It does this by selectively retaining wanted water and other substances, and excreting unwanted water and other substances in urine. Urine formation occurs by the processes of filtration, reabsorption, and secretion.

Filtration. The process of filtration begins at the glomerulus. The renal arteries bring blood to the kidneys; the smaller branches of these arteries bring blood to the glomerulus of each nephron. The capillaries of the glomerulus are porous, and as the blood passes through the glomerular capillaries, some of the constituents of the blood are actually filtered out. The red blood cells and the proteins are too large to be filtered, and remain in the capillary, but most of the remaining plasma constituents can be filtered. The fluid that is filtered out of the glomerulus into the Bowman's capsule is called the glomerular filtrate.

Reabsorption. The glomerular filtrate then enters the second segment of the nephron, the tubule. The tubule actively and passively reabsorbs substances that the body wants to retain. These substances include varying amounts of water and electrolytes (Na^+, K^+, Cl^-, and HCO_3^-), and all of the glucose and amino acids. Reabsorption occurs mostly in the proximal convoluted tubule but also in the distal and collecting tubules. Almost 99% of the glomerular filtrate is reabsorbed by the tubules. Only 1% of the glomerular filtrate remains unabsorbed by the tubules, to form the fluid waste called urine (Smeltzer & Bare, 1996).

Secretion. In addition to reabsorbing substances, the tubules secrete some substances to rid them from the body. Varying amounts of H^+ ions and K^+ ions are secreted, as well as ammonia, creatinine, uric acid, and some other metabolites. Urine then consists of the 1% of unreabsorbed glomerular filtrate plus some secreted substances. By forming urine, the kidney successfully accomplishes its major role of regulating the volume and composition of the ECF.

Process of Urination

Several words are used to describe the process of excreting urine from the body, including urination, voiding, and **micturition**. In adults, the emptying of the bladder usually occurs when the bladder is stretched or distended by about 250 to 400 mL of urine. Smaller amounts of urine trigger bladder emptying in children. When the volume of urine in the bladder reaches the range of 250 to 400 mL, the pressure of that amount stretches the detrusor sufficiently to begin to force the bladder neck to open. This sensation of stretch in the detrusor is transmitted to sacral segments of the spinal cord; reflex motor action is transmitted back to the detrusor muscle to cause it to contract. The detrusor contraction causes even more stretch and pressure, and it is usually at this point that the person perceives a full bladder and the need to urinate. This reaction of bladder stretch, leading to bladder contraction and the perceived need to void, is called the micturition reflex. The micturition reflex is an involuntary spinal cord reflex.

In children younger than 3 years of age, the micturition reflex leads to spontaneous urination. Beyond 3 years of age, however, most people have learned to postpone urination until the time and place is more socially acceptable; this is because the act of urination is ultimately controlled by higher nerve centers in the brain. The person can consciously decide to postpone voiding by keeping the external sphincter, a skeletal muscle, contracted in a closed position. This effectively keeps urine from being released, even in the presence of the micturition reflex. When the person decides the time and place is right for voiding, the external sphincter can consciously be relaxed, permitting urine to flow from the bladder. The emptying of the bladder also involves the contraction of abdominal muscles and the relaxation of pelvic floor muscles. The amount of urine emptied is usually in the range of 250 to 400 mL per void. All but 5 to 10 mL of urine is typically emptied from the bladder (Guyton, 1995).

Characteristics of Normal Urine

Common characteristics of urine include amount, color, clarity, and odor. Many factors can produce normal variations among different people, or even variations at different times for the same person.

Volume. The average amount of urine per void for an adult is approximately 250 to 400 mL. Urinary output can vary greatly, depending on intake and other fluid losses. A catheterized client should drain a minimum of 30 mL of urine per hour. Urine output less than 30 mL per hour can indicate inadequate blood flow to the kidneys.

Color. The color of urine ranges from a light yellow, to a darker yellow, to a dark yellow–brown, called amber. The client's state of hydration alters the color. Urine may be almost colorless if it is very dilute secondary to a high fluid intake. Urine may be dark amber or orange–brown if it is very concentrated secondary to a decreased fluid intake. Medications may also alter the color of urine. The urine may appear dark reddish brown or streaked with blood if a woman is menstruating.

Clarity. Urine is normally transparent. Freshly voided urine should appear clear, without sediment. Urine draining from a retention catheter should appear clear and without sediment in the tubing, but may contain occasional mucus shreds. Urine that has been sitting unemptied in a urinal or collecting device for an hour or more may normally appear cloudy secondary to separation or settling of urinary constituents.

Odor. The odor of freshly voided urine is typically described as aromatic. Generally, the more dilute the urine, the fainter the odor, and the more concentrated the urine, the stronger the odor. Urine that has been sitting unemptied for a long period of time may have a strong ammonia odor. Medications and certain foods may alter the odor of urine. A strong, offensive odor is not normally present in urine free of infection.

Normal Pattern of Urinary Elimination

Many people have a routine pattern associated with urinary elimination. Most people void four to six times a day. Typically, people void soon after getting out of bed in the morning. Many people tend to void within an hour after mealtime and once again before bedtime. Variations in the pattern of fluid intake have a direct effect on the routine pattern of voiding.

The total amount of urine voided during a 24-hour period usually ranges from 1,200 to 1,500 mL. Each void should contain a minimum of approximately 200 mL and a maximum of 500 mL.

Factors Affecting Normal Urinary Elimination

Many factors can affect normal urinary elimination. Fluid intake, loss of body fluid, dietary intake, body position, and psychological factors all can affect normal urinary patterns.

Fluid Intake. The amount of fluid ingested by a person is the most influential factor in determining urine output. If all other factors are held constant, a complementary relationship exists between fluid intake and urine output. If a person increases the volume of fluid intake there will be an associated increase in the volume of urine output. Conversely, a decrease in fluid intake will cause a corresponding decrease in urine output. This relationship is hormonally controlled.

Several hormones, the most important of which is antidiuretic hormone (ADH), play significant roles in the reabsorption of water in the tubules of the nephron. The name "antidiuretic" implies its function, which is to prevent **diuresis**, or the excretion of water. ADH is secreted by the hypothalamus and released by the posterior pituitary in the brain. Increased plasma osmolarity stimulates the release of ADH (this is discussed in detail in Chapter 36). When ADH is present, the distal tubule of the nephron becomes more permeable to water. The release of ADH causes more water to be reabsorbed by the kidney, thus producing a more concentrated urine. When fluid intake is increased, ADH release is suppressed. In the absence of ADH, the renal tubules become relatively impermeable to water, and little water is reabsorbed. This produces increased volume of dilute urine.

Not only does the amount of fluid intake have an effect on the amount of urine produced, but it also influences the frequency of urination. If fluid intake is greatly increased, frequency of voiding increases because the bladder fills more quickly. Conversely, if fluid intake is low, voiding frequency decreases.

Loss of Body Fluid. When a person loses a great deal of body fluid, the kidneys increase reabsorption of water from the glomerular filtrate to maintain the proper osmolarity of the ECF. This saving of water to regulate the concentration of solutes in the ECF results in decreased urine output. Increased loss of body fluids can occur with vomiting, diarrhea, excessive diaphoresis secondary to fever or exercise, excessive wound drainage, extensive burns, or blood loss from trauma or surgery.

Nutrition. Diet may affect urinary elimination. If the diet contains a high percentage of foods that have a high water content (eg, fresh fruits and vegetables), urine volume will be greater than if these foods are ingested on a limited basis. If large quantities of salty foods are ingested without increasing water intake, urine output will decrease and be more concentrated.

Alcohol or foods containing caffeine (such as coffee, tea, cola, and chocolate) also affect urinary output. Alcohol and caffeine both contain a diuretic and increase urine output.

Body Position. Body position plays an important role in the ability to empty the bladder completely with each voiding. The typical body position for urinary elimination in men is the upright standing position. Some men find it difficult to empty their bladder fully into a urinal while lying flat in bed. Commonly, this alters the voiding pattern so that voiding is more frequent, with less volume. The normal position for voiding in women is the sitting position. If a woman must use a bedpan while flat in bed, she also may be unable completely to empty her bladder.

Psychological Factors. Because the release of urine from the bladder is ultimately under voluntary conscious control, the process of voiding can be influenced by anything that causes one to think about voiding. If another person talks about the need to void, one may also feel the urge to void. If one reads a chapter about urinary elimination, one may need a bathroom break before finishing. If one hears running water, the need to void may be intensified. Pouring warm water over a client's inner thigh or perineal area may stimulate voiding; giving a client a cold bedpan may temporarily prevent voiding.

Stress or anxiety can have an effect on urinary elimination. In a stressful or anxious situation, a person can experience a strong urge to urinate. Stress can also cause the reverse problem of urinary retention. A person's muscles become so tense that relaxation of the perineal muscles does not occur, thus inhibiting voiding.

Privacy for voiding is an important psychological factor to consider. Many people are unable to relax their perineal muscles if they feel they have inadequate privacy. Women, in particular, have been culturally trained to require more privacy for voiding. Women's public restrooms always have private stalls for elimination, whereas men's public restrooms have open rows of receptacles for urinary elimination. People have varying requirements of privacy for voiding.

Lifespan Considerations

Newborn and Infant

The kidneys of the fetus begin functioning and the fetus voids urine in utero from about the third month after conception. The newborn, therefore, may have urine in his or her bladder at birth and should be able to void within the first 24 hours after birth. The first voiding may be of slightly pink-tinged urine. The pinkish color is caused by an accumulation of uric acid crystals. It is important to note the first voiding after birth to verify that urine formation and elimination are adequate. The kidneys at birth are still not fully developed; Bowman's capsule and the tubules are still refining their respective filtering and reabsorption abilities. It is likely that the newborn will void small amounts (15–30 mL, up to 30–40 times a day) of a dilute, light yellow-colored urine. As the infant grows, he or she is able to void in slightly larger amounts at slightly less frequent intervals. The color of the urine remains pale yellow throughout infancy. The total amount of urine voided in a 24-hour period depends on total fluid intake and fluid losses from other sources. The average urine output for the newborn or infant is about 500 to 600 mL in 24 hours. Table 41-1 gives the normal ranges of daily urine output during the lifespan.

An infant has no voluntary control of urinary elimination. The sacral spinal cord segments innervating the bladder are not yet mature. The bladder will empty in reflex fashion after a degree of bladder stretch has occurred.

Serious alterations in urinary elimination may be caused by congenital malformations of the urinary tract or the central nervous system. Urinary tract infections (UTIs), which are more common in the female infant than the male infant, can also cause disruption of normal urinary function.

Toddler and Preschooler

It is during toddlerhood and the preschool years that a child usually achieves voluntary urinary continence. During this time, a child becomes physiologically and psychologically capable of this task. Sometime between 12 to 18 months, the myelinization of the sacral spinal segments that control the bladder becomes complete, and a child can then perceive bladder fullness. A good indicator of the maturation of the spinal cord is when a toddler can walk independently.

Even though a toddler can perceive bladder fullness by age 18 months, he or she may not choose voluntarily to hold the urine in the bladder and delay voiding. Sometime between 2.5 to 3 years, most children can perceive a full bladder *and* voluntarily delay voiding. Children also need a sufficient vocabulary to communicate the need to urinate, be able to access toilet facilities, and have sufficient fine motor control to loosen or remove necessary clothing (Fig. 41-4). In the American culture, most parents sense their child's readiness to begin toilet training at age 2.5 to 3 years. They notice that the child is voiding less frequently (longer periods of diaper dryness) and is able to acknowledge in words that he or she does feel bladder fullness. Sometimes toddlers need to experience some outdoor play time without a diaper to see visually what happens when they experience bladder fullness followed by urethral relaxation and bladder emptying. They begin to understand cognitively the relationship between bladder fullness and voluntary bladder emptying, and are ready for toilet training. Children in the American culture usually achieve daytime urinary continence by 3 years of age; boys may take longer to achieve daytime continence. Nighttime continence may not occur until 4 or 5 years of age.

Table 41-1 • Normal Ranges for Daily Urine Output During Lifespan

Age (years)	Output (mL)
Newborn–2	500–600
2–5	500–800
5–8	600–1,200
8–14	1,000–1,500
14 and over	1,500

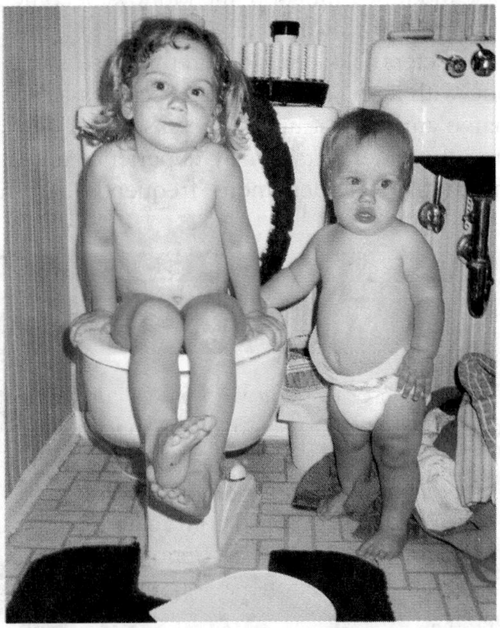

Figure 41-4 • *Sometimes toddlers learn about toileting from their older siblings. (From Jackson, D.B., & Saunders, R.B. (1993).* Child health nursing: A comprehensive approach to the care of children and their families. *Philadelphia, J.B. Lippincott.)*

Child and Adolescent

School-age children have achieved both daytime and nighttime urinary continence. These children and adolescents are approaching the urinary elimination habits of adults; they void straw-colored urine six to seven times a day. The amount of urine output is greatly influenced by the amount of oral fluid intake; Table 41-1 lists the average ranges of urine output in a 24-hour period. A small percentage of school-age children continue to experience involuntary urinary incontinence, which is termed enuresis. Parents often seek advice from healthcare providers when nocturnal enuresis occurs past 7 years of age. Specific nursing interventions for the management of nocturnal enuresis are discussed later in this chapter.

Adult and Older Adult

In late middle age, men may experience altered urinary elimination related to prostatic hypertrophy, and women may experience altered urinary elimination related to weakened perineal muscles (cystocele or rectocele).

As a result of cardiovascular changes that occur with aging, there is usually decreased perfusion to the kidneys in the older adult. This decreased arterial flow to the renal arteries is a gradual change that results from decreased cardiac muscle strength, which reduces cardiac output to the periphery, and a decrease in the elasticity of the peripheral blood vessels. Over time, owing to decreased arterial perfusion, there is a progressive decrease in kidney function; the kidneys become a less effective regulator of the body's ECF.

The ureters, bladder, and urethra lose some muscle tone with aging. The bladder becomes less able to hold large amounts of urine (decreased bladder capacity), and the older person may experience an urgency to empty the bladder more frequently of smaller amounts of urine. The urge to void may be sensed only when the bladder is at the limit of its capacity, which diminishes the ability voluntarily to delay voiding (Turner & Plymat, 1987). Uninhibited bladder contractions can further increase the sense of urgency. These factors place older people at risk for incontinence. Nocturia is a frequent complaint in older adults, and urinary retention is also more common in the older adults. This predisposes older adults to UTIs. Women may experience stress incontinence as they age, related to weakened perineal muscles. Older men eventually experience urinary hesitancy and difficulty starting the urinary stream, related to prostatic hypertrophy.

Factors Associated With Altered Urinary Elimination

- Obstruction of urine flow: renal calculi, prostatic enlargement, tumors, structural abnormalities
- Infection
- Hypotension
- Neurologic injury: spinal cord injury, cerebral vascular accident (stroke), brain tumor
- Decreased muscle tone: aging, multiple pregnancies, obesity
- Medications
- Surgery: anesthesia, edema, immobility
- Pregnancy
- Urinary diversions

Altered Urinary Function

Potential for Altered Urinary Function

Many factors can predispose a person to disruption of normal patterns of urinary elimination (see the accompanying display). Obstruction of urine flow, UTIs, hypotension, neurologic injury, medications, surgery, pregnancy, and urinary diversion all affect urinary function.

Obstruction of Urine Flow

Obstruction of the normal flow of urine can lead to problems in urinary elimination, and, when severe, can cause kidney damage. Urinary obstruction can be caused by structural abnormalities within the urinary tract, urinary tumors or other tumors that press against the urinary tract, renal stones, or prostatic enlargement. Obstruction can also occur when a client has a catheter or tubes in place to drain urine, and they become plugged or kinked.

One of the complications of obstruction within the urinary system is hydronephrosis. Hydronephrosis is the distention of the kidney pelvis with urine secondary to the increased resistance caused by obstruction to normal urine flow. Unrelieved hydronephrosis can cause renal cell atrophy and necrosis, which can cause permanent kidney damage.

Urinary stasis also occurs secondary to urinary obstruction. The stagnant urine proximal to the obstruction provides a good growth medium for microorganisms, and thus fosters the development of UTIs.

Infections of the Urinary Tract

Urinary tract infections are usually caused by microorganisms normally found in the gastrointestinal tract. The microorganisms commonly responsible for UTIs are of the Enterobacteriaceae species, including *Escherichia coli, Klebsiella,* and *Proteus* (Conti & Eutropius, 1987). These microorganisms typically gain access to the urinary system via the urethral meatus. Hence, the most common UTIs are infections of the urethra (urethritis) or bladder (cystitis). Urethritis and cystitis are classified as lower UTIs, whereas infections of the ureters (ureteritis) and the kidney pelvis or tubule system are classified as upper UTIs. Upper UTIs occur less frequently, but are more serious, because kidney damage and renal failure may result.

Normally the urinary tract is sterile, except at the urethral meatus. In the healthy person, bacteria tend to be flushed away during the act of voiding. Infection occurs when microorganisms from the surrounding perineal skin or anal opening find their way to the urinary meatus and ascend the urethra. Women are more susceptible to lower UTIs because of the short length of the female urethra and the proximity of the vagina and anus to the urinary meatus. Men are less susceptible to lower UTIs because of the longer length of the male urethra, and also because of the antibacterial properties of prostatic secretions (Conti & Eutropius, 1987).

Other factors that can increase the incidence of UTIs include incorrect wiping of the anal area after a bowel movement, sexual intercourse, which can bring perineal microorganisms into closer contact with the urinary meatus, and any procedure that places an object in the urethra or bladder for diagnostic or therapeutic reasons. The longer a catheter remains in the bladder, the greater the chance of nosocomial infection (Resnick, 1993).

Infections of the urinary tract can disrupt the normal pattern of urinary elimination in a number of ways. Voiding becomes painful and more frequent. The person with a UTI often experiences urgency, a subjective feeling of being unable voluntarily to delay the urge to void. Urine becomes abnormal, containing pus (pyuria) and blood (hematuria). Ultimately, if the infection ascends to the kidney, renal damage can occur and possibly result in renal failure.

Hypotension

It is important to maintain adequate blood perfusion to the kidneys to ensure urine formation. When arterial blood pressure drops too low, the renal arteries do not have enough pressure to cause glomerular filtration. Inadequate circulating volume or inability of the heart to pump adequately can decrease blood flow to the kidneys. Decreased circulating volume can occur after surgery, trauma, or when the client has severe loss of fluids, such as from diarrhea or vomiting. When urine output drops below 30 mL per hour for 2 consecutive hours, decreased perfusion of blood to the kidneys and other vital organs must be suspected.

Neurologic Injury

Neurologic injury after a stroke or spinal cord injury can cause disruption in normal patterns of urinary elimination. Injury (by trauma, hemorrhage, or tumor) to the frontal lobes of the brain, which control the voluntary nature of voiding, can lead to incontinence.

The micturition reflex occurs at the sacral level of the spinal cord. If the spinal cord is injured at the sacral level or above, the person will experience a change in control of urinary elimination. A person may experience reflex voiding, which results in incontinence. This occurs because as soon as the bladder is stretched to a certain degree, a reflex contraction of the bladder occurs, resulting in loss of urine. This condition is called reflex neurogenic bladder. If the reflex arc itself is injured, the bladder may fill without the bladder stretch contraction mechanism working, resulting in urinary retention. This condition is called autonomous neurogenic bladder.

Decreased Muscle Tone

Weakened abdominal and perineal muscles can impair bladder contraction and control of the external urinary sphincter. Abdominal and perineal muscles can become weak because of obesity, multiple pregnancies, stretching during childbirth, menopausal atrophy due to decreased estrogen, and chronic constipation. A cystocele is the protrusion or herniation of the bladder into the vaginal canal; it produces symptoms of stress incontinence, frequency, dribbling, and an inability to empty the bladder completely.

Continuous bladder drainage with a catheter can also cause decreased bladder tone. Continuous bladder drainage prevents the bladder from ever getting full; thus, stretch of the bladder musculature is limited, promoting bladder atrophy. After the removal of a catheter, some clients experience dribbling and difficulty with urinary control. This is usually temporary, lasting until bladder tone returns.

Pregnancy

Pregnancy can cause an alteration in urinary elimination. The increasing size and weight of the growing uterus can exert pressure on the bladder, a common cause of frequency in pregnant women. Compression of the bladder by the uterus may also lead to obstruction of urinary flow and incomplete emptying of the bladder. During the early postpartum period, a woman is also prone to altered urinary function. Trauma from vaginal delivery causes swelling in the perineal area, which can obstruct the flow of urine.

Surgery

Postoperative clients should be able to void within 10 hours after surgery. Some clients have postoperative difficulty voiding for a number of reasons. Often, postoperative clients are volume depleted because of limited fluid intake and loss of blood and fluid during surgery. The stress of surgery triggers the release of ADH, which decreases urinary output. During the immediate postoperative period, clients often are unable to get up and use the bathroom. Using a bedpan or urinal in a supine position often impedes normal urinary patterns. Many medications used to control postoperative pain have urinary retention as a side effect. This is especially true when opioids are administered epidurally for pain control.

Surgery involving the urinary system, intestines, or reproductive organs predisposes a client to urinary retention. Trauma to tissues can cause edema, which can potentially obstruct the flow of urine. The use of a retention catheter is indicated after any surgery on the urinary tract.

Anesthesia can also affect urinary elimination. Anesthetic agents slow the glomerular filtration rate, reducing urinary output. People receiving a spinal or regional block during surgery are at increased risk for postoperative urinary problems because these agents impair the sensory and motor impulses that control micturition. Until the anesthesia has worn off, the client will be unable to perceive bladder fullness and will not be able to initiate voiding. This can cause urinary retention.

Medications

Medications can be given therapeutically to affect urinary elimination, and medications administered for other reasons can have side effects that influence normal urinary patterns. Some medications also change the color of urine.

Medications classified as diuretics are administered to increase urine output. They accomplish this by affecting the reabsorption of sodium and water in the tubules of the nephron. Commonly used diuretics include chlorathiazide, hydrochlorathiazide, furosemide, spironolactone, and triamterene. People with edema or a propensity toward development of edema are candidates for diuretic therapy. Cholinergic medications (eg, Urecholine [bethanechol; Merck Sharp & Dohme, West Point, PA]) may be given to promote voiding because they stimulate contraction of the detrusor muscle.

Side effects of medications used to treat other health problems can adversely affect urinary elimination. The risk of urinary retention is increased with medications having anticholinergic effects. Belladonna alkaloids, phenothiazines, tricyclic antidepressants, and antihistamines are examples of such drugs. Narcotics can decrease glomerular filtration rate and decrease the sensation of bladder fullness.

Some medications can change the color of urine. For example, pyridium causes the urine to turn bright orange, and amitriptyline turns urine blue–green.

Urinary Diversion

A urinary diversion is a surgical procedure in which the normal pathway of urine elimination is altered. The ureters are rerouted from a diseased or damaged urinary system to a new outlet, called a stoma, created surgically on the client's abdomen. The diversion may be permanent, as with cancerous conditions that require removal of the bladder (cystectomy). In other conditions, such as trauma or severe chronic UTIs, the diversion may be temporary to promote healing.

Urinary diversions alter normal urinary elimination because the person no longer has control over voiding. Although the person is able to engage in all normal activities, adjustment to the urinary diversion and learning to manage it may take some time.

Four types of urinary diversions are the ileal conduit (or ileal loop), the Kock pouch diversion, the ureterostomy, and the vesicostomy (Fig. 41-5).

Ileal Conduit. The procedure known as an ileal conduit or ileal loop involves removing a small segment of the ileum and then reattaching the two portions of the intestine that have been severed. One end of the removed section is sutured closed to form a conduit for urine collection and passage; the other end is brought out through the abdominal wall to form a stoma. The stoma usually protrudes 0.5 to 0.75 inch above the abdominal skin. The ureters are then implanted into the conduit so that urine flows from the kidneys into the conduit (through the ureters), and out through the stoma. The client is fitted with and uses a stoma appliance to collect urine. The ileal conduit is the most common type of urinary diversion.

Kock Pouch Diversion. The Kock pouch diversion is similar to the ileal conduit except that it requires no external appliance to collect urine. Instead, a pouch is formed by taking a 60- to 70-cm segment of ileum, which will hold urine inside the body. The urine is prevented from leaking out of the pouch through the stoma by an outlet nipple valve, which is created using intussuscepted portions of the ileal segment (the tissue is folded back against itself in such a way that the path of fluid is obstructed). Reflux of urine from the pouch back into the ureters is prevented with a similar inlet nipple valve. Urine is removed from the internal pouch on a scheduled basis, usually four to six times a day, by inserting a catheter through the stoma, through the outlet valve, and into the pouch.

Ureterostomy. The ureterostomy urinary diversion has the ureters diverted from their normal attachment in the bladder to the client's abdominal wall or flank. Like the ileal conduit, a stoma is created, one or two depending on whether one ureter has been connected to the other before being brought to the body's sur-

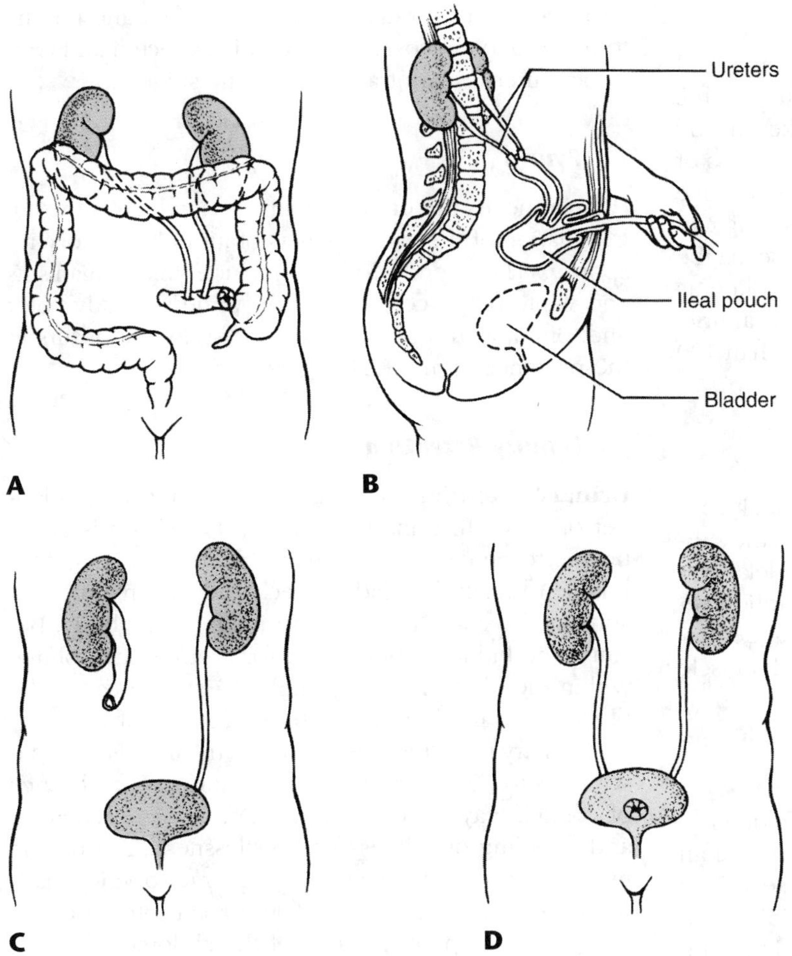

Figure 41-5 • *Urinary diversions: (A) Ileal conduit. (B) Kock pouch. (C) Ureterostomy. (D) Vesicostomy.*

face. Urine drains continuously from the ureters out through the stoma, which necessitates the use of an appliance to collect urine.

Vesicostomy. The vesicostomy urinary diversion involves suturing closed the neck of the bladder, bringing forward the anterior wall of the bladder to the abdomen, and then forming a tube and stoma from a portion of the anterior bladder wall. Urine drains continuously from a portion of the bladder through the exit tube and stoma, so a urinary diversion appliance must be worn. A continent vesicostomy is similar to the Kock pouch diversion, however, in that it can be created by forming an outlet nipple valve from intussuscepted portions of the anterior wall. The client is routinely catheterized or performs self-catheterization to remove urine.

Manifestations of Altered Urinary Function

Disruption of normal patterns of urinary elimination can be seen in the following signs and symptoms: dysuria, polyuria, oliguria, urgency, frequency, hematuria, urinary retention, incontinence, and enuresis. The nurse plays a significant role in detecting abnormal patterns of urinary elimination, as well as in preventing such problems.

Dysuria

Dysuria means painful voiding. Pain is often associated with UTIs and is felt as a burning sensation during urination. Any bladder inflammation or trauma, or inflammation of the urethra can cause dysuria. Dysuria may occur temporarily after sexual activity, and is often associated with sexually transmitted disease in both men and women. Some medications can cause dysuria. Painful voiding should be referred to a physician because there are many causes of dysuria.

Polyuria

Polyuria is the formation and excretion of excessive amounts of urine in the absence of a concurrent increase in fluid intake. Urine output of greater than 2,500 to 3,000 mL in 24 hours is considered polyuria. Untreated diabetes insipidus and diabetes mellitus can greatly increase urine output. Ingestion of diuretics, caffeine, and alcohol also results in polyuria.

Oliguria

Oliguria is the formation and excretion of decreased amounts of urine, or urinary output less than 500 mL in 24 hours. A severe decrease in fluid intake, or any disease state or injury that leads to an excessive loss of body fluids, can cause oliguria. For example, excessive vomiting, diarrhea, diaphoresis, burns, or bleeding can decrease urine output. People with renal disease maybe oliguric. As the kidney approaches complete failure as a functioning organ, the person may become anuric. **Anuria** is the formation and excretion of less than 100 mL of urine in 24 hours.

Urgency

Most adults can delay emptying the bladder until it contains 250 to 400 mL of urine. Urgency describes the subjective feeling of being unable voluntarily to delay the urge to void. Urgency implies a strong micturition reflex due to inflammation or irritation of the bladder, incompetent urethral sphincter, weak perineal muscle control, or psychological stress.

Frequency

Voiding at frequent intervals is known as frequency. This occurs when a person voids more frequently than the normal pattern, without a significant increase in fluid intake. Each void usually contains less than 250 mL of urine. Frequency not associated with increased fluid intake can be related to other factors, such as UTIs or pressure on the bladder from pregnancy. Frequency and urgency often occur together.

Nocturia

Voiding during normal sleeping hours is called nocturia. If a person voids before going to bed, it should be possible to sleep for 7 to 8 hours without feeling a strong micturition reflex. Ingestion of large amounts of fluids before bed, especially those containing alcohol or caffeine, may promote nocturia. People with medical conditions such as congestive heart failure may also experience nocturia. When lying supine, edema decreases as fluid enters the circulation. This increases blood flow to the kidneys and thus increases glomerular filtration and urine output.

Hematuria

Hematuria indicates blood in the urine; it can be gross (visible on visual examination) or occult (not visible on visual examination). Occult blood may change the color of urine from normal clear yellow or amber to a cloudy or hazy yellow or amber. As the number of red blood cells increases, the urine may become bright red in color. Pathologic causes of hematuria include UTIs, urinary tract tumors, renal calculi, poisoning, and trauma to the urinary mucosa. Hematuria is expected and temporary after urinary tract or prostatic surgery.

Pyuria

Pyuria means the urine contains pus, which is the accumulation of the end-products of an inflammatory response. These end-products include microorganisms and white blood cells. Pus gives urine a cloudy color and, often, a strong, unpleasant odor. Pyuria occurs in the presence of any UTI.

Urinary Retention

Urinary retention is the inability to empty the bladder of urine. In urinary retention, the person is either unable to perceive the growing bladder fullness, or is unable to relax the bladder neck and external urethral sphincter to allow passage of urine from the body. Because the kidneys continue to form urine, the volume within the bladder grows, until, in extreme cases, the bladder can hold up to 2,000 to 3,000 mL of urine.

Urinary retention often involves the inability to void within 8 to 10 hours of the last voiding. The absence of voiding may be followed by suprapubic discomfort, and a feeling of fullness and restlessness. The person may or may not perceive a strong urge to void. Bladder distention of more than 600 mL can often be palpated in the suprapubic area of the abdomen.

Urinary retention with overflow is the loss of small amounts of urine from an overdistended bladder. As the bladder becomes overdistended with urine, it no longer responds to bladder stretch as a stimulus to initiate detrusor contraction and voiding. The bladder can maintain only a certain degree of overdistention before excess urine is eliminated in small amounts at frequent intervals. The small amounts of urine that are voided are known as "overflow."

Complications of urinary retention include the loss of bladder tone secondary to the excessive stretch of the detrusor muscle fibers. Even after the primary retention is relieved, it may take a period of weeks for the bladder/stretch—bladder/emptying response to return to normal. The accumulation of urine in the bladder also leads to stasis of urine, which predisposes the person to UTI and calculus development. Bladder distention can also lead to hydronephrosis as the urine backs up into the ureters and kidney.

People at risk for development of urinary retention include those with neurologic impairment, such as spinal cord injury or brain lesions. Postoperative clients may experience temporary urinary retention until edema subsides and spinal anesthesia wears off. After vaginal delivery of a baby, swelling of the urinary meatus is a common occurrence that may cause a temporary obstruction to the outflow of urine.

Incontinence

Urinary incontinence is the involuntary loss of urine from the bladder. Five types of urinary incontinence are identified by patterns of uncontrolled voiding and related causative factors. The five classifications are stress, urge, reflex, functional, and total incontinence. The accompanying Therapeutic Dialogue addresses urinary incontinence.

Stress Incontinence. The sudden, involuntary loss of small amounts (less than 50 mL) of urine that accompanies a sudden increase in intraabdominal pressure is called stress incontinence. Examples of activities that increase intraabdominal pressure are coughing, sneezing, laughing, lifting, and jumping.

Factors associated with stress incontinence include a weakening of the pelvic floor muscles, high intraabdominal pressure, damage to the bladder neck, or side effects of medications. The pelvic floor muscles can be weakened by the stretching that occurs during childbirth. Women who have experienced a long and difficult labor and delivery or who have experienced multiple childbirths are most likely to have weakened pelvic muscles. Estrogen is necessary to maintain the normal tone of reproductive organs and associated musculature; therefore, postmenopausal women who have decreased estrogen levels may suffer from stress incontinence (Agency for Health Care Policy and Research, 1992). Obesity or pregnancy can cause high intraabdominal pressure. Obese, postmenopausal women who have had multiple pregnancies are most likely to experience stress incontinence. Another cause of stress incontinence is direct trauma, which may occur as a result of a fractured pelvis or during genitourinary surgery.

Urge Incontinence. The involuntary loss of urine after a strong feeling of the need to urinate is termed urge incontinence. The person with urge incontinence is unable simultaneously to perceive a full bladder and hold urine until the bathroom is reached. Urge incontinence is often accompanied by frequency, dysuria, and nocturia.

Factors associated with urge incontinence include UTIs, the use of diuretics, the consumption of fluids containing caffeine or alcohol, or an increase in fluid intake. An overdistended bladder can precipitate urge incontinence. Some clients experience urge incontinence

Therapeutic Dialogue
Urinary Incontinence

Scenes for Thought

Mrs. Clements is a 55-year-old woman who has been referred for complaints of incontinence of urine for 3 months. You are scheduled to perform a history and physical.

Effective

Nurse: *Good morning, Mrs. Clements. Please sit down so we can talk a while before I do your physical. (Acknowledge the client, give simple directions) What can I do for you this morning? (Open-ended question)*
Client: *You can help me stop wetting myself.* Client looks down at her lap.
Nurse: *You look worried about that. (Observing behavior accurately)*
Client: *Yes, I am.* Client looks up with relieved face. *Before my mother died last year she had to wear adult diapers; she always smelled and had bladder infections, and it was awful for her and for everyone else. I don't want to get that way.*
Nurse: *So what you would like is for me to help you figure out a way to deal with the wetting problem so you don't have to live the way your mother did. Is that right? (Stating what you understand the client wants and checking with her)*
Client: *Yes! That would be great.*
Nurse: *Okay. why don't we start with some questions, and then I'll do a physical and we can go from there. (Give client some idea of what you're planning to do)*

Less Effective

Nurse: *Good morning, Mrs. Clements. How are you today? Please sit down so I can ask you about your history. (Nurse asks about age, address, number of children, and other items on the assessment sheet)*
Client: *(Answers all questions quietly)*
Nurse: *I understand that you have an incontinence problem. Many women your age have that kind of difficulty, and I'm sure we can fix you up so you'll be just fine.*
Client: *My mother's doctor told her that years ago, but she never got better.* Looks down at her lap.
Nurse: *Well, we'll just see what we can do for you here. Could you undress and put on this gown? I'll be back in a minute to do your physical. (Leaves room, closing the door quietly)*

Critical Thinking Challenge

• *Critique what the nurse did that was effective in the first scene.* • *Consider how you think the client felt.* • *Determine what was less effective about the second scene.* • *Consider how you think the client felt in the second scene.* • *Although each nurse spent the same amount of time with the client, analyze how the second nurse could have been more effective.*

for a short period of time after an indwelling catheter has been removed. They have become accustomed to an empty bladder, and need time to accommodate the usual degree of bladder distention.

Reflex Incontinence. An involuntary loss of urine that occurs at somewhat predictable intervals when a specific bladder volume is reached is called reflex incontinence. The person is unable to sense bladder fullness because of neurologic impairment, and the bladder simply empties when a certain degree of bladder stretch has been reached. Bladder emptying occurs at the sacral reflex level, because the connection to the cerebrum allowing voluntary inhibition of voiding is impaired. Reflex incontinence is seen in the client with neurologic impairment, such as spinal cord lesion, cerebrovascular accident, or brain tumor.

Functional Incontinence. Functional incontinence involves the inability or unwillingness of a person with normal bladder and sphincter control to reach the bathroom in time to void. Environmental barriers, disorientation, or physical limitations can contribute. The amount of urine that is lost is typically large.

Many factors can interfere with the ability to reach the toilet in time. A poorly lit, cluttered room may obstruct easy access to the bathroom. Raised side rails or a call bell that is out of reach can contribute to functional incontinence in the hospitalized client. Sensory or cognitive factors are also associated with functional incontinence, because confusion, disorientation, and sedatives or side effects of medications can impair cognitive functioning. Motor deficits, such as impaired gait and loss of fine motor control needed to release necessary clothing, can also contribute.

Total Incontinence. The continuous, involuntary, unpredictable loss of urine from a nondistended bladder is termed total incontinence. The designation is sometimes used when the observed incontinence does not fit any other incontinence category and does not respond to usual incontinence treatment methods.

Factors associated with total incontinence include a specific neurologic lesion in the brain or spinal cord, traumatic or surgical injury to the genitourinary area or spinal cord, or a congenital malformation within the urinary tract or spinal cord.

Enuresis

Enuresis is involuntary voiding with no underlying pathophysiologic origin, after the age that bladder control is usually achieved. By the time most children are 4 or 5 years of age, they can control urinary elimination during both the day and night. Enuresis beyond the age of 5 years is typically nocturnal. Nocturnal enuresis is called bedwetting by most parents. Involuntary voiding during sleep can occur during daytime naps, but is more frequent during longer periods of sleep at night.

Factors associated with nocturnal enuresis include small bladder capacity, sound sleeping, stress and anxiety at home or school, UTIs, and family history of nocturnal enuresis.

Impact of Urinary Dysfunction on Activities of Daily Living

Individual Considerations

The elimination of fluid wastes from the body is an important function of daily living. The inability to do this properly has serious psychological and social implications. Incontinence can lead to social isolation because many people fear that bladder incontinence will prove embarrassing in social situations (Talbot, 1994). Sometimes this limits trips outside the home or limits social encounters to close friends only, who will understand if incontinence should occur. The loss of control over this basic body function can create feelings of anxiety or fear, whether in the 8-year-old with enuresis, or the 80-year-old in whom a bladder control problem has developed.

Planning should assist in maintaining normal urinary elimination whenever possible. Clothing should be chosen that is easy to get on and off and does not require dry cleaning. Some people may need to choose styles that will hide protective pants. If the location of the bathroom is upstairs or difficult to access, a urinal or bedside commode can help promote urinary continence. Adequate hygiene is important for people with alterations in urinary function. Adequate bathing after incontinence will decrease odor and prevent skin breakdown. Adequate washing may be difficult for the elderly, those who are cognitively impaired, or the child who has to get to school on time.

Family Considerations

Alterations in urinary elimination may place an extra financial burden and care responsibilities on the family or designated caregiver. Protective pants and special equipment such as ostomy supplies can be financially burdensome for a family, especially if the cost is not covered by insurance. Frequent trips to the physician and required medications can add to the financial burden and the caregiving burden. Frequently, extra energy and time must be spent washing clothing and bedding. If it is a child who is experiencing nocturnal enuresis, sleep is usually disrupted for the parent who gets up to help the child with these tasks.

Frequent uncontrolled incontinence in the older person often contributes to the family's decision to seek institutional care. For many people, a move to an extended care facility drastically affects independence in the tasks of daily living. As the percentage of the aged population increases, the impact on society at large is considerable.

Assessment

Functional assessment allows the nurse to collect subjective and objective data regarding normal urinary status and risk factors that can contribute to urinary dysfunction, and to identify dysfunctional urinary patterns. The nurse can collect such information by asking direct questions, watching for subtle nonverbal cues, performing physical assessment, and evaluating information gathered in diagnostic and laboratory tests.

Subjective Data

The collection of subjective information from the client (or other significant person) about urinary status usually begins with obtaining a detailed history. The nurse should ensure client privacy, and be sensitive to feelings of embarrassment the client may experience during the discussion of urinary function.

Functional Pattern Identification

It is often easier for the client to describe alterations in urinary elimination pattern than to describe normal urinary elimination. Normal patterns of elimination can be affected by many factors in daily living, so that some people have difficulty recognizing their own normal pattern within daily variation.

Specific questions regarding when the last voiding occurred, how many times per day urination usually occurs, whether each void contains a small, medium, or large amount of urine, and whether the client often wakes during the night to void, help the nurse identify normal patterns of urinary elimination. The nurse may have to clarify the term "urinating" by using other words the client may be more familiar with, such as voiding, peeing, passing water, or "going potty." The data the nurse gathers from such questions can then be analyzed to evaluate whether the client's typical pattern falls within expected parameters of the healthy child or adult.

Risk Identification

A nursing history also allows the nurse to identify factors that could potentially alter urinary elimination. Information should be elicited concerning previous renal or urinary tract problems, such as kidney failure, renal calculi, or UTIs. If one of these conditions is present, the nurse should obtain a history of the condition and how it was treated and resolved. The nurse should question the client about any previous genitourinary surgery, such as prostatic surgery or repair of a cystocele. Other acute or chronic medical problems, such as congestive heart failure or neurologic injury, should be evaluated in terms of their impact on normal patterns of urinary function.

Data should be elicited about recent changes in daily routine concerning exercise, food, or fluid intake. A significant change in oral intake or the consumption of beverages containing alcohol or caffeine should be noted. Medications that can alter urinary output or function, such as diuretics or anticholinergics, should also be indicated.

Motor or cognitive dysfunction that could impede successfully getting to a bathroom should be evaluated. Visual impairment or communication difficulties could also affect the ability to reach the bathroom in a timely manner in a new environmental setting. The general ability to understand and follow directions should be assessed so that teaching can be individualized for the client.

Dysfunction Identification

The collection of subjective data can also help the nurse identify dysfunctional patterns of urinary elimination. An open-ended question such as, "Have you noticed any problems with voiding lately?" is often a good way to begin. If the client responds by indicating no urinary difficulties, clarify the meaning of his or her response by asking more specific questions, such as:

Do you have any pain or burning with urination?
Have you noticed any pink or reddish color in your urine?
Do you feel you are able to empty your bladder completely every time you urinate?
Do you accidentally lose any urine when you sneeze or cough?
Do you have any difficulty stopping or starting your urinary stream?

Such questions are useful because alterations in normal urinary function often occur gradually and are perceived as normal by the client. For example, an older man may have had difficulty starting his urinary stream for the past 10 years as a result of prostatic enlargement, and does not view this as a urinary problem.

Abnormal patterns of voiding such as polyuria, oliguria, or anuria are important to document, as well as hematuria, dysuria, frequency, or urgency. When any of these are present, the nurse should question the client as to the length of time the problem has persisted, and when it first began.

If the client does indicate a chronic problem with urinary function, such as stress incontinence or a urinary diversion, the nurse should question the client regarding individual management of the problem. At this time, the nurse can also ask the client how he or she would like things handled during hospitalization. For example, the woman who manages her stress incontinence by wearing sanitary napkins at home may want to continue doing so while hospitalized for an acute appendectomy.

When a problem in urinary elimination is identified, the nurse should assess the client's support system. Because urinary elimination problems often are stressful, the support of family and friends is often helpful and necessary for the client.

Objective Data

Assessment of Urine

Assessment of urine is best done when the client does not void directly into the toilet, but rather into a urine collection device (urinal for men; bedpan for women), or when a retention catheter is in place. When assessment of the urine is important, the nurse may have to request that the client void into one of these devices. A "hat" is a device that can be placed in between the toilet and the toilet seat to catch urine (see Fig. 36-8). Using a hat permits the client to void normally in the toilet, but still allows for visual inspection or measurement of urine.

Assessment of urine includes visual inspection for color, clarity, and the presence of blood or mucus, and noting the odor of the urine. The amount of urine should be assessed for each void, as should the total urine output over a 24-hour period. The 24-hour output can be compared to the intake, and any significant difference noted. Trends of increasing or decreasing output should be evaluated.

Assessment of Urinary Retention

To assess a client for urinary retention, the nurse should examine the client's voiding pattern. If the client's intake and output (I & O) are being monitored, a written record of the time and amount of each void is maintained. When examining this flowsheet, the nurse can determine the pattern of voiding and the balance of overall I & O. Within a 24-hour period, the I & O is usually within 200 to 300 mL. The absence of voiding during any 8-hour period or the frequent voiding of small amounts of urine (50–100 mL) per void suggest urinary retention or urinary retention with overflow voiding.

When a client's I & O is not being monitored, it is important to obtain subjective information regarding urinary elimination at least once every 8 hours. Question the client as to whether voiding has occurred and whether any difficulty in voiding was experienced. Risk factors, such as anticholinergic medications, surgery, vaginal delivery, or prostatic hypertrophy should be considered. Physical assessment of the lower abdomen is indicated for any client in whom urinary retention is suspected. When urinary retention is suspected, catheterization can determine the amount of urine remaining in the bladder immediately after voiding. This is referred to as **postvoid residual**.

Noninvasive Urine Volume Monitoring. Noninvasive technology is now available to estimate urine volume in the bladder. A portable ultrasound device measures urine volume using a probe that is attached to a machine that contains a screen capable of visualizing the bladder with ultrasound. Lubricating jelly is placed on the lower abdomen, and the probe is moved until a clear outline of the bladder is present on the screen. Two separate readings are taken, from which the machine computes the volume of urine. Accuracy of estimating bladder volumes using noninvasive ultrasound has been documented by research (Chan, 1993).

Portable bladder ultrasound allows the nurse to obtain measurements at the bedside or in the home. Bladder ultrasound can be used to measure postvoid residual, thus avoiding the necessity of in-and-out catheterization. This reduces infection risk and is more cost effective (Chan, 1993). Bladder ultrasound equipment is usually available only on specialized units (rehabilitation or neurology) where clients frequently have problems with urinary retention.

Physical Assessment

Inspection. The nurse inspects the client's lower abdomen when the client's history or recent voiding pattern indicates that urinary retention is a potential urinary alteration. When the client is lying in a supine position, a bulge in the central lower abdomen just above the symphysis pubis can be noted if the bladder is distended. When the bladder contains less than 500 mL, no bulge will be present. When the bladder holds more than 700 mL, the bulge may be observed extending in the direction of the umbilicus. It may not be easy to observe a distended bladder in an obese person.

It is not necessary to inspect the client's perineal area routinely, unless the client complains of severe dysuria and the presence of purulent drainage. When there are no specific complaints, the nurse can examine the urinary meatus when performing perineal hygiene for the client unable to meet his or her own hygiene needs. The nurse should always inspect the urinary meatus when inserting or removing a urinary catheter. If healthy, the skin surrounding the urinary meatus is nonreddened, moist, and without discharge. Smegma, an accumulation of white, odorous secretions from sebaceous glands found under the labia minora in women and under the foreskin in men, is normal, and is not discharge from the urinary meatus. Abnormal findings on inspection of the perineum are reddened, inflamed skin surrounding the urinary meatus, and purulent discharge.

Percussion. Percussion of the lower abdomen follows inspection to determine the presence of a distended bladder. Percussion should begin at the umbilicus and proceed downward toward the symphysis pubis. If the bladder is empty or contains less than 150 mL of fluid, a hollow note will be heard, the normal sound expected over the abdomen. Percussion over a distended bladder will produce a duller sound. Urine, being liquid, is denser than the mixture of air and fluid in the small intestines, and therefore produces a duller sound. The closer the dull sound is to the umbilicus, the greater the degree of bladder distention. Percussion is the most reliable element of the physical assessment in evaluating the degree of bladder distention.

Palpation. Palpation is the final component of physical assessment of the lower abdomen to assess for bladder distention. As with percussion, palpation should start at the level of the umbilicus and move in a downward direction toward the symphysis pubis. The fingertips of both hands should be used to palpate deeply in an attempt to feel the top edge of the bladder. When the bladder contains more than 150 mL of urine, the edge of the bladder will feel smooth and rounded. The top edge of the distended bladder should be at the same level of the abdomen where percussion changed from a hollow to a dull sound. Even though palpation of the bladder must be deep to feel the edge of the bladder, it should be done gently. Palpation may cause discomfort and stimulate voiding. Table 41-2 gives a comparison of normal and abnormal findings during physical assessment of the lower abdomen.

Diagnostic Tests and Procedures

The nurse is responsible for collecting urine specimens for laboratory examination. Some urine tests are performed by the nurse, whereas others require that the urine be sent to a laboratory for more sophisticated examination. The nurse is also involved in preparing the client for diagnostic procedures that help identify pathologic urinary conditions. The nurse is responsible for client teaching and preparation before such procedures, as well as for assisting with procedures and providing the client with postprocedure care.

Collection of Urine Specimens. The nurse is responsible for collecting urine specimens for a number of different types of tests. Different tests require different collection procedures. Special considerations may be required during collection of urine from an infant or small child. Guidelines for these procedures are given in Procedure 41-1, "Collecting Urine Specimens."

Random Specimen. Random urine specimen collection is used when sterile urine is not required. The clean specimen can be collected in a urinal, bedpan, hat, or directly into a specimen cup. The urine should not be contaminated with feces or toilet paper. If a woman is menstruating, this should be noted on the specimen. The specimen should be properly labeled and promptly sent to the laboratory, or used for a test to be made at the bedside.

Clean-Catch or Midstream Specimen. A clean-catch or midstream-voided specimen is used when a specimen relatively free of microorganisms is required. A sterile specimen cup or sterile bedpan or urinal is used to collect the urine specimen. The urinary meatus should be cleansed of the organisms normally found on the skin surrounding the meatus. Women need to be instructed to clean the perineal area well with soap and water or an antiseptic before voiding. Cotton balls with soap or antiseptic should be used only once, wiping from front to back to avoid contamination from the anus. This cleansing is usually repeated three times with different cotton balls. Men should clean the end of the penis in a circular motion starting at the tip. The client is then asked to void a small amount of urine into the toilet, stop the urinary flow, and then void midstream urine into the specimen container. Obtaining a midstream urine specimen decreases the chance that the sample will be contaminated with microorganisms from the perineal skin or vaginal secretions. The sample is not acceptable if contaminated with stool, vaginal secretions, or menstrual blood.

The container should be properly labeled and immediately transported to the laboratory. If the specimen cannot be taken to the laboratory immediately, it must be refrigerated. Changes in the urine begin to occur within an hour if it is left unrefrigerated. Multiplying bacteria may split urea, which produces a more alkaline urine. One researcher questions the importance of meatal cleansing and holding labia apart during urine collection because these factors did not seem

(text continues on page 1194)

Table 41-2 • Comparison of Normal and Abnormal Findings on Physical Examination of Lower Abdomen for Bladder Distention

Normal	Abnormal
Inspection	
No distention	Bulging above symphysis pubis
Percussion	
Hollow	Dull
Palpation	
Bladder not palpable	Smooth, round edge of bladder can be felt

Procedure 41-1
Collecting Urine Specimens

Purpose

1. Obtain a noncontaminated urine specimen for routine analysis or diagnostic studies that include culture and sensitivity tests.

Assessment

- Determine client's ability to understand directions and to obtain specimen independently.
- Identify purpose for obtaining specimen to guide selection of best method for obtaining specimen.
- If collecting specimen from indwelling urinary system, assess tubing for sampling port.

Equipment

Disposable gloves.
Container, label.
For collecting sterile urine specimen from indwelling catheter: Betadine or alcohol swab, 10 mL syringe with 23- to 25-gauge needle, sterile specimen container.
For collecting midstream urine specimen: cleansing solution, towel, specimen container.
For collecting a specimen from a child without urinary control: cleansing solution, towel, pediatric urine collection bag, diaper.

Procedure

Collecting Sterile Specimen From an Indwelling Catheter

1. Explain procedure to client.
2. Wash hands. Put on disposable gloves.
   Rationale: Handwashing prevents transmission of microorganisms.
3. Position client so that catheter is accessible.
4. Allow urine to collect in tubing by clamping or bending tubing (2 mL of urine is sufficient for a culture and sensitivity specimen).
   Rationale: Fresh urine is needed for accurate test results.

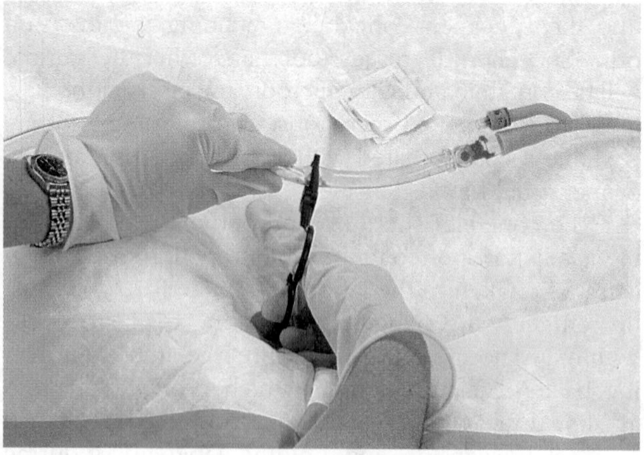

Step 4 • *Clamp tubing to allow urine to collect. (Photo © B. Proud.)*

5. Cleanse the aspiration port of the drainage tubing with alcohol or Betadine swab.
   Rationale: Alcohol or Betadine prevents microorganisms from entering the drainage tubing.
6. Insert needle into aspiration port. Draw urine sample into syringe by gentle aspiration. Remove needle.

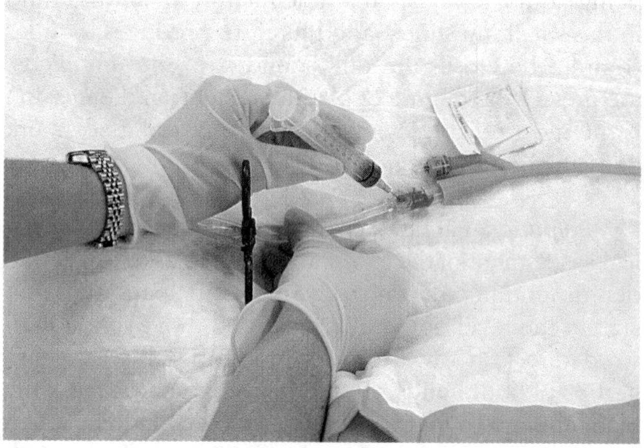

Step 6 • *Aspirate urine sample into a syringe. (Photo © B. Proud.)*

7. Transfer urine from syringe into a sterile specimen container.
   Note: Hospital policy may allow specimen to be transported to laboratory in syringe with sterile cap on syringe in place of needle.
8. Label the container. Date and time laboratory requisition.
   Rationale: Incorrect identification of specimen could cause diagnostic or therapeutic error.
9. Send specimen to laboratory within 15 minutes or place in specimen refrigerator.
   Note: If specimen is for microbiology testing, it *must* be sent *immediately* and not refrigerated.
   Rationale: Microorganisms grow quickly in urine, especially at room temperature. Refrigeration retards bacterial growth.
10. Dispose of all contaminated supplies. Wash hands.
11. Document procedure and observations.

Procedure

Self-Collecting Midstream Urine Specimen for a Woman

1. Instruct client how to cleanse urinary meatus and obtain urine specimen
   a. (Client) Wash hands.

b. Separate labia minora and cleanse perineum with cleansing agent, starting in front of the urethral meatus and moving swab toward the rectum.
Rationale: Cleansing in this manner prevents spread of micro-organisms from the rectum to the urinary meatus.
c. Begin to urinate while continuing to hold labia apart. Allow first urine to flow into toilet.
Rationale: First urine washes microorganisms and cellular debris out of meatus.
d. Hold specimen container under the urine stream and collect sample.
e. Remove specimen container, release hand from labia, seal container tightly, and finish voiding. Wash hands.

2. (Nurse) Put on disposable gloves to receive specimen container from the client. Clean and rinse outer surface of container with disinfectant.
Rationale: Steps are taken to prevent transfer of microorganisms to other healthcare workers from possible urine spillage outside containers.
3. Label the container. Date and time laboratory requisition.
Rationale: Incorrect identification of specimen could cause diagnostic or therapeutic error.
4. Send specimen to laboratory within 15 minutes or place in specimen refrigerator.
Note: If specimen is for microbiology testing, it *must* be sent *immediately* and not refrigerated.
Rationale: Microorganisms grow quickly in urine, especially at room temperature. Refrigeration retards bacterial growth.
5. Dispose of all contaminated supplies. Wash hands.

Procedure

Self-Collecting Midstream Urine Specimen for a Man

1. Instruct client how to cleanse urinary meatus and obtain urine specimen.
   a. (Client)Wash hands.
   b. Cleanse end of penis with cleansing agent. If man is not circumcised, instruct him to retract foreskin to expose urinary meatus before cleansing and throughout specimen collection.
   c. Begin to urinate, allowing urine to flow into toilet.
   Rationale: First urine washes microorganisms and secretions from urethra before collecting specimen.
   d. Pass specimen container into urine stream and collect sample.
   e. Remove container, seal tightly, and finish voiding.
2. Follow steps 2 to 5 above.

Procedure

Collecting a Specimen From a Child Without Urinary Control

1. If parents are present, explain procedure to them.
2. Position child gently on back. Put on disposable gloves. Remove diaper.
3. Clean perineal–genital area gently with soap and water, followed by antiseptic.
4. For a girl: Separate labia and cleanse from front of urethral meatus toward the rectum. Rinse with sterile water and dry with cotton balls.
Rationale: Cleansing removes lotions, powders, fecal matter, as well as decreases the numbers of microorganisms present on the skin. Drying the area thoroughly facilitates adhesion of the urine collection bag.
5. For a boy: Cleanse the penis and scrotum. If boy is not circumcised, retract foreskin and cleanse. Rinse with sterile water and dry with gauze or cotton balls.
Rationale: Same as for a girl.
6. Remove paper backing from adhesive of collection bag.

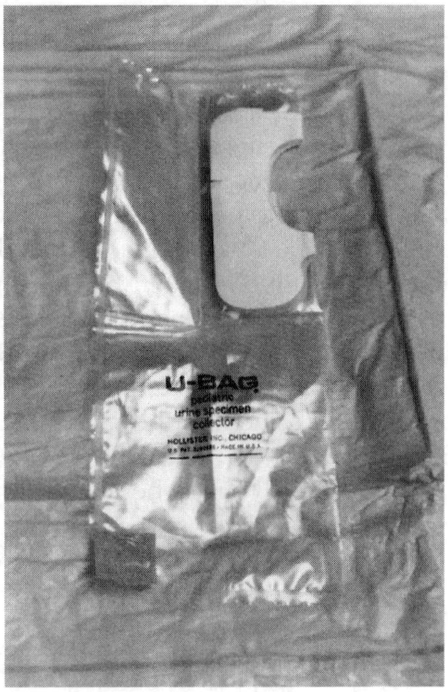

Step 6 • *Remove paper backing.*

7. Spread the child's legs widely apart.
Rationale: Separates and flattens skin folds to increase adhesion of bag and decreases chances of leaking.
8. Apply collection bag over child's perineum, covering penis and scrotum on boy, and urinary meatus and vagina of girl. Press adhesive to secure, starting at the perineum and working outward.

(continued)

Rationale: Securing adhesive from the center toward the outside decreases wrinkling and subsequent leaking of urine.

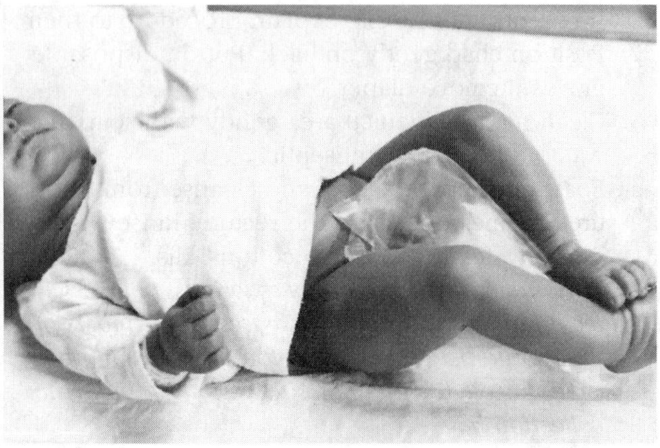

Step 8 • *Apply urine collection bag over child's perineum.*

9. Place a diaper on the child loosely.
   Rationale: Helps to hold the urine collection bag in place.
10. Remove gloves, wash hands.
11. Check the collector for urine every 15 minutes.
    Note: Parents can check child for urine specimen.
12. When urine specimen is obtained, glove again, and gently remove collection bag from the skin and empty urine into specimen container.
13. Tighten lid and cleanse outside of container if contaminated with urine.
    Rationale: Cleansing the outside of container prevents spread of microorganisms.
14. Label the container. Date and time laboratory requisition.
    Rationale: Incorrect identification of specimen could cause diagnostic or therapeutic error.
15. Send specimen to laboratory within 15 minutes or place in specimen refrigerator.
    Note: If specimen is for microbiology testing, it *must* be sent *immediately* and not refrigerated.
    Rationale: Microorganisms grow quickly in urine, especially at room temperature. Refrigeration retards bacterial growth.
16. Dispose of all contaminated supplies. Wash hands.
17. Document that specimen was collected and sent.

significantly to affect the bacterial contamination of the specimen (Winslow, 1993).

Twenty-Four–Hour Specimen. A 24-hour urine specimen is required to measure accurately kidney excretion of certain substances. The nurse is responsible for explaining the procedure to the client and for taking steps to ensure that *all* urine is saved. Inadvertent discarding of even a small amount of urine invalidates the test results, necessitating that collection of urine be started all over again. A sign over the client's bed and on the bathroom door helps alert all hospital personnel and family members that all urine must be saved. A large container for urine collection is usually provided by the laboratory. A preservative may be added to this container to prevent the breakdown of certain urinary constituents.

Often a 24-hour sample is started early in the morning after the client's first void. The nurse should instruct the client to void until the bladder is completely empty. This voided urine should be discarded and the time noted as the beginning of the 24-hour period during which all urine must be saved. The client may void into any clean urinary container (bedpan, hat, urinal), but care must be taken to avoid contamination with stool or toilet paper. All urine is then emptied into the 24-hour collection container, taking care not to splash, because the added preservative can be caustic. The large container should be refrigerated or placed in a bucket of ice during the 24 hours of collection. At the end of the 24 hours, the client should be asked to empty his or her bladder, and this urine is added to the collection container. The container is then labeled and sent to the laboratory.

Specimen From Catheter. Obtaining a specimen from a catheter may be necessary when the client is unable to void or already has a catheter in place. Urine collected in this manner is sterile. When obtaining urine from a catheter, it is important to maintain strict asepsis at all times to prevent entry of microorganisms into the bladder.

When catheterization is necessary to obtain urine, an in-and-out catheterization is performed. This means the catheter is left in place only long enough to obtain the specimen (see Procedure 41-4 later in the chapter). The sterile urine is permitted to flow into the specimen container, and then the container is properly labeled and sent to the laboratory.

When the client already has a retention catheter in place, the specimen is obtained by using a syringe to draw urine from a self-sealing port in the catheter (see Procedure 41-1). The specimen port of the catheter is cleansed with alcohol or Betadine. A small-gauge needle (eg, 23- or 25-gauge) is inserted into the port and the necessary amount of urine is withdrawn into the syringe. Once the urine is obtained, it is usually transferred to a specimen container, labeled, and sent to the laboratory. It may be necessary to clamp the catheter tubing just below the specimen port for 20 to 30 minutes with a rubber band or screw clamp to allow enough urine to collect in the tubing so that a specimen can be obtained. This is especially true if more than a few milliliters of urine is needed in the specimen.

Urine should not be collected from the catheter drainage bag. This urine is not considered sterile because the collection system has been opened to drain urine at different intervals. Also, as the urine sits for long periods of time in the drainage bag, growth of bacteria can occur.

Collecting Urine From Children. Collecting urine from infants and children may necessitate special attention if the child has not yet achieved control of voiding. Catheterization is often difficult, and not recommended because of the small meatal opening and the trauma to the young child. Plastic collection devices are a more acceptable method of collecting urine from an infant or young child. Clear plastic bags with adhesive material can be attached over the child's urethral meatus (see Procedure 41-1). The child's perineal area is washed and dried thoroughly before application of the bag. Bags should be applied according the manufacturer's instructions, and care taken to avoid trauma to the delicate meatus of the young child.

Collecting specimens from children who have achieved bladder control may also be challenging. Often children find it difficult to start their stream on command. Drinking a glass of water, running a faucet, and permitting the parent to help the child obtain the urine specimen may increase the chances of success.

Urine Tests. Common tests that are routinely performed on urine by the nurse include specific gravity, pH determination, and assessing for the presence of glucose, protein, ketone bodies, or occult blood. The most common laboratory tests of urine include the urinalysis, culture and sensitivity, and 24-hour assays for different urinary constituents.

Specific Gravity. Specific gravity is the weight or concentration of urine as compared to water. Specific gravity can be measured using a urinometer. The urinometer is calibrated to float at the 1.000 mark in distilled water. To test for specific gravity, urine is placed in a test tube and the urinometer is gently spun and allowed to float in the urine (see Procedure 41-2, "Testing Specific Gravity of Urine"). The specific gravity is read where the meniscus of the urine hits the urinometer marking. The more concentrated the urine, the higher the float will rise in the urine, and the higher the specific gravity reading. Normal specific gravity of urine is 1.010 to 1.025 g/mL. A low specific gravity usually occurs because of overhydration or a pathologic condition that affects the kidneys' ability to concentrate urine. A high specific gravity occurs because of fluid volume deficit.

Reagent Strips. Reagent strips (or dipsticks) are available to measure the amount of certain substances such as glucose, protein, or ketones in the urine. Such strips can also be used to determine urinary pH or the presence of occult blood. The instructions for proper use of the various reagent strips are clearly printed on the container and should be followed precisely to ensure accurate results. The procedure usually involves dipping the reagent strip into the urine sample and comparing any color changes to the color chart provided on the container. Timing is crucial for the accurate interpretation of results for some tests, such as testing for glucose or ketones. Assessment of the urine by reagent strips is ordered by the physician when he or she wants to monitor closely certain parameters on high-risk clients (eg, assessing pregnant women for protein in their urine), or to monitor continually the urine status for each voiding. The nurse may independently decide to use reagent strips when necessary for comprehensive assessment of high-risk clients.

Urinalysis. Urinalysis is one of the most common screening tests performed on urine. A urinalysis provides data about the color, turbidity, pH, and specific gravity of the urine, as well as indicating the presence of protein, glucose, ketones, red blood cells, white blood cells, bacteria, and casts in the urine. The collection of a urine specimen for urinalysis is routine for all hospitalized clients. The test can be performed on any random specimen of 20 to 30 mL of urine. Although the specimen can be collected at any time during the day, the first voided morning specimen is preferred. The first urine voided in the morning is ordinarily more concentrated because the client is usually without fluids during the night. The influence of diet and activity is minimized. All these factors make the first voided specimen more likely to reveal any abnormalities that are present. Table 41-3 presents a concise summary of the parameters tested in a urinalysis, the range of acceptable normal values, and the clinical significance of abnormal values.

Urine Culture and Sensitivity. Culture and sensitivity tests can be performed on the urine to identify any microorganism causing a UTI, and to identify those antibiotics that can effectively kill the organism. The culture allows the bacteria to grow and multiply over a period of at least 48 hours. After 24 hours of growth, the laboratory is able to make a preliminary identification of the organism. Another 24 to 48 hours may be necessary to conduct the definitive analytic tests that identify the exact microorganism responsible for the infection. After identification of the organism, the laboratory can test to see which antibiotics inhibit growth of the organism. If an antibiotic inhibits bacterial growth, the bacteria is said to be sensitive to the antibiotic. If the antibiotic does not inhibit bacterial growth, the organism is considered resistant. The purpose of performing a culture and sensitivity is to ensure effective antibiotic therapy in the treatment of UTIs.

Twenty-Four–Hour Specimens. Twenty-four–hour urine specimens may be used to measure kidney excretion of certain substances. Some substances excreted by the kidney are not excreted at the same rate throughout the day. A single random specimen may give

Procedure 41-2
Testing Specific Gravity of Urine

Purpose

1. Evaluate the extent to which urine is being concentrated in the kidney.
2. Monitor the client's hydration status in response to therapies such as intravenous fluids and drugs (mannitol, antidiuretic hormone).

Assessment

- Assess client's ability to collect urine specimen. Determine alternate methods of specimen collection, if necessary.
- Assess related clinical signs/symptoms of hydration status:
  - Intake and output records.
  - Daily weight.
  - Vital signs.
  - Serum electrolytes.
  - Skin turgor, mucous membranes.
  - In infants, position of fontanel.

Equipment

Urinometer (hydrometer).
Glass cylinder.
20 mL freshly obtained urine.
Clean, disposable gloves.

Procedure

1. Wash hands, put on clean, disposable gloves.
   Rationale: Protects against microorganisms being transferred from urine specimen to nurse's hands.
2. Make sure urinometer is on flat surface. Pour urine into glass cylinder until it is one-half to three-quarters full.
   Rationale: Flat surface ensures accurate measurement. Urinometer will not float unless glass cylinder is at least one-half full. Over filling will result in spillage when urometer is placed.
3. Place urinometer into the cylinder. Gently spin stem of urinometer.
   Rationale: Prevents the urinometer form adhering to the side of the cylinder.
4. Place cylinder on flat surface at eye level. When twirling stops, read where the urine level meets the calibrated urinometer at the base of the meniscus.
   Rationale: The concentration of dissolved solutes in the urine affects the depth at which the urinometer floats.
5. Discard urine, wash equipment with soap and water, allow to air dry. Discard gloves.
   Rationale: Prevents growth of microorganisms in equipment in between users.
6. Document findings in the client record.

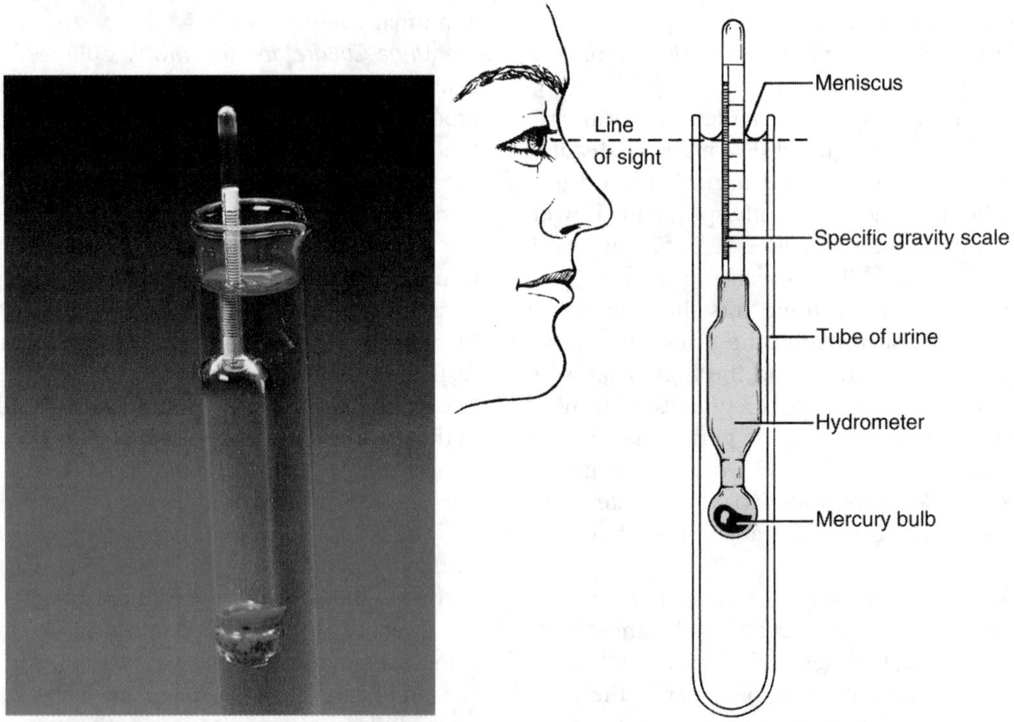

Step 4 • *Place urometer into cylinder and read measurement where base of meniscus meets the calibrated urometer.*

Table 41-3 • Urinalysis Parameters

Parameter	Normal Values	Clinical Significance of Variations
Color	Light yellow–amber	Almost colorless: ↑ fluid intake; Dark color: ↓ fluid intake; Pink, red, dark brown: red blood cells in urine; pink, orange, red, brown, blue–green: medications or foods
Turbidity	Clear	Hazy, cloudy, smoky: urine specimen allowed to stand at room temperature; red blood cells, white blood cells, bacteria, mucus threads: mucosal irritation secondary to indwelling catheter
pH	Normal: 6 Range: 4.6–8	< 6: Diet high in meat or some fruits (cranberries); metabolic acidosis (diabetes mellitus, starvation); respiratory acidosis (emphysema) > 6: Diet high in vegetables and citrus fruits; urinary tract infections; metabolic alkalosis (vomiting, prolonged diuretic therapy); respiratory alkalosis (hyperventilation)
Specific gravity	Range: 1.015–1.025	< 1.015: ↑ Fluid intake, diuretic therapy, diabetes insipidus, renal diseases > 1.025: ↓ Fluid intake; ↑ fluid loss (vomiting, diarrhea, fever); Antidiuretic hormone secretion (trauma, stress)
Protein	None-trace	Present in severe stress, renal disease, preeclampsia of pregnancy
Glucose	None	Present in diabetes mellitus
Ketones	None	Present in diabetes mellitus, ketoacidosis, starvation
Microscopic examination: high–power field		
Red blood cells	0–3	> 3: Urinary tract infection, bleeding, urinary tract trauma, anticoagulant therapy
White blood cells	0–5	> 5: Urinary tract infection
Bacteria/yeast	None–few	Few: contamination from perineal skin Many: urinary tract infection
Casts (precipitation or clumping of protein substances)	None–occasional	Many: possible renal diseases

incomplete, inaccurate results about these urinary solutes. Some of these substances include total urine protein, creatinine, urobilinogen, uric acid, electrolytes, and hormones. To evaluate accurately the presence and amount of these substances, all urine excreted by a client during a 24-hour period is collected and sent to the laboratory for examination.

Blood Test. Small samples of blood can be analyzed in the laboratory to screen for kidney disease. Two of the more commonly performed tests are blood urea nitrogen (BUN) and serum creatinine.

Blood urea nitrogen measures the amount of urea nitrogen in the blood. Urea, the major nitrogenous end waste product of metabolism, is formed in the liver. Urea is carried in the bloodstream from the liver to the kidneys for excretion. When the kidney is diseased, it is unable to excrete urea adequately, and urea begins to accumulate in the blood, causing the BUN to rise. Normal BUN is 8 to 25 mg/100 mL. Because other factors, such as high dietary intake of protein, fluid deficit, infection, gout, or excessive breakdown of protein stores, can also elevate BUN, it is not a highly sensitive indicator of impaired renal function.

Serum creatinine is a more sensitive indicator of renal function. Creatinine is the waste product formed from the breakdown of skeletal muscle tissue; its formation is not influenced by diet or other factors. As creatinine is formed, it is carried in the bloodstream to the kidneys for filtration and excretion. Damage to a large number of nephrons prevents efficient excretion of creatinine and causes the build-up of creatinine in the blood. An elevated serum creatinine is indicative of impaired renal function. When the BUN and serum creatinine are both elevated, it is a reliable indicator of kidney dysfunction.

Creatinine clearance is a combination blood and urine test that measures the rate at which creatinine is cleared from the blood by the kidneys. Creatinine is excreted in the urine by the process of glomerular filtration. Creatinine is not secreted by the kidney tubule, nor is it reabsorbed anywhere in the kidney tubule. Therefore, its excretion is an accurate measure of the glomerular filtration ability of the kidney. To compute the creatinine clearance, a measurement of the creatinine level in the blood, the creatinine level in the urine, and the amount of urine produced in a set period of time (usually 24 hours) is needed. A decreased creatinine clearance value indicates renal impairment.

Diagnostic Procedures. The physician can order many diagnostic urologic procedures to understand better the functioning of the client's urinary system, and to identify any abnormalities. The nurse prepares the client physically and psychologically for these tests, monitors the client during and after the procedure, and uses the information obtained to individualize the plan of care for the client.

X-ray Examination. X-ray examination can provide helpful information concerning the status of the urinary tract. The two most commonly performed x-ray examinations for this purpose are the flatplate of the abdomen to visualize the kidneys, ureters, and bladder (KUB) and the intravenous pyelogram (IVP).

KUB is helpful in detecting malformations in the size or shape of the kidneys, ureters, or bladder, and to detect the presence of any stones that could obstruct the flow of urine. This x-ray procedure is painless and requires no special care before or after the procedure.

An IVP is an x-ray that visualizes the urinary system by the use of a radiopaque (contrast) dye. The dye is injected intravenously and x-rays are taken at set intervals. This permits visualization of the dye as it is excreted by the kidneys, emptied into the ureters, and finally deposited in the bladder. An x-ray is also taken immediately after the client voids to check if the bladder is completely emptying. The procedure takes about 1 hour to complete. Special preparations before the procedure include clear liquids or a light meal the evening before the test; nothing by mouth after midnight (although sometimes clear fluids are permitted); and enemas and laxatives to clear the colon of feces, because fecal contents can interfere with visualization. The nurse should also check for any history of allergy to iodine (x-ray dye) before beginning preparation for the test.

Several other tests are helpful in visualizing the urinary system and detecting abnormalities of the kidney or bladder. They include computed axial tomography scan, magnetic resonance imaging, renal scan, and abdominal ultrasound. During these procedures, various types of energy are directed over the abdomen. Computer technology converts the information into visual pictures of the kidney. Client preparation varies with each test. There may be some discomfort associated with maintaining body position during the procedure, but the procedures themselves are not painful.

Cystoscopy. Cystoscopy involves the insertion of a tube into the bladder for the purpose of direct visualization. A cystoscope is a flexible tube that can be inserted into the urethra and guided into the bladder. A light at the end of the cystoscope allows the physician to look for abnormalities such as tumors, stones, or structural problems. Specialized instruments can be passed through the cystoscope to remove small stones or to take tissue biopsies. Radiopaque dye may be injected for subsequent kidney x-rays; this is known as a retrograde pyelogram. The client needs to sign a consent form before the cystoscopy. After the procedure, the nurse needs to assess for hematuria, urinary retention, dysuria or bladder spasms, and any signs or symptoms of UTI. A retention catheter may be left in place for a short period of time after the cystoscopy.

Urodynamic Studies. Urodynamic studies are used to detect abnormalities in bladder function or voiding. These procedures (uroflowmetry, cystometrograms, and urethral pressure profile) measure pressure (from the bladder, urethra, and within the abdomen), urinary flow, and striated muscle activity. The procedures require no special preparation before testing. Urodynamic studies usually are not painful, but the client may experience some intermittent discomfort during the procedure.

Nursing Diagnoses

Accepted North American Nursing Diagnosis Association (NANDA) nursing diagnoses involving alterations in urinary elimination include Urinary Retention and five types of Urinary Incontinence: Stress, Urge, Reflex, Functional, and Total. The nurse uses data from the assessment of urinary elimination to determine the presence or risk for any of these disruptions in normal urinary elimination patterns.

Diagnostic Statement: Stress Incontinence

Definition

Stress Incontinence is the state in which an individual experiences a loss of urine of less than 50 mL occurring with increased abdominal pressure (NANDA 1994).

Defining Characteristics

Major characteristics are reported or observed dribbling with increased abdominal pressure.

Minor characteristics are urinary urgency; urinary frequency (more often than every 2 hours) (NANDA, 1994).

Related Factors

Related factors are degenerative changes in pelvic muscles and structural supports associated with increased age; high intraabdominal pressure (eg, obesity, gravid uterus); incompetent bladder outlet; overdistention between voidings; weak pelvic muscles and structural supports (NANDA, 1994).

Diagnostic Statement: Urge Incontinence

Definition

Urge Incontinence is the state in which an individual experiences involuntary passage of urine occurring soon after a strong sense of urgency to void (NANDA, 1994).

Defining Characteristics

Major characteristics are urinary urgency; frequency (voiding more often than every 2 hours); bladder contracture/spasm.

Minor characteristics are nocturia (more than twice per night); voiding in small amounts (less than 100 mL) or in large amounts (more than 550 mL); inability to reach toilet in time (NANDA, 1994).

Related Factors

Related factors are decreased bladder capacity (eg, history of pelvic inflammatory disease, abdominal surgeries, indwelling urinary catheter); irritation of bladder stretch receptors causing spasm (eg, bladder infection); alcohol; caffeine; increased fluids; increased urine concentration; overdistention of bladder (NANDA, 1994).

Diagnostic Statement: Reflex Incontinence

Definition

Reflex Incontinence is the state in which an individual experiences an involuntary loss of urine, occurring at somewhat predictable intervals when a specific bladder volume is reached (NANDA, 1994).

Defining Characteristics

Major characteristics are no awareness of bladder filling; no urge to void or feelings of bladder fullness; uninhibited bladder contraction/spasm at regular intervals (NANDA, 1994).

Related Factors

A related factor is neurologic impairment (eg, spinal cord lesion that interferes with conduction of cerebral messages above the level of the reflex arc) (NANDA, 1994).

Diagnostic Statement: Functional Incontinence

Definition

Functional Incontinence is the state in which an individual experiences an involuntary, unpredictable passage of urine (NANDA, 1994).

Nursing Research
Urinary Elimination

Selected Nursing Research Studies

Charbonneau-Smith, R. (1993). No-touch catheterization and infection rates in selected spinal cord injured population. *Rehabilitation Nursing, 18,* 296–299.

Dillie, C. M., Kirchhoff, K. T. (1993). Decontamination of vinyl urinary drainage bags with bleach. *Rehabilitation Nursing, 18,* 292–295.

Moore, K. M., Kelm, M., Sinclair, O., & Cadrain, G. (1993). Bacteria in intermittent catheterization users: The effects of sterile versus clean reused catheters. *Rehabilitation Nursing, 18,* 306–309.

Skoner, M. (1994). Self-management of urinary incontinence among women 31 to 50 years of age. *Rehabilitation Nursing, 19,* 339–343.

Possible Topics for Nursing Inquiry

- What are the major predictors for gerontologic incontinence?
- Does complete urinary drainage of amounts in excess of 1,000 mL adversely affect blood pressure and heart rate?
- For which population group is bladder credé effective to enhance complete bladder emptying?
- How frequently is perineal care performed for clients having indwelling catheters? Does the frequency of perineal care affect the incidence of urinary tract infections for clients with indwelling catheters?
- Does the use of a leg bag drainage system increase the incidence of infection for clients with indwelling catheters?

Defining Characteristics

Major characteristics are urge to void or bladder contractions sufficiently strong to result in loss of urine before reaching an appropriate receptacle (NANDA, 1994).

Related Factors

Related factors are altered environment; sensory, cognitive, or mobility deficits (NANDA, 1994).

Diagnostic Statement: Total Incontinence

Definition

Total incontinence is the state in which an individual experiences a continuous and unpredictable loss of urine (NANDA, 1994).

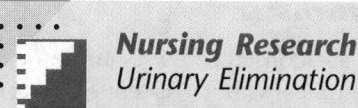

Defining Characteristics

Major characteristics are constant flow of urine occurring at unpredictable times without distention or uninhibited bladder contractions/spasm; unsuccessful incontinence-refractory treatments; nocturia.

Minor characteristics are lack of perineal or bladder filling awareness; unawareness of incontinence (NANDA, 1994).

Related Factors

Related factors are neuropathy preventing transmission of reflex indicating bladder fullness; neurologic dysfunction causing triggering of micturition at unpredictable times; independent contraction of detrusor reflex due to surgery; trauma or disease affecting spinal cord nerves; anatomic (fistula) (NANDA, 1994).

Diagnostic Statement: Urinary Retention

Definition

Urinary Retention is the state in which an individual experiences incomplete emptying of the bladder (NANDA, 1994).

Defining Characteristics

Major characteristics are bladder distention; small, frequent voiding or absence of urine output.

Minor characteristics are sensation of bladder fullness; dribbling; residual urine; dysuria; overflow incontinence (NANDA, 1994).

Related Factors

Related factors are high urethral pressure caused by weak detrusor; inhibition of reflex arc; strong sphincter; blockage (NANDA, 1994).

Related Nursing Diagnoses

The client with altered urinary elimination can experience other problems, such as Impaired Skin Integrity and Fluid Volume Deficit. Psychological stress due to problems with urinary elimination can result in Anxiety or Ineffective Individual Coping. Sleep Pattern Disturbance and Sexual Dysfunction can also result. Knowledge Deficit is also common in the client with urinary dysfunction because new treatment regimens will have to be learned to prevent or cope with problems with urination.

Outcome Identification and Planning

After nursing diagnoses and related facts have been established, the nurse and client plan for realistic outcomes and how to meet those outcomes. Outcomes for the client with urinary dysfunction should be individualized depending on client assessment data. General client goals might encompass the following:

Client will strengthen or maintain adequate perineal muscle control.
Client will reestablish control over voiding.
Client will verbalize understanding of procedures necessary to promote optimal urinary function.

Examples of some nursing interventions to meet these outcomes are listed in the accompanying display and discussed in the following section.

Implementation

The nurse plays a significant role in preventing and managing urinary dysfunction. Client teaching can inform the general population as well as each individual client how urinary problems can be prevented. The nurse also implements specific measures to promote optimum urinary elimination, such as comfort measures, catheterization, and administering medications. Specialized knowledge is required to care for the client with a urinary diversion or one who is undergoing renal dialysis. Individual plans of care are developed for people with special urinary problems such as urinary retention, incontinence, or enuresis.

Planning

Examples of Nursing Interventions Used in Common Urinary Problems

Urinary Retention

- Verbal prompting
- Physiologic positioning for voiding
- Running water
- Bladder credé
- In-and-out catheterization
- Intermittent catheterization

Urinary Incontinence

- Bladder training
  - Regulating fluid intake
  - Voiding schedule
  - Abdominal and perineal muscle strengthening
- External and indwelling catheters
- Protective pants

Nursing Interventions to Promote Health and Urinary Function

Client Teaching

Client teaching is important in promoting optimum health and urinary function. All clients should be taught the importance of adequate fluid intake, how to avoid UTIs, and measures to maintain adequate perineal muscle tone.

Promoting Fluid Intake. Educating people regarding the importance of adequate fluid intake is a significant nursing intervention. Normally, an adult should drink between six to eight glasses or about 1,500 to 2,000 mL of fluid per day. Fluid intake may have to increase proportionally with any excessive loss of body fluid.

Fluid intake should be spaced throughout the waking hours to prevent transitory dehydration. Fluid intake may be restricted before bed to avoid waking during the night. Water is a preferred fluid because excessive intake of caffeine, glucose, or sodium can alter urinary elimination.

Adequate fluid intake serves two functions: adequate urine production will flush microorganisms out of the urinary system, thus decreasing the chance of infection or obstruction from stones, and producing large amounts of urine will help to distend and stretch the detrusor muscle, preventing atrophy. For these reasons, adequate fluid intake is helpful in preventing UTI and maintaining bladder tone.

Preventing Urinary Tract Infection. In addition to maintaining adequate fluid intake, other measures can prevent UTI. Adequate perineal hygiene is important in preventing contaminating microorganisms of the anus or vagina from entering the urethra. Women should be instructed at an early age always to wipe from front to back after urinary or fecal elimination. Voiding immediately after sexual intercourse also helps to prevent bacteria from entering the woman's urinary tract. Adequate perineal care is important during the postpartum period and during menstruation. Men and women should be reminded of the importance of washing hands carefully with soap and water whenever the perineal area or body fluids are touched.

The nurse can also teach the signs and symptoms of UTIs, namely fever, flank pain, dysuria, frequency, urgency, pyuria, or hematuria. Teaching is especially important after any instrumentation of the bladder. Some people may be embarrassed to contact their physician about urinary problems, so the importance of prompt treatment for potential UTIs should be stressed.

Promoting Optimum Muscle Tone. Loss of perineal and abdominal muscle tone can contribute to urinary retention and incontinence. Promoting regular exercise of these structures can prevent loss of tone. Kegel exercises involve tightening of the perineal and anal muscles. This should be done several times per hour, and incorporated into activities of daily living so that lifelong habits can be formed. Kegel exercises are discussed in Chapter 52. Another muscle-strengthening exercise involves having the client voluntarily stop and start the stream of urine when voiding. Exercise instruction is especially important during the postpartum period. Client teaching concerning weight reduction for the obese person is also helpful in improving muscle tone.

Client Teaching
Urinary Elimination

Instruct the client as follows:

- *Drink between 6 to 8 glasses of fluid per day.*
- *Increase oral fluid intake to promote sufficient urine flow and prevent urinary stasis and infection.*
- *If you experience incontinence, restrict your intake of coffee, tea, or alcohol. The diuretic effect of these liquids may result in unpredictable voiding.*
- *(Female clients) Wipe the perineum in a front-to-back motion to prevent the introduction of microorganisms from the anal area into the urinary meatus, which can cause urinary tract infection.*
- *Learn the signs and symptoms of urinary tract infections: frequency, urgency, dysuria, flank pain, hematuria, or pyuria.*
- *Practice Kegel exercises.*
- *Keep urinary drainage bags below the level of the bladder so gravity can assist the outflow of urine from the bladder. Do not lay on or kink tubing because this might also obstruct the flow of urine.*
- *If you have just had a catheter removed, dribbling small amounts of urine for a short time is not uncommon.*
- *If urinary dribbling persists beyond 24 hours, increase oral fluid intake and use perineal strengthening exercises.*
- *Intermittent self-catheterization in the home is done as a clean procedure. A mirror can be used to help visualize the urinary meatus for female clients.*

Measures to Promote Voiding

Illness and hospitalization can disrupt a person's usual routine of urinary elimination. Unfamiliar and sometimes uncomfortable medical procedures, loss of privacy, strange surroundings, and anxiety concerning medical diagnosis or prognosis are just a few of the factors that may disrupt usual urinary elimination habits. In addition to promoting an adequate fluid intake, there are a number of comfort measures that the nurse can use to promote urinary elimination and to assist the client in maintaining his or her usual normal pattern:

- Provide a private setting for voiding.
- Allow adequate, unhurried, and uninterrupted time for voiding.
- If nursing assistance is needed for voiding, assess the client's usual voiding times (such as when awakening, before meals, and at bedtime), offer assistance at those times in particular, and be available for assistance at in-between times.
- Promote relief of physical discomfort and anxiety-producing situations. These may increase muscle tension and inhibit the relaxation needed for urination. Provide medications for pain as ordered, and emotional support and reassurance.
- Aid the client in assuming a comfortable and, if at all possible, physiologic position for voiding. This is a sitting or squatting position for women and a standing position for men.
- If the client has difficulty starting to urinate, it may be helpful for the nurse to provide sensory stimuli that act either by promoting relaxation or by the concept of suggestion. These stimuli include pouring warm water over the perineum, running water from the faucet, having the client relax in a warm bath, placing the client's hands in warm water, stroking the inner thighs, providing music or reading material, and offering a beverage.

Urinary Collection Devices

Urinary collection devices to promote normal urinary elimination are the toilet, bedside commode, urinal, and bedpan.

Toilet. For clients who are ambulatory, the typical procedure for urinary elimination involves walking to and from the bathroom and using the toilet for voiding, with assistance provided by the nurse as necessary. For some clients who have difficulty sitting down on and arising from a conventional-height toilet, a raised or elevated toilet seat can be attached, so that the client has a decreased distance to lower and raise himself or herself. Based on previous assessment, necessary comfort measures should be provided for the client using the bathroom, and opportunity given after voiding for the client to wash his or her hands. This may be a good time to instruct the client about hygiene techniques.

Bedside Commode. If the client is unable to ambulate as far as the bathroom, but can transfer out of bed to a chair, then a commode may be the device of choice for urinary elimination. A commode is a straight-backed armchair, frequently with locking wheels, with a toilet-like seat and receptacle for urine and feces. Some commodes are made with their own receptacles; others have a place for attaching a conventional bedpan. Many commodes have a flat seat covering the toilet seat, so that it may also be used as a chair. Commodes can be rented for use at home if access to the bathroom (eg, upstairs) or ambulation is difficult during recovery from acute illness or during chronic illness. Before assisting the client to the commode, the nurse must assess whether the client can safely transfer independently and, if not, just how much support he or she needs. If the client is at risk for falling, it may be necessary for the nurse or caregiver to remain with the client or to stand just beyond the privacy curtains while he or she urinates. Other comfort measures must be provided as needed, and the client should be provided with a means of handwashing after voiding.

Urinal. When a male client is confined to bed, he may use a urinal as a convenient collection device for urine (Fig. 41-6). Although urinals are made in a number of designs, and some urinals are designed specifically for women, it is typically the man who uses the urinal. Assisting the client to stand at the bedside when voiding while using the urinal is physiologically advantageous. Sometimes, however, this is contraindicated, and consequently the client is positioned in bed in as close to an upright position as feasible. In most instances the client is able to place and hold the urinal himself. If he is unable to do so, then the nurse may need to hold the urinal in place while the client urinates, or place the urinal and then leave the client alone for a few moments. When the client has completed voiding into the urinal, he will typically place it on the

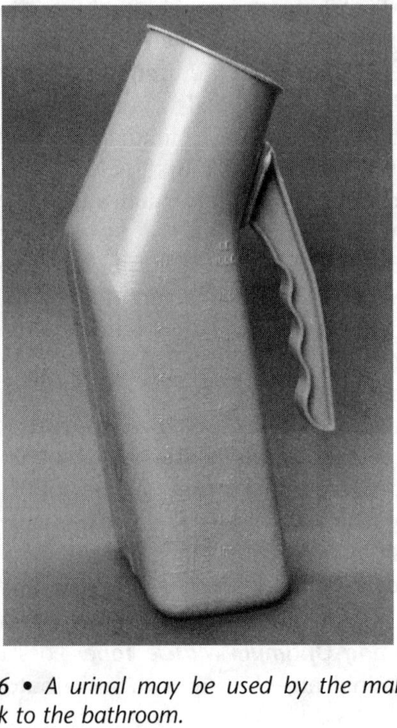

Figure 41-6 • *A urinal may be used by the male when he cannot walk to the bathroom.*

overbed table or hang it on the side rail of his bed. To avoid having the urinal bumped or knocked and the contents spilled, and to avoid any embarrassment that may be caused by having the client's urine clearly visible at the bedside, it is important that the nurse remember to empty and rinse the urinal in a timely manner. Once again, it is also important for the nurse to provide comfort measures as needed and a means of handwashing after voiding.

Bedpan. For female clients confined to bed, the bedpan is the collection device frequently used for urinary elimination. Typically, the male client uses the urinal for urine elimination and the bedpan for bowel elimination, and the female client uses the bedpan for both. Two types of bedpans are commonly available (see Chapter 32): the first, called a fracture pan, is smaller and flatter; the second, known as a regular bedpan, is rounded somewhat like a toilet seat and has a higher back. Fracture pans are used primarily for clients who have physical limitations or have difficulty lifting their buttocks onto the bedpan. Fracture pans are also used for clients whose medical complications contraindicate lifting onto a regular bedpan.

Some clients who are confined to bed can independently use the bedpan for urinary elimination. The bedpan should be kept within easy reach, along with toilet paper or other means of cleaning the perineum after urination. The nurse may need only to ensure privacy, to empty and clean the bedpan in a timely manner, return the bedpan to the client, and provide supplies for handwashing.

For many clients confined to bed, however, more assistance by the nurse is required. Having to use a bedpan for urine elimination may be an embarrassing, uncomfortable, and tiring procedure. Some clients may say that they feel it requires less energy to get up to use a commode than to get onto and off a bedpan. The positioning may be awkward, particularly if the client is unable to sit erect. It may feel as if she is sitting in a precarious position on top of the bedpan. In addition, complete emptying of the bladder may be inhibited when the client must attempt to urinate in a more recumbent position, leading to urinary retention.

Measures to promote urinary elimination for clients who must use a bedpan for urination include many of the previously noted comfort measures. Privacy must be ensured and the client placed in a comfortable, physiologic position for voiding if at all possible. Often it is helpful for the nurse to elevate the head of the client's bed to a Fowler's position and to place a small supportive pillow or rolled towel under the small of the back. It may also be helpful to have the client flex her knees and hips to provide as close to a normal position for voiding as possible. Warming the bedpan under running tap water just before placing it frequently helps to promote relaxation and avoid the muscle-contracting sensation of bare skin on cold metal or plastic. The nurse may find it helpful to place a small amount of talc or cornstarch on the seat of the bedpan to facilitate sliding the bedpan under the client and removing it after voiding. It may also be a prudent measure to place extra absorbent pads under the client and bedpan during the procedure to prevent soiling of the bed linen if the bedpan tips when being removed. For specific guidelines about assisting a client onto and off of a bedpan, refer to Procedure 32-7, "Using a Bedpan."

In timing or scheduling the use of the bedpan, toilet, urinal, or commode, the nurse must assess each client as to the amount of assistance required. Some clients are capable of monitoring their own elimination needs and will request assistance as necessary. For other clients, however, this is not the case. Some clients may feel the need to urinate but have difficulty communicating that need, or have awareness of the need to urinate and be able to communicate that need, but have difficulty using the collection devices independently. Others may have difficulty controlling urinary elimination, and may need assistance in planning and implementing a regular schedule of times for urinary elimination, frequently at 2-hour intervals. No matter what the difficulty, however, it is important for the nurse to approach the client in a calm, matter-of-fact manner and to provide appropriate comfort measures as necessary for promotion of optimal urinary elimination.

Nursing Interventions for Altered Function

The nurse can use many therapeutic nursing interventions to assist the client with altered urinary function. External catheters, protective pants, or indwelling catheters can be used for incontinent clients if bladder training in unsuccessful.

Bladder Training

Bladder training is the major independent nursing intervention used to treat urinary incontinence. Bladder training involves regulation of fluid intake and establishment of regular voiding times, assisting the client in the ability to postpone voiding despite a sensation of urgency. Additional techniques such as biofeedback, electrical stimulation, and pelvic muscle exercises may also be used to retrain the bladder (Agency for Health Care Policy and Research, 1992).

Sufficient fluid intake is important for the success of a bladder training program. The bladder requires at least 200 mL volume to initiate the micturition reflex. A fluid intake of at least 2,000 mL daily is recommended to provide sufficient hydration to allow the normal bladder stretch–contraction reflex to occur. The nurse and the client together should decide on the daily fluid volume goal. Most fluids should be taken during daytime hours, decreasing intake of fluids as bedtime approaches. Fluids with a diuretic effect such as coffee, tea, cola, or alcohol are best avoided during bladder retraining.

Establishing and maintaining a voiding schedule is the most challenging aspect of bladder training. Several options are available, and if one is unsuccessful another may be tried.

- Traditional bladder retraining starts with scheduled voidings. The client is asked to void at scheduled times (usually every 2 hours) and suppress the urge to void before the scheduled time. The time interval is gradually increased to every 4 hours.
- Habit retraining schedules the client's voiding in an attempt to approximate the client's usual voiding pattern.
- Timed voiding is the continuous use of an unchanged, fixed voiding schedule (usually every 2 hours).
- Prompted voiding involves the use of regular checks to see if the client perceives the urge to void. Sometimes just the reminder or suggestion of the need to void is sufficient stimulus to initiate voiding. Prompted voiding can prevent incontinence when there is difficulty perceiving bladder fullness.

It is important that the client and all people responsible for the client's care be aware of the method of bladder retraining and the schedule. It is often helpful if the schedule is posted above the client's bed or at the bedside, and data recorded. The success of bladder retraining depends on consistency over time, because the bladder is being retrained to respond to a normal micturition reflex. Refer to the Nursing Plan of Care near the end of this chapter for an example of a bladder retraining schedule.

Muscle-strengthening exercises are the third part of a bladder retraining program. Kegel exercises to strengthen the pubococcygeal muscles and exercises such as sit-ups to strengthen the abdominal muscles are helpful in promoting optimum urinary control.

Habit Training

Habit training does not actually retrain the bladder but may be helpful in preventing episodes of incontinence. Verbal cues or prompts are given to a client to encourage voiding. This is usually done at scheduled intervals such as every 2 hours. Positive reinforcement is given when voiding occurs after verbal cuing. Habit training is especially helpful in cognitively impaired clients who may postpone voiding until incontinence occurs. Success of habit retraining often depends on how willing and diligent the caregiver is in consistently providing prompts on schedule.

External Catheters and Protective Pants

For some clients bladder or habit training may not be satisfactory because of an inability to control voiding. These may be elderly clients with some form of cognitive dysfunction, unconscious clients, or others with extreme weakness. Clients who are unable to control urination need assistance with urine collection. They also need frequent cleansing or bathing to remove odors and to maintain clean, dry, and intact tissues in the perineal area.

Condom Catheter. An external catheter (condom catheter, or "Texas" catheter) is sometimes used for male clients unable to control voiding. External catheters have a much lower risk of UTI than indwelling catheters and may decrease the risk of fecal contamination for the incontinent client. Condom catheters have also been shown effectively to control odor associated with incontinence (Lyder, et al., 1992). The external catheter comprises a condom that is placed on the penis and attached to tubing that inserts into a closed collection bag. The collection bag may be similar to the type used for indwelling catheters, or for clients who are more mobile, it may be a bag that attaches securely to the leg. When applying or removing an external catheter, it is important to follow carefully the specific directions of the manufacturer or agency policy. For general guidelines on applying and removing an external catheter, see Procedure 41-3, "Applying a Condom Catheter." The external catheter should be removed daily to cleanse the penis and surrounding tissues, and to assess the skin for any edema or areas of excoriation. The client's leg bag or larger urine collection bag should also be emptied at least every 8 hours or more frequently as needed.

Protective Pants. For female clients unable to control urination, a device such as an external catheter has not been developed. As an alternative to indwelling catheterization, some female clients as well as some male clients use protective pants. Also known as incontinent briefs, protective pants are typically disposable, waterproof briefs lined with soft, absorbent material. The briefs are open at the sides with tape or Velcro closures to facilitate application for clients who are confined to bed or have difficulty moving, turning, or pulling on clothes. It is important to change the protective pants frequently to avoid odor and to prevent skin irritation from prolonged exposure to moisture. The client should bathe daily. Each time the protective pants are changed, the perineal area should be cleansed and examined for any areas of irritation.

Urinary Catheterization

Urinary catheterization involves inserting a small tube, called a catheter, through the urethra into the bladder,

Procedure 41-3
Applying a Condom Catheter

Purpose

1. Provide a means of collecting urine and controlling incontinence without the risk of infection that an indwelling urinary catheter imposes.

Assessment

- Identify clients who require control of incontinence.
- Assess mental status of client to determine ability to cooperate with procedure.
- Inspect penis for irritation or areas of skin breakdown from previous incontinence.
- Determine client's activity level and need of leg bag or continuous drainage system for urine collection.

Equipment

Soap, warm water, towel
Commercially packaged condom catheter with adhesive.
Disposable gloves.
Urine collection bag with drainage tubing or leg bag with straps.

Procedure

1. Close room door or bedside curtain. Explain procedure to client.
   Rationale: Provides privacy and encourages cooperation.
2. Wash hands.
3. Assist client to supine position with only genitalia exposed.
   Rationale: Provides client comfort and privacy.
4. Put on disposable gloves. Wash genitals with soap and water. Towel dry.
   Rationale: Removes secretions to prevent skin breakdown. Catheter adheres best if skin is thoroughly dry.
5. Trim or shave excess pubic hair from base of penis, if necessary.
   Rationale: Excess hair adheres to the condom adhesive, interferes with a good seal, and is uncomfortable when condom is removed.
6. Apply thin film of skin protector on penis shaft (usually found in commercially packaged condom catheter kits). Allow to dry for 30 seconds.
   Rationale: Protects sensitive penile skin from irritation and provides better adherence to the adhesive liner.
7. Peel paper backing from both sides of adhesive line and wrap spirally around penis shaft.
   Rationale: Spiral wrap prevents a constricting tourniquet effect of the adhesive strip on the penis that could impede circulation.

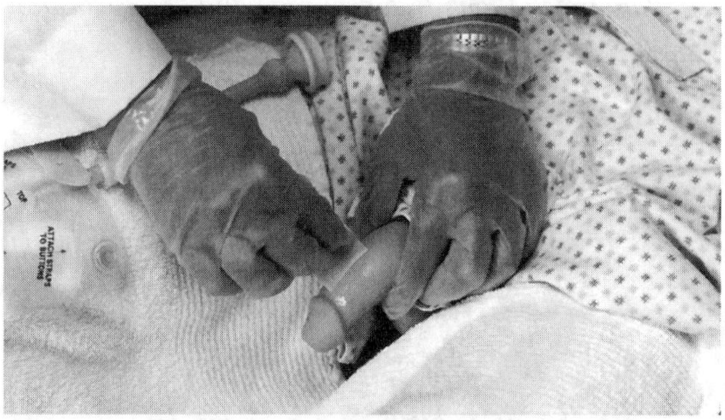

Step 6 • *Apply skin protector to penis shaft.*

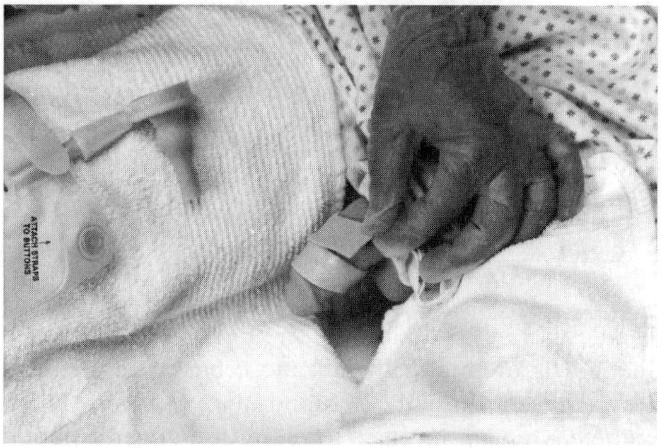

Step 7 • *Wrap adhesive spirally around penis.*

8. Place funnel end of pre-rolled condom against the glans of penis. Unroll the sheath the length of the penis, over the adhesive liner.
   Note: Some brands of condom catheters are held in place with a velcro strap over the condom catheter.

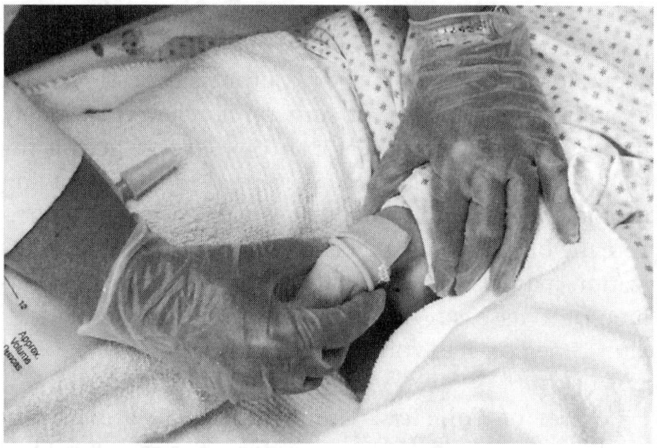

Step 8 • *Unroll condom sheath over adhesive liner.*

(continued)

9. Attach funnel end of condom to collection system. Secure system below level of condom, avoiding kinks or loops in the tubing.
   Rationale: Allows free drainage and observation of color and quantity of urine.

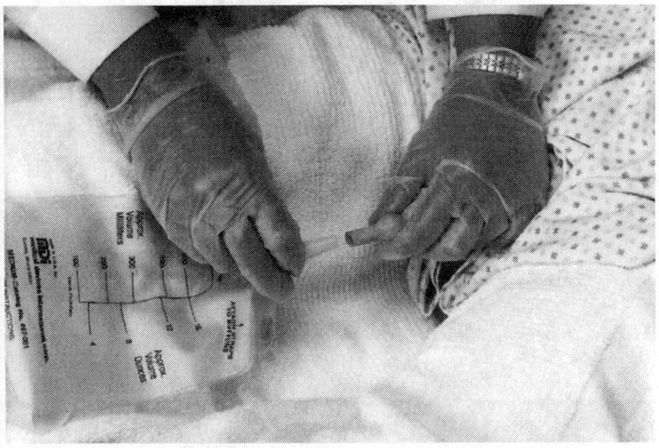

Step 9 • *Attach funnel end of condom to collection system.*

10. Discard used supplies and wash hands.
11. Observe penis 15 to 30 minutes after application of condom, for swelling or changes in skin color.
    Rationale: Swelling or discoloration of penis indicates condom it too tight and should be removed and reapplied in a larger size.
12. Document procedure and observations.

Lifespan Considerations

- Condom catheters are not indicated for use in children.
- Young men might experience an erection as the penis is grasped for condom application.
- When penis is grasped in older men, it may retract into lower abdominal skinfolds, making application difficult.

Home-Care Modification

- Clients using condom catheters at home should be taught how to empty and care for their drainage collecting bag. In addition, the client should be taught how to attach his condom to a leg bag to allow physical activity without fear of embarrassment from urine incontinence.

to allow urine to drain out. The most frequently used method is urethral catheterization, but urine can also be removed through a suprapubic catheter. When catheters remain in place to drain urine over a period of time, they are referred to as **indwelling** (or retention) **catheters**. When a urethral catheter is inserted temporarily to empty urine from the bladder and then removed, it is referred to as an in-and-out catheterization. If in-and-out catheterization is performed on a routine, scheduled basis for a particular client, it is known as intermittent catheterization.

Indications for Catheterization. A urethral catheter may be inserted when the client is experiencing difficulty with urination, such as with incontinence or urinary retention. A catheter may also be inserted when accurate assessment of urinary output is necessary, such as after trauma, burns, or surgery. Surgical clients may have a catheter in place for a few days to permit tissues to heal and edema to subside. For clients having urologic surgery, the catheter provides a means to irrigate the bladder or instill bladder medications. Catheterization may also be necessary to collect a urine specimen or to assess how much urine is left in the bladder after a person has voided.

Types of Catheters. Urinary catheters are usually made of rubber, plastic, or nylon. A straight rubber catheter with only one lumen is used for in-and-out and intermittent catheterization procedures. When an indwelling catheter is required, a double-lumen catheter known as a Foley is most commonly used (Fig. 41-7). A Foley catheter contains one lumen to remove the urine, and a second, smaller lumen to inflate a balloon that keeps the catheter from falling out of the bladder. The balloon is located near the insertion tip of the catheter and can be inflated and deflated with a syringe. A third type of catheter, a triple-lumen indwelling catheter, is inserted when a client requires an indwelling catheter not only to remove urine from the bladder but also for the administration of medications or irrigating fluid. A triple-lumen catheter is usually used after urologic or prostatic surgery (Fig. 41-8). A coudé catheter has a curved tip that permits easier insertion, especially as the catheter passes urethral narrowing, such as that caused by prostatic hyperplasia. Silver-impregnated or coated catheters may be commonly used in the future because they delay the incidence of bacteriuria and prevent ureteral entry of microorganisms (Pinkerman, 1994).

Urinary catheters are available in different sizes. The selection of the proper size is important to aid in the prevention of trauma to urethral tissues. A catheter smaller than the external meatus should be used to minimize trauma. Catheters are sized on the French scale of numbers, according to the diameter of the lumen. On this scale, the larger the lumen size, the larger the French number. Available adult sizes range from #14 to #22, with sizes #18 and #20 commonly used for men, and sizes #16 and #8 commonly used for women.

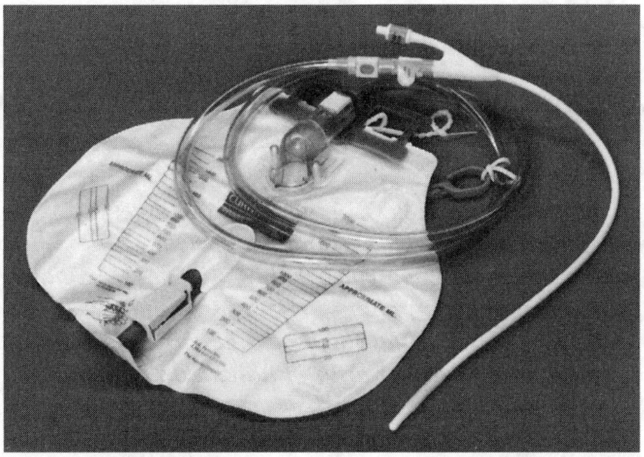

Figure 41-7 • A Foley catheter and drainage bag.

Catheterization. To avoid introducing microorganisms into the urinary system, which is sterile, aseptic technique must be used whenever a urinary catheter is inserted. Procedure 41-4, "Inserting a Straight or Indwelling Urinary Catheter," outlines the correct technique for catheterization.

The male client can be positioned in a supine or semi-Fowler's position. The female client is often placed in a dorsal recumbent (supine with knees flexed) position for catheterization. An alternative, especially for the client who has limited hip mobility, is the side-lying position (see Procedure 41-4). This position is more comfortable for the weak client who may have difficulty keeping legs flexed and spread apart to permit visualization. The side-lying position also permits excellent visualization of the urinary meatus.

Risks of Catheterization. Any break in sterile technique during catheter insertion carries with it the risk of infection to the bladder, ureters, and, eventually, kidneys. In addition, with an indwelling catheter, the risk of infection continues and increases as long as the catheter remains in place. The risk of infection is especially significant if the catheter remains in place longer than 72 hours. The indwelling catheter must be connected to a closed drainage bag to prevent the migration of microorganisms up the inside of the catheter lumen to the bladder. What still can occur, even with

(text continues on page 1213)

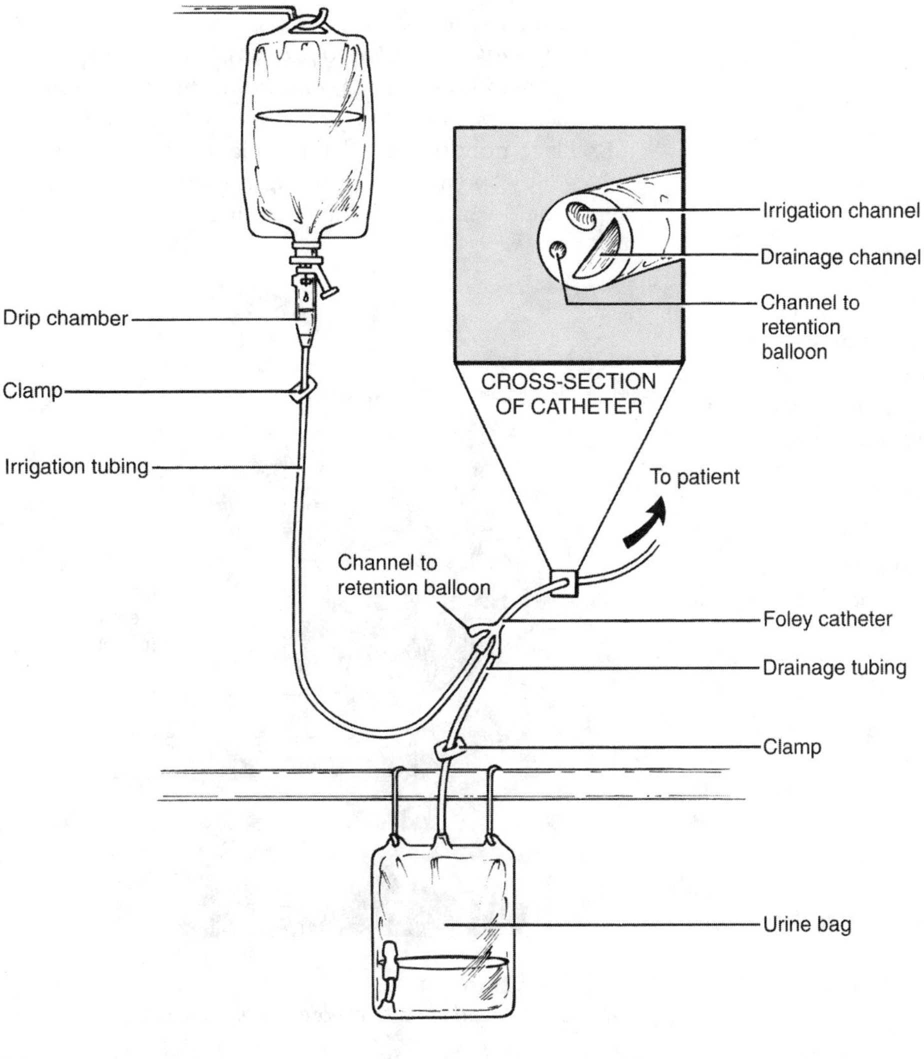

Figure 41-8 • Closed irrigation system showing the triple-lumen catheter.

Procedure 41-4
Inserting a Straight or Indwelling Urinary Catheter

Purpose

1. Monitor urinary function, prevent or relieve bladder distention.
2. Provide continuous bladder drainage.
3. Obtain sterile urine specimens.
4. Measure residual urine.
5. Provide a means for irrigating the bladder with fluids or medication.

Assessment

- Reason(s) catheterization has been ordered.
- Client for bladder distention.
- Client's physical ability to tolerate positioning.

Equipment

A light source.

Prepackaged, sterile catheterization kits that usually include the catheter (the most commonly used adult indwelling catheter is the Foley catheter, size 16 French with a 5 mL balloon), cotton balls, lubricant, disposable forceps, cleansing Betadine solution, specimen cup, gloves and drapes, and drainage bag.

Extra catheter and sterile gloves.

Procedure

1. Explain the procedure and rationale to client.
Rationale: The client who understands the procedure is more apt to relax, which facilitates the procedure and is more comfortable for the client.
2. Provide the client with opportunity to perform personal perineal/penile hygiene. Assist client as necessary.
Rationale: Strict asepsis must be maintained to reduce the possibility of introducing a urinary tract infection. Initial cleansing rids body of gross contamination.
3. Wash your hands.
Rationale: Handwashing prevents transfer of microorganisms.

Procedure

Inserting Catheter for a Woman

1. Position in dorsal recumbent position (supine with knees flexed). Externally rotate thighs. Side lying is an alternative position.
Rationale: Allows for visualization of the urinary meatus.
2. Drape legs to midthigh with bath blanket.
Rationale: The blanket provides privacy and prevents chilling, which aid in patient relaxation.
3. Set up light source.
Rationale: Adequate lighting and correct positioning are crucial for clear visualization of the urinary meatus.
4. Open the catheterization tray.
5. Slide sterile drape under client's buttocks, grasping corners of drape. Ask client to lift hips so drape can be slid under.
Rationale: The drape provides a large sterile field.
6. Don sterile gloves.
Rationale: This is a sterile procedure.
7. Open sterile lubricant and lubricate catheter tip. Open cleansing solution and pour over half of the sterile balls. Open the sterile specimen container. Inflate balloon with prefilled syringe to check for defective balloon. Aspirate fluid back into syringe and leave attached.
Rationale: Attention to preparation of tray decreases chances of contaminating sterile hands or equipment before procedure is completed.
8. Place nondominant hand on labia minora and gently spread to expose urinary meatus. Visualize exact location of meatus. During cleansing and

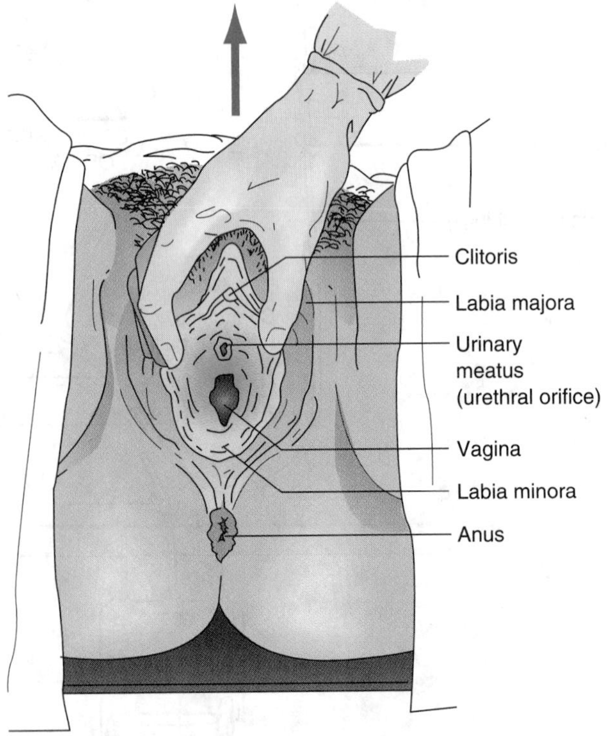

Step 8 • *Spread labia to expose urinary meatus.*

catheter insertion, do not allow labia to close over meatus until after the catheter is inserted. (This hand is now considered contaminated.)
Rationale: If labia closes over the meatus before catheter insertion, the meatus is considered contaminated and must be recleansed.

9. Using sterile hand, pick up antiseptic solution-saturated cotton ball with sterile forceps.
Rationale: Using forceps during cleaning protects sterile hand from contamination.
10. Cleanse the urinary meatus with one downward stroke. Discard the cotton ball. Repeat this step three to four times. Place dry cotton ball over vagina.
Rationale: Cleansing from front to back avoids introducing microorganisms from the rectum to the urinary meatus. Cotton ball over vagina allows for easier identification of urinary meatus.

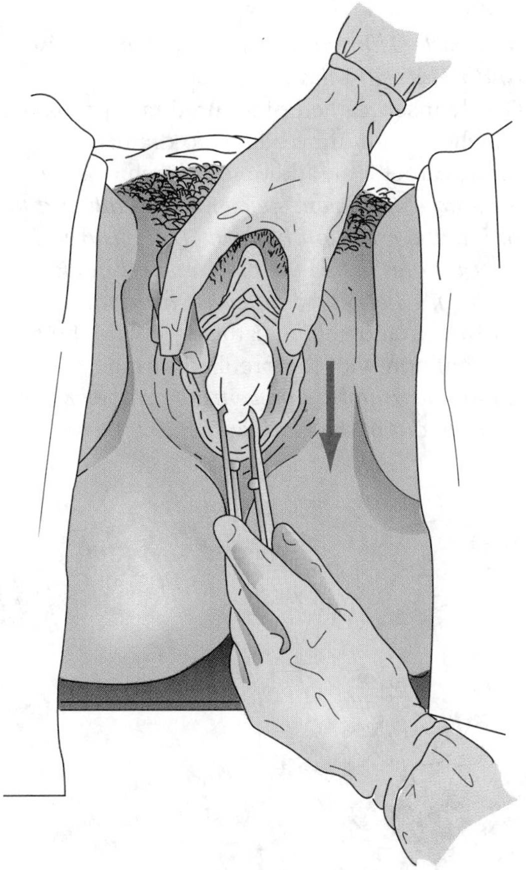

Step 10 • *Cleanse urinary meatus with downward strokes.*

11. Use forceps and two dry cotton balls to dry the meatus.
Rationale: Drying the meatus decreases the slipperiness of the tissues, aids visualization of the meatus, and prevents introducing the cleansing solution into the meatus.
12. With sterile hand, pick up the catheter approximately 3 inches from the tip and dip into sterile lubricant. Place distal catheter end into sterile basin.
Rationale: Lubricant facilitates catheter insertion and reduces urethral trauma.
13. Gently insert catheter into urethra (approximately 2 inches) until urine begins to drain. If no urine appears, have client cough, or reposition catheter by rotating. Have client take slow, deep breaths during catheter insertion.
Rationale: Coughing increases intraabdominal pressure and may assist urine flow. When the client takes slow, deep breaths, the external sphincter relaxes.
14. Insert the catheter an additional 1 inch or 2.5 cm.
Rationale: Sufficient space must be allowed to inflate the retention balloon. This ensures the balloon inflates inside the bladder and not inside the urethra, where it would cause trauma.
Note: If the catheter enters the vagina by mistake, leave it there as a landmark. Insert a second catheter into the meatus.
15. Obtain urine specimen in sterile container, if ordered.
16. If using a straight catheter: allow bladder to empty, then remove the straight catheter.
17. If using an indwelling catheter: inflate the retention balloon with the prefilled syringe.

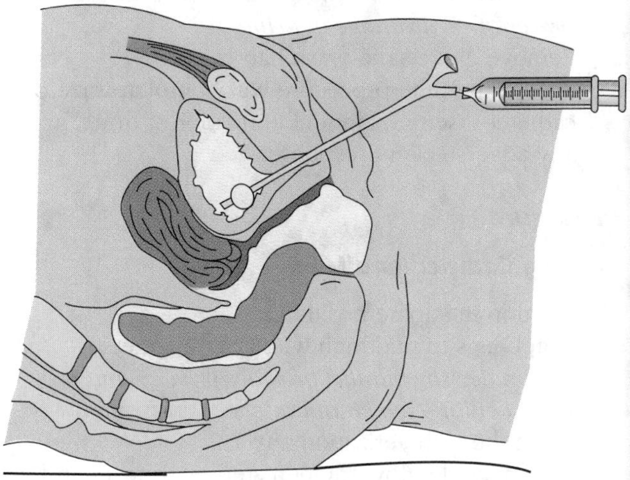

Step 17 • *Inflate retention balloon with prefilled syringe.*

18. Check to ensure placement by gently pulling on catheter.
Rationale: If resistance is felt, the catheter balloon is properly inflated in the bladder.
19. Connect distal end of catheter to drainage bag.
Note: In some kits the catheter is already connected to the drainage unit. Some nurses prefer to connect equipment before catheter insertion.

(continued)

20. Tape the catheter securely with 1-inch tape to inner thigh, with enough give so it will not pull when moving the legs.
   Rationale: Securing the tape reduces urethral friction and irritation during client movement.

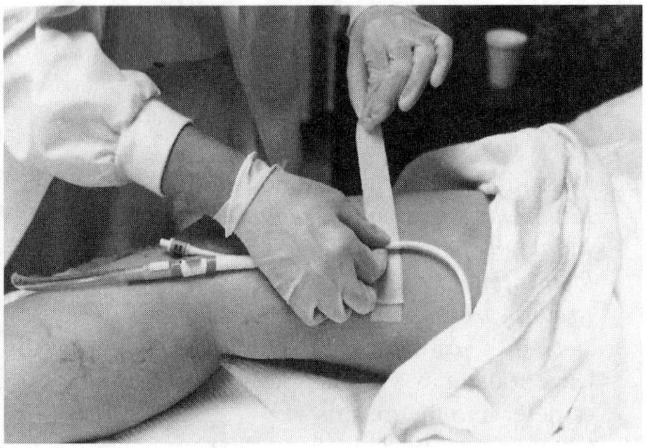

Step 20 • *Tape catheter securely to thigh.*

21. Attach drainage bag to bed frame, ensuring that tubing does not fall into dependent loops or that side rails do not interfere with drainage system.
   Rationale: Dependent loops fill with urine and can prevent free drainage of urine.
22. Remove gloves and wash hands.
23. Record the time procedure was complete, size of catheter inserted, amount and color of urine, and any adverse client responses.

Procedure

Inserting Catheter for a Man

1. Position in supine position.
2. Drape legs to midthigh with bath blanket.
   Rationale: The blanket provides privacy and prevents chilling, which aid in client relaxation.
3. Open the catheterization tray.
4. Put on sterile gloves. Open sterile lubricant and lubricate catheter liberally. Open cleansing solution and pour over half of the sterile balls. Open the sterile specimen container. Inflate balloon with prefilled syringe to check for defective balloon. Aspirate fluid back into syringe and leave attached.
   Rationale: Attention to preparation of tray decreases chance of contaminating sterile hands or equipment before procedure is completed.
5. Place the fenestrated drape over the client's genitalia.
6. With your nondominant hand, hold the penis at a 90-degree angle to his body. If the client is not circumcised, pull back the foreskin with this hand to visualize the urethral meatus. (This hand is now considered unsterile.)
   Rationale: Holding the penis at a 90-degree angle is important to straighten the urethra and allow for nontraumatic catheter insertion.
7. Using the sterile hand, pick up antiseptic solution-soaked cotton ball with sterile forceps.
   Rationale: Using forceps during cleaning protects sterile hand from contamination.
8. Cleanse the urinary meatus with one downward stroke or use a circular motion from meatus to base of penis. Discard the cotton ball. Repeat this step at least three to four times.
   Rationale: Cleaning from meatus outward helps keep insertion site as clean as possible.
9. Use forceps to pick up one dry cotton ball to dry the meatus.
   Rationale: Drying the meatus prevents introduction of cleansing solution into meatus, which could cause discomfort.
10. With sterile hand, pick up the catheter approximately 3 inches from the tip and lubricate catheter generously. Place distal catheter end into sterile basin.
   Rationale: Lubricant facilitates catheter insertion and reduces urethral trauma.
11. Gently insert catheter into urethra (approximately 8 inches) until urine begins to drain.
12. Insert catheter an additional 1 inch or 2.5 cm.
   Rationale: Sufficient space must be allowed to inflate the retention balloon. This ensures the balloon inflates inside the bladder and not inside the urethra, where it would cause trauma.
13. If using an indwelling catheter, inflate the retention balloon with the prefilled syringe.
   Rationale: Inflation prevents the catheter from slipping out of the bladder.

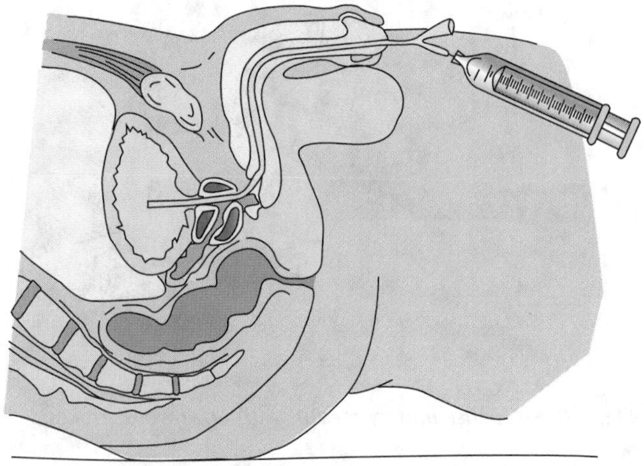

Step 13 • *Inflate retention balloon with prefilled syringe.*

14. Check for placement by gently pulling on catheter.
   Rationale: If resistance is felt, the catheter balloon is properly inflated in the bladder.
15. Connect distal end of catheter to drainage bag if necessary.

16. Tape the catheter securely with 1-inch tape to the abdomen.
    Rationale: Securely taping the catheter prevents trauma to the penile–scrotal junction and reduces friction and irritation of the urethra from catheter movement.

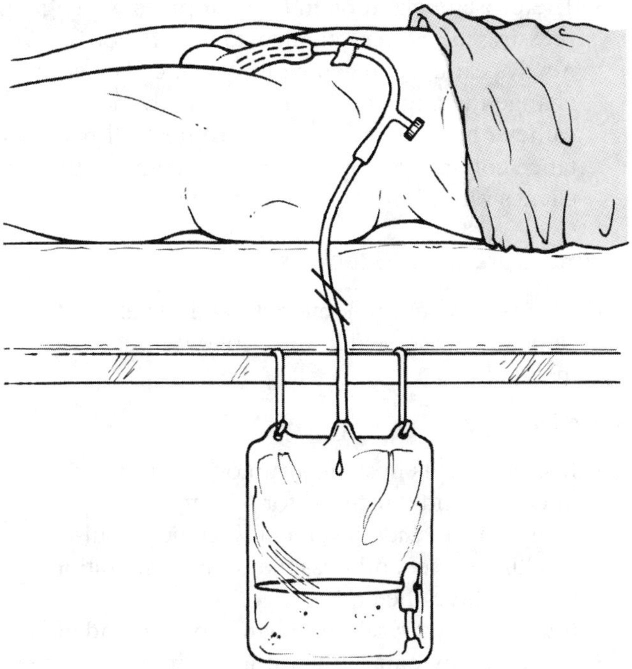

Step 16 • *Tape catheter securely to abdomen.*

17. In the uncircumcised male, gently replace the foreskin over the glans.
    Rationale: If the foreskin is left retracted, it can cause constricting edema and impair circulation to the penis.
18. Attach drainage bag to bed frame, coiling tubing to ensure that tubing does not fall into dependent loops.
19. Wash hands.
20. Record the time procedure was complete, size of catheter, amount and color of urine, and any adverse client responses.

Procedure

Removing an Indwelling Catheter

1. Wash your hands.
2. Don clean, disposable gloves.
   Rationale: Handwashing and use of gloves prevent transfer of microorganisms from client's urine to the nurse.
3. Clamp the catheter (optional).
   Rationale: Clamping prevents urine collected in catheter from leaking onto bed after removal.
4. Insert hub of syringe into balloon inflation tube of catheter and draw out all liquid. Size of balloon is indicated on catheter; most commonly, less than 10 mL are used. Larger balloons (30 mL) may be used after prostatic or urologic surgery.
   Rationale: The balloon must be completely deflated to prevent trauma to the urethra as catheter is removed.

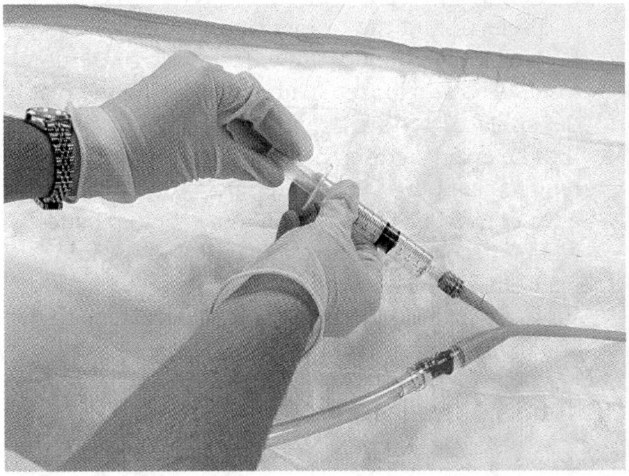

Step 4 • *Insert hub of syringe into balloon inflation tube. (Photo © B. Proud.)*

5. Ask client to breathe in and out deeply. Pinch gently and remove catheter as client exhales.
   Rationale: Breathing provides distraction and exhalation prevents tightening of abdominal and perineal muscles as catheter is withdrawn. Pinching catheter prevents leakage of urine.

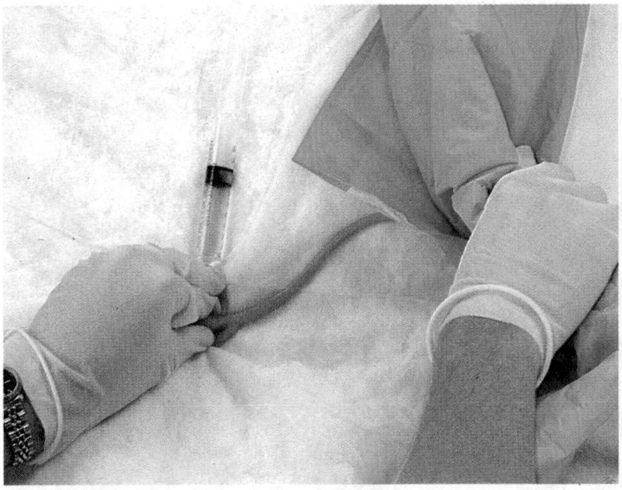

Step 5 • *Gently remove catheter as client exhales. (Photo © B. Proud.)*

6. Assist client to cleanse and dry genitals.
7. Measure and document urine in drainage bag and time of catheter removal.
8. Wash hands.

(continued)

Safety Alert

- Strict adherence to sterile technique is necessary to prevent introduction of microorganisms into the urinary tract.
- Trauma and pain are minimized by preprocedure client teaching to gain cooperation, adequate lighting for visualization of the urethral meatus, and selection of the proper size of catheter. Distraction techniques are useful during insertion to reduce catheter resistance by relaxing the bladder sphincter.
- If catheterizing a distended bladder, some agencies require clamping the catheter after 700 mL of urine have drained. Wait 30 to 60 minutes before completing decompression. Removing all of the urine may cause a shift in intraabdominal pressure and sufficient shift of blood from central circulation to the abdominal vessels that the client becomes dizzy.

Lifespan Considerations

Children

- Catheterization can be a frightening, painful procedure for a small child. It should be completed in the treatment room so the child's bed remains a "safe" area.
- An assistant may be necessary to help the child remain still during the procedure.
- Locating the urethral meatus on young girls takes extra care because the vaginal opening is more anterior than in grown women.
- A variety of sizes of catheters are available for use in children.

The Older Woman

- The labia of women atrophy after menopause. The skin folds can feel loose and slippery when cleansing before insertion.

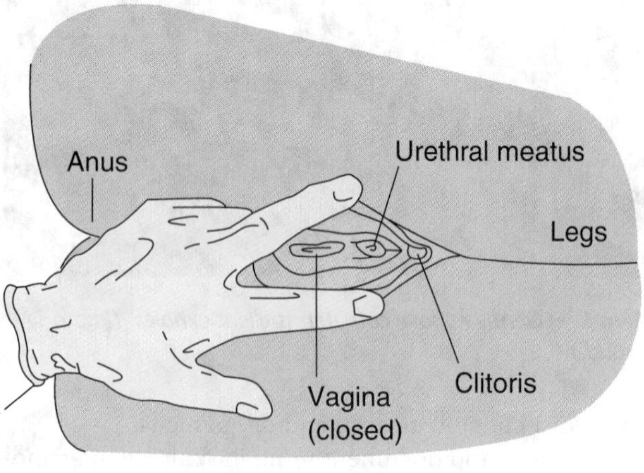

- Arthritis and other age-related musculoskeletal conditions may make it difficult for the older woman to maintain position for insertion without an assistant. Side-lying position often is more comfortable.

The Older Man

- The prostate gland often hypertrophies with aging, pressing in at the urethral–bladder junction. Always catheterize gently; if resistance is met, change the angle of the penis and advance catheter again, or use a coudé catheter. If resistance continues, stop the procedure and notify the client's physician.

Home-Care Modifications

- Clients may return home with an indwelling catheter. Home health nurse follow-up is recommended.

Infection

- Instruct clients in signs/symptoms of urinary tract infection, and directions for who to notify. Symptoms include fever, chills, cloudy, foul-smelling urine, and possible burning sensation around the catheter.
- Clients should wash their hands before and after touching any part of their urinary drainage system.
- Cleansing of the urinary meatus and catheter should be done with warm water and soap at least twice a day. The uncircumcised man should retract the foreskin and cleanse the entire glans well.
- Intermittent self-catheterization in the home is usually done using clean technique.
- To help prevent infection with long-term catheter use, 1 g ascorbic acid per day may be ordered to acidify the urine. Cranberry juice is also recommended to lower urine pH, but six to eight glasses per day are necessary to accomplish this. Vitamin C may also be used.

Urinary Drainage Bags

- Small bags that attach to the leg are available to increase independence in the ambulating patient.
- Bed-hanging, larger-volume collection bags are used at night.
- Check and follow home agency guidelines for changing the catheter and collecting tubing and drainage bags.

the use of a closed drainage system, is the migration of microorganisms from the meatus up the outside of the catheter and drainage tubing toward the bladder. Manipulation of the catheter, especially advancing the catheter into the bladder after it has been originally placed, can increase infection risk (Pinkerman, 1994).

Another risk of urethral catheterization is trauma to the urethral tissues, which can also contribute to an eventual infection. Men are particularly at risk for tissue trauma because of the length and the curvature of the male urethra. Particular care must be taken to insert the catheter along the normal contour of the urethra to avoid trauma to the tissues. For men in particular, the normal curve of the urethra can be straightened somewhat by elevating the penis to a position perpendicular to the body.

A third risk of urethral catheterization, both in-and-out and indwelling, involves removing a large amount of urine from the bladder at one time. When the urinary bladder is distended with urine beyond 400 to 500 mL, compression of the blood vessels in the bladder wall occurs. If the bladder is quickly emptied of amounts greater than 700 mL by catheterization, those blood vessels that have been compressed dilate and fill with blood. This can lead to a sudden decrease in the overall circulating blood supply, and can cause the client to feel faint. As a response to this risk, and as a precautionary measure, if urine is still flowing after 700 mL have been removed from the bladder, the catheter is typically clamped for 30 to 60 minutes to allow the vessels in the bladder wall to accommodate. The tubing is then unclamped to complete the removal of urine. One study (Bristoll, 1989) with a small sample (six clients) indicated that rapid bladder decompression may not have clinically significant adverse physiologic effects. More research into this area is needed. Another risk of rapid bladder decompression is submucosal hemorrhage in the bladder that has been chronically overdistended (Williams, et al., 1993).

Care of Indwelling Catheters. Because the presence of an indwelling urethral catheter increases a client's risk for acquiring a UTI, special care must be taken by nursing personnel to minimize that risk. The catheter, drainage collection tubing, and bag comprise a closed drainage system that preferably should not be disconnected except to change to a new closed system. The retention catheter and collection bag and tubing should be changed as frequently as necessary, as indicated by the presence of increasing sediment in the urine and along the catheter tubing (Roe, 1985). The drainage collection bag should be emptied through the outlet port at the bottom of the bag at least every 8 hours, more frequently if necessary, because pooled urine is an excellent growth medium for microorganisms.

To prevent pulling or kinking of the catheter, it should be taped securely to the body in a fashion that keeps the catheter securely in place, but with enough slack to allow movement by the client. The catheter should be taped to the inner aspect of the thigh of the female client or to the lower abdomen of the male client. It is important to tape the catheter to the abdomen of the male client rather than the leg to prevent irritation at the penile–scrotal angle. In addition, sometimes a water-soluble lubricant is applied to the meatus to decrease irritation of the urethra.

The drainage collection bag and tubing should be kept below the level of the bladder to maintain proper drainage and prevent pooling or backflow. Most collection bags have a one-way valve at the insertion of the tubing into the collection bag that also prevents backflow. The collection bag should be attached to the frame of the bed not the side rail, and it should not rest on the floor. The tubing should be coiled on the bed and attached to the bed linens in such a way that there are no dependent loops. The collection bag and tubing come equipped with means to attach both the collection bag to the bed frame and the tubing to the bed linens.

The perineal area and the catheter should be cleansed at least twice daily to remove normal secretions and to help prevent infection. Because specific directions for catheter care vary among agencies, it is important to check agency policy. Most agencies suggest the use of soap and water for cleansing, but some recommend the use of povidone–iodine for cleansing, followed by the application of iodophor ointment to the meatus. In either case, the perineal area is cleansed thoroughly, the meatus washed carefully, and the area rinsed and dried thoroughly. To avoid bringing organisms from the rectum forward toward the meatus, it is important to cleanse the perineal area from front to back in the woman. During catheter care, the client is assessed for any complaints of perineal irritation or burning, and the area is inspected for redness or excoriation. The color of urine in the tubing and the presence or absence of mucus is noted.

When caring for the client with an indwelling catheter, it is important for the nurse to monitor I & O and encourage adequate oral intake. Foods such as meats, eggs, whole-grain breads, cranberries, prunes, and plums should be encouraged, because they tend to produce acid urine. An acidic urine environment may inhibit the growth of certain microorganisms and decrease the incidence of infection.

Urinary Catheter Irrigation. The purpose of catheter irrigation is to cleanse the lumen of the catheter tubing to promote patency of the tube. The purposes of irrigation of the urinary bladder include the instillation of solution to help remove mucus, blood clots, or other tissue in the bladder (particularly after genitourinary surgery), and the application of medication to the bladder wall. A physician's order is required before either procedure is performed. In addition, the physician will prescribe the type and amount of solution to be administered and either the closed or open method of irrigation.

The closed method of irrigation is performed without disrupting the closed drainage system using a triple-lumen indwelling urethral catheter (see Fig. 41-8). One lumen is used to inflate the balloon of the catheter to keep it securely inside the bladder, one lumen is used for the removal of urine into a closed drainage system, and the third lumen is connected to a container of sterile irrigating solution. The specified type and amount of irrigating solution is administered via a continuous drip at a rate prescribed by the physician or by written protocol. The catheter lumen used for the removal of urine can be clamped until the prescribed solution has been instilled, and then opened to allow drainage, or it can be left open to allow outflow of urine throughout the procedure (Fig. 41-9). Throughout the closed method of irrigation, the catheter and drainage tube remain connected to decrease the risk of entry of microorganisms into the system, which could cause an infection. See Procedure 41-5 for a description of continuous bladder irrigation.

The open method of irrigation, which is associated with an increased risk of UTI, is performed with the double-lumen indwelling urethral catheter. After cleansing the junction between the urethral catheter and the drainage tubing, and using sterile technique, the catheter and the drainage tubing are disconnected. Using a sterile syringe, usually an asepto syringe, the prescribed type and quantity of solution is administered slowly, either by gravity or gentle pressure, into the catheter tubing. The irrigating solution is then allowed to drain by gravity from the catheter. This procedure may be repeated depending on the amount of solution to be instilled and the physician's order. After completion of the irrigation, the catheter and drainage tubing are connected again. Care must be taken throughout the procedure to maintain sterile technique because of the increased risk of UTI associated with this procedure.

With both the closed and open methods of catheter and bladder irrigation, it is important to assess the re-

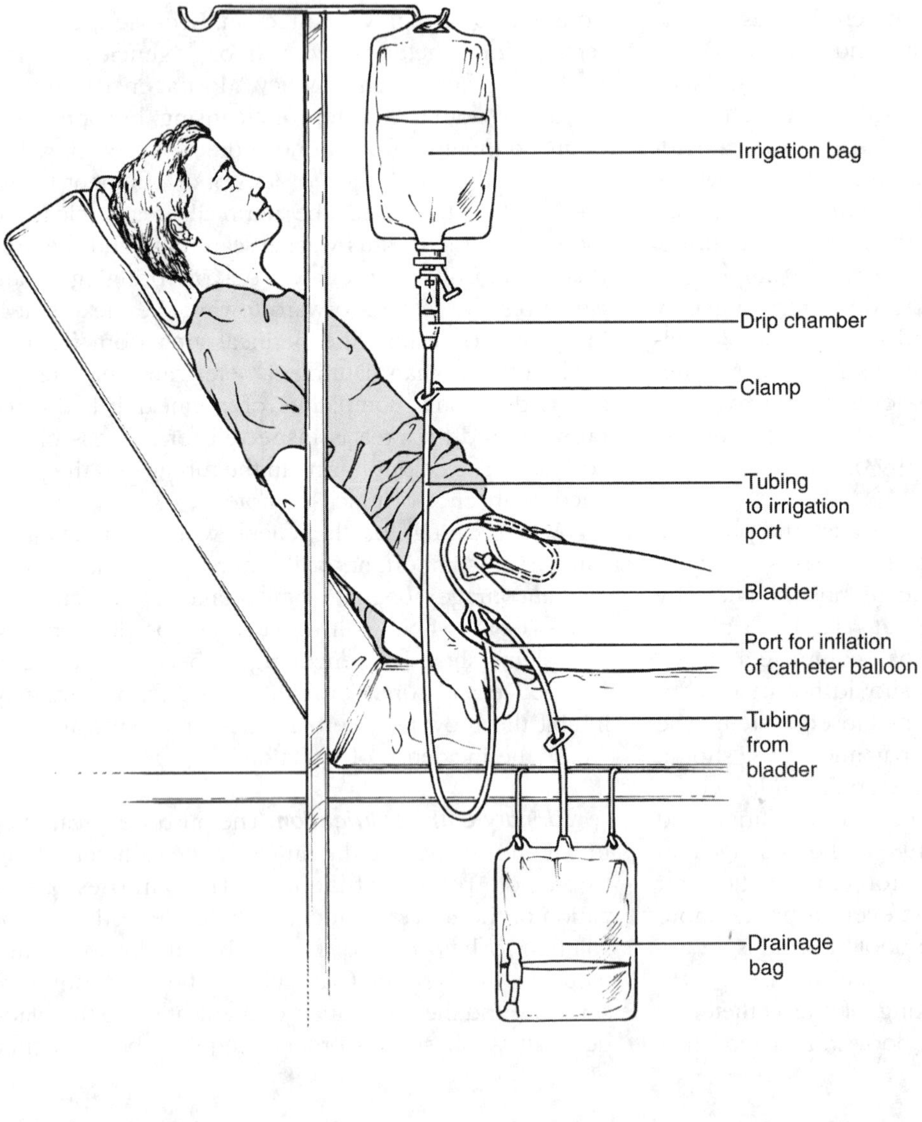

Figure 41-9 • *Irrigating an indwelling catheter using continuous bladder irrigation (CBI).*

Procedure 41-5
Performing Continuous Bladder Irrigation

Purpose

1. Maintain patency of the urethral catheter by removing blood clots and cellular debris.
2. Instill medications into the bladder.

Assessment

- Review chart for physician's order for type of solution and irrigation rate.
- Determine purpose of irrigation.
- Assess type of catheter already present. Continuous bladder irrigation requires use of a three-way retention catheter.
- Assess urine for amount, color, and presence of mucus, sediment, or blood clots.
- Assess client for bladder distention, spasms, or pain.

Equipment

Sterile irrigating solution.
Infusion tubing.
IV pole.
Three-way retention catheter—present in client's bladder.
Sterile drainage bag and tubing.
Clean, disposable gloves.

Procedure

1. Close room door or pull curtains around bed, and drape client with bath blanket.
   Rationale: Provides privacy.
2. Explain procedure to client.
   Rationale: Reduces anxiety and increases cooperation.
3. Don disposable clean gloves. Empty and record amount of urine in drainage bag. Dispose of soiled gloves.
   Rationale: Provides for accuracy of intake and output record before and during bladder irrigation.
4. Wash your hands.
   Rationale: Reduces transmission of microorganisms.
5. Connect sterile tubing to irrigation solution using aseptic technique. Hang solution container on IV pole.
6. Flush fluid through tubing, maintaining sterility of the distal end. Close the flow clamp.
   Rationale: Expels air from the tubing.
7. Connect input port of the three-way catheter to the irrigating tubing. The other port is connected to the drainage tubing.
8. Open the flow clamp on the irrigation tubing and adjust the drip as ordered.
   Note: If a flow rate is not specified, adjust the rate to keep the urine clear of mucus and blood clots (about 40–60 drops/minute).
   Rationale: Maintains patency of the catheter.
9. Tape the catheter securely with 1-inch tape (for woman to inner thigh, for man to the abdomen).
   Rationale: Prevents trauma to urethra.
10. Assist client to comfortable position.
11. Inspect the drainage for color, clarity, and amount.
    Rationale: Observation assesses for evidence of increased bleeding or infection.
12. Wash hands and document procedure and observations.
13. Measure and record intake and output every 2 hours or per agency protocol.
    Note: The drainage includes both irrigation solution and urine. Actual urine output is calculated by subtracting the amount of irrigation infused from the amount of drainage obtained.

sponse by the client to the procedure. Any complaints of pain or discomfort should be noted, as well as the quantity, color, and characteristics of the fluid draining out of the bladder. In addition, note whether the amounts of solution entering the bladder and flowing from it seem to be in appropriate proportions. In most circumstances, the irrigation procedure is painless.

Removal of Indwelling Catheter. The removal of the indwelling urethral catheter is a simple procedure using medically aseptic technique (see Procedure 41-4). Care must be taken to avoid trauma to the urethra and discomfort for the client. In addition, the client must be informed about what many clients frequently experience after catheter removal. After assembling the necessary equipment (an absorbent pad, disposable gloves, a 10- or 30-mL syringe depending on the size of the catheter balloon, and wash cloth, soap, and towels for perineal care), explain the procedure and position the client to allow visualization of the perineum. Remove the tape that has secured the catheter tubing to the client's body. Put on gloves. Insert the syringe into the entry port of the lumen of the catheter that was used to fill the balloon, and then aspirate all fluid from the balloon. Avoid using scissors to cut this portion of the tubing to remove the fluid, because this prevents an accurate assessment of whether the balloon is completely empty. If the tubing is obstructed and it has been cut with scissors, aspiration of remaining fluid is difficult, and trauma to the urethra may occur.

After aspirating the fluid from the balloon, instruct the client to inhale deeply, and then remove the catheter slowly and carefully. As the catheter is removed, pinch the tubing to prevent dribbling of urine onto the client's bed linens, and then allow the urine to drain into the collection bag. Wrap the catheter in towels, then measure and record the amount of urine remaining in the collection bag at the time of catheter removal.

After removing the catheter, assess the perineum and meatus for any signs of redness or irritation, and then provide perineal care. Inform the client that it is not uncommon to experience some amount of dribbling of urine after catheter removal, particularly if the catheter has been in place for several days. Clamping the catheter for periods of 2 to 4 hours in attempt to regain tone, before indwelling catheter removal, is no longer thought to be effective to increase bladder tone (Resnick, 1993).

The client should be encouraged to drink plenty of liquids to distend the bladder, and should expect to void within the next 6 to 8 hours. The nurse must continue to assess the client's I & O, note the time of catheter removal, and also the time 8 hours later when the client is due to void. If the client has difficulty reestablishing voluntary control of urination, the physician should be notified, because it may become necessary to reinsert the catheter or perform an in-and-out catheterization.

Suprapubic Catheter. A suprapubic catheter (Fig. 41-10), designed exclusively for suprapubic catheterization, is a narrow-lumen tube with a curl at the distal end that helps keep the catheter from being expelled by the bladder. It is inserted by the physician into the client's urinary bladder from an abdominal entry point just above the symphysis pubis. Suprapubic catheterization can be performed with the client in his or her hospital bed under local anesthesia, or it can be performed in the operating room with the client under general anesthesia and in conjunction with bladder or vaginal surgery.

In addition to the curl at the distal end of the tubing, which helps to keep the catheter from being expelled, suprapubic catheters are also kept in place by sutures at the abdominal entry point or by a form of body retention seal, which is a part of each catheter. The catheter tubing is then connected to a closed urinary drainage system. When the suprapubic catheter is to be removed, the sutures or body retention seal are removed and, as the catheter is guided out of the bladder, the bladder muscles contract over the entry site and seal off the opening made into the bladder. The abdominal entry point is then cleansed and a sterile dressing applied according to agency policy.

Advantages of suprapubic catheterization include association with a lower rate of UTI then with urethral catheterization, and potential increased comfort for the client. In addition, when a client has a suprapubic catheter, it can be easier to evaluate bladder emptying and residual urine (urine remaining in the bladder after voiding). The catheter is first clamped, and the client voids normally. After voiding, the catheter is then unclamped and the amount of residual urine assessed.

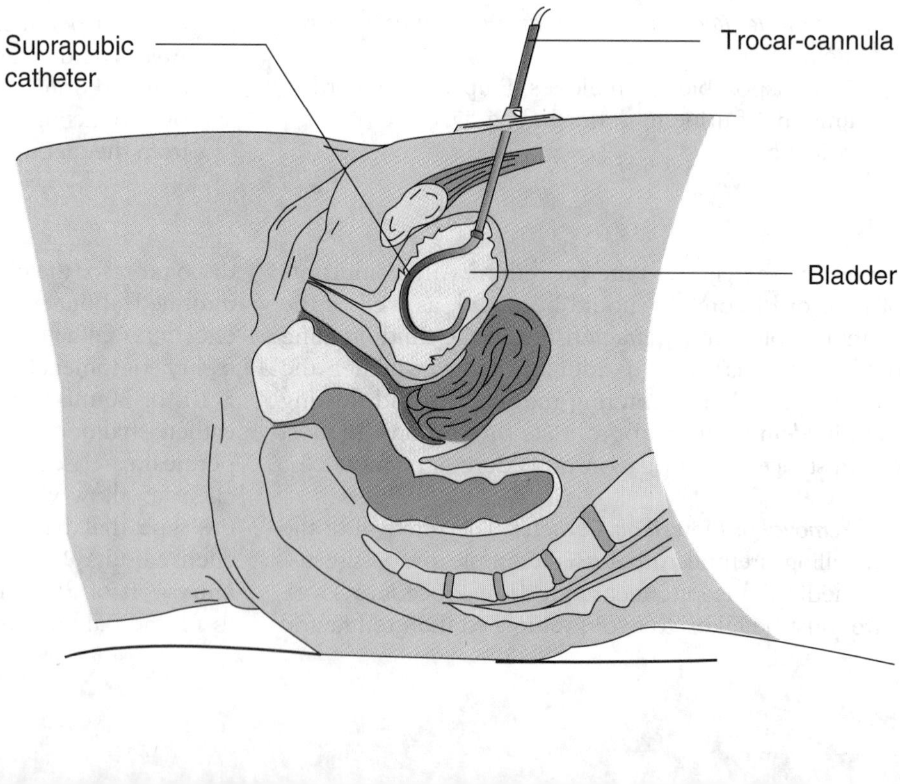

Figure 41-10 • Suprapubic catheter.

This avoids the need for catheterization to assess residual urine volumes after the indwelling catheter is removed.

Complications that can occur with suprapubic catheters include obstruction of urine flow from the bladder due to accumulation of sediment or clots, or the bladder wall closing over the catheter tip. The small lumen size of the suprapubic catheter also increases the incidence of tube kinking and obstruction. The catheter can become dislodged or trauma to the bladder wall can occur during suprapubic catheter insertion. Nursing assessment of a client with a suprapubic catheter includes frequent observations of the client's urine as to its color, clarity, and quantity. In addition, the nurse must assess the client's fluid intake, temperature status, level of comfort, and condition of the abdominal insertion site.

Intermittent Catheterization

Intermittent catheterization involves the introduction and removal of a catheter into the bladder to permit drainage of urine at routine intervals, usually every 4 or 6 hours. Intermittent catheterization is used most commonly by spinal cord-injured or neurologically impaired clients who are not able to void. The incidence of UTI is less with intermittent catheterization than if a retention catheter is used (Webber-Jones, 1991). Intermittent catheterization also permits the client with chronic neurogenic bladder greater control and independence in self-care. Intermittent catheterization can be performed with clean or sterile technique, but when done in the home setting it is almost always performed using clean technique. This enables the client to self-catheterize. A mirror helps the female client visualize the meatal opening. To locate the meatus without a mirror, she is instructed to place the index finger of her nondominant hand on the clitoris and the third and fourth fingers at the vagina, directing insertion of the catheter between these two landmarks. For the quadriplegic client, a caregiver is taught the procedure. Some healthcare providers recommend using a sterile catheter; others permit reuse after cleaning. Moore and colleagues (1993) did not demonstrate a significant difference in infection rates when sterile versus reused clean catheters were used for intermittent catheterization.

A no-touch method of intermittent catheterization has been demonstrated to decrease the rate of urinary infection (Charbonneau-Smith, 1993).

Leg Bags

Leg bags are smaller drainage units that can be attached to the leg and worn under clothing. Leg bags are helpful when the client must return home with a catheter or urinary drainage system (eg, condom catheter, nephrostomy tube, or suprapubic catheter) in place. Often the leg bag is used during daytime hours, enabling the client to participate in normal daily activities without having to carry a large urinary drainage bag. The leg bag contains a smaller volume of urine, so it must be emptied often. This is done by opening a clamp on the system and allowing urine to flow in the toilet or appropriate container.

Clients should be taught how to change from one drainage system to another, as illustrated in Figure 41-11. First have the client gather equipment and wash his or her hands. If the nurse is doing this for the client, clean gloves should be worn. Wipe the connecting area with an alcohol wipe, using friction, before disconnecting tubing from the collection system. Recap the old drainage system and connect the leg bag, keeping all ends sterile. Once connected, the bag can be attached to the leg using the rubber straps provided with the drainage unit.

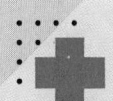

Safety Alert
Catheterization

- Avoid applying a condom catheter too tightly because this can interfere with blood flow to the distal end of the penis. Remove condom catheters daily to inspect penile skin for signs of decreased circulation or skin breakdown.
- Maintain strict asepsis during urethral catheter insertion or irrigation to decrease the incidence of urinary tract infection.
- Attach urinary drainage bags to bed *frames* and never to bed rails to prevent accidental pulling and extreme tension on the tubing when the side rails are raised up and down. This can result in mucosal damage.
- Frequently monitor clients receiving continuous bladder irrigation. Empty the urinary drainage bag when approximately 1,000-mL full; a bulging bag of urine can cause a back pressure, preventing proper outflow of urine, which can cause urinary retention and unrelieved bladder distention.
- Securely tape and take care not to kink tubing under the client when repositioning in bed. Catheter or drainage bag tubing that is kinked or flattened when the client lies on it can prevent proper outflow of urine and lead to urinary retention.

Bladder Credé

Bladder credé involves manually compressing the walls of the bladder with the hands. This technique is helpful in promoting complete bladder emptying, especially in clients who have neurologic impairment that contributes to urinary retention. Hands are placed on the abdomen below the umbilicus and above the sym-

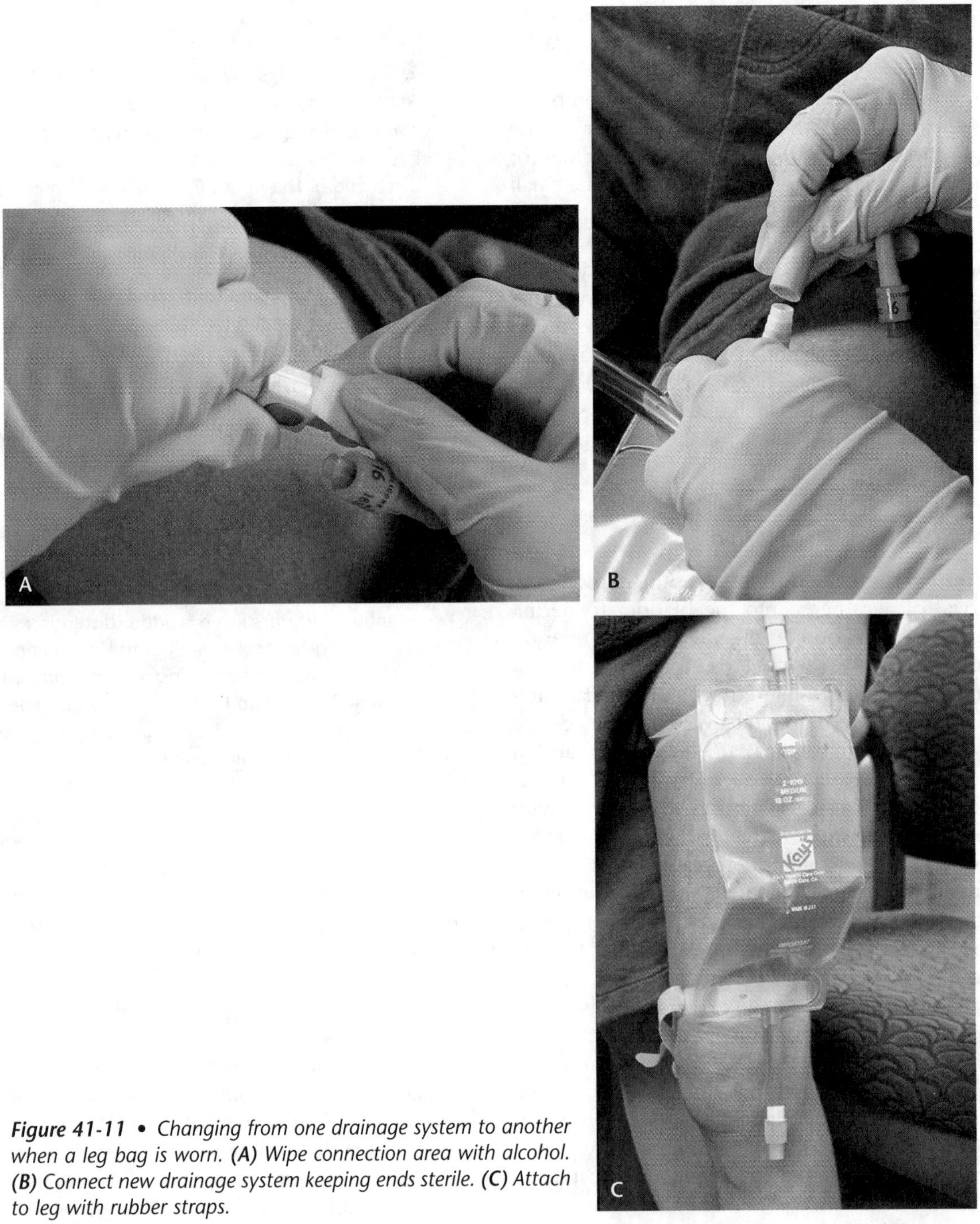

Figure 41-11 • *Changing from one drainage system to another when a leg bag is worn.* ***(A)*** *Wipe connection area with alcohol.* ***(B)*** *Connect new drainage system keeping ends sterile.* ***(C)*** *Attach to leg with rubber straps.*

physis pubis, with the fingers pointed down toward the bladder. As the hands are pressed into the bladder, the client tightens the perineal muscles and performs the Valsalva maneuver (holds breath while bearing down).

Medications

Medications can be prescribed for urinary retention and urinary incontinence, with varying degrees of success. Cholinergic drugs such as Urecholine can be given to strengthen detrusor muscle contraction, improving voiding during periods of acute urinary retention, if obstruction is not present. Alpha-Adrenergic blockers such as prazosin (Minipress; Pfizer Laboratories, New York, NY), normally given as an antihypertensive agent, can relax the bladder sphincter. Anticholinergic medications increase bladder capacity and sphincter tone and are sometimes used to treat urinary incontinence. For the postmenopausal woman, oral or vaginal estrogen therapy can improve vaginal atrophy associated with incontinence.

Urinary Diversion

Although specific nursing care must be individualized according to the specific urinary diversion performed, there are many principles guiding general care of the urinary diversion. Accurate assessment of fluid I & O, color of the urine, and the presence of sediment or blood clots is important. The stoma should also be carefully inspected for color and skin integrity around the stoma.

During the postoperative period after a urinary diversion, special considerations are necessary. Sometimes the physician has placed special splinting catheters, called stents, inside the ureters to keep them patent and maintain urine flow during the initial postoperative period. The stents protrude out of the stoma, and urine should flow out of both stents and also from the stoma. The stents are usually removed after 5 to 10 days. The nurse should assess the stents and make sure they are not accidentally dislodged.

Frequently a referral is made to an enterostomal therapist, a nurse who is a specialist in the care of clients with urinary or bowel diversions. Often the enterostomal therapist assesses the client before surgery, marking the recommended stoma site on the client's abdomen. After surgery, the enterostomal therapist fits the client's stoma with the appropriate appliance, provides wound care to the stoma site, and begins to teach the client about stoma care. If the client has a continent urinary diversion, instruction in self-catheterization is also needed.

The nurse also offers emotional support to both the client and family members. Often a urinary diversion has been performed because of serious medical problems with which the client and family may need assistance understanding and accepting. Urinary diversion may alter body image or impair self-esteem. Learning independent management of the stoma takes time and practice. Teaching sessions should be individualized for each client and include family or significant others when appropriate.

Renal Dialysis

Renal dialysis involves using a semipermeable membrane to remove fluid, electrolytes, and other waste products from the body that are normally removed by healthy kidneys. It is used in acute renal failure to allow the kidneys time to heal and help prevent further complications of the disease process. In instances of irreversible renal failure, dialysis is necessary to sustain life. Dialysis may be performed as a temporary or permanent measure, depending on the renal impairment. Hemodialysis and peritoneal dialysis are two types of renal dialysis.

Peritoneal Dialysis. When waste products, electrolytes, and excessive fluid are removed from the body using the peritoneum as diffusing membrane, it is referred to as peritoneal dialysis. A solution called dialysate is infused into the peritoneal cavity by means of a catheter. The dialysate contains water, glucose, and normal serum electrolytes. As dialysate is instilled, waste products from the blood diffuse across the semipermeable peritoneal membrane into the dialysate solution. In this way, diffusion filters from the blood high levels of electrolytes, fluid, and waste products. Because the dialysate contains glucose in higher concentration than the blood, excess fluid is drawn from the blood by the process of osmosis. Blood remains free of toxins and excessive fluid for a period of time, until once again dialysis is necessary to return the body to homeostasis.

The nurse observes and records the amount and color of the dialysate that is returned. Typically dialysate drainage is initially bloody, but should quickly clear to become straw colored. Vital signs are monitored frequently, as well as changes in mentation or level of comfort. Nursing interventions for the client undergoing peritoneal dialysis include assisting with the placement of the peritoneal catheter, caring for the abdominal wound at the catheter insertion site, and administering and withdrawing the dialysate solution prescribed by the physician. Additional nursing responsibilities include assessment and implementation of any teaching the client may need regarding the dialysis procedure.

Hemodialysis. Hemodialysis is the removal of fluid, electrolytes, and waste products from the body via access to the circulating blood. During hemodialysis, the client's blood is pumped from an artery into the dialysis machine. Here, the blood flows through a dialyzer, which serves as a semipermeable membrane, and is bathed by dialysate solution. As blood flows through the semipermeable membrane, waste products and electrolytes diffuse into the dialysate. Excess fluid is removed by a process called ultrafiltration, which provides a hydrostatic pressure gradient. After passing through the dialyzer, the blood is returned to the body through venous access.

Special catheters are used for arterial and venous access for hemodialysis and, once inserted, they can be left in place for many dialysis procedures. In between dialysis procedures, heparinized normal saline is injected into the catheter to prevent clotting. The catheter is then capped and covered with a sterile dressing. Care must be taken not to dislodge the catheter because direct arterial access can result in extensive bleeding. Grafts connecting the venous and arterial circulation can also be performed and serve as an access route for hemodialysis. Blood pressure monitoring or any invasive techniques should always be performed on the unaffected arm.

Nursing interventions for the client undergoing hemodialysis are similar to interventions for the peritoneal dialysis client. Careful monitoring is essential. The client undergoing hemodialysis is weighed before the procedure is begun and afterward to assess the quantity of fluid removed. Fluid and electrolyte status is closely monitored by measuring I & O, serum electrolytes, lung sounds, and weight changes. Clients may report symptoms of dizziness, diaphoresis, and nausea. Adverse reactions include headache, increased blood pressure, decreased pulse rate, and marked neurologic changes.

Community-Based Nursing

Urinary dysfunction, especially chronic conditions, is managed by the person in the home with assistance and support from the family. Even in acute situations such as urologic surgery, the client is discharged earlier from the acute care facility or ambulatory surgical center, often with catheters or special tubes in place. The role of the nurse changes from that of direct care provider to teacher, promoting and enabling the client to be successful in self-care and management. All clients should be taught to recognize the symptoms of infection and given clear guidelines regarding when to contact a healthcare provider.

Care of specialized equipment at home will not be necessary for all discharged clients. However, some clients will be sent home with devices to manage a temporary or permanent alteration in urinary elimination. Clients and their families may need to be taught the correct methods to care for indwelling urethral or suprapubic catheters, how to manage urinary diversion devices, or how to perform intermittent straight catheterization. Standardized teaching plans are often prepared for common procedures with appropriate audiovisual aids to assist in teaching the care of complex home care equipment. Urinary procedures in the home, such as self-catheterization, are performed using clean technique. When clients are sent home with an indwelling catheter, the nurse instructs the client on how to use a leg bag for drainage, changing back to a drainage unit at night. Vinyl drainage bags and leg bags can be decontaminated with household bleach. Dillie and Kirchhoff (1993) recommend a 10% bleach solution for daily cleaning of the interior of the drainage bag. The drainage bag should be agitated twice with the bleach solution, rinsed well between cleanings, and then hung to air dry.

Sometimes adjustments in the home environment may be necessary to promote optimal self-management. A bedside commode can be rented if ambulating or easy access to the bathroom is difficult, or a raised toilet seat may be installed for clients with mobility limitations. Bathroom remodeling may be necessary in some situations (eg, doorways too narrow to accommodate wheelchair entry).

It is possible that clients or their families will not be able to master the care of specialized equipment or techniques quickly. Contacts with resource people in the community for follow-up and home management may be necessary, especially if the client has recently learned self-catheterization, has a new urinary diversion, or will have dialysis in the home. Nurses can visit clients in their homes on a routine basis to assess progress in the management of their healthcare needs. These nurses can be associated with the discharging hospital, but are more likely to be associated with a city or county health agency, or with an independent home healthcare agency. The hospital-based nurse should be involved in the decision to make referrals to community agencies.

The home healthcare nurse evaluates the client's progress, assesses for signs and symptoms of any deteriorating condition requiring physician referral or hospitalization, and continues to provide individualized client teaching and emotional support.

Evaluation

Specific outcome criteria are the evaluative tools used to measure the attainment of client goals; nursing interventions are the management tools used to achieve the goals. Examples of outcome criteria are listed below. Some criteria may be appropriate for more than one goal. It is important to identify specific outcome criteria that will uniquely measure the attainment of the *client's* goal.

Goal

Client will maintain strengthened or adequate perineal muscle control.

Possible Outcome Criteria

- Client performs Kegel exercises five times per day during postpartum period.
- Client accurately verbalizes purpose of Kegel exercises after teaching session and repeats 2 days later.

Goal

Client will reestablish control over voiding.

Possible Outcome Criteria

- Client remains continent for 2-hour intervals over next 48 hours.
- Client voids four to five times a day, remaining continent for 48 hours before discharge from rehabilitation.
- By next home visit, caregiver reports client recognizes the urge to void in time to use the toilet or commode.

Goal

Client will demonstrate understanding of procedures necessary to promote optimal urinary function.

Possible Outcome Criteria

- Client verbalizes steps in intermittent self-catheterization by the end of the teaching session.

Nursing Plan of Care
The Client With Urge Incontinence

Nursing Diagnosis

Urge incontinence related to decreased bladder capacity and tone secondary to indwelling catheter post-operatively as manifested by strong urinary urge with incontinence, frequency, dribbling, and nocturia.

Client Goal

Client will reestablish control over voiding.

Client Outcome Criteria

- Client remains continent for 2-hour intervals over next 48 hours.
- Client verbalizes the importance of fluid intake and complies with prescribed intake.
- Client will demonstrate Kegel exercises after teaching session.

Nursing Intervention	*Scientific Rationale*
1. Measure and record I & O.	1. Data are used to assess for pattern of urinary output, relationship of intake to episodes of incontinence, relative overall fluid balance, success of bladder training.
2. Percuss and palpate lower abdomen after an incontinent episode. Straight catheterize for postvoid residual volume (PVR), if necessary.	2. Assessment is made to rule out urinary retention and overflow incontinence as the primary urinary alteration.
3. Teach client perineal muscle-strengthening exercises and tell him or her to perform them 10 times every 2 to 3 hours during the day.	3. These exercises strengthen skeletal perineal muscles and increase voluntary contraction of urethral sphincter.
4. Work with client to develop acceptable regimen. Increase fluid intake to 1,500 to 2,000 mL per day, concentrating most fluid intake during day.	4. Adequate hydration is necessary to cause bladder filling and trigger the normal stretch/contraction response.
5. Post fluid intake schedule by the bedside.	5. Concentration of most fluids during daytime hours will decrease nocturia.
6. Begin bladder training routine:	
6a. Assist client, as necessary, to bathroom to void every 2 hours during daytime, every 4 hours at night. Decrease between-voiding intervals to 1.5 hours if client is initially unable to consistently remain continent for the longer intervals.	6a. This regimen allows bladder to refill between voidings and gradually retrains the normal bladder stretch/contraction response.
6b. Encourage the client to "hold" his or her urine if he or she experiences the urge to void before the next scheduled voiding time.	6b. Suppressing urge to void assists in retraining of voluntary contraction of external urethral muscles.
6c. Increase between-voiding intervals by 0.5 hours after client has successfully remained continent for 24 hours	6c. Gradual retraining is aimed at achieving fewer voids with larger amounts, a more normal pattern.
7. Post voiding schedule in client's room. Change prn. Include details of current voiding schedule at change of shift report.	7. Communication increases client and staff compliance.

- Client practices proper self-catheterization technique during teaching sessions and twice in the next 48 hours.
- Client demonstrates proper application of stoma appliance before discharge.
- Client demonstrates use of leg bag before discharge.

Key Concepts

- Normal kidneys, ureters, bladder, and urethra are important for normal urinary function.
- Filtration, reabsorption, and secretion are processes involved in urine formation.
- The voluntary process of micturition is stimulated by stretch of the detrusor muscle as the bladder fills with urine.
- Two hundred fifty to 400 mL of clear, yellow, aromatic urine per void is considered normal.
- Kidneys mature and voluntary control over urinary elimination is achieved as the child approaches 3 to 4 years of age; kidney function declines in the elderly owing to normal age-related changes.
- Many factors, such as fluid intake, loss of body fluid, dietary intake, body position, and psychological state can affect normal urinary elimination.
- Potential alterations in urinary function can be caused by obstruction, infection, hypotension, neurologic injury, decreased muscle tone, pregnancy, surgery, medications, or diversions in structures of the urinary tract.
- Manifestations of altered urinary function include dysuria, polyuria, oliguria, urgency, frequency, nocturia, hematuria, pyuria, urinary retention, urinary incontinence, and enuresis.
- Physical assessment of urinary function includes inspection of urine, and percussion and palpation of the bladder for residual urine.
- Diagnostic tests and procedures that are helpful in identifying urinary dysfunction include urine analysis, urine for culture and sensitivity, specific gravity, BUN, creatinine, cystoscopy, and urodynamic studies.
- There are six approved NANDA nursing diagnoses that identify problems in urinary function.
- Nursing measures to promote normal urinary function include adequate fluid intake, preventing UTIs, and promoting optimum perineal muscle tone.
- Nursing interventions for urinary retention include bladder credé, in-and-out catheterization, and intermittent catheterization.
- Nursing interventions for urinary incontinence include bladder training, use of external and internal catheters, and the use of protective pants.
- Self-management of many urologic problems occurs in the home setting with adequate support from the family, community, and healthcare provider.

Critical Thinking Challenges

Return now to the situation concerning John that was presented in the beginning of the chapter. Using information learned in the chapter, reflect on the following questions.

1. *Identify risks that could alter urinary function for your client.*
2. *Analyzing the data provided, determine what alteration in urinary function is suggested.*
3. *Reflect on your own feeling about the client's statement and possible ways you could respond to John.*
4. *Construct appropriate client teaching for when an indwelling catheter is removed, and plan how you will individualize this teaching for your client.*
5. *Consider what data are essential to collect to identify if your client is voiding adequately after the catheter removal.*

References

Agency for Health Care Policy and Research. (1992). *Clinical practice guidelines for urinary incontinence in adults* (AHCPR 92–0038). Rockville, MD: U.S. Department of Health and Human Services.

Bristoll, S. L. (1989). The mythical danger of rapid urinary drainage. *Am J Nurs, 89,* 344–345.

Chan, H. (1993). Noninvasive bladder volume measurement. *J Neurosci Nurs, 25,* 309–312.

Charbonneau-Smith, R. (1993). No-touch catheterization and infection rates in selected spinal cord injured population. *Rehabilitation Nursing, 18,* 296–299.

Conti M. T., & Eutropius, L. (1987). Preventing UTI's: What works? *Am J Nurs, 87,* 307–309.

Dillie, C. M., & Kirchhoff, K. T. (1993). Decontamination of vinyl urinary drainage bags with bleach. *Rehabilitation Nursing, 18,* 292–295.

Guyton, A. C. (1995). *Textbook of medical physiology* (9th ed.). Philadelphia: W. B. Saunders.

Lyder, C. H., McCray, G., & Singh, M. K. (1992). Efficacy of condom catheters in controlling incontinence odor. *Applied Nursing Research, 5,* 186–187.

Moore, K. M., Kelm, M., Sinclair, O., & Cadrain, G. (1993). Bacteria in intermittent catheterization users: The effects of sterile versus clean reused catheters. *Rehabilitation Nursing, 18*, 306–309.

North American Nursing Diagnosis Association (NANDA). (1994). *NANDA Nursing Diagnoses: Definitions and Classifications 1992–1993*. Philadelphia: Author.

Pinkerman, M. L. (1994). Indwelling urinary catheters: Reducing infection risks. *Nursing94, 24*, 66–68.

Resnick, B. (1993). Retraining the bladder after catheterization. *Am J Nurs, 93*(11), 46–49.

Roe, B. (1985). Catheter care: An overview. *Int J Nurs Stud, 22*(1), 45–56.

Smeltzer, S.C., & Bare, B.G. (1995). Brunner and Suddar this textbook of medical and surgical nursing. Philadelphia: J.B. Lippincott.

Talbot, L. A. (1994). Coping with urinary incontinence: Development and testing of a scale. *Nursing Diagnosis, 5*(3), 127–132.

Turner, S., & Plymat, K. (1988). As women age: Perspectives on urinary incontinence. *Rehabilitation Nursing, 13*, 132–135.

Webber-Jones, J. E. (1991). Performing clean, intermittent self-catheterization. *Nursing91, 21*(8), 56–59.

Williams, M. P., Wallhagen, M., & Dowling, G. (1993). Urinary retention in hospitalized elderly women. *Journal of Gerontological Nursing, 19*(2), 7–14.

Winslow, E. H. (1993). Myth of the clean catch. *Am J Nurs, 93*(8), 20.

Bibliography

Bates, B. (1995). *A guide to physical examination* (6th ed.). Philadelphia: J. B. Lippincott.

Carpenito, L. J. (1995). *Nursing diagnosis: Application to clinical practice* (6th ed.). Philadelphia: J. B. Lippincott.

Cooper, C. (1993). What color is that urine specimen? *Am J Nurs, 93*(8), 37.

Lewis-Abney, K., & Lien-Gieschen, T. (1994). Content validation of impaired skin integrity and urinary incontinence in the home health setting. *Nursing Diagnosis, 5*(1), 36–42.

Mattheson, M. K. (1994). *Pharmacotherapeutics: A nursing process approach* (3rd ed.). Philadelphia: F. A. Davis.

National Institutes of Health. (1988). Consensus development conference statement: Urinary incontinence in adults. 7(5).

Palmer, M. H., Bone, L. R., Fahey, M., et al. (1992). Detecting urinary incontinence in older adults during hospitalization. *Applied Nursing Research, 5*, 174–180.

Rainville, N. C. (1994). The current nursing procedure for intermittent urinary catheterization in rehabilitation facilities. *Rehabilitation Nursing, 19, 330–333*.

Skoner, M. (1994). Self-management of urinary incontinence among women 31 to 50 years of age. *Rehabilitation Nursing, 19*, 339–343.

Stark, J. (1994). Interpreting BUN/creatinine levels: It's not as simple as you think. *Nursing94, 24*(9), 58–61.

Wyman, J. F., Elswick, R. K., Ory, M. G., et al. (1993). Influence of functional, urological, and environmental characteristics on urinary incontinence in community-dwelling older adults. *Nurs Res, 42*, 270–275.

Bowel Elimination

Key Terms	Learning Objectives

Key Terms

Borborygmi
Colostomy
Constipation
Defecation reflex
Diarrhea
Distention
Enema
Flatus
Gastric lavage
Gavage
Guaiac
Ileostomy
Impaction
Peristalsis
Sigmoidoscopy
Stoma
Suppository

Learning Objectives

Upon completion of this chapter, the student will be able to do the following:

- *Understand the process of defecation.*
- *List factors that influence bowel elimination.*
- *List and describe the manifestations of altered bowel elimination.*
- *Recognize age-related differences in bowel elimination.*
- *Describe appropriate subjective and objective data to collect to assess bowel function.*
- *Identify nursing diagnoses relating to altered bowel elimination.*
- *Describe independent and collaborative nursing interventions to promote normal bowel function.*
- *Discuss appropriate community-based care for clients with altered bowel function.*

42

You are working in a nursing home and caring for a 76-year-old woman who has breast cancer with bone metastasis. For the last few weeks she has been receiving increasing doses of morphine to control her back pain. Her appetite is poor, and she spends most of the day in bed. At change of shift report, you learn that she has not had a bowel movement for 7 days and she has an order for an enema. When you go in to assess her and explain that she needs an enema, she replies, "Please leave me alone. Can't you see how tired I am and how much I hurt?"

In previous chapters you learned about nutrition, activity, and medications. Those topics and the discussion in this chapter will help you understand factors that contribute to normal and altered bowel function. As you expand your knowledge base, you may want to review information from the chapters on ethical and legal concerns and communication before considering the situation given here and the related Critical Thinking Challenges exercise at the end of this chapter.

The elimination of waste from the bowel is an essential function of the human body. Defecation is the process by which the solid waste products of digestion, known as feces or stool, are eliminated from the bowel. The major nursing responsibilities associated with bowel elimination include assessing bowel function, promoting normal bowel health and function, and intervening to manage alterations in bowel function.

Such responsibilities span many age groups and different health settings. For example, the nurse might teach new parents about the color and consistency of stool to expect from their newborn, or help a family cope with an older parent in whom fecal incontinence has recently developed. The nurse who works in industry may develop an education program to alert workers to the symptoms of colorectal cancer. In acute care settings the nurse is responsible for working independently and collaboratively to assess and manage bowel function. For example, the nurse may assess the resumption of bowel motility during the postoperative period for a client who has had colon surgery; individualize a bowel management program for a client who has had a stroke; and teach a client how to manage and adjust to a new colostomy. The nurse should have adequate knowledge of normal bowel function and factors that can alter normal function to provide optimum care for all clients.

Normal Bowel Function

Structures of the Gastrointestinal Tract

The final formation of feces occurs in the lower portion of the gastrointestinal tract, the large intestine. The type and amount of food and fluids ingested have a definite effect on the amount and consistency of the waste produced. Food and fluids enter the mouth; the food is mixed with salivary enzymes, and the process of digestion begins (Fig. 42-1). The bolus of food is propelled to the pharynx, down the esophagus, and into the stomach, where secretions from the stomach further break down and digest the food.

From the stomach, the slurry of food enters the small intestine. This hollow, tube-like organ made of smooth muscle is approximately 2.5 cm (1 inch) wide and 6 m (20 feet) long. It has three anatomic divisions: the duodenum, the jejunum, and the ileum. About 3 to 10 hours are required for the contents to leave the small intestine and enter the large intestine. The large intestine also is composed of smooth muscle and is about 6 cm (2.5 inches) wide and 1.5 m (5 feet) long in the average adult. The large intestine consists of the cecum, colon, rectum, and anus. Muscle fibers within the intestine are both circular and longitudinal; this permits circumferential and lengthwise changes in size and shape that promote intestinal motility.

At the junction of the ileum and the cecum is the ileocecal valve, which serves two purposes: 1) to retard movement of semidigested food into the large intestine, thus allowing more time for the small intestine to absorb nutrients; and 2) to prevent the backflow of fecal contents from the large intestine into the small intestine.

The colon, the major portion of the large intestine, has four parts, the ascending, transverse, descending, and sigmoid colons (see Fig. 42-1). The rectum is the portion of the large intestine that immediately follows the sigmoid colon. The rectum is about 10 to 12 cm (4 inches) long. The rectum is normally empty, but is capable of considerable distention (expansion) to accommodate stool. The anus, the last portion of the large intestine, serves as an exit passageway for the feces. It is about 5 cm (2 inches) long and has two sphincters, the internal sphincter and the external sphincter (Fig. 42-2). The internal anal sphincter is smooth muscle that lies within the anus and is under involuntary neural control. The external sphincter surrounds and extends beyond the internal sphincter and is made of striated muscle; it is under voluntary neural control. Both sphincters are normally in a contracted (closed) position.

Normal Function of the Intestine

Motility

Two types of movements, segmentation and peristalsis, occur within the intestine and are responsible for assisting with absorption and transportation of waste products over the full length of the intestines (Fig. 42-3). During segmentation, alternating contraction and relaxation of the intestinal smooth muscle occur. Segmentation mixes the products of digestion in the small intestine, thereby exposing partially digested food to all surface areas of the bowel. This type of movement slows the passage of intestinal contents to permit more complete digestion and absorption of nutrients. Segmental contractions in the large intestine are sometimes referred

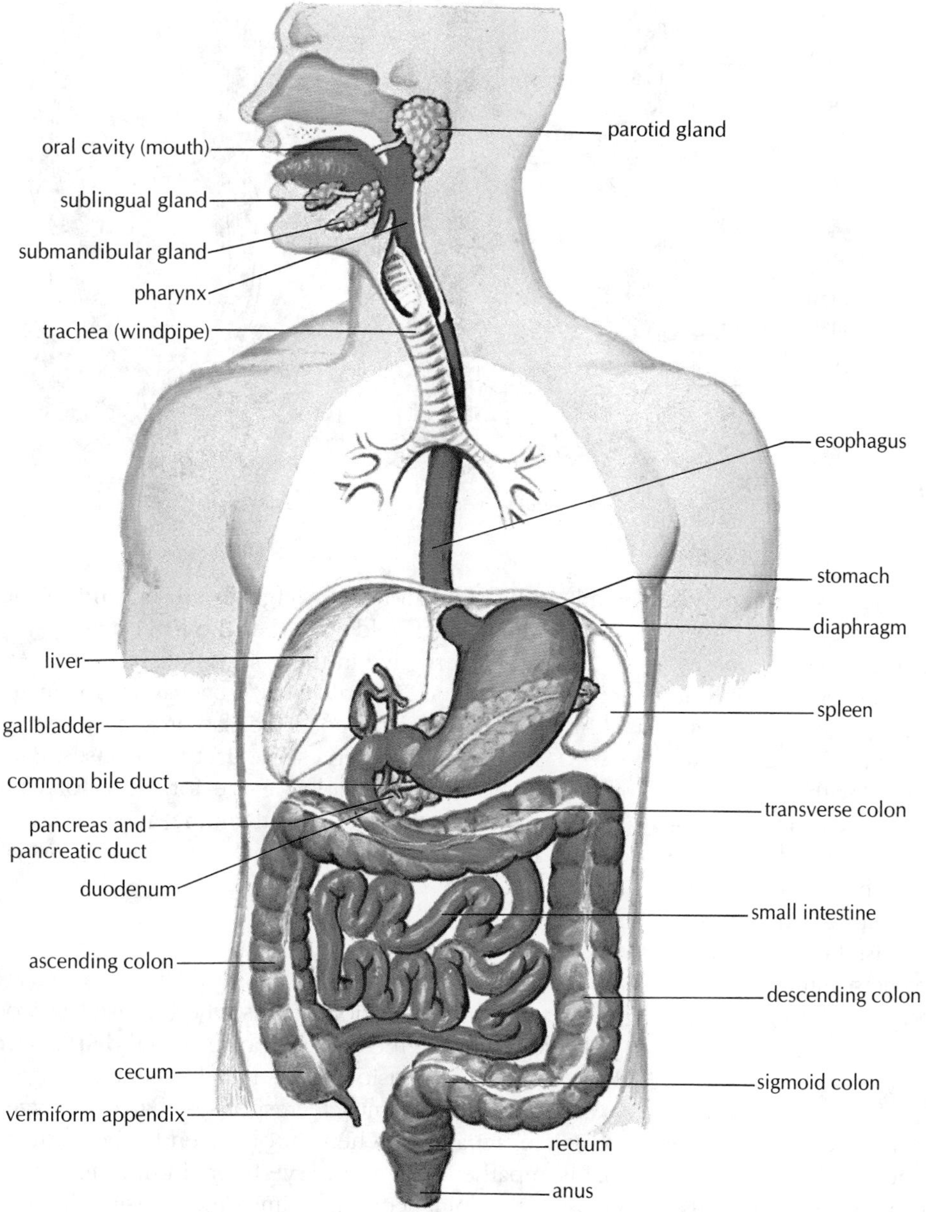

Figure 42-1 • *Anatomic structures of the gastrointestinal tract.*

to as haustral contractions (each segment within the large intestine is a haustrum). Intestinal motility is more sluggish in the large intestine than the small intestine.

The second type of movement, **peristalsis**, propels the intestinal contents along the entire length of the small and large intestines. Peristalsis is reflexively induced by the walls of the intestine. Peristalsis is particularly stimulated when partially digested food enters the duodenum from the stomach; this strong contraction of colonic smooth muscle serves to propel fecal contents from the transverse colon to the sigmoid colon and the rectum. This duodenocolic reflex is especially strong when food or fluids enter the duodenum after several hours of not eating, especially about 15 minutes after breakfast (Guyton, 1991).

Nervous system input affects the rate of intestinal motility. The intestine is supplied by parasympathetic and sympathetic nerve innervation. Sympathetic stimulation slows down peristalsis and delays passage through the intestine, whereas parasympathetic stimulation increases bowel motility and emptying.

Absorption

Partially digested food (also known as chyme) empties from the stomach into the small intestine. It is in the small intestine that the digestive process is completed and the absorption of nutrients and fluids begins. Most absorption of nutrients and electrolytes occurs in the duodenum and jejunum, but some vitamins, iron, and fluid are absorbed in the ileum.

Approximately 1,500 mL of chyme enter the large intestine each day. Here the final absorption of nutrients, especially the absorption of fluid and electrolytes,

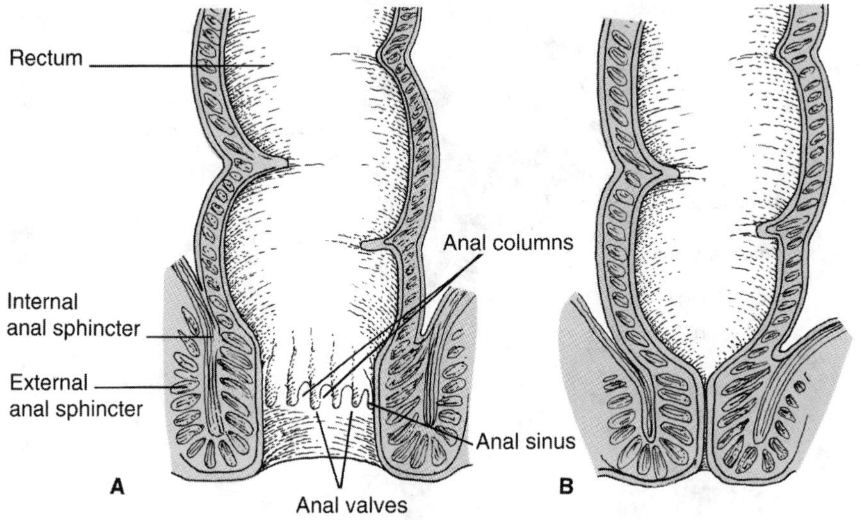

Figure 42-2 • *Anal sphincter.* ***(A)*** *Open position.* ***(B)*** *Closed position.*

occurs. The amount of absorption that occurs depends on the speed at which the intestinal contents move through the colon; the longer that intestinal contents remain in the colon, the greater the absorption of fluid and electrolytes. Reabsorption mainly occurs in the ascending and transverse colon. Sodium is actively absorbed; chloride is passively absorbed with the sodium. Therefore, an osmotic gradient exists, causing the absorption of water. The intestinal contents that enter the ascending colon are liquid. When the contents leave the transverse colon, they are semisolid and mushy and can be called feces. Although the distal colon's principal function is storage of feces, some sodium, chloride, and water will continue to be absorbed during storage.

Mucus and Vitamin Production

The large intestine secretes mucus, which protects the walls of the large intestine from digestive acids and from acids formed by bacteria within the feces. Mucus also lubricates the contents of the colon, thereby decreasing the chance of mechanical trauma to the intestinal wall as the stool moves through the distal end of the colon. Mucus also holds together the fecal mass.

Many bacteria live in the colon. Bacilli such as *Escherichia coli* and *Enterobacter aerogenes* predominate, although normally some cocci are also present (Ganong, 1993). Some of the bacteria serve useful purposes. Bacterial activity is responsible for the formation of vitamins, including vitamins K, B_{12}, thiamine, and riboflavin. Gases are also formed in the colon as a by-product of bacterial activity.

Defecation

The process of defecation begins when peristalsis propels feces into the rectum and causes rectal **distention** (stretching or expansion). This rectal distention begins a series of smooth muscle responses that can trigger bowel evacuation. When stool distends the rectum, parasympathetic afferent nerve fibers in the sacral segment of the spinal cord are stimulated, causing, in turn, contraction of the descending and sigmoid colon, rectum, and anus and relaxing the internal anal sphincter.

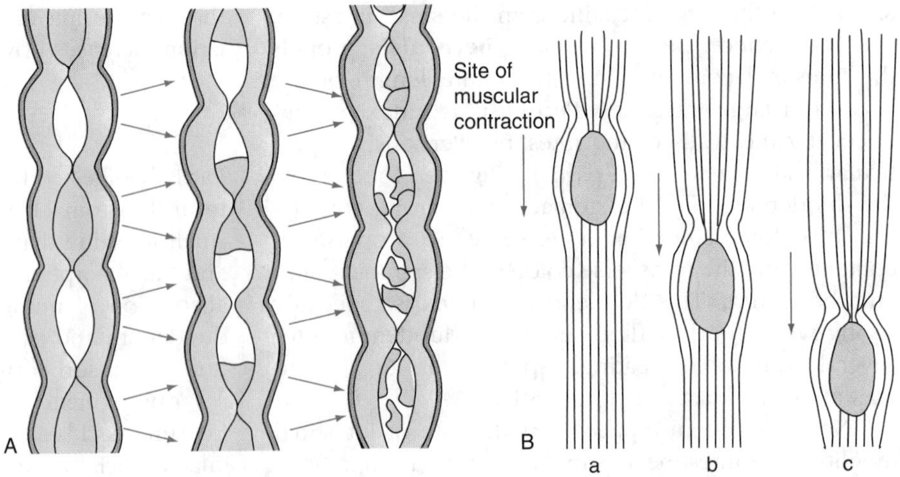

Figure 42-3 • *Intestinal motility.* ***(A)*** *Segmentation in small intestine.* ***(B)*** *Progressive peristalsis in large intestine.*

This stimulus–response sequence is a sacral reflex, not under voluntary control; it is called the **defecation reflex**. Defecation will automatically occur unless the external anal sphincter (a striated muscle under voluntary control) remains contracted. In the presence of the defecation reflex, the external anal sphincter can remain contracted until the person decides that the time and place for defecation is appropriate. At that time, the person can voluntarily relax the external anal sphincter. Defecation is assisted by taking a deep breath against a closed glottis (to move the diaphragm down), contracting the abdominal muscles (to increase intraabdominal pressure), and contracting the pelvic floor muscles (to push the feces downward). These actions are called the Valsalva maneuver. A strong defecation reflex can successfully evacuate stool from the descending colon to the anus.

Characteristics of Normal Feces

The feces consist of 75% water and 25% solids. The solids include bacteria, undigested fiber, fat, inorganic matter, and some protein. Cellulose is the major undigested fiber left in the feces after digestion and absorption have occurred. If dietary fiber intake is small, less stool is produced daily. The fat in feces is from unabsorbed dietary fatty acids, fat formed by bacteria, and fat in the sloughed epithelial cells.

The normal color of feces is brown, which results from the chemical conversion of bilirubin, an orange or dark yellow bile pigment, into urobilin and stercobilin (brown pigments) by intestinal bacteria and enzymes. The characteristic odor of feces comes from solids produced by bacterial decomposition of proteins in the intestine. Hydrogen sulfide, a gas produced by bacterial activity, also contributes to fecal odor. The feces normally have a soft consistency and cylindrical form that approximates the shape of the rectum. Between 150 and 300 g of feces is produced daily.

Table 42-1 compares normal and abnormal feces.

Normal Bowel Pattern

The normal bowel elimination pattern is highly individualized. The frequency of defecation can normally range from one or two bowel movements per day to one bowel movement every 2 to 3 days. Normal stool is characteristically soft, formed, and brown. The color may be affected by the food ingested; for example, beets may give stool a reddish color. Ingesting certain medications can also affect the color and consistency of stool.

Factors Affecting Normal Bowel Elimination

Many factors affect normal bowel elimination. Diet and fluid intake, body position, activity and exercise, privacy, and lifestyle changes can all change normal bowel patterns.

Diet and Fluid Intake

Diet influences bowel elimination. The 25% of feces that is solid contains a combination of bacteria, inorganic material, some fat and protein, and the undigested residue of food. It is the undigested residue that adds bulk to feces, and this comes chiefly from food with a high cellulose or fiber content. Cellulose or fiber is contained in plant foods. Examples of foods in the high-fiber category are fresh fruits and vegetables with the skins and outer coverings intact, and cereal grains without the outer covering of bran removed. A person who consumes approximately 800 g of any combination of

Table 42-1* • *Characteristics of Normal and Abnormal Feces

Characteristic	*Normal*	*Abnormal*
Frequency	Variable Usual range: 1–2 per day to 1 every 2–3 days	Dependent on usual pattern Guideline: $>$ 3 per day; $<$ 1 every 3 days
Color	Brown	Black, tarry Reddish–brown, maroon Clay-colored Yellow–green
Consistency	Soft, formed	Hard Loose, liquid High mucus content
Shape	Cylindrical	Narrow, pencil-thin
Amount	100–300 g/day	$<$ 100 g/day $>$ 300 g/day
Odor	Aromatic; pungent	Foul; objectionable

fruits, vegetables, and grains will most likely have sufficient bulk in the stools to allow for easy defecation. Fatty acids slow the digestive process, which affects the intensity of the defecation reflex. For this reason some professionals recommend a fat-free breakfast.

Because 75% of the feces is water, fluid intake also has a great deal of influence on stool consistency. Although the kidneys have a more direct role in regulating body fluid balance, the intestines also play a role in the absorption of fluid. The ascending colon in particular absorbs water as the fecal contents pass through the large intestine. The body cells' need for water is a higher priority than stool consistency. When the body needs to conserve fluid, more water will be absorbed from the large intestine to meet bodily needs. A fluid intake of approximately 1,500 to 2,000 mL per day is necessary to meet the cells' needs and have enough left over to promote a soft stool consistency. Storage time in the large intestine also affects stool consistency. The longer feces remain in the large intestine, the more water will be absorbed; the result is a harder, drier stool. Conversely, feces that do not spend sufficient time in the large intestine will be watery and a source of fluid loss for the person.

Body Position

A sitting or semisquatting position is the most advantageous position for defecation. This position allows gravity to assist in eliminating feces and also makes it easier to contract the abdominal and pelvic muscles, thereby applying external pressure to the large intestine and encouraging evacuation of its contents.

Activity and Exercise

Physical activity and regular physical exercise promote muscle tone and facilitate peristalsis. Strong abdominal and perineal muscles are needed to increase intraabdominal pressure during defecation. Muscle tone is lost when activity decreases or neurologic impairment results in loss of neurologic control.

Privacy

Most people require a certain degree of privacy to feel psychologically comfortable defecating. Deferring defecation until one reaches a toilet is considered essential for everyone past the age of 3 or 4 years. Although part of the defecation reflex is involuntary, the external anal sphincter is under voluntary control. Most people learn to ignore the urge to defecate until the time and place for defecation is appropriate.

Lifestyle

Many people develop a pattern with respect to the timing of bowel elimination. For many people, ingesting food or fluid first thing in the morning stimulates an urge to defecate. Over time, a pattern of bowel elimination every morning can be established and is considered a normal pattern of bowel elimination for that person. Some people are ritualistic, using the same method to promote a regular pattern of bowel elimination, whereas other people have no set pattern except to respond to the defecation urge whenever it occurs.

Lifespan Considerations

Newborn and Infant

The newborn usually evacuates stool between 24 and 48 hours after birth. This stool, which is softly formed and dark greenish, is called meconium. Meconium is the partially dried intestinal secretions that accumulated in the infant's large intestine before birth.

By about the third day after birth, the characteristics of the newborn's stool begin to reflect the type of milk in the diet. If the neonate is fed breast milk, the stools will be bright yellow, soft, and unformed; they will have an unobjectionable odor. If the neonate is fed formula, which is usually cow's milk, the stools will be dark yellow or tan, slightly more formed than the stools associated with breast milk, and will have a strong, somewhat objectionable odor. The digestive and absorptive capacities of the gastrointestinal system are not mature at birth. The intestinal contents pass through the system more quickly than in the older child and adult, producing less firm stool. Stools become firmer as the infant's gastrointestinal system matures and as he or she ingests more solid foods.

Frequency of bowel elimination varies among newborns and infants, as it does in adults. Stool may be passed with every feeding, or just once a day, or even only once every 3 days. As the infant becomes older, he or she may seem to have bowel movements in a more regular or identifiable pattern. The infant cannot control bowel elimination until the central nervous system becomes more mature.

Toddler and Preschooler

The duodenocolic reflex is strong in toddlers and preschoolers. Any ingestion of food may stimulate a bowel movement, and toddlers and preschoolers may normally have more than one bowel movement per day. Water absorption in the large intestine does not occur as quickly in the toddler and preschooler as it does in the older child and adult; therefore, the consistency of the toddler's and preschooler's stool may normally be loose.

The toddler is curious about the products his or her body produces. It is not unusual that at some time during toddlerhood smearing or playing with feces will occur. It is appropriate to let the toddler know that smearing feces is not an acceptable practice. In a matter-of-fact manner that does not threaten the child's self-esteem, encourage an alternative substance, such as modeling clay or fingerpaints.

Privacy for bowel movements is a value learned early in one's culture. Young toddlers who are not yet toilet trained will sense the urge to defecate and then may hurry to another room or hide behind a couch or other piece of furniture to squat down for a bowel movement. The older preschooler who has mastered the voluntary control of bowel movements usually prefers the privacy of his or her own bathroom at home, rather than public restrooms.

It is during toddlerhood, usually between 22 and 36 months, that a child is ready to learn voluntary control of bowel elimination. By this time, the central nervous system has developed to a point where voluntary control of bowel movement is possible. At some time between 12 and 18 months, the myelinization of the sacral spinal cord segments, which control the anus, becomes complete. When this occurs, the toddler can recognize that stool is present in the rectum. A good indicator of spinal cord maturation is the toddler's ability to walk independently.

Successful bowel training—deferring defecation until reaching an acceptable waste receptacle—usually will not occur before the age of 22 months. Until that age, a toddler's rectum and colon cannot hold large amounts of feces. Training is easier when the number of daily bowel movements decreases to one or two. Also before the age of 22 months, many toddlers do not have sufficient vocabulary to communicate the need to defecate, and would not remember to do so before actually defecating. A toddler also needs to understand that he or she has control over certain bodily functions. A child is seldom ready for bowel training until he or she can sense rectal distention, is able and willing momentarily to defer defecation, *and* can communicate the need to defecate. In the American culture, most parents believe that children are emotionally, socially, and physically mature enough to begin toilet training for bowel movements somewhere between the age of 22 and 36 months, and most children attain bowel control before 4 years of age. Bowel control is usually achieved before bladder control.

Child and Adolescent

School-age children are bowel trained and are approaching the bowel elimination habits of adults. Stools are brown and softly formed. Consistency and frequency of bowel movements depend on intake of sufficient fluids, dietary fiber, and the amount of daily exercise. School-age children, including adolescents, may choose to defer defecation until they are in the privacy of their own bathroom at home. Often children of this age delay elimination because they are enjoying an activity such as playing with friends. Continuous practice of this bowel habit puts the child at risk for a decreased responsiveness of the bowel to rectal distention and may contribute to constipation.

Adult and Older Adult

By the time a person reaches adulthood, a bowel elimination pattern that is normal or typical has developed. Bowel elimination pattern depends on diet, fluid intake, and level of activity. Deviations from typical daily routine can result in short-term alterations in bowel elimination. A return to the typical daily routine usually ensures a return to the typical bowel elimination pattern.

Because gastrointestinal motility slows with aging, frequency of bowel movements commonly decreases. Intestinal contents remain in the large intestine for a longer time, resulting in greater absorption of fluid from the feces. Older adults need to increase the amount of fluids and high-fiber foods in the diet to prevent the formation of a harder stool. Weakened pelvic muscles and decreased activity level also lead to constipation in older adults.

Because of physiologic changes that occur in the gastrointestinal tract with aging, older adults are at risk for thinking they are constipated when in fact they are experiencing symptoms associated with normal aging. Some people have a strong belief that a daily bowel movement is essential to health. Therefore, when normal age-related bowel changes occur, the older person may resort to a laxative to restore the "normal" pattern of daily bowel evacuation. Long-term use of laxatives can lead to a decreased ability of the large intestine to respond to rectal distention; the laxative-dependent bowel will empty only with the chemical stimulation from the laxative. Unfortunately, this type of laxative abuse is common among older adults. It is far better to educate the older person to recognize that decreased frequency of bowel movement is usually a normal result of aging and to encourage a change in dietary habits and an increase in activity to prevent a change in stool consistency. With aging, the strength of the striated external sphincter muscles decreases and leads to decreased sphincter control, which increases the possibility of fecal incontinence.

Altered Bowel Function

Potential for Altered Bowel Function

Many factors have the potential to disrupt normal bowel patterns. Typically, more than one factor may be involved before disrupted bowel function becomes apparent. The nurse assesses the potential risk for bowel dysfunction by assessing the presence of the following:

Nursing Research
Bowel Elimination

Selected Nursing Research Studies

Dunn, K. L., & Galka, M. L. (1994). A comparison of the effectiveness of Therevac SB and Bisacodyl suppositories in SCI patients' bowel programs. *Rehabilitation Nursing, 19,* 334–338.

Munchiando, J., & Kendall, K. (1993). Comparison of the effectiveness of two bowel programs for CVA patients. *Rehabilitation Nursing, 18,* 168–172.

Passmore, A. P., Wilson-Davis, K., Stoker, C., & Scott, M. E. (1993). Chronic constipation in long stay elderly patients: A comparison of lactulose and a senna-fibre combination. *British Medical Journal, 307,* 679–671.

Rodriques-Fisher, L., Bourguignon, C., & Good, B. V. (1993). Dietary fiber nursing intervention: Prevention of constipation in older adults. *Clinical Nursing Research, 2,* 464–477.

Ross, D. S. (1993). Subjective data related to altered bowel elimination pattern among hospitalized elder and middle-aged persons. *Orthopedic Nursing, 12*(5), 25–32.

Possible Topics for Nursing Inquiry

- Does biofeedback therapy decrease stress-induced diarrhea?
- Does the use of videotaped instruction, rather than written instruction, increase client compliance with stomal self-management?
- Do perineal muscle-strengthening exercises help decrease incidence of fecal incontinence in alert geriatric clients?
- Does the ingestion of apple juice in adult populations increase the incidence of diarrhea episodes?
- Does right side-lying position versus left side-lying position affect the effectiveness of enema administration?
- Incidence of independent initiation of a bowel training program for high-risk clients among nursing staff.

inadequate diet, food intolerances, inadequate fluid intake, ignoring the urge to defecate, lifestyle changes, immobility, medications, diagnostic procedures, general surgery, or surgical interventions creating a fecal diversion.

Dietary Factors

A person whose diet is deficient in adequate fiber generally has less frequent bowel movements and stools with less bulk, and may experience some difficulty in bowel elimination. On the other hand, ingesting large amounts of certain foods, such as fresh fruits, may produce loose stools.

Food intolerances also may alter bowel function. Many people have difficulty digesting lactose (the sugar contained in milk products). The breakdown of lactose into its component sugars, glucose and galactose, requires a sufficient quantity of the enzyme lactase in the small intestine. If a person is lactase deficient, alterations of bowel elimination, including the formation of gas, abdominal cramping, and diarrhea, can follow the ingestion of milk products.

Some people cannot digest gluten, a protein found in wheat, rye, barley, and buckwheat. For these people, ingesting gluten-containing food results in the retention of carbohydrates and fats, which cannot be digested and absorbed through the intestine. The person experiences abdominal distention and a bloated feeling, along with a diarrhea of bulky, greasy stools.

For people without a food intolerance, the ingestion of certain specific foods can still alter normal bowel patterns. Over time and with experience, a person may recognize that the ingestion of a particular food results in uncomfortable bowel elimination. For example, for some people, eating hot, spicy foods speeds peristaltic transit through the gastrointestinal tract. This can result in loose or watery stools, sometimes accompanied by abdominal cramping, and usually with a burning sensation in the anal area as the stool exits.

Fluid Intake

An average fluid intake of 1,500 to 2,000 mL per day is necessary to maintain normal bowel patterns. Usually this means people should drink six to eight glasses of water or other fluids daily. Some fluids are obtained through solid foods, as well as through the metabolism of food. When a person loses excessive water—for example, from a high fever, profuse diaphoresis, or other abnormal drainage—usual fluid intake may not be sufficient. When fluid intake is inadequate, stools become harder and more difficult to pass. However, ingestion of large amounts of fruit juices may predispose some people to diarrhea.

Ignoring the Urge to Defecate

The defecation reflex and the urge to defecate subside after a few minutes if the initial urge is ignored. The feces then remain in the rectum until another mass colonic movement propels more stool into the rectum; this may not occur for several hours or more. While the feces remain in the colon and rectum, water continues to be absorbed from the feces by the intestinal mucosa. A harder and drier stool that may be more difficult to evacuate results. Eventually, if the person continually denies the defecation reflex, recognition of the urge to defecate becomes more difficult, and the defecation reflex weakens and subsides in time. Rather than relying on inherent body signals to initiate defecation, a person in this situation may have to depend on alternative methods. Stimulating a weak defecation reflex by the Valsalva maneuver, the persistent use of laxatives or enemas, or manual disimpaction of stool are examples of alternative methods.

Fear of Pain

People who experience pain during defecation may choose to deny the urge to defecate, which can lead to constipation. People at risk for delaying defecation because of pain include those with rectal or anal abnormalities, including hemorrhoids or fissures, after anal or perineal surgery and those clients with chronic constipation.

Hemorrhoids are enlarged or varicose veins in the anal canal. Pain and rectal bleeding are sometimes associated with hemorrhoids, and these may lead to frequent denial of the defecation reflex to avoid pain. An anal fissure is an ulcerous crack or split in the anal mucosa. Bleeding and pain occur as the stool passes the fissure.

Lifestyle Changes

Alterations in a person's lifestyle or pattern of daily living can have an effect on bowel elimination. Vacations or travel often change daily routine enough to cause alterations in bowel elimination. Lifestyle changes that cause either acute or chronic feelings of anxiety, anger, fear, depression, excitement, or other strong emotions can lead to an altered bowel elimination pattern as well. Any acute stress or change in a person's lifestyle can increase bowel motility and mucus secretion. The result may be a sudden increase in frequency of bowel movements, with the stool containing large amounts of mucus. Hospitalization, a career change, a disruption in personal or family relationships, and anticipation of final exams are just a few examples of situations that can stimulate acute stress. Chronic exposure to stress can slow bowel activity, resulting in decreased frequency of bowel movements. Chronic depression is an example of a chronic stressor that slows bowel activity and frequency of bowel movements.

Immobility

Any limitation of normal or usual physical activity can increase the risk of constipation. Decreased physical activity of the large skeletal muscle groups slows overall body activity, including colonic peristalsis. Weakened abdominal and pelvic muscles are not as effective in assisting normal defecation.

Medications

Laxatives, stool softeners, and enemas are medications that are administered to promote stool evacuation. Antidiarrheal medications can be given to decrease stool frequency. Side effects of many medications can increase the person's risk for bowel elimination problems. Examples of these types of drugs include narcotics and iron preparations (constipation), antibiotics (diarrhea), and antacids (constipation or diarrhea).

Diagnostic Procedures

Some radiologic and endoscopic procedures require cleansing fecal material from the large bowel before the procedure. The thorough cleansing of the large bowel alters the normal pattern of elimination for 2 or 3 days after the test. When the person resumes his or her usual diet, the normal bowel elimination pattern usually reemerges. If barium is administered as a test agent, the stools after the procedure will appear chalky white or tan until all of the barium has been eliminated from the gastrointestinal tract. Barium hardens if it remains in the colon and causes impaction of stool. Laxatives are commonly ordered after the diagnostic test to facilitate barium removal.

Surgery

Surgical intervention can place the client at risk for altered patterns of bowel elimination. General anesthetics may slow gastrointestinal motility, and clients who have undergone a surgical procedure using general anesthesia usually experience a period of decreased bowel functioning for 1 to 2 days postoperatively.

Clients who have had abdominal surgery, especially surgery on a portion of the gastrointestinal tract, will require 3 or 4 days for bowel activity to return to normal. These clients are usually given preoperative laxatives or enemas to cleanse the large intestine of feces. In addition, their diet may be restricted to low-residue (low-fiber) food for 1 or 2 preoperative days. During surgery, the bowel is exposed to air and manipulation, leading to further decreased bowel motility.

Postoperative use of narcotic analgesics, reduced activity, and fear of pain further inhibit normal bowel motility. Postoperative clients are not allowed food and fluids orally until there is evidence of the return of active bowel motility.

Fecal Diversion

The presence of all or part of the large intestine is not necessary to maintain life. In some clients, cancer or other conditions, such as inflammatory bowel disease, require the surgical removal of all or part of the colon, rectum, and anus. In such cases, the proximal portion of the remaining bowel may be redirected through the abdominal wall to the abdominal skin surfaces. The portion of the intestine brought through the abdominal wall is known as a **stoma**. When this surgery is performed, it is referred to as a fecal diversion, because the normal route for feces is altered. Fecal diversions can be

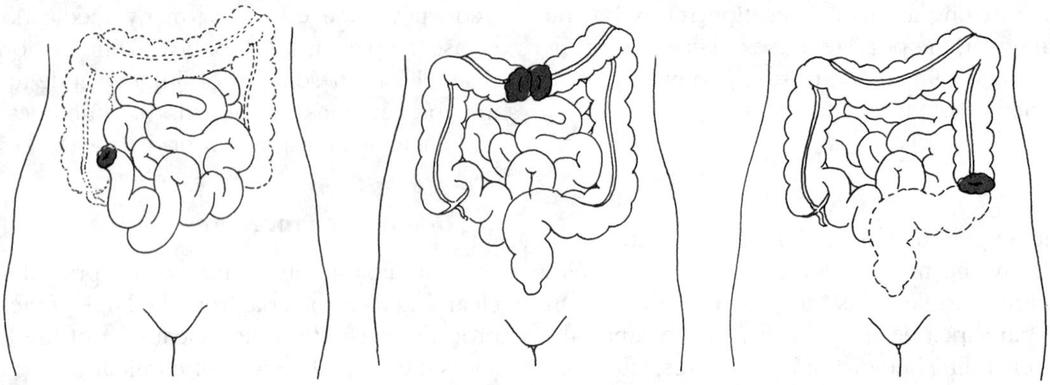

Figure 42-4 • Intestinal diversions: ileostomy, transverse colostomy, sigmoid colostomy.

permanent or temporary. Which bowel segment is used to form the stoma depends on the location of the bowel abnormality. For example, if the person has rectal cancer, the segment of bowel removed will be the cancerous rectum. The healthy, noncancerous sigmoid colon, which is the segment of the bowel just proximal to the rectum, can be used to form the stoma. A bowel diversion surgery that brings a segment of the large colon out to the abdominal skin is called a **colostomy**. It is also possible that the entire length of the large colon is so diseased that the next healthy proximal segment of intestine is the ileum. When a portion of the ileum is used to make the stoma on the abdomen, the procedure is called an **ileostomy**. Figure 42-4 illustrates fecal diversions.

People with colostomies or ileostomies have altered bowel elimination. These people evacuate feces through a stoma. The consistency of the stool is affected by the length of functioning intestine that remains after the surgery. When an ileostomy is created, the large intestine is no longer available to absorb water from the stool. Thus, stool produced from an ileostomy is liquid and contains large quantities of electrolytes. In a person with a descending colostomy, in which only the rectum has been removed, stool that is soft in consistency is produced, and elimination may be controlled with daily colostomy irrigations. This may permit a pattern of bowel evacuation similar to that experienced before surgery.

Modern surgical methods aim for as little disruption of normal bowel patterns as possible despite fecal diversion. For example, in one kind of surgery, an ileoanal reservoir is constructed and an ileal pouch is attached to the anal canal, bypassing the large intestine. This permits a person to evacuate feces, usually five to six times a day, through the anus (Wilson, 1993). A Kock pouch or continent ileostomy is another recent development in fecal diversions. A pouch is made from 30 cm of ileum and an outlet valve is constructed. Although this procedure requires a stoma, feces can be drained at the client's convenience rather than continually into an external pouch, as occurs in the traditional ileostomy.

Manifestations of Altered Bowel Function

Common manifestations of altered bowel function include constipation, fecal impaction, diarrhea, fecal incontinence, flatulence, and abdominal distention. The nurse works independently and collaboratively with other healthcare team members to identify and treat these bowel problems.

Constipation

Constipation is the infrequent, sometimes painful passage of hard, dry stool. This occurs when stool moves through the large intestine too slowly or remains in the large intestine too long. Constipation is defined relative to the person's normal defecation pattern and involves a change in stool consistency (harder and drier than usual) and a change in defecation frequency (less than usual). Ingesting inadequate dietary fiber can lead to constipation. A diet with a large quantity of refined foods or other low-residue foods is likely to be deficient in bulk-producing fiber. A diet low in natural fiber results in a less bulky stool, which encourages sluggish colonic movement and distention. In addition, a fluid intake of less than 1,000 mL per day also contributes to drier stool formation and leads to constipation.

People who consistently delay bowel evacuation risk development of constipation. Unreasonable privacy requirements, unavailability of toilet facilities during travel, an unwillingness to interrupt other activities, and embarrassment about using a bedpan are just a few reasons why people might delay bowel evacuation. Other factors that contribute to constipation are decreased physical activity, and chronic stress. Continual use of laxatives to trigger bowel evacuation weakens natural bowel responses to fecal distention, resulting in chronic constipation. Medications used for other purposes may produce side effects that decrease gastrointestinal activity, which also contributes to constipation. Finally, one of the physiologic changes that occurs with aging is the slower motility of the gastrointestinal tract. The older adult is physiologically predisposed to development of constipation.

Fecal Impaction

A **fecal impaction** is the accumulation of hardened feces in the rectum (Fig. 42-5). The word "impaction" implies that the stool is lodged or stuck in the rectum: there is an inability to voluntarily evacuate the stool. A fecal impaction is usually the result of untreated and unrelieved constipation. As stool remains in the rectum and sigmoid colon, water is absorbed from the stool, making it drier, harder, and more difficult to pass. More feces continue to be made and accumulate in the colon proximal to the impacted stool. The rectum and large colon are capable of considerable distention to accommodate large amounts of stool.

Fecal impaction is suspected when there is a history of an absence of a regular bowel movement for several days (3–5 days or more), followed by the passage of liquid or semiliquid stool. The person is typically incontinent of the liquid stool, complaining of an inability to perceive urge. The passage of liquid stool usually does not relieve the reported rectal and abdominal fullness. The passage of semiliquid stool results from the seepage of unformed fecal contents around the impacted stool in the rectum; the pressure from the large volume of accumulated fecal contents forces liquid feces to the anus. This liquid or semiliquid stool is not diarrhea, but is sometimes confused with it. Fecal impaction is confirmed by detecting hardened stool in the rectum on digital palpation.

Symptoms similar to those experienced with constipation are also present—a subjective feeling of rectal and abdominal fullness or bloating, an urge to defecate but an inability to pass stool, and a generalized feeling of malaise. Loss of appetite, and nausea or vomiting, are typical as well. Abdominal distention is usually apparent.

The causes of fecal impaction are usually the same as those of constipation. Frequent denial of the urge to defecate, inadequate dietary fiber or fluids, and laxative abuse causing impaired colonic motility are typical. A nontypical cause of fecal impaction is the hardening of barium, a radiopaque substance used in radiologic examination of the gastrointestinal tract. Clients who have swallowed barium or received a barium enema should be monitored for complete evacuation of barium after the radiologic procedure. Some healthcare protocols require using laxatives for 1 or 2 days after the procedure to ensure complete evacuation of the white, chalky barium from the gastrointestinal tract.

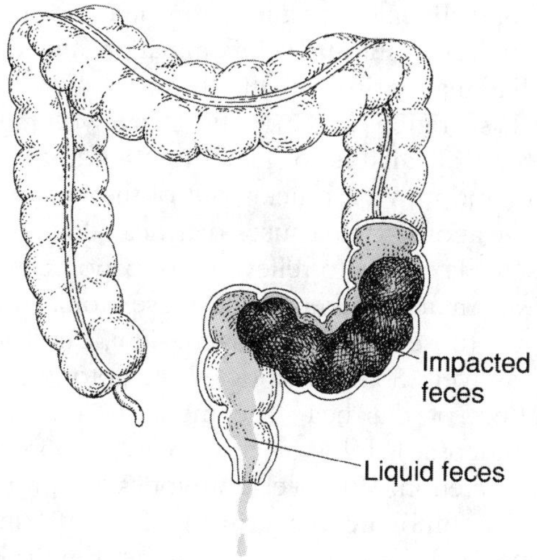

Figure 42-5 • *Fecal impaction in the sigmoid colon. Liquid stool may pass around hard fecal plug.*

People with fecal impactions need medications or special treatments to remove the impacted stool. Laxatives, enemas, or manual removal of the stool are possible measures.

Diarrhea

Diarrhea is manifested by frequent evacuation of watery stools. Diarrhea is usually associated with increased gastrointestinal motility and, therefore, a rapid passage of fecal contents through the lower gastrointestinal tract. The feces do not remain in the colon long enough for the usual amount of water to be absorbed, resulting in the evacuation of feces with a high water and electrolyte content. It is the consistency of the stool (less formed and more watery than normal) that is more definitive of diarrhea than the increased frequency of defecation. In diarrhea, increased frequency usually, but not always, accompanies the change in stool consistency. In addition to having a high water content, diarrhea stools may also have increased mucus; both of these factors contribute to increased volume. The extra volume and the rapidity with which it reaches the rectum cause rectal distention, resulting in the intense urge to defecate. Diarrhea stools may vary in color from light brown to yellow to green.

Diarrhea is often accompanied by abdominal cramping and an intense urge to evacuate fecal contents, nausea (with or without vomiting), and a painful burning sensation at the anus. Diarrhea stool is usually acidic, and it is this high acid content that causes anal soreness. Frequent passage of acidic stools can cause inflammation of the skin surrounding the anus, and result in bleeding and breakdown of the perianal tissue.

The causes of diarrhea are many and varied. Any disease that inflames the intestinal tract can lead to diarrhea. Specific microorganisms or the toxins they produce can cause intestinal inflammation and diarrhea. The inflammation irritates the intestinal mucosa to increase its secretions and motility. A large volume of water becomes available to flush the offending organism or toxin and move it quickly out of the body.

Medications can cause diarrhea. For example, overuse of laxatives to relieve constipation can lead to diarrhea. Antacids taken to decrease stomach acidity, especially those containing magnesium, can lead to diarrhea as well. Some antibiotics are notorious for the side effect of diarrhea. The medication irritates the bowel mucosa, leading to an increase in bowel motility and secretion. Moreover, antibiotics can promote diarrhea by inhibiting the growth of normal intestinal flora. Normal intestinal flora inhibit the growth of *Clostridium difficile.* When broad-spectrum antibiotics are administered and normal flora altered, *C. difficile* can proliferate and release toxins that cause antibiotic-associated diarrhea (Anand, et al., 1994).

Lifestyle changes causing acute stress and anxiety can result in episodes of diarrhea. Acute stress may increase parasympathetic stimulation of the large intestine. The stimulation increases colonic motility, decreasing the transit time of the feces through the intestines. In addition, intense parasympathetic stimulation increases mucus secretion; the diarrhea stools associated with high stress usually have a high mucus content. In severe stress, the excessive volume of mucus itself stimulates a defecation reflex. A stool with little fecal material but much mucus is possible.

While traveling, some people experience diarrhea after ingesting food or water from an unfamiliar locale. Often a water-borne foreign strain of *E. coli* causes the intestinal inflammation and consequent symptoms known as traveler's diarrhea.

Additional diarrheal responses may be precipitated by lactase deficiency, gluten intolerance, or a specific food allergy. For example, apple juice may cause chronic diarrhea in some children; parenteral tube feedings may cause a high osmotic load and precipitate a diarrheal response.

Fecal Incontinence

Fecal incontinence is the involuntary elimination of bowel contents often associated with neurologic, mental, or emotional impairments. Clients with injury to the cerebral cortex may have difficulty perceiving a distended rectum or initiating the motor responses required to inhibit defecation voluntarily. People who have sustained sacral spinal cord injury or have neurologic diseases that impair the nerve supply to the rectum and anal sphincters (eg, multiple sclerosis) may also be unable to initiate the natural defecation reflex.

Clients who are disoriented or confused may have lost the social inhibition that prevents immediate fecal evacuation. In the absence of voluntary contraction of the external anal sphincter, the immediate evacuation of the rectum follows rectal distention.

Diarrhea predisposes a person to fecal incontinence. Sometimes the volume of feces is so large and the defecation urge so intense that the person cannot maintain sphincter contraction long enough to access toilet facilities and remove the necessary clothing.

Flatulence

Flatus is the accumulation of gas in the gastrointestinal tract. Gas enters the gastrointestinal tract from three sources: swallowed air, bacterial action in the large intestine, and diffusion from the blood.

Excessive swallowing of air sometimes occurs with anxiety, rapid food or fluid ingestion, improper use of drinking straws, ingestion of large amounts of carbonated beverages, gum chewing, candy sucking, and smoking. Swallowed air is usually eliminated by burping or belching.

Gases produced by bacterial activity in the large intestine are eliminated through the anus. About 7 to 10 L of gases is produced each day, but only 0.6 L is expelled as flatus (Guyton, 1991). When larger than usual quantities of flatus are expelled, it is most often a result of increased colonic motility secondary to intestinal irritation. The colonic activity propels the gases toward the anus before they have time to be absorbed by the intestinal mucosa. Certain foods tend to produce more gas than others. Cabbage, onions, and legumes (beans) often increase the amount of flatus produced in the intestine. Many other high-fiber foods that are recommended to promote normal bowel elimination can cause excess flatus production when the intake of these high-fiber foods is not introduced into the diet gradually.

Distention

An accumulation of excessive amounts of flatus or liquid or solid intestinal contents causes abdominal **distention**. Subjectively, the person complains of abdominal fullness and discomfort and the inability to pass flatus or stool. Visual inspection of the abdomen reveals a distended or a convexly stretched abdomen. Depending on the amount of flatus and fluids in the intestines, the abdomen can appear only slightly distended or taut and stretched. Auscultation of bowel sounds may indicate either hypoactive bowel sounds or a combination of hypoactive and hyperactive bowel sounds. Percussion of the distended abdomen reveals tympanic sounds over areas of the abdomen filled with excessive gas and a duller sound over areas filled with fluid or solid contents.

Bowel obstruction that blocks the passage of flatus and intestinal chyme or feces is a primary cause of abdominal distention. Paralytic ileus, abdominal infections, and abdominal tumors are types of bowel obstructions that produce distention.

Long periods of bed rest or relative inactivity can slow peristalsis and lead to accumulated flatus in the large intestine. Peristalsis also slows after surgery with general anesthesia. In particular, bowel surgery in which the bowel is manipulated will cause decreased peristalsis after surgery, with abdominal distention as a possible consequence. Constipation and fecal impaction may lead to abdominal distention as well.

Impact of Bowel Dysfunction on Activities of Daily Living

Individual Considerations

The excretion of solid waste is an important bodily function around which independent and acceptable behaviors have evolved in most cultures. People who have difficulty with independent toileting or adequate bowel control may experience consequent anxiety, social censure, and alterations in self-concept.

Altered bowel function can potentially alter social relationships. For some, the fear of sudden episodes of loose stool necessitates staying close to bathroom facilities, calling in sick to work, or avoiding social obligations outside the home. For others, related hospitalizations and decreased work efficiency can cause significant financial strain and family stress.

Alteration in bowel function can affect sexual function. The fear of loose stool or flatus during sexual activity can cause much anxiety and decrease sexual spontaneity, and the changes caused by ostomy surgery frequently require both partners to undergo an adjustment period. Decreased energy reserves related to bowel dysfunction can also negatively affect sexual function.

Nutritional status is affected by altered bowel function. For example, constipation causes bloating, which decreases appetite. Diarrhea often necessitates rest of the gastrointestinal tract by eliminating all oral intake or limiting intake to clear fluids. The person with altered bowel function may be unable or unwilling to shop for or prepare food. Blood loss associated with frequent diarrhea can further deplete energy levels. Interference with restful sleep can occur when frequent night wakings are necessary, and pain and discomfort can also contribute to exhaustion.

Family Considerations

Significant or chronic bowel alterations in a person can affect the entire family. For example, family members may have to assume additional responsibility, including physical care of the person with bowel dysfunction. If the person is experiencing serious related stress, family dynamics may also be stressed. If bathroom facilities are limited within the home, stress may occur if facilities are in constant demand by one family member with bowel dysfunction. Family members, especially adolescents, can be embarrassed by unpleasant bowel-related odors. Financial strain may occur from inability to work or high medical costs. When an ostomy is performed, many adjustments are necessary. In older family members, assistance may be needed with ostomy care, or cleansing after episodes of fecal incontinence.

Assessment

Asking questions about a person's bowel habits is potentially an embarrassing situation for the client and the beginning nursing student. Bowel elimination is considered a private function; however, the nurse who intends to give the best possible nursing care must get factual information both from the client's perspective and through direct observation. The nurse should keep in mind that bowel elimination is a vital part of human functioning; it is therefore essential that the nurse have a sufficient database to form a plan of care. If the nurse uses a matter-of-fact approach in interaction with the client, the client's embarrassment can often be eased.

Subjective Data

A focused functional assessment of bowel elimination includes obtaining subjective data from the client by asking a series of purposeful questions, and making a mental note of the client's nonverbal communication, such as facial expression, body language, and tone of voice. On first interaction with a client, this information is usually collected by conducting a nursing history. In later interactions with the client, the nurse may focus on important considerations for that specific client.

Collection of subjective data assists the nurse in identifying the client's functional bowel pattern, determining factors that place the client at risk for development of bowel dysfunction, and recognizing actual, current dysfunctional patterns.

Functional Pattern Identification

To determine the client's current bowel elimination pattern, the nurse needs to obtain the following information from current medical records, the client, or significant others.

What is the client's usual pattern of bowel elimination?
What are the usual characteristics of the client's stool?
Which aids, if any, does the client routinely use for defecation?

When was the client's last bowel movement?
What are any recent changes in the client's normal bowel pattern?

Risk Identification

The nursing history includes information that identifies factors placing the client at risk for development of alterations in normal bowel elimination function. Areas of risk to be assessed include dietary factors, such as adequacy of fiber and water intake; ignoring the urge to defecate; factors or conditions that may alter the client's mobility pattern; diagnostic procedures, especially those involving the use of radiographic contrast material such as barium; surgical procedures; fear of pain on defecation; and lifestyle changes.

A client needs good teeth to chew high-fiber foods such as fresh fruits and vegetables. Poor dentition with concomitant chewing difficulty may lead to an insufficient intake of this food group and place the client at risk for constipation. Some clients who have difficulty chewing or swallowing may be placed on a liquid diet administered through a feeding tube, and these clients may be at risk for constipation or diarrhea.

Dysfunction Identification

To determine whether the client has a bowel elimination dysfunction, it is necessary to assess his or her beliefs about "normal" bowel function. Some people believe that a normal bowel pattern is a bowel movement every day; they may further believe that a laxative or enema is necessary to correct any deviations from this pattern. A person's concept of whether he or she has a bowel elimination dysfunction usually depends on the person's beliefs about "normal" bowel elimination and whether his or her current pattern fits these beliefs. Although a client may believe he or she has an altered bowel elimination pattern, the nurse's analysis of the data may differ. Understanding the client's beliefs about normal bowel patterns helps direct subsequent nursing interventions.

Dysfunctional patterns can be identified as significant differences from the client's normal pattern or a pattern that is outside the standards for bowel function. For instance, if a person usually has a bowel movement each day and states the absence of stool for the last 5 days, the nurse may identify a dysfunctional pattern of bowel elimination. Also, a dysfunctional pattern may be identified if a client states he or she normally has a bowel movement every 3 weeks, because this does not fall within normal bowel status.

Objective Data

Objective data about the client's bowel elimination pattern are gathered through physical assessment and diagnostic and laboratory testing. Objective data augment subjective data gathered in determining the client's current pattern of bowel function, risk for bowel dysfunction, and actual bowel problems.

Physical Assessment

Visual inspection of the feces and physical assessment of the abdomen and perirectal area provide objective data on the client's bowel elimination status. The physical examination techniques used are inspection, auscultation, percussion, palpation, and measurement of abdominal girth. A comparison of normal and abnormal findings on physical examination of the abdomen and perirectal area is given in Table 42-2.

Inspection. The abdominal examination begins with inspection. The nurse observes the abdomen for contour and symmetry. The abdomen's contour is normally convex (ie, slightly rounded). The abdomen may be flat in a muscular or athletic person. An abdomen that appears hollow or scaphoid is not normal and may be associated with malnutrition. An abdomen that appears more than slightly rounded is called protuberant or distended; an abdomen may be protuberant because of excess subcutaneous fat, pregnancy, or accumulated fluid or gas. The nurse notes any signs of obvious asymmetry, comparing the contour of the right side of the abdomen with the left side of the abdomen, and the upper quadrants with the lower quadrants. The normal abdomen shows no obvious asymmetry.

Auscultation. Auscultation of the abdomen must be performed before percussion or palpation. Percussion or palpation of the abdomen may stimulate intestinal activity and therefore change the quality or frequency of bowel sounds. If the client has a nasogastric or intestinal tube connected to suction, the suction should be shut off temporarily so that the sound of suction is not misinterpreted as bowel sounds. Bowel sounds, which are a result of peristalsis throughout the intestine, are heard through the stethoscope as a bubbling or gurgling noise. Everyone has heard his or her stomach "growl" without the benefit of a stethoscope. These loud bowel sounds are termed **borborygmi**. Bowel sounds heard through the stethoscope sound similar, only quieter. The diaphragm of the stethoscope should be placed on the client's abdomen. If the client complains of pain in the abdomen, the stethoscope should be placed on the painful quadrant last. Normally, bowel sounds are heard in each of the quadrants within 5 to 15 seconds of placing the diaphragm on the abdomen; infrequent bowel sounds suggest decreased gastrointestinal peristalsis and motility. Hypoactive bowel sounds in a client with previously normal bowel sounds suggest the risk for a developing bowel elimination problem, such as constipation or perhaps an obstruc-

Table 42-2 • Normal and Abnormal Findings on Physical Examination of the Abdomen and Perirectal Area

Examination	Normal	Abnormal
Abdomen		
Inspection		
Contour	Convex or flat	Hollow or scaphoid; distended
Symmetry	Symmetric	Asymmetric
Auscultation	Bowel sounds in all quadrants every 5–15 seconds	Bowel sounds absent in all quadrants Hypoactive bowel sounds—every 15–30 seconds Hyperactive bowel sounds—continuous or more than every 5 seconds Absent bowel sounds—no sounds in 1–2 minutes
Percussion	Hollow, tympany in LUQ (stomach)	Dull, tympany in quadrants other than LUQ
Palpation	Soft	Firm distention Presence of mass
Perirectal		
Inspection	Intact, nonreddened skin	Excoriated, reddened skin Hemorrhoids Bleeding
Palpation	No stool or only soft, brown stool present in rectum	Presence of hard stool Bleeding

LUQ, left upper quadrant.

tion. Hypoactive bowel sounds in a client previously without bowel sounds suggest that intestinal peristalsis is returning.

An absence of bowel sounds means that the nurse has listened in each of the four quadrants for at least 1 to 2 minutes and heard no bowel sounds; it is the rare clinical nurse who has the time to listen to a client's abdomen for 8 minutes. Clinically, most nurses define absent bowel sounds as no sounds heard within 30 seconds for each quadrant. This method requires the nurse to auscultate bowel sounds for only 2 minutes to document absent bowel sounds. A client who has undergone abdominal surgery may have hypoactive or absent bowel sounds for 1 to 3 days postoperatively. Bowel sounds should gradually resume, indicating that normal peristalsis has begun. A continued absence of bowel sounds beyond 72 hours may signal paralytic ileus, a condition in which the bowel is temporarily paralyzed and distention occurs.

Abnormal bowel sounds also include hyperactive sounds; continuous bowel sounds or sounds heard more frequently than every 5 seconds can be termed hyperactive. Clients with diarrhea usually have hyperactive, high-pitched bowel sounds, which indicate hypermotility in the intestines. A client with a bowel obstruction may have a combination of hypoactive and hyperactive bowel sounds, with hypoactive bowel sounds below the level of the obstruction and hyperactive bowel sounds above the level of the obstruction.

A time-efficient method for charting the findings of auscultation during an abdominal examination is to make a small drawing of a simple cross to define the four abdominal quadrants. Plus or minus signs are placed in each of the quadrants to represent the presence or absence of bowel sounds heard during auscultation. Documentation and interpretation can be done quickly and easily with this method of charting. Samples of this type of charting appear in Figure 42-6.

Percussion. Percussion is used to identify air, fluid, or solid masses in the abdomen. Percussion is usually used when an abnormality has been identified during

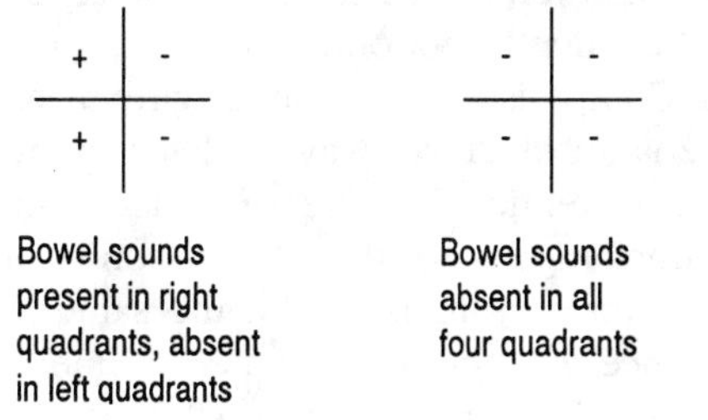

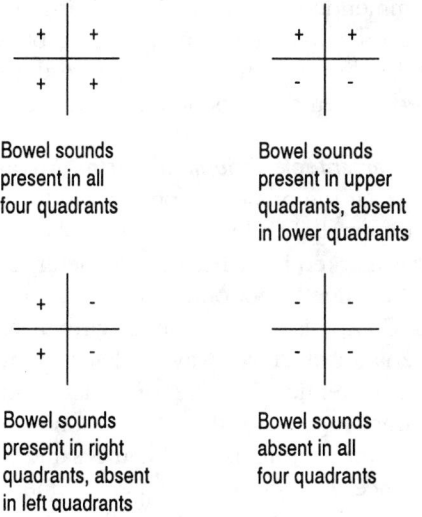

Figure 42-6 • *Charting findings from auscultation of bowel sounds.*

inspection or auscultation. The nurse begins percussion in the quadrant that was first auscultated. It is normal to hear a high-pitched, hollow sound, called tympany, over the left upper quadrant (LUQ). The stomach is in the LUQ and contains more air than the small and large intestines. The normal percussion sound heard in the other three quadrants is a hollow sound that is not quite as high-pitched as tympany, reflecting a mixture of air and fluid in the intestines. When an abdomen is abnormally distended with air (or gas), tympanic percussion notes may be heard throughout the abdomen. When an abdomen contains an excess fluid accumulation, duller, lower-pitched sounds are heard over the fluid-filled areas. A mass or feces in the large intestine would produce a dull sound.

Palpation. Palpation is the last physical assessment technique used in examining the abdomen. If the history indicates problems in normal bowel elimination, or if abnormal findings have been observed during inspection, auscultation, or percussion, the nurse may wish to use light palpation. In light palpation, the examiner uses the warmed fingertips of one hand to press on the abdomen firmly enough so as not to cause a tickling sensation to the client, but gently enough so as not to cause discomfort. The nurse palpates all quadrants of the abdomen in a systematic manner. Instructing the client to flex the knees during this part of the examination often helps the client to relax abdominal muscles and results in less discomfort. From light palpation, the nurse can determine the firmness or softness of the abdominal muscles, the relative degree of abdominal distention, or possibly abdominal masses.

A special technique called deep palpation is also part of the abdominal physical examination. During deep palpation, the examiner uses both hands and special techniques to assess deep abdominal masses and specific abdominal organs such as the liver and spleen. It is recommended that beginning nursing students not perform deep palpation independently. If possible, they should take the opportunity to observe the technique performed by a more experienced practitioner.

Measurement of Abdominal Girth. An assessment technique that the nurse can perform independently is the measurement of abdominal girth. A plastic tape measure that is marked in inches or centimeters is wrapped around the client's abdomen and the measurement recorded. Comparison of abdominal girth measurements over time is an objective way of determining whether abdominal distention is increasing, decreasing, or remaining unchanged. For the comparison of abdominal girth measurements to be valid, the same abdominal circumference must be measured each time. The nurse marks an "X" with a marking pen on the client's abdomen at the point of greatest distention, ensuring that any subsequent measurement will be from the same location.

Perirectal Examination. Examination of the perirectal area completes the physical assessment. The client needs to be side-lying with one or both knees flexed forward. The nurse needs disposable examination gloves and a packet of water-soluble lubricant.

The nurse inspects the perianal integument. The normal finding is perianal skin intact without excoriation or redness. There should be no evidence of bleeding, and hemorrhoids will not normally be present.

Examples of abnormal inspection findings include excoriation (red, bleeding, tender skin), hemorrhoids, and bleeding. Excoriated perianal skin can be caused by the frequent evacuation of diarrhea stools. Another abnormal finding is hemorrhoids, which may result from the evacuation of hard, constipated stools over time. Blood at the perianal skin is also an abnormal finding. If the person has recently evacuated a constipated stool past hemorrhoids, it is possible to see bleeding.

Palpation of the rectal area is the next part of the physical assessment. To perform a digital examination of the rectum, the nurse needs to separate the client's buttocks, and insert the lubricated index finger of the gloved hand into the client's anus and rectum. The nurse directs the finger toward the client's umbilicus and feels the sides of the rectal wall and at the tip of the finger for stool in the rectum. If any stool is felt, the nurse determines whether it is hard or soft. To help the client relax the anal sphincter, the nurse may slightly distract the client by directing him or her to inhale deeply at insertion and to exhale as the nurse quickly assesses the rectum.

Sometimes, as the nurse's finger enters the rectum, the client may exhibit a temporary loss of sphincter control and will involuntarily release stool from the rectum. This is especially true for the weak older client and for infants and small children. For these clients, the nurse places a disposable pad under the client's buttocks before performing the digital examination.

The normal finding during the digital examination is the absence of hard stool in the rectum. A comparison of normal and abnormal findings on physical examination of the abdomen and perirectal area appears in Table 42-2.

Diagnostic Tests and Procedures

Two laboratory tests are commonly performed on stool specimens for diagnostic purposes: the guaiac, or Hemoccult, test and the stool culture. Other diagnostic procedures include radiologic examinations and endoscopic examinations. The nurse assists with these procedures and uses information gained to develop a plan of care.

Collecting Stool Specimens. Whether a stool specimen is tested by the nurse or the laboratory technician, it is commonly the nurse's responsibility to collect it.

First the nurse must explain to the client the need for a stool sample. If the client can walk to the bathroom, a clean bedpan or other container used for obtaining specimens should be placed on the toilet. If the client cannot ambulate to the bathroom, the nurse ensures that a bedpan or bedside commode is readily available in the client's room. When obtaining a specimen for stool culture, the nurse informs the client that it is best if urine is not mixed with the stool in the bedpan. The male client can easily use a urinal to prevent this from occurring, but it will be more difficult for the female client. The nurse may need to have two bedpans ready in the room, one to be used for urine and the second to be used for the stool specimen.

Hemoccult Test. "Heme" refers to blood, and "occult" means hidden or not visible on inspection. Testing the stool for hidden blood is called a **guaiac** (Hemoccult) test. The nurse can easily perform this diagnostic test. A small amount of stool is placed on a card or slide made especially for this purpose, and a few drops of a chemical developer are then placed on the slide. The nurse then observes for a color change. Blue is a positive diagnostic finding, indicating the presence of blood in the stool sample. No color change or any color other than blue is a negative diagnostic finding, indicating the absence of blood in the stool sample. Guaiac testing is a simple procedure, as explained in Procedure 42-1, but the nurse should be sure to read the instructions that accompany the test slide and follow them every time for accurate results.

The stool is tested for occult blood to check for pathologic sources of bleeding from the gastrointestinal tract. Gastrointestinal bleeding could be caused by peptic or small intestinal ulcers or tumors of the gastrointestinal tract. If blood is on the surface of the stool, it is likely to be secondary to bleeding from hemorrhoids and is not occult. If blood is mixed in the stool mass itself, its likely source is intestinal. When collecting a stool specimen for occult blood, a stool sample obviously contaminated by hemorrhoidal blood should not be used.

Other false-positive results on a Hemoccult test can occur if a client has recently taken medications known to irritate the gastric mucosa. People who routinely take aspirin or other nonsteroidal antiinflammatory drugs or steroidal medications should avoid taking these medications for 3 days before a stool specimen is collected. The ingestion of rare red meat in large quantities for 3 days before guaiac testing can also cause a false-positive result. False-negative results can occur if the client has taken more than 2 to 4 g of vitamin C in 24 hours before the test.

Stool Culture. The other laboratory test performed on stool is a culture for specific infectious organisms. The stool normally has a high bacteria count as a result of normal intestinal flora. A stool culture is performed to distinguish atypical intestinal organisms present in the stool sample. Examples of atypical infectious organisms that might be cultured from a stool sample would be *Salmonella* or *Shigella* species. When these organisms are present in the intestine, they usually cause diarrhea; specific antibiotics are necessary to kill the offending organism and stop the diarrhea. A special kind of stool culture sometimes necessary is the testing of the stool for ova (eggs) and parasites. A stool specimen should be sent to the laboratory soon after the client defecates (ie, while the stool is still warm), where it can be tested for specific parasitic organisms or their eggs, such as *Giardia lamblia* or *Entamoeba histolytica* that could cause diarrhea.

Radiologic Procedures. Several diagnostic tests aid in identifying specific pathologies associated with alterations in bowel elimination. These tests are either radiologic (x-ray) procedures, using barium as a contrast medium, or are performed by the healthcare provider using specialized instruments that provide a direct view of the lower gastrointestinal tract.

The small and large intestines can be visualized by x-ray imaging if a radiopaque substance, such as barium, is swallowed or instilled in the rectum. The small bowel x-ray procedure is usually done in conjunction with the x-ray of the upper gastrointestinal tract. The client must swallow barium, a white liquid with a chalky taste. The radiologist then monitors the progress of the barium from the esophagus though the ileum. Still x-ray films can be taken at any time as the barium progresses through the gastrointestinal system. The lower gastrointestinal tract can be radiologically visualized by instilling the barium through the rectum. The term *barium enema* is often used for this procedure. The radiologist can visualize the colon as the barium travels from the rectum back toward the ascending colon.

The purpose of these two radiologic procedures is to visualize the segments of the small and large bowel and detect abnormalities in shape, motility, and functioning. Examples of abnormal findings are tumors, diverticula, obstruction, or filling defects.

For best results and maximum visualization, the bowel must be as free as possible from fecal contents. Clients need to take a combination of oral and rectal laxatives the day before and the morning of the procedure; tap-water enemas can sometimes be substituted for the laxative regimen. The client's oral intake is also restricted, usually beginning at midnight on the day of the test. The client is NPO (allowed no food or fluids by mouth) until the procedure is finished; oral medications are also withheld until the procedure is completed if withholding the medications will not pose an adverse risk for the client. The nurse is responsible for informing the client about the preparatory regimen and purpose of the procedure, and may also be responsible

Procedure 42-1
Assessing Stool for Occult Blood

Purpose

1. Screen clients who have or who are at risk for gastrointestinal bleeding.
2. Screen for early-stage colon cancer.

Assessment

- Review client's medical and drug history for risk factors for gastrointestinal bleeding.
- Assess client's understanding of need for the procedure and his or her ability to cooperate.
- Note client's dietary history and need for any modifications before the test. Rare meats can cause false-positive test results for occult blood. Some physicians may restrict red meat for 72 hours before the test.

Equipment

Bedpan, bedside commode, or toilet hat to catch stool.
Disposable exam gloves.
Tongue blade or wooden applicator stick.
Prepackaged Hemoccult cardboard slide, developing solution or Hematest tablets, guaiac filter paper, and several drops of water.

Procedure

1. Ask the client to void before collecting the stool specimen.
   Rationale: Urine mixed with stool sample could dilute stool sample so occult blood is not detected. If urine has red blood cells, the test results might be positive, but the source would be masked.
2. Assist client onto bedpan, commode, or to bathroom. Provide privacy; leave call bell handy.
3. Once the client has passed stool and is clean and comfortable, don disposable gloves and obtain small amount of stool with a tongue blade or wooden applicator.

Procedure

Hemoccult Slide Test

1. Open flap of slide and apply a very thin smear of stool onto first window.
   Rationale: The guaiac filter paper is very sensitive to blood content, so only a small sample is needed.

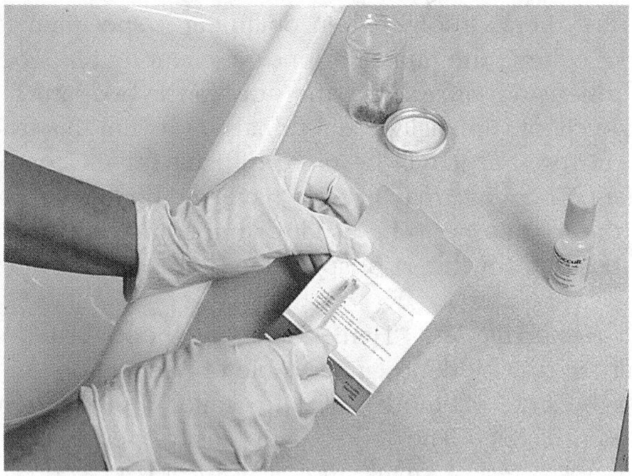

Step 1 • *Apply a thin smear of stool on Hemoccult slide.*

2. Using second applicator, obtain a second sample from a different area of the stool. Smear thinly on second window of slide.
   Rationale: Blood may not be equally distributed throughout stool sample. Testing findings from one area may not reveal blood in another area.
   Note: Physicians typically order three different stool samples to be tested.
3. Close slide cover. Open flap on reverse side and apply two drops of Hemoccult developing solution onto each window.
   Rationale: The developing solution penetrates the stool sample to react chemically with the blood.

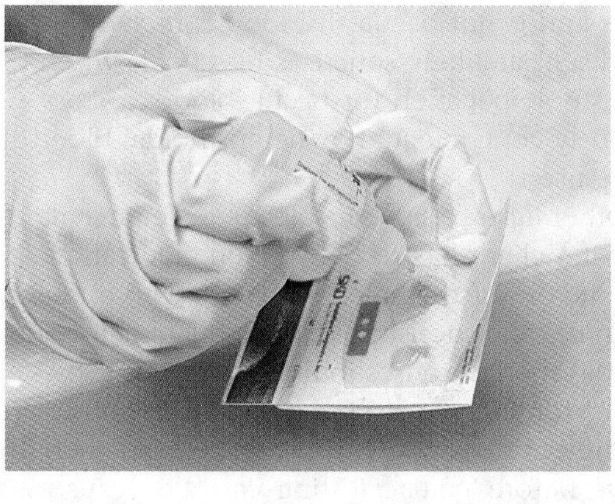

Step 3 • *Apply Hemoccult developing solution on slide window.*

4. Wait 30 to 60 seconds. Read test results.
   Rationale: Test results are positive, indicating the presence of blood, if the filter paper has a bluish tint. Test findings are negative if there is no color change.

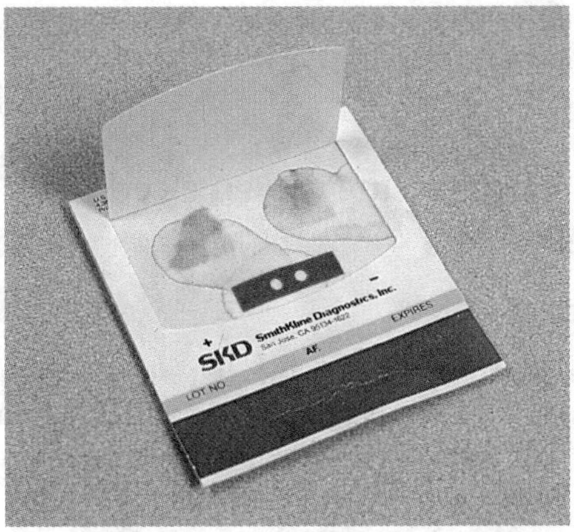

Step 4 *• Blue discoloration indicates the presence of occult blood.*

Test With Hematest Tablets

1. Apply small smear of stool onto guaiac filter paper.
   Rationale: Guaiac paper is highly sensitive to blood, so only a thin smear is needed.
2. Place Hematest table on stool sample.
3. Apply two to three drops of water onto Hematest tablet. Hold paper so water runs onto it.
   Rationale: Hematest tablet contains a solid developing solution that dissolves with addition of water.
4. Read test results within 2 minutes by observing color of guaiac paper.
   Rationale: Test is positive if filter paper has a bluish tint. Test is not valid after 2 minutes.
5. Remove gloves, wash hands, and document findings.

Lifespan Considerations

Infants and Children

- A child who is not toilet trained cannot cooperate with stool specimen collection. The specimen can be obtained from a diaper if it is not contaminated with urine.
- If the child has watery diarrhea, place a plastic liner inside the diaper and use a cotton swab to obtain the specimen.

Home-Care Modifications

- If client will collect stool sample at home, instruct client to prepare slide with sample, close cardboard flap, write name on slide, and return to the office or clinic for specimen developing.

for administering the laxatives or enemas and for maintaining the client's NPO status.

When the client returns from the procedure, he or she may again eat and drink. The nurse must be aware that barium left in the bowel after the procedure can harden and become extremely difficult to eliminate. Therefore, the nurse should encourage the client to take a laxative such as milk of magnesia, 1 ounce for 1 or 2 days after the test, until the client passes no more white-colored, barium-containing stool.

Endoscopic Examination. Endoscopic examination of the large colon is another means of detecting abnormalities. A flexible fiberoptic instrument called a proctoscope or a sigmoidoscope is advanced through the anus and rectum up to a distance of 65 cm; the procedure is called proctoscopy or **sigmoidoscopy**. The lower segment of the colon can be directly visualized by the physician. The bowel is examined for severe inflammation or for tumors. Sometimes the barium enema test does not offer sufficient diagnostic information about the sigmoid colon and rectum, and sigmoidoscopy is necessary. During this procedure, the client must be in a knee-to-chest position, which is an uncomfortable and somewhat embarrassing position for most people. Clients also feel the urge to defecate when the fiberoptic probe is inserted into the rectum, another embarrassing feeling for most people. For clients who are too weak to be examined in the knee–chest position, a side-lying position with the upper leg flexed (Sims' position) can be used, although this position makes visualization of the sigmoid colon more difficult.

The nurse's responsibilities include educating the client before the procedure. The nurse explains the purpose of the examination, the position necessary for the procedure, and sensations likely to be felt during the procedure. The nurse explains dietary restrictions and test preparations as well. For example, the client may be allowed only clear liquids the evening before and the morning of the test. Laxatives, a rectal suppository, or a small-volume enema may also be required to clean the lower colon of stool before the procedure. After the procedure, the client will likely be tired and perhaps hungry and thirsty; the nurse offers rest, food, and fluids.

The upper portion of the large colon can also be directly visualized by a fiberoptic probe. The colonoscope, a flexible fiberoptic instrument, can be advanced up to 180 cm to the ileocecal valve. The purpose of this procedure is to directly visualize a greater segment of the large colon, again observing for severe inflammation or tumors along the entire length of the large colon.

Again, client preparation is an important nursing responsibility. The client alters his or her diet; clear liquids may be recommended for up to 3 days (72 hours) before the procedure. Laxatives are necessary for 1 or 2 days before the test so that the entire length of the colon is cleared of feces, and a small-volume enema is necessary the morning of the procedure. Colonoscopy takes longer and produces more discomfort than sigmoidoscopy or proctoscopy; therefore, the client is given intravenous medications to control pain, to reduce bowel spasm, and to produce light anesthesia. The client is in the Sims' position for the procedure. Afterward, the client needs rest but must be closely monitored by the nurse for signs of rectal bleeding or the onset of continuous, dull abdominal pain, possibly indicating colonic perforation.

The client must sign a consent form before an endoscopic procedure. A biopsy (retrieval of a small piece of colon mucosa or tumor for analysis) or polypectomy (complete surgical removal of a colonic lesion) can be done during endoscopy.

Nursing Diagnoses

Specific information from the nursing assessment assists the nurse in identifying potential and actual problems in the area of bowel elimination. North American Nursing Diagnosis Association (NANDA) nursing diagnoses concerning bowel elimination include Colonic Constipation, Perceived Constipation, Diarrhea, and Bowel Incontinence. Before 1988, Altered Bowel Elimination was an accepted nursing diagnosis, but was found to be too broad for clinical use (Carpenito, 1995)

Diagnostic Statement: Colonic Constipation

Definition

Colonic Constipation is the state in which an individual's pattern of elimination is characterized by hard, dry stool that results from a delay in passage of food residue (NANDA, 1994).

Defining Characteristics

Major characteristics are decreased frequency; hard, dry stool; straining at stool; painful defecation; abdominal distention; palpable mass.

Minor characteristics are rectal pressure; headache, appetite impairment; abdominal pain (NANDA, 1994).

Related Factors

Related factors are less than adequate fluid intake; less than adequate dietary intake; less than adequate fiber; less than adequate physical activity; immobility; lack of privacy; emotional disturbances; chronic use of medications and enemas; stress; change in daily routine; metabolic problems (eg, hypothyroidism, hypocalcemia, hypokalemia) (NANDA, 1994).

Diagnostic Statement: Perceived Constipation

Definition

Perceived Constipation is the state in which an individual makes a self-diagnosis of constipation and ensures a daily bowel movement through abuse of laxatives, enemas, and suppositories (NANDA, 1994).

Defining Characteristics

Characteristics are expectation of a daily bowel movement with the resulting overuse of laxatives, enemas, and suppositories; expected passage of stool at the same time every day (NANDA, 1994).

Related Factors

Related factors are cultural–family health beliefs; faulty appraisal and impaired thought processes (NANDA, 1994).

Note: A sudden change in normal bowel status, together with inadequate knowledge, can motivate a person to overuse medical therapies to ensure a daily evacuation of stool. This is more likely to occur if the person tends to be obsessive–compulsive in behavior or has a long-held belief that deviation from a stool every day is unhealthy (Carpenito, 1995).

Diagnostic Statement: Diarrhea

Definition

Diarrhea is a state in which an individual experiences a change in normal bowel habits characterized by the frequent passage of loose, fluid, unformed stools (NANDA, 1994).

Defining Characteristics

Characteristics include abdominal pain; cramping; increased frequency; increased frequency of bowel sounds; loose, liquid stools; urgency. Change in stool color is another possible characteristic (NANDA, 1994).

Related Factors

Related factors are inflammation or infection; treatments such as medications or tube feedings; and altered situations such as stress or ingestion of certain foods (Carpenito, 1995).

Therapeutic Dialogue
Constipation

Scenes for Thought

Helen Palumbo is a 79-year-old woman who comes to the clinic for a check-up every 6 months or so. She is a busy, active, and pleasant woman who is interested in all aspects of life and is committed to staying healthy so she can continue to enjoy it.

Effective

Nurse: *Hi, Mrs. Palumbo, I'm glad to see you. How are you feeling?*
Client: *Hello, there, Maryjo. I'm doing fine except I think I'm a little constipated.* She whispers this last word.
Nurse: *Tell me a little more about that. (Listens attentively.)*
Client: *Well, I usually go every morning, but over the last few months I only go every 2 or 3 days, and I'm worried about that.* She looks worried.
Nurse: *What worries you about that?*
Client: *Well, when I was in my twenties I had a fistula. I had to put off having my first baby because of it. And then 5 years ago I had diverticulitis and it put me in the hospital for a week with antibiotics. It wasn't fun, I can tell you. So if I get constipated I'm worried about getting sick again, or putting strain on my fistula scars. You see?* Looks hopeful that you do see. *So I give myself little enemas and that relieves me.*
Nurse: *Yes, I understand why you're concerned. Let me ask you a few questions about nutrition and fluids, and I'll examine your abdomen, then we can talk more about some things you might do. Is that okay with you?*
Client: *Whatever you say, I always learn something new when I come here.* Big smile.
Nurse: *(After the assessment.) Well, you seem to be drinking lots of fluids, which is wonderful, you tell me you go every 2 to 3 days, and you have no gas or pain in the abdomen. I wonder if maybe your definition of constipation and mine are different.*
Client: *What do you mean?*
Nurse: *My definition of constipation is hard, dry stool that passes after 3 days or more and is accompanied by gas, bloating, and pain, maybe even nausea.*
Client: Looks horrified. *No, I don't get that!*
Nurse: *I know. Lots of people believe that if they don't go every day they're constipated and so they use laxatives and enemas, and these can make it worse. From your description, it sounds as though your bowel function is fine for a healthy woman your age. You have none of the symptoms of constipation, I can tell you. (Smiles.)*
Client: Smiles back. *Good, I'm glad.*
Nurse: *Be sure to call me if you have any questions at all. You know I'm happy to talk to you anytime.*
Client: *Thank you so much. I will.* Looks relieved and beams happily as she briskly leaves the office.

Less Effective

Nurse: *Hi, Mrs. Palumbo, I'm glad to see you. How are you feeling?*
Client: *Hello, there, Barbara. I'm doing fine except I think I'm a little constipated.* She whispers this last word.
Nurse: *Tell me a little more about that. (Listens attentively.)*
Client: *Well, I usually go every morning, but over the last few months I only go every 2 or 3 days, and I'm worried about that.* She looks worried.
Nurse: *You certainly look worried. But, you know, a woman your age is bound to slow down in some areas, even though you're still active and busy. Your bowel is slowing down and so you don't need to evacuate every single day.*
Client: Looks doubtful. *Really?*
Nurse: *Absolutely. I have many senior patients who are perfectly fine even though they don't have a movement every day. They drink enough fluids, eat enough fruits and vegetables, exercise, and do just fine. And I know from our last visit that you're doing all those things. Tell you what: If you have any questions, you give me a call, but I think you're doing great, Mrs. Palumbo.*
Client: *Well, okay. I guess I'm just being silly. I'll call you if anything new comes up.* Smiles and says goodbye.
Nurse: *Great! I'll talk to you then. (Smiles.)*

Critical Thinking Challenges

• Compare and contrast the different determinations Maryjo and Barbara made, as shown by their different responses to Mrs. Palumbo. • Infer what Mrs. Palumbo needed from her nurse. • If you were the nurse, what changes would you have made in Maryjo's conversation with Mrs. Palumbo? • In Barbara's?

Diagnostic Statement: Bowel Incontinence

Definition

Bowel Incontinence is the state in which an individual experiences a change in normal bowel habits characterized by involuntary passage of stool (NANDA, 1994).

Defining Characteristics

The defining characteristic is involuntary passage of stool (NANDA, 1994).

Related Factors

Related factors include gastrointestinal disorders; metabolic disorders; nutritional disorders; endocrine disorders;

infectious processes; tube feedings; fecal impaction; change in dietary intake; adverse effects of medications; high stress levels (NANDA, 1994).

Related Nursing Diagnoses

The impact of dysfunctional bowel status can contribute to or cause many potential or actual problems for the client. Emotionally, altered bowel function can cause Anxiety, Self-Esteem Disturbance, or Ineffective Individual Coping. Knowledge Deficit is often present as a person learns to cope with new treatment modalities. Pain can result from constipation, diarrhea, or abdominal distention. Alteration in bowel status can disrupt physiologic homeostasis by contributing to Fluid Volume Deficits, Altered Nutrition, Decreased Cardiac Output, and Impaired Skin Integrity with increased chance for infection. Interference with sleep patterns and sexual activity can also occur.

Outcome Identification and Planning

After nursing diagnoses and related factors have been established, the nurse and client identify outcomes and interventions. The direction of planning for bowel function depends on the time frame established to achieve the outcomes. Short-term goals are intended to be achieved within hours or days; a long-term goal is more realistic when the problem will take longer than 2 or 3 days to resolve. The overall outcomes for clients with bowel elimination pattern disturbances are

The client will demonstrate a normal pattern of bowel elimination without evidence of constipation, diarrhea, fecal incontinence, or distention.

The client will not experience preventable complications or adverse consequences from altered bowel elimination.

The client will participate in a program to maintain and promote an acceptable pattern of bowel elimination.

The time frame for the client to achieve a normal pattern of bowel elimination depends on the particular alteration involved. For example, constipation can usually be relieved in 1 or 2 days, whereas relief of diarrhea or incontinence is not always achievable in this time frame. The etiologic factors associated with the dysfunction also dictate the realistic time frame in which an outcome can be accomplished.

The potential complications from bowel elimination dysfunction vary with the specific alteration involved. Some potential complications include the following: an alteration in cardiac output as a result of constipation and straining at stool; an alteration in cardiac output as a result of vagal nerve stimulation during digital rectal examination; fluid volume and electrolyte deficit resulting from diarrhea; impaired skin integrity resulting from diarrhea or incontinence; fear, anxiety, and possible altered coping accompanying unpredictable diarrhea; impaired social interaction or social isolation; self-care deficit; and an alteration in health maintenance when clients cannot manage their bowel elimination dysfunction.

Promoting an acceptable bowel elimination pattern is, realistically, a long-term goal; in actual clinical practice, however, it is often subject to short-term management. Client teaching is a major management tool for achieving this goal. Examples of nursing interventions for various bowel problems are listed in the accompanying display and discussed in the following section.

Planning

Examples of Nursing Interventions Used in Common Bowel Problems

Constipation

- Increase fluid intake
- Increase dietary fiber
- Increase activity and exercise
- Provide laxatives
- Provide suppositories
- Administer enemas
- Initiate bowel management program

Diarrhea

- Treat underlying cause
- Provide bowel rest; limit oral intake
- Administer antidiarrheal medications

Fecal Incontinence

- Initiate bowel management program
- Provide fecal collection devices

Flatulence and Distention

- Administer antiflatulence medication
- Increase activity
- Place rectal tubes
- Administer return-flow enemas
- Provide nasogastric decompression

Fecal Diversion

- Assist in obtaining stoma appliances and fecal collection devices.
- Teach client self-care measures for ostomies.

Implementation

Nursing Interventions to Promote Health and Function

Client Teaching

Client teaching is an important nursing intervention for assisting clients to maintain normal bowel elimination. The nurse teaches the client to promote a normal, acceptable bowel pattern through adequate diet, fluid intake, and exercise. The nurse also teaches the client to avoid common causes of bowel elimination problems such as laxative abuse, food intolerances, excessive stress, and ignoring normal body signals (see the accompanying display).

Diet. The nurse should assist the client with planning a diet containing sufficient daily intake of high-fiber foods because dietary fiber is necessary to provide bulk to stool. The nurse can offer the client a list of high-fiber foods, which include fresh or cooked fruits and vegetables with their skins, whole-grain breads and cereals, and fruit and vegetable juices. The client's food preferences should be discussed. The nurse can assist the client in selecting foods from a list, identifying those foods that he or she will most likely incorporate into his or her lifestyle. A dietitian can be consulted for a more extensive list of high-fiber foods and recipes using these ingredients. Unprocessed bran flakes can be added to cooked or processed cereals; the client should start with small amounts (1 or 2 teaspoonfuls) to determine whether bran causes any intestinal irritation or flatulence. Unprocessed bran can absorb eight times its weight in water. An acceptable amount of bran is added gradually to the diet to achieve an acceptable bowel elimination pattern. The daily intake of about 800 g of high-fiber foods (eg, any combination of five or six servings of fruit or vegetables, and whole-grain bread or cereal) is encouraged. A sandwich with two slices of whole-grain bread, served with a large fresh vegetable salad and two pieces of fruit would provide about five servings of fiber.

Fluids. Intake between 1,500 and 2,000 mL of fluids per day promotes a normal bowel elimination pattern. The nurse should discuss with the client his or her fluid preferences and find a way to encourage the intake of about 8 to 10 glasses of fluid per day.

Some fruit and vegetable juices provide not only fluid but bulk because of their high pulp or fiber content. A glass of prune juice is equivalent to more than one serving of the dried fruit, has high magnesium content, and is an excellent source of fluid to promote bowel elimination. Hot fluids, such as coffee, tea, or hot water with lemon juice may also increase intestinal motility.

Client Teaching
Optimal Bowel Function

Instruct the client as follows:

- *Drink eight glasses of water per day, increase fiber in your diet, and increase daily exercise to maintain normal bowel patterns.*
- *Don't introduce high-fiber foods into the diet too quickly; such an action may cause excessive gas or diarrhea.*
- *Avoid using drinking straws when flatulence or abdominal distention is a problem.*
- *If you take loperamide (Imodium) or diphenoxylate (Lomotil) for diarrhea, be cautious about driving or other activities that require mental alertness. These medications may cause drowsiness.*
- *Empty an ostomy pouch when it is one-quarter to one-third full because the weight of a full pouch can break the appliance seal.*
- *Change a colostomy pouch when the bowel is least likely to emit stool—for example, first thing in the morning before eating or drinking.*

Activity and Exercise. A sufficient amount of daily exercise is necessary to promote general muscle tone. Exercise also encourages normal smooth muscle functioning, which is important for normal intestinal functioning. If a client has a relatively sedentary lifestyle, the nurse can explore reasonable alternative ways for him or her to incorporate additional activity in his or her lifestyle. Walking is an excellent exercise in which most people (even hospitalized clients) can participate. The nurse can encourage isotonic or isometric exercises to increase abdominal muscle tone. An example of these exercises is the alternate contraction and relaxation of the abdominal muscles for about 8 to 10 repetitions. The many variations of sit-up exercises isometrically tone and strengthen the abdominal muscles. The nurse assists the client on bed rest to perform range-of-motion exercises until he or she can perform more independent activities.

Bowel Habits. Many people recognize that their bodies have a regular time for bowel elimination; some people have a bowel movement every day, some twice a day, and some once every 2 days. Some people have a bowel movement at the same time of day or after a certain regular stimulus. The duodenocolic reflex is a strong reflex, especially when food or hot liquid is ingested after a period of fasting, such as after a night's sleep. For some people, ingesting breakfast or a cup of coffee, tea, or any liquid is stimulus enough to activate the duodenocolic reflex. The nurse teaches clients to heed their body signals and stresses that ignoring the urge to defecate can lead to constipation.

Nursing Interventions for Altered Bowel Function

Nurses have important responsibilities in managing altered bowel function. Nursing interventions are individualized to reestablish optimal bowel function and treat common bowel alterations such as constipation, diarrhea, flatulence, abdominal distention and related problems. Fecal impaction, neurologic impairment (requiring bowel training), fecal incontinence, and stoma care and irrigation required by fecal diversion surgery are more complex bowel problems that nurses independently or collaboratively manage. Constipation is treated with laxatives, suppositories, enemas, and, if chronic, a bowel management program. Diarrhea is managed by treating the underlying cause, bowel rest, and antidiarrheal medications. Fecal incontinence is managed by instituting a bowel-training program and using fecal collection devices. Flatulence is treated by increasing activity, administering medications, using rectal tubes, and administering return-flow enemas. Persistent abdominal distention may require decompression by nasogastric intubation. Other nursing interventions may involve those to relieve fecal impaction, to facilitate bowel training, and to care for the stoma and client after fecal diversion surgery.

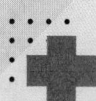

Safety Alert
Bowel Elimination

- Never leave a client on a toileting device without a mechanism for summoning assistance; straining with defecation can lead to cardiac arrhythmias or vertigo and thus potential falls and injury.
- Do not administer a laxative to client with undiagnosed abdominal pain; the resultant increase in peristalsis can rupture an inflamed bowel and cause peritonitis.
- Never administer more than three large-volume tap-water enemas in succession; excess absorption of the hypotonic solution by colonic mucosa leads to fluid and electrolyte imbalance.
- Use warm water (100° to 105°F, 37.7° to 40.5°C) for enemas. Cold water may lead to a decrease in temperature; hot water can cause burns to intestinal mucosa.
- Use the hooking motion of the index finger during manual disimpaction of stool carefully to avoid perforation of the rectum.
- Teach clients to exhale slowly during defecation, to avoid the Valsalva maneuver. This will avoid alterations in venous return and intracranial pressure, which can be dangerous for selected clients.

Medication Use

Laxatives. Usually oral laxatives are the treatment of choice for constipation because these medications promote evacuation of hardened stool from the bowel. Table 42-3 presents some common agents, such as oral laxatives and stool softeners, to relieve constipation. Oral laxatives take longer to evacuate stool than do laxatives given rectally, but are preferred by most clients for their ease of administration and the more gradual effect on intestinal motility.

Laxatives may be given in the form of a rectal suppository. A **suppository** is a medication prepared in a base (eg, glycerin) that, when inserted into the rectum, melts and can be absorbed for systemic or local effects. Many suppositories are used to promote bowel evacuation, but other drugs that do not affect bowel status (such as aspirin) can be administered in suppository form. A suppository is administered when a quick (15-60 minutes) effect is desired.

To administer a rectal suppository, the nurse needs the medication, a packet of water-soluble lubricant, and a pair of disposable gloves. If the client cannot ambulate independently to the bathroom, the nurse also places a bedside commode or bedpan close by before administering the suppository. Placement of disposable underpads on the bed may be advisable whenever the client's motor or mental abilities are compromised.

The client should assume a side-lying position. With gloved hands, the nurse removes the outer wrapper from the suppository and covers the suppository with lubricant. While separating the client's buttocks, the nurse locates the anus and inserts the suppository past the internal sphincter. For the adult, the internal sphincter is at approximately 4 inches, or at the end of the nurse's index finger. The nurse should guide the suppository with his or her index finger, aiming in a slightly upward direction toward the umbilicus. The pointed or rounded end of the suppository is inserted first, with the suppository resting on rectal mucosa. A suppository melts at body temperature and releases its medication as it rests against the rectal mucosa. The nurse should be sure the suppository is not inadvertently deposited into stool that might be present in the rectum because this prevents absorption by the rectal mucosa.

Antidiarrheal Agents. Medications that act directly on the intestine to slow bowel motility or to absorb excess fluid in the bowel are called antidiarrheals. Table 42-4 lists the antidiarrheal agents most commonly administered. Absorbents and bulk-forming agents change the consistency of the stool to relieve diarrhea; they cause few adverse systemic effects and are considered safe for general use. Opiates and antispasmodics act systemically to decrease intestinal motility. Antidiarrheal agents are contraindicated when viral or bacterial in-

Table 42-3 • Common Agents Used to Relieve Constipation

Agent	Action
Stool Softeners	
Surface-active agents	
Docusate sodium (*DOSS, Colace) Docusate calcium (Surfak)	↓ Surface tension of feces in colon → softer and bulkier stool
Laxatives	
Mechanical stimulation of colon	
Osmotic agents	
Magnesium hydroxide (Milk of Magnesia [MOM]) Magnesium citrate (Citro-Nesia) Magnesium sulfate (Epsom salts)	↑ Bulk in LGI by the osmotic action of the mineral salt to attract water → rectal distention (mechanical stimulation of defecation reflex)
Other bulk-forming agents	
Psyllium (Metamucil) Effer-syllium	Nonabsorbable fibers attract water in LGI → rectal distention (mechanical stimulation of defecation reflex)
Lubricant Mineral oil (Fleet Mineral Oil, Nujol)	Lubricates and softens stool in colon → easier evacuation of stool
Chemical stimulation of colon Castor oil Phenolphthalein (Ex-Lax) Bisacodyl (Dulcolax) Cascara sagrada Senna (Senokot) Aloes	Chemical properties of medication stimulate LGI to ↑ peristalsis → evacuation of colon contents
Suppositories	
Glycerin (Osmoglyn)	Attracts water and softens stool
Bisacodyl (Dulcolax)	Chemically stimulates LGI to ↑ peristalsis
Small-Volume Enemas	
Phosphate/biphosphate (Fleet Enema, Phospho-Soda)	Osmotically attracts water to ↑ colonic distention
Oil retention	Lubricates and softens stool in rectum

*Trade names in parentheses.
LGI, lower gastrointestinal tract.

fections cause diarrhea, because diarrhea is a protective mechanism to shed the microorganism from the body.

Medications may also be used to relieve the underlying problem. For example, antibiotics are administered when an infectious microorganism causes diarrhea. Steroids may be given to decrease the inflammation in the exacerbation of a chronic inflammatory bowel disease.

Antiflatulent Agents. Antiflatulent agents, such as simethicone, are used to relieve gas. Simethicone coalesces gas bubbles in the intestine; it does not prevent the formation of gas but does allow gas to pass from the gastrointestinal tract either by belching or anal expulsion. Antiflatulent medication is usually given in combination with an antacid. Suppositories that increase intestinal motility can also relieve accumulated intestinal flatus.

Enemas

An **enema** is the cleansing of a portion of the large bowel by insertion of fluid rectally. Enemas can be small volume, containing a laxative medication (approximately 150 mL), or large volume, containing only ordinary tap water or saline solution (up to 1,000 mL for the adult). Procedure 42-2 gives the steps in administering an enema.

Small-Volume Enemas. Small-volume enemas are commercially prepared and usually administered when

Table 42-4 • Medications Used to Relieve Diarrhea

Agent	Action
Absorbents	
Kaolin/pectin (*Donnagel) Attapulgite (Kaopectate) Bismuth subsalicylate (Pepto Bismol)	Absorbs excess fluid and bowel irritants; provides soothing effect to irritated bowel
Bulk-Forming Agents	
Psyllium (Metamucil, Effer-syllium)	Attracts water to absorb excess fluid
Opiates	
Paregoric Codeine	↓ Intestinal motility ↑ Intestinal water and electrolyte absorption
Synthetic Opiates	
Lopermide (Imodium)	↓ Intestinal motility
Diphenoxylate/atropine (Lomotil)	↓ Intestinal motility ↑ Intestinal water and electrolyte absorption
Antispasmodics	
Atropine Tincture of belladonna	↓ Intestinal motility

*Trade names in parentheses.

an oral laxative fails to produce sufficient stool return or when a rapid evacuation is preferred. The laxative solution is hypertonic, osmotically drawing water from colonic mucosa to cause water retention in the lower colon, and it also increases peristalsis. The volume of fluid itself distends the rectum to trigger a defecation reflex.

An oil retention enema is a small-volume enema containing a quantity of mineral oil. The mineral oil softens any hardened stool that is in the rectum, making the stool easier to pass. An oil retention enema is usually given only when a fecal impaction is suspected.

Small-volume enemas come from the manufacturer in disposable containers with prelubricated tips. When administering a small-volume enema, the nurse must use disposable gloves, place underpads on the bed as necessary, and have a bedpan, commode, or bathroom accessible. The client should be side-lying, with bed in low position. The client usually experiences the urge to defecate within 5 to 10 minutes after administration of the enema.

Large-Volume Enemas. Large-volume enemas cleanse the bowel of stool by distending the bowel with up to 1,000 mL fluid for the adult (15–60 mL are recommended for an infant; 240–360 mL for a child). Warm tap water or saline solution is used as the cleansing agent; saline solution is the only fluid recommended for infants and children. The large volume of fluid instilled into the bowel causes distention and stimulates the defecation reflex. The large-volume enema can be used as a treatment for constipation or as a method of cleansing the bowel before bowel x-rays or surgery.

The nurse needs to gather the necessary equipment, including an enema bucket or bag connected to plastic tubing, disposable gloves, disposable underpads for the bed, water-soluble lubricant, and the solution. A bedpan, commode, or access to a toilet should also be available. The client is positioned as for administration of a suppository or small-volume enema. The nurse flushes or primes the tubing with the solution all the way to the tip of the tubing to prevent air from inadvertently being instilled into the rectum; air will cause the client discomfort. The nurse inserts the lubricated tip of the tubing approximately 4 inches, aiming toward the umbilicus, and slowly instills the solution into the client's rectum. Care must be taken not to insert the tubing too far or to advance the tubing forcefully because this could injure mucosal tissue or, in extreme situations, perforate the intestine.

The nurse controls the amount and speed of the fluid instillation by opening and closing the tubing clamp and by adjusting the height of the enema bucket. Opening the clamp and raising the bucket increase the rate of flow of the solution into the rectum. Conversely, closing the clamp or lowering the enema bucket decreases the rate of flow. If the client complains of abdominal discomfort and cramping, the nurse momen-

Procedure 42-2
Administering an Enema

Purpose

1. Relieves gas, constipation, or fecal impaction.
2. Cleanses the bowel in preparation for diagnostic or surgical procedures.
3. Evacuates feces in clients with hemiplegia, quadriplegia, or paraplegia.
4. Delivers medication.

Assessment

- Assess client's past and present elimination history: presence of hemorrhoids, external and internal.
- Review healthcare provider's order, and determine the purpose for the enema to guide selection of the solution.
- If constipation or impaction is suspected, palpate abdomen for distention, and perform digital rectal exam.
- Determine client's understanding of purpose of enema, what to expect during the procedure, and how he or she can help.
- Assess client's developmental level and whether additional assistance is needed to hold the client while the enema is administered.

Equipment

Enema container with appropriately sized tubing (adults—size 22–32 Fr, children—size 14–18 Fr, infants—size 12 Fr, or a bulb syringe).
Possible solutions: Normal saline, tap water, soap solution, medications, commercially prepared bulb enema.
Disposable gloves and water-soluble lubricant.
Personal hygiene items: soap, towel, water.
Waterproof bed protector.
Clean bedpan or commode, and toilet paper. Children may use potty chair or diaper.

Procedure

1. Assemble the needed equipment in one place; then provide privacy by closing curtains or room door.
   Rationale: Speeds the procedure, reduces embarrassment for the client, and increases his or her ability to relax.

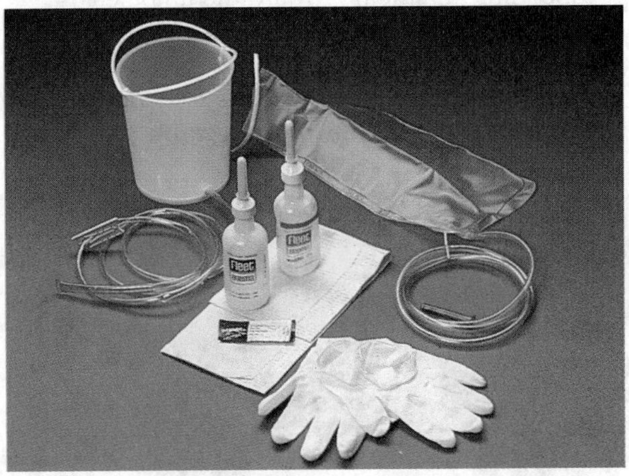

Step 1 • *Assemble equipment.*

2. Have client lie on left side (Sims' position) with right knee flexed. Children and adults with poor sphincter control may be placed in dorsal recumbent position on a bedpan.
   Rationale: Sims' position improves retention of enema by allowing solution to flow along the natural sigmoid colon curve.
3. Put on disposable gloves.
4. Place waterproof towel under client's buttocks.
   Rationale: Soiling of linen is prevented.
5. Cover client with bath blanket, exposing only the rectum.
   Rationale: Blanket provides privacy, warmth, and increases ability to relax.

Procedure

Large-Volume Enema

1. See steps 1 to 5.
2. Fill enema bag with 750 to 1,000 mL lukewarm solution (105° to 110°F, for child—500 mL or less, 100°F). Check temperature of solution with bath thermometer or by pouring some over your inner wrist.
   Rationale: Intestinal mucosa can be damaged if solution is too warm. Cold solutions are difficult to retain and can cause abdominal cramping.
3. Open clamp on tubing and flush solution to remove the air. Reclamp tubing.
   Rationale: Air in the rectum causes discomfort.
4. Lubricate 2 to 3 inches of the tip of rectal tube with water-soluble lubricant.

(continued)

Rationale: Insertion is smoother and minimizes trauma with lubrication.

5. Separate the buttocks to visualize the anus. Observe for external hemorrhoids, ask client to take a slow, deep breath. Gently insert the rectal tube, directing the tip toward the umbilicus (adult—3–4 inches, child—2–3 inches, infant—1–1.5 inches).
   Rationale: Prevents injury to the intestinal mucosa by directing the tube along the natural bowel curve.

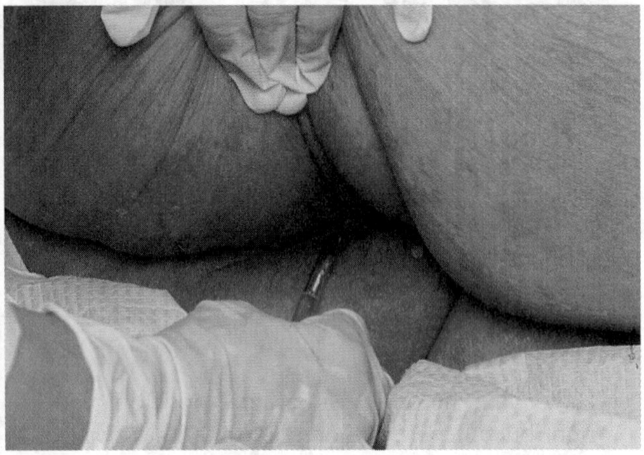

Step 5 • *Raise buttocks and insert tubing into anus.*

6. Continue holding the tube in the rectum. With other hand open the clamp and allow solution to slowly enter the client. Raise container 18 inches above the anus, allowing solution to flow slowly over 5 to 10 minutes. If client complains of cramping or pain, have client breathe deeply and lower bag until the sensation stops.
   Rationale: Slow instillation reduces client discomfort from bowel distention and cramping, thereby allowing a greater volume of solution to be retained.

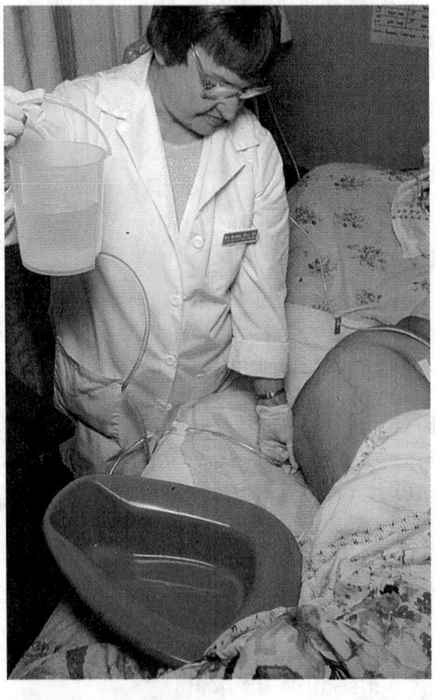

Step 6 • *Raise enema solution about 18 inches above rectum and instill slowly.*

7. Reclamp tubing when desired amount of solution has infused.
   Rationale: Clamping prevents air from entering the rectum.
8. Remove tube gently and have client squeeze buttocks together firmly for several minutes.
   Rationale: The urge to defecate caused by tube removal will decrease as sphincters are contracted.
9. Have client retain solution as long as possible.
   Rationale: Longer retention enhances peristalsis and evacuation of bowel contents.
10. Assist client to bathroom, commode, or bedpan. Place call bell within reach. Provide privacy until all of the solution has been expelled.
11. Visually inspect character of the feces and solution.
    Rationale: If enemas are ordered "until clear" as preparation for diagnostic testing, it is essential to assess expelled solution for fecal material. Allow client to rest, then repeat as necessary.
12. Assist client into comfortable position.
13. Assist with cleansing as needed. Provide materials for client to wash hands. Open windows or provide air freshener if needed. Clean and dispose of equipment as necessary. Remove gloves and wash hands.
    Rationale: Spread of microorganisms is prevented, and client comfort is increased.

Procedure

Small-Volume Enema

1. See Steps 1 to 5 at beginning of Procedure.
2. Remove protective cap from prelubricated catheter tip. You may add more lubricant if necessary.
   Rationale: Allows smooth insertion of the rectal tip and minimizes trauma to the mucosa.
3. Separate the buttocks to visualize the anus. Observe for hemorrhoids and gently insert rectal tip into rectum. Advance 3 to 4 inches in an adult, directing the tip toward the umbilicus.
   Rationale: Prevents injury to the intestinal mucosa by following the natural curve of the bowel.
4. Squeeze bottle to empty contents into the rectum and colon (approximately 240 mL of solution).
   Rationale: Prepackaged solutions are usually hypertonic and require only small volumes to stimulate defecation. Not to be used in children!

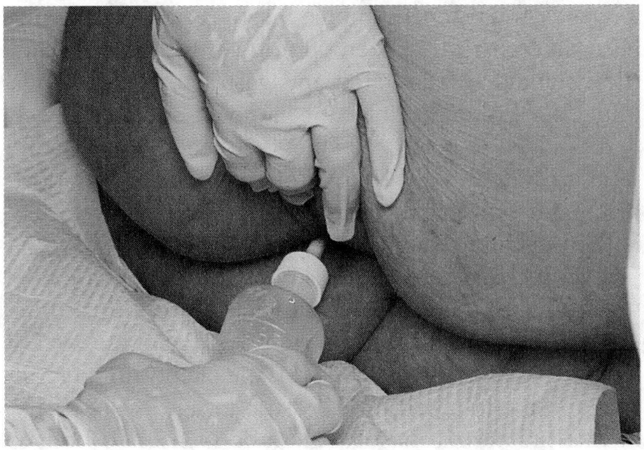

Step 4 • *Squeeze small enema container to insert fluid into rectum.*

5. Maintain pressure on the enema container until you withdraw it from the rectum.
   Rationale: Releasing the pressure while the container is still in the rectum will cause the liquid to be drawn back into the container.
6. Continue same as with large-volume enema.

Lifespan Considerations

Infants and Children

- Children who are not toilet trained are incontinent. Other children may be unable to control their rectal sphincter sufficiently to retain enema solutions. Administer with the bedpan in place.
- For children under 2 years of age, the healthcare provider should order the amount of solution to be administered.
- Children and infants do not usually receive tap water or prepackaged hypertonic enemas because fatal water intoxication or circulatory depletion could occur.

Older Adults

- If adult is incontinent, place clean, dry, waterproof linen under his or her buttocks until enema solution has been expelled and buttocks are cleaned. The skin of older adults macerates easily from prolonged contact with moisture. Check frequently for newly expelled stool and clean as necessary.

Home-Care Modifications

- Clients should be taught not to rely on enemas to maintain bowel regularity. Enemas *do not* treat the cause of irregularity, and if used frequently can result in dependence on enemas for defecation because they can disrupt normal elimination reflexes.

tarily stops the flow of solution. To cleanse the bowel successfully of stool, the average adult needs to tolerate approximately 350 to 500 mL of solution instilled before expelling the enema. When the client cannot tolerate any more solution per rectum, the nurse stops the enema and assists the client as necessary to the bedpan, commode, or toilet.

A large-volume enema can be repeated up to three times in succession. Guidelines for repetition include the statement that the client feels there is more stool in the bowel that needs to be evacuated, large pieces of stool in the enema returns, and the water in the enema returns is heavily stool-colored. A step-by-step guide is given in Procedure 42-2.

Return-Flow Enemas. The return-flow enema is used to relieve accumulated flatus. The nurse uses the same equipment as for the large-volume enema; however, only 300 to 500 mL of warm tap water is necessary. The nurse proceeds in the same way as for the large-volume enema. When the client indicates he or she feels abdominal discomfort or cramping, the nurse lowers the enema reservoir (the bag or bucket) and allows the water to return through the tubing into the reservoir. Flatus will also return, as evidenced by the bubbling of the water in the bucket. The nurse continues to repeat the procedure until there is no more evidence of expelled flatus, or the client reports relief. This procedure may take 15 to 20 minutes to be effective. The return-flow enema can be repeated as necessary.

Rectal Tubes

A rectal tube, which is a short piece of plastic tubing similar to the tubing used for large-volume enemas, may be used if increased activity or medication does not relieve flatulence. The nurse inserts the lubricated tip of the tube about 4 inches into the client's rectum and leaves it in place for 15 to 20 minutes or until the client reports relief. The gas in the rectum can pass from the rectum through the tube and into a collecting device, such as a bag. Abdominal pain is the predominant adverse consequence of flatulence. It is wiser to relieve the cause of the pain by using antiflatulence agents or rectal tubes than to administer pain medications. Narcotic analgesics in particular slow intestinal motility and compound the problem.

Nasogastric Intubation

Nasogastric intubation may be ordered by the healthcare provider for a variety of bowel problems, among them distention, gastric decompression, gastric analysis, gastric lavage, or gastric gavage.

Gastric Decompression. Gastric decompression may be accomplished through nasogastric intubation, in which the nurse inserts the nasogastric tube, assesses the client during the period of intubation, and provides nursing care that ensures proper tube function and client comfort. A nasogastric tube is a thin, pliable plastic tube that can be inserted into a client's nose and advanced into the stomach (Fig. 42-7). Decompression relieves the stomach and intestines of pressure caused by accumulated gastrointestinal air and fluid. The nasogastric tube is connected to suction to facilitate decompression of the stomach contents. (Refer to Procedure 42-3, "Inserting a Nasogastric Tube," for a detailed description of the technique.) Gastric decompression is indicated for a bowel obstruction, paralytic ileus, or when surgery is performed on the stomach or intestine. In each situation, potential or actual accumulation of fluid and gas in the intestine can cause abdominal distention, discomfort for the client, and serious physiologic alterations. The tube usually remains in place until normal bowel function resumes, as evidenced by active bowel tones on auscultation.

Gastric Analysis. Gastric analysis can be accomplished by testing stomach contents aspirated through a nasogastric tube. The nurse inserts a nasogastric tube in a client who has been NPO for 6 to 8 hours. Gastric contents are aspirated and gastric acidity is determined. A histamine injection is given subcutaneously to stimulate stomach secretions. Stomach contents are then aspirated every 10 to 20 minutes until three posthistamine samples are obtained. The nasogastric tube is then usually removed.

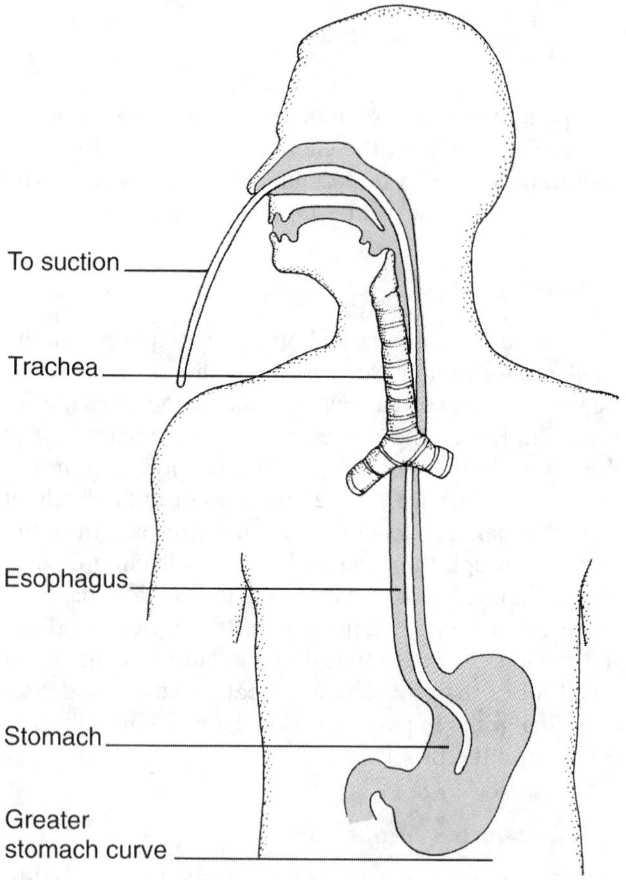

Figure 42-7 *• Proper placement of the nasogastric tube.*

Gastric Lavage. **Gastric lavage** is the irrigation of the stomach. In cases of accidental poisoning and accidental or intentional drug overdoses, swift removal of stomach contents is necessary. If the client cannot swallow an emetic medication, gastric lavage is necessary. In this situation, a nasogastric tube is inserted both to aspirate gastric contents and to instill a rinsing solution (usually normal saline) into the stomach to dilute the toxic substances. Clients with gastric bleeding are sometimes treated with an iced saline lavage, which involves instilling and aspirating iced saline solution through the nasogastric tube to empty the stomach of blood and slow the bleeding at its source.

Gastric Gavage. In clients who cannot obtain adequate nourishment orally, **gastric gavage** delivers liquid food into the stomach through the nasogastric tube. This type of feeding is also called enteral nutrition. Nasogastric tubes for feeding are intended to be used for a longer time than nasogastric tubes used for decompression or lavage. They are narrower and made of a more pliable material. Nasogastric feeding tubes and the nursing care associated with enteral nutrition are discussed in Chapter 37.

Equipment

Nasogastric Tubes. The two most commonly used nasogastric tubes are the single-lumen (one channel) Levin tube and the double-lumen (two channels) gastric sump tube (Fig. 42-8). The Levin tube is sized according to the French method; sizes 14 to 18 Fr are typical adult sizes, with a length of 120 cm (48 inches). The Levin tube is plastic or rubber and can be used for gastric decompression, analysis, lavage, or gavage. Small openings at the tip end of the tube allow for fluid flow in or out of the tube, and markings at specific points on the tube serve as measurement guidelines for the length of tube to be inserted.

The double-lumen gastric sump tube is clear plastic and also sized according to the French method. Gastric sump tubes are the preferred tube for decompression. The larger lumen is connected to suction and a drainage container to collect the aspirated gastric contents, and the smaller second lumen terminates in a blue vent, often called the tube's "pigtail." The blue vent is always open to the air, providing continuous atmospheric air irrigation. Markings along the length of the tube serve as guides for depth of insertion. Both lumens have openings at the tip end to allow for fluid or air flow in and out of the tube.

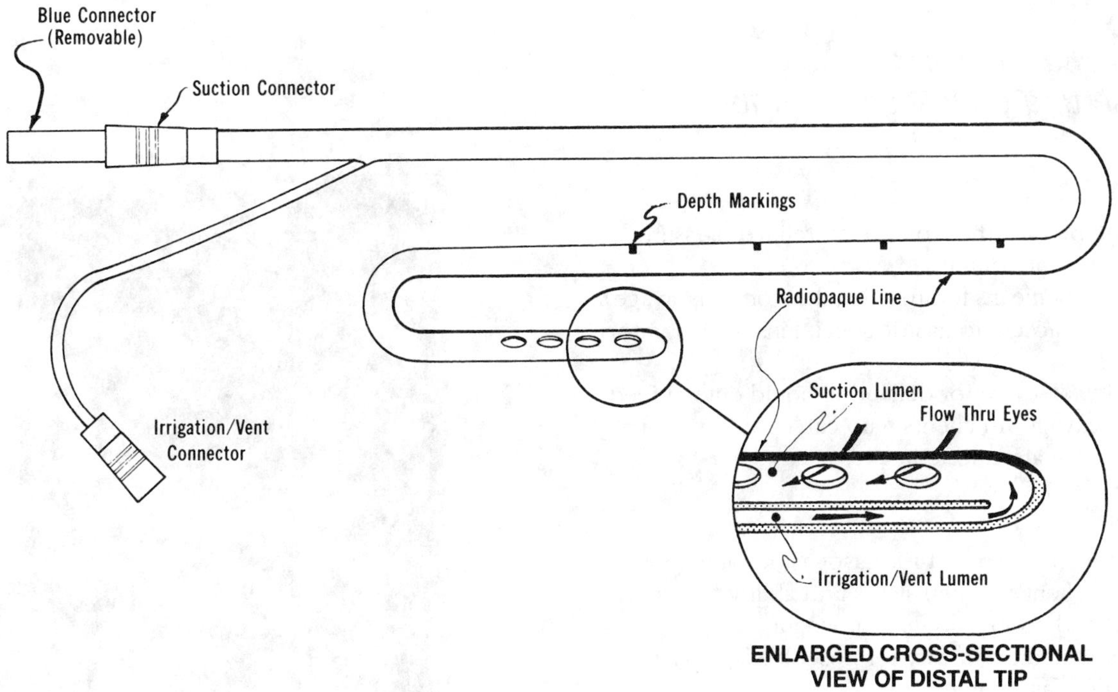

Figure 42-8 • *Double-lumen gastric sump tube. (Courtesy of National Catheter Co., Argle, N.Y.)*

Nasointestinal Tubes. When intestinal decompression for mechanical or nonmechanical bowel obstruction is the desired outcome, a longer tube capable of advancing the length of the intestine is used. As with nasogastric tubes, single- or double-lumen tubes are available.

The Harris tube (6 feet) and the Cantor (10 feet) are single-lumen tubes intended for intestinal decompression. Both tubes have mercury-weighted bags attached to the tip of tube. The weight of the mercury assists the tube in passing from the pylorus of the stomach into the duodenum. The weighted tip and the natural peristalsis of the intestine keep the tube advancing through the intestine.

The Miller-Abbot is a double-lumen, 10-foot tube. One lumen drains or decompresses the intestine; the second lumen is used to inflate the balloon at the tip of the tube with mercury. Therefore, the double-lumen tube allows for insertion of the mercury after the tip of the tube has passed through the nose and into the stomach.

Nasointestinal tubes are inserted in the same manner as nasogastric tubes. When the tip of the tube has reached the stomach, the tubing is not taped to the client's nose. The client can be positioned on the right side, allowing gravity and the mercury bag to enhance passage of the tube into the duodenum. In a few hours, passage of the tube into the small intestine should be verified by x-ray. If the tube has not advanced on its own, it can be advanced manually from the stomach into the duodenum under fluoroscopy by the healthcare provider or radiologist. Client activity, position changes in bed, or ambulation encourage increased intestinal peristalsis and self-advancement of tube along the length of the intestine. Markings along the length of the tube help to estimate progress of the tube through the intestine.

Nasointestinal tubes can be attached to a bag positioned below the client's torso to achieve a drainage of intestinal contents by gravity. Suction, either continuous or intermittent, can also be applied and contents emptied into a collecting device.

Suction. Subatmospheric or negative pressure is applied to nasogastric tubes to pull air or fluid out of the stomach. Most healthcare facilities have wall outlet suction at the client's bedside. A suction regulator is inserted into the wall unit. The suction gauge can be set at millimeters of mercury of pressure: 20 to 40 mm Hg = low suction; 80 to 120 mm Hg = high suction. Suction can be regulated as continuous or intermittent.

Intermittent suction provides for suction at preset time intervals—up to 60 seconds—followed by set intervals of no suction. Connecting tubing is attached between the client end of the nasogastric tube and a collecting device. The collecting device is connected by tubing to the suction regulator. In healthcare facilities without wall outlet suction, portable suction units are available. These portable units usually provide only for intermittent suction at a "low" or "high" setting.

Continuous suction greater than 25 mm Hg can lead to irritation of the gastric mucosa if the mucosa are inadvertently "sucked" against one of the openings at the

Procedure 42-3
Inserting a Nasogastric Tube

Purpose

1. Decompresses the stomach to relieve pressure and prevent vomiting.
2. Provides a means for irrigating the stomach (lavage).
3. Provides access to gastric specimens for laboratory analysis.
4. Provides a route for delivering liquid enteral feedings (gavage) in clients who can't swallow or ingest adequate calorie intake.

Assessment

- Identify client's need for nasogastric intubation.
- Assess client's mental status and ability to understand and cooperate with procedure.
- Review medical history for nosebleeds, deviated septum, nasal surgery.
- Assess nostrils for size, lesions, obstructions, or deformities.
  Note: Have client breathe through one nostril while occluding the other. The tube should be inserted through the most patent nostril.

Equipment

Nasogastric tube of appropriate size (Adult: 14–18 Fr, Infant/child: 5–10 Fr).
Water-soluble lubricant.
20- to 50-mL syringe with catheter tip or adapter.
Glass of tap water with straw.
Towel, stethoscope, disposable gloves.
Hypoallergenic tape.

Procedure

1. Identify client and explain procedure.
   Note: Insertion is not painful, but it is uncomfortable because the gag reflex is usually stimulated.
   Rationale: Client is more cooperative when the procedure is understood.
2. Provide privacy by closing curtains or room door.
3. Raise bed to high-Fowler's position, cover chest with towel, and place emesis basin nearby.
   Rationale: Elevated head protects against aspiration.
4. Wash hands, and put on gloves.
5. Determine length of tubing to be inserted by measuring nasogastric tube from tip of ear lobe to tip of nose, then to tip of xyphoid process. Mark tubing with adhesive tape or note striped markings already on the tube.
   Rationale: This measure determines approximate length of esophagus from nares to stomach, which varies among clients.

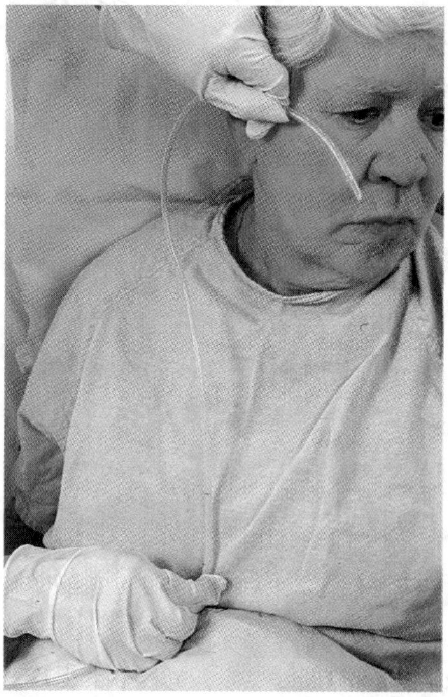

Step 5 • *Measure proper tube length to insert.*

6. Lubricate tip of tube with water-soluble lubricant.
   Rationale: A water-soluble lubricant will be reabsorbed if tube inadvertently enters the lung. Never use an oil-based lubricant because respiratory complications may ensue.
7. Gently insert tube into nostril. Advance toward posterior pharynx.
   Rationale: Following natural contour prevents trauma to nasal mucosa.
8. Have client tilt head forward and encourage client to drink water slowly. Advance tube without using

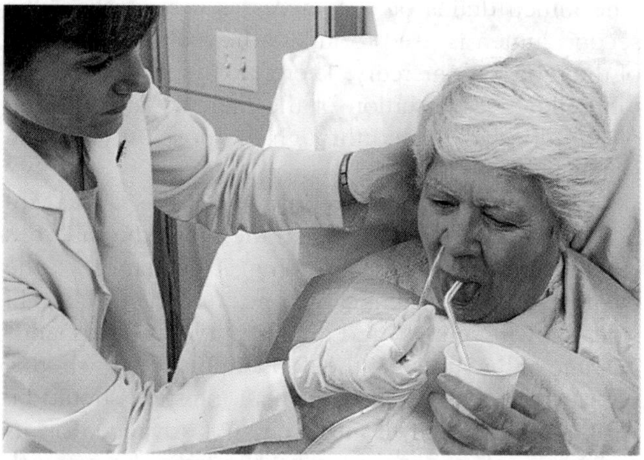

Step 8 • *Advance tube as client swallows water.*

force as client swallows. Advance tube until desired insertion length is reached.
Rationale: Forward tilt of head facilitates passage of tube into esophagus and not the larynx. Swallowing moves epiglottis over the larynx and facilitates tube passage.

9. Temporarily tape the tube to the client's nose; then assess placement of the tube:
   a. Aspirate gastric content with 20- to 50-mL syringe.
   Rationale: Gastric content is yellow to green and usually present in amounts greater than 10 mL.
   b. Auscultate over epigastrium while injecting 10 to 20 mL air into nasogastric tube.
   Rationale: Bubbling is heard if tube is in stomach.

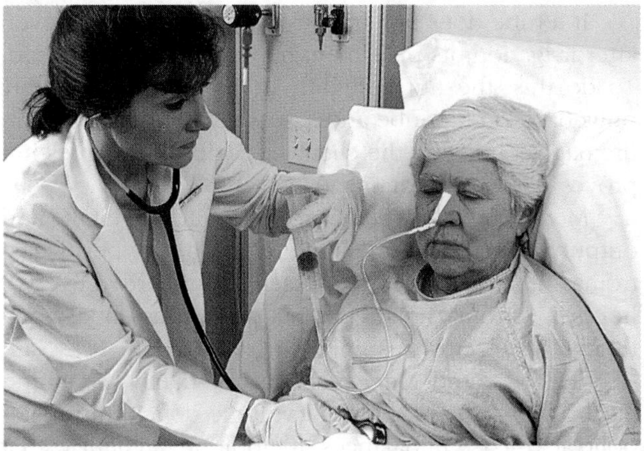

Step 9 • *Check proper tube placement.*

10. If placement in stomach is not verified, untape tube, advance tube 5 cm, and repeat assessment in Step 9.
11. Secure tube by taping to bridge of client's nose. Anchor tubing to client's gown.
Rationale: Correct taping prevents the tube from dislodging or pulling and traumatizing the nostril.

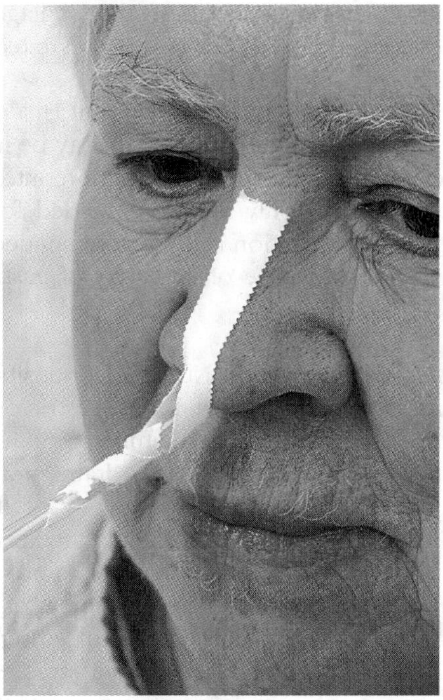

Step 11 • *Securely fasten tube to nose.*

12. Clamp end of tubing or attach to suction, as ordered by healthcare provider.
13. Wash hands, provide for client's comfort, and remove equipment.
14. Establish and document a nursing plan for daily care of the nasogastric tube:
   a. Inspecting nostril for irritation.
   b. Cleanse nostril frequently.
   c. Changing adhesive as required to prevent skin irritation or pressure sores on nostril from the tube.
   d. Increase frequency of oral care because clients with nasogastric tubes often mouth breathe and may be NPO.

Lifespan Considerations

Infants

- Measurement of tube length in children younger than 1 year of age is from the tip of the nose to the ear lobe, then to point halfway between xyphoid process and umbilicus.

tip of the nasogastric tube. Gastric irritation is most likely to occur when a single-lumen Levin tube is connected to medium or high suction. The blue air vent of a double-lumen sump tube is designed to minimize gastric irritation associated with suction pressure; the blue air vent is left open to the air, allowing air under atmospheric pressure to flow continually into the stomach. As long as the air vent is patent, air will continuously irrigate the distal tip of the tube, keeping the gastric mucosa from tightly adhering to the larger outlets of the suction lumen. To be effective as an air vent, the pigtail must be kept at a level above the client's stomach; otherwise, gravity allows gastric contents to flow out of the air vent. Whenever gastric contents or the irrigation fluid enters the air vent, it must be cleared with 5 to 10 mL of air to reestablish air irrigation. Some gastric sump tubes come with an antireflux valve. When the antireflux valve is firmly in place in the blue air vent of the double-lumen sump tube, spillage of gastric contents from the blue pigtail is prevented regardless of pigtail position.

Low continuous suction (30–40 mm Hg) is recommended for double-lumen tubes, but may be increased as needed to stimulate flow of gastric contents. Low intermittent suction only is recommended for single-lumen tubes. High suction is not recommended for single-lumen tubes because of high risk of gastric irritation.

Nursing Considerations. Nursing responsibilities involved in caring for clients with nasogastric or nasointestinal tubes include placing the tube accurately, monitoring for adequate suction to drain stomach or intestinal contents, maintaining patency of the tube, monitoring and recording the client's intake and output, and providing adequate skin (nares) and oral care.

Accurate Placement. Accurate placement of the tube is important to ensure client safety. Inserting a nasogastric tube is a nursing procedure. Before inserting the tube, the nurse explains its purpose and lets the client know that discomfort may be felt as the tube passes along the back of the throat (initiating the gag reflex). Clients usually experience transient nausea, and some clients vomit at this point. Once the tip of the tube passes the gag reflex, the client can assist in advancing the tube down the esophagus by swallowing. The nurse gently guides the tube with each client swallow to the predetermined mark on the tube (see Procedure 42-3).

Accurate placement is verified by x-ray, aspirating gastric contents, and auscultating the LUQ with a stethoscope for a "burp" as 5 to 10 mL of air is instilled by syringe into the tube.

Maintaining Suction. Maintaining suction is important when nasogastric tubes are used for gastric decompression. The nurse uses the lowest suction that will achieve successful drainage, checks the suction gauges every 4 hours for proper setting, and observes the drainage tubing every hour to make sure that gastrointestinal contents are flowing in the direction of the collection container. To test suction, the nurse may temporarily disconnect the tubing at the junction between the nasogastric and drainage tubing to hear the "whoosh" of suction and feel the suction at his or her fingertip. The nurse replaces any nonfunctioning suction units.

Maintaining Tube Patency. Tube patency is important to ensure proper functioning of the inserted tube. Occasionally thick or solid particles of gastrointestinal contents plug the holes of a nasogastric or nasointestinal tube; the tube then ceases to drain gastrointestinal contents, even with properly functioning suction. When a tube clogs, minimal drainage appears in the tubing or collecting receptacle. The client may begin to complain of nausea, which does not occur with a properly functioning system. The abdomen may appear distended.

The nurse can irrigate the tube with about 20 mL of water (Surratt, et al., 1993) to dislodge particles or viscous gastrointestinal contents from the tip of the tube. When large volumes of irrigant are instilled, such as during gastric lavage, normal saline solution should be used to prevent fluid and electrolyte shifts that can occur when a hypotonic solution is used. Using water when only a small amount of irrigant is necessary helps reduce costs (Surratt, et al., 1993). Nasogastric irrigation is a clean rather than a sterile procedure because the gastrointestinal tract is not sterile. A physician's order is required for irrigation after gastric surgery. When irrigating a double-lumen nasogastric tube, the nurse can instill irrigant in either lumen. If using the blue air vent, the nurse need not disconnect suction during irrigation, but must remember to clear the air vent with 10 mL of air after the procedure. Air clears the blue lumen of fluid and restores continuous air irrigation. The nurse ensures that the antireflux valve in the blue air vent is replaced after irrigation.

If a tube does not appear to be draining well even after irrigation, its placement may need to be checked. To do this, the nurse slightly advances or alternately pulls back on the tube and assesses for any increase in drainage. Changing the client's position sometimes improves nasogastric drainage.

Monitoring Intake and Output. Monitoring intake and output (including the volume, color, and type of gastrointestinal drainage) is assessed and recorded every 8 hours. Gastrointestinal contents contain essential body fluids and electrolytes, including water, H^+, K^+, Na^+, Cl^-, HCO_3^- and Mg^{2+}. Losing too many fluids and electrolytes can lead to fluid volume deficit and metabolic acid–base imbalances. In addition, a client with a nasogastric or nasointestinal tube for decompression will usually be NPO. Any fluids swallowed would be immediately returned via the tube; any food swallowed would eventually clog the tube. Clients with nasogastric or nasointestinal tubes will receive intravenous therapy to supply needed fluids and electrolytes. It is the responsibility of the nurse to measure and record all intake and output and monitor fluid and electrolyte status. Some newer tubes permit stomach decompression as well as intestinal feedings via a double-lumen tube system.

Providing Nasal and Oral Care. Nasal and oral care is an important nursing concern during a client's intubation. Skin irritation and breakdown at the nares (nostrils) can be prevented by appropriately taping the tube and providing frequent skin care. Applying a water-soluble lubricant to the nostrils provides moisturizing relief to dry skin. Using an oil-based lubricant (eg, petroleum jelly) can inadvertently result in oil particles being aspirated into the lungs, leading to lipid pneumonia.

To prevent constant tension and pulling on the tube, the nurse can secure the tube to the client's gown (channeling it through tape or a safety pin). The nurse should ensure enough slack so the client can turn his or her head from side to side without pulling on the tubing.

Frequent oral hygiene can prevent the consequence of dry mouth associated with nasogastric intubation. Clients usually become mouth breathers with a tube in the nose. Sucking on ice chips or hard candies, if approved by the healthcare provider, can also provide some relief.

The nurse encourages clients who can brush their teeth to do so frequently. An oral swab soaked in a solution of one-half water and one-half mouthwash is refreshing to many clients. Using lemon-glycerin oral swabs or swabs soaked in full-strength mouthwash should be avoided. The immediate relief provided by the swab is sometimes followed by rebound dryness. The nurse offers lubricant for the lips to prevent drying and cracking.

Administering Medication. The nurse can administer medication intended for oral consumption through a nasogastric tube. A liquid form of the medication is preferred, but many tablets can be crushed, mixed with water, and safely administered through the tube. All nasogastric medication administration should be followed with water to clear the tube and ensure that the medication has reached the stomach. The tube should remain clamped for a 30-minute period following medication administration to permit absorption via the gastric mucosa.

Fecal Impaction Removal

Removal of fecal impactions is a nursing responsibility. Manual removal of an impaction can be a cause of embarrassment for the client. The nurse explains the purpose and necessity of the procedure, telling the client before beginning what will be done. The nurse proceeds in a matter-of-fact manner to reduce anxiety and embarrassment for the client.

The equipment necessary for manual removal of fecal impaction includes plenty of disposable gloves, a gown, packets of water-soluble lubricant, several disposable underpads to protect the bed and floor, two bedpans, and a commode if the client is capable of transferring to it. It is possible for the large intestine to distend to hold a large amount of stool, and because the nurse cannot accurately predict the volume before beginning the procedure, it is best to be prepared to remove a large quantity of stool. The nurse should wear an impermeable or disposable gown because some stool is likely to spill or splash during the procedure. The odor of the stool can be strong, and an open window or other form of ventilation should be provided.

The nurse begins the procedure with the client in the side-lying position. The double-gloved, lubricated index finger is inserted into the rectum. With a gentle hooking motion of the index finger, the nurse removes some of the stool from the rectum. The removal of stool begins slowly, but as the hardened stool that is blocking the lumen of the rectum is removed, the remaining stool is usually loosely formed and will pass quickly. The bedpan should be ready to place under the client so that he or she can evacuate stool into it if possible; the stool may come so quickly that the client is unable to control its evacuation. The nurse continues to remove stool manually until he or she can no longer feel stool at the fingertip, and the client is not voluntarily evacuating any more stool. The nurse removes and disposes of collected stool and soiled linens, and provides hygiene care for the client. Removal of a fecal impaction is a tiring procedure for the client, so the nurse provides uninterrupted time and a restful environment after the procedure.

Nursing interventions to prevent complications in the management of fecal impaction include effective yet gentle insertion of the gloved index finger into the client's rectum when performing digital examination and manual removal of stool. Excess vagal stimulation during digital examination and removal of stool can precipitate cardiac arrhythmias in weak clients or those with cardiovascular disease. Forceful pressure against the rectal mucosa can damage the bowel tissue.

Bowel Training

A long-term approach to controlling bowel elimination may be necessary, especially for clients who are in the rehabilitation phase of a neurologic impairment (eg, paralysis, stroke, head injury). These clients are at high risk for constipation or fecal incontinence, or both. (Bowel training is not appropriate for clients with inflammatory bowel disease, infection, or lactose intolerance.)

A standard bowel-training program aims to maintain a soft stool consistency and develop a routine method of stool evacuation. The routine is repeated at the same time of day with the same techniques to train and control the bowel's evacuation time. An example of a standard bowel-training program for neurologically impaired clients appears in Figure 42-9. A common bowel-training program includes using stool softener twice a day, a bulking agent daily, a suppository (glycerin or bisacodyl [Dulcolax; Boehringer Ingelheim, Ridgefield, CT]), usually given after breakfast, followed by toileting and digital stimulation (McLane & McShane, 1992). Bowel training may require weeks to months of persistence before success is attained. Reassurance and verbal expressions of confidence in the client contribute to success of the program. Client teaching about normal bowel function and factors to promote a soft stool are helpful.

For clients with anal sphincter control that is weak but not lost, a variation of the classic bowel-training program is implemented. Stool softeners and an increase

Date	Time	Related Meal or Fluid	Time and Type of Suppository	Comments: How, Where, Level of Independence
8/10	0800	Breakfast containing fiber	0830 Suppository with digital stimulation	Can transfer independently to bedside commode

1. Time bowel program to occur 20 to 30 minutes after eating a meal or at least drinking some warm fluid.
2. Begin program by inserting a well-lubricated suppository past the external and internal anal sphincters.
3. 0 to 20 minutes after inserting suppository, transfer patient to commode or toilet (unless the program is to be done in bed).
4. At 15-minute intervals starting approximately 30 minutes after suppository insertion, perform rectal massage or digital stimulation. This is done by gently inserting a well-lubricated gloved finger into the anal canal. Then using a gentle circular motion the rectal wall is stretched to help stimulate the defecation reflex. The rectal stretching must be done gently and slowly to prevent trauma and to allow enough stimuli for the reflex emptying to occur.

Figure 42-9 • *Classic bowel-training program.*

in dietary fiber are used to maintain a soft stool, but instead of relying on the routine use of suppositories and digital stimulation, emphasis is placed on the client recognizing the body's own defecation signals. Careful assessment and documentation of incontinent episodes are performed for several days. From then on, the client is assisted to the toilet at a time that has been identified as "routine." The time often coincides with a duodenocolic mass movement after eating. The intent is to establish a regular defecation time in synchrony with the client's natural physiologic function.

Pelvic floor exercises, biofeedback, and abdominal massage have been used by some healthcare providers to promote regular stool evacuation. When performing pelvic floor exercises, the client alternately contracts and relaxes anal sphincter and puborectal muscles 25 to 30 times 3 times a day for a brief time lasting about 3 or 4 seconds (McLane & McShane, 1992).

Biofeedback is used to help clients recognize rectal distention and provide a visual cue as to the effectiveness of pelvic muscle contraction. Abdominal massage stimulates peristalsis. The abdomen is massaged starting at the right iliac fossa, moving along the large colon and proceeding from the ascending to the transverse and descending colon (Emly, 1993)

Fecal Collection During Incontinence

In cases where bowel training is unsuccessful or when fecal incontinence is considered intractable, a drainable fecal collector may be used. The drainable fecal collector is similar to an ostomy appliance. It consists of a collecting pouch and a skin-protective barrier designed to adhere firmly to the perineum, anal cleft, and inner surfaces of the buttocks. If a formed stool collects in the pouch, the drainage outlet can be cut off with scissors, the stool emptied, and the end of the pouch resealed with a plastic clamp.

Just as diapers are considered appropriate management for the nontoilet-trained infant or child, protective pants, called incontinent briefs, are sometimes used for intractable fecal incontinence in the adult.

Stoma Management

Stoma management consists of a group of nursing interventions that may be necessary after fecal diversion surgery. Nursing responsibilities for clients with stomas include stoma assessment and management of feces collection via an ostomy appliance or through stoma irrigation. Many healthcare facilities have enterostomal therapists, nurses with specialized training, to assist clients and support other nurses in the care of clients with fecal diversions.

Stoma Assessment. After surgery, the stoma and abdominal incision may be covered with a sterile dressing. When removing the dressing or when changing appliances over the stoma, the nurse should assess the stoma for color and position. Ideally, the stoma should be a healthy pink; a dusky pink or bluish tint (cyanosis) suggests inadequate circulation to the stoma. The stoma must remain pink and healthy to function properly. The stomal mucosa must remain on the abdominal surface. If the stoma retracts, feces may potentially enter the abdominal cavity and cause peritonitis. The stoma should also be inspected for bleeding and drainage.

Fecal Collection. Clients with ileostomies or colostomies that continuously drain liquid stool will need an ostomy appliance (pouch or bag) over the stoma at all times. A large selection of ostomy appliances is commercially available; a common type of ostomy pouch is featured in Figure 42-10. Usually when the enterostomal therapist visits a new ostomy client, he or she inspects the condition of the stoma and discusses the methods for feces collection. The diameter of the stoma must be measured accurately for an appliance with the correctly sized opening to obtain proper fit. An opening that is too small may constrict the stoma and restrict circulation, whereas an opening that is too large will allow stool to leak onto the abdominal skin. The enzymatic juices contained in the liquid stool will cause maceration and eventual skin breakdown. The back surface of the ostomy appliance contains a sticky substance that will adhere to the abdominal skin. Also the appliance is usually taped for extra security.

The ostomy pouch should be emptied of fecal contents when it is about one-fourth to one-third full. If the pouch becomes too full, the weight of fecal contents will disrupt the seal, causing the stool to leak. The odor of the stool may be strong and offensive, especially to the client with a new stoma. In such cases, the nurse can spray a deodorant in the room before emptying the pouch. The bottom of the pouch has an opening secured by a clip, which is removed to empty the pouch into the toilet. The appliance can also be emptied into a bedpan or other collecting device laid on the bed if the client cannot get out of bed. As with all procedures in which the nurse handles feces or other bodily fluids, disposable gloves are worn.

Emptying an ostomy pouch is a clean, not a sterile, procedure. The pouch should be rinsed with clean, warm tap water after emptying. A large (60-mL) syringe works well for this purpose. Air is eliminated by compressing the pouch and reapplying the clip to close the pouch. Then the pouch is checked for leaks from the stomal area, and the condition of the stoma is assessed. If the ostomy appliance leaks fecal contents where it is

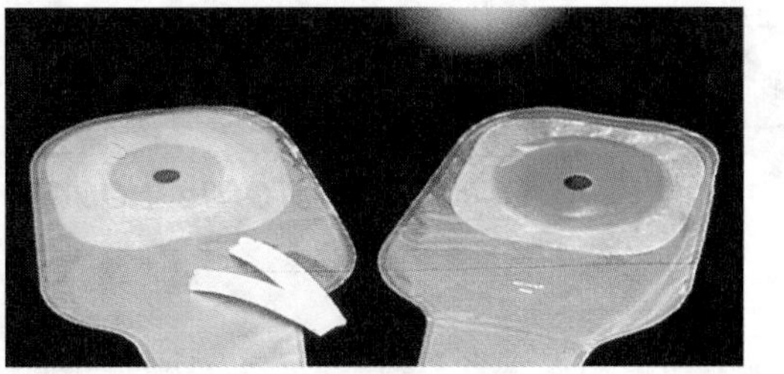

Figure 42-10 • *One-piece drainable ostomy pouch with clamp. (Courtesy of Hollister, Inc., Libertyville, Il.)*

attached to the skin, the entire bag needs to be removed and replaced. The nurse or client cleanses the abdominal skin surrounding the stoma, inspects the stoma's appearance, gently dries the abdominal skin, and applies a new ostomy pouch. The latter is described in Procedure 42-4.

If the ostomy is continuously draining fecal material, the pouch change will need to be quick and well planned. A sterile or clean gauze 4 × 4 pad may be placed temporarily over the stoma to collect a small amount of fecal contents as the skin is dried and the new pouch is secured. The gauze pad must be removed before clipping the bottom of the pouch shut.

Stomal Irrigation. Bowel training to achieve a predictable evacuation of stool from a sigmoid colostomy can be assisted by stomal irrigation, because the bowel can be trained to evacuate feces only at times of irrigation. Stomal irrigation is similar to giving a large-volume enema through the stomal opening instead of through the anus. More specialized equipment is necessary, but the principle of instilling fluid into the colon to cause distention and resultant elimination is the same. Figure 42-11 shows typical irrigation equipment, including irrigating sleeve with belt, and water container connected to irrigating catheter with cone and lubricant. Procedure 42-5 gives specific guidelines. The evac-

(text continues on page 1264)

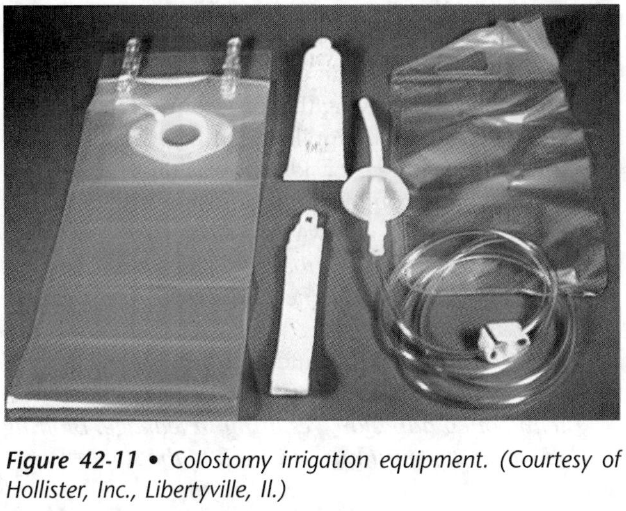

Figure 42-11 • *Colostomy irrigation equipment. (Courtesy of Hollister, Inc., Libertyville, Il.)*

Procedure 42-4
Applying a Fecal Ostomy Pouch

Purpose

1. Contains drainage and odors for the comfort of the client and allows accurate assessment of output.
2. Protects the peristomal skin from excoriation.
3. Provides visualization of the stoma and sutures during the postoperative period.

Assessment

- Observe color and amount of drainage from stoma.
- Assess existing pouch for leakage and note appearance of stoma and incision to determine need to change pouch. A pouch does not have to be changed if it is not leaking and if the skin barrier is intact.
- Inspect condition of peristomal skin for erythema, excoriation, ulceration, or fistulas before selecting type of skin barrier to apply.
- Note presence of skin folds, creases, scars, and abdominal softness or firmness before selecting pouch.

Equipment

A clean, drainable pouch and clamp, skin barrier, and disposable gloves.
Warm water, wash cloth and towel, mild soap.
Plastic disposal bag for old pouch.
Hypoallergenic paper tape.

Procedure

1. Provide privacy.
2. Don disposable gloves. The client may perform the procedure without gloves, as shown in the photos accompanying this procedure.
3. Gently remove old appliance. If disposable, discard. If reusable, set aside for washing.
4. Wash skin thoroughly around stoma with skin cleanser or soap and water.
   Rationale: Bacteria in the fecal secretions can cause infection in the incisional area and irritate the skin.
5. Rinse skin thoroughly and blot dry.
   Rationale: Soap residue or dampness can interfere with pouch adhesion, resulting in leakage. Blotting the area dry minimizes trauma to the stoma.

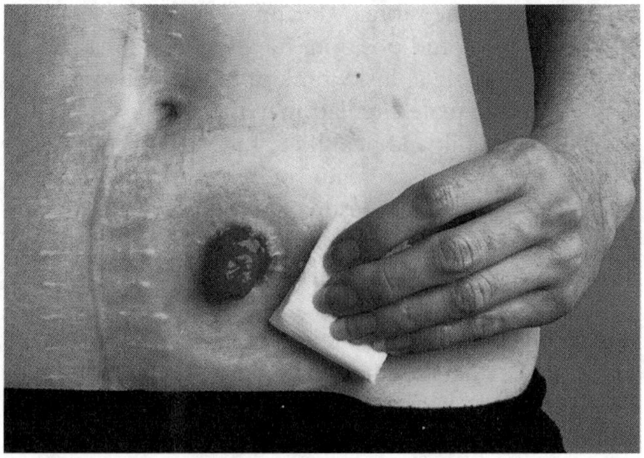

Step 5 • Wash area around stoma and pat dry.

6. Observe condition of peristomal skin, the stoma, and the sutures. Teach the client to make these observations daily.
   Rationale: Allows monitoring for complications. The stoma is at risk for necrosis during the first postoperative week, as evidenced by dark color and lack of bleeding. The peristomal skin is at risk for breakdown from irritating fecal secretions. Infection is more easily corrected if detected early.
7. Prepare clean pouch: measure stoma and trace circle ⅛-inch larger than stoma on the adhesive paper backing. Cut the stoma pattern.
   Rationale: Pattern cut slightly larger than barrier avoids risk of paper cuts to stoma and ensures a tight seal with the barrier.

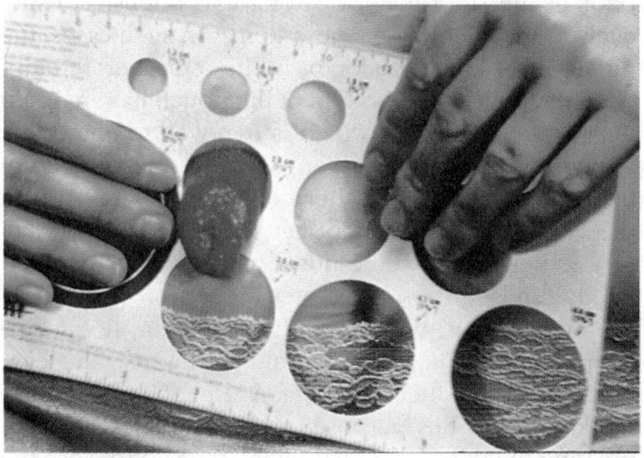

Step 7 • Measure stoma size to ensure proper fit. (Courtesy of Hollister, Inc., Libertyville, Il.)

8. Prepare skin barrier: measure stoma and cut hole in barrier the same size as the stoma. Be sure edges are rounded.
   Rationale: Close fit of barrier around stoma prevents fecal secretions from contacting and irritating the skin.

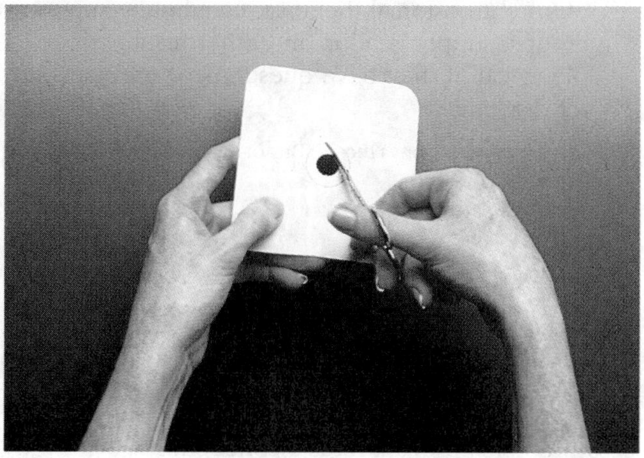

Step 8 • *Cut wafer to proper size.*

9. If stoma is located in an abdominal crease or the skin is irregular, use a paste barrier to fill the irregularity.
   Rationale: Minimizes leakage by providing a smooth surface for applying the skin barrier.
10. Apply protective skin barrier.
    a. Peel paper backing off wafer and center stoma in hole.

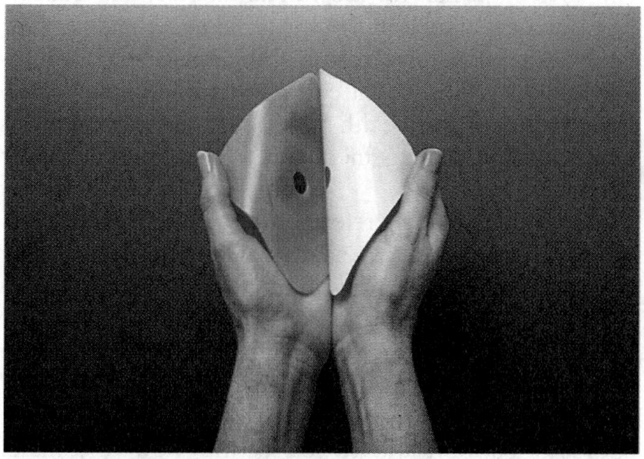

Step 10A • *Remove backing from skin barrier.*

    b. Place on abdomen, pressing lightly over all areas of the barrier to promote adhesion with skin surfaces.
    Rationale: A tight fit will prevent leaking and protect the skin underlying the appliance.

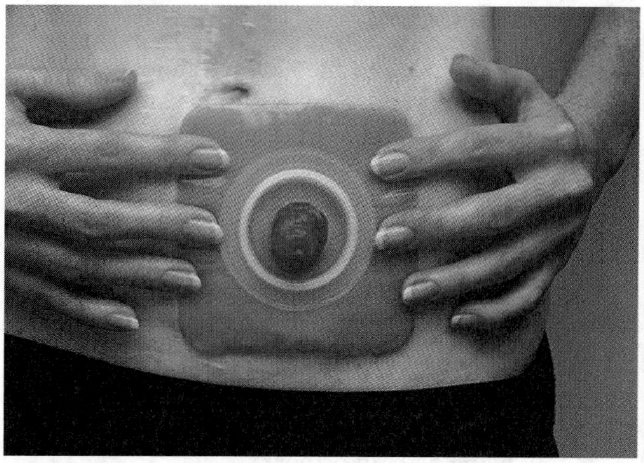

Step 10B • *Center hole over stoma and apply light pressure to ensure adherence to skin.*

11. Attach drainable pouch to skin barrier. Some equipment attaches by means of a plastic flange that snaps in place; other models adhere through self-adherent tape that is exposed after protective paper backing is removed. Tug gently or inspect for secure fit.
    Rationale: If pouch is not securely attached to protective barrier, leakage could occur, especially as weight from collected feces increases.

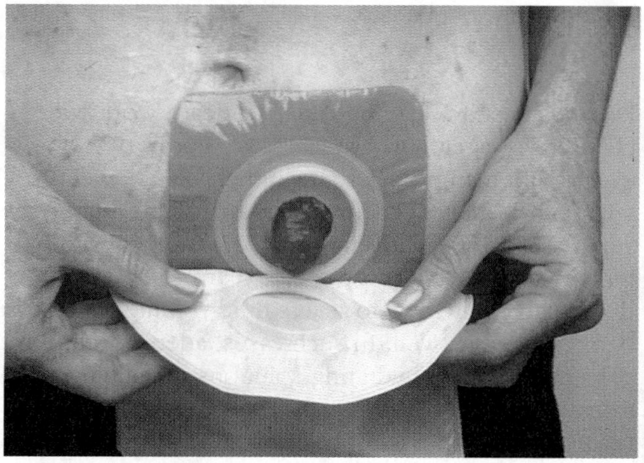

Step 11 • *Apply drainable pouch to skin barrier.*

12. Frame every edge of the faceplate with hypoallergenic tape to provide reinforcement. This is called "picture framing."
13. Fold over bottom edge of pouch and clamp.
14. Dispose of old appliance. Clean and store any reusable supplies.
15. Wash hands.
16. Document noted observations.

(continued)

Lifespan Considerations

- The very young and the elderly often are not able to perform their own ostomy care. Any client who is not able to change his or her pouch independently should have a caregiver instructed in this procedure.
- Postoperative necrosis of the stoma occurs more commonly in obese clients. The healthcare provider should be notified immediately if this is seen.
- New ostomy clients often experience the stages of grief as they try to adjust to their new body image. Good nurse–client communication is essential to help the client develop a positive attitude about living with an ostomy.
- Young children and infants adjust more readily to lifestyle changes from ostomies than do adolescents and adults.

Home-Care Modifications

- Client should have the name and phone number of an enterostomal therapist, community support groups, supply vendor, and other resource people to call if they have questions or problems after discharge.

Photos courtesy of ConvaTec, a Bristol-Myers Squibb Company, Princeton, NJ.

uation of the colon at predictable times allows the client a sense of control over his or her body and environment. Clients who have sigmoid ostomies and who have achieved reliable bowel training may not need to wear a fecal collection pouch at all times. Some can wear a specialized covering over the stoma between bowel evacuations. The covering protects the stoma from irritation by clothing.

Because a stomal irrigation is essentially an enema, it can be administered to relieve constipation or to cleanse the bowel before diagnostic procedures or tests.

Community-Based Care

Diarrhea is still a leading cause of death worldwide in children younger than 4 years of age (Porth, 1994); however, it and many other acute and chronic bowel problems can be managed in the home setting under the supervision of a healthcare provider. The viral and bacterial infections that cause severe diarrhea and that predispose the individual to severe fluid volume deficit can be controlled as well. In such cases, adequate fluid replacement with rehydrating solutions containing electrolytes is important. Fortunately, various world relief organizations provide rehydrating solutions to decrease mortality from diarrhea. In developed countries solutions such as Pedialyte or GatorAid can be purchased and used in the home during acute episodes of diarrhea.

To develop a teaching plan that meets the client's unique needs, the nurse needs to consider features of the client's home environment that could affect optimal bowel management. For example, does the client have adequate access to toilet facilities? If the client has to use a walker or wheelchair for mobility, will these devices fit through the bathroom doorway? Are there any steps that need to be negotiated to get to the bathroom? Is there someone available to assist the person to the bathroom or with special interventions such as enema administration? Sometimes the use of a bedside commode at home can help a person with mobility or access problems prevent fecal incontinence.

Are there any financial constraints? Does the client have health insurance, and does it cover the necessary medications or special equipment? If the assessment data disclose potential problems with financial or social support resources, a social worker should be consulted as soon as possible. The social worker is knowledgeable about the many community agencies available for assistance and can begin contacting the community agencies that will best meet the client's unique needs.

Clients or their families may need assistance and advice in managing specialized equipment and techniques. Clients with recent ostomies (ostomates) and clients at high risk for fecal incontinence, particularly, will need assistance in the home management of their bowel alterations. Enterostomal therapists are often responsible for most client education about ostomy care; however, the home health nurse must reinforce the concepts of stoma management and be available to answer questions.

The client can be referred to ostomy organizations within the community. Usually a member of an ostomy organization who also has an ostomy, and who has satisfactorily adjusted to the necessary lifestyle changes, can visit with the new ostomate. The first visit can be arranged before hospital discharge or can occur when the client is at home. The "old" ostomate can be a source of support and advice for the "new" ostomate.

Home-health nurses routinely visit clients in their homes to assess and assist their progress in managing healthcare problems. These nurses can be associated with the discharging hospital, but more likely are associated with a city or county health agency or with an independent home healthcare agency. The hospital-based nurse should be involved in the decision to make referrals to community agencies and in the communi-

Procedure 42-5
Irrigating a Colostomy

Purpose

1. Schedules the evacuation of stool from the colon if the colostomy is in the sigmoid or descending position.
2. Cleanses the colon before a procedure or surgery.

Assessment

- Assess permanence of colostomy and location along the large intestine.
- Complete abdominal assessment. Palpate abdomen for distention. Auscultate for bowel sounds.
- Assess current frequency and character of stool. Assess bowel habits before colostomy.
- Assess stoma for complications (ie, prolapsed stoma, peristomal hernia).
- Assess client's mental status, understanding of the procedure, and ability to learn the procedure.
- Assess client's manual dexterity and physical ability to tolerate sitting upright for long periods.

Equipment

Irrigating catheter with cone, irrigating sleeve with belt.
Water container, warm water.
Water-soluble lubricant, personal care items.
New appliance and skin barrier.
Clean, disposable gloves.

Procedure

1. Prepare client by explaining procedure.
2. Plan appropriate time for procedure. (Approximately 1 hour after a meal, when client will be uninterrupted for 45 minutes.)
   Rationale: Coordinate irrigation with normal time of duodenocolic reflex after meals.
3. Assist to comfortable position. Have ambulatory client sit on toilet. Have client on bed rest lie on side.
4. Close bathroom door or bed curtains.
   Rationale: Provides privacy and encourages client relaxation and cooperation.
5. Don gloves.
   Rationale: Prevents contact with body substances.
6. Remove and discard used pouch. Clean stoma and surrounding skin with warm water and soft cloth.
7. Apply irrigating sleeve. Place sleeve into toilet. If procedure is done in bed, place sleeve in bedpan.
8. Fill container with 500 to 1,000 mL warm water (105° to 110°F).
   Rationale: 500 to 1,000 mL water is needed to distend the colon sufficiently to trigger peristalsis. Cold water may cause cramping; hot water may damage the mucosa.
9. Connect cone to irrigating tube and run water through entire length of tubing.
   Rationale: Flushes air from the tubing.
10. Apply water-soluble lubricant to cone tip.
    Rationale: Prevents trauma to the stoma.
11. Insert cone firmly into stoma toward direction of bowel lumen. Stoma may have to be digitally inspected with a gloved, lubricated finger before irrigation to determine direction of bowel lumen.
    Rationale: The stoma is easily traumatized. Inserting cone toward bowel facilitates introduction of the irrigating solution.

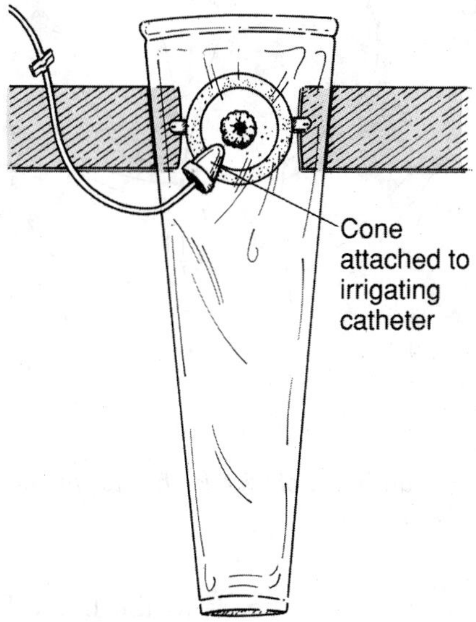

Step 11 • *Insert cone into stoma.*

12. Slowly begin flow of water into stoma, readjust position of cone gently with increasing firmness until there is no leakage around cone.
    Rationale: A tight seal is necessary to distend the bowel with water sufficiently to stimulate peristalsis and bowel evacuation.
13. Adjust height of water container to deliver 1,000 mL water in 10 to 15 minutes. The bottom of the container should be even with the client's shoulder if he or she is in sitting position. If client complains of cramps, slow or temporarily stop infusion without removing cone.

(continued)

Rationale: Too-rapid instillation can result in cramping, weakness, vertigo, or syncope.

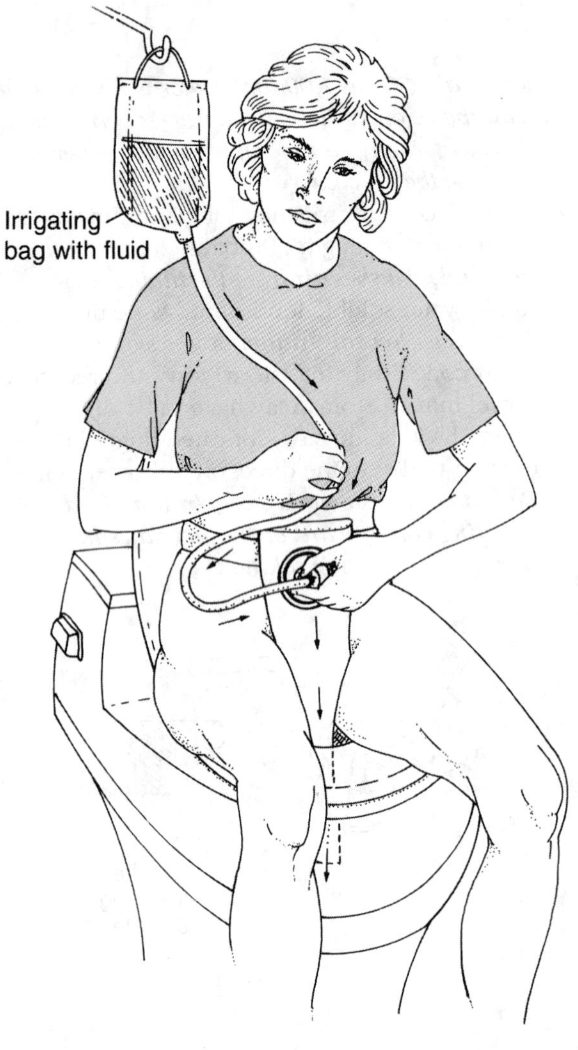

Step 13 • *Adjust height of irrigating bag to prevent cramping.*

14. Clamp tubing and remove cone, closing top of sleeve. Small gush of fluid should return into sleeve, followed by intermittent spurts. If return is slow, pour warm water over stoma, massage abdomen, or have client drink a warm liquid.
    Rationale: Once bowel is sufficiently distended to stimulate defecation, contraction of muscles with peristalsis should result in intermittent spurts of fluid and feces.
15. When most feces and water have been evacuated, dry and seal bottom of sleeve. Small amounts of fecal return may continue for another 20 to 45 minutes.
    Rationale: Wearing closed sleeve allows patient to ambulate while preventing leakage.
16. Remove and dispose of gloves, but reglove before beginning following steps.
17. When bowel evacuation has ceased, remove sleeve and set aside for cleansing.
18. Clean stoma and skin with warm water.
19. Apply skin barrier and new pouch.
20. Rinse sleeve with soap and water. Air dry.
    Rationale: Some sleeves are disposable, but most are intended for reuse.
21. Remove and dispose of gloves.

Lifespan Considerations

- Infants and children must have a healthcare provider's orders to determine when to irrigate and amount of irrigant.

Home-Care Modifications

- Bowel training can take weeks to months. It is easy for the client and family to grow discouraged with the process. Long-term support from a home health nursing service may be required.

cation of nursing care needs to the home healthcare agency. The home healthcare nurse evaluates the client's progress, assesses for signs and symptoms of any deteriorating condition requiring referral to the healthcare provider, or hospitalization, and continues to provide individualized client teaching and emotional support.

Evaluation

Expected outcomes are the evaluative tools used to measure the attainment of client goals. Nursing interventions are the management tools used to achieve the goals. Examples of outcomes are listed in the following. Note that some criteria are appropriate for more than one goal; it is important to identify specific outcome criteria that will most uniquely measure the attainment of the individual client's goal.

Goal

The client will demonstrate a normal pattern of bowel elimination without evidence of constipation, diarrhea, fecal incontinence, or abdominal distention.

Possible Outcome Criteria

- Client has a bowel movement within 24 hours and then every other day during rehabilitation.
- Client has a decrease in loose stools from four to five per day to one to two per day within 2 days.
- Client demonstrates a stool consistency changing from liquid to semisoft within 24 hours.
- Client has a bowel movement every morning after suppository and digital stimulation during rehabilitation.

Nursing Plan of Care
The Client With Constipation

Nursing Diagnosis
Constipation related to immobility manifested by straining and inability to pass stool for 3 days.

Client Goal
Client will demonstrate a normal pattern of bowel elimination.

Client Outcome Criteria
Client has a formed brown stool within 24 hours and every 1 to 2 days during rehabilitation.

Nursing Intervention	*Scientific Rationale*
1. Notify dietitian to increase high-fiber foods in client's meals.	1. High-fiber foods increase the amount of bulk in the lower gastrointestinal tract and result in softer, easier-to-eliminate stools.
2. Increase fluid intake to 2,000 mL/day.	2. A fluid intake of 2,000 mL in 24 hours is necessary to promote the formation of soft stools.
3. Assist client to ambulate (within medically prescribed guidelines) at least three times daily.	3. Increased physical activity promotes increased gastrointestinal motility.
4. Assist client to bedside commode or toilet. Fit commode or toilet with raised seat if needed.	4. The sitting position enlists gravity to promote bowel elimination. A raised seat may be necessary to increase client comfort in sitting.
5. Provide privacy but do not compromise client safety.	5. Many people require a degree of privacy during bowel elimination.
6. Inspect client's abdomen and auscultate for bowel sounds every shift.	6. Inspection and auscultation provide essential data about bowel elimination status.
7. Administer stool softeners and laxatives as necessary per bowel management program	7. Daily administration of stool softeners can prevent constipation for clients in high-risk groups. Laxatives can stimulate the evacuation of bowel contents on an as needed basis.
8. Record client's bowel movements in the client's record.	8. Documentation provides essential data about client's current bowel elimination pattern.

Client Goal
Client will participate in a program to maintain and promote an acceptable pattern of bowel elimination.

Client Outcome Criteria
After teaching session, client identifies at least three methods to be used to promote a normal bowel elimination pattern.

Nursing Intervention	*Scientific Rationale*
1. Teach client about methods to promote normal bowel elimination: high-fiber diet; increased fluid intake; increased physical activity; avoiding denial of defecation reflex; use of stool softeners; sitting position for bowel movements.	1. Increased knowledge leads to increased compliance and more successful outcomes.
2. Plan with client for daily routine after discharge with respect to bowel elimination. Discuss client's likes/dislikes/intolerances of high-fiber foods and types of fluids. Discuss plans for physical activity within medically prescribed restrictions.	2. Individualized plan promotes compliance and successful outcomes.

- Client has an absence of hardened stool in rectum on digital examination during each home visit.

Goal

The client will exhibit no preventable complications or adverse consequences from altered bowel elimination.

Possible Outcome Criteria

- The perianal skin remains intact throughout hospital stay.
- After a teaching session, the client verbalizes the importance of exhaling during defecation.
- Throughout hospitalization, the client washes hands after bowel movements.
- The client expresses satisfaction with success of bowel training program within 1 week.

Goal

The client will participate in a program to maintain and promote an acceptable pattern of bowel elimination.

Possible Outcome Criteria

- The client eliminates softly formed, brown stool every 1 to 2 days.
- The client identifies methods to increase dietary fiber at next appointment.
- The client requests assistance to toilet at scheduled time during the day.
- The client drinks 1,500 mL of fluid per day, as evidenced on chart each day.
- The client demonstrates correct ostomy bag application by discharge.

Evaluation includes assessing the client and comparing the client's current condition to the established outcome criteria as a measure of goal attainment. Continuation, modification, or termination of the nursing plan of care are implemented based on the systematic evaluation of client progress.

Key Concepts

- Defecation, the process of eliminating feces from the body, is initiated by reflexes in response to intestinal distention.
- Defecation is under voluntary neural control.
- Many lifestyle habits affect stool consistency and the pattern of bowel elimination.
- Physiologic alterations of the intestines can adversely affect bowel elimination.
- The manifestations of altered bowel elimination are constipation, fecal impaction, diarrhea, incontinence, flatulence, and abdominal distention.
- The characteristics of feces and bowel elimination patterns change during the lifespan.
- Altered bowel elimination can be a source of physiologic, psychological, and social distress.
- A focused nursing assessment of bowel elimination includes client history, inspection of stool characteristics, and physical examination of the abdomen and perirectal area.
- The nurse has collaborative responsibilities in laboratory analysis of the feces and other diagnostic procedures.
- The nurse can diagnose and collaboratively treat altered bowel elimination.
- Discharge planning considers the home environment and the unique learning needs of the client and family.
- Continuation, modification, and termination of nursing strategies are based on systematic evaluation of client response to therapy.

Critical Thinking Challenges

Return to the situation at the beginning of the chapter that describes the 76-year-old woman with metastatic bone cancer and a bowel elimination problem. Consider how you would respond to the following statements, applying the information you have gained in this chapter.

1. *Examine factors that could contribute to the client's constipation.*
2. *Reflect on how you feel when you must ask clients questions about elimination or perform procedures such as enemas.*
3. *Appraise possible factors that may have influenced the woman's refusal to have an enema.*
4. *Consider ethical and legal factors in determining how to respond to the client.*
5. *Critique the use of therapeutic communication in responding to this client.*

References

Anand, A., Bashey, B., Mir, T., & Glatt, A. E. (1994). Epidemiology, clinical manifestations, and outcome of *Clostridium difficile*-associated diarrhea. *Am J Gastroenterol, 89,* 519–523.

Carpenito, L. J. (1995). *Nursing diagnosis: Application to clinical practice* (6th ed.). Philadelphia: J. B. Lippincott.

Emly, M. (1993). Abdominal massage. *Nursing Times, 89* (1), 34–36.

Ganong, W. F. (1993). *Review of medical physiology* (15th ed.). Los Altos, CA: Lange Medical Publications.

Guyton, A. C. (1991). *Human physiology and mechanisms of disease* (5th ed.). Philadelphia: W. B. Saunders.

McLane, A. M., & McShane, R. E. (1992). Bowel management. In G. Bulechek & J. C. McCloskey (Eds.), *Nursing intervention: Essential nursing treatments* (2nd ed.). Philadelphia: W. B. Saunders.

North American Nursing Diagnosis Association (NANDA). (1994). *NANDA nursing diagnoses: Definitions and classification 1995–1996.* Philadelphia: Author.

Porth, C. M. (1994). *Pathophysiology: Concepts of altered health states.* Philadelphia: J. B. Lippincott.

Surratt, S., Ryan, A. B., Hallenbeck, P., et al. (1993). Trouble shooting a sump tube. *Am J Nurs, 93* (1), 42–47.

Wilson, R. E. (1993). Patient teaching for ileoanal reservoir. *Journal of Enterostomal Nursing, 20* (5), 199–203.

Bibliography

Doughty, D. B. (1994). What you need to know about inflammatory bowel disease. *Am J Nurs, 94* (7), 24–30.

Fischbach, F. (1996). *A manual of laboratory diagnostic tests* (5th ed.). Philadelphia: J. B. Lippincott.

Gurevich, I. (1994). Your patients don't need diarrhea, too! *RN, 57* (4), 52–55.

Hu, T., et al. (1990). The cost effectiveness of disposable versus reusable diapers: A controlled experiment in a nursing home. *Journal of Gerontological Nursing, 16* (2), 19–24, 36–37.

Kaltreider, D. L., et al. (1990). Can reminders curb incontinence? *Geriatric Nurse, 11* (1), 17–19.

Luz, R.A., et al. (1990). Ethnic differences in physiological responses associated with the Valsalva maneuver. *Res Nurs Health, 13 (1), 9–15.*

McConnell, E. A. (1990). Assessing abdominal pain in postoperative patient. *Nursing 90, 20* (3), 86–88.

McConnell, E. A. (1994). Managing nasoenteric decompression tube. *Nursing 94, 24* (3), 18.

Williams, S. G., et al. (1990). Constipation in the long-term facility. *Gastroenterological Nursing, 12,* 179–182.

Sleep and Rest

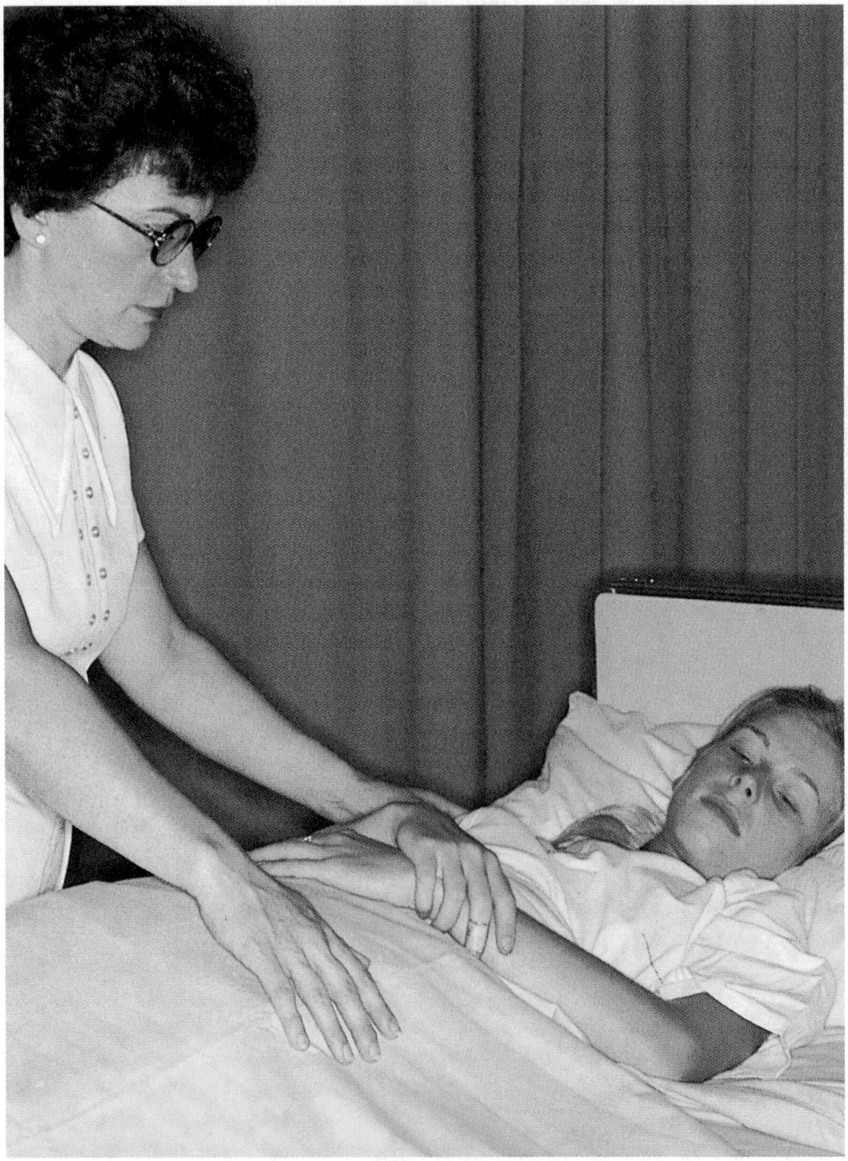

UNIT XI

Unit XI examines the sleep and rest area of human function. It is one that, for the most part, is taken for granted unless it becomes problematic. Yet adequate rest, sleep, and relaxation are essential for maintaining healthy function and critical for restoring and supporting health. Additionally, it is an area of function that presents client needs for which nurses intervene on a daily basis.

The single chapter in this unit considers the principles and concepts surrounding sleep and rest. Normal sleep and rest vary greatly from client to client. Additionally, many clients experience sleep pattern disturbances while in a healthcare facility. To help the client adequately meet his or her sleep and rest needs, it is essential for the nurse to carefully assess normal sleep patterns as well as nighttime routines. In addition, nurses need to assist clients in maintaining normal patterns of function whenever possible. Using a nursing process format, this chapter explores nursing interventions to promote health and function as well as the many independent nursing interventions for sleep pattern disturbances.

Meeting clients' sleep and rest needs is essential for normal, healthy function in all areas.

43
Sleep and Rest

Sleep and Rest

Key Terms

Chronotherapy
Circadian rhythms
Fatigue
Hormonal dysynchrony
Hypnotics
Hypopnea
Insomnia
Narcolepsy
Parasomnias
Rest
Sleep
Sleep apnea
Sleep latency
Sleepiness

Learning Objectives

Upon completion of this chapter, the student will be able to do the following:

- *Describe the five stages of sleep.*
- *Identify factors that affect sleep and rest.*
- *Describe normal patterns of sleep and rest throughout the lifespan.*
- *Conduct an assessment interview regarding usual sleep patterns, risk for disturbance, and problems.*
- *Develop a daily schedule with an individual, incorporating his or her unique needs and patterns for sleep and rest.*
- *Discuss interventions to promote rest and sleep.*
- *Develop a nursing care plan for a person with sleep pattern disturbance.*

43

Normal Sleep/Rest Function
Normal Physiologic Function
- Electrophysiologic Approach
- Neurotransmitter Balance
- Hormonal Approach

Characteristics of Normal Sleep/Rest
- Awareness of Need
- Restoration and Protection
- Psychological Function
- Circadian Rhythms

Normal Sleep/Rest Pattern
Factors Affecting Sleep and Rest
- Need
- Environmental Stimuli
- Nutrition and Metabolism
- Elimination Patterns
- Exercise and Thermoregulation
- Vigilance
- Lifestyle and Habits

Lifespan Considerations
Altered Sleep/Rest Function
Potential for Altered Sleep
- Distractions
- Illness
- Medications and Chemicals
- Mood States

Manifestations of Altered Sleep Function
- Insomnia
- Narcolepsy
- Sleep Apnea
- Sleep-Related (Nocturnal) Myoclonus
- Altered Sleep–Wake Patterns
- Parasomnias

Impact of Sleep Dysfunction on Activities of Daily Living
- Individual Considerations
- Family Considerations

Assessment
Subjective Data
- Functional Pattern Identification
- Risk Identification
- Dysfunction Identification

Objective Data
- Physical Assessment
- Diagnostic Tests

Nursing Diagnosis
Diagnostic Statement: Sleep Pattern Disturbance
- Definition
- Defining Characteristics
- Related Factors

Related Nursing Diagnoses
Outcome Identification and Planning
Implementation
Nursing Interventions to Promote Health and Sleep/Rest Function
- Environment Modification
- Provision of Intimacy and Security
- Sleep Rituals
- Managing Individual Sleep Needs

Nursing Interventions for Altered Function
- Rest
- Use of Medications
- Use of Consistent Routine

Community-Based Nursing
Evaluation
Key Concepts
Critical Thinking Challenges

You are the invited speaker to a high school biology class. When given a choice of health-related topics, the students chose sleep. The teacher has asked you, as a community health nurse, to lead a class discussion on this topic. He tells you that some of the questions they submitted are: "why do we sleep? how much is enough? why do parents think it is so important to get up early? I get so uptight when I can't get to sleep, is there anything I can do? How come I sometimes walk in my sleep?" The teacher also confides in you that he is worried about a couple of students: one who always seems to be dozing off in class even though he claims to get 9 to 10 hours of sleep most nights; and several high achievers who tend to stay up late at night after night studying, then come dragging into class the next morning. He asks you to include some discussion of different kinds of sleep problems like the ones he has observed among the students.

You have acquired a broad base of knowledge about the nursing profession and nursing care. In this chapter you will learn about sleep and rest as a normal function of the body, and how the nurse can promote adequate sleep. When you have completed the chapter, you will have expanded your knowledge about the necessity of sleep and rest in performing other functions of the body. The Critical Thinking Challenges at the end of the chapter will help you organize your thinking about sleep and rest

One-third of human life is spent sleeping. Periods of rest may account for another major portion of the lifespan. However, the significance and mechanisms of this function remain largely a mystery. Sleep has long been assumed to have a restorative function, and until recently was thought to be a passive state of decreased stimulation. It is now known that active physiologic processes are involved. Sleep and rest are important in health and illness, although the relationships are not clearly understood.

Normal Sleep/Rest Function

Sleep is a naturally occurring altered state of consciousness characterized by decreased awareness and responsiveness to stimuli. It is distinguished from abnormal states of consciousness by being readily reversible. With **rest**, awareness of the environment is maintained but motor or cognitive response is decreased. Whereas sleep is a total body system phenomenon, the state of rest may involve the total system or only a part. Thus, the person sunbathing on a beach during summer vacation may be experiencing a generalized state of rest associated with decreased mental and physical activity, whereas a person with an injured arm in a sling is resting that body part but otherwise may be relatively active mentally and physically.

Normal Physiologic Function

The physiology of sleep can be discussed in relation to three basic research approaches, each of which has provided building blocks for developing concepts relating to mechanisms and functions of sleep.

Electrophysiologic Approach

Polygraph recordings of electrophysiologic changes in brain waves (electroencephalogram; EEG), eye movements (electrooculogram; EOG), and muscles (electromyogram; EMG) show five sleep stages. The first four stages are classified as non-rapid eye movement (NREM) sleep, in contrast to the other stage, REM or paradoxical sleep, in which rapid eye movement is characteristic (Table 43-1).

Stage 1. Stage 1 is the transitional stage between drowsiness and sleep, indicated by a shift from alpha waves to low-voltage, fast theta waves on the EEG. Muscles relax, respirations become even, and pulse decreases. This stage usually lasts only a few minutes, and if awakened, the person may say he or she was not asleep.

Stage 2. Stage 2 is still a relatively light sleep from which the person is easily wakened. Bursts of sleep spindles appear on the EEG (Fig. 43-1). Rolling eye movements continue and snoring may occur.

Stages 3 and 4. Stages 3 and 4 constitute "deep" sleep, sometimes termed slow-wave sleep or delta sleep after characteristic waves seen on EEG (see Fig. 43-1). These two stages are differentiated primarily by the amount of delta waves, and are usually discussed together (Robinson, 1993). During slow-wave sleep the muscles are relaxed, but tone is maintained, respirations are even, and blood pressure, pulse, and temperature decrease, as do formation of urine and oxygen consumption of muscle. These are the stages during which snoring, sleepwalking (somnambulism), and bedwetting (enuresis) are most likely to occur. Stronger stimuli are required to awaken people during these stages. Dream content tends to be realistic and may be without plot; these are the dreams in which one drives to work or phones a friend and, when awakened, wonders if it was really done!

REM Sleep. REM sleep closely resembles wakefulness except for very low muscle tone, indicated by a reduction in amplitude of the EMG (Fig. 43-2). The rapid eye movements from which it receives its name are documented through EOG recording, but may also be noted by careful observation of tiny eye movements detectable through the closed lids. The brain waves as recorded on EEG are similar to those of the awake state (see Fig. 43-1). Blood pressure and pulse rate show wide variations, and may fluctuate rapidly. Respirations are irregular and oxygen consumption increases. Thermoregulation is lost. Vaginal secretions increase in women, and erections may occur in men. Dreams occurring during REM sleep tend to be vivid and implausible, often including a sense of being unable to move.

Sleep Rhythm. Electrophysiologic recordings of nocturnal sleep show a rhythmic pattern of approximately 90-minute cycles during which people progress in sequence through the sleep stages. The usual pattern is fairly rapid progression through stages 1 to 4 and then back through stages 3 and 2, from which REM is then entered (Fig. 43-3). During the early part of the night, periods of slow-wave sleep (stages 3 and 4) are longer. In contrast, the time spent in REM during the first cycle may be only 3 to 4 minutes, whereas toward morning it may be as much as 45 minutes, balanced with shorter periods of slow-wave sleep in which stage 4 may not

Table 43-1 • Characteristics of the Sleep Stages

Stage	Physiologic Correlates	Biochemical Correlates	EEG	Dreaming	Sleep Disorders	Subjective Awareness	Rebound
1 Light	Muscle relaxation Rolling eye movements Respiration even ↓ pulse		Gradual loss of alpha waves			Floating Idle images If awakened, may say was not asleep	No
2 Transition to REM	Eyes may appear to roll		Bursts of sleep spindles Sharp slow waves			Awakens easily May report was thinking or day-dreaming	No
3 Deep—slow-wave	Muscles very relaxed but tone maintained Respirations even	Growth hormone Serotonin	Delta (slow-wave) May show responses to outside stimuli but person not aware Spindles present	Less dramatic, more realistic May lack plot	Somnambulism Night terrors Enuresis	Requires stronger stimuli to waken	No
4 Deep—slow-wave	BP ↓, T ↓, P ↓ ↓ urine secretion ↓ O_2 consumption of muscle Snoring may occur						Yes, priority
REM	Lowest muscle tone Fasciculations ↑ BP, ↑ P. fluctuating respiration ↑ vaginal secretion ↑ cerebral blood flow ↑ O_2 consumption	Episodic cortisol and ACTH Catecholamine	Desynchronized Extremely active Similar to wakefulness	Content vivid Full-color Auditory Implausible settings Frequently involve paralytic component	Nightmares	Difficult to awaken except with significant stimuli	Yes

EEG, electroencephalogram; REM, rapid eye movement; ACTH, adrenocorticotropic hormone.

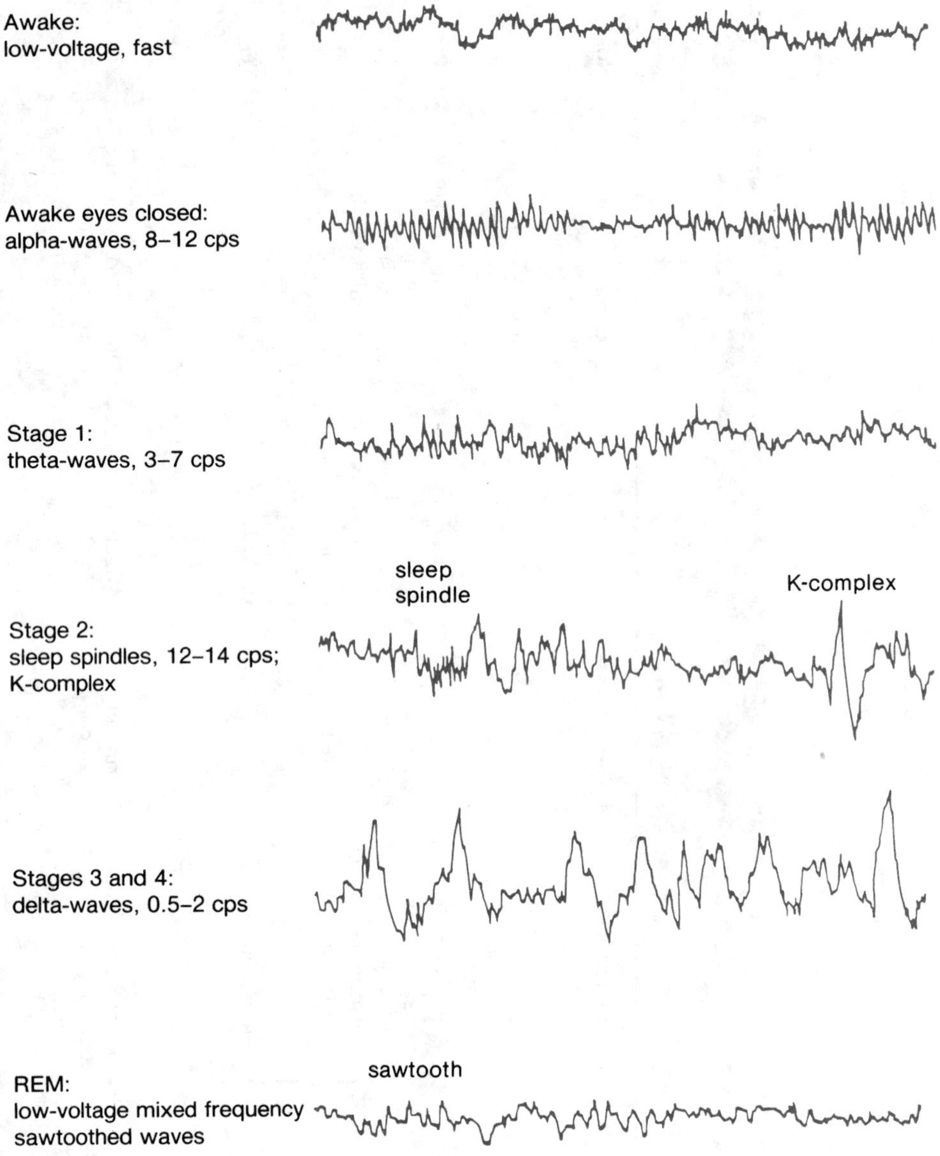

Figure 43-1 • Characteristic electroencephalogram wave forms by sleep stage. (Courtesy University of Washington School of Nursing, Sleep Laboratory.)

be present. If awakening occurs, the cycle begins again with stage 1. If the awakening was brief, the tendency is to reenter the type of cycle from which the person was aroused. Thus, an early morning awakening may be followed by return to one or more cycles in which a high percentage of REM is present. In situations where REM deficiency is suspected, it is therefore more helpful for the nurse to encourage clients to return to sleep immediately after an early awakening than to plan on napping in the afternoon.

Neurotransmitter Balance

Sleep is an active process involving the reticular activating system (RAS) and a dynamic interaction of neurotransmitters. The RAS consists of a network of interconnecting neurons in the medulla, pons, and midbrain, with projections to the spinal cord, hypothalamus, cerebellum, and cerebral cortex. It literally fills in the spaces in the brain stem among the major tracts, bringing in sensory messages and relaying motor ones. Thus, it is in a strategic location for stimulation from a wide variety of inputs. The RAS includes the ascending facilitatory area, which is intrinsically active, and a less well understood bulbar inhibitory area, which appears to be particularly involved in decreasing muscle tone during REM sleep (Porth, 1994).

As with other parts of the nervous system, communication between neurons primarily involves the release of specific neurotransmitters from axon terminals and their attachment to specific receptors on other cells. Serotonin is a major neurotransmitter associated with sleep. Produced in the Raphe nuclei in the brain stem, this neurotransmitter is derived from its precursor, tryptophan, a naturally occurring amino acid. Serotonin is thought to decrease the activity of the RAS, thereby in-

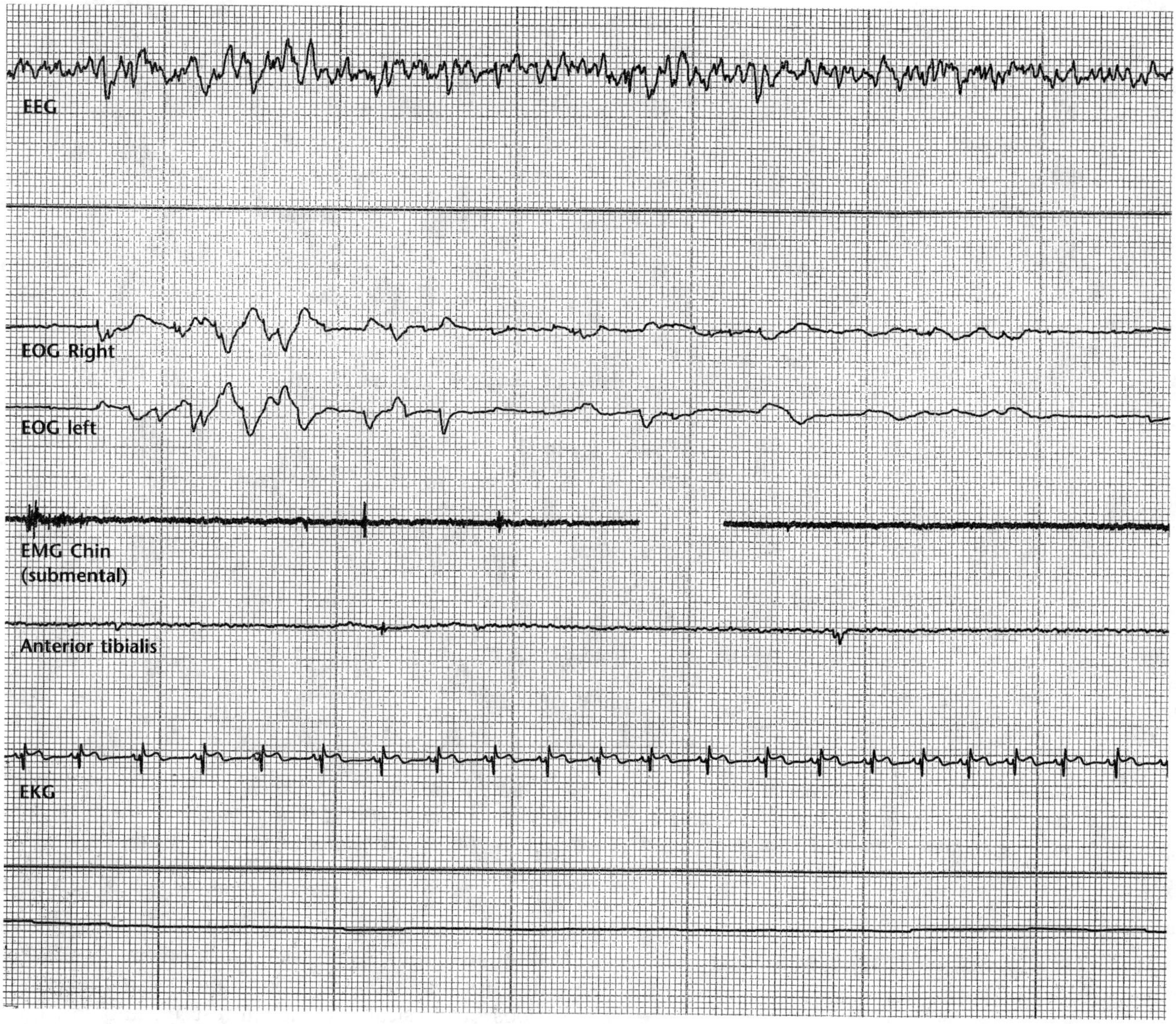

Figure 43-2 • *REM sleep on polygraph recording. Note the rapid, low-amplitude waves on the EEG, eye movements on EOG, and minimal muscle activity on EMG. (Courtesy of Alberta Lung Association Sleep Center, Calgary, Alberta, Canada.)*

ducing and sustaining sleep. Another neurotransmitter, the catecholamine norepinephrine from the locus ceruleus (also in the brain stem), appears to be required for REM sleep. The role of acetylcholine and other neurotransmitters is less well understood (Robinson, 1993).

Hormonal Approach

Sleep–wake patterns appear to be affected by and to affect certain hormone levels. Melatonin from the pineal gland is secreted in enormous quantities during sleep. Its apparent rhythm-setting function seems to be closely related to darkness and light. It takes 2 weeks of altered sleep time before secretion of melatonin again matches with the sleep period. Adrenocorticotropic hormone secretion from the pituitary is high during the early part of the sleep period, and levels of cortisol, its target hormone from the adrenal cortex, rise toward the end of the nocturnal sleep period. This pattern also remains stable in relation to clock time in spite of variations in sleep time (eg, shift work), unless these changes are sustained for up to 2 weeks.

Growth hormone and prolactin levels are closely tied to actual sleep time, changing immediately in relation to variations in the sleep period. Secretion of both hormones increases early in the sleep period.

The significance of this **hormonal dysynchrony**, in which hormonal levels adjust at different rates to alterations in the timing of the sleep period, is not clearly understood but is an important research area, particularly in relation to shift work and jet travel.

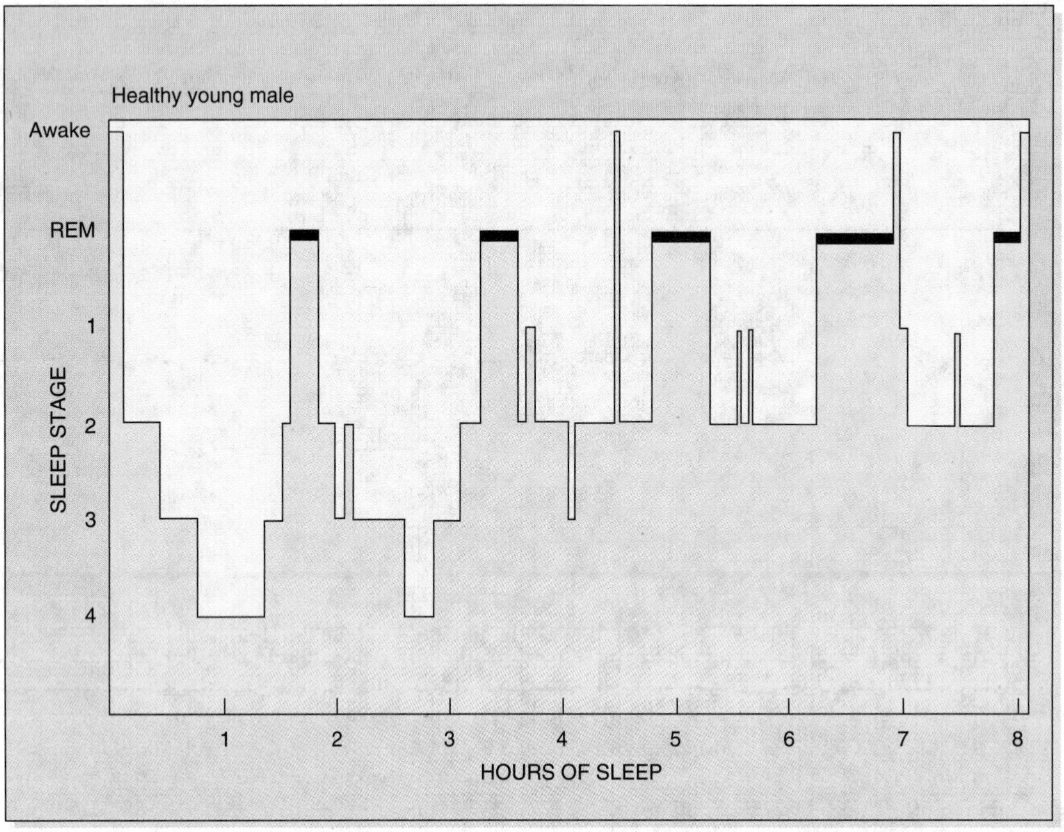

Figure 43-3 • *Typical sequence of sleep stages in a young, healthy adult man. Progression occurs through a sequence of 1-2-3-4-3-2 and into REM. Note increased amount of REM sleep and absence of stage 4 toward end of sleep period. (Courtesy University of Washington School of Nursing, Sleep Laboratory.)*

Characteristics of Normal Sleep/Rest

Awareness of Need

Awareness of the need for sleep and rest is most commonly associated with the states of sleepiness and fatigue. These states often overlap. **Sleepiness** refers to an urge of varying intensity to go to sleep. It may occur in response to too little or too much sleep, or lack of adequate sensory stimulation. **Fatigue** is a subjective state of weariness in which physical activity is accompanied by intense or rapid tiring. It is a common human response to illness, suggesting the need to conserve energy through rest and sleep.

Restoration and Protection

Sleep and rest are believed to have restorative and protective functions (Hodgson, 1991). Oswald (1987), the leading proponent of the restorative theory, has provided research evidence that shifts in the hormonal balance facilitate physical restoration through the processes of anabolism (synthesis of cell constituents) during sleep. Horne (1988), on the other hand, suggests that the main purpose of sleep may be energy conservation for parts of the body other than the brain. Periods of physical and mental rest are known to reduce metabolic rate and the sense of fatigue.

Psychological Function

Psychological functions of sleep are thought to include:

- Sorting and discarding of neurophysiologic data. Much of short-term memory is filled with inconsequential detail that is sifted through and discarded. A person can usually remember what was eaten for breakfast that day or how long the bus took to come, but a month later those data will probably be beyond recall (unless something special happened that day).
- Character reinforcement and adaptation. The REM stage of sleep in particular appears to be important for mental and emotional stability. Through REM dreaming, a reprocessing of knowledge and memories is thought to occur. An increased need for REM sleep has been found in people experiencing stress, worry, or new learning situations (Hodgson, 1991).

Circadian Rhythms

Biologic rhythms that follow a cycle of about 24 hours are termed **circadian rhythms** from the Latin words *circa* (about) and *dies* (day) (Porth, 1994). The sleep–wake cycle is an example, and is closely linked with other circadian rhythms such as body temperature. While a person sleeps, core body temperature drops, often reaching the 24-hour low around 4:00 AM. When the sleep period shifts, for instance when the person moves to another time zone, temperature fluctuations also shift to match the new sleeping patterns after a week or so. The superchiasmatic nucleus, located above the optic chiasm in the anterior hypothalamus, has been found to provide the "clock" for most circadian rhythms, including the sleep-wake cycle (Harrington, et al., 1994). It receives direct input from the retina regarding environmental cues as to darkness and light.

In situations where environmental cues to time are largely removed, circadian rhythms are maintained, but duration may extend to 25 or more hours and may become less synchronized. Experimental conditions typically involve controlled artificial light and removal of all indicators of time. Nurses are sometimes involved with people who have established life patterns in which environmental cues to time are decreased to the point at which erratic sleep and temperature cycles develop (Robinson, 1993). People living alone without regular occupational or social contact are at risk. Although rare, some people have natural circadian rhythms extending to 50 hours or more (Wirz-Justice & Pringle, 1987).

Normal Sleep/Rest Pattern

The well-rested person is mentally alert, energetic, and spontaneous. Daytime activity, even of a monotonous nature, is maintained with a minimum of drowsiness.

The range of "normal" sleep duration is great. Short sleepers, that is, those who sleep for less than 6 hours in 24, tend to be efficient, hardworking people. Winston Churchill required little nighttime sleep, relying instead on his ability to take brief but renewing naps. Long sleepers, that is, those who sleep for more than 9 hours in 24, have a higher percentage of REM sleep, and there is some suggestion that as a group they are more creative. Albert Einstein was a long sleeper.

The range of normality with respect to sleep patterns is also broad. Generally, most people require 10 to 30 minutes to fall asleep; this period of time required to fall asleep is called **sleep latency**. A regular sleep latency of less than 5 minutes suggests excessive sleepiness. Sleep latency of longer than 30 minutes may be accompanied by some sense of frustration with the time taken to get to sleep.

Changes of position during sleep typically occur 20 to 40 times during the night in all but the elderly (De Koninck, et al., 1992). For people with impaired physical mobility, the normally unconscious act of changing positions during sleep may require awakening, conscious planning and effort, or the assistance of the bed partner or care provider. The institutional norm of turning clients every 2 hours scarcely meets the physiologic norm of natural position changes during sleep. Such simple interventions as the use of satin sheets have been found to help people with impaired physical mobility turn more easily.

One to two awakenings per night are common for young adults; the frequency and duration of awakenings tends to increase with age. The final awakening is often spontaneous, even in North American society, where alarm clocks symbolize the precision of occupational and educational schedules. The well-rested person generally awakens with a sense of refreshment and energy for the day.

Daytime naps and rest periods are infrequent among North American adults and older children, except as associated with illness, pregnancy, or "catching up" on a day off. In warmer climates, however, the midday rest period is a cultural expectation. Rest breaks in the more industrialized nations have tended to be associated with the use of stimulants such as the caffeine in coffee or the nicotine in cigarettes. The value of mini-rests in the form of stretching exercises, focusing thoughts or vision on a pleasant scene away from the work station, or going for a walk have been recognized more recently.

Factors Affecting Sleep and Rest

Need

The need for sleep and rest fluctuates according to developmental, individual, and situational variables. Developmental variables are discussed in the section on Lifespan Considerations. Individual variations occur in relation to total sleep need and in relation to preferred schedule. Numerous situational variables are superimposed on developmental considerations, need, and individual variables affecting sleep and rest patterns (Shaver & Giblin, 1989).

It has been hypothesized that humans may require less sleep than they have habitually. Horne (1988) suggests that there are two forms of sleepiness: "*core sleepiness*, associated with the loss of core sleep and reflected in impaired cerebral functioning, and *optional sleepiness*, associated with the loss of optional sleep and mostly affecting motivation" (p. 312). This concept of lower sleep need is supported by studies that have shown that students in the latter part of the 20th century average 1.5 hours less sleep per day than their counterparts in 1910 (Hauri, 1982). The unresolved question is whether this represents less need for sleep or a chronic state of sleep deprivation, or lack of sleep.

More recently, it has been hypothesized that much of the population in industrialized nations may be chronically sleep deprived.

It is important that people attune themselves to their own specific patterns rather than aiming for the mythical standard of 8 hours a night. As a general rule, the person who falls asleep fairly quickly on going to bed, awakens feeling refreshed, and functions with minimal daytime sleepiness can be assumed to be getting adequate sleep.

Individual variations also occur as to the preferred portion of the 24-hour period used for sleeping. Morning people are those who awaken early and easily, feel at their best in the early part of the day, and who prefer to retire early in the evening. Evening people find they function best later in the day, and are often wide awake and looking for activity late in the evening. Adjustments to variations in the timing of the sleep period, as occur with shift work, seem to be more readily tolerated by evening people (Monk, 1994).

Environmental Stimuli

Reduction of environmental stimuli, particularly light and noise, facilitates sleep. People vary in their sensitivity to different stimuli, and appear to vary in the intensity and degree of fluctuation of sensory input required. Some people seem to require a slight elevation of sensory input, sleeping better when surrounded by low-level noise such as a radio playing, after drinking coffee, or after exercising.

Awakening or a lightening of sleep pattern often occurs when the bed partner changes position or snores. Presence of the habitual partner may provide a sense of security; absence of the habitual partner may be disturbing. As discussed in the next section, the nature, quality, and present state of the relationship may be factors that contribute to the effect of the presence or absence of the partner. For those who habitually sleep alone, the presence of another person may be disturbing.

Nutrition and Metabolism

Hunger disturbs the sleep of some people, whereas others have difficulty sleeping after a large meal. Ingestion of L-tryptophan, a precursor of serotonin found in protein foods such as milk, beef, eggs, wheat flour, and corn, has been found to decrease sleep latency and increase stage 4 sleep (Robinson, 1993). Sleep patterns tend to be disturbed during periods of either rapid weight loss or gain.

Elimination Patterns

The need to void is one of the most frequent internal stimuli to disturb sleep among the general population. Children can be assisted in establishing the habit of voiding as part of bedtime preparations. Limiting fluid intake after supper may decrease this nocturnal stimuli.

Exercise and Thermoregulation

Habitual exercise contributes to deeper and longer sleep. In physically fit people, light-intensity exercise seems to decrease sleep latency and intensive exercise increases the proportion of slow-wave sleep (Horne & Staff, 1983). The basis for increased slow-wave sleep after vigorous exercise may be related to an increase in core body temperature. Passive heating, as in a sauna or tub of warm water, especially in the evening, has been shown to produce effects similar to those of vigorous exercise on the amount of slow-wave sleep (Bunnell, et al., 1988). These findings suggest a promising area for nursing research regarding the value of a warm bath for enhancing the quality of sleep. The relationships between exercise and sleep are more complex than they may first appear, however. Contrary to what might be expected from the previous discussion, bed rest also increases slow-wave sleep by mechanisms not understood.

Vigilance

Another factor affecting sleep is the perceived need to maintain vigilance. Parents and others in protective roles seem able to establish a variable noise threshold in which they may respond to the faintest sound of a toddler changing position in the next room, and yet sleep through a thunderstorm. Hospital clients, such as those recently disconnected from cardiac monitoring equipment, may deliberately prevent themselves from entering the deeper stages of sleep for fear of succumbing to a complication that might go unnoticed by nursing staff.

Lifestyle and Habits

Certain bedtime rituals become such a habitual part of preparation for sleep that to interfere with them is to interfere with sleep itself. Some rituals, such as a warm bath or a snack, may have a physiologic basis. The effectiveness of bedtime habits is also linked with decreasing arousal. Participation in a repetitive routine such as putting out the dog, winding the clock, and changing into night attire become associated with the expectation of sleep.

Lifestyle patterns influencing the sleep-wake schedule, such as time of rising, are closely linked with societal and occupational expectations. A regular time of rising is one of the most effective means of improving sleep quality and synchronizing circadian rhythms with clock time. Toddlers who are having difficulty settling into a bedtime routine can be helped by maintaining an early and consistent rising time and being allowed to stay up in the evening until they are sleepy enough to settle with quieting activities. Adults who have difficulty getting to sleep should also be encouraged to maintain a consistent rising time, going to bed later if necessary, rather than laying awake for long periods.

Lifespan Considerations

Developmental variations in sleep patterns are evident. Circadian rhythms develop in the first few months of life, are well established through childhood and adulthood but gradually decrease with advancing age. The polyphasic two-to-one ratio of sleep to wakefulness characteristic of infants gradually shifts to the biphasic one-to-two ratio of adulthood.

Newborn and Infant

Two major sleep states can be observed in newborns. Quiet sleep is characterized by closed eyes, regular respirations, and absence of eye and body movements. Active sleep is manifested by eye movements observable through the closed lids, other body movements, and irregular respirations. Of the three waking states—quiet awake, active awake, and crying—quiet awake would seem to correspond to a state of rest in adults. Newborns sleep an average of 16 to 17 hours per day, divided into about seven sleep periods distributed fairly evenly day and night (Fig. 43-4).

Infants' sleep patterns differ from those of adults in that the sleep cycle is shorter (50–60 minutes), the proportion of active or REM sleep is higher (approximately 50%), and the initial stage is active rather than NREM (Keefe, 1987). Between 1 and 2 months of age, NREM sleep becomes differentiated into stages 1 to 4 (Robinson, 1993).

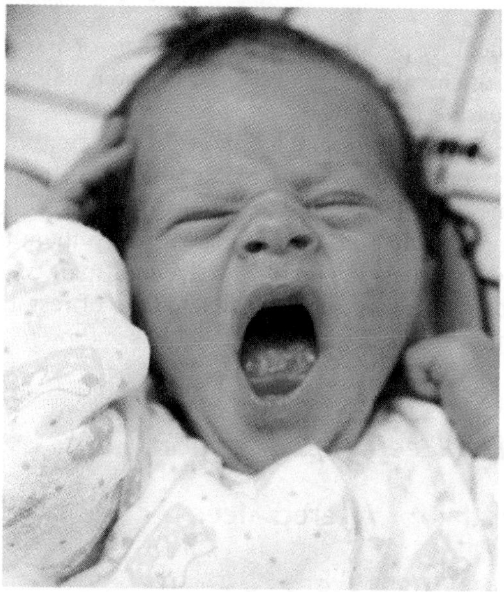

Figure 43-4 • *Infants establish sleep–wake cycles that fit their environment.*

One of the infant's major adaptive tasks is to establish sleep-wake patterns compatible with the environment. Most infants are sleeping through the night by 3 months, but nocturnal awakenings continue to be frequent during the latter half of the first year (Trilling, 1989).

The number of sleep periods continue to drop from four to five per 24-hour day at 3 months of age to one nighttime period and two naps at 6 months. Total sleep time averages 14 to 15 hours, but there is wide variability among infants (Anders, 1994).

Toddler and Preschooler

By 1 year of age, napping has usually been reduced to once or twice a day. Some sleep disturbance is observed in almost all children between 1 and 2.5 years of age; it is thought to be related to the rapidly developing mental abilities of the child. Getting the child to fall asleep is the most frequently reported problem, but frequent awakenings and occasional night terrors may also occur (Gates, et al., 1989). Total sleep time drops from an average of 13 to 14 hours at age 2 to 12 hours by the end of the fifth year, mainly because of the elimination of the afternoon nap. REM sleep drops to about 30%, which is still higher than for adults. The percentage of slow-wave sleep is also higher through childhood, whereas the amount of stage 1 sleep is less.

Child and Adolescent

Sleep and rest needs fluctuate somewhat for school-age children and adolescents in relation to growth spurts and activity patterns. REM content gradually drops to about 20% at puberty. Adolescents actually require slightly more rest than they did before puberty. The cardiovascular and respiratory systems mature less rapidly than other systems, contributing to fatigue from inadequate oxygenation.

Adult and Older Adult

Adults vary widely in the number of hours of sleep that they require and in their preferred portion of the 24-hour period for sleeping. By middle age, the frequency of nocturnal awakenings tends to increase, and the satisfaction with the quality of sleep tends to decrease. Situational variables, such as job-related stress, parenting responsibilities, and illness probably account for much of the variation seen among people in early to middle adulthood (Verran, et al., 1988).

As people age, the amount of stage 4 sleep decreases significantly (Fig. 43-5). The intranight distribution of REM sleep becomes more even and the per-

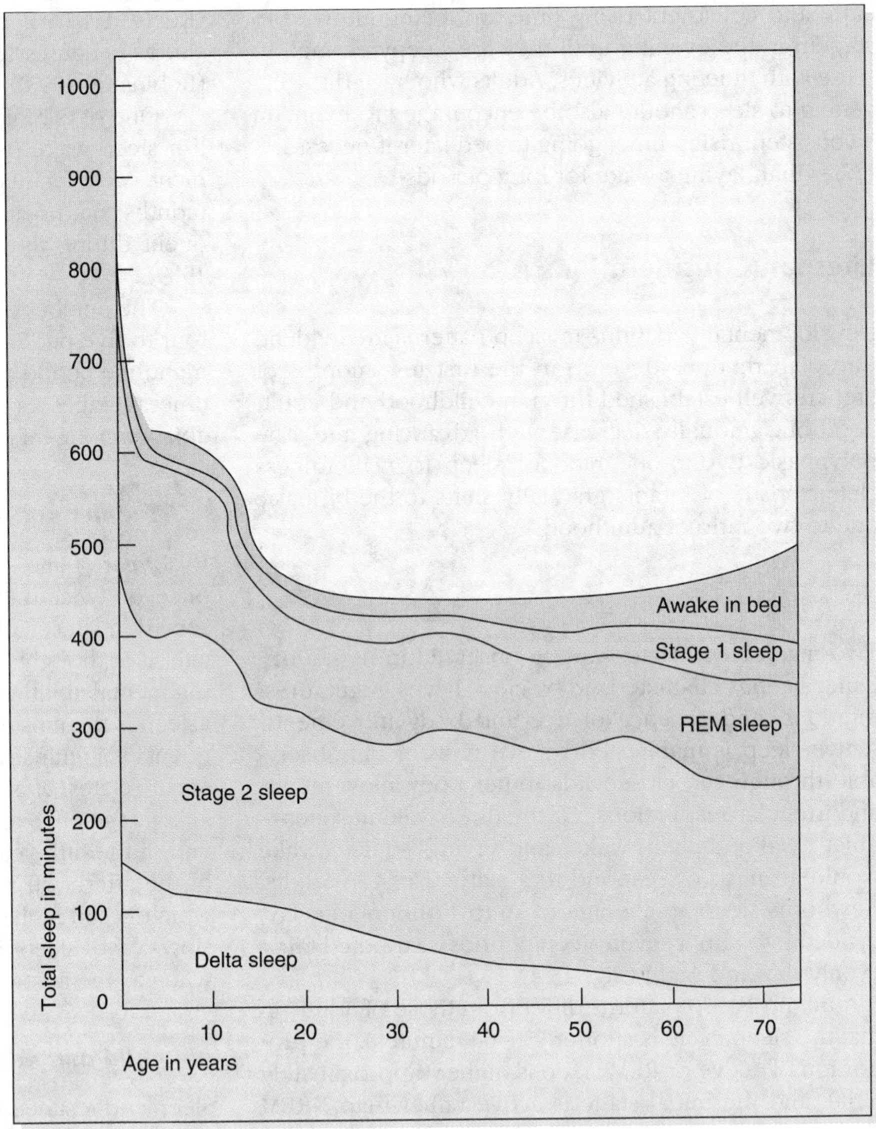

Figure 43-5 • *Schematic representation of the changes in sleep stages by age. Note that elderly spend more time in bed than adults but have less deep sleep. (Adapted with permission from Williams, R.L., Karacen, I., & Hursch, C.J. (1994).* Electroencephalography (EEG) of human sleep: Clinical applications. *New York: Wiley)*

centage decreases. Older men tend to have decreased stage 3 sleep as well and have more difficulty maintaining sleep toward the end of the sleep period (Robinson, 1993). Circadian rhythms become less prominent with increasing age. Sleeping patterns may become polyphasic, with a shorter nocturnal period plus daytime naps. Core body temperature may no longer show the usual circadian changes. If external cues to time also decrease, as with institutionalization, the cognitively impaired elderly may develop sundowner's syndrome, characterized by nocturnal wakefulness and agitation. It is thought that this may be related to a drop in stimulation level to the point at which the cognitively compromised client can no longer maintain contact with reality.

Time spent napping and time in bed increase with advancing age (Robinson, 1993). Daytime napping does not appear to interfere with nighttime sleep for these older adults. Total time in bed gradually increases because of napping, longer sleep latency, increases in the number and length of awakenings, and general fatigue. Even healthy people older than 85 years of age show a significant increase in total sleep time and usually change to an earlier bedtime.

Older adults frequently express concern about taking longer to fall asleep, awakening more frequently, daytime sleepiness, and needing longer to adjust to changes in schedule. The nurse can help them to recognize that these changes are a natural part of aging, and to establish or maintain a schedule of rest and activity that meets their individual needs and preferences.

Altered Sleep/Rest Function

Potential for Altered Sleep

Distractions

Noise. People chronically exposed to high noise levels have less slow-wave and REM sleep with more stage 1 and awakenings than their counterparts who live in quieter neighborhoods (Roehrs, et al., 1994). Women and older people are more likely to be awakened by noise. As might be expected, the awakening threshold varies with the stage of sleep, with stage 1 being the most vulnerable.

Noise levels recorded in a critical care unit between 10:15 PM and 3:00 AM ranged from 72 to 75 decibels, the equivalent of a noisy office (Snyder-Halpern, 1985). In subsequent testing with volunteer subjects, critical care unit noise from mechanical sources (eg, suction machines, alarms) was even more disturbing than sounds from staff and clients. Nurses can modify the noise level in hospital environments by keeping equipment noise to a minimum, avoiding unnecessary conversation, and closing doors when possible. The use of ear plugs can be suggested in home environments where noises in the same room (eg, partner snoring) or outside (eg, traffic) are disturbing sleep.

Light. Control of light is usually adequate in home environments. This is not true for shift workers and young children during summer evenings in the northern latitudes. In acute care environments, control of light becomes a nursing responsibility often overlooked in the complexity of meeting other client needs.

Temperature. The benefits of cool versus moderate sleeping room temperatures are matters of personal preference; however, it has been shown that excessive warmth or cold increases restlessness (Roehrs, et al., 1994). During REM sleep, thermoregulation is impaired and shivering does not occur.

Environment. Generally, in a new environment sleep latency is increased; total sleep time and proportion of REM are decreased. Those who have chronic difficulties sleeping may associate certain objects in the environment, such as their bed, with poor sleep. These people report sleeping better away from home. In the hospital environment, certain objects in the room may be associated with pain. If a sleeping room doubles as a work area, the room may become associated with work rather than sleep. Objects of play in the child's room may disturb the child's sleep and rest.

Caregiving. The frequent awakenings associated with parenting may contribute to chronic sleep pattern disturbance. It is not unusual to hear mothers speak of never getting more than an hour's sleep at a time over a period of 1 or more weeks when caring for a sick child or a colicky baby. The associated REM deprivation may make coping even more difficult. Likewise, caregivers of people with advanced disease in the home may become chronically sleep deprived (Hodgson, 1991).

Caregivers are among the most frequent disturbers of sleep in institutional settings. In critical care environments, clients are awakened frequently for various assessments and treatments. Where possible, these activities should be clustered to provide periods of 1.5 to 2 hours of undisturbed sleep time. The nurse may have to assume a client advocacy role in coordinating interruptions from the many disciplines involved in client care.

Disruptions in Relationships. Disruptions in primary relationships are commonly associated with sleep pattern disturbance. Bereaved people often report the night period as their most difficult. Children who are away from home are frequently homesick at bedtime. Marital discord may contribute to sleep disturbance in children as well as in the involved adults. Security needs are heightened at bedtime for people of all ages.

Shift Work. Frequent changes in the sleep-wake schedule, such as occur with shift work, contribute to shorter and more fragmented sleep and a high incidence of fatigue (Roehrs, et al., 1994). The dysynchrony of trying to sleep at times when the body's circadian rhythm is set for wakefulness is thought to be the main reason for the disturbed sleep. Fatigue is secondary to the disturbed sleep. Nurses are among the 20% of the population in industrialized countries involved in shift work, as are many of the people for whom they care (Monk, 1994). Research on the effectiveness of various shift schedules has been inconclusive, suggesting the need for further investigation.

Illness

During acute and chronic illness, clients are particularly vulnerable to loss of stage 3 sleep. Conditions involving pain have long been known to disturb sleep. Current research indicates that body system disturbances also have an effect on sleep, and vice versa. Ventilatory responses to hypoxia and hypercapnia decrease during REM sleep. Although diaphragmatic function is essentially unchanged during REM sleep, the intercostals and other accessory muscles lose substantial activity (Johnson & Remmers, 1984). Thus, the pattern of frequent arousals seen in people with chronic obstructive lung disease may be the body's adaptation to maintain adequate oxygenation. Hypnotics should be used cautiously, if at all, in people experiencing ineffective breathing patterns or impaired gas exchange. Often, low doses of oxygen are required by these clients at night.

The pain and discomfort of angina or dyspnea occurring during the night can disturb sleep. Circadian variations in blood pressure, heart rate, and platelet aggregation around the time of wakening may be associated with the observed frequency of myocardial infarction and stroke from cerebral thrombus formation that occur in the latter part of the nighttime sleep period or within the first hours of wakening (George, 1994).

People with a history of seizure activity risk increased occurrence of seizures after sleep deprivation or with variable sleep habits. Sleep may be disturbed by seizure activity; some epileptic clients have seizures only at night. The recording of brain waves during sleep is an important method for diagnosing the site of abnormal electrical activity.

Hormonal changes contribute to a variety of sleep pattern disturbances. Hyperthyroidism causes fragmented short sleep with an excess of the slow-wave stages, whereas hypothyroidism seems to cause excessive sleepiness with a lack of slow-wave sleep. The tremendous fatigue often reported after hysterectomy may be related to the loss of estrogen. Administration of estrogen to postmenopausal women has been shown to decrease sleep latency (Driver & Taylor, 1993). In contrast, progesterone enhances ventilatory responses.

Skin conditions such as eczema have been shown to contribute to sleep onset delay, frequent awakenings, and reduction of stages 3, 4, and REM during the first part of the night. The itching and discomfort associated with hives, insect bites, and other skin lesions also disturb sleep.

Hospitalization as a result of illness adds a number of additional factors that may disturb sleep. In a survey of 143 adult clients on medical-surgical units, "difficulty finding a comfortable position" and "pain" were identified as the most common stimuli disturbing sleep in hospital. Anxieties arising from the illness and hospitalization, such as those related to tests and surgery, diagnosis, and impact on family and job, were other frequently identified reasons for disturbed sleep (Fig. 43-6).

Medications and Chemicals

Sleep patterns are vulnerable to disturbance from medications taken to facilitate sleep, alcohol, medications used to treat other conditions, and other chemicals (Nicholson, et al., 1994). **Hypnotics**, or "sleeping pills," the very medications used to decrease sleep latency and improve sleep maintenance, are among those medications most prone to disturb sleep architecture. REM sleep is most vulnerable.

Alcohol is probably the oldest and most commonly used chemical for promoting sleep. A moderate single dose causes early onset of sleep but increases wakefulness in the last half of the night. With acute intoxication, REM sleep is suppressed; slow-wave sleep may initially increase. Abrupt withdrawal in the heavy drinker may trigger massive REM rebound. Recovered alcoholics continue to have decreased slow-wave sleep and gross cycle disturbance even after 1 or 2 years of abstinence. Other medications also affect sleep patterns. Morphine,

	% 10 20 30 40 50 60 70 80 90 100
Difficulty finding a comfortable position	XXXXXXXXXXXXXXXXXXXXXX
Pain	XXXXXXXXXXXXXXXXXXXX
Worry about test/surgery	XXXXXXXXXXX
Worry about family, job, managing at home	XXXXXXXXX
Worry about diagnosis/ getting well	XXXXXXXXX
Discomfort from dressing, cast, etc.	XXXXXXXXX
Being awakened for treatments	XXXXXXXXX
Noise from other patients	XXXXXXXX
Too much light	XXXXXXXXX
Fear of dislodging tubing	XXXXXXXX
Lack of exercise	XXXXXXX
Temperature	XXXXXX
Noise from TV/radio	XXXXXX
Unfamiliar environment	XXXXXXX
Disrupted habits	XXXXXX
Noise from nursing station	XXXXXXX
Uncomfortable bed	XXXX
Napping	XXX
Sleeping alone	XXX

Figure 43-6 • *Percentage of clients identifying selected stimuli as disturbing to sleep in hospital. (From Reimer, M.A. (1985).* Nursing interventions perceived by patients and their nurses as facilitating nocturnal sleep in hospital. *Unpublished manuscript.)*

for example, increases the time spent awake during the sleep period and shortens total sleep time by decreasing both REM and stages 3 and 4. Antidepressants suppress REM sleep also. Dilantin, used in the treatment of epilepsy, may contribute to insomnia.

The effects of caffeine on the central nervous system (CNS) may last for up to 14 hours, delaying sleep onset and affecting sleep patterns even in those who believe that they are not affected by it (Zarcone, 1994). The half-life of caffeine in the elderly is even longer, making them particularly vulnerable to its effects. Nicotine, another mild CNS stimulant, accounts for the poorer sleep observed in heavy smokers compared with nonsmokers.

Mood States

Anxiety frequently delays sleep onset. The tension associated with psychological stress may also contribute to maintenance or early-awakening insomnia. Depression usually results in disturbed sleep. Both the depression and sleep pattern disturbance may be linked to neurotransmitter imbalance. The depressed person is also more likely to be distressed by poor sleep.

Manifestations of Altered Sleep Function

Signs and symptoms associated with sleep deprivation are fatigue, headache, nausea, increased sensitivity to pain, decreased neuromuscular coordination, general irritability, and inability to concentrate. Eventually, disorientation and hallucinations may occur with the breakthrough of "mini-sleeps," which further interfere with functioning.

Selective disruption of specific stages of sleep results in distinct symptom patterns. Those deprived of REM sleep become agitated and impulsive, whereas deprivation of slow-wave sleep results in withdrawal and vague physical complaints. Tolerance of musculoskeletal pain in particular is significantly decreased after deprivation of slow-wave sleep. When deprived of stage 1, 2, or 3 sleep, the body makes no effort to recover those specific stages, but there seems to be a mechanism that gives priority to recovering stage 4 sleep and REM as soon as the opportunity is given.

Insomnia

Insomnia is a perceived difficulty in sleeping. The persistent insomnia experienced by those who refer to themselves as insomniacs reflects a pattern of perceived difficulty with sleeping over months to years. Patterns of insomnia can also be classified as onset insomnia (prolonged sleep latency), maintenance insomnia (multiple awakenings), and early-awakening insomnia. When polygraph recordings of insomniacs have been compared with those of self-defined good sleepers, both have been found to be within normal range. Insomniacs consistently underestimated total sleep time but were accurate in identifying the pattern of insomnia and actually underestimated the number of awakenings. Thus, the problem of insomnia appears to be more of a lack of quality than quantity (Hauri, 1994).

Narcolepsy

Narcolepsy is a disorder of excessive daytime sleepiness characterized by short, almost irresistible daytime sleep attacks, usually of 10 to 15 minutes' duration, and abnormal manifestations of REM sleep. Onset usually occurs in adolescence. Narcolepsy is thought to be a disturbance between REM sleep and wakefulness-triggering systems, in which REM sleep intrudes into wakefulness (Carskadon & Dement, 1994). Most narcoleptics go almost immediately into REM sleep at the beginning of the sleep period. Episodes of profound weakness during intense emotion, called cataplexy, are reported by 70% of narcoleptics. Other common signs related to disturbed REM mechanisms include episodes of feeling paralyzed when falling asleep or awakening, and vivid hallucinations (Bergstrom & Keller, 1992).

Sleep Apnea

Sleep apnea refers to recurrent periods of absence of breathing for 10 seconds or longer, occurring at least five times per hour. Three types of sleep apnea are recognized: obstructive, central, and mixed (Robinson, 1993).

Obstructive Sleep Apnea. Obstructive sleep apnea involves collapse of the upper airway in spite of respiratory effort. With sleep, the muscles of the upper airway relax, occluding an airway that may be already narrowed because of obesity, jaw structure, or enlarged soft tissue structures. With arousal, voluntary control of the upper airway muscles is restored, relieving the obstruction. Some people do not become completely apneic, but recurrent periods of very shallow breathing (**hypopnea**) have a similar effect (Stewart, 1991).

The person, often a heavy-set man, may be partially roused up to a couple of hundred times a night. Symptoms are excessive daytime sleepiness, and bed partner reports of apneic periods, heavy snoring, and restless sleep. Common treatments include continuous positive airway pressure applied through a nose mask and surgical reconstruction of the upper airway with removal of most of the uvula, posterior portion of the soft palate, and tonsils. Current developments include laser-assisted pharyngoplasty and various dental splints. Weight control, relief of nasal congestion, and avoidance of sleeping on the back may be effective in milder cases.

At least 1% of the adult male population has obstructive sleep apnea. About 5% of the most severely affected of these clients fit the classic description of pickwickian syndrome, but obesity is not always present nor are all clients male. Occasional apneic periods occur normally during sleep stage transitions. Such apneas are not of concern. However, people who have frequent apneas exceeding 20 seconds at a time and occurring most nights, with or without snoring or excessive daytime sleepiness, should be encouraged to seek assessment for possible obstructive sleep apnea.

Central Apnea. Central apnea during sleep occurs because of neurogenic failure to trigger respiratory effort. It is most commonly seen with neurologic conditions such as stroke or brain stem involvement. Severely affected clients may require ventilatory support at night.

Mixed Apnea. Mixed apnea, a combination of the two preceding types of sleep apnea, is especially common in the elderly. Manifestations and treatment are similar to those for obstructive sleep apnea.

Use of hypnotics, alcohol, or antihistamines by clients with sleep apnea can be dangerous. Duration of apneic spells may increase because responsiveness to change in oxygen desaturation is already reduced. Drugs that may induce drowsiness are more likely to do so in people who are already chronically sleep deprived. Sleep apnea essentially results in chronic sleep deprivation because of the frequency of mini-arousals and the lack of slow-wave and REM sleep.

Sleep-Related (Nocturnal) Myoclonus

The periodic leg movements of sleep-related (nocturnal) myoclonus involve repetitive dorsiflexion of the foot and flexion of the knee during sleep at a rate up to once every 15 to 20 seconds. The resultant mini-arousals disrupt sleep, leading to excessive daytime sleepiness, or in some cases insomnia. Frequency tends to increase with age. Up to 45% of community-living people older than 65 years of age report having periodic leg movements (Bliwise, 1994).

Altered Sleep–Wake Patterns

Altered sleep–wake disorders include transient disruptions, such as the jet lag syndrome, and persistent disorders, such as delayed sleep phase syndrome. Jet lag tends to be worst after west-to-east travel across time zones, and affects poor sleepers and the elderly more than good sleepers (Graeber, 1994; Roehrs, et al., 1994). Delayed sleep phase syndrome is a less common but more problematic mismatch of personal circadian rhythm with societal expectations. Some people who function best by going to bed in the early hours of the morning and sleeping into the afternoon find occupations and partners to match. Other people with this disorder find that the continued struggle to rise hours earlier than their internal clock dictates is not made easier by simple treatments such as establishing a consistent rising time. These people can be helped to achieve a phase shift through **chronotherapy**, in which they progressively delay sleep onset by 2 hours per week until they eventually work around to a more functional schedule.

Parasomnias

Parasomnias are activities that are normal during waking but abnormal during sleep, such as sleepwalking (somnambulism), talking, and bedwetting (enuresis). These usually occur during slow-wave sleep and are most frequent in children. There is often a family history of similar behaviors.

Occasional episodes of sleepwalking in children are fairly common, usually beginning before age 10 and stopping by age 15 years. Behavior during a sleepwalking episode may be semipurposeful, such dressing or going to the bathroom, but lacking in coordination and appropriateness, such as voiding in the closet. Occurrence in adults is frequently associated with stress and anxiety. Parents and family members may need assistance in providing a safe environment to decrease the potential for injury.

Night terrors, another type of parasomnia, are repeated, sudden awakenings accompanied by screaming, acute anxiety, and disorientation (Gates, et al., 1989). They occur mainly among children, and are associated with incomplete arousal from slow-wave sleep early in the night. They are different from nightmares, or bad dreams that occur during REM sleep.

Attempts to awaken people from the parasomnias of slow-wave sleep should be discouraged. Help in the event of night terrors or somnambulism should be given only to the extent that it is accepted, and the person should be encouraged to return to sleep as the event subsides.

Enuresis is not limited to slow-wave sleep, although almost two-thirds of all episodes occur in the first third of the night. The prevalence decreases from 30% at age 4 to 10% at age 6 and 3% at age 12 years (American Sleep Disorders Association, 1990). Enuresis is less common in girls and tends to disappear earlier.

Impact of Sleep Dysfunction on Activities of Daily Living

Individual Considerations

Sleep pattern dysfunction affects most activities of daily living to a varying degree. Closely linked to quality of life is the sense of feeling well rested and refreshed, with energy available for activity. Thus, adequacy of sleep and rest directly affects and is affected by the activity and exercise pattern. Lack of sleep impairs coping and cognitive responses.

Therapeutic Dialogue
Sleep and Rest

Scenes for Thought

Joanna and Paco Estevez are parents of two small children, one of whom is just 3 weeks old. Their older child, Theresa, is 3 years old. Paco works nights, and Joanna has recently returned to work at her day shift job as a nurse's aid in a large nursing home. You, Emily Arana, are a community health nurse and are at their home for a follow-up visit because the Estevez family uses your clinic for their health-care needs.

Effective

Client: *Oh, hello. I'm glad you came early, Ms. Arana. The kids are both asleep and so is Paco. We can talk in peace for a little while.* Sits on sofa in living room and motions to sit down.
Nurse: *Sounds like it's been busy around here lately. (Settles onto sofa and sits attentively.)*
Client: *You got that right! Enrique isn't sleeping through the night yet, and Theresa wakes up, too. Plus she has a cold so she isn't feeling too good. And Paco isn't around to help much since he's working nights, so it gets pretty hairy around here at 2 A.M.* Smiles a tight little smile.
Nurse: *How about you? (Good eye contact.)*
Client: *I do what I can do.* Shrugs wearily. *I had to go back to work after the baby came home or lose my job, and I have to get up at 5 to get the kids ready to take to my mother's so she can take them while I work. So I don't get much rest. Or much time with Paco. I really hate this night shift he's on. But it's extra money and it won't be forever. He's put in for a shift change so we can have some sort of a normal life, but it won't come through for a while.* Yawns. *Sorry! I didn't mean to yawn in your face!*
Nurse: *No problem. You have lots of reason to be tired. What are you doing to try and get more rest? (Looking concerned. Open-ended question.)*
Client: *I try to snatch here and there. Paco takes the night feedings on his nights off so I can sleep all the way through at least 2 nights a week. Other than that, I wait for the baby to grow a bit more so he'll sleep through and for Theresa's cold to get better.* Shrugs again with a resigned look.
Nurse: *Would you be willing to discuss a few things that might help both kids move along faster so you can sleep through the night sooner?*
Client: Looks surprised. *Sure! I didn't know there was anything else I could do for them.* Baby begins to cry. Joanna rushes to get him so Paco won't wake. She returns. *Let me just change him and get a bottle and then we can talk!* Looks eager.

Less Effective

Client: *Oh, hello. I'm glad you came early, Ms. Arana. The kids are both asleep and so is Paco. We can talk in peace for a little while.* Sits on sofa in living room and motions to sit down.
Nurse: *Sounds like it's been busy around here lately. (Settles onto sofa and sits attentively.)*
Client: *You got that right! Enrique isn't sleeping through the night yet, and Theresa wakes up, too. Plus she has a cold so she isn't feeling too good. And Paco isn't around to help much since he's working nights, so it gets pretty hairy around here at 2 A.M.* Smiles a tight little smile.
Nurse: *And I understand you're working, too. Day shift?*
Client: *Yes.* Wearily. *I had to go back or lose the job. I leave the kids with my mother all day until I get off at 3 P.M. She lives close by.* Yawns. *Sorry! I didn't mean to yawn in your face!*
Nurse: *No problem. And is your husband able to help or is he too tired? (Beginning to open bag and take out assessment equipment.)*
Client: *He helps on his days off. He's really good with both of them.* Watching the equipment emerge. Sounding a little defensive.
Nurse: *I'm sure he is, having had three brothers and sisters of his own to take care of. Maybe I could see the baby now and see how he's doing. Do you think Theresa will be up soon? Then I can look at her, too, and see what we can do for her cold. What do you think?*
Client: *Sure, you start on the baby, and I'll see if Theresa's about to wake up.* Pauses to get a clean towel for the baby to lie on and goes in to the bedroom. Yawns again.

Critical Thinking Challenge

• Determine the factors affecting this family's sleep and rest patterns. • Detect how the nurse in the first dialogue elicited additional information from the client. • Explain what information the nurse in the second dialogue missed out on. • Formulate your ideas of what consequences further sleep deprivation may have for this family.

Family Considerations

Role performance and social interactions may become disrupted in the presence of sleep pattern dysfunction. Irritability and impaired concentration accompany sleep deprivation. Snoring often disturbs the bed partner, who not infrequently seeks the refuge of another bedroom. The excessive sleepiness associated with disorders such as sleep apnea pose serious safety risks for those driving and operating hazardous machinery.

Assessment

Sleep pattern disturbances in health and illness are frequent sources of concern to people. It is easy in the hospital situation for nurses to become preoccupied with assessments and treatments associated with the presenting illness. Likewise, in community practice, the diabetic's foot care or the new mother's ability to breastfeed may overshadow the concerns those people have regarding unsatisfactory sleep or inadequate rest.

However, the professional nurse can play a pivotal role in helping people assess and meet their needs for sleep and rest.

Subjective Data

The single most important criterion for adequacy of sleep and rest is the client's statement. The state of feeling rested is a highly subjective one. As discussed earlier, individual requirements for sleep vary widely. Besides the sense of feeling rested, people usually consider the congruency between their expectations and experience in relation to total sleep time, time in bed before sleep onset, number of awakenings, and time of final awakening. The history is the most important component of assessment of sleep and rest.

Functional Pattern Identification

Determine the person's usual sleep and rest patterns through questions such as:

How many hours of sleep do you usually get?
What time do you usually go to bed? Get up?
What helps you get to sleep?
What makes it hard for you to sleep?
How do you feel when you awaken?
How much sleep do you believe you should be getting?
What helps you relax?
How often do you nap? Take rest periods?

Risk Identification

Look for developmental and situational changes (environmental, physical, social) that may increase the need for or interfere with sleep and rest. Assess caffeine, nicotine, and alcohol intake, and involvement in shift work.

Dysfunction Identification

Validate with the person whether getting adequate sleep and rest is perceived as a problem. If a problem is identified, determine whether it is chronic or situational, what has helped, and what has made it worse. In situations of chronic disturbance it may be useful to interview the sleep partner as well. Questions should be directed toward elaboration of the presenting concern. For example, if the person is concerned about daytime sleepiness, the nurse should inquire about a history of snoring, awakenings accompanied by gasping, apneic periods that may have been observed by the partner, restlessness, and impact on activities associated with work, driving, and social interactions.

Having the person keep a sleep diary may be useful as an assessment and as an intervention. By giving the person responsibility for monitoring his or her own health pattern, the nurse may help the person recognize patterns and related factors. Young and middle-aged adults in the habit of sleeping late on days off sometimes express concern about sleep disturbances at the beginning of their work week, which they may attribute to job stress. Reviewing a sleep diary maintained for a couple of weeks may help them realize that when they average out total sleep time they are meeting their perceived requirements.

Objective Data

Physical Assessment

Observe for circles under the eyes, yawning, nodding, and slowness of response. Irritability, impaired concentration, and word-finding difficulties may be indicative of sleep pattern disturbance but may also occur because of other problems.

Adequacy of rest after activity is often measured through return of heart rate and other physiologic parameters to baseline levels (Alteri, 1984). The nurse should monitor vital signs after client- or caregiver-initiated activity for return to baseline resting levels in the severely compromised client.

Diagnostic Tests

People with severe sleep problems or excessive daytime sleepiness should be referred to a sleep laboratory for more thorough investigation. Polygraph recordings can be made, including evaluation of other parameters such as oxygen saturation and periodic leg movements. Home monitoring has the advantage of familiar surroundings and is being used more for screening. It is important that results of home monitoring are interpreted by a qualified sleep specialist.

Nursing Diagnosis

To formulate the nursing diagnosis, the nurse clusters the data, sifting out the incidental from the significant. For example, in this author's investigation of presleep rituals, 72% of the respondents reported habitually watching television before going to bed, yet only 26% of them considered this activity important in getting to sleep (Reimer, 1985). Thus, the absence of a television in a client's hospital environment may be of little significance. However, the same client's seemingly casual comment regarding how the children at home are managing "without a disciplinarian around" may be a significant clue to sleep-disturbing anxiety. Diagnostic statements should be as specific as possible.

Nursing Research
Sleep and Rest

Selected Nursing Research Studies

Becher, P. T., Chang, A., Kameshima, S., & Bloch, M. (1991). Correlates of diurnal sleep patterns in infants of adolescent and adult single mothers. *Research in Nursing and Health, 14*(2), 97–108.

Edwards, G. B., & Schuring, L. M. (1993). Pilot study: Validating staff nurses' observations of sleep and wake states among critically ill patients, using polysomnography. *American Journal of Critical Care, 2*(2), 125–131.

Jimmerson, K. R. (1991). Maternal, environmental, and tempermental characteristics of toddlers with and toddlers without sleep problems. *Journal of Pediatric Health Care, 5*(2), 71–77.

Johnson, J. E. (1991). Progressive relaxation and the sleep of older non-institutionalized women. *Applied Nursing Research, 4*(4), 165–170.

Possible Topics for Nursing Inquiry

- What are the long-term effects of chronic sleep deprivation?
- Does a warm tub bath change the quality and quantity of sleep?
- How long does it take a client's vital signs to return to resting baseline after having an occupied bed made?

Diagnostic Statement: Sleep Pattern Disturbance

Definition

Sleep Pattern Disturbance is disruption of sleep time (that) causes discomfort or interferes with desired lifestyle (North American Nursing Diagnosis Association [NANDA], 1994).

Defining Characteristics

Of the defining characteristics for sleep pattern disturbance, the following four characteristics are critical for making the diagnosis:

- Verbal complaints of difficulty falling asleep
- Awakening earlier or later than desired
- Interrupted sleep
- Verbal complaints of not feeling well rested.

In other words, the length of time it takes to fall asleep, the time of awakening, and the number of arousals during the night are not sufficient to make the diagnosis. The person must be expressing difficulty with these aspects of sleep and about not feeling refreshed after sleep.

Other major defining characteristics are ones that the nurse can observe:

- Changes in behavior and performance (increasing irritability, restlessness, disorientation, lethargy, or listlessness)
- Physical signs (mild fleeting nystagmus, slight hand tremor, ptosis of eyelid, expressionless face, dark circles under the eyes, frequent yawning, or changes in posture)
- Thick speech with mispronunciation and incorrect words (NANDA, 1994).

Related Factors

Sensory alterations may have affected this change in functional health status. Internal sensory alterations such illness or psychological stress may be affecting the state of arousal, the ability to relax, or even the balance of the neurotransmitters that contribute to changing sleep stages. External sensory alterations from environmental changes or social cues may also affect sleep patterns by way of modifying sensory input from changes in levels of light, noise, or social stimulation (NANDA, 1994).

Related Nursing Diagnoses

Fatigue, in the NANDA classification, is defined as "an overwhelming sustained sense of exhaustion and decreased capacity for physical and mental work" (Cox, et al., 1993, p. 407). Some defining characteristics such as irritability and impaired concentration are shared, but Cox and associates suggest that Fatigue is a subjective state that persists in spite of an apparently adequate quantity of sleep (Cox, et al., 1993). Ineffective Individual Coping may be the more appropriate nursing diagnosis if there is evidence that the client has a normal sleep pattern but wants to sleep more as a way of trying to avoid or cope with stress. Activity Intolerance can also be confused with Sleep Pattern Disturbance unless one listens carefully to the cues. The person with Activity Intolerance will complain of lack of energy but not of inadequate sleep. Other diagnoses such as Altered Rest, which appears in NANDA Taxonomy I (Carroll-Johnson & Paquette, 1994) but has not been approved as part of the standard list, may be clinically useful as parts of diagnostic statements.

Outcome Identification and Planning

After the nursing diagnoses and related factors are identified, client goals and interventions are planned. Client goals for sleep pattern disturbance are specifically

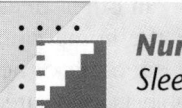

Planning

Examples of Nursing Interventions Used in Common Sleep Problems

- Identify factors affecting the quality of sleep.
- Minimize stimuli by having a darkened, quiet room with low lights.
- Encourage sleep rituals, such as a gentle backrub, plumping of pillows, and eliminating distracting sound.
- Relieve discomfort through position changes, pain medications, or other measures.
- Reduce factors affecting safety by having call light near at hand, bed in the lowest position, and using a nightlight.
- Encourage contact with family or other significant others who provide the client with a sense of intimacy and security.

stated in terms such as "minutes before sleep onset," "hours of unbroken sleep," or "verbal statement of feeling refreshed on wakening." Examples of specific client goals are

Client will report fewer problems with falling asleep.
Client will report feeling more rested.
Client will demonstrate physical signs of being rested.

Involving people in setting their own goals for sleep and rest is a useful way of helping them explore what is realistic for their developmental stage, lifestyle, and state of health.

Counseling may be high on the priority list of nurses in helping clients establish periods of adequate sleep and rest. The nurse may need to meet with family members and caregivers to address environmental needs and to teach caregiving practices for comfort. Examples of nursing interventions commonly used in promoting sleep and rest are listed in the accompanying display and discussed in the next section of the chapter.

Implementation

Nursing Interventions to Promote Health and Sleep/Rest Function

Environmental modifications, provision of intimacy and security, sleep rituals, and variables in sleep needs are among the nursing interventions to promote health and sleep.

Environment Modification

The nurse can encourage clients to reserve the sleeping room for sleep whenever possible (Engle-Friedman, et al., 1992). Children should learn to play in other areas. Opportunities should be provided for the home care, hospitalized, or residential client to get out of his or her room during the day when feasible. Objects associated with work, conflict, pain, or sleeplessness should be removed.

Establish a quiet, darkened environment modified according to the person's preferred level (eg, low light may be a source of comfort for children or those in a strange environment). Children often need to be reminded to go to the bathroom before going to bed. Fluids may need to be restricted in the evening. Simple relaxation exercises can be taught for use at bedtime. People with impaired physical mobility should be assisted with voiding before retiring and made comfortable in the bed. Some older male clients appreciate having a urinal within reach.

Provision of Intimacy and Security

A bedtime hug for a child, the shared bed of a marriage partner, and an enjoyable evening with a friend are a few ways in which people enhance sleep quality for one another (Fig. 43-7). If social isolation is suspected as a related factor in Sleep Pattern Disturbance, the nurse may need to assist the person in making social contacts. A favorite blanket or stuffed animal are other ways of enhancing security.

In the institutional setting, a backrub provides the warmth of human touch as well as physical relaxation. Arranging for family members to sit at the bedside may be helpful. Assurance of frequent checks by nursing staff, prompt response to the call bell, and a caring manner can do much to allay the fears of the anxious client. Prayer and reading scripture often facilitates a sense of peacefulness and subsequent sleep onset. Other people may find meditation helpful. A sensitive assessment of the person's values and beliefs (see Chapter 53) helps the nurse maximize strengths.

Client Teaching
Sleep and Rest

Instruct the client as follows:

- *Get up at the same time each day. Avoid sleeping in on days off.*
- *Eat sensibly and regularly. If used to a bedtime snack, keep up the habit. Otherwise skip it.*
- *Avoid alcohol and caffeine. Their effects linger to disturb sleep.*
- *Exercise daily but not too late in the day. Enjoyable activities will enhance the benefits for sleep and rest.*
- *Set your mind at rest before going to bed with relaxing music, a good book, or valued companionship.*
- *Enjoy what sleep you get. Needs vary, and you really can get by on very little sleep.*

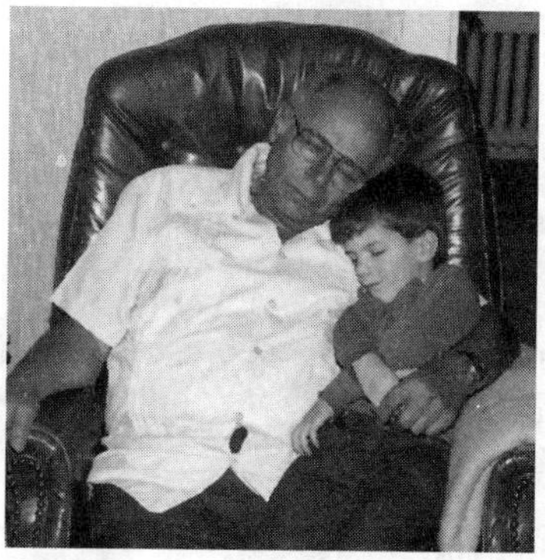

Figure 43-7 • *Sometimes naps are taken in unplanned places if the environment is right.*

Sleep Rituals

Rituals play an important role in facilitating sleep. Whether it is the bedtime story for the toddler or a cup of tea for the elderly couple, the regular association of certain activities with the end of the waking period is one of the most effective ways of creating the expectation of sleep.

A routine of "settling" clients in institutional settings can provide a similar marking of the end of the day. Assisting with washing of hands and face, a gentle massage, plumping of pillows, and provision of an extra blanket may be incorporated. The nurse can use this time as an opportunity to help clients focus on small goals accomplished during the day, the visit of a loved one, or whatever else is helpful to settle the mind as well as the body.

Managing Individual Sleep Needs

People should be helped to assess their individual sleep needs and to anticipate developmental changes. Middle-aged and older people can be helped to realize that shorter unbroken sleep periods are normal for their age. Likewise, insomniacs (and potential ones) may benefit from the assurance that they can function on relatively little sleep (Engle-Friedman, et al., 1992). Parents may need anticipatory guidance regarding the wide variability in sleep needs of individual children.

Nursing Interventions for Altered Function

In spite of major advances in medical therapeutics, rest remains one of the most common symptomatic treatments for a wide variety of disease conditions. "Rest the affected part" is a standard intervention for almost any condition.

Rest

The person who has suffered myocardial ischemia as a result of a blood clot is placed on a strict regimen of restricted activity. To maintain a resting state for the heart once the initial period of pain has subsided challenges the nurse's creativity. The client is helped to realize that although he or she may "feel great," the damaged heart needs further rest, with a gradual return to the previous or a decreased activity level. The nurse also has a major role in helping such clients make more lasting lifestyle changes to incorporate more rest and relaxation.

Research on the amount of rest required after various activities provides a basis for nurses to make decisions in implementing care. Alteri (1984) studied 10 male clients 8 to 20 days after myocardial infarction to determine the length of time required for vital signs to return to the preactivity baseline. Climbing one flight of stairs required 7 minutes to recover, a 10-minute walk on a level surface required 10 minutes to recover, and showering required 30.5 minutes to reach the preactivity baseline. She also found that participants consistently expressed the feeling that they had recovered long before their vital signs returned to normal.

Maintaining traction to "rest" a client's fractured femur or instilling eye drops temporarily to paralyze and thus rest the eye after surgery are further examples of ways in which nurses help clients meet situationally induced changes in rest requirements.

Use of Medications

Hypnotics may be useful as a short-term intervention during situationally induced sleep pattern disturbance. Other interventions should be tried first, however. When hypnotics are ordered prn (as necessary) in the hospital environment, the nurse has the responsibility of deciding with the client if and when they should be

Safety Alert
Sleep and Rest Within a Healthcare Facility

- Keep the call bell within reach, the bed in low position, and the nightlight turned on to prevent falls in hospital.
- Remove extra equipment and position chairs and tables to leave easy access to the bed and bathroom.
- Encourage clients to seek assistance when getting up, especially at night if they are at risk for dizziness (eg, postoperatively or after sedation), or have impaired mobility.
- Keep a urinal at the bedside of male clients. It may avoid a fall on the way to the bathroom.
- Putting siderails up may keep a client from rolling out but not necessarily from crawling out of bed.
- Hypnotics and alcohol should be used cautiously, if at all, by people with impaired gas exchange or sleep apnea.

Nursing Plan of Care
The Client With Sleep Pattern Disturbance

Nursing Diagnosis

Sleep Pattern Disturbance related to positional discomfort secondary to low back pain and manifested by wakening every 1 to 2 hours to turn, difficulty getting back to sleep, and expressed feelings of inadequate rest.

Client Goal

Client will use a sleep pattern that allows him to feel well rested.

Client Outcome Criteria

- Client has periods of 3 to 4 hours of undisturbed sleep within 2 days, as observed by the nurse.
- Client expresses feeling more rested by the end of this week.

Nursing Intervention	Scientific Rationale
1. Offer backrub at bedtime and during the night when assisting with turns.	1. Muscle tension increases pain and arousal; backrubs help relaxation.
2. Assess mattress comfort with client.	2. Adequate support is important in reducing back pain, but too firm a surface can cause more wakenings and more stage 1 sleep.
3. Keep radio with earphones within reach during the night.	3. Some people find low-level stimuli help them get to sleep, especially because they mask strange sounds of hospital environment.
4. Alternate supine position with side-lying when assisting with position changes (unless contraindicated or uncomfortable for client).	4. Poor sleepers have been found to spend more time on their backs with the head straight. This position may be more comfortable for some clients with back pain, however.
5. Increase activity during the day. If client is on bed rest, arrange to take bed to sunroom.	5. Daytime activity and change of environment help in cueing sleep–wake patterns.
6. Cluster assessments and treatments required during the night to coincide with times when the client is already awake for position change.	6. Sleep cycles average 90 minutes. A sleep latency of 20 to 30 minutes means that clients should be given up to 2 hours of undisturbed time whenever possible.

taken. In making decisions and teaching clients regarding the use of hypnotics, the nurse should consider the following principles:

- All hypnotics require judicious use because they interfere with normal sleep architecture to some degree. REM sleep is most vulnerable. Therefore, signs of selective stage deficit may be evident, even though total sleep time has increased through hypnotic use. Clients can be taught that a night or two of increased dreaming (REM rebound) after the drug is discontinued is not unusual. Tapering withdrawal in long-term users can prevent REM rebound.
- All hypnotics impair waking function as long as they are pharmacologically active. Perception of daytime drowsiness and impairment of psychomotor skills fades more rapidly than do the actual effects (Nicholson, 1994). Therefore, people in the community environment who are taking hypnotics should be taught about the half-life of the drugs and warned to avoid driving or handling machinery while the drug is in their system. Safety precautions should also be taken in home and hospital when those who have taken a hypnotic need to get up to the bathroom at night.
- The effectiveness of hypnotics decreases over a 4-week period, so long-term users are probably being affected more by expectation of sleep associated with taking a pill than by the active drug. It is therefore important to teach these people alternative sleep-promoting strategies and prepare them for the possible short-term rebound effects that may follow withdrawal (Kripke, et al., 1979).

- Hypnotics are most appropriately used for insomnia of recent origin, such as after a situational crisis. The smallest effective dose should be taken, and then only for a few nights or intermittently as required (Nicholson, 1994).
- Certain people are at increased risk from the use of hypnotics. The time required for the elderly to metabolize long-acting benzodiazepines is increased. Arousal because of decreased oxygen levels is depressed after the administration of hypnotics. Therefore the nurse must use particular caution in administering ordered hypnotics to the elderly or to those whose pulmonary function is compromised.

Table 43-2 shows how knowledge of the specific properties of each hypnotic can help the nurse determine implications for assessment and teaching. The chart is not intended to be exhaustive, but rather to highlight the need for nurses to be knowledgeable about the hypnotics clients are taking.

Sleep pattern disturbance is often associated with periods of high anxiety or depression and therefore the nurse will also encounter clients who are on anxiolytic or sedative antidepressants that have the effect of improving sleep. Most of the anxiolytics are also benzodiazepines, but of the long-acting type such as Lorazepam (Ativan). The action of antidepressants on sleep may be direct, through their modulation of neurotransmission, especially serotonin, as well as indirect through treating the underlying depression (Nicholson, 1994).

Use of Consistent Routine

The single most important intervention for chronic sleep pattern disturbance may be to establish a consistent rising time. Getting up is subject to voluntary control, whereas falling asleep usually is not. Slightly decreasing the time in bed solidifies sleep and, along with a consistent rising time, will finally lead to more regular times of sleep onset.

Counseling regarding the maintenance of routines may be required for the socially and occupationally isolated. For the acutely ill client, the nurse can enhance cueing by turning lights down at night, keeping window drapes open during the day when possible, and providing verbal cueing regarding time of day.

Community-Based Nursing

Clients often underestimate their needs for rest when recovering from illness or surgery. The nurse may need to help them plan for periods of rest and for energy conservation. Assessment of, and suggestions for correction or adaptation to, environmental conditions may be necessary. The sleep and rest needs of the home caregiver must also be considered when ill or immobile clients need assistance during the night. Respite care may be an option, or the caregiver may need counseling about his or her sleep and rest needs.

Table 43-2* • *Selected Hypnotics: Their Properties and Nursing Implications

Hypnotic	Properties	Nursing Implications
Benzodiazepines		
Flurazepam (Dalmane)	Onset rapid (17 minutes) Half-life 74–160 hours	Good for onset and maintenance insomnia maximum effectiveness not until third night Less rebound effect because of a long half-life but more hangover
Temazepam (Restoril)	Onset 1–2 hours Half-life 9–12 hours	Poor for onset insomnia Most effective for maintenance or early-wakening insomnia Hangover effect Safer for elderly people
Other		
Zopiclone (Imovane)	Short-acting Half-life 4–6.5 hours	Good for onset and maintenance insomnia Less suppression of slow-wave sleep than the benzodiazepines

Evaluation

The nurse evaluates the degree to which sleep pattern disturbance or inadequate rest has been resolved according to the client goals initially established. Examples of outcome criteria for the client goals are listed below.

Goal
Client will report fewer problems with falling asleep.

Possible Outcome Criteria
- Within 7 days, client reports decrease in sleep latency to 10 to 15 minutes.
- Within 7 days, client reports less anxiety regarding falling asleep.

Goal
Client will report feeling more rested.

Possible Outcome Criteria
- Within 10 days, client verbalizes feeling less fatigued.
- As observed by nurse by tenth day, client nonverbally demonstrates increased restfulness (less dozing, more animation in activity).

Goal
Client will demonstrate physical signs of being rested.

Possible Outcome Criteria
- By seventh day, client has decrease in circles under the eyes, excessive yawning, or slowness of response.
- Within 10 days, client reports to nurse that he or she feels rested after activity.

Validation should occur with the client particularly for this functional health pattern because of the subjectivity and individual variations in what it takes to have adequate rest and satisfying sleep.

Key Concepts

- Sleep is a naturally occurring, altered state of consciousness characterized by awareness and responsiveness to stimuli, and by being readily reversible.
- Rest is a physical and emotional state of decreased muscle and cognitive activity.
- Sleep and rest have restorative, protective, and energy-conserving functions.
- Psychological functions of sleep include reprocessing of memories and character reinforcement.
- The two main types of sleep are NREM (quiet sleep) and REM (rapid eye movement sleep).
- NREM sleep consists of four stages: stage 1, transitional; stage 2, light; stages 3 and 4, and deep, slow-wave sleep.
- REM sleep is similar to wakefulness in terms of brain activity, but muscle tone is low and vital signs fluctuate widely.
- Adults progress through stages 1-2-3-4-3-2-REM in 90-minute cycles.
- Infants have sleep cycles that last about 50 minutes.
- Guidelines for evaluating adequacy of sleep are awakening with a feeling of being refreshed and the absence of daytime sleepiness.
- Factors affecting sleep and rest include environmental stimuli, nutrition, exercise, illness, and hospitalization.
- Common disorders of sleep include disorders of initiating and maintaining sleep (insomnia), excessive daytime sleepiness, disorders of the sleep–wake cycle, and parasomnias.
- Sleep patterns change throughout the lifespan, with the very young and the very old requiring the most sleep.
- Anticipating changes in sleep patterns and needs for rest can contribute to promotion of a healthy balance between rest and activity, and a recognition that sleep pattern changes are developmentally normal.

Critical Thinking Challenges

Now that you have completed this chapter on sleep and rest, turn back to the situation at the beginning of the chapter. Consider the following questions.

1. *Recall the first thoughts that came to your mind when you initially read the situation.*
2. *Spend a few moments imagining yourself back in high school. Reflect on the quality and quantity of sleep you used to get and what you believed about sleep.*
3. *Develop your priorities in teaching this class.*
4. *Discuss ways in which the sleep needs and experiences of these high school students are affected by their developmental stage. Consider these needs from a holistic perspective.*

References

Alteri, C. A. (1984). The patient with myocardial infarction: Rest prescriptions for activities of daily living. *Heart Lung, 13,* 355–359.

American Sleep Disorders Association. (1990). *The International Classification of Sleep Disorders: Diagnostic and coding manual.* Rochester, NY: Author.

Anders, T. F. (1994). Infant sleep, nighttime relationships, and attachment. *Psychiatry, 57,* 11–21.

Bergstrom, D. L., & Keller, C. (1992). Narcolepsy: Pathogenesis and nursing care. *Journal of Neuroscience Nursing, 24*(3), 153–157.

Bliwise, D. L. (1994). Normal aging. In M. H. Kryger, T. Roth, & W. C. Dement (Eds.), *Principles and practice of sleep medicine* (2nd ed.) (pp. 26–39). Philadelphia: W. B. Saunders.

Bunnell, D. E., Agnew, J. A., Horvath, S. M., et al. (1988). Passive body heating and sleep: Influence of proximity to sleep. *Sleep, 11,* 210–219.

Carroll-Johnson, R. M., & Paquette, M. (1994). *Classification of nursing diagnoses: Proceedings of the tenth conference.* Philadelphia: J. B. Lippincott.

Carskadon, M. A., & Dement, W. C. (1994). Normal human sleep: An overview. In M. H. Kryger, T. Roth, & W. C. Dement (Eds.), *Principles and practice of sleep medicine* (2nd ed.) (pp. 16–25). Philadelphia: W. B. Saunders.

Cox, H., Hinz, M., Lubno, M., et al. (1993). *Clinical applications of nursing diagnosis* (2nd ed.). Baltimore: Williams & Wilkins.

De Koninck, J., Lorrain, D., & Gagnon, P. (1992). Sleep positions and position shifts in five age groups: An ontogenetic picture. *Sleep, 15,* 143–149.

Driver, H. S., & Taylor, S. R. (1993). Dealing with sleep disorders: Sleep patterns in women with regard to the menstrual cycle, pregnancy, and menopause. *Journal of the Society of Obstetricians and Gynecologists of Canada, 15*(7), S17–S19.

Engle-Friedman, M., Bootzin, R. R., Hazlewood, L., et al. (1992). An evaluation of behavioral treatments for insomnia in the older adult. *J Clin Psychol, 48*(1), 77–90.

Gates, D., et al. (1989). Night terrors: Strategies for family coping. *Journal of Pediatric Nursing, 4*(1), 48–53.

George, C. F. (1994). Cardiovascular disease and sleep. In M. H. Kryger, T. Roth, & W. C. Dement (Eds.), *Principles and practice of sleep medicine* (2nd ed.) (pp. 835–846). Philadelphia: W. B. Saunders.

Graeber, R. C. (1994). Jetlag and sleep disruption. In M. H. Kryger, T. Roth, & W. C. Dement (Eds.), *Principles and practice of sleep medicine* (2nd ed.) (pp. 463–470). Philadelphia: W. B. Saunders.

Harrington, M. E., Rusak, B., & Mistlberger, R. E. (1994). Anatomy and physiology of the mammalian circadian system. In M. H. Kryger, T. Roth, & W. C. Dement (Eds.), *Principles and practice of sleep medicine* (2nd ed.) (pp. 286–300). Philadelphia: W. B. Saunders.

Hauri, P. (1982). *The sleep disorders: Current concepts* (2nd ed.). Kalmazoo, MI: Upjohn.

Hauri, P. (1994). Primary insomnia. In M. H. Kryger, T. Roth, & W. C. Dement (Eds.), *Principles and practice of sleep medicine* (2nd ed.) (pp. 494–499). Philadelphia: W. B. Saunders.

Hodgson, L. A. (1991). Why do we need sleep? Relating theory to nursing practice. *J Adv Nurs, 16,* 1503–1510.

Horne, J. A. (1988). *Why we sleep.* New York: Oxford University Press.

Horne, J. A., & Staff, L. H. (1983). Exercise and sleep: Body-heating effects. *Sleep, 6*(1), 36–46.

Johnson, M. W., & Remmers, J. E. (1984). Accessory muscle activity during sleep in chronic obstructive pulmonary disease. *J Appl Physiol, 57,*1011–1017.

Keefe, M. (1987). Comparison of neonatal nighttime sleep–wake patterns in nursery versus rooming-in environments. *Nurs Res, 36,* 140–144.

Kripke, H., Simons, R., Garfinkel, L., et al. (1979). Short and long acting sleeping pills: Is increased mortality associated? *Arch Gen Psychiatry, 36,* 103–116.

Monk, T. H. (1994). Shift work. In M. H. Kryger, T. Roth, & W. C. Dement (Eds.), *Principles and practice of sleep medicine* (2nd ed.) (pp. 471–476). Philadelphia: W. B. Saunders.

Nicholson, A. N. (1994). Hypnotics: Clinical pharmacology and therapeutics. In M. H. Kryger, T. Roth, & W. C. Dement (Eds.), *Principles and practice of sleep medicine* (2nd ed.) (pp. 355–363). Philadelphia: W. B. Saunders.

Nicholson, A. N., Bradley, C. M., & Pascoe, P. A. (1994). Medications: Effect on sleep and wakefulness. In M. H. Kryger, T. Roth, & W. C. Dement (Eds.), *Principles and practice of sleep medicine* (2nd ed.) (pp. 364–372). Philadelphia: W. B. Saunders.

North American Nursing Diagnosis Association (NANDA). (1994). *Nursing diagnoses: Definitions and classification 1995–1996.* Philadelphia: Author.

Oswald, I. (1987). The benefit of sleep. *Holistic Medicine, 2,* 137–139.

Porth, C. (1994). *Pathophysiology: Concepts of altered health states* (4th ed.). Philadelphia: J. B. Lippincott.

Reimer, M. (1985). *Nursing interventions perceived by patients and their nurses as facilitating nocturnal sleep in hospital.* Unpublished manuscript.

Robinson, C. (1993). Impaired sleep. In V. K. Carrieri, A. M. Lindsey, & C. M. West (Eds.), *Pathophysiological phenomena in nursing* (2nd ed.) (pp. 390–417). Philadelphia: W. B. Saunders.

Roehrs, T., Zorick, F., & Roth, T. (1994). Transient and short-term insomnia. In M. H. Kryger, T. Roth, & W. C. Dement (Eds.), *Principles and practice of sleep medicine* (2nd ed.) (pp. 486–493). Philadelphia: W. B. Saunders.

Shaver, J. L. F., & Giblin, E. C. (1989). Sleep. *Annual Review of Nursing Research, 7,* 71–93.

Snyder-Halpern, R. (1985). The effect of critical care unit noise on patient sleep cycles. *Critical Care Quarterly,* 41–51.

Stewart, A. (1991). The sleep apnea/hypopnea syndrome. *Canadian Nurse, 87*(10), 25–27.

Trilling, J. S. (1989). Nighttime waking in children: A disease of civilization. *Family Systems Medicine, 7*(1), 17–29.

Verran, J. A., et al. (1988). Do patients sleep in the hospital? *Applied Nursing Research, 1*(2), 95.

Wirz-Justice, A., & Pringle, C. (1987). The non-entrained life of a young gentleman at Oxford. *Sleep, 10,* 57–61.

Zarcone, V. P. (1994). Sleep hygiene. In M. H. Kryger, T. Roth, & W. C. Dement (Eds.), *Principles and practice of sleep medicine* (2nd ed.) (pp. 542–546). Philadelphia: W. B. Saunders.

Bibliography

Balsmeyer, B. (1990). Sleep disturbances of the infant and toddler. *Pediatric Nursing, 16,* 447–452.

Brugne, J. R. (1994). Sleep, wakefulness and the nurse. *British Journal of Nursing, 3*(2), 68–71.

Clore, E. R., & Hibel, J. (1993). The parasomnias of childhood. *Journal of Pediatric Health Care, 7*(1), 12–16.

Coco, P. (1990). Bereavement questions and answers . . . various sleep pattern disturbances related to grief. *Advances in Clinical Care, 5*(2), 44.

Cosnett, J. E. (1992). Charles Dickens: Observer of sleep and its disorders. *Sleep, 15,* 222–226.

Culver, B. H. (1989). Pulmonary responses to sleep. *Respiratory Care, 34,* 510–516.

Davis-Sharts, J. (1989). The elder and critical care: Sleep and mobility issues. *Nurs Clin North Am, 24,* 755–767.

Jensen, D. P., & Herr, K. A. (1993). Sleeplessness. *Nurs Clin North Am, 28,* 385–405.

Johnson, J. E. (1993). Progressive relaxation and the sleep of older men and women. *Journal of Community Health Nursing, 10*(1), 31–38.

Kedas, A., et al. (1989). A critical review of aging and sleep research. *Western Journal of Nursing Research, 1*(2), 95.

Knapp, M. (1993). Night shift: The restorative sleep specialists. *Journal of Gerontological Nursing, 19*(5), 38–42.

Littrell, K., et al. (1989). Promoting sleep for the patient with a myocardial infarction. *Critical Care Nursing, 9*(3), 44, 46–49.

Roberts, A. (1990). Senior systems . . . older patients and their medication . . . sleep and sleep difficulties in later life: Part 46. *Nursing Times, 86* (11): *Systems of Life* No. 181:61–64.

White, M. A., et al. (1988). Distress and self-soothing bedtime behaviors in hospitalized children with non–rooming-in parents. *Matern Child Nurs J, 17*(2), 67–77.

Cognition and Perception

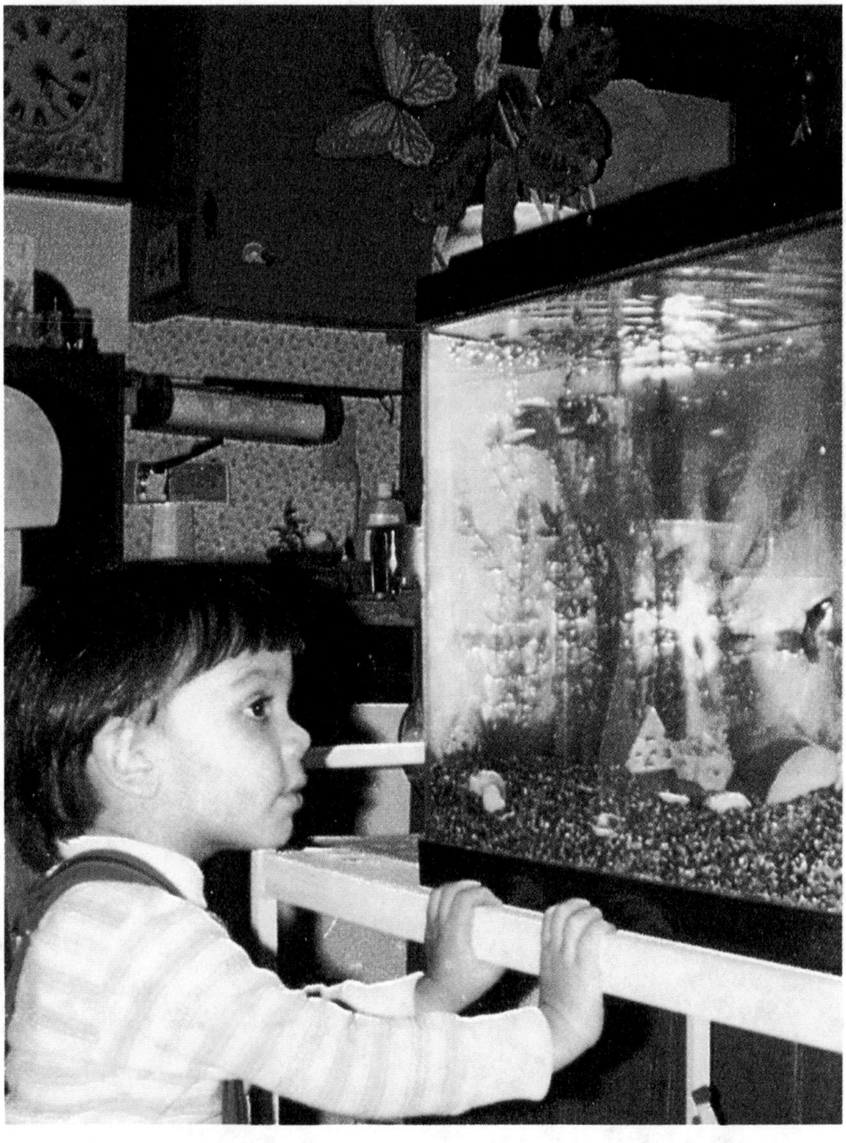

UNIT XII

Cognition and perception affect many other aspects of function; they are of particular concern in the elderly population. Unit XII explores these areas of human function and the nursing responsibilities associated with them.

Chapter 44 considers all aspects of pain perception and comfort. Pain relief is a primary nursing responsibility that involves both independent nursing actions and nursing interventions resulting from physician's orders. Pain relief techniques include physical pain relief techniques, cognitive pain relief techniques, behavioral pain relief techniques, pharmacologic management, and invasive medical management. Holistic nursing care is essential for meaningful interaction with the environment. The challenge for the nurse is to avoid both deprivation and overload. Many elderly clients enter the healthcare system with decreased sensory function, although this may not be the reason they seek healthcare. The final chapter in this unit explores cognitive processes. Normal cognitive function is necessary to meaningfully process information. Many clients who enter a healthcare facility have altered processes to some degree. The nurse must be able to meet the needs of clients who cannot always make their needs known.

The chapters in this unit discuss issues relating to how well a client perceives stimuli and interacts with his or her environment. As the population ages, the number of clients with these nursing care needs will increase.

Pain Perception and Comfort

Key Terms

Acute pain
Allodynia
Biofeedback
Contralateral stimulation
Chronic pain
Endogenous
Exogenous
Hyperalgesia
Malignant pain
Neural plasticity
Neuropathic pain
Nociceptors
Pain threshold
Pain tolerance
Spinal dorsal horn
Suffering
Titration
Transcutaneous electrical nerve stimulation

Learning Objectives

Upon completion of this chapter, the student will be able to do the following:

- *Explain how pain sensation is transmitted.*
- *Outline how pain transmission is facilitated or inhibited.*
- *Describe the four sensory pain components that must be included in the nursing database.*
- *Examine nonpharmcologic methods of pain relief based on individual needs.*
- *Describe the types, actions, and side effects of analgesics.*
- *List nursing implications for various classes of drugs used for pain management.*
- *Develop a nursing plan of care for surgical clients with problems related to pain.*

44

You are a home care/hospice nurse caring for an older client who was diagnosed 3 months ago with non–small-cell cancer of the left lung. The client's history is positive for lung cancer (father died from it) and smoking one to two packs of cigarettes per day for 50 years. At diagnosis, staging revealed metastases in the right lung, bilateral kidneys, and the sixth cervical vertebra. The client reports pain in the left shoulder, upper arm, and the right upper thigh. The client rates the pain as 6 on a 0-to-10 scale and describes it as dull and aching, but the client is unable to provide further description of its quality. The shoulder pain is reported as constant but increases with particular movements. The right leg pain is present only when the client ambulates and when she turns onto the left side when in bed. Ability to tolerate activity has diminished since radiation treatments began. Before treatment, the client was out of bed 14 to 16 hours per day, but now the client is out of bed 3 to 5 hours per day.

You have studied the nursing process and medications. When you combine these with the information about pain in this chapter, you will have a broader knowledge base for caring for clients suffering from pain. You will learn how to assess pain, which is different to different people. You will learn a variety of therapies to help the client manage pain. When you have completed the chapter, you will be able to address the Critical Thinking Challenges at the end of the chapter.

Pain, one of the most complex human experiences, is an invisible phenomenon influenced by the interaction of affective (emotional), behavioral, cognitive, and physiologic-sensory factors. Because pain is a highly individual experience, the basis for pain management by the nurse is simply the client's description of pain. Pain exists whenever the person says it does (McCaffery & Beebe, 1989).

Normal Function of Pain

Pain serves a protective function. It alerts the person to potentially harmful stimuli and elicits escape, immobilization, and other behaviors to protect uninjured tissue. Pain is one of the most common and compelling reasons that people seek healthcare. Understanding the mechanisms of pain processing and the phenomenon of pain helps the nurse to intervene effectively.

Structures Related to the Pain Process

Pain is perceived in the brain as a result of complex processing of stimuli from a site of injury or potential injury. The perception of pain sensation is the result of many different inputs.

Peripheral Structures

Sensory receptors of pain, or **nociceptors,** are free nerve endings in the tissue that respond to tissue-injuring stimuli (*noxious stimuli*). Receptors that respond to noxious temperature changes (*thermoreceptors*), chemicals (*chemoreceptors*), or pressure (*mechanical receptors*) transmit a pain signal if the stimuli are sufficiently strong.

Nociceptors are found in the skin, blood vessels, subcutaneous tissue, muscle, fascia, periosteum, viscera, joints, and other structures (Woolf, 1994). Nociceptors are located on two types of peripheral nerve cells (A-delta fibers and C-fibers) that are responsible for transmitting pain sensations from the tissues to the central nervous system (Fig. 44-1). A-delta fibers give rise to bright, sharp, well-localized pain that is immediately associated with the injury. Slow-conducting C-fibers cause a second pain sensation that is dull, poorly localized, and persistent after injury.

The difference between pain from A-delta and C-fiber activation can best be described as first versus second pain. For example, if a sharp object falls on your foot, a fast, sharp pain alerts you to the injury. This is caused by stimulation of the A-delta fibers. After the object is moved from the foot, a burning, dull, aching sensation persists and is caused by stimulation of the C-fibers.

Central Structures

Ascending Pathways. Signal transmission from the peripheral nociceptive fibers to the brain is complex. Signals carried by A-delta fibers and C-fibers travel along the fibers from peripheral tissues through the dorsal root of the spinal cord and terminate in the dorsal horn of the spinal cord (Meyer, Campbell, & Raja, 1994). Signals communicate with local interneurons (excitatory and inhibitory) and neurons with long axons (*projection cells*) that ascend to the brain by way of several crossed and uncrossed pathways. The spinothalamic tract appears to be the most important pathway for pain sensation. It is a crossed pathway located in the white matter of the anterolateral quadrant of the spinal cord (see Fig. 44-1). The spinothalamic tract transmits sensations of pain and temperature and crudely localized touch. The spinothalamic tract enters the brain stem and terminates principally in the thalamus, where other neurons convey the information to the sensory cortex. Projection cells in other pathways play a role in activating descending control of dorsal horn neurons (Woolf, 1994).

Descending Pathways. Several pathways convey information from the brain to the spinal dorsal horn (Fields & Basbaum, 1994). Pain perception can be modulated by this information from the brain. Descending in the lateral white columns, a third of corticospinal tract neurons terminate on neurons in the spinal dorsal horn and modify afferent nociceptive information (ie, allow the brain to pay selective attention to certain stimuli and to ignore other painful stimuli).

Normal Physiology of Pain

The afferent nociceptive message (to the central nervous system and brain) is subject to modulation (both enhancement and inhibition) at all levels of the nervous system. Modulation at the peripheral nerve, the spinal cord, and several brain sites influences pain perception. The capacity for modulation helps to explain the tremendous variability in pain experienced by people with similar types of injury.

Peripheral Modulation

Nociceptors usually are stimulated by mechanical, chemical, or thermal events that injure tissue (Meyer, et al., 1994). Injured cells and tissue-repair mechanisms release one or more chemical substances that bind to

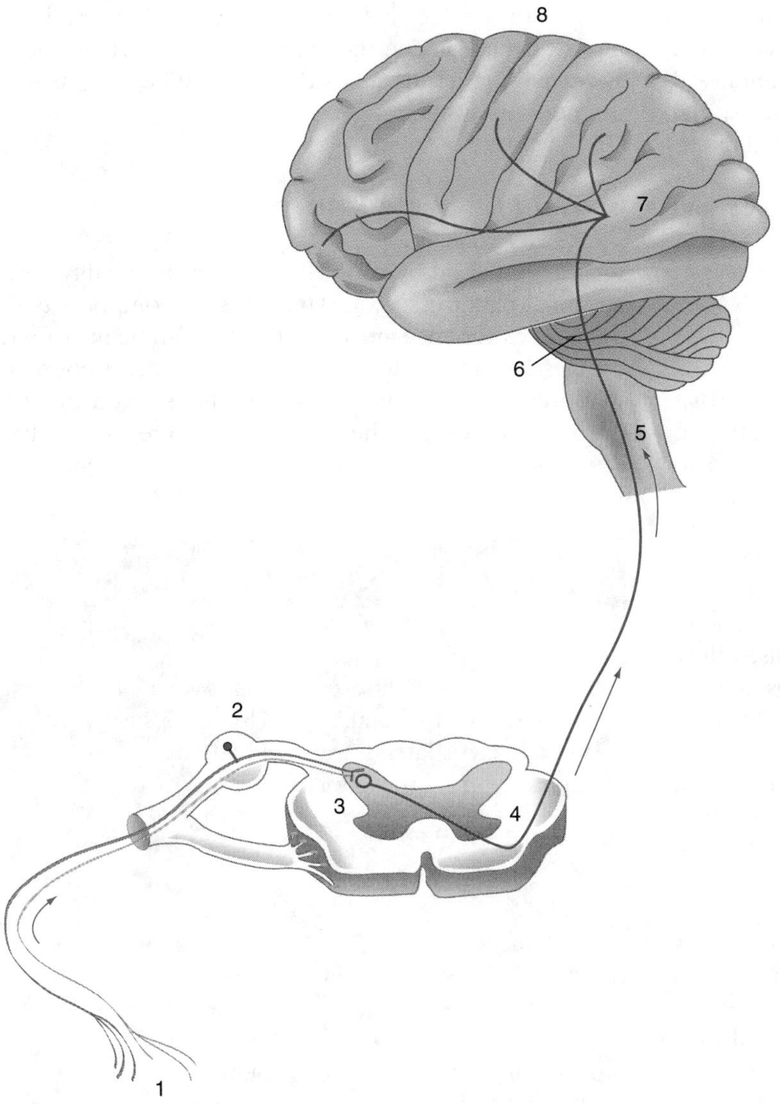

Figure 44-1 • *Pain stimuli are transmitted from pain receptors (1) via sensory nerves into the dorsal root ganglia (2). The impulse enters the spinal cord, and synapses terminate on neuron cells in the substantia gelatinosa (3). Signals then cross the cord and ascend in the spinothalamic tract (4), through the reticular formation (5) and areas of the midbrain (6) to the thalamus (7) and cortex (8). Pain is perceived somewhere in the brain.*

peripheral nociceptors and activate the nerve fiber (cause an action potential). Some chemicals activate the nerve fiber, and others sensitize the nerve to be activated with a smaller stimulus than usually required (Levine & Taiwo, 1994). These chemicals cause A-delta and C-fibers to be excited and transmit an action potential toward the spinal cord. Presence of these chemicals increases the amount of pain perceived. Blocking release or production of these chemicals, some of which are part of the inflammatory response, is one peripheral mechanism to inhibit pain perception. Another way to inhibit pain is through blockade of the sodium channels on the A-delta or C-fibers to prevent transmission of the action potential to the spinal cord, such as by use of local anesthetic agents.

Spinal Cord Modulation

One of the most important areas for pain modulation is the **spinal dorsal horn**, where complex processing of messages occurs (Woolf, 1994). Input to dorsal horn excitatory interneurons releases neurotensin and glutamate, both of which have the potential to facilitate pain sensation (Yaksh & Malmberg, 1994). Input to inhibitory interneurons and from descending neurons releases a number of neurochemicals that have inhibitory effects on pain sensations. These neurochemicals bind to several types of receptors (Yaksh & Malmberg, 1994). The opioid receptors are sites where **endogenous** (produced by the body) opioids and **exogenous** (administered to the person) opioids bind and are important to inhibition of pain perception. Three groups of endogenous opioids have been identified: enkephalins, endorphins, and dynorphins. Their exact roles throughout the nervous system are under investigation, but they contribute to analgesia and side effects produced by opioids.

Spinal Reflexes

Some sensory impulses that enter the spinal cord produce a reflex response through motor neurons in the spinal ventral horn with fibers to a muscle near the pain site. The muscle then contracts in a protective action (for instance, a pinprick causes immediate withdrawal of the extremity). Pain may be enhanced by these spinal reflexes through an effect on the injured tissue. For example, trauma may provoke an efferent (motor) reflex that produces muscle spasm in the injured area and causes more pain.

Pain Theories

Many theories have been developed to describe the complex phenomenon of pain. The *gate control theory,* developed by Melzack and Wall (1965), was the first to incorporate some aspects from other theories and to present the notion of pain modulation at the spinal cord and brain levels. According to this theory, dorsal horn cells act as a gate, closing to prevent nociceptive impulses from reaching the brain or opening to allow impulses to be transmitted to the brain (Fig. 44-2). In simple terms, when the gate is open, pain impulses flow through, and pain is felt. When the gate is closed, pain impulses are stopped. Opening the gate is influenced by the A-delta and C-fibers, and closing the gate is influenced by the activity of the large A-alpha and A-beta fibers, the reticular formation in the brain stem, other brain sites, and the cerebral cortex (Melzack & Wall, 1965; Wall & Melzack, 1994).

The gate control theory emphasizes sensory, emotional, behavioral, and cognitive dimensions of pain as playing a role in modulation of the physiologic dimension. The theory stimulated much of the research to understand what is now known about normal processing of nociceptive information and the altered processing that occurs in persistent, unrelieved pain states. Many of the mechanisms suggested by the gate control theory are specifically known today, others are still being investigated. The theory, however, provided ideas about pain relief therapies that act in different parts of the nervous system.

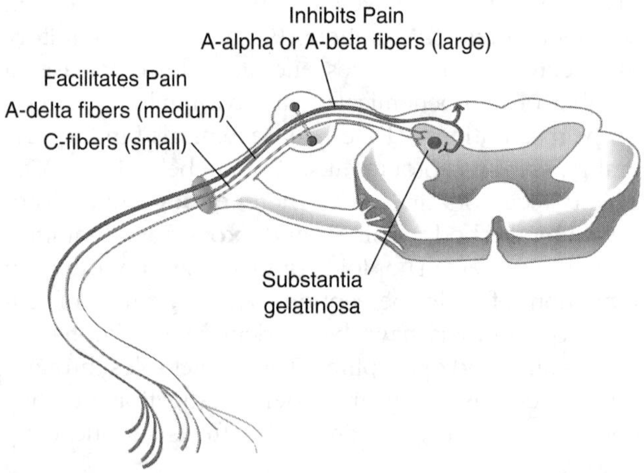

Figure 44-2 • *In the gate control theory, small fibers carry pain impulses (opening the gate) that may be modulated by other sensations from the large fiber, thus closing the gate to the transmission of pain.*

Sensory Characteristics of Pain

Pain is described by its location, intensity, quality, and temporal pattern (see display). Sensory components of the pain experience are subjective but can be measured using standardized tools. One person's description of pain intensity may differ from another's, even though the pain stimuli are the same; this difference emphasizes the role of pain modulation in the unique per-

Descriptions of Pain

Location	
Localized versus diffuse	Right versus left
Proximal versus distal	Upper versus lower
Medial versus lateral	Phantom
Anterior versus posterior	Referred
Intensity	
Mild	
Slight	Severe
Moderate	Excruciating
Quality	
Aching	Sickening
Annoying	Stabbing
Burning	Tender
Exhausting	Terrifying
Gnawing	Throbbing
Heavy	Tight
Intense	Tiring
Nagging	Torturing
Sharp	Unbearable
Shooting	
Temporal Pattern	
Acute	Intermittent
Chronic	Spasmodic
Constant	Transient
Associated Characteristics	
Anger and aggression	Muscle spasms
Anorexia	Nausea and vomiting
Anxiety	
Depression	Regression
Fatigue	Visual disturbance
Fear	Withdrawal

sonal experience. There are, however, some commonalities in location, quality, and temporal pattern when similar types of pain are experienced.

Location

Superficial pain that emanates from the skin or from tissues close to the surface is usually localized, and the client's pain location report matches the location of tissue damage. However, when pain originates from internal organs, the location reported may not be localized in the area of tissue damage. For example, pain from the abdominal or pelvic organs (liver, spleen, kidney, bladder) may be referred to areas far distant from the site of tissue damage (Fig 44-3). If referred pain is not considered when evaluating pain location report, therapy could be misdirected.

Intensity

Pain intensity indicates the magnitude or amount of pain perceived. Terms used to describe pain severity include none, mild, slight, moderate, severe, and excruciating. Pain intensity also may be described on a numeric scale: for example, on a scale of 0 to 10, 0 would be no pain, and 10 would be pain as bad as it could be.

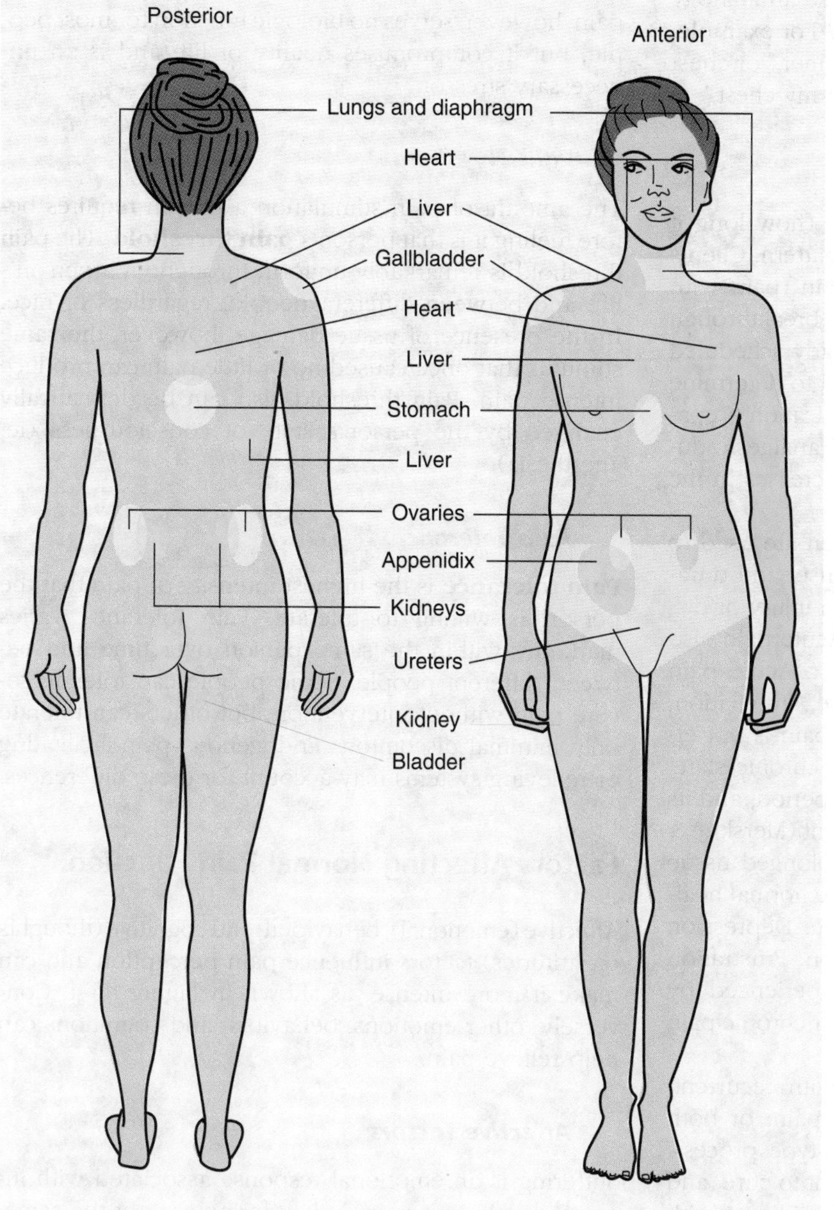

Figure 44-3 • *Common referred pain sites. These anterior and posterior views of the body show where a client might feel pain referred from various visceral organs.*

Pain intensity may vary among clients, depending on their previous experience with pain, personal expectations, ability to be distracted or to concentrate on other things, level of consciousness, and activity level. Fear of the consequences of reporting pain intensity may cause clients to minimize their reported pain. Level of activity also influences pain intensity. A person may have no pain at rest or when lying still but have severe pain with the slightest movement, such as shifting positions or deep breathing.

Quality

Pain quality is how the pain feels to the client or words that describe the nature of the pain. When presented with a list of verbal descriptors, clients frequently use words such as those listed in the display. Without a list of descriptors, many clients find it easier to use an analogy than to find words that describe the pain. For example, a headache may be "pounding like a hammer," or chest pain may be "like an elephant sitting on my chest."

Temporal Pattern

Pain onset (when it starts) and duration (how long it lasts) are components of temporal pain pattern. Clients may have pain all the time, incident pain (pain with movement or specific procedures), or breakthrough pain (pain that returns before the regularly scheduled analgesic dose). Pain pattern can be used to determine the appropriate dosing schedule and medication preparation. Return of pain before the end of analgesic duration of a drug suggests the need for increases in the amount or frequency of the drug.

The terms "acute" and "chronic" often are used to designate the two main types of pain onset and duration. **Acute pain** occurs abruptly after an injury or disease and persists until healing occurs. Acute pain also may be associated with anxiety and fear. Acute pain consistently increases during wound care, ambulation, coughing, and deep breathing. If acute pain is not effectively managed, it may progress to a chronic state.

Chronic pain lasts for a prolonged period, and its cause is not amenable to specific treatment (Merskey & Bogduk, 1994). It is associated with prolonged tissue pathology or pain that persists beyond the normal healing period for an acute injury or disease. Depression related to chronic pain is not uncommon. Frustration and fear also are common feelings experienced by clients when no identifiable cause for their chronic pain can be determined.

Malignant pain is a third type, with recurrent, acute pain episodes, persistent chronic pain, or both associated with a progressive malignant-type process. The etiology for malignant pain is resistant to cure, and the pain may be described as intractable. Clients with malignant pain often describe it as all-consuming and interfering with their quality of life. Examples of causes of malignant pain are arthritis or cancer. Like chronic and acute pain, malignant pain often increases at night.

Normal Function of Pain Perception

Although pain is a great source of human misery, initially it serves an important biologic purpose: It helps to minimize injury and is often a protective mechanism to prevent injury. For instance, pain makes a person pull a hand away from a hot stove, and right lower abdominal pain warns the person of a possible diseased appendix, prompting early medical intervention. People who are born without the ability to feel pain do not usually survive past early childhood: Death occurs because of the lack of warning of injury or disease and the delay of prompt treatment. Persistent, unrelieved pain, however, serves no biologic function for most people, but it compromises quality of life and is an unnecessary stressor.

Pain Threshold

The amount of pain stimulation a person requires before feeling it is that person's **pain threshold.** The pain threshold is remarkably uniform throughout a person's life and between different people, regardless of race. In the presence of tissue damage, however, the same stimulus that once caused no or little pain can produce intense pain. Pain threshold also can be dramatically changed by the person's state of consciousness (ie, anesthesia).

Pain Tolerance

Pain tolerance is the highest intensity of pain that the person is willing to tolerate. Pain tolerance varies markedly within the same person over time and between different people. Some people can tolerate severe pain without intervention, but others can tolerate only minimal discomfort. Endogenous pain-facilitating or relieving systems may account for these differences.

Factors Affecting Normal Pain Function

Affective (emotional), behavioral, and cognitive (thoughts or attitudes) factors influence pain perception and can make it more intense, as shown in Figure 44-4. Conversely, other emotions, behaviors, and cognitions can help relieve pain.

Affective Factors

Suffering is an emotional response associated with increased pain, but pain and suffering are not the same. **Suffering** is associated with events that threaten the in-

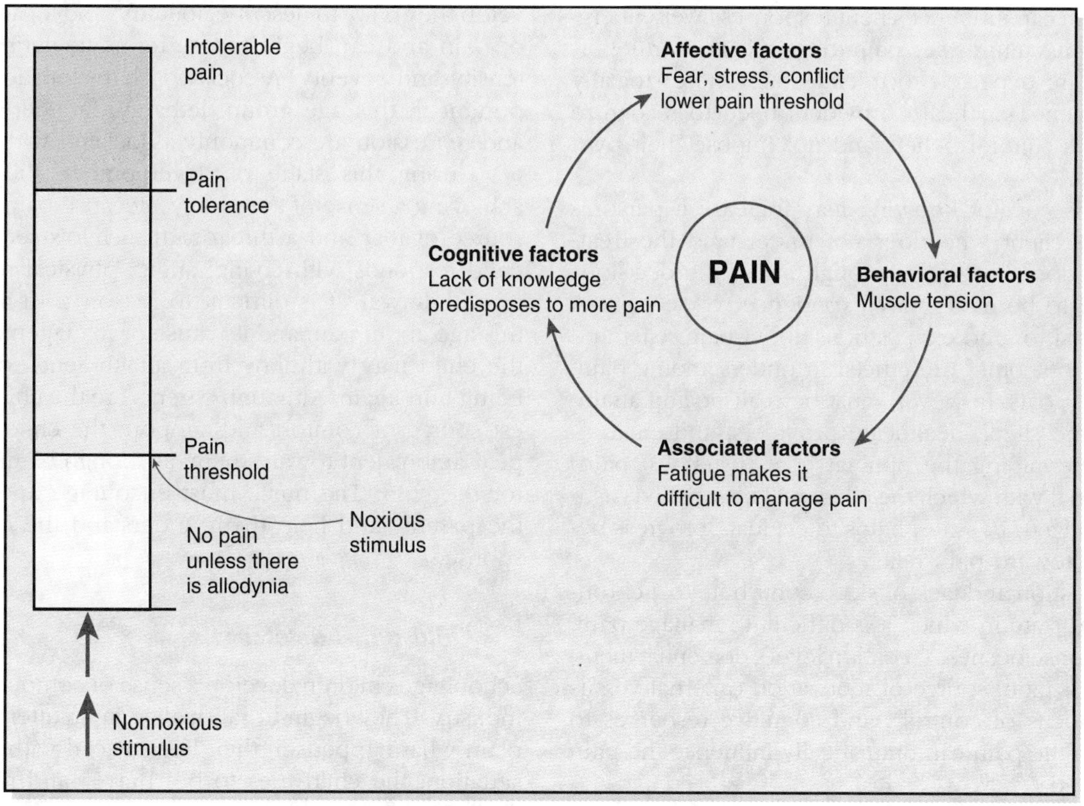

Figure 44-4 • *Factors affecting normal pain function. Pain is a normal function of the body. It warns the body of injury and disease. Factors can lower the pain threshold and pain tolerance, and a cycle of pain can follow.*

tactness of a person (Cassell, 1989), whereas pain is associated with events that threaten tissue (Merskey & Bogduk, 1994). People can suffer with no pain, have pain with no suffering, or have pain and suffering at the same time (Ferrell, 1993). Assessments and treatments for pain and suffering can be quite different.

Clients with unrelieved pain often have concurrent emotional responses, such as anger, fear, anxiety, sadness, or depression that can intensify pain perception. Emotions such as joy and pleasure may decrease the amount of pain perceived. Emotional factors can play a powerful role in pain perception. Helping clients understand the link between emotions and pain perception is an important role for nurses in all care settings.

Behavioral Factors

Many different behaviors are associated with pain; some aggravate the pain, but others alleviate it. Clients with pain notice that certain activities can cause pain to be noticed or increased. These activities often are avoided, but this avoidance may not be in the client's best long-term interest. Pain may interfere with usual behaviors that bring the client joy and satisfaction. When many activities are prevented by cancer pain, the client may experience increased emotional distress, such as anxiety. Clients also engage in a number of behaviors to control their pain (reduce pain, prevent pain onset, reduce pain duration, and tolerate the pain). For example, watching television or talking with friends, staff, or family members helps to distract clients from their pain and can be effective in helping to control it. How clients comply with or adjust analgesic therapy plans also is an important aspect of pain behavior.

Emotional responses to pain, such as fear and anxiety, increase muscle tension, which increases pain perception and intensity. Fear of the unknown also may worsen pain because of the tension and anxiety that the client brings to the situation. For instance, a toddler fearing an injection will cry and tense his or her muscles, thus intensifying the pain. It is not uncommon for aggressive behavior to be a way of "fighting back" against the pain. At the other extreme, the person in pain may withdraw from it by minimizing interaction with the environment and other people. Regression to earlier stages of development may occur.

Pain can be fatiguing, and fatigue can predispose the client to pain. What might be tolerable to a well-rested person may be intolerable to a fatigued person.

Cognitive Factors

Meanings associated with a disease (eg, cancer) and pain, along with beliefs, attitudes, and expectations about them can influence client responses (Weisenberg, 1994). Many cultures see pain tolerance as a virtue; often men are expected to tolerate pain more stoically than women. Healthcare providers need to recognize the client's cultural beliefs and not impose their own judgments.

A sense of not knowing may increase a person's pain. The client who does not understand the treatments or does not know enough about the decisions that need to be made may experience worse pain. A client's goal for and expectations about pain relief and treatment outcomes are crucial in understanding pain. Treatment goals, however, must be realistic and attainable for the client, healthcare providers, and environment. Determining the optimal goal (usually 0 pain) and the goal with which the client will be satisfied (usually 1–4 on a 0–10 scale) helps to evaluate progress being made toward pain relief.

Exhaustion and lack of sleep contribute to a chronically tired state in which it is difficult to manage pain. Level of consciousness (sedation level), dementia, memory of past pain, source of motivation (internal versus external locus of control), and cognitive resources to cope with the pain can dramatically influence the pain experienced.

Coping with pain includes cognitive and some behavioral activities. In general, when clients actively engage in behaviors to cope with the pain, they are less likely to be debilitated by it. Clients who focus on how terrible the pain is (coping by catastrophizing) are more likely to have functional and emotional problems related to the pain. Examples of coping strategies are listed in the accompanying display on the next page.

Lifespan Considerations

Newborn and Infant

A neonate or infant cannot verbally report pain. Although it was formerly believed that newborns' neurophysiologic systems were too immature to transport pain impulses, researchers have learned that newborns can perceive pain, although measuring it is difficult. Neonates respond to pain with increased sensitivity at birth with whole body movement (Fitzgerald, 1994). Within 3 seconds of a heel lance, the newborn begins to cry and cries for an average of 3 minutes, with a heart rate of 50 beats/min over baseline (Owens, 1986).

As infants develop more motor control, they try to pull or roll away from the pain and show general physical resistance. The behavioral or emotional reactions of the parents or the nurse may influence the infant's response. Endogenous pain inhibition develops after birth when large fibers become myelinated (Fitzgerald, 1994).

Toddler and Preschooler

Toddlers cannot identify the pain they are experiencing or its source. Older toddlers and preschoolers develop the ability to describe, identify, and locate sources of pain and can begin to use terms to define the intensity and severity. Associated characteristics are important in this age group: lethargy, fatigue, anorexia, and regression are commonly associated with pain.

During this stage of development, the child is achieving a sense of autonomy. Because pain can be a source of fear and a threat to the child's security, the child responds with crying, anger, physical resistance, or withdrawal. It is difficult to reason with a child of this age about pain and its cause or management; thus, the child may withdraw from attachments for fear of being hurt again. Although parents are the child's greatest source of comfort and support, the child may appear ambivalent toward them, as though blaming them for the pain. The nurse must encourage and support the parents and help them understand the child's response.

Child and Adolescent

School-age children develop a sense of competence and industry. They begin to rationalize in an attempt to explain what happens in their lives. Faced with a painful situation, the child tries to be "brave" and rationalize the pain; he or she is more responsive to explanations about the pain than a younger child. School-age children can identify the specific location, intensity, quality, and temporal pattern of pain (Savedra, Holzemer, Tesler, Ward, & Wilkie, 1993). If pain persists, the school-age child may temporarily regress to an earlier stage of development in an attempt to handle the situation. For example, the young school-age child may temporarily lose bladder control and may revert to comfort measures, such as thumb-sucking, nail-biting, and favorite toys.

Because adolescents are developing an identity and personal independence, their physical appearance and abilities are important. When coupled with concern about peer relationships, adolescents demonstrate careful self-control and may be reluctant to acknowledge pain. To recognize or "give in" to pain may seem a sign of weakness. For example, a high-school football player

Children Learn by Familial Role Modeling

- What pains are and are not appropriate to talk about
- Appropriate and inappropriate behavior when in pain
- What circumstances cause pain and should be avoided
- Methods to avoid or relieve pain
- Reasons we experience pain (eg, punishment, testing, bad thoughts)
- Possible consequences of pain

Examples of Pain Coping Strategies

Active Cognitive Coping Strategies

Reinterpreting the Pain Sensation

I don't think of it as pain but rather as a dull or warm feeling.
I try not to think of it as my body but rather as something separate from me.
I pretend it's not a part of me.

Diverting Attention From the Pain

I try to think of something pleasant.
I count numbers in my mind or run a song through my mind.
I play mental games with myself to keep my mind off the pain.
I replay in my mind pleasant experiences in the past.

Ignoring the Pain

I don't think about the pain.
I tell myself it doesn't hurt.
I pretend it's not there.
I just go on as if nothing happened.

Coping Self-Statements

I tell myself to be brave and carry on despite the pain.
I tell myself that I can overcome the pain.
I tell myself I can't let the pain stand in the way of what I have to do.
No matter how bad it gets, I know I can handle it.

Passive Cognitive Coping Strategies

Praying/Hoping

I know someday someone will be here to help me, and it will go away for awhile.
I pray to God it won't last long.
I try to think what everything will be like after I've gotten rid of the pain.
I have faith in doctors that someday there will be a cure for my pain.

Catastrophizing (associated with severe emotional distress and functional status)

It's terrible, and I feel it's never going to get any better.
I worry all the time about whether it will end.
I feel my life isn't worth living.
I feel I can't stand it anymore.

Behavioral Coping Strategies

I do anything to get my mind off the pain.
I do something active, like household chores or projects.
I try to be around other people.
I leave the house and do something, such as going to the movies or shopping.

From: Rosenstiel, A. K., & Keefe, F. J. (1983). The use of coping strategies in low back pain patients: Relationship to patient characteristics and current adjustments. *Pain, 17,* 33–44.

may know that his knee is injured, but he may prefer to deny the pain in an effort to be a "team player" and not let down his team, coach, or school.

Adult and Older Adult

Adult responses to pain vary. For some adults, like adolescents, giving in to pain may be a sign of weakness or failure; hence, they may ignore the normal warning function of pain. Other adults may respond to the warning and take appropriate action, such as making lifestyle changes and getting a medical check-up. Fear of what the pain may indicate prevents some adults from taking action.

The older adult presents other problems, often because of misconceptions about the effects of aging on pain perception. An older person who is well instructed in the use of pain measurement tools and without diseases (eg, diabetes) affecting the nervous system tends to report pain intensity similar to younger people (Harkins, Price, Bush, & Small, 1994). In the presence of decreased sensation associated with peripheral nerve disease (diabetic neuropathy), however, an older person is likely not to sense pain. Older age is associated with chronic health problems, increased risk for musculoskeletal pain, depression, and limitations in activities of daily living. Increased pain intensity has been noted, particularly when adequate treatment is not provided for chronic and recurrent pain. Treatment of pain in the older person is as likely to be successful as treatment in a younger person.

A condition that would produce acute pain in some younger people may remain virtually undetected in some older people until complications occur. For example, an older person experiencing a myocardial infarction may complain of excess gas, an upset stomach, or extreme fatigue rather than the crushing chest pain identified by younger adults. In this situation, the complication of congestive heart failure may be the first indicator of the older person's primary problem. However, pain is the most frequent presenting symptom of acute myocardial infarction in older (61%) and younger (77%) clients (McDonald, Baillie, Williams, & Ballantyne, 1983). The frequency of silent myocardial infarctions in older people has been overestimated.

Altered Function Resulting in Pain

Initially pain is a normal protective function, but persistent, unrelieved pain serves no useful purpose (Woolf, 1994). Unrelieved pain can be harmful to recovery, lead to abnormal anatomic and genetic changes, and interfere with quality of life. Pain even can kill (Liebeskind, 1991). Recent findings indicate that chronic pain can lead to early death and decreases in natural killer cell activity (an immune response). Processes such as peripheral and central sensitization and regenerative neuronal growth produce pathophysiologic pain that leads to some of the detrimental effects of pain.

Potential for Altered Function: Nervous System Plasticity

Allodynia and hyperalgesia are two types of dynamic nervous system plasticity (nervous system adaptation after pain). These abnormal sensations occur with tissue injury that lead to inflammation. **Allodynia** is an enhanced sensation of pain produced by an innocuous stimulus, such as light touch. **Hyperalgesia** is an enhanced sensation of pain produced by a noxious stimulus. For example, inflamed pharyngeal tissue produces allodynia type pain on swallowing, and micturition produces allodynia type pain when a person has a urinary tract infection. Swallowing very hot fluid would produce hyperalgesic pain in inflamed pharyngeal tissue. Plasticity in the peripheral and central nervous systems are involved with these types of pain.

Peripheral Sensitization

Allodynia and primary hyperalgesia result from adaptation in the peripheral nervous system, or peripheral sensitization (Coderre, et al., 1993). Three characteristics of sensitization are a decrease in the threshold at which the nerve is activated, an enlarged response to noxious thermal or chemical stimuli, and ongoing spontaneous activity in the A-delta and C-fibers. Additionally, a decreased response to non-noxious mechanical stimuli by A-beta fibers (eg, touch) is a characteristic of sensitization (Meyer, et al., 1994). An example of peripheral sensitization is pain produced by the weight of bed linens or clothing (light pressure) in a person with a sunburn.

Central Sensitization

Allodynia and secondary hyperalgesia result from adaptation in the central nervous system, or central sensitization. This type of sensitization is important not only in pain from tissue injury (inflammation), but also in chronic pain. It is characterized by enhanced pain to non-noxious mechanical stimuli (touching) but not thermal stimuli (Meyer, et al., 1994). Touch causes pain because continuous or very frequent C-fiber input to the dorsal horn enables dorsal horn receptors (*N*-methyl-*D*-aspartate [NMDA] and neurokinin, which are normally inactive) to become hyperexcitable and project the pain signal to the brain (Woolf, 1994). Although this sensitization may promote healing by encouraging immobilization of an injured body part, it may continue after the injury is healed and help explain some chronic pain states.

Regenerative Neuronal Growth

Injured peripheral nerve axons produce pathophysiologic pain by generating impulses at abnormal sites (ectopic) along their course, such as at sites of injury. Cut nerves produce pathophysiologic pain by growing a neuroma at the cut end. Nearby intact afferent nerves are triggered to sprout when nerves are injured. Neuromas and nerve sprouts are other sources of ectopic impulses. Nerve fibers that have lost some of their myelin due to injury or disease processes (diabetic neuropathies, heavy metal neuropathies, multiple sclerosis) also produce spontaneous neural discharge. All these ways for nerves to send messages to the spinal cord without ongoing tissue injury may help to explain pain reported by people whose injuries have appeared to heal (ie, people with chronic pain; Devor, 1994). Recent evidence indicates that norepinephrine released by the sympathetic nervous system, which normally does not excite nociceptors, can do so if they have been injured (Sato & Perl, 1991).

Injuries sufficient to cause nerve cell death produce changes in the spinal dorsal horn, including attempts at regeneration in other cells to maintain lost connections. Large myelinated fibers (A-beta fibers) particularly have been shown to sprout and make connections in areas where C-fibers terminate (Woolf, 1994). Such connections could dramatically alter central processing of touch signals. Such changes can be long term and result in genetic expression within nervous tissue (Dubner & Basbaum, 1994).

Manifestations of Pain

Physiologic and behavioral responses occur in the person in pain. Observers consider these responses indicators of pain, but for the person with pain, some of these responses represent dangerous effects of the pain. Absence of these responses *does not* indicate a client has no pain or has less intense pain than he or she reports.

Physiologic Responses

Observable physiologic signs of acute pain include changes in blood pressure, heart rate, respiratory rate, and metabolic responses. Commonly observed responses in acute pain are usually absent in persistent and chronic pain because adaptation occurs (Bonica, 1990). It is not clear how long it takes for adaptation to occur; therefore, lack of elevation in vital signs cannot be used as a reliable indicator of the presence or magnitude of persistent pain. Furthermore, other reasons for alterations in physiologic responses must be considered (eg, effects of drug therapy lowering blood pressure in the presence of severe pain; Puntillo & Wilkie, 1991).

Increased Blood Pressure. The increase in blood pressure that may accompany acute pain is believed to be due to overactivity of the sympathetic nervous system. Peripheral vasoconstriction is an adaptive response, as the blood shifts away from the periphery (skin, extremities) to the heart and lungs when the body perceives a threat. The increased blood pressure also increases the work of the heart and can lead to coronary artery vasoconstriction and potential for myocardial ischemia (Cousins, 1994). Decreased peripheral circulation can be dangerous to people undergoing vascular grafting procedures.

Increased Heart Rate. The increased heart rate is the body's attempt to increase the available oxygen and circulating fluid volume to the tissues determined to be in danger as a result of pain. The shunting of blood from the periphery to the vital organs (brain, heart, liver, kidney) is an effort to preserve the body's life-support systems.

Increased Respiratory Rate. An increase in the respiratory rate is an effort to increase the amount of oxygen available to the heart and circulation. Increased respiration also helps eliminate carbon dioxide from the circulation. Unrelieved pain classically includes rapid and shallow breathing that is inefficient to meet oxygen needs, which results in hypoxemia. The rapid, shallow breathing is corrected with effective pain relief (Cousins, 1994).

Neuroendocrine and Metabolic Responses. Unrelieved pain produces a catabolic state, that is, stored energy is consumed to provide energy to vital organs and injured tissue. These responses also are known as the stress response, which is capable of producing widespread metabolic effects. Some of these effects include generalized increase in metabolism and oxygen consumption and increased blood glucose, free fatty acids, blood lactate, and ketones (Bonica, 1990). These effects are related to the degree and duration of tissue damage and can last for days.

Behavioral Responses

Observable behavioral signs of acute and chronic pain include verbal, vocal, or nonverbal responses. As with physiologic signs, behavioral responses often adapt with time (Table 44-1).

Verbal Responses. Verbal behavioral responses to pain are subjective and are the most dependable indicator of pain. Therefore, the client's report should be believed and not dismissed if it varies from other objective information.

Vocal behavioral responses include crying, grunting, moaning, and groaning. In people without verbal abilities (eg, preverbal children, cognitive impaired clients) vocal responses may provide important clues about the presence of pain but does little to indicate where or what kind it is, how much there is, or how it changes with time.

Nonverbal Responses. Common nonverbal behavioral responses are rubbing painful areas, frowns and grimaces, and increased muscle tension that occurs with guarding and immobilization. Increased muscle tension shown by guarding is part of the body's fight-or-flight response and is a reaction to protect against further pain. Prolonged muscle tension, however, contributes to impaired muscle metabolism, muscle atrophy, and significantly delayed normal muscle function (Cousins, 1994). Nonverbal behaviors often give a clue about pain location, but verbal reports indicate more clearly its lo-

Table 44-1 • Objective Behavioral Indicators of Pain

Type of Indicator	Examples
Verbal Behavior	
Vocalization	Moaning, groaning, grunting, sighing, gasping, crying, screaming
Verbalization	Praying, counting, swearing or cursing, repeating nonsensical phrases
Nonverbal Behavior	
Facial expression	Grimacing, clenching teeth, tightly shutting lips, gazing/staring, wrinkling forehead, tearing
Body actions	Thrashing, pounding, biting, rocking, rubbing, stretching, shrugging, rotating body part, shifting weight
Behaviors	Massaging; immobilizing; guarding; bracing; eating or drinking; applying pressure, heat, cold; assuming special position or posture; reading; watching television; listening to music; crossing legs

These behaviors may signal presence of pain, but absence of behavior does not signal lack of pain.

cation, intensity, quality, and temporal pattern (onset, duration, changes with time and activity).

Impact of Pain on Activities of Daily Living

Individual Considerations

Unrelieved pain generally causes decreased energy, which affects all aspects of daily living. The client in pain often finds it difficult to perform basic daily activities. People who have difficulty with independent living may experience anxiety or alterations in self-concept. Basic hygiene activities (bathing, dressing, eating, grooming) may be mildly or severely affected, depending on the location and degree of pain. Household activities also may be difficult to perform. Persistent pain can interfere with the person's ability to concentrate on work or school. Pain may be increased with physical activity, such as leisure activities, walking, or driving.

A person with pain finds it difficult to fall asleep or stay asleep. The resulting lack of sleep contributes to fatigue, which predisposes the client to more pain. Pain also can be fatiguing. Sleep, however, does not indicate pain relief. After experiencing pain for an extended time, the client becomes too tired to talk or cry and falls asleep. Clients in pain may close their eyes and appear to be asleep but actually may be conserving energy or focusing on something else to make the pain bearable.

Family Considerations

Clients with pain may focus on finding pain relief and thus be unable to explore outside interests and relationships. This may alter family and social relationships, and persistent, unrelieved pain can lead to family conflict and deterioration (Faucett & Levine, 1991). Decreased energy also hinders sexual functioning. The impact of pain on family members should not be ignored. Family members assume tremendous responsibilities in assisting clients with pain (Ferrell, Cohen, Rhiner, & Rozek, 1991). There are many decisions and ethical conflicts in which family members participate as they deal with unrelieved pain (Taylor, et al., 1993).

Assessment

An accurate diagnosis of the cause of pain is the cornerstone of management. Without an accurate diagnosis, it is impossible to select the best therapy. Ongoing assessment also is important for implementing an effective pain management plan. The nurse obtains facts from the client and from direct observation. The nurse may find it difficult to remain objective and nonjudgmental, but *pain occurs whenever the client says it does* (McCaffery & Beebe, 1989). The client is the expert about how the pain feels (Wilkie, Olsson, & Metcalf, 1993). Direct observation may corroborate client report but must not be used to dismiss that report.

Pain assessment information should be documented in an accessible location. Even the best pain assessment conducted by one nurse is of limited value unless the information is shared with other nurses and other healthcare professionals responsible for the client's care. Until documentation forms are available in all healthcare settings, the progress notes and flow sheets can be used to document pain measurement information.

Subjective Data

Functional Pattern Identification

To determine the sensory pain, the nurse needs information from the client, the person expert about the pain sensation. The nurse needs answers to these questions about pain perception:

- Where is the pain located?
- What is the magnitude or intensity (level) of the pain?
- What level of pain would the client like to have?
- What level of pain would the client be willing to tolerate?
- How does the pain feel to the client; how is it described (its quality)?
- How does the pain change with rest, activity, or time (its temporal pattern)?

Pain location and intensity are the most important aspects of sensory pain in critical care. Other aspects can be assessed when the client's condition is stable. For ongoing assessment, pain intensity is assessed routinely, and the other aspects are assessed if the pain has changed.

When asked about pain, some clients deny it unless it is severe. These same clients will report that they hurt a lot or have a great deal of discomfort. For this reason, it is important for nurses to inquire about the client's meaning of *hurt, discomfort,* and *soreness* to determine if a person has pain (Gaston-Johansson, Albert, & Fagan, 1990). Conducting a pain assessment is simple when the nurse uses tools to measure the sensory pain experience.

Location. Because clients initially are inclined to describe where the pain or discomfort is located, it is logical and efficient to start with measurement of pain location. Pain location is measured by using a drawing of a body outline and asking the client to mark all the places where pain is perceived (Fig. 44-5). The marks are made as big as or small as the pain is perceived in those places. Body outlines have been used successfully with children as young as 8 years (Savedra, et al., 1993) and adults older than 85 years (Wilkie, Williams, Grevstad, & Mekwa, 1995). Alternatively, a client can be asked to point to the places where the pain is felt, but pointing may be inconvenient or embarrassing.

Intensity. Pain intensity is measured with the use of a scale. Nurses evaluate pain intensity at rest, with various activities, and when painful procedures are performed. Wilkie, Olsson, & Metcalf (1993) describe a script to use when giving directions to use such a numbered scale.

> "I need to know how much pain you have. Because I can't feel your pain, I want you to use a scale to let me know how much pain you have right now. The numbers between 0 and 10 represent *all* the pain a person could have. Zero means no pain and 10 means pain as bad as it could be. You can use *any* number between 0 and 10 to let me know how much pain you have right now. **Call** your pain a number between 0 and 10 so I will know the intensity of the pain you feel now."
>
> *Note*: Use the phrase "call your pain" rather than "rate your pain" because clients have difficulty knowing what is expected of them when asked to rate their pain. They easily "call" their pain a number.*

The number given by the client is recorded for comparison with the number representing the amount of pain the person wants and is able to tolerate and with future pain intensity measurements. These numbers provide a perspective on how the pain intensity fluctuates with time (they also show a temporal pattern). If clients are unable to call their pain a number, they can select an intensity word from one of the tools to report pain intensity.

Children as young as 8 years can use a 0-to-10 number scale, although most children prefer to use a graphic rating scale, as shown in Figure 44-5, to report pain intensity (Tesler, et al., 1991). Alternatively, a child can be asked to select the number of poker chips (Hester, Foster, & Kristensen, 1990) or faces (Beyer & Aradine, 1987) that reflects his or her pain.

Quality. The most widely used measure of pain quality is the McGill-Melzack Pain Questionnaire (Fig. 44-6). It includes a list of verbal descriptors from which the client selects the one word per group that best describes the pain. Supplying the list makes the task easy for clients who do not know how to describe the quality of the sensation. Clients who would use other words will supply that information as they select words from the list. If clients have pain in more than one site, they often will select two words per group and indicate that one word describes one site and the other word another site. Words in groups 1 to 10 represent sensory qualities of pain. Words in groups 11 to 15 represent affective qualities of pain. Group 15 words are evaluative qualities, and words from groups 16 to 20 are miscellaneous words (sensory, affective, and evaluative). A total pain quality score is obtained by counting the number of words selected. Children also are able to use descriptors to describe their pain (Savedra, et al., 1993; Wilkie, et al., 1990). Research findings indicate that complex pain quality, as reflected by a large number of words, is associated with increased client attempts to engage in pain-control behaviors (Wilkie, Keefe, Dodd, & Copp, 1992).

* Copyright 1990, Wilkie, D. J.; reprinted with permission.

CODE ____________

DATE ____________

ADOLESCENT PEDIATRIC PAIN TOOL (APPT)

INSTRUCTIONS:

1. Color in the areas on these drawings to show where you have pain. Make the marks as big or small as the place where the pain is.

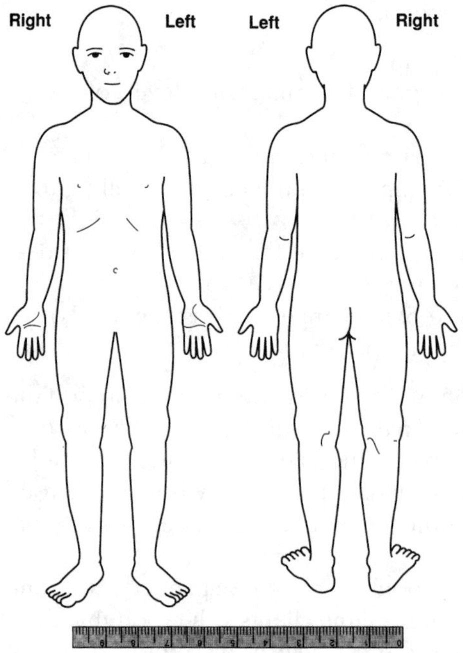

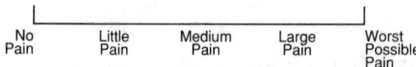

2. Place a straight, up and down mark on this line to show how much pain you have.

No Pain — Little Pain — Medium Pain — Large Pain — Worst Possible Pain

3. Point to or circle as many of these words that describe your pain.

1
annoying
bad
horrible
miserable
terrible
uncomfortable

2
aching
hurting
like an ache
like a hurt
sore

3
beating
hitting
pounding
punching
throbbing

4
biting
cutting
like a pin
like a sharp knife
pin like
sharp
stabbing

5
blistering
burning
hot

6
cramping
crushing
like a pinch
pinching
pressure

7
itching
like a scratch
like a sting
scratching
stinging

8
shocking
shooting
splitting

9
numb
stiff
swollen
tight

10
awful
deadly
dying
killing

11
crying
frightening
screaming
terrifying

12
dizzy
sickening
suffocating

13
never goes away
uncontrollable

14
always
comes and goes
comes on all of a sudden
constant
continuous
forever

15
off and on
once in a while
sneaks up
sometimes
steady

If you like, you may add other words:

____

____

____

For office use only.

BSA: ______
IS: ______

#S(2-9) ______ /37= ______ %
#A(10-12) ______ /11= ______ %
#E(1,13) ______ /8 = ______ %
#T(14,15) ______ /11= ______ %

Total ______ /67= ______ %

Figure 44-5 • *Adolescent Pediatric Pain Tool. (Courtesy of Savedra, Tesler, Holzemer, & Ward © 1992.)*

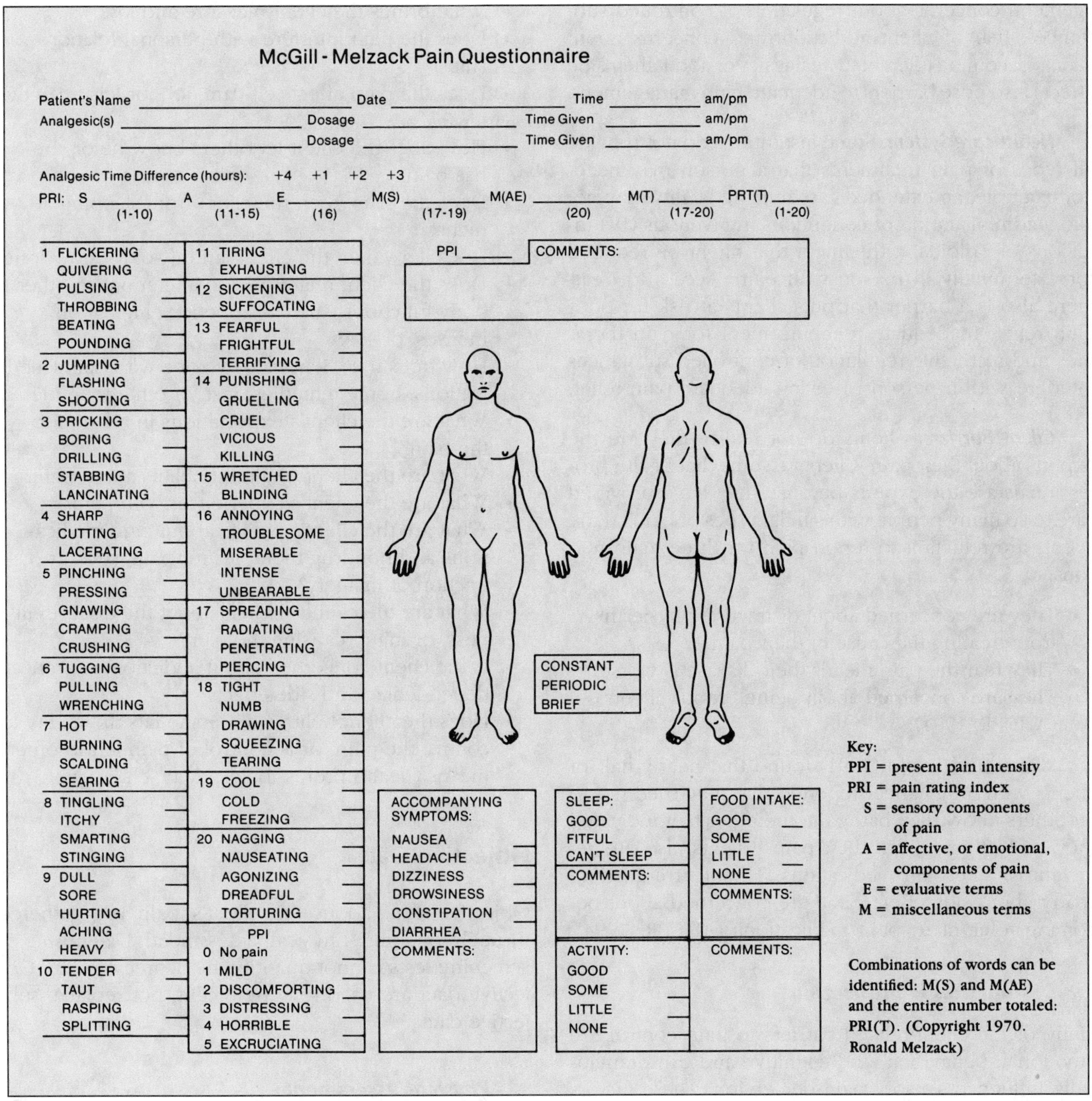

McGill - Melzack Pain Questionnaire

Patient's Name ________ Date ________ Time ________ am/pm
Analgesic(s) ________ Dosage ________ Time Given ________ am/pm
________ Dosage ________ Time Given ________ am/pm

Analgesic Time Difference (hours): +4 +1 +2 +3

PRI: S ____ (1-10) A ____ (11-15) E ____ (16) M(S) ____ (17-19) M(AE) ____ (20) M(T) ____ (17-20) PRT(T) ____ (1-20)

1 FLICKERING, QUIVERING, PULSING, THROBBING, BEATING, POUNDING
2 JUMPING, FLASHING, SHOOTING
3 PRICKING, BORING, DRILLING, STABBING, LANCINATING
4 SHARP, CUTTING, LACERATING
5 PINCHING, PRESSING, GNAWING, CRAMPING, CRUSHING
6 TUGGING, PULLING, WRENCHING
7 HOT, BURNING, SCALDING, SEARING
8 TINGLING, ITCHY, SMARTING, STINGING
9 DULL, SORE, HURTING, ACHING, HEAVY
10 TENDER, TAUT, RASPING, SPLITTING
11 TIRING, EXHAUSTING
12 SICKENING, SUFFOCATING
13 FEARFUL, FRIGHTFUL, TERRIFYING
14 PUNISHING, GRUELLING, CRUEL, VICIOUS, KILLING
15 WRETCHED, BLINDING
16 ANNOYING, TROUBLESOME, MISERABLE, INTENSE, UNBEARABLE
17 SPREADING, RADIATING, PENETRATING, PIERCING
18 TIGHT, NUMB, DRAWING, SQUEEZING, TEARING
19 COOL, COLD, FREEZING
20 NAGGING, NAUSEATING, AGONIZING, DREADFUL, TORTURING

PPI
0 No pain
1 MILD
2 DISCOMFORTING
3 DISTRESSING
4 HORRIBLE
5 EXCRUCIATING

PPI ____ COMMENTS:

CONSTANT
PERIODIC
BRIEF

ACCOMPANYING SYMPTOMS: NAUSEA, HEADACHE, DIZZINESS, DROWSINESS, CONSTIPATION, DIARRHEA
COMMENTS:

SLEEP: GOOD, FITFUL, CAN'T SLEEP
COMMENTS:

ACTIVITY: GOOD, SOME, LITTLE, NONE

FOOD INTAKE: GOOD, SOME, LITTLE, NONE
COMMENTS:

COMMENTS:

Key:
PPI = present pain intensity
PRI = pain rating index
S = sensory components of pain
A = affective, or emotional, components of pain
E = evaluative terms
M = miscellaneous terms

Combinations of words can be identified: M(S) and M(AE) and the entire number totaled: PRI(T). (Copyright 1970. Ronald Melzack)

Figure 44-6 • *McGill-Melzack Pain Questionnaire.*

Temporal Pattern. The duration of pain is described by terms such as brief, momentary, transient, rhythmic, periodic, intermittent, continuous, steady, or constant. The client is asked the date or time the pain started and how long the pain lasted to measure pain onset and duration. Assessing when the pain began (onset) is important in determining whether the client's pain is acute, recurrent, or chronic. Adaptations can be made to the graphs to show how pain changes with time of day or activity level.

Risk Identification

Pain management is often suboptimal (Agency for Health Care Policy and Research [AHCPR], 1994). Together, health professionals, the healthcare system, and client-related barriers to pain management add to the risk of poor pain control. These factors are discussed in the following section.

Health Professionals. Poor assessment of pain is a leading risk factor for poor pain control. Nurses and physicians may not know a client has pain because of poor assessment. The nurse's attitudes toward pain may contribute to poor assessment. If the nurse and client perceive pain differently, major conflicts and increased pain may result. The nurse who assumes that a client will always report pain may be contributing to the client's discomfort; specific and careful questioning about pain is necessary. Inadequate knowledge of pain management, concerns about regulation of controlled substances, fear of client addiction, and concerns about clients becoming tolerant to analgesics or about their side effects also pose barriers to adequate pain management.

Healthcare System. Some institutions do not provide all types of pain treatments that a person may need. For example, an extended care nursing facility may not allow administration of continuous intravenous (IV) infusions of opioids, a treatment that might be required for a terminally ill person with pain. Access to treatment also is a barrier that puts clients at risk for poor pain relief. Inadequate reimbursement for pain therapies and restrictive regulation of controlled substances interfere with a person receiving adequate pain relief.

Client Barriers. Clients do not realize they are the experts about their pain. Clients assume that health professionals are the experts because they have provided care to so many people with similar types of pain. Many clients are reluctant to report pain for three main reasons:

- They are concerned about distracting physicians from treating the cause of their pain.
- They fear the pain means their disease is worse.
- They are concerned about being "good" clients (AHCPR, 1994).

Wilkie and Keefe (1991) found that nearly half of clients with lung cancer reported that they tried not to let others know they had pain; the other half indicated they told others about their pain. Clients also are reluctant to take pain medications. They fear addiction, worry about side effects, and are concerned about becoming tolerant to pain medications (AHCPR, 1994).

Dysfunction Identification

Many of the client-related barriers to pain control are emotional, behavioral, and cognitive and can dramatically influence sensory pain perception. These factors must be assessed if initial pain therapies do not provide the degree of pain relief expected. There are few clinically useful measurement tools for these factors. The Memorial Pain Assessment Card (Fishman, et al., 1987) measures general mood, and the Brief Pain Inventory (AHCPR, 1994) measures pain interference with mood and activities. Additionally, the McGill Pain Questionnaire (Melzack, 1975) measures affective and evaluative pain qualities and includes interview questions about activities that increase or relieve pain. To obtain additional information, the nurse relies on interview questions and active listening skills. Some of the following questions are helpful to gain access to the client's personal pain experience:

- Does the client feel anxious, upset, depressed, sad, fearful, or angry?
- What brings the client pleasure and joy?
- Does the pain interfere with personal relationships?
- Does the pain affect self-care, job, or leisure activities?
- How does the client let others know he or she has pain?
- Does the pain keep the client from sleeping at night?
- Does it awaken the client, and if so, for how long?
- Does the client relate pain to alterations in other body functions, such as appetite, elimination, menses, or sex?
- How does the client usually cope with pain (medications, home remedies, rest, or other therapies)?
- What are the client's expectations in relation to the pain?
- What are the client's cultural beliefs about pain?
- What are the client's experiences with pain?
- What are the client's beliefs about pain medications and nondrug therapies for pain, such as distraction or imagery?
- What are the client's beliefs about the disease, illness, or injury causing the pain?
- Is the client concerned about addiction, tolerance, dependence, and side effects?
- Does the client believe he or she has the ability to control the pain, or is control of pain left to other means (health professionals, deity, chance)?

Objective Data

Objective data about the client's pain are gathered through ongoing physical assessment. Diagnostic or screening tests cannot quantify the degree of pain. Objective data are used to supplement, not replace, subjective data.

Physical Assessment

Physiologic responses to pain are the result of the activation of the sympathetic nervous system. With acute pain, the general responses observed are tachycardia, elevated blood pressure, increased respiratory rate, diaphoresis, and gastric distress. With chronic pain, these responses may be modified or absent.

Vital Signs. Assessing the client's vital signs is important for obtaining baseline information, particularly before a potentially painful procedure or situation. The sympathetic nervous system responses to acute pain are evident with diaphoresis and increases in heart rate, respiratory rate, and blood pressure. For clients who have difficulty expressing pain or cannot do so, the vital sign readings and comparisons may be useful for acute pain evaluation.

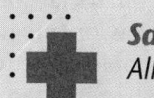

> **Safety Alert**
> *Alleviating Pain*
>
> - Thoroughly assess the client (ie, past experience with drugs, medical and surgical history, client expectations) before any interventions for pain are instituted.
> - Carefully monitor the client's level of consciousness, respiratory rate and quality, and vital signs before and after drugs are given.
> - Gain knowledge and become skillful at safely administering pharmacologic and nonpharmacologic pain-relief methods.
> - Research potential interactions before giving any analgesic.
> - Before applying heat or cold therapies, consider the client's sensory function, age, level of consciousness, intellectual ability, health problems, and the condition of the affected skin surface.
> - Ensure that equipment functions correctly.
> - Know the agency's policy about assessment, evaluation, and use of pain-relief methods.

A common misconception is that objective, physiologic responses are less likely to be manipulated than self-reports. This belief is unfounded. Lack of elevation in the vital signs must not be interpreted as an indication that pain is not present (McCaffery & Ferrell, 1992). Many factors influence heart rate, blood pressure, and respiratory rate and may obscure these physiologic responses to pain (Puntillo & Wilkie, 1991).

Associated Characteristics. Related symptoms may give additional clues about pain. Nausea and vomiting, anorexia, or withdrawal are common with pain. The presence of these symptoms should be assessed for potential for or presence of pain. Relieving the pain also may relieve these associated characteristics. For example, relieving pain may allow the client to relax and rest, thus diminishing fatigue.

Physical Expressions of Pain. The nurse observes the client's facial expressions and body movements. Wincing, frowning, and grimacing can indicate pain, but lack of these expressions does not mean that a client has no pain. People with chronic pain are likely *not* to show these facial expressions of pain. The most common facial expression associated with chronic pain in a group of clients with lung cancer was movement of the lower eyelid to make a squinting appearance (Wilkie, 1995). In general, these clients with chronic pain had a mask-like appearance and little spontaneous movement of facial muscles. If nurses expect to see wincing, frowning, and grimacing when a person has pain, they are likely to misdiagnose many people.

Body movements may represent protective actions to decrease the pain. Body movements may increase with pain and include rubbing, splinting, guarding, immobilizing, or elevating the painful extremity or changing positions frequently. For example, a woman in labor rhythmically rubs her abdomen. As pain increases, total body activity decreases, and eventually the client lies still and is quiet if pain is not relieved. Splinting, guarding, and immobilization by a person in pain protects the client from pain but can be harmful. This decrease in activity may delay recovery (eg, when the postoperative client refuses to ambulate, turn, cough, or deep-breathe and subsequently develops atelectasis, thrombopheblitis, or a pulmonary embolus).

Pain evokes emotional responses that may be expressed as depression, anger, fear, anxiety, sadness, excitement, denial, or regression. A wide range of verbal responses (moaning, sighing, screaming, crying, and repetition of words or phrases) can be a result of pain. However, such restlessness, moaning, and grimacing can be misleading: the client may not be in pain but may be disoriented, hypoxic, or febrile or having a medication reaction. Unrelieved pain also leads to disorientation or confusion that clears with appropriate pain management (Coyle, Breitbart, Weaver, & Portenoy, 1994).

Any of these expressions of pain may be absent in stoic clients or those with prolonged chronic pain. Lack of pain expression does *not* mean lack of pain, because clients adapt physically and psychologically to pain (McCaffery, 1979). Therefore, nurses must actively solicit information about pain; they must observe accurately, listen, and never judge or jump to conclusions.

Diagnostic Tests and Procedures

Although tests cannot quantify the degree of pain, procedures can validate painful events (eg, an electrocardiogram shows a myocardial infarction after chest pain). Other diagnostic tests relate to the specific pain source. For example, a bone scan is used to diagnose that cancer has spread to the bone, a frequent cause of pain in the person with cancer.

Nursing Diagnoses and Client Goals

There are two accepted North American Nursing Diagnosis Association (NANDA) nursing diagnoses related to altered comfort: Pain and Chronic Pain.

Diagnostic Statement: Pain

Definition

Pain is a state in which an individual experiences and reports the presence of severe discomfort or an uncomfortable sensation (NANDA, 1994). As previously

Nursing Research
Pain

Selected Nursing Research Studies

Beck, S. L. (1991). The therapeutic use of music for cancer-related pain. *Oncology Nursing Forum, 18,* 1327–1337.

Gaston-Johansson, F., Albert, M., & Fagan, E. (1990). Similarities in pain descriptions of four different ethnic-culture groups. *Journal of Pain & Symptom Management, 5,* 94–100.

Savedra, M. C., Holzemer, W. L., Tesler, M. D., Ward, J. A., & Wilkie, D. J. (1993). Assessment of postoperative pain in children and adolescents using the Adolescent Pediatric Pain Tool. *Nursing Research, 42,* 5–9.

Wilkie, D. J., Keefe, F. J., Dodd, M. J., & Copp, L. A. (1992). Behavior of clients with lung cancer: Description and associations with oncologic and pain variables. *Pain, 51,* 231–240.

Possible Topics for Nursing Inquiry

- Do clients experience more or less respiratory depression if usual postoperative opioids are given on a regularly scheduled versus prn basis?
- If clients report using active pain-coping strategies, does client education in the use of imagery result in improved client acceptance of the strategy and more effective pain relief?
- If clients fear addiction to opioids, does client education about the occurrence of addiction increase the number of analgesic doses accepted by the client and reduce pain intensity?

defined from a multidisciplinary perspective, "pain is an unpleasant sensory and emotional experience associated with actual or potential tissue damage, or described in terms of such damage" (Merskey & Bogduk, 1994, p. 210).

Defining Characteristics

Several clinical cues point to this nursing diagnosis. One of the following subjective or objective characteristic must be present.

Subjective. There is communication (verbal or coded) of pain descriptors (NANDA, 1994). The client reports the location, intensity, quality, and temporal pattern of the experienced pain.

Objective. There may be guarding behavior that protects the injured area from movement. The client appears to have a narrow focus within himself or herself. The client has an altered perception of time, has impaired thought processes, or withdraws from social contact. The client engages in distraction behavior (moaning, crying, pacing, seeking out other people or activities). The client appears restless (fixed or scattered movement) with a facial mask of pain in which the eyes lack luster; there is a "beaten look," or a grimace. The client's muscle tone may alter from listless to rigid. The autonomic responses (not seen in chronic stable pain) may be present, including diaphoresis, blood pressure and pulse change, pupillary dilation, and increased or decreased respiratory rate (NANDA, 1994).

Presence of these behaviors may confirm but cannot rule out the possibility that the client has pain. Similarly, absence of these behaviors must not negate the client's report that pain is present or its intensity, quality, or pattern. Many clients do not look like they have pain when their pain is quite severe.

Diagnostic Statement: Chronic Pain

Definition

Chronic pain is the state in which the individual experiences persistent or intermittent pain that lasts for more than 6 months (NANDA, 1994). Many pain experts argue that 6 months is an arbitrary time frame and recently have defined chronic pain "as a persistent pain that is not amenable, as a rule, to treatments based upon specific remedies, or to the routine methods of pain control such as non-opioid analgesics" (Merskey & Bodguk, 1994).

Defining Characteristics

Many clinical cues point to this nursing diagnosis. To make this diagnosis, the person must report that pain has existed for more than 6 months; this report may be the only assessment data present (NANDA, 1994).

Several minor characteristics may be present but are not required for this diagnosis (NANDA, 1994):

- Discomfort and emotions, such as anger, frustration, or depression, may be present because of the situation.
- Anorexia and weight loss may be associated with the chronic pain.
- Insomnia may result from the constant pain.
- The client may show a facial mask of pain, reflex abnormalities, or guarded movements. (Guarded movements may result in muscle spasms.)
- There may be color changes, redness, swelling, and heat in the painful area

Related Factors

Chronic physical or psychosocial disability increases chronic pain (NANDA, 1994). Many neural changes (**neural plasticity**) are likely to be factors in continued pain (Coderre, et al., 1993), but other affective, behavioral, and cognitive factors contribute to chronic pain experienced by the person.

Related Nursing Diagnoses

Although Pain and Chronic Pain are the obvious nursing diagnoses for the person in pain, assessment may indicate that the client has other problems related to the pain. For instance, Anxiety, Ineffective Individual Coping, Ineffective Family Coping, Altered Health-Maintenance, Impaired Home Maintenance Management, and Sleep Pattern Disturbance may be related to pain. If the client suffers from chronic pain, additional nursing diagnoses may be defined, including Self Care Deficit, Self Esteem Disturbance, Hopelessness, Impaired Physical Mobility, Sexual Dysfunction, and Spiritual Distress. If the client is taking medications for pain, other nursing diagnoses may be evident, such as Constipation and Altered Thought Processes.

Outcome Identification and Planning

After the nursing diagnoses and related factors are identified, goals and nursing interventions can be designed. The overall goal in pain management is for the client to seek interventions that maximize his or her pain relief and quality of life. Specific goals for the client in pain follow:

Client will report no new pain sites and reduced pain intensity and pain quality complexity. (This goal could be unrealistic in clients with progressive disorders associated with pain, such as cancer or arthritis.)

Client will monitor and report changes in pain location, intensity, quality, and pattern.

Client will identify and avoid emotional, behavioral, and cognitive factors that precipitate pain.

Client will identify and use cognitive and behavioral techniques to decrease or cope with pain

Care of the person in pain involves a four-step process:

1. Assess sensory pain.
2. Provide pain therapy.
3. If relief is not as expected, assess emotional, behavioral, cognitive, and physiologic aspects of pain.
4. Revise plans for therapy to meet needs

Although physicians prescribe many pain management techniques, the nurse is responsible for assessing, administering, monitoring, and evaluating the effectiveness of these techniques and initiating independent nursing measures for pain relief. Using the four-step process allows the physician and nurse to plan optimal pain relief collaboratively before or soon after it is experienced or to control persistent pain as much as possible.

The accompanying display outlines some of the nursing interventions used in planning individualized care for the client with pain. A realistic goal for the client in acute and chronic pain is to reduce pain to the level the client indicates he or she is able to tolerate. Complete elimination of acute pain is possible during recovery and healing. The client with chronic pain needs to learn that no interventions will cure the cause of the pain, that it may not be eliminated entirely, and that it may recur. Adapting daily activities to control the pain effectively may be a goal for this client.

Because results are not always predictable, confidence and enthusiasm on the nurse's part increase the chances that a pain-relief measure will be successful. If the client knows that numerous methods are available, he or she will not be devastated if one is less than totally effective.

Implementation

Based on sensory data, appropriate therapies (pharmacologic and nonpharmacologic) are provided by the healthcare team. The nurse has many important roles in providing the therapies. One essential role is monitoring the client's response to the therapy. If the cause of the pain is eliminated with treatment, the pain disappears. If the cause of the pain cannot be eliminated, the pain intensity should decrease to the level the client desires or at least to the level the client indicates he or she is willing to tolerate. Pain quality often diminishes, and the pain pattern may change. It is not unusual for some therapy adjustments to be needed before these improvements are seen. If the degree of pain relief expected is not achieved, however, then an in-depth assessment of all the factors that contribute to the pain is needed.

Nursing Interventions to Promote Health and Function

Clients can be taught ways of anticipating and managing painful procedures or situations. This decreases anxiety and fear and allows clients to become active participants in preventing pain and promoting recovery. Recognizing pain-inducing situations and factors is the first step in preventing pain. For instance, many procedures performed routinely produce pain (blood pressure, needle stick for blood tests, inserting an IV or urinary catheter). Preparation, including premedication, is indicated for all painful procedures, even if they pro-

Planning
Examples of Nursing Interventions Used in Common Pain Problems

Preventing Pain

- Encourage appropriate use of body position and mechanics during work and recreation.
- Assist the client in identifying factors that precipitate or aggravate pain.
- Provide comfort measures for the client on bed rest, such as eliminating wrinkles in sheets, avoiding constrictive clothing, and changing positions.
- Provide careful skin hygiene to prevent pain from pressure, excoriation, or irritation.
- Give anticipatory explanation of the amount of pain that can be expected during a procedure or activity.

Acute Pain

- Measure the client's pain location, intensity, quality, and temporal pattern.
- Formulate a plan of managing pain with the client.
- Use pharmacologic methods of pain control judiciously; give adequate medication to relieve pain; use medication when pain begins, so analgesics can be most effective; and monitor effectiveness of medication.
- Promote periods of uninterrupted rest after pain relief measures.
- Teach the client to minimize pain by splinting the area in pain with a pillow before activities, such as moving or coughing.
- Encourage the use of distraction by focusing on pictures, reading, music, guided imagery, or hypnosis.
- Promote the use of cutaneous stimulation, such as massage, heat and cold, acupuncture or acupressure, and contralateral stimulation.

Chronic Pain

- Measure the client's pain location, intensity, quality, and temporal pattern and assess affective, behavioral, and cognitive responses to the pain.
- Encourage the client to maintain a log of factors relating to pain, such as activities that precede pain, length and duration of pain, and therapies used to relieve pain.
- Use pharmacologic methods on a time-contingent basis.
- Teach the client to use distraction, cutaneous stimulation, and relaxation techniques alternately, and monitor for pain-relief effects.
- Promote a schedule of rest and activity during the day to minimize pain.
- Refer to appropriate resources and support services for evaluation.

duce only mild pain. If a client is scheduled for a potentially painful procedure, the nurse can discuss techniques (relaxation exercises, deep breathing, distraction) that will add to the effect of analgesic therapies to decrease the pain and improve coping mechanisms.

Chronic pain can be prevented or minimized. For example, someone who gets migraine headaches may be aware that certain foods, such as chocolate, induce a migraine. Increased knowledge about the ways that sports or other recreational activities can aggravate pain allows the person to modify his or her activities to prevent pain and promote function. Adequate warm-up activities to stretch muscles and limber up joints before sporting activities help prevent pain during and after the activity. Using appropriate posture and mechanics at work can help preserve function and prevent pain by avoiding strained muscles and other types of injury.

Clients with chronic pain can be taught lifestyle changes to avoid precipitating pain and dysfunction. For instance, the client with chronic lower back pain should be taught proper lifting and bending techniques and exercises to decrease muscle contraction and increase back muscle strength (see Chap. 29). The client can be taught to use analgesics effectively and alternate pain-relief measures.

Nursing Interventions for Altered Comfort

Nursing management of pain includes physical, cognitive, behavioral, and pharmacologic measures. Being familiar with these techniques and the types of pain for which they are effective helps the nurse decide which ones to use, when to initiate them, what outcomes to expect, and how to teach them to clients (Rhiner, Ferrell, Ferrell, & Grant, 1993).

Physical Pain Relief Techniques

Positioning and Hygiene. For clients who spend many hours in bed, the bed and the client's position may contribute directly to pain. Sheets tend to bunch up, creating pressure and discomfort. Tightening sheets regularly or changing them, if needed, can make the client more comfortable. Repositioning the client on a regular schedule also can help promote comfort. Pressure areas created by lying in one position too long can be painful. If not contraindicated, backrubs can contribute to relaxation and comfort. Giving a backrub also allows the nurse to spend a few minutes with the client, listening attentively and continuing the ongoing pain assessment.

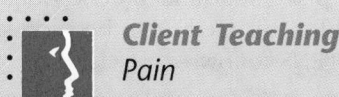

Client Teaching
Pain

Instruct the client as follows:

- *Monitor where you have pain, how much pain you have (use a 0–10 scale), how your pain feels, and how your pain changes with activity and time. Report this information to your nurse and healthcare provider.*
- *When visiting your healthcare provider, take a list of all your medications, so the physician knows what you are taking and how often.*
- *If you have an unusual reaction, contact your healthcare provider.*
- *When pain occurs, write down any events you think may be related.*
- *Anticipate painful events, and alter your behavior to prevent or minimize pain.*
- *Ask if you are allowed to drive a car or operate machinery while taking your medication.*
- *Keep the drugs away from children.*
- *Tell your healthcare provider if you are breast-feeding or think you may be pregnant.*

Any constrictive item contributes to pain. This includes gowns that twist or bind, support hose, or wrist restraints. Gowns must be the correct size for the client and should be checked for comfort whenever the client's position is changed. Restraints and support hose must be removed regularly to assess pressure on the skin and other problems that may cause pain.

Areas of irritation or excoriation may be sources of pain. Clients who require a bedpan or who are incontinent of urine or stool are at risk for skin impairment and pain if perineal hygiene is not carefully managed. Skin that may be exposed to secretions from gastrostomy sites, ileostomies, or colostomies also is at risk for impairment.

Cutaneous Stimulation. Cutaneous stimulation relieves acute or chronic pain. Techniques such as pressure, massage, vibration, heat, cold, and plain or menthol ointments are safe and effective (Woolf & Thompson, 1994). All these methods have the added benefit of distracting and relaxing the client; they also help to establish or extend the nurse-client relationship. The analgesic effects of these therapies are thought to be caused by activation of large A-beta fibers and inhibition of smaller A-delta and C-fibers, thus closing the gate to pain impulses. The exact mechanism by which this gating occurs has not been established but may be through endorphin release. If a person has allodynia, these types of therapies may be inappropriate because they would dramatically increase pain sensation.

The effects of cutaneous stimulation are variable and unpredictable, and patience is required while various methods are tried and adjusted. For some clients, the pain is relieved until long after stimulation; others find that their pain returns to pretreatment levels immediately after therapy. In others, stimulation may not relieve pain or may actually cause further pain when the therapy is abandoned. A technique should be tried more than once before deciding that it does not work.

Cutaneous stimulation should be moderate in frequency and duration, and its use should be determined by the extent of pain relief. Areas that can be used are the skin over or near the pain site, trigger or acupuncture points, and peripheral nerves.

Massage. Massage, or rubbing a painful area, may relax muscles and reduce tension (Haleman, 1994), but it is contraindicated over broken skin, mucous membranes, or rashes. Massage can be performed with counterirritants, such as mustard plasters, poultices, and liniments. Menthol products are the most common over-the-counter irritants, but the smell of menthol may

Nursing Care Guidelines
Physical, Cognitive, and Behavioral Pain Therapies

- Consider nonpharmacologic therapies when
  - Anxiety is augmenting pain levels and physiologic response.
  - Client wants more active participation in pain management.
  - Client or physician wants to decrease or eliminate use of medications.
  - Pharmacologic or invasive methods are not producing adequate pain relief.
  - Family and friends want to be involved.
  (When in doubt about the safety of a method or legality of independent nursing action, obtain the physician's order.)
  - Communicate on the plan of care/or tell all health team members, family, and friends what technique will be used, its purpose, how it is individualized to the client's preferences and needs, and when to use the technique. This will reinforce the technique.
- Anticipate client needs by starting measures before the pain begins. Practice techniques before they are needed if possible (ie, preoperatively, before the procedure).
- Recognize the importance of the nurse–client relationship on the client's willingness to try and to have confidence in the technique.
- Appreciate that a combination of methods that allows for flexibility often is most efficient.

From McCaffery, M. (1979). *Nursing management of the patient with pain.* Philadelphia: J.B. Lippincott.

be offensive to some clients. Most menthol products contain methyl salicylate, which is absorbed through the skin to cause the analgesic effect. The immediate sensation of warmth or coolness may last for hours. The sensation may be intensified by increasing the strength of the menthol, prolonging the massage, and ensuring that pores are open. If the ointment relieves the pain, wrapping the painful area in plastic will prolong relief.

Heat and Cold. Heat and cold may be used to reduce muscle spasm and decrease pain (Lehmann & de Lateur, 1994). Except for decreasing muscle spasm and reducing pain, heat and cold have opposite effects on the body. Heat (from a hot water bottle, heating pad, moist pad, warm bath, or the sun) should not be used within 24 hours of an injury because it increases blood flow, edema, and bleeding at a site; after 24 hours, it is especially effective for joint and muscle pain. Cold (from crushed ice in a towel, ice bag, reusable gel pack, frozen paper cup of ice, bag of frozen peas, and Popsicles) decreases the inflammatory response, blood flow, and edema and relieves chronic migraines and back pain. Precautions when using heat or cold stimulation include the following:

- Do not use heat for pain prior to medical diagnosis of its cause.
- Do not use it over areas of impaired circulation.
- Avoid extremes of temperature, which can cause burns or frostbite.
- Do not use heat over a new injury; it may cause increased bleeding and edema.
- Discontinue use if stimulation increases pain.

Contralateral Stimulation. In **contralateral stimulation**, the opposite area is stimulated with pressure, massage, cold, heat, or menthol to relieve pain (for instance, the left hand is stimulated when the right hand is painful). It is effective when the painful area cannot be reached because of a cast or bandages, when the affected skin is too sensitive to touch, or when phantom pain is present. Contralateral massage may be useful for muscle cramps, spasms, or itching. The precautions are the same as for heat and cold and for massage.

Transcutaneous Electrical Nerve Stimulation. **Transcutaneous electrical nerve stimulation** (TENS) is used as an adjunct in the overall management of acute and chronic pain. The TENS unit consists of a palm-sized, lightweight, battery-operated stimulator that generates a mild electrical impulse. Two to four electrodes are taped to the skin near or over a pain zone, and the client controls the electrode output to produce a pleasant sensation that relieves pain. The location of the electrodes and the voltage, frequency, and duration of the stimulus are determined by the spinal dermatomes most likely affected by the pain and the client's response. Tingling, buzzing, or vibrating sensations are initially felt, and some clients find them unpleasant or intolerable. Correct electrode placement and precise output adjustment are essential for this method to be successful. The advantages of TENS follow:

- It appears to produce increased blood flow.
- It may allow the client to decrease or eliminate pain medications.
- It does not produce dependence.
- It does not interfere with the client's daily activities.

Skin problems are the major adverse side effect. Skin irritation can be caused by tape irritation or an allergy to the tape or the gel; using hypoallergenic tape, a stockinette-type dressing, or a belt may help. Rashes from the gel may be remedied by changing to another gel, using cortisone cream by itself or mixed with the gel, rotating the electrode sites, and cleaning the electrodes daily with soap and water.

The client must use TENS only as the physician has prescribed; using TENS for new pain could lead to a delay in diagnosis and treatment. TENS should not be used by clients who have pacemakers because it may interfere with or inhibit the output of some demand-type pacemakers. Electrodes should not be placed over the eyes, over the carotid sinus (could precipitate a vasovagal reaction), and over the anterior neck or mouth areas (could cause spasms and the danger of airway closure). Safety has not been proven for the first trimester of pregnancy, but TENS has been used on the lower back during childbirth (McCaffery, 1979).

Increased pain has been reported in some clients after TENS; this is thought to be due to histamine release. The pain can be abolished by changing the frequency stimulation to 80 Hz or below 106 Hz (Woolf & Thompson, 1994). TENS is thought to produce analgesia by stimulating A-beta fibers to block A-delta and unmyelinated C-fibers, thus blocking noxious stimuli from the periphery by stimulating endorphins in the dorsal horn (Woolf & Thompson, 1994).

Cognitive Pain Relief Techniques

Cognitive therapies target beliefs, attitudes, expectations, control, and cognitive coping with pain. The major cognitive pain relief measures are anticipatory guidance and distraction, including guided imagery and hypnosis.

Anticipatory Guidance. Fear and dread may enhance or precipitate pain. The nurse can help by giving an honest explanation of what the client can expect. Sharing information about what the client will feel (sensory) and about the procedure is more effective than procedure information alone (Johnson, 1972; Johnson, Nail, Lauver, King, & Keys, 1988). Even if the nurse says that there probably will be pain, the client can usually man-

Therapeutic Dialogue
Pain Medication

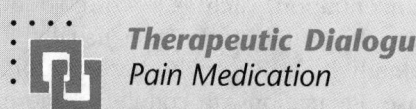

Scenes for Thought

As you walk down the hall of the hospital unit you hear quiet moaning. You go into room 410 and see Kathy Goodman lying on her side with her face to the wall. Her body is restless, and she is breathing erratically. Her roommate tells you (a little irritably) that she's been that way for the last 10 minutes. You note that she had varicose vein surgery yesterday and that she is 42 years old.

Effective

Nurse: *Ms. Goodman, I'm Linda Norman, the charge nurse. Can you tell me what's happening? (Standing by the bed.)*
Client: *My leg hurts.* She is grimacing and gasps as she turns over to look at you.
Nurse: *Has it gotten worse recently?*
Client: *No, it's just constant unless I move. So I don't move.*
Nurse: *I'll just run and get your chart so I can see when you had your last pain medication. (Does so.) Okay, you're about due for more medication, but maybe we can get you an increase until your pain decreases and you start to heal a little.*
Client: *No! I don't want to take more.*
Nurse: *I'm surprised to hear you say that. Could you explain?*
Client: Looks down. *I don't want to get too dependent on the pain pills.*
Nurse: *(Silent attention.)*
Client: *The last time I had my veins stripped the nurses would give the pain pills only every 4 hours and no more. They said it wasn't allowed because I'd get addicted. So I don't want any more.* Looks down.
Nurse: *I see.*
Client: *So I'll just have to deal with it.* Begins to close her eyes and settle her body stiffly into position.
Nurse: *Can I help in any way?*
Client: Opens her eyes wearily. *How?*
Nurse: *Well, first I need to examine your leg and ask you a few questions. Then we might be able to add a nonnarcotic pain pill to the ones you have to provide some overlap. When narcotics are used for medical purposes, such as your surgery pain, very few people become addicted—actually only four in 12,000 according to several studies. I also can teach you some relaxation techniques that might help relax you and reduce the pain. How do those options sound?*
Client: Thinking about it. *They might work. Worth a try, anyway.*
Nurse: *I thought you might be interested. Let's get started. (Begins to turn down the covers over the bed cradle covering her affected leg.)*

Less Effective

Nurse: *Ms. Goodman, I'm Liz Newman, the charge nurse. Can you tell me what's happening? (Standing by the bed.)*
Client: *My leg hurts.* She is grimacing and gasps as she turns over to look at you.
Nurse: *Has it gotten worse recently?*
Client: *No, it's just constant unless I move. So I don't move.*
Nurse: *I'll just run and get your chart so I can see when you had your last pain medication. (Does so.) Okay, you're about due for more medication, but maybe we can get you an increase until your pain decreases and you start to heal a little.*
Client: *No! I don't want to take more.*
Nurse: *But you seem to be in such pain! Besides (whispering) I think your roommate is really concerned for you and maybe a bit annoyed?*
Client: Looks embarrassed. *Oh, I didn't know I was bothering her. Are the pills safe for me to take? Someone told me I could become, you know, addicted.* Her body is tense.
Nurse: *As long as you're in such pain, you won't become addicted to them. We're careful about that. I'll bet they'll help.*
Client: Reluctantly. *Okay.*
Nurse: *Great! I'll get them to you right away. (Goes out in a hurry.)*
Client: Looks over at roommate as if to speak but then remains silent. Roommate doesn't make eye contact. Kathy's body remains tense.

Critical Thinking Challenge

• Relate Kathy's body language to her pain. • Explain the relationship between pain and stress. • Detect what the first nurse taught Kathy. • Compare and contrast what the second nurse taught her. • Propose other ways that Kathy could be helped to handle her pain. • Explain what happened by the end of the second dialogue to contribute to Kathy's tension. • Describe each nurse's manner in talking to Kathy.

age the pain better knowing what to expect and how to manage it. Anticipatory guidance can be used along with analgesics to prevent pain as much as possible.

The nurse can teach the preoperative client how to cope with postsurgical pain and how to improve mobility, because early ambulation and pulmonary hygiene are important after surgery. The nurse and client must recognize that most of these activities increase pain. Some techniques to relieve pain associated with these activities include the following:

Premedicating with an analgesic prior to painful activity; amount of time before the activity depends on the peak action of the drug

Splinting the incision with pillows to provide external immobilization and decrease muscle tension at the site

Positioning techniques, such as moving side to side, transferring to the side of the bed and to the chair, and proper walking posture

Distraction. Distraction is useful when clients are undergoing brief periods of sharp, intense pain, such as dressing changes, wound debridement, biopsy, or incident pain from shifting positions. The pain relief tends to be temporary, lasting only through the distraction exercise (ie, the Lamaze method for the woman in labor). Complex stimuli are useful for mild to moderate pain, but as the intensity of pain increases, the stimuli must be simplified.

Distraction may be visual (reading, looking at pictures), auditory (playing an instrument, listening to music), or tactile (stroking a pet, rocking). It is more effective if the distraction is something the client enjoys doing. Listening to music was shown to be an effective way to control cancer pain (Beck, 1991).

Guided Imagery. Guided imagery is a technique in which the person focuses on a pleasant, relaxed mental image as a way to decrease the intensity of pain or as a substitute for pain. The image of a healing ball of energy that reduces pain is sometimes used.

Hypnosis. Hypnosis heightens a person's susceptibility to suggestion and alters the subject's state of consciousness. It blocks the awareness of pain through suggestions or by substituting another feeling for pain, altering the meaning of pain, increasing the tolerance for pain, and in extreme cases, dissociating the perception of the body from the person's awareness (Syrjala, Cummings, & Donaldson, 1992). In general, about 20% of hypnotized clients with moderate to severe pain achieve total relief. Cancer clients with severe mucositis pain in the mouth and throat from bone marrow transplant therapy obtained excellent analgesia with hypnosis and required less pain medication than clients not using hypnosis (Syrjala, et al., 1992). Common myths about hypnosis limit its acceptance. It can be expensive and time-consuming, and practitioners require advanced training.

Behavioral Pain Relief Techniques

Behavioral therapies target actions under control of the client, such as muscle tension. Relaxation, meditation, and biofeedback are several of the techniques effective in controlling pain.

Relaxation. Relaxation techniques are useful pain-relief measures. Most call for a combination of a quiet environment, a comfortable position, a passive attitude, and a focus of concentration, such as a word, sound, or breathing pattern. Relaxation techniques usually are initiated independently by a nurse who has additional training in their use. Relaxation can counteract the effects of the fight-or-flight response and promote mental and physical freedom from tension and stress. Physical and mental tension can aggravate any pain; they may actually cause conditions such as headaches and back pain. Relaxation therapies promote a sense of detachment: The client feels a sense of control over the pain in a particular body part. Other benefits of relaxation include the following:

- It enables the client to fight fatigue and sleep restfully, thus increasing energy.
- It complements other pain-relief techniques.
- It allows the client to cope more effectively with the same intensity of pain.
- It improves the client's mood and flexibility.
- It produces physiologic changes (decreased muscle tension, increased blood flow, decreased heart and respiratory rate).

Relaxation training is not without problems. Many clients require booster sessions to refamiliarize themselves with procedures they may have forgotten. Some clients with chronic pain may resort to excessive use of relaxation procedures to escape from normal stresses of daily living: The technique itself becomes a debilitating pain behavior.

Meditation. Meditation is a technique in which the person focuses on a single thought or sound. *Transcendental meditation* is a popular form. *Yoga* is a combination of meditation and stretching exercises. *Progressive relaxation* is a technique of discriminating between tension and relaxation of specific muscles from head to toe. In *autogenics,* or passive progressive relaxation, the person repeats certain phrases silently to induce relaxation without discriminating between tension and relaxation. Autogenics can be useful with a cardiac client because tensing the muscles might add work for the heart; visualizing relaxation of muscles could decrease pain.

Biofeedback. In **biofeedback**, the client learns voluntary control over autonomic functions, such as heart rate, hand temperature, and muscle tension. Electrodes are placed on the client's body, and auditory or visual feedback (ie, lights, sounds, digital or graphic readings) provides the client with information about muscle relaxation, heart rate, blood pressure, and skin temperature. After baseline data are obtained, the client is taught relaxation and deep-breathing exercises. The relaxation decreases pain by decreasing anxiety and increasing the client's sense of control over pain. With practice, the client learns to call on the skills at will. This technique is helpful in clients with hypertension, muscle tension, tension headaches, migraines, temporal mandibular joint syndrome, insomnia, chronic pain, and stress-related disorders. Motivation is an important component in its success, because it requires extensive training.

Pharmacologic Management

Analgesic medication is the most common approach to pain management. Although analgesics are ordered by the physician, the nurse is responsible for giving the drugs, evaluating their effectiveness, and notifying the physician if the relief obtained is inadequate. The accompanying display gives an overview of the nurse's responsibility in the use of analgesics.

Analgesics may be separated into three major groups: nonopioid, opioid, and adjuvant. Their actions and nursing implications are given in Table 44-2. These analgesics are discussed in the following section.

Nonopioid analgesics: Used for mild to moderate pain, they alter pain perception by diminishing peripheral soup ingredients (peripheral sensitizing or activating substances) and by other mechanisms.

Opioid analgesics: Used for moderate to severe pain, they alter pain perception by binding to opioid receptors in the central and peripheral nervous system.

Nurses' Responsibility in the Use of Analgesics

- In hospitals, the nurse usually determines if and when an analgesic is given. Because analgesics are usually ordered prn, the nurse must judge how often the analgesic is given.
- Often the nurse must select the appropriate analgesic when more than one is prescribed. With various drugs and various routes of administration, the nurse needs to know about the drugs' potency, absorption, and pharmakokinetics.
- The nurse should have sound pain assessment skills to evaluate the effectiveness of the analgesic after each administration.
- The nurse is the health team member most likely to observe side effects from the analgesic. Close observation minimizes the risk for the client.
- The nurse must report promptly and accurately to the physician when a change in medication is needed.
- In home care, in office and clinic settings, and after discharge, the nurse is responsible for advising the client about analgesic use.

From McCaffery, M. (1979). *Nursing management of the patient with pain*. Philadelphia: J.B. Lippincott.

Three Reasons Pain Is Undertreated With Opioids

- Fear of causing respiratory depression
- Fear of causing addiction
- Clinicians' lack of basic pharmacologic knowledge

From Agency for Health Care Policy and Research (1994). Management of cancer pain. (Clinical practice guideline). Rockville, MD: U.S. Department of Health and Human Services.

Adjuvant analgesics: These are chemically and pharmacologically diverse drugs that act by various mechanisms to relieve pain or to enhance the analgesic effects of opioids

Nonopioid Analgesics. Nonopioid analgesics include aspirin, nonsteroidal anti-inflammatory drugs (NSAIDs), and acetaminophen. Aspirin and the NSAIDs have strong anti-inflammatory actions in peripheral tissue. Aspirin and other NSAIDs are generally effective for pain related to tissue damage. Also, these drugs have antiprostaglandin effects in the central nervous system (Weissman, 1991; Yaksh & Malmberg, 1994). The analgesic action of acetaminophen is unclear, but it also appears to act through central nervous system mechanisms. These drugs are used as single-agent therapy principally for mild pain but can be combined with opioids to improve pain control for mild, moderate, and severe pain. Because aspirin, several NSAIDs, and acetaminophen are so readily available without prescription, their effectiveness is often underestimated (Wilkie, 1993).

Opioid Analgesics. The opioid analgesics are a group of naturally occurring and synthetic agents that can relieve moderate to severe pain in the conscious state. Opioids are used for postoperative or trauma analgesia and are the mainstay of pain management for cancer. Research findings also indicate that opioids can be used for long-term management of chronic nonmalignant pain (Portenoy, 1990).

Opioid agonists are drugs that bind to specific opioid receptors to produce analgesia; morphine is the prototype (Jaffee & Martin, 1990). *Opioid antagonists* block the opioid receptors or displace the agonists from these sites; naloxone is the prototype. Opioid antagonists can reverse the depressant effects of opioids and are used to treat acute opioid overdoses. *Opioid agonist-antagonists* are drugs that bind to opioid receptors but exert effects only at certain receptors. Use of an opioid agonist-antagonist drug in a person dependent on an opioid agonist can precipitate acute withdrawal syndrome.

Table 44-2 • Drug Actions and Nursing Implications

Category/Drug	Action	Nursing Implications
Nonopioids		
Acetylsalicylic acid (ASA)	Analgesic: Blocks prostaglandin synthesis, thus decreasing sensitivity of peripheral pain receptors to mechanical or chemical activation. Antipyretic: Decreases outflow of vasoconstrictor impulses from hypothalamus, thus promoting vasodilation, sweating, and heat loss. Anti-inflammatory: Decreases capillary permeability and leakage of fluid into surrounding tissues; interferes with release of enzymes. Other actions decrease platelet aggregation.	Because gastric irritation is the major side effect of ASA, it should be given on a full stomach (although this delays absorption and pain relief). Stomach upset can also be avoided by taking enteric-coated ASA, which isn't absorbed until it reaches the intestine. Over several days or after several doses, ASA may cause ringing in the ears (tinnitus). This reflects damage to the auditory nerve and means the dose should be reduced immediately. ASA should never be given with oral anticoagulants, methotrexate, probenecid, or sulfinpyrazone because significant drug interactions will occur.
Acetaminophen	Analgesic and antipyretic: Elevates the pain threshold and reduces sympathetic outflow from hypothalamic temperature-regulating center. Weak antidiuretic action. Exerts no significant anti-inflammatory effect and does not produce gastric erosion, inhibition of platelet aggregation, or prothrombin depression.	Must be used with caution in people with known liver disease because it may cause liver toxicity. Daily dosage should not exceed 5,000 mg. Chronic use is associated with analgesic nephropathy.
Corticosteroids (eg, hydrocortisone, prednisone, dexamethasone)	Anti-inflammatory: Stabilize tissue membranes, and inhibit capillary dilation and permeability. Block synthesis of leukotrienes and prostaglandins.	Give with food or milk and urge clients to advise physician if gastric irritation persists, as drug can cause gastric ulceration. Supplemental antacids may alleviate the distress. Inform clients to notify physician if excessive weight gain, edema, hypertension, muscle weakness, bone pain, sore throat, fever, cold, infection, mood changes, or visual disturbances occur. Observe diabetics closely during steroid therapy, as hyperglycemia or loss of blood sugar control could occur.
Nonsteroidal anti-inflammatory drugs (NSAIDS) (eg, ibuprofen, naproxen, tolmetin, indomethacin)	Analgesic, anti-inflammatory, and antipyretic effects: Block synthesis and possibly release of prostaglandins. The principal advantage of these drugs is a somewhat lower incidence of the milder forms of GI distress that commonly occur with high-dose salicylate use (excluding indomethacin).	Observe clients with a history of GI problems for signs of gastric pain, nausea, cramping. Stop drug if symptoms persist. Reversible and preventable renal insufficiency is associated with most of the NSAIDs. Clients most at risk for this problem are those with congestive heart failure, renal disease, cirrhosis with ascites, and those over 60. Some clients may respond to only one of the several available nonsteroidal agents. Try different derivatives at 2- to 3-week intervals before concluding that this type of drug is ineffective.
Opioid Antagonist		
Naloxone	Binds to all the opioid receptors, but does not produce any effect on them. If an opioid agonist is bound to the receptor, this drug will displace the agonist and thereby counteract the agonist effect.	The drug of choice to counteract respiratory depression induced by opioids. Large doses will reverse the analgesic effects of opioids as well as the respiratory depression and could cause seizures.

(continued)

Table 44-2 *(Continued)*

Category/Drug	*Action*	*Nursing Implications*
Opioid Agonist–Antagonists		
Pentazocine, nalbuphine, butorphanol, dezocine	Bind to several types of opioid receptors, but produce a morphine-like action only at certain receptors (eg, agonist pain relief effect at kappa receptors). No morphine-like action is produced by binding at the mu or delta receptors (antagonist-like effect). If the receptor is dependent on agonist binding, withdrawal effects may be produced.	May precipitate withdrawal in people who have been receiving agonist opioids, antagonize the analgesic effects, and provide poor pain relief. Side effects include hallucinations.
Opioid Agonist		
Naturally occurring opium alkaloids (morphine, codeine) Semisynthetic derivates (hydromorphine, oxycodone, oxymorphone) Entirely synthetic derivates (meperidine, fentanyl, methadone)	Bind to opioid receptors in the peripheral and central nervous systems and produce pain-relieving effects at mu, delta, and kappa receptors. Agonist drugs alter perception and response to pain, may produce CNS depression (sedation and respiratory depression), and usually decrease gastric motility.	Morphine provides satisfactory pain relief in about 70% of clients with moderate to severe pain. However, if morphine fails to relieve pain or produces side effects (ie, nausea), better pain relief with fewer side effects may be achieved by changing to another opioid. Meperidine, although effective in many clients with acute pain, must be used cautiously because of possible CNS toxicity, hallucinations, seizures, and disorientation, especially in clients with renal or hepatic dysfunction. Poor oral absorption and short duration of action preclude its use in chronic pain. Methadone is useful in managing severe chronic pain, such as cancer pain, because it is only mildly sedating after the initial 2–5 days, has a long duration of action, and is absorbed well from the GI tract. Side effects include drowsiness, nausea, respiratory depression, CNS depression, and constipation.

Combining opioid and nonopioid analgesics is logical and effective, because pain is attacked by two different mechanisms. This approach allows better pain control without increasing the opioid dose. When the drugs are combined into one tablet, however, caution is needed to avoid excessive doses of the nonopioid. For example, total daily acetaminophen dosage should not exceed 4,000 to 5,000 mg, or liver damage is possible (American Pain Society, 1992). The opioid in most of the combination products (Percodan or Percocet), however, can be increased to as high a dose as is needed to provide pain relief.

Generally, intramuscular or subcutaneous administration of an opioid is appropriate for only a few days because subcutaneous and muscle tissue can quickly become irritated. Oral opioids are useful for the client in prolonged pain and with a functioning gastrointestinal tract. Transdermal fentanyl (a synthetic opioid) patch is now available for clients with cancer pain who cannot tolerate oral analgesics. This method of opioid delivery through the skin has an analgesic action with a slow onset (12–18 hours) and long duration (48 hours; Portenoy, et al., 1993). Clients with a stable temporal pattern to their pain are most likely to benefit from the patch. In cancer pain management, continuous subcutaneous infusions of opioids has been effective for months (MacMillan, Bruera, Kuehn, Selmser, & Macmillan, 1994). Severe cancer pain and postoperative pain also can be controlled by injecting opioids or combinations of opioids and local anesthetics directly into the epidural or intrathecal spaces, known as spinal analgesia (Wilkie, Vivenzo, & Puntillo, 1991).

The frequency with which a client receives an opioid for pain is often left largely to the nurse's discretion. This approach, however, should not preclude preventive pain relief. Because clients may not request an analgesic, the nurse should assess pain and determine if the client could benefit from one. With constant pain, opioids are given at fixed intervals before the pain returns (that is, before the analgesia wears off). Thus, the client's anticipation of pain is eliminated, and the client's anxiety decreases, controlling the vicious cycle of increasing pain with anxiety (see Fig. 44-4). This method may contribute to decreased pain and a decreased need for analgesia.

Respiratory Depression. Respiratory depression with opioid use is uncommon and is easily observed and treated with an opioid antagonist, such as naloxone. Resiratory depression occurs most often after acute administration of an opioid and is associated with other signs of central nervous system depression. Maximal respiratory depression occurs within 7 minutes of IV administration, within 30 minutes of intramuscular administration, within 60 minutes of oral administration, and within 24 hours of epidural or intrathecal administration.

When giving the initial opioid dose to a sleeping person, the nurse should closely observe the client for pain relief and respiratory depression (rate and depth). Awake clients do not succumb to respiratory depression (American Pain Society, 1992). The nurse also should monitor clients with a decreased respiratory reserve of effort (eg, those who have undergone thoracic or upper abdominal surgery). Because breathing causes considerable pain in these clients, they often do not breathe deeply, and this can lead to atelectasis and pneumonia. In these clients, opioids may actually increase respiratory activity by relieving the pain associated with breathing (Cousins, 1994).

Clients in respiratory depression, usually defined as less than 8 breaths per minute, can initially be treated by directing the client to "breathe now" and "breathe deep" (American Pain Society, 1992). If the client cannot follow instructions or is apneic, artificial ventilation is needed until naloxone, the opioid antagonist of choice for treating respiratory depression, is given. Small doses of naloxone can be given safely without causing withdrawal symptoms or counteracting all the analgesic effect of the opioid.

Addiction. Opioids can produce addiction, a psychological condition characterized by a drive to obtain and take substances for other than the prescribed value (AHCPR, 1994). Despite recent studies clearly indicating that medical use of opioids rarely leads to drug abuse or addiction, fear of addiction is still a major barrier to effective use of opioids in clients with pain. Less than 0.1% of clients who receive opioids as part of their medical treatment regimen become addicted; that is, 4 out of nearly 12,000 clients became addicted (Porter & Jick, 1980). Nurses can share these numbers with clients to help them reduce their concern about addiction.

Dependence. Dependence develops in most clients who receive opioids regularly for more than 10 days; it is an expected physiologic response to ongoing exposure to opioids (AHCPR, 1994). A person who is dependent on opioids responds to abrupt discontinuation or to administration of an opioid antagonist with characteristic withdrawal symptoms: anxiety, nervousness, irritability, diarrhea, and alternating chills and hot flashes. A prominent withdrawal sign is "wetness," including salivation, lacrimation, rhinorrhea, profuse perspiration, and gooseflesh. At the peak of withdrawal, clients may experience nausea and vomiting, abdominal cramps, insomnia, and rarely multifocal myoclonus. Abstinence symptoms usually occur within 6 to 12 hours and peak at 24 to 72 hours after cessation of morphine; a delayed onset is seen with drugs with long half-lives, such as methadone.

To prevent withdrawal syndrome, an opioid is discontinued by reducing the dose with a taper schedule. For example, to withdraw from morphine, calculate the 24-hour dose, decrease it by 50%, and give 25% of it every 6 hours. After 2 days, reduce the daily dose by an additional 25% every 2 days until the 24-hour oral dose is 30 mg/d, then discontinue the morphine (American Pain Society, 1992). Clonidine is useful for counteracting the side effects of withdrawal.

Tolerance. Tolerance develops when a dose of an opioid becomes less effective on repeated administration; larger doses are needed to produce the original effect. Tolerance is *not* addiction, but involves physiologic changes related to drug metabolism, the nervous system's adaptation to the drug action, or other factors. Intermittent use of opioids does not usually lead to significant tolerance. Not all clients experience tolerance. The need for an increase in the analgesic dose may reflect other factors, such as disease progression (eg, cancer progression) or new pathology (eg, pulmonary embolus). Do not ignore the client's reports of increased pain. It should be treated while the cause is pursued. One of the ways tolerance is managed is by drug titration to balance desired effects and side effects to maintain client comfort. Other approaches include changing to another drug in the same class or adding a nonopioid drug, such as ibuprofen. There is no ceiling effect for opioid agonist drugs. As tolerance increases, doses can be increased; doses as large as 1,654 mg IV morphine per hour have been administered (37,536 mg per day).

Side Effects. Other side effects of opioids are constipation, nausea and vomiting, and sedation. Constipation is the most common and most problematic adverse effect. Opioids act at multiple sites in the gastrointestinal tract and spinal cord to reduce intestinal secretions and decrease peristalsis. Tolerance to constipation does not develop at the same rate as tolerance to the other side effects. Clients taking routine doses of an opioid should drink at least 2 L of fluid daily, get daily exercise, eat a high-fiber diet, and take daily laxatives.

Nausea and vomiting are caused by delayed gastric emptying, stimulation of the medullary chemoreceptor zone and resultant stimulation of the nearby vomiting center, and stimulation of the vestibular part of the ear. Substituting an equianalgesic dose of another opioid may reduce or stop nausea and vomiting, or an antiemetic may be given with the opioid. Metoclopramide is an effective antiemetic for opioid-induced nausea because it increases gastric emptying. Many clients become tolerant to this side effect in a few days if it is not severe.

Sedation and drowsiness, which occur in most clients receiving opioids, are useful in some clinical situations, such as before anesthesia. Excessive sedation may be countered by reducing the dose and increasing the interval between doses. In addition, other central nervous system depressants should be discontinued, such as sedative-hypnotics and antianxiety agents, which potentiate the sedative effects of opioids. However, fatigue and insomnia may be caused by the pain itself; an opioid dose may allow the client to sleep. In the client taking regular opioids, drowsiness may occur for the first 2 or 3 days but is usually temporary (AHCRP, 1992; 1994). Psychostimulants, particularly methylphenidate, dramatically improve opioid-induced sedation (AHCPR, 1994).

Precipitous Death. Some individuals believe that administering large doses of morphine constitutes assisted suicide or euthanasia. It is not uncommon for health professionals, clients, and family members to be concerned about the effect of sufficient pain relief on precipitating the death of a terminally ill person. Relieving pain, even if it hastens death in a terminally ill person, is the ethical and moral obligation of the professional nurse; it is not euthanasia or assisted suicide (American Nurses Association [ANA], 1992). When consistent with the client's wishes, the position of the ANA is, "Nurses should not hesitate to use full and effective doses of pain medication for the proper management of pain in the dying client. The increasing titration of medication to achieve adequate symptom control, even at the expense of life, thus hastening death, is ethically justified" (ANA, 1992, p. 14).

Patient-Controlled Analgesia. Patient-controlled analgesia (PCA), in which clients give themselves doses of opioid analgesics, allows clients to become more involved in their own care (AHCPR, 1992). Clinical studies show that it is safe and effective and that selected clients tend to take only as much drug as they need for pain control (AHCPR, 1992). The small, frequent IV doses given in PCA systems relieve pain without excessive sedation because they do not produce the wide variations in blood levels of analgesics with conventional therapy (Fig. 44-7).

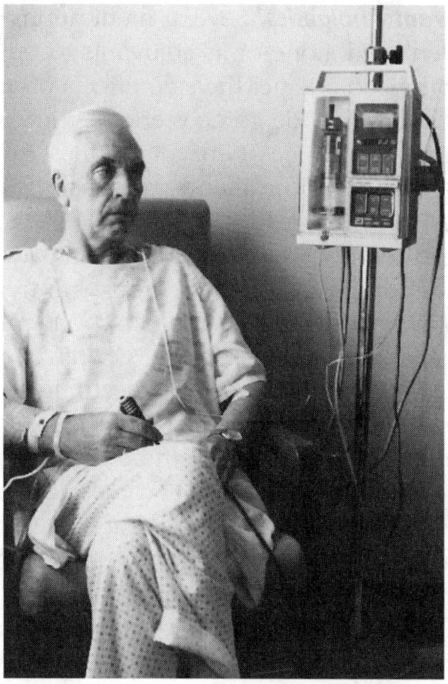

Figure 44-7 • *Patient-controlled analgesia (PCA) allows the client to self-administer only as much medication as needed to control pain.*

The PCA system has a safety feature to prevent accidental overdoses. Even if the client pushes the button for another dose, the device cannot deliver another full dose until the correct amount of time, as preset by the physician, has elapsed. This lock-out time should not be so long that the client must wait in pain between doses, however. In clients with severe acute or prolonged pain that cannot be controlled by any other route, a continuous IV or subcutaneous infusion may be used in addition to the PCA approach. This method provides a steady blood level of the analgesic.

Postoperative Pain. The accompanying display shows guidelines on the nursing management of acute postoperative pain. Unfortunately, too often these guidelines are not used in the treatment of pain in adults (Maxam-Moore, Wilkie, & Woods, 1994) or children (Tesler, Wilkie, Holzemer, & Savedra, 1994).

Nursing Care Guidelines
The Person With Acute Postoperative Pain

- Assess the client's physiologic, affective, behavioral, and cognitive response to pain, both verbal and nonverbal.
- Give narcotics around the clock, not prn, for the first 36 hours after surgery.
- Give analgesics before or as soon as pain returns.
- Give analgesics before activities, such as ambulation or incentive spirometer use.
- Individualize the drug and dosage.
- Monitor and record the client's response using a pain scale routinely.

From Agency for Health Care Policy and Research (1992). Acute pain management: Operative or medical procedures and trauma. (Clinical practice guideline). Rockville, MD: U.S. Department of Health and Human Services.

Adjuvant Analgesics. Several medications are analgesic when used alone or as adjuvants to opioid analgesia, or they counteract the side effects of analgesics. Adjuvant drugs include corticosteriods, tricyclic antidepressants, antihistamines, benzodiazepines, caffeine, anticonvulsants, local anesthetics, and psychostimulants (AHCPR, 1994; American Pain Society, 1992).

Corticosteroids are useful for inflammation-related pain. These drugs are used for short-term treatment in young, otherwise healthy clients with sports-related pain that does not respond to NSAIDs (Chapman & Bonica, 1983). Corticosteroids also can be useful for various inflammatory conditions (such as active rheumatoid arthritis and ulcerative colitis) and can be injected at the site of inflammation or given by other routes. Corticosteroids provide a range of other effects that are useful in the treatment of cancer pain, such as mood elevation, antiemetic activity, and appetite stimulation (AHCPR, 1994). In clients with cancer, corticosteroids, particularly those with mineralocorticoid-sparing activity (dexamethasone), have been used for more than 6 months without adverse effects outweighing their useful effects.

Antidepressant drugs are effective analgesics, especially in clients with pain from nerve damage (**neuropathic pain**). These drugs potentiate the analgesic effect of opioids and have innate analgesic properties; they provide analgesia in people who are not depressed and in those who are depressed. In addition to pain relief, which occurs within 1 to 2 weeks, these drugs elevate mood and improve sleep. The most widely reported experience has been with amitriptyline, the tricyclic antidepressant of choice, even though it produces side effects (dry mouth, constipation, urinary retention, and orthostatic hypotension) related to its anticholinergic activity. To minimize side effects, small (10–25 mg) doses at bedtime are recommended (AHCPR, 1994). Safety is a major concern in clients taking this drug; they may fall because of the orthostatic hypotension. Encouraging adequate hydration and resting in a sitting position before shifting from a reclining to a standing position are important nursing interventions to assist clients to tolerate this effective drug.

Other adjuvant drugs interfere with nerve conduction (anticonvulsants and local anesthetics), block histamine in the peripheral soup (antihistamines), or reduce anxiety (benzodiazepines, antihistamines). Caffeine increases analgesia when given with aspirin-like drugs (American Pain Society, 1992). Psychostimulants, such as dextroamphetamine or methylphenidate, improve opioid analgesia and decrease sedation (AHCPR, 1994).

Older Clients. Older clients are more susceptible to drug effects and may more readily experience confusion, excessive sedation, or respiratory depression from opioids. With age, the liver and kidneys become less efficient at metabolizing and clearing drugs from the system, and this can lead to accumulation of the drug in older clients. Because older clients tend to take more drugs, there is an increased risk of drug interactions. Therefore, **titration** (adjusting the dosage based on the client's response) is mandatory.

Use of Placebos. Placebos historically have been used in selected situations to differentiate psychological pain from nociceptive or neuropathic pain. Pain relieved by a placebo was considered to be psychogenic. Now it is clearly known that a positive placebo response does not prove that a client's pain is psychogenic. Placebos act through endogenous opioids and are reversed by naloxone, just like morphine's effects are reversed by naloxone (Levine, Gordon, & Fields, 1978). Use of a placebo without the client's knowledge is considered unethical nursing practice. A placebo, however, can be used with client consent to determine if a particular therapy is effective. When placebos are used in this manner, it is essential that the client have access to other analgesics if they request additional pain relief.

The nurse who explains the drug's effects optimistically to the client may find that the drug works more effectively. This approach is thought to maximize the placebo response and minimize emotional and cognitive factors that influence pain perception.

Invasive Medical Management of Pain

When intractable pain cannot be controlled by analgesics and other nonpharmacologic approaches, as in advanced cancer or excessive pain with tic douloureux (trigeminal neuralgia), surgical intervention to interrupt pain pathways may be necessary (Rosomoff, Papo, & Loeser, 1990). Table 44-3 summarizes common invasive interventions. Proper client and family teaching is essential before any surgical procedure. They must understand the procedure, risks, possible complications, and possible duration of pain relief.

Community-Based Nursing

Increasingly, pain management is occurring through case management. Such care crosses a variety of healthcare settings. Economic trends suggest that even cancer clients with pain will soon be managed without hospitalization. Pain experts agree that a combination of pharmacologic and nonpharmacologic strategies provides the best management in all healthcare settings (AHCPR, 1994).

Home pain management is critical in determining the functional ability and quality of life of clients with chronic pain. Chronic pain may immobilize clients and hinder their daily activities, relationships, sleep, and appetite. Family members often provide complex symp-

Table 44-3* • *Invasive Pain Management Interventions

Technique	Advantage	Limitations/Precautions	When Used
Nerve roots or pathway interrupted or destroyed: Neurectomy—peripheral sensory nerves; Sympathectomy—sympathetic ganglia; Rhizotomy—dorsal root ganglia; Cordotomy—anterolateral spinothalamic tract	May decrease or eliminate pain	May leave permanent damage (ie, paralysis, loss of control of the elimination process and sensation) or more severe pain	Intractable pain (ie, advanced cancer or tic douloureux [trigeminal neuralgia])
Nerve blocks (injected with anesthetic to interrupt nerve pathway)	May decrease or eliminate pain	Pain relief variable	Intractable pain (ie, celiac block for gastrointestinal malignancy)
Alcohol injections through transnasal or transphenoid approach of pituitary gland	Nontraumatic, easily performed, inexpensive	Pain relief variable; complications are signs of pituitary inactivation: hypopituitarism, steroid deficiency, decreased libido	Intractable pain from bony metastases from breast and prostate that are estrogen-sensitive
Injections of opioids, local anesthetics, or clonodine into central nervous system through a catheter placed in either the epidural space (space just outside dura mater; analgesic must filter through dura throughout the cerebrospinal fluid [CSF] and spinal cord) or subarachnoid space (contains the CSF)	Catheters can be left in place for months or years. Client or caregiver can give injections or have intermittent or continuous pump placed to deliver drugs. This allows independence and allows client to go home and into community. May decrease or eliminate pain.	Preservative-free opioid is used to avoid damage to spinal cord or nerve roots. A pump increases the cost of therapy. Preservative-free opioids are costly. Complications may include nausea/vomiting, urinary retention, pruritus, myoclonus, and respiratory depression, which naloxone can reverse. Close nursing monitoring for somnolence and respiratory depression for the first 24 hours is imperative.	Acute pain (ie, postoperative thoracic or abdominal surgery, postcesarean section, phantom pain), chronic intractable pain

tom management; ambulatory and home-health nurses assess the interventions and test new interventions.

It is the nurse's responsibility to teach pain management to the client and family as early as possible in the course of care and to anticipate the length of time pain will be experienced. The postoperative client needs information on the healing process and should be encouraged to maintain his or her pain at the lowest level possible, get adequate rest and nutrition, avoid fatigue, and increase mobility. These factors affect client comfort and enhance recovery. The client should know how long recovery should take so that medical intervention can be sought if complications occur.

Clients taking analgesics must understand the correct dosage and common side effects and how to avoid or manage them. They should know that analgesics initially may produce changes in judgment, perception, and coordination when doses are increased, but these effects clear in a few days. Clients should be cautioned not to drive or operate machinery until these cognitive effects have cleared. Clients with cancer often drive safely when they require huge doses of morphine (more than 1000 mg/d) to control their pain (Hill, 1991) because they are adjusted to the side effects. Breastfeeding mothers need to know whether the drug is present in their milk and whether it may affect the infant. At

Nursing Plan of Care
The Client Experiencing Pain

Nursing Diagnosis

Pain related to abdominal surgical incision manifested by verbal report of pain (9 on a 0–10 scale) and nonverbal communication of pain.

Client Goal

Client will experience pain level no greater than 2 (on a 0–10 scale) (number able to tolerate)

Client Outcome Criteria

- Client reports location, intensity, quality, and temporal pattern of pain and appropriate relief measures for pain.
- Client reports pain immediately at each occurrence.
- Client states pain is minimized at onset of analgesic effect and relieved at peak effect of analgesic therapy.

Nursing Intervention	Scientific Rationale
1. Evaluate preoperative comprehensive pain assessment.	1. The most important component of pain is an ongoing, accurate, thorough pain assessment.
2. Assess level of pain every 2 hours for first 24 hours using a self-rating scale of 0 to 10. Also assess location, quality, and temporal pattern if these have changed since initial assessment.	2. To obtain data about how this person reports pain intensity.
3. Provide optimal pain relief with prescribed analgesics.	3. Optimal pain relief decreases anxiety and fear, both of which increase pain. Goal is to use a preventive approach to avoid severe pain.
a. Individualize medication regimen. Collaborate with physician to prescribe opioid around the clock instead of prn in the first 36 hours to maintain opioid blood levels and provide good pain relief.	a. Ongoing assessment of severity of pain before and pain relief after medication is important. This identifies if the drug or dose is sufficient for the client's pain.
b. Assess response to medications.	b. Respiratory depression, constipation, nausea, vomiting, and dry mouth can be caused by opioids.
c. Monitor for and minimize common side effects of medications (specify).	
4. Solicit techniques that have previously been helpful.	4. Individual techniques that a client has used in the past enhance pain relief.
5. Establish a trusting relationship.	5. An effective nurse–client relationship enhances all pain-relief measures because it conveys "I care—you can trust me."
6. Instruct client to report pain promptly so that relief measures can be instituted before severe pain occurs. Use therapeutic approaches for the prevention of severe pain, not the relief of severe pain.	6. Relief measures are instituted based on client's verbal report of pain and regular client assessments. This also informs client of the expectation to communicate when in pain, because many ethnic and cultural influences often discourage or prohibit expression of pain.
7. Allow rest periods during day and periods of uninterrupted sleep at night when possible. Keep environment quiet.	7. Rest facilitates comfort and sleep, reduces stress, relieves muscle tension, and increases relaxation. Fatigue may enhance pain by lowering pain tolerance.

(continued)

Nursing Plan of Care
The Client Experiencing Pain (continued)

8. Collaborate with client to initiate the appropriate noninvasive pain relief measure(s). a. Instruct in distraction technique (specify). Example: Engage in conversation or turn radio on to favorite station during abdominal dressing change. b. Instruct in cutaneous stimulation (specify). Example: Give backrub after turning and before bedtime. c. Instruct in relaxation techniques (specify). Example: Relax muscles when turning.	8. Attention is focused away from pain, and increased pain tolerance results. a. Skin stimulation closes the gate to pain impulses by stimulating endorphins. b. Change of position increases circulation and decreases muscle tension.

home, analgesics must be kept in safe, childproof bottles away from children or others.

Evaluation

An important part of the nurse's role in pain management is accurately evaluating the effectiveness of pain-relief measures by observing and questioning the client. The nurse never assumes that nursing interventions have been successful. Depending on the results, the measures may be modified or an alternate approach tried.

Specific outcome criteria are used to measure the attainment of client goals. Although some examples of outcome criteria are presented, it is essential to develop outcome criteria for each client.

Goal

The client will report a pain intensity level at or less than he or she states is tolerable.

Possible Outcome Criteria

- At the time of therapy onset, the client calls the pain intensity a lower number (0–10) than that reported when the therapy was administered (at 5 minutes for IV morphine).
- Client states at the time of peak effect for the therapy that the pain intensity level is 0 on a scale of 0 to 10 (at 20 minutes for IV morphine).
- Within the duration of effect for the therapy administered, the client will perform self-care activities to the extent of his or her ability (within 20 minutes and 2 to 4 hours of the IV morphine dose).

Goal

The client will identify factors that precipitate pain.

Possible Outcome Criteria

- At the next appointment, client describes factors that precipitate pain.
- At the next appointment, client describes thoughts and feelings that aggravate pain.
- On the next home visit, client reports behaviors that aggravate the pain.

Goal

The client will use techniques that decrease pain.

Possible Outcome Criteria

- At the next appointment, client identifies the medication regimen that optimally controls pain.
- Within 24 hours, client describes at least one behavioral intervention that helps to control pain.

Key Concepts

- Pain is a subjective experience that occurs whenever the client says it occurs.
- Initially, pain minimizes injury and warns of disease. Persistent pain has no purpose.
- All pain-relief measures are based on a thorough ongoing assessment.
- Sedation does not always indicate pain relief.
- Because clients may not always report pain, the nurse must assess for pain regularly.
- Clients of all ages experience pain, but the way they express it differs with age, the type of pain, and their ability to cope with the pain.
- The nurse should be able to recognize physiologic, verbal, and nonverbal ways of expressing pain.

- Lack of pain expression does not mean lack of pain.
- Cognitive and behavioral pain-relief measures can augment the effectiveness of pharmacologic or invasive methods.
- The nurse's optimistic attitude about expected pain relief helps produce a positive result.
- Educating the client and family about pain reduces anticipatory fear and anxiety, thereby decreasing the client's pain.
- Using a preventive approach for pain relief is more beneficial than waiting until pain becomes severe.
- All routes of opioid administration are effective for mild, moderate, and severe pain, but intramuscular and IV routes act faster.
- Combining nonopioid, opioid, and adjuvant drugs with nonpharmacologic methods produces excellent analgesia because pain is relieved through different methods.

Critical Thinking Challenges

Now that you have added pain perception and pain management to your knowledge base, turn again to the situation at the beginning of the chapter. Apply what you have learned to your client with lung cancer by addressing the challenges that follow.

1. *Give your opinion of the client's reports of pain and immobility.*
2. *Reflect on your feelings about the client's health history and present condition. Infer what the client's thoughts and feelings may be.*
3. *Outline additional assessment data you need to develop a plan for managing this person's pain.*
4. *Explain the rationale for using pharmacologic and nonpharmacologic methods of pain relief for this client.*
5. *Plan at least two health-promotion activities that would be helpful for this client.*

References

Agency for Health Care Policy and Research (1994). *Management of cancer pain.* (Clinical practice guideline). Rockville, MD: U.S. Department of Health and Human Services.

Agency for Health Care Policy and Research (1992). *Acute pain management: Operative or medical procedures and trauma.* (Clinical practice guideline). Rockville, MD: U.S. Department of Health and Human Services.

American Nurses Association (1992). *Compendium of position statements on the nurse's role in end-of-life decisions* (M-30). Washington, DC: Author.

American Pain Society (1992). *Principles of analgesic use in the treatment of acute pain and chronic cancer pain: A concise guide to medical practice* (3rd ed.). Skokie, IL: Author.

Beck, S. L. (1991). The therapeutic use of music for cancer-related pain. *Oncology Nursing Forum, 18,* 1327–1337.

Beyer, J. E., & Aradine, C. R. (1987). Patterns of pediatric pain intensity: A methodological investigation of a self-report scale. *The Clinical Journal of Pain, 3,* 130–141.

Bonica, J. J. (Ed.) (1990). *The management of pain* (Vols. 1–2) (2nd ed.). Philadelphia: Lea & Febiger.

Cassell, E. J. (1989). The relationship between pain and suffering. In C. S. Hill & W. S. Fields (Eds.), *Advances in pain research and therapy* (11th ed.) (pp. 61–70). New York: Raven Press.

Chapman, C. R., & Bonica, J. J. (1983). *Acute pain.* Upjohn Scope. Kalamazoo: The Upjohn Company.

Coderre, T. J., Katz, J., Vaccarino, A. L., et al. (1993). Contribution of central neuroplasticity to pathological pain: Review of clinical and experimental evidence. *Pain, 52,* 259–285.

Cousins, M. (1994). Acute and postoperative pain. In P. D. Wall & R. Melzack (Eds.), *Textbook of pain* (3rd ed.) (pp. 357–385). New York: Churchill Livingstone.

Coyle, N, Breitbart, W., Weaver, S., & Portenoy, R. (1994). Delirium as a contributing factor to "crescendo" pain: Three case reports. *Journal of Pain and Symptom Management, 9,* 44–47.

Devor, M. (1994). The pathophysiology of damaged peripheral nerves. In P. D. Wall & R. Melzack (Eds.), *Textbook of pain* (3rd ed.) (pp. 79–100). New York: Churchill Livingstone.

Dubner, R., & Basbaum, A. I. (1994). Spinal dorsal horn plasticity following tissue or nerve injury. In P. D. Wall & R. Melzack (Eds.), *Textbook of pain* (3rd ed.) (pp. 225–241). New York: Churchill Livingstone.

Faucett, J. A., & Levine, J. D. (1991). The contribution of interpersonal conflict to chronic pain in the presence or absence of organic pathology. *Pain, 44,* 35–43.

Ferrell, B. R. (1993). To know suffering. *Oncology Nursing Forum, 20,* 1471–1477.

Ferrell, B. R., Cohen, M. Z., Rhiner, M., & Rozek, A. (1991). Pain as a metaphor for illness part II. Family caregivers' management of pain. *Oncology Nursing Forum, 18,* 1315–1321.

Fields, H. L., & Basbaum, A. I. (1994). Central nervous system mechanisms of pain modulation. In P. D. Wall & R. Melzack (Eds.), *Textbook of pain* (3rd ed.) (pp. 243–257). New York: Churchill Livingstone.

Fishman, B., Pasternak, S., Wallenstein, S. L., Houde, R. W., Holland, J. C., & Foley, K. M. (1987). The Memorial Pain Assessment Card: A valid instrument for the evaluation of cancer pain. *Cancer, 60,* 1151–1158.

Fitzgerald, M. (1994). Neurobiology of fetal and neonatal pain. In P. D. Wall & R. Melzack (Eds.), *Textbook of pain* (3rd ed.) (pp. 153–163). New York: Churchill Livingstone.

Gaston-Johansson, F., Albert, M., & Fagan, E. (1990). Similarities in pain descriptions of four different ethnic-culture groups. *Journal of Pain & Symptom Management, 5,* 94–100.

Haleman, S. (1994). Manipulation and massage for the relief of back pain. In P. D. Wall & R. Melzack (Eds.), *Textbook of pain* (3rd ed.) (pp 11251–1262). New York: Churchill Livingstone.

Harkins, S. W., Price, D. D., Bush, F. M., & Small, R. E. (1994). In P. D. Wall & R. Melzack (Eds.), *Textbook of pain* (3rd ed.) (pp 769–784). New York: Churchill Livingstone.

Hester, N. O., Foster, R., & Kristensen, K. (1990). Measurement of pain in children: Generalizability and validity of the Pain Ladder and the Poker Chip Tool. In D. C. Tyler & E. J. Krane (Eds.), *Pediatric pain. Advances in pain research and therapy* (Vol. 15) (pp. 79–84). New York: Raven Press.

Hill, C. S. (Speaker) (1991). *My word against theirs: Narcotics for cancer pain control* (Video cassette). Norwalk, CT: The Purdue Frederick Co.

Jaffee, J. H., & Martin, W. R. (1990). Opioid analgesics and antagonists. In A. G. Gilman, T. W. Rall, A. Nies, & P. Taylor (Eds.), *Goodman and Gilmans' the pharmacological basis of therapeutics.* New York: Pergamon Press.

Johnson, J. E. (1972). Effects of structuring clients' expectations on their reactions to threatening events. *Nursing Research, 21,* 499–503.

Johnson, J. E., Nail, L. M., Lauver, D., King, K. B., & Keys, H. (1988). Reducing the negative impact of radiation therapy on functional status. *Cancer, 61,* 46–51.

Lehmann, J. F., & de Lateur, B. (1994). Ultrasound, shortwave, microwave, laser, superficial heat and cold in the treatment of pain. In P. D. Wall & R. Melzack (Eds.), *Textbook of pain* (3rd ed.) (pp. 1237–1249). New York: Churchill Livingstone.

Levine, J. D., Gordon, N. C., & Fields, H. L. (1978). The mechanism of placebo analgesia. *Lancet, 2,* 654–657.

Levine, J., & Taiwo, Y. (1994). Inflammatory pain. In P. D. Wall & R. Melzack (Ed.), *Textbook of pain* (3rd ed.) (pp 45–56). New York: Churchill Livingstone.

Liebeskind, J. C. (1991). Pain can kill. *Pain, 44,* 3–4.

Maxam-Moore, V. V., Wilkie, D. J., & Woods, S. L. (1994). Analgesics for cardiac surgery clients in critical care: Describing current practice. *American Journal of Critical Care, 3,* 31–39.

McCaffery, M. (1979). *Nursing management of the client with pain.* Philadelphia: J. B. Lippincott.

McCaffery, M., & Beebe, A. (1989). *Pain: Clinical manual for nursing practice.* St. Louis, MO: C. V. Mosby.

McCaffery, M., & Ferrell, B. R. (1992). How vital are vital signs? *Nursing, 22,* 42–46.

McDonald, J. B., Baillie, J., Williams, B. O., & Ballantyne, D. (1983). Coronary care in the elderly. *Age Aging, 12,* 17–20.

MacMillan, K., Bruera, E., Kuehn, N., Selmser, P., & Macmillan, A. (1994). A prospective comparison study between a butterfly needle and a Teflon cannula for subcutaneous narcotic administration. *Journal of Pain and Symptom Management, 9,* 82–84.

Melzack, R. (1975). The McGill Pain Questionnaire: Major properties and scoring methods. *Pain, 1,* 277–299.

Melzack, R., & Wall, P. (1965). Pain mechanisms: A new theory. *Science, 150,* 971–979.

Merskey, H., & Bogduk, N. (1994). *Classification of chronic pain: Descriptions of chronic pain syndromes and definitions of pain terms.* Seattle: IASP Press.

Meyer, R. A., Campbell, J. N., & Raja, S. N. (1994). Peripheral neural mechanisms of nociception. In P. D. Wall & R. Melzack (Eds.), *Textbook of pain* (3rd ed.) (pp. 13–44). New York: Churchill Livingstone.

North American Nursing Diagnosis Association. *NANDA Nursing diagnoses: Definition and classification* 1995–1996. Philadelphia.

Owens, M. E. (1986). A crying need. Infants perceive pain. *American Journal of Nursing, 86* (1), 73–94.

Porter, J., & Jick, H. (1980). Addiction rare in clients treated with narcotics. *New England Journal of Medicine, 302,* 123.

Portenoy, R. K. (1990). Chronic opioid therapy in nonmalignant pain. *Journal of Pain and Symptom Management, 5* (Suppl. 1), S46–S62.

Portenoy, R. K., et. al. (1993). Transdermal fentanyl for cancer pain: Repeated dose pharmacokinetics. *Anesthesia, 23,* 207–214.

Puntillo, K. A., & Wilkie, D. J. (1991). The assessment of pain in the critically ill. In K. A. Puntillo (Ed.), *Pain in the critically ill: Assessment and management* (pp. 45–64). Rockville, MD: Aspen.

Rhiner, M., Ferrell, B. R., Ferrell, B. A., & Grant, M. M. (1993). A structured nondrug intervention program for cancer pain. *Cancer Practice, 1,* 137–143.

Rosomoff, H. L., Papo, I., & Loeser, J. (1990). Neurosurgical operations on the spinal cord. In J. J. Bonica (Ed.), *The management of pain* (Vol. II) (pp. 2067–2081). Philadelphia: Lea & Febiger.

Sato, J., & Perl, E. R. (1991). Adrenergic excitation of cutaneous pain receptors induced by peripheral nerve injury. *Science, 251,* 1608–1610.

Savedra, M. C., Holzemer, W. L., Tesler, M. D., Ward, J. A., & Wilkie, D. J. (1993). Assessment of postoperative pain in children and adolescents using the Adolescent Pediatric Pain Tool. *Nursing Research, 42,* 5–9.

Syrjala, K. L., Cummings, C., & Donaldson, G. W. (1992). Hypnosis or cognitive behavioral training for the reduction of pain and nausea during cancer treatment: A controlled clinical trial. *Pain, 48,* 137–146.

Taylor, E. J., Ferrell, B. R., Grant, M., et al. (1993). Managing cancer pain at home: The decisions and ethical conflicts of clients, family caregivers, and homecare nurses. *Oncology Nursing Forum, 20,* 919–927.

Tesler, M. D., Savedra, M. C., Holzemer, W. L., Wilkie, D. J., Ward, J. A., & Paul, S. M. (1991). The word-graphic rating scale as a measure of children's and adolescents' pain intensity. *Research in Nursing and Health, 14,* 361–371.

Tesler, M. D., Wilkie, D. J., Holzemer, W. L., & Savedra, M. C. (1994). Postoperative analgesics for children and adolescents: Prescription and administration. *Journal of Pain and Symptom Management, 9,* 85–95.

Wall, P. D., & Melzack, R. (Eds.) (1994). *Textbook of pain* (3rd ed.). New York: Churchill Livingstone.

Weisenberg, M. (1994). Cognitive aspects of pain. In P. D. Wall & R. Melzack (Eds.), *Textbook of pain* (3rd ed.) (pp. 275–289). New York: Churchill Livingstone.

Weissman, G. (1991). The actions of NSAIDs. *Hospital Practice, 26,* 60–76.

Wilkie, D. J. (1995). Facial expression of pain in lung cancer. *Analgesia, 1,* 91–99.

Wilkie, D. J. (1993). Pharmacological management of cancer pain: Summary-of-the-science. *Journal of the National Cancer Institute, 85,* 1117–1120

Wilkie, D. J., Holzemer, W. L., Tesler, M., Ward, J. A., Paul, S. M., & Savedra, M. C. (1990). Measuring pain quality: Validity and reliability of children's and adolescents' pain language. *Pain, 41,* 151–159.

Wilkie, D. J., & Keefe, F. J. (1991). Coping strategies of clients with lung cancer-related pain. *The Clinical Journal of Pain, 7,* 292–299.

Wilkie, D. J., Keefe, F. J., Dodd, M. J., & Copp, L. A. (1992). Behavior of clients with lung cancer: Description and associations with oncologic and pain variables. *Pain, 51,* 231–240.

Wilkie, D. J., Olsson, G. L., & Metcalf, C. L. (1993). *Essentials of pain management: A nursing handbook.* Seattle, WA: Optioncare.

Wilkie, D. J., Williams, A. R., Grevstad, P., & Mekwa, J. (1995). Coaching persons with lung cancer to report sensory pain: Literature review and pilot study findings. *Cancer Nursing, 18,* 7–15.

Wilkie, D. J., Vivenzo, K., & Puntillo, K. (1991). Point: Registered nurses should administer and monitor spinal analgesia within the state-defined scope of practice—The California perspective. *Nurse Anesthesia, 2,* 6–9.

Woolf, C. J. (1994). The dorsal horn: State-dependent sensory processing and the generation of pain. In P. D. Wall & R. Melzack (Eds.), *Textbook of pain* (3rd ed.) (pp. 101–112). New York: Churchill Livingstone.

Woolf, C. J., & Thompson, J. W. (1994). Stimulation-induced analgesia: Transcutaneous electrical nerve stimulation (TENS) and vibration. In P. D. Wall & R. Melzack (Eds.), *Textbook of pain* (3rd ed.) (pp. 1191–1208). New York: Churchill Livingstone.

Yaksh, T. L., & Malmberg, A. B. (1994). Central Pharmacology of nociceptive transmission. In P. D. Wall & R. Melzack (Eds.), *Textbook of pain* (3rd ed.) (pp. 165–200). New York: Churchill Livingstone.

Bibliography

Carroll, D., & Bowsher, D. (1993). *Pain: Management and nursing care.* Oxford: Butterworth-Heinemann.

Culpepper-Morgan J. A., Inturrisi, C. E., Portenoy, R. K., Foley, K., Houde, R. W., Marsh, F., & Kreek, M. J. (1992). Treatment of opioid-induced constipation with oral naloxone: A pilot study. *Clinical Pharmacology and Therapeutics, 52,* 90–95.

Empting-Koschorke, L. D., Hendler, N., Kolodny, A. L., & Kraus, H. (1990). Non-drug management of chronic pain: What today's pain clinics have to offer. *Client Care, 24* (1), 165–168.

Ferrell, B. R., McCaffery, M., & Rhiner, M. (1992). Pain and addiction: An urgent need for change in nursing education. *Journal of Pain and Symptom Management, 7,* 117–124.

Green, P. E. (1993). America responds to cancer pain: A survey of state pain initiatives. *Cancer Practice, 1,* 65–71.

McCaffery, M., Ferrell, B., O'Neil-Page, E., & Lester, M. (1990). Nurses' knowledge of opioid analgesic drugs and psychological dependence. *Cancer Nursing, 13* (1), 21–27.

McGuire, D. B., Yarbro, C. H., & Ferrell, B. R. (1995). *Cancer Pain Management* (2nd ed.). Boston: Jones & Barlett.

Miaskowski, C., Niles, R., Brody, R., & Synold, T. (1994). Assessment of client satisfaction utilizing the American Pain Society's Quality Assurance Standards on Acute and Cancer-Related Pain. *Journal of Pain and Symptom Management, 9,* 5–11.

Morris, D., Wilkie, D. J., & Fanslow, J. Registered Nurses' knowledge of opioid analgesic pharmacology. Submitted.

Puntillo, K. A., & Weiss, S. J. (1994). Pain: Its mediators and associated morbidity in critically ill cardiovascular surgical clients. *Nursing Research, 43,* 31–36.

Ready, L. B., & Edwards, W. T. (Eds.) (1992). *Management of acute pain: A practical guide.* Seattle, WA: International Association for the Study of Pain.

Wilkie, D. J., Lovejoy, N., Dodd, M., & Tesler, M. (1990). Cancer pain intensity measurement: Concurrent validity of three instruments-finger dynamometer, pain intensity number scale, visual analogue scale. *Hospice Journal, 6,* 1–13.

Wilkie, D. J., Savedra, M., Holzemer, W. L., Tesler, M. P. (1990). Use of the McGill Pain Questionnaire to measure pain: A meta-analysis. *Nursing Research, 39,* 36–41.

Sensory Perception

Key Terms	Learning Objectives
Delusion *Hallucination* *Perception* *Reticular activating system* *Sensation information* *Sensoristasis* *Sensory deprivation* *Sensory overload* *Stress*	*Upon completion of this chapter, the student will be able to do the following:* • *Associate stress and sensoristasis with the sensory/perceptual process.* • *Describe the five senses and their activity in sensory perception.* • *Summarize factors affecting normal sensory perception.* • *Specify how sensory overload, deprivation, and deficit can occur, and consider interventions for each.* • *Relate behavioral manifestations of altered sensory function to their cause.* • *Identify clients at risk in a healthcare setting and in the home.* • *Discuss safety in relation to sensory dysfunction.*

45

Patrick Matthews, an active and popular college baseball star, was admitted for a retinal detachment after being hit in the head by a baseball. He talked a great deal to the staff about his concerns, and the staff all commented on what a likable person he was. After surgery, he was put on bed rest, and both eyes were bandaged. He was given a private room to minimize distractions and overstimulation. After the first day, Patrick stopped putting on his call light, did not engage in conversation with the nurses, and refused to contact his family and friends. On the second night after his surgery, Patrick showed signs of having hallucinations that a roommate was talking to him, and delusions that he was being poisoned through his meals. You have been assigned to give nursing care to Patrick the next morning.

You have studied about many physical problems in previous chapters. In this chapter, you will add sensory perception to your knowledge base. As you study about sensory function, you will be able to relate to Patrick's condition. When you have finished the chapter, Critical Thinking Challenges at the end of the chapter will help you use your knowledge base in addressing Patrick's care.

Because of today's fast pace, people often feel they do not have time to deal fully with one demand before the next one is nipping at their heels. The average American has daily exposure to 65,000 more stimuli (demands) than ancestors of 100 years ago (Schafer, 1992). Human beings uniquely deal with these demands through senses and higher cognitive processes (the latter is discussed in Chapter 46).

Sensing stimuli is basic to human functioning, growth, and development. Any alteration in sensory function places a person at risk for more serious mental and physical health deficits unless coping takes place.

Nurses encounter clients with preexisting sensory alterations and those with new alterations because of the stress of illness. Assessment of sensory function and risk factors for sensory alterations is necessary for all clients but especially for older adults who frequently have visual and hearing impairment.

Normal Sensory Perception Function

Normal Sensory Perception

Sensory perception depends on the sensory receptors, reticular activating system (RAS), and functioning nervous pathways to the brain. Awareness of stimuli is influenced by the RAS. Stimuli are received through the five senses: sight, hearing, touch, smell, and taste. Kinesthetic and visceral senses are stimulated internally.

Sensory Awareness

Awareness of the world depends on the RAS, located between the nerve centers of the medulla oblongata in the brain stem. The RAS is responsible for bringing together information from the cerebellum and other parts of the brain and from the sense organs. It is stimulated by sensory, visceral, kinesthetic, and cognitive input (Lee, 1991b). Multiple stimuli received by the senses reach the RAS, which selects certain impulses to be conducted to the cerebral cortex of the brain to be perceived.

When the nervous system is oriented to a stimulus and receptive toward it, the neurons of the RAS arouse the brain, facilitating information reception (Vander, Sherman, & Luciano, 1993). The RAS is highly selective; for example, a parent may be awakened in the middle of the night at the slightest murmur of an infant in a bedroom down the hall but may sleep through the sound of loud traffic noises outside the bedroom window. Destruction of the RAS produces coma and an electroencephalograph pattern characteristic of sleep (Vander, et al., 1993).

Input by Senses

Sensory function begins with reception of stimuli. The senses receiving stimuli externally are vision, hearing, smell, taste, and touch. Receptor organs are the eyes, ears, olfactory receptors in the nose, tastebuds of the tongue, and nerve endings in the skin. The kinesthetic and visceral senses receive stimuli internally. Receptors are nerve endings in the skin and body tissues. The kinesthetic sense influences awareness of the placement and action of body parts, whereas visceral stimuli affect awareness related to the body's large interior organs. Vision, hearing, smell, and taste are termed special senses. Touch, kinesthetic (or proprioceptive) sensation, and visceral sensation are termed somatic senses (Vander, et al., 1993).

After stimuli are received, they are perceived with the help of the RAS. Sensory **perception** is a conscious process of selecting, organizing, and interpreting sensory stimuli and depends on intact and functioning sense organs, nervous pathways, and the brain. (Chapter 46 provides more information on cognitive function.)

Characteristics of Normal Sensory Perception

Characteristics of normal sensory perception are the normal measures in quality and quantity of the special and somatic senses. Characteristics of normal vision are visual acuity at or near 20/20, full field of vision, and tricolor vision (red, green, blue). The characteristic of normal hearing is auditory acuity of sounds at an intensity of 0 to 25 dB, at frequencies of 125 to 8,000 cycles per second. The characteristic of normal taste is discrimination of sour, salty, sweet, and bitter; that of normal smell is discrimination of primary odors, such as camphoraceous, musky, floral, pepperminty, ethereal, pungent, and putrid. The characteristics of somatic senses include discrimination of touch, pressure, vibration, position, tickling, temperature, and pain (Vander, et al., 1993).

Normal Sensory Pattern

A normal pattern of sensory perception is common to all human beings in that the person sees, smells, hears, tastes, feels, and responds to stimuli adequately. Normal patterns differ among people, however.

Sensoristasis

Each person has his or her own comfort zone or a zone of optimum arousal (Schafer, 1992). This comfort zone varies from person to person and is the range at which a person performs at his or her peak. **Sensoristasis** is a state of optimum arousal—not too much and not too little. The RAS is viewed by some theorists as a monitor for sensoristatic balance.

Adaptation

Beyond the point of sensoristasis, sensory adaptation occurs. Sensory receptors adapt to repeated stimulation by responding less and less, and eventually, the brain will not perceive constant stimulation, as in background traffic noise. Varied and irregular stimuli will still be perceived, however.

Two necessary time periods are crucial in helping a person deal with new stimuli, lead time and afterburn (Schafer, 1992). Lead time is the time each person needs to prepare for an event emotionally and physically. Afterburn is the time needed to think about, evaluate, and come to terms with the activity after it happens. The necessary amount of lead time and afterburn is different for each person. Lead time and afterburn help a person process stimuli so that he or she is not overwhelmed and can respond appropriately.

Factors Affecting Normal Sensory Perception

Environment

Sensory stimuli in the environment affect one's sensory perception. For example, a consistently noisy environment, such as a school cafeteria, may cause a teacher not to notice the noise, but the same teacher may perceive a loud television set very differently in his or her own home, which is usually quiet.

Therapeutic Dialogue
Sensory Dysfunction

Scenes for Thought

Charlie Brisco is 27 years old and is in the ICU following a car accident in which he sustained internal injuries and many lacerations on his face and arms. He has an IV, urinary catheter, heart monitor, and nasogastric tube. The pumps and monitors give off soft beeps. The ICU has been a busy, noisy place since Charlie was admitted. You have been his primary nurse since that time.

Effective

Nurse: *Hi, Charlie. How're you doing? (Checking the IV and NG tube pumps.)*
Client: *Who are you?! What are you doing with those machines?!* Sits up in the bed abruptly, wincing with pain, looking frightened.
Nurse: *(Turns to look at him, stands still with arms at side and hands open.) I'm Georgia, Charlie. I'm your nurse.*
Client: *Georgia? I don't know you! Where's my mom? What did you do with her?* Looking frightened.
Nurse: *She's right there, Charlie. Do you see her standing at the desk there?*
Client: *Oh. Yeah.* Focusing on his mother. Slumps back on the pillows. *Sorry.* Starts to cry but tries to hide it from you. *I get confused.*
Nurse: *I can see that.*
Client: *Yeah.* Closes his eyes wearily. *And I can't sleep too good.*
Nurse: *I know. I was wondering if you had a portable cassette player at home.*
Client: *Yeah. Why?*
Nurse: *Well, how about using it to shut out the noise of the ICU with some music. Not loud music, though, something mellow.*
Client: *Yeah, that would be good.* Shifts in bed, wincing.
Nurse: *You look uncomfortable.*
Client: *I am.*
Nurse: *Okay, I'll get you some more pain pills, and I'll talk to your mom about the cassette player, too. You can tell her what tapes to bring later.*
Client: *Okay. Thanks.* Closes his eyes and lies still.

Less Effective

Nurse: *Hi, Charlie. How're you doing? (Checking the IV and NG tube pumps.)*
Client: *Who are you?! What are you doing with those machines?!* Sits up in the bed abruptly, wincing with pain, looking frightened.
Nurse: *(Turns to look at him, then continues to check the equipment.) I'm Gigi, Charlie. I'm your nurse.*
Client: *Gigi? I don't know you! Where's my mom? What did you do with her?* Looking frightened.
Nurse: *She's right over there, Charlie, at the desk. See her? Sounds like you need a little sedative to calm you down. I'll go get it right now.*
Client: *Mom! Mom! Where are you?!* Now struggling to sit up in bed.
Nurse: *(Gets sedative and calls for help to restrain Charlie so he won't dislodge his tubes.)*

Critical Thinking Challenge

• Name and explain some of the factors that contributed to Charlie's sensory dysfunction. • Decide if this dysfunction was sensory overload or deprivation and give your reasons. • Describe the relationship between traumatic events and pain and sensory dysfunction. • Appraise how each nurse related to Charlie and summarize the outcomes.

Previous Experience

Previous experience affects sensory perception in that people become more alert to stimuli that evoke a strong response. For example, a person may drive to work by the same route each day, noticing little along the way. A person may listen to the radio inattentively until a favorite song is played, then listen to every word. A new experience, such as hospitalization, may cause a client to perceive a barrage of threatening new stimuli.

Lifestyle and Habits

Lifestyle affects sensory perception. One person may enjoy a lifestyle of abundant stimulation, surrounded by many people, frequent changes, bright lights, and noise, whereas others may prefer less contact with crowds, less noise, and a slow-paced routine. People with different lifestyles perceive stimuli differently.

Cigarette smoking causes atrophy of tastebuds, decreasing sensory perception of taste. Chronic alcohol abuse may lead to peripheral neuropathy, a functional disorder of the peripheral nervous system that results in sensory impairment.

Illness

Certain illnesses affect sensory perception. Diabetes and hypertension cause changes in tiny blood vessels and nerves, leading to visual deficits and decreased sensation of touch in the extremities. Cerebrovascular disorders impair blood flow to the brain, possibly blocking sensory perception in the brain. Pain, fatigue, and stress caused by illness also affect perception of stimuli.

Medications

Some antibiotics, including streptomycin and gentamicin, can damage the auditory nerve, impairing hearing. Central nervous system depressants, such as narcotic analgesics, decrease awareness and impair perception of stimuli.

Lifespan Considerations

Sensory perception is a crucial consideration in the very young and in older adults.

Newborn and Infant

Sensory perception is rudimentary at birth and requires repeated stimulation for the nervous system to mature and discrimination within the senses to develop. The newborn and infant receive most stimulation by touch; they need to feel objects in the environment and learn to feel comfortable with their own bodies in space. They respond to holding, cuddling, soothing, rocking, and changing position. The newborn sees only gross patterns of light and dark or bright colors, but vision becomes more discriminating as the infant develops.

Toddler and Preschooler

A child's growth, development, and attachment are directly linked with sensory stimulation. Vision is fundamental to the growth of the mind, but full acquaintance with the world includes exploration with all the senses (Gesell & Ilg, 1949). As the child grows, he or she reacts to a world of people and things (Gesell & Ilg, 1949); lack of meaningful stimulation can lead to developmental and motor delays (Lee, 1991a). Successful adaptation to change occurs when stimulation is not too much or too little.

The toddler is an explorer, learning through investigation of the environment by seeing, hearing, touching, tasting, and smelling. The preschooler seeks in more organized play to perceive and respond to stimuli through the senses, as in singing and story telling.

Child and Adolescent

Children and adolescents experience rapid changes in their world, and learning occurs at an accelerated pace. Reading and listening to school lessons dominate a child's day. School-age children and adolescents are learning to make independent responses based on what is perceived through the senses, such as crossing the street when the light turns green or reporting a fire when smelling smoke.

Adult and Older Adult

Adults' sensory perception function is at its peak; however, as people reach middle age, they begin to notice certain changes in their sensory system. Eyesight diminishes, sounds become more muffled, and the other sensory systems deteriorate. Marked decrements in sensory/perceptual behaviors begin as people approach 60 to 70 years of age (Creditor, 1993). This reduction in efficiency means that older people cannot process sensory input as rapidly as they did when they were young (Creditor, 1993; Lee, 1991b); because of this slowing, they need more time to deal with stimulating events.

Altered Sensory Function

Potential for Altered Sensory Function

If a person experiences more sensory stimulation than he or she is used to or can make sense of, distress and sensory overload may occur. On the other hand, if a person experiences less than the usual stimulation, that person is below his or her optimum state of arousal and may be at risk for sensory deprivation.

Reactions to sensory overload or sensory deprivation are special challenges that nurses frequently encounter in themselves and clients. Sensory overload and deprivation can lead to perceptual, cognitive, and decisional problems. It is often difficult to separate where one area begins and another ends. For example, when a person's senses are bombarded with seeing, feeling, and hearing too much information at one time, it may be difficult to perceive accurately, think clearly, or make a good decision.

When the RAS is overwhelmed with input, a person may experience sensory overload and feel confused, anxious, and unable to take constructive action. When the RAS fails to recognize a stimulus because it is below the threshold level or lacks relevant meaning to the person, sensory deprivation may occur, and the person experiences boredom, depression, restlessness, and vivid sensual imagery, including hallucinations (Lee, 1991b; McFarland & Thomas, 1991).

Sensory Overload

Sensory overload occurs when a person is unable to process or manage the intensity or quantity of incoming sensory stimuli. The person feels overwhelmed by the excessive input from the environment and does not feel in control (McFarland & Thomas, 1991; Lee, 1991b). For example, when a woman having a routine check-up is told she may have a malignant breast tumor, she may not be able to process additional stimuli correctly because of shock. She may not perceive additional information about scheduling a biopsy and surgical options.

Nurses need to understand that routine activity in the health setting can contribute to sensory overload in their clients. Such occurrences fall into three main categories: internal factors, information, and environment.

Internal Factors. Internal factors, such as thinking about impending surgery or the meaning of a medical diagnosis, can contribute to anxiety and cognitive overload so that the person cannot process additional stimuli (Fig. 45-1). Pain, medication, lack of sleep, worry, and brain injury also can contribute to a person's vulnerability to sensory overload.

Information. Imparting information to a client may lead to sensory overload. Some examples include teaching a client about a procedure, informing a client about a diagnosis, making requests of a client, or helping the client solve a problem.

The Environment. The environment of the healthcare agency provides a higher than usual amount of sensory stimulation. A client newly admitted to the hospital, for example, may have to cope with adjusting to

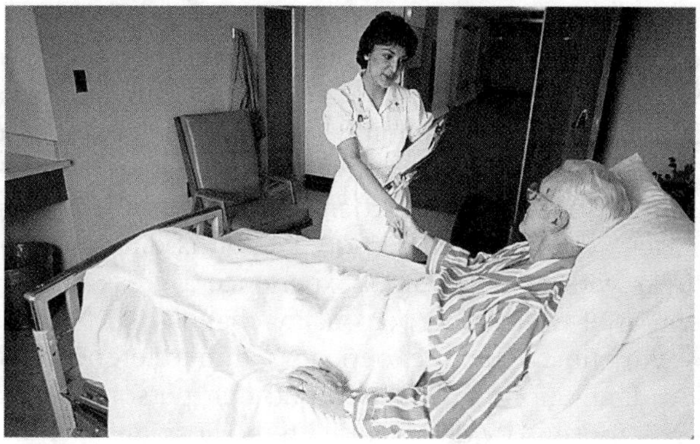

Figure 45-1 • *Anxiety related to medical diagnosis, prognosis, and treatment can contribute to sensory overload.*

a new roommate, having the television on more than usual, bright lights, paging systems, unexpected intrusions, meeting a variety of staff, having the bed move up and down at someone else's bidding, waiting for someone to answer the call light, uncontrolled pain, and having strangers touch and probe private areas of the body. Clients in intensive care units often exhibit symptoms of sensory overload because of the high degree of light, noise, and activity around the clock (Fig. 45-2) (Geary, 1994).

Sensory Deprivation

Although **sensory deprivation** can be thought of as the opposite of sensory overload, they have many elements in common; think about the paradoxical statement, "The silence was deafening." Sensory deprivation generally means a lessening or lack of meaningful sensory stimuli, monotonous sensory input, or an interference with the processing of information (Lee, 1991b; McFarland & Thomas, 1991).

Sensory deprivation (understimulation) can be just as disruptive as sensory overload. Cognitive and emo-

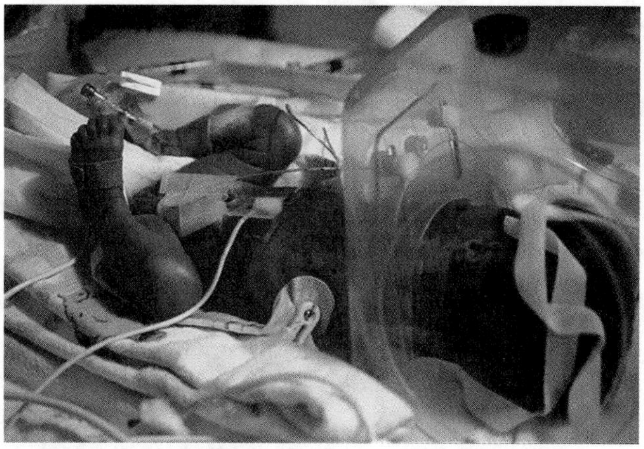

Figure 45-2 • *Lights and frequent activity may cause sensory overload in a premature newborn in the neonatal intensive care unit.*

tional deterioration can occur when stimuli are reduced below a person's optimum level of stimulation (Schafer, 1992). One common source of sensory deprivation is a sudden decrease in stimuli when a person moves from a fast- to a slow-paced environment (Schafer, 1992). Each person's tolerance of and reaction to a lessening or lack of meaningful sensory stimuli is different, but clients with extreme cases experience a gross misperception of events and personality changes.

Any time a client experiences an interference with or a diminution of sensory input, that person may be at risk for sensory deprivation. In the hospital, such occurrences fall into two general categories: altered sensory reception and deprived environments.

Altered Sensory Reception. Altered sensory reception occurs in such conditions as spinal cord injury, brain damage, changes in receptor organs, sleep deprivation, and chronic illness. The person does not receive adequate sensory input because of an interference with the nervous system's ability to receive and process stimuli. This inability also can lead to secondary problems, as in the following example:

Ralph Wilson suffered a spinal cord injury in an automobile accident, leaving him paraplegic. One day he decided to sneak a cigarette while no one was looking. He accidentally dropped the lighted match on his knitted slipper and burned his foot because he could not feel the heat when his slipper began to smolder.

Older people are especially susceptible to sensory deficits, as shown in the following example:

Cassie Taylor stopped attending her senior citizen group. She began to spend most of her time sitting alone. She became more depressed, ate less, and began to show signs of confusion. Nurses who observed these actions were able to intervene to assist her to increase her socialization and communication with others.

Deprived Environments. Deprived environments can have a negative effect on a person's sensoristasis. A person who is immobilized for any reason or is in isolation is being deprived of the usual amount of stimulation and may show manifestations of sensory deprivation (Fig. 45-3). Consider Patrick Matthews' circumstances as presented in the situation at the beginning of this chapter.

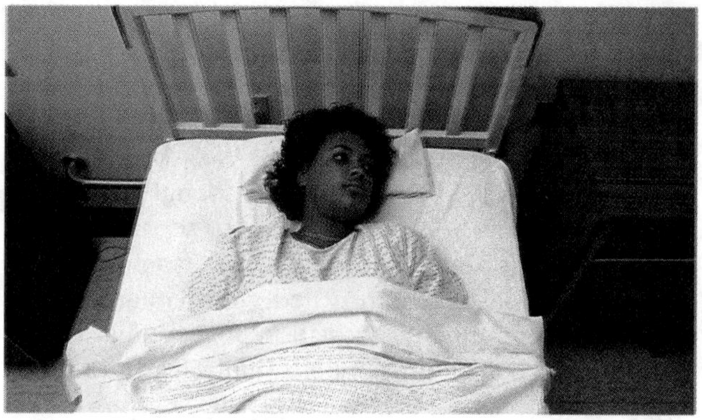

Figure 45-3 • *Isolation and lack of mobility may contribute to sensory deprivation.*

Patrick's verbal communication with the staff and his family diminished dramatically shortly after his hospitalization. He could not see. Because he did not have visual senses, he experienced perceptual distortions. He misinterpreted sounds outside his room. He changed from being a likable, open person to being angry and suspicious.

Patrick was showing signs of sensory deprivation. He was used to being active and having a stimulating life. Suddenly his environment was nonstimulating and quiet. To compensate for temporary loss of sight, his senses of hearing and taste became more acute, leading to misinterpretations of sounds and taste of food. His personality changed drastically.

Sensory Deficit

Sensory deficit is impaired function in sensory reception or perception. The deficit may be blindness due to disease of the eyes, such as glaucoma. In this example, reception is affected. Spinal cord injuries and strokes cause loss of tactile sensation. This affects perception because of disruption in nerve pathways or the brain.

Compensation for the deficit usually occurs when loss of function is gradual. The person often changes behavior to adapt to sensory deficit, such as turning a functioning ear toward a speaker to hear, or measuring temperature of bathwater with a thermometer if there is decreased sensation of the extremities. Physiologic compensation occurs as well, with the remaining senses becoming more acute. For example, a blind person may develop a more acute sense of smell or hearing.

A sudden loss of sensory perception through a sensory deficit may cause total disorientation. Compensation does not occur immediately. A sensory deficit may be temporary or permanent because of illness or treatment (Glide, 1994). Temporary bandaging following eye surgery may render a client totally unable to care for himself or herself. Nasal packing that temporarily eliminates the sense of smell affects taste and may lead to anorexia. The client with sudden loss of lower extremity sensation through a spinal cord injury in a motor vehicle accident will be at risk for injury to the lower extremities.

Manifestations of Altered Sensory Function

Anxiety

Altered sensory perception frequently leads to anxiety, just as anxiety can further lead to additional altered sensory perception. An older woman with poor hearing who lives alone may be anxious about going to bed at night because she might not hear a smoke alarm, the phone ringing, or someone trying to break into the house. Anxiety stems from not being able to interact fully with the environment due to sensory deficit, fear of embarrassment when trying to communicate with others, or misinterpretation of information perceived through the senses.

Cognitive Dysfunction

Disturbances in remembering, reasoning, and problem-solving may occur with sensory overload. Decision-making may be irrational or dysfunctional. Other common behaviors indicative of cognitive dysfunction include disorientation; verbalizing disconnected thoughts; complaining of too much going on, sleeplessness, and fatigue; an inability to think; and poor work performance (Gordon, 1994). Sensory deprivation causes a reduction in mental capabilities as well (Toffler, 1970). Mind wandering occurs, along with fantasy activity. The person may have difficulty concentrating and thinking logically.

Hallucinations and Delusions

Hallucinations are sensory impressions that are based on internal stimulations and have no basis in reality. Hearing voices when no one is there is a typical auditory hallucination. **Delusions** are beliefs that are not based in reality and reflect an unconscious need or fear (eg, believing the hospital food is poisoned). Both hallucinations and delusions have been documented in cases of sensory deprivation, sensory overload, and sensory deficits, such as hearing and vision loss (Lee, 1991b). For example, an older woman is suddenly hospitalized. Her glasses are misplaced, and the battery is weak in her hearing aid. She may not understand why strange people come into her room at night. She may have difficulty with toileting, so she soils her bed. Her sensory deficits cause her to misinterpret stimuli and distort reality. She has delusions that she is in a prison, the nurses are guards, and other prisoners are trying to take advantage of her; she hallucinates that her dead sister is telling her to join her in heaven.

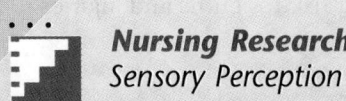

> ### *Nursing Research*
> *Sensory Perception*
>
> **Selected Nursing Research Studies**
>
> Janken, H. K., & Cullinan, C. L. (1990). Auditory sensory/perceptual alteration: Suggested revision of defining characteristics. *Nursing Diagnosis 1*(4): 147–154.
>
> Kennedy, B. R., Williams, C. A., & Pesut, D. J. (1994). Hallucinatory experiences of psychiatric patients in seclusion. *Archives of Psychiatric Nursing, 8*(3), 169–176.
>
> Jairath, N., & Cambell, H. M. (1990). Two mental status assessment methods: An evaluation. *Journal of Ophthalmic Nursing and Technology, 9*(3), 102–105.
>
> **Possible Topics for Nursing Inquiry**
>
> - Does location of the room make a difference in sensory overload or deprivation?
> - Will assisting the client to gain a sense of control related to the environment reduce the risk of sensory overload?
> - What nursing interventions are most successful in reducing symptoms of sensory deprivation overload?

Depression and Withdrawal

Depression may result from sensory deficits or sensory deprivation. Helplessness and loss of self-esteem lead to depression and withdrawal. The client who is on isolation precautions may show signs of poor appetite, sleeplessness, and loss of interest in activities or interaction with others as he or she becomes depressed, leading to further sensory deprivation.

Impact of Dysfunction on Activities of Daily Living

Individual Considerations

Sensory perception dysfunction may have profound effects on activities of daily living (ADLs). Visual deficits cause problems with self-care activities as basic as dressing, toiletry, and preparing meals. Hearing deficits restrict people from watching television, listening to the radio, and answering the telephone; safety hazards exist for deaf pedestrians. People with taste and smell deficits may lose interest in eating. Those with sensory deficits of touch are at risk for burns and injuries to the extremities.

Family Considerations

Moving around outside the home may be impossible without special aids or someone's help. Many jobs are prohibited for people with sensory deficits, and driving may not be allowed. This restricts the environments in which they may move about safely and makes them dependent on others. If the affected person is the breadwinner, that may mean a reduction in or loss of income. People with cognitive dysfunction from sensory overload or deprivation may exhibit poor judgment and problem-solving during everyday activities, which increases the necessity for family members to monitor activities and decisions. All of these concerns place more stress on the family to cope with sensory dysfunctions.

Assessment

Nursing assessment should explore the client's sensory perception through subjective and objective data collection. Assessment for sensory perception focuses on the client, the environment, and interaction between the client and others. Subjective data include normal sensory function identification, identification of risk factors, and identification of dysfunctional sensory perception. Family and friends may provide helpful data about changes in the client's behavior that indicate problems in sensory perception. Objective data are collected by physical examination of the neurologic system and special senses and by diagnostic tests.

Subjective Data

Functional Pattern Identification

To determine a client's normal functional pattern of sensory perception, the nurse first asks a general question, such as "How do you spend a typical day?" This question can give the nurse a feel for the level of stimulation the client usually experiences on a daily basis and the client's response to that stimulation.

The nurse should next assess how the client responds to change. Because change and stress can affect perception, it is useful to find out how the client manages these. Asking, "Have there been any recent changes in your life?" can lead to an informative discussion of the degree of complexity of the changes and the client's responses.

Next an investigation of the client's living and social situation and available modes of transportation give the nurse a better idea of the degree of complexity of the client's life and the level of independence. The following questions provide important information about the client's daily functioning: "With whom do you live?" "Do you prepare your own (your family's) meals?" "When you want to go someplace, how do you get there?"

Finally, questioning can center on the person's lifestyle and habits. If the client's usual diet consists of highly spiced foods, a change in menu may seem dull and uninteresting; it may affect the client's appetite because it does not meet the usual needs of the client in the area of gustatory stimulation. Determine how much alcohol the person drinks daily or weekly, how much sleep the person is used to, and the usual time the client retires and arises. Also determine educational level, hobbies and interests, and what jobs the person holds or has held. Table 45-1 gives examples of general and specific questions to elicit information about the client's interaction with his or her environment.

Risk Identification

To collect data about risk factors for sensory perception dysfunction, the nurse elicits information about the client's age, culture and language, level of activity, medical history, and medications. When a person is hospitalized, the nurse assesses the degree of stimulation in the environment in light of the client's experiences. Some risk factors in the hospital environment are listed in the accompanying display.

Nursing Assessment
Risk Factors for Sensory Perception Dysfunction in the Healthcare Environment

Sensory overload

Room close to nurse's station	______
ICU or intermediate unit	______
Bright lights	______
Use of mechanical ventilator	______
Use of ECG monitor	______
Use of oxygen	______
Use of IVs	______
Other equipment	______
Roommate	______
Frequent treatments	______

Sensory Deprivation

Private room	______
Eyes bandaged	______
Bed rest	______
Sensory aid not available (hearing aid, glasses)	______
Isolation precautions	______
Few visitors	

Table 45-1 • General and Specific Questions About the Client and Environment

General Question	Specific Questions
How do you spend a typical day?	Do you go to school? Do you work outside the home? Do you watch TV, listen to the radio, read the newspaper? How often do you talk to friends and family?
Have there been any recent changes in your life?	Have you experienced any changes, such as loss of a loved one, change of a job, a friend moving away, new baby in the house? How are you adjusting to the change?
What are your living arrangements like?	With whom do you live? What is the size of your home? Do you cook and care for family members? Do you live in a neighborhood? How convenient is shopping? Do you have transportation?
What are your interests and habits?	What are your hobbies? Are you involved in sports? Do you smoke, and if so, how much? Do you drink alcohol, and if so, how much? Do you use any recreational drugs? How much sleep do you need; how much do you get? Do you like to go out? What types of food do you eat?

Older clients are more at risk for sensory deficits because of normal physiologic changes of aging, especially in hearing and vision. Clients with cultural and language barriers may be at risk for sensory deprivation. The nurse should ask about the client's level of activity; immobilization due to physical disability restricts the client from his or her usual amount of stimulation. The medical history includes present illness, any chronic illnesses, past hospitalizations, accidents, and surgeries. A history of sensory deficits, such as visual and hearing impairment, places the client at risk for sensory deprivation. A history of illnesses, such as diabetes, hypertension, stroke, or spinal cord injury, also places the client at risk for sensory deficits. The client's experience with the healthcare environment determines the effect of stimulation on the client. Lack of experience with an intensive care unit or isolation precautions may place the client at risk for sensory overload or deprivation during hospitalization. Medications for which the nurse should assess include central nervous system depressants, such as narcotic analgesics and sedatives, and large doses of antibiotics that may affect hearing.

Dysfunction Identification

During the nursing assessment, the nurse collects data about actual sensory perception problems. The nurse must determine if the client has difficulty with vision, hearing, smell, taste, and touch. If problems are identified, the nurse should determine when the problem started, its severity, and what the client has done about it. This information is useful in helping the client adapt to his or her environment.

The nurse also should determine whether the client is anxious, depressed, withdrawing from social contact, or having difficulty concentrating, making decisions, or remembering. Has the client ever experienced hallucinations or delusions? This information will uncover any manifestations the sensory dysfunction may have caused.

Objective Data

Physical Assessment

The focus of the physical assessment is to determine if the senses are impaired. The following must be assessed: hearing, vision, taste, smell, touch, somatic senses, and mental status. Mental status data can be collected as the nurse takes the client history. Mental status data should include level of consciousness, orientation, attention span, memory, and cognitive skills. See Chapter 21 for more information on assessment.

To collect objective data about the sensory system systematically, the nurse first inspects, then performs

Table 45-2 • Physical Assessment of Sensory Function

Sense	Technique for Assessment
Vision	Use Snellen chart to measure visual acuity (or have client read newspaper, menu, or whatever is available). Test visual fields.
Hearing	Whisper numbers in each ear, while occluding the other; ask client to repeat. Perform Weber and Rinne tuning fork tests. Observe client's conversation with others.
Smell	With eyes closed, have client identify three odors, such as coffee, tobacco, and cloves, one nostril at a time, while occluding the other nostril.
Taste	With eyes closed, have client identify three tastes, such as lemon, salt, and sugar, waiting 1 minute and giving sips of water in between. Have client close eyes for all tests.
Somatic sensation	Test light touch of extremities with a wisp of cotton. Test sharp and dull sensation using the point and blunt end of a pin. Test two-point discrimination using two pins held close together. Test hot and cold sensation using test tubes filled with warm and cold water. Test vibration sense using a tuning fork over joints. Test position sense by moving the client's fingers or toes. Test stereognosis by giving the client a common object (quarter, paperclip) to identify by feel.

simple tests. The nurse inspects the head for any abnormalities of the eyes, ears, nose, or mouth and inspects the extremities for any burns or injuries. Table 45-2 lists tests used to assess sensation.

Diagnostic Tests and Procedures

The nurse needs to be aware of several laboratory findings. Electrolyte imbalances; alterations in blood chemistry, such as elevated ammonia or blood urea nitrogen; and toxic levels of drugs that affect the central nervous system can alter sensoristasis (Kim, McFarland, & McLane, 1987; McFarland & Wasli, 1986). Special visual and auditory acuity tests also may be ordered. Neurologic tests, such as nerve conduction studies, computed tomographic scanning of the brain, and cerebral angiography, may be performed to determine the cause of sensory deficits.

Nursing Diagnoses

The accepted North American Nursing Diagnosis Association (NANDA) nursing diagnosis for sensory overload, deprivation, and deficit is Sensory/Perceptual Alterations. These may include visual, auditory, kinesthetic, gustatory, tactile, or olfactory alterations. The nurse uses data from the assessment to determine the presence or risk of any of these disruptions in normal sensory/perception function.

Diagnostic Statement: Sensory/Perceptual Alterations

Definition

Sensory/perceptual alteration is a state in which an individual experiences a change in the amount or patterning of oncoming stimuli, accompanied by a diminished, exaggerated, distorted, or impaired response to such stimuli (NANDA, 1994).

Defining Characteristics

Defining characteristics include disorientation to time, place, or person and altered ability to think abstractly or in concepts. A change in problem-solving abilities; a reported or measured change in sensory acuity, such as vision or hearing; a change in behavior pattern, either increased or decreased; anxiety; restlessness; irritability; apathy; or a change in usual response to stimuli may be defining characteristics. Body image alteration or altered communication patterns also characterize this nursing diagnosis.

Other possible characteristics include complaints of fatigue, alteration in posture, change in muscular tension, inappropriate responses, and hallucinations (NANDA, 1994).

Related Factors

Excessive or insufficient environmental stimuli; altered sensory reception, transmission, or integration; endogenous (electrolyte) or exogenous (eg, drugs) chemical alterations; and psychological stress are related factors (NANDA, 1994).

Related Nursing Diagnoses

Other nursing diagnoses may be identified for the client with sensory alterations. The following are possible problems: Impaired Environmental Interpretation Syndrome, Body Image Disturbance, Chronic Low Self Esteem, Diversional Activity Deficit, Fatigue, Altered Growth and Development, Risk for Injury, Risk for Poisoning, Self Care Deficits, and Sleep Pattern Disturbance. If the sensory alterations are the result of spinal injury, additional nursing diagnoses may be the following: Dysreflexia, Impaired Home Maintenance Management, Altered Role Performance, or Impaired Skin Integrity.

Outcome Identification and Planning

After the nursing diagnoses and related factors are identified, client goals and nuring interventions are planned. Client goals are individualized but focus on achieving optimal sensory function. The client goals for Sensory/Perceptual Alterations are the following:

The client will demonstrate an understanding of contributing factors by reducing or eliminating them.
The client will demonstrate an understanding of interventions and rationale by using this information as foresight in maintaining sensoristasis.
The client will achieve sensoristasis through a decrease in the symptoms of sensory overload or deprivation.
The client will demonstrate achievement or maintenance of self-care.
The client will maintain safety.

Planning will revolve around the client's ability to function on a perceptual level. Client teaching, procedure preparation, provision of stimulation or stimulation reduction, and safety are major issues. Examples of nursing interventions commonly used in problems with sensory overload and deprivations are listed in the accompanying display and discussed in the following section.

Implementation

Nursing Interventions to Promote Sensory Health and Function

Nurses can promote sensory function of clients by preparing them for appointments and procedures and by providing effective interactions with the client.

Client Teaching

Nurses can promote sensory health and function by teaching clients at risk ways to prevent sensory loss and by teaching general health measures to healthcare consumers. Teaching topics include frequent eye examinations and close control of chronic illness, such as diabetes. Some client teaching suggestions are given in the accompanying display.

Teaching healthcare consumers the importance of sensory function and the roles of sensory receptors and the central nervous system in receiving and perceiving stimuli is important. Preventing sensory dysfunction will enable the person to interact with the environment at an optimal level. Yearly eye examinations, more often if problems arise, help promote optimal visual function. Other measures to prevent visual dysfunction include avoiding eyestrain and eye infection or injury. Hearing loss may be prevented by prompt recognition and treatment of ear infections and childhood immunization against illnesses such as rubella.

Client Teaching
Sensory Perception

Instruct the client as follows:

- *Obtain routine medical check-ups.*
- *Seek early attention for any potential sensory problems to prevent sensory misperceptions.*
- *Obtain a yearly eye examination (more frequently if problems arise) to prevent visual sensory deficits.*
- *Increase or reduce sensory stimulation as necessary to have an optimal balance in sensory perception.*
- *If you have diabetes or high blood pressure, maintain tight control of blood sugar and blood pressure through self-monitoring, medication compliance, diet, and medical follow-up to avoid related sensory disturbances.*
- *Seek medical attention for signs of ear infections in your children to avoid hearing problems that interfere with perception.*
- *Provide regular immunizations for your children, and maintain a record to prevent auditory and other sensory losses.*

Planning

Examples of Nursing Interventions Used in Common Sensory Problems

Sensory Deprivation

- Encourage use of sensory aides, such as eyeglasses or hearing aids.
- Identify barriers to communication and sensory perception.
- Address the client by name, and touch the client during communication.
- Communicate frequently with the client to maintain meaningful interactions.
- Modify the environment to provide meaningful sensory stimulation.
- Promote uninterrupted periods of sleep and rest.
- Provide a structured routine and activities.

Sensory Overload

- Address the client by name, and introduce yourself.
- Provide orienting cues such as clocks, calendars, and windows.
- Support accurate interpretations of perceptions.

Internal Factors

- Provide time for the client to discuss his or her thoughts. Correct misperceptions.
- Orient the client, when indicated, to person, place, and time.
- Provide for rest and sleep periods to prevent exhaustion.
- Provide for the possibility of increasing the dose and frequency of pain medication until pain management can be achieved through other means.
- Help the client use stress-reduction behaviors to relieve anxiety.

Imparting Information

- Introduce new information gradually to allow time for the client to process the meaning.
- Speak in a slow, unhurried manner.
- Keep medical jargon to a minimum.
- Use several sensory pathways whenever possible rather than overloading one pathway (ie, state your name *and* wear a name tag)
- Have the client repeat information, so you know the client has a correct understanding.
- Provide for frequent undisturbed rest periods

Reducing Environmental Stimuli

- Dim lights, or provide dark glasses.
- Avoid loud noises, or provide ear plugs.
- Refrain from bumping the bed or moving or touching the client unnecessarily.
- Turn off the TV set.
- Ask staff to hold conversations out of hearing range.
- Request other personnel not to disturb the client for unessential tasks (ie, housekeeping).
- Encourage the client to use earphones to listen to soothing music or relaxation tapes to block out other noises.
- Plan a routine of care so the client knows when and what to expect (post the schedule for the client wherever possible).
- Limit visitors as necessary.
- Reduce noxious odors: Empty commode or bedpan immediately after use, keep wounds clean and covered, use room deodorizer when indicated, and provide good ventilation.
- Provide a private room until the client can tolerate a roommate.

The older adult who is at risk for sensory loss due to physiologic changes of aging should be taught to have routine check-ups and seek attention for any developing problems. He or she may delay medical attention, fearing that hearing loss is inevitable, when simple ear irrigation may dislodge impacted cerumen and restore hearing. Clients with chronic illnesses, such as diabetes and hypertension, should be taught the importance of close control of blood sugar and blood pressure, respectively. Control can help prevent tactile and visual dysfunction. Self-monitoring of blood sugar or blood pressure, compliance with medications, diet control, and medical follow-up are essential.

Procedure Preparation

A primary concern of the nurse is to prevent symptoms of sensory overload for the client. The client is especially at risk for sensory overload when unfamiliar procedures are taking place. Overstimulation can be prevented by preparing the client before a procedure, using a technique called **sensation (sensory) information.** The purpose of this intervention is to alleviate distress responses of the client to threatening stimuli and improve the client's coping through stimulation of the cognitive processes. The technique involves objectively and specifically describing to a client, in serial order, what they typically will see, hear, smell, taste, or feel (tactile) in a particular situation (rare or atypical events are not to be included), from the client's point of view, not the observer's (Horsley & Crane, 1981; Sime, 1985).

The nurse must have a good understanding of this technique before using it. In general, sensation information is useful when a client feels threatened by a procedure. The client must make that appraisal, not the nurse. Clients who indicate a high level of anxiety before a procedure seem to benefit more than those with low levels of anxiety. Finally, the nurse should determine what client outcomes are desired. Sensation information will not help the client achieve new coping skills, but it may enhance his or her current coping mechanisms (Sime, 1985).

Other interventions to help prevent sensory overload include educating a client about why a procedure will be done, who will do it, and how long it will take. Helping a client gain a sense of control by interventions, such as establishing a schedule for routine care, providing a calendar and clock, and allowing choices whenever possible, also can reduce the risk of sensory overload (Lee, 1991).

Nurse–Client Interaction

Nurse-client interaction needs to be individualized to promote sensory health function. Clients at risk for sensory deprivation may need frequent interaction initiated by the nurse, while others may not. In any case, the nurse should provide appropriate stimuli, such as addressing the client by name, introducing and reintroducing oneself as necessary, explaining all activities, and when leaving, acknowledging when the nurse will return. Length, frequency, and content of interactions should be based on individual needs. Talking to the client, showing the client equipment or articles used in care, encouraging the client to smell and taste food that is served, and touching the client are appropriate stimuli while interacting with him or her (Fig. 45-4).

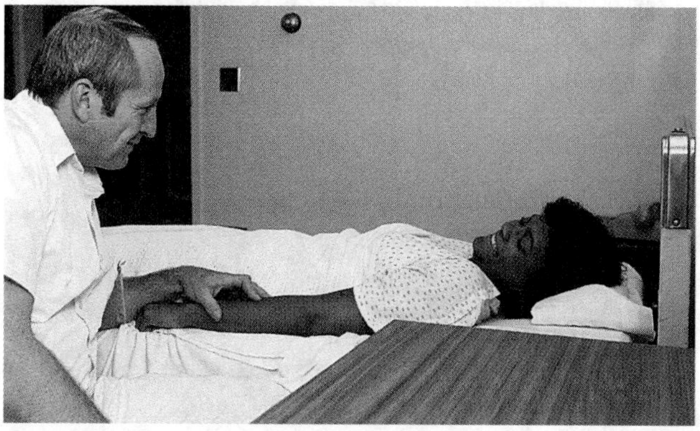

Figure 45-4 • *The simple act of touching a client or talking or listening may provide sensory stimulation.*

Nursing Interventions for Altered Sensory Function

Nursing interventions for clients with altered sensory function may focus on enhancing or reducing stimulation to minimize sensory deprivation or sensory overload, respectively. Sensory aids can be provided to minimize a client's sensory deficit. Nurses must intervene to provide safety for the client who is at risk for injury due to sensory dysfunction.

Stimulation Provision

Provision of meaningful external stimuli can help a client overcome sensory deprivation or sensory deficit. Stimulation can be provided by playing the television or the radio occasionally, playing music for brief periods, encouraging the use of a clock and calendar, encouraging the client to dress for the day's activities, putting up colorful pictures, encouraging visitors, opening the drapes, and turning on lights. The bed or chair should be placed so the client can see or hear activities in the area and when someone enters the room.

Frequent interaction with the client also may help. Discussing scheduling of care and placement of equipment, encouraging self-care activities, providing tactile stimulation through back rubs, combing and brushing the client's hair (or encouraging the client to do so), reading to the client, speaking slowly and clearly, and identifying yourself verbally and with a name tag are meaningful interactions. It also may be necessary to reorient the client frequently to person, place, and time. Because the client may be having difficulties concentrating, he or she may need repeated direction to accomplish even simple tasks. The nurse must add stimulation slowly so that the client is not overwhelmed; he or she also should include a variety of stimuli and keep the amount of sensory input at a moderate level. Orienting the client to the environment can help the client avoid experiencing misinterpretations. Visiting the client often and letting him or her know when the nurse will return helps the client overcome a feeling of isolation. Providing a calendar and a clock to assist in keeping track of time helps keep the client in touch with activities in the environment. A roommate for a client experiencing sensory deprivation can help a great deal. Preparation for any procedure that may add to the sensory deprivation, such as being restricted to bed rest, gives the client time to think of alternatives to sensory stimulation (McFarland & Thomas, 1991).

The nurse can encourage clients to provide self-stimulation. Self-stimulation, such as singing, reading, and talking into a tape recorder and playing it back, can be helpful. Encouraging maximum use of the available senses can help a person adjust. Self-care and activity also are self-stimulation.

A client can use up restless energy and prevent symptoms of sensory deprivation by using physical movement. Encouraging the client to move around in the bed or walk around the room, sit in a chair, do ADLs as independently as possible, and do exercises in the room or in bed provide stimulation to the client's senses.

Stimulation Reduction

If the client is experiencing sensory overload, interventions will focus on reducing stimulation. Nursing care can include reducing sensory overload when imparting information, reducing environmental stimuli, and assisting the client to deal with internal factors (see the display on nursing interventions to reduce sensory overload in the Planning section of this chapter). Reducing extraneous noise, lights, room clutter, interruptions, pain, and stress all reduce stimulation.

Clients in sensory overload may neglect their ADLs to the point that they need assistance. Such assistance can be problematic because it can add to sensory overload. With this in mind, the client should be assisted only with the immediately essential ADLs (eg, moving, eating, toileting, and resting); additional tasks can be added as the client is able to cope.

Sensory Aids

When a client experiences a sensory deficit, sensory aids help promote optimal function of that and other available senses (eg, hearing aids in good working order, clean eyeglasses, good oral hygiene). In addition to providing actual physical and situational sensory aids, the nurse should enlist significant others whenever possible to assist the client in dealing with the deficit. Suggestions for sensory aids are listed in the accompanying display. Sensory aids can be used in the healthcare environment and taught to clients for use at home. When one sense is lost, sensory aids can be used for other senses to enhance general stimulation. For example, a blind client should be encouraged to savor the aroma, taste, and texture of food.

Safety

Implementing safety precautions is another nursing intervention for clients with sensory perception dysfunc-

Nursing Care Guidelines
Sensory Aids

Vision

- Eyeglasses with the proper prescription, cleaned and in good repair
- Adequate room lighting, drapes open
- Sunglasses or window shades to reduce glare
- Literature with large print
- Uncluttered environment, no furniture rearranging
- Clock with large numbers
- Telephone dial with large numbers
- Magnifying glass
- Bright, contrasting colors in environment
- Color coded dials on appliances, medication bottles, and so forth
- Braille, recorded books, seeing-eye dog, and so forth, as necessary

Hearing

- Hearing aid in good repair with working battery
- Speaking slowly and distinctly in full view of client, no mouth covering or gum chewing
- Avoidance of background noise
- Amplified phone ringer, doorbell, smoke alarm, and so forth
- Head set for telephone communication
- Closed-caption television

Smell

- Fresh food served for meals
- Fresh flowers or fragrance in the room
- Others wearing light perfume or fragrance
- Notice of environmental smells

Taste

- Fresh food, seasoned appropriately, not overcooked or overprocessed to preserve texture
- Foods served at appropriate temperature and time of day
- Note smell and taste of food
- Sips of water between foods
- No mixing of foods

Touch

- Therapeutic touch
- Massage (self or nurse)
- Turning and repositioning
- Hairbrushing and grooming (self or nurse)
- Activity around environment
- Amount of pressure individualized to client's comfort level
- Clothing of various textures

Safety Alert
Sensory Dysfunction

- When assisting a visually impaired client with ambulation, stand on the client's hand-dominant side, about 1 ft in front of him or her. Have him or her grasp your arm with the nondominant hand, and use the client dominant hand to feel around him or her for barriers or landmarks.
- Maintain an uncluttered environment for a visually impaired client.
- Organize self-care articles within client's reach and orient him or her to their location.
- Make sure the nurse call system is operating and within reach.
- Never rearrange furnishings without orienting the client.
- Do not rely on a hearing-impaired client to notify you of an alarm from an IV pump or malfunctioning cardiac monitor. Teach the client to visually identify kinked IV tubing or a loose ECG lead, and check these clients frequently.
- Test the temperature of bath or basin water before a client with altered tactile sensation bathes.
- Teach a client with altered taste and smell to avoid ingesting outdated food by checking expiration dates on food packages and visually inspecting the food for color and texture.

tion. Sensory deficits and the cognitive effects of sensory deprivation or sensory overload place the client at risk for injury from the environment. The nurse should implement actions such as assisting clients with ambulation, use of bed siderails, night lights, and call system and frequent or continuous observation as necessary.

The nurse must teach clients with sensory deficits how to ensure safety at home. For example, clients with decreased sensation to temperature in the extremities should have their hot water heater temperature adjusted and must test water temperature with a thermometer before bathing. They should be taught to inspect their legs and feet for any injuries or pressure sores they cannot feel. Clients with a decreased sense of smell should be taught the danger of using gas and chemicals. For example, cleaning with ammonia in a confined space such as a bathroom may cause the client to be overcome by fumes before he or she can smell them. A client may not smell a gas leak in the home, but if a stove or gas heater is not working properly, it should be reported promptly. Food should be inspected for freshness, because the client may not smell spoiled meat or dairy products. Clients with hearing and visual deficits need to take additional safety precautions as well. See Chapter 29 for more information on safety.

Community-Based Nursing

With rising costs and shorter hospital stays, a client may be discharged while still adjusting to his or her condition. This may be a new or worsening sensory deficit or an illness or treatment that causes sensory deprivation or sensory overload. Planning should be initiated as soon as possible to help the client adjust to sensory dysfunction. Planning includes client teaching, enlisting the help and cooperation of family and friends, assembling sensory aids and equipment, contacting home-health services, and locating additional support groups as needed.

The client's home environment should be assessed to determine what will be needed to help the client adapt to his or her sensory dysfunction. The nurse can teach the client and family how to interact in the home environment, using other senses and sensory aids to adapt and remain safe. The client may need much help during the adaptation process, but eventually he or she may become independent. At first, the client may need help with basic care and hygiene; however, ongoing nursing assessment will determine the need for further interventions.

Because family roles may change suddenly (eg, the breadwinner becomes the care receiver), family members may need as much help and support as the client for their own issues and concerns. Social services may be enlisted to help with financial problems related to the client's sensory dysfunction. Occupational therapy is a referral that can help the client adapt. Nurses are in a unique position to assess the client's needs before discharge and organize services that can continue the client's care after discharge.

Evaluation

Evaluation of the care of a client with sensory/perceptual dysfunction is based on the goals that were designed for that client. Outcome criteria are reviewed to determine if goals were achieved. For a client with sensory/perceptual alteration, was sensoristasis achieved? Were contributing factors to sensory dysfunction reduced or eliminated? Can the client describe the interventions and rationale so that this information can be used in the future to deal with sensory dysfunction? Was self-care maintained? Was safety maintained? Examples of positive outcome criteria for a client at risk for sensory overload follow.

Goal

The client will demonstrate an understanding of contributing factors by reducing or eliminating them.

Possible Outcome Criteria

- Client uses ear plugs and eye shades during sleep for the next 3 nights.

Nursing Plan of Care
The Client with Sensory/Perceptual Alterations

Nursing Diagnosis

Visual Sensory/Perceptual Alteration related to temporary decrease in visual sensory input manifested by fear of body-image alteration, irritability, withdrawal, and misinterpretation of sensory stimuli

Client Goal

Client will demonstrate an understanding of the sensory deprivation experience.

Client Outcome Criteria

- Within 8 hours, client accurately describes this eye injury and expected medical outcome (ie, full visual recovery).
- During hospitalization, client freely discusses problems with the staff, asking appropriate questions.
- Before discharge, client describes his or her behavioral changes and relates them to temporary deficit.
- Before discharge, client explains his or her behavior changes to family.

Nursing Intervention	Scientific Rationale
1. Introduce self from doorway before entering room and explain reason for being there.	1. This action avoids startling the client and prevents misperceptions.
2. Post schedule for day on wall for all staff, visitors, and family to follow. Review schedule with client for input.	2. A schedule assists the client to know what is going to happen and helps the client with orientation and anxiety reduction.
3. As rapport and trust build, invite the client to share his or her concerns about recovery; answer questions and correct misconceptions.	3. By getting the concerns out in the open, the nurse can help the client separate fears from reality.
4. Encourage client to identify his or her frustrations and anxieties related to being temporarily "blind" and to ask questions about his or her environment.	4. Orienting client to his or her environment provides reassurance and a variety of sensory stimulation.
5. Hold a conference with the client's family to promote mutual discussion of the experience. Encourage client to teach the family what he or she understands about sensory deprivation.	5. The nurse can evaluate the understanding of sensory deprivation and do additional teaching related to concerns of family about home management.

Client Goal

Client will demonstrate achievement of sensoristasis through a decrease in the symptoms of sensory deprivation.

Client Outcome Criteria

- Before discharge, client uses various sensory pathways to increase sensory variation.
- Before discharge, client reports no difficulty related to misperceiving sensory stimuli.
- During hospitalization, client visits with family, and friends for a minimum of 15 minutes per visit.

Nursing Intervention	Scientific Rationale
1. Schedule 5-minute conversations every hour on the hour while awake for the first 24 hours.	1. Regular conversations provide cognitive and sensory stimulation gradually and at a time the client can count on, so the client is not overwhelmed.

(continued)

Nursing Plan of Care *(Continued)*
The Client with Sensory/Perceptual Alterations

2. Orient to any noises that can be misinterpreted (eg, the air-conditioner thermostat on the wall, the noises from the pneumatic-tube system [especially loud at night], the chimes indicating a fire drill, the sound of the food cart being wheeled in at meal times).	2. Awareness of specific sounds helps the client stay focused in reality.
3. After the first 24 hours, on day and evening shifts, a minimum of two and maximum of four staff per shift, other than assigned caretakers, should talk with the client for a minimum of 10 minutes. Post a schedule in the front of the client's chart to sign up for these social visits.	3. This helps build trust, reduce anxiety, provide cognitive stimulation, and sensory variation.
4. Teach the client about the importance of gradually increasing input from other sensory pathways when vision is temporarily unavailable; include teaching about; self-stimulation, such as counting, singing, and using a tape recorder to talk into; isometric exercises; tactile stimulation; auditory variation, gustatory and olfactory stimulation.	4. The client needs information about management of sensory deficit, how to increase stimulation gradually, and prevention of further sensory deprivation or overload.

- Client limits television and radio use to 1 to 3 hours per 8-hour period for next 48 hours.
- Client asks appropriate questions about care before and during treatment in next 24 hours.

Goal

The client will demonstrate an understanding of interventions and rationales by using this information as foresight.

Possible Outcome Criteria

- During next 24 hours, client describes procedures to nurse before they are done, including what he or she might see, hear, feel, smell, or taste; client gives rationale for procedure and asks questions.

Goal

The client will achieve sensoristasis through a decrease in the symptoms of sensory overload or deprivation.

Possible Outcome Criteria

- Client demonstrates ability to concentrate by listening to explanation of medications, asking appropriate questions, and repeating medication schedule every time medication is given in next 24 hours.
- Client sleeps 5 to 7 hours each night without awakening every night.
- Client is oriented to person, place, and time during visiting hours for remainder of day as reported by nurse.
- Client listens to relaxation tape with earphones when housekeeping personnel are cleaning room.

Goal

The client will maintain safety.

Possible Outcome Criteria

- Client accurately uses safety devices, such as side rails, night light, and call system consistently.
- Client reports absence of injuries.

Goal

The client will maintain self-care.

Possible Outcome Criteria

- Client bathes and performs adequate oral care daily.
- Client performs toileting independently and safely.
- Client ambulates in hall three times a day.
- Client feeds self food and liquid for next 3 meals.

Key Concepts

- Senses include vision, hearing, taste, smell, and touch. Senses related to touch are the somatic senses of kinesthesia, or position sense, and visceral, or deep sensation.

- The RAS controls arousal and awareness to stimuli.
- Sensoristasis refers to a person's optimum state of arousal through stimulation.
- Adaptation occurs when stimulation is constant.
- Sensory perception generally decreases over 60 to 70 years of age.
- Altered sensory function can occur due to sensory overload, sensory deprivation, or sensory deficits. Sensory overload occurs when a person is unable to process the intensity or quantity of incoming stimuli, as in an intensive care unit. Sensory deprivation is a lack of meaningful stimuli, often occur ring when a client is on isolation precautions.
- Sensory deficits that occur gradually often bring about behavior changes and sharpening of other senses to help the person adapt.
- Anxiety, cognitive dysfunction, depression, and hallucinations and delusions are manifestations of sensory perception dysfunction.
- Nursing assessment of sensory perception function includes subjective information about the client and his or her usual environment and physical examination for vision, hearing, taste, smell, and the somatic senses of touch, pressure, position, vibration, pain, and temperature.
- Client goals for the nursing diagnosis of Sensory/Perceptual Alterations include achieving sensoristasis, reducing contributing factors, describing intervention and rationales, achieving self-care, and maintaining safety.
- Client teaching about eye examinations and treatment of ear infections may help promote sensory function.
- Preparing clients for procedures should include sensory experiences to prevent sensory overload.
- Nurses must provide appropriate stimulation for clients, while reducing excess stimulation for sensory deprivation or overload, respectively.
- Sensory aids may be physical, such as glasses, hearing aids, large-print books, and sound amplifiers, or situational, such as speaking directly in front of a hearing-impaired client or encouraging a client to smell and taste food.
- Safety must be maintained while the client is hospitalized by assisting with ambulation and care, using side rails, night lights, call system, and frequent observation.

Critical Thinking Challenges

Now that you have added sensory perception to your knowledge base, turn to the situation concerning Patrick Matthews at the beginning of the chapter. Plan his care by using the following questions.

1. *List information you have and further information you think you will need.*
2. *Identify your specific concerns about communicating with Patrick.*
3. *Considering the information you have and your concerns, describe how you feel about being assigned to Patrick.*
4. *Identify the sources of sensory perception disturbance you believe are critical for Patrick.*
5. *Clarify the priority considerations in determining your nursing care.*

References

Creditor, M. C. (1993). Hazards of hospitalization of the elderly. *Annals of Internal Medicine, 118*(3), 219–223.

Geary, S. M. (1994). Intensive care unit psychosis revisited: Understanding and managing delirium in the critical care setting. *Critical Care Nursing Quarterly, 17*(1), 51–63.

Gesell, A., & Ilg, F. (1949). *Child Development.* New York: Harper Brothers.

Glide, S. (1994). Maintaining sensory balance. *Nursing Times, 90*(17), 33-34.

Gordon, M. (1994). *Nursing diagnosis: Process and application* (3rd ed.). St. Louis: C.V. Mosby.

Horsley, J. A., & Crane, J. (1981). *Distress reduction through sensory preparation.* New York: Grune & Stratton.

Kim, M. J., McFarland, G. K., & McLane, A. M. (1987). *Pocket guide to nursing diagnosis* (2nd ed.). St. Louis: C.V. Mosby.

Lee, J. H. (1991a). An experimental study of the effects of sensory stimulation on the early growth and development of Korean low-birth-weight infants. *Journal of Pediatric Nursing, 6*(2), 144-145.

Lee, K. A. (1991b). Sensory overload, sensory deprivation, and sleep deprivation. In M. L. Patrick, S. L. Woods, R. F. Craven, et al. (Eds.), *Medical–surgical nursing: Pathophysiological concepts* (2nd ed.). Philadelphia: J.B. Lippincott.

McFarland, G. K., & Thomas, M. D. (1991). *Psychiatric mental health nursing: Application of the nursing process.* Philadelphia: J.B. Lippincott.

McFarland, G. K., & Wasli, E. L. (1986). *Nursing diagnoses and process in psychiatric mental health nursing.* Philadelphia: J.B. Lippincott.

North American Nursing Diagnosis Association (1994). *NANDA nursing diagnoses: Definitions and classification 1995–1996.* Philadelphia: Author.

Schafer, W. (1992). *Stress management for wellness* (2nd ed.). New York: HB College Publications.

Sime, A. M. (1985). Sensation information. In M. Snyder (Ed.), *Independent nursing interventions.* New York: John Wiley.

Toffler, A. (1970). *Future shock.* New York: Random House.

Vander, A. J., Sherman, J. H., & Luciano, D. S. (1993). *Human physiology: The mechanisms of body function* (6th ed.). New York: McGraw-Hill.

Bibliography

Barry, P. D. (1994). *Mental health and mental illness* (5th ed.). Philadelphia: J.B. Lippincott.

Baradel, J. G. (1985). Humanistic care of the client in seclusion. *Journal of Psychosocial Nursing and Mental Health Services, 2,* 9–14.

Grazier, S. (1988). The loneliness barrier ... clients in isolation. *Nursing Times, 84*(41), 44–45.

Kee, C. C. (1990). Sensory impairment: Factor X in providing nursing care to the older adult. *Journal of Community Health Nursing, 7*(1), 45–52.

Rogers J. C., et al. (1987). Maude: A case of sensory deprivation. *American Journal of Occupational Therapy, 41,* 673–676.

Thomas, K. A. (1989). How the NICU environment sounds to a preterm infant. *Maternal–Child Nursing Journal, 14,* 249–251.

Cognitive Processes

Key Terms	Learning Objectives

Key Terms

Attention
Cognition
Comprehension
Confusion
Consciousness
Delirium
Delusions
Dementia
Hallucinations
Intelligence
Judgment
Memory
Perceiving
Reality orientation
Sundown syndrome

Learning Objectives

Upon completion of this chapter, the student will be able to do the following

- *Identify the components of cognitive and thought processes.*
- *Describe the characteristics of normal cognition.*
- *Identify the cognitive factors that are a part of each of the stages of the lifespan.*
- *Recognize factors that affect normal cognitive function.*
- *Describe components of potential altered cognition.*
- *Identify manifestations of altered cognitive processes.*
- *Use the nursing process in the care of the person experiencing altered cognitive processes.*
- *Appreciate the types of resources available to families of people with altered cognitive processes.*

46

You are a nurse working on a general surgical floor of the hospital. A new client is admitted after surgical repair of a broken hip. She appears agitated and confused despite a pain control regimen of morphine. Her daughter, Donna, comes in to visit and looks acutely anxious. Donna tells you that her mother has been residing in a nursing home for 16 months. Two nights ago, her mother got up to go to the bathroom, fell, and broke her hip. The daughter says she thinks the nurses at the nursing home had ignored her mother's call light because "Mother would never get up at night without calling the nurse." While you are talking with the daughter, the mother is moaning, pulling at her intravenous tubing, and intermittently calls for "Dorothy."

In previous chapters, you learned about pain perception and sensory perception. This chapter expands your knowledge about perception as organized and recognized by the senses and the brain. After you have learned more about cognition, you will be able to recognize and plan care for clients with cognitive dysfunction such as the woman in the situation above. The Critical Thinking Challenges at the end of the chapter will help you use thinking skills in working with this client.

In any practice setting, nurses may work with people experiencing temporary or irreversible impairment of cognitive function. The nurse plays a central role in identification of people at risk for and experiencing cognitive impairment, as well as in the ongoing assessment of the impact of cognitive impairment on self-care and safety. Nursing interventions are focused on preventing, minimizing, or restoring contributing factors, compensating for deficits, and promoting optimal function. Planning and evaluating nursing care require an understanding of normal cognition, factors that place a person at risk for cognitive impairment, and effective interventions that can be individualized.

Normal Cognitive Function

Cognition is the systematic way in which a person thinks, reasons, and uses language. Each instant of awareness can be defined as a thought, and awareness itself can be defined as consciousness. **Attention** is the aspect of consciousness that enables one to concentrate on and take in specific sensory stimuli. **Memory** is the capability of recalling a thought at least once and usually again. **Learning** is the capability of the nervous system to store memories. The cerebral cortex coordinates consciousness, thoughts, memory, and learning. All four functions are inseparable (Guyton, 1991).

Anatomic Structures Involved in Cognition

For information to be processed, the person must be able to perceive the information. Perception of information from the environment begins when the information enters the person's awareness through the senses, and the four cognitive processes of consciousness, thinking, memory, and learning all play roles in the further processing of that information. Intact structure and functioning of the sensory receptors, the afferent nervous pathways, and the cerebral cortex are required for a person to be able to take in information through the senses, and to assimilate and interpret that information in the cerebral cortex.

The eyes and ears are the major means of sensory input. The eyeball (Fig. 46-1), a mobile, spherical structure located in the orbit of the skull, is composed of the sclera (the white, outer, fibrous layer), the choroid (the vascular layer), and the retina (the neural layer). The interior chambers are filled with clear media (the aqueous and vitreous humors) through which light is transmitted to the retina. Visual stimuli are sensed by the rods and cones of the retina and carried to the visual cortex of the brain by the optic nerve and optic tract.

The ear (see Fig. 46-1) consists of the external ear (the auricle and the external acoustic meatus or ear canal), the tympanic membrane, the middle ear (the ossicles and the eustachian tube), and the inner ear (the cochlea, vestibule, and semicircular canals). Sound is transmitted through the auricle and ear canal to the tympanic membrane, which vibrates freely. The vibration is transmitted to the ossicles (malleus, incus, and stapes), which continue the transmission to the labyrinth or inner ear. The vibration moves through the fluid of the inner ear to the apex of the cochlea and the organ of Corti. In response to vibration, hair cells of the organ of Corti generate nerve impulses that are carried to the auditory cortex in the brain by the acoustic nerve.

The reticular formation is a diffuse cluster of neurons that extends from the brain stem and projects upward and throughout the cerebral cortex and downward into the spinal cord (Guyton, 1991). Its location is illustrated in Figure 43-1. The reticular formation is essential for maintaining wakefulness (it is also referred to as the reticular activating system [RAS]), and controls portions of vital cardiovascular and respiratory reflexes (McCance & Heuther, 1994). The nervous system, including the cranial nerves (see Chapter 21), must be intact for full cognition. In most people, language centers are in the left hemisphere of the brain; these are illustrated in Figure 48-1.

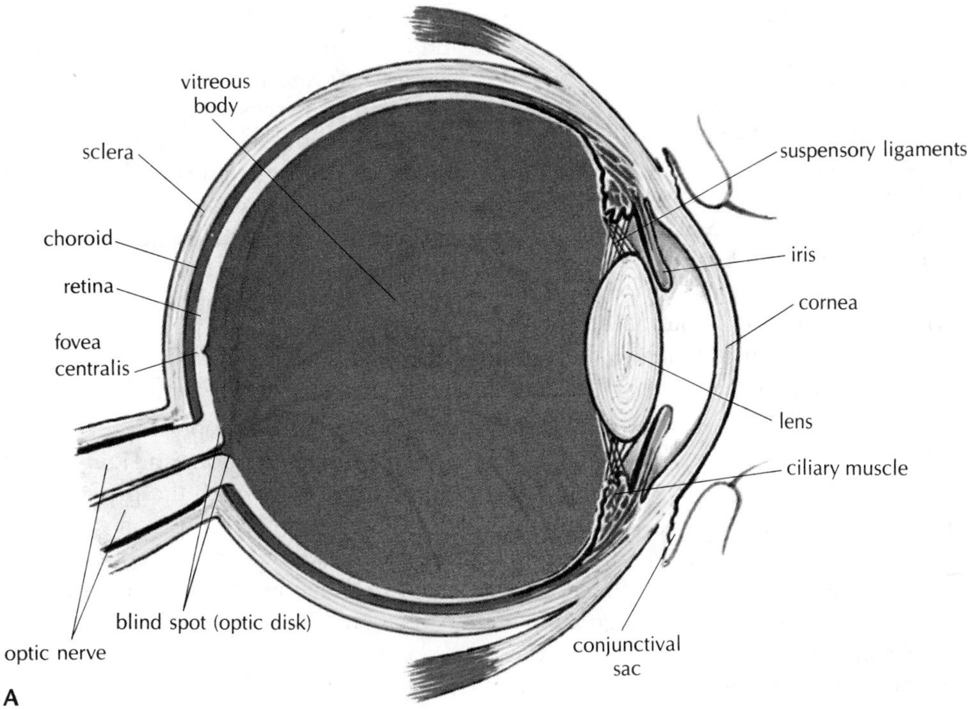

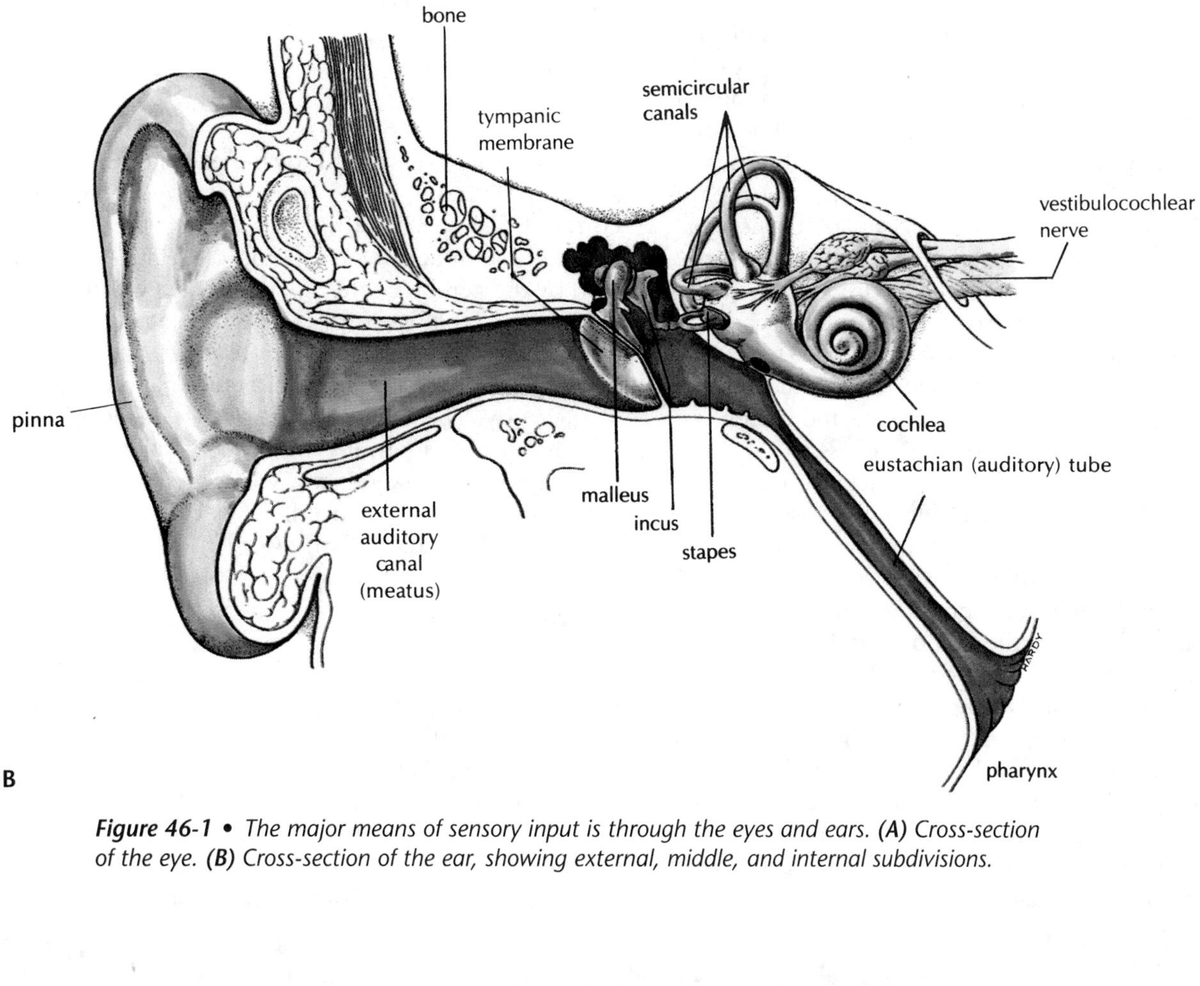

Figure 46-1 • *The major means of sensory input is through the eyes and ears.* ***(A)*** *Cross-section of the eye.* ***(B)*** *Cross-section of the ear, showing external, middle, and internal subdivisions.*

Normal Physiologic Function

Perception of Information

Perception of information includes the sensing and interpretation of stimuli from the external and internal environments. Perception depends on functioning sensory receptors, neurotransmission, and central processing.

Sensory receptors can be classified into three groups: exteroceptors (external sensors), proprioceptors (position sensors), and interoceptors (internal sensors). Neurotransmission occurs when the stimuli to the sensory receptors are converted to neural impulses and transmitted to the appropriate area of the brain for central processing and translation.

Exteroceptors. The exteroceptors respond to stimuli from the external environment and include the receptors for vision and hearing, and the somatic receptors for pain, touch, and pressure in the skin. Vision allows people to perceive and learn about their world from the time of birth throughout life, assuming it remains intact. Vision permits abstract concepts to be linked with concrete objects, thus aiding the learning and memory processes. Hearing, also present from birth, links concepts with frequency, intensity, and duration of sounds. Both vision and hearing enable the person to enhance awareness of the environment and experiences to amplify cognitive development.

Vision requires the brain-related functions of photoreception, visual sensation, and perception for full function. The primary visual cortex, located in the calcarine fissure area of the occipital lobe, is the location where visual sensation is first experienced. The nearby associational visual cortex, along with previous learning, adds meaningfulness to the visual perception.

Sound is the external stimulus to which the ear responds. Nerve impulses from the organ of Corti are carried to the primary and associational auditory cortex of the brain's temporal lobes (Guyton, 1991). These areas of the brain are necessary for sound to be meaningful, and for integration of past experience and current auditory information in the hearing process.

Somatic sensors in the skin are activated by touch, pressure, heat, cold, or chemicals in the tissue. The resulting nerve impulses enter the spinal cord through the posterior roots. Depending on the sensation, the impulse is transmitted to the brain through either the dorsal column system or the spinothalamic system. The dorsal column transmits sensory information that must be transmitted rapidly, incorporates fine gradations of intensity, and is discretely localized. The spinothalamic system carries information that lacks fine gradations, has less exact localization, or does not need rapid transmission. From the spinal cord, sensory information is transmitted through the thalamus to the somatosensory cortex in the brain's parietal lobes.

Taste is a function of the taste buds of the tongue, and includes sweet, sour, salty, and bitter components. The sensation of taste is transmitted via the seventh and ninth cranial nerves to the brain stem. Ascending fibers carry the impulses to the taste area of the sensory cortex. Smell is a function of the olfactory cells located in the upper nose, and is the least understood of the special senses. The olfactory cells are actually projections from the brain itself. Taste and smell seem to be closely related, because diminished function in one usually affects the function of the other (McCance & Heuther, 1994).

Proprioceptors. Proprioceptors are located in the inner ear, muscles, tendons and joints. Proprioceptive sensations have to do with the physical state of the body, including the relative position of the different parts of the body, and the sensation of movement. The proprioceptive function of the inner ear is discussed in detail in Chapter 33.

Interoceptors. Interceptors are located in and respond to stimuli from the viscera of the body and the deeper tissues such as bone. Sensations relate to changes in the internal environment. With the exception of visceral pain receptors, the interoreceptors operate at a reflex level. That is, sensory signals elicit reflex responses that enable the visceral organs to control their activities without involvement of consciousness (Guyton, 1991).

Consciousness

Consciousness, a state of awareness and full responsiveness to stimuli, relies on an intact RAS and cerebral cortex. Level of arousal is mediated by the RAS, and the perception and interpretation of stimuli are mediated by the cerebral cortex. The RAS is divided into facilitatory and inhibitory areas. The facilitatory area is intrinsically active, provides arousal to the cerebral hemispheres, and produces an increase in muscle tone in the body. The inhibitory area causes a decrease in muscle tone, and permits decreased activity and sleep after prolonged wakefulness. When the facilitatory and inhibitory areas are balanced, the person is neither excited nor inhibited, but conscious.

Thoughts

Each thought results from a momentary pattern of stimulation of many parts of the nervous system at the same time. This stimulation involves, most importantly, the cerebral cortex, thalamus, limbic system, and the upper reticular formation of the brain stem. The stimulated areas of the limbic system, thalamus, and reticular formation give thought its crude nature, such as pleasure, displeasure, pain, and comfort. The stimulated area of the cortex determines discrete characteristics of thought (what is seen in the visual field), discrete patterns of sensation (texture of objects), and other specific characteristics (Guyton, 1991).

Memory

Memory is the process by which information and experiences are stored and retrieved. Physiologically, memories are caused by changes in nerve transmission from one neuron to the next as a result of previous neural activity (learning). Plasticity, the tendency of synapses and neural circuits to change as a result of activity, allows for the formation of new synaptic pathways. These new pathways are called memory traces, and once established can be activated to reproduce the memories (Guyton, 1991).

Memory is subdivided into three basic types based on the time span between stimulus presentation and memory retrieval. Immediate memories last for a few seconds to a few minutes, and may be caused by local reverberating neural impulses. Short-term memories may last for minutes or weeks, but will be lost unless converted to long-term memories. Physiologically, short-term memories involve changes in the strength of the synaptic connections, which may be attributed to changes in neurotransmitter or intracellular chemicals. Long-term memories, those that can be recalled for an indefinite period of time, are stored at the same site as short-term memories, but require the activation of previously inactive genes and the expression of new proteins (for example, there may be an increase in number of cell membrane channels) (Kandel & Hawkins, 1992).

The hippocampi, located within both temporal lobes, and part of the limbic system, play a role in determining which memories get committed to long-term memory. The ability to retain some things and forget others is essential to intelligent behavior. Assimilating experiences and new information is a process involving memory. The hippocampi play a vital role in retaining new knowledge and preventing dissipation of the information.

Characteristics of Normal Cognition

The characteristics of normal cognition, including intellectual function, perception of reality, orientation, communication, judgment, and recall, are revealed in many aspects of daily life. Integrated cognitive function is required to allow people to perform the processes necessary to carry out activities of life.

Intelligence

Intelligence is the measurable product of intellectual functioning. Intellectual function consists of memory, comprehension, and concentration. Memory was discussed previously. Comprehension is a part of learning and involves grasping the meaning of the stimulus. Concentration is the ability to screen out extraneous stimuli to focus on a task. People depend on intellectual function to be able to learn in school settings, in vocational surroundings, and in their living environments. Society evaluates and values people in terms of intellectual function abilities.

Reality Perception

Perception of reality, or **reality orientation**, includes the awareness of time, place, situation, and self. It is the knowledge of how the self and the environment interact on the continuum of time, and transform sensory information into meaning (Schuster & Ashburn, 1992). Reality perception is complex and depends on functioning sensory receptors, neurotransmission, and intact central processing. People with sensory impairments, such as blindness or hearing deficit, may compensate by increasing the acuity of other senses.

Orientation

Orientation is the basic process by which people know their location in the dimensions of time and place. Orientation also includes the ability to know who one is as a person and in relation to other people. People tend to take these abilities for granted until they experience confusion about orientation. On a simple level, one can become confused about one's orientation, or experience *disorientation,* when on vacation and awakening in a new setting, and momentarily forgetting where one is.

Communication

Communication involves the use of language to store, process, and transmit thought content. Language development depends on a nurturing environment during childhood, when language is developed, and can be affected by sociocultural experiences throughout life. Language uses words, and words vary in use and meaning, depending on a person's age, education, culture, socioeconomic background, and geographic region.

Judgment

Judgment, or insight, the process of reasoning, is the ability to process incoming stimuli and determine the complex meanings associated with the many aspects of a situation. For example, a person driving down the street may see a truck blocking the road ahead. The person determines that the truck is an obstacle and that evasive action is required to prevent a crash. The term "insight" is often used to express perceptions people make about behavior or feelings. For example, recognizing that a craving for chocolate when studying for exams is an indicator of stress is an insight. The correlation between craving and studying and the recognition of being anxious about doing well in school lead to the insight. This is an example of a complex reasoning process.

Recall and Recognition

Recall and recognition are abilities used to retrieve the information from the long- and short-term memory. Recall involves the ability to retrieve information directly or by relating it to other information (eg, seeing a person and "recalling" his or her name accurately). Recognition is the ability to relate accurately something currently in the environment with what is in the memory (eg, seeing a rose and "recognizing" it as a type of flower). People depend on these abilities to perform in school, on the job, and in everyday life. Recall and recognition are cognitive characteristics that can be developed and that need to be practiced to keep them actively useful.

Normal Cognition

Cognition is the sum of the various thinking processes through which knowledge is gained, stored, manipulated, and expressed. Cognition enables the person to interact with the environment in a meaningful and purposeful way. Cognitive function consists of attending, perceiving, thinking, learning, and remembering, by which a person comprehends. Normal cognitive function requires integration of these processes.

Attending

Attending is the process of concentrating on a specific stimulus without being distracted by other, irrelevant stimuli in the environment (Strub & Black, 1993). The capability to concentrate is a cortical function of the frontal lobe of the brain. Attending contrasts with alertness—an alert but inattentive person will be attracted to any stimulus in the environment.

Perceiving

Perceiving is the process of receiving and interpreting the sensory stimuli that function as a basis for understanding, knowing, or learning. In perceiving, a person uses the integrated information obtained through vision, hearing, touching, taste, or smell in concert with past experiences to create understanding or make sense of the environment. An example of perceiving is hearing a phone ring, seeing the phone, touching and holding the receiver, listening to the person speaking, interpreting the meaning in the cerebral cortex, and responding in an appropriate manner. The integration of the motor activities involved in handling the phone, the sensory activities of seeing and hearing, and the central perceptual activities of interpretation results in a meaningful interaction.

Thinking

Thinking is the process of sorting, organizing, and categorizing information to form mental concepts or perceptions. "Thinking" is forming ideas or arriving at conclusions; "reasoning" is following a logical sequence of thought, starting with what is known and proceeding to a conclusion. A person is capable of different types of thinking. Concrete thinking involves objects or groups of things that can be perceived by the senses. An example of concrete thinking is the proof of the arithmetical proposition that $1 + 1 = 2$ by attaching the numbers to objects, such as apples. Abstract thinking is a higher-level thinking that involves a thought or idea apart from any material object. For example, the idea of beauty is a value attributed to a flower but is not a concrete object in itself. A maxim, such as "People who live in glass houses shouldn't throw stones," is an example of how abstract thinking is required for a veiled or abstract truth to be interpreted from the use of concrete objects and terms.

Learning

Learning is the process of acquiring knowledge, and, as such, is a multidimensional process that depends on symbols, language, classifications, concepts, and other concrete operations, along with abstract functions. **Comprehension** is the capacity for understanding and reasoning. (A complete discussion of the concept and process of learning is beyond the scope of this chapter.) For learning to be useful, the person needs to develop strategies for organizing the information in the memory so that it can be recalled as needed.

Remembering

Memory is a complex biochemical storage system that is not yet completely understood. Experiences, ideas, and images are chemically coded and integrated for later retrieval (Freiberg, 1992). The content of long-term memory, which is the storehouse of a person's knowledge, depends on the perceived value and significance of the past event. Specific significant life events, such as weddings or the birth of a child, hold greater value and memory potential. Immediate and short-term memory, also known as working memory, are easily affected by emotional stress (Foreman, 1992). The reason some items are moved from short- to long-term memory is not clear, but is probably related to the perceived value of the information and its relation to other memories.

Therapeutic Dialogue
Safety Related to Memory Loss

Scenes for Thought

Carmen Morales (see Chap. 40) has returned for her blood pressure check but this time has brought her grandmother, Rosa Gomez, to be checked, too. Mrs. Gomez, aged 84, is a smiling little woman who affectionately pats your hand as you greet her. Carmen tells you that "Abuelita" is having some trouble with her memory, and the family is worried that she might be unsafe at home because she tends to forget to turn off the stove, has trouble with the household appliances, and is getting irritable when the children make noise after school. This problem has been occurring over the last 2 months. Mrs. Gomez has no physical problems except controlled high blood pressure and occasional constipation.

Effective

Nurse: *Mrs. Gomez, you've heard what Carmen and I have been talking about?* She nods, smiling brightly. *What do you think about that?*
Client: *I lose my memory sometimes, but it's nothing to get worried about. I'm old. I'm supposed to lose my memory sometimes.* She continues to smile.
Nurse: *You expect that your memory will be lost as you grow older?*
Client: *Sure. My parents didn't live to be very old, but I remember my grandmother not remembering things very well by the time she was 70! So I'm doing fine.* Gives a little laugh.
Nurse: *I'm wondering if you can think of times that you have more trouble remembering than other times.*
Client: Sits and concentrates for a minute. *I think it's when there's too much commotion in the house or when I don't get enough sleep. Then I can't remember things very well.* Turns to Carmen. *That's when I forgot to turn off the stove, querida mia, and it was only once, you know. Yes, it's when there's a lot to distract me from my work.*
Nurse: *I understand. You said you don't get enough sleep sometimes? Tell me a little more about that, please.*
Client: *Certainly. I sometimes have to go to the bathroom in the middle of the night. Then it's hard for me to get back to sleep all alone in that big bed. My husband died 2 years ago, and it's still hard for me to sleep in that big bed.* She doesn't smile now.
Nurse: *You're still missing him, I can see that. I guess it helps to take care of the family the way you do.*
Client: *Yes, it does help. And I want to do the best I can for them. I don't want them to worry about me, or send me away.* Looks at Carmen with tears in her eyes.
Carmen: *No, Abuelita, we don't want to send you away, we just want you to be safe and comfortable. Don't cry, don't cry.* She puts her arm around her grandmother.
Nurse: *I think if we three talk together we can come up with some ways to help you get better sleep, Mrs. Gomez. And there are some tricks I can think of to help you remember things better. Let's work together on this. What do you say?*
Client: *I would be happy to! Thank you very much!* Squeezes your hand and smiles.

Less Effective

Nurse: *Mrs. Gomez, you've heard what Carmen and I have been talking about?* She nods, smiling brightly, *What do you think about that?*
Client: *I lose my memory sometimes, but it's nothing to get worried about. I'm old, I'm supposed to lose my memory sometimes.* She continues to smile.
Nurse: *It's true that as we get older our memories get a little worn out (patting her hand), but Carmen is worried about your safety while you're taking care of the cooking and cleaning and so on. I'm thinking that it would be a good idea for you to see one of the geriatric nurse specialists here in the clinic. He could talk with you, maybe run some tests, work with you on your memory and so forth. He's very good, very caring, and has lots of experience with people your age. What do you think?*
Client: *Am I sick or something? Why do I need a specialist?* Looks at Carmen anxiously.
Carmen: *It's okay, Abuelita, we'll go see what this other nurse has to say. I'm sure he can help us with your memory.* Rises to leave. *Come on, Abuelita, let's go and make the appointment.*
Client: *Okay, querida, if you say so. But I don't understand all this fuss over a little memory loss.* Grumbles on her way out.

Critical Thinking Challenge

Although Mrs. Gomez ultimately received effective care in both dialogues, detect what made the second dialogue "less effective" from the client's point of view • Explain what factors the second nurse never found out about • Describe the relationship between anxiety and cognitive processes.

Factors Affecting Normal Cognitive Function

Cognitive processes can be affected by physiologic, emotional, or environmental factors. Whether these factors affect normal cognition or thought processes depends on the interaction of person and environmental factors. Person factors include blood flow, nutrition, fluid and electrolyte balance, sleep and rest, and the ability to organize environmental stimuli. Environmental factors include the amount and kind of stimuli and demands in the environment. Environmental stimuli can range from too little or meaningless stimulation, through optimal stimulation, to too much or disorganized stimulation.

Adequate Blood Flow

All cells require a continuous oxygen supply and a stable extracellular environment of fluid and electrolytes to function optimally. Oxygenation depends on respiratory and circulatory function and hemoglobin production. During respiration, oxygen enters the alveoli, diffuses across capillary membranes to enter the pulmonary venous system, and binds with hemoglobin. Oxygen, bound to hemoglobin in the arterial blood, is transported to brain cells. The brain accounts for 20% of the total oxygen uptake of the body, and requires a constant, ample supply to support brain cell life.

Nutrition and Metabolism

Nutrition affects normal cognitive function because the brain cells need glucose for metabolic energy and other nutrients for optimal functioning. The efficiency with which oxygen is delivered to the cells is related to hemoglobin production, which requires an adequate dietary intake of iron. The brain, which consumes 25% of the glucose used by the body, requires a steady supply of glucose. Vitamins and minerals are essential for effective neurologic functioning and neurotransmitter activity.

Fluid and Electrolyte Balance

The brain cells require a constant extracellular environment of fluid and electrolytes for optimal function. In the brain, as elsewhere, cellular processes depend on the active and passive movement of water and charged particles across cell membranes (see Chapter 36). The brain is protected by the blood–brain barrier, a shield that prevents or delays the entry of certain substances from the blood into the cerebrospinal fluid or interstitial spaces of the brain. The blood–brain barrier protects the brain cells from substances other than normal fluid and electrolytes, which could damage sensitive nerve cells. Maintenance of a dynamic state of fluid balance and electrolyte levels provides the ideal internal environment for neurologic function.

Sleep and Rest

Sleep has a restorative function, allowing the person to regain energy for cognitive functions, such as attending, perceiving, thinking, learning, and remembering (see Chapter 43). Rapid eye movement (REM) sleep seems to be particularly important for mentally restoring the person for efficient cognitive functioning.

Organization of Environmental Stimuli

The basic cognitive processes of perceiving, thinking, learning, and remembering depend on the ability to receive and organize stimuli. The amount of stimuli in the environment, either increased or decreased, can influence normal cognition. For example, one student preparing for exams in an environment of noisy students, television, and loud music may find it difficult to organize the stimuli and study effectively. At the same time, another student may find that some background noise assists with concentration, depending on the level of distraction.

Perceptual ability, which contributes to cognitive functioning, declines as a normal part of aging as sense organ functions diminish. For example, the older person needs more light to see an object, has more problem with light glare, and experiences loss of accommodation for near objects (presbyopia). Hearing diminishes, especially in the high-frequency range, and acuity of sense of touch declines. These normal changes affect the ability to organize incoming stimuli.

Lifespan Considerations

Cognitive development is a complex process affected by physiologic health and the quality of the social and physical environment. The rate at which a person proceeds through the usual stages of cognitive development can be strongly affected by the environment. People need emotional security, human interaction, and a variety of sensory experiences to develop optimally. Jean Piaget is the most widely recognized theorist in cognitive development, although the work of other theorists, such as Erikson (1963) and Havighurst (1972), contributes to the understanding of cognitive development throughout the lifespan.

Newborn and Infant

The newborn and infant are in the sensorimotor period, in which sensory experience is the major developmental task (Piaget, 1969). The infant interacts with the environment through the five senses and learns to modify his or her behavior in response to environmental stimuli. The infant's language skills are not developed, and thoughts or needs are expressed through behavior.

The cognitive developmental work of infancy is carried out through exploration of the environment and through play. The infant learns to connect some behaviors with expected responses. For example, moving a toy in a certain way may cause a pleasing sound to occur. The infant may have learned that through play, but, with repetition and maturity, is able to remember and repeat the action to have it occur at will. In the same manner, an infant begins to assimilate language, linking specific words and sounds with an object of meaning, such as "Mama" or "bottle." Providing stimulation through varied objects, different sounds, and face-to-face communication and interaction enhances cognitive development (Freiberg, 1992).

Toddler and Preschooler

The young child develops object permanence and begins to label familiar items. The child learns that an object has permanence and constancy, and gives the object a name, using it to represent the object to others (Piaget, 1969). Perceptual ability in vision and hearing is necessary to obtain an understanding of the environment as a basis of thinking. Language and cognition develop side by side. The preschool-age child is concrete in thinking patterns and demonstrates pronounced egocentrism, or self-concern. The world is viewed from the child's point of view only, and in a concrete manner.

The process of reasoning begins as the young child tries to make sense of the world. When two events occur simultaneously, the child thinks one caused the other (transductive reasoning). Because of this, the preschooler thinks his or her thoughts are all-powerful. For example, if a child spilled his or her milk and later fell and scraped a knee, he or she might interpret the pain associated with the abrasion as punishment for spilling the milk. More significantly, the child may interpret parental divorce as punishment for his or her "bad" thoughts or behavior. Because adults find this thinking so absurd, they may underestimate its seriousness to a preschooler.

As a part of cognitive development, the young child develops confidence in abilities and gains independence through the encouragement of parents in each new area of learning (Erikson, 1963). Positive, nurturing play environments that encourage imaginative play, interaction, questioning, and use of language and symbols, while reinforcing earlier knowledge, will foster cognitive development in the preschooler (Fig. 46-2).

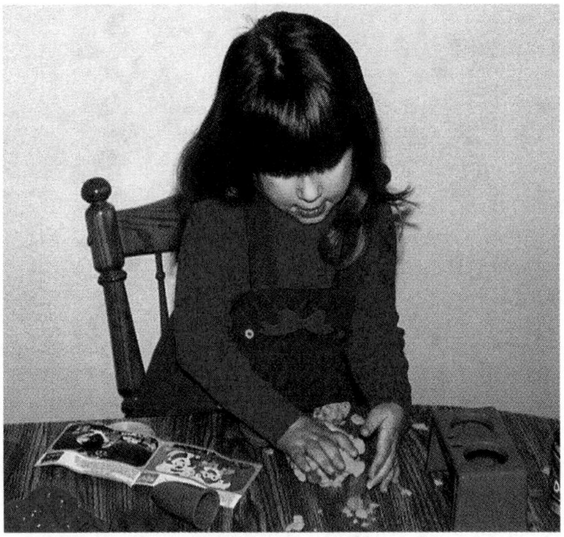

Figure 46-2 • *Play activities that incorporate imagination and creativity help to develop cognitive abilities in preschoolers.*

Child and Adolescent

The school-age child can carry out complex mental operations such as addition, subtraction, grouping, classifying, and ordering (Piaget, 1969). The multiple dimensions of objects and symbols are understood and represented mentally, and the child can encode stimuli for later retrieval. The school-age child understands conservation, or the idea that the properties of an object can stay the same even if the object is altered in certain ways. For example, if an equal volume of fluid is poured into two differently shaped containers, the preschool-age child will perceive that the volume of water has changed, whereas the school-age child will see a change in shape but a constant volume. This shift in comprehension indicates the ability to incorporate abstract thinking with concrete processes. At this age, the child receives great pleasure in accomplishments that result from new learning and thinking skills (Erikson, 1963). Learning and play environments that reward the achievements of the child contribute positively to cognitive development.

Adolescence is a particularly difficult time for the development of thinking processes because it is a time of enormous emotional stress from a variety of sources, including the struggle to develop a sense of separateness from parents and a strong need to identify with a peer group (Erikson, 1963). Abstract reasoning and logical judgment are two functions that the adolescent develops with increasing maturity.

During adolescence, the person develops the ability to think abstractly and perform complex processes in his or her head. The adolescent is able to hypothesize situations and solutions as well as conceptualize abstract ideas (Piaget, 1969). Classification, serialization, spatial abilities, verbal skills, and abstract relationships are cognitive capacities being developed by the adolescent. Providing opportunities for independent thinking and decision-making encourages increased maturity in cognitive development.

Adult and Older Adult

Throughout young and middle adulthood, the person is steadily gaining in rational thinking abilities, formal and informal educational opportunities, career development, and life experiences. As the adult feels progressively more competent with cognitive management of life, the less rigid and more flexible he or she is able to become. Making decisions and adjusting to changes are managed with less life disruption. Creativity and

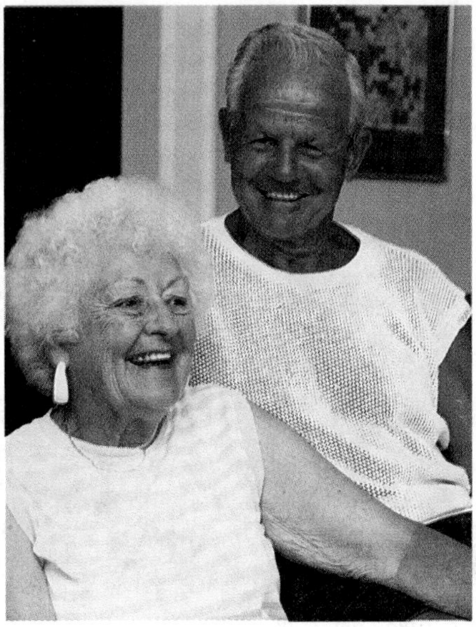

Figure 46-3 • With aging, adults can continue to use wisdom and cognitive abilities in all aspects of life.

productivity in work contribute to continual cognitive development and innovative use of integrated abstract and concrete thinking.

Aging is part of the life-long developmental process (Fig. 46-3). The fastest-growing segment of the population consists of those older than 85 years of age. Aging is a time when people may feel an attainment of purpose or accomplishment in an area of expertise (Erikson, 1963). Although the older adult still faces developmental tasks such as retirement and change in relationships (Havighurst, 1972), he or she is also a repository of knowledge, wisdom, and cognitive competence. Seeking opportunities to continue to use the accumulated knowledge of a lifetime by volunteering or consulting assists in maintaining cognitive abilities.

As a person ages, cognitive function remains relatively unchanged in the absence of trauma or specific dysfunction, although processing of information may require more time. Although problems with thought processes are more common in older adults, they are usually related to a decrease in coping reserves or to a specific problem, and are not a normal part of aging. Age-associated memory impairment is a mild memory impairment that does not significantly interfere with activities of daily living. Items forgotten are usually relatively unimportant. People can learn memory techniques to compensate for benign forgetfulness.

Altered Cognitive Function

Cognition is a complex process. Multiple, varied stimuli are perceived, organized, and integrated with previous knowledge and experience. The outcome of this process is an appropriate, adaptive behavioral or emotional response. Anything that interrupts this complex process can result in impaired thinking and abnormal behavioral or emotional responses. Clinically, altered cognitive function or cognitive impairment may be manifested as acute confusion (delirium) or as chronic, irreversible confusion (dementia). Acute confusional states result from physiologic alterations or person–environment imbalances and are reversible with appropriate, timely intervention. Chronic confusion results from diffuse shrinkage and destruction of brain tissue related to degenerative processes or blockage of cerebral blood vessels. A third category of altered cognitive function results when acute confusion is superimposed on chronic dementia.

Potential for Altered Cognition

Cognitive function is affected by physiologic, psychological, and environmental stress. Altered cognition often results from multiple interacting factors, rather than from a single causative factor. Any physiologic abnormality that affects the cellular environment can interfere with brain function and produce altered cognition, ranging from mild mental clouding, through disorientation and acute confusion, to coma (Porth, 1994). Physiologic abnormalities contribute to some kinds of dementia, such as multi-infarct and AIDS-related dementias.

With aging, the older person usually experiences a need for more time to perform mental operations, although this does not interfere with either the ability to learn new things or to carry out activities of daily living. Although the brain undergoes some degenerative changes, with the ventricles enlarging slightly and brain weight decreasing, significant cognitive impairment in an older person is never normal but is an indication of a disorder.

Inadequate Blood Flow

The brain depends on oxygen and glucose for energy metabolism. Any interruption in blood flow to brain cells causes cellular hypoxia and results in changes in function. A chronically inadequate blood supply to the brain causes cell dysfunction and deterioration of mental processes (Porth, 1994). Any disease process that interferes with alveolar ventilation, pulmonary circulation, cardiac function, cerebral blood flow, or the production of normal hemoglobin can result in hypoxia and altered cognition.

Altered Nutrition and Metabolism

People with inadequate nutrition often have low hemoglobin levels (anemia). Abnormal hemoglobin can be produced in people with specific genetic disorders, such as sickle cell anemia. Disorders that impair metabolic processes and oxygen use, such as hypothermia and hypothyroidism, can also cause altered cognition (Porth, 1994). Inadequate intake of glucose or impaired use of glucose by the body will limit the quantity of glucose available for the metabolic demands of the brain.

Fluid and Electrolyte Imbalance

Disturbances in the concentration and balance of intracellular and extracellular water and electrolytes can cause cellular dysfunction, which can be manifested by changes in cognition. Such disturbances can have a variety of causes, including abnormal losses of body fluids, dietary deficiencies, acute and chronic disease, and the effects of medication. Although any disturbance in fluid or electrolyte balance can cause **confusion** (impairment of cognitive processes), a few disturbances are more common (Porth, 1994). They are hyponatremia and hypernatremia (variations in the serum sodium level), hypercalcemia (elevated serum calcium level), and hypoglycemia and hyperglycemia (abnormal serum glucose levels).

Accumulated metabolic by-products, the end products of metabolism, if not eliminated from the body, can be toxic to central nervous system function. Impaired function of the kidney, liver, or both together can impair the ability to break down and excrete such potential toxins. Ammonia, a by-product of protein metabolism, is converted by the liver into urea, which is excreted by the kidney. Liver or kidney dysfunction can interfere with this process and cause elevated ammonia levels, producing a delirium known as hepatic encephalopathy.

Infectious Processes

Infectious processes of the central nervous system, including encephalitis and brain abscesses, and the subsequent inflammatory response of nerve cells are obvious causes of altered cognition. The human immunodeficiency virus can invade the central nervous system, causing acute infection and the AIDS dementia complex. Infections elsewhere in the body can also cause mental status changes. Any person with a severe infection in the circulation (eg, bacteremia, septicemia) may experience central nervous system effects, including lethargy and confusion. Common sources for bacteremia or septicemia include the urinary tract, the respiratory system, and any open wounds (Porth, 1994). Altered cognitive function in an older person may be the earliest indication of an infectious process.

Inadequate Sleep and Rest

Lack of sleep, or sleep deprivation, can cause various disruptions, including irritability, decreased calculation and problem-solving skill, poor concentration, or impaired memory. Everyone has experienced feeling dull and slow after having a sleepless night or staying up too late. Rotating shifts can cause similar problems, particularly if the person has to change shifts frequently without adequate time to adjust to a new sleep pattern. These changes in normal sleep patterns may result in inadequate amounts of REM sleep, which may impair both learning and memory as well as decreasing the subjective feeling of being rested.

Inability to Organize Incoming Stimuli

Emotional stress or physical discomfort can lead to disorganized thinking, memory impairment, and poor judgment. A person learning of an injury to a loved one, finding out about a failed exam, or planning a wedding can have difficulty maintaining the usual level of cognitive performance. Concentration and problem-solving are also difficult when a person is in pain, has a full bladder, or experiences other discomfort. These sometimes minor everyday problems can combine and accumulate, creating enough stress to impair thinking.

Psychological disorders, such as depression, interfere with cognitive function and can contribute to altered thought processes. Psychological and emotional disorders can interfere with sleep, rest, and nutrition, as well as affecting cognitive functions directly.

Environmental Stress. The stress of an unfamiliar environment can affect the basic cognitive processes of orientation and arousal, which depend on the ability of the cerebral cortex to receive and organize incoming stimuli (Kane, et al., 1994). There are numerous stimuli in any environment, some of which are attended to and some ignored. Through a complex perceptual process, habituation or familiarization occurs to routine background stimuli, such as the feel of clothing and the tick of a clock. As a result, the person is not "overloaded" with meaningless input. The brain can also conjure up input when none is available. People experiencing inadequate sensory input are at risk for cognitive dysfunction as the brain attempts to stimulate itself (see Chapter 45 for a complete discussion of sensory function).

Hospitalization removes people from familiar surroundings and daily activities that provide orienting cues, placing them in an environment of strange noises, sights, feelings, and procedures (Fig. 46-4). All of these unfamiliar stimuli demand attention because habituation has not had time to develop. This state of sensory overload can overwhelm the person's ability to find meaning, and a state of perceptual dysfunction occurs. There are plenty of stimuli present, but none of them makes any sense.

Pharmacologic Agents. Pharmacologic agents, or medications, that primarily act on the central nervous system, such as anticonvulsants, antidepressants, antianxiety agents, antipsychotics, narcotics, and hypnotics,

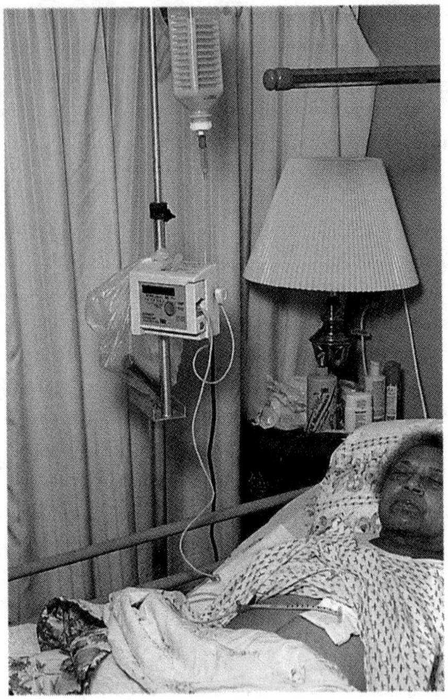

Figure 46-4 • Older adults may be at risk for cognitive dysfunction related to unfamiliar environments and procedures.

can impair thinking and cause confusion. Discontinuing or decreasing the dosage of these medications will often improve cognitive function within a few days. Medications commonly prescribed to manage agitated or confused behavior, such as haloperidol and the benzodiazepines, may cause a paradoxical increase in confusion in some people, especially older adults.

Drugs that do not have primary pharmacologic effects on the central nervous system can also cause confusion, either alone or in combination with other drugs (Kane, et al., 1994). The mechanism is variable and not always well understood. In some cases, such as with strong diuretics, the drug predisposes the person to another physiologic cause of confusion—hyponatremia. In practice, it is wise to consider almost any medication as a possible contributing factor to altered cognition.

Toxicity states can occur with overdose of a medication or alcohol, and cause confusion. Overdosage of drugs that at normal levels have no central nervous system effects can potentially cause significant mental status changes. Overuse of drugs affecting the central nervous system alone or in combination with alcohol will also impair thinking

Degenerative Processes

Any process contributing to degeneration of the cells of the brain may ultimately affect cognitive function. Causes of degeneration may be related to an organism (viral or bacterial infection), aging, or unknown sources. Degeneration can produce impaired judgment, insight, planning, memory, and problem-solving. Potential impairments range from mild disability to severe dysfunction that may be incompatible with normal cognition.

It is important to clarify the terms used to describe degenerative processes related to cognition. Senility, which literally means the process of aging, is a term used in common language to describe cognitive impairments that are mistakenly thought to be a normal part of the aging process. Actually, significant memory and problem-solving impairment is not a part of normal aging, but rather indicates a pathologic process (Kane, et al., 1994). The terms "senile dementia" and "organic brain syndrome" have no place in current nursing practice.

Dementia is a clinical syndrome involving progressive impairment of intellectual function and memory, which is not associated with disturbance in level of consciousness, and which interferes with social or occupational functioning. People with dementia experience a gradual decline in all cognitive processes, as contrasted to acute confusion, in which dysfunctions may be reversible (Table 46-1). Potential causes for dementia include trauma, circulatory interferences, genetic predisposition, alterations in neurotransmitters, and infectious agents. The most common form of dementia is Alzheimer's type, which is a primary neuronal degeneration of unknown cause. It occurs at all ages of adulthood, but increases in incidence with aging, affecting 5% to 10% of people older than 65 years of age, and 20% of people older than 75 years (Katzman, 1987; Reifler, et al., 1986)

Manifestations of Altered Function

Disorganized Thinking

A person experiencing disturbed thought processes or disorganized thinking does not interact appropriately with others or with the environment, and may have an altered perception of reality. Thinking, learning, reasoning, and remembering do not occur in an orderly fashion. Disorganized thinking may be manifested by inappropriate interactions and conversations with others, talking or gesturing to oneself, performing inappropriate activities, or bizarre behavior. Regression, hallucinations, and delusions are common manifestations of disorganized thinking. Disorganized thinking occurs in schizophrenia and affective disorders. It may also occur in acute confusion and, less commonly, in dementia of the Alzheimer's type.

Cognitive impairment frequently interferes with perception of reality, which is based on life experience, personal relationships, and environment. When thought processes become altered, it may be difficult for the person accurately to separate altered perceptions from reality. **Delusions** (fixed false beliefs) and **hallucinations** (perceptions arising from the person's own thoughts) are examples of altered perceptions of reality. Both of these responses are attempts to cope with

Table 46-1 • Differences Between Confusion and Dementia

Feature	Acute Confusion	Dementia
Onset	Rapid, often at night	Insidious
Duration	Hours to weeks	Months to years
Course	Fluctuates over 24 hours; worse at night; lucid intervals	Relatively stable
Awareness	Impaired	Usually normal
Alertness	Reduced or increased; tends to fluctuate	Usually normal
Orientation	Always impaired, at least for time	Variable, often impaired
Memory	Immediate and recent impaired	Recent and remote impaired
Thinking	Disorganized; may be dreamlike	Impoverished; poor in abstraction
Perception	Illusions and hallucinations (especially visual) common	Misperceptions uncommon; usually normal
Sleep–wake cycle	Always disrupted; daytime drowsiness and nighttime agitation and restlessness	Fragmented sleep
Physical illness or drug toxicity	Either or both always present	Often absent

Source: Lipowski, Z. J. (1992). Delirium and impaired conciousness. In J. G. Evans & T. F. Williams (Eds.). *Oxford Textbook of Geriatric Medicine.* Oxford, England: Oxford University Press.

or manage stresses or physiologic dysfunctions that impair cognition.

In disorganized thinking, the content of the person's speech may not make any sense in the context of the conversation, or a sentence may contain multiple unrelated ideas. Interactions with people with disorganized thinking are difficult because these people are unable to follow a logical sequence or respond in a rational, predictable way. The client who ignores the meal tray but tries to eat the tissue box with a spoon, or who asks to go to the bathroom but resists assistance to get out of bed, displays impaired reasoning processes. People with chronic disorganized thinking related to mental illness require specialized nursing management, a subject beyond the scope of this chapter.

Impaired Thought Processes

Judgment, insight, planning, and problem-solving can be affected by abnormal levels of arousal, attention span deficits, and memory impairments. Most people with impaired thought processes have aspects of all three elements, and the severity can fluctuate.

Altered Level of Arousal. Arousal is a person's level of reactivity to incoming stimuli. Levels of arousal may be categorized as alert, lethargic, obtunded, stuporous, and comatose (Strub & Black, 1993). Alert means the person is awake and fully aware of incoming stimuli. Lethargic describes the client who is not fully awake and tends to drift off to sleep when not actively stimulated. Obtunded describes the client who is difficult to arouse, and when aroused is confused. Stupor (and semicoma) describes the client who responds only to persistent and vigorous stimulation. Coma describes the client who is completely unresponsive to incoming stimuli. Arousal does not imply the ability to focus attention.

Altered Attention. Attention span and concentration are easily impaired by stress and illness. People with a short attention span are highly distractible and cannot screen out competing stimuli. These people will not be able to stay on a conversational topic, or will stop in midsentence to look out the window to watch a bird. This distractibility interferes with the ability to learn new things and to perform activities of daily living.

Disorders of arousal and attention are major features of acute confusion. Clients, particularly older clients with chronic cognitive impairment or reduced physiologic reserve, are at risk for acute confusion during acute illness or hospitalization, or after surgical intervention (Neelon & Champagne, 1992). Acute confusion impairs the ability to reason, follow directions, concentrate, and remember. The sleep–wake cycle is often disrupted, and inappropriate behavior may be experienced. Delirium, Sundown syndrome, and intensive care unit (ICU) psychosis are conditions manifested by acute confusion.

Delirium. **Delirium** is an acute organic mental syndrome characterized by global cognitive impairment, disturbance of attention, reduced level of consciousness, increased or reduced psychomotor activities, and disturbed sleep–wake cycle (American Psychiatric Association, 1994). Delirium is caused by one or more organic factors; medications and metabolic disorders are the most common causative factors. Predisposing factors include aging, dementia, systemic illness and infection, sensory impairment, and addiction to alcohol or other drugs. Delirium has an acute onset, is often unrecognized, and, if the underlying defect is not corrected, can lead to death.

Sundown Syndrome. **Sundown (or Sundowner's) syndrome** is a state of disorientation and agitation that occurs at night in institutionalized people who are oriented during the day. It is a temporary state of confusion that cycles with the sun (Beel-Bates & Rogers, 1990). The exact cause is unknown, but it is likely that the person's tenuous hold on reality requires a certain level of sensory input (Kane, et al., 1994). At night there is less light, less activity, and fewer caregivers, resulting in less availability of orienting stimuli. The syndrome is often associated with a disturbance in sleep–wake patterns as well.

ICU Psychosis. ICU psychosis has been defined as a reversible global clouding of consciousness with poor attention span and impaired cognitive processes. It is usually manifested 2 to 5 days after entering the intensive care environment and resolves a few days after leaving, although some clients may experience a longer term dysfunction. The ICU is a particularly risky sensory environment owing to the constant activity level, noises from machines and alarms, frequent intrusive procedures, and lack of difference between day and night because of lights and routines, all of which provide the client with little meaningful input (Foreman, 1992). Adverse psychological responses to the ICU environment, ranging from mild (apathy, depression) to severe behavioral manifestations (combativeness, acute confusion), afflict up to 80% of older adults in ICUs (Foreman, 1992).

Memory Impairment. Memory impairment is a concern for old and young alike. Long-term memory, that which has been accumulated over many years, is less affected by situational and emotional stress. Significant impairment of long-term memory usually indicates a central nervous system disorder or a severe confusional state. Short-term memory, that which is of recent events, is much more sensitive to stress. For example, hospitalized clients may have little recall of conversations with healthcare professionals because the stress of illness and coping interfere with the usual functioning of memory.

Impact of Dysfunction on Activities of Daily Living

Individual Considerations

Memory, judgment, problem-solving, and the ability to process sensory stimuli appropriately are essential to the performance of any activity. For example, brushing one's teeth requires remembering where the supplies are and how the procedure is done, as well as deciding when to do it. Mild cognitive impairment can be compensated for with written reminders, posted schedules, occasional supervision, and change in occupation or living situation. When cognitive impairment interferes with the ability to perform essential activities safely and appropriately, continued independent living is threatened. This is the critical outcome of impaired cognitive function—the loss of independence, altered self-concept, and impaired role performance.

Everyone has an individual lifestyle that requires a unique set of skills to maintain. For instance, the daily life of a woman juggling child care and a career in a large city requires skills that are different from those needed by a migrant worker. Social support networks are also individual and may mitigate the impact of cognitive impairment on daily living. For example, the mild memory impairment of an older woman living with her husband in a retirement community may have little impact on daily living, whereas the same degree of memory loss may have major lifestyle implications for a single person employed at a low-income job.

Family Considerations

When healthcare professionals talk about activities of daily living, they are usually referring to basic individual skills that are essential to personal safety and hygiene, such as dressing, toileting, feeding, mobility, and bathing. The next level of skills (instrumental activities of daily living) includes complex tasks necessary to meet survival needs and maintain a healthy environment. Shopping, cooking, arranging transportation, managing money, and following medical regimens are examples of such instrumental or complex skills, and these skills may require dependence on family members or significant others. Impaired cognition and thought processes interfere with the ability to accomplish and manage consistently activities needed to carry out daily life within a family situation. Alterations in thought processes become critical when the impact on daily living is perceived to be a problem by the affected person, family, or significant others.

Assessment

Functional assessment is an essential aspect of nursing care for clients with actual or potential alterations in cognitive function. Assessment of cognitive function identifies clients with alterations in cognitive processes, and assessment of other functional patterns describes the client's ability to function safely within his or her environment. Determining how a person functions and the quality of his or her social and physical environment guides the development of outcome criteria and nursing interventions.

Subjective Data

Subjective information about cognitive function and its impact on other functional patterns is often available from many sources. Gathering subjective data about cognitive ability is a time-consuming process that usually involves multiple brief, planned interactions with a variety of people. It is helpful to keep a general assessment framework in mind (the accompanying display is an example) so that key areas are not forgotten. The situation can be especially complex when the client is hospitalized and unknown to the staff. Nurses, physicians, and social workers may individually gather information from many sources, which is shared collaboratively. Nurses are in the best position to gather data related to the client's normal pattern of function, the areas of risk, and the areas of actual dysfunction. It is important that all healthcare team members document essential subjective data so a consistent assessment can be made and a collaborative approach developed.

Functional Pattern Identification

When assessing thought processes, the nurse gathers information about the client's usual cognitive function

Nursing Assessment
Thought Processes

Current Cognitive Function

- Objective tool—Mini-Mental Status or Pfeiffer
- Subjective evaluation
  Attention
  Ability to answer questions
  Appropriateness of affect

History and Time Course of Cognitive Impairment

- Previous difficulties with thinking or perception
- When current symptoms began and how they evolved; include information from family and friends

Presence of Contributing Factors

- Chronic or acute illness
  Laboratory abnormalities
  CNS disorders
  Multisystem disease
- Use/abuse of medications
  Drugs with CNS effects
  Drugs with CNS side effects
  Drugs with potential for toxicity
  Use of recreational drugs or alcohol
- Sensory impairment
  Vision
  Hearing
- Quality of environment
  Family support
  Frequency and number of social contacts
  Availability of transportation
  Adequacy of financial resources
  Nutritional status
  Living situation
- Presence of psychological stressors
  Bereavement
  Major life change
  Lack of financial resources
  Family crisis
  Loss of independence
  Serious illness
- Family history of dementia or mental illness

Current Functional Status

Ability to perform activities of daily living
Amount of assistance currently available in the home
Ability to exercise good judgment
Safety of home environment

Physical Assessment

- Respiratory function
  Rate, rhythm, depth of normal respirations
  Lung and breath sounds
- Cardiovascular function
  Rate, rhythm, and quality of heartbeat
  Carotid pulses and presence of bruits
- Nutrition
  Adequacy of protein, iron, sodium, and calcium intake
  Adequacy of fluid intake
  Previously identified nutritional disorder
- Sleep and rest
  Restfulness after a night's sleep
  Changes in life events, patterns, or current environment
- Motor activity
  Agitation or withdrawal from activity
  Recent patterns of increased or decreased mobility
  Muscle tone and strength
- Activities of daily living
  Level of independence in hygiene and home maintenance
  Problem-solving abilities, such as money management, use of telephone, and interactions with needed services

and its impact on everyday living. Cognitive changes are often nonspecific and most obvious to those who know the affected person well. For this reason, it is important to elicit information from family and friends as well as from the client.

Information about cognitive function is best obtained in a systematic, hierarchical manner. Consciousness, the most basic cognitive process, is assessed first and described in terms of the intensity of stimulus used and the nature of client response. Next, the client's ability to pay attention must be evaluated before more complex cognitive functions. The abilities to use language and memory are assessed next because they are basic to reasoning and problem-solving.

The significance of any cognitive impairment lies in the relationship between the impairment and function in daily living, not in the impairment itself. For example, an older woman may tell the nurse she does not remember the names, dosages, and purposes of her medications. On the surface, it may seem that she would have a problem with medication management without that information. With further questioning, the nurse learns that she identifies her pills by color, uses a medication management system that has pills grouped in daily dosage units, and that her granddaughter, a registered nurse, oversees her medication management. This woman and her family have developed an effective system to compensate for a mild cognitive deficit.

Detecting mild to moderate cognitive impairment on interview or during casual conversation can be difficult. People who are aware of and embarrassed by their poor memory can become expert at giving vague answers and steering the conversation into "safe" territory. It is advisable to use a formalized approach to cognitive testing (such as the Folstein or Pfeiffer mental status examinations) if an impairment is suspected. A nonjudgmental, warm, and friendly demeanor is important to put the person at ease.

Assessing perception of reality includes determining the person's orientation to time, place, and person. This is sometimes referred to as "orientation × 3." To assess these data, the nurse asks questions pertaining to time: the year, the day, the date, and approximate time of day. Place is determined by asking the client questions related to city or location. Person is assessed by asking the client for his or her name. Orientation usually becomes dysfunctional in that order, with time orientation showing deficit first, and deficits in orientation as to the client's own identity being the last and most severe form of dysfunction in orientation.

Levels of consciousness and orientation are not by themselves adequate assessments of cognitive function. Comprehensive assessment includes the use of a mental status questionnaire (such as Folstein's mini-mental status examination) and a behavioral rating scale (such as the Clinical Assessment of Confusion-A or the NEECHAM Confusion Scale) (Vermeersch, 1992).

In assessing reality, it is important to clarify what is going on in the environment that may be contributing to the indications of disorganized thinking. An older woman may be calling for her son and not understanding why he will not come in to see her when she saw him go by her door. In exploring what may be going on in the environment, the nurse may realize that the woman did not have her glasses on and that the man who walked by her door had the same build and similar clothes to her son's. As a result, she misperceived the information she had. If a nurse is not thorough in assessment, it might lead to the wrong conclusion about the client, attaching a label of "confused" when there is actually a difficulty with perception. The nurse needs to be careful that his or her personal perceptions of reality do not overshadow the ability to monitor another person's perception of reality.

With older people, it may be easy to dismiss changes in mentation as being a "normal part of aging." Clients and families need to understand that cognitive impairments are never "normal," and, if a person is experiencing changes, these changes should be evaluated by a healthcare professional. The earlier families intervene by reducing environmental stressors, adjusting diet, or seeking care for diagnosed problems, the less likely it is that the client will experience a major confusional state or other cognitive problems.

Risk Identification

Risk identification is the process of assessing for physiologic, psychological, and environmental factors that increase the likelihood of experiencing impaired thought processes. The degree of risk from each category will depend on the individual client and setting. A nurse working in an acute care setting will focus on physiologic variables, with some attention to environmental concerns. A community health nurse making a home visit to an older client will include a detailed assessment of social and psychological support systems, as well as physiologic assessment.

The presence of multiple risk factors does not always lead to dysfunction. Individual strengths and resources can enable a person to withstand multiple stressors. An important part of a nursing assessment is the identification of existing and potential coping resources. Interventions can then be designed to support and develop these resources. An example is an older woman with sensorineural hearing loss who is in rehabilitation after hip replacement. Risk factors for this client include altered perceptions related to an unfamiliar environment, altered sleep and rest, and a hearing deficit. These environmental stresses and risk factors usually manifest as a shortened attention span, irritability, impaired sense of time, and, possibly, confusion. During the assessment, the nurse learns that the woman's hearing aid is at home and that she has several family members and supportive friends. Having a family member bring in the hearing aid and some familiar items from home and encouraging frequent contact will decrease the risk of dysfunction.

Medications can be a primary risk factor for altered thought processes, either alone or in combination with other drugs or substances. Clients and their families need to know the expected actions of medications, potential side effects, potential interactions, and indications of toxicity. Many instances of altered cognitive function can be traced directly to the addition of a new medication, toxic levels of a usual medication, or unexpected interactions with other substances. Clients and families need to be alert to subtle changes in cognition and mental status in relation to their pharmacologic therapies.

As part of the assessment process, the nurse obtains a detailed medication history from primary or secondary sources. The medication history includes all medications (prescribed, over-the-counter preparations, home remedies, and others) taken by the client. Medications recently added and those recently stopped should be noted. Information about the amount of alcohol consumed must also be obtained.

Some physiologic functions that may increase the risk of cognitive impairment are assessed subjectively as well. Subjective assessment of sleep and rest determines if the client felt rested after a night's sleep, experienced delay in falling asleep, awoke frequently during the night, or experienced disturbing dreams. When the client is unable to provide this information, the family is asked about the usual sleep–wake pattern. The impact of impaired cognitive function on activities of daily living may be assessed subjectively by questioning the client and family, or objectively, by direct observation of client abilities. Each method of assessment provides different information, and both may be indicated. Inquiry about the client's usual function at home provides information about the client's capability in a familiar environment; however, some clients exaggerate their capabilities, and direct observation may be more reliable.

Dysfunction Identification

Information gathered in the functional pattern identification and the risk identification is analyzed to determine if dysfunction is present for a specific client. When identifying the presence of dysfunction, it is vital to document assessed data in clear terms that are well understood by others. Instead of using vague terms like "slightly confused" or "poor attention span," the nurse should describe the behaviors associated with the deficits precisely, using anecdotes when appropriate. Phrases like "oriented to self only," "needs verbal cueing to wash face," and "when given toothbrush, combed hair with it" provide clear information for identifying dysfunction.

Objective Data

The physical assessment skills of inspection, palpation, percussion, and auscultation, along with diagnostic tests, are essential in identifying the physiologic causes of potential or actual cognitive impairment. Direct observation of the client may provide clues to impaired thought processes.

Physical Assessment

Assessment of physiologic function provides clues as to the source of altered thought processes. Because the earliest clinical signs of changes in the levels of oxygen, electrolytes, and metabolic by-products are lethargy, mild confusion, and impaired thinking, it is important to assess those components. Assessment of these functions requires skill in the physical examination and laboratory evaluation. Physical functions to be assessed are listed in the display on Nursing Assessment for Thought Processes.

Observation. Observation is a useful means for identifying clues to impaired thinking. A disheveled appearance, disorganized speech, and abnormal movements are obvious indicators of dysfunction, especially when they represent a change in status from baseline. Difficulty maintaining eye contact, a tendency to tell the same story over and over, disproportionate responses to stress or stimuli, and emotional lability can also indicate difficulty with thought processes. At times, these behavior changes can be subtle, and repeated observation for consistency or inconsistency of behaviors is necessary to identify dysfunction. The assessment of cognitive function in infants and young children is complicated by several factors. Because the child's language skills are not fully developed, and there is difficulty expressing thoughts, observation of behavior becomes the primary data source.

Diagnostic Tests and Procedures

Physiologic Tests. The physiologic causes of confusion can be the result of disorders of multiple systems. Their diagnosis and management require multiple tests and procedures, from simple urinalysis to highly technical scans. Tests such as weight, vital signs, serum electrolytes, complete blood count, cultures, and measures of oxygen saturation are used by nurses to identify potential contributors to impaired cognition. Monitoring these parameters allows the nurse to identify imbalances and plan early interventions to prevent complications.

Arterial Oxygen. Arterial oxygen level is best determined by measuring arterial blood gases. An oxygen partial pressure greater than 60 mm Hg reflects adequate oxygenation. A noninvasive technique for assessing oxygenation is pulse oximetry, which measures oxygen saturation (the percentage of hemoglobin that is bound to oxygen). A saturation of 90% correlates with a partial pressure of 60 mm Hg, given a normal level of hemoglobin. If a low (less than 90%) value is determined, oxygen therapy and further evaluation may be indicated.

Electrolytes. Electrolytes can be measured to determine their contribution to altered cognition. A serum sodium level less than 135 mEq/L or greater than 145 mEq/L may result in cognitive impairment. Mild confusion can progress to agitation or confusion, with hallucinations or delusions, followed by stupor and coma, if the condition is untreated. Because brain cells can adapt to slow changes, severity of symptoms is related to how rapidly the sodium level drops.

An elevated level of serum calcium can cause severe defects in neuromuscular activity, with cognitive manifestations of lethargy or decreased level of consciousness. When the total serum calcium exceeds 14 mg/dL (normal level is 8.5-10.5 mg/dL), confusion is common, and further increases in the calcium concentration may result in coma or death.

Serum Glucose. Serum glucose levels below 70 mg/dL typically cause shakiness or nervousness but can progress to cause altered cognition. Although the determination of serum glucose from venipuncture is the most accurate method of measurement, the widespread availability of capillary blood glucose monitoring has promoted more reliable self-assessment of serum glucose.

Ammonia and Urea. Ammonia and urea are potentially toxic by-products of protein metabolism. In health, amino acids are converted to carbohydrate in the liver by the removal of ammonia. Ammonia is converted to urea in the liver and excreted by the kidney. Liver failure can interfere with this process and cause elevated ammonia levels; high blood ammonia levels are toxic to brain cells. Kidney failure can cause an elevated blood urea nitrogen level and can produce confusion, although the mechanism is poorly understood.

Toxic Levels of Drugs. Toxic levels of drugs can result from an impaired ability to metabolize or excrete the drug. Serum levels of many drugs can be measured to determine therapeutic and toxic ranges. People with impaired hepatic or renal function are at risk for drug toxicity and require dosage reduction and regular monitoring of drug levels. Drug and toxicologic screening is indicated for suspicion of drug overdose or toxic exposure.

Tests of Cognitive Function. Intellectual function consists of short- and long-term memory, comprehension,

Mini-Mental State Examination

Orientation

What is the (year) (season) (date) (day) (month)? **5**____

Where are we: (state) (county) (town) (hospital) (floor)? **5**____

Registration

Name 3 objects: 1 second to say each. Then ask the client all 3 after you have said them. Give 1 point for each correct answer. Then repeat them until he learns all 3. Count trials and record. (trials________). **3**____

Attention and Calculation

Serial 7's (begin with 100 and count backwards by 7). 1 point for each correct answer. Stop after 5 answers. Alternatively, spell "world" backwards. **5**____

Recall

Ask for the 3 objects repeated above. Give 1 point for each correct answer. **3**____

Language

Name a pencil, and watch. (2 points)

Repeat the following: "No, ifs, ands, or buts." (1 point)

Follow a 3-stage command: "Take a paper in your right hand, fold it in half, and put it on the floor." (3 points)

Read and obey the following: Close your eyes. (1 point)

Write a sentence. (1 point)

Copy design. (1 point) **9**____

Total Score **30**____

Assess level of consciousness along a continuum:

____

Alert Drowsy Stupor Coma

Adapted from Folstein, M. F., Folstein, S. E., & McHugh, P. R. (1975). "Mini-Mental state": A practical method of grading the cognitive state of patients for the clinician. *J Psychiatric Res, 12,* 189–198. Copyright 1975, Pergamon Press, Ltd.

and concentration. These are straightforward abilities, easily tested and converted to objective measurements with standardized tools. Intelligence or IQ tests attempt to measure intellectual function. These tests rely on measuring verbal ability and vocabulary with a structured questioning format. They are standardized to the vocabulary and cultural experience of white, middle-class Americans, and have questionable validity when administered to other ethnic and socioeconomic groups. It is important to remember that standardized tests of verbal ability are not sensitive to sociocultural differences, and so should not be used to assess "normality" for all groups. The primary usefulness of standardized tests is that each person using them assesses the same information, thus providing a common base of information and quantification for comparison.

Because of their limited attention span, it is difficult for children to cooperate with tedious assessment procedures. Assessment tools used with children focus on the observation of behavior, especially behavior elicited by a standard set of stimuli.

Standardized tools are available for the objective assessment of mental status. Two examples are the Pfeiffer Short Portable Mental Status Questionnaire (Pfeiffer, 1975) and the Mini-Mental Status Exam (Folstein, et al., 1975) (see the two accompanying displays). A score of 7 or less on the Pfeiffer or 20 or less on the Mini-Mental Status Exam indicates significant cognitive impairment. These tools are most useful when given on an ambulatory basis to healthy people repeatedly over time, allowing identification of changes from baseline. Administering these tools during an acute confusional state can help quantify daily changes, but without a premorbid baseline and in the presence of physiologic imbalance, little can be determined about the client's change from baseline function. There is a specific battery of tests used to diagnose dementia.

Behavioral Observation Scales. Two new instruments have been designed to measure behavioral aspects of acute confusion in hospitalized clients. The NEECHAM Confusion Scale is an observational scale designed to detect unobtrusively cues to the onset of acute confusion and to monitor recovery (Neelon & Champagne, 1992). The Clinical Assessment of Confusion-A scale is a 25-item observational scale that assesses cognition, general behavior, motor activity, orientation, and psychotic or neurotic behaviors (Vermeersch, 1992).

Nursing Diagnoses

The accepted North American Nursing Diagnosis Association (NANDA) nursing diagnoses for a client with cognitive impairment are Acute Confusion, Chronic Confusion, Impaired Memory, and Altered Thought Processes. Each of these diagnoses describe alterations in cognitive function that interfere with daily living. These nursing diagnoses are classified by NANDA within the taxonomic pattern of Knowing.

Pfeiffer Mental Status Questionnaire

1. What is today's date?________
2. What day of the week is it?________
3. What is the name of this place?________
4. What is your telephone number?________ If none, what is your address? ________
5. How old are you?________
6. When were you born?________
7. Who is the President of the U.S. now?________
8. Who was the President before him?________
9. What is your mother's maiden name?________
10. Subtract 3 from 20 and keep going down to 0. ________

Total numbers of errors________

From Pfeiffer, E. (1975). A short portable mental status questionnaire for the assessment of organic brain deficit in elderly patients. *J Am Geriatr Soc, 23,* 433–443.

Diagnostic Statement: Acute Confusion

Definition

Acute Confusion is the abrupt onset of a cluster of global, transient changes and disturbances in attention, cognition, psychomotor activity, level of consciousness, and/or sleep–wake cycle (NANDA, 1994).

Defining Characteristics

Of the defining characteristics or clinical cues that point to this nursing diagnosis, one of the following major characteristics must be present:

- Fluctuation in cognition
- Fluctuation in sleep–wake cycle
- Fluctuation in level of consciousness
- Fluctuation in psychomotor activity
- Increased agitation or restlessness
- Misperceptions
- Lack of motivation to initiate and/or follow through with goal-directed or purposeful behavior (NANDA, 1994)

An additional minor defining characteristic is the presence of hallucinations (NANDA, 1994).

Related Factors

Related factors show a patterned relationship with the nursing diagnosis and may be described as antecedent to, associated with, related to, contributing to, or abetting the diagnosed condition (NANDA, 1994). Factors identified by NANDA as related to Acute Confusion include age older than 60 years, dementia, alcohol abuse, drug abuse, and delirium (NANDA, 1994).

Etiologic factors for Acute Confusion can be physiologic, environmental, and emotional in nature. Physiologic factors include alterations in oxygenation and biochemical components, genetic disorders, and dementias. Environmental factors include change in surroundings or routine, or loss of significant others; altered sensory input (too much or too little); abuse or misuse of alcohol or drugs; and fear of the unknown. Emotional factors include anxiety, depression, grief, family conflict, or separation. Most often, the etiology of acute confusion is multifactorial (ie, the presence of more than one etiologic factor is common).

Nursing Research *Cognitive Processes*

Selected Nursing Research Studies

Faux, S. A. (1993). Siblings of children with chronic physical and cognitive disabilities. *Journal of Pediatric Nursing,* 8, 305–317.

Foreman, M. D., Theis, S. L., & Anderson, M. A. (1993). Adverse events in the hospitalized elderly. *Clinical Nursing Research,* 2, 360–370.

Harvath, T. A. (1994). Interpretation and management of dementia-related behavior problems. *Clinical Nursing Research,* 3, 7–26.

Scherubel, J. C., & Tess, M. M. (1994). Measuring clinical confusion in critically ill patients. *Journal of Neuroscience Nursing,* 26(3), 146–150.

Possible Topics for Nursing Inquiry

- What nursing interventions permit the greatest independence for the client with altered thought processes and allow safety for the client?
- What nursing situations place the elderly client at risk for cognitive dysfunction?
- What is the relationship between a person's coping behavior and potential for reversible cognitive changes?

Diagnostic Statement: Chronic Confusion

Definition

Chronic Confusion is an irreversible, long-standing and/or progressive deterioration of intellect and personality characterized by decreased ability to interpret environmental stimuli and decreased capacity for intellectual thought processes, and manifested by disturbances of memory, orientation, and behavior (NANDA, 1994).

Defining Characteristics

Of the defining characteristics or clinical clues that point to this nursing diagnosis, one of the following major characteristics must be present:

- Clinical evidence of organic impairment
- Altered interpretation/response to stimuli
- Progressive/long-standing cognitive impairment (NANDA, 1994)

Additional minor defining characteristics include no change in level of consciousness, impaired socialization, impaired memory (short term or long term) and altered personality (NANDA, 1994).

Related Factors

Factors identified by NANDA as related to Chronic Confusion include Alzheimer's disease, Korsakoff's psychosis, multi-infarct dementia, and cerebral vascular accident (NANDA, 1994).

Diagnostic Statement: Impaired Memory

Definition

Impaired Memory is the state in which a person experiences the inability to remember or recall bits of information or behavioral skills. Impaired memory may be attributed to pathophysiologic or situational causes that are either temporary or permanent (NANDA, 1994).

Defining Characteristics

Of the defining characteristics or clinical cues that point to this nursing diagnosis, one of the following major characteristics must be present:

- Observed or reported experiences of forgetting
- Inability to determine if a behavior was performed
- Inability to learn or retain new skills or information
- Inability to perform a previously learned skill
- Inability to recall factual information
- Inability to recall recent or past events (NANDA, 1994)

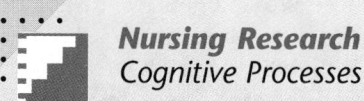

Related Factors

Factors identified by NANDA as related to Impaired Memory include acute or chronic hypoxia, anemia, decreased cardiac output, fluid and electrolyte imbalance, neurologic disturbances, and excessive environmental disturbances (NANDA, 1994).

Diagnostic Statement: Altered Thought Processes

Definition

Altered Thought Processes is a state in which a person experiences a disruption in cognitive operations and activities (NANDA, 1994).

Defining Characteristics

Of the defining characteristics or clinical cues that point to this nursing diagnosis, one of the following major characteristics must be present:

- Inaccurate interpretation of environment
- Cognitive dissonance (disorganized thinking)
- Distractibility
- Memory deficit or problems
- Egocentricity (self-centered or existing only as created in the mind)
- Hypervigilance or hypovigilance (attention dysfunction)
- Inappropriate reality-based thinking (NANDA, 1994)

Related Factors

NANDA is developing related factors (NANDA, 1994).

Related Nursing Diagnoses

Related diagnoses, such as Impaired Environmental Interpretation Syndrome, may be antecedent to the presenting diagnosis. The range of other factors that can affect cognition encompasses a multitude of nursing diagnoses. For example, Altered Nutrition: Less Than Body Requirements, Hypothermia, Hyperthermia, Altered Tissue Perfusion (Cerebral), Fluid Volume Excess, Fluid Volume Deficit, Decreased Cardiac Output, Impaired Gas Exchange, Fatigue, Sleep Pattern Disturbance, and Pain are nursing diagnoses that can have direct pathophysiologic effects on cognition. Social Isolation, Dysfunctional Grieving, Anxiety, and Fear are nursing diagnoses related to environmental or emotional factors that may adversely affect cognition.

Consequences of Impaired Memory, Acute Confusion, or Chronic Confusion may include the following nursing diagnoses: Self-Care Deficits, Self-Esteem Disturbance, Altered Role Performance, and Impaired Home Maintenance. Nursing care extends to the family of the client with altered thought processes. Nursing diagnoses that might be relevant for families include Knowledge Deficit, Ineffective Denial, Anticipatory Grieving, Compromised Family Coping, and Caregiver Role Strain.

Outcome Identification and Planning

After nursing diagnoses and related factors are identified, the nurse and client or family plan outcomes and interventions. In many cases, because of the client's dysfunction, planning will be done with the family or support people. The goals of nursing intervention for a client with altered cognition focus on prevention and early recognition of the disturbance, reversal of contributing factors, and the provision of an environment that compensates for existing impairments, does not predispose to new impairments, and protects the client from harm. Goals need to be individualized, taking into consideration the client's history, areas of risk, evidence of dysfunction, and related objective data. Examples of client goals for the client with Acute Confusion include

The client will express a realistic perception of reality.
The client will demonstrate return to previous level of cognition.
The client will have absence of injury related to the confusion.

Examples of client goals for the client with Chronic Confusion include

The client will experience adequate support to compensate for deficits.
The client will participate in a safe, protected environment.

Examples of client goals for the client with Impaired Memory include

The client will use memory aids to compensate for deficits.
The client will participate safely in his or her home environment.

Examples of some nursing interventions that can be used in planning are outlined in the accompanying display and discussed in the following section.

Implementation

Appropriate nursing interventions will vary with the specific nursing diagnosis and its behavioral manifestations. Preventing, reversing, or slowing the progression of dysfunction, along with providing for client safety and dignity, are central goals of nursing care.

Planning
Examples of Nursing Interventions Used in Common Problems of Confusion

Acute Confusion

- Orient client to environment.
- Introduce self and others to the client.
- Provide physical contact (eg, hand on arm) when communicating with the client.
- Reduce extraneous noise, light, and other distractions.
- Provide reality orientation with calendars, clocks, and other cues.
- Explain procedures, sounds, and equipment to the client.

Chronic Confusion

- Establish a stable, structured environment.
- Employ reality orientation and memory cues consistently.
- Provide for safety within the environment.
- Encourage the client and family to accept the client's level of functioning.
- Use the client's name frequently.
- Establish physical contact with the client during communication.
- Refer the client and family to resources and support services.

Nursing Interventions to Promote Cognitive Health and Function

Instituting preventive measures and recognizing persons at risk for experiencing cognitive impairment are relevant activities for nurses in the community and in acute, long-term, and home-care settings. Promoting a healthy lifestyle, improving memory, and maintaining learning skills are particularly useful interventions for healthy cognitive functioning.

Healthy Lifestyle Promotion

Primary prevention of cognitive impairment involves maximizing brain reserve and minimizing brain damage across the lifespan (Nolan & Blass, 1992). Maximizing brain reserve begins with adequate prenatal and early childhood nutrition and educational experiences. Preventing brain damage through the prevention of accidents, injuries, and toxic exposures will prevent cognitive impairment. Because cognitive function is influenced by so many physiologic, social, and psychological factors, achievement of many of the national objectives for health promotion and disease prevention identified in *Healthy People 2000* (United States Department of Health and Human Services) will promote healthy cognitive function.

Maintaining a lifestyle that includes adequate nutrition, rest, regular exercise, stress management, and social activity is essential. A balanced diet with sufficient protein, iron, and other nutrients is required for cells to function optimally. Serum imbalances of water, sodium, calcium, and glucose can be prevented through adequate fluid intake throughout the day, in conjunction with a balanced diet. For people who have known dysfunctions that may place them at risk for some serum imbalances, such as a person with diabetes mellitus, teaching the importance of regulation of the dysfunction, recognizing early indications of imbalances, and initiating preventive dietary or fluid therapy are primary interventions. Chapters 36 and 37 present complete discussions of interventions for promoting fluid and electrolyte balance and balanced nutrition.

Oxygen perfusion to brain cells is enhanced through the practice of regular exercise. Regular exercise enhances cardiovascular conditioning, improves circulation throughout the body, and contributes to a sense of well-being and refreshment (see Chapter 33 for a more complete discussion of the benefits of exercise). Encouraging people to develop the habit and practice of vigorous exercise contributes positively to cognitive functioning. Depending on the person, the exercise may range from energetic walking to more active sports.

Equally important as getting sufficient exercise is having adequate sleep and rest. Inadequate sleep or interrupted sleep cycles usually results in loss of REM sleep manifested by fatigue and, if prolonged, may produce forgetfulness, confusion, and disorientation. Encouraging people to maintain regular sleep patterns will assist them in obtaining sufficient sleep and in feeling rested when they are awake. Counseling the person to create an environment that is conducive to rest and sleep is an important consideration. Chapter 43 presents additional nursing interventions for promoting sleep and rest.

Stress management can contribute to healthy cognition through minimizing distractions, improving rest, and enhancing concentration. Stress is managed by developing effective coping skills that allow the person to channel stress in a way that is productive or that dissipates the resulting tension. Exercise, as previously discussed, is one type of coping skill that the nurse can encourage. Chapter 51 presents a variety of coping skills and mechanisms from which the nurse can draw in assisting the person with stress management.

Cognitive skills have been developed throughout life. These skills, like all others, need to be practiced regularly to be maintained. Social interaction is one such skill in which the person needs to participate for a variety of reasons, including enjoyment of human contact, stimulation of conversation, and confirmation of personhood. Nurses can use social interaction on a one-on-one basis with the client and can encourage opportunities for social interaction with others in informal group situations. These interactions can provide feedback to the client related to reality orientation, self-concept, and sensory perception.

The person with a chronic illness who is functionally able to live in the community can easily become socially isolated and sensorily deprived at home. Any person who depends on others for mobility, is isolated, and has a poor social support system is at risk for development of cognitive dysfunction. Preventive interventions that the nurse can use include referral for home nursing care and providing information about community services. Examples of community services that the nurse can incorporate in preventive interventions include subsidized transportation, senior centers, adult day care, congregate meal programs, community mental health centers, and volunteer opportunities.

Prompt and effective medical care for infections and other treatable conditions will preserve optimal cognitive function. Treatable conditions associated with cognitive decline include high blood pressure, high cholesterol, diabetes, stroke, and sleep disturbances. Affective disorders (depression, schizophrenia, bipolar disorders) and alcohol consumption can impair cognition.

For people with sensory impairments, there are a number of assistive devices the nurse can recommend that can help maintain and promote cognitive function. People who have hearing difficulties can often be fitted with hearing aids. Telephone companies can provide equipment to assist with communication, and television now offers "closed caption" programs with printed captions that permit hearing-impaired people access to cognitive stimulation from televised programs. Talking books and other services from public libraries help supplement cognitive input for the visually impaired.

Memory Improvement

The fear of losing one's cognitive abilities is often focused on concerns about the quality of memory. Fatigue, stress, and illness may temporarily reduce the efficiency with which a person is able to store information in or retrieve it from the memory. The nurse can reassure the client that, in most situations, there is no organic basis for simple, occasional forgetfulness, and that reducing stress, relieving fatigue, or recovery from illness may eliminate the temporary memory difficulty.

For people with minimal memory problems, memory training programs or devices may be a beneficial intervention. Memory training programs focus on the personal abilities and compensatory capabilities of the person to stimulate cognitive function. The nurse can encourage the person to participate in memory training or to use principles of memory enhancement. Focusing attention deliberately on the information to be remembered helps to reduce stress and minimize distractions. Using both visual and auditory senses provides two important sources of perceptual input for cognition. Making lists, using mnemonic devices (formulas or patterns of letters to aid in remembering), and developing other association techniques can assist the person with remembering tasks or information. The regular practice or rehearsal of retrieving information from the memory helps maintain the skill of retrieval. For example, doing crossword puzzles regularly helps many people rehearse the skill of knowledge and information retrieval from the long-term memory.

Maintenance of Learning Skills

Developing the skill for learning is nearly as important as the actual knowledge learned. These learning skills, developed in childhood, need to be practiced, reinforced, and used throughout life. The nurse can strengthen these skills when teaching. People learn better when the relevance of the information is apparent; for example, if a person has experienced side effects of a medication, the learning related to potential effects of other medications has increased relevance because of the desire to prevent problems in the future.

Learning is increased when it is meaningful and linked with previous learning. To illustrate, if the nurse wants to teach an automobile mechanic about the importance of exercise, associating various body parts with analogous parts of an automobile may increase the meaningfulness. As another example, for a person needing to learn about medications, the classifications and generic names of drugs will not be as meaningful as the color, shape, and size of the medication and the frequency with which it is to be taken.

Simplicity, clarity, and relevance are important considerations when teaching older clients. The nurse should center on a single topic at a time to allow focused attention. Minimizing noise and other environmental distractions assists in the learning process. Providing learning materials and approaches that use vision, hearing, and touch will help the older person obtain perceptual input from several sources.

Nursing Interventions for Altered Cognitive Function

When a diagnosis of impaired cognitive function is made, the nurse can intervene to help identify causative factors, to restore or improve cognitive function, to protect the client from injury, and to help the family cope. The nurse has both an independent and a collaborative role in identifying clients at risk for acute confusion, modifying or structuring the environment, and initiating appropriate teaching for the client and family. The nurse, as the healthcare professional with the most client contact, is in the best position to monitor changes in cognitive function, to communicate these to the healthcare team, and to intervene as appropriate.

Cognitive deficits may be acute and reversible or chronic and irreversible, or an acute insult may exacerbate a chronic deficit. Nursing interventions designed to improve function include similar measures and activities for clients with each of these deficits. The major focus of nursing care is restoring physiologic balance, while creating an environment that provides appropriate sensory stimulation, adequate assistance with activities of daily living, and protection from physical injury.

Fluid Intake and Nutrition

Because shifts in nutrients, electrolytes, and fluids contribute to cognitive changes, monitoring the food and fluid intake of clients is an essential nursing intervention. People who are ill often do not feel like eating and may not find food appealing. Clients should be allowed to choose foods they particularly like, with supportive encouragement and monitoring so that the diet is reasonably well balanced.

Similarly, clients may not experience thirst even when increased fluid intake is needed. Keeping fluids within easy reach of the client, along with reminders to drink, are simple approaches. Fluid intake and output records are useful to observe for a pattern of fluid intake. The most accurate guideline for the adequacy of food and fluid intake is regular measurement of body weight. For clients at risk for fluid imbalances, a regular schedule of weighing will need to be established.

Clients and families will need health teaching regarding the factors that place them at risk for food and fluid imbalances. The diabetic who may have fluctuations in serum glucose needs to understand appropriate diet and medication management. The person who is taking diuretics requires an understanding of the effects and side effects of the medication, and that water should not be withheld unless specifically prescribed by the physician or nurse practitioner. Clients who have any identified risk factors for the development of cognitive dysfunction should receive health teaching related to the problem, along with supportive nursing care.

Clients with chronic confusion need particularly close monitoring of food and fluid intake. With the loss of judgment, some clients do not respond to the normal signals from appetite, thirst, or satiety, so that they may not eat or drink unless reminded, may overeat, may eat inappropriate things, or may forget how to perform the mechanical process of eating. Sitting with these clients while they eat, reminding them to eat, and assisting them with the mechanics of eating may be useful interventions. For some clients, socialization opportunities when eating at a table with others may help to reinforce desired behaviors and activities. For others, a quiet environment free of distractions is required at mealtime.

Mobility

Isolated or withdrawn clients should be encouraged to move around for several reasons. The physical activity of moving stimulates improved ventilation and improved cardiovascular function, with improved oxygenation of the brain as a result. Not only is oxygenation improved, but the person also generally feels better physically and personally. Socialization is often one aspect of increased mobility. As a person moves around more, even on a hospital unit, contact with other people is increased. Contact with other people and varied environments provides more stimulation and reinforcement of reality.

Selectively providing sensory stimulation for all of the senses is an important consideration, particularly for those clients with chronic confusion. In addition to hearing and seeing, the nurse should make use of touch through personal contact and varied fabric textures, taste through varieties of food and beverages, and smell through food and flowers (Fig. 46-5). While providing stimulation, it is important to avoid overstimulating the client with chronic confusion. Overstimulation can result in apparently purposeless behaviors such as wandering, agitation, and aggression. Recognizing signs of overstimulation (inability to maintain eye contact, increased or decreased verbalizations, or attempts to avoid or retreat from the situation) and reducing the level of stimulation may prevent these behaviors.

Safety

A person with altered cognitive function is at risk for injury and requires nursing intervention to ensure safety.

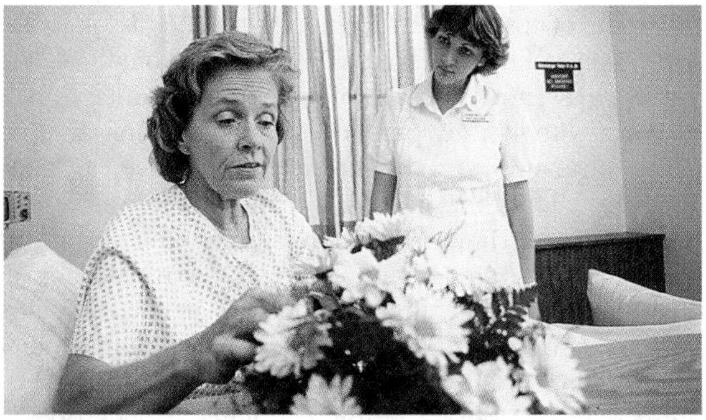

Figure 46-5 • *Vision, smell, and touch stimulate the client's cognitive processes and help the client maintain touch with reality.*

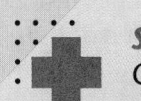

Safety Alert
Confusion

- Supervise clients with confusion during ambulation and other activities because they may have altered judgment as to where they are.
- Be sure that the environment is free from unnecessary obstructions to prevent potential falls.
- Provide structure and predictable routine whenever possible to minimize distractions and potential accidents.
- Provide adequate lighting for safe ambulation within the environment.

For example, when a person is hospitalized, the location is unfamiliar, routines are strange, and the person is ill. This client may temporarily lose orientation and think he or she is at home or somewhere else and be at risk for falling while trying to get out of bed or while going to the bathroom. Safety measures such as orienting the client to the room, the nurse call system, and the lights help to prevent accidents and injuries. Safety is discussed in Chapter 29.

Safety becomes a primary concern for the client with progressively impaired judgment. In an institutional setting, safety measures for the client with chronic confusion involve having the bed at the lowest level; frequent observations to assist the client in getting out of bed; supervision of wandering behavior; and providing secured locks or alerting systems for elevators and doors that allow security for the clients and avoid accidental wandering away. Monitoring of behavior may allow the identification of relationships and temporal patterns that can be used to understand the nonverbal client's needs.

Physical or chemical restraints generally are not useful in maintaining safety. Studies have demonstrated that agitated behaviors tend to increase after the application of restraints (Werner, et al., 1989), the desire for wandering behaviors becomes intensified (Rader, 1991), and falls are not prevented (Janelli, 1989). Many long-term care facilities are becoming more creative in their management of safety, providing innovations such as an enclosed courtyard with unlimited access for the clients with dementia so that they can wander within a protected confine.

Clients with chronic confusion may become upset and distressed by changes in routine and environment. For this reason it is beneficial for the care environment to be as predictable as possible. This includes having meals, baths, treatments, and other activities at regular times with as many familiar staff people as practical. If changes are necessary, remember that the client with chronic confusion needs additional support and reassurance as an essential element of nursing care.

Therapeutic Communication

Therapeutic communication means that the nurse respects the individuality of clients and uses modes of communication to convey that respect. Therapeutic communication can be used in assessment to obtain accurate information, but it is equally important in ongoing interactions between the nurse and the client. These communication techniques are presented in detail in Chapter 20, and the student needs to be familiar with, if not skillful in, using them.

Therapeutic communication enables the nurse to reevaluate and to intervene consistently using as accurate client-based information as possible. Regular use of these communication techniques allows the nurse to detect cognitive changes whenever they occur, so that interventions are as free from personal bias on the part of the nurse as they can be.

Understanding verbal and nonverbal responses is important in caring for people with chronic confusion. For example, the client who repeatedly calls for "Mama" may be expressing a need for nurturing and affection. The client who takes food from the plate of another may be communicating that he or she is still hungry (Stolley & Buckwalter, 1992). Nonverbal communication can be used to express positive regard through touch, facial expression, and eye contact. Finally, the client without other means of communication may express distress or dislike through nonverbal behaviors, including spitting, turning away, or striking out. The importance of nonverbal communication may be heightened as other cognitive abilities decline.

Therapeutic communication with clients with chronic confusion may be enhanced by assuming a non-threatening posture, for example, sitting at eye level with the client. Explain what you are going to do in a calm, friendly tone of voice. Avoid using commands or asking "why" questions. Do not try logically to convince a resistive client to comply with your requests; leaving the area for a few minutes and returning is often more successful.

Reality Orientation

Reality orientation is a nursing technique used to assist the client in restoring awareness of reality. A hallmark in reinforcing reality for hospitalized clients is to provide those environmental cues on which people depend for orientation to time and place. Having the change in lighting match the usual day and night cueing is helpful. Clients who are in specialized units with few windows and lights have greater difficulty relying on environmental cues.

Clocks and calendars that allow the client to know the date, day of the week, and time of day are important sources of input for reality orientation. Additional interventions that can promote reality orientation include allowing uninterrupted sleep periods when possible and encouraging visits from family and friends. Contact with familiar objects, such as family photographs, a favorite chair, or special books, is also useful in maintaining contact with reality.

Allowing the client the maximal advantage in relation to sensory–perceptual data is equally important in reinforcing reality. If the client normally wears glasses or a hearing aid, the nurse ensures these are available. Glasses must be clean and hearing aids adjusted correctly. If the information that the client takes in is as accurate as possible, interpreting and responding to reality is easier.

Although clients with irreversible changes such as dementia will not return to previous levels of cognitive functioning, the nurse needs to assist the client in maintaining existing levels of function for as long as possible. Nonconfrontational reality orientation is an appropriate intervention, and a variety of modalities can be used to accomplish this, such as clocks, calendars, lighting cycles, or personal contact. However, attempts verbally to orient a client with dementia to time, place, or person are often futile and may exacerbate behavioral problems. Attempts to understand and respond to the covert meaning of the client's utterances are more effective. The nurse can assist the family in understanding how to work with the family member through teaching (see the accompanying display).

Socialization Therapies

Socialization therapies can take many forms, such as music, recreation, and reminiscence. The purpose of these therapies is to encourage the client to expand contact with other people in social settings in an effort to increase cognitive stimuli. For some people, the contact within usual social groups, such as Senior Citizen Centers, volunteer groups, church groups, or recreation groups, may provide beneficial stimulation.

For clients who are at risk for being isolated or who may require a more protected environment, reality orientation groups or day-care centers provide the same type of human contact and stimulation. Developing an ongoing relationship with the people who staff these groups or centers provides continuity of care and consistent support for cognitive function.

In reminiscence therapy, the client uses recall of the past to assist in clarifying meaning in the present or reconciling conflict. It is a particularly useful therapy for older clients in that it contributes to successful aging through maintaining self-esteem and reinforcing cognitive function. This therapy requires facilitation by a nurse or other health professional who is skilled in group process and in reminiscence therapy.

Recreation therapy involves using recreation or hobbies to increase meaningful experiences and contact with other people. It is another way of using familiar objects or abilities from the past to help the person ascribe meaning. Although recreation therapy may be prescribed and directed by another health professional, the nurse also may use recreation or hobbies appropriate to the individual client to stimulate cognitive function. Activities that elicit pleasant memories may be used to engage the chronically confused or withdrawn client. Examples are the review of a personal scrapbook or photograph album.

Music therapy makes cognitive contact with the person through the familiarity of music. The music may be in the background, used for exercise, or may be used in group sings. Both the music itself and the socialization and recreation inherent in group opportunities for music are stimulating for the client. Some therapists may use music in a specific, prescriptive fashion; however, nurses can use music as a part of nursing care as deemed appropriate. Although selected music may provide therapeutic cognitive stimulation, it must be individualized to the client's preferences, and the risk of overstimulation must be kept in mind.

Family Support

Clients with acute confusion, and their families, are often anxious and fear chronic confusion. The nurse can reassure the client and family that, in most cases, cognitive function will improve with time. Families can be encouraged to participate actively in the planning and care of the client, with the goal of preventing or minimizing altered thought processes through collaboration in the interventions previously discussed.

Many clients with chronic confusion live at home and are cared for by family members. Although caring for a family member with chronic confusion is extremely

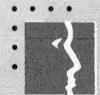

Client Teaching
Reality Orientation

- *Use cues for reality data, such as clocks, calendars, verbal reminders.*
- *Address the client by name often to strengthen personal identification.*
- *Do not reinforce references to nonreality, as in hallucinations or delusions.*
- *Speak clearly and in short, simple statements.*
- *Maintain a predictable routine or schedule for the client.*
- *Promote the addition of familiar objects in the room.*
- *Encourage visits and meaningful interaction with family and friends.*
- *Positively reinforce small changes in behavior that indicate increasing orientation to reality.*
- *Promote continuity of care by having familiar staff with the client whenever possible.*

difficult, family caregivers often receive inadequate training for the task (Hall, et al., 1995). Teaching family caregivers about the nature and progression of chronic confusion, along with techniques for managing the behavioral manifestations, may reduce caregiver exhaustion and delay institutionalization.

Nurses may also provide care and support to family members directly. Families have a difficult time adjusting to the fact that their loved one is losing or has lost all memory of them and their lives together. The grief process begins before the death of the client with dementia. In essence, the person that the family once knew and interacted with is no longer present mentally, but still is present physically. The nurse can use nursing interventions that aid the family in their grief process, as discussed in Chapter 50.

Community-Based Nursing

Because of shorter hospital stays, clients may be discharged before cognitive function has returned to normal. Careful discharge planning is imperative. The planning may need to include teaching family caregivers effective techniques in communicating with and caring for their care recipient. Support groups, such as the Alzheimer's Disease and Related Disorders Association, can be beneficial for caregivers and families by putting them in contact with others who share similar experiences.

Home Care

Home-care services, which include nurses and homemakers, can be arranged before the client is discharged. Medicare and some health insurance will assist in the cost of these services. Home care eases the transition from the protected setting of the hospital, with its many staff people, to the home, where there are fewer people to call on.

Return to home may be useful in reversing the dysfunction of the mildly cognitively impaired client, as a result of the return to a familiar environment and customary routines. The person who has a more severe impairment may require more frequent home visits for nursing care and homemaking.

If impaired cognitive function interferes with the ability to perform higher-level skills (such as managing medications and home maintenance), support systems usually can be created to promote safety and independence. For people with minor memory impairment, there are many ways to support and compensate for memory function, such as making lists of medications to take, things to do, or appliances to turn off. Maintaining organization in the home and in routines provides a predictable environment with fewer distractions, so that the memory functions more effectively. For people with moderate memory impairment, resources like chore service, volunteers, subsidized van service, Meals on Wheels, grocery delivery, and increased family involvement can be arranged.

Day and Respite Care

Day care and respite care are two useful support services for irreversibly cognitively impaired people and their family caregivers. Fatigue is a constant companion of caregivers of progressively impaired family members. One means of managing that fatigue is having access to services that allow the caregiver some time away from caregiving, while providing the impaired person with health and rehabilitative services. The caregiver can feel that the impaired family member is benefiting from the alternative care, and, at the same time, the caregiver can have much-needed rest and personal time.

Day Care. Day care is an alternative to residential long-term care. It can provide assistance for the caregiver who must work, while furnishing the client with a structured atmosphere for socialization, rehabilitation services, and healthcare. People with severe cognitive impairment have poor judgment and inadequate problem-solving skills, are at risk for injuring themselves and others, and are vulnerable to becoming victims of crime. The availability of a safe environment and constant supervision during the day benefits the client and the caregiver, and delays the need for institutional care.

Respite Care. Respite care provides care for the client for periods ranging from several days up to 1 or 2 weeks. This allows the caregiver to rest, handle business matters, or take a trip without excessive concern about the family member's care. If the caregiver can have regular periods of respite, it is easier to cope with the stress of continual caregiving.

Long-Term Care

Often a person with a progressive cognitive impairment or dementia will need the more consistent support of a long-term care setting, in which there is 24-hour supervision of care, structured environment, and extended health services. Caregivers need the support and reinforcement of nurses and healthcare providers as the decision for admission to long-term care is made. This is not a decision that families make easily or casually. Families should be supported and assured that they have made the right decision, whatever that decision ultimately is.

Admission to long-term care can be a very positive move for the client. The client will have contact with more people, objects, and situations, all of which provide increased stimulation. The full-time care allows the client's environment to be structured and predictable, which may actually increase the level of cognitive functioning, even if this is temporary. The actual process of relocation can be stressful, but the client can be helped in coping with it through diligent orientation and unhurried repetition. A caring attitude on the part of the professional caregivers is essential for both the client and family.

Evaluation

Specific outcome criteria are the means of measuring the achievement of client goals. Examples of outcome criteria for cognitive function in the client with reversible confusion are listed here. Outcome criteria need to be individually personalized to the particular client so that they will measure the attainment of the specific client's goals.

Goal

The client will express a realistic perception of reality.

Possible Outcome Criteria

- By discharge, client identifies orientation to time, place, and person.
- Within 2 days, client participates appropriately in self-care activities.

Goal

The client will demonstrate return to previous level of cognition.

Possible Outcome Criteria

- By discharge, client performs previous activities of daily living, as acknowledged by spouse.
- By discharge, client demonstrates ability to carry out the intellectual functions of which he or she was capable at appointments 6 months ago.

Nursing Plan of Care
The Client With Altered Thought Processes

Nursing Diagnosis

Altered Thought Processes related to biochemical imbalances and sensory deprivation manifested by lack of orientation to place and time and inability to manage activities of daily living (ADLs).

Client Goal

Client will regain baseline cognitive function.

Client Outcome Criteria

- Client will be oriented to self, place, and time during course of care.
- Client's family will state that client's mental status has returned to pre-illness level.

Nursing Intervention	*Scientific Rationale*
1. Assess and record mental status every shift.	1. Regular assessment promotes recognition of changes in condition and allows determination of effectiveness of interventions.
2. Reorient as necessary. Provide orientation cues such as a clock, calendar, and a sign with room number.	2. Frequent reorientation and use of cues compensates for the short-term memory loss that occurs with cognitive impairment.
3. Encourage client to be out of bed for meals when possible. Establish a consistent bedtime routine.	3. Providing an ADL routine that is similar to that followed at home can help minimize the strangeness of hospital environment.
4. Assign consistent caregivers when possible.	4. Minimizing the number of caregivers allows the client to recognize staff and feel comfortable with their care.
5. Encourage family and friends to visit; put cards and flowers where client can see them.	5. The ability to recognize family and friends persists even in state of severe confusion. Presence of loved ones can be reassuring and can minimize the negative effects of the illness experience.
6. Encourage client to participate in ADLs as much as possible.	6. Performing ADLs helps the client regain a sense of control and gives the nurse an opportunity to assess functional ability.

Goal

The client will have absence of injury related to confusion.

Possible Outcome Criteria

- Within 48 hours, client reports absence of falls related to cognitive dysfunction.
- Within 1 week, client reports absence of bruises, cuts, abrasions, or other signs of injury or harm.

Goal

The client will experience adequate support to compensate for deficits.

Possible Outcome Criteria

- Before discharge, client demonstrates adequate nutrition, safety, and mobility.
- Before discharge, client receives support services as needed to offset needs presented by cognitive deficits.

Goal

The client will participate in a safe, protected environment.

Possible Outcome Criteria

- During hospitalization, client demonstrates the absence of injury from environmental hazards.
- During hospitalization, client demonstrates relaxed behavior and other indications of comfort with the environment.

Evaluation includes assessing the client's cognitive function and comparing the client's progress with the individually established outcome criteria as a measure of the client's goal attainment. The nursing care plan for the client with altered thought processes is continued, modified, or concluded based on this systematic evaluation of the individual client's functioning.

Key Concepts

- Cognition is the process of knowing, thinking, and learning; it is the complex processing of information by which sensory input, past experiences, awareness, and emotions are integrated and made meaningful for the person, enabling him or her to interact with the environment in a purposeful way.
- To provide comprehensive nursing care, nurses need to be aware of factors affecting normal cognitive function, such as physiologic state, infectious processes, medications, personal and environmental stressors, and affective states.
- Manifestations of altered cognition include disorganized thinking, attention deficits, memory impairment, and impaired thought processes.
- For the person with altered thought processes, activities of daily living are disrupted, and the amount of support in the living situation must be assessed.
- The nurse needs to determine how a person functions, along with assessing the quality of the social and physical environment, to guide the development of the nursing process.
- Identifying risk factors for impaired thought processes will assist the nurse in defining the actual dysfunction and the appropriate interventions.
- Thorough assessment of physiologic and psychosocial function is essential in identifying causes of altered thought processes.
- The nursing diagnosis of Acute Confusion is defined as the abrupt onset of reversible disturbances in attention, cognition, psychomotor activity, level of consciousness, and/or sleep–wake cycle. The nursing diagnosis of Chronic Confusion is defined as an irreversible, long-standing, and/or progressive deterioration of intellect and personality. The nursing diagnosis of Impaired Memory is defined as the inability to remember bits of information or behavioral skills.
- Nursing goals should focus on restoring physiologic balance while providing an environment that supports function, does not cause new impairments, and protects the client from harm.
- If the nurse is aware of potential risk for dysfunction, preventive interventions will concentrate on minimizing those factors and supporting the client and caregivers.
- Among many supportive interventions for the impaired client is reality orientation, used to reinforce and restore awareness of reality.
- People with altered cognitive processes require careful discharge planning and home care, with referral for families to long-term care, day care, or respite care, as appropriate.

Critical Thinking Challenges

Your knowledge base now includes information about pain, sensory perception, and cognition. Using this information, apply your thinking skills to the woman who had hip surgery at the beginning of the chapter. Now look at the following questions.

1. *Describe your immediate impressions of this situation.*
2. *Reflect on what information in the scenario, as well as what knowledge and values of your own, contributed to these impressions.*
3. *Given the situation as presented, formulate plans for your nursing intervention and rank your priorities.*

4. *Organize your plans for assessing the client's cognitive function.*

References

American Psychiatric Association (1994). *Diagnostic criteria from DSM-IV.* Washington, DC: Author.

Beel-Bates, C. A., & Rogers, A. E. (1990). An exploratory study of sundown syndrome. *J Neurosci Nurs, 22* (1),51–52.

Erikson, E. H. (1963). *Childhood and society* (2nd ed.). New York: Norton.

Folstein, M., Folstein, S., & McHugh, P. (1975). Mini-mental status. *J Psychiatr Res, 12,* 189–198.

Foreman, M. (1992). Adverse psychologic responses of the elderly to critical illness. *AACN Clinical Issues, 3* (1), 64–72.

Freiberg, K. (1992). *Human development: A lifespan approach* (4th ed.). Boston: Jones and Bartlett.

Guyton, A. C. (1991). *Basic neuroscience: Anatomy and physiology* (2nd ed.). Philadelphia: W. B. Saunders.

Hall, G. R., Buckwalter, K. C., Stolley, J. M., et al. (1995). Standardized care plan: Managing Alzheimer's patients at home. *Journal of Gerontological Nursing, 21,* 37–47.

Havighurst, R. J. (1972). *Developmental tasks and education* (3rd ed.). New York: David McKay.

Janelli, L. M. (1989). Physical restraints: How little we know. *Nursing Homes, 38* (10), 10–12.

Kandel, E. R., & Hawkins, R. D. (1992). The biological basis of learning and individuality. *Sci Am, 267* (3), 78–86.

Kane, R., Ouslander, J., & Abrass, I. (1994). *Essentials of clinical geriatrics* (3rd ed.). New York: McGraw-Hill.

Katzman, R. (1987). Alzheimer's disease: Advances and opportunities. *J Am Geriatr Soc, 35,* 69–73.

McCance, K. L., & Heuther, S. E. (1994). *Pathophysiology: The biologic basis for disease in adults and children* (2nd ed.). St. Louis: Mosby.

Neelon, V. J., & Champagne, M. T. (1992). Managing cognitive impairment: The current bases for practice. In S. G. Funk, E. M. Tornquist, M. T. Champagne, & R. A. Wiese (Eds.), *Key aspects of elder care: Managing falls, incontinence, and cognitive impairment.* New York: Springer.

Nolan, K. A. & Blass, J. P. (1992). *Preventing cognitive decline. Clinics in Geriatric Medicine, 8*(1), 19–34.

North American Nursing Diagnosis Association. (1994). *NANDA Nursing diagnoses: Definitions and classification 1995–1996.* Philadelphia: Author.

Pfeiffer, E. (1975). A short, portable mental status questionnaire for the assessment of organic brain deficit in elderly clients. *J Am Geriatr Soc, 23,* 433–443.

Piaget, J. (1969). *The psychology of the child.* New York: Basic Books.

Porth, C. (1994). *Pathophysiology: Concepts of altered health states* (4th ed.). Philadelphia: J. B. Lippincott.

Rader, J. (1991). Modifying the environment to decrease use of restraints. *Journal of Gerontological Nursing, 17* (2), 9–13.

Reifler, B., Larson, E., Teri, L., et al. (1986). Dementia of the Alzheimer's type and dementia. *J Am Geriatr Soc, 34,* 855–859.

Schuster, C., & Ashburn, S. (1992). *The process of human development* (3rd ed.). Boston: Little, Brown & Co.

Stolley, J. M. & Buckwalter, K. C. (1992). Confusion management. In G. M. Bulechek and J. C. McCloskey (Eds.), *Nursing interventions: Essential nursing treatments,* 2nd edition. Philadelphia: W. B. Saunders.

Strub, R. L., & Black, F. W. (1993). *The mental status examination in neurology* (3rd ed.). Philadelphia: F. A. Davis.

Vermeersch, P. E. H. (1992). Clinical assessment of confusion. In S. G. Funk, E. M. Tornquist, M. T. Champagne, & R. A. Wiese (Eds.), *Key aspects of elder care: Managing falls, incontinence, and cognitive impairment.* New York: Springer.

United States Department of Health and Human Services. (1991). Healthy people 2000: National health promotion and disease prevention objectives. Washington, DC: United States Department of Health and Human Services, Public Health Service.

Werner, P., Cohen-Mansfield, J., Braun, J., et al. (1989). Physical restraints and agitation in nursing home residents. *J Am Geriatr Soc, 37,* 1122–1126.

Bibliography

Divela, A. L., Kongas, S. P., Saviaro, P., Pahkala, K., Kesti, E., et al. (1993). Five year prognosis for dysthymic disorder in old age. *International Journal of Geriatric Psychiatry, 8* (11), 939–947.

Holden, U. (1994). Dementia in acute units: Agression. *Nursing Standard, 9* (11), 37–39.

Miziniak, H. (1994). Persons with Alzheimer's: Effects of nutrition and exercise. *Journal of Gerontological Nursing, 20* (10), 27–32, 46-47.

Rantz, M. J., McShane, R. E. (1994). Nursing home staff perception of behavior disturbance and management of confused residents. *Applied Nursing Research, 7* (3), 132–140.

Sullivan-Marx, E. M. (1994). Delirium and physical restraint in the hospitalized elderly. *Image the Journal of Nursing Scholarship, 26* (4), 295–300.

Weinrich, S., Sarna, L. (1994). Delirium in the older person with cancer. *Cancer, 74* (Suppl), 2079–2091.

Self-Perception and Self-Concept

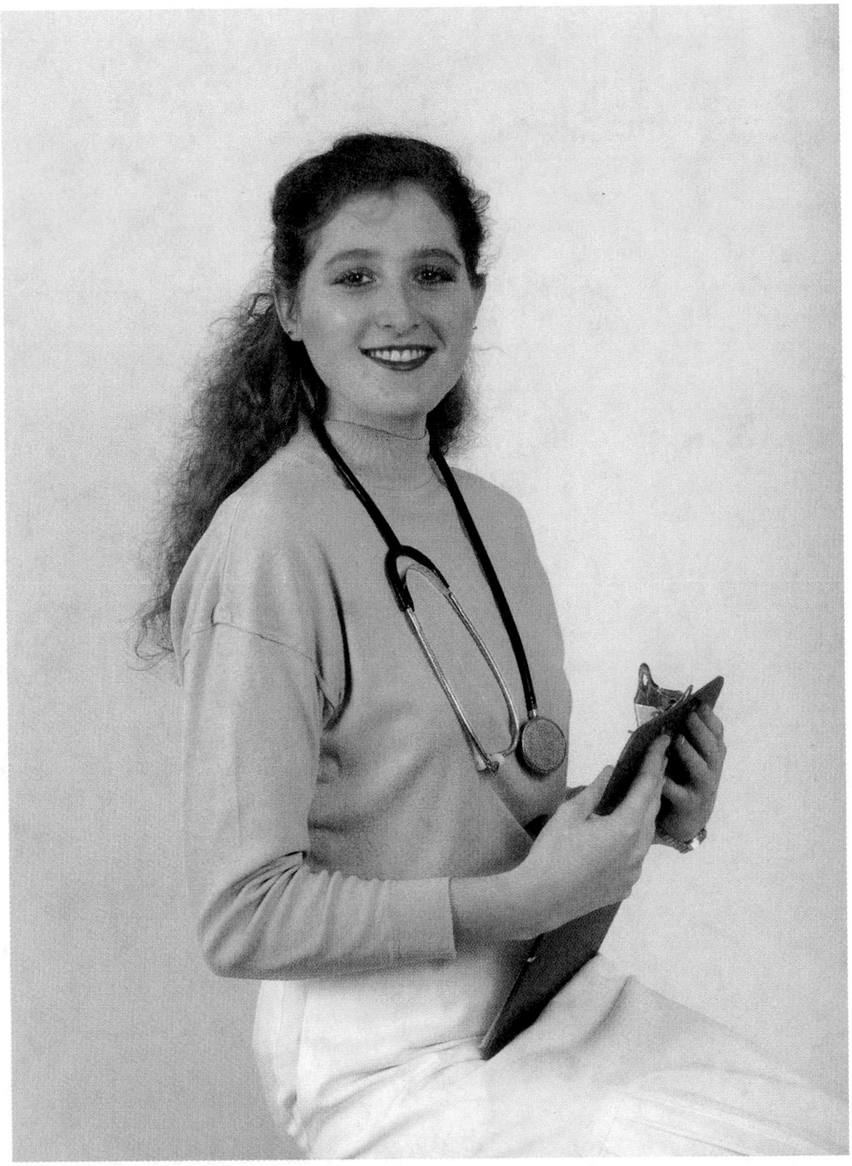

UNIT XIII

Unit XIII discusses the self-perception and self-concept areas of human function. Beginning at birth, a person's perception of himself or herself affects actions and pursuits throughout a lifespan. People tend to act in accordance with their internal self-perception. Therefore, a client's self-concept affects all aspects of client care.

The content in the single chapter in this unit focuses on the principles and concepts of self-perception, with an eye toward helping the nurse understand the effect self-perception has on a client's sense of worth and, ultimately, the choices he or she makes. A client's self-concept can be a strength and can positively influence other areas of function. Conversely, a negative self-concept can result in self-esteem disturbances, body image disturbances, altered role performances, or personal identity disturbances. Such client responses greatly interfere with normal function and affect all activities of daily living. Using a nursing process format, this chapter presents an introductory discussion of self-concept as a client need requiring nursing attention. An understanding of how human responses affect self-concept and the impact of self-concept on the client's responses allows the nurse to incorporate this awareness into all aspects of client care. This chapter emphasizes nursing interventions to promote health and function to maximize client strengths. Additionally, a beginning discussion of altered function and appropriate nursing interventions helps the nurse provide sensitive, holistic care.

The nurse's sense of self affects his or her provision of care to his or her clients. This unit addresses the nurse's needs as well.

47
Self-Concept

Self-Concept

Key Terms	Learning Objectives
Body image Identity Role Self Self-concept Self-esteem Self-evaluation Self-expectation Self-knowledge Self-perception Social self	Upon completion of this chapter, the student will be able to do the following: • Describe the normal function of self and self-concept. • Define self-concept, self-perception, self-knowledge, self-expectation, social self, and self-evaluation. • Discuss factors affecting self-concept. • Identify potential factors for altered self-concept. • Identify manifestations of altered self-concept. • Discuss how self-concept develops throughout the lifespan. • Apply theory to assess for self-concept functioning. • Plan care for a person with an altered self-concept.

47

You are a nurse working in a well-baby clinic. A 31-year-old married woman brings in her 3-month-old child for a scheduled appointment. While you are weighing the baby, the mother talks about feeling tired and fat and says, "these breasts are too big." She tells you she misses the baby when she goes to her part-time job but sure feels better now that she is back to aerobics class. When you ask about the baby, she smiles and tells you how happy she and her husband are to have him. She describes how much more rewarding caring for her own child is than babysitting her nieces and nephews, and wonders if she'll ever feel rested again.

In the previous unit you learned about cognition and perception. In this chapter you will study about one's perception of self. When you have added self-concept to your knowledge base you should be able to understand and plan for the care of the 31-year-old mother and her family. The Critical Thinking Challenges at the end of the chapter will help you consider how you can care for this client.

People adapt to changes in life. As they do, their body image, role performance, self-esteem, and personal identity evolve. Self-concept is dynamic and is influenced by experiences and expectations. A sound self-concept is a prerequisite for mental health. Nursing responsibilities associated with self-concept include self-knowledge, assessment of self-concept, promotion of adequate self-concept functioning, and intervening when self-concept is at risk or altered. If the nurse possesses a healthy self-concept, he or she will be better equipped to deal with the client's unique and varied needs. Conversely, if the nurse's self-concept is dysfunctional, he or she will be unable to meet the client's needs. In fact, the task of coping with such a nurse may actually add to the work of the client.

Normal Function of Self

The concept of self has been examined by many disciplines because of its importance in understanding human behavior. **Self** is elusive and can be defined variously; it may be defined as a person's unique dimensions, potential, and purposes (Rogers, 1961). **Self-concept** is the mental image one has of oneself; it is the person's meaning when stated as "I" or "me." Self-concept is the frame of reference that influences how one handles life situations and relationships. Esteem and self-actualization are the highest needs in Maslow's hierarchy of human needs. Self-concept is critical to both.

Characteristics of Normal Self-Concept

People with a healthy self-concept exhibit a clear sense of self and others; they have an understanding of who they are in the real world. They can and do distinguish themselves as separate individuals, with strengths and weaknesses. These people acknowledge their emotions and have energy available to bring meaning into life. The person with a healthy self-concept has a realistic view of others and an ability to relate to them in a satisfying manner, including the capacity for intimate and loving relationships. The person with a healthy self-concept is able to deal with the realities and problems of life with appropriate coping behaviors.

Self-Concept and Self-Perception

Whereas self-concept is the mental image of self, **self-perception** is a filtering process (Gary & Kavanagh, 1991) that evaluates events and enters them in the subconscious. Such filtering "prevents feelings of guilt, anxiety, and unworthiness from surfacing" (Gary & Kavanagh, 1991). How one perceives oneself has several dimensions: self-knowledge, self-expectations, social self, and self-evaluation.

Self-Knowledge. **Self-knowledge** or self-awareness involves a basic understanding of oneself, a cognitive perception. It is a consciousness of one's abilities: cognitive, effective, and physical. Self-knowledge involves basic facts (age, weight, sex) and qualities (sincere, athletic, intelligent) related to who one is.

Self-Expectation. **Self-expectation** involves the "ideal" self—the self a person wants to be. It is the setting of goals for present and future. If they are realistic goals, the person may attain them; however, unrealistic goals can be defeating. Self-expectation is based on the limits of the person's awareness. For instance, the person who watches glamorous shows on television may have as goals to be thin, beautiful, popular with the other sex, and wealthy with a beautiful home and expensive car. The person who spends time reading may have knowledge as an expectation. Self-expectation is influenced by significant others. If a mother pushes a son to be a physician, the son may have this as an expectation, or may set up an expectation of failure because of lack of interest.

Social Self. One never fully knows how others see one's self. One can only guess, and the guess may be far from reality. Conversely, people tend to wear masks in their social obligations; they tend to hide the true self. The "religious" self may be different from the party goer. A person may hide feelings of aggression when being interviewed, but show aggression later on the job. **Social self** is how one sees oneself in relation to social situations, including behavior and interaction with others.

Self-Evaluation. **Self-evaluation** is the conscious assessment of the self, leading to self-respect or self-worth. "Have I met my expectations? Do I like what I see in the mirror? what I know? how I act?" Self-evaluation involves the aforementioned dimensions. It also involves self-esteem, which is discussed shortly.

Normal Functional Self-Concept Patterns

The mental image of one's self comprises body image, self-esteem, personal identity, and role performance. The whole of self represents more than the total of the four components. The instance of the mother and 3-month-old infant can be used to clarify the dynamic of these components. The woman's body image and role performance have clearly changed with pregnancy and motherhood; these components then influence identity—motherhood must be incorporated—and self-esteem. If her self-concept is healthy, she will be able to make the necessary changes to cope with and adapt to the dynamics of self.

Positive Body Image

The human body is the physical manifestation of self in the real world. How one pictures one's body and how one feels about one's body describes **body image.** Body image includes the total conscious and unconscious disposition toward one's body. It is the unifying concept behind feelings about one's size, sex, and sexuality; the way one looks; the way one's body functions; and whether one's body can help one accomplish goals. Sexual satisfaction is positively correlated with positive body image (Berscheid, et al., 1973).

Body image is influenced by culture and social experience. In American culture, influenced by the media, beauty, health, and youth are valued. Each person has a picture of how he or she hopes he or she might look, an idealized body image. In addition, each person has an awareness of how he or she really looks, a mirrored image. When the real image is close to the ideal image, the person experiences positive regard for self. These positive feelings about body image are part of self-esteem.

Self-Esteem

Self-esteem is the judgment that one makes regarding one's self. It is the result of self-evaluation of worth. Self-esteem is affective in nature, but it is made up of both thoughts and feelings. Stanwyck (1983, p. 11) defined self-esteem as "how I feel about how I see myself." Two sources for esteem are the self and others (Fig. 47-1). Self-esteem develops throughout childhood and adolescence, to become more stable in adulthood.

Early in life, the child accepts the parents' evaluation as his or her own. Then the child incorporates others' appraisals and expectations to form a self-ideal, and then slowly begins self-evaluation. The person emerges into adulthood with a basic or core self-esteem. Coopersmith (1967) identified antecedents of high self-esteem: parental acceptance, clear expectations, limitations, and freedom to express opinions. From these four antecedents, fundamental criteria by which people's self-appraisals are made have been proposed. These include

- Power, the ability to influence people and events—the sense that my opinion counts and will be listened to
- Meaning, the sense of being valued and worthwhile—my existence matters to others
- Competence, the ability to achieve personal goals—personal success
- Virtue, behaving in a manner consistent with personal values—adherence to a moral or ethical standard

Core self-esteem is the person's consistent, overall appraisal of self. The person acts in ways or perceives events in ways that tend to support his or her level of self-esteem. Although core self-esteem is relatively stable, people do change their perceptions of self based on current experience. Such an example is the woman described at the beginning of this chapter. This changing self-esteem has been called functional or situational self-esteem (Norris, 1992).

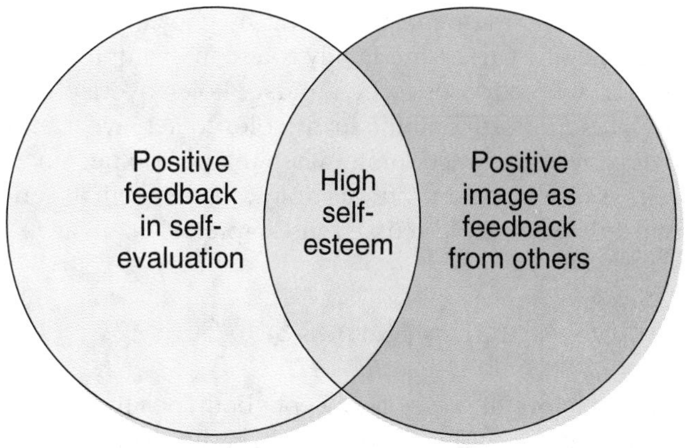

Figure 47-1 • High self-esteem develops when there is positive feedback from both self and others.

The person with adequate self-esteem has learned to cope with personal deficiencies and to maximize strengths; this person is self-accepting. The person with high self-esteem accepts others, experiences less anxiety, and functions effectively in social situations.

Strong Personal Identity

Identity is an organizing principle of the self, the awareness that one is a distinct individual separate from others. The person with a strong sense of personal identity has integrated self-esteem, body image, and various roles into an integrated, whole self-concept. This whole or "I" is not associated with any one aspect of the person. Identity provides the person with a sense of continuity through time. "I am not the person I was yesterday, but there are similarities and consistency that provide links for today and the future."

The concept of boundaries is central to identity. Actual body boundaries (this is my hand; that is your hand) and ego boundaries, (this is my thought or feeling, not your thought or feeling) must be intact for a person to have personal identity. The person must be able to differentiate self from others to possess mental health.

Role Performance

A person fills many roles in a lifetime. **Role** is defined as the expected characteristic behavior of a person in a social position. Roles are ascribed or assumed. A role is ascribed when the person has no choice. An example of an ascribed role is daughter; because the person is born female, she becomes a daughter. A role is assumed when the person selects it by choice. Assumed roles include career and family roles; an example is the person who chooses to be a nurse. Roles overlap and the person must combine many roles to achieve a unified pattern for functioning. When the person perceives self as adequate in various roles, self-esteem is enhanced. Roles are discussed in Chapter 49.

Factors Affecting Normal Self-Concept

Many factors affect self-concept, both positively and negatively, including biologic make-up; coping and stress tolerance; culture, values, and beliefs; previous experience; and developmental level.

Biologic Make-Up

One's biologic make-up comprises many characteristics that affect self-concept. Sex, height, weight, skin color, and attractiveness or unattractiveness are set characteristics that are self-perceived and perceived by others to help form self-concept (Fig. 47-2). These factors also affect what a person experiences. For example, men often have more opportunities to play competitive sports, enhancing self-concept, whereas women may be barred from playing certain sports. The woman who is athletically inclined may perceive her sex and abilities as inferior, thus damaging her self-concept. Likewise, someone who is black in a predominantly white society may have difficulty securing a positive self-concept if others' perceptions are discriminatory. However, a person who is tall, slender, and attractive may easily develop a positive self-concept because these are favorably perceived qualities.

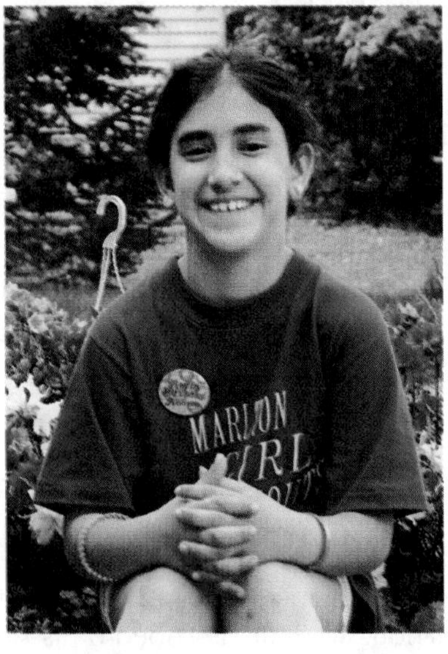

Figure 47-2 • One's sex, skin color, hair color, and eye color affect self-perception and perception by others.

Culture, Values, and Beliefs

Children grow up internalizing the culture, values, and beliefs to which they are exposed. The degree to which they can subscribe to those norms affects self-concept. The media provide daily lessons on the norms of American culture. Dietary, childbearing, health, and religious practices are norms that may vary among ethnic groups in the American culture, however. Integration of cultural practices and American beliefs can lead to a healthy self-concept. An adolescent who cultivates an interest in ethnic music and dance but still shares a love of rock music with his peers will have a strong identity and self-esteem.

Coping and Stress Tolerance

Coping and stress tolerance influence self-concept. People who are able to adapt to stress and resolve conflicts through coping tend to develop healthy self-concepts. Internal resources, such as a sense of humor and productivity under pressure, as well as external resources, such as strong support groups, enhance coping. A single mother who has a strong family support group may master the roles of parenthood, financial provider, and activist for women's rights, enhancing self-esteem and likewise strengthening performance in these roles. Poor stress tolerance may lead to crisis, however, and damaged self-concept.

Previous Experience

Because self-concept is a complex, ever-changing personal perspective on the person's relationship with the world, self-concept is affected by one's previous experiences with the world.

Experiences include opportunities for success and failure. If the person meets with success, he or she begins to feel self-esteem and role satisfaction, and begins to expect success. The person also learns what and who he or she can influence. These experiences teach the person expectancies (Rotter, 1966). An expectancy is a belief that one's behavior will lead to a given response. Two expectancies that are incorporated into the self are expectancy for success and locus of control. Expectancy for success means the person has a belief that personal behavior will lead to something desired. Locus of control can be internal or external. A person with external locus of control perceives that outcomes happen because of luck, chance, or the influence of powerful others; a person with internal locus of control believes that personal behavior influences outcome, and that he or she can achieve desired results. These expectancies develop from life experiences, and influence the self. For instance, if a person believes that luck brought about an outcome, that person would not feel increased esteem because of the outcome, whereas a person with internal locus of control would. A person with strong internal locus of control may be threatened by illness because it shakes belief in personal control; however, self-concept can be preserved by the person's belief that subsequent health-seeking behavior will bring about wellness.

Experience also allows the person to develop and use coping strategies. As the person experiences stress in life, he or she uses the coping skills that fit with his or her view of self and the world. The person who is able to use health coping mechanisms that worked in the past will reinforce self-esteem with future successful coping.

Developmental Level

Developmental level influences self-concept from infancy through older adulthood. Whereas the newborn has no separate sense of self and the young child is learning that his or her identity is separate from others, the adolescent must deal with body image changes. Each developmental level brings unique experiences that can reinforce or alter self-concept, as discussed more fully in the previous section. Accomplishment of key tasks at each level enhances self-concept.

Illness

Positive self-concept is usually based on a healthy self; self-esteem and body image can be adversely affected by acute and chronic illness, trauma, or surgery. Even physical changes associated with normal aging may alter self-concept. Successful coping during illness, however, may enhance self-esteem. For example, a person with cancer who tolerates chemotherapy can hold down a job, becomes closer to the family, and may emerge feeling emotionally stronger, more resourceful, and with a more positive self-concept than before the illness.

Lifespan Considerations

Each stage of development implies special considerations. Knowledge of these considerations helps the nurse plan and implement appropriate interventions that foster the development of positive self-concept.

Theorists in lifespan development were discussed in Chapter 16 and in Table 16-1. Prominent for theories regarding development of self-concept are Freud (1920/1966), Piaget (1969), Erikson (1963), Havighurst (1972), and Kohlberg (1969). Sullivan (1953) discussed an interpersonal theory. Four of these theorists (Freud, Sullivan, Erikson, and Havighurst) and their theories related to development of self-concept are listed in Table 47-1.

Newborn and Infant

The newborn has an undifferentiated self; the newborn does not experience a separate existence from others. The mother's self-concept, her sense of competence in the new mothering role, and the amount and intensity of anxiety she feels are transmitted to the newborn (Fig. 47-3). When the mother is reasonably calm, and communicates warmth and acceptance to the baby, the basis for a positive self-concept is established.

The family as well as the newborn experience dramatic changes during the neonatal period. These changes have the potential to affect the self-concept of the neonate. The mother shifts from being pregnant and having a pregnant body to not being pregnant. If the mother chooses to breastfeed, she has further body image changes, and concerns about milk production, sexuality, and competence. If she chooses not to breastfeed, she may experience guilt or doubt concerning the mothering role. During this same time the mother is shifting in existing roles and developing new roles.

The father also experiences shifts in roles and development of new roles; his new relationships must be integrated into his identity. Relationships with others are altered during this time. An extended family may either help or confuse role transition. Friends may treat the couple differently. Siblings of the newborn experience shifts in role also. Healthy acceptance and working through changes during this period set the stage for positive self-concept development. The infant begins to understand self as a separate body, and that feelings (eg, hunger) are his or her own. As the infant begins to distinguish self from others, self-concept begins to develop. As the infant interacts with meaningful others, he or she begins to read the wants of others.

For example, when Mom smiles and plays patty-cake, Mom smiles even more when the infant smiles and makes noises. Thus the infant begins to learn social role expectations. During this stage the child learns

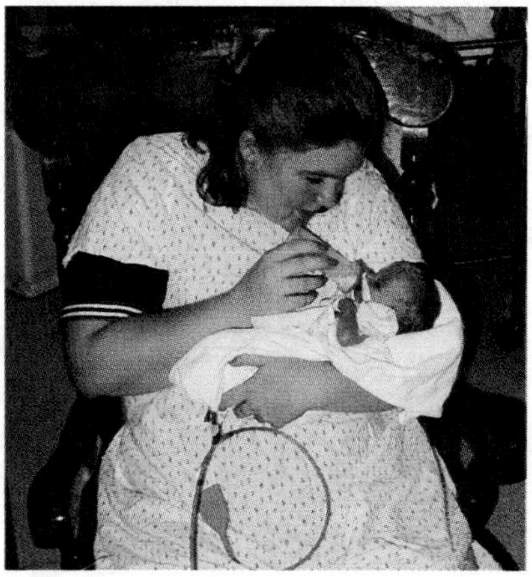

Figure 47-3 • *The identity of a newborn is integrated with the identity of the mother.*

Table 47-1 • *Theories of Self-Concept Development*

	Freud: Psychodynamic (1920/1966)	***Sullivan: Interpersonal (1953)***	***Erickson: Ego (1963)***	***Havighurst: Tasks (1972)***
Newborn/ Infant	Oral stage, 0–3 months; child is undifferentiated from mother	Infancy: beginning self-concept formed; security = good me; anxiety = bad me; Overwhelming anxiety or deprivation = not me	Trust vs. mistrust; adequate mothering helps infant establish trust in self and others	Task: establishes physiologic stability
Infant	3 months to 1.5 years; child begins to distinguish his or her body from objects (people and things) in the environment	Infant has no separateness from caretaker		
Toddler	Anal stage; personal identity pronounced "I"; role performance in family learned	Early childhood: beginning differentiation; if relationship adequate, child begins to integrate good me, bad me, and not me into self-concept	Autonomy vs. shame; Personal identity: body image and self-esteem develop as child experiences self-control through exploration in the world	Tasks: learns body image through walking, talking, control of waste
Pre-schooler	Phallic stage; sex role, body image and personal identity become more clearly differentiated		Initiative vs. guilt; beginning role established through sexual identity development and family relationships	Learns own sex role and identity through above tasks
School-age child	Latency; role performance is primary work of this stage; body image problems may manifest if previous stages not resolved successfully	Juvenile; the process of individuation occurs as peer relationships develop. The individual learns competition, compromise, and collaboration	Industry vs. inferiority; socialization and competence are developing, helping continued growth of self-concept	Tasks: learns physical skills for games; roles (ie, sex, student, and friend); values
Adolescent	Genital stage; body image is altered as the individual establishes self as sexual being; separation from parents leads to enhanced sense of identity; role choices are made	Identity, body image, and role continue to develop or be redfined as individuation progresses	Identity vs. role confusion; search for self	Tasks: acceptance of body and sex role; independence from parents; occupational preparation and other roles learned (ie, marriage, citizen)
Adult	Individual works on conflicts/lack from previous developmental stages		Intimacy vs. isolation; primary task role related: acquisition of love, sexual fulfillment and closeness	Tasks: marriage, parenting, occupation
			Generativity vs. self-absorption; as person concerns self with next generation(s), new sense of identity develops, increasing self-comfort and integration of varied roles	Tasks: adjusting to physiologic changes; role with aging parents

(continued)

Table 47-1 • (continued)

	Freud: Psychodynamic (1920/1966)	Sullivan: Interpersonal (1953)	Erickson: Ego (1963)	Havighurst: Tasks (1972)
Older Adult			Integrity vs. despair; individual accepts personal accomplishments or feels decreased worth; body image changes as the person experiences physical alterations associated with old age (eg, decreased sensory acuity)	Tasks: adjusts to decreased physical strength, retirement, possible death of self or spouse, decreased income

to sit, stand, and possibly walk. This managing of body allows the infant to experience the world in different ways, and teaches the child body boundaries. Bodily control helps to establish a beginning sense of separateness from others. Through play, the infant learns to control aspects of the environment. For instance, early during this stage the infant bats at objects, such as colorful items on a mobile. Later, the infant grasps items, and toward the end of this phase may be able to stack two blocks. This play helps the child during the earliest stages of acquiring identity, just as social control (eg, smiles) helps the child with beginning roles.

In addition, the infant begins communication through symbols, that is, a smile means good, a cry means bad, "ma-ma" is associated with the mothering one, and the infant begins to respond to his or her name. The infant accomplishes these developmental tasks through interaction with caregivers and through exploration.

Toddler and Preschooler

The toddler has a rudimentary body image. Although the toddler knows self as separate from others, there is no clear definition of where the body ends. The child may not want to flush the toilet after defecating; the stools are part of the child. The child is not aware of specific influences, only general feelings or thoughts. However, the toddler understands others' responses to behavior; thus, excessive punishment leads to bad feelings and praise leads to good feelings. Gradually these feelings become incorporated into the toddler's self-concept.

Self-concept continues to develop actively during preschool years. The preschooler's sense of self becomes more defined as he or she realizes that he or she is separate and unique. During this stage of development, the child exhibits great sexual curiosity; the child is aware that he or she is different from others. In addition to this sense of sexual self, the preschooler's body image is incorporating both spatial relationships and increased coordination of his or her body (Fig. 47-4).

The preschooler's sense of how he or she relates to others is more defined than in previous stages. The child's roles in the family and the world are beginning to take shape. During this stage, the child may share in older siblings' accomplishments or perceive himself or herself as not as good because he or she cannot achieve the same things. If a new baby is added to the family, the preschooler may respond with anger, jealousy, or regression. The family's response to the child's reaction influences his or her role performance and self-esteem.

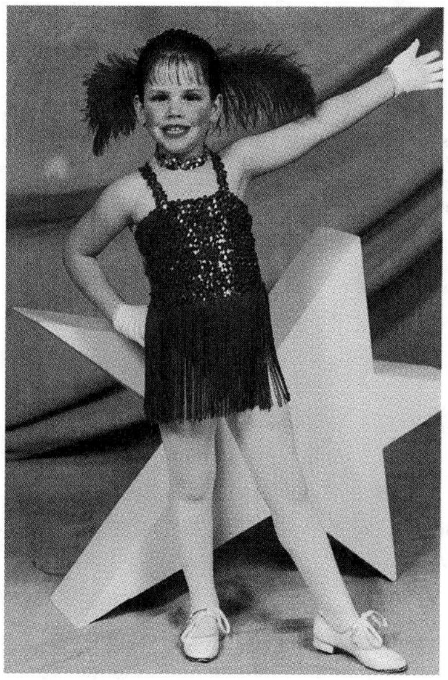

Figure 47-4 • *This preschooler's body image is incorporating both spatial relationships and increased coordination as she performs in a tap dancing recital.*

Because of the preschooler's amount of curiosity, he or she learns body parts and names as well as attitudes about his or her body and self. If the preschooler's questions are discounted, met with great anxiety, or if the child is given misinformation, the child may develop a negative self-concept or poor body image.

Child and Adolescent

The school experience can strongly reinforce or alter the child's body image, sense of self, and identity. Teachers and peers become important influences on self-concept. Basically, the child compares self to peers and measures looks, abilities, and social self with them. Because of the rapid change and growth of this stage, the child's self-concept remains quite flexible, and changes are very individual. Figure 47-5 illustrates the flow of a child's self-concept development from 6 to 12 years of age.

Through life experiences, children "place values on feelings and on themselves as individuals, and they make decisions about how to behave. When significant others accept an individual's expression of feelings, the self grows and thrives, and the individual feels valued and loved simply for existing. Thus the self and its feelings become part of the developing self-concept . . ." (Gary & Kavanagh, 1991).

The adolescent experiences remarkable changes. The body grows rapidly, and secondary sex characteristics and hormones appear. Both necessitate rapid change in the adolescent's view of self. The adolescent must incorporate these changes to establish a coherent body image. Peers and role models such as sports or media stars strongly influence self-concept. Clothes, hairstyles, and the way the person moves are extensions of body image that are influenced by peers. Sexual changes and peer group expectations regarding sexual behavior may lead to a sexually active role.

As the adolescent seeks added responsibility, the parents need to learn new methods of parenting. Striving for independence can be felt as a conflict for all family members. The adolescent may act in ways that seem to be in direct opposition to values and expectations of the family. This behavior occurs because the adolescent's chief developmental task is to develop and define personal identity. Near the end of adolescence, the person chooses a career or a career path that will influence self-concept for the rest of life. In American society, *what* the person does is often seen as *who* the person is. Occupation determines status, economic freedom, and much about lifestyle.

Adult and Older Adult

Adults continue to modify self-concept. The young adult moves away from the conforming peer group with a strong sense of self, a struggled-for personal identity. This is modified through life experiences.

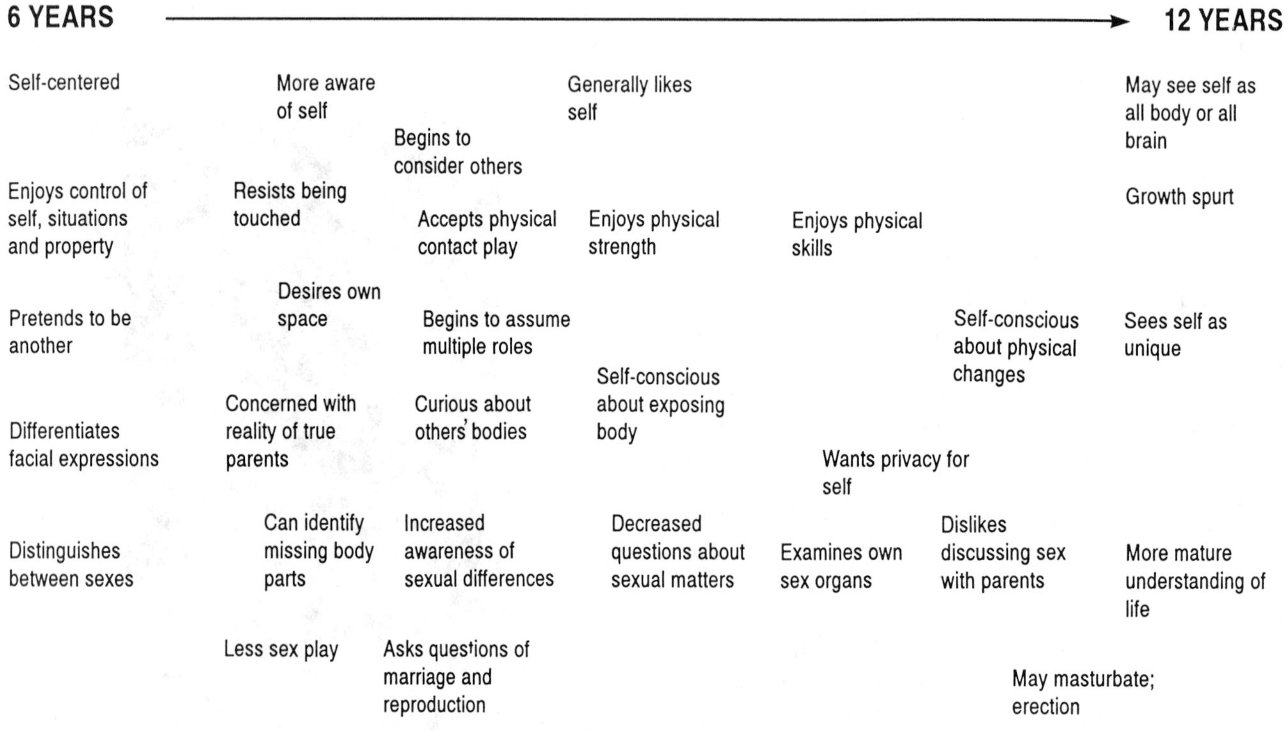

Figure 47-5 • Self-concept development on a continuum from age 6 to 12 years. Attributes are approximate on the continuum. Although there is general consistency in development, each child is unique.

Common life experiences for early adulthood include forming intimate relationships, choosing a career, establishing a home base, and starting a family. Much of assumed role formation happens early in the adult stage of life.

During the fourth and into the fifth decade the person may question the fit of the identity chosen and experienced. The person may examine the meaning of self and contemplate the parts of self not previously explored. Roles and options taken and those discarded are examined as the person looks for more meaning in life. This process has been called an "authenticity crisis" by Sheehy (1974). The outcome of this authenticity crisis is renewal or resignation. With renewal, the person emerges from the crisis with an expanded sense of self. If resignation is the outcome of the crisis, the person's self remains defined by the narrow constraints of the roles he or she participates in. The sixth and early seventh decades leave the person living with the outcome of the authenticity crisis.

Retirement requires extraordinary changes in role performance and self-esteem. Because career roles have much to say about who a person is, the retired person is often described by who he or she *was*, implying the person no longer has value. Devaluing the person in this manner greatly affects self-esteem. Most older Americans live independently in their own homes. Independence and self-care have been correlated with higher self-esteem and life satisfaction (Public Health Service, 1987).

Physical changes such as decreased strength, lost skin turgor, and decreased sensory acuity affect body image in later life. Because of America's valuation of youth, lowered self-esteem is experienced with the changed body image. Sensory changes also affect personal identity. If the environment does not provide feedback, the person may have difficulty determining what is or is not part of self.

When an older person accepts self, the person has found meaning in life. If contributions in the form of perspectives are accepted by others, especially younger members, self-esteem is enhanced. If the older person is treated as if he or she has no more to contribute, self-esteem is damaged.

Altered Self-Concept

In addition to understanding normal self-concept functioning, the nurse must be aware of factors that place people at risk for dysfunctional self-concept, and manifestations of that dysfunction. Potential for altered self-concept function may arise from stressful life events, inadequate coping, incomplete developmental tasks, role transition, and illness, trauma, or surgery. Manifestations of altered function include self-care deficit, emotional and behavioral changes, anxiety and depression, and self-destructive behavior.

Potential for Altered Self-Concept

Stressful Life Events

Most people face numerous stressors in daily life, many occurring simultaneously. Common stressors are financial difficulties, problems on the job, change or loss of a job, relationship concerns, sexuality concerns, divorce, moving, making new friends, loss of a loved one, competition, and making an important decision. Stressful events often challenge the person's identity and self-esteem. One stressor may be so intense as to paralyze the person and damage self-concept, but more often, cumulative stress wears away at self-concept (see Chapter 51). For example, a young couple marries and must move to another city where the husband found a job. They have difficulty buying a house because of the high cost of living in the new area, and immediately have financial difficulties. The wife would like to start a family, but must take a job for which she feels overqualified. They have difficulty making new friends and are overwhelmed by the numerous decisions that have to be made while starting their life together. The husband begins to feel that he is not a good provider and cannot afford the lifestyle he would like. The couple experiences stress in their relationship, and both may feel that self-esteem and identity are damaged.

Inadequate Coping

Inadequate coping can lead to self-concept dysfunction. In the above example, the young couple overwhelmed by stressful life events needs strong coping skills to maintain intact self-concepts. However, lack of support systems and an inability to prioritize and problem-solve contribute to further problems. Some people with inadequate coping develop defensive self-esteem. Defensive self-esteem is a protective mechanism in which the person reports high self-esteem in order to deny negative personal information. The person defends the self against hurt, failure, or anxiety through denial, grandiosity, or projection, and has a high need for social approval.

Incomplete Developmental Tasks

Incomplete developmental tasks can lead to self-concept dysfunction. Adolescence is a particularly difficult time because of the many physical, emotional, and sexual changes occurring during this period. Adolescents must make decisions about the future, are seeking independence from their parents, and are pressured by peer groups. Body image and identity are not secure, but depend on others' perceptions. Self-esteem is fragile.

When a person has disturbed personal identity, he or she has difficulty stating who he or she is. This person may be unable to differentiate personal thoughts and feelings from those of others. This component of self-concept can be affected by changes in role or body image that are occurring during developmental transition. Relationships are affected by decreases in amount or quality of social interaction. If developmental tasks are not completed, self-concept dysfunction occurs, and may lead to incomplete tasks at a later developmental level.

Role Transition

Multiple role transitions are made in a lifetime. Two types of role transition are developmental and situational. Developmental role transitions are commonly associated with aging and growth, such as the transition from student to wage earner. Situational transitions are associated with change in relationships, such as the death of a spouse, changing one's status from married to widowed. Either type of role transition can prompt role problems.

Common problems associated with role are role ambiguity, role strain, and role conflicts. Role ambiguity occurs when the person lacks knowledge of role expectations; this fosters anxiety and confusion. An example of role ambiguity is assuming a new job without an orientation to expected performance and responsibilities. Role strain occurs when the person perceives himself or herself as inadequate or unsuited for a role. This can occur in any role, or because of numerous roles. One example is a contemporary woman fulfilling roles of wife, lover, mother, employee, and professional, and feeling that she is not fulfilling any role the way she feels that she should. Role conflict is related to expectations concerning the role. Role conflict can be described as intrapersonal, interpersonal, or interrole. Intrapersonal role conflict exists when role expectations conflict with the person's personal values, such as a nurse being asked to assist with an abortion when she feels it is an immoral act. Interpersonal role conflict exists when the person's expectations differ from some significant other's; for example, an adolescent might want to play in a rock band, but his or her parents value intellectual pursuits. Interrole conflict exists when a person is expected to fulfill two or more roles simultaneously. In the case of the death of a spouse, a widow may become sole wage earner for the family, a single parent, and the caretaker of the house. She may be unsure what is expected of her in a new job, her role as wage earner may conflict with parenting responsibilities, and the combination of roles may be overwhelming. Self-concept can be damaged by such role transitions.

Illness, Trauma, and Surgery

Illness, trauma, or surgery produces stress and role strain, reduces self-esteem, and alters body image. Altered body image occurs when the person experiences a disruption in the perception of the body image. Obviously, if the person has an actual loss of a body part or function, he or she will have a disrupted body image until the change is incorporated. Feelings associated with disturbed body image include helplessness, hopelessness, powerlessness, fear of others' reactions, and anger.

Amputation, mastectomy, burns, and facial trauma cause significant change in body structure and appearance. Cardiac disease, which limits activities, renal disease requiring dialysis, and a colostomy all change the function of the body. The ability to retain an intact self-concept in the face of illness, trauma, and surgery varies among people. The person's perception of the alteration and the importance he or she places on the body part or function affected influences body image dysfunction. For example, an athlete who places great importance on his or her long, strong legs for running would be devastated by a neurologic illness that produces weakness, placing him or her in a wheelchair. The athlete experiences decreased self-esteem as well as change in body image.

Manifestations of Altered Function

Manifestations of self-concept dysfunction range from subtle emotional and behavioral changes to full-blown, self-destructive behaviors. Manifestations may occur as an immediate reaction to self-concept dysfunction, or may be revealed years after self-concept development has been altered.

Self-Care Deficit

People with dysfunctional self-concept may exhibit self-care deficit. People with chronic disease may disregard special diet instructions, not take medications, and not keep follow-up appointments. The hospitalized client may avoid participation in medical and nursing treatment. Self-care deficit may also be characterized by poor personal hygiene, disregard for health maintenance activities, inappropriate exposure or concealment of parts of the body affected by disease, and lack of health-seeking behavior. The person may refuse to acknowledge health concerns or express feelings of not being worth special care or concern. For example, a middle-aged diabetic woman with an amputated leg keeps her lower body covered by a blanket, even in warm weather. She rarely combs her hair or puts on makeup, and she frequently misses appointments and eats sweets because she feels she is "not worth it."

Emotional and Behavioral Changes

Emotional changes with self-concept dysfunction include feelings of depersonalization, hopelessness, helplessness, alienation, fear of rejection, anger, sadness,

Nursing Research
Self-Concept

Selected Nursing Research Studies

Dukes, R. L., & Martinez, R. (1994). The impact of gender on self-esteem among adolescents. Adolescence, 29, 105–115.

Goodman, S. H., Cooley E. L., Sewell, D. R. & Leavitt, N. (1994). Locus of control and self-esteem in depressed, low-income African-American women. Community Mental Health Journal, 30, 259–269.

Killeen, M. R. (1993). Parent influences on children's self-esteem in economically disadvantaged families. Issues in Mental Health Nursing, 14, 323–336.

Mock, V. (1993). Body image in women treated for breast cancer. Nursing Research, 42, 153–157

Possible Topics for Nursing Inquiry

- What nursing interventions permit the greatest reinforcement of positive self-worth and self-concept for the client with altered body image?
- What nursing interventions place the elderly client at risk for altered self-concept?
- What is the relationship between a person's coping behavior and successful adaptation to altered body image?

shame, guilt, inadequacy, worthlessness, and suspicion of others. Emotional responses may be blunted or inappropriately intense.

Behavioral changes that indicate self-concept dysfunction include lack of interest in activities, inability to make decisions, withdrawal from social situations, isolation, refusal to look in the mirror, refusal to look at an affected body part or discuss a limitation, avoiding responsibility, showing hostility toward others, refusal to make eye contact, and negatively verbalizing about self. Behavior may become more dependent on or independent of others, including healthcare providers. A woman who has undergone cancer chemotherapy and has lost her hair and undergone significant weight loss may show emotional and behavioral manifestations of self-concept dysfunction. She may refuse to look in the mirror, assume independence in bathing and dressing to prevent others from seeing her body, avoid eye contact with the staff, refuse visitors by saying she is tired, and seem emotionally apathetic.

Anxiety and Depression

Anxiety and depression are two common psychological disturbances that are manifestations of self-concept dysfunction. Whenever there is a change in body image, problems with roles or identity, and low self-esteem, the person is threatened. This threat is often the cause of great anxiety, and is frequently followed by the grieving process. Negative body image has also been related to depression (Cronan, 1991) and to eating disorders (Wolf, 1991). Low self-esteem is frequently evident in major psychiatric disorders such as depression. An older man who has recently experienced loss of a job, loss of a wife, and loss of good health may show signs of depression.

Self-Destructive Behavior

Substance abuse (drugs, alcohol), sexual promiscuity, gambling, and overeating can be manifestations of self-concept dysfunction. These self-destructive behaviors numb the pain of self-hate and perpetuate the belief that the person with low self-esteem is a loser (Briggs, 1987). These self-destructive behaviors are addictive behaviors, giving immediate gratification only. The person with low self-esteem and negative self-image finds it difficult to change self-destructive behaviors because he or she has difficulty seeing himself or herself in a more positive light. A 40-year-old male alcoholic who attributes loss of a job, financial insecurity, and injuries in a car accident to bad luck is an example of a person with self-destructive behavior and a self-concept dysfunction.

Impact of Dysfunction on Activities of Daily Living

Individual Considerations

Alteration of self-concept may have an impact on the simplest activities of daily living (ADLs). People with low self-esteem or altered body image may try to avoid social situations and minimize interactions with others. They may not attend to hygiene needs or keep up their appearances. They may show little interest in recreational activities. Those people with altered body image often have difficulty moving in the environment until they incorporate the change psychologically. They may not maneuver well if the body image change involves a disfigured, amputated, or dysfunctional limb, despite physical rehabilitation.

People with identity dysfunction also lose interest in self-care activities, and often cannot make personal decisions. People with role dysfunction often place excessive demands on themselves to perform daily activities, and are self-deprecating when they cannot meet these demands. The quality of ADLs suffers in people with self-concept dysfunction, and there is a concurrent loss of enjoyment and productivity.

Family Considerations

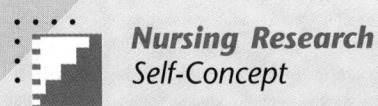

When an individual suffers from an illness or exhibits a self-concept dysfunction, family members are often influenced. Family members may need to assist the individual to perform ADLs or have to change the living situation to accommodate adaptive equipment or other assistive devices. Members may also need to fulfill new role responsibilities. Often family members will feel helpless or guilty for an emotional response to the changes in the family or to the "sick" member. All of these changes require integration in each family member's self-concept.

> ***Safety Alert***
> *Body Image*
>
> - Supervise clients with body image disturbance during activities of daily living and other activities, because they may have altered judgment related to the affected body part.
> - Maintain an environment that encourages use of physical strengths without creating potential safety problems.
> - Provide a structured and predictable setting for children with altered body image that will support the child's self-concept and self-worth.
> - Provide an environment in which a child with an altered body image related to physical disability can risk physical activity without injury.

Assessment

The nurse who assesses the client's self-concept is better equipped to implement the nursing process. This allows the nurse to assist the person in strengthening self-concept. At times, the client's self-concept will be an identified strength that the nurse uses to enhance interventions for other nursing diagnoses. The nurse collects subjective data in the areas of functional pattern identification, risk identification, and dysfunction identification. The nurse also is alert to objective signs of self-concept dysfunction.

Subjective Data

Collection of subjective data assists the nurse in identifying the client's self-concept functioning, as well as assisting in identifying risk factors or disturbed self-concept. Data are collected by asking purposeful questions during the initial interactions while collecting a nursing history, or as part of a focused assessment after caring for immediate needs.

Functional Pattern Identification

Gordon (1987) suggests the following questions be asked about self-concept when doing a nursing history:

How would you describe yourself?
Most of the time, how do you feel about yourself?
Are you experiencing changes in your body or the things you can do?
Is this a problem for you?
Have you or are you experiencing changes in the way you feel about yourself or your body?
Do you find things frequently make you feel angry, anxious, frustrated, afraid, sad, or annoyed? If so, what helps?

Further assessment of roles and relationships is discussed in Chapter 49.

Risk Identification

When assessing a person for risk of self-concept dysfunction, the nurse must consider developmental stage, previous experience, intensity of a stressor or threat, and self-expectations. Certain developmental stages are more risky than others. If the client is an infant, what are the self-concepts of the parents? Is the client an adolescent who has had a body image change? Does the change affect sexuality? Assessment of previous experience should include past problems with self-concept and history of unsuccessful coping mechanisms, and lack of resources and support. Intensity of a stressor may help identify risk. Is the client threatened by a role? By an illness or body image change? How important is good health or performance of a role? How serious is an illness or change in body function?

Assessment of the difference between the real self and the ideal self can also identify risk. What are the client's expectations? How far is he or she from meeting these expectations? Are expectations unrealistic?

Dysfunction Identification

Dysfunction identification also involves assessment of the client's thoughts and feelings. People who do not possess a healthy self-concept are less able to cope with life. These people often express feelings of inferiority, self-doubt, and self-dislike. Does the client verbalize negative feelings, such as "I don't like myself"; "I'm so ugly now"; "I'm worthless"; or "I'm a terrible mother?" Why does the person feel this way? In what area is the person having a problem—self-esteem, role function, personal identity, or body image?

Objective Data

Objective data about the client's self-concept are gathered through direct observation. These data include behavioral manifestations such as lack of eye contact, and physical observations such as a missing body part or function. The person may try to conceal a body part, for example by bandaging an arm scarred by burns after the burns have healed. The person may exhibit anxious behavior such as hand-wringing and shallow breathing, or grief behavior such as weeping.

Although some behaviors may be easily observed, assessing the meaning of these behaviors may be more difficult. For instance, if the person hides a body part, does this manifest body image disturbance or extreme need for privacy? These data are clues and must be judged with the subjective data to determine risk for or actual disturbances in self-concept. Ongoing observation of the client's behavior helps identify changes in the self-concept.

Nursing Diagnoses

North American Nursing Diagnosis Association (NANDA)-approved nursing diagnoses to be considered in caring for clients with dysfunctional self-concept are Body Image Disturbance, Self-Esteem Disturbance, Situational

Therapeutic Dialogue
Self-Concept

Scenes for Thought

Gwen Jacobs is 12 years old and comes to your clinic for her school sports physical accompanied by her mother.

Effective

Nurse: *Hi, Gwen, I'm Becky Thomas, the nurse practitioner. I'll be doing your physical today. What sport are you trying out for this year?*
Client: *All of them.* Looks at you with curiosity. *I thought only doctors did physicals.*
Nurse: *Actually, nurses do physicals, too. What sports do you particularly like? (Checking head, eyes, ears, nose, and throat [HEENT])*
Client: *I like soccer and softball the best. I want to play them in high school too.*
Nurse: *Good for you. You really look strong, especially your leg muscles. You've been playing sports a long time? (Warming up the stethoscope for heart and lung assessment.)*
Client: *Yes, since I was little.* Looking at the stethoscope. *Are you going to listen to my heart with that?*
Nurse: *(Stopping to look at her.) Yes. And your lungs, too. Any problems?*
Client: Looking down at the floor. *Do I have to take my gown off?*
Nurse: No. *I can examine your heart this way (showing her how the drape will continue to cover her chest) and I'll listen to your lungs through your back. Is there something that worries you about being examined?*
Client: No. Blushing.
Nurse: *I wonder if you might be a little embarrassed about being examined. (Listens to heart sounds under the gown.)*
Client: *Yeah.* Looks guilty.
Nurse: *I understand. I have a daughter your age, and she's also pretty shy about my seeing her body. She says it's because it's changing so fast, and she doesn't understand it all. (Listens to lung sounds.)*
Client: *Yeah.* Looks interested. *Does she play sports, too? The hardest part is taking a shower after gym. Everybody always looks. I hate it.*
Nurse: *Not an easy time, I imagine. Could you lie down, please? (Examines abdomen.)*
Client: Big sigh. *Yeah. Are you almost done?* Giggles. *That tickles!*
Nurse: *Almost. (Finishes exam.) I'm going to leave the room so you can get dressed, and then you and your mom and I can sit and talk for a little bit. If you or your mom have any questions you want to ask me I can answer them then. Okay?*

Less Effective

Nurse: *Hi, Gwen, I'm Barbara Thompson, the nurse practitioner. I'll be doing your physical today. What sport are you trying out for this year?*
Client: *All of them.* Looks at you with curiosity. *I thought only doctors did physicals.*
Nurse: *Actually, nurses do physicals, too. What sports do you particularly like? (Checking HEENT)*
Client: *I like soccer and softball the best. I want to play them in high school too.*
Nurse: *Good for you. (Asks mom a question, continues to do exam, taking out stethoscope.)*
Client: *Are you going to listen to my heart with that?* Looking at stethoscope.
Nurse: *Sure am. (Opens gown and listens to heart sounds.)*
Client: Blushes and hunches shoulders as if to hide chest from view.
Nurse: *Okay, now I'll listen to your lungs from the back. Breathe in for me. (Completes exam. Gwen is silent.) Okay, now that I'm done, I can see you look pretty healthy, Gwen. All the normal milestones are being reached, Mrs. Jacobs, including some breast development. If you need any information about menstruation or anything like that, the clinic has some terrific pamphlets I could give you. Otherwise, we'll see her for her next exam next year. Hope you have a good year, Gwen. Win a lot of games! (Smiles and leaves the room.)*
Client: Blushing. *I hope we don't get her again! Let's go, Mom, I'm going to be late for practice.*

Critical Thinking Challenge

• Explain the relationship between body image and self-concept • Interpret how you think Gwen would describe herself. • Compare and contrast how each nurse talked to Gwen and her response to each. • Describe how Becky used self-disclosure to help Gwen. • Identify to whom Barbara was primarily talking.

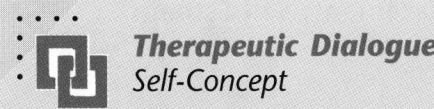

Low Self-Esteem, Chronic Low Self-Esteem, Personal Identity Disturbance, and Altered Role Performance.

Diagnostic Statement: Body Image Disturbance

Definition

Body Image Disturbance is disruption in the way one perceives one's body image (NANDA, 1994).

Defining Characteristics

Of the defining characteristics or clinical cues that point to the diagnosis of Body Image Disturbance, one of the following major characteristics must be present:

- Not looking at or touching a body part
- Hiding or overexposing body part (the person may or may not be aware of this behavior)
- Trauma to nonfunctioning part
- Change in social involvement (the person changes the amount or quality of interaction with others—especially family or friends)
- Change in ability to estimate spatial relationship of body to environment (the person may bump into items in the environment, or bend, stoop, or move unnecessarily)

Verbalization of any of the following:

- Change in lifestyle
- Fear of rejection or reaction by others
- Negative feelings about body
- Feelings of helplessness, hopelessness, or powerlessness
- Preoccupation with the change or loss (the person discusses the change or loss to the exclusion of all or almost all else)
- Focus on past strength (the person overfocuses on the past)
- Emphasis on remaining strengths and heightened achievement (the person places undue emphasis on strengths or achievements)
- Extension of body boundary to incorporate environmental objects (the person verbalizes feelings that the bed, chair, or other object is part of their body)
- Personalization of part or loss by name (the person names the missing/injured part or loss)
- Depersonalization of part or loss (the person uses impersonal pronouns ["it"] to talk about missing/injured part or loss)
- Refusal to verify actual change (the person is unable to describe the actual loss or injury)

Related Factors

There are a variety of etiologic or contributing factors that may affect this change in functional health status. They may include amputation of a body part; brain injury that has the effect of altering perception of the body; surgery; colostomy; urinary diversion; congenital deformity; eating disorders; morbid obesity; trauma with altered body part—structure or function; chronic illness that results in change of structure or function; body scheme/perceptual disorders; change in lifestyle; depression; trauma (eg, rape); cultural or spiritual differences; developmental or age-related factors (NANDA, 1994).

Diagnostic Statement: Self-Esteem Disturbance

Definition

Self-Esteem Disturbance is negative self-evaluation/feelings about self or self-capabilities, which may be directly or indirectly expressed (NANDA, 1994).

Defining Characteristics

Defining characteristics include self-negating verbalization; expressions of shame/guilt; evaluates self as unable to deal with events; rationalizes away/rejects positive feedback and exaggerates negative feedback about self; hesitant to try new things/situations; denial of problems obvious to others; projection of blame/responsibility for problems; rationalizing personal failures; hypersensitive to slight or criticism; grandiosity (NANDA, 1994).

Diagnostic Statement: Self-Esteem Disturbance: Chronic Low

Definition

A state in which an individual has long-standing negative self-evaluation/feeling about self or self-capabilities (NANDA,1992).

Defining Characteristics

Of the defining characteristics or clinical cues that point to this diagnosis, one of the following major must be present:

Long standing or chronic self-negating verbalizations (the person discounts, minimizes, or criticizes self, personal ideas, or accomplishments), expressions of shame or guilt, evaluation of self as unable to deal with events, rejection of positive feedback or exaggeration of negative feedback, or hesitance to try new things or situations (the person says "I can't" in relation to new experiences).

The following minor characteristics may be present but are not required for this diagnosis. The minor characteristics include frequent lack of success in work or other life events (the person may not excel, quit, or fail at school or work or in relationships), overly conforming or dependent on others' opinions, lack of eye contact, passive or nonassertive, indecisive, seeks excessive reassurance (NANDA, 1992).

Diagnostic Statement: Self-Esteem Disturbance: Situational Low

Definition

Negative self-evaluation or feelings about self, which develop in response to a loss or change in an individual who previously had a positive self-evaluation (NANDA, 1992).

Defining Characteristics

Of the defining characteristics or clinical cues that point to this diagnosis, one of the following characteristics must be present: episodic occurrence of negative self-appraisal in response to life events in a person with a previous positive self-evaluation or verbalization of negative feelings about the self (the person expresses feeling of helplessness, uselessness, or extreme self-doubt).

The following minor characteristics may also be present but are not required for this diagnosis. These characteristics may include self-negating verbalizations (the person makes statements such as "I can't" or "I'm no good" when describing self), expressions of shame or guilt, evaluation of self as unable to handle situations or events (the person expresses feelings of fear of failure or inability when discussing situations or events), or difficulty making decisions (NANDA, 1992).

Diagnostic Statement: Personal Identity Disturbance

Definition

Personal Identity Disturbance is inability to distinguish between self and nonself (NANDA, 1994).

Defining Characteristics

Defining characteristics have yet to be developed by NANDA.

Diagnostic Statement: Altered Role Performance

Definition

Altered Role Performance is disruption in the way one perceives one's role performance (NANDA, 1994).

Defining Characteristics

Change in self-perception of role (the person perceives the role to have changed or that his or her ability to perform the role has changed); denial of role (the person denies that he or she has taken on or been assigned a role [eg, a child denies that he is a brother after a new sibling is born]); change in others' perception of the role; conflict in roles; change in physical capacity to resume role; lack of knowledge of role (the person lacks either knowledge of role expectation or skills to meet the role expectation necessary to fulfill the role); change in usual patterns of responsibility (the person's usual pattern of fulfilling the role changes, ie, time available, broadened expectations, etc.) (NANDA, 1992).

Related Factors

Related factors have yet to be developed by NANDA.

Related Nursing Diagnoses

When making a diagnosis related to disturbed self-concept, the nurse must also consider diagnoses with common defining characteristics. Often these are inherent in dysfunctional self-concept. Among these diagnoses are Anxiety, Ineffective Individual/Family Coping, Defensive Coping, Fear, Altered Family Process, Anticipatory Grieving, Hopelessness, Powerlessness, Social Isolation, and Altered Thought Processes.

Outcome Identification and Planning

After nursing diagnoses and related factors have been identified, the plan of care is developed. Planning focuses on either promotion of a healthy self-concept or change of the altered self-concept. The following general areas may be included in the formulation of client goals:

Client will integrate a realistic body image.
Client will express positive feelings about self or self capabilities.
Client will distinguish between self and nonself.
Client will perform capably.

Client goals will become more specific and differ according to the defining characteristics that apply to each client. The client and nurse plan together to identify goals and interventions. Some interventions used in planning are listed in the accompanying display and discussed in the following section.

Implementation

Interventions to promote self-concept include identifying strengths, maintaining a sense of self, and assisting development. Interventions used for altered self-con-

Planning
Examples of Nursing Interventions for Common Body-Image Problems

- Identify the client's concerns regarding changed body image.
- Provide opportunities to openly discuss feelings related to body image.
- Listen attentively and nonjudgmentally to concerns.
- Demonstrate unconditional acceptance of the client's altered body image.
- Accept the client's coping mechanisms for adjusting to the altered body image.
- Promote independent decision-making in as many areas as possible.
- Assist the client as needed with hygiene and personal grooming.
- Encourage client to participate in care of affected body part.
- Provide opportunities for success in personal care or in resuming normal activities of daily living.
- Teach family to focus on the client's abilities, rather than the body image change.
- Refer the client and family to appropriate support groups.

cept function include establishing and maintaining a therapeutic relationship, self-evaluation, and behavioral change. Nurses can incorporate these interventions into routine nursing care.

Nursing Interventions to Promote Health and Function

Identification of Strengths

Nurses can promote positive self-concept in their clients by assisting them in identifying strengths (Fig. 47-6). The continued use of internal and external resources helps strengthen identity, role performance, self-esteem, and body image. Various personal strengths include good sense of humor, good communication skills, good problem-solving ability, a nice smile, strong health maintenance patterns, strong values, a hobby, strong social support systems, a stable marriage, enjoyment in work, and a good education. When presented with stressors such as illness or loss of a loved one, the nurse can point these strengths out to the client to reinforce self-concept. The client should be encouraged to cultivate these strengths and use them in the coping process whenever the self is threatened.

Sense of Self

Nurses must treat clients in a respectful, personal manner to help them maintain a sense of self. By respecting the client's individuality, the nurse promotes a positive self-concept. Nurses should pay special attention to their verbal and nonverbal interactions with all clients. Appropriate interventions include introducing oneself to the client, addressing the client by name, speaking respectfully, maintaining the client's privacy, explaining all procedures and nursing activities, and paying attention to the client's emotional responses.

Development of Self-Concept

The following discussion and Table 47-2 give nursing interventions that assist development and promote self-concept.

Neonatal Period. The nurse's role in anticipatory guidance during the neonatal period is to assist the family in adapting to their new roles and the self-concept related to these roles. Most often, this is accomplished through a therapeutic relationship that allows for exploration of expectations and provides support to deal with anxiety. The nurse educates the family about parental roles, body changes, emotional changes, and family role expectations. When this is done early, it provides care that minimizes disturbances in self-concept for all members of the family, including the newborn.

Infancy. The nurse teaches the parents of the infant about the child's need for movement, stimulation, and safety. If a child has an acute or chronic illness during this period, an environment that facilitates continued development is crucial. This means having activities that are age- and health-appropriate, providing safety and security. The parents need to provide as much care as possible for the hospitalized infant. Assisting the parents to decrease their anxiety (to cope with the hospitalization) will assist the infant to feel more secure, foster trust, and promote continued self-concept development.

Toddlerhood. The toddler needs an environment that allows practice of newly developing skills, especially movement-related skills. These skills allow body image and esteem to develop positively. Education for the family includes the knowledge that repetitive positive input and allowing the toddler to explore support the development of a favorable self-concept. Hospitalization or illness during toddlerhood affects the development of self-concept. The nurse supports the toddler and family by helping the toddler maintain self-control.

Preschool. During the preschool years, the nurse educates the family about normal development and supports their establishing an effective environment that fa-

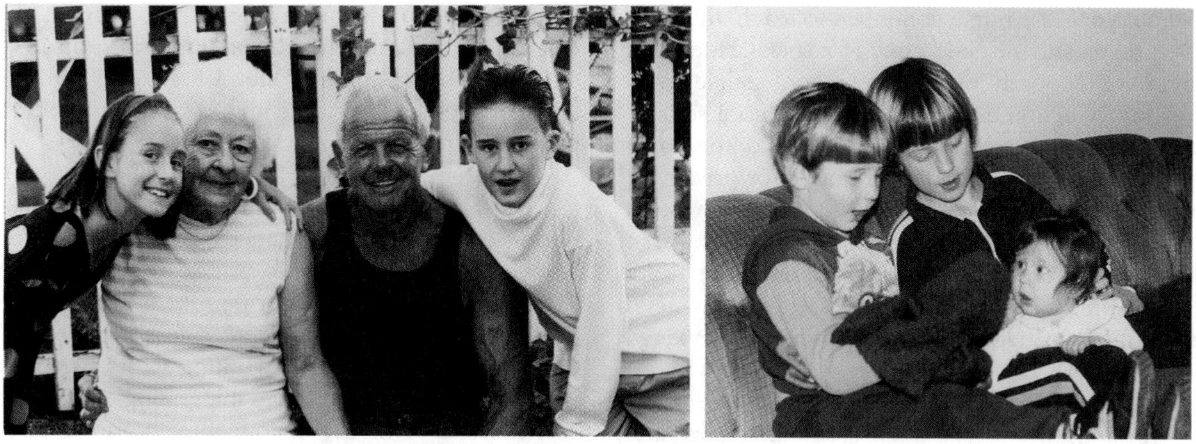

Figure 47-6 *• Families give stability and strength when there are changes. Strengths may come from intergenerational relationships or sibling relationships.*

cilitates growth. Because the child has increased sexual feelings, the preschooler fears damage to his or her body; therefore the preschooler needs support and education concerning health maintenance behaviors, such as personal hygiene and healthcare visits. This can be accomplished through visits to healthcare providers with other family members, or through supportive treatment of the child during routine examinations. Hospitalization or serious illness in the preschooler is especially difficult. The preschooler has many fantasies about punishment, abandonment, or physical harm. The nurse combats these fantasies by including the preschooler in decisions as much as possible. In addition, the family should stay with the child as much as possible. The nurse must remember that the family may respond to the child's hospitalization with guilt, helplessness, and anxiety. The family will need assistance with these feelings to aid the child.

Table 47-2 • Developmental Interventions to Promote Self-Concept

Developmental Level	Intervention
Newborn	Assist family in adapting to new roles by establishing therapeutic relationship and educating members.
Infancy	Teach family about infant's need for movement, stimulation, safety.
	Encourage parents to help provide physical care and security to hospitalized infant.
Toddler	Allow toddler to develop skills through exploration.
	Support family and help toddler maintain self-control.
Preschool	Teach preschooler and family health maintenance behaviors.
	Encourage family to stay with the child if hospitalized, and let the child make some decisions about care.
School age	Allow privacy.
	Teach parents of need for socialization and belonging.
	Allow liberal visitation and age-appropriate activities if hospitalized.
Adolescent	Educate adolescent about sexual health, drug and alcohol use.
	Educate family about identity and body image changes.
	If hospitalized, offer choices in care to maintain autonomy.
Adulthood	Use therapeutic relationship to support the adult and significant other, if hospitalized.
	Support decisions made in relationships and work role.
Older adult	Treat older adult with respect and allow independence and individuality if hospitalized.
	Help older adult integrate loss of spouse, job, social support network, health, and the like

School Age. The nurse continues to teach and help parents understand the child's need for socialization and belonging. Frequently, it is the school nurse who teaches reproduction and health in the school setting. If the child is hospitalized during this period, the nurse must be cognizant of the changing need for privacy in this age group, as well as the child's need to know that he or she still belongs to the family and peer group. In addition, the school-age child needs information about his or her illness and treatments. Parents again need support and help dealing with their fear and anxiety.

Adolescence. The nurse supports the adolescent and family through the process of assuming roles and establishing independence. The nurse teaches the family about the developmental process and why individual family members may have intense feelings during this period. The adolescent experiments as he or she makes choices to establish identity. Health teaching for the adolescent includes information concerning birth control, AIDS, and sexually transmitted diseases. A further concern is drug use and alcohol abuse. The adolescent needs to know the ramifications of choosing drugs or alcohol as a coping style. The adolescent may need assistance to learn and practice alternate coping behaviors.

Often adolescents are hospitalized on the pediatric unit, which may contradict the person's view of himself or herself as an independent, grown-up person. Offering the adolescent choices regarding care helps the adolescent maintain some autonomy. Feedback about the adolescent's strengths and weaknesses helps him or her establish a realistic self-concept.

Adulthood. The nurse assists the adult with role satisfaction primarily in intimate relationships and occupation. Interventions include use of a therapeutic relationship, structuring the environment to provide for successes, and allowing the person time and support while exploring the meaning of life. A feeling of generativity enhances self-concept. The nurse continues to offer support to significant others.

Older Adult. Older people do not seek care as "old" people but as people with needs. Loss of independence associated with aging often brings loss of self-esteem. The nurse approaches older people as adults and supports appropriate independence and self-care, which enhances self-concept. In working with older people, the nurse's role is to assist in integrating changes, most often loss, into their self-concept. The nurse also enhances the older adult's self-concept by using respect and allowing individuality. Allowing the client to keep personal belongings, listening to stories told by the client, respecting privacy, explaining procedures, and allowing the client extra time to accomplish tasks are some of the interventions aimed at older adults (Fig. 47-7).

Nursing Interventions for Altered Self-Concept

Therapeutic Relationship

Nurses intervene with clients with altered self-concept through a therapeutic relationship. To develop a therapeutic relationship, the nurse must demonstrate great self-awareness and effective communication. The nurse establishes rapport with the client by conveying a sense of friendship and trust. When the nurse shows empathy, the client feels that the nurse understands his or her feelings and will care for his or her needs. Once the relationship is established, the nurse uses thera-

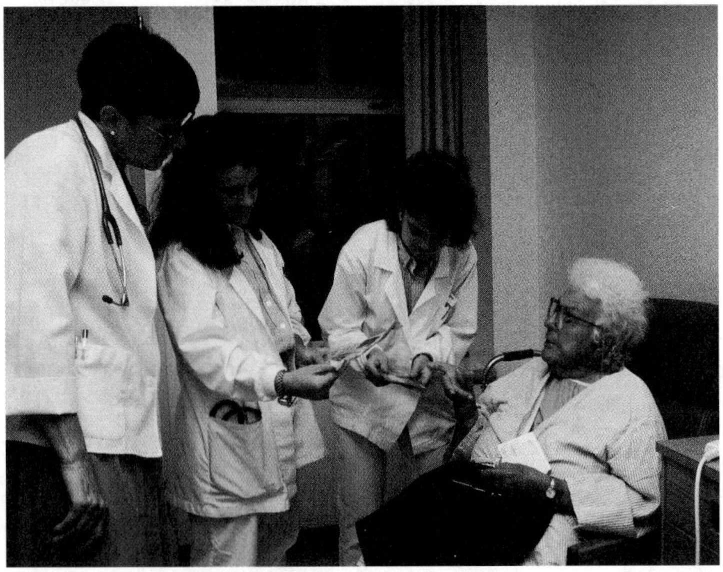

Figure 47-7 • *An older client tells her story through family pictures and mementos. (Courtesy of Seattle University School of Nursing.)*

peutic communication techniques, such as active listening, reflection, and reality-based feedback. Through therapeutic communication, the nurse assists the client with defining self-concept problems and attempting to problem-solve.

Self-Evaluation

Nursing interventions that assist the client with positive self-evaluation can help change poor self-concept. People with low self-esteem frequently put themselves down and act in ways that perpetuate negative self-evaluation. To break this cycle, the client needs help in realistically evaluating the self, and developing more positive thoughts and feelings about the self. Emphasis is placed on positive attributes rather than negative behavior. The nurse can assist the client to point out tasks or accomplishments that deserve positive feedback. The nurse offers praise honestly and encourages the client to make positive self statements. The nurse should also be a model for the client by acting confident, making positive statements, and accepting compliments.

Behavioral Change

Nursing interventions aimed at changing behavior also assist the client with self-concept problems. General measures that bring about behavioral changes include accepting responsibility for self, defining realistic goals, using resources to enact change, and rewarding positive outcomes. The nurse can help the client accept responsibility for self by suggesting the client make "I" statements that reflect his or her thoughts and feelings. For example, for a client with role performance problems, instead of saying, "nothing ever goes right," a more active statement might be "I can't get the hang of my new job." This is the first step in realizing that the client may have the power to change behavior.

In helping the client define realistic goals, the nurse assists the client in evaluating expectations. If expectations are unrealistic or the discrepancy between the real self and the ideal self is too great, behavior will not change. Goals should be specific, such as "I will ask my boss for a 2-week training period on the new computer system." The nurse helps the client identify resources to accomplish goals, including, for example, a computer training department at the office, night school courses, or someone to help around the house so the client can temporarily devote more time to work.

The client will be more likely to change behavior if he or she feels he or she will be rewarded for more positive behavior. The nurse can point out rewards, such as a feeling of greater competence, less time spent at the office, greater productivity, and praise by others. By assisting the client with problem-solving, his or her role performance should improve, and self-concept will be strengthened.

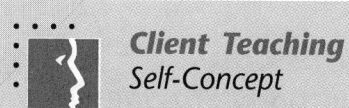

Client Teaching
Self-Concept

Instruct the client as follows:

- *State views and opinions. They have worth and validity.*
- *Identify strengths and develop them further.*
- *Learn how to use strengths for successful coping.*
- *Explore the meaning of life and develop a value system.*
- *Think positively about one's self.*
- *Set realistic goals for one's self.*
- *Learn about community resources and how to use them.*
- *Develop an interest in people and their personalities.*

Community-Based Nursing

The client with self-concept disturbance often requires psychosocial assistance beyond basic nursing. The nurse assists the client to recognize difficulties and accept additional therapy. Afterward, the nurse and client can initiate plans for additional care. The goals of discharge planning are effective teaching and referral.

The teaching plan may include where and how to use community resources, such as support groups, or individual teaching concerning stages of loss. Referral may be to a specialized support group such as a group for mastectomy clients, or may be for therapy through a psychiatric nurse specialist, psychologist, or psychiatrist. The physician should be consulted regarding ambulatory referrals. If the client is to receive home-health follow-up, communication about the plan of care to the home-health nurse is essential. For example, home care for the client after mastectomy should include interventions to help incorporate a change in body image and strengthen self-esteem, if those problem areas were identified while the client was hospitalized. Interventions that have worked should be described in a home-health referral for continuity of care.

Evaluation

Specific outcome criteria are the evaluation tools used to measure the attainment of goals in self-concept. If the nurse asks what the client hopes to see or hear if the interventions chosen are effective, goals will be behavioral in nature. The nurse then asks under what circumstances the client will exhibit that behavior, and by when. Such goals are measurable. Because the nurse and client (in most cases) established goals and outcome criteria, they can discuss whether these criteria have been met. Outcome criteria for client goals discussed earlier in the chapter could be the following:

Nursing Plan of Care
The Patient With Body Image Disturbance

Nursing Diagnosis
Body Image Disturbance related to change in physical appearance manifested by client's refusal to look at body.

Client Goal
Client will express improved perception of physical appearance.

Client Outcome Criteria
- Client discusses his or her physical changes within 2 days of surgery.
- Client demonstrates participation in activities of daily living within 3 days.
- Client uses coping skills to prepare for changes in physical appearance within 3 days.
- Client views affected body part within 1 week of surgery.

Nursing Intervention	Scientific Rationale
1. Assess client's strengths that will positively affect body image, such as family relationships.	1. Assessment of factors in the client that can contribute to improved body image builds on the client's strengths.
2. Provide opportunities to discuss altered appearance and self-worth.	2. Stating feelings verbally often helps to clarify and provide perspective for the client.
3. Assist with grooming.	3. When client is unable physically or emotionally to groom self, the nurse's care activities indicate the nurse's concern for the client's welfare and help to establish rapport.
4. Encourage the client to participate in self-grooming and to strive for independence.	4. Encouraging participation in self-care provides a sense of control.
5. Encourage identification and use of positive coping strategies.	5. Use of coping strategies that have worked effectively for the client aids in successful coping with body image.
6. Encourage client to cultivate positive coping strategies.	6. Use of internal and external resources helps strengthen self-esteem and body image.
7. Provide a mirror for the client to view self. The client may want to do so in privacy.	7. Client must view physical changes before he or she can integrate them into a realistic body image.
8. Provide information and education regarding the altered appearance, support groups, and other resources.	8. Individualized education and information meet the unique needs of the client.

Goal
Client will integrate a realistic body image.

Possible Outcome Criteria
- Client speaks about his or her body within 2 days after surgery.
- Client views self in mirror within 3 days after surgery.
- Client assists with dressing changes within 4 days after surgery.

Goal
Client will express positive feelings about self.

Possible Outcome Criteria
- Client establishes eye contact with nurse during conversation within 2 days.
- Client lists negative attitudes and their effect on self by discharge.
- Client verbalizes feelings of success with self-care activities by discharge.
- Client verbalizes strategies to support self-care and positive feelings related to self in the community.

Goal
Client will distinguish between self and nonself.

Possible Outcome Criteria

- Client identifies feelings of depersonalization as related to illness within 2 days.
- Client states realistic expectations for discharge within 5 days.
- Client expresses feelings of hope and power over own life within 7 days.

Goal

Client will perform capably.

Possible Outcome Criteria

- Client expresses interest in caring for newborn within 1 day.
- Client identifies three coping strategies to help assume new role within 2 weeks.
- Client performs basic care of newborn successfully within 24 hours and more complex care within 2 weeks.
- Client verbalizes who the client will contact for social support when home, before discharge from center.

Key Concepts

- Self-concept is the mental image one has of one's self.
- Characteristics of normal self-concept include the dimensions of self-perception: self-knowledge, self-expectation, social self, and self-evaluation.
- Positive body image, self-esteem, strong personal identity, and role performance are normal patterns of self-concept.
- Factors that affect normal self-concept include biologic make-up; culture, values and beliefs; coping and stress tolerance; previous experience; developmental level; and illness.
- Several factors place a person at risk for altered self-concept, including stressful life events, inadequate coping resources, incomplete developmental tasks, role transition, and illness, trauma, or surgery.
- Manifestations of altered self-concept include self-care deficit, emotional and behavioral changes, anxiety and depression, and self-destructive behavior (such as alcoholism, drug abuse, and sexual promiscuity).
- NANDA-approved nursing diagnoses to be considered in caring for clients with dysfunctional self-concept are Body Image Disturbance, Situational Low Self-Esteem, Chronic Low Self-Esteem, Personal Identity Disturbance, and Altered Role Performance.
- Personal strengths the nurse can encourage the client to cultivate to promote positive self-concept include good sense of humor, good communication skills, strong health maintenance patterns, a hobby, strong social support systems, enjoyment in work, and a good education.
- Loss of independence associated with aging may bring loss of self-esteem; therefore, the nurse should treat older adults with a sense of respect and individuality.
- Nurses help clients with low self-esteem by assisting them with realistic self-evaluation and development of more positive thoughts and feelings about themselves.
- Nurses can also help bring about behavioral change in clients with altered self-concept by assisting them to accept responsibility for themselves, define realistic goals, use resources to enact change, and reward positive outcomes.

Critical Thinking Challenges

Now you have learned about self-concept and studied your own self-concept. Adding this to your knowledge base of nursing care, you are now ready to help clients with self-concept concerns. Turn back to the situation at the beginning of the chapter and consider the following:

1. *Describe your immediate impressions.*
2. *Think about the information provided as well as your own experience, knowledge, and beliefs. Consider how these influence your impressions.*
3. *Analyze how the mother feels and how the infant feels.*
4. *Consider additional assessment data that you might need to collect.*
5. *State possible nursing diagnoses for this family and identify some desired outcomes.*
6. *Given your assessment, nursing diagnoses, and outcome identification, plan interventions that may be appropriate.*

References

Berscheid, E., Walster, E., & Bohrnstedt, G. (1973). Body image. *Psychology Today,* Nov., 119–131.

Briggs, D. C. (1987). Your child's self-esteem: The key to life. In E. Shiff (Ed.), *Experts advise parents.* New York: Delacorte Press.

Ciseaux, A. (1980). Anorexia nervosa: A view from the mirror. *Am J Nurs, 80,* 1468–1474.

Coopersmith, S. (1967). *Antecedents of self esteem.* San Francisco: Freeman.

Cronan, L. (1993). Management of the patient with altered body image. *British Journal of Nursing, 21, 257–261.*

Erikson, E. (1963). *Childhood and society* (2nd ed.). New York: W. W. Norton.

Freud, S. (1920/1966). *Lectures on psychoanalysis.* (J. Strachey, ed. and trans.). New York: W. W. Norton.

Gary, F., & Kavanagh, C. K. (1991). *Psychiatric mental health nursing.* Philadelphia: J. B. Lippincott.

Gordon, M. (1987). *Manual of nursing diagnosis* (2nd ed.). New York: McGraw-Hill.

Havighurst, R. (1972). *Developmental tasks and education* (3rd ed.). New York: David McKay.

Kohlberg, L. (1969). Stage and sequence: The cognitive developmental approach to socialization. In D. A. Goslin (Ed.), *Handbook of socialization: Theory and research.* Chicago: Rand McNally.

Noles, S., Cash, T., & Winstead, B. (1985). Body image, physical attractiveness, and depression. *J Consult Clin Psychol, 53,* 88–94.

Norris, J. (1992). Nursing intervention for self esteem disturbances. *Nursing Diagnosis, 3,* 48–53.

Norris, J., & Kunes-Cornell, M. (1985). Self-esteem disturbance. *Nurs Clin North Am, 20,* 745–761.

North American Nursing Diagnosis Association (NANDA). (1994). *Nursing diagnoses: Definitions and classification 1995–1996.* Philadelphia: Author.

Piaget, J. (1969). *The psychology of the child.* New York: Basic Books.

Public Health Service. (1987). *Personnel for health needs of the elderly through the year 2020.* Sept. 1987.

Rogers, C. R. (1961). *On becoming a person.* Boston: Houghton Mifflin.

Rotter, J. B. (1966). Generalized expectancies for internal versus external locus of control reinforcement. *Psychology Monographs, 80,* 1–28.

Sheehy, G. (1974). *Passages.* New York: E. P. Dutton.

Stanwyck, D. (1983). Self esteem through the life span. *Family and Community Health, 6*(2), 11–28.

Sullivan, H. (1953). *The interpersonal theory of psychiatry.* New York: W. W. Norton.

Wolf, N. (1991). *The beauty myth: How images of beauty are used against women.* New York: Morrow.

Bibliography

Carrigan, J. T. (1994). The psychosocial needs of patients who have attempted suicide by overdose. *J Adv Nurs, 20,* 635–642.

Davidhizar, R., & Shearer, R. A. (1994). Is adapting to others codependency or flexibility? *Today's OR Nurse, 16*(5), 41–43.

Heidrich, S. (1994). The self, health, and depression in elderly women. *Western Journal of Nursing Research, 16,* 544–555.

McKivergin, M. J., & Daubenmire, M. J. (1994). The healing process of presence. *Journal of Holistic Nursing, 12*(1), 65–81.

Smith, M. E., & Hart, G. (1994). Nurses' responses to patient anger: From disconnecting to connecting. *J Adv Nurs, 20,* 643–651.

Roles and Relationships

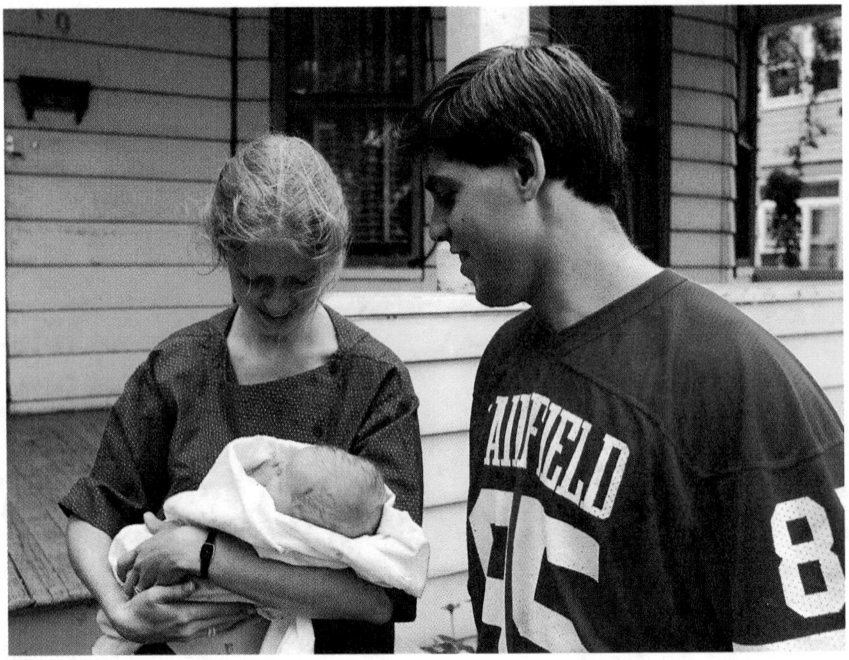

UNIT XIV

A person's roles and relationships make up the fabric of his or her life responsibilities. These areas of psychosocial function have a significant impact on health and wellness, and conversely, on other areas of function. Unit XIV explores roles and relationships.

Chapter 48 discusses the concept of communication as both a human need and a form of social interaction essential in any human relationship. Nurses need to be able to assess a client's ability to communicate his or her needs to provide holistic nursing care. Most importantly, nurses need to know how to intervene for a client who has impaired verbal communication and cannot readily make his or her needs known. The chapter emphasizes nursing interventions to promote health and function as well as those for altered function. Chapter 49 considers families and their relationships. As healthcare focuses more on self-responsibility, nurses need to understand and assess family functioning, so they can involve families as the primary source of client support. This chapter provides a beginning discussion of family concepts, featuring holistic nursing interventions to promote family health and function, and discusses sources of support for altered family function. The final chapter discusses loss and grieving. Any loss a client experiences threatens his or her roles and relationships. Conversely, the loss of a client produces stress and requires adaptation for the family. Death of a client or of a client's loved one requires nursing interventions to promote health and function as well as those to facilitate coping.

This unit focuses on the universal human need for and influence of relationships with others. Both are interwoven with a person's health and well-being.

Communication: Social Interaction

Key Terms	Learning Objectives

Key Terms

Anomia
Aphasia
Articulation
Coma
Communication
Dysarthria
Language
Laryngectomy
Nonverbal communication
Phonation
Resonance
Tracheostomy
Tracheotomy

Learning Objectives

Upon completion of this chapter, the student will be able to do the following:

- *Identify the areas dominant for language in the left hemisphere of the brain.*
- *Describe the components of speech and language.*
- *Contrast verbal and nonverbal communication.*
- *Summarize development of language and communication during the lifespan.*
- *Identify common causes of altered communication.*
- *Explain the differences between types of aphasia.*
- *Discuss the effect of dysfunctional communication.*
- *Use subjective and objective data in assessing speech and language capabilities.*
- *Provide interventions facilitating communication.*
- *Discuss socialization needs of people with altered communication.*
- *Discuss referrals available to people with communication dysfunction.*

48

You are making a home visit with an older couple for whom English is not their first language. The husband, who has had a cerebrovascular accident, has trouble expressing himself. You notice that he becomes short-tempered with his wife when she doesn't understand his request. Because of the language barrier, you are having difficulty understanding what the wife is trying to tell you about her husband and his needs. The wife is tearful, wringing her hands, and pacing about the room.

You learned about communication in earlier chapters of this text. The importance of communication in the nurse–client relationship (therapeutic relationship) was discussed in Chapter 20. Written communication as part of nursing process was discussed in Chapter 14. This chapter discusses the functioning of people through communication in their roles and relationships with others. When you have finished this chapter, you should have a strong knowledge base on communication. You will be able to plan for the care of the couple mentioned in the situation at the beginning of the chapter. The Critical Thinking Challenges at the end of the chapter will help you in thinking through a nursing plan.

Communication brings people together while it sets them apart from one another: it allows individuals to be unique.

The combination of speech and language, along with the senses of vision and hearing, allows humans to receive, interpret, and express ideas, feelings, and needs.

Normal Communication

Communication is the interchange of information between at least two people. There are various types of communication and several elements to the communication process (see Chapter 20). There must be a message delivered from one person (the sender or source) to another (the receiver) (see Fig. 20-2). The message must get the attention of the receiver. Sometimes the sending and receiving of messages occur simultaneously, and the messages must be separated out. Once a message has been received it must be interpreted. Interpretation is based on language abilities, cultural influences, cognitive function, and past experiences.

Structures of the Communication Centers

Speech production is a motor activity that requires the coordination of laryngeal and respiratory structures to produce the sound patterns of speech. To understand how motor activity and interpretation are coordinated by the brain, one must look at how the brain functions in relation to speech and language. The brain is divided into two sides, or hemispheres, which are connected and work closely together to monitor and regulate the body's functions. The left hemisphere has been found to be dominant for language function in approximately 90% to 99% of right-handed people (Fig. 48-1). Similarly, in left-handed people, the left hemisphere is dominant for language function 50% to 75% of the time. In addition, the left hemisphere develops those functions that are closely related to speech and language, including arithmetic ability, verbal ideation and abstraction, and interpretation and understanding of speech.

Production and Coordination of Communication

Speech and vocalization involve the respiratory system, the speech control centers in the cerebral cortex, and the structures of the mouth and nose. Speech is basically composed of the functions of phonation (achieved by the larynx) and articulation (achieved by the mouth).

Phonation. **Phonation** is the process by which humans create vocal sound. Sounds are made when air from the lungs is forced through the oral cavity or nasal passages during exhalation. As forced air moves past the vocal cords (larynx), the vocal folds vibrate.

The vocal pitch, volume, and quality or timbre of phonation are produced at this site. The pitch of the voice can be changed by stretching or relaxing the vocal cords or by changing the mass of the vocal cords' edges by contracting the thyroarytenoid muscles. The volume of the voice is controlled, in part, by the amount of air being forced through the larynx. To force the air through the larynx, the lungs must recoil by means of constriction of the rib cage and contraction of the diaphragm.

Articulation. **Articulation** refers to the enunciation of words and sentences. It is affected by the lips, the tongue, and the soft palate. The movement of the

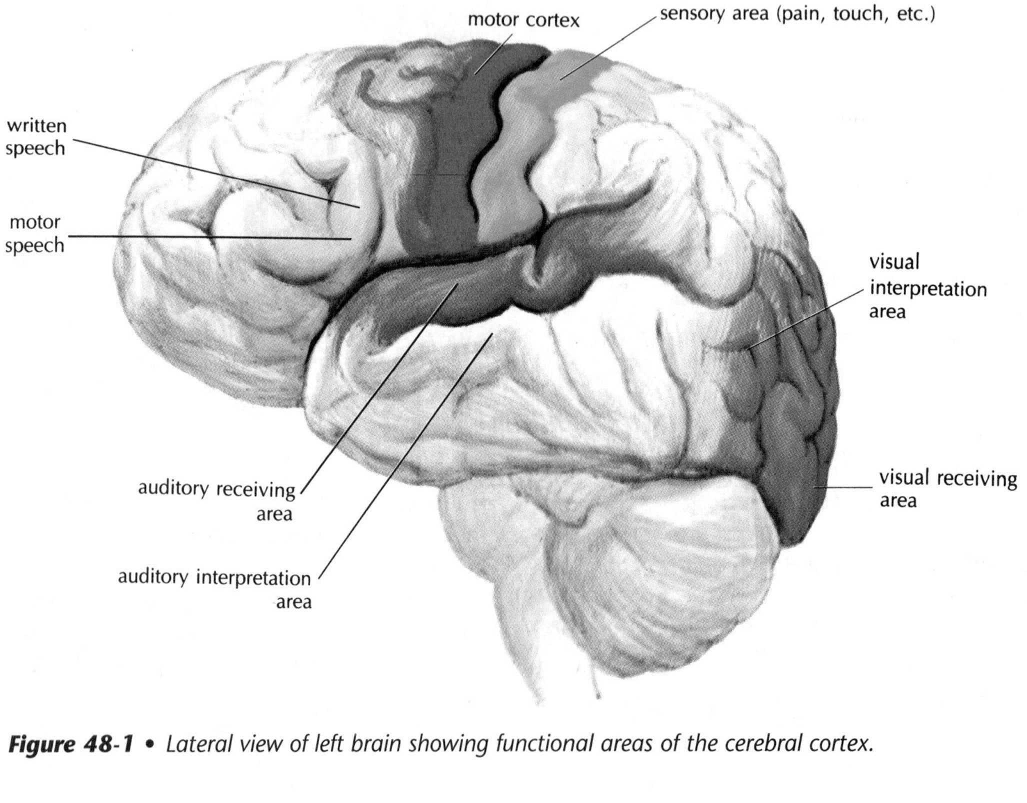

Figure 48-1 • *Lateral view of left brain showing functional areas of the cerebral cortex.*

tongue against the palate, the teeth, and the muscles of the mouth and face influences the sound that is made. The lips and the surrounding muscles provide the vault and assist the oral cavity in making rapid changes in shape and size for sound formation and articulation.

The major organs of resonance include the mouth, nose, associated nasal sinuses, pharynx, and the chest. **Resonance** refers to echoing or resounding of sound through various passages. The amount of resonance is reflected in the tone and timbre of the voice. The function of the resonators is demonstrated by the change in voice quality when a person has a severe head cold with congestion.

Cortical Control. In addition to vocalization, speech involves the formation in the mind of the thoughts, words, and meanings to be expressed. Thought formation and word choice occur in the sensory areas of the brain. The motor aspect of vocalization is controlled by Broca's area of the dominant hemisphere of the motor cortex. The patterns for control of the larynx, lips, mouth, respiratory system, and other muscles of articulation are controlled by this area of the cortex. The muscular movements that control the actual emission of sound are activated by the facial and laryngeal regions of the motor cortex. Dysfunction or destruction of this region of the cortex can cause either total or partial inability to speak.

Normal Function of Communication

Communication is essential to social interaction. It enables a person to relate to people in his or her family and community (Fig. 48-2). The communication may revolve around home, work, play, and study. Communication helps a person identify and express roles in those relationships. For instance, a father may discipline a child, an instructor may give instructions for an assignment, or a student may ask questions for clarification of studies.

Communication aids not only in developing the function of social interaction but also supplies a means of expression for other healthy functioning: coping behaviors, self-concept, and expression of values and belief (including communication with a higher being).

Characteristics of Normal Communication

Communication does not occur in a vacuum but is influenced by many factors. It involves both verbal and

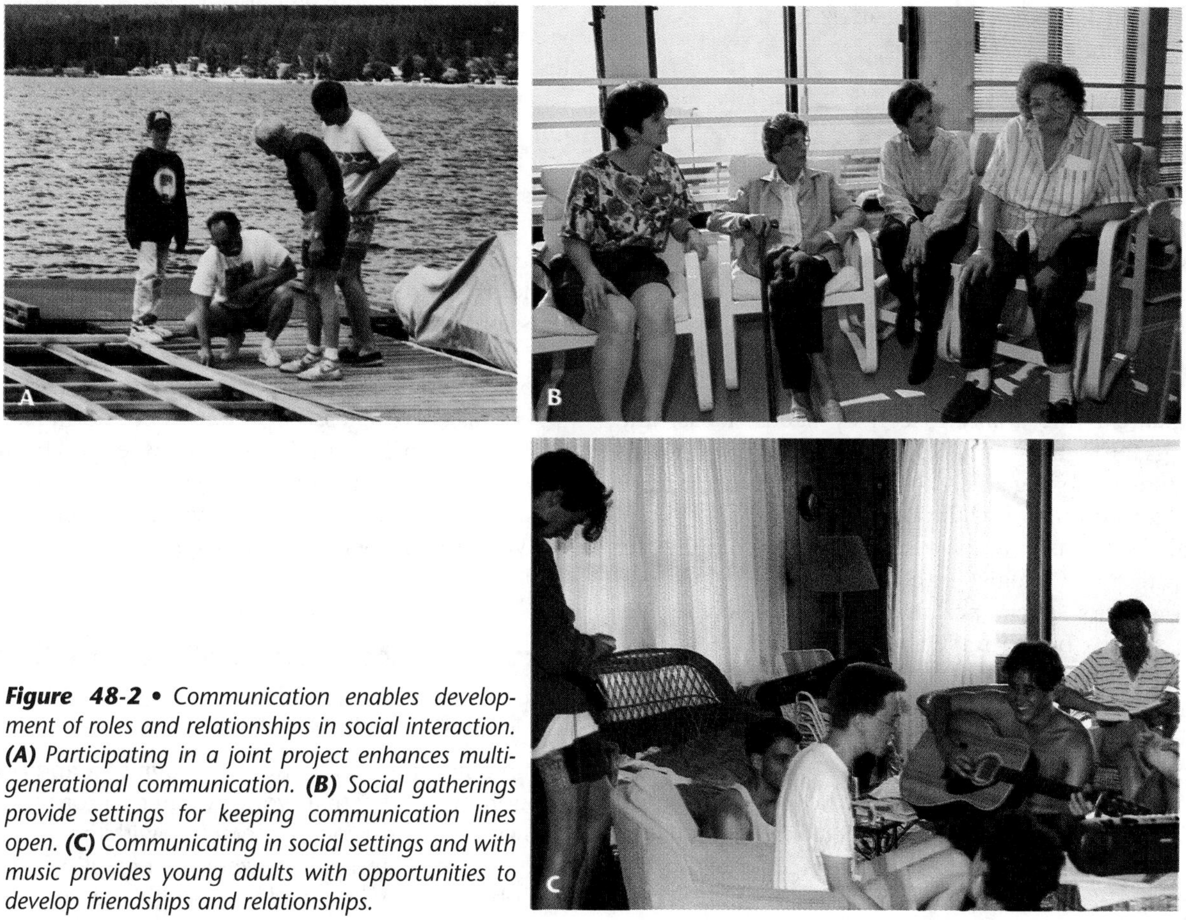

Figure 48-2 • *Communication enables development of roles and relationships in social interaction.* ***(A)*** *Participating in a joint project enhances multigenerational communication.* ***(B)*** *Social gatherings provide settings for keeping communication lines open.* ***(C)*** *Communicating in social settings and with music provides young adults with opportunities to develop friendships and relationships.*

> **Prerequisites to Adequate Speech Production**
>
> ***Intact Structures for the Physical Production of Sound***
>
> - Larynx
> - Respiratory structures
> - Oral cavity structures
> - Nasal cavity structures
>
> ***Functioning Structures for the Physical Reception of Sound***
>
> - Discriminating auditory apparatus
> - Receptive speech center
>
> ***Maturation of the Central Nervous System***
>
> - Myelination of major neural pathways
> - Growth in functional capacity of the cerebral cortex
> - Functioning speech control center in the cerebral cortex
>
> ***Cognitive Maturation***
>
> - Adequate intellectual ability
> - Ability to process thoughts
>
> ***Psychological Stimulation***
>
> - Verbal and nonverbal human interaction
> - Environmental stimulation
>
> From Broadwell, D., & Saunders, R. (1993). *Child health nursing: A comprehensive approach to the care of children and their families.* Philadelphia: J. B. Lippincott.

nonverbal exchanges, which occur simultaneously during a conversation (see Chapter 20).

Verbal Communication: Language

Language is the ability to convey needs, ideas, and feelings through the systematic use of symbols. Humans are unique in being able to use symbolic codes to communicate abstract ideas through a highly refined verbal language (Schuster & Ashburn, 1992). The biophysical interaction and integration of the brain, neural system, and organs of speech permits humans not only to produce sounds but to remember what they said in the past and to speak about the future. From early times, humans have sought ways to communicate through the verbal symbols of speech, encoding meaning to certain sounds and usages.

The next step was to convert those verbal sounds to a written format that could be deciphered readily by all the members of the group. Pictographs were among the earliest forms of written language, using line drawings or depictions of objects or events to communicate meaning. Hieroglyphics were a sophisticated form of pictographs that combined language and pictures.

Verbal language evolved into special sounds, tones, and inflections peculiar to groups of people. These languages began to take on territoriality, ultimately dividing people into cultures and nations. These languages united the people who used the same language; at the same time, it separated people from others who spoke a different language. Speaking, writing, and reading of the language of the group were taught to pass the culture and the language on to future generations.

As civilization evolved, printing by mechanical means further promoted language and allowed people to learn to speak and understand increasing numbers of languages. Books, newspapers, and journals enhanced the spread of information through various languages. Development of the electronic media, beginning with the radio, has promoted the spread of communication throughout the world using satellites, television, telephones, and sophisticated combinations.

Nonverbal Communication

Nonverbal communication is the exchange of messages without using verbal language. Types of nonverbal communication were discussed in Chapter 20 and include such things as eye contact, facial expressions, body posture and movement, gestures, and touch. Nonverbal expression is more likely to be involuntary and less likely to be consciously controlled. Therefore, it is usually a more accurate picture of a person's true intent in communication.

Touch is one of the most effective means of expressing oneself nonverbally. Touch can be used to convey a variety of messages. Touch has many different meanings and, because of its personal nature, understanding its true meaning may be difficult. Tactile expressions are shaped by familial, regional, class, and cultural influences. Age and sex also play a role in developing meanings that are associated with touch.

Physical closeness between client and nurse is an essential part of nursing. There is an exceptional amount of touching in the nurse–client relationship. The use of touch in family relationships is even more personal and conveys a more personal message.

Factors Affecting Normal Communication

Cognition and Perception

Communication is influenced by cognition and by perception of the external world. Cognition, or the act of knowing, occurs through interaction with the world, formal education, and culturalization. Perception refers to the obtaining of knowledge through the senses. The senses of vision and hearing directly affect cognition and the ability to communicate.

Vision allows the person to see the initiation of and response to interaction with another person. The eye transmits electrical impulses from the retina through the optic nerve to the brain, where the impulses are translated into images and meanings. This process of visual perception in communication begins in infancy when an infant responds to the caregiver's presence, facial expressions, and other nonverbal behavior. As the person continues through life, communication is affected by the visual feedback that is provided by expression and body language. The same words or phrases can mean different things when linked with different expressions that are visually detected by the listener.

Hearing is another primary avenue of perception. The ear carries sound that has been collected in the outer ear through the middle ear to the inner ear. The sound waves are converted to nerve impulses and sent to the brain by way of the auditory nerve. The impulses are translated into meaning, based on the pitch, loudness, and duration of the sound. The expression of meaning and emotion is conveyed through pitch, loudness, tonal quality, and inflection. Beginning in infancy, changes in inflection, pitch, and tonal quality clearly convey meaning even without distinguishable words. In turn, the infant understands meaning based on what is heard in spoken tone variation. Throughout life, the person listens to the meaning and emotion conveyed in speech for a portion of the meaning contained in the words being spoken.

People who have dysfunction of hearing or vision may also have the potential for altered cognition or knowing. If cognition is impaired, communication lacks clarity. The person who is visually impaired loses the information obtained through facial expression and body language, and the person who has a hearing impairment may have little or no perception of tone variation.

Self-Concept

The perception held of one's self is called self-concept. The way a person feels about himself or herself in relation to the world is conveyed in the person's communication. If a person feels competent and successful and in control of his or her life, the quality of communication reflects that confidence and security.

People who feel disadvantaged or less competent are likely to believe they have little control over their lives. Their self-concept is apt to be correspondingly less confident. If a person sees the self as less able to compete in a given arena (school, work, or play), the person's communication reflects that lack of confidence as well.

The manner in which a person communicates to others usually is mirrored back. If a person communicates confidence and security, that is the response that is received from others. Conversely, if the person communicates insecurity and feelings of lack of control or inadequacy, the responding communication reflects the person's concept of self.

Whether there is any validity in the person's concept of self is a separate question. As a person matures, he or she realizes that people vary in personal skills and that one can compensate for other areas. This adaptation and adjustment leads to a balanced self-concept and more confident communication.

Culture, Values, and Beliefs

Comprehension and meaning vary among cultures, and communication is often inhibited or blocked as a result. Words and their meanings carry different nuances and significance depending on a person's culture, values, and beliefs.

Although these differences may be particularly noticeable among immigrant groups, they also hold true for groups from different regions within the same country. For example, the same language and some of its meanings may sound different to and be comprehended differently by a person from the southeastern United States than by a person from northeastern states (Ahmann, 1994; Rothenburger, 1990).

Language barriers, whether they are the result of foreign languages or varying dialects of the same language, can result in anxiety, fear, and frustration for people who need to communicate on a daily basis, and especially where healthcare is required. Because communication involves body language along with verbal language, the meaning of body position and expression can further facilitate or impede communication. Although putting an arm around the shoulder of one person may indicate caring and concern, for a person of another culture that act may be a violation of privacy and an intrusion that blocks communication rather than facilitating it.

A person's values regarding what personal thoughts and feelings are appropriate to share with others also affect communication. In this culture, women tend to be more comfortable in communicating feelings than men. This culture values stoicism and emotional reserve in men, so men are less likely to communicate personal thoughts and responses. This reluctance to communicate may actually interfere with effective communication if actual understandings and needs are not shared.

Lifespan Considerations

Each phase of development brings with it unique aspects related to language and communication. Although it is not possible to discuss these complex phenomena completely in this chapter, some interesting points are highlighted here.

Therapeutic Dialogue
Communication and Social Interaction

Scenes for Thought

You, a community health nurse, have been visiting the family of Georgia and Stuart Keene, parents of three, including Stuart, Jr., aged 4 years, who was premature at birth and is now somewhat developmentally delayed. The other children are Kristen, aged 7, and Janine, aged 10 years. Mr. Keene is at work as a city bus driver. Mrs. Keene is at home to meet you today because it is her day off from her part-time job at the public library.

Effective

Nurse: *Hi, Mrs. Keene, how are you today? (Walks in the door she holds open for you to enter.)*
Client: *Hello, Patty. I'm fine. Glad to see you.* She looks well rested and happy.
Nurse: *You look fine, much more rested than last month. (Both of you sit down together at the kitchen table.)*
Client: *Yes, things are going much better these days. Stuart's just got a promotion at work, which he's pleased about, and little Stuart is having a fine time in his new preschool. He comes home every day with something new he's made or some new story he's made up that the teacher copied down for him. It's wonderful to watch him.* Beaming proudly.
Nurse: *I'm glad to hear it. You're obviously delighted by all this.*
Client: *Yes, it's working out very well. The other thing that Stuart and I feel good about is that little Stuart's school has a special group for parents, and we've made some friends there. It's so important not to feel alone when you have a special-needs kid. Not only are they a support to us, but they're becoming real friends, you know, like getting together for a movie or visiting each other with all the families for a cook-out.*
Nurse: *I can see how important this is to you. How are the girls doing with all this socializing?*
Client: *They seem to be loving it. Janine, especially, is coming out of her shell a little. There are a couple of other girls her age with brothers with little Stuart's problems and they get together on the phone and talk and have a great time. It's been a comfort to both girls to know they aren't the only ones with a preemie brother.*
Nurse: *That's great, especially since they were feeling a little isolated and jealous at the beginning. I'm so glad it's working out better. And I'm glad for you and your husband, too. You both expressed a need for some connections with other families. I'm actually wondering if you need my services anymore because Stuart seems to be coping very well physically (looks at his chart) and socially, and you are too. What do you think?*
Client: Looks thoughtful and then a little sad. *I think you're right, although I'll miss our talks, and I know Stuart will miss you, too.*
Nurse: *I'll miss coming here too. It's been wonderful to see all the great changes. (They reminisce about the first time they met when Stuart was just home from the hospital, and continue to say goodbye.)*

Less Effective

Nurse: *Hi, Mrs. Keene, how are you today? (Walks in the door she holds open for you to enter.)*
Client: *Hello, Jeannette. I'm fine. Glad to see you.* She looks well rested and happy.
Nurse: *You* look *fine, much more rested than last month. (Both of you sit down together at the kitchen table.)*
Client: *Yes, things are going much better these days. Stuart's just got a promotion at work, which he's pleased about, and little Stuart is having a fine time in his new preschool. He comes home every day with something new he's made or some new story he's made up that the teacher copied down for him. It's wonderful to watch him.* Beaming proudly.
Nurse: *That's great. Sound's like everything's going well for him. How's he doing physically? (Taking out chart and writing notes.)*
Client: *Just fine. No earaches or colds since last month. The vitamins you changed him to are working fine, too; he actually asks me for them now. The school is helping him with some of the motor things, too, like climbing and swinging. He's doing fine.*
Nurse: *Well, it's a far cry from the beginning when we weren't sure what kind of life he'd have. Looks like he really doesn't need my services, do you think? (Closing up the chart and putting the pen away.)*
Client: *Oh! I guess not, but I know he'll miss seeing you.* Looks a little surprised and sad.
Nurse: *And I'll miss the little fella, too. I'll come back when he's home from school so I can say goodbye, okay? Let's see when a good time would be. (Takes out the calendar and confers with Mrs. Keene on dates and times.)*

Critical Thinking Challenges

• Decide who Patty thought was her client and who Jeannette thought was her client. • Explain the importance of the information that Patty elicited from Mrs. Keene about the social aspects of their lives. • Contrast this to Jeannette's approach. • Evaluate the difference and give your reasons. • Describe what you think the relationship was between each nurse and Mrs. Keene.

Newborn and Infant

The newborn and infant are totally dependent on others for their needs; a lower form of communication is designed to make these needs known to the caregiver. Crying is a form of communication. The newborn's needs must be met promptly, gently, and consistently to lay a foundation of basic trust.

Bonding is essential to the development of basic trust. The primary caregiver is the infant's lifeline. Through this consistent relationship, the infant learns to differentiate self from others, to communicate, and to relate to others. Even young infants respond differently to strangers (Emde, et al., 1976; Field, et al., 1984). Around the age of 9 months, infants become more fearful of strangers, especially if strangers are intrusive. The nurse should approach babies in a gentle but secure manner, allowing time for the baby to become accustomed to the nurse. Touch is an important factor in communicating with infants.

Language skills begin with cooing, smiling, and crying and progress to vocalizations that express various emotional states (Hetherington & Parke, 1993). During the babbling period, sounds are produced that form the basis of any language. As the baby matures, he or she begins to understand language and uses words to communicate. A baby's first words usually are spoken at the end of the first year. The baby also uses gestures such as pointing or tugging at an adult.

Toddler and Preschooler

Children vary in their rate of language acquisition, but there is a uniformity in the way all children acquire language. Language is acquired not only in terms of learning principles but through biologic, environmental, and cognitive factors. A serious change or interruption in any part of these can affect a child's acquisition of language (Harrison, 1990).

By the time an infant becomes a toddler, he or she has transformed vocalizations and gestures into words to express himself or herself. At 3 years of age, a child has about 900 words in his or her vocabulary, and can form simple sentences (Hetherington & Parke, 1993).

Another means of expression for children is play. Through play, children learn, explore their environment, develop socially, and learn to cope with stressful situations. Opportunities for play include age-appropriate toys, playmates, and a safe environment.

Child and Adolescent

Children and adolescents are social beings who seek out and need relationships with peers. As they move into the teenage years, they adopt the norms and language uses of their peer group. Communication with peers takes priority over communication with adults. Yet at the same time, children and adolescents need adult guidance and protection. During illness, peer relationships provide support and companionship.

Adult and Older Adult

Adults depend on communication for dealing instrumentally with the world, managing careers and vocations, maintaining relationships, and carrying out their various roles. Communication conveys thoughts, feelings, and the innermost aspects of the human experience.

As a person ages, communication becomes increasingly challenged. Diminished vision and hearing are common and can interfere with effective communication. Because these senses usually diminish gradually, older adults develop compensatory mechanisms for adapting to the changes and to the resulting effect on communication.

Altered Communication

Communication can be impaired by anything that alters brain functioning (such as interrupted circulation, trauma, pressure, or drugs) or impairs articulation and phonation. When there has been an interruption or damage to the speech centers of the brain, communication, both spoken and written, is impaired. The impairment may

Nursing Research
Impaired Communication

Selected Nursing Research Studies

Buckwalter, K. C., Cusack, D., Kruckeberg, T., & Shoemaker, A. (1991). Family involvement with communication-impaired residents in long-term care settings. *Applied Nursing Research, 4*(2), 77–84.

Loughrey, L. (1992). The effects of two teaching techniques on recognition and use of function words by aphasic stroke patients. *Rehabilitation Nursing, 17*(3), 134–137.

Mahoney, D. F. (1992). Hearing loss among nursing home residents: Perceptions and realities. *Clinical Nursing Research, 1,* 317–332.

Possible Topics for Nursing Inquiry

- What are indicators of role alterations in people with impaired verbal communication?
- What form of communication is most effective in dealing with clients in a coma?
- What nursing interventions contribute to effective communication with clients experiencing temporary loss of verbal speech?

be either temporary or permanent, depending on the degree of injury. Temporary dysfunction in communication results from reversible injuries to the speech and cognition centers of the brain or to the organs of speech. Permanent impairment in communication occurs when the speech centers of the brain or the organs of speech have been irreversibly injured.

Temporary or permanent interruptions in communication abilities affect relationships with others. Clear communication facilitates a person's carrying out the various roles with family, coworkers, and others. Relationships depend on communication and the interchange of information. When communication is altered, the ability to carry out usual roles becomes less effective.

Potential for Altered Communication

Impaired Speech Apparatus

Functional impairment of the speech apparatus of the larynx, the ability to move air, the use of the tongue and the oral pharynx, and the innervation to each of these structures may alter communication. Cancer of the throat is probably the major risk for impaired phonation. If detected early, cancer of the larynx can be treated with radiation or surgery limited to the exact site; however, extensive malignancies require removal of the whole larynx and the creation of a permanent tracheostoma (external opening to the trachea). Neurologic impairment or muscular dysfunction also have the potential for affecting communication.

Disturbed Articulation

Incoordination or decreased movements of muscles required for articulation can be related to cortical, cerebellar, or cranial nerve dysfunction or from effects of drugs such as alcohol, sedatives, or other medications.

People who have a high cervical (C2, C3 quadriplegia) injury have a permanent tracheostomy and cannot speak because no air will be forced through the vocal cords. They also require ventilatory support. Other neurologic conditions, such as amyotrophic lateral sclerosis, multiple sclerosis, and myasthenia gravis, may also lead to inability to speak because of loss of muscle function. These conditions may also necessitate a tracheostomy or ventilatory assistance, depending on the severity of the disease. Clients with these diseases have lost the muscle function needed for them to breathe on their own.

Cortical Control Interference

Any substance or event that clouds the sensorium or interferes with usual cortical functioning alters many normal functions, including communication.

Drug Use. Pharmacotherapeutic agents of many types can inhibit or interfere with higher cortical functions. These agents include prescription drugs, alcohol, and illicit drugs. In the early stages or with moderate to heavy dosages, the person may experience impairment in motor control of speech (slowness and slurring) and in comprehension and expression (inability to think of the correct word or response).

Overdosage of drugs potentially can inactivate the speech centers of the brain along with the motor activity required to carry out communication. The degree of damage to these centers determines whether the altered communication is temporary (until the effects of the drug wear off) or permanent. An example of controlled drug use that temporarily interferes with communication is administration of an anesthetic agent, which when appropriately controlled is metabolized by the body in an expected period of time, after which the client's communication abilities return.

Stroke. In the United States, approximately 500,000 people per year have a stroke; approximately 144,000 of those die. Seventy-two percent of those who suffer a stroke are older than 65 years of age; it affects all races, both sexes, and all socioeconomic levels (American Heart Association, 1994). Approximately 20% of all surviving stroke victims need the specialized services of a speech pathologist to help them regain communication skills. The other 80% have only minor or temporary damage to the language centers of the brain (Gresham & Weiss, 1993). The location of the insult and the extent of damage affect the pattern and severity of the speech impairment.

Head Trauma. About 7 million head injuries are estimated to occur annually in the United States, with about 500,000 people admitted to the hospital (Rosenthal, et al., 1990). Most seriously injured clients have major disabilities. Because there are rarely specific injury sites, classification of brain injury and prediction of outcome are difficult. The study of communication disorders secondary to head trauma is in the initial stages. The more severe the head injury, the more likely there is an interruption in communication. Communication problems in head-injured clients are usually compounded by impairments in cognitive function, such as behavior, memory, orientation, and attention.

Coma. **Coma** or **comatose** describes people who do not communicate or make meaningful responses to stimuli and who do not open their eyes to stimuli. This rapid change in level of consciousness can occur from slow-growing mass lesions (eg, chronic accumulation of fluid or tumor), metabolic problems (eg, alterations in serum glucose), or from trauma (eg, rupture or occlusion of a blood vessel, bleeding, or edema). Altered communication may be either temporary or permanent, depending on the severity of damage from whatever is causing the comatose condition. The person may recover with little or no long-term effects on communication, or may have to learn alternate methods of communication.

Manifestations of Altered Communication

Aphasia

Aphasia is the complete or partial loss of all language modalities, including an understanding of speech (auditory comprehension), reading, speaking, writing, arithmetic, and expression through pantomime. It is an acquired dysfunction of communication that is the result of brain damage, but it does not affect intelligence. Aphasias are produced mostly through damage to the cortical language areas of the dominant left hemisphere (see Fig. 48-1). Rarely, an injury affects one isolated area of speech, but usually all speech and language functions are affected. Aphasia could develop in anyone who incurs a brain injury or insult. The most common cause of aphasia is related to an interruption in circulation as a result of a cerebral vascular accident (stroke). Approximately 85,000 new cases of aphasia occur in the United States each year from stroke alone (Albert & Helm-Estabrooks, 1988a). Significant improvement in speech and communication occurs in the first 6 months and can continue up to 18 months after the onset of aphasia (Nicholas, et al., 1993).

The manifestation of speech impairment depends on the location and the extent of damage and can range from slight slurring of speech to total loss of communication. Aphasia has been described and categorized based on lesion location and linguistic deficit (Albert & Helm-Estabrooks, 1988a, 1988b; Mitchell, et al., 1988). The four most common types of aphasia are expressive (Broca's), receptive (Wernicke's), anomic, and global (Table 48-1).

Expressive Aphasia. Expressive aphasia (also called Broca's, motor, and nonfluent aphasia) is characterized by limited speech that is slow and halting with great effort, reduced grammar, and poor articulation. The person knows what he or she wants to say, but cannot find the words needed. Problems with word retrieval are called **anomia**. In expressive aphasia, the person's speech often sounds like a telegraph message, consists of isolated or small groups of words, and lacks tone or inflection.

Because intellect is not necessarily impaired, aphasic clients know what they want to say but are unable to say it correctly. This leads to an extreme sense of frustration and anger. Sometimes the anger shows in physical behaviors, such as pushing objects or people away and shouting. Often the anger is directed at those people who are closest to the client. This behavior makes it difficult for the spouse or significant others to understand what is happening to the client.

Writing is also affected and can be as severely, or more severely, impaired than speech.

Receptive Aphasia. Fluent aphasia (also called Wernicke's, sensory, and receptive aphasia) is characterized by speech that is well articulated, has good melody, and has a normal or slightly faster rate. The major manifestations are impaired auditory comprehension and feedback and fluent or hyperfluent, well-articulated, paraphasic speech. Such clients have difficulty understanding spoken and written words. They talk a great deal, but they often do not make sense and their speech lacks specific content. Their ability to read, write, listen, concentrate, or follow instructions is impaired; the level of severity is usually consistent with or worse than the speech impairment.

The client is unaware of the language impairment and appears euphoric in relation to their language problems. They display little frustration because they are unaware of any problem.

These clients also have a host of symptoms referred to as a right hemisphere syndrome. They often display a neglect of the paralyzed side of their body, even to the point of not knowing that their left arm or leg is really theirs. Behaviorally, these clients are impulsive, lack insight into their deficits, and have poor judgment. Often they are said to have inappropriate behavior, when actually their behavior is a result of their injury. The combination of these symptoms and behaviors

Table 48-1 • Expression and Comprehension With Major Types of Aphasia

Types of Aphasia	Oral Expression	Written Expression	Comprehension
Expressive (Broca's or motor)	Nonfluent, telegraphic	Limited	Usually good
Receptive (Wernicke's or sensory)	Fluent, speech well articulated, disorganized content	Impaired	Impaired
Anomic	Speech fluent, talks around the subject	Variable, mild to severe impairment	Variable, mild to severe impairment
Global	Speech very poor, meaningless recurrent sounds	Severely impaired	Severely impaired

makes language rehabilitation and rehabilitation in general difficult.

Anomic Aphasia. Anomic or amnesic aphasia is characterized predominantly by word-finding problems of a milder nature than expressive aphasia. The speech is fluent and grammatically correct. The communication difficulties arise in using the correct names for particular objects, people, places, or events. If the client cannot remember the correct name, they talk about the subject until the listener understands what they mean. Auditory comprehension is generally good, although the levels of reading and writing impairment are variable and can range from mild to severe. Behaviorally, these clients display anger, frustration, and depression in ways similar to clients with expressive aphasia.

Global Aphasia. Global aphasia results from severe and extensive damage to all language areas (Broca's and Wernicke's) of the brain. These clients have no consistent functional skills in any of the language modalities. They cannot speak or understand speech, nor can they read or write. Some clients' speech consists of meaningless, recurrent sounds.

Dysarthria

Dysarthria is a totally separate speech disorder. **Dysarthria** refers to a group of speech disorders that result from a disturbance of motor control, weakness, paralysis, or incoordination of the oral musculature. The disorder is a result of damage to the central or peripheral nervous system. Clients with dysarthria usually have normal auditory comprehension and can select and order words correctly. They do not have a language problem but rather a motor speech disorder. This disorder causes them to have difficulty saying words and sounds precisely with appropriate stress, loudness, pitch, and control. The result is speech that is described as "slurred," "heavy," or unclear. There are numerous types of dysarthria. The specific type depends on the site of the neurologic lesion.

Total Loss of Speech

Cancer of the larynx is the most common cause of loss of functioning of the larynx. A **laryngectomy** is the result. Clients who have had a total laryngectomy have had the larynx removed and also the tissues in the area known as the Adam's apple. After the larynx is removed, there is no ability to produce sound and, thus, no ability to speak. The loss of speech is permanent.

Clients who have had a permanent **tracheostomy** (incision through the neck to create a permanent opening in the trachea) have the same difficulty communicating as the client with a laryngectomy (Fig. 48-3). Some may be able to "mouth" words; others may be able only to blink their eyes in response to yes or no questions. Intellectual functions are not impaired, however.

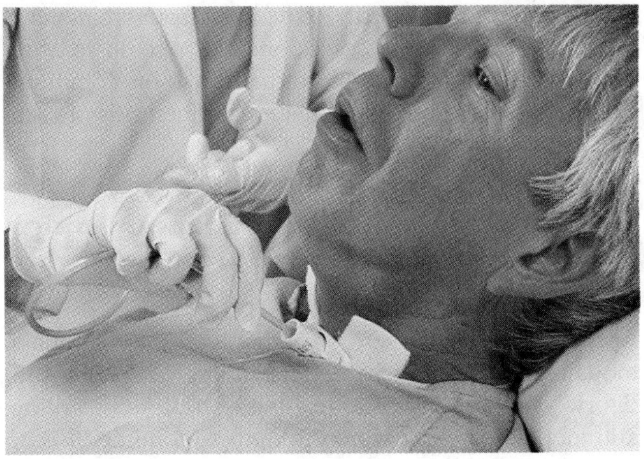

Figure 48-3 • *The presence of a tracheostomy tube alters verbal communication.*

Loss of function of the larynx can occur temporarily if a **tracheotomy** is required for emergency care and respiratory ventilation. With a tracheotomy, air is diverted through the tracheotomy tube to outside of the body without passing through the larynx. To have laryngeal speech, the person would need to block the tracheotomy tube and allow air to pass through the larynx. After the emergency has subsided and before the temporary tracheotomy tube is removed, this is the action that is used to produce speech. Ultimately, with the removal of the tracheotomy tube, the person can resume usual laryngeal speech.

Impact on Activities of Daily Living

Individual Considerations

The ability of the person to perform activities of daily living and to participate in usual roles and relationships depends on the degree of impairment to communication. For example, a person whose career depends on speech production and written expression finds that role impaired if he or she has an aphasic dysfunction. People with altered communication may become frustrated with trying to express what they need in relation to hygiene, nutrition, and activities. The affected person may experience problems with continence directly as a result of the difficulty of communicating the need to urinate or defecate.

Some types of aphasia interfere with more than communication. With a specific type of brain damage, the person may also neglect one side of the body. The person may need reminding and assisting in grooming the neglected side of the body and in communicating needs related to that side of the body. Eating may be a problem as well if the person is unable to see or is unaware of half of the food that is presented.

Because communication is inseparably integrated with perceptual processes, many people with a communication dysfunction are not able to be independent. These people need support for their activities of daily living through the provision of a structured environment and around-the-clock assistance.

Family Considerations

Relationships depend on an interchange of ideas, thoughts, and feelings. The person with altered communication is unable to convey ideas, thoughts, and feelings as clearly, resulting in less intimacy and clarity. When this occurs with friends and acquaintances, they often find it easier to end the relationship or to make it more distant rather than try to bridge the communication problem. Families usually work hard to maintain communication and relationships, although it often becomes a strain on that relationship as well.

Home maintenance activities such as banking, food shopping, paying bills, and meal preparation are difficult, if not impossible for a person alone, because these instrumental activities require the communication skills of arithmetic, reading, writing, and spelling. Depending on the degree of dysfunction, the person may be able to do light meal preparation and light housekeeping tasks, but may be unable to do heavy housecleaning and laundry without the assistance of family.

Assessment

The ability to communicate is vital to survival. Without communication, a person's physical and psychological health suffers. When encountering a client with a communication problem, the nurse must rapidly assess the client's communication difficulties and take appropriate steps to intervene. It is particularly important when assessing a client with communication difficulties to remain attentive and be patient when the person is attempting to communicate (Braverman, 1990; McClenahan, et al., 1990). This places the person at ease and encourages the client to initiate communication.

Subjective Data

The collection of subjective information helps the nurse identify the normal pattern of communication and relationships for the client, any risk factors that may predispose the client to alterations in roles and relationships related to communication dysfunction, and any actual dysfunctions in communication, roles, and relationships. If the client cannot communicate, family or friends may need to provide data regarding communication patterns and abilities.

Functional Pattern Identification

The nurse usually begins the assessment of a person's communication status and ability by obtaining or reviewing his or her history. In this process, the nurse gains an understanding of the person's normal communication and roles and any factors that may predispose the person to altered communication and relationships.

To determine the client's current communication pattern, the nurse needs to obtain data from the client and significant others. An assessment of the client's ability to communicate should include not only asking questions, but an assessment of general level of alertness, appropriateness, and emotional state. Assessment of the person's speech patterns and comprehension ability is an important component of the subjective data.

General assessment can begin with an evaluation of how the client seems to feel about the dysfunction and how the family and significant others view the alteration in communication. Does the client seem distressed by the inability to communicate, or does the client appear unconcerned or unaware of a difficulty in communication? Does the communication impairment pose a problem for the spouse or significant other? Is there a disturbance in the person's roles and relationships as a result of the altered communication? Among the questions that the nurse needs to ask are those listed in the accompanying display. Answers to these questions aid the nurse in determining the client's previous patterns of communication. To determine the type of communication disorder that the client is experiencing, the nurse needs to assess verbal expression, written expression, comprehension, and nonverbal expression. Table 48-1 defines the expected comprehension and verbal and written expression for the four major types of aphasia.

Communication abilities to assess for in the major types of aphasia are also delineated in the display. Answers to these questions aid the nurse in determining the degree of the client's communication dysfunction. As the nurse clarifies the alterations in communication, the presence of or potential for disturbances in roles and relationships becomes apparent. This information assists in developing an individual plan of care.

Risk Identification

The client's history and observed dysfunction may give the nurse information as to whether communication is altered and whether roles and relationships are affected. Clients with brain damage from stroke or head injury, impaired speech apparatus (eg, laryngectomy or tracheotomy), and other temporary dysfunctions such as

Nursing Assessment
Initial Assessment Concerns About Communication

Is the person able to speak at all?
If so, is the speech intelligible and appropriate to the situation?
Does the person use gestures or point in an effort to communicate?
Is the person literate?
How much formal education does the person have?
Is the person able to speak another language?
Can the person understand and follow simple one-step commands?
Did the person have a speech difficulty before this most recent difficulty?
Was the person previously an active conversationalist, or did he or she prefer to listen?

Assessment for Major Types of Aphasia

Verbal Expression

Does the person speak easily, fluently?
Is the content appropriate in context?
Does the person initiate speech on his or her own?
Is the speech telegraphic (short, choppy)?
Is the speech organized?
Does the verbal output contain recurrent sounds?
Does the person name objects correctly?
Does the person repeat words and phrases easily?

Written Expression

Can the person write own name and address correctly?
Can the person produce a short narrative written paragraph?
Does the written product have appropriate meaning?

Comprehension

Does the person give any indication of hearing impairment?
Does the person answer simple, open-ended questions appropriately?
Does the person answer yes/no questions in appropriate context?
Can the person correctly point to an object that has been named?
Does the person respond appropriately to simple commands?

Nonverbal Expression

Observe for the type of effect (sign of emotion):
- Flat—no sign of emotion
- Labile—wide fluctuation in emotions

Observe gestures for appropriateness to the situation.
Observe for the integrated context of voice tone, emotional expression, body movement.

drug overdosage and comatose states are at greatest risk for communication impairment. The presence of pathophysiologic factors such as cerebral, neurologic, respiratory, or auditory impairments, and laryngeal infection or edema places the person at high risk for altered communication. Other factors for which the nurse needs to assess are endotracheal intubation, pain medication, oral–facial deformities, and speech problems such as stuttering or lisping, or a language barrier. The inability to communicate clearly and effectively places the person at risk for interruption of roles and relationships (Fig. 48-4). Last, factors such as shyness and lack of privacy and support can be significant barriers to communication and cannot be ignored as causes for impaired communication and altered relationships.

Dysfunction Identification

The nurse can use the subjective data collected to help identify role and relationship dysfunctions related to communication impairment. Actual communication impairments demonstrate aspects of impaired verbal, written, and nonverbal expression and comprehension. The client or family can provide information regarding the degree of difference from normal patterns of communication. Subjective data need to be validated with objective information gained through the physical assessment and the evaluation of diagnostic results before the actual diagnosis is made.

Objective Data

In addition to gathering subjective data, the nurse also collects objective data concerning the client's communication abilities through physical assessment of the client and reviewing related tests.

Physical Assessment

The mouth, tongue, and facial muscles are required to form and articulate words correctly. The client with altered communication related to impaired motor functioning or brain damage needs to have a thorough assessment of the muscles and organs of speech. Table 21-3 lists assessment methods for cranial nerves.

The tongue receives its motor innervation from the twelfth cranial nerve (hypoglossal). Motor control of the

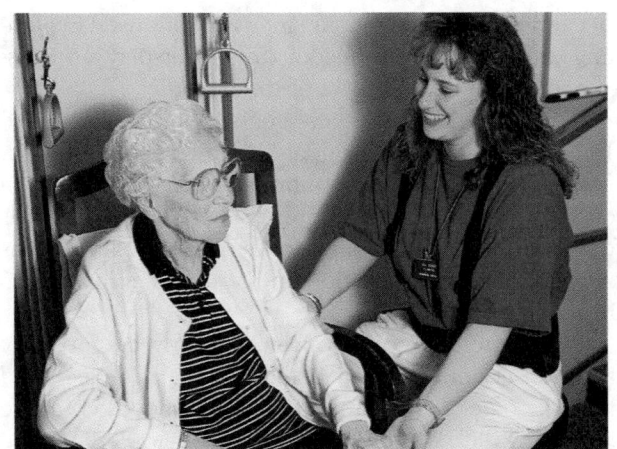

Figure 48-4 • *An older person with impaired verbal communication may be at risk for sensory deprivation.*

tongue can be assessed through instructing the client to protrude his or her tongue. If there is damage to the hypoglossal nerve, the tongue deviates to the side of the weakness as a result of the strong side pushing the tongue forward unopposed.

The muscles of the face are innervated by the fifth (trigeminal) and seventh (facial) cranial nerves. The motor function of these nerves can be assessed by noting symmetry of facial movement when the client is asked to show teeth, purse lips, and frown. When the client's face is at rest, asymmetry of the forehead or cheeks should be noted, along with facial drooping or drooling. A palpable change in the muscle mass of the face may be identified that corresponds with a change in symmetry.

The muscles of swallowing and the gag reflex are supplied by the ninth (glossopharyngeal), tenth (vagus), and eleventh (accessory) cranial nerves. The larynx is supplied by the tenth cranial nerve alone. Motor weakness of the soft palate contributes to difficulty in swallowing (dysphagia). Swallowing difficulties may be identified by history as well as by physical assessment. To test for swallowing, the client should be asked to swallow chips of ice. The ice gives some substance for the client to manipulate in the mouth, yet if he or she is unable to swallow successfully, it introduces only water.

The presence of the gag reflex can be assessed by lightly touching a tongue blade to one side of the palatal arch and then the other. An absence of the gag reflex can be caused by nerve damage.

Impairment in the use of the larynx is immediately obvious in the presence of an endotracheal tube or tracheostomy or a ventilator. Because the movement of air bypasses the laryngeal function, the client is unable to communicate verbally. The nurse needs to assess if the client is able to use other modes of communication, such as gestures, codes using eye blinks or hands, or written notes.

Indications of motor impairment validate communication alterations observed in the subjective data. Linking the identified objective and subjective data assists in defining the specific problem and appropriate care.

Diagnostic Tests and Procedures

The client with altered communication is evaluated by a speech pathologist, who does a detailed assessment of speech, expression, and comprehension. The results of this assessment contribute to the plan of care and to establishing communication with the client.

Nursing Diagnoses

The accepted North American Nursing Diagnosis Association (NANDA) nursing diagnosis for a client with communication problems is Impaired Verbal Communication. The diagnosis can be further divided into specific categories based on the cause and defining characteristics.

Diagnostic Statement: Impaired Verbal Communication

Definition

Impaired Verbal Communication is the state in which an individual experiences a decreased or absent ability to use or understand language in human interaction (NANDA, 1994).

Defining Characteristics

The client is unable to speak dominant language that is the person's first language (eg, English, Spanish); speaks or verbalizes with difficulty; or does not or cannot speak. Stuttering; slurring words; having difficulty forming words or sentences; or having difficulty expressing thought verbally are also characteristics. The client exhibits inappropriate verbalization (saying things out of context or with wrong meanings), dyspnea (difficulty breathing), and disorientation as to time, place, or person (NANDA, 1994).

Related Factors

Related factors that may contribute to the client's diagnosis include decrease in circulation to the brain from interference to vascular circulation; or brain tumor. Physical barriers (tracheostomy, intubation) that prevent normal air movement through the vocal cords; anatomic defect, such as cleft palate, that mechanically interferes with speech; or psychological barriers (psychosis, lack of stimuli) may be related to the communication problems. In addition, cultural differences, in which culture defines the meaning of the communication, and developmental or age-related factors may limit communication (NANDA, 1994).

Related Nursing Diagnoses

Because communication alterations may interfere with roles and relationships, related nursing diagnoses include Altered Family Processes, Altered Parenting, Parental Role Conflict, Altered Role Performance, Impaired Social Interactions, Social Isolation, and Grieving. The specific disturbances in roles and relationships determines which, if any, of these related diagnoses are appropriate to consider.

Outcome Identification and Planning

After nursing diagnoses and related factors have been identified, the nurse and client (or family) make plans for care. Examples of nursing interventions used in planning are listed in the accompanying display and discussed in the next section of the chapter.

The formulation of client goals should include both short-term and long-term goals. Short-term goals are directed at establishing a communication system that allows the client to have basic needs met. Long-term goals focus on the client's ability to live with the limitations of impaired communication and accept the changes in lifestyle and self-concept.

The potential complication with any diagnosis of impaired communication is that the client's basic and immediate needs may go unmet. These needs could be essential to life or could be fairly routine. Perhaps the most traumatic complication is the social isolation that comes from being unable to express one's thoughts, feelings, or emotions. This inability to express one's self often manifests itself in anger, rage, depression, or withdrawal. These behaviors may also be seen in the spouse, family, or significant others who have also lost the ability to communicate and are experiencing an interruption in relationships.

Planning
Examples of Nursing Interventions for Common Communication Problems

Impaired Verbal Communication

- Establish a calm, structured environment.
- Maintain a consistent approach with the client, using a normal tone of voice.
- Address the client by name and speak to person as an adult.
- Ask the client to repeat words that are unclear.
- Allow the client adequate time for response and for speech.
- Ask only questions that require short answers.
- Promote use of alternate means to express self, such as gestures, pointing to pictures or a wordboard, or writing.
- Teach family to communicate with the client at appropriate rates of speed and only one person at a time.

Impaired Hearing Ability

- Limit environmental interferences by minimizing noise from equipment, loudspeakers, and visitors.
- Establish contact with the client to focus the client's attention before speaking.
- Speak slower and distinctly without excessive loudness.
- Use visual cues along with speech to enhance understanding.
- Assist the client in referral for or in obtaining assistive listening devices.

Comprehension Deficits

- Orient the client to time, place, and person.
- Establish a calm, structured environment and routine.
- Keep distractions at a minimum.
- Remove unnecessary items from the client's visual field so that he or she can focus on the task at hand.
- Turn off the television or radio.
- Monitor the client for safety. Do not overestimate the client's abilities.
- Address the client by name and introduce yourself when entering room.
- Ask questions or give information in small segments.
- Listen patiently to content and context of responses.
- Redirect the client frequently to the task at hand. It may be necessary to move into the client's visual field to get his or her attention.
- Break tasks into small steps.
- Use auditory and visual cues. Repeat the names of objects as they are touched.
- Gently correct errors.
- Reorient frequently.
- Encourage socialization activities that are not overstimulating.
- Limit the number of visitors at one time.
- Instruct family and visitors to have only one person talk to the client at one time; do not carry on more than one conversation.

Examples of short-term goals for the client with impaired verbal communication include

The client will communicate basic needs.
The client will demonstrate improved ability to express self.
The client will demonstrate increased ability to understand.
The client will verbalize experiencing less frustration with communication.

Implementation

A central focus of nursing implementation for the client with impaired verbal communication is preventing alterations in roles and relationships and supporting effective relationships. Relationships are affected by the ability to communicate effectively thoughts, feelings, needs, and other intimate aspects of life. When one's ability to understand other people's communications and to respond verbally to those communications is disrupted, the usual relationship with those people is also disrupted. Nursing interventions need to reflect recognition of those relationships and of their importance to the client as an individual.

Nursing Interventions to Promote Health and Function

Through general health promotion, the nurse provides guidance for optimum health and communication and helps minimize dysfunctional relationships. Client teaching revolves around the causes of impaired communication. Prevention of cerebrovascular disease and accidents causing trauma to the brain or muscles of the speech organs are high on the agenda.

Client Teaching

Preventing cardiovascular disease, which can lead to cerebrovascular disorders, has several aspects that each person can personally influence. Prevention initially involves exercise and a low-fat diet (see Chapters 33 and 37). A dietitian should be consulted to help the client plan menus, change recipes, and learn to read labels on food. A regular program of exercise should be developed after consultation with a physician. Serum cholesterol should be monitored regularly to determine the effects of following a low-fat diet and an exercise program. Clients who have high blood pressure should be encouraged to maintain their current medication regimen, to check their blood pressure routinely, and to follow up with their physician.

Smoking increases the chance of heart disease and throat cancer. The nurse can educate the client about the numerous health risks associated with smoking. Clients should be encouraged to quit, and often find that support of some type is useful. Early warning signs of throat cancer are nagging cough and chronic hoarseness. Awareness of the warning signals can be helpful for early detection or prevention.

> **Client Teaching**
> *Health Promotion*
>
> *Instruct the client as follows:*
> - *Stop smoking to prevent cerebrovascular disease.*
> - *Wear seatbelts to avoid head injury.*
> - *Use helmets for biking and skateboarding to prevent head trauma.*
> - *Swim with a buddy in case help is needed and to prevent injury.*
> - *Do not dive into shallow or unknown waters to prevent spinal cord injury.*
> - *Avoid alcohol and drug use to protect cerebral function.*
> - *Eat a low-fat diet to minimize the occurrence of cardiovascular disease.*
> - *Plan a regular regimen of exercise to promote cardiovascular fitness.*
> - *Monitor blood pressure and serum cholesterol regularly to avoid vascular disorders.*
> - *Continue taking prescribed medications unless the physician has been consulted.*

The most frequent causes of communication impairment in young adults are brain injuries and spinal cord injuries. Eighty percent of spinal cord injuries occur before the age of 40 years (Porth, 1994). Motor vehicle accidents account for nearly half of all head injuries in the 15- to 24-year-old age group (National Safety Council, 1994). The brain-injured adult can experience aphasia or dysarthria; spinal cord-injured clients could require a temporary or permanent tracheostomy depending on the level of their injury.

Drug use contributes to the potential for impairment in communication and relationships. Experimenting with drugs (eg, alcohol, marijuana, cocaine) may begin during school-age years and adolescence and may impair school roles and family relationships. Programs of drug education are increasing in numbers and in community support. Nurses need to serve as role models by actively supporting these programs.

Because of their age, young adults tend to engage in sports and activities that may place them at greater risk for injury. Yet this group is often resistant to preventive education. A public safety awareness program stressing helmet use with motorcycles, use of seatbelts, use of proper protective sports equipment, and the avoidance of alcohol and drugs may help in reducing injuries. Prevention programs that start in the elementary schools may be the most effective in preventing unsafe behavior.

Nursing Interventions for Altered Communication Function

The plan of care developed by the nurse assists the client with the ability to express needs and feelings to the nurse, family, and others. Nursing interventions need to be directed toward maintaining communication and relationships (Adkins, 1991).

Orientation to Surroundings

The nurse needs to have special consideration for the client who has difficulty with understanding, such as those with fluent or Wernicke's aphasia. The client who is experiencing impaired communication may also be experiencing some confusion related to this unfamiliar state. Maintaining a structured environment assists the client in adapting to this alteration and in reestablishing communication. The presence of a calendar and a clock large enough to be seen by the client and kept current assists the client in orientation to time.

A structured routine minimizes the number of factors on which the client must focus. Sequenced events, a consistent daily schedule, a calendar, and frequent orientation to the schedule contribute to structure for the client. Predictability in the environment allows the client to conserve energy for the communication impairment and its related relationship difficulties.

The nurse must orient these clients to person, place, and time. To assist with orientation, ask the client why he or she is in this healthcare facility, or where he or she is, gently correcting a false answer. Encourage the person to look to the affected side by approaching from the affected side and calling the client's name. Refer to the client's body parts on the affected side, having the client rub or touch the affected side. When the client is eating, encourage the client to look for food on the tray on the affected side and make sure that food is not pocketed in the affected cheek. Keep the client oriented to task by constantly cueing him or her to what he or she is doing. The client may be impulsive and have poor judgment; therefore, do not take the client's word that he or she can do an activity; watch him or her do it.

Alternative Communication Methods

The nurse needs to develop a plan of care that provides the client with Broca's or nonfluent aphasia with an effective, efficient means with which to communicate. The client who has difficulty speaking may benefit from having others use gestures and facial expressions to give additional clues. Encourage the client to use any means available to express himself or herself. Other methods of communication that may be helpful include offering the client pictures at which to point, having the client use gestures, or letting the client show you what he or she wants. The client's writing and reading skills may be impaired along with speech, and therefore these skills may not be useful alternatives.

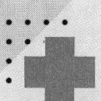

> **Safety Alert**
> *Altered Communication*
>
> - Remove clutter or unnecessary items from the client's room or bed table.
> - Orient client to surroundings.
> - Place call button within client's reach.
> - Encourage the client to use any means available to express self and needs.
> - Develop a system for signaling emergencies.
> - Be sure you understand the client's method for communication.
> - Do not pressure the client if he or she is tired.
> - Do not allow clients to perform activities by themselves unless you have observed them perform the activity and are sure they can perform the activity alone safely.
> - Keep the tracheostomy stoma clean and clear.

If it is difficult to understand what the client has said, be honest and let the client know. Ask the client to try again and perhaps use gestures to assist with understanding. If the client tries again and you still do not understand, take a rest, and come back to it in a few minutes. Do not pressure the client; some symptoms get worse if the client is fatigued, upset, or anxious. Be alert to the client's daily schedule, and allow for adequate rest at night and naps during the day.

For clients who have lost the ability to produce sound because of a laryngectomy, communication may be restored through the use of sophisticated electronic or computer communication devices or an electronic larynx. In these cases, it is useful for the nurse to know how to use these devices.

As a result of increasingly sophisticated computer technology, "adaptive computing" (professional services and the technology that make computing technology accessible for people with disabilities) has become more common. Clients with disabilities, such as visual, mobility, hearing, learning, and communication disorders, may benefit from computer adaptations (Merrow & Corbett, 1994).

The Client With a Laryngectomy. Clients who are to undergo a laryngectomy should address the issue of communication before surgery. The clients should be given a choice of how they wish to communicate—by wordboard, flashcards, or writing. This method should be delineated explicitly in the care plan. It would be beneficial for the client to practice lip speaking (forming words with the mouth). By addressing before surgery how the client wishes to communicate, the anxiety level is greatly reduced. The nurse also needs to watch the speaker's lips, because articulation should not be affected by surgery. The client should be referred to a speech therapist for either esophageal speech or an electronic larynx. If the client already is using esophageal speech, extraneous environmental noise should be eliminated because esophageal speech is quieter and less intelligible than normal speech. The client who uses esophageal speech has a low-pitched monotone with no melody to phrases. The client also has no air reservoir, so there are short burps of speech. Gestures may enhance speech and communication. Learning to use esophageal speech or an electronic larynx can be frustrating, yet, once the client has adapted to using a new communication system, there are few restrictions on his or her ability to perform activities of daily living.

Clients with a laryngectomy need to learn a new breathing system as well as how to keep the stoma open and clean. Clients may shower using a stoma shield, but they cannot swim. If there are no other physical difficulties, the client should be able to return to work and home management (Keith & Darley, 1994).

The Client With a Tracheostomy. The client who has a temporary tracheostomy or is temporarily intubated should be reassured that he or she will be able to talk again once the tube is removed. Often the client is hoarse for a period of time after tube removal. While the client is intubated, a temporary communication system should be agreed on by the nurse and client, using whatever means are available.

The client who has a permanent tracheostomy and is ventilator dependent may have limited resources to implement a communication system. Often these clients have neuromuscular or neurologic diseases, which limit their ability to use gestures, write, or point. Lip speaking or an eye blink are usually the only means of communication (Connolly & Shekleton, 1991). The Passy-Muir valve, a speaking valve for tracheostomies, is one alternative for enhancing communication skill in children with long-term tracheostomies (Jackson & Albamonte, 1994).

The Client With Dysarthria. The client who has impaired verbal communication related to dysarthria has slow, slurred speech that is difficult to understand. To facilitate communication with these clients, the nurse should face the client to read his or her lips. Communication could be augmented by gestures, written messages, a communication board, or flashcards. The client should be encouraged to slow speech, to speak louder, and to take a breath between sentences. Ask the client to repeat words that are unclear. If the client appears fatigued, ask only questions that require short answers. Some of these clients may have highly specialized computer equipment for communication, but this is an exception more than the norm. Establishing a specific care plan and a routine for delivering care reduces the amount of time the client would otherwise need to explain his or her care to others.

Environmental Restrictions

The number of visitors with whom the client has to communicate may add to the level of frustration for the client with impaired verbal communication. Increased numbers of people and noise in the environment can interfere with cognitive function and understanding. A quiet environment allows the client to focus on understanding and on speaking or communicating.

The nurse may find that environmental restrictions are advantageous in assisting communication with the client. Be aware of excessive noise levels caused by equipment, loudspeaker systems, or other clients. Limit the number of visitors present at any given time. Teach visitors how to communicate with the client, such as only one person speaking at a time and avoiding carrying on another conversation simultaneously in the room.

Coping Measures

The nurse can assist the client with Broca's or nonfluent aphasia in coping with impaired communication by explaining to the client what happened, that they had a stroke, that the stroke causes language problems, and that anger and sadness are normal reactions. Clients need to understand and be prepared for wide emotional swings (lability), which are common and decrease with recovery. The nurse should remain calm and not show a negative reaction to the outburst if it occurs, but rather give calm, quiet reassurance and support.

The client who understands what has occurred but has great difficulty in expressing self may be at risk for depression. A depressed client may refuse therapy and food and ignore family and friends. Sometimes reassurance is not enough to overcome depressive feelings. The physician needs to be consulted if depression is suspected so that other therapy may be used.

Community-Based Nursing

Planning for maintaining relationships despite alterations in communication begins the day the nurse first assesses the client. In planning for healthcare for such a client, the nurse may consider referrals to a speech pathologist for communication deficits and cognitive evaluation and training. Referral should be made to occupational therapy to plan for activities of daily living, and to physical therapy for mobility evaluation and training. The nurse's thorough assessment provides the physician with an understanding of the necessity of the referrals. The family must be included in assessment and planning (see the accompanying display).

Family Teaching
Clients With Expression Deficits

Instruct the client's family as follows:

- Anticipate the client's needs by asking if he or she needs something so that the client will be less frustrated with trying to communicate.
- Use one- or two-word phrases and simple word commands to simplify the communication process.
- Use gestures with demonstrations to help clarify meaning.
- Encourage the client to speak by allowing him or her enough time to speak so that he or she may regain confidence in speaking.
- Acknowledge the frustration the client displays so that his or her feelings are validated and understanding is expressed.
- Give positive feedback to attempts at speech to encourage the client's efforts.
- Ignore profanity, understanding that it represents an expression of communication disorder.
- Delay conversation with the client if fatigue is apparent because fatigue interferes with communication and speech.
- Speak to the client on an adult level because cognition may be unaffected even with impaired communication.

Because the stay as an inpatient may be short, evaluation of nursing interventions and teaching may not be accomplished in the hospital. Therefore, it is necessary to ensure follow-up through a public health or visiting nurse referral, or to an appropriate clinic or community program. These programs need to adapt the client's care plan based on the needs he or she develops when back in the community.

Community self-help groups, such as Stroke Clubs, The Multiple Sclerosis Society, The National Spinal Cord Injury Society, and The International Association of Laryngectomies, can be beneficial to the client and family in reestablishing and maintaining relationships through communication. These groups offer clients support and provide them with tips to make role adjustment easier and to improve the quality of relationships.

Evaluation

Outcome criteria are the evaluative tools used to measure goal attainment. Nursing interventions allow clients to attain goals. Nursing interventions must be specific to the client goal, although some nursing interventions are applicable to more than one goal.

Goal

The client will communicate basic needs.

Possible Outcome Criteria

- Client demonstrates improved ability to express needs by practicing using a new method (gestures, writing, blinking, or electronic device) with nurse.

Goal

The client will demonstrate improved ability to express self.

Possible Outcome Criteria

- Client engages in spontaneous social interactions and conversations with healthcare personnel and family as observed by nurse before discharge or transfer to home or long-term care.

Goal

The client will demonstrate increased ability to understand directions.

Possible Outcome Criteria

- Client demonstrates an understanding of simple, one-step commands by following through with the given command at the next teaching session with the nurse.

Goal

The client will verbalize experiencing less frustration with communication.

Possible Outcome Criteria

- Client verbalizes to nurse a decrease in frustration with communication problems.
- Client expresses a decrease in feelings of isolation and depression.

The evaluation of the effect of nursing interventions on client goals includes an assessment of the client in relation to the outcome criteria. Continuation, modification, or termination of nursing interventions depends on the assessment. This process may be ongoing depending on the cause of the communication impairment.

Key Concepts

- Disorders in communication can markedly disrupt the quality of life for the person affected and the person's family.
- Speech problems, when they occur, usually result in long-term difficulties and role disruptions, which may never be completely resolved.

Nursing Plan of Care
The Client With Impaired Verbal Communication

Nursing Diagnosis

Impaired Verbal Communication related to decreased cerebral circulation manifested by difficulty in speaking and in expressing comprehension/understanding.

Client Goal

Client will establish an effective means of communication.

Client Outcome Criteria

- Client demonstrates improved ability to express himself or herself.
- Client demonstrates improved ability to understand within 1 week.
- Client experiences decreased frustration with communication.

Nursing Intervention	*Scientific Rationale*
1. Assess the client's ability to comprehend, speak, read and write • Ask simple questions. • Ask the client to repeat single words and sentences. • Have the client name simple objects. • Ask the client to write his or her name or copy a sentence. • Have the client read words or phrases.	1. These exercises help the nurse determine the specific form of aphasia. The specific type of aphasia must be identified before a care plan can be developed.
2. Create an atmosphere that is quiet, relaxed, and supportive.	2. Tension decreases comprehension and inhibits the motor programming for articulation.
• Remove or decrease any extraneous noise.	• Extraneous stimuli decrease attention.
• Speak to the client in a normal tone of voice.	• Increasing the loudness of your speech does not increase comprehension. Hearing loss is not part of the aphasia syndrome.
• Speak on an adult level.	• Aphasia does not affect intelligence.
• Listen to the client and wait for him or her to attempt to communicate.	• Rushing the client by interrupting, finishing sentences, or appearing hurried increases his or her frustration and makes speech even more difficult.
• Establish and maintain eye contact.	• Allows the client to make use of both verbal and nonverbal cues to help in comprehension.
• Assume that the client can understand. Do not talk about the client in his or her presence.	• Shows your client basic respect. Intelligence is not affected by aphasia. Talking about the client in his or her presence is upsetting.
• Delay conversation when the client is tired or frustrated.	• People with aphasia become easily fatigued. Attempting conversation when the client is fatigued makes it more difficult.
3. Use techniques that increase comprehension. Be a role model. • If the client wears glasses or a hearing aid, encourage their use. • Modify your speech. Speak slowly, using adult language. • Do not change the subject rapidly or ask multiple questions in succession. • Match your verbal and nonverbal behavior.	3. These techniques enhance communication and decrease frustration for the client.

(continued)

Nursing Plan of Care *(continued)*
The Client With Impaired Verbal Communication

Nursing Intervention	Scientific Rationale
4. Use techniques that enhance communication.	
• Phrase questions so they can be answered with yes or no responses.	• Simple questions can facilitate communication, but an aphasic client may be confused by verbal symbols and may say yes but nod his or her head no.
• In a group, have only one person talk at a time.	• The client will become more confused if they need to follow a multisided conversation.
• Encourage the use of gestures, pantomime, pictures, writing, or flash cards. Write key words on cards.	• Approaching the client through whatever sense is stronger helps facilitate communication.
• Rephrase message to validate client the response. If you do not understand the client, be honest and attempt the message again.	• Pretending you understand when you do not will frustrate the client even more.
5. Encourage and use techniques to improve speech. • Have the client slow the rate of speech and say each word clearly. • Encourage the use of short phrases. • Explain when words are not clear. • Avoid topics that are controversial. • If the client makes an error do not correct. • Give positive feedback for attempts at communication.	5. Use of these techniques decreases frustration at communication attempts.
6. Acknowledge the client's frustration. • Explain that the stroke caused language difficulty and that feelings of frustration are normal. • Maintain a calm, positive attitude. • Use reassurance and touch to communicate your understanding. • Encourage and use a sense of humor. • Allow tears. • Ignore profanity, recognize it for what it represents. • Allow the client to make choices about his or her care.	6. Understanding the client's frustration and communicating this understanding permits the client to accept the situation and learn to work through the speech difficulties.
7. Initiate health teaching and referrals. • Consult a speech therapist. • Teach family and significant others techniques for improving communication.	7. Early intervention and treatment can reduce the frustration and isolation that accompanies aphasia.

- Establishing an effective communication system and maintaining relationships are priorities.
- In adults, the main cause of impaired communication is brain damage. Other major causes are cancer and neurologic disorders.
- Aphasia is the inability to express oneself. The four types are expressive, receptive, anomic, and global aphasia.
- Dysarthria is not an aphasia, but is a speech disorder related to difficulty in articulation.
- The plan of care involves collaboration of nursing, speech therapy, and other disciplines, as needed.

Critical Thinking Challenges

Communication involves relationships. You now have a strong knowledge base about communication as social interaction and as a nurse–client therapeutic relationship. Using this knowledge about communication and your knowledge about nursing care in general, you should be able to plan care for clients who have problems communicating. Turn back to the situation at the beginning of the chapter and consider the following:

1. *Identify the communication barriers present in this situation.*
2. *Discern how the wife may be feeling. Contrast how the husband may be feeling compared to his wife.*
3. *Describe your own feelings as you observe this couple and try to communicate with them.*
4. *Based on those analyses, identify additional information for which you need to assess.*
5. *With that additional assessment information, list nursing interventions that may be appropriate for this couple.*

References

Adkins, E. R. (1991). Nursing care of clients with impaired communication. *Rehabilitation Nursing, 16* (2), 74–76.

Ahmann, E. (1994). "Chunky stew": Appreciating cultural diversity while providing health care for children. *Pediatric Nursing, 20,* 320–324.

Albert, M., & Helm-Estabrooks, N. (1988a). Diagnosis and treatment of aphasia: Part I. *JAMA, 259,* 1043–1047.

Albert, M., & Helm-Estabrooks, N. (1988b). Diagnosis and treatment of aphasia: Part II. *JAMA, 259,* 1205–1210.

American Heart Association. (1994). *Heart and stroke facts: 1994 statistical supplement.* Dallas: Author.

Braverman, B. (1990). Eliciting assessment data from the patient who is difficult to interview. *Nurs Clin North Am, 25,* 743–750.

Connolly, M., & Shekleton, M. (1991). Communicating with ventilator dependent patients. *Dimensions of Critical Care Nursing, 10,* 115–122.

Emde, R. N., Gaensbauer, T. J., & Harmon, R. J. (1976). Emotional expression in infancy: A biobehavioral study. *Psychological Issues, 10* (37), 1–2000.

Field, T. M., Cohen, D., Garcia, R., & Greenberg, R. (1984). Mother–stranger face discrimination by the newborn. *Infant Behavior and Development, 7,* 19–25.

Gresham, G. E., & Weiss, C. J. (1993). The role of speech therapy in stroke rehabilitation. *Heart Disease and Stroke, 2,* 49–52.

Harrison, L.L. (1990). Minimizing barriers when teaching hearing-impaired clients. *Am J Matern Child Nurs, 15,* 113.

Hetherington, E. M., & Parke, R. D. (1993). *Child psychology: A contemporary viewpoint* (4th ed.). New York: McGraw-Hill.

Jackson, D., & Albamonte, S. (1994). Enhancing communication with the Passy-Muir valve. *Pediatric Nursing, 20,* 149–153.

Keith, R. L., & Darley, F. L. (1994). *Laryngectomee rehabilitation* (3rd ed.). Austin, TX: PRO-ED.

McClenahan, R., Johnston, M., & Densham, Y. (1990). Misperceptions of comprehension difficulties of stroke patients by doctors, nurses, and relatives. *J Neurol Neurosurg Psychiatry, 53,* 700–701.

Merrow, S. L., & Corbett, C. D. (1994). Adaptive computing for people with disabilities. *Computers in Nursing, 12,* 201–209.

Mitchell, P. H., Hodges, L. C., Muwaswes, M., & Walleck, C. A. (1988). *AANN's neuroscience nursing.* Norwalk, CT: Appleton & Lange.

National Safety Council. (1994). *Accident facts.* Itasca, IL: Author.

Nicholas, M. L., Helm-Estabrooks, N., & Ward-Lonergan, J. (1993). Evolution of severe aphasia in the first two years post onset. *Arch Phys Med Rehabil, 74,* 830–836.

North American Nursing Diagnosis Association (NANDA). (1994). *Nursing diagnoses: Definitions and classification 1995–1996.* Philadelphia: Author.

Porth, C. (1994). *Pathophysiology: Concepts of altered health states* (4th ed.). Philadelphia: J. B. Lippincott.

Rosenthal, M., Griffith, E. R., Bond, M. R., & Miller, J. D. (1990). *Rehabilitation of the adult and child with traumatic head injury* (2nd ed.). Philadelphia: F. A. Davis.

Rothenburger, R. (1990). Transcultural nursing: Overcoming obstacles to effective communication. *AORN J, 51,* 1349–1354, 1357–1363.

Schuster, C. S., & Ashburn, S. S. (1992). *The process of human development* (3rd ed.). Philadelphia: J. B. Lippincott.

Bibliography

Davies, P. (1993). Diagnosing hearing loss in children. *Nursing Standard, 7* (35): 33–36.

Erber, N. P. (1994). Communicating with elders. *Journal of Gerontological Nursing, 20* (10): 6–10.

Kravitz, L., Selekman, J. (1992). Understanding hearing loss in children. *Pediatric Nursing, 18,* (6):591–594.

Riesch, S. K., Tosi, C. B., Thurston, C. A., Forsyth, D. M., Kuenning, T. S., Kestly, J. (1993). Effects of communication training on parents and young adolescents. *Nursing Research, 42* (4):254.

Ripich, D. N., Wykle, M., Niles, S. (1995). Alzheimer's disease caregivers: The focused program. A communication skills training program helps nursing assistants to give better care to patients with disease. *Geriatric Nursing, 16* (1):15–19.

Families and Their Relationships

Key Terms

Anticipatory guidance
Blended family
Cohabitated family
Communal family
Dysfunctional family
Extended family
Family-centered care
Nuclear family
Single-parent families
Social isolation
Role strain

Learning Objectives

Upon completion of this chapter, the student will be able to do the following:

- *Describe variations in normal family relationships and roles.*
- *Identify factors affecting family and social relationships.*
- *Describe manifestations of dysfunctional families.*
- *Associate the impact of dysfunction with individual and family activities.*
- *Differentiate subjective and objective data needed to assess altered family and social relationships.*
- *Identify nursing diagnoses and related goals commonly used with altered family and social relationships.*
- *Discuss nursing interventions to promote family relationships.*
- *Discuss nursing interventions for the dysfunctional family.*
- *List family-centered healthcare services in your community.*

49

You are the home care nurse coordinator conducting the final hospital discharge planning meeting for an adolescent single mother and her son, born 8 weeks prematurely (preterm). The adolescent mother is accompanied by her mother, the grandmother of the newborn. The newborn will need to continue on an apnea monitor after discharge. The grandmother holds the infant. She explains that her daughter is "afraid to take the baby home because he's so little and floppy.

She's afraid she'll break his neck or something." The young mother sits quietly with her head down. She does not look at you or the baby. When you ask if the apnea monitor has been delivered, the grandmother immediately replies that it has. "But," she continues, "I don't think the baby really needs all this stuff. Anyone can tell when a baby is not breathing."

In previous chapters you learned about the relationship among individuals, the family, and the community; about health promotion and disease prevention; and about client teaching. This chapter expands this knowledge base by delving into the nuances of social relationships within the family and the nurse's responsibility in using family strengths to help families cope. The situation above gives you a chance to apply your knowledge about health and wellness to dysfunctional families. The Critical Thinking Challenges at the end of the chapter will help you apply your knowledge base to the care of the adolescent single mother, her newborn, and the newborn's grandmother with whom they live.

Two hundred years ago, children were raised in extended families that encompassed several generations of family members living in close proximity. Large families were desired; members were interdependent, and socialization was accomplished as traditions passed from one generation to the next. Significant social, demographic, and economic trends, including increases in higher education, diverse employment opportunities, and economic independence of women, have changed family life (Glick, 1994). At the end of the 20th century, family structures are more varied than in the past. The small, traditional family unit known as the nuclear family remains prominent. However, more than one-third of family units now consist of children living with a single parent (Fig. 49-1). There are also blended types of families, extended families, cohabitated families, communal families, and other variations. Increased lifestyle options have established new family norms with a concurrent need for nurses to focus on helping individuals and families to adapt to their varied family units.

Although nurses deal with the individual, those individuals are integral parts of families. The adolescent single mother, her mother, and the newborn present such a situation. You can see in this situation how families influence the health perceptions and practices of their members. Nurses must understand the importance of family functioning to affect positively the health status of the individual. Nurses practicing **family-centered care,** which means caring for the client and family as a unit, recognize the positive aspects of diversity and facilitate client/caregiver/professional collaboration (Ahmann, 1994).

Normal Family Function

A family is a social group whose members share common values, occupy specific positions, interact with each other over time, and have diverse strengths and needs. Family members bear and rear children, engage in economic and political cooperation, and care for the ill and aged.

Characteristics of a Normal Family

Although there is no one true "normal" family model, families have some common structural and functional characteristics. Family structure is described by who the members are and what their relationships are to one another. Function is what the family does. Structure and

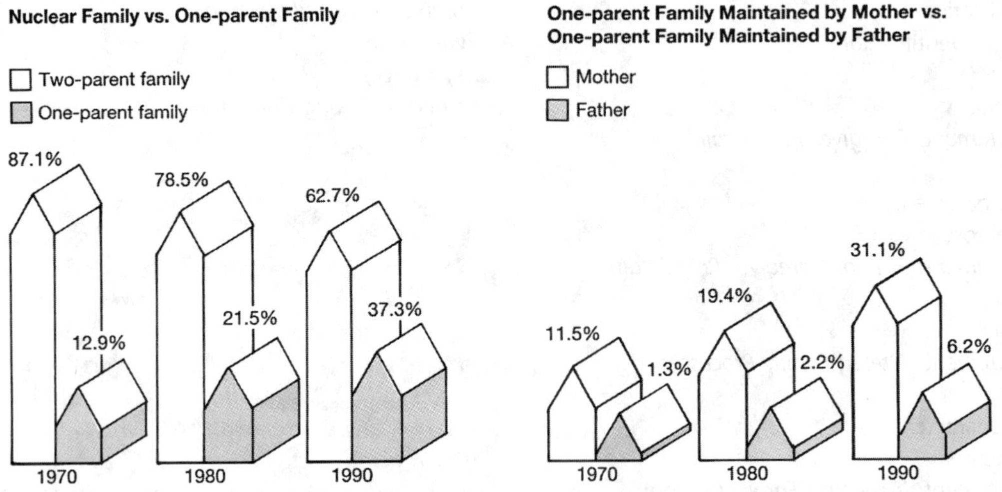

Figure 49-1 • *The changing American family.*

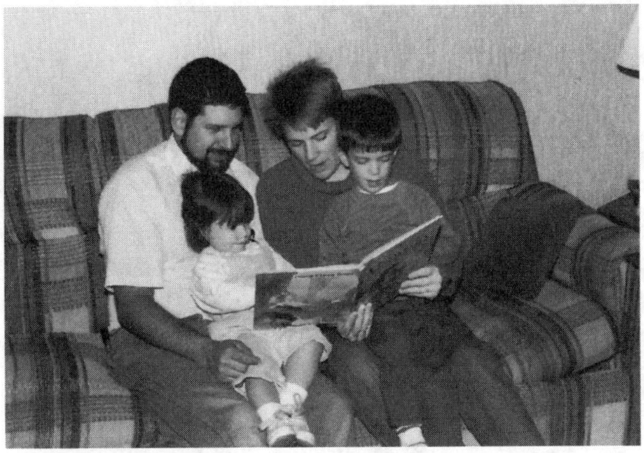

Figure 49-2 • The nuclear family consists of the married husband and wife and one or more children, living together in one household.

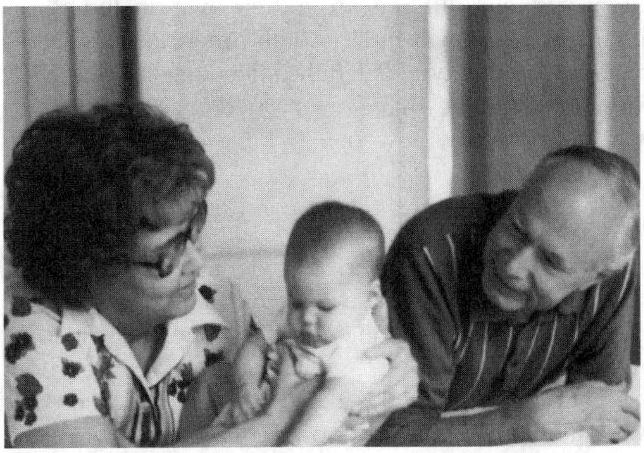

Figure 49-3 • As part of the extended family, grandparents contribute to nurturing young children.

function vary from one family to another, as well as within a family over time.

Family Structure

Although the traditional structure of the family in America is that of the nuclear family, a variety of family structures exist today. Family members do not always live together in one household but are linked together by relationships.

Nuclear Family. The **nuclear family** includes a married adult man and woman and their children (Fig. 49-2). Members live under the same roof, usually until the children leave home to work and support themselves or to attend college. In 1990, 26% of the nation's 93.3 million households were composed of a married couple and children younger than 18 years of age (United States Bureau of the Census, 1990). Variations in the nuclear family include couples remaining childless or older children moving back in with parents after a period of independence. Traditional roles in the nuclear family have been the man as breadwinner outside the home, and the woman as responsible for physical provision of the home and children. The number of traditional families remained stable over the last 20 years, ranging from 24.2 million to 26 million (United States Bureau of the Census, 1990). But in 64% of nuclear families with children younger than 18 years of age, both parents work outside the home (United States Bureau of the Census, 1990).

Extended Family. Members of the **extended family** include the nuclear family as well as grandparents, aunts, uncles, and cousins (Fig. 49-3). They may or may not live under the same roof, and exert a varying amount of influence on one person. The extended family often consists of three or more generations.

Single-Parent Families. **Single-parent families**, composed of one parent and one or more children, are growing because of high separation and divorce rates (see Fig. 49-1). There were 9.7 million single parents in the United States in 1990, 41% more than 10 years earlier. Death of a spouse, desertion, and unwed pregnancy or adoption also result in single-parent families. These families may experience financial strain and an overburdened parent owing to lack of support systems. Women head more single-parent families than men, by a margin of 5:1 (United States Bureau of the Census, 1990).

Blended Family. Members of a **blended family** (or stepfamily) include children living with one birth parent and one nonbirth parent, as well as the offspring of a nonbirth parent. Each member faces the challenge of forming new relationships with the new members.

Cohabitated Family. **Cohabitated family** structure includes people living together without the formal or legal bond of marriage. Couples include men and women living together as a trial to marriage or as an alternative to marriage, or gay or lesbian couples. Cohabitated families may include children.

Communal Family. A **communal family** includes a number of members who share a common bond such as religious affiliation, ideology, economic needs, or a situation such as attending college. Membership may be short-term, creating instability in the family unit.

Other Families. Still other variations in family structure exist, including commuter marriages, in which one member may live away from the rest of the family part of the time to work or go to school. Caring for foster children or adopted children is another way to include children in a family. Many families have adopted children of a race different from their own, including orphans from southeast Asia, South America, and eastern Europe. Another type of family unit is single adults living alone because they have not married or are older adults who have been widowed.

Family Function

Although family function is not identical in all families, all families exist to meet some common goals. The usual functions of families involve physical and economic provisions of care, sexual intimacy, reproduction, education, socialization (including communication), as well as nurturing and support for problem-solving and goal-setting. Besides the physical bonds of family relationships, members experience emotional bonds. Emotional bonds provide support and security for members, fostering growth and development.

Physical Provision. Physical provision of care is a common need for all members of the family but is greater for those who are more dependent because of age or illness. Physical provision includes food, clothing, shelter, and healthcare. A normal, functioning family should have some members providing comfort and safety for others. Certain members cook, clean, shop for food and clothing, and possibly feed and bathe other members. Those being cared for and those doing the caring may change owing to situations such as maturation or illness.

Economic Provision. One or more family members contribute monetary funds to provide basic necessities such as food and clothing, as well as luxuries and provisions for the future, such as college tuition. Families usually share the funds earned by members. Two-career families are increasingly common because of today's economic climate and standard of living. About 67% of the female population in the United States participates in the work force (United States Bureau of the Census, 1990).

Sexual Intimacy. Most couples in families need sexual intimacy. This includes married and cohabitating men and women, and gay and lesbian couples. Sexual intimacy is a basic human need and developmental concern that can be met within a family.

Reproduction. Reproduction is not a function of all families; it is more often a choice rather than a given in family life. Couples may postpone childbearing, eliminate it, or be unable to accomplish it. Alternate methods of having children such as adoption, foster parenthood, use of donor sperm, and surrogate mother programs exist to fulfill a family's desire for children.

Education. Education, whether formal or informal, is a function of all families. Parents discipline children, teach them how to begin to care for themselves and get along in the world, and send them to school for formal education. Older members share with younger members information they have learned through living, and younger members in turn teach older members about the changing world. Education not only involves information, but techniques for problem solving and coping, as well as attitudes and values. Education is an ongoing and lifelong function in many families.

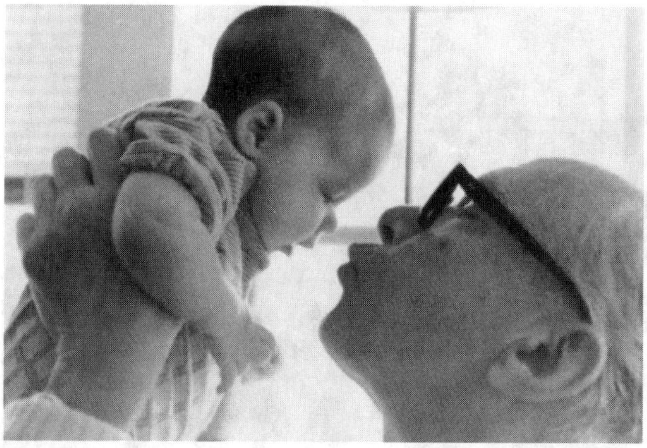

Figure 49-4 • Grandparents participate in the socialization of infants.

Socialization. Socialization is a function in all families, especially in close extended families (Fig. 49-4). Gathering together at the dinner table or converging for holiday celebrations are prime opportunities for socialization in the family. Through socializing, family members learn to get along, learn appropriate behavior in various situations, and express culture, tradition, and religious beliefs.

Nurturing and Support. Families provide nurturing and support to members, from initial bonding at birth to old age and death. Nurturing and support may be provided through the emotional tasks of love, belonging, and affection, as well as through the provision of safety and security for growth (Fig. 49-5). Caplan (1990) describes ten support functions of the family and social groups. These include providing information, providing feedback, transmitting attitudes, beliefs, and values, guiding problem-solving, providing practical services, providing a safe, comfortable environment, providing standards, helping establish identity, assisting in emotional development, and fostering mutual support by family and community professionals.

Normal Functional Family Pattern

A normal functional family meets the family's developmental tasks and guides family members in accomplishing tasks according to their age and developmen-

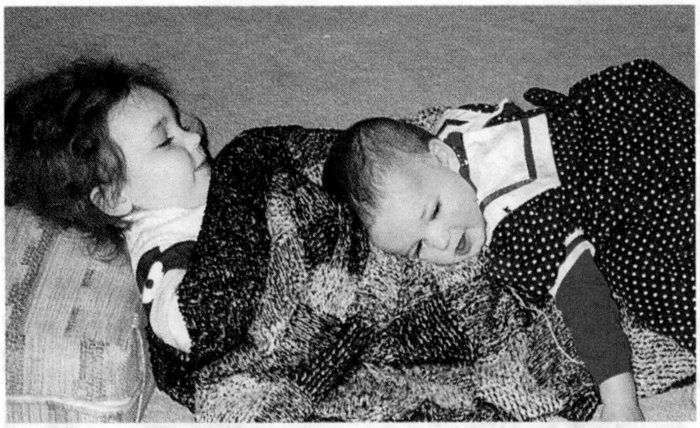

Figure 49-5 • Siblings provide socialization and comfort for each other. (Jackson, D.B., & Saunders, R.B. [1993]. Child health nursing: a comprehensive approach to the care of children and their families. Philadelphia, J.B. Lippincott.)

tal level. Family development is discussed in Chapter 17, and Table 17-1 presents the developmental cycle of stages and tasks.

Factors Affecting Normal Family Function

Factors in addition to age that may affect family and social relationships include cultural beliefs, economic status, lifestyle, previous life experience, and external stressors such as illness of a family member.

Culture, Values, and Beliefs

Cultural traditions have an impact on the family as it functions in Western society. Components of a sociocultural dimension include ethnic patterns, language, food customs, patterns of communication, role expectations, healthcare beliefs, childrearing practices, availability of extended family support, and religious beliefs and practices. The nurse may encounter much variation in family structure and function among different cultures; each of these variations can have an affect on the person's health status. For example, the extended family is basic to Native American society; children and the elderly are valued, and childrearing is a group endeavor. The extended family is essential as a support system to help families cope when stressors such as illness occur.

The African American or black population has traditionally had families with a matriarchal focus, often involving several generations in childrearing (Thomas, 1993). A strong sense of kinship with the extended family is valued, and the church provides financial, spiritual, and social support (Thomas, et al., 1994). With Mexican Americans, machismo, or the emphasis on proving masculinity through sexual potency, has historically been a predominant cultural value. Women have had lower status than men, but family unity is strongly supported. Haitian individuals conceptualize the presence of signs and symptoms of illness as "ill health" only if they are incapacitated; healthy family members are those who continue to function (DeSantis, 1993).

Asian American families continue to stress traditional values of loyalty and obedience to parents. The value placed on education has perhaps accounted for the rising middle-class status accorded many Asian families. Elders, men, and "professionals" have high status within the family. Traditional submissiveness of women has created a significant role conflict for more recent generations of Asian American women, although reduced authoritarianism and an increasing role for fathers can be found in contemporary society (Wang, 1993). Strict control of social interactions is still valued to avoid "loss of face."

Religious customs also dictate how children grow up in families. The bar or bat mitzvah is considered the "rite of passage" in the Jewish religion. Strict fundamentalist religions rear children with corporal punishment combined with an emphasis on manifest love. Mormons emphasize self-discipline and strong family ties. Families pass down attitudes about male and female roles and childrearing through the generations; they also pass on beliefs and practices about health, illness, and healthcare. Even those people born and raised in traditional American society may exhibit behavior arising from a variety of cultural beliefs.

Economic Resources

A clear economic influence on family and social relationships can be observed as people with marginal incomes struggle to survive. Economic constraints often create problems in maintaining a family's lifestyle after divorce or a change in employment, or with a change from two wage-earners to one. Resentment toward society or toward other members of the family for forcing a below-standard lifestyle may arise. According to Parette (1993), functioning in single-parent families will be difficult when they have limited support, without psychological and economic resources.

Lifestyle

The mobility of families can affect relationships as parents move from job to job and children move from school to school. Support people and friendships change. Lack of extended family support systems due to geographic distance can increase the strain on parents after relocation. The need to have two incomes has created the "latch-key" practice in childrearing, in which children are responsible for their own care and supervision after school. The family's lifestyle in terms of rest and relaxation, nutrition, smoking, drug and alcohol use, and exercise influences the health status of all the members and the choices the children will make as they become adults.

Previous Life Experience

Previous life experience greatly affects a family's functioning. Children learn about relationships almost exclusively from their parents and early family life. They will carry beliefs to their own future families about how to form relationships, how to make decisions and solve problems, what are accepted roles for men and women, how to raise children, how to use resources, and how to show affection (Fig. 49-6). Some coping strategies, such as taking an alcoholic beverage to numb mental pain and stress, may have been accepted in a person's previous life experience and yet destroy present family relationships.

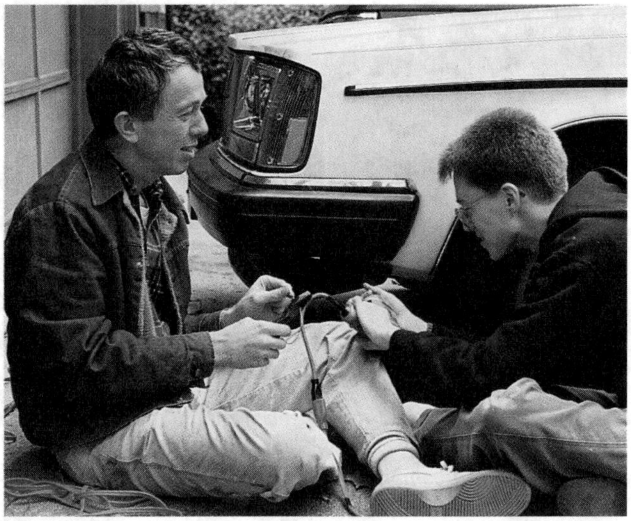

Figure 49-6 • *A father and son share mutual interests in their lifestyle, providing both education and socialization. (Jackson, D.B., & Saunders, R.B. [1993]. Child health nursing: a comprehensive approach to the care of children and their families. Philadelphia, J.B. Lippincott.)*

Coping and Stress Tolerance

Any stress on the entire family or an individual member greatly affects functioning. Acute or chronic illness of a member may alter roles and relationships within the family. For example, in a family with a seriously ill father, the mother may become the primary economic provider and a child may provide care and nurturing for the father in the home setting. Other stresses, such as loss of a family member, involvement in a natural or manmade disaster, or an accident, also alter family functioning. Some families have the ability to grow as the result of a crisis, whereas others experience dysfunction; some families live with constant stress, and others experience little change or stress.

Lifespan Considerations

An understanding of normal growth and development can be a reference point for understanding families.

Newborn and Infant

A process of infant–parent attachment or bonding after birth is critical to family development. Factors that affect the process of attachment may include availability of both parents after birth, flexibility of schedules, feelings about the birth, comfort in parenting roles, emotional responsiveness of infant and parents, financial security, other demands such as care of another child, and presence of supportive others. The situation at the beginning of the chapter includes cues to the mother's and grandmother's bonding that can influence their ability to care for the infant.

By 8 months of age the infant usually becomes attached to the primary caregiver, developing "trust," as described in Erikson's (1963) classic theory of development. The process of socialization can be supported by an interactive family environment. If there are changes in the infant's environment, such as illness of the primary caretaker or of the infant, necessitating separation, inconsistencies can impede the infant's development.

Toddler and Preschooler

Beginning to walk imparts mobility, and increasing cognitive ability adds curiosity. Protection from harm is an important focus for these adventurous years. At the same time, the development of self-control characteristics can strain family interactions as parent–child power struggles, often accompanied by temper tantrums, become the norm. Promoting independence within established limits should be encouraged to develop "autonomy" (Erikson, 1963). Sibling rivalry may escalate as the egocentric toddler resents the dominance of older children and the attention given to younger children in the family. Despite the power struggle, the toddler remains attached to the parent, and from 18 to 24 months of age, severe separation anxiety may be noted when the mother or primary caregiver leaves the child. Hospitalization or a disability involving separation at this time may be especially traumatic. Role changes necessitated by the need to care for a disabled family member in the home may decrease the parent's contact time with the toddler, who may then regress into an earlier developmental stage.

Psychosocial development escalates during the preschool years. Identification with the role of man or woman is developed as the preschooler interacts differently with the parent(s). The parent of the opposite sex becomes a focus for love, whereas aggression may be directed toward the parent of the same sex. Consistent involvement with people of both sexes enhances the preschooler's development.

Associative play, with interaction but little organization, evolves into cooperative play as the child nears school age. Cooperative play, along with preschoolers' generally increasing social skills, helps them to develop mutually supportive roles with siblings, even though rivalry continues.

The preschool years are crucial for development of "initiative," the ability to begin actions independently (Erikson, 1963). Stable family relationships can enhance the development of creativity. The preschooler can be prepared for changes through playing out feelings and focusing attention on the event one part at a time. The family should reassure the children that changes are not their fault.

Significant others can expand the socialization process as the preschooler develops an ability to separate from home and family. The preschooler still needs both independence and security. Fear of separation remains and may be reinforced by parental anxiety.

Child and Adolescent

The school years are a time of change for both the child and the family. A need for association with peers, usually of the same sex, is enhanced. The role of "best friend" takes on importance. Family atmosphere continues to provide a sense of security as the child moves away from obvious signs of dependence on parents. Sibling rivalry is still present but continues to resolve unless parents make comparisons among children for differing levels of ability.

Children's perceptions of their own abilities are significant as they seek to accomplish the task of "industry" (Erikson, 1963) and avoid feeling inferior. Fears of illness, injury, punishment, and death of self or significant others are evidenced during this age period. Phobias and ritualistic "good luck" behaviors may be used as adaptive mechanisms by the child. Parental understanding, rather than denial of phobias, is important.

In some cultures, puberty, after completion of identifiable "rites of passage," signals the assumption of adult roles. American culture is not as clear in defining the steps for transition into adulthood. To the extent that independence is desirable, alterations in family and social relationships are normal and inevitable in adolescence. Psychosocial development is closely related to changes in physical development during adolescence. Peer group identity is strongly desired; the adolescent strives to look and act like the group. Stability in the home environment and supportive relationships with significant others can help an adolescent avoid "role confusion" (Erikson, 1963).

Adult and Older Adult

According to Erikson (1963), the chief developmental tasks of the adult period are "intimacy," involving commitment to others, and "generativity," focusing on productivity. An adult's development is strongly influenced by both social and job-related concerns. Critical life junctures such as marriage, cohabitation, becoming a parent, career advancement, and mobility affect the development of both intimacy and generativity.

A decision to remain single does not exclude development of intimate relationships. Nevertheless, the young adult usually leaves a family of origin, often to form a family of procreation. Social relationships with peers remain important for the young adult's feeling of identity. The need for peer group support may be intertwined with such serious problems as substance abuse, sexually transmitted diseases, unwanted pregnancies, and abortion. The family's acceptance is necessary to help in dealing with these serious health problems.

In the middle years, relationships with children gradually change as children develop independence, and relationships with a significant partner change as each matures. Menopause in the woman and climacteric in the man can precipitate crises in the family, requiring role adjustment. Relationships with aging parents may result in conflict, frustration, or anger as the older adults become more dependent. Family support is needed to help the older adult achieve "ego integrity" and avoid "despair" (Erikson, 1963). Changes in family structure occur as children leave home (and sometimes return), as death occurs, and as new relationships are formed. Changes related to retirement, death of a family member, and decreasing social contacts alter family and social structure because usual roles must be changed.

Altered Family Function

Potential for Altered Function

Acute and chronic illness, traumatic experiences, and substance abuse all potentially alter family function. Family function may be only mildly altered and affect just some of the members, or the entire family may be thrown into crisis. Family bonds may actually be strengthened by a crisis, however, when members become more committed to common goals of the family. Table 49-1 lists common stressors that contribute to altered family function.

Acute Illness

Acute illness may place sudden demands on the family. The ill member often looks to the family for validation that he or she is sick; with validation from the family, the ill member can seek healthcare. Roles may be changed as the ill member becomes dependent on other members for physical care, nurturing, and economic security. The ill member's self-esteem may drop as he or she feels less value as a member of the family.

Other members may temporarily sacrifice their own needs to provide for the needs of the ill member. Needs

Table 49-1 • Sources of Family Conflict

Source	Problem Areas
Finances	Lower socioeconomic status; income inadequate to meet needs; disagreement on money management
Occupation	Unemployment; semiskilled status, task-sharing when both adults working
Culture/religion	Mixed religious or cultural background; in-laws; disagreement on childrearing practices
Education	Incongruent levels of education, especially if school dropout
Residence	Mixed rural/urban background; relocation for benefit of only one family member; isolated
Sexual	Dissatisfaction with intimacy level; disagreement on family planning
Substance abuse	Difference in values; physical/psychological changes due to chemical addiction
Social ties	Dissimilar selection of friends; single versus couple focus in friendships
Situational	Fatigue; loss; illness; separation, trauma, disaster
Developmental	Change in family stage (Duvall, 1977); change in individual stage (Erikson, 1963)

such as sexual intimacy may go unmet. Problems arise when role adjustments are not made and family or individual needs go unmet. In some situations, the caregiver role changes from an "ordinary exchange of assistance among people standing in close relationship to one another to an extraordinary and unequally distributed burden" (Pearlin, et al., 1990, p. 583). One member in particular may feel overburdened by the situation. For example, when a construction worker is unemployed while receiving treatment for fractured vertebrae, his wife may have to go to work full time to provide for the family economically. The children may have to assume more responsibility for meeting their own needs, and housework may be left undone. The wife tries to fit in around her work schedule support of her husband, meal preparation, and chauffeuring the children. She is anxious about her husband's condition, as well as about how the children are managing without her presence. Consequently, her own physical needs for sleep and nutrition, as well as the family's need for nurturing, may go unmet. Depending on the severity of the illness and how suddenly it occurred, the family may need increased nurturing at this time. Stability of the family structure is essential when one or more members is absent or incapacitated, as with the ill husband and working wife. However, some flexibility is needed to share roles and still meet needs such as economic provision and physical care.

Chronic Illness

Because chronic illness is of longer duration, it can influence the family to a greater extent than acute illness. The course of chronic illness may require both individual and family adaptation to changes in lifestyle and roles, and often may result in an increasing degree of dependence on others. Actions by family or significant others can be supportive, but behaviors such as overprotection can be problematic.

Because of the inherent dependency of children, their illness provokes yet other adjustments in the family. The birth of an infant with a congenital defect or the diagnosis of a child with a chronic illness or developmental disability is traumatic and may result in severe stressors to family relationships. The ability of a family to function will influence the child's ability to develop and cope, and will affect the course of the illness or disability (Bond, et al., 1994). A congenital birth defect that would initially be stressful but is ultimately correctable could have less impact on family and social relationships than would a chronic illness or developmental disability requiring lengthy family involvement with treatment.

Common stressors with regard to childhood illness include exhaustion, anxiety, needing help from relatives and friends, alterations in social contacts or travel abilities, concern about sibling needs, and financial concerns (Ahmann, 1994). Family roles, responsibilities, and social relationships change to meet the needs of the family system as well as the ill child and family members.

Parents with disabled or chronically ill children often express negative feelings about themselves, such as guilt, inadequacy, failure, rejection, and helplessness (Leff & Walizer, 1992). Denial may be necessary initially as a family struggles with the initial shock of the child's illness or disability, but after the problem is acknowledged, the goal is simply to function as a "normal" family.

Traumatic Experiences

Trauma, because of the stress and disruption of normal interactions it entails, can alter family relationships. Traumatic experiences can be physical, such as a gunshot wound, or emotional, such as robbery; can involve one person or many; and can be caused by humans (eg, surgery) or nature (eg, flood).

Personal involvement or having a family member or significant other involved in a disaster, such as severe fire, flood, hurricane, or car, train, or plane accident, is associated with loss of control and role change. The role of the survivor is fraught with conflicts. Family members may experience guilt over ideas that they were responsible or that they should have been the victim. One family member may blame another for contributing to the event. The victim may experience difficulty concentrating as the event is relived, or may move from numbness to awareness of the event. The entire family will need support.

Substance Abuse

The consequences for the family of coping with substance abuse are multiple. For each person afflicted with alcoholism, there are family members who also suffer social and emotional problems associated with the alcoholic's lifestyle disruption. The alcoholic and possibly the family will deny that there is a problem with alcoholism. A spouse or child often becomes an "enabler," one who keeps the family functioning, even on a dysfunctional level. The enabler takes over tasks the alcoholic cannot accomplish, cares for the alcoholic, and makes excuses for them to "cover their tracks." This enables the alcoholic to keep drinking and contributes to the deterioration of the family unit.

Drug abuse also alters family function. Economic destruction may play a greater role in the family of a drug abuser than in that of an alcoholic, owing to the higher cost of illegal drugs compared with alcohol. Because drug use is less socially acceptable than alcohol use, the drug abuser and family may be isolated from the community. The threat of drug testing in the workplace may prevent the drug abuser from holding a job, and further disrupts family economic security. Arrest and incarceration may completely disrupt the family unit.

Both alcohol and drug abuse may lead to physical problems from the effects of the substance, as well as injury incurred while intoxicated. Chronic liver disease, poor nutrition, and eventual heart failure are common in alcoholics. Intravenous drug abusers suffer from frequent infections, hepatitis, and possibly AIDS. Family dynamics are further altered by these illnesses.

Manifestations of Altered Family Function

Manifestations of altered family function include structural, functional, and developmental changes (Wright & Leahey, 1994). Examples of structural changes are separation and divorce; functional changes include role strain and abuse; developmental changes may be manifested as social isolation and emotional problems in children. Separation and divorce may be solutions, as well.

Separation and Divorce

Divorce or separation may be a positive solution to a dysfunctional family situation or a manifestation of the families' altered function. A **dysfunctional family** is not able to create and maintain a system to nurture and support its members. A major interruption in the developmental process occurs when the family unit is broken by separation or divorce. An ever-increasing number of families are being thus affected. The most common form involves the mother and children forming a family unit, while the father moves into a separate environment. A problem that can lead to further dysfunction is role overload for the custodial parent. Shared custody has been attempted to reduce the strain on a single parent, but there is no single solution best for all families.

Remarriage after divorce accounts for one-third of all marriages in the United States (United States Bureau of the Census, 1990). Blended families thus formed are also at risk for dysfunction as ties to previous marriages are maintained or broken, and extended family ties are questioned.

Role Strain

Role strain is a manifestation of altered family function when changes in roles are chosen or forced on family members by changing events or developments in the family. For example, when a husband becomes chronically ill and unable to work, the wife may become the primary economic provider. She may experience role strain because she must combine the role of caretaker with wife, mother, and employee roles. The husband may experience stress as he gives up his role as economic provider and spends more time at home. Children may be reassigned tasks as well, including some physical care for the father.

Giving up familiar roles and taking on new roles may be chosen, as in the case of a two-career family deciding to suspend or temporarily give up the wife's career for her to stay home and raise children. Family developmental stages call for changing roles periodically; however, role strain develops when family members cannot adapt and needs are not met. Inherent decision-making power influences role strain. Altered roles and resultant role strain can further impede interactions within the family and between the family and society.

Abuse

Family abuse and violence are social problems of increasing significance. Abuse may be physical, sexual, emotional, or economic. It may be aimed at the spouse, children, older parents, or grandparents. Factors that contribute to abuse in families include unemployment, substance abuse, chronic illness, inadequate housing, and lack of education and other resources. Family abuse is not limited to lower socioeconomic levels, however, and it is often passed down through the generations in a family; an abused child often grows up to abuse members of his or her own family. The number of child maltreatment cases reported in the United States is about 330 per 1,000 population (United States Bureau of the Census, 1990).

Abusive family dysfunction is often manifested in parenting behaviors. There may be a lack of attachment (bonding), evidenced by failure to care for the physical or emotional needs of a child or by verbalized resentment or indifference toward the parenting role. Evidence of neglect or physical abuse may be noted, as well as "failure to thrive." Rigidity in role expectations may be present in both parents, inhibiting flexibility in meeting the child's needs.

Sexual abuse of children is another area of concern. Emotional turmoil escalates when the abuse is not reported or, if reported, is ignored to avoid shaming a family member. The child is often confused about the appropriateness of the abuser's behavior and may feel he or she is to blame.

Older adults are also victims of abuse. As they become physically dependent, they may be neglected or verbally and financially abused by their own children. Immobility or sensory disabilities may prevent them from seeking help.

Social Isolation

Social isolation may result when family members are separated, when there is poor communication within families, or when a family or its members are not accepted by others. Isolation can be physical or psychological. Separation may result from hospitalization, job commitment, or going away to college. Today, many young nuclear families or single adults are separated from their extended families because they have been forced to seek employment elsewhere. They may feel isolated in a new town without the usual family support. Daily demands of a job, parenting, home maintenance, college studies, and finances may overburden the person or family members involved. They may not know where to turn for support if they have depended on family in the past. Geographic distance or desire to be independent may make family contact difficult, worsening isolation.

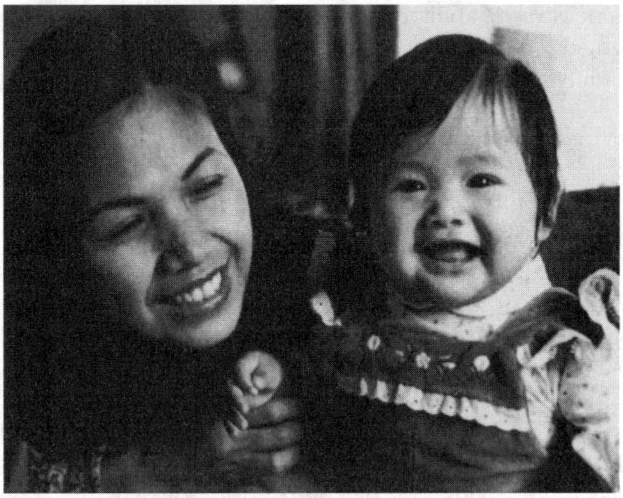

Figure 49-7 • *Many ethnic groups feel rejected by society. In the past, one such group has been Mexican Americans. However, because of their entrance into politics, new perspectives on their culture, and new opportunities, Mexican Americans have come out of isolation and into the "American" culture.*

Older adults are facing their final years away from their children and grandchildren, and may be living alone after their spouses are deceased. They may feel isolated by a society that values youth.

Poor communication within a family can isolate individual members. Consider the following example. After the loss of a child, the parents try quickly to get back into a normal routine. If they do not involve the sibling in funeral activities and do not cry or talk about their child's death, in an attempt to spare the sibling from pain, the remaining child, who is confused about death, thinks the parents must blame her for the other's death and are punishing her by not involving her. She feels guilty and imagines that her parents do not love her. She becomes isolated from the family and from friends as well.

Another form of isolation that families and their members experience occurs when they are not accepted socially or fear such rejection. They may be discriminated against because of race, color, religion, or ethnic origin (Fig. 49-7), or because of stigma associated with illnesses such as AIDS. Fear of isolation by the community, in the workforce, or by others causes further tension within the family.

Emotional Problems in Children

A variety of emotional and developmental problems can be manifestations of a dysfunctional family. Parenting may suffer whenever family function is altered. Problems with bonding and attachment may arise, and children may have difficulty with emotional development. Depending on the age of the child when family conflict arises, psychosocial development is arrested at that level. For example, if family tension arises while a child is an adolescent and the family does not function adequately, the adolescent may not complete the task of establishing "identity" (Erikson, 1963). He may be left confused, indecisive, and unable to make plans for the future. He may not satisfactorily complete successive tasks of intimacy and generativity.

The ability of the family to teach, nurture, educate, and socialize offspring is important, according to many developmental models. Emotional problems are often displayed by behavior inappropriate for age or situation. Acting out may occur in the form of temper tantrums, poor school performance, or sexual promiscuity. See Chapter 16 for more information on development.

Impact of Family Dysfunction on Activities of Daily Living

Family dysfunction can have an impact on the individual's activities of daily living as well as the family's.

Individual Considerations

Accomplishing the routine activities of daily living, such as preparing meals, eating, sleeping, taking medications, and so on, often becomes problematic when a person becomes ill. Issues often center around required assistance with tasks as well as changing roles and lifestyle. To examine changes in one family member related to illness, consider the following example. A 42-year-old single mother is diagnosed with lung cancer after repeated colds and a bout with pneumonia. The client will have to decide what kind of treatment (surgery, radiation, chemotherapy) to choose, and then adjust to the side effects of the treatment (eg, dressing changes, nausea, tiredness, hair loss). The need for treatment will determine whether she takes a leave of absence from her teaching job or just a few weeks of sick leave. Changes in daily activities are inevitable.

Family Considerations

Continuation of family functioning in activities of daily living becomes a significant focus as members alter their normal patterns to meet the client's needs and altered roles. In the immediate crisis after the diagnosis of lung cancer, decisions as to how to share the diagnosis with 15- and 11-year-old daughters, and whether to ask the grandmother to come and "keep house" during the period of treatment have to be made. Family relationships will change as usual roles are adjusted. Someone must continue the cooking, cleaning, chauffeuring of children to activities, and so forth. Who in the family will make decisions about discipline, spending money, organizing the home? What will be the financial impact of an extended illness? As the illness moves from an acute to a chronic stage, what options are available for extended care? The grandmother may need to return to her own job. Will friends be available to support the family? Will they feel comfortable continuing to interact with a "cancer client?" The nurse must be able to identify the effect of an illness on both the individual and the family. Assessing strengths as well as limitations of the family can help them to develop a realistic perspective for coping with their problems (Carpenito, 1993).

Assessment

Family functional assessment can be accomplished in terms of structure, function, development, communication, and support. Subjective and objective data should be recorded. Subjective data are gathered by interviewing the client and family members to explore their strengths and needs, and objective data are gathered by observing family interactions as well as by performing the physical examination. Functional patterns, risks, and family dysfunction are identified through nursing assessment. This serves as a basis for making nursing diagnoses and formulating interventions in collaboration with the client and family.

Subjective Assessment

Functional Pattern Identification

A structural and functional assessment can incorporate gathering data on the composition of the family and the ability of the family to meet its daily living needs, such as food, shelter, health maintenance, and so forth, along with its patterns of communication and support. Areas such as love and belonging, emotional stability, and sociocultural needs or interactions within the family and with society are also examined. The developmental assessment considers the ways in which a family changes within its own life cycle (Wright & Leahey, 1994).

Function, communication, and support can also be noted in family interaction patterns in terms of the roles each member assumes. Assessment would include but not be limited to a study of the relationships between husband and wife or parent and child; role relationships of cohabitating members could also be included in an interactional study of family structure and function in meeting individual and group needs. Communication patterns would be considered the key to an interactional approach.

Work roles and responsibilities in current life situations are subjective assessment factors related to the actual and perceived roles of family members. Client identification of satisfaction or disturbances in family, work, or social relationships, and responsibilities related to these roles should also be assessed. Assessment guidelines for family function are summarized in a display in Chapter 17.

Risk Identification

History-taking to identify areas of risk or potential problems can use both open-ended and focused questioning. Questions related to potential sources of stress in the areas of roles, finances, lifestyle, previous experience, and general health can help identify risk. A general question such as "What are the potential sources of stress in your family?" can be followed by specific questions such as those given in the accompanying assessment display.

Developmental stage of the family should also be taken into account when assessing a family's risk for dysfunction. For example, the birth of a child is a critical point in family development. Perinatal information can be gathered through open-ended questions such as "How did you feel when you realized you were pregnant?" Further information can be obtained with direct questions such as "Who is available to help you after the baby is born?" Reaction to the birth will depend on multiple factors, such as whether the pregnancy was planned or desired; whether the child is the first, second, or third (and so forth); whether there is physical space for an additional child; whether the family finances are adequate; whether resource persons are available; and whether the relationship between partners was of short or long duration before the birth.

Characteristic risk factors for potential alterations in parenting include unrealistic expectations of self or a child, lack of an appropriate role model, history of a parent having been abused as a child, inability to complete the bonding process, an inadequate support sys-

Nursing Assessment
Family Social Relationships

Family Structure and Function

- Description of client's family unit—age, sex, etc.
- Client's responsibilities in the household?
- Persons responsible for decision within client's household
- Management of finances?
- Ways in which family responsibilities are distributed?
- Pattern of eating, sleeping, and health practices?

Family/Social Interaction

- Most significant person in client's life?
- Availability of significant others to client?
- Any other people that client can turn to if necessary?
- Number of friends?
- Client's socialization with friends, neighbors, relatives?
- Description of client's neighborhood, neighbors.

Indicators of Change

- Any major change in client's role(s) or responsibilities (explain)?
- Client's anticipated future changes in the coming years.
- Preparations made for these changes?
- Any family stressors—how are they being handled?

Parental Role Function (If Person Is a Parent)

- Client's relationship with his or her children? Parents?
- Any plans to expand his or her family?
- Comparison of parenting patterns to those of client's parents (eg, discipline) (explain)?

Occupational Role Factors

- Client's occupation (include work role and responsibilities)?
- Hours worked per week—interference from work with other aspects of client's lifestyle?
- Ability of client's income to maintain client's lifestyle?

Leisure Time Management

- Usual activity pattern? Joint activities?
- Vacations taken and frequency?
- Client's plans for retirement—if retired, is client enjoying it?

Cultural Factors

- Ethnic/religious background.
- Similarity of family values.
- Relatives' childrearing practices.

Adapted from University of Scranton Guide to Care Plan Assessment.

tem, the presence of stress, a skill or knowledge deficit, growth and developmental delay in a child, and unmet psychosocial needs of a child or parent.

Dysfunction Identification

Dysfunctional family functioning can be identified when there is a significant difference from an effective pattern of functioning. Inability to express or accept emotions, lack of respect or support for other family members, and inability to adapt to change are contributing factors for alterations in family functioning.

When a child is ill, the parental role as caretaker alters. This may be evidenced by verbalization of feelings of inadequacy, guilt, anxiety, failure, helplessness, and powerlessness. Parents may also express concerns about the effect of the child's illness on siblings and the financial burden of illness. Noncompliance with treatment may be manifested in situations involving denial, when parents refuse to acknowledge that there is a problem. Denial may be used as a mechanism to maintain or restore "normality" in family life but can indicate dysfunction if it deters a family from dealing with the situation.

Objective Data

Objective data for assessing family function include observation of family interactions and individual members' behaviors, as well as the physical examination. Behavioral signs of family dysfunction may include labile emotions, withdrawal, irritability, poor sleeping and eating, inability to concentrate, and dependency. The nurse should observe family communication patterns. How do members relate to each other, and how effectively do they communicate? Observation includes who does the talking, who remains silent, whether they listen to one another, how disagreements are handled, how decisions are made, and what is communicated nonverbally. Observation of who visits the ill person, how often, and how the client responds can also help the nurse assess the family.

Physical assessment includes inspection, palpation, auscultation, and percussion, performed systematically. While assessing physical health, the nurse looks for family dysfunction clues. The nurse should pay special attention to injuries or bruises, which may indicate physical abuse; enlarged liver and other signs of chronic alcoholism; track marks indicating intravenous drug injection; nasal inflammatory symptoms of cocaine abuse; signs of stress such as weight loss, fatigue, and impaired cognitive function; and multiple acute and chronic physical problems.

Nursing Diagnoses

Careful assessment of members and the family as a whole is needed to identify actual or potential problems. As suggested in the situation at the beginning of the chapter, the nurse will work with the family to make a diagnosis by eliciting the members' perceptions of needs, goals, and expectations. The North American Nursing Diagnosis Association (NANDA) has identified the following accepted nursing diagnoses in family problems: two diagnoses of Caregiver Role Strain (Risk for and Actual); Altered Family Processes; Compromised

---

Nursing Research
Family Relationships

Selected Nursing Research Studies

Hall, L., Gurley, D., Sachs, B., et al. (1991). Psychosocial predictors of maternal depressive symptoms, parenting attitudes, and child behavior in single-parent families. *Nursing Research, 40*, 214–220.

Jocono, I., Hicks, G., Antonioni, C., et al. (1990). Comparison of perceived needs of family members between registered nurses and family members of critically ill patients in intensive care and neonatal intensive care units. *Heart and Lung, 19*, 72–78.

Payne, J. A. (1993). The contribution of group learning to the rehabilitation of spinal cord injured adults. *Rehabilitation Nursing, 18*, 375–379, 427–428.

Zabielski, M. T. (1994). Recognition of maternal identity in preterm and full-term mothers. *Matern Child Nurs J, 22*(1), 2–36.

Possible Topics for Nursing Inquiry

- Do nurses who use the family APGAR screening tool to evaluate family functioning develop more family-centered diagnoses?
- Does including family members in group learning situations increase client compliance?
- Is there a relationship between socioeconomic status and nurses' use of referral as an intervention in families dealing with chronic childhood illnesses?
- Does providing weekly telephone contact with a professional nurse make a difference in caregiver stress levels?

Ineffective Family Coping; Disabling Ineffective Family Coping; two diagnoses for Altered Parenting (Risk for and Actual); and Parental Role Conflict.

Diagnostic Statement: Caregiver Role Strain

Definition

Caregiver Role Strain is a a caregiver's felt difficulty in performing the family caregiver role (NANDA, 1994).

Defining Characteristics

Of the defining characteristics or clinical cues that denote this nursing diagnosis, one of the following major characteristics is required to be present, and it must be reported by the caregiver:

- Caregiver reports shortage of resources needed to provide care. (Although the caregiver desires to care for the client, because of other responsibilities or lack of support from other family members, caregiving may require more time, money, emotional strength, or physical energy than is available.)
- Caregiver has difficulty in doing specific caregiving activities. (The caregiver lacks the needed knowledge, strength, developmental readiness, or confidence in ability to provide care such as bathing, toileting, and managing pain.)
- Caregiver expresses emotional or psychological difficulty in caring for the client. (The caregiver worries about uncertain needs and ongoing care, or may feel loss, stress, nervousness, anger, or depression owing to the client's previous relationship or present dependency.) (NANDA, 1994).

Related Factors

There are numerous etiologic or contributing factors that may lead to or place a caregiver at risk for role strain. They revolve around four categories: pathophysiologic/physiologic, developmental, psychosocial, and situational.

Pathophysiologic/physiologic factors include illness severity; addiction or codependency; premature birth or congenital defect; discharge with significant home care needs; caregiver's health; unpredictable course or instability in the care receiver's health; or the caregiver is female.

Developmental factors include caregiver not developmentally ready for caregiver role; and developmental delay or retardation of care receiver or caregiver.

Psychosocial factors include psychological or cognitive problems in care receiver; marginal family adaptation or dysfunction; caregiver's marginal coping patterns; past history of poor relationship between caregiver and care receiver; caregiver is spouse; care receiver exhibits deviant, bizarre behavior.

Situational factors include abuse or violence; situational stressors that normally affect families; duration of time required for caregiving; inadequate physical environment for providing care; family/caregiver isolation; lack of respite for caregiver; inexperience with caregiving; caregiver's competing commitments; complexity/amount of caregiving tasks (NANDA, 1994).

Diagnostic Statement: Risk for Caregiver Role Strain

Definition

Risk for Caregiver Role Strain is a caregiver's vulnerability for felt difficulty in performing family caregiver role (NANDA, 1994).

Risk Factors

Related factors for Caregiver Role Strain, listed earlier, become risk factors in this diagnostic statement.

Diagnostic Statement: Altered Family Processes

Definition

Altered Family Processes is the state in which a family that normally functions effectively experiences a dysfunction (NANDA, 1994).

Defining Characteristics

Of the defining characteristics or clinical cues that denote this nursing diagnosis, one of the following major characteristics is required to be present:

- Family system unable to meet physical, emotional, security, or spiritual needs of its members. (Although the family continues to function in meeting most of their requirements, for some reason such as lack of resources or poor communication, at least one of the areas of need—physical, emotional, security, or spiritual—is not satisfied.)
- Family unable to adapt to situational or developmental change. (The family may not be able to understand the change, to alter roles, or to express need or accept help from others or the community to adapt to the change.)
- Inappropriate family interaction. (The family may be unable to communicate or make decisions, or may not demonstrate respect or acceptance of individual members' ideas, feelings, and actions, or

may inappropriately direct their energy.) (NANDA, 1994.)

Related Factors

Two etiologic or contributing factors may be associated with alterations in the process of family functioning: situation transition or crisis, such as job loss, surgery, or trauma, which requires families to deal with unexpected events; and developmental transition or crisis, such as birth of a preterm infant or need to care for an aging parent, which increases the complexity of the family's normal pattern of functioning (NANDA, 1994).

Diagnostic Statement: Ineffective Family Coping: Compromised

Definition

Ineffective Family Coping: Compromised is the state in which a usually supportive primary person (family member or close friend) is providing insufficient, ineffective, or modified support, comfort, assistance, or encouragement that may be needed by the client to manage or master adaptive tasks related to his or her health challenge (NANDA, 1994).

Defining Characteristics

Defining characteristics or clinical cues that point to this diagnosis include both subjective and objective factors, one of which must be present.

Subjective characteristics are the following:

- Client expresses or confirms a concern or complaint about significant other's response to his or her health problem. (The client has knowledge of the effectiveness of care provided by others.)
- Significant person describes preoccupation with personal reaction to client's illness, disability, or to other situational or developmental crises. (The significant person may be experiencing fear, anticipatory grief, guilt, or anxiety.)
- Significant person describes or confirms an inadequate understanding or knowledge base. (A knowledge deficit interferes with effective assistive or supportive behaviors.) (NANDA, 1994.)

Objective characteristics include:

- Significant person attempts assistive or supportive behaviors with less than satisfactory results (The effectiveness of care can be determined from observation of the client's physical or emotional condition.)
- Significant person withdraws or enters into limited or temporary personal communication with the client at the time of need. (Altered communication may indicate the personal discomfort being experienced by the significant person.)
- Significant person displays protective behavior disproportionate to the client's abilities or need for autonomy. (Either overprotective behavior or neglect of the client can interfere with effective care.) (NANDA, 1994).

Related Factors

Several etiologic or contributing factors may result in compromised family coping behaviors. They may include inadequate or incorrect information or understanding on the part of a significant person, which may result in incompetent care; temporary preoccupation by a significant person who is trying to manage his or her own emotional conflicts and personal suffering, resulting in an inability to perceive or act effectively with regard to client's needs; temporary family disorganization, role changes, or other situational or developmental crises or situations the significant person may be facing that limit the resources available for helping the client; little support provided by client, in turn, for significant person, which may inhibit motivation to provide care; and prolonged disease or disability progression that may exhaust supportive capacity of significant people (NANDA, 1994).

Diagnostic Statement: Ineffective Family Coping: Disabling

Definition

Ineffective Family Coping: Disabling is the behavior of a significant person (family member or other primary person) that disables his or her own capacities and the client's capacities effectively to address tasks essential to either person's adaptation to the health challenge (NANDA, 1994).

Defining Characteristics

Of the defining characteristics or clinical cues that identify Ineffective Family Coping: Disabling, one of the following must be present:

- Neglectful care of the client with regard to illness treatment or physical, emotional, or spiritual needs. (Neglect can still be present even if the client's appearance is clean and orderly.)
- Distortion of reality regarding the client's health problem. (This may be noted as denial of its existence or severity, or intolerance, rejection, abandonment, or desertion of the client, or carrying on usual routines that disregard the client's needs.)

- Psychosomaticism. (The significant person may take on illness signs of the client or show prolonged over-concern for client.)
- Impaired individualization. (The significant other may limit meaningful life for client or self or neglect relationships with other family members; eventually agitation, depression, aggression, or hostility may result.)
- Decisions and actions by family that are detrimental to economic or social well-being. (This may be seen as the client develops feelings of isolation, helplessness, and inactive dependence.) (NANDA, 1994.)

Related Factors

Etiologic or associated factors may have contributed to the family's inability to cope. These may include significant person has chronically unexpressed feelings of guilt, anxiety, hostility, or despair that inhibit development of a trusting relationship and effective problem-solving; incompatible coping styles of the significant person and client or among significant people, which limits their ability to dealing with adaptive tasks; highly ambivalent family relationships, which has the effect of inhibiting their ability to function supportively; and inconsistent handling of family's resistance to treatment, which tends to solidify defensiveness as it fails to deal adequately with underlying anxiety (NANDA, 1994).

Diagnostic Statement: Altered Parenting

Definition

Altered Parenting is the state in which a nurturing figure(s) experiences an inability to create an environment that promotes the optimum growth and development of another human being (NANDA, 1994).

Defining Characteristics

Of the defining characteristics or cues, one of the following major characteristics must be present to define "Actual" Altered Parenting:

- Physical or psychological trauma. (This may be noted as obvious signs of abuse or inappropriate caretaking behaviors such as inadequate feeding, or may be suggested by a history of child abuse or frequent accidents/illnesses, or repeated "runaway" behavior).
- Lack of parental attachment behaviors. (Inappropriate visual, tactile, or auditory stimulation may be noted; the parent may have child call himself or herself by first name instead of traditional titles such as "mom" or "dad"; or the parent may verbalize resentment or negative perception of child's gender, physical characteristics, and body functions; abandonment may result.)
- Neglect and inattention to infant/child needs. (This may be revealed in noncompliance with health appointments for self or child, a lag in growth and development, or the child receiving care from multiple caretakers without consideration for the child's needs.)
- Observed or verbalized role inadequacy. (The parent may be using inappropriate or inconsistent discipline practices, or may verbalize that he or she cannot control child, or may compulsively seek role approval from others.) (NANDA, 1994.)

Related Factors

There are several etiologic or contributing factors that may contribute to Altered Parenting. They may include lack of an available role model or an ineffective role model, which limits the person's parenting skill development; physical or emotional abuse of parent, which may threaten his or her own survival; lack of support between/from significant other(s) that limits coping ability; unmet social, emotional, or maturational needs of person that may result in parental role inadequacy; interruption in bonding process that may occur with mental or physical illness such that the parent and child do not have an opportunity to develop a trusting relationship and may lack role identity; lack of knowledge or limited cognitive functioning resulting in unrealistic expectations; unrealistic expectations for self, infant, or partner, resulting in frustration and inappropriate parenting behaviors; presence of stress (financial, legal, recent crisis, multiple pregnancies, cultural move), which may be expressed as abuse or neglect of the child; and a child may show no response or inappropriately respond to parents, which may discourage positive relationships (NANDA, 1994).

Diagnostic Statement: Risk for Altered Parenting

Definition

Risk for Altered Parenting is the state in which a nurturing figure(s) is at risk of experiencing an inability to create an environment that promotes the optimum growth and development of another human being (NANDA, 1994).

Defining Characteristics

The presence of risk factors such as those listed earlier under Altered Parenting are indications that the family is at risk for altered parenting. Especially critical are inattention to the infant's or child's needs and inappropriate caretaking behaviors.

Related Factors

Related factors are the same as those discussed earlier for Altered Parenting.

Diagnostic Statement: Parental Role Conflict

Definition

Parental Role Conflict is the state in which a parent experiences role confusion and conflict in response to crisis (NANDA, 1994).

Defining Characteristics

Of the defining characteristics or clinical cues that indicate this nursing diagnosis, one of the following major characteristics must be present:

- Parent verbalizes concerns or feelings of inadequacy about providing for the child's physical or emotional needs. (This occurs in response to a crisis such as hospitalization or the need to care for an ill child at home.)
- Demonstrated disruption in caretaking routines. (The family is not able to maintain their normal pattern of behavior during a crisis situation.)
- Parent expresses concern about changes in family. (These changes can include alterations in parental role, family functioning, family communication, or family health related to the crisis situation.)

Minor defining characteristics may also be present, but are not required for this diagnosis. They may include

- Parent(s) expresses concern about perceived loss of control over decisions relating to their child
- Reluctance to participate in usual caretaking activities even with encouragement and support
- Verbalize/demonstrate feelings of guilt, anger, fear, anxiety, or frustration about effect of child's illness on family process (NANDA, 1994).

Related Factors

Parental role conflict may be associated with several etiologic or contributing factors. They may include separation from the child due to illness of the parent or child, specialized care center policies, or change in marital status; intimidation with invasive or restrictive treatments such as isolation or intubation that provokes anxiety in the parent; home care of a child with special needs such as apnea monitoring that causes feelings of inadequacy in the parent; and interruptions of family life caused by the home care regimen, which may result in limited time for caring for other children and lack of respite for caregivers (NANDA, 1994).

Related Nursing Diagnoses

When a family is dysfunctional, other problems may arise for its members. Related nursing diagnoses include Anxiety; Decisional Conflict; Fear; Anticipatory or Dysfunctional Grieving; Chronic or Situational Low Self-Esteem; Powerlessness; Altered Role Performance; Impaired Verbal Communication; Impaired Social Interaction; Social Isolation; Relocation Stress Syndrome; Spiritual Distress; and High Risk for Violence (Self-Directed or Directed at Others).

Outcome Identification and Planning

After the nursing diagnoses and related factors are identified, client goals and nursing interventions are planned. Goals are designed to identify the general and specific changes that the client and family think will demonstrate that the situation has improved. Client- and family-centered care goals are often derived from identification of the contributing factors and are designed to indicate specific, discernible behaviors. General goals can be identified for family functioning and then individualized for each client situation. Common client- and family-centered goals for families experiencing problems include:

Client and family will identify instances in which intrafamily communication has been achieved.
Client and family will demonstrate awareness of other members' needs for physical care, economic security, education, and nurturing.
Client and family will demonstrate knowledge of effective coping mechanisms.
Client and family will demonstrate achievement of the developmental stages of the individual and family.

When using family-centered care, the nurse in the situation at the beginning of the chapter will need to review and clarify expectations with both the mother and the grandmother before proceeding to interventions. Implementation is most effective when the client, family, and nurse have collaboratively set goals and developed interventions.

Nurses plan with the client, the family, or both to promote healthy family patterns and function or to assist directly in meeting the needs of the dysfunctional family. Planning will be influenced by motivation and educational needs. Examples of nursing interventions commonly used in family care are listed in the accompanying display and discussed in the following section.

Planning
Examples of Nursing Interventions Used in Family-Centered Care

Family Coping

- Identify decision-making style in the family.
- Encourage open discussion among family members.
- Identify coping mechanisms within the family.
- Teach communication skills for expressing concerns.
- Support use of counseling for the family to improve communication.
- Identify self-help and support groups appropriate for the family dysfunction.
- Refer to parenting groups or classes if needed.

Problem-Solving Needs

- Clarify the actual conflict among the participants.
- Assist participants in identifying contributing factors.
- Correct and clarify misconceptions.
- Provide concrete feedback based on nursing observations.
- Assist participants in developing solutions.
- Support decision-making among participants.

Implementation

To promote family function, the nurse supports, reinforces, teaches, and gives anticipatory guidance. Interventions for the dysfunctional family include referral, counseling, and help with problem-solving. The more members of the family the nurse can involve, the more family-centered the care, and the greater the potential impact on the family.

Nursing Interventions to Promote Family Health and Function

The emphasis is on prevention of family dysfunction. The family can be supported by identifying strengths and reinforcing positive behaviors and resources. These strengths and resources are key areas to assess and can be included in your first visit with the family described at the beginning of this chapter.

Reinforcement of Family Strengths

From information obtained in the assessment, the nurse can help the client and family identify their own areas of strength. These could include effective communication, good parenting practices, mutual support of members, flexible roles, general stability, healthy coping mechanisms, and presence of good support systems (Fig. 49-8). Identification of strengths will help the family realize that it has resources to draw from for daily functioning, as well as for when crises develop. Focus is on the strengths rather than weaknesses of the family. The nurse can point out examples of strengths, such as the ability of a husband to take a leave of absence to care for the children while the wife is undergoing treatment for her illness, or the spiritual support provided by the family's clergy or spiritual consultant. The client and family should be encouraged to think of examples of strengths they have used when faced with problems in the past and how these strengths can be drawn on if needed. It is important to identify both individual and family strengths.

Support

The nurse can support the client and family in actions that promote family functioning. The nurse acts as a support system by listening to and educating the client and family. With serious or chronic illnesses, close bonds may be formed between the nurse and client and family, so they may naturally look to the nurse for emotional support. The nurse also helps them identify other sources of support in their lives. These may include extended family, religious affiliations, work groups, peers, and community groups. Once identified, contact with support groups can be strengthened to help the family function. The family should be assured that use of support systems is a strength rather than weakness.

Client Teaching
Family Relationships

Instruct the client as follows:

- *Identify your family's strengths and use them when dealing with family problems.*
- *Seek outside support when there are problems. Outside support is a strength rather than a weakness.*
- *Use clear communication, clarify ideas, and listen to one another.*
- *Use positive (rather than negative) coping mechanisms to deal with family stress.*
- *Use problem-solving techniques to work through your problems: recognize general problem area; gather information pertaining to it; define specific problem(s); discuss means of solving the problem(s); decide on which means you will use and set goals; periodically evaluate your progress and make further plans.*

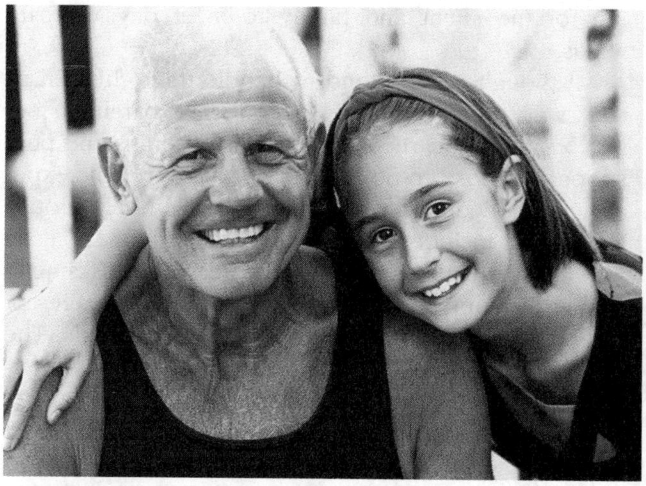

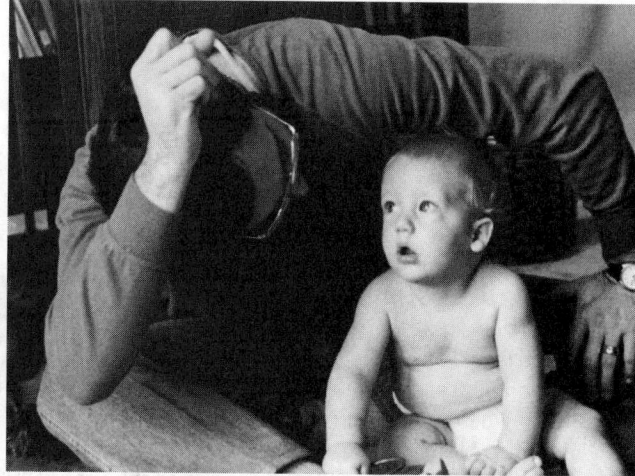

Figure 49-8 • *Sources of strength and support come in various relationships, such as grandfather and granddaughter or father and son.*

Anticipatory Guidance

Anticipatory guidance is a technique that combines teaching and support. Rather than focusing on what has happened in the course of an illness, the nurse prepares the client and family for what is going to happen, and why. A proven example of anticipatory guidance is childbirth preparation. Anticipatory guidance is especially helpful for developmental issues. Family development and child development can be fostered by guiding the family through what is expected to occur and what actions can be helpful. Specific information should be taught, so the family knows what to expect (Fig. 49-9). See Table 16-2 for a list of developmental tasks and parental focuses that can be used to guide the childrearing family. Developmental aspects are discussed in more detail in Chapter 16. General nursing interventions using anticipatory guidance include:

- Provide a safe and accepting environment for discussion.
- Offer anticipatory information of expectations for child development.
- Identify a positive support system for parents to contact if problems arise.
- Provide opportunities to observe parent–child interactions.
- Discuss parenting strategies and alternatives if problems arise.

Caregivers need to be helped to understand the child's development and express their feelings about their own parenting roles. Opportunities for physical and emotional contact need to be provided. Culturally based child-care practices can also be important. For example, if a grandmother is afforded a primary responsibility in advising the family, it is appropriate to support this cultural tradition unless the advice is injurious. Teaching should be directed toward all people who are involved in the child's care.

Nursing Interventions for Altered Family Function

If altered family functioning has been identified, interventions focus on adopting behaviors that will return the family to positive outcomes and improve the problem. The nurse can help the family with problem-solving, offer referrals, and facilitate family counseling if necessary.

Problem-Solving

Nurses can help dysfunctional families attain goals by assisting them in problem-solving. Interventions

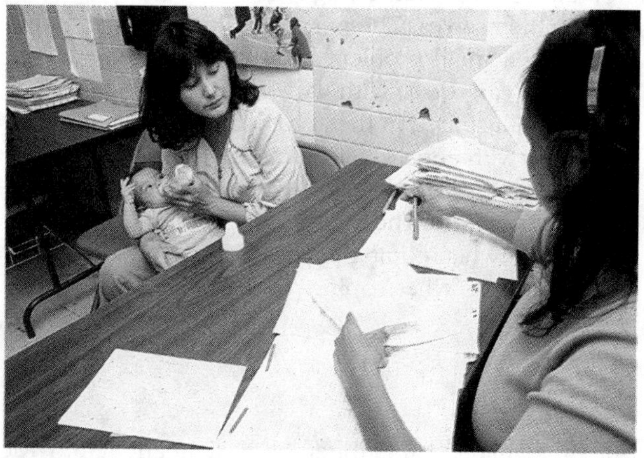

Figure 49-9 • *Anticipatory guidance is an important aspect of nursing responsibilities. Families who understand the developmental aspects of their children can better cope with the impact of certain tasks.*

Safety Alert
Family Care

- If you suspect child abuse, notify the police or local child protective services agency. Tell the family that you are acting as an advocate for the child, and you are legally responsible to report your suspicion.
- Enlist the help of social services to assist the family.
- Find resources for child care, paying medical bills, and providing other basic needs while a parent is hospitalized.
- Refer an abused spouse to the police or temporary shelter when safety is threatened.
- Point out the deleterious effects of alcohol or drug abuse on the person and family, and refer the person to a substance abuse treatment program.

aimed at resolving a family conflict must first identify the willingness of participants to acknowledge a problem and their ability to communicate. Communication practices, such as allowing each member to speak, listening, and expressing feelings as well as facts, should be stressed. Nursing interventions to foster problem-solving would then include:

- Clarify the conflict with participants
- Help participants identify contributing factors
- Correct misconceptions
- Provide concrete feedback based on nursing observations
- Assist participants to develop solutions
- Support decision-making among participants.

The nurse should focus on helping the participants develop self-awareness and identify a working method to solve problems. The family should be led through problem-solving while being taught how to conduct the process themselves. The nurse should guide the family in solving a small problem first, providing reassurance that they can deal with larger problems. Problem-solving is illustrated in the accompanying display.

Along with improving communication and problem-solving, coping mechanisms should be strengthened (see Chapter 51). The nurse can assist the family in identifying what coping mechanisms worked in the past, as well as what coping mechanisms can be detrimental.

Referral

The nurse may be able to refer the client and family for help in areas of dysfunction within the agency. Members of the social service department or spiritual ministry may help families with unmet needs. Clinical nurse specialists, nutritionists, and physical and occupational therapists may provide information and training for the client and family to meet physical care needs.

Although people tend to handle their children as they were treated themselves, effective parenting behaviors can be learned. Professional referrals and peer support groups can be sources of help to people experiencing difficulty in a parenting role. Self-help groups for parents include Parents Without Partners, La Leche League International, and Parent Effectiveness Training. Numerous support groups listed in the blue pages of phone books are valuable resources for referrals. The Association for the Care of Children's Health, an international organization located in Bethesda, Maryland, can provide information and a comprehensive list of support groups, their activities, and resources.

Other referrals the nurse may have to initiate are those to psychiatric programs, police, drug and alcohol treatment programs, social workers, department of child protective services, and shelters for battered women. When a family is in crisis, the nurse is obligated to ensure the safety of individual members through notification and referral to the appropriate groups. Evidence of suspected child abuse necessitates notification of the police and referral to appropriate agencies.

Ongoing counseling may be necessary for families with chronic stressors such as chronic illness, substance abuse, loss of family member, role strain, or separation or divorce. Family or marital counseling focuses on members interacting with one another rather than on counseling any one person. Roles and relationships are examined, communication and problem-solving are fostered, and bonds are strengthened. Nurses can be instrumental in leading clients and families to counseling if members are unable to overcome dysfunction within the family without outside help.

Community-Based Nursing

Dysfunctional family relationships often must be dealt with in the home environment, placing stress and additional responsibility on family members. When the causative factor is illness, it is necessary to assess the home environment for supports and barriers to provision of appropriate care and quality of life. Family members can differ in their willingness to assume additional responsibilities. Referral to social agencies such as home health care providers may be needed to ensure adequate support for a person or family.

Healthcare planning should address specific needs, types of assistance and equipment needed, who needs to be taught what, and alternative support availability. Teaching family members techniques of care to meet physical needs can assist in adaptation to the role of caregiver. Teaching should also include signs of risk factors for complications to promote confidence in caring for a client at home. Providing the family with the

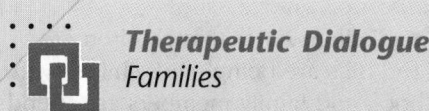

Therapeutic Dialogue
Families

Scenes for Thought

The Loeman family (Ronald and Marilyn, aged 50, Jeff, aged 18, and Stefanie, aged 14 years) are in the hospital visiting Mr. Loeman, Ronald's father, aged 84 years, who lives with them. Mr. Loeman, an otherwise healthy person, has been admitted for a replacement of his pacemaker and is doing well at this time, 2 days postoperatively. He, his family, and you, his nurse, are sitting in the unit's solarium chatting.

Effective

Ronald: *Dad looks great, doesn't he, Mr. Ballard?* Beaming at his father and patting his shoulder.
Nurse: *He does seem to be recovering well after the surgery. How do you feel today, Mr. Loeman? (Sitting next to the wheelchair).*
Mr. L: *Wonderful, wonderful! Why do all of you keep asking me that and treating me like I'm a baby?* Grumpily.
Marilyn: *Now, Dad, don't start that. We're just concerned about you, you know that.* Smiling tightly and throwing significant looks at her husband.
Jeff: *Mom, Stef and I are going to the cafeteria for a soda.* Starts to leave with his sister.
Ronald: *Not now, Jeff. Stay and visit with Opa for a little while. We've only been here 5 minutes.* Sternly.
Mr. L: *Never mind, Ronald. Let them go. I'll see them later. Here, Jeff, have a soda on me.* Hands him a few dollars. The children quickly leave.
Ronald: *You spoil them, Dad.* Exasperated.
Mr. L: *And why not? They're my only grandchildren. When I go they won't get much, but at least they'll think of me fondly.* Looks sad, defiant, and angry. *Mr. Ballard, wheel me back to my room. I'm tired.*
Nurse: *Sure, Mr. Loeman. Is it okay with you if I talk to Ronald and Marilyn while you rest? (Continues to sit next to him.)*
Mr. L: *What are you going to talk to them about?* Suspiciously.
Nurse: *What they need to do to help you recover when you're discharged tomorrow. Would you rather stay and participate? Or would you like to rest in bed and participate while you're resting?*
Mr. L: Thinking about it. *I'd rather rest in bed and listen to you all in my room. I'm tired.*
Nurse: Good idea. *Let's go. I'll get us all some juice on the way. (Wheels Mr. L. to his room. He looks tired but more relaxed. Ronald and Marilyn look surprised at how easily the decision was accomplished. They make a mental note to try it at home with Mr. L.)*

Less Effective

Ronald: *Dad looks great, doesn't he, Mr. Boren?* Beaming at his father and patting his shoulder.
Nurse: *He does seem to be recovering well after the surgery. How do you feel today, Mr. Loeman? (Sitting next to the wheelchair).*
Mr. L: *Wonderful, wonderful! Why do all of you keep asking me that and treating me like I'm a baby?* Grumpily.
Nurse: Now, now, *Mr. Loeman, your family are all here to see you because they love you. You were looking forward to seeing them this morning, remember? (Gives his hand a reassuring pat.)*
Jeff: *Mom, Stef and I are going to the cafeteria for a soda.* Starts to leave with his sister.
Ronald: *Not now, Jeff. Stay and visit with Opa for a little while. We've only been here 5 minutes. Sternly.*
Mr. L: *Never mind, Ronald. Let them go. I'll see them later. Here, Jeff, have a soda on me.* Hands him a few dollars. The children quickly leave.
Nurse: *That's sweet, Mr. Loeman. I'll bet they really appreciate you. (Smiles at Ronald and Marilyn. They smile weakly back.)*
Mr. L: *Mr. Boren, wheel me back to my room. I'm tired.*
Nurse: *Sure, Mr. Loeman. (To Ronald and Marilyn.) I'll be right back. I'll just get him settled.*
Mr. L: *What are you going to talk to them about?* Suspiciously.
Nurse: *Just about how to help you recover when you go home tomorrow. Don't you worry, we'll take good care of you. Here's your room, now. (Helps Mr. L. into bed. Marilyn and Ronald silently watch them go.)*

Critical Thinking Challenge

• Analyze the effect Mr. L's illness has on his family (individually and collectively). • Detect and examine how the stress shows up. • Construct what the family must be like at home together. • Detect what indicates this is a dysfunctional family. • Compare and contrast how the two nurses facilitated and hindered family coping.

name and phone number of someone to contact with questions can ease client and caregiver anxiety in the home setting. An interdisciplinary approach should include referrals to social workers, counselors, spiritual advisors, community resource centers, and self-help support groups as needed.

Examples of self-help and support groups that are often community based include Alcoholics Anonymous, Al-Anon, Al-Ateen, Narcotics Anonymous, cancer support groups, Compassionate Friends, stroke support groups, and Alzheimer support groups. These groups can help the family work out problems by providing information and emotional support. Parenting groups also are available.

Case management, a means of coordination and ongoing evaluation of care, is used to help the client and family deal with the complex healthcare system. Kaufman (1992) suggests that case management includes identifying, coordinating, and evaluating the provision of services, including cost, quality, and continuity. People must be connected to outside resources and support systems, as well as assisted to maximize their own strengths in caring for the client at home. Family members, neighbors, and community organizations can form a "family-centered" network of care ((Bond, et al., 1994). Their goal is to provide as "normal" a lifestyle as possible, with the client and family in partnership with the nurse case manager and other professional healthcare providers. If the caregivers, client, and family members are not in agreement, the case manager needs to remain nonjudgmental and show acceptance of the differences. Family-centered care is facilitated by encouraging everyone's active involvement; asking questions about each family member's knowledge and understanding of past and present situations as well as expectations about the future should help to define problems and suggest solutions. In the situation at the beginning of the chapter, questions addressed to the mother, grandmother, and anyone else involved in the infant's care could facilitate optimal home care.

Evaluation

Evaluation is an ongoing process of determining progress toward the stated goals that were described in the outcome identification phase. For alterations in family function, expected outcome criteria would focus on client and family communication, family needs, use of coping mechanisms, and family development. The following are examples of possible outcome criteria for general goals.

Goal

Client will identify instances in which intrafamily communication has been achieved.

Possible Outcome Criteria

- By discharge, each family member engages in conversation while visiting client, as observed by nurse.
- By discharge, other members listen while family member is talking, as observed by nurse.
- Client relates that content of conversations includes feelings within 48 hours.
- Client identifies nonverbal communication as being consistent with verbal messages within 48 hours.
- Client expresses use of alternatives such as telephone and letter writing when personal visits are not possible during hospital stay.

Goal

Client or family will demonstrate awareness of other members' physical care, economic security, educational needs, and nurturing.

Possible Outcome Criteria

- Within 48 hours, client states that children are being cared for, bills are being paid, children are attending school, and family members are attending social functions.
- Within 48 hours, family members display affection toward one another, as observed by nurse.

Goal

Client will demonstrate knowledge of effective coping mechanisms.

Possible Outcome Criteria

- During first counseling sessions, client discusses family coping mechanisms that worked in past.
- During first counseling session, client states coping mechanisms that were detrimental in past.
- By discharge, client verbalizes coping mechanisms that he or she will use in future.

Goal

Client will demonstrate achievement of developmental stages of the family.

Possible Outcome Criteria

- Client exhibits appropriate parenting behaviors (holds infant, maintains eye contact, smiles at infant) by discharge.
- Client maintains family contact by displaying pictures of children in room within 48 hours.
- Client discusses children with spouse within 48 hours.

Key Concepts

- Although the traditional nuclear family is common, many other family structures exist, including extended families, single-parent families, and blended families.
- Families function in their own unique ways, but usually have common goals. Some needs for which families provide include physical and economic provision of care, sexual intimacy, reproduction, education, socialization (including communication), as well as nurturing and support for problem-solving and goal-setting.
- Factors that affect family function include culture, economics, lifestyle, previous life experience, and stress and illness.
- Families and their relationships change in reaction to both acute and chronic illness. Roles may be redefined to meet individual and family needs.
- Common manifestations of altered family function include separation, divorce, role strain, abuse, social isolation, and emotional problems in children.

Nursing Plan of Care
The Infant and Family With Altered Parenting

Nursing Diagnosis

Altered Parenting related to anxiety, lack of knowledge, money, and paternal support manifested by developmental delay in infant; mother crying easily; verbalized inadequacy of knowledge, finances, and husband.

Family Goal

Child will experience nurturance as caregiver(s) increase parenting skills.

Family Outcome Criteria

- Mother demonstrates decreased anxiety with increased confidence in caretaking behaviors within 1 month.
- Infant demonstrates progress in development within 1 month.
- Family seeks external resources within 2 weeks.

Nursing Intervention	*Scientific Rationale*
1. Assess mother's knowledge of child-care techniques by questioning and observation. Be nonjudgmental. Encourage expression of feelings.	1. Verbal responses can be validated by objective data. Need to identify without provoking resentment.
2. Reinforce positive caregiving and focus on positive behaviors.	2. Reinforcement encourages mother and decreases anxiety.
3. Role-model effective stimulation techniques (low cost), such as having mother explore body parts, use colors, talk to and hold infant.	3. Stimulation is important for developmental growth. Sounds, body parts, and color are recognizable by 6 months.
4. Explore with mother ways to involve all family members in meeting infant needs consistently and securely.	4. By decreasing passivity infant can be helped to trust. Likelihood of compliance increased if all members involved.
5. Initiate a plan to develop parenting skills by providing information and alternative opportunities for mother–child interaction with feedback.	5. Information on realistic expectations and solutions can promote effective coping. Practice reinforces.
6. Explore possible sources of support. Offer to make initial contacts. Fear of authorities may inhibit initiating action.	6. Support needs to be ongoing for change to be maintained.
7. Refer for home visit care.	7. Continuity of care includes assessment and support.

- Both objective and subjective data are useful for assessment of family dysfunction. Assessment seeks to identify normal family patterns of function, families at risk for dysfunction, and actual dysfunction.
- Outcome identification and planning focus on the family members and the family unit when caring for dysfunctional families. Goals applying family-centered care involve improved communication and coping mechanisms, fulfilled needs of the family, and accomplished development of the family.
- A multidisciplinary approach is useful in interventions for altered family and social relationships. Interventions to promote family functioning include reinforcement of family strengths, support, and anticipatory guidance. Interventions for the dysfunctional family may include referral, problem-solving, and counseling.
- Evaluation of nursing care is accomplished by comparing outcomes with criteria established during the planning stage.

Critical Thinking Challenges

You have now increased your knowledge base of the family and social relationships. Review the situation at the beginning of the chapter, and answer the following questions.

1. *Analyze your initial feelings about this family's ability to care for the newborn at home.*
2. *Plan how you will elicit the family's perception of needs, goals, and outcomes.*
3. *Compare and contrast the differences in the mother's, grandmother's, and your perception of the situation.*
4. *Summarize key areas that should be assessed when you visit the family within 48 hours after discharge.*
5. *Recommend ways to facilitate family-centered care, particularly if there are disagreements about the home care plan.*

References

Ahmann, E. (1994). Family-centered care: Shifting orientation. *Pediatric Nursing*, 20, 113–117.

Bond, N., Phillips, P., & Rollins, J. A. (1994). Family-centered care at home for families with children who are technology dependent. *Pediatric Nursing, 20,* 123–130.

Caplan, G. (1990). Loss, stress, and mental health. *Community Mental Health Journal, 26,* 27.

Carpenito, L. J. (1993). *Nursing diagnosis: Application to clinical practice* (5th ed.). Philadelphia: J. B. Lippincott.

DeSantis, L. (1993). Haitian immigrant concepts of health. *Health Values: Achieving High Level Wellness, 17*(6), 3–16.

Duvall, E. (1977). *Marriage and family development* (5th ed.). Philadelphia: J. B. Lippincott.

Erikson, E. (1963). *Childhood and society.* New York: Norton.

Glick, P. C. (1994). American families: As they are and were. In A. Skolnick & J. Skolnick (Eds.). *Family in transition* (8th ed.) (pp. 91–104). New York: HarperCollins.

Kaufman, J. (1992). Case management services for children with special health care needs: A family-centered approach. *Journal of Case Management, 1*(2), 53–56.

Leff, P., & Walizer, E. (1992). *Building the healing partnership.* Cambridge, MA: Brookline.

North American Nursing Diagnosis Association (NANDA). (1994). *Nursing diagnoses: Definitions and classification 1995–1996.* Philadelphia: NANDA.

Parette, H. P. Jr. (1993). High-risk infant case management and assistive technology: funding and family enabling perspectives. *Matern Child Nurs J, 21,* 530–564.

Pearlin, L., Mullan, J., Semple, S., et al. (1990). Caregiving and the stress process: An overview of concepts and their measures. *The Gerontologist, 30,* 583–594.

Thomas, D. D. (1993). Minorities in North America: African-American families. In J. L. Paul & R. J. Simeonsson (Eds.). *Children with special needs: Family, culture, and society* (2nd ed.) (pp. 122–138). Philadelphia: Harcourt Brace Jovanovich.

Thomas, S. B., Quinn, S. C., Billingsley, A., et al. (1994). The characteristics of northern black churches with community outreach programs. *Am J Public Health, 84,* 575–579.

United States Bureau of the Census. (1990). *Statistical abstract of the United States: 1990.* Washington, DC: Author.

Wang, T. M. (1993). Families in Asian cultures: Taiwan as a case example. In J. L. Paul & R. J. Simeonsson (Eds.). *Children with special needs: Family, culture, and society* (2nd ed.) (pp. 165–178). Philadelphia: Harcourt Brace Jovanovich.

Wright, L. M., & Leahey, M. (1994). *Nurses and families: A guide to family assessment and intervention* (2nd ed.). Philadelphia: F. A. Davis.

Bibliography

Basolo-Kunzer, M. (1994). Caring for families of psychiatric patients. *Nurs Clin North Am, 29*(1), 73–79.

Danielson, C., Hamel-Bissell, B., & Winstead-Fry, P. (1993). *Families, health, and illness.* St. Louis: C. V. Mosby-Year Book.

Ebersole, P., & Hess, P. (1990). *Toward healthy aging: Human needs and nursing response* (3rd ed.) St. Louis: C. V. Mosby.

Groce, N., & Zola, I. (1993). Multiculturalism, chronic illness, and disability. *Pediatrics, 91,* 1048–1055.

Hostler, S. L. (1991). Family-centered care. *Pediatr Clin North Am, 38,* 1545–1560.

Koroloff, N. M., & Friesen, B. J. (1991). Support groups for parents of children with emotional disorders: A comparison of members and non-members. *Community Mental Health Journal, 27,* 265–279.

Mayers, A., & Spiegel, L. (1992). A parental support group in a pediatric AIDS clinic: its usefulness and limitations. *Health Social Work, 17*(3), 183–191.

McCord, B. (1993). *Family profile.* Millersville, MD: The Coordinating Center for Home and Community Care.

McGonigel, M., Kaufmann, R., & Johnson, B. (Eds.). (1991). *Guidelines and recommended practices for the Individualized Family Service Plan* (2nd ed.). Bethesda, MD: Association for the Care of Children's Health.

Nugent, K., Hughes, R., Ball, B., et al. (1992). A practice model for a parent support group. *Pediatric Nursing, 18*(1), 11–16.

Pokorni, J. (1992). *Promoting family collaboration.* Videotape and study guide. Lawrence, KS: Learner Managed Designs.

Zambelli, G. C., & DeRosa, A. P. (1992). Bereavement support groups for school-age children: Theory, intervention, and case example. *Am J Orthopsychiatry, 62,* 484–493.

Loss and Grieving

Key Terms	Learning Objectives
Anticipatory grief *Bereavement* *Dysfunctional grief* *Grief* *Hospice* *Loss* *Mourning*	*Upon completion of this chapter, the student will be able to do the following:* • *Define selected terms related to loss and grief.* • *Identify the normal function of grief.* • *Analyze the advantages and limitations of using a stage model of grief to guide practice with clients who have experienced a loss or who are anticipating a loss.* • *Identify the common manifestations of grief.* • *Compare grief reactions after various types of losses.* • *Compare children's and adults' understanding of death and grief reactions.* • *Identify variables that influence normal grieving.* • *Discuss the effects of multiple losses on the grief process.* • *Apply the nursing process to grieving clients.* • *Differentiate between normal grieving and dysfunctional grieving.* • *Identify nursing interventions that would be appropriate at different points in the grief process.* • *Discuss the role of hospice programs in facilitating the grief process.*

50

You are a nurse working for a family practice physician. A woman comes to the office for a routine check-up because she "has no energy and is tired all the time." On taking her history, you learn that the woman's husband died 6 months ago, that her oldest child is preparing to leave for college, and her youngest child is entering first grade. The woman confides that she has been "having trouble coping" since her husband died, that she has lost all interest in things, including her children, that she has difficulty sleeping, and that she has lost 20 pounds in the past 6 months.

In previous chapters, you have built a knowledge base related to taking care of physical and emotional needs of clients and their families. One of the greatest emotional feelings is that of grieving and loss. As you pursue the profession of nursing, you will meet many people who are feeling loss. You will need to pull together your knowledge and understanding of people to work with those who have suffered a loss and are grieving. This chapter adds this consideration to your knowledge base. The Critical Thinking Challenges at the end of the chapter will help you apply what you have learned.

Loss and grief are universal experiences; each person experiences various losses from birth until death. These losses vary in importance, from insignificant losses that cause minor and brief distress, to major losses that cause intense and long-lasting distress. Grief is a normal response to loss: it is the price that humans pay for becoming attached to people, objects, or beliefs.

Normal Grief

Normal Grief Pattern

Grief has several important functions:

- To make the outer reality of the loss into an internally accepted reality
- To sever the emotional attachment to the lost person or object
- To make it possible for the bereaved person to become attached to other people or objects.

Although grief is often very painful, it is both normal and necessary. In contrast, inability to grieve is abnormal.

Characteristics of Normal Grief and Loss

Loss and Grief

Loss is a normal part of the human experience. Some losses are the result of normal development, whereas other losses are the result of nonnormative events. Whether a loss is the result of an expected developmental event or an unexpected, nonnormative event, grief is a necessary and normal reaction to loss. The presence of grief indicates attachment to the lost object or person (Fig. 50-1). Through the grief process the person is able to sever attachment to the lost person or object and become attached to other people or objects.

Loss. **Loss** is defined as the experience of parting with an object, person, belief, or relationship that is valued; the loss necessitates a reorganization of one or more aspects of the person's life. Losses range from minor ones, such as the loss of a wallet, which necessitates only minor adjustments, to major ones, such as the death of a loved one, which necessitates major adjustments. The intensity and duration of grief depend on numerous factors, including the significance of the loss, the person's personality, and the availability of support.

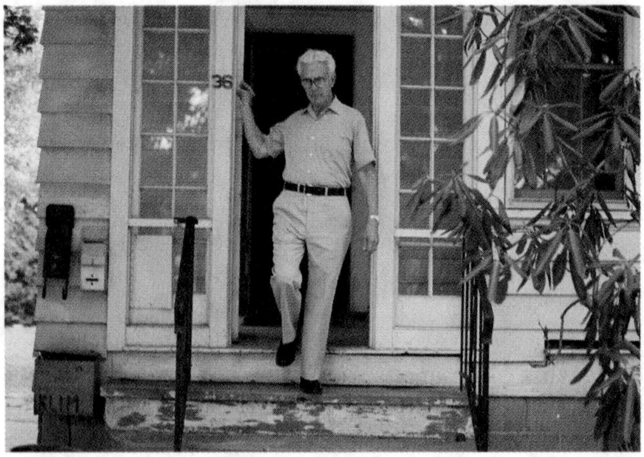

Figure 50-1 • Loss is a normal part of the human experience. Sometimes it means living alone in grief.

Losses are part of the normal developmental cycle. At birth, the newborn loses the warmth and security of the mother's womb. Later, the infant loses the comfort and gratification of the mother's breast. When a sibling is born, the child loses his or her place as the baby or the youngest in the family. Physical losses, such as loss of teeth, follow. Each loss has both negative and positive aspects. For example, by no longer being the youngest in the family, the child gains certain rights and responsibilities, but the child also loses the undivided attention of his or her mother and the special privileges attached to being the youngest in the family.

Many developmental milestones that are ordinarily perceived as desirable events have a component of loss to them. Graduation from high school signifies completion of a major portion of the adolescent's education, and a movement into the world of adults, with its greater freedoms and choices, but it also means the loss of important peer and teacher relationships, and the loss of the routine and security of the high school environment. Marriage is usually perceived as a gain of love, status, and security, but it may also result in a number of losses, such as loss of freedom, loss of individuality, and loss of the single lifestyle.

Individual patterns of coping with losses are established early in life. Parents often want to protect children from experiencing the pain of loss; however, such protection interferes with the child's development of skills to cope with loss. The person who has learned in childhood that loss is a natural part of life and that grief is a normal response to loss will be better prepared to cope with major losses later in life. On the other hand, a major loss or too many minor losses early in life often has a harmful effect on the child's personality development and on the child's ability to cope with losses and develop intimate interpersonal attachments.

Types of Loss. Losses may be categorized in a number of ways: objective versus subjective; actual versus perceived; material versus psychological; or expected versus unexpected. An objective loss is one that is readily recognized by others as a loss, whereas a subjective loss is one that is not readily apparent to others but is perceived by the person as a loss. A material loss is a loss of some tangible object or possession, whereas a psychological loss is a loss of something that has no physical form but has important symbolic meaning.

Objective or material losses include loss of a body part; loss of body function (paralysis); loss of money; loss of job (retirement); or loss of home (relocation, fire, or disaster). Subjective or psychological losses include loss of a relationship (by death, divorce, or termination of a friendship); loss of hope; loss of a dream; loss

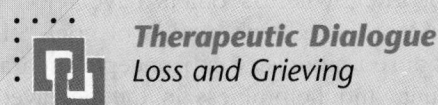

Therapeutic Dialogue
Loss and Grieving

Scenes for Thought

Maureen O'Hagan is 48 years old and had a simple mastectomy 2 months ago. She is married with two grown children and runs her own business. She is returning to the clinic for a check of her operative site. You note that she looks pale and tired even though she is dressed well and is wearing makeup.

Effective

Nurse: *Hi, Ms. O'Hagan. I'm Rosalie Brady, the clinical nurse specialist. I'm going to check your mastectomy site today and see how you're doing in general.*
Client: *Fine.* Gives a small smile just to be polite.
Nurse: *So how are you doing? (Showing concern, using good eye contact)*
Client: *I...I'm not too sure, actually. I have no pain, the arm feels fine, the scar is okay, but I don't seem to be back to my normal self yet. My husband is beginning to complain about our not having sex like we used to. I don't get it.* Looks confused, annoyed and depressed.
Nurse: *I'm checking your chart and all your blood work is fine. How have you been eating and sleeping? (Assessment of the physical signs of grief)*
Client: *Not too well. I can't get to sleep very easily, and then I wake up in the middle of the night with dreams I can't remember. And I have no appetite.*
Nurse: *It sounds like you've been going through a difficult time. You're having trouble with sleep, disturbing dreams, fatigue, appetite loss, decreased sex drive, and not feeling like yourself. Is there anything else you want to add? (Summarization, open-ended question)*
Client: *Uh, well, yes, but it's stupid.* Looks embarrassed.
Nurse: *Oh? (Continues with good eye contact and interested posture)*
Client: *I, ah, thought about driving into a wall one day last week. Quickly. I would never do it, but I got worried when I thought about that. Besides, what does it have to do with feeling tired and everything else?*
Nurse: *I think you haven't finished grieving for the loss of your breast. (Said gently)*
Client: After a short silence. *Oh. So you think I'm depressed? And that I haven't accepted that the breast is gone?*
Nurse: *Let's talk some more about it. I know some ways to help you feel better. Would that be okay?*
Client: *Well, maybe. I'm willing to try.*

Less Effective

Nurse: *Hi, Ms. O'Hagan, I'm Natalie Whorley, the clinical specialist on your case. How are you doing?*
Client: *Okay, I guess.*
Nurse: *Good! Any pain in the incision or in the muscles underneath? (Client shakes head no.) How about your general health? Any problems there? (Looking at client and chart)*
Client: *Well, I haven't been eating or sleeping too well since the operation.* Looks down at her hands.
Nurse: *Really? Your lab work looks good. I wonder what the problem is. Do you have any ideas?*
Client: *Not really.*
Nurse: *Well, let me see about getting you some sleep medication to relax you. Getting enough sleep usually makes people feel better right away. Okay? (Writes in chart and leaves the room. Ms. O'Hagan sighs.)*

Critical Thinking Challenges

• *Compare and contrast the signs to which Rosalie paid attention and Natalie missed.* • *Propose the stage of grief Ms. O'Hagan might be in. Give your reason.* • *Analyze her potential support system.* • *Specify other assessment factors to be considered.* • *Select interventions you would use if you were Rosalie.*

of a sense of immortality; or loss of a sense of invulnerability.

Many losses have both material and psychological components. For example, loss of a job results in the material loss of income, but it may also result in numerous psychological losses, such as loss of status, loss of self-esteem, loss of relationships with coworkers, loss of meaning for living, and loss of structure in daily routines. Loss of health may be objectively observable to the person and to others, or it may be unobservable to self or others. Loss of health often precipitates many other losses, such as loss of ability to work or to perform in one's marital or parental role, or inability to continue in social and recreational activities. Loss of health may be a precursor to loss of life, and therefore loss of health may initiate grieving for the person's anticipated death.

Loss of the breast by surgery provides an example of the complex interaction of the various types of loss. Loss of the breast has both objective and subjective components; the removal of the breast results in physical loss of a body part, but it may also result in some loss of function (inability to nurse a child or decreased strength in the arm) or loss of self-image, or perceived loss of potential for dating or for marriage, and thus the loss of the anticipated future. Although the objective loss is the same—loss of the breast—the significance of the loss varies greatly from person to person based on the subjective meaning of the loss as perceived by the person. Thus, objective losses are often accompanied by subjective losses. However, subjective losses may occur in the absence of an objective loss. The significance of the loss is determined by the individual's perception of the loss and the meaning he or she ascribes to the loss. An example of such a loss is presented in the accompanying Therapeutic Dialogue.

Infection with the human immunodeficiency virus is another example of an illness that results in multiple losses. Infected people often experience multiple intrapersonal, social, and economic losses long before they experience loss of health, or terminal illness. Concurrently, their families also face multiple losses, such as loss of hope for the future, loss of the loved one that they previously knew, and loss of their own freedom as they become caregivers for their ill family member or friend (Brown & Powell-Cope, 1991, 1993; Rolland, 1990).

Grief. **Grief** is the characteristic pattern of psychological and physiologic responses a person experiences after the loss of a significant person, object, belief, or relationship. Grief encompasses the entire range of physical, psychological, cognitive, and behavioral responses to a loss, and incorporates the loss into the personality and makes resolution of the loss possible.

Bereavement is a state of desolation that occurs as the result of a loss, particularly the death of a significant other. Bereavement manifestations are the person's total response to a loss and include emotional, physical, social, and cognitive responses.

Mourning encompasses the socially prescribed behaviors after the death of a significant other. Such behaviors vary from culture to culture. Mourning behaviors are socially conventional bereavement behaviors, and do not necessarily indicate the presence or absence of grief. Examples include wearing black clothing, or a black veil or arm-band.

Types of Grief. Two major types of normal grief have been identified: conventional grief, which occurs after a loss, and anticipatory grief, which occurs in anticipation of a loss.

Anticipatory grief is the characteristic pattern of psychological and physiologic responses a person makes to the impending loss (real or imagined) of a significant person, object, belief, or relationship. Although there is little agreement on the exact nature of anticipatory grief (Fulton & Gottesman, 1980; Rando, 1986), there is general agreement that anticipatory grief facilitates coping with loss when the loss actually occurs. Forewarning of a loss should not be confused with anticipatory grief, because it is possible to be forewarned of a loss and not engage in anticipatory grief.

Models of Grief

Normal grief is a multifaceted response to loss. Many researchers and theorists have attempted to describe the characteristics of normal grief and the grief process. Professionals from many disciplines, including nursing, have developed models of grief. Some have proposed stage models of grief, whereas others have rejected stage models and proposed task models of grief. Still others have proposed models of subconcepts such as bereavement guilt, and helpfulness in the bereaved. Each of these models provides a framework for understanding the grief process; which model a practitioner chooses to use will influence the nursing process.

Models of grief are useful in guiding nursing care of people experiencing loss. These conceptual models provide understanding of the normal grief process and can be used to provide directions for interventions. They are also useful in helping to identify grief reactions that are outside the normal range.

Some of the problems that arise from use of grief models result from the inappropriate application of these models, not from limitations in the models themselves. There are no clear-cut stages of grief, nor are there any exact timetables; furthermore, people tend to move back and forth from one stage to another. It is inappropriate and insensitive to expect everyone to conform to a specific model, and to imply that the client or the staff has failed if the client does not conform to the model.

Many models of grief have been developed (Miles & Demi, 1994); some of these are outlined in the display and discussed in the following paragraphs. Three popular stage models of grief are those proposed by Engel (1964), Kübler-Ross (1969), and Parkes (1986).

Whereas Engel and Parkes applied their models primarily to the bereaved, Kübler-Ross applied her model primarily to the dying, which may account for some of the differences between the models. All three saw shock and denial as the first reaction; however, there is little similarity between the models' subsequent stages.

Kübler-Ross' model has gained wide acceptance in nursing and other disciplines, probably because she was a pioneer in developing sensitive, compassionate care for the dying. Her work provided the impetus for increased attention to the needs of the dying and the bereaved, and had an influence on the later development of hospice programs. However, nurses must critically evaluate the relevance of Kübler-Ross' theory to their nursing practice (Carr, 1993).

Engel's Model. Engel (1964), one of the first to study grief, proposed six phases of the grief process: 1) shock and disbelief, 2) developing awareness, 3) restitution, 4) resolving the loss, 5) idealization, and 6) outcome. In the shock–disbelief stage, the survivor either refuses to accept the loss or shows intellectual acceptance of the loss but denies the emotional impact. Developing awareness occurs as the reality and meaning of the loss penetrate the person's consciousness. The numbness of the first phase is replaced with feelings of intense psychological pain, often expressed through crying and anger. The next phase, restitution, consists of the work of mourning and includes the various funeral and reli-

Models of Grief

Popular Early Models

Engel's Model

1. Shock and disbelief
2. Developing awareness
3. Restitution
4. Resolving the loss
5. Idealization
6. Outcome

Kübler-Ross' Model

1. Denial
2. Anger
3. Bargaining
4. Depression
5. Acceptance

Parkes' Model

1. Numbness
2. Yearning
3. Disorganization
4. Reorganization

Nursing Models of Grief

Murphy (1983)

Organized variables that influence bereavement responses

Richter (1984)

Interpersonal support, religious–spiritual belief, and interpersonal coping are resources that, when combined with caring approach of the nurse, can promote health after bereavement

Dimond (1981)

Complexity of grief and the interrelatedness of many intervening factors with bereavement processes and outcomes

Demi (1984)

Incorporates the stage theory of grief, crisis theory, and stress theory

Miles and Demi (1983–1984)

Bereavement guilt

Rigdon, Clayton, and Dimond (1986)

Helpfulness in the aged bereaved

Grief Cycle Model for Use With Bereaved and Other Types of Losses

1. Shock
2. Protest
3. Disorganization
4. Reorganization

gious rituals. The next phase, resolving the loss, occurs intrapsychically as the grieving person focuses energy on thoughts of the deceased. In the phase of idealization, first, all negative feelings toward the deceased are repressed, then, through identification, the survivor incorporates certain characteristics of the deceased into his or her own personality. Gradually, the grieving person's psychological dependence on the deceased diminishes and his or her interest in new relationships returns. According to Engel, the resolution of grief takes 1 year or more.

Kübler-Ross' Model. Kübler-Ross (1969) proposed five stages of grief: 1) denial, 2) anger, 3) bargaining, 4) depression, and 5) acceptance. The denial stage is similar to that proposed by Engel. Anger in the second stage may be directed toward fate, God, family members, healthcare providers, or others. Bargaining occurs as the client seeks to delay the dreaded event; the client bargains with God for more time, and, in return, promises to do something to repay God for this favor. Depression occurs when the client acknowledges the reality and inevitability of his or her impending death. In the fifth and final stage, acceptance, the client comes to terms with the loss, begins to detach himself or herself from supportive people, and to lose interest in worldly activities.

Parkes' Model. Parkes (1986) proposed four stages of grief in his model: 1) numbness, 2) yearning, 3) disorganization, and 4) reorganization. In the numbness stage, the bereaved survivor is so overwhelmed by the trauma that denial must be used as a psychological defense. This stage usually is of brief duration. The next stage, yearning, is characterized by intense psychological distress, with thoughts focusing on the deceased. The yearning stage generally lasts several months. The disorganization stage follows, and is characterized by severe depression, social withdrawal, and lack of interest in people and activities. Reorganization usually begins 6 to 9 months after the loss, and is characterized by a gradual renewal of interest in people and activities, and return of a sense of meaning in life. Parkes proposed that this progression through the stages of grief (after the death of a significant other) normally takes 2 or more years.

Nursing Models. Several nurses have also developed models of grief. Murphy (1983) organized the variables that influence bereavement responses into a model of grief. Richter (1984) proposed relationships between the variables that affect grief and health outcomes; in this model, interpersonal support, religious–spiritual belief, and interpersonal coping are resources that, when combined with the nurse's caring approach, can promote health after bereavement. Dimond's (1981) model indicated the complexity of grief by showing the interrelatedness of many intervening factors with bereavement processes and outcomes. Demi (1984) proposed a model of grief that incorporates the stage theory of grief, crisis theory, and stress theory.

Nurses have also developed models of grief subconcepts. Miles and Demi (1983–1984; Demi & Miles, 1994) developed a theory of bereavement guilt, and Rigdon and colleagues (1987) developed a theory of helpfulness in the aged bereaved. Each of these models is useful in guiding practice in specific types of bereavement situations.

Grief Cycle Model. The grief cycle model (Fig. 50-2), which was derived from Parkes' (1986) theory of grief, provides a model that can be used to guide practice with the bereaved. It can also be used, with minor modifications, to guide practice with people who have experienced other types of loss. The grief cycle model assumes that, before a major loss, the person is functioning on a relatively unchanging level.

Shock. When a loss occurs, the first reaction is shock; concurrent with shock is a drop to a lower level

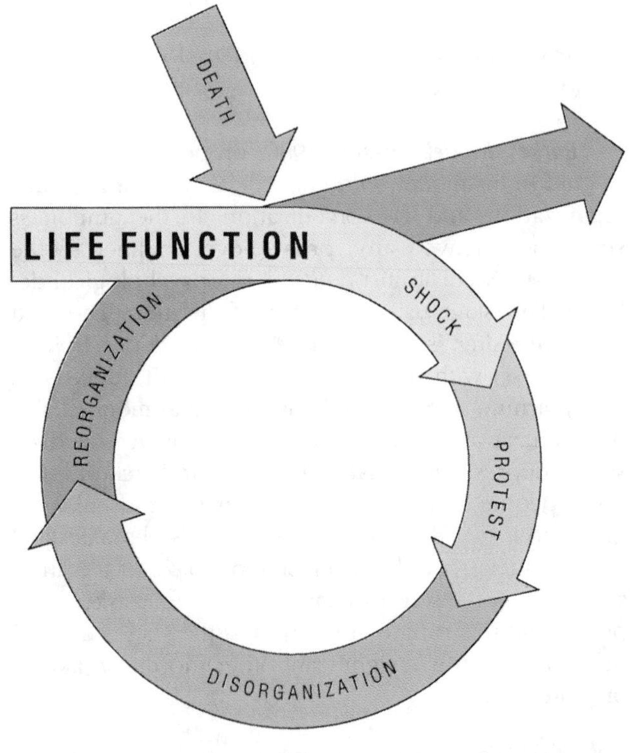

Figure 50-2 • Grief cycle. (From Demi, A. [1981]. Bereavement support group: Leadership manual. *Littleton, CO: Grief Education Institute.*

of functioning. The shock stage may last several hours to several days. The most common manifestations of the shock stage are listed in Table 50-1. People vary greatly in their responses to loss; some of the manifestations listed are polar opposites, such as hyperactivity and underactivity. Thus, not all of these characteristics are exhibited simultaneously by one person.

Protest. The second stage, protest, generally starts in the first week and continues through the third month. The person continues to drop in his or her level of functioning. During this period there is intense physical and psychological distress. The common characteristics of this stage are listed in Table 50-1.

Disorganization. The disorganization stage starts around the third month and continues for 3 to 6 months. The person continues to drop in his or her level of functioning and sinks to the lowest level of functioning during this stage. This stage is characterized by feelings of depression and social withdrawal. The manifestations of this stage are listed in Table 50-1.

Reorganization. The reorganization stage starts at approximately the sixth month and usually continues for at least 1 year, but may continue for a much longer period of time. Many people will continue in this phase for the rest of their lives. The major characteristics of this stage are listed in Table 50-1. During reorganization, the person gradually increases his or her level of functioning. People who have sufficient resources during this period are likely to continue to improve their level of functioning and often emerge from the grief cycle at a higher level of functioning than before the loss. On the other hand, people who experience many stressors during the grief period, and who have limited resources are often unable to recover fully from the grief experience, and thus will continue to function at a lower level than before the loss.

Caution must be used to prevent interpreting the grief cycle model too literally. In reality, the stages are not as discrete as the model implies, and there is much individual variation in the grief process. It is helpful to use the model as a general guide, however, while keeping in mind the fact that people may vary greatly in their responses to loss and still fall within the normal response range.

Comparison of Grief Reactions by Types of Loss

Only a few researchers have attempted to compare reactions to types of losses. Parkes (1986) compared grief reactions after the loss of a significant other by death with loss of a limb by amputation, and Fried (1962) compared reactions to death of a spouse with reactions to the loss of a home through relocation. Both of these researchers found a number of similarities in grief reactions after these diverse losses.

Table 50-1 • Major Functional Manifestations During Grief

Category	*Shock Stage*	*Protest Stage*	*Disorganization Stage*	*Reorganization Stage*
Cognitive	Slowed thinking Disorganized thinking Blocking of thoughts Wish to join deceased Thoughts of suicide	Preoccupation with thoughts of deceased Searching for deceased Dreams (pleasant or unpleasant) Hallucinations Concerns about health and safety of others Continued death wishes	Difficulty making decisions Aimlessness Loss of interest in people Loss of interest in work Loss of interest in usual activities Life perceived as meaningless Focus on memories and reminders of deceased	Realistic memory of deceased Comfortable when remembering deceased Return to previous level of ability
Denial	Denial of the reality of the loss Denial of the significance of the loss			
Emotional	Blunted affect Emotional outbursts May appear unaffected Euphoria Numb emotionally Feeling of unreality	Sadness Anger Guilt Relief Anxiety Yearning for deceased Presence of deceased felt	Depression Loneliness Meaninglessness Decreased self-esteem Apathy	Feels life has meaning Able to experience pleasure
Physical	Numbness Hyperactivity Underactivity Immobility	Pain in heart Sleep problems Appetite problems Weight loss Neglect of appearance Fatigue Lethargy	Continued sleep and appetite problems Restlessness Decreased sexual interest/satisfaction Aimless activity Decreased resistance to illness Accident prone Poor health habits Increased alcohol intake Increased drug use Increased tobacco use	Renewed vigor Restoration to previous level of health Improved health habits Sexual drive renewed
Social	Passive Unaware of others Focus on supporting others	Dependent on others Help and advice of others sought	Withdrawn Contact with other people avoided Initiative severely diminished Interest in social activities absent	New or renewed social relationships New or renewed activities Development of close relationship with at least one other person

Parkes (1986) found a similar pattern of reaction in amputees and in widows. The first reaction was the gradual process of realization, then a stage of alarm, and next an urge to search and recover the lost loved object. The process was less obvious in the amputee than in the widow, but it was nevertheless present. One of the problems for the amputees was that society did not expect them to mourn the loss of a leg, and thus they received little support in their grieving process. The bereaved were preoccupied with thoughts of the deceased, while the amputees were preoccupied with thoughts of their altered body image. Both groups of subjects pined painfully for the world that was no longer theirs. The widowed envied other couples, and the amputees envied intact people. Both groups of people felt anger at physicians and nurses.

Parkes found that, at 1 year after surgery, 26% of the amputees were still depressed and withdrawn, and most were making little use of their prosthesis. Parkes concluded that the psychosocial transition from intact person to amputee is a time-consuming process similar to the transition from married status to widowhood.

Two researchers investigated the effect of loss of one's home by relocation (Fried 1962; Marris, 1975). Fried (1962) studied Boston slum dwellers after their forced geographic relocation and found that although their reactions to the loss of their homes varied widely, the general pattern was congruent with a grief reaction. Common manifestations were feelings of loss, continued longing, depressive feelings, displaced anger, and idealization of the lost place. Marris (1975) studied Nigerian slum dwellers and found similar effects after their relocation. Marris proposed that the loss of one's home was as devastating as the death of a family member.

Loss: Crisis or Transition

Some theorists propose that a major loss results in a life crisis, whereas others propose that a major loss results in a life transition. Caplan's (1964) and Lindemann's (1944) early conceptualizations of bereavement as a life crisis were oversimplifications. Crisis theory (Caplan, 1964) is based on the following propositions:

- The psychobiologic forces for change during a crisis operate for a relatively short period of time (a few weeks).
- The outcome of a crisis is not predetermined but rather is determined by the balance of stressors and resources available during the crisis.
- During a crisis, a person has a heightened desire for help.
- During a crisis, the person is more susceptible to the influence of others.

In the intervening years, Caplan (1974) realized the inappropriateness of the proposition that a major loss can be resolved in a few weeks. Consequently, he developed a life transition theory, in which he proposed that there are several crisis periods during the course of mourning, which are more appropriately perceived as life transition periods than as a single crisis. He recognized that some people will continue the psychological work of mourning for the rest of their lives and still be within the normal range of grieving.

Factors Affecting Normal Function

Many factors influence people's reactions to loss, the course of the grief process, and the ultimate recovery from grief. These factors include characteristics of the loss itself, personal resources, personal stressors, sociocultural resources, and sociocultural stressors.

According to crisis theory (Caplan, 1964), the outcome of a loss experience is not predetermined, but rather is determined by the balance of stressors and resources present during the grief period. Thus, a person who has few stressors and many resources is likely to be able to cope well with a loss, whereas a person who has many stressors and few resources is likely to have difficulty coping with a loss.

Characteristics of the Loss

People have a tendency to ascribe their own values and feelings to others, and thus incorrectly assume that a specific loss is or is not traumatic to a specific person without first ascertaining the meaning of the loss to that person. Loss of a finger would have very different meanings to a classical guitarist and to a manual laborer. Divorce may be extremely undesired and cause intense grief in one person, or it may be welcomed and thus cause little or no grief reaction in another.

When it is a loved one who is lost, regardless of the mode of loss (eg, death, divorce, or separation), numerous aspects of the relationship affect the grief process. These aspects include such factors as the intensity of the relationship, the symbolic meaning of the relationship, the public recognition of the relationship, the amount of ambivalence in the relationship, and the availability of others to fulfill some of the roles of the lost person (Doka, 1989).

The circumstances under which the loss occurred also affect the grief process. A loss that occurs under violent or frightening conditions is much more difficult to cope with than a loss that occurs under more peaceful conditions. For example, a death that occurs as a result of homicide or suicide is usually more stressful than a death from natural causes. Another stressor is the perception that the grieving person in some way caused or contributed to the loss. For example, when a parent buys a child a bicycle and the child is maimed or killed in a bicycle accident, the parent may blame himself or herself for the accident.

Personal Resources and Stressors

Each person enters a loss situation with a unique combination of personal resources and stressors. What is a resource for one person may be a stressor for another. For example, health status may be either a resource or a stressor: the person who has good nutrition, good health habits, and a generally high level of wellness has a major advantage over the person who has poor nutrition, poor health habits, both chronic and acute diseases, and a history of emotional illness.

Personal resources and stressors that influence response to a loss include coping skills, previous experiences with loss, emotional stability, spiritual beliefs, physical health, individual developmental stage, family developmental stage, and socioeconomic status.

Research indicates that socioeconomic status is one of the major factors related to ability to cope with loss. People with higher levels of education, higher income, and higher job status tend to have better outcomes after a major loss. This may not be a causal relationship, but rather may be the result of the fact that people who are healthier mentally and physically are more likely to be in higher socioeconomic classes.

Additional factors that may influence outcomes are the number of other crises that the person experienced in the time periods preceding and after the loss. Other losses may produce a pile-up effect that may overwhelm the person's capacity to cope with these multiple stressors.

Sociocultural Resources and Stressors

The sociocultural resources and stressors that influence grief reactions also vary widely from person to person. Sociocultural resources include the social support that is available from family, friends, coworkers, and formal institutions (Fig. 50-3). Absence of these social supports creates additional stressors for the grieving person. In some instances, the presence of these supports can also be stressors, particularly if the resource people are not able to empathize with the grieving person. The overall sociocultural environment influences outcomes. If a community is able to deal with loss and has reasonable expectations of the survivors, this reduces stress; however, if the community tends to blame the survivors for their plight (as in the case of AIDS), or if the community has unrealistic expectations, the grieving person will have much more difficulty coping with the loss.

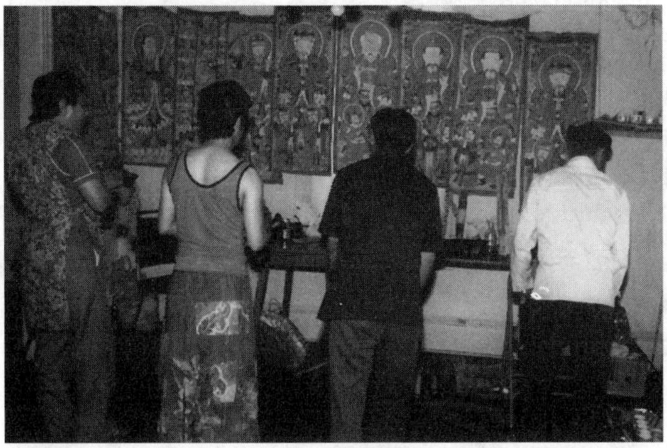

Figure 50-3 *• A Mien shaman and his assistants present offerings to the gods at a grandmother's home after her death in a hospital. (Photo courtesy of Marjorie A. Muecke, Seattle, WA.)*

Lifespan Considerations

The interaction of grief and the life cycle is complex. Grief may interfere with the achievement of developmental tasks, and developmental tasks may interfere with the grieving process. Thus, the person's developmental stage must be considered when assessing reactions to loss and planning interventions.

The impact of a traumatic event depends heavily on the developmental stage during which the event occurs. Children's reactions to loss differ markedly from adults' reactions, both in their specific characteristics and in their duration. Children tend to grieve in a piecemeal fashion. Losses are so painful to the young that they are able to endure distressing emotions for only brief periods of time; they grieve for intermittent periods of time, but their grief work extends over many years. Because children's distressing emotions are often expressed as anger or behavior problems, these signs are often not recognized as grief manifestations. The overwhelming need for love and security promptly motivates the child to search for and find a replacement for the lost loved person or loved object.

Newborn and Infant

To develop a concept of life and death, of being and nonbeing, one has to have cognitive function and have begun the socialization process. The newborn, thus, has no concept of life and death.

The ability to sense alterations in existence during the cycles of wakefulness and sleep is likened to a beginning understanding of the physical states of "being" and "nonbeing." The game of "peek-a-boo," ironically, an old English game meaning "alive or dead," introduces the child to the death-related concepts of absence and presence. The child's delighted reaction represents relief from the terror of being briefly separated from physical reality (Waechter, et al., 1985).

As the infant develops, he or she begins to distinguish the primary caregiver from other people. The infant responds to the mother's or father's voice and face. The infant's concept of death or loss is related to feelings of separation anxiety. This occurs when the mother is out of sight during early infancy, but levels off when the infant learns (as in peek-a-boo) that the mother still exists although she cannot be seen. Nevertheless, this recognition that mother will return initiates another realization that the mother *may not* return. Thus, the developmental task of developing a sense of trust works to nullify the anxiety that the caregiver will not return. Other characteristics of grief and loss in the infant are given in Table 50-2.

Toddler and Preschooler

Cognitive powers are evidenced by 18 to 24 months. Cognitive meaning intensifies the toddler's experience of separation anxiety. The developmental task of developing a sense of autonomy occurs during toddlerhood. This task helps the toddler break the tie with mother. She can now be out of sight for some time without the toddler being unduly concerned. However, because the toddler vacillates between being independent and being clinging, the separation still gives the toddler a fear of maternal loss or abandonment. Other characteristics of grief and loss in the toddler are given in Table 50-2.

Preschoolers develop an increasing awareness of themselves as separate physical and emotional beings. With this deepening awareness of "self" comes the vague realization that one's identity may cease to exist. Although preschoolers sense their own vulnerability and begin to make the distinction between being alive and dead, they still cannot grasp the finite limits imposed by death (Waechter, et al., 1985).

Preschoolers develop their concepts from their experiences. If the child watches television, many life concepts may develop from what they see. People die and reappear in another show, and this is how the preschooler sees death. The preschool child has some beginning cognitive understanding of death but perceives death as reversible, avoidable, and occurring in degrees.

Preschoolers think of death as a long sleep. They cannot differentiate infinite and finite. The death of a

Table 50-2 • Characteristics of Children Across the Lifespan Regarding Loss and Death Concept

Developmental Age	Developmental Task	Characteristics and Concepts
Infant	To develop a sense of trust	Dependent on those around him or her to meet his or her basic needs No intellectual capacity to comprehend death Experiments with concepts of absence/presence and being/nonbeing Anxiety separation from primary caregiver
Toddler	To develop a sense of autonomy	Less dependent, learning to separate from primary caregiver Egocentric Fully explores concepts of absence/presence and being/nonbeing May misinterpret illness as punishment for being bad Fears abandonment or separation from family
Preschooler	To develop a sense of initiative	Expanding his or her social environment Egocentric, influenced by magical thinking Death concept involves a temporary departure or sleep Fears family separation
School-aged child	To develop a sense of industry	Less egocentric; views world from an external point of view Death concept is well equated with old age and violence Death is personified Concept evolves rapidly until aware that death is irreversible, permanent Fascinated with physiologic phenomena and death rituals May believe in spiritual continuation Fears own possible death
Adolescent	To develop a sense of identity	Working toward being independent and self-sufficient Looking toward the future, establishing career, and personal life goals Moving into adulthood Death is viewed as a universal, inevitable process that is permanent

pet or a family member plays an important part in developing a concept of death, although their cognitive ability does not allow a clear understanding. At first they ask straightforward questions but later begin to develop an aversion to it.

Psychoanalysts believe that children cannot complete the work of mourning until they have a realistic concept of death. Because it is generally agreed that preschool-aged children have a very limited understanding of death, they are unable to complete mourning until they are older. Table 50–2 provides more information on the preschooler.

Child and Adolescent

The school-aged child gradually develops a more realistic concept of death. In the early school years, the child perceives death as unnatural, reversible, and avoidable; the child may also personify death (eg, perceives death to be a person or an animal). At about 9 years of age, the child's concept of death matures, and the child perceives death realistically as irreversible, universal, inevitable, and natural.

Society reinforces concepts of life and death. By school age, children have usually been touched by death in some way (ie, a family member, classmate, friend's family, a pet, or a news story). Some children live in violent neighborhoods where death is common, and some live in abusive families where injury and hospitalization may occur. The modern school curriculum includes discussions about war and death if these are prominent in the news or a traumatic local event occurs. The religious institution teaches about spiritual life and heaven and hell. Christian denominations observe the death, birth, and resurrection of a savior. The school child eventually realizes that death is an event no one escapes. See Table 50-2 for further characteristics of children regarding loss and grief.

As age increases, the child's understanding of death becomes more realistic. A high level of cognitive development allows the adolescent to view life and death with an adult understanding. Adolescents begin to develop a philosophy of life and death. "Nevertheless, the thought of one's own death is extremely overwhelming, and consequently, is suppressed. Adolescents are already in the midst of a developmental crisis during which they experience constant change" (Waechter, et al., 1985). Adolescents generally have the capacity to mourn fully, but they are at greater risk for poor outcomes than adults because of the numerous other stressors and developmental changes they experience during this stage of the life cycle (Hogan, 1994).

Adult and Older Adult

In contrast to children, adults tend to grieve more intensely and more continuously, but for a relatively shorter period of time. Furthermore, adults usually do not seek an immediate replacement for the lost loved person, but rather move toward this after achieving some resolution of their grief.

Young adults often experience many losses within a short period of time, which makes them particularly at risk for poor outcomes. They may experience the death of a family member for the first time in their lives, or the ending of their schooling and consequent separation from peers, or broken relationships, or failure in their attempt to achieve a satisfying job. The suicide rate for 20- to 24-year-olds is second only to the rate for the aged. Special attention must be given to meet the needs of this at-risk group.

Middle-aged adults who have a relatively stable lifestyle and adequate support systems generally cope well with loss; however, an untimely loss, such as the death of a child or the death of a spouse, may be extremely stressful, because this is perceived as out of the normal sequence of events.

Older adults are at higher risk in general than other adults for poor outcomes after major losses. Older adults often experience numerous losses, sequentially or simultaneously. At a time when their stressors are the highest, their resources are often the most meager. Deaths of relatives and friends, retirement, impaired health of self or family members, and decreased economic resources are all common stressors for the older adult. As their social network shrinks because of deaths and illnesses of family members and friends, they have fewer support networks available to them. Thus, older adults may need to rely more on healthcare providers to assist them in coping with their losses.

Altered Grieving

Dysfunctional grief is grief that falls outside the normal response range and may be manifested as exaggerated grief, prolonged grief, or absence of grief. In dysfunctional grief, the grieving person often becomes stuck in one stage of the grief process and is unable to progress to the next stage or stages. Furthermore, the grieving person expends so much energy either repressing the grief or dealing ineffectively with the grief that little time or energy is left to invest in normal growth and development.

Potential for Altered Grieving

The potential for altered function is affected by the stressors and resources that the person experiences during the loss, by the piling up of stressors that occurred before the loss, and by the accumulation of resources before the loss. If the stressors outweigh resources, then the person is at risk for altered functioning. Particularly at risk are those with several concurrent losses, few support systems, poor coping skills, and previous unresolved losses.

Manifestations of Altered Grieving

In a study of bereavement experts' perceptions of "grief that falls outside normal parameters," Demi and Miles (1987) found that more than 30 different terms were commonly used to label dysfunctional grief. The most commonly accepted terms were pathologic grief, unresolved grief, dysfunctional grief, and prolonged grief. Many symptoms that have been considered abnormal or dysfunctional were identified as components of the normal grief process. At 1 year after bereavement, most experts believed that the grief manifestations listed in the accompanying display were within normal parameters.

Bereavement experts reported that they consider almost all bereavement manifestations to be normal during the early stages of grief but consider most of the manifestations to be abnormal if they continue beyond 3 years after bereavement. Some of the symptoms considered normal during the early bereavement period but abnormal if present beyond 3 years are listed in the display.

Normal and Abnormal Grief Manifestations

Normal at 1 Year Postbereavement

- Excessive or persistent expression of affect
- Inability to experience joy
- Clinical symptoms of depression
- Inability to form new relationships
- Inability to speak of the deceased without intense emotion
- Hearing or seeing the deceased
- Feelings of emptiness or meaninglessness

Abnormal if Present Beyond 3 Years

- Leaving the deceased's room and belongings intact
- Reporting physical symptoms similar to those the deceased had before death
- Talking about the loss as if it just happened
- Inability to remember or talk about the deceased
- Being preoccupied with thoughts of the deceased
- Talking or acting as if the deceased were still alive
- Experiencing physical illness that seems to be related to the loss

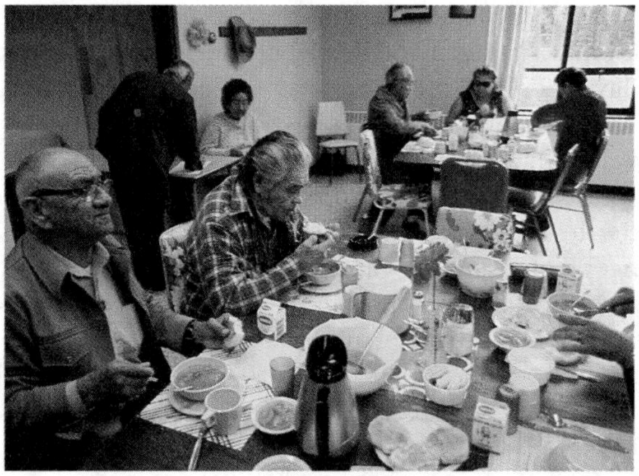

Figure 50-4 • *Families who live at a distance worry about whether their grieving father or mother is getting good nutrition. They can feel more secure if they know the parent is involved in a food program or a social group. (Source: USDA.)*

Impact of Grieving Dysfunction on Activities of Daily Living

Dysfunctional grief leads to dysfunction in everyday life activities. This dysfunction may be manifested by individual family members or by the family as a whole.

Individual Considerations. The person may be too tired or too depressed to concentrate on daily household chores or personal hygiene. Crying, loss of appetite, and sleep disturbance add to the grieving dysfunction and loss of energy. The adult may no longer be able to maintain a job or provide a safe and healthy home atmosphere, and the child may be unable to keep up with schoolwork. Individual family members may not be able to carry out their family or work roles.

Family Considerations. The family as a whole is also greatly affected by the grief experience. Because members in the family are unable to carry out their individual roles, the family is unable to carry out its roles of nurturing and protecting (Fig. 50-4). The family life cycle stage that the family is in at the time it experiences the loss greatly affects family functioning (Demi, 1989). Families are particularly vulnerable when they are gaining or losing family members through normal development. That is, if the family is in the stage of child-bearing or child-launching, it is often more difficult to cope with a loss. In addition, if one or both of the parents are deeply involved in grieving, they may not be able to carry our their parental roles.

Assessment

Questions about losses (actual and anticipated) need to be incorporated into the assessment of every client. Frank physical illness may be the result of a loss, actual or anticipated; often the client does not connect the presenting symptom with the loss. On the other hand, physical illness or accident may result in loss, both actual and anticipated. Some clients recognize the effect of loss or anticipated loss, whereas others completely deny the loss and its meaning. The skillful nurse will recognize the relationship of loss to health status and will help the client recognize and acknowledge this connection also.

Subjective Data

Nurses must be cautious not to interpret a single behavior as dysfunctional grief. Many behaviors previously thought to be dysfunctional are being recognized as normal components of grief. Observation and assessment of a grieving person at a single point in time is not a good way to assess the normality of the grief response. A much better way to assess the normality of a grief response is to follow the grieving person over time and observe whether grief manifestations are increasing, remaining the same, or diminishing. Furthermore, one must assess the entire constellation of grief manifestations and not overemphasize any specific symptom.

To distinguish between a normal grief reaction and a dysfunctional grief reaction, one must assess the severity of the symptoms and the pattern of change over time. Many of the symptoms previously reported as signs of dysfunctional grief are believed to be normal components of the grief process and therefore are not discussed here. Data to be collected are listed in the display.

Functional Pattern Identification

Historical events that should be assessed include the nature of the relationship with the deceased and the circumstances of the loss. When interviewing a client, it is helpful to start the interview with some general, nonthreatening questions before moving in to ask questions about the loss. However, a major factor in understanding the loss reaction is assessing the relationship to the lost person/object. The nurse needs to know:

- What was the physical and psychological significance of the lost person/object?
- Was the loss unexpected or expected?
- Did the survivor contribute or perceive that he or she contributed to the loss?

The nurse also needs to assess the client's personal resources and personal stressors. Personal resources are strengths within the person that contribute to a healthy pattern of grieving. Personal stressors are limitations within the person that may inhibit healthy grieving. Personal stressors and resources include personality characteristics, coping skills, communication skills, physical health status, spirituality, and previous experi-

Nursing Assessment

Subjective Data Collection in Loss and Grieving

- Nature of the loss:
- Meaning of the loss to the client:
- Client's usual pattern of coping with loss:
- Availability of resources:
- Other stressors (preceding or concurrent with loss):
- Physical symptoms:
  - Sleep patterns
  - Appetite
  - Tightness in throat and chest
  - Heart palpitations
  - Pain in chest
  - Frequent sighing
- Emotional symptoms:
  - Sadness
  - Guilt
  - Anger
  - Relief
  - Anxiety
  - Loneliness
  - Wishing to die
  - Suicidal ideation:
- Substance Use:
  - Alcohol
  - Illegal drugs
  - Prescribed drugs
  - Caffeine
  - Nicotine
- Social behavior:
  - Ability to function in roles (family, work, and social roles)
- Cognitive behavior:
  - Preoccupation with thoughts of loss
  - Searching for lost person/object
- Spiritual:
  - Loss of faith
  - Anger at God

ences with loss. To assess personal stressors and resources, one needs to know the following:

- Does the client have a history of emotional illness?
- What coping behaviors does the client usually use?
- How well does the client communicate with others?
- What previous losses has the client experienced?
- How did the client cope with these previous losses?
- Are any of these previous losses still unresolved?
- Does the client have any physical health problems?
- What are the client's spiritual beliefs, and how do they influence his or her reactions to loss?

The nurse also needs to assess sociocultural resources and stressors. Sociocultural resources are the assets that are available to the client from the interpersonal environment, and include social support, practical support, and cultural traditions and customs. Sociocultural stressors are strains and tensions exerted on the client by the social and cultural systems. Adequate social support is a key factor in the prevention of dysfunctional grieving. Family members, peers, friends, coworkers, and employers can function as either resources or stressors. Cultural traditions also may be either resources or stressors. For example, if the cultural tradition dictates a long mourning period and the bereaved person is ready to move into the reorganization stage of grief, this may create feelings of conflict. However, it is more likely that sociocultural expectations will be that the bereaved person stop grieving and get "back to normal" long before the bereaved person is capable of doing so. To assess sociocultural stressors and resources, the following questions need to be asked:

- What social supports are available to the grieving person?
- Does the grieving person perceive these supports as helpful?
- What are the traditional rituals for dealing with this type of loss?
- To what extent did the grieving person participate in the sociocultural rituals, and how satisfied were they with the rituals?
- Do any of the social and cultural traditions conflict with needs of the grieving person?

Risk Identification

The risk for dysfunctional grief can be identified through analysis of the resources and stressors that the client is experiencing. Clients with many stressors and few resources are at greatest risk. The severity of the loss and the degree of anticipation of the loss also affect risk. Losses that affect many aspects of the person's life and losses that are unanticipated are more stressful. The nurse must always keep in mind the client's perception of the loss; what is perceived as a minor loss by one person may be perceived as a major loss by another.

Physical health and psychosocial adjustment are intricately intertwined. The bereaved are known to be at greater risk for mortality and morbidity than are comparable nonbereaved people. Research reveals that the greatest increases in mortality after bereavement have been the result of suicide, accidents, and homicide (Kaprio, et al., 1987). In addition, men are particularly at risk for dying of cardiovascular disease. This increased risk of mortality is greatest in the first month after bereavement, remains elevated throughout the first year of bereavement, then drops to normal range by the end of the second year of bereavement (Kaprio, et al., 1987).

Dysfunction Identification

It is difficult to identify dysfunction based on a single contact with a client. People with normal grief may display many diverse and intense signs and symptoms. Nurses must avoid inappropriately placing a label of dysfunctional grief on a normal process. Generally, dysfunction can be identified only after several contacts with the client over an extended period of time. If a person remains in complete denial of the loss or if the person's grief symptoms continue unabated over a long period of time, the person is likely to be experiencing dysfunctional grief.

Objective Data

Grief may manifest itself in many diverse physiologic and psychological signs that are directly observable. Many of these signs are identical to the signs of depression; consequently, it is very difficult to differentiate between normal grieving and depression. Currently, there is no laboratory test to assess the presence of grieving, but there are a few paper-and-pencil tests that are helpful in assessing grief symptomatology, such as the Grief Experience Questionnaire (Sanders & Mauger, 1979), the Bereavement Experience Questionnaire (Demi & Schroeder, 1985), the Impact of Event Scale (Zilberg, et al., 1982), the Texas Inventory of Grief (Faschingbauer, et al., 1977), and the Beck Depression Inventory (Beck, 1972).

Physical Assessment

Many of the subjective manifestations of grief have concomitant objective manifestations:

- Dejected physical appearance
- Slowed motor function

- Weeping
- Outbursts of anger
- Emotional blunting
- Unkempt appearance
- Sleep disturbance
- Appetite disturbance (excessive weight loss or gain)
- Preoccupation with thoughts of that which was lost

Nursing Diagnoses

Anticipatory Grieving and Dysfunctional Grieving are the two approved nursing diagnoses relevant to loss and grief (McLane, 1987). A number of nurses believe that another diagnostic category should be added, Normal Grieving (Carpenito, 1992). The rationale for adding this diagnosis is that normal grieving results in numerous physical, emotional, and social consequences that can be ameliorated through nursing interventions.

Diagnostic Statement: Anticipatory Grieving

Definition

Anticipatory Grieving is the intellectual and emotional responses and behaviors by which individuals work through the process of modifying self-concept based on the perception of potential loss (North American Nursing Diagnosis Association [NANDA], 1994).

Defining Characteristics

Among the defining characteristics are the following: potential loss of significant object; expression of distress at potential loss; denial of potential loss; guilt, anger, sorrow, or choked feelings; changes in eating habits; alterations in sleep patterns, or alterations in activity level; altered libido; altered communication patterns (NANDA, 1994).

Related Factors

Related factors have yet to be developed for this diagnosis.

Diagnostic Statement: Dysfunctional Grieving

Definition

Dysfunctional Grieving is extended, unsuccessful use of intellectual and emotional responses by which individuals attempt to work through the process of modifying self-concept based on the perception of loss (NANDA, 1994).

Defining Characteristics

The defining characteristics or clinical cues that point to this nursing diagnosis include verbal expression of distress at loss; denial of loss; expression of guilt or expression of unresolved issues; anger, sadness, or crying; difficulty in expressing loss; alterations in eating habits, sleep patterns, dream patterns, activity level or libido; idealization of lost object; reliving of past experiences; interference with life functioning; developmental regression; labile affect; and alterations in concentration or pursuits of tasks (NANDA, 1994).*

Related Factors

A variety of etiologic or contributing factors may contribute to development of this altered pattern of grieving. The major etiologic factors include perceived object loss (object loss is used in the broadest sense). Objects may include people, possessions, a job, status, home,

* Caution must be exercised in using these characteristics to diagnose Dysfunctional Grieving because many of the characteristics are components of the normal grief process (Demi & Miles, 1987).

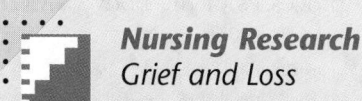

Nursing Research
Grief and Loss

Selected Nursing Research Studies

Brown, M. A., & Powell-Cope, G. (1993). Times of loss and dying in caring for a family member with AIDS. *RINAH, 16*, 179–191.

Fraser, S., et al. (1990,. Survivors' recollections of helpful and unhelpful emergency nurse activities surrounding sudden death of a loved one. *Journal of Emergency Nursing, 16*(1), 13–16.

Lang, A., & Gottlieb, L. (1993). Parental grief reactions and marital intimacy following infant death. *Death Studies, 17*(3), 233–255.

Sowell, R. L., Bramlett, M. H., Guildner, S. H. et al. (1991). The lived experience of survival and bereavement following the death of a lover from AIDS. *Image, 23*, 89–94.

Possible Topics for Nursing Inquiry

- What are the long-term effects of specific nursing therapies with grieving children?
- Do specific nursing activities provide definable support for families of terminally ill clients?
- What coping mechanisms do critical care nurses employ when caring for critically ill clients?

ideals, and parts and processes of the body (NANDA, 1994).

Related Nursing Diagnoses

In addition to the diagnoses of Anticipatory Grieving and Dysfunctional Grieving, clients who have experienced a major loss may also be found to have the nursing diagnoses based on functional health given in Table 50-3.

Outcome Identification and Planning

After the nursing diagnoses and related factors are identified, client goals and nursing interventions are planned. Development of client goals centers around the stage of grief the client is in and whether the grief is normal, anticipatory, or dysfunctional. The client should have input in deciding what personal needs are at the moment. Short-term and long-term goals are needed. The following client goals are samples of what may need to be addressed with this client.

The client will move toward resolution of diverse emotions.
The client will accept the reality of the loss.
The client will reinvest emotional and physical energy in meaningful people and activities.

Planning will evolve around the phase or stage in which the client is. It may vary from emotional support, to counseling, to finding a support group, and includes dignified care of the body after death. Some of the interventions used in various phases of grief are listed in the accompanying display; the next section of this chapter describes their implementation.

Table 50-3 • Sample Nursing Diagnoses Related to Grief and Based on Functional Health

Functional Health Area	*Nursing Diagnoses*
Health perception and health management	Altered Health Maintenance Risk for Injury Altered Growth and Development Noncompliance
Nutrition and metabolism	Altered Nutrition: Less than body requirements
Activity and exercise	Activity Intolerance Diversional Activity Deficit Impaired Home Maintenance Management
Sleep and rest	Sleep Pattern Disturbance
Cognition and perception	Altered Thought Processes Knowledge Deficit Acute Confusion Decisional Conflict
Self-perception	Anxiety Fear Hopelessness Powerlessness Body Image Disturbance Self-Esteem Disturbance
Roles and relationships	Altered Family Processes Risk for Loneliness Altered Parenting Social Isolation
Sexuality and reproduction	Sexual Dysfunction
Coping and stress tolerance	Ineffective Individual Coping Impaired Adjustment Ineffective Family Coping; Compromised Risk for Suicide
Values and beliefs	Spiritual Distress

Planning

Examples of Nursing Interventions Used in Helping Clients Move Through Grief Stages

Interventions During Shock Phase

- Help client mobilize a support system.
- Protect client from physical harm
- Have a family member present when notifying client of a loss.
- Have someone drive client home.
- Help client establish coping behaviors used in past.
- Encourage client to participate in mourning rituals.

Interventions During Protest Phase

- Encourage expression of diverse feelings (sadness, loneliness, anger, guilt, resentment, relief).
- Encourage remembering and talking about that which was lost.
- Provide anticipatory guidance regarding the normal grief process.
- Provide role models who have successfully coped with similar loss.
- Encourage client to use existing support systems.
- Identify new support systems.
- Discourage use of alcohol, drugs, and caffeine.
- Promote appropriate sleep habits.
- Promote good nutrition.
- Refer for complete physical examination.
- Encourage participation in religious rituals.
- Encourage use of previous healthy coping behaviors.
- Introduce new coping behaviors.

Interventions During Disorganization Phase

- Continue interventions begun in shock phase.
- Refer client to self-help groups.
- Refer client for individual or group counseling.

Interventions During Reorganization Phase

- Refer client for career counseling.
- Refer client to educational programs.
- Refer client to social activity programs.

Implementation

Nurses have many opportunities to provide care for grieving people because of their frequent contact with people experiencing a major loss. Because grief can be both devastating and long-lasting, the opportunities occur throughout the grief process. Because dysfunctional grieving is beyond the scope of the beginning student, only normal grieving is discussed in this chapter.

Nursing Interventions to Promote Health and Normal Grieving

Nursing interventions to promote normal grieving should occur before the loss occurs or before it is anticipated to occur.

Client Teaching

Loss education should begin in early childhood. Nurses should prepare parents for loss education. Preschoolers should be taught about the normality of loss and grief through exposure to naturally occurring events. A visit to a nursing home, the death of a distant relative, the death of a goldfish, the loss of a favorite toy, or the loss of a friend all provide opportunities to discuss the natural life cycle and loss in nonthreatening ways. The parent or other relative who can talk about loss honestly and openly, in terms that the child can understand, will help the child establish a healthy attitude toward loss and will serve as a role model for the child.

Loss education should continue throughout childhood and adolescence. Nurses should continue their role in educating parents about ways to help children deal with grief and loss (see the display). Parents should be encouraged to include children in mourning rituals; however, children should never be forced to participate in such rituals. Parents should also be encouraged to allow children to express their diverse feelings about various losses. Gradual exposure to loss and death situations concurrent with appropriate preparation and support will prepare the child to cope with losses later in life.

Nurses should also be directly involved in education of children about grief and loss. Nurses should incorporate grief education naturally into their contacts with children in various healthcare settings, such as schools, hospitals, physicians' offices, and clinics.

Working Through Grief Stages

Nursing interventions for grieving should be based on the client's present stage of grief. The following discussion and the display in the Planning section list these interventions. Further interventions are found in the Nursing Plan of Care at the end of the chapter.

During the shock phase, nursing interventions should focus on protecting the client from physical

Client Teaching
Preparing Children for Death

Instruct the parent as follows:

DOs:

- *Know your own feelings and beliefs.*
- *Be honest.*
- *Begin at the child's level.*
- *Include child in family rituals related to death and mourning.*
- *Encourage expression of feelings.*
- *Provide security and stability.*
- *Encourage remembrance of deceased.*
- *Recognize that children grieve differently from adults.*
- *Expect the child to alternate between grieving and normal functioning.*
- *Talk openly about death and feelings it generates.*
- *Introduce death concepts into conversation naturally.*

DON'Ts:

- *Praise stoicism.*
- *Encourage forgetting of the deceased.*
- *Force the child to participate in grief and mourning rituals.*
- *Emphasize the likeness of the child to the deceased.*
- *Compare the child to the deceased.*
- *Use euphemisms.*

harm and on getting the client to accept the reality of the loss. During this phase, the nurse should help the client mobilize normal support systems; for example, the nurse should help the client contact family members and tell them about the loss. Clients may act out impulsively or may have decreased reaction times, and therefore effort must be taken to prevent the client from self-harm (suicide attempts) and from accidents. It usually is helpful to have a family member present when the client is notified of a loss, or an anticipated loss, and to have this person drive the client home; this is particularly important when the loss is unanticipated. Clients should be encouraged to use coping behaviors that have been helpful to them in the past, such as participation in religious activities, or talking with a friend or relative (Fig. 50-5). If the loss was a death, clients should be encouraged to participate in funeral and mourning rituals.

During the protest phase, nursing interventions should focus on getting the client to express thoughts and feeling about the loss and maintaining the client's normal health status. Interventions include those listed in the display in the Planning section.

During the disorganization phase, emphasis should be placed on getting the client to accept the reality of the loss and to begin reorganization of his or her life. Interventions instituted during the shock phase should be continued. Additional interventions are included in the display in the Planning section.

During the reorganization phase, emphasis should be placed on helping the client to continue reorganizing his or her life, and to find new or renewed meaning in life. Some losses, such as the death of a spouse, or a spinal cord injury or blindness, require a major reorganization of many life activities, whereas other losses, such as reproductive sterility or amputation of a finger, may require reorganization in only a few areas. Clients who experience a greater degree of life reorganization may need additional interventions (see the display in the Planning section).

Support Groups

Common problems for those experiencing loss are intense emotional distress, lack of social support, and prolonged grief. To prevent these problems from occurring, clients should be encouraged (early in the grief process) to participate in befriender programs or self-help support groups. Befriender programs, such as the Widow-to-Widow program (Silverman, et al., 1974) and the Reach-to-Recovery program for mastectomy clients, provide one-to-one support by nonprofessionals who have experienced a similar loss and have made a satisfactory recovery from the loss. These befriender programs provide role modeling, education, and emotional support. Self-help support groups serve the same functions as befrienders; however, the help is less individualized and is primarily provided in a group setting. Furthermore, the support group is composed of people in various stages of recovery from their grief.

Care of the Deceased

Nursing care continues after the death of the client. Concern for dignity in the care of the body as well as sensitivity to the needs of the deceased client's family are within nursing's responsibility. Immediately after the client's death has been certified, family members may

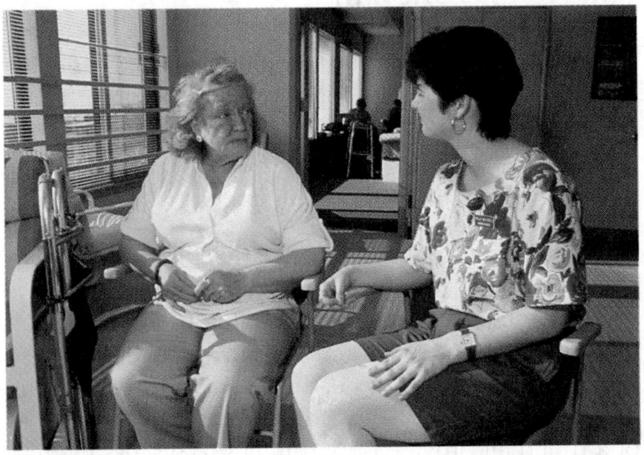

Figure 50-5 *• Individuals can find comfort in their relationships with others, whether it is a friend, relative, or healthcare professional.*

wish to spend some time alone with the client's body. In an effort to limit exposure to the disturbing sight of equipment and medical supplies, the nurse should remove unneeded items, and clean, position, and cover the client. Allowing the family time alone with the client may be an important step for them in the grief process. Some families may appreciate the presence of a nurse, spiritual leader, other family members, or friends. Other families may feel comforted by spending this time alone. Religious and ethnic beliefs and customs should be observed as far as possible.

The physical care of the body includes bathing as needed to remove drainage and secretions. The client's eyelids should be gently closed. Dentures (if any) can be inserted in the mouth, and a rolled towel or washcloth placed under the chin to help keep the mouth closed. The body needs to be aligned as normally as possible before rigor mortis develops (about 4 to 6 hours after death). Jewelry and other valuables need to be removed and given to the family along with other personal belongings, and their disposition should be noted in the medical record.

When the client's body has been prepared and the family leaves, the nurse should place appropriate identification tags on the wrist and ankle of the client's body. The body is then taken to the hospital's morgue, or is removed from the room by the mortician.

If there have been special instructions from the client's family regarding donor use of the client's organs, the nurse will need to take immediate measures to preserve the donor organs, either by notification of the appropriate medical teams or by placement of ice packs. When an autopsy is desired, the physician will request written permission from the family. Although the general aspects of care after death remain the same in all facilities, each individual facility may have specific guidelines and policies of which the nurse needs to be aware.

Nursing Interventions for Altered Grieving

Clients experiencing dysfunctional grief need professional help to resolve problems. This help generally takes one of two forms: individual therapy, or professionally led support groups. This type of help may be prescribed, in addition to self-help. Professional support is particularly important if the client has inadequate support systems. Many nurse–therapists specialize in grief therapy.

Community-Based Nursing

When a client has experienced a major loss, or is anticipating such a loss, adequate discharge planning and follow-up are essential. Because the grief process extends over a long period of time, the severity of the client's grief may not be obvious during hospitalization. Nurses may misperceive the client's shock and denial, and conclude that the client is "unaffected by the loss." Actually, the client who appears unaffected by a loss is particularly in need of follow-up care, because he or she may have a delayed grief reaction (Fig. 50-6).

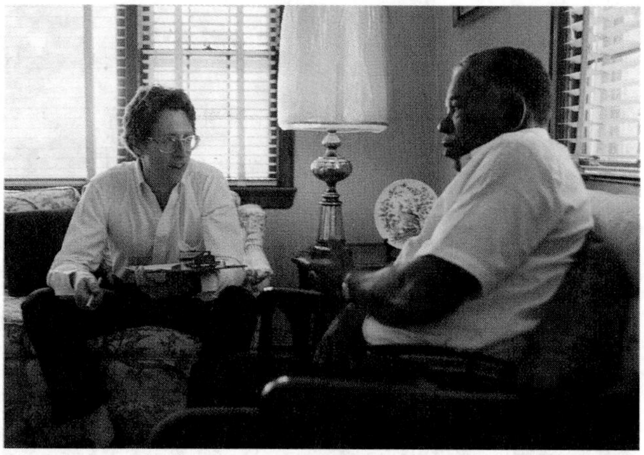

Figure 50-6 • *The community-based nurse provides comfort with a follow-up visit.*

Referral

Discharge planning should include referral to befriender programs, self-help groups, professionally led support groups, public health nurses, or hospice programs, depending on the clients' specific needs and the community resources. Widow and widower groups may help when the client is ready for such a program. Pastoral counselors and other clergypeople are helpful resources to many. Clients should also be encouraged to continue their contact with their primary healthcare provider (physician or nurse), because the grief process often decreases resistance to disease and exacerbates existing illnesses.

Hospice Programs

Hospice programs are particularly important resources for the terminally ill and their families. **Hospice** refers to both a place where people can go to receive care when they are terminally ill and to a philosophy of care for the terminally ill. The goal of the hospice program is to promote the highest possible quality of life for the client and family throughout the terminal illness and at the time of death.

There are two major types of hospice programs, inpatient programs and home care programs. All hospice programs are based on the principles listed in the accompanying display.

One of the unique aspects of hospice care is the attention given to the dying client's grief and to family members' grief. Hospice caregivers assist the client in coping with numerous losses and in facing impending

Principles of the Hospice Program

- The quality of life is more important than the quantity of life.
- The family is the unit of care.
- Many of the needs of the dying client can be met at home.
- Hospice services must be available 24 hours per day. Because client's needs cannot always be met in the home, appropriate inpatient services must be available.
- Because of the complex needs of dying clients and their families, services are provided by an interdisciplinary team.
- Interventions focus on the management of physical and psychosocial needs of clients and family members.

death. They also facilitate anticipatory grieving of family members and provide bereavement care after the client has died. Thus, hospice programs are important community resources that contribute to continuity of care for grieving clients.

Evaluation

This section lists some general goals and outcome criteria for a grieving client that can be used as a guide for evaluation. However, the nurse must constantly keep in mind the fact that evaluation must be individualized based on the client's specific needs and goals. Thus, these goals and outcome criteria are presented as suggestions, to be amended based on knowledge about the specific client.

Goal

The client will recognize and express diverse emotions.

Possible Outcome Criteria

- Within 7 days, client expresses diverse emotions, such as sadness, anger, guilt, loneliness, or relief.
- Within 14 days, client states that experienced emotions are normal components of the grief process.

Goal

The client will move toward resolution of diverse emotions.

Possible Outcome Criteria

- Within 6 months, client states decreased frequency and intensity of painful emotions.
- Within 9 months, client expresses decreased frequency of preoccupation with thoughts of the lost loved one/object.

Goal

The client will recognize reality of the loss.

Possible Outcome Criteria

- Within 4 weeks, client discusses the loss and its meaning.
- Within 4 weeks, client discusses potential life changes necessary because of the loss.
- Within 6 months, client disposes of articles no longer needed (eg, paraplegic gives away skis, widow gives away deceased spouse's clothing).
- Within 12 months, client plans for major life changes to accommodate the loss (eg, selling home, taking new job).

Goal

The client will recognize need for help and seek help appropriately.

Possible Outcome Criteria

- Within 24 hours, client reaches out to family and friends for emotional and practical help.
- Within 2 months, client uses family and friends for social support.
- Within 6 months, client uses community resources for support.
- Within 12 months, client assumes major responsibility for self.

Goal

The client will retain or regain physical health status.

Possible Outcome Criteria

- Client does not use sleeping pills, alcohol, caffeine, tobacco, or tranquilizers as crutches to ease the pain.
- Within 3 months, client follows prescribed medical regimen and adheres to healthful behaviors.
- Within 12 months, client states that he or she has returned to normal eating, sleeping, and exercise habits.

Goal

The client will reinvest emotional and physical energy in meaningful people and activities.

Possible Outcome Criteria

- Within 9 months, client participates in new activities.
- Within 12 months, client reports making necessary changes in social, recreational, and occupational spheres.

(text continues on page 1491)

Nursing Plan of Care
The Client Who Is Grieving

Nursing Diagnosis

Grieving (normal) related to actual loss of significant person manifested by expression of unresolved issues. (During the shock stage)

Client Goal

Client will move toward resolution of diverse emotions.

Client Outcome Criteria

- Client cognitively accepts the reality of death within 1 week.
- Client participates in funeral and mourning rituals within 1 week.
- Client expresses emotional affect in discussion, facial expressions, and reactions within 72 hours.
- Client uses family and friends for social support in resolving emotional responses within 1 week.

Nursing Intervention	*Scientific Rationale*
1. Encourage mourner to see deceased and allow mourner to touch or hold the deceased, if desired.	1. Cognitive recognition of the reality of death is necessary before beginning to work on acceptance of the emotional significance of the death.
2a. Provide anticipatory guidance regarding physical appearance of the deceased. b. Encourage mourner to participate in grief and mourning activities that are congruent with their sociocultural and spiritual/religious beliefs.	2. Cognitive acceptance of the death is facilitated by participating in funeral and mourning rituals.
3. Notify the family members of the death in person in a private setting whenever possible.	3. Trauma of notification of the death can be eased by sensitive attention to family members' needs.
4. Encourage mourner to express diverse feelings (eg, guilt, sadness, relief, numbness, anger).	4. Open expression of feelings facilitates gradual resolution of these feelings; some feelings are perceived as socially unacceptable.
5. Encourage mourner to talk about the deceased and to ask questions about the death.	5. Preoccupation with thoughts of the deceased is a normal part of the grief process; talking about the deceased's life and death begins breaking emotional bonds with the deceased.
6. Provide anticipatory guidance on the grief process, including common thoughts, feelings, and behaviors; emphasize that there is no one right way to grieve.	6. Most people have little knowledge about the normal grief process, and it is reassuring for them to know that what they are experiencing is normal.
7. Assist mourner with making decisions regarding urgent postdeath responsibilities; help mourner contact family members and other support persons.	7. Bereaved person is often in crisis and needs the emotional and practical support from family and other support systems.
8. Protect the mourner from deliberate or unintentional harm, (eg, inquire about suicidal thoughts; encourage mourner not to drive own car immediately after learning of the death).	8. Bereaved are at greater risk of mortality and morbidity, particularly from accidents and suicide.

(continued)

(During the protest stage)

Client Goal

Client will begin acceptable transition to life without deceased.

Client Outcome Criteria

- Client recognizes and accepts emotional feelings as acceptable within 2 months.
- Client begins transition to new roles within 2 months.
- Client experiences minimal deterioration of physical health during first 3 months after death of loved one.

Nursing Intervention	*Scientific Rationale*
1. Encourage mourner to remember and talk about both the negative and positive memories of the deceased. Use counseling skills of empathy, warmth, and positive regard Facilitate reality testing. Assess need for individual or family who have numerous counseling.	1. The process of breaking bonds with the deceased continues over an extended period of time. Counseling skills can be used to elicit unrecognized thoughts and feelings. Bereaved people who have numerous stressors and few resources benefit from professional therapy.
2. Teach support people about the emotional needs of the bereaved.	2. Adequately prepared support people can augment professional services or may be the only intervention needed.
3. Provide appropriate reading materials on the grief process.	3. Identification with other bereaved people can be therapeutic.
4. Reinforce use of healthy coping skills.	4. During a crisis, a person may be too overwhelmed to use his or her usual coping skills; therefore, the nurse must help them remember these skills.
5. Assess for suicidal ideation.	5. Transition to new roles is a major stressor for the bereaved; role models and education on the new roles facilitates ease in role transition.
6. Encourage client to assume some new roles, to relinquish other roles, and to allow support people to fill some of the deceased's roles. Provide role models for new roles (eg, widow-to-widow befriender) Recommend participation in self-help or mutual help support groups.	6. The death of a significant other precipitates role changes. Clients often do not know how to function in new roles; role models can show them how to function.
7. Teach problem-solving skills related to new roles.	7. New roles require diverse problem-solving skills.
8. Provide appropriate reading materials on practical aspects of role transition (eg, financial management, automobile maintenance, child care, home maintenance).	8. Seeing things in written form helps to reinforce ideas and knowledge; books become references.
9. Encourage complete physical assessment.	9. The risk of increased mortality and morbidity is highest during the early bereavement period but continues throughout the first year of bereavement.
10. Promote good health habits (eg, nutrition, rest, avoidance of alcohol and tobacco).	10. Good health habits and early identification of health problems may prevent serious illness.

(continued)

(During the disorganization stage)

Client Goal

Client will reinvest emotional and physical energy in meaningful people and activities.

Client Outcome Criteria

- Client emotionally accepts the loss within 9 months, as disclosed by client.
- Client experiences improved functioning in new roles within 9 months.
- Client discusses with nurse a search for new meaning in life within 9 months.
- Client/family verbalizes experiencing increased family cohesiveness within 9 months.

Nursing Intervention	Scientific Rationale
1. Assist client in decision-making regarding disposal of deceased's belongings.	1. During the disorganization state the client recognizes the emotional significance of the loss and begins to accept the meaning of the loss.
2. Support client's expression of grief (eg, cemetery visits, memorial services, visiting places of special meaning to deceased)	2. Activities focusing on the unresolved grief can facilitate resolution of the loss.
3. Normalize thoughts and feelings.	3. Same as above.
4. Use role-play to work through unresolved issues.	4. Same as above.
5. Encourage client to express thoughts and feelings through writing.	5. Same as above.
6. Enhance previous coping skills.	6. New roles continue to cause stress; effort must be directed toward strengthening bereaved's intrapersonal and interpersonal competence.
7. Introduce additional coping techniques.	7. Same as above.
8. Support independent problem-solving skills.	8. Same as above.
9. Keep support systems mobilized.	9. Same as above.
10. Encourage to delay major decisions until out of acute grief.	10. Same as above.
11. Support client's reevaluation of the meaning of his or her life.	11. The death of a loved one leads the bereaved to question the meaning of life.
12. Encourage participation in spiritual/religious activities.	12. Same as above.
13. Encourage client to participate in social and recreational activities.	13. Same as above.
14. Teach family members that each person expresses grief differently and resolves his or her grief at a different speed.	14. The family functions as a system; death of a family member affects all parts of the system.
15. Encourage open family communication about the loss and the feelings engendered.	15. Each subsystem affects other subsystems and the system as a whole.
16. Identify and reinforce the strengths of each family member.	16. Strengthening any part of the system has a positive effect on the other subsystems and on the system as a whole.
17. Encourage family members to provide support to each other.	17. Same as above.
18. Mobilize extra family support systems.	18. Friends, coworkers, and others can supplement support received from family members.

(continued)

Nursing Plan of Care
The Client Who Is Grieving *(continued)*

(During the reorganization stage)

Client Goal

Client will increase level of physical, emotional, social, and spiritual functioning (previous level or higher level of functioning)

Client Outcome Criteria

- Client resolves emotional reactions to the loss within 2 years.
- Client reports satisfaction with new roles within 2 years.
- Client reports finding new meaning in life within 2 years.
- Client reports achievement of personal growth within 2 years.
- Client reports improved coping skills within 2 years.

Nursing Intervention	*Scientific Rationale*
1. Avoid unrealistic expectations for mourner to recover quickly.	1. Resolution of grief after the death of significant other often takes 2 to 5 years. By the end of the first year, the bereaved should have resolved the major portion of his or her grief but will continue to reexperience grief on anniversaries.
2. Remind client that it is normal for grief feelings to be rekindled by trigger events such as holidays and anniversaries.	2. Same as above.
3. Support renewal of old friendships/interests and development of new friendships/interests.	3. Meeting with friends and finding new activities eases the emotional loss and gives new meaning to life.
4. Use gentle confrontation to deal with unresolved feelings toward deceased.	4. It is important to deal with all feelings before the grief period can end.
5. Facilitate recognition of own strengths and limitations.	5. Knowing yourself aids in acceptable functioning.
6. Encourage continued participation in support group.	6. Support is still needed from people with similar problems.
7. Support continued involvement in religious, social, and recreational activities.	7. By the end of second year, bereaved should have found a satisfactory level of health and functioning.
8. Praise client for satisfactory achievement of roles.	8. By the end of second year, bereaved should be functioning satisfactorily in roles.
9. Encourage reevaluation of diverse meanings in life.	9. The search for meaning continues for a long period of time after resolution of other aspects of grief.
10. Support changes in client's behavior and lifestyle.	10. The crisis of bereavement often produces profound personal growth.
11. Reinforce use of a variety of coping skills.	11. Bereaved people often report greatly increased coping skills after resolution of grief and also report a sense of confidence that since they managed to handle their grief satisfactorily, they will be able to handle any other stressor satisfactorily.

- Within 12 months, client identifies renewal of old friendships and development of new friendships.
- Within 24 months, client expresses sense of satisfaction with life and a sense of meaning in life.

Evaluation is an ongoing process that includes assessing the client and comparing the client's status to the outcome criteria. During this process the nurse must keep in mind the long-term nature of grief and that progress toward these outcomes may be very slow, but nevertheless, within the normal range. The nurse must use astute clinical judgment to determine if the client is making satisfactory progress toward the goals; if the client is not making satisfactory progress, then the nursing care plan must be revised.

Key Concepts

- Loss is a universal experience, and grieving is a normal response to loss.
- Models of the grief process provide direction for nursing assessment.
- The grief process is similar regardless of the type of loss experienced.
- A major loss results in a long-term life transition.
- The characteristics of the loss, personal resources and stressors, and sociocultural resources and stressors affect the normal grief process.
- The outcome of a loss experience is not predetermined, but rather is determined by the balance of stressors and resources present during the grief period.
- Risk of dysfunctional grieving can be identified through analysis of the stressors and resources that the client is experiencing.
- Response to loss is influenced by the person's stage of development.
- Physical health and psychosocial adjustment during the grief process are intricately intertwined.
- Nursing interventions should be based on knowledge of the long-term nature of the grief process.
- Many grief manifestations, identified in the literature as dysfunctional, are considered to be components of the normal grief process.
- Caution should be used in labeling a client as having dysfunctional grieving.
- Discharge planning must consider the long-term nature of the grief process.
- Hospice programs are important community resources that provide family-focused support for clients who are experiencing grieving.

Critical Thinking Challenges

You have expanded your knowledge base to include an understanding of loss and the grieving process. Now turn back to the situation of the widow at the beginning of the chapter and consider the following questions.

1. *From the information provided, consider possible nursing diagnoses for this woman.*
2. *Plan additional information you need to make a thorough assessment of this woman and her family.*
3. *Plan actions you should take to assist this woman.*
4. *Examine other resources (professional and nonprofessional) you think could be mobilized to assist this woman and her family. Propose how these resources would be used.*

References

Beck, A. (1972). *Depression: Causes and treatment.* Philadelphia: University of Pennsylvania Press.

Brown, M. A., & Powell-Cope, G. M. (1991). AIDS family caregiving: Transitions through uncertainty. *Nurs Res, 40,* 338–345.

Brown, M. A., & Powell-Cope, G. (1993). Times of loss and dying in caring for a family member with AIDS. *RINAH, 16,* 179–191.

Caplan, G. (1964). *Principles of preventive psychiatry.* New York: Basic Books.

Caplan, G. (1974). Foreword. In I. Glick, R. Weiss, & C. M. Parkes (Eds.), *The first year of bereavement* (pp. vii–xi). New York: John Wiley & Sons.

Carpenito, L. (1992). *Nursing diagnosis: Application to clinical practice* (5th ed.). Philadelphia: J. B. Lippincott.

Carr, C. A. (1993). Coping with dying: Lessons that we should and should not learn from the work of Elizabeth Kübler-Ross. *Death Studies, 17*(1), 69–83.

Demi, A. (1984). Hospice bereavement programs: trends and issues. In S. Schraff (Ed.), *Hospice: The nursing perspective* (pp. 131–151). New York: National League for Nursing.

Demi, P. (1989). Death of a spouse. In R. Kalish (Ed.), *Coping with the losses of middle age* (pp. 218–248). Newbury Park, CA.

Demi, A., & Miles, M. (1987). Parameters of normal grief: A Delphi study. *Death Studies, 11,* 397–412.

Demi, A., & Miles, M. (1994). Bereavement guilt: A conceptual model with application. In I. Corless, B. Germino, & M. Pittman (Eds.), *Dying, death, and bereavement* (pp. 171–188). Boston: Jones & Bartlett.

Demi, A., & Schroeder, M. (1985). *Bereavement experience questionnaire.* Paper presented at Measurement of Clinical and Educational Nursing Outcomes Conference, New Orleans, LA.

Dimond, M. (1981). Bereavement and the elderly: A critical review with implications for nursing practice and research. *J Adv Nurs, 6,* 461–470.

Doka, K. (1989). *Disenfranchised grief.* Lexington, MA: Lexington Books.

Engel, G. (1964). Grief and grieving. *Am J Nurs, 64*(9), 88–100.

Faschingbauer, T., DeVaul, R., & Zisook, S. (1977). Development of the Texas Inventory of Grief. *Am J Psychiatry, 134,* 696–698.

Fried, M. (1962). Grieving for a lost home. In L.J. Duhl (Ed.), *The environment of the metropolis.* New York: Basic Books.

Fulton, R., & Gottesman, A. (1980). Anticipatory grief: A psychosocial concept considered. *British Journal of Psychiatry, 137,* 45–54.

Hogan, N. (1994). Things that help and hinder adolescent sibling bereavement. *Western Journal of Nursing, 16*(2), 146–148.

Kaprio, J., Kaskenvuo, M., & Rita, H. (1987). Mortality after bereavement. *Am J Public Health, 77,* 283–287.

Kübler-Ross, E. (1969). *On death and dying.* New York: Macmillan.

Lindemann, E. (1944). Symptomatology and management of acute grief. *Am J Psychiatry,* 101, 141–148.

Marris, P. (1975). *Loss and change.* Garden City, NY: Doubleday.

McLane, A. (1987). *Classification of nursing diagnoses.* St. Louis: C. V. Mosby.

Miles, M. S., & Demi, A. S. (1983–1984). Sources of guilt in bereaved parents: Toward the development of a theory bereavement guilt. *Omega, 14,* 299–314.

Miles, M., & Demi, A. (1994). Historical and contemporary theories of grief. In I. Corless, B. Germino, & M. Pittman (Eds.), *Dying, death, and bereavement* (pp. 83–-106). Boston: Jones & Bartlett.

Murphy, S. A. (1983). Theoretical perspectives on bereavement. In P. L. Chinn (Ed.), *Advances in nursing theory development* (pp. 191–206). Rockville, MD: Aspen.

North American Nursing Diagnosis Association (NANDA). (1994). *Nursing diagnoses: Definitions and classification* 1995–1996. Philadelphia: NANDA.

Parkes, C. M. (1986). *Bereavement: Studies of grief in adult life* (2nd ed.). New York: International Universities Press.

Rando, T. (1986). *Loss and anticipatory grief.* Lexington, MA: Lexington Books.

Richter, J. M. (1984). Crisis of mate loss in the elderly. *Advances in Nursing Science, 6*(4), 45–53.

Rigdon, I., Clayton, B., & Dimond, M. (1987). Toward a theory of helpfulness for the elderly bereaved: An invitation to a new life. *Advances in Nursing Science, 9*(2), 32–43.

Rolland, J. S. (1990). Anticipatory loss: A family systems developmental framework. *Family Process, 29,* 229–244.

Sanders, C., & Mauger, P. (1979). *A Manual for the Grief Experience Inventory.* Tampa, FL: University of Florida.

Silverman, P., MacKenzie, D., Pattipas, M., et al. (1974). *Helping each other in widowhood.* New York: Health Sciences.

Waechter, E. H., Phillips, J., & Holaday, B. (1985). *Nursing care of children* (10th ed.). Philadelphia: J. B. Lippincott.

Zilberg, N., Weiss, D., & Horowitz, M. (1982). Impact of event scale: A cross validational study and some empirical evidence supporting a conceptual model of stress response syndromes. *J Consult Clin Psychol, 50*(3), 407–414.

Bibliography

Beaton, J. L., et al. (1990). Life and death decisions: The impact on nurses. *Canadian Nurse,* 86(3), 18–19, 21–22.

Cecchini, J. A. L. (1990). Reach out and touch . . . dealing with dying patients and their families. *Imprint, 37*(1), 73.

Claxton, J. W. (1993). Paving the way to acceptance: Psychological adaptation to death and dying in cancer. *Professional Nurse, 8*(4), 206.

Cooley, M. E. (1992). Bereavement care: A role for nurses. *Career Nursing, 15*(2), 125–129.

Cowles, K. V., & Rogers, B. L. (1991). The concept of grief: A foundation for nursing research and practice. *RINAH, 14,* 119–127.

Curry, L. C., & Stone, J. G. (1992). Moving on: Recovering from the death of a spouse. *Clinical Nurse Specialist, 6*(4), 180–190.

Davis, B. (1993). Sibling bereavement: Research-based guidelines for nurses. *Seminars in Oncology Nursing, 9*(2), 107–113.

Farrar, A. (1992). How much do they want to know? Communicating with dying patients. *Professional Nurse, 7*(9), 606–610.

Gifford, B. J., et al. (1990). Supporting the bereaved. *Am J Nurs, 90*(2), 48–55.

Glass, B. C. (1993). The role of the nurse in advanced practice in bereavement care. *Clinical Disease Specialists, 7*(2), 62–76.

Hallal, J. C., & Walsh, M. B. (1992). Loss bereavement and care of the dying patient. In *Gerontological nursing: Care of the frail elderly* (pp. 434–451). St. Louis: C. V. Mosby.

Heiney, S. P., Hasan, L., & Price, K. (1993). Developing and implementing a bereavement program for a children's hospital. *Journal of Pediatric Nursing, 8*(6), 385–391.

Hunt, M. (1992). "Scripts" for dying at home . . . displayed in nurses,' patients,' and relatives' talk. *J Adv Nurs, 17,* 1297–1302.

Hutti, M. H. (1992). Parents' perceptions of the miscarriage experience. *Death Studies, 16*(5), 401–415.

Jones, P. S., & Marinson, I. M. (1992). The experience of bereavement in caregivers of family members with Alzheimer's disease. *Image, 24,* 172–176.

Lambert, J. W., Delmer, C. M. (1993). Model of family grief assessment and treatment. *Death Studies, 17*(1), 55–67.

Longman, A. J. (1993). Effectiveness of a hospice community bereavement program. *Omega, 27*(2), 165–175.

McCain, N. L., & Gramling, L. F. (1992). Living with dying: Coping with HIV disease. *Issues in Mental Health Nursing, 13*(3), 271–184.

McClelland, M. L. (1993). Our unit has a bereavement program. *Am J Nurs, 93*(1), 62.

Mendyka, B. E. (1993). The dying patient in the intensive care unit: Assisting the family in crisis. *AACN Clinical Issues in Critical Care, 4*(3), 550–557.

Parry, J. K., & Thornwall, J. (1992). Death of a father. *Death Studies, 16*(2), 173–181.

Rosen, S. L. (1990). Stillbirth: What the nurse should and should not do. *Imprint, 37*(1), 65–67.

Schoefeld, D. J. (1993). Talking with children about death. *Journal of Pediatric Healthcare, 7*(6), 267–274.

Steele, L. (1992). Risk factor profile for bereaved spouses. *Death Studies, 16*(5), 87–99.

Sweeting, H. N., & Gilhooly, M. L. M. (1990). Anticipatory grief: A review. *Soc Sci Med, 30,* 1073–1080.

Trolley, B. C. (1993). Kaleidoscope of aid for parents whose child died by suicidal and sudden, non-suicidal means. *Omega, 27*(3), 239–250.

Trunnell, E. P., Caserta, M. S., & White, G. L. (1992). Bereavement: Current issues in intervention and prevention. *Journal of Health Education, 23*(5), 275–280.

Walsh, F., & McGoldrick, M. (1991). *Living beyond loss: Death in the family*. New York: W. W. Norton.

Coping and Stress Management

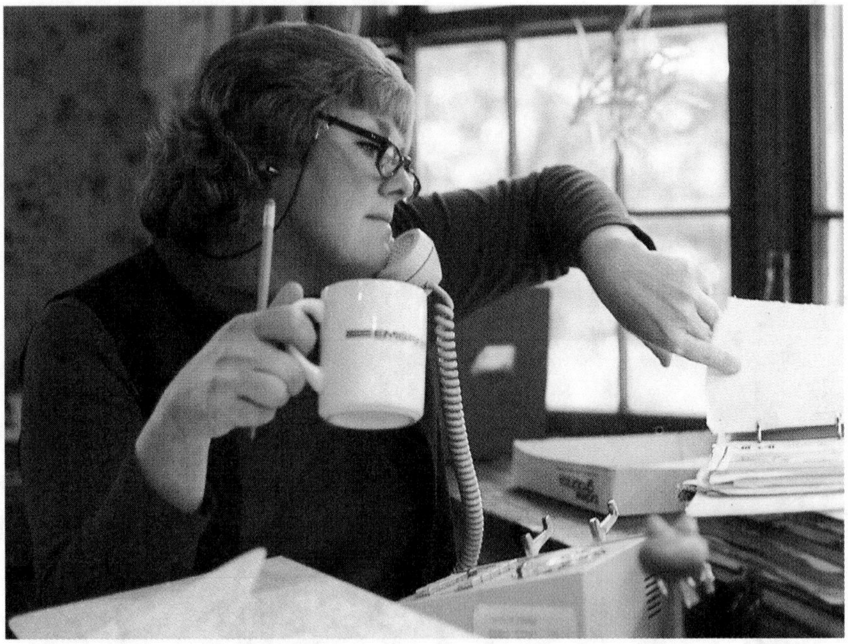

UNIT XV

Stress and its necessary coping and adaptions are daily facts of life for clients and nurses. Stress affects how clients perceive and meet needs and has an impact on every other area of function. Unit XV discusses the coping and stress tolerance area of function.

The single chapter in this unit explores theories and concepts about stress and the many factors that affect coping stress tolerance. Using the nursing process as a framework, the chapter emphasizes assessment for stressors and previous coping patterns and interventions to maximize effective stress management. Nursing interventions are particularly important in this area of human function because the degree to which the client manages stress tolerance and coping can be either health promoting or illness producing. The chapter focuses on holistic nursing interventions to promote health and function and also details the many independent nursing interventions that can be used for a client who has ineffective coping.

The content covered in this unit provides the knowledge base and skills needed to assist or support clients in reducing or managing stress through effective coping and also assists the nurse as he or she manages the stress of daily life.

Stress, Coping, and Adaptation

Key Terms	Learning Objectives

Adaptation
Burnout
Coping
Coping mechanism
Fight-or-flight response
General adaptation syndrome
Homeostasis
Local adaptation syndrome
Mental health
Stress
Stressor

Upon completion of this chapter, the student will be able to do the following:

- *Describe the three stages of the general adaptation syndrome.*
- *Identify physiologic signs and symptoms of stress.*
- *Identify psychological responses to stress.*
- *List examples of biophysical and psychosocial stressors.*
- *Give examples of mediating variables that affect a person's ability to cope with stress.*
- *Identify stress management techniques that the nurse can use to help a client adapt to stress*

51

While caring for an older woman with chronic mental health problems, you interview her 46-year-old daughter. She tells you that the client has been married for 51 years to a man who has had quadruple cardiac bypass surgery, recurrent kidney and bladder cancer, and a long history of alcoholism, although he is not drinking currently. In assessing the client's home situation, you learn that the client and her husband live in their own home, but the daughter cooks and takes meals to them, takes them to their many healthcare appointments, handles their finances, and provides most of their support. The daughter is married, has three children, and works full-time. She states that she frequently feels torn between her responsibilities to her parents and to her family, who feel neglected. Although you began the interview to learn more about your client, you find you are learning more about the daughter's conflicts.

In previous chapters you learned about health and wellness, human needs, self-perception, communication, and more. This chapter adds information about stress, coping, and adaptation to your knowledge base. After you have completed the chapter you should be able to give care to both the mother and daughter in the situation above. The Critical Thinking Challenges at the end of the chapter will help you think through problems dealing with stress and coping.

Stress is a complex phenomenon, which some people define as a stimulus or a response that causes physical or emotional tension. Stress is inherent to life. It is essential, yet problematic. Stress can be the stimulus for constructive change and positive growth, or it can result in illness, disease and, possibly, death. Coping is a problem-solving process that a person uses to manage the stresses or events with which he or she is presented. Coping with stress successfully requires adaptation (the process by which the human system modifies itself to conform to the environment). Therefore, the ability to cope with and adapt to stress is a crucial determinate of human well-being.

The major nursing responsibilities associated with assisting a client to cope with and adapt to stress include assessing the client's ability to cope with the stressors in the environment; identifying risk factors that could lead to ineffective coping; promoting effective coping and stress management; and implementing nursing interventions to manage ineffective coping when it occurs. In addition, nurses must recognize and cope effectively with stress in their own lives.

Normal Coping and Adaptation to Stress

Throughout history, humans have experienced stressful lives. Like all organisms, they face demands from the environment that necessitate changes in them to ensure survival. For many years, this adaptive process was assumed to occur as a series of starts and stops, in which constancy and stability were thought to prevail until some danger or threat occurred. Faced by the danger, the organism changed in some way, and then entered another period of stability until another circumstance resulted in the demand for change. In actuality, both the organism and the environment are involved in a process of continual change.

Normal Function of Stress and Coping

Today more than ever, people live in a world full of change, one that requires many adjustments. Some of these adjustments are made with little effort, and some are made subconsciously. Other adjustments require major efforts to accomplish. These demands, changes, adjustments, and efforts constitute what we mean when we talk about stress, coping, and adaptation.

Homeostasis

Walter B. Cannon (1935), an American physiologist, created the term **homeostasis** to refer to the coordinated physiologic processes that maintain most of the steady states in the organism. He applied the term mainly to the self-regulation of physiologic processes within the body, such as heart rate, blood pressure, body temperature, and fluid and electrolyte balance. Today, the concept of homeostasis has been expanded to include external as well as internal environments and psychosocial as well as physiologic balance.

Physiologic Homeostasis. Physiologic homeostasis denotes the condition in which the internal environment of the body is relatively constant. This relative constancy, which is essential for the survival and proper functioning of cells, is maintained through continual changes in such internal physiologic processes as heart rate, blood pressure, body temperature, fluid and electrolyte balance, blood glucose concentration, and blood oxygen level.

Although homeostasis is simple in principle, it is wonderfully complex in actuality. Numerous interrelated control mechanisms involving virtually all tissues and organs of the body interact to maintain the delicate homeostatic balance. Neuroendocrine integration functions in a central role. The neuroendocrine response comprises the activities of the autonomic nervous system and the endocrine system, mediated by the hypothalamic–pituitary–adrenal axis.

In general, the nervous system regulates the rapid muscular and excretory activities of the body, whereas the endocrine system regulates mainly the slower-reacting metabolic functions. Other important regulatory mechanisms are governed by the renal, cardiovascular, respiratory, gastrointestinal, and musculoskeletal systems.

Autonomic Nervous System. The autonomic nervous system plays a major role in homeostatic control. The autonomic nervous system regulates the visceral functions of the body involving the smooth muscles of the blood vessels and digestive tract, cardiac muscle, and glands of the digestive organs, liver, pancreas, and adrenal medulla. The two divisions of the autonomic nervous system are the parasympathetic and sympathetic nervous systems. The parasympathetic system, which is generally responsive to an internal need for restoration and conservation, promotes digestion and elimination. The sympathetic system, which functions as an emergency system, responds to sudden demands or threats. The resulting physiologic changes prepare the body for increased energy expenditure. Some of the sympathetic responses include increases in heart rate, blood glucose level, blood flow to skeletal muscles, and mental arousal.

Endocrine System. The endocrine system is another important homeostatic regulatory mechanism. The functions of five major endocrine glands are involved: pituitary, adrenal, thyroid, parathyroid, and pancreas. The endocrine glands secrete chemical substances called hormones, which are specific mediators that alter cell activity some distance from their source. Figure 51-1 shows the location and function of specific endocrine glands that affect the body's adaptation to stress.

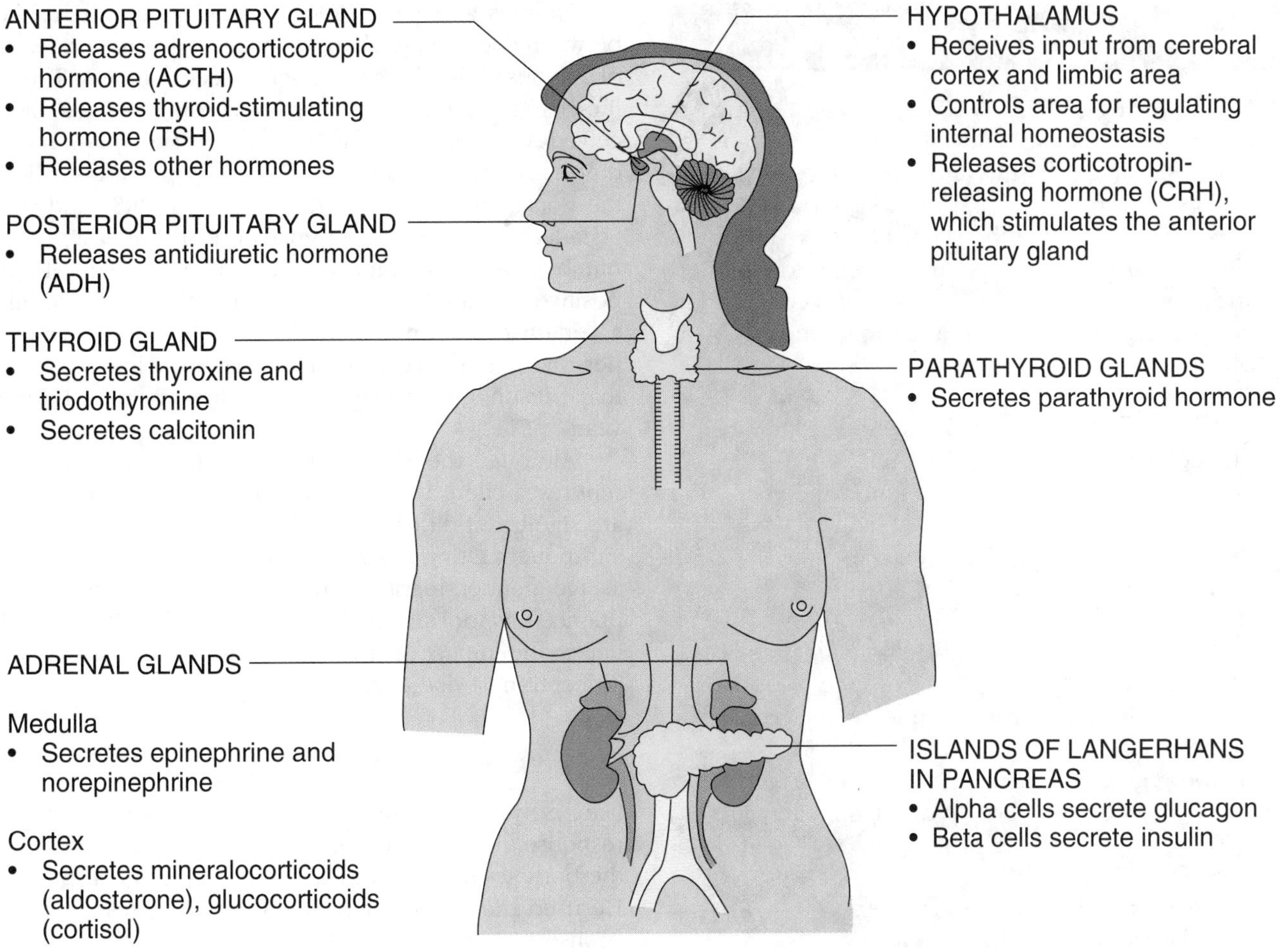
ANTERIOR PITUITARY GLAND
• Releases adrenocorticotropic hormone (ACTH)
• Releases thyroid-stimulating hormone (TSH)
• Releases other hormones
POSTERIOR PITUITARY GLAND
• Releases antidiuretic hormone (ADH)
THYROID GLAND
• Secretes thyroxine and triodothyronine
• Secretes calcitonin
ADRENAL GLANDS
Medulla
• Secretes epinephrine and norepinephrine
Cortex
• Secretes mineralocorticoids (aldosterone), glucocorticoids (cortisol)
HYPOTHALAMUS
• Receives input from cerebral cortex and limbic area
• Controls area for regulating internal homeostasis
• Releases corticotropin-releasing hormone (CRH), which stimulates the anterior pituitary gland
PARATHYROID GLANDS
• Secretes parathyroid hormone
ISLANDS OF LANGERHANS IN PANCREAS
• Alpha cells secrete glucagon
• Beta cells secrete insulin

Figure 51-1 • *Location of specific endocrine glands that affect the body's adaptation to stress.*

Psychosocial Homeostasis. Psychosocial homeostasis refers to a state of mental or emotional well-being. **Mental health** is typically defined in terms of a person's mastery of interpersonal relationships, as well as role fulfillment and achievement in the realms of work, family, and community. In addition, the person must have a positive sense of self-esteem and self-worth.

Human beings are open systems, constantly interacting with the environment. Several approaches address helping the person maintain a state of dynamic equilibrium, or psychological homeostasis. For instance, Maslow's hierarchy of human needs (see Chapter 2) should be met to maintain equilibrium.

Levine and Scotch (1970) report that various broad sociocultural phenomena, derived from sociologic, anthropologic, and epidemiologic data, can serve as sources of stress. These sources include

- Differences between the structure of the person's family and the structure of families that predominate in the social environment
- Varying aspects of the life cycle of families
- Role conflict
- Work-related stressors
- Social isolation
- Socioeconomic class and race.

Lazarus (1981) developed the Everyday Hassles Scale to help identify and rank everyday stressful events (see the accompanying display). The scale contains both "hassles" that create stress and "uplifts" that promote a sense of well-being. People may have different awarenesses of hassles and uplifts. Knowing the nature of potential psychosociologic stressors, however, provides the means of anticipating possible problems and the related psychological reactions.

Characteristics of Normal Coping and Adaptation

Stress is normal. People talk about the stress in their lives on a daily basis. Work, relationships, family, school, and illness all are possible sources of stress. Even though stress is a term in common usage, the concept is difficult to define. The term **stress** means different things at different times to different people. Stress may be considered a stimulus, or it may be considered

Lazarus's Everyday Hassles Scale

The following scale rank orders "hassles," which contribute to stress, and "uplifts," which contribute positively to stress management, as evaluated by several middle-aged client groups. The nurse may determine the client's hassles and uplifts for purposes of providing anticipatory guidance. Individual clients may perceive hassles and uplifts differently from the groups studied by Lazarus.

Hassles (Rank Ordered)

1. Feeling concerned about weight.
2. Worrying about health of a family member.
3. Worrying about rising cost of living.
4. Dealing with home maintenance.
5. Having too many things to do.
6. Misplacing or losing things.
7. Doing yard work or outside home maintenance.
8. Worrying about property, investment, or taxes.
9. Worrying about crime.
10. Feeling concern about physical appearance.

Uplifts (Rank Ordered)

1. Relating well to spouse or lover.
2. Relating well with friends.
3. Completing a task.
4. Feeling healthy.
5. Getting enough sleep.
6. Eating out.
7. Meeting responsibilities.
8. Visiting, telephoning, or writing someone.
9. Spending time with family.
10. Taking pleasure in one's home.

Adapted from Lazarus, R. S. (1981). Little hazards can be hazardous to your health. *Psychology Today, 15*(7), 58–62.

a response to a particular stimulus. A broader concept of stress encompasses many interacting factors, such as stimulus, response, appraisal of the threat, and coping styles (Mason, 1975 and 1975b).

Stress as a Stimulus

When viewed as a stimulus, stress is defined as an event or set of events causing a disrupted response (Lazarus, 1992). In 1953, Wolff described disease states resulting from life stress caused by disruption in lifestyles and relationships, deprivation of human needs, and failure to act in ways to eliminate the cause of the distress.

Holmes and Rahe (1967) studied the relationship between specific life changes, such as divorce or death of a spouse, and the subsequent onset of illness. These life-change events were rated according to their perceived stressfulness and the degree of adaptation required. Holmes and Rahe (1967) developed tools called the Social Readjustment Rating Scale (SRRS) and the Schedule of Recent Experiences (SRE) to measure the number and magnitude of life-changing events, both positive and negative, experienced by the subject within a certain time frame. They found that the higher the person's cumulative score, the greater the likelihood of that person incurring a serious illness within 1 to 2 years.

Although the SRE has been used extensively, current researchers advise caution in its use, because there are significant differences in a person's perception and subsequent rating of stressful life events. Variables such as age, gender, marital status, and ethnic origin can influence this tool's results. Thus, a critical factor in evaluating the impact of stressful life events is the person's perception of that event.

Stress as a Response

Hans Selye, the author of several books on the stress response, defined stress as "the nonspecific response of the body to any demand upon it" (Selye, 1974, p. 27). He used the theoretical framework that stress is a response to a certain stimulus.

Selye used the term "stressor" to differentiate between the stress-producing agent and the response to stress. A **stressor** is the stimulus or agent that evokes a stress response in the person; it is anything that places a demand on the person for change or adaptation. Stressors may be biophysical, psychological, or sociocultural.

Stressors can be viewed by the person as positive or negative. Selye (1974) referred to pleasant events as *eustress* from the Greek prefix *eu*, meaning good or positive. One example of such a stressor might be going to college, which the person views as positive and desirable, but is also stressful, because it involves changes in one's routine and requires adaptation to those changes. Negative or undesirable events are referred to as *distress*. Examples of such a stressor might include being fired from a job, having an argument with a close friend, or being hospitalized. Pleasurable events seem to evoke the same physiologic reactions as negative stressors.

Selye (1974) termed this undifferentiated physiologic reaction "nonspecific response," meaning that the body goes through a number of biochemical changes and readjustments without regard to the nature of the stress-producing agent. Because the physiologic response to the stressful agent seemed to be universal in all organisms, he referred to this pattern of defense as the general adaptation syndrome. The following section discusses these changes and readjustments. They are also outlined in Figure 51-2.

General Adaptation Syndrome. The nonspecific response to stress is termed the **general adaptation syndrome** (GAS). The GAS is a generalized adaptive response to states of stress, and consists of three stages: alarm, resistance, and exhaustion (Selye, 1974, p. 38).

Alarm Reaction. The alarm reaction, also called the **fight-or-flight response** is the body's initial response to stress, in which its defenses are alerted and the person is prepared for "fight or flight." This preparation involves the secretion of hormones and the response of target organs.

The hormones epinephrine and norepinephrine, secreted by the adrenal glands, trigger an increase in blood pressure and in the heart and respiratory rates, which increases oxygen availability and blood flow to the muscles to prepare for defense by either fight or flight. Increased mental alertness and pupillary dilation to improve visual acuity are additional effects of the hormonal influence. Epinephrine increases the blood glucose level, and cortisol, also secreted by the adrenals, stimulates the process of gluconeogenesis (the conversion of proteins and fats into glucose by the liver), making additional energy available to the skeletal muscles of the body. The conversion of proteins and fats to simpler substances (glucose) is known as a catabolic process (Vander, 1993).

In the alarm reaction, the body prepares to react to the stressor with which it has been presented. This stage may last only a few minutes or may continue for several hours. A stress situation that is longer-lasting or in which a more serious threat is perceived causes the body to move to the next stage, the stage of resistance.

Stage of Resistance. In the stage of resistance, the body attempts to adapt to the stressor and mobilizes coping mechanisms. Stabilization occurs in the heart

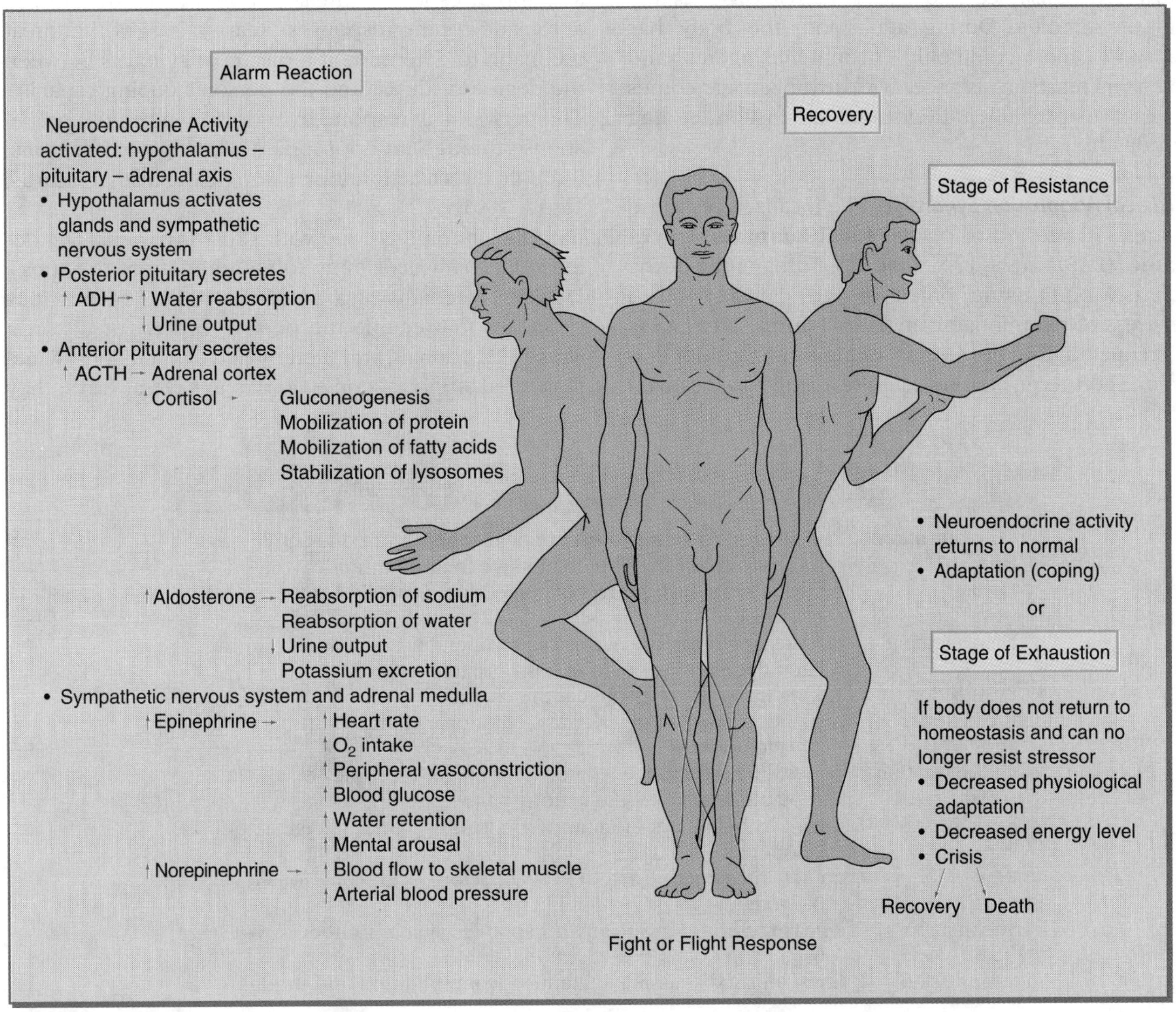

Figure 51-2 • *General adaptation syndrome.*

and respiratory rates, blood pressure, and hormone levels. The body begins coping with the new state of adaptation, trying to return to normal function.

If the stressor has not been removed or if the effects of the stressor lead to continued inability to adapt, then the body's attempt to return to normal will be incomplete, and the attempt at physiologic adaptation will not return the body to its previous homeostatic state.

Stage of Exhaustion. When the body can no longer resist the stressor or cannot maintain its adaptation, it moves to the stage of exhaustion. In this stage the body's ability to respond to the continuing stress is diminished or depleted. If the body has sufficient energy stores for continued adaptation, then rest, recovery, and return to normal may be the end result. If the adaptation is not adequate or if the body cannot mobilize a further defense, exhaustion ensues, and death may be the outcome.

Finite Adaptability. According to Selye (1974), the GAS demonstrates that the body's adaptability, or adaptation energy, is finite. He compared the three stages of the GAS to the human lifespan. In childhood, there is lowered resistance and excessive response to any kind of stimulus. During adulthood, the body has adapted to most commonly encountered agents, and there is increased resistance. With advanced age comes a loss of adaptability and eventual exhaustion, ending with death.

Local Adaptation Syndrome. The localized response to stress is referred to as the **local adaptation syndrome** (LAS). In the LAS, a localized area of the body, such as a body tissue, organ, or part, can respond to the stress of pain, inflammation, or trauma. The LAS is differentiated from the GAS by being localized (not systemic), short-term, adaptive, and restorative to localized homeostasis. The LAS has three stages as well; however, they occur locally, rather than generally, as in the GAS. During the LAS, the following changes occur:

Blood vessels dilate in the stressed area.
Fibrous connective tissue proliferates to prevent spread of potential pathogens into the blood stream.
Cells proliferate to repair or replace damaged tissue.
Chemical substances are secreted from the blood and connective tissue to neutralize toxins and destroy any bacteria present (Selye, 1974).

Psychosociologic Response. A person's response to stress is influenced by his or her use of coping strategies, or coping skills. When stressful events are successfully managed by effective coping, the person experiences personal growth and improved problem-solving abilities. A person who is most successful in coping tends to be flexible and to use a variety of strategies to adapt to new situations and stressors.

Cognitively, a person perceives an event or stressor, appraises it as a threat or non-threat, and calls on automatic coping responses. Reappraisals of the threat are made to determine if a discrepancy exists between the degree of threat and the person's coping capacity. The person may respond by reducing the emotional response through an appropriate discharge of emotions, through direct actions, or through defenses (Lazarus, 1991a, 1991b).

One attempt to cope with stress involves using defense mechanisms simply to withdraw from the stress. Defense mechanisms are self-protective, unconscious processes that enable the person to deny or distort a stressful encounter, and thereby decrease anxiety (Wineman, et al., 1994). People do this in several ways: they

Table 51-1 • Common Defense Mechanisms

Compensation	The attempt to achieve respect or recognition in one activity as a substitute for inability to achieve in another endeavor.
Denial	Refusing to believe or accept something as it is but rather as one wishes it to be.
Displacement	Transferring emotion away from the person or situation that incited the emotion to an inappropriate person or object.
Introjection	Taking into one's personality the characteristics of another.
Projection	Attributing one's own thoughts, emotions, characteristics, or motives to another.
Rationalization	Concealing the motive for behavior by giving some socially acceptable reason for the action.
Regression	Return to behaviors more appropriate to an earlier stage of development.
Repression	Immersing something in the subconscious or unconscious level of thought.
Sublimation	Release of libido in socially acceptable behavior rather than using it to obtain sexual gratification.
Suppression	Consciously dismissing something from the mind and thoughts.

may use denial or they may increase time spent sleeping, daydreaming, and fantasizing. Table 51-1 lists and defines the common defense mechanisms. If the stress is more than the person can or wants to deal with, one method of coping is to withdraw to an activity that is comforting and nonstressful. For example, while one is sleeping, one can avoid stress or delay responding to it, assuming that the stress does not keep one awake. Daydreams and fantasies allow the person to withdraw mentally to a more pleasant, less stressful scene.

Normal Pattern of Coping and Adaptation

Coping successfully with stress requires adaptation, or the process of the person's effort to manage internal and external demands. Coping is usually described as a problem-solving process or strategy by which the person manages the out-of-the-ordinary events or situations with which he or she is presented. Although coping may be entirely cognitive, it is more likely to be a psychophysiologic activity involving an integration of the mind and body. As such, it is a major process in the successful response to stress and crucial to the person's continued growth and adaptation.

Lazarus (1991a) described two types of coping processes: problem-oriented (manipulation of the person–environment relationship that is the source of stress) and emotion-focused (regulation of stressful emotions). Examples of both are given in the accompanying display.

Bell (1977) divided **coping mechanisms** (activities or measures for managing stress) into two groups, long-term and short-term. Long-term coping mechanisms are positive, constructive ways of dealing with stress and can be effective over long periods. Short-term coping methods are temporary measures that reduce stress and tension; however, if used over long periods of time, they may have a detrimental effect on the person, and lead to maladaptive behavior. Examples are given in the display.

Examples of Coping Strategies

Examples of Problem-Oriented Coping Mechanisms

- Making a time schedule for studying and sticking to it
- Applying for a job at another company because your current position is too demanding
- Trying to find out more about an illness, such as diabetes, so it can be managed better

Examples of Emotion-Focused Coping Mechanisms

- Accepting sympathy and understanding from a friend in the loss of a family member
- Releasing tension after a hard day at work by meditating, crying, or taking a walk
- Blaming someone else—for example, a spouse or teacher—for the situation you are in

Examples of Long-Term Coping Mechanisms

- Working out the stress through physical exercise
- Talking with others about a problem (friend, counselor)
- Relying on belief in a higher power
- Seeking additional information about a situation
- Drawing on past experience
- Developing alternative plans for handling the situation

Examples of Short-Term Coping Mechanisms

- Smoking
- Alcohol use
- Overeating
- "Pill-popping"
- Excessive coffee intake

Factors Affecting Normal Coping and Adaptation

Over a lifetime, many events and situations occur as a normal part of living. Although these events are within the realm of normal living, they still may produce stress, requiring a person to cope and adapt to them. Among these events are transitions or changes, such as attending school, moving, marrying, and childbearing, and lifestyle factors, such as nutrition, exercise, and fitness.

Roles and Relationships. For a child who has felt secure and has experienced only minimal stress, attending school for the first time can be filled with real or perceived stress, with which the child must cope. On an extended scale, the student who moves to new schools and various levels of education (middle school, high school, college) learns to cope and adapt to the stresses related to each new situation with increasing maturity (Sorensen, 1994).

In a mobile society such as the United States, many families experience frequent moving and relocation for career purposes as a way of life. Each move has its own unique stresses related to closure of family life in one community and beginning of family life in a new community. The relocation involves not only physical relocation but also separation from the family's emotional ties and support systems within the community. Most families can develop these relationships in time in their new community, but it is usually a stressful time, even when everything goes well.

As people mature and move into the developmental tasks of adult life, the transitions related to those events require adequate coping and adaptation. The selection of a mate, marriage, and childbearing are examples of those transitional events. Usually, the marriages of young adults are happy occasions. Even so, families are faced with the stresses of decisions relating to the actual event, to the new alliance, and to separation from the previous parent–child relationship. The newlyweds face the stresses of changing their previous relationships with their families, developing the new marriage relationship, and making decisions relating to day-to-day life. When a child is born, new stresses accompany the expansion of the family, even when the baby is anticipated with great delight. There are now new demands on both marriage partners in terms of emotions, dependencies, time, and money. Childbearing demands a new set of coping strategies to adapt successfully (Hall, 1994).

Nutrition and Metabolism. Today, more and more people are concerned about the quality of their dietary intake. They are concerned not only with total caloric intake but with the nutritional value of the food. When the body has adequate nutrients and does not experience the malnutrition of being either undernourished or overfed, the nutritional resources give the body more reserve with which to respond to stress. Imbalances in the intake of essential nutrients can enhance or even exaggerate the stress response. A person who is poorly nourished as a result of overeating or undereating may be less well prepared to face a stressful situation.

Activity and Exercise. When adequate nutrition is combined with a regular exercise program, the resulting fitness benefits the person physiologically and psychologically. The benefits of exercise include improved cardiovascular conditioning, weight control, muscle tone, and sense of well-being. Because many chronic illnesses have some relation to one or more of these factors, exercise programs can be effective in decreasing these outcomes of stress. Regular patterns of exercise provide people with a ready outlet for stress before it becomes prolonged or chronic.

A person who is fit usually has developed lifestyle habits that provide an outlet for stress on a regular basis. The exercise routine permits the person to cope with the normal, day-to-day stresses so that adaptation occurs in smaller increments. This modulated approach to the daily stresses of life prevents the accumulation of many little things to a point where the person can no longer cope.

Sleep and Rest. To be rested and relaxed, a person needs a pattern of adequate sleep. When a person is anticipating stress or experiencing stress, it is particularly important to be rested and relaxed. The busy schedules of many people leave little time for adequate rest and sleep, which therefore compromises their ability to manage stress.

Safety and Security. The amount of threat perceived compared to the degree of security a person feels affects the response to stress. For example, if a student is failing a class in school and feels very insecure about how his or her parents will react, the student will experience greater stress than if he or she felt secure about the support and understanding of his or her parents. Similarly, the effect of other stress-producing situations, such as giving birth, acute illness, or role changes, depends on the person's perception of the event and the presence of adequate support and effective coping mechanisms.

Previous Experience. Past experience with stressors can influence the response and adaptation to current stressful encounters. Responses to stressors may be learned, often from other family members. For instance, a fear of heights may develop in a child because the father also had this phobia.

Previous exposure to a stressful situation may also help the person to cope with similar situations. For example, a person who has been hospitalized before may find the experience much less stressful than the client who has never been hospitalized.

Lifespan Considerations

Newborn and Infant

The newborn and infant depend largely on reflex responses for coping with their environment and the stresses that are presented. For example, if a newborn is hungry, he or she will cry and be physically active as a means of reflexively coping with the situation and attempting to do something about it. The parent learns to respond to the infant's communication and participates in a mutual coping adaptation by giving the infant food. With continuing development, the infant gradually learns new coping strategies to fit various situations, although these usually are limited to reflex and sensory functions, and responses to stress may be excessive.

At this stage of development, the infant depends totally on the parent for physiologic needs, safety, and loving attachment. These needs, if met, ameliorate the effect of stress and provide the basis for coping.

Toddler and Preschooler

During the toddler and preschool stages of development, the child's physical development becomes more stable. The child learns to develop strategies for coping with relatively simple events, such as not getting something that he or she wants exactly when he or she wants it. Learning to handle a slight delay in getting wants and needs met may seem like a small accomplishment, but it sets a pattern that the child can apply to other situations later in life.

Parents and family members are a key part of the child's frame of reference in terms of handling stress and adapting to situations (Fig. 51-3). Because the child is developing coping strategies, the child may still experience excessive response to stressful situations. He or she depends on parents for safety and limit-setting to define the boundaries within which stress can be handled.

Child and Adolescent

The school-age child is expanding his or her world, moving out of the totally protected realm of home into the experience of school and interactions with others. Classroom situations, structured play, and interactions with other children and adults present new stresses. The child must learn to adapt to these stresses and to cope with new experiences and rules. At this age, the child can identify stressors, begin to reason with parents and others about how to cope with them, and draw from past experience to develop new approaches.

During adolescence, the person moves toward achieving emotional independence from the parents, develops a sexual identity, acquires values, and achieves socially responsible behavior. Achieving these tasks is stress-producing in itself, requiring the adolescent to use the coping strategies developed thus far and to develop new ones continually (Puskar, et al., 1993). Physiologically, the adolescent has adequate reserves for responding to stress. Psychological maturation, however, is a primary task of adolescence, requiring behavioral adaptations and development of new coping mechanisms. Although separation from parents is in progress, the adolescent still needs the security and boundaries provided by parents and family.

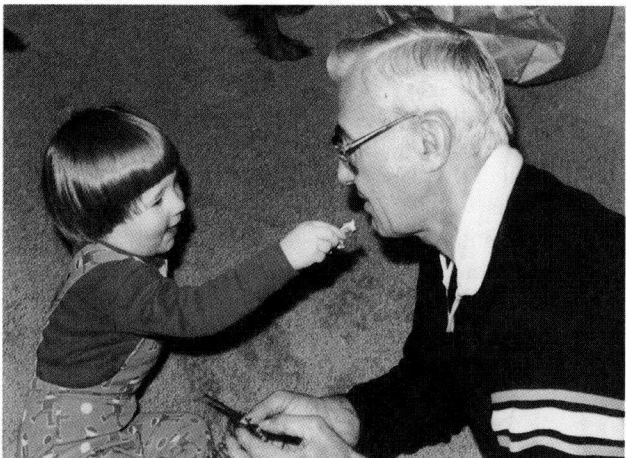

Figure 51-3 • *Play activities between a child and a grandparent promote the child's learning and coping strategies.*

Adult and Older Adult

Adults are relatively stable physiologically and able to handle stress efficiently in most cases. However, the various demands of adulthood (occupation, lifestyle, relationships, family, and the like) impose more stress on a daily basis. The adult draws on coping skills developed throughout life and develops new ones. Previous exposure to a stressful situation may help the person to cope with similar situations in a more adaptive manner. For example, as mentioned earlier, a person who has been hospitalized before may find the experience much less stressful than the client who has never been hospitalized. For parents, bringing a new baby into the home may present stress, and having that same child grow up and leave home may present stress on another level. These stresses may stimulate positive change and growth.

As a person ages, stress does not decrease. Among the stresses of aging are retirement, decline in physical energy, decrease in financial potential, loss of family and friends, and, possibly, relocation. Older adults must adapt to these stresses and changes at the same time that their individual reserves and strength are declining. When the GAS is initiated in the older adult, there is much more concern that the stage of exhaustion may end in death, rather than rest and recovery.

Altered Coping and Adaptation to Stress

In addition to being knowledgeable about the function of stress and the factors that affect stress and coping, the nurse needs first to differentiate normal coping with stress from altered coping situations. Then the nurse can identify the manifestations of these responses and their impact on clients.

Potential for Altered Coping

The same factors that create stress in day-to-day living, and can be considered normal, may have other facets posing the potential for altered coping and adaptation. These include such *transition factors* as involuntary relocation, hospitalization, divorce, loss, or domestic abuse and such *lifestyle factors* as fatigue, illness, or death.

Involuntary Relocation

Even under the best of circumstances, relocation can be stressful, but when the move is involuntary, the potential for stress increases greatly. For example, although

Nursing Research
Stress and Coping

Selected Nursing Research Studies

Cayse, L. N. (1994). Fathers of children with cancer: A descriptive study of their stressors and coping strategies. *Journal of Pediatric Oncology Nursing, 11*(3), 102–18.

D'Avanzo, C. E., Frye, B., & Froman, R. (1994). Stress in Cambodian refugee families. *Image: The Journal of Nursing Scholarship, 26*(2), 101–105.

Godbey, K. L., & Courage, M. M. (1994). Stress-management program: Intervention in nursing student performance anxiety. *Archives of Psychiatric Nursing, 8*(3), 190–199.

Ryan-Wenger, N. M., & Copeland, S. G. (1994). Coping strategies used by black school-age children from low-income families. *Journal of Pediatric Nursing, 9*(1), 33–40.

Wineman, N. M., Durand, E. J., & Steiner, R. P. (1994). A comparative analysis of coping behaviors in persons with multiple sclerosis or a spinal cord injury. *Res Nurs Health, 17,* 185–194.

Possible Topics for Nursing Inquiry

- What are early indicators of ineffective coping in adolescents of single-parent families?
- What are effective coping strategies in clients who have experienced disfigurement due to surgery?
- What nursing interventions can be used to minimize ineffective coping in clients who require frequent procedures and treatment?

moving may be necessary for career reasons, moving may be disruptive and stressful, especially for families that may be fragile in some way (eg, a disabled child, health problems, disturbed adolescents). Many of these families have developed needed and useful support systems in their present community. A move in such cases may well interfere with coping strategies, preventing adaptation.

In another example, an older person may face the realization that living independently is no longer an option, but may choose to deny it. Family or other support systems may have to help the older person make the decision to move to an environment offering improved safety and more support for daily living activities. This involuntary relocation can produce overwhelming stress and altered coping for the older person (Kammer, 1994).

Another form of involuntary relocation is hospitalization. A person is not admitted to a hospital without a specific health reason, either physiologic or psychological. Depending on the problem, the person may experience a mild amount of stress or a great amount, both of which require using coping skills and patterns to manage the problem. The health problem may overwhelm the person's previous patterns of coping, leading to or adding to a dysfunctional state of stress.

Dysfunctional Families

Although families can be a great source of support, they can also be a source of distress and altered coping. Many marriages end in separation and divorce, which can be amicable or bitter. Divorce, particularly in families with dependent children, is a stressful situation that can lead to altered coping, which in turn requires new adaptation strategies. Children in particular feel the stress of the loss of a secure environment and may respond with altered coping and adaptation, either behaviorally or physically. Adolescents are particularly vulnerable to instability, which can lead to serious consequences from the resultant altered coping.

Stresses from other sources often have their outlet in the family. When individual coping strategies are inadequate, that outlet may take the form of physical abuse. The abuse of one spouse by another (usually the wife by the husband) or the abuse of a child by a parent are often the outcome. In the United States, increased public awareness of domestic abuse has led to the increased availability of service agencies and support groups.

Dysfunctional Lifestyles

Inadequate nutrition, rest, exercise, and fitness can predispose the person to fatigue, illness, and perhaps death. A person who has a lifestyle pattern of poor nutrition, insufficient rest, and irregular exercise is prone to experience altered coping and adaptation as a result of inadequate physiologic reserves. In these circumstances, the person may overreact psychologically to stress-producing situations, as in the domestic abuse described above, and the neuroendocrine response may be compromised, as well.

Dysfunctional Defense Mechanisms

Coping mechanisms may keep the person from dealing realistically with stress. Daydreams, increased sleeping, denial, or fantasies can be dysfunctional coping mechanisms when the person resorts to them rather than confronting the stress and actively problem-solving. Although defense mechanisms help the person to avoid pain, modify strong emotions, or relieve anxiety, overuse can be self-defeating and interfere with productive coping and adapting.

Sensory Deficits

Deficits or impairments in the senses can alter the person's ability to cope with and respond effectively to stress. Sensory deficits in vision and hearing interfere with the ability to interact with the environment and with other people. It becomes increasingly difficult to make judgments when under stress, to know what coping options exist, or to adapt to changes that challenge sensory–perceptual abilities. Inability to see or hear accurately can lead to misperception and the potential for altered coping.

Manifestations of Altered Coping

Altered coping may be manifested in various ways, including use of alcohol and drugs, excessive smoking, increased sleeping, overeating, avoidance and withdrawal, daydreaming and fantasizing, and illness. Table 51-2 presents additional examples of expressions of stress.

Addictive Behaviors

Alcohol has long been used as a means of altering reality and awareness. The phrase "crawling into a bottle" illustrates the attempt to withdraw from stress and problems by ingesting alcohol. In recent years, excessive use of drugs, both prescription and "street" drugs, has joined alcohol use as a way of escaping stress. The results of excessive alcohol and drug use are addiction, dependency, psychological problems, physiologic consequences, and, probably, more stress and less effective coping. Adolescents are at particular risk for substance abuse as a result of their vulnerable stage of development.

Smoking is also an addictive behavior, with nicotine being the addictive substance. People, particularly adolescents, typically begin smoking in an effort to portray a certain image (older, macho, or more sophisticated), and end up being addicted and finding it difficult to stop. When stressed, people commonly increase the amount of smoking, both to handle the stress via the nicotine and to provide a physical outlet by having something to do with their hands when they are upset. Smoking is an ineffective coping strategy for stress. Physiologic alterations, including respiratory and cardiovascular disorders, are the end result of chronic smoking.

The use of food can become addictive in much the same way as smoking, in that the person seeks the immediate pleasure of food to avoid the discomfort caused by stress. The problem of overeating has no simple cause or explanation. As with sleeping and daydreams, food offers many people a pleasurable escape from stressful situations. The behavior may work over the short term; however, over the long term, overeating leads to obesity, which has significant health consequences. People exhibiting stress and altered coping through substance abuse or overeating require a comprehensive treatment program to address their coping and adaptation problems.

Physical Illness

Prolonged stress and exposure to the effects of the neuroendocrine hormones can lead to physiologic dysfunction. Selye (1974) found that, as a result of prolonged stress, the adrenal glands enlarge, lymphatic structures (thymus, spleen, and lymph nodes) atrophy (shrink), and the stomach develops deep ulcerations. These effects indicate an overstimulation of the adrenals, a decline in immune system function, and an increased risk for cell and tissue damage. Although controversy continues over the exact relationship of stress to illness, evidence exists that a person can mediate his or her heart rate and blood pressure through effective

Table 51-2 • *Psychosocial and Physiologic Expressions of Stress*

Psychosocial Expressions		*Physiologic Expressions*
Behaviors	*Emotions*	
Crying	Anger, anxiety	Back, neck, or shoulder pain
Decreased motivation	Nervousness	Breathing irregularities
Decreased self-esteem	Moodiness, depression	Elevated blood pressure
Decreased intellectual processes	Emotional instability	Change in appetite
Forgetfulness	Irritability	Stuttering, trembling
Impulsive behavior	Fears, phobias	Jaw tension
Inability to make decisions	Feeling out of control	Sexual dysfunction
Learning disabilities	Frustration	Constipation or diarrhea
Poor concentration	Feelings of worthlessness	Irregular heartbeat
		Muscle cramps, spasms
		Stomach, digestive disorders
		Sweating, skin problems
		Tension headaches
		Insomnia or fatigue

application of coping strategies. Increased blood pressure and heart rate are manifestations of the effect of the adrenal hormones.

Anxiety and Depression

Stress can cause anxiety, a subjective reaction to a real or imagined threat. The sense of uneasiness or dread may range from mild to severe, and may be manifested by lack of sleep, poor nutrition, excessive caffeine intake or smoking, or physical illness.

The extreme response to prolonged stress may be depression and suicide. People with poor coping mechanisms or inadequate support may see suicide as a desirable way to end stress and depression. Because of the inherent instability of the teenage years, adolescents who are experiencing various kinds of stress have a higher rate of suicide than the general population.

Violent Behavior

People with poor impulse control or with inadequate coping mechanisms may respond to stress through acting out in violent or abusive ways. For example, a man who has a stressful situation at work may come home and behave violently with his wife or children as an outlet for the stress. Wife battering and child abuse are common violent behaviors related to altered coping.

Impact of Coping Dysfunction on Activities of Daily Living

Individual Considerations

Manifestations of stress and altered coping can interfere with the person's activities of daily living (ADLs). The use of addictive substances, such as alcohol, drugs, and nicotine, to handle stress ultimately leads to more problems, not only with stress management, but with the simple activities that are a part of daily living. The outcomes of alcohol and drug use contribute to cognitive impairments, making personal hygiene and school and work performance difficult. Smoking and other substance use diverts income to support those activities instead of the needs of the person or household.

Family Considerations

As stress becomes prolonged or overwhelming, it can dominate the awareness of the person, or the person may try to withdraw from it. In either event, routine activities, such as home maintenance, food preparation, cleaning, and personal hygiene and grooming, may become less important. If that occurs, stress may actually increase as a result both of the changes in ADLs and of the further compromise of the person's reserves, thus creating additional stress for the family members.

Stress may interfere with individual employment and family finances if it prevents optimal performance in school or work or the attempt to secure a position. Although some stress may heighten performance, excessive stress may severely impair it, adversely affecting the person and, ultimately, the family.

Assessment

Many clients with health problems are faced with many stressors and have varying ways of coping with them. It is important that the nurse have an understanding of the methods or strategies used by the client so that nursing care can be individualized appropriately.

Subjective Data

The focused functional assessment of coping and adaptation includes obtaining subjective data from the client through a series of purposeful questions and interviews, and through observation and mental notation of the client's nonverbal communication, such as body position, facial expressions, gestures, and voice and speech. Examples of these interview questions are given in the accompanying display. The nursing history is one of the earliest sources of these data, and in continued interactions, the nurse becomes increasingly focused in the specific considerations for that particular client.

Subjective data assist the nurse in identifying the client's functional coping and adaptation patterns and strategies, determining factors that place the client at additional risk for ineffective coping, and perceiving any actual dysfunction that may be present.

Functional Pattern Identification

To assess the client's coping and adaptation pattern, the nurse needs to obtain information from the client, family members or significant others, and healthcare providers. Because the client may have many stressors with which to cope or adapt, it is helpful to determine the source of stress, whether physiologic, psychological, environmental, or sociocultural (Fuller & Schaller-Ayers, 1994).

Physiologic Stress. Because physiologic stress produces a physiologic response, the nurse needs to ask about these responses, particularly fatigue, adequacy of sleep, appetite, bowel elimination patterns, and level of physical activity. Assessment of physical responses to stress is discussed more fully in the section on Objective Data. Changes in normal patterns of these or other physiologic activities may be an expression of ineffective coping.

Psychological Stress. Psychological stress is generated from the person's thoughts and feelings about spe-

Nursing Assessment
Interview Guide: Stress and Stress Responses

Stressors

Major changes/losses in the past year ____________________
Situations that cause stress: At the present time ____________________
In the past ____________________

Perception of Stressors/Stress

What does this problem/stressor/loss mean to you? ____________________
Have stressful situations been good or bad for you? ____________________
How have stressful situations affected you? (physically and emotionally) ____________________

Coping Strategies

How do you relieve tension and deal with stress? ____________________

Talk to others _____	Try to solve the problem _____	Blame someone else for the problem _____
Try to forget _____	Try to relieve tension with alcohol _____ drugs _____ overeating _____	Seek help _____
Do something to get mind off problems _____	Go to sleep _____	Other (describe) _____
Pray _____	Accept the situation _____	_____
Do nothing _____		_____

Is there someone you rely on to help you solve problems? ____________________
Is there something the nurse can do to make hospitalization (clinic visits, home visits, etc.) less stressful?

Resolution of Stress

Do you usually solve your problems? ____________________
Do the methods you just described for relieving tension usually help? ____________________

From Fuller, J., & Schaller-Ayers, J. (1994). *Health assessment: A nursing approach,* (2nd ed.). Philadelphia: J. B. Lippincott.

cific events or perceptions of events. For a person facing a health problem or hospitalization, stresses may relate to loss of personal control or a sense of powerlessness over the situation. The client may exhibit behavioral responses such as denial, ambivalence, suspicion, hostility, regression, depression, or withdrawal. Asking the client to express his or her concerns, identify problems, and describe feelings experienced with specific problems is a beginning approach to obtaining information for both the client and the nurse. In helping the client to clarify stressful feelings and problems, the nurse enlists the client's participation in establishing a basis for purposeful nursing interventions.

Environmental Stress. Environmental stress may be related to relocation or unfamiliarity with the setting. The change in surroundings, with new sounds, smells, and sights may produce stress for a client. In a hospital or long-term care facility, there is also a loss of privacy, change in daily activities, and change in the level of sensory stimulation (either more or less). The nurse should ask questions that elicit the client's response to the environment, define sources of stress for the client, and disclose areas that both the nurse and the client think may be amenable to mutual planning.

Sociocultural Stress. Sociocultural stress may be related to family, financial, career, and spiritual concerns. The nurse needs to elicit information about specific concerns the client may have about the care of the family during hospitalization; whether his or her job or career will be affected; what kind of financial support is available from job, insurance, or spouse; and how the current situation affects spiritual beliefs and values. This information alerts the nurse to the type of planning and collaboration that may be necessary for this client.

Risk Identification

The nursing history includes collected information identifying factors that place the client at risk for ineffective coping and adaptation. Risk assessment areas include transition factors, such as moving and relocation, situations involving separation (eg, divorce, child custody, prison, and hospitalization), and lifestyle factors, such as fatigue, malnutrition, and illness.

Many of the factors that place a client at risk for ineffective coping may actually be positive factors in relation to long-term outcomes, but that does not eliminate the possibility that ineffective coping may occur in the short term. For example, a woman leaving an abusive marriage may have very positive outcomes as an end result, but she may be at risk for ineffective coping during the transitional period when she is adapting to her new situation and reestablishing herself, and perhaps her children, in a new life.

Some risk factors are directly related to the reason for a client's health problem. If a client has a history of an eating disorder, such as anorexia or bulimia, the resulting malnutrition may predispose the client to related health problems. In caring for the client, the nurse needs to identify specific risk situations that may be present for the client.

Dysfunction Identification

To determine whether the client has a coping dysfunction, it is necessary to assess the client's beliefs about normal levels of stress and usual coping behaviors or strategies. Some people have a high tolerance for stress and are so accustomed to living with an elevated level of stress that what may be identified as extremely stressful by another person is considered as rather ordinary. In addition, correspondingly wide variations in coping behaviors and strategies are exhibited by different people. To gain the most accurate understanding, the nurse should avoid inserting his or her bias and personal coping expectations into the assessment and stay open to learning how the client identifies the situation.

Dysfunctional patterns can be identified as significant differences from the client's normal behavior for coping with stress and as coping and adaptation patterns that are outside the range of normal for a particular client. For example, the person who usually handles job stress by doing hard physical activity in a gym but who now reports that his or her response to job stress has become fatigue and excessive sleep, has identified a dysfunctional coping pattern.

Objective Data

Physical Assessment

With activation of the autonomic nervous system and the endocrine system, physiologic responses may occur and be observed in the physical assessment. Because there may be many other reasons for some of the responses, the nurse must be careful not to assume that the cause of some physical findings is stress alone, when there may be other contributory causes.

Cardiovascular System. The cardiovascular system is the target system for the effects of epinephrine and norepinephrine, which include increased heart rate, vasoconstriction of peripheral organs, and increased oxygen consumption by the heart. The manifestations of prolonged stimulation by these hormones may include

- An increase in the resting heart rate related to direct stimulation of the myocardium; the client may describe a "pounding in the chest" or palpitations
- An increase in systolic blood pressure related to peripheral vasoconstriction
- Arrhythmias related to ischemia (tissue oxygen deprivation in the face of increased energy demand), noted in an irregular heartbeat or in rhythm changes
- Angina, or chest pain, and ischemia-related changes in the electrocardiogram
- Migraine headaches related to vasoconstriction.

Respiratory System. The respiratory system is affected by norepinephrine, which leads to an increased breathing rate and to bronchiolar dilation. Hyperventilation accompanied by a feeling of "air hunger," dizziness, and tingling in the hands and feet are usually the most common physical manifestations.

Gastrointestinal System. The gastrointestinal system is a common target system in stressful situations. Whereas nervous system activity usually slows motility, people experiencing stress often report loss of appetite, nausea, vomiting, and increased peristaltic activity. Increased peristalsis is manifested by increased bowel sounds, increased secretion of hydrochloric acid in the stomach, and increased number of bowel movements. The increase in hydrochloric acid may also contribute to the nausea and vomiting, and, in combination with cortisol, to gastrointestinal ulcer formation.

Musculoskeletal System. The musculoskeletal system responds to stress by exhibiting increased tenseness in the larger muscles, and shakiness and tremor in smaller muscles. The muscle tenseness is related to the GAS—the "fight-or-flight" response preparing the body to protect itself. Prolonged tenseness can lead to muscle spasm, particularly in the back.

Integumentary System. The skin, or integumentary system, manifests the peripheral effects of norepinephrine and epinephrine by being diaphoretic (moist) and cool, and by exhibiting smooth muscle tenseness ("making the hairs stand on end").

Diagnostic Tests and Procedures

No simple laboratory tests can determine the amount of stress. However, stress-related hormones (epinephrine, norepinephrine, and cortisol) can be detected

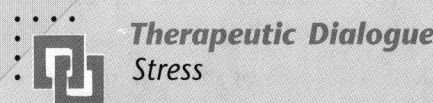

Therapeutic Dialogue
Stress

Scenes for Thought

Kathleen O'Brien, an RN and one of the staff on the clinic team, is sitting in the staff break room alone one morning, looking sad and preoccupied. Jean enters, looking for a cup of coffee and a little break from the hectic morning.

Effective

J: *Hi, Kathleen, how are you doing?*
K: *Okay, I guess.* No eye contact. Looking at the floor.
J: *(Sitting down next to her.) You don't seem okay. Anything wrong?*
K: Giving an embarrassed smile. *I just don't seem to have my usual energy, that's all.*
J: *I noticed you've seemed a little tired. What do you think is going on?*
K: *Just stressed out, I guess.* Looks down again.
J: *You mean more stressed than usual? Are the kids and George okay?*
K: *Yes, thank goodness.*
J: *How about school? Are you still taking two courses at night?*
K: *Yes. I'm doing alright.*
J: *(Silence)*
K: Taking a deep breath. *I guess the only thing that's changed is my brother Tom. He was diagnosed with a malignant brain tumor last week. And the cancer is already in his bowel and liver.* Tears in her eyes. *And I feel so helpless. My other brothers are looking to me to help them and Tom and his family to handle the shock and the sorrow, and I guess I'm feeling a little overwhelmed.*
J: *I guess so! Who's supporting you? (Putting her hand on Kathleen's.)*
K: *George has been wonderful and helps all he can.* Squeezes Jean's hand and sighs. *It's a matter of finding enough time to keep up my schoolwork and talk on the phone to all the people calling about Tom. And I haven't been for a run in weeks.* Sighs again.
J: *Is there anything I can do to help?*
K: *No, but thanks. Just talking about it to someone who'll listen is comforting.*
J: *Let me know if you need a change in your schedule for anything, including a chance to exercise. And come talk to me anytime. (Puts an arm around her shoulder.)*
K: *Thanks. I appreciate that.*

Less Effective

J: *Hi, Kathleen, how are you doing?*
K: *Okay, I guess.* No eye contact. Looking at the floor.
J: *(Sitting down next to her.) You don't seem okay. Anything wrong?*
K: Giving an embarrassed smile. *I just don't seem to have my usual energy, that's all.*
J: *I've noticed. It's been pretty hectic around here lately and we're all tired out, including me! Are you getting enough rest with your busy schedule? (Concerned tone of voice.)*
K: *Not really. Finals are coming up at school, and I've been working on those.* No eye contact.
J: *Well, if there's anything I can do to help, let me know. I've got to get back to my meeting. See you later.*
K: *Okay. Thanks.* Gets up and walks back to her desk to prepare for her next client.

Critical Thinking Challenges

• Examine psychosocial expressions of stress Kathleen exhibited. • Suggest what you think prevented her from being able to cope with all the stressors at this time. • List who and what her resources are, and give reasons. • Determine whether the second nurse responded to her own stressors. • Propose what you would do to reduce your stress level if you were Kathleen.

through laboratory tests, and from their existence a stress state can be inferred. Objective data about the client's coping and adaptation are gathered by means of structured interviews and coping and stress assessment tools. These types of laboratory tests are evaluated with other data related to measuring stress. These tools attempt to identify and quantify stressors and coping patterns, as described in the section on Subjective Data. Formal assessment tools include instruments such as the SRRS (Holmes & Rahe, 1967); Everyday Hassles Scale (Lazarus, 1981); Interview Guide: Stress and Stress Responses (Fuller & Schaller-Ayers, 1994); and the Stress Audit (Miller, et al., 1991). These assessment tools are discussed throughout this chapter. Using these instruments helps identify behaviors and feelings that may relate to the amount of stress and the corresponding vulnerability to illness and dysfunction. The scales, which turn subjective factors into objective numbers, may be used by the nurse in some situations, or they may be used by a psychosocial clinical nurse specialist, a consultant, or a psychologist. The interview guide can be employed usefully by all nurses.

Nursing Diagnoses

Several categories of diagnoses related to coping and adaptation are currently approved as nursing diagnoses. These diagnoses include Impaired Adjustment; Defensive Coping; Ineffective Denial; Ineffective Family Coping: Disabling; Ineffective Family Coping: Compromised; Family Coping: Potential for Growth; Potential for Enhanced Community Coping; Ineffective Community Coping; Relocation Stress Syndrome; Post-Trauma

Response; and Risk for Violence: Self-Directed or Directed at Others. One diagnosis is presented in this text: Ineffective Individual Coping.

Diagnostic Statement: Ineffective Individual Coping

Definition

Ineffective Individual Coping is the impairment of adaptive behaviors and problem-solving abilities of a person in meeting life's demands and roles (North American Nursing Diagnosis Association [NANDA], 1994).

Defining Characteristics

Defining characteristics include verbalization of inability to cope or inability to ask for help (critical); inability to meet role expectations; inability to meet basic needs; inability to problem-solve (critical); alteration in societal participation; destructive behavior toward self or others; inappropriate use of defense mechanisms; change in usual communication patterns; verbal manipulation; high illness rate; and high rate of accidents (NANDA, 1994).

Related Factors

Related factors are situational crises, maturational crises, and vulnerability (NANDA, 1994).

Related Nursing Diagnoses

In addition to the previously mentioned nursing diagnoses related to Ineffective Individual Coping, Dysfunctional Grieving and Post-Trauma Response may also be related to ineffective coping. When a person moves beyond normal grieving (see Chapter 50), continued inability to cope with a loss leads to dysfunctional grieving in connection with ineffective coping. A trauma victim has been exposed to extraordinary stress or to repeated stresses, usually with threats to personal safety; in the period after the trauma, the person may reexperience the traumatic event, resulting in manifestations of ineffective coping.

Outcome Identification and Planning

After nursing diagnoses and related factors have been established, the client and nurse work together to identify goals and interventions. Goals for the client with ineffective individual coping need to be individualized, taking into consideration the client's history, areas of risk, evidence of dysfunction, and related objective data. Examples of client goals include

The client will identify sources of stress in his or her life.
The client will identify usual personal coping strategies for stressful situations.
The client will define the effect of stress and coping strategies on ADLs.

For the client who has related nursing diagnoses and more complex problems with stress, coping, and adaptation, the goals need to be adjusted accordingly, along with the time frame in which they can be realized. Examples of some of the interventions that can be used in planning are listed in the accompanying display and discussed in the following section.

Implementation

The nurse can intervene independently or collaboratively to help restore function. The nurse can assist the client in recognizing signs and symptoms of stress, identifying the sources of distress, and choosing an appropriate and safe course of action. The client may be unable to recognize that muscle tension, or feelings such

Planning

Examples of Nursing Interventions Used for Common Stress Problems

Ineffective Individual Coping

- Identify the client's coping mechanisms that are ineffective.
- Encourage discussion of behaviors that are counterproductive to coping.
- Explore the effects that ineffective coping have on the client's health.
- Reinforce decisions and efforts to alter coping mechanisms.

Stress Management

- Identify factors that relate to or precipitate increased stress in the client.
- Explore with the client positive and negative behaviors for managing stress.
- Discuss alternative strategies for stress management, such as exercise, music, reading, relaxation, or imagery.
- Reinforce behaviors that produce positive stress management.
- Refer to resources or groups that can assist the client in stress management decisions.

as depression and anxiety, are related to stress. Because the stress response is highly complex and individual, the management of that response must also be individualized. Similarly, stress management techniques that are effective for one person may not be helpful for another. The nurse can assist the client in finding the techniques that are most effective.

The nurse also has a significant role in identifying people at risk for ineffective coping and initiating appropriate teaching to promote optimal health.

Nursing Interventions to Promote Health and Function

Helping the client recognize and manage stress is an important aspect of health maintenance and disease prevention. Learning to adapt to stress requires self-appraisal and recognition of one's own manifestations of stress; this is true for nurses as well as clients.

Stressor Reduction

The nurse needs to be sensitive to client responses that assist the nurse in recognizing stress, its source, and its meaning to the client. By clarifying these parameters, the nurse and the client are formulating an approach either to reducing the stressor or removing it entirely. Through health education, which leads to learning the cause of stress, the client can develop strategies for coping and adapting. The person is continually appraising his or her symptoms, with respect to their significance for well-being and survival, and coping accordingly (Lazarus, 1994).

For example, the working mother who is tired from putting in overtime and does not have enough time to spend with her family may find herself feeling angry, excessively fatigued, and short-tempered with her children. She may be helped to realize that the mood changes she is experiencing are stress induced, and that coping strategies may include changing jobs to accommodate better her family's needs as well as her own, asking her spouse for help, or hiring part-time help.

Addressing Perfection

Faulty perceptions in one's belief system can contribute to the stress response. Often, perfectionistic "shoulds, oughts, and musts" only enhance the person's response to stress. An example is the person who tells himself or herself: "I must never make a mistake" or "I should always clean the house before going to work." Helping the client realize that a desire for perfection or unrealistic self-expectations are stress inducing is an important nursing intervention. Being realistic about self-expectations and remembering that relationships

---

Nursing Care Guidelines

Stress Management for Nurses

Nursing practice often involves working in a stressful environment, caring for clients in noisy or overcrowded spaces, visiting homes or situations that are depressing, adjusting to various work shifts, and being understaffed. Nursing literature describes two conditions that commonly affect nurses: burnout and tedium.

Burnout results from working with people who are demanding and needy, which often produces conflict within the nurse and leads to depleted energy and low morale. *Tedium* results from environmental factors that create conflicts or place demands on the nurse. Burnout and tedium are often characterized by physical and emotional depletion, negative self-concept, negative attitudes, and feelings of helplessness and hopelessness.

Nurses must be aware of their own stress levels. The nurse must first recognize his or her personal stress and its manifestations. Recognizing that increased fatigue, anger, disorganization, or other behavior changes may be related to an increased level of stress is one step. Noting changes in lifestyle factors, such as smoking, eating behaviors, or alcohol or other substance use, may provide further evidence of personal stress.

Once the nurse can recognize the ways in which he or she responds to stress, the nurse can then attend to the times when stress is most pronounced and to the situations that stimulate a stress response. Once this is done, the nurse can take positive action to prevent, manage, and alleviate stress so that effective coping strategies can be instituted.

Suggestions for Stress Management

- Get out of bed 15 minutes earlier to have more time to prepare for the day.
- Establish a regular program of exercise and activity to focus energy expenditure.
- Eliminate or restrict the amount of alcohol, caffeine, and other mood-altering substances as a means of managing stress.
- Learn to accept failure, your own and others, and turn it into a constructive experience.
- Develop techniques for assertiveness to have more feelings of personal control.
- Develop support systems among colleagues and friends to bolster personal resources.
- Have an optimistic view of the world, believing that most people are doing the best they can.

are more important than things or tasks can help reduce stress.

Supportive Internal Messages

The internal dialogue whereby a person describes and interprets the world is referred to as self-talk, or internal messages. Internal messages have a definite impact on one's daily functioning and self-concept. A constant stream of negative self-messages can lead to generalized feelings of inferiority and self-doubt. Instead of being defeated by negative internal messages, one can learn to control them by substituting supportive messages to help cope with difficult situations. Changing internal messages involves these three steps:

- Identifying what one says when the situation occurs (self-talk).
- Evaluating how rational or irrational these messages are.
- Replacing the negative messages with supportive coping statements and integrating them into daily life (Nakagawa-Kogan, 1994; Nakagawa-Kogan, et al., 1979).

For example, a person interviews for a job but is not hired. Instead of saying, "I blew it, I'm a failure; I'll never get the job I want," the person learns to restructure negative thoughts into supportive self-statements such as, "I feel disappointed that I didn't get this job. I know I presented myself well. I have the ability to get the job I want." The nurse can encourage the client to examine internal messages and practice rephrasing those that are negative or irrational.

Another behavioral strategy useful for gaining control over self-defeating thoughts is called "thought stopping." Thought stopping can be accomplished by using the following technique:

- Say "stop," inwardly or out loud, when a negative or self-defeating thought crosses the mind (eg, "I'll never be able to find a job").
- Substitute a positive, assertive statement for the negative thought (eg, "I have the skills needed to get the job I want").
- If using the word "stop" is ineffective, place a rubber band around the wrist and snap it whenever negative, unwanted thoughts occur.

Assertiveness

Another useful technique for changing one's behavior in response to a stressful encounter is assertiveness. Assertive behavior enables the person to act in his or her own best interests, to stand up for himself or herself, to express his or her feelings openly and honestly, and to exercise his or her rights without infringing on the rights of others. Assertiveness is a learned behavioral skill that requires practice. A nurse who recognizes a person who has difficulty expressing feelings or getting his or her needs met might suggest that this person enroll in a class or workshop in assertiveness training.

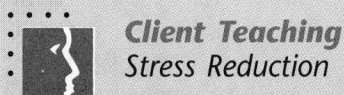

> **Client Teaching**
> *Stress Reduction*
>
> *Instruct the client as follows:*
> - *Exercise to release tension in muscles.*
> - *Get adequate sleep and rest to reenergize the body.*
> - *Eat a balanced diet to give energy for body and mind.*
> - *Manage time appropriately to increase sense of control and organization.*
> - *Be assertive to increase self-esteem and personal control.*
> - *Learn relaxation techniques (breathing, progressive relaxation, or visualization) to release tension and quiet the mind.*
> - *Do something for others to get your mind off yourself and boost your self-esteem.*
> - *Laugh to release tension and relax mind and body.*
> - *When you are experiencing an unusual amount of stress, take extra precaution while operating motor vehicles because you may be easily distracted.*
> - *Be aware of alcohol intake and the amount of smoking because it may be easy to overdo them as a result of stress.*
> - *If eating is a coping mechanism, keep a journal of food intake so that when you are experiencing stress, any extra food consumption will be easily recognized.*
> - *If specialized types of stress reduction and coping strategies are to be used, be sure that you learn them from expert clinicians.*

Lifestyle Changes

Adequate rest and nutrition are important components of a person's personal resources in managing stress and effective coping. Everyone is more capable of handling the stressful events of daily life if the body is not fatigued or malnourished. Encouraging the client to get adequate sleep and nutrition, to limit or eliminate smoking, to cut down on coffee consumption, and avoid depending on "pill-popping" (such as aspirin or tranquilizers) will promote healthier management of stress.

Exercise

A technique that helps counter the effects of the stress response is physical activity or exercise. Vigorous physical exertion helps to release tension from the muscles and is a natural outlet when the body is in a fight-or-flight state of arousal. Of the broad categories of exercise, two are aerobic exercise and low-intensity exer-

Health Benefits of Exercise

- Improves muscular strength, endurance, and flexibility
- Improves cardiovascular efficiency
- Lowers resting heart rate
- Reduces blood cholesterol levels
- Reduces general anxiety and depression
- Reduces chronic fatigue and insomnia
- Lowers body weight by burning calories and suppressing appetite
- Increases absorption and use of food
- Improves appearance and self-image

cise. Aerobic exercise involves sustained activity of the large muscle groups and places an increased demand on the cardiopulmonary system. Examples of aerobic exercise include running, bicycling, swimming, cross-country skiing, brisk walking, and rowing.

Low-intensity exercise is not vigorous and provides little benefit to the cardiovascular system. However, it can increase muscle strength and flexibility and prepare the sedentary person for more vigorous aerobic exercise. Examples include calisthenics, slow walking, gardening, and housecleaning.

A regular program of exercise is an important component of health. For the client, exercise may take the form of active or passive range of motion, either encouraged or performed by the nurse. Examples of benefits of exercise are shown in the accompanying display.

Relaxation Techniques

Another method of decreasing physiologic arousal is through relaxation techniques. The physiologic reactions of the GAS, described earlier in this chapter, activate all body systems. During this state, muscle tension and heightened awareness begin to compete with a state of relaxation. The body has the ability to elicit the "relaxation response," which is in direct opposition to the responses of the GAS. The relaxation response was first described by the Harvard researcher, Dr. Herbert Benson (1976). He discovered that meditation brought about an integrated set of physiologic changes, in opposition to the fight-or-flight response, including lowered oxygen consumption, heart rate, respirations, and blood lactate.

Several techniques have been shown to elicit the relaxation response, including deep breathing, progressive relaxation, autogenics, visualization, meditation, yoga, and biofeedback. Some selected advanced stress management techniques are presented in Table 51-3.

Deep Breathing. Breathing is an important element of the relaxation response. As stress and tension mount during the day, breathing becomes shallow and irregular, and the heart rate accelerates. Poorly oxygenated blood contributes to lethargy, tension, and depression. When a person is relaxed, breathing slows and deepens, and the heart rate returns to normal. Because breathing is the easiest physiologic system to control, a person can use slow, deep breathing to trigger the relaxation response. In fact, many relaxation techniques begin by having the person slowly inhale and exhale for a few minutes.

As an incentive to practice deep breathing, a person might associate it with something commonly done during the day, such as answering the phone or looking at the clock. Frequently, the act of taking a few deep breaths before a stressful situation can decrease fear and anxiety, allowing for a more relaxed frame of mind.

Progressive Relaxation. Progressive relaxation consists of systematically tensing and relaxing various muscle groups in the body, moving from head to toe. Many people do not realize that their muscles are in a state of chronic tension. Progressive relaxation provides a method of identifying particular muscle groups and distinguishing between sensations of tension and tranquility. The steps involved in doing progressive muscle relaxation are shown in the display on Progressive Muscle Relaxation Technique.

There are other specialized forms of relaxation techniques that require training, expertise, and supervised practice for the nurse to be skillful in using them with clients.

Nursing Interventions for Altered Function

Many of the techniques that promote healthy coping function can also be used for situations of altered function. An advantage of using techniques for controlling stress and promoting effective coping when one is well is that the person then has the skill to use these techniques when altered function exists.

Relaxation Training

The nurse may encounter many stressful situations, not only in institutional but in home and community settings, in which it is appropriate to teach, or to remind the client to use, relaxation techniques. Such situations include

- Before and after diagnostic tests or treatments
- During childbirth
- After surgery to help manage postoperative pain
- During recovery from a myocardial infarction
- While calming an anxious or agitated person
- Before a painful procedure, such as an intramuscular injection or inserting an intravenous line

It is becoming a common practice in institutional and community settings to have relaxation tapes avail-

Table 51-3* • *Selected Advanced Stress Management and Relaxation Techniques

Autogenic training	A systematic technique teaching the body and mind to respond to verbal commands, allowing the person to achieve a deep state of relaxation through self-suggestion (or self-hypnosis).
Visualization and imagery	An attempt to affect an unconscious process by using a conscious suggestion, or a mental picture of the desired change.
Affirmations	Strong, positive, feeling-rich statements about a desired change to reinforce and increase the effectiveness of visualization; can be done silently, aloud, in writing, or chanted. For example, a person with a strong sense of time urgency might use this affirmation: "I am relaxed and centered. I have plenty of time for everything."
Meditation	A traditional Eastern religious technique to achieve mental and physical relaxation. Four elements include a quiet place; a comfortable position; an object to dwell on, such as a word or symbol; and a passive attitude.
Biofeedback	A specialized relaxation technique in which the person learns to monitor physiologic processes, feed back a measure of that function, and exert control over autonomic functions. Information, such as heart rate, muscle tension, and finger temperature, is translated into an auditory or visual signal that the person senses, and through these signals the person learns to discriminate between tension and relaxation.
Therapeutic touch	The use of touch to reduce anxiety and stress, relieve pain, and provide comfort.
Massage	The manipulation of soft issue, generally with the hands, to provide stimulation and relaxation and to reduce stress and anxiety.
Yoga	A form of exercise (usually combined with meditation) to foster relaxation, mental alacrity, and good health.

able for clients' use. Relaxation tapes may be purchased, or the client may want to make his or her own personal recording. Taking a few deep breaths before a procedure can decrease the client's anxiety. For example, before a painful procedure or intramuscular injection, ask the client to take two or three slow, deep breaths. Usually clients will experience less discomfort if they are relaxed and calm, both physically and emotionally.

Environmental Modifications

The nurse needs to be aware of stressors in the environment and make changes and adjustments whenever possible to reduce sensory overload and to assist the client with coping and adaptation. For the hospitalized client, the environment, which affords little privacy and is unfamiliar, may be the source of the stress. Increased noise levels, constant lights, and unfamiliar procedures all contribute to stress.

The nurse may be instrumental in making modifications in the environment that assist the client in managing the stress of the situation and in coping with the environment. Organizing nursing care to decrease disturbance to the client, having as few extra lights on as possible, and keeping down the conversational noise in the hallways are a few examples. In the home, encouraging the family to create a room or space in which the client can control the noise level and stimuli may be helpful (Tyler and Ellison, 1994).

Crisis Intervention

An acute health problem, illness, loss, or trauma may precipitate a crisis in a person's life. A crisis suggests a situation in which usual coping strategies are ineffective, and the person is disorganized or unable to problem-solve appropriately. To resolve a crisis, the client needs assistance from family, friends, clergy, and health-

Progressive Muscle Relaxation Technique

Progressive relaxation is a self-taught or instructed exercise that involves learning to constrict and relax muscle groups in a systematic way, beginning with the face and finishing with the feet. This exercise may be combined with breathing exercises that focus on inner body processes. It usually takes 15 to 30 minutes and may be accompanied by a taped instruction that directs the person concerning the sequence of muscles to be relaxed.

1. Wear loose clothing; remove glasses and shoes.
2. Sit or recline in a comfortable position with neck and knees supported; avoid lying completely flat.
3. Begin with slow, rhythmic breathing.
   a. Close your eyes or stare at a spot and take in a slow deep breath.
   b. Exhale the breath slowly.
4. Continue rhythmic breathing at a slow, steady pace and feel the tension leaving your body with each breath.
5. Begin progressive relaxation of muscle groups.
   a. Breathe in and tense (tighten) your muscles, and then relax the muscles as you breathe out.
   b. Suggested order for tension–relaxation cycle (with tension technique in parentheses).
      Face, jaw, mouth (squint eyes, wrinkle brow)
      Neck (pull chin to neck)
      Right hand (make a fist)
      Right arm (bend elbow in tightly)
      Left hand (make a fist)
      Left arm (bend elbow in tightly)
      Back, shoulders, chest (shrug shoulders up tightly)
      Abdomen (pull stomach in and bear down on chair)
      Right upper leg (push leg down)
      Right lower leg and foot (point toes toward body)
      Left upper leg (push leg down)
      Left lower leg and foot (point toes toward body)
6. Practice technique slowly.
7. End relaxation session when you are ready by counting to three, inhaling deeply, and saying, "I am relaxed."

From Carpenito, L. J. (1995). *Nursing diagnosis: Applications to clinical practice* (6th ed.). Philadelphia: J. B. Lippincott.

care providers, including nurses. Adequate support during the crisis and its resolution can help the client realistically perceive the problem or stress and relearn or reinstitute coping strategies.

Community-Based Nursing

A person who is convalescing from a stress-producing situation is increasingly vulnerable to other stresses and to ineffective coping. It is at this time that continued support for coping and adaptation are particularly important (Fig. 51-4). Support groups can be effective at this time. These groups can be informal, such as family, friends, and spiritual sources, or they can be formal, for example, the Alzheimer's Disease and Related Disorders Association, which is composed of people who have family members with Alzheimer's disease, a progressive senile dementia. A group such as this can be particularly helpful for someone experiencing the stress associated with caring for a person with that diagnosis, and can offer many useful ideas for coping strategies and effective adaptation.

There are many support groups that offer that type of assistance for many specialized problems and needs. It is useful for the nurse to be aware of these groups and to develop networks with other healthcare professionals to link clients with them appropriately.

Evaluation

Specific outcome criteria are the evaluative tools for measuring the attainment of client goals. Nursing interventions are the means for achieving the goals. Examples of the outcome criteria are listed in the following. Outcome criteria need to be specifically tailored to the individual client so that the criteria will uniquely measure the attainment of client's goals.

Nursing Plan of Care
The Client With Ineffective Individual Coping

Nursing Diagnosis
Ineffective Individual Coping related to situational crises manifested by inability to manage stressors.

Client Goal
Client will identify cause of current problems and usual personal coping strategies for stressful situations.

Client Outcome Criteria
- Client verbalizes feelings related to present emotional state within 24 to 48 hours.
- Client identifies recent stressful life events or sources of stress during first week.
- Client identifies signs and symptoms of current stress.
- Within one week, client identifies current coping patterns and consequences of such behavior.

Nursing Intervention	Scientific Rationale
1. Assess causative and contributive factors by discussing with client (ie, loss, grieving, inadequate support, recent life changes).	1. Assessment of causative factors provides the nurse with information on which to develop a treatment plan.
2. Assess the person's present coping status: Determine onset of symptoms and correlation with recent life changes Assess for risk of self-harm.	2. Identification of current coping skills helps the nurse to assess adequacy/inadequacy of coping.
3. Encourage the client to evaluate the effectiveness of current coping skills.	3. Personal understanding of coping skills and outcomes reinforces use of acceptable coping or encourages the client to look for alternatives in coping.

Client Goal
Client will demonstrate appropriate coping strategies.

Client Outcome Criteria
- Client makes environmental changes to reduce stress within 1 to 3 months.
- Client practices several new coping skills (ie, relaxation techniques, assertiveness, exercise, talking about feelings, thought stopping, affirmations).
- Client assesses effectiveness of social support network and, if inadequate, take steps to correct lack of support within 1 to 3 months.

Nursing Intervention	Scientific Rationale
1. Assist client to problem solve in a constructive manner.	1. Development of healthy coping strategies helps to eliminate or reduce stress and decrease possibility of chronic illness.
2. Help client identify problems in environment that are stressful. Discuss how to change them, if this is possible.	2. Client may need help in knowing how to make necessary changes.
3. When there are problems the client cannot control directly, help him or her identify stress-reducing techniques that can be used.	3. In addition to identifying techniques, the client needs to understand them and learn proper skills for their usefulness.
4. Assist client in identifying social support network. Encourage client to develop this support if it is helpful Assist client in finding support groups to meet his or her needs.	4. People need external as well as internal resources for coping.

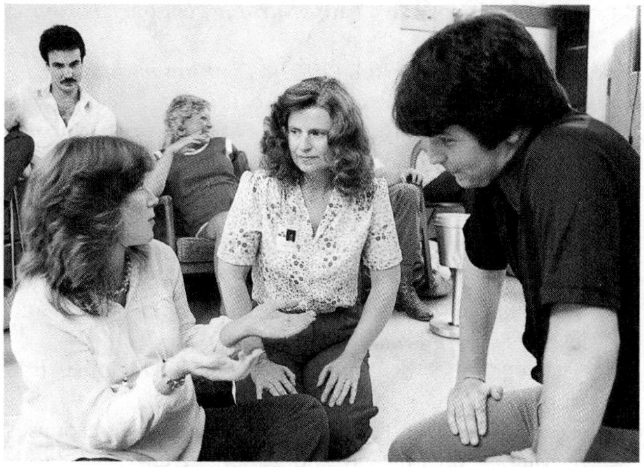

Figure 51-4 • Support groups provide opportunities to explore or make lifestyle changes.

Goal

The client will identify sources of stress in his or her life.

Possible Outcome Criteria

- The client defines events that create personal stress by listing them before next meeting with the nurse.
- The client demonstrates anticipation of stressful situations by discussing them with the nurse before they occur.
- The client identifies the difference between positive and negative sources of stress in the next discussion with the nurse.

Goal

The client will identify usual personal coping strategies for stressful situations.

Possible Outcome Criteria

- The client names at least 10 personal coping patterns.
- The client describes techniques used to reinforce previous responses or to establish new responses in the next teaching session with the nurse.
- The client consciously initiates effective stress-management techniques during a stressful period, as observed by the nurse.

Goal

The client will define the effect of stress and coping strategies on ADLs.

Possible Outcome Criteria

- The client identifies specific ADLs affected by stress by describing them to the nurse at the first home visit.
- The client describes how specific coping strategies interfere with or promote ADLs after the next teaching session with the nurse.
- The client demonstrates new coping skills effective in managing stress and assisting ADLs to the visiting nurse at the next home visit.

Evaluation includes assessing the client and comparing the client's current progress with the individually established outcome criteria as a measure of the client's goal attainment. The nursing care plan is continued, modified, or concluded based on this systematic evaluation of the individual client.

Key Concepts

- Stress, an inherent part of life, may have positive or negative effects.
- Coping with stress successfully requires adaptation, or a change, in response to stress.
- Homeostasis consists of coordinated physiologic processes that maintain most of the steady states in the person.
- The multisystem response to stress is referred to as the general adaptation syndrome (GAS). The three stages of GAS are alarm reaction, stage of resistance, and stage of exhaustion.
- The local adaptation syndrome (LAS) is a localized expression of the three stages of the GAS.
- The physiologic response to stress is mediated by the hypothalamic—pituitary—adrenal axis.
- Coping is a problem-solving process that the person uses to manage the stresses or events with which he or she is presented.
- Altered coping may be manifested by use of alcohol and drugs, excessive smoking, increased sleeping, withdrawal, and illness.
- Manifestations of altered coping can interfere with the person's effective management of ADLs.
- A focused nursing assessment of coping and adaptation includes the history of the client's previous coping methods, areas of risk for ineffective coping, and identification of a coping and adaptation dysfunction.
- Nursing interventions include assisting the client to develop effective coping strategies to promote healthy adaptation to stress, and supporting the client in using those strategies in unusually stressful situations.
- Community-based care needs to include the use of support people or groups to maintain effective coping strategies.

Critical Thinking Challenges

Building on what you have learned in this and previous chapters, apply your strengthened knowledge base to handling the situation at the beginning of the chapter. Consider care of the mother and daughter by thinking through the following:

1. *Clarify how you will proceed with this assessment.*
2. *Identify factors that cause stress to the people in the situation.*
3. *Identify factors that affect the coping behaviors of the daughter.*
4. *Explore factors that place this family at risk for dysfunctional coping.*
5. *Describe manifestations of altered coping behavior.*
6. *Based on the accumulated information, plan your nursing interventions.*

References

Bell J. M. (1977). Stressful life events and coping methods in mental-illness and wellness behaviors. *Nurs Res, 26,* 136–141.

Benson, H. (1976). *The relaxation response.* New York: Avon Books.

Cannon, W. B. (1935). Stressors and strains of homeostasis. *Am J Med Sci, 189,* 1.

Fuller, J., & Schaller-Ayers, J. (1994). *Health assessment: A nursing approach* (2nd ed.). Philadelphia: J. B. Lippincott.

Hall, W. A. (1994). New fatherhood: Myths and realities. *Public Health Nurs, 11,* 219–228.

Holmes, T. H., & Rahe, R. H. (1967). The social readjustment and rating scale. *J Psychosom Res, 11,* 213–218.

Kammer, C. H. (1994). Stress and coping of family members responsible for nursing home placement. *Res Nurs Health, 17* (2), 89–98.

Lazarus, R. S. (1981). Little hazards can be hazardous to your health. *Psychology Today, 15* (7), 58–62.

Lazarus, R. (1991a). Cognition and motivation in emotion. *Am Psychol, 46,* 352–367.

Lazarus, R. (1991b). Progress on a cognitive-motivational-relational theory of emotion. *Am Psychol, 46,* 819–834.

Lazarus, R. S. (1992). Coping with the stress of illness. *WHO Regional Publications European Series, 44,* 11–31.

Levine, S., & Scotch, N. (1970). *Social stress.* Chicago: Aldine Publishing.

Mason, J. W. (1975a). A historical view of the stress field, Part 1. *J Human Stress, 1,* 6–12.

Mason, J. W. (1975b). A historical view of the stress field, Part 2. *J Human Stress, 1* (2), 22–36.

Miller, L. H., Smith, A. D., & Mehler, B. L. (1991). *The stress audit.* Brookline, MA: Biobehavioral Association.

Nakagawa-Kogan, H. (1994). Self-management training: Potential for primary care. *Nurse Practitioner Forum, 5* (2), 77–84.

Nakagawa-Kogan, H., et al. (1979). *Training manual for the management of stress response program.* Seattle, WA: University of Washington, School of Nursing, Psychosocial Nursing Department.

North American Nursing Diagnosis Association (NANDA). (1994). *NANDA nursing diagnoses: Definitions and classification 1995–1996.* Philadelphia: Author.

Puskar, L. R., Lamb, J. M., & Bartolovic, M. (1993). Examining the common stressors and coping methods of rural adolescents. *Nurse Pract, 18* (11), 50–53.

Selye, H. (1974). *Stress without disease.* Philadelphia: J. B. Lippincott.

Sorensen, E. S. (1994). Daily stressors and coping responses: A comparison of rural and suburban children. *Public Health Nurs, 11,* 24–31.

Tyler, P. A., & Ellison, R. N. (1994). Sources of stress and psychological well-being in high-dependency nursing. *J Adv Nurs, 19,* 469–476.

Vander, A. J. (1993). *Human physiology: The mechanisms of body function* (6th ed.). New York: McGraw-Hill.

Wineman, N. M., Durand, E. J., & McCulloch, B. J. (1994). Examination of the factor structure of the Ways of Coping Questionnaire with clinical populations. *Nurs Res, 43,* 268–273.

Wolff, H. G. (1953). *Stress and disease.* Springfield, IL: Charles C Thomas

Bibliography

Beaton, R. D., Egan, K. J., Nakagawa-Kogan, H., & Morrison, K. N. (1991). Self-reported symptoms of stress with temporomandibular disorders: Comparisons to healthy men and women. *J Prosthet Dent, 65,* 289–293.

Brashares, J. J., & Catanzaro, S. J. (1994). Mood regulation expectancies, coping responses, depression, and sense of burden in female caregivers of Alzheimer's patients. *J Nerv Ment Dis, 182,* 437–442.

Eccles, A. M. (1990). Using humor to relieve stress. *Point of View, 27* (1), 8–9.

Everly, G. S., & Lating, J. M. (1994). *Psychotraumatololgy: Key papers and core concepts in post-traumatic stress.* New York: Plenum Press.

Gilligan, B. (1993). A positive coping strategy: Humour in the oncology setting. *Professional Nurse, 8,* 231–233.

Hahn, W. K., Brooks, J. A., & Hartsough, D. M. (1993). Self-disclosure and coping styles in men with cardiovascular reactivity. *Res Nurs Health, 16,* 275–282.

Humphrey, J. H. (1994). *Human stress: Current selected research, 1986–1993* (Vols. 1–5). New York: AMS Press.

Maslow, A. (1954). *Motivation and personality.* New York: Harper Brothers.

Pelletier, K. (1977). *Mind as healer, mind as slayer.* New York: Dell.

Pepin, J., Ducharme, F., Kerouac, S., et al. (1994). The development of a research program based on a conceptual model for the discipline of nursing. *Canadian Journal of Nursing Research, 26* (1), 41–53.

Rahe, R. H. (1993). Acute versus chronic post-traumatic stress disorder. *Integrative Physiological and Behavioral Science, 28* (1), 46–56.

Roberts, S. J. (1994). Somatization in primary care: The common presentation of psychosocial problems through physical complaints. *Nurse Pract, 19* (5), 47, 50–56.

Ryan-Wenger, N. M. (1994). Coping behavior in children: Methods of measurement for research and clinical practice. *Journal of Pediatric Nursing, 9* (3), 183–195.

Selye, H. (1982). History and present status of the stress concept. In L. Goldberger & S. Breznitz (Eds.), *Handbook of stress.* New York: Free Press.

Smith, J. G. (1990). *Cognitive–behavioral relaxation training.* New York: Springer.

Troop, N. A., Holbrey, A., Trowler, R., & Treasure, J. L. (1994). Ways of coping in women with eating disorders. *J Nerv Ment Dis, 182,* 535–540.

Sexuality and Reproduction

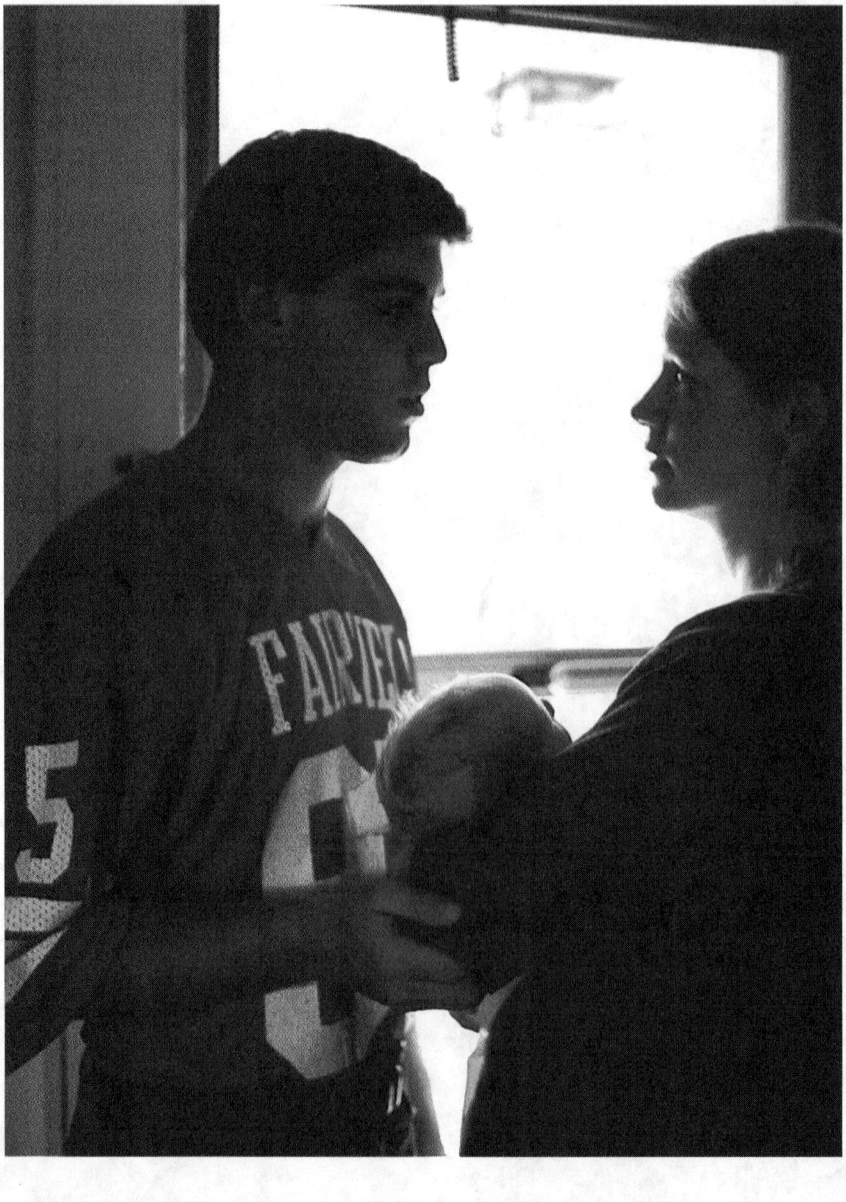

UNIT XVI

Unit XVI discusses the sexuality and reproduction area of human function. Sexuality is a basic human need and one that concerns many clients when illness threatens their normal function. It is also a subject that creates discomfort for many nurses.

The single chapter in this unit explores the physiologic and psychosocial components of sexuality. The discussion encourages nurses to explore their own feelings about sexuality. This is particularly important because normal function varies. Additionally, nurses may find themselves in situations in which they must generate the conversation. The content in this chapter helps the nurse learn to avoid being judgmental when assessing and interviewing in this area of function. Holistic nursing interventions and empathetic caring are essential for effective care for clients with sexuality needs. The chapter offers nursing interventions that promote health and function as well as a beginning discussion of holistic nursing interventions for clients with altered function.

A feeling of sexuality, a need for sexuality, and a variety of expressions of sexuality permeate the client's very being because it is integral to the human makeup. The nurse helps the client meet these needs and expressions in health and illness.

Human Sexuality

Key Terms

Bisexual
Climacteric
Clitoris
Dyspareunia
Foreskin
Heterosexual
Homosexual
Human sexual response
Impotence
Masturbation
Menarche
Menopause
Orgasm
Prepuce
Premature ejaculation
Sexuality
Transsexual
Vaginismus

Learning Objectives

Upon completion of this chapter, the student will be able to do the following:

- *Describe the anatomy of the male and female reproductive systems.*
- *Discuss sexual expression; sexual orientation; gender identity and roles; menstruation; and conception, pregnancy, and birth.*
- *Compare the male and female sexual response cycles.*
- *Relate sexuality to all stages of the life cycle.*
- *Identify factors that affect normal sexual functioning.*
- *Describe common risks and alterations in sexuality.*
- *Understand the nursing process as it relates to people with altered sexual functioning.*
- *Perform breast self-examination or testicular self-examination.*

Ruth F. Craven and Constance J. Hirnle: FUNDAMENTALS OF NURSING, Second Edition. © 1996 Lippincott-Raven.

52

You are a nurse working in a women's health practice. A woman comes in for a routine examination (Pap smear/pelvic exam, annual exam). While you are preparing her for the examination, she tells you she is very nervous about it and she always has difficulty "relaxing" when she has a pelvic examination. She is worried the examiner will not be able to insert the speculum. She is unmarried and not involved currently in a sexual relationship.

You have built a wide range of knowledge in the previous chapters. In this chapter you will study how sexuality functions in the makeup of the individual. By the time you have finished the chapter, you should be able to discuss intelligently sexuality, reproduction, and other sexual matters with your clients. Your knowledge base of this important human need will help you understand the woman discussed in the situation above and help you consider the Critical Thinking Challenges at the end of the chapter.

Although there is marked openness in the media regarding sexual matters, some individuals are hesitant to discuss sexuality and sexual matters. The nurse's challenge is complex in today's social context of more open sexual expression combined with more fears of sexually transmitted diseases.

Most nurses see clients in settings not directly related to sexuality. The nurse, however, may be confronted in any setting with clients' concerns regarding their sexuality. Sexual issues, then, should be part of the client history. Although some common problems can be dealt with in the healthcare facility, more advanced problems require specially trained personnel. Each nurse must be aware of his or her own personal attitudes and personal expertise and limitations. These should not interfere with care given.

Normal Human Sexuality

Sexuality includes function of the sexual organs plus a person's perceptions of his or her own functioning and sexual expression and preference. Human sexual response is highly variable and greatly influenced by many factors. These may include psychological, emotional, and cultural factors, and values and moral views, as well as comfort with one's body and quality of one's relationship with the other person, assuming one is involved in a relationship. A person not involved in a sexual relationship may very well still regard himself or herself as a sexual being with a sexual identity.

Anatomy of the Reproductive Systems

Although sexuality is not synonymous with reproduction, the reproductive organs are involved in human sexual response. For purposes of clarity, the male and female reproductive systems are discussed separately.

Male Reproductive System

The male reproductive system, as illustrated in Figure 52-1, is composed of both external and internal organs. The external organs include the penis and scrotum. The penis is a cylindrical, pendulous, erectile organ. It is composed of the shaft and glans. The shaft contains the urethra, the outlet for urine from the urinary bladder. The glans is the cone-shaped head of the penis; it is covered with loose skin called the **prepuce** or **foreskin**. In the uncircumcised man, the glans can be retracted for intercourse and cleaning. In the circumcised man, the glans is exposed because the foreskin has been removed surgically. The scrotum is the loose, pouchlike sac that contains the testes. The testes are the male gonads, reproductive glands that produce male cells, or spermatozoa, and testosterone, the male hormone.

The internal organs include the prostate gland and seminal vesicles. These are glands that produce and store most of the seminal fluid. The combination of seminal fluid and spermatozoa forms semen, the secretion discharged from the urethra during orgasm.

Female Reproductive System

The female reproductive system includes external and internal organs, as illustrated in Figure 52-2. External genitalia include the mons pubis, labia majora, labia minora, clitoris, urethral meatus, Skene's and Bartholin's glands, and the vaginal orifice. Collectively, these external anatomic parts are referred to as the vulva.

The mons pubis is a pad of fatty tissue that lies over the bony prominence called the symphysis pubis. The labia are the fleshy borders of the external genitalia. The labia majora lie on either side of the vaginal opening, forming the lateral borders. The labia minora are thinner folds that lie just inside the labia majora.

The **clitoris** is a small erectile body lying just above the urinary meatus and partially covered by the meeting of the labia minora. The clitoris corresponds to the male penis in its physiologic function of orgasm. Skene's glands lie inside of and on the posterior of the urethra, and Bartholin's glands are small mucous glands on the lateral wall of the vestibule of the vagina.

The internal genitalia include the ovaries, fallopian tubes, uterus, and vagina (see Fig. 52-2). The ovaries are two almond-shaped bodies lying on either side of the pelvic cavity, which contain ova and female hormones, specifically estrogen and progesterone. Fallopian tubes are narrow ducts of about 4.5 inches (11.4 cm) in length. They extend laterally on either side of the uterus and terminate in finger-like projections near but not touching the ovaries.

The uterus is a muscular, pear-shaped organ that lies between the sacrum and the symphysis pubis. It consists of three areas: the fundus or upper portion; the cavity, which is hollow; and the lower end, the cervix, which connects the uterus to the vagina. The uterus is an expandable organ.

The vagina is a musculomembranous tube that forms a passageway from the uterus to the vulva. It is located between the urinary bladder and the rectum.

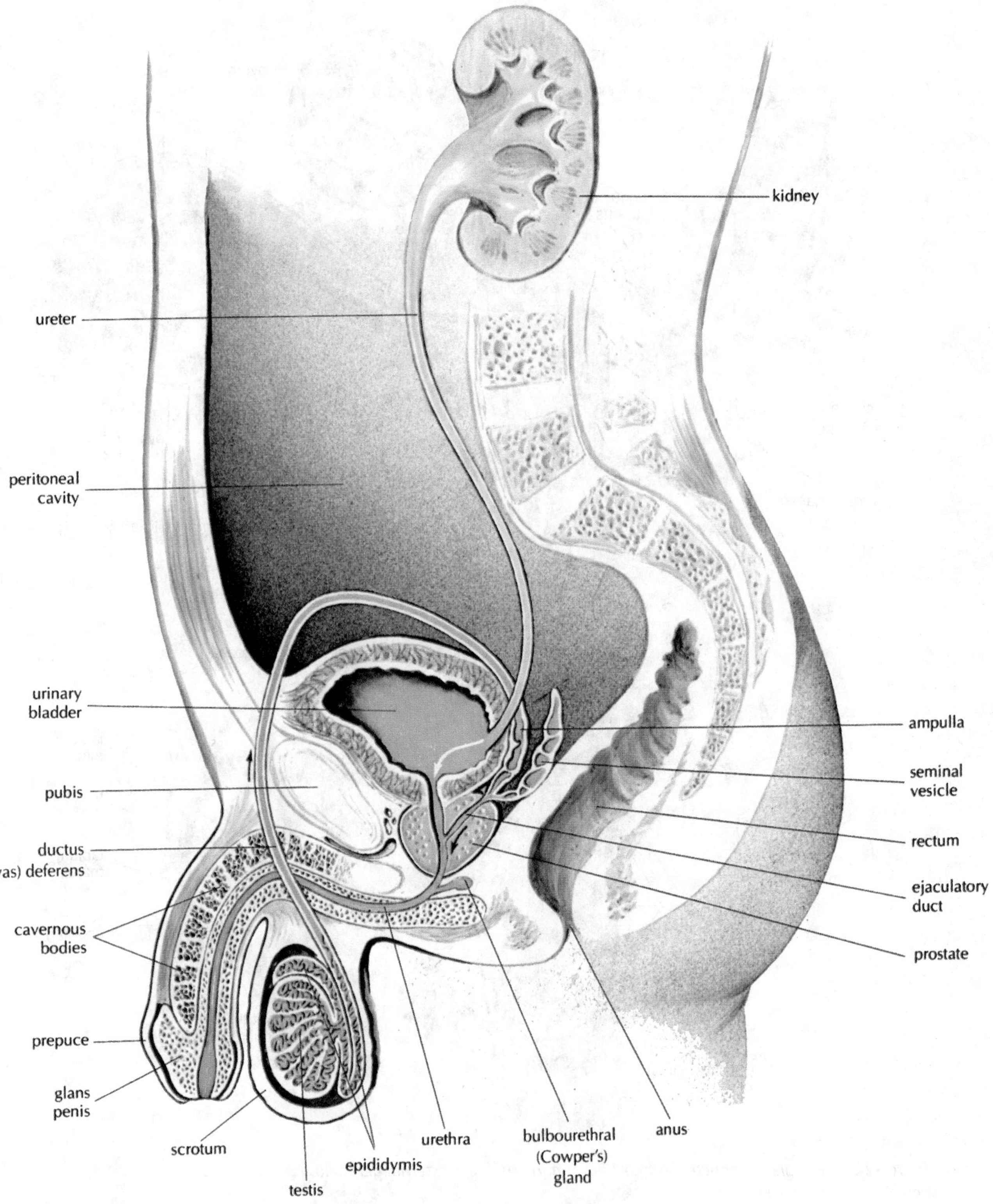

Figure 52-1 • *Male genitourinary system. The black arrows indicate the course of spermatozoa through the duct system; the single white arrow indicates the course of urine.*

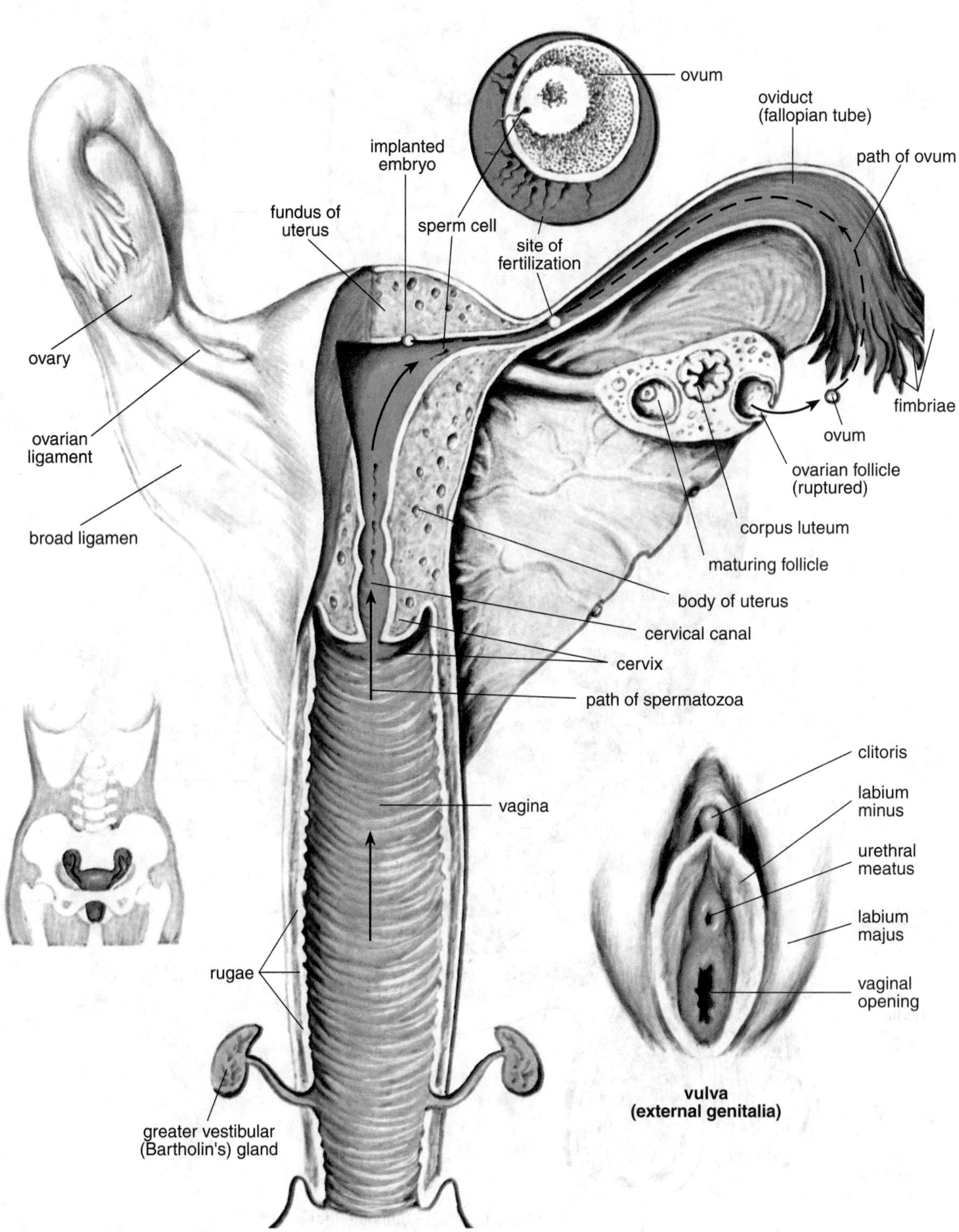

Figure 52-2 • *Female reproductive system showing internal and external genitalia. Fertilization is shown in the top portion of the art.*

The vagina represents a potential space—that is, the walls of the vagina, which are normally in contact, will stretch for sexual intercourse or the birth of a baby.

Breasts. The female breasts are considered organs of reproduction because they are directly influenced by the reproductive hormones, estrogen and progesterone, and because they are organs of lactation. Also called the mammary gland, each breast is composed of fatty and glandular tissue and consists of 15 to 20 lobes (Fig. 52-3). Each lobe drains through a lactiferous duct that opens on the tip of the nipple. The nipple is surrounded

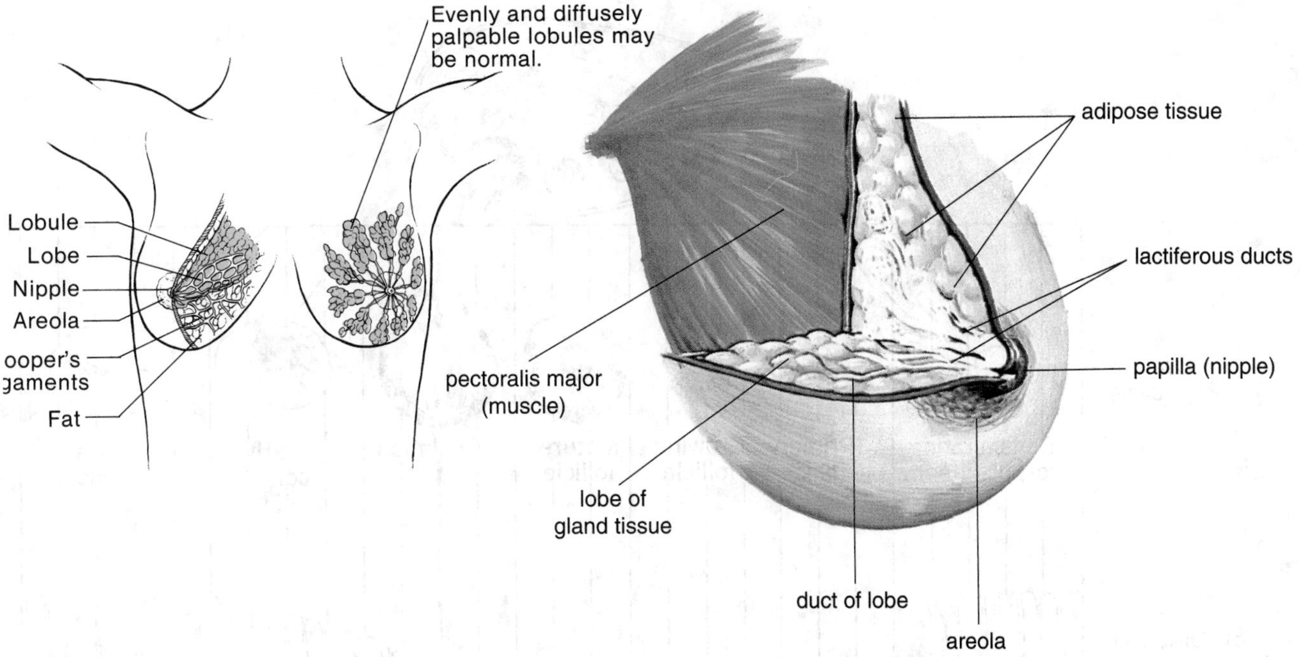

Figure 52-3 • *Breast structure. (From: [Left], Fuller, J., Schaller-Ayers, J. (1994). Health assessment: A nursing approach, 2nd ed. Philadelphia, J.B. Lippincott; [Right], Memmler, R. L., Cohen, B. J., & Wood, D. I. (1996). (Structure and Function of the human body, 6th ed. Philadelphia: J.B. Lippincott.)*

by a circular, pigmented area called the areola; the color of the areola is a pale to deep pink. Breast size varies from woman to woman and throughout the lifespan.

Normal Function of Male and Female Reproductive Systems

The male reproductive system is responsible for the generation, maturation, and ejaculation of spermatozoa. The female reproductive system is responsible for cyclic maturation and release of an ovum, and preparation of the uterus for implantation of a fertilized ovum, should fertilization occur. Reproduction is only one part of sexuality. Human beings can be sexual—can engage in sexual relationships—without the occurrence of reproduction.

Sexual Expression

Sexual expression varies among people. Various positions for coitus and stimulation may be used, without any particular one being considered "normal." The frequency of sexual expression also varies, with no determined "normal" frequency. In addition, the amount and kind of **foreplay** (activity before sexual intercourse) may vary greatly. Some people engage in **masturbation** (self-stimulation), whether it is mutual masturbation with a partner or masturbation without a partner. Others choose **celibacy** (abstention from sexual intercourse), although they still consider themselves to be sexual beings.

Menstruation and Ovulation

Menstruation is a physiologic process that occurs in women and is essential to their reproductive function. Sexual expression can occur in the absence of menstruation (eg, a woman with Turner's syndrome or a woman who has gone through menopause). Because of its direct connection with reproduction, however, it is appropriate to discuss menstruation in this chapter. Menstruation is a cyclic, periodic discharge of a bloody fluid from the uterus through the vagina during the reproductive years of a woman's lifetime. The length of a cycle may vary from woman to woman and even within one woman. The cycle repeats itself approximately every 28 days, although much variation can occur and still be considered normal.

Menstruation depends on the interplay of various hormones (Fig. 52-4). The hypothalamus secretes gonadotropin-releasing hormone, which stimulates the pituitary gland to secrete follicle-stimulating hormone and luteinizing hormone (see Fig. 52-4A). These hormones stimulate the ovaries to produce estrogen and progesterone, which are necessary for stimulation of the target organs (vagina, breast, uterus) in preparing the body for a possible pregnancy. If pregnancy does not occur, the levels of estrogen and progesterone fall, menses ensues, and the feedback mechanism begins again with a new menstrual cycle.

The menstrual cycle is discussed in terms of the ovarian cycle and the endometrial or uterine cycle. The ovarian cycle consists of the follicular phase, the ovu-

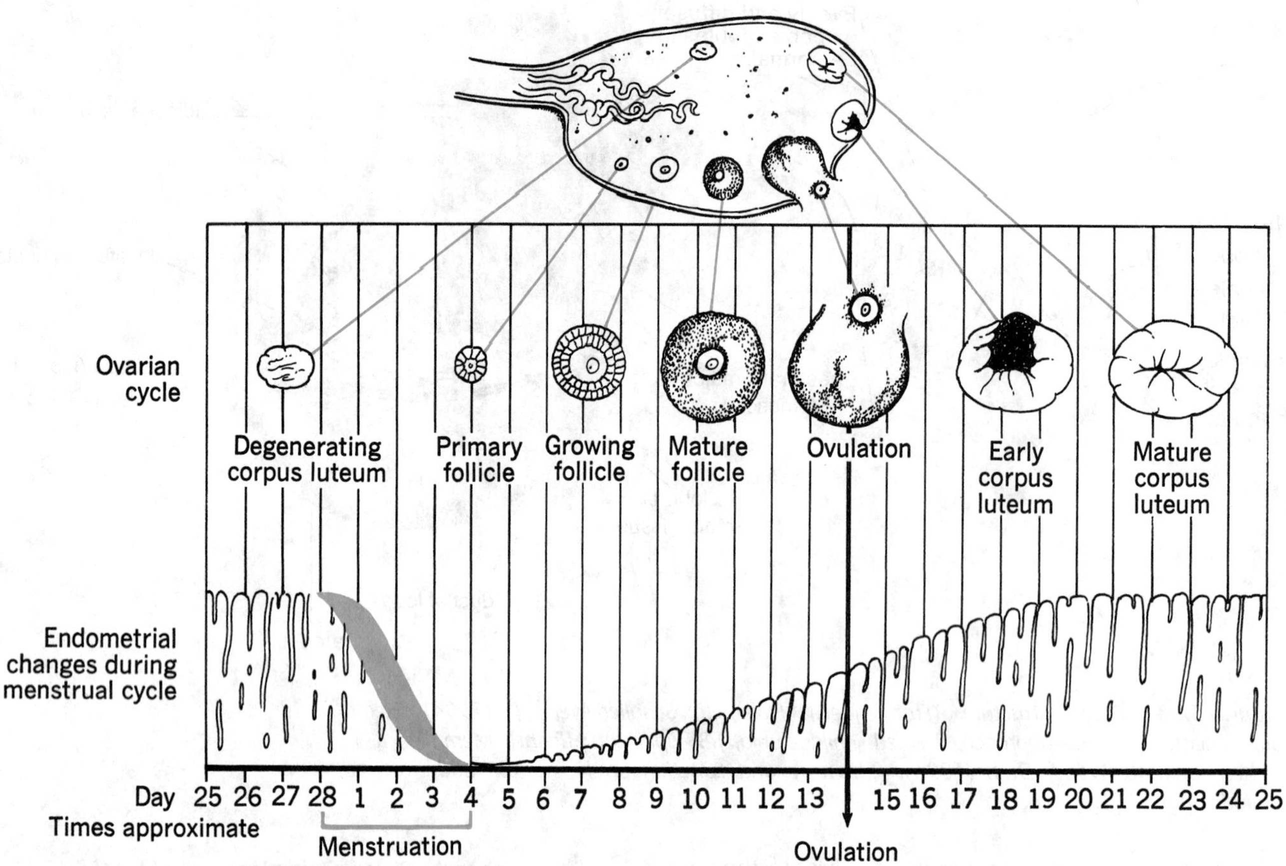

Figure 52-4 • *Schematic representation of one ovarian cycle and the corresponding changes in thickness of the endometrium. The ovarian cycle includes the changes within the corpus luteum and follicle. The endometrial changes indicate the thickness of the endometrium just before the onset of menstruation and its thinness just as menstruation ends.*

latory phase, and the luteal phase (see Fig. 52-4B). The follicular phase is estrogen-dominant; during this phase the follicles mature, with usually only one follicle reaching full maturity. This follicle, or oocyte, ruptures from the ovary at the time of ovulation. At this point the estrogen level loses its dominance and progesterone becomes the dominant hormone during the second half of the cycle, or the luteal phase. During this phase, the progesterone levels become elevated, preparing the uterus for possible implantation and maintenance of a fertilized ovum.

The endometrial or uterine cycle is divided into the proliferative and secretory phases (see Fig. 52-4C). The proliferative phase refers to the proliferation of the endometrium, or uterine lining, as the dominant hormone, estrogen, influences such growth. During the secretory phase, which is progesterone-dominant, the endometrial glands continue to grow, becoming edematous and dense, in preparation for implantation and maintenance of a fertilized ovum.

Hormones also affect the uterus at the cervical level (see Fig. 52-4D). Under the influence of estrogen, the cervical mucus becomes more watery, alkaline, and stretchy, resembling the quality of egg whites. This quality is conducive to sperm survival, thus preparing for the possibility of conception.

Conception, Pregnancy, and Birth

For conception and reproduction to occur, several complicated factors must be in full operation. First, the man must produce fully matured spermatozoa in enough numbers and with enough motility to penetrate the cervix and ascend the uterus and fallopian tubes. This transportation occurs by way of cervical mucus, which becomes alkaline and thus receptive to the sperm. When the spermatozoa reach the fallopian tubes, they undergo capacitation, a process in which the surface characteristics of the sperm change, releasing enzymes that enhance their ability to penetrate the ovum.

The occurrence of ovulation must correspond to the process described earlier, because there is a time period of only a few days in which the woman can be impregnated. In ovulation, a mature follicle is released from the ovary into one of the fallopian tubes. The fimbriae or finger-like projections at the end of each fallopian tube assist in extracting the ovum from the ovary and bringing it into the fallopian tube.

Fertilization of one ova with one spermatozoon normally occurs in the outer third of the fallopian tube (see Fig. 52–2). After fertilization occurs, the fertilized ovum undergoes several cell divisions and moves down toward the uterus, where it implants in the uterine wall.

The first 2 weeks after fertilization are critical; many pregnancies do not continue beyond this point because of a defective ova or spermatozoon or because of hormone imbalances. If a pregnancy continues in spite of these complex factors and potential risks, the embryo develops rapidly. The average length of pregnancy, counted from the time of conception, is approximately 267 days or 38 weeks, but may vary by about 2 weeks in either direction.

Birth is a normal process that occurs in three stages of labor. Although the initiation of labor and birth is not entirely understood, labor involves stimulation by hormones that cause the uterus to contract, thus pushing the fetus through the birth canal after a number of hours of labor.

Milk Production

With pregnancy, the breasts undergo physiologic and anatomic changes. They enlarge and become more sensitive. The nipples enlarge, becoming darker, and the sebaceous glands in the areola hypertrophy. Later in pregnancy (during the second half), colostrum may begin to be secreted by the alveolar cells. Colostrum is a yellowish fluid, considered a precursor to actual milk, containing important nutrients for the newborn.

Milk production occurs under the influence of prolactin, glucocorticoids, insulin, and parathyroid hormone. Estrogen and progesterone actually inhibit milk production, and thus, at birth, with the delivery of the placenta, the levels of estrogen and progesterone fall dramatically.

Characteristics of Normal Sexuality

Sexual Orientation

It is essential that, when working with clients, nurses understand and appreciate that various forms of sexual orientation exist. As mentioned earlier in the section on Sexual Expression, there is not one "normal" way of being in relation to sexuality and sexual orientation. Some people are **heterosexual**, relating sexually to members of the opposite gender. Others are **bisexual**, relating to both men and women in a sexual way. Others are **homosexual**, relating sexually to members of the same gender. Still others may abstain totally from sexual relations, either permanently or temporarily.

Gender Identity and Roles

One's gender identity and corresponding roles that one takes on influence sexuality. It is important for the nurse to understand the person's perception of his or her gender, and what that gender means to the person in terms of identity and roles.

Sometimes actual biologic gender does not coincide with gender identity; this is so in the case of people who are **transsexuals**. A man who is a transsexual views himself as a woman trapped in a man's body, and the reverse is true for a female transsexual. Social roles are often very confusing for transsexuals. Some may marry and have families, but others may never do so. Some seek medical intervention in the form of hormones and surgery to change their physical gender.

Sexual Response

The human sexual response was first studied scientifically by Masters and Johnson (1966). They found that humans undergo four distinct phases of sexual response, as outlined in Table 52-1. These phases are referred to as excitement, plateau, orgasm, and resolution. The excitement phase begins as a result of various stimuli, both physiologic and psychological. If there are no distracting stimuli, this phase will continue and will intensify as the person begins the plateau phase, in which there is increased sexual tension. If this sexual tension continues, still without distracting stimuli, **orgasm**, or the involuntary climax of this tension, occurs. During orgasm the person experiences involuntary contractions and release of the vasocongestion that occurs in the phases leading to orgasm. The resolution phase refers to the period after orgasm, in which physiologic changes occur that allow the body to return to its preexcitement state. These phases will be discussed more specifically as they are experienced by both men and women. It is important to note, however, that other researchers have defined the sexual response pattern in slightly different ways (Lauver & Welch, 1990). Kaplan (1979), for example, defines the sexual response cycle according to three phases, consisting of desire, excitement, and orgasm. Because Masters and Johnson's work is considered "classic" and because much of the sexual response research is based on their work, this chapter presents detailed descriptions of both the male and the female sexual response cycle according to the work of Masters and Johnson.

Male Sexual Response. Masters and Johnson (1966) found one pattern of sexual response in men, although

Table 52-1 • Phases of the Human Sexual Response Cycle

Phase	Changes in Man	Changes in Woman
Excitement	Rapid penile erection Partial elevation of testes Increased size of testes Nipple erection	Enlargement of clitoris Vaginal lubrication Expansion of vagina Enlargement of breasts Nipple erection Sex flush
Plateau	Thickening of circumference of penis Continued increase in size of testes Fluid from Cowper's glands Sex flush Muscle contraction Hyperventilation Increased heart rate Increased blood pressure	Retraction of clitoris Increased size of labia minora Elevation of uterus Muscle contraction Hyperventilation Increased heart rate Increased blood pressure
Orgasm	Expulsive contractions of urethra Ejaculation	Contractions of orgasmic platform Possible gushing of fluid
Resolution	Rapid loss of vasocongestion Decreased size of penis Decreased size of testes Descent of testes into scrotum Refractory period	Return of clitoris to normal size and position Decreased size of orgasmic platform Relaxation of vagina No refractory period

Adapted from Masters, W. H. & Johnson, V. E. (1966). *Human sexual response.* Boston: Little, Brown, & Co.

according to Woods (1984), it is unlikely that male sexual response occurs without variation. This predominant pattern, as described by Masters and Johnson, and Woods, includes a rapid excitement phase, a short plateau phase with orgasm occurring immediately, and a resolution phase, which includes an obligatory refractory period.

Excitement. The excitement phase is characterized by rapid erection of the penis, with tensing and thickening of the scrotal skin and elevation of the scrotal sac. In addition, there is shortening of the spermatic cords, resulting in partial elevation of both testes toward the perineum. The vasocongestion that occurs during this phase is responsible for the erection of the penis, as well as the thickening of the scrotal skin and the elevation of the scrotal sac. The testes increase in size as they are partially elevated. The man may experience nipple erection during the excitement phase. During the excitement phase it is not unusual for the man partially to lose his penile erection and regain it. He is also subject to distractions that may interfere with this phase.

Plateau. The plateau phase involves a thickening of the circumference of the penis at the coronal ridge, and an increase in size of the testes by about 50% more than their nonstimulated size (Woods, 1984). A couple of drops of fluid appear at the urethral meatus. This fluid is produced from Cowper's glands, and contributes to lubrication. In addition to being mucoid-producing lubrication, this fluid may contain some active spermatozoa. The man may experience nipple erection, and a sex flush, characterized by a maculopapular rash over the epigastric area, may appear during the latter part of the plateau phase. The plateau phase also consists of an increase in voluntary and involuntary muscle contraction, hyperventilation, increased heart rate, and elevated blood pressure.

Orgasm. Orgasm is the climax of the plateau phase and consists of expulsive contractions of the entire length of the urethra. The initial three or four contractions are the strongest, and they subsequently decrease. Concurrently, the force of ejaculation is greatest with the first several contractions and decreases thereafter. Ejaculation can be viewed as composed of two stages (Woods, 1984). The first stage consists of expulsion of seminal fluid substrate from the seminal vesicles into the prostatic urethra. The second stage consists of expulsion of the seminal fluid from the prostatic urethra to the urethral meatus.

Resolution. The fourth and final phase, resolution, occurs immediately after orgasm and consists of an initial rapid loss of vasocongestion with an accompanying decrease in the size of the penis. The scrotum becomes less congested, and the testes descend back into the scrotum and decrease to their preexcitement size. Disappearance of the sex flush and of nipple erection, if they occurred, is apparent.

Men experience an obligatory refractory period, during which they are unable to be restimulated to erection. The length of this period varies individually.

Female Sexual Response. Although they found only one response pattern in men, Masters and Johnson (1966) found some variability in the patterns of sexual response among women. Some women experience a plateau phase with several peaks, without actually experiencing orgasm. Others experience a definite orgasm, and still others experience multiple orgasms. Masters and Johnson believe that many other patterns in addition to these three exist in women's sexual response.

Excitement. The excitement phase in women consists of enlargement of the clitoris and vaginal lubrication occurring in response to vasocongestion. The vaginal space expands in the inner one-third portion, and the uterus may become elevated. The vaginal orifice opens as the labia majora and minora either separate or move away slightly. The woman may also experience nipple erection and enlarging of the breasts. She may experience a sex flush, similar to that described earlier for men.

Plateau. The plateau phase involves retraction of the clitoris under the clitoral hood. The labia minora increase in size as a result of vasocongestion, and the vagina itself expands in width and depth. Full elevation of the uterus with concurrent rising of the cervix occurs. Nipple erection may continue, and the sex flush, if it has occurred, may spread. There is an increase in both voluntary and involuntary muscle contraction, and hyperventilation, increased heart rate, and increased blood pressure occur.

Orgasm. The orgasmic platform, or the outer third of the vagina and the labia minora, is the location of primary response during the orgasmic phase. Contractions occur very quickly and strongly in this area during orgasm. After the initial three to six contractions, the intensity and frequency of the contractions decrease. The woman experiences an increased respiratory rate, increased heart rate, and increased blood pressure. Controversy exists as to whether women experience an expulsion of fluid during orgasm. Some research reports that women have described feeling that there was a gushing of fluid along with orgasm (Belzer, 1981).

Resolution. The resolution phase includes a return of the clitoris to normal size and position. Vasocongestion dissipates, with resulting decrease in size of the orgasmic platform and relaxing of the vagina.

The woman does not have an obligatory refractory period and may experience multiple orgasms in a short period of time.

Normal Sexual Functional Pattern

People have a basic human need to be loved. Sexuality involves much more; it also affects self-esteem, roles and relationships, values and beliefs, and coping. The World Health Organization (1975) has defined sexual well-being as the following three elements:

- A capacity to enjoy and control sexual behavior in accordance with a social and personal ethic
- Freedom from fear, shame, guilt, false beliefs, and other psychological factors inhibiting sexual response and impairing sexual relationships
- Freedom from organic disorder, disease, and deficiencies that interfere with sexual and reproductive functions.

Factors Affecting Sexuality

Human sexual response is highly variable and greatly influenced by many factors. These may include health management, roles and relationships, cognition and perception, culture, values and beliefs, self-concept, coping and stress tolerance, and previous experience. As described previously, not all people are involved in sexual relationships, but they still regard themselves as sexual beings. One's sexuality or experiences with sexuality can also affect other areas of one's life. For example, in the Critical Thinking situation posed at the beginning of this chapter, it may be that this woman who is worried about her upcoming pelvic examination has had sexual difficulties in the past that might be the cause of vaginismus.

Health Management

Managing one's health influences one's sexuality. Sleep, rest, adequate nutrition, and positive mental outlook all contribute to pleasure in one's sexual life.

Roles and Relationships

The quality of a person's relationship with a sexual partner has a strong influence on the quality of the sexual relationship. Love and trust may be key factors in facilitating one's comfort with sexuality and sexual relations with the person with whom one shares mutual love and trust. The experience of a sexual relationship is often greatly influenced by the relationship one has with the person with whom one engages in sex. Again, referring to the situation posed at the beginning of the chapter, it is incumbent on the nurse to understand how the quality of a person's relationships, particularly sexual relationships, may influence subsequent sexual difficulty (eg, this woman may have been betrayed in a trusting relationship, which could be contributing to her difficulty with pelvic exams).

Cognition and Perception

Psychological factors include such aspects as certain mental images being triggered in the mind, leading to sexual arousal. One's emotional state may have a great influence on one's sexual response. For example, someone who is depressed may be less sexually arousable or less concerned with sex overall than someone who is not depressed.

In addition, one's knowledge or lack of knowledge regarding sexuality will influence sexual functioning; misperceptions about sexuality often adversely affect one's sexual functioning.

Again, with regard to the Critical Thinking situation, cognition and perception must be considered.

Culture, Values, and Beliefs

Cultural factors include society's predominant views of sexuality, with those views comprising the social context within which people experience sexuality. Values and morals also have a great impact on one's sexuality. Subscribing to particular values related to sexuality, such as whether one condones sex outside of marriage, is directly related to one's own sexuality. Religious beliefs may affect a person's views of contraception, abortion, and sex education. The woman described at the beginning of the chapter may be from a particular culture or ethnic group whose values may influence her perceptions of a pelvic examination, particularly one done by a male healthcare provider.

Self-Concept

One's view of self has a direct impact on one's sexuality. A person who feels decreased self-esteem and lacks confidence in himself or herself may experience a negative effect on his or her sexual functioning. The person may have a decreased sexual drive or, conversely, may attempt to compensate for this negative self-concept by overemphasizing involvement in sexual relations. The area of one's self-concept must be taken into account when analyzing the Critical Thinking situation posed at the beginning of this chapter.

Coping and Stress Tolerance

A person's level of tolerance for stressful situations and ways of coping with these situations influence self-concept, and, in turn, influence sexual functioning. As noted in the preceding paragraph, one's sexual functioning is affected by one's self-concept. Again, coping and stress tolerance are important considerations in understanding the Critical Thinking situation.

Previous Experience

Previous experience with sexuality or ideas about sexuality influences one's current sexual functioning. For example, a woman who has been sexually abused in the past will, most likely, have repercussions from that experience that negatively affect her current sexual functioning. A more subtle example is that of a man or woman who has grown up with many cultural taboos related to sexuality, and finds it difficult later on to engage in a healthy sexual relationship. Previous experience is an essential area that needs to be explored to understand the situation described.

Lifespan Considerations

Rynerson (1990) has outlined the stages of the life cycle with reference to sexuality, incorporating the earlier work of Woods and Stamer (1984), who adapted the work of Mims and Swenson (1980). This section examines sexuality at each developmental stage of life, emphasizing physiologic, emotional, and social aspects of sexuality. Figure 52-5 shows couples at two ends of the spectrum of male–female relationships.

Prenatal

At fertilization, when the ovum and spermatozoon unite, the chromosomal formation is determined. The sperm carries either an X or a Y chromosome to combine with the X chromosome supplied by the ovum. An XX combination becomes a female and an XY combination becomes a male at about the fifth or sixth week of prenatal life. Hormonal influences play an important part in determining gonadal sex. In addition to the presence of an XY zygote, androgens must be present and cells must be sensitive to androgens for male genitalia to form. Lack of sensitivity to androgens, even in the presence of an XY genotype, will lead to development of female genitalia.

If genetic errors occur that lead to ambiguous genitalia, parents will have difficulty assigning gender to their newborn. Under normal circumstances, parents automatically interact with their child according to the child's gender. Problems such as ambiguous genitalia or lack of particular sex hormones may create serious problems for parents in relating to their child as male or female, and may create serious problems for the child as he or she grows up.

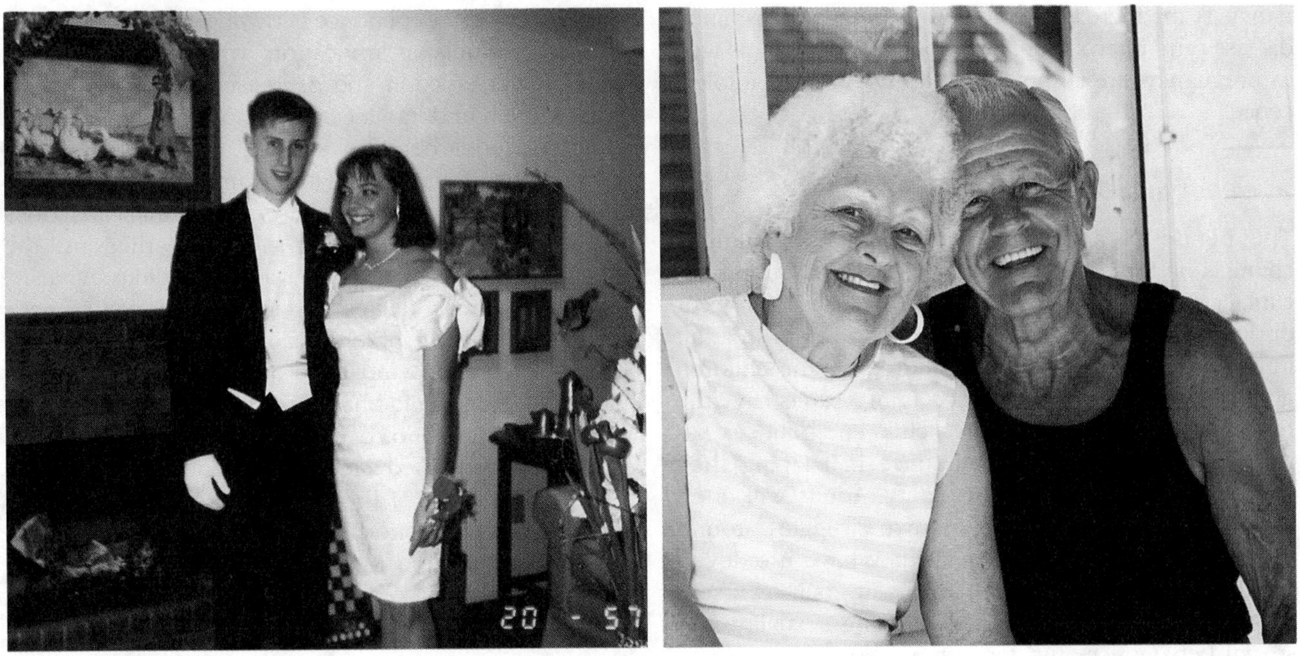

Figure 52–5 • Expressions of sexuality from two aspects of the lifespan. A key aspect of adolescent development is learning to develop relationships. In older adulthood, warmth, intimacy, and companionship are comfortable aspects of sexuality.

Newborn and Infant

It is particularly important for parents to touch and cuddle their newborn and infant. This is considered crucial for normal psychosexual development. The development of trust should occur in this period, paving the way for future healthy interpersonal relationships. Parents normally relate to their infants as either male or female, which has consequences for later development. Because infants are very sensitive to touch, it is common for them to explore their own bodies, often their own genitalia, and it is important for parents to recognize this as a normal developmental process.

Toddler and Preschooler

As a child becomes a toddler, learning to walk and gaining independence from parents, he or she begins to explore his or her body even more. The toddler begins to develop a concept of his or her own body, and sexual identity is part of this body image. The toddler may engage in masturbation, and parents need to be reassured that this is normal behavior and, in fact, healthy for normal development.

As a child becomes preschool-age, he or she begins to engage in further exploration of the body. Playing with friends as well as exploring one's own body is normal. A child at this age will be curious about body parts, and may often ask questions related to such things as where babies come from, breast-feeding, and physical differences between grown men and women and young boys and girls.

Child and Adolescent

During elementary school age, children continue to learn certain sex role behaviors and usually maintain friendships with same-sex friends. Children continue to learn about anatomy of their bodies, particularly their genitals, and continue to engage in masturbation, a normal and healthy activity. Rynerson (1990) notes that experimentation in both heterosexual and homosexual roles is a normal part of childhood and adolescence.

Adolescence is a turbulent time, after the relative calmness of the school-age stage of psychosexual development. The adolescent not only copes with development of identity and independence from parents, but concurrently experiences a surge of hormonal changes, leading to the physiologic changes of puberty.

A key point in the development of the adolescent girl is the beginning of menstruation. The first menstrual period is termed **menarche**. The accompanying development of breasts and of an adult female shape and proportions coincide with puberty. Adolescent girls become concerned with these physical changes, often equating them with acceptance, confidence, and popularity as well as with sexual identity.

Adolescent boys begin to experience such things as nocturnal emissions. The adolescent boy assumes a masculine sexual identity and behaviors based on role models and on personal expectations. At this age, boys are often competitive in all areas of life and, particularly, in sexual activity.

The adolescent's engagement in sexual experimentation is not without consequences. Adolescent pregnancy is an increasing problem. Sexually transmitted diseases and interpersonal relationship conflicts, as well as pregnancy, are common occurrences during adolescence.

Adult and Older Adult

The period of adulthood, between the tumultuous changes of adolescence and the later years during the climacteric, spans about 35 years. Many changes occur during this time, such as becoming involved in an adult intimate relationship, raising children, letting children go, and beginning to experience aging. Adults have the responsibility of educating their children about sexuality, and they have much influence in shaping their children's attitudes toward sexuality. Adults will often continue to grapple with their own struggles around sexuality and sexual behavior if they have not developed a high enough comfort level with their own sexuality. Many myths persist surrounding sexuality and sexual behavior; many stereotypes abound, and some people fear certain aspects of sexuality, such as homosexuality. Adults, therefore, often also need guidance from healthcare professionals, as they struggle with their own conflicts regarding values and beliefs about sexuality.

During adulthood, many women and their mates experience pregnancy. Although this can also occur during adolescence, it is more predominant during adulthood. Pregnancy poses many developmental issues related to sexuality. In addition, it may pose sexual difficulties between partners, owing to fear of sexual intercourse during pregnancy or contraindication of sexual intercourse due to high-risk conditions during pregnancy. For couples who wish to become pregnant but are unable to because of infertility problems, sexual issues may arise as well, caused by the need for them to have sexual intercourse according to a rigid schedule.

The **climacteric** refers to the period of time in which changes occur in the transition from middle age to old age. During this period, both men and women experience changes that are significant in their lives and their sexuality. This term more commonly refers to the transition that women experience as they begin to lose their reproductive function and approach cessation of their menstrual cycles. **Menopause** is the permanent cessation of menstrual activity. It normally occurs between the approximate ages of 40 and 55 but may be surgically induced.

Certain physiologic changes occur as a result of decreasing amounts of estrogen in women during the climacteric. Some women require estrogen replacement, which is controversial. Physiologic changes occur in men also. Specific effects can be noted in relation to the sexual response cycle, as described by Masters, Johnson, and Kolodny (1988). During the excitement phase, women experience slower onset of and decreased amounts of lubrication, whereas men experience slower erection and decreased firmness of erection. Women undergo a certain amount of atrophy, and thus the clitoris becomes smaller, and men may need more direct genital stimulation during the excitement phase. During the plateau phase, the vaginal canal does not increase in size as much as it did earlier, and the uterus does not become as elevated as it did previously. Men experience a decrease in the amount of Cowper's gland secretion, are able to maintain an erection longer before ejaculation, and have decreased testicular elevation. The orgasmic phase may become shortened for women and may not occur for men, as their need to ejaculate is decreased. Men also experience a decreased force and volume of the ejaculate. Men experience a longer refractory period, and both men and women experience more rapid return to nonengorgement of the genitals.

Altered Sexual Function

Certain conditions directly related to sexuality have a direct influence on a person's ability to engage in mutually satisfying sexual relations. Conditions other than those mentioned in this section also may have a direct impact on sexuality.

Potential for Altered Sexuality

Many factors can predispose a person to disruption of normal patterns of sexuality. Such factors are pregnancy, infertility, and abortion; alterations in gender identification; environment; illness; and surgery.

Pregnancy, Infertility, and Abortion

Pregnancy clearly alters sexual functioning. Although sexual intercourse is not contraindicated during a normal, low-risk pregnancy, sexual drive is often affected. It is common for women to have a decreased sexual drive during the first trimester, when they are fatigued and may feel nauseated. In addition, they may worry about miscarriage during the first trimester, and thus fear having sexual intercourse. During the second trimester, many women experience a surge of energy and a corresponding increase in sexual drive. The third trimester may again be a time of decreased sexual drive as the woman's abdomen grows, making it difficult to have sexual intercourse comfortably. It must be noted, however, that there is much variation in this pattern, and not all women respond in the same way. Men may also vary in their sexual desires. Some men find their pregnant wives sexually attractive, whereas others are apprehensive about having sexual relations with their pregnant wives for fear of harming their wives or the fetuses.

Infertility is often a stressor on a couple's sexual relationship. Infertile couples must have sex on a rigid schedule, according to when the woman is ovulating. Sex becomes programmed and loses its spontaneity. In addition, couples feel that they are having sex for a specific purpose rather than for enjoyment and mutual satisfaction. They often feel that they are being judged for how well they have sex, in that pregnancy will symbolize "successful" sex and lack of pregnancy will symbolize "failure." Many couples report that normal sexual relations resume after time has elapsed or infertility treatments are discontinued.

Women who have experienced unwanted pregnancies and subsequent abortions may feel apprehensive about having sexual intercourse. They may be fearful of having another unwanted pregnancy, they may not trust their contraceptive method, or they may continue to misuse or not use contraception while having sexual intercourse.

Alterations in Gender Identification

Alterations in gender identification may have a significant or insignificant effect on one's sexual functioning. Some transsexuals marry and have children and function in their socially prescribed sexual roles, while feeling trapped in those roles and experiencing much unhappiness. Other transsexuals do not function in socially prescribed roles.

Environment

Environment can have a large impact on one's sexual functioning. A hospitalized client, particularly one undergoing long-term hospitalization, may find it inhibiting to have sexual relations with a partner or to masturbate within the confines of a hospital room. Lack of privacy becomes a major issue. The same is true for people in nursing homes. Environment is a factor for people who are not hospitalized. Living in crowded conditions may preclude privacy. Fears about environmental pollutants affecting fertility may influence sexuality.

Illness

Illness poses a threat to normal sexual functioning. A person with cardiac problems may fear overexertion from engaging in sexual relations. Although this fear may not be based on physiologic principles, it can still be inhibiting to both sexual partners. A person with a sexually transmitted disease may fear transmitting the disease to a partner, or conversely, a person may fear contracting a sexually transmitted disease from a partner. Although safer sex guidelines may be followed, this fear can often inhibit sexual relations.

Pain and disorders of the joints may make normal sexual intercourse uncomfortable. Motor vehicle accidents have created a sizable population with spinal cord injuries (paraplegia and quadriplegia). People with any of these problems must find alternate methods of sexual functioning.

Medication

Some medications affect the ability to perform sexually. Rogers (1990) discusses these medications according to the categories of prescription drugs, over-the-counter drugs, and social drugs. Many conventional therapeutic drugs may adversely affect sexual functioning. Such drugs are antihypertensives, antipsychotic tranquilizers, antidepressants, neurotransmitters, and hormones. Social drugs that can affect sexuality and sexual response include alcohol, opiates, marijuana, sedative–hypnotics, cocaine and amphetamines, amyl nitrite, LSD, cantharides, and yohimbine.

Surgery

Examples of surgical procedures that have an effect on sexuality are cesarean births, hysterectomy, and mastectomy. Women who have cesarean births may experience a longer recovery period than women who have vaginal births, and may feel less desire to resume sexual relations. A woman who has had a cesarean birth may also feel that she was a "failure" during the labor and birth process, even though this is an irrational thought. Such thoughts may affect her sexual functioning.

A woman who has had a hysterectomy may feel that her femininity has been adversely affected. Again, this is irrational in the sense that women with hysterectomies are certainly able to engage in sexual intercourse and have orgasms, but the meaning of the hysterectomy to the woman may be so negative that it adversely affects her sexual functioning.

A woman who has had a mastectomy may also feel that her femininity has been adversely affected, particularly in a society in which the breasts are highly emphasized as sexual objects. A woman's view of herself may be negatively affected by having had a mastectomy, and this, in turn, will often negatively affect her sexual functioning.

Manifestations of Altered Sexuality

Alterations in normal patterns of sexuality can be seen in the following manifestations: sexual abuse, inhibited sexual desire, impotence, premature ejaculation, inability to ejaculate, organic dysfunction, dyspareunia, and vaginismus. The nurse can play a key role by assessing alterations in sexuality and assisting in prevention

Therapeutic Dialogue
Sexuality

Scenes for Thought

Richard Meyers and his wife Aileen are both in their sixties and have been healthy and active until Richard's car accident 3 months ago. At that time, he sustained a comminuted fracture of his right femur that had to be reduced surgically. He still needs crutches to help him ambulate and sometimes has pain in his right leg. You, Maddie Hines, his clinic health nurse, have been visiting the family since Richard was discharged from the hospital.

Effective

Nurse: *Good afternoon, Mr. Meyers. How are you this week? (Sitting down at the kitchen table with him.)*
Client: *Glad to see you Maddie. Who would've thought a broken leg would cause a body such trouble!* Laughing a little.
Nurse: *Are you having trouble? (Good eye contact. Smiling but not laughing with him so as to pay attention.)*
Client: *Well, I'm still having trouble negotiating around the house. The furniture and rugs and all are still in my way, even though you helped us move them.* Sighs. *I'm just having trouble with those crutches.*
Nurse: *(After assessing client's ability to maneuver and making some suggestions.) Is there something else that's causing you trouble, Mr. Meyers?*
Client: *Uh,* looking to see where his wife is, *I am having some trouble in the bedroom.* Looks embarrassed but determined to talk about this.
Nurse: *Okay, tell me a little more. (Sitting quietly.)*
Client: *It's the positioning of this darned leg. It hurts when Aileen and I try to, uh, get close, and then she gets worried and I get annoyed and it all goes to heck!* Sounds frustrated.
Nurse: *Frustrating, huh.* He nods. *Let me ask you a few questions first so I can find out what you're used to and then we can talk about modifications you and your wife might want to try. (Assesses usual sexual habits and practices, including willingness to experiment with new positions and effective use of analgesics. Then suggests two different positions that would afford pleasure without undue pain on the affected leg.)*
Client: *That sounds doable, Maddie. I think we'll start out with some dinner and flowers. I'm going to call my son and see if he can help me arrange a dinner here tomorrow night. Aileen's worked hard these last weeks. She deserves it. Then we'll see what we can manage after that.* Said with a wink. Looks eager to start planning.
Nurse: *How romantic! Sounds like you two are going to have a great evening. I'm glad we were able to talk about this.*
Client: *Me too, me too.* Big smile.

Less Effective

Nurse: *Hi, Mr. Meyers. How are you today? (Sitting next to him at the kitchen table.)*
Client: *Glad to see you, Maddie. Who would have thought a broken leg would give a body such trouble!* Laughs a little.
Nurse: *Well, it wasn't just a broken leg, you know. It was pretty severe. What's giving you trouble? (Good eye contact. Smiles.)*
Client: *I'm still having trouble negotiating around the house. The furniture and rugs are still in my way even though you helped us move them.* Sighs. *I'm just having trouble with those crutches.*
Nurse: *(After assessing client's ability to maneuver and making some suggestions.) There, that should work better, don't you think?*
Client: *Yes, that's fine. Could I ask you about something else?* Looks embarrassed but determined.
Nurse: *Sure. (Sitting quietly.)*
Client: *Um, I seem to be having some trouble in the bedroom.*
Nurse: *What kind of trouble? (Looks skeptical about this subject.)*
Client: *It's the positioning of this darned leg. It hurts when Aileen and I try to, uh, get close, and then she gets worried and I get annoyed and it all goes to heck!* Sounds frustrated.
Nurse: *Oh, I see. Let me tell you about a few things you might try to alleviate the pain that would work for you. (Settles in for a teaching session.)*
Client: *I don't know about trying anything new. We're pretty happy with the way we do it.* His turn to look skeptical.
Nurse: *Don't worry, these will work just fine. Other orthopedic clients have told me they were happy with the way things worked out. (Talks to him about two or three ways to alleviate pain and pressure on his leg during sex. Says she'll bring pamphlets on the subject next time.) What do you think? (Smiles brightly at him.)*
Client: *Well, I suppose they're worth a try. I'll let you know. Now, I wonder if you could take my pressure. I've felt it was a little high lately. (They go on to other subjects, both feeling vaguely unfinished.)*

Critical Thinking Challenges

• The client in both dialogues received the same information. Discern what was more effective about the first dialogue. • Distinguish what Maddie did the first time that made it effective for the client's sexual needs. • Analyze your thoughts about a couple in their sixties, seventies, or eighties having sex. • List effects pain has on a person's desire to have sex.

of problems as well as coping with problems that exist.

Sexual Abuse

Some people manifest altered sexual functioning by being sexually abusive to others, whether it be children, spouses, acquaintances, or unknown people. Sexual abuse results in sexual problems for the abused person as well.

Inhibited Sexual Desire

A lack of or inhibited sexual desire can be subjective. Because there is no "normal" for frequency of sexual relations, it is difficult to determine what frequency reflects a decreased or inhibited sexual desire. A key feature is when the person's partner is not satisfied with the frequency of sexual relations. Thus, relationships play an important role in discussing sexual dysfunctions. Often, inhibited sexual desire in one partner goes hand-in-hand with inhibited desire in the other partner, although it is more common for the desires of each partner to be incongruent, and hence it is viewed as a problem. Many factors contribute to inhibited sexual desire, among them physical factors such as taking certain medications, neurologic problems, hormonal imbalances, as well as psychological factors such as depression and interpersonal difficulties. Sometimes it is quite difficult to determine whether depression is a result of inhibited sexual desire or if it is, in fact, a cause of inhibited sexual desire and consequent marital problems. In addition, a history of sexual abuse or incest, pain with intercourse, or vaginismus may be factors leading to inhibited sexual desire.

Impotence

Impotence, the inability to attain or maintain an erection long enough to have satisfactory sexual intercourse, is troubling to a man. Most cultures highly value a man's "virility," and erectile dysfunction is a manifestation of his "failure to perform" as a man. Impotence can be primary or secondary. Primary impotence refers to a man who has never been able to achieve an erection necessary for intercourse; secondary impotence refers to a man who in the past has been successful in attaining and maintaining erection, but who has subsequently experienced difficulty in this area.

Causes of impotence, whether primary or secondary, can be physiologic, psychological, or a combination of both. Certain manifestations may indicate the probability that the problem is secondary to a physiologic factor or a psychological factor. For example, if a man is able to attain erection in certain sexual situations but not others, or if he has erections during sleep or has experienced periods in which he had no erection difficulties, the problem is probably the result of psychological factors. If erection is not possible in any of these situations, however, the problem is probably a physiologic one.

Ejaculatory Dysfunction

Premature Ejaculation. **Premature ejaculation** is a relatively recent phenomenon, according to Hogan (1985). This is not because the condition itself has occurred only recently, but because in the Victorian era, women predominantly viewed sex as something to endure; the sooner the sex act was over, the better. Today, however, with women desiring sexual satisfaction as well, it is often unacceptable if a man ejaculates early and does not allow for the woman to reach orgasm. Premature ejaculation is a relative definition, depending on the subjective responses of both partners, that is, whether both partners are satisfied. It is a condition in which the man is unable to maintain an erection long enough for satisfactory intercourse to occur. It is believed that premature ejaculation is caused by anxiety on the part of the man and fear of failure in the sex act.

Inability to Ejaculate. Inability to ejaculate actually refers to inability to ejaculate in the vagina. This condition is not as common as premature ejaculation. The cause of ejaculatory incompetence may be primary or secondary. Primary causes include psychological disturbances; secondary causes may be related to interpersonal problems with one's sexual partner, or organic causes such as lumbar sympathectomy or antiadrenergic drugs, such as guanethidine or methyldopa (Hogan, 1985).

Orgasmic Dysfunction

Difficulty achieving orgasm is common in women. Historically, orgasm was differentiated according to vaginal or clitoral orgasm, with vaginal orgasm considered to be the more mature, according to psychoanalytic thought. Masters and Johnson (1966) have found that this dichotomy is misleading, however, because orgasm occurs through vaginal or clitoral stimulation. In addition, it has been found that the Grafenberg spot, in the anterior portion of the vagina halfway between the vaginal opening and the cervix, is another area capable of stimulation to orgasm. Difficulty with attaining orgasm may be caused by lack of information, lack of adequate stimulation, or problems in an intimate relationship. Sometimes women feel pressure to have an orgasm to please their partners, and some partners feel pressure to "bring" their female partner to orgasm so that they will know they have been "successful" in the sex act. This kind of pressure may inhibit the woman's ability to attain an orgasm.

Dyspareunia

Dyspareunia, or painful intercourse, is thought to occur regularly in 1% to 2% of adult women (Masters, et al., 1988). These researchers estimate that 15% of adult women occasionally experience pain with intercourse. Dyspareunia is commonly caused by organic problems, including lack of adequate lubrication at the opening to the vagina or within the vaginal walls, usually because of inadequate sexual arousal, drugs (antihistamines, certain tranquilizers, marijuana, alcohol), or estrogen deficiency. In addition, vaginal infections may lead to painful penetration on intercourse. Barrier methods of contraception may be irritating to the vagina, causing painful intercourse. Pelvic diseases may also cause pain.

Vaginismus

Vaginismus is involuntary contraction of the muscles surrounding the vaginal orifice, such that penetration may be impossible and very painful. This is an uncommon condition, occurring in about 2% to 3% of women (Masters, et al., 1988). There usually is no concurrent anatomic abnormality, and rarely is there a physiologic abnormality, although these must be ruled out. Vaginismus usually is the result of psychological problems, namely fear of penetration due to a negative association with it, such as rape and sexual abuse, or fear of men or of sexual intercourse. The woman develops a conditioned reflex in certain situations (eg, attempted sexual intercourse or during a pelvic examination) in which her vaginal muscles involuntarily contract, precluding penetration.

Impact of Sexual Dysfunction on Activities of Daily Living

Because sexuality is integral to one's life, any sexual dysfunction can have a major impact on activities of daily living. This impact is felt on both an individual level and a family level.

Individual Considerations

Emotionally, one may suffer from a decrease in self-esteem and in self-confidence. The consequences are that a person may have less emotional energy to concentrate on important aspects of daily living, or may be slow and careless in accomplishing daily, routine tasks. Physically, although a person may function normally, one's view of the physical self may be adversely affected. In turn, one's view of one's psychological and emotional self can have profound negative effects.

Family Considerations

Sexual difficulties often lend themselves to interpersonal difficulties. An individual's altered sexual functioning likely does not occur in isolation. Often such alterations are correlated with interpersonal problems. In fact, some sexual difficulties may be symptoms of underlying problems within a marital relationship. On the other hand, marital difficulties may result from sexual dysfunction.

Assessment

Functional assessment involves the nurse collecting subjective and objective data regarding normal sexual function, risk factors for sexual dysfunction, and any present sexual dysfunction(s). Such an assessment is made by asking direct questions, observing nonverbal behavior, and evaluating information obtained through physical assessment and diagnostic and laboratory tests.

The content of the history is also important, although the technique and approach influence the content obtained. Hogan (1985) includes a thorough outline of important content to elicit in a sexual history. This outline is reproduced as an example of necessary information (Table 52-2); however, it is essential to point out that not all clients need to be questioned on all areas in this outline. The nurse must assess which areas are appropriate for the individual client with whom he or she is working.

Subjective Data

Subjective data are gathered through a careful nursing history. Although the data elicited in a sexual history are important, the approach used in eliciting the data is often equally, if not more, important. The process of interacting with a client around his or her sexual concerns provides an excellent opportunity for the nurse to put the client at ease, encourage the client to ventilate any pent-up feelings, and listen actively to any concerns the client may have. If a sexual history is approached in a humane, open manner, it can have therapeutic value as well as being a source for essential information. Nonverbal cues can be noticed as well.

The nurse should know the slang terms for sexual functions and organs (Hogan, 1985; Poorman, 1988). Some professionals believe that it is beneficial to use the client's terminology to communicate better; however, others believe that professionals should use formal terminology so clients know that the professional is, indeed, a professional. What is clear is that professionals should be sure they understand what their clients are saying, clients need to understand what the professionals are saying, and professionals should clarify terminology with the clients if they are not sure they are communicating correctly.

Table 52-2 • Data to be Collected by Nursing History for All Clients

Data	Significance of Data	Nursing History Question
Age	Identifies period in life cycle.	In what year were you born; month, day?
Sex	Each sex may react differently to life events. Highlight gender identity problems.	[Usually is evident by dress, otherwise. What sex do you consider yourself to be?
Education, occupation	Sexual practices may be related to education–socioeconomic class; change in occupation may contribute to role disturbances	How far did you go in school? What do you do for a living? What change has there been in your ability to do your job?
Significant others	Other sources of support, stable or otherwise.	What people do you consider most helpful right now? In what way? Are they available?
Quality of relationship with significant others	Relationship may be supportive, negative, or punitive, and these affect ability to cope with sexual problems.	Are there any differences in the way you get along with these people since you have been ill or hospitalized (or recently)?
Interests, hobbies	Indicates other support systems and avocational interests that contribute to self-esteem.	What do you do with your free time? What leisure and work activities are important to you? How are these being affected now?
Spiritual/religious/ philosophical beliefs	Sexual practices may be related to beliefs. Guilt may occur if religious beliefs are compromised. Conflict and anxiety may be experienced by client if different practices are suggested by nurse.	With what religious denomination are you affiliated? Can you describe any spiritual or other beliefs that are helpful to you now? Do you have or want the support of a clergyman (minister, priest, rabbi)?
Health problems, medical conditions. surgical procedures in the past and anticipated in the future; medication therapy	Some medical problems, surgical treatment, or medications result in sexual dysfunction (physiologic changes). Anxiety over outcome or change in body image may lead to functional problems.	What illness and/or surgery have you had in the past? Did they affect your usual way of living or work? Did they affect sexual function? Do you expect this illness/hospitalization will have effects on your usual way of living or work? In what ways? What medications do you take?
Changes in role relationships and ability to carry out the usual sexual role	Change in ability to carry out what is perceived as the usual sexual role may cause anxiety, depression, and sexual dysfunction.	What difference has there been in your functioning in the family? Describe. Can you do your usual tasks or jobs? Describe. Have there been any changes in your relationship with the way you get along) with others (male, female, significant others)?
Potential changes in ability to carry out usual sexual role	Expectations of problems may cause problems (self-fulfilling prophecy).	What changes do you expect after you get home (or in the future)?
Change in perception of self as male or female due to illness or life events	Anxiety and sexual dysfunction may result from threat to gender identity	How do you expect this illness (or life event) to affect how you see yourself as a man/woman?
Existing or potential sexual dysfunction	Elicits problems (sexual dysfunction).	Has there been or do you expect to have any changes in sexual functioning (sex life) because of (illness, life events)? Describe.

Note: Wording of the questions is changed depending on educational level of the client.
From Hogan, R. (1985). *Human sexuality: A nursing perspective* (2nd ed.) (pp. 162–163). New York: Appleton-Century-Crofts.

A technique in interacting with clients is to ask less sensitive questions initially, gradually progressing to more sensitive areas. For example, initial questions such as "When did you begin menstruating?" are much less threatening than such questions as "What is your sexual orientation?" or "How satisfied are you with your sex life?"

Functional Pattern Identification

Specific questions regarding the client's normal functional status will yield information about functional patterns. The nurse must approach the client in an open manner, asking open-ended, nonjudgmental questions. Some examples are: "How often do you masturbate?" instead of saying, "Do you ever masturbate?" The first question allows the person permission to state that he or she masturbates, whereas the second question may suggest a more judgmental attitude to a "yes" answer.

Assessment of the client's psychosocial status is part of the sexual history, but it is discussed separately to reinforce the importance of doing such an assessment. Often, assessing a problem with sexuality is highly subjective because it depends on the client's perspective on the problem or potential problem. For example, an assessment of inadequate frequency of sexual relations is meaningless unless it is placed within the context of the client's perceptions of what adequate frequency means to him or her. Psychosocial assessment includes the client's perception(s) of his or her sexuality. In addition, it includes an assessment on the part of the health-care provider, based on data elicited, of the client's psychosocial functioning. Outlook on life, social support, role relationships, and family functioning are all aspects of a psychosocial assessment.

Risk Identification

A careful history should reveal clues to the nurse about those clients at risk for altered sexual function.

Pregnancy, Infertility, and Abortion. Although pregnancy is usually a time of anticipation, that is not always the case. Unwanted pregnancies occur and can create many problems for the people involved. Although unwanted pregnancies are more common among adolescents, they can occur in adult years as well. In assessing the pregnant woman, the nurse needs to be careful not to let personal assumptions influence the assessment. The nurse should phrase questions to determine what the pregnancy means to this woman, how she feels about it, how her partner feels (if she has a partner), and what her plans are.

When a pregnancy is lost, either by miscarriage or voluntary termination, the nurse needs to assess the effect of the loss on the individual woman. In both voluntary and involuntary abortion, a sense of loss is usually present. Sensitive assessment will assist the client and nurse in planning the type of support from which the client can receive the greatest benefit.

The nurse should be particularly sensitive to the stress placed on infertile couples. Assessing the feelings of both spouses is essential; there may be guilt, self-blame, or other feelings that are present and affecting the situation. Inquiring about past illnesses, infections of the reproductive system, and previous nonterm pregnancies may provide useful assessment and counseling information.

Alterations in Gender Identification. For clients experiencing alterations in gender identification, the nurse needs to be tactful and discerning in assessment. Although the beginning nurse will not have many opportunities to work with these clients, it is useful to be aware of the assessment needs, including the client's feelings about self, how others regard the client, the treatments and medications, and other feelings that may be present in this situation.

Environment. Lack of privacy, especially that which occurs in acute and long-term care, is a concern. Sensitive assessment of the client's response to the environment is essential. Because acute-care settings involve relatively short stays, long-term care settings are where the nurse will particularly encounter and need to assess the effect of the environment on sexuality. Assessing the need for privacy for the client is a necessary part of nursing assessment in nursing homes and other long-term care settings.

Illness. Assessment of present illness, past illnesses, chronic conditions, and medications is an integral part of assessing sexuality. Illness may have created some constraints on sexual relations or on sexual performance. Attentive assessment by the nurse may reveal areas of previously unspoken concern that can be dealt with (Schover, 1988). Careful assessment may reveal misconceptions about the advisability of having sexual relations, as with clients with cardiac problems. Obtaining this information may assist the nurse and the client in planning further assessment or counseling.

If the illness the client is concerned about is a sexually transmitted disease, the nurse needs to do a diligent assessment of the person's feelings regarding the diagnosis, fears related to the consequences, and anxiety about future sexual relations. A nonjudgmental approach to assessment will support the client in clarifying and focusing on the aspects of greatest concern.

Surgery. Surgical procedures that relate to the reproductive organs often create sexual concern. Procedures such as prostate resection, mastectomy, and hysterectomy may initiate apprehension regarding sexuality, desire, disfigurement, and future sexual relations. Thoughtful questioning and listening as part of the assessment may alert the nurse to areas of anxiety as well as to misunderstandings.

Dysfunction Identification

Dysfunctional patterns can be identified as those significantly different from the client's or couple's normal patterns, such as a difference in desires for frequency of sexual intercourse, lack of interest, or anger, which may indicate an underlying problem. If a problem is detected, an approach to discovering important data regarding that problem is suggested by Annon (1976), and includes eliciting information in several areas. These areas include a description of the current problem, the onset and course of the problem, the client's perception of what has caused the problem and what prevents the problem from being alleviated, any past treatment and the outcome of that treatment, whether it was medical, professional, or self-treatment, and the client's current expectations and goals of treatment.

Objective Data

Objective data consist of information elicited from physical examination and from diagnostic tests and procedures. This combination yields data important in the nurse's overall functional assessment.

Physical Assessment

A thorough physical examination is important. It should include a complete, systematic, head-to-toe examination, with specific focus on the genital organs or any infectious process that might be a result of sexual activity or might impair sexual activity. Privacy should be provided and careful draping used. Instruments should be warm. Gloves must be worn during physical examination of the genitals.

Physical examination includes inspection and palpation, as described in Chapter 21. The role of the nurse in examination of the genitals varies with nursing preparation and the type of healthcare facility. The nurse may perform the assessment or assist another clinician.

Examination of Male Genitalia. The nurse helps the male client into a position for examination of the penis, scrotum, and testicles. A side-lying position with the knees bent exposes the genitals for examination. Genitals are inspected and palpated. Distribution of hair in the area is observed.

Careful attention to any skin masses, lesions on the skin, discharge from the penis, or anal/rectal abnormalities is essential. Attention to absence or atrophy of the testicles and the presence of the foreskin or of circumcision is also important. The location of the urethra will indicate whether or not hypospadias exists; hypospadias is an abnormal congenital opening of the urethra on the undersurface of the penis rather than the center of the glans penis. Male breasts are observed for deviations from normal. Although rare, breast cancer can occur in men.

> **Safety Alert**
> *Gynecologic Examinations*
>
> - Use sterile equipment for gynecologic examinations to avoid introducing organisms into the vagina.
> - Always wash hands and wear gloves when assessing or performing hygiene in the perineal area. This limits the spread of organisms from the nurse to the client and from the client to the nurse.
> - Handle equipment or dressings used in the perineal region appropriately. Limit the spread of contact with body substances.

Examination of Female Genitalia. The female client is helped into the lithotomy position. The nurse ensures that the client is comfortable. External genitalia are inspected for normal and abnormal characteristics, including hair distribution and development of the genitals.

A complete pelvic examination is necessary, and includes checking for pelvic masses, pelvic tenderness, vaginal discharge, other signs of infection, and vaginal or vulvar lesions. The pelvic examination is conducted in two parts: a speculum examination and bimanual palpation. The speculum examination views the vagina and cervix. The speculum is a two-bladed instrument that, after its insertion in the vagina, is expanded for viewing. It is helpful if the client relaxes to minimize discomfort. The speculum should be warmed before insertion. Samples and smears for culture are taken while the speculum is in place. As the speculum is withdrawn, the clinician views the vaginal walls.

In bimanual palpation, the clinician places the index and middle fingers of one hand into the vagina, while placing the other hand on the lower abdomen. The cervix, ovaries, and uterus are palpated by this method.

A breast examination is included with the assessment of the reproductive organs. The breast examination is discussed in Chapter 21 and illustrated in Figure 21-21. The clinician checks for size, symmetry, contour, color, lesions, and nipple discharge. This is also a good time to teach the woman how to do a breast self-examination, which is discussed in the section on Nursing Interventions to Promote Health and Function in this chapter.

Table 52-3 • Diagnostic Tests and Procedures of the Reproductive Systems

Test/Procedure	Description
VDRL (Venereal Disease Research Laboratories)	Blood test to detect syphilis ♂ ♀
Chlamydia culture	Cervical culture to detect *Chlamydia*
Gonorrhea culture	Cervical culture to detect gonorrhea
Wet preparation (KOH—potassium hydroxide) (NS—normal saline)	Slide preparation from vaginal secretions to detect *Candida, (Monilia), Gardnerella, Trichomonas* ♀
Pap smear	Slide preparation from endocervical secretions to detect cellular changes in cervix, cervical cancer ♀

Diagnostic Tests and Procedures

In conjunction with the physical examination, certain diagnostic tests are often performed. Blood work to detect anemia or infection may routinely be ordered. Cultures to detect sexually transmitted diseases such as gonorrhea or chlamydial infection may be indicated. For women, a Pap smear would probably be done if one had not been done within the past 6 months to 1 year. Depending on the nature of the problem or potential problem, certain other tests may be performed at the discretion of the healthcare provider. A summary of various diagnostic tests and procedures is given in Table 52-3.

Nursing Diagnoses

The North American Nursing Diagnosis Association (NANDA)-approved nursing diagnoses in the area of sexuality are Sexual Dysfunction and Altered Sexuality Patterns. Also included in this pattern is Rape-Trauma Syndrome, although this diagnosis will not be discussed in this chapter because it is beyond the scope of the information presented here. The nurse uses data from the assessment of sexual function to determine the presence of or risk for any of these alterations in normal sexual functioning.

Diagnostic Statement: Sexual Dysfunction

Definition

Sexual Dysfunction is the state in which an individual experiences a change in sexual function that is viewed as unsatisfying, unrewarding, or inadequate (NANDA, 1994). The definition of Sexual Dysfunction is subjective in that how one person perceives the degree of satisfaction in their sexual life may be different from how another person perceives such satisfaction. In other words, this diagnosis depends on the assessment made by the individual.

Defining Characteristics

The defining characteristics that contribute to this diagnosis are found mostly in the client's verbalization of the problem. For example, a client may verbalize that he or she is experiencing a change in fulfilling his or her perceived sex role. The client may perceive limitations imposed by disease or therapy, conflicts involving values, alteration in achieving sexual satisfaction, inability to achieve desired satisfaction, or alteration in relationship with significant other. In addition, the client may seek confirmation of his or her desirability and may experience a change of interest in self and others (NANDA, 1994). These defining characteristics reflect the subjective nature of this diagnosis. These defining characteristics also reflect the importance of thorough and sensitive history-taking on the part of the nurse to elicit these perceptions, which often are difficult to verbalize.

Related Factors

Several factors may be the cause of or may contribute to sexual dysfunction. Any change in sexuality, whether it be a biologic, a psychological, or a sociologic change, may lead to sexual dysfunction. For example, recent surgery, pregnancy, childbirth, drug use, disease process, trauma, radiation, and anomalies can be contributing factors. Ineffectual or absent role models may contribute, as well as physical and psychosocial abuse. Such abuse indicates the presence of harmful relationships, which can lead to vulnerability, values conflict, lack of privacy, and lack of a reliable significant other. Misinformation or lack of knowledge also contributes to sexual dysfunction (NANDA, 1994). All of these related factors either contribute to or are influenced by sexual dysfunction in an individual or couple.

Nursing Research
Sexuality

Selected Nursing Research Studies

Barclay, L., Bond, M., & Clark, M. (1992). Development of an instrument to study the sexual relationship of partners during pregnancy. *Australian Journal of Advanced Nursing, 10*(2), 14–21.

Kau, M. (1991). Sexual behaviour and knowledge of adolescent males in the Molop region of Bophuthatswana. *Curatonia: South African Journal of Nursing, 14*(1), 37–40.

Smook, K. (1992). Nurses' attitudes towards the sexuality of older people: An investigative study. *Nursing Practice, 6*(1), 15–17.

Wall-Haas, C. L. (1991). Nurses' attitudes toward sexuality in adolescent patients. *Pediatric Nursing, 17*(6), 549–547.

Wilson, P. S., & Dibble, S. L. (1993). Rehabilitation nurses' knowledge of and attitudes toward sexuality. *Rehabilitation Nursing Research, 2*(2), 69–74.

Possible Topics for Nursing Inquiry

- What are cultural indicators of sexual activity among adolescents?
- How does the sexual health concept of a specific ethnic group affect compliance with treatment programs?
- What factors have a relationship with access to sexual health information and education?

Diagnostic Statement: Altered Sexuality Patterns

Definition

Altered Sexuality Patterns is the state in which an individual expresses concern regarding his or her sexuality (NANDA, 1994). Similar to Sexual Dysfunction, this diagnosis is also very subjective, depending on the person's own self-perception. One person's sexual concerns may be very different from another person's sexual concerns, making it difficult to determine objective data to define this pattern. Again, it is essential that the nurse interact sensitively in obtaining a sexual history to elicit Altered Sexuality Patterns.

Defining Characteristics

The major point in determining defining characteristics is that these are "reported" difficulties, again emphasizing the subjective nature of the diagnosis. These reports are best elicited through sensitive history-taking. These reported difficulties include any limitations or changes in sexual behaviors or activities (NANDA, 1994).

Related Factors

Similar to the diagnosis of Sexual Dysfunction, the related factors for the diagnosis of Altered Sexuality Patterns include those that both contribute to and result from the actual diagnosis, or pattern. Such factors include lack of knowledge or skills regarding alternative responses to health-related transitions, meaning that often clients do not have the knowledge or the skill to respond to transitions in their own health in other ways (ie, in ways that are not necessarily disruptive to their sexual lives). These health-related transitions are brought on by changes in body function or structure, illness, or certain medical diagnoses. Additional contributing factors are lack of privacy, which may lead to disruptions in sexual life; lack of a significant other (or impaired relationship with a significant other), which leads to lack of sexual activity with another person; ineffective or absent role models, which leads to difficulty in making sexual decisions; conflicts with sexual orientation, leading to conflicts in sexuality; and fear of potential consequences of sexual activity, including pregnancy and sexually transmitted diseases (NANDA, 1994).

Related Nursing Diagnoses

Other diagnoses may be relevant to clients with sexual difficulties. Such diagnoses are Altered Family Processes, Rape-Trauma Syndrome, Altered Role Performance, Ineffective Individual or Family Coping, and Spiritual Distress.

Outcome Identification and Planning

After the nursing diagnoses and related factors are identified, client goals and nursing interventions are planned. Common goals for the client or couple with sexual dysfunction should be individualized, depending on client assessment. General goals for most clients include:

The client/couple will recognize symptoms of sexual dysfunction.

The client/couple will decrease symptoms of altered sexual functioning.

The client/couple will express satisfaction with level of sexual functioning.

Planning will evolve around the client's motivation to be healthy. The nurse uses educational interventions to teach about self-care and responsible sex. Examples of nursing interventions commonly used in caring for clients with sexuality needs are listed in the accompanying display and discussed in the next section of this chapter.

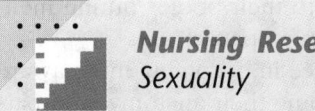

Planning
Examples of Nursing Interventions Used in Common Problems With Sexuality

- Explore feelings and fears related to sexuality.
- Discuss the client's expectations in regard to sexuality.
- Assist the client in becoming more aware of own body.
- Teach self-examination techniques.
- Encourage sex education and responsible sex.
- Promote open communication between the client and partner.
- Support appropriate counseling for the client or partner.

Implementation

The nurse plays a key role in assisting clients with any of the diagnoses listed earlier. At times, however, the nurse may need to refer clients to other healthcare providers, for example if a major sexual dysfunction is noted.

Nursing Interventions to Promote Health and Function

Concerns about sexual issues may or may not be obvious to the nurse. Clients may enter the healthcare system for a primary problem unrelated to sexuality. Nurses must put clients at ease, develop rapport, and allow clients to discuss any issues of concern.

Client Teaching

Anticipatory guidance is a major role of the nurse. Nurses assist clients in anticipating outcomes and consequences, as well as helping them to devise plans to cope with or manage such outcomes and consequences (Fig. 52-6).

Self-Awareness. Nurses can assist people in becoming more aware of their bodies and how their bodies function. Exploring and understanding the body are essential in assisting both men and women to achieve healthy sexual relationships. Women need assistance in understanding their anatomy. The use of a mirror during a pelvic examination is one way of beginning this process; a second way is encouraging women to examine themselves with a mirror. Understanding the anatomy of their genitals may help women understand how their bodies respond to sexual stimulation and what helps them to achieve orgasm. Women need to understand what happens to their bodies during menstruation, pregnancy, and menopause.

Men also need assistance in becoming more aware of their bodies. Understanding their anatomy, and particularly what kind of stimulation causes them to have an erection, will assist them in developing healthy sexual relationships.

Self-Examination. As part of developing awareness of their own bodies, men and women need assistance in learning techniques of self-examination. Men should be taught to perform testicular self-examination and women to perform breast self-examination, as illustrated in the accompanying displays.

Kegel Exercises. Self-awareness for the woman also involves control of the muscle of the pelvic floor. The nurse can teach the simple steps necessary during assessment or in a teaching situation. The exercises involve contraction and release of the pubococcygeus muscle, which is contracted when one prevents urine flow or a bowel movement. Muscles always work better when they are in good shape. Muscle tone can be restored in about 6 weeks of regular practice of the Kegel exercises. Benefits of Kegel exercises are increased vaginal lubrication during sexual arousal, enhanced sexual excitement, stronger gripping of the base of the penis, more rapid postpartum recovery of the pelvic floor muscles, increased flexibility of episiotomy scars, and relief of constipation (May & Mahlmeister, 1994). Kegel exercises are also used in bladder training. Steps of the Kegel exercises are listed in the accompanying display.

Sex Education. Parents of preschool children need guidance in becoming comfortable answering questions, as well as in volunteering information that may not have been directly asked for by their children. Dur-

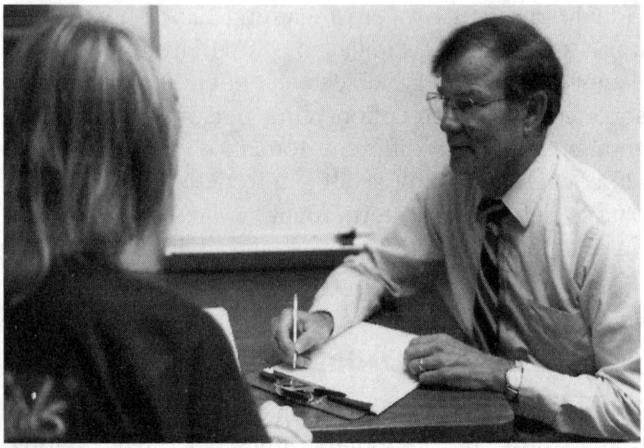

Figure 52-6 • *School or clinic nurses help young people understand the consequences of their sexual activities. (Courtesy of Overlake Hospital Medical Center, Bellevue, WA.)*

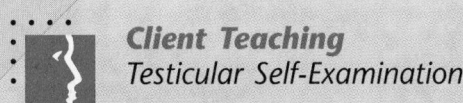

Client Teaching
Testicular Self-Examination

What Can I Do?

Your best hope for early detection of testicular cancer is a simple 3-minute monthly self-examination. The best time is after a warm bath or shower, when the scrotal skin is most relaxed.

Roll each testicle gently between the thumb and fingers of both hands. If you find any hard lumps or nodules, you should see your doctor promptly. They may not be malignant, but only your doctor can make the diagnosis.

After a thorough physical examination, your doctor may perform certain x-ray studies to make the most accurate diagnosis possible.

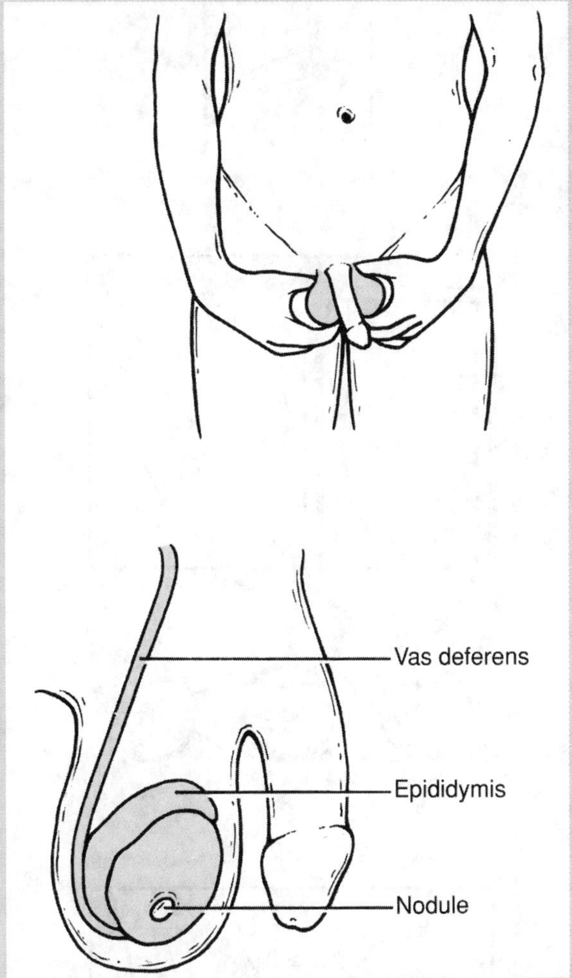

ing adolescence, both the adolescent and the parents need guidance. Adolescents need reassurance that their confusing and conflicting feelings are often normal, and they need to be treated with patience as they vacillate between wanting to be taken care of and wanting to assert their independence. Parents need assistance in dealing with the mood swings and unpredictability of their adolescents. They need reassurance and support regarding their approach to their adolescent children. In addition, parents need help in maintaining their own intimate relationship with one another during a turbulent time, one that often points out their own aging as their children are growing older.

Responsible Sex. Teaching men and women to participate in responsible sex is important. Specifically, advising limiting the number of sexual partners and advising the use of condoms in a nonmonogamous relationship are very important. If the nurse can present, in a nonjudgmental manner, the importance of limiting sexual contacts, he or she should do so. If such a discussion is going to defeat the purpose of the counseling or teaching session, however, the importance of hygiene and condom use must be stressed. Condoms should always be used in nonmonogamous relationships and male homosexual relationships, and in other relationships that have the potential for AIDS transmission. Much has been said in the media about "safe sex," and the nurse should build on this groundwork. Potential sexual partners need to be encouraged to talk openly with one another about how to have safer sex, and to be honest with one another about any history of sexually transmitted diseases.

As part of responsible sex teaching, the nurse teaches clients about the prevention of sexually transmitted diseases. Some sexually transmitted diseases are easily treatable, whereas others are not (eg, herpes). Currently, AIDS is considered incurable and ultimately fatal. The importance of teaching about prevention of sexually transmitted diseases cannot be overemphasized.

Contraceptive Use

Decisions regarding family size and spacing are possible largely because of the variety of birth control methods available. Child spacing, limitation of family size, and timing of the first birth are recognized as preventive health measures (May & Mahlmeister, 1994). Health measures must be addressed especially in the adolescent, because of the rise in adolescent pregnancy and births (see Fig. 52-6).

Men and women need to become aware of various contraceptive methods available to them. It is the nurse's responsibility to be familiar with the various contraceptive methods: their advantages and disadvantages, contraindications, effectiveness, safety, and cost. The best method is the one the couple decides is most comfortable for them to use and will use consistently and correctly.

No perfect contraceptive method exists, but there are several good methods, each with advantages and disadvantages. It is beyond the scope of this text to dis-

Client Teaching
Breast Self-Examination

Why Do The Breast Self-Exam?

There are many good reasons for doing the breast self-exam (BSE) each month. One reason is that breast cancer is most easily treated and cured when it is found early. Another is that if you do BSE every month, it will increase your skill and confidence when doing the exam. When you get to know how your breasts normally feel, you will quickly be able to feel any change. Another reason is that it is easy to do.

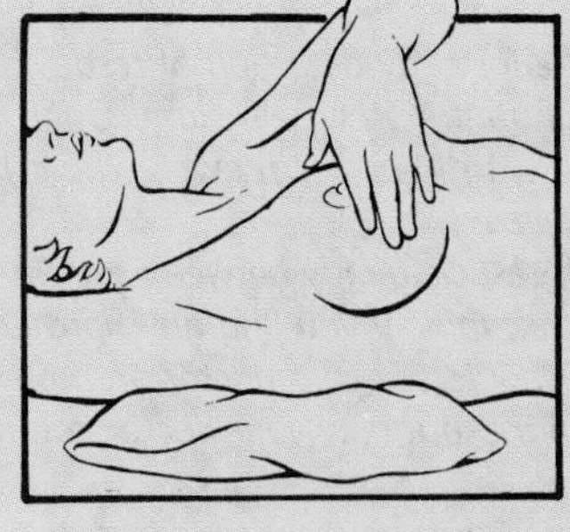

When To Do BSE

The best time to do BSE is about a week after your period, when breasts are not tender or swollen. If you do not have regular periods or sometimes skip a month, do BSE on the same day every month.

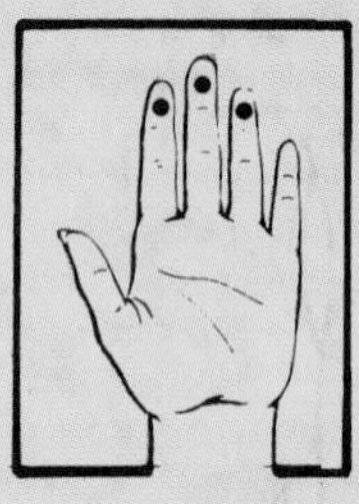

Now, How To Do BSE

1. *Lie down and put a pillow under your right shoulder. Place your right arm behind your head.*
2. *Use the finger pads of your three middle fingers on your left hand to feel for lumps or thickening. Your finger pads are the top third of each finger.*
3. *Press firmly enough to know how your breast feels. If you're not sure how hard to press, ask your health-care provider, or try to copy the way your healthcare provider uses the finger pads during a breast exam. Learn what your breast feels like most of the time. A firm ridge in the lower curve of each breast is normal.*
4. *Move around the breast in a set way. You can choose either the circle (A), the up-and-down line (B), or the wedge (C). Do it the same way every time. It will help you make sure that you've gone over the entire breast area and to remember how your breast feels each month.*
5. *Now examine your left breast using right hand finger pads.*
6. *If you find any changes, see your doctor right away.*

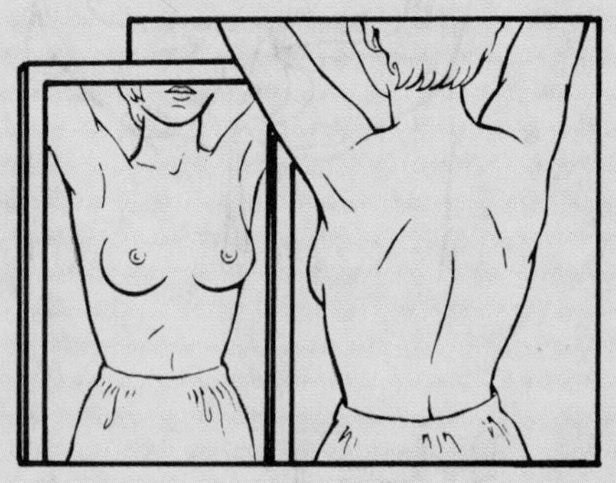

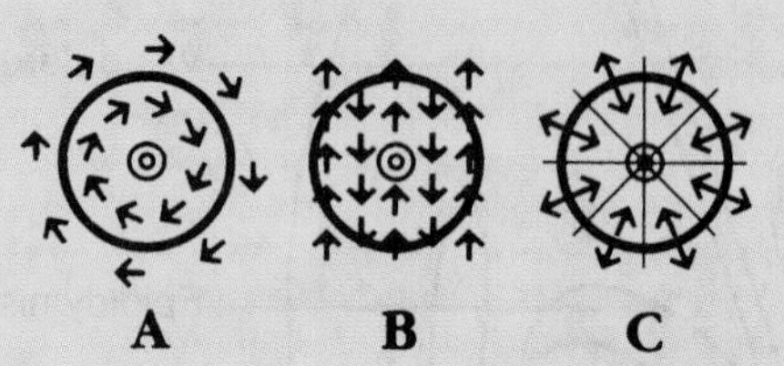

For Added Safety

You might want to check your breasts while standing in front of a mirror right after you do your BSE each month. See if there are any changes in the way your breasts look: dimpling of the skin, changes in the nipple, or redness or swelling. You might also want to do an extra BSE while you're in the shower. Your soapy hands will glide over the wet skin, making it easy to check how your breasts feel.

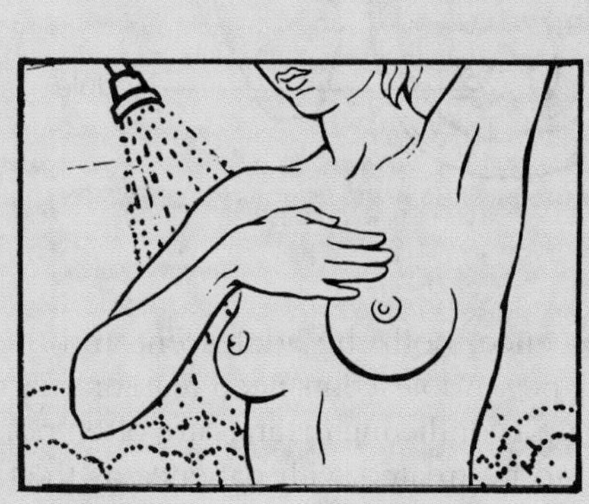

***Remember:** BSE could save your breast—and save your life. Most breast lumps are found by women themselves, but, in fact, most lumps in the breast are not cancer. Be safe, be sure.*

Client Teaching
Kegel Exercises

1. *Locate the muscles surrounding the vagina by sitting on the toilet and starting and stopping the flow of urine.*
2. *Test the baseline strength of the muscles by inserting a finger in the opening of the vagina and contracting the muscles.*
3. *Exercise A—Squeeze the muscles together and hold the squeeze for 3 seconds. Relax the muscles. Repeat.*
4. *Exercise B—Contract and relax the muscles as rapidly as possible 10 to 25 times. Repeat.*
5. *Exercise C—Imagine sitting in a pan of water and sucking water into the vagina. Hold for 3 seconds.*
6. *Exercise D—Push out as during a bowel movement, only with the vagina. Hold for 3 seconds.*
7. *Repeat exercises A, C, and D 10 times each, and exercise B once. Repeat the entire series three times a day.*

From May, K. L, & Mahlmeister, L. R. (1994). *Comprehensive maternity nursing: Nursing process and the childbearing family* (3rd ed.). Philadelphia: J. B. Lippincott.

cuss them in detail, but they are summarized in the accompanying display and in the following sections.

Natural Family Planning. Fertility awareness is used in natural family planning. Currently there are four methods available, all using some period of abstinence (periodic abstinence). The *calendar rhythm* method uses calculations of menstrual cycles and fertile and infertile periods. The *temperature* method uses the rise in basal body temperature to determine ovulation. The *cervical mucus* method involves training the woman by a professional in the differentiation of dryness, moistness, and wetness at the vaginal introitus, and differentiation of types of mucus. The *symptothermal* method combines the other techniques. These methods are acceptable to couples who follow the tenets of certain religions. Disadvantages are that the methods require motivation, time, keeping consistent daily records, and abstinence for long periods of time. Miscalculations can occur in any of the methods, and they do not allow for spontaneous sex.

Hormonal Methods. Hormonal methods provide the most effective birth control (after surgery), and they are easy to use. They use estrogen and progestin in various combinations, and are introduced by various means into the female body. Oral contraceptives ("the pill") are the most commonly used, despite years of controversy about them. Mini-pills and postcoital pills are also used. Oral contraceptives and mini-pills are taken daily. Postcoital pills are used "the day after" coitus. After being used in Europe for years, a progestin implant was accepted and introduced to the United States in 1991. Capsules are inserted under the skin of the forearm, and are effective for 5 years. Hormonal methods allow for spontaneous sex and less stress and anxiety. There are side effects to these methods, and they can become expensive if used for a lengthy period of time. For those women taking daily pills, remembering to take each pill is critical to the success of the method.

Intrauterine Devices. Intrauterine devices (IUDs) are also controversial. Some IUDs were taken off the market in the 1970s and 1980s. Two remain: Progestasert and ParaGard (Copper T). In this contraceptive method, a small device is inserted in the uterine cavity, where it remains until removed by a healthcare worker. The exact mechanics for contraception are not clearly understood. Women who use the IUD must be carefully screened, because there are a number of contraindications. Women who use the IUD must learn danger signals to report to their healthcare worker. Infection and ectopic pregnancy are the major considerations.

Barrier Methods. Chemical and mechanical barriers are popular with women who cannot or prefer not to use the pill or IUD. Barrier methods are readily available, and some can be bought over the counter. Mechanical barriers include diaphragms, cervical caps, and condoms. Diaphragms and cervical caps are prescribed and fitted by a professional; both fit over the cervix. The diaphragm must be used with spermicide. In both cases, the woman has to learn correct insertion meth-

Client Teaching
Human Sexuality

Instruct the client as follows:

- *Use condoms to help prevent AIDS and other sexually transmitted diseases.*
- *Do not use a condom more than once because there is danger of spillage of semen.*
- *Seek professional help if you have unusual pain or bleeding from any sexual activity. Only a healthcare provider can determine the cause.*
- *Consult with a healthcare provider if medications interfere with sexual functioning. Do not stop the medication on your own; different treatment may be necessary.*
- *Perform regular breast or testicular self-examinations.*
- *Discuss safe sex with your partner.*
- *Learn all you can about your body and how it functions.*
- *Discuss sexual concerns with your partner and a healthcare provider.*

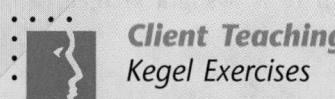

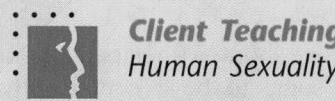

Contraceptive Methods

- Abstinence
- Coitus interruptus (withdrawal)
- Natural family planning
- Hormonal methods
- Intrauterine devices (IUDs)
- Mechanical barriers: diaphragm, cervical cap, condom
- Chemical barriers: foam, cream, jelly, suppositories
- Elective abortion
- Surgical sterilization

ods and must plan ahead for sexual encounters, because the devices must be inserted before intercourse. Both seem to be highly effective. Their use may result in discomfort to one or both partners. Infection, including toxic shock syndrome, is among the side effects.

The major form of male birth control is the condom, which ranks in popularity second only to the pill as a contraceptive method. The ability to block sexually transmitted diseases is an advantage of this method.

Foams, creams, jellies, and suppositories are chemical barriers. These vaginal spermicides act in two ways, blocking and killing sperm. Chemical barriers are bought without prescription and have few, if any side effects; that is their advantage. However, there is some question regarding possible harm to an already implanted embryo.

Elective Abortion. Elective abortion (therapeutic abortion) is considered by some to be a contraceptive method, although this remains controversial. There are several methods for performing an abortion. The rate of complications, such as infection, bleeding, and uterine or cervical trauma may be extremely high in illegal abortions.

Coitus Interruptus. Coitus interruptus, withdrawal of the penis just before ejaculation, has been used for centuries. Although no expense is involved in its use and there are no medical side effects, the effectiveness is not high because of difficulty in using the method.

Surgical Sterilization. Surgical sterilization may be done for both men and women. Female sterilization includes tubal ligation (cutting and tying of the fallopian tubes so ova cannot pass through) and tubal cauterization (cauterizing or burning the tubes so that ova cannot pass through). Vasectomy is the male form of surgical sterilization. Vasectomy involves cutting the vas deferens, preventing sperm from being ejaculated in the semen. Although both male and female sterilization are considered permanent, there is a slight chance of reversing each.

Nursing Interventions for Altered Function

A holistic approach addresses both physical and psychological issues related to sexual dysfunction. Each client must be aided in living as full a life as possible, even in the presence of dysfunctions. This is accomplished through counseling and educating regarding a specific problem area, treating a specific problem if appropriate, promoting activities of daily living, referral to appropriate resources, and home management.

Levels of Activities of Daily Living

One of the nurse's responsibilities is to assist clients in achieving and maintaining a level of daily living that reaches their potential. Nurses can be instrumental in suggesting ways of improving clients' levels of activities of daily living despite their sexual dysfunction. For example, nurses play a key role in counseling older adults regarding sexuality and the fact that it is possible for older adults to maintain an active sex life. The nurse gives guidance on modifications, such as using lubricants to counteract the effect of decreased lubrication in women, and to engage in more foreplay to allow more stimulation of the man so that he can more easily have an erection. Also, older adults can be helped to discover alternative forms of sexual expression such as physical closeness and caressing, in addition to sexual intercourse (see Fig. 52-5).

Counseling

When treating a person with a nursing diagnosis of Sexual Dysfunction, the nurse should direct his or her intervention toward educating and counseling the client and his or her partner regarding various patterns of human sexual response. By talking with the client and allowing the client to describe and ventilate his or her feelings, the nurse will have a clearer sense of the client's perspective on the sexual dysfunction. In this way, the nurse will discover what the dysfunction means to the client and how the client is responding to it, enabling the nurse to develop interventions that are individualized for that client.

The PLISSIT Model. One specific technique that nurses can use in working with clients with altered sexual functioning is the PLISSIT Model. The PLISSIT Model was developed by Annon (1976), and is based on learning principles. The acronym stands for the following:

P = permission-giving, LI = limited information, SS = specific suggestions, and IT = intensive therapy.

Using this approach, nurses begin with nonthreatening actions: permission-giving and limited information. If the client continues to need further therapy or has more serious problems, specific suggestions will be recommended, and, possibly, intensive therapy will be warranted. The belief, according to this model, is that many sexual problems are a result of lack of education, and, therefore, applying learning principles may help alleviate many sexual problems. Table 52-4 gives the principles of the PLISSIT model with examples of how it may be used.

Referral

Nurses may refer clients for further counseling if they deem that to be appropriate. In addition, nurses may refer clients to organizations that educate and provide support to people regarding sexuality.

Community-Based Nursing

Much of the nurse's work with clients suffering from sexual dysfunction involves ambulatory settings or, if clients are hospitalized, assisting clients in preparing for discharge.

Discharge Planning

Questions regarding sexual functioning are common as clients prepare to return home. Such questions may be common after birth, cesarean section, hysterectomy, or other surgery. The nurse should be prepared to give guidance in such sexual matters. Clients may be referred for group therapy in instances that seem appropriate.

Home visits by nurses may be appropriate to assess how well the client is doing. Nurses can reinforce specific treatment protocols that may have been prescribed for clients. In addition, nurses can assess how well clients are after the treatment protocols, and can

Table 52-4 • Principles of the PLISSIT Model* With Examples

Acronym	Definition	Example
P =	Permission-giving (allowing client to say what is on his/her mind without value judgments communicated by nurse.)	The client says, "I need to practice birth control. Too many pregnancies are tiring me out physically and emotionally. But I'm not sure if birth control is right." The nurse may reply, "Some people practice birth control, while others choose not to. It is an individual choice."
LI =	Limited Information (giving/providing the client with information, but not too much information that would be overwhelming.)	After further questions, the nurse says, "A variety of contraceptives exist, each having advantages and disadvantages. People choose contraceptives that are best for their personal situation."
SS =	Specific Suggestions (giving specific advice to the client in an attempt to solve the client's problems or alleviate concerns/worries.)	The nurse gives specific information regarding a variety of contraceptives: advantages, disadvantages, contraindications, side effects, effectiveness, cost, and procedures for each.
IT =	Intensive Therapy (providing more in-depth, perhaps long-term treatment, if problems are not solved with specific suggestions.)	If the client has had several (planned or unplanned) abortions, she may need intensive, professional help related to using a specific contraceptive; dealing with grief, guilt, self-blame, or other emotional results; fitting for a specific method.

*The PLISSIT Model provides an organized approach to the client, based on teaching–learning principles.

Nursing Plan of Care
The Client With Sexual Dysfunction

Nursing Diagnosis

Sexual Dysfunction related to inability to conceive as manifested by altered sexual satisfaction.

Client Goal

The client/couple will restore normal sexual functioning.

Client Outcome Criteria

- Client/couple verbalizes increased satisfaction in sexual relationship within 3 months of treatment, as measured by their self-evaluation.
- Client/couple verbalizes to healthcare provider that they are more relaxed and feeling better within 6 months.

Nursing Intervention	*Scientific Rationale*
1. Encourage client and partner to discuss their current patterns of sexual behaviors, with acknowledgment by the nurse that the client's complaints are understandable	1. If the partners are able to discuss their current patterns of sexual behavior and these patterns are acknowledged by the nurse as normal, the couple may feel more relaxed and less concerned about their new sexual patterns.
2. Suggest possible ways for the couple to attain and maintain a close physical relationship even without sexual intercourse if they are uncomfortable with it.	2. If permission is given to have close physical contact without sexual intercourse, the couple may feel more relaxed and less pressured to have unspontaneous sexual intercourse.
3. Give couple permission to "take a vacation" from infertility at times in an effort to restore their previous sexual relationship.	3. Permission to take a vacation from infertility may help restore some spontaneity into their sexual relationship.

answer any questions that clients may have regarding the treatment. Most important, the nurse serves as a supportive person with whom the client can develop a trusting relationship. When clients are being followed for sexual problems, many personal issues often are raised as well, and the supportive presence of the nurse is important for the client's well-being.

Ambulatory Settings

Education is a prominent nursing role related to sexuality issues. Such teaching can take place in a variety of settings. The school, walk-in clinics, a family planning office, and the mall are examples of settings in which the nurse may be involved in discussing sexual issues. Teaching may be as simple as creating wall posters, as informal as a one-to-one counseling session, or as formal as a video presentation.

The nurse may function independently, particularly in the area of anticipatory guidance.

The nurse must be nonjudgmental, allowing clients to ventilate their feelings, concerns, and fears. Rapport, truth, and respect should be the characteristics of such teaching. Often, nurses can clear up misconceptions and dispel myths that may be interfering with a person's sexual relationship or acceptance of his or her own sexuality.

Clients may approach the nurse for information and counseling regarding family planning; therefore, the nurse needs a working knowledge of family planning and contraceptives. Some nurses may work in family planning clinics, where their major responsibility is assistance in family planning and contraceptive methods. The adolescent may approach the school nurse for counseling. Sex education needs to be encouraged by nurses. It is also appropriate for nurses to become involved at the community level. By supporting and encouraging sex education in the schools, nursing is taking a stance in support of educating people about their own bodies and sexuality.

Evaluation

Specific outcome criteria are used to evaluate attainment of client goals related to sexuality. These criteria may be different from criteria related to ordinary physiologic problems, in that the nurse can observe results in many physiologic problems, but in most instances relies on the client/couple's verbal report of goal achievement in sexuality. Examples of possible outcome criteria for sexuality are listed here. Criteria may be similar because there is some overlap in goals.

Goal

The client/couple will recognize symptoms of sexual dysfunction.

Possible Outcome Criteria

- Client describes male and female reproductive anatomy after next teaching session with the nurse.
- Within 6 months, client/couple describes normal sexual functioning to nurse, as learned in teaching session.
- Client identifies specific symptom experiences, including etiology and treatment, as client talks with nurse in next 6 months.

Goal

The client will have decreased symptoms of altered sexual functioning.

Possible Outcome Criteria

- Within 6 months, client verbalizes to nurse that symptoms are decreasing.
- Within 1 year, client and partner report satisfaction with sexual relationship.

Goal

The client/couple will express satisfaction with level of sexual functioning.

Possible Outcome Criteria

- Within 6 months, client states success in using alternate method of sexual functioning.
- Within 6 months, client reports satisfaction with level of sexual functioning.
- Within 1 year, client's partner reports satisfaction with level of sexual relationship.

Key Concepts

- Nurses require a valid understanding of the reproductive system, sexuality, and sexual orientation, because sexual health is a holistic approach to human health.
- Sexuality includes function of the sexual organs, individual perceptions of functioning, sexual expression, and preferences.
- Sexual activity is highly individual, with wide variation in expression.
- Reproduction depends on the establishment of the menstrual cycle in women and spermatozoa production and motility in men.
- Sexual orientation may be heterosexual, homosexual, or bisexual.
- Human sexuality appears in a variety of forms across the lifespan.
- Factors affecting normal sexual function include health maintenance; roles and relationships; cognition and perception; culture, values, and beliefs; self-concept; coping and stress tolerance; and previous experience.
- Sexual function may be altered by pregnancy, infertility, and abortion; altered gender identification; environment; illness; surgery; or medications.
- Altered sexuality may be manifested by sexual abuse; inhibited sexual desire; impotence; ejaculatory dysfunction; orgasmic dysfunction; dyspareunia; or vaginismus.
- Functional assessment by the nurse includes subjective and objective data regarding normal sexual function, risk factors, and sexual dysfunction.
- Teaching includes self-awareness, self-examination, Kegel exercises, sex education in general, responsible (safe) sex, and contraceptive use.
- Nursing interventions for altered function include guidance in increasing levels of activities of daily living, ensuring privacy, counseling, and referral as necessary.
- The nurse functions independently in areas of teaching and anticipatory guidance, and refers clients with major sexual dysfunction to specialists.

Critical Thinking Challenges

Sexuality is one of the basic human needs and an important function of the individual. Now that you have added sexuality to your knowledge base about nursing and nursing care, turn to the situation at the beginning of the chapter. Study the situation again and consider the following questions.

1. *Reflect on your own feelings and impressions about this situation and distill the possible explanations for your feelings, impressions, and reactions.*
2. *Propose additional information you would attempt to elicit from this woman, and give your rationale.*
3. *Plan what information you would give to the examiner before the examination.*
4. *Describe what interventions you would use to make this woman more comfortable before and during the examination.*
5. *Develop a plan for follow-up activities appropriate for this woman.*

References

Annon, J. S. (1976). *The behavioral treatment of sexual problems, vol. 1: Brief therapy.* Philadelphia: J. B. Lippincott.

Belzer, E. (1981). Orgasmic expulsions of women: A review and heuristic inquiry. *Journal of Sex Research, 17*(91), 1–12.

Hogan, R. (Ed.). (1985). *Human sexuality: A nursing perspective* (2nd ed.). New York: Appleton-Century-Crofts.

Kaplan, H. S. (1979). *Disorders of sexual desire.* New York: Simon & Schuster.

Lauver, D., & Welch, M. B. (1990). Sexual response cycle. In C.I. Fogel & D. Lauver (Eds.), *Sexual health promotion.* Philadelphia: W. B. Saunders.

Masters, W., & Johnson, V. (1966). *Human sexual response.* Boston: Little, Brown & Co.

Masters, W., Johnson, V., & Kolodny, R. (1988). *Human sexuality* (3rd ed.). Boston: Little, Brown & Co.

May, K. A., & Mahlmeister, L. R. (1994). *Comprehensive maternity nursing* (3rd ed.). Philadelphia: J. B. Lippincott.

Mims, F. H., & Swenson, M. (1980). *Sexuality: A nursing perspective.* New York: McGraw-Hill.

North American Nursing Diagnosis Association (NANDA). (1994). *Nursing diagnoses: Definitions and classification 1995–1996.* Philadelphia: Author.

Poorman, S. C. (1988). *Human sexuality and the nursing process.* Norwalk, CT: Appleton & Lange.

Rogers, A. (1990). Drugs and disturbed sexual functioning. In C. I. Fogel & D. Lauver (Eds.), *Sexual health promotion.* Philadelphia: W. B. Saunders.

Rynerson, B. (1990). Sexuality through the life cycle. In C. I. Fogel & D. Lauver (Eds.), *Sexual health promotion.* Philadelphia: W. B. Saunders.

Schover, L. R. (1988). *Sexuality and chronic illness.* New York: Guilford Press.

Woods, N. F. (1984). Human sexuality: A holistic perspective. In N. F. Woods (Ed.), *Human sexuality in health and illness* (3rd ed.). St. Louis: C. V. Mosby.

Woods, N. F., & Stamer, A. F. (1984). Sexuality throughout the life cycle: Prenatal life through adolescence. In N. F. Woods (Ed.), *Human sexuality in health and illness* (3rd ed.). St. Louis: C. V. Mosby.

World Health Organization. (1975). *Education and treatment in human sexuality: The training of health professionals.* Technical Report Series No. 572. Geneva: Author.

Bibliography

Benson, R. C. (1987). *Current obstetric and gynecologic diagnosis and treatment* (6th ed.). Los Altos, CA: Appleton-Lange.

Dirubbo, N. E. (1987). The condom barrier. *Am J Nurs, 87*(10), 52.

Speroff, L. (1987). Which birth control pill should be prescribed today? *Contemporary OB/GYN, 29*(3), 102.

Yoos, L. (1987). Adolescent cognitive and contraceptive behaviors. *Pediatric Nursing, 13*(4), 247.

Values and Beliefs

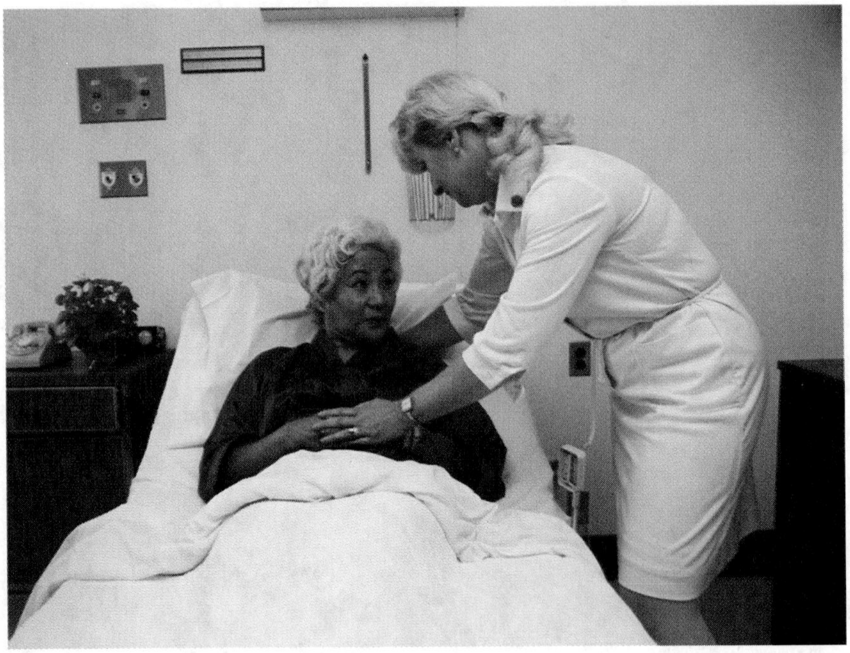

UNIT XVII

The values and beliefs area of human function includes those aspects of a person that guide his or her actions and choices. It is this function that governs what a person perceives as important in life. Unit XVII searches these values and beliefs.

An earlier chapter, Chapter 16, discusses the principles and concepts related to values and values clarification. Chapter 53, Spiritual Health, builds on that foundation, exploring the concept of spiritual health. Spirituality encompasses more than just religious beliefs and practices, and meeting a client's spiritual needs is the essence of providing holistic nursing care. Using a nursing process format, this chapter provides a beginning discussion of assessment factors about a client's spirituality. In this way, the nurse can adequately begin to understand and evaluate a client's spirituality needs. Likewise, the chapter presents an introductory discussion of nursing interventions to promote health and function as well as those for the client with spiritual distress.

The content of this unit focuses on spirituality from the perspective of meeting a client's needs for this area of function. By providing this emphasis, the nurse is truly able to incorporate holistic care into every facet of his or her client encounters.

Spiritual Health

Key Terms	Learning Objectives

Key Terms

Agnosticism
Atheism
Faith
Holism
Spiritual dimension
Spiritual need
Spiritual well-being
Spirituality
Theism

Learning Objectives

Upon completion of this chapter, the student will be able to do the following:

- *Explore philosophic questions about life.*
- *Discuss his or her personal spiritual journey.*
- *Identify spiritual needs in self and others.*
- *Identify major local religious faiths and their traditions.*
- *Incorporate spiritual assessment questions into nursing assessment appropriate to age and situation.*
- *Use appropriate nursing diagnoses in writing a plan of care for clients with spiritual problems.*
- *Plan how to use self in spiritual support.*
- *Develop a resource library of "spiritual" literature.*

53

You are a nurse working in a daytime drug rehabilitation program. One of the clients, a cocaine user, tells you he was notified that his younger brother attempted suicide by jumping from a building. The client tells you that the night before the suicide attempt, the brother had called and asked to go skiing, but the client (on a "high") said "no." The subsequent suicide attempt was unsuccessful and the brother is now in serious condition, suffering from paraplegia. The client also learned that this is the second suicide attempt in a month. No one had told the client previously because he was "stoned" all the time. The client also confides in you that when he visited with his brother the evening before, "I tried to pray, but nothing would come."

By now you have developed a sound knowledge base of human health and function, including such things as holism, culture, ethics, individual and family, values, and the nurse–client relationship. When you complete this chapter, you will be able to relate spiritual health and function to the "whole" person. You will understand some of the significance of your client's concerns about not being able to pray. The Critical Thinking Challenges at the end of the chapter will guide you in your nursing considerations of the client in this situation.

The nurse has the opportunity to participate in any client's spiritual health by promoting spiritual well-being and providing the climate for spiritual healing. All people have a spiritual component or dimension that can be developed; however, the ways in which a person's spirituality is expressed depend on the person's family background, society, culture, and particular religion.

As the nurse begins to think about spiritual care, his or her own family background, culture, and religion become integral parts of the nurse–client interaction. For this reason, the nurse must step back and examine his or her own spirituality, values, and beliefs. Often, this examination leads to reflection on some deeper philosophic questions such as: Who am I? Why am I here? What am I doing? Why am I doing it? How can I justify these things? Reflecting on these questions aids in developing the nurse's philosophic base from which to think more clearly about nursing and health. For example, what one believes about the spiritual dimension is reflected in one's relationship to people.

Normal Spiritual Function

"The **spiritual dimension** is a quality that goes beyond religious affiliation, that strives for inspiration, reverence, awe, meaning and purpose, even for those who do not believe in any god. The spiritual dimension tries to be in harmony with the universe, strives for answers about the infinite, and comes into focus when the person faces emotional stress, physical illness, or death" (Murray & Zentner, 1985, pp. 474–475).

Although all people have this dimension within their being, not all have the same depth or intensity of it in their lives. **Spirituality** is the quality or essence that pervades, integrates, and transcends one's biopsychosocial nature.

Fromm (1968) commented on what it means to be human: "If man were satisfied to spend his life making a living, there would be no problem . . . [however] there is a sphere characteristic of man which one can call the trans-survival or trans-utilitarian sphere . . . He [man] is the only case of life being aware of itself" (p. 68).

Both Assagioli (1971), a psychotherapist, and Tillich (1969), a theologian, describe the human need for synthesis with the Supreme Being or Supreme Other. It appears that all humans have a spiritual dimension, the potential to strive toward unity and a higher consciousness in order to locate meaning and purpose in life.

Characteristics of Normal Spirituality

The major characteristics of normal spirituality include a sense of wholeness and harmony within one's self, with others, and with God, or one's higher power as one defines it. The person, according to his or her developmental level, experiences and projects personal security, a strong identity, and a sense of hope. However, this does not mean that the person is totally satisfied with life or has all the answers, for as one's life normally unfolds, there are many situations in which one may experience anxiety, helplessness, or confusion. During these times it is important that the nurse recognize that these experiences of difficult situations often generate spiritual questions, and that assisting a client with the ensuing spiritual struggle is a valid and important aspect of maintaining health and giving healthcare.

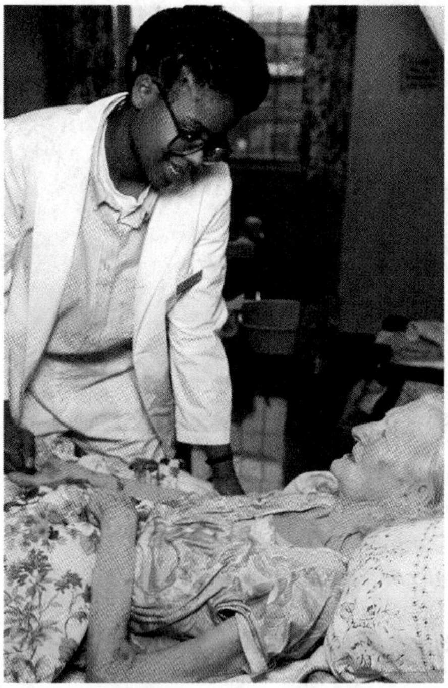

Figure 53-1 • *In spiritual care, the nurse addresses both the physical and spiritual needs of the client.*

Holism

Holism, as discussed in Chapter 15, was defined as the position of reviewing the universe as a system of harmonious interconnectedness rather than a sum of isolated parts. Holism not only integrates mind–body, but emphasizes spirit. Brallier (1978) states that, "Holistic practitioners take the spiritual aspects seriously. They believe that man is more than a clump of well organized cells, that man has a spirit and that this spark of life energizes the body" (p. 645).

A holistic approach is grounded in the recognition that the spiritual struggle is a valid and important aspect of health and healthcare (Fig. 53-1). It is the integrating factor of "previously compartmentalized constructs of physical body, rational mind, emotional psyche, and intuitive spirit" (Ruffing-Rahal, 1984, p. 12).

Spiritual Need

Definitions of spiritual need vary according to the author's belief system. In summarizing the various definitions of spiritual need, it appears that a **spiritual need** represents a normal expression of a person's inner being that seeks meaning in all experience and a dynamic relationship with self, others, and to the supreme other as defined by the person. Spiritual needs are derived through affective experiences of faith, hope, love, and positive experiences that serve as catalysts of synthesis and meaning. A list of the spiritual needs identified so far in the literature includes trust, forgiveness, love and relatedness, faith, creativity and hope, meaning and purpose, and grace.

Spiritual Quest

Life may be looked on as a spiritual quest, not only to answer the philosophic questions given at the beginning of this chapter, but to seek a higher level of consciousness or a deeper awareness of spiritual life. For example, the Twelve-Step program of Alcoholics Anonymous identifies recovery as a spiritual journey; members of this group practice a spiritual discipline to live in a more meaningful way, day by day. Recovery begins "through a 'leap of faith' which says that there is no meaning to be found other than that which is beyond one's self; that which transcends man's ability to know—that which is God" (Kreidler, 1984, p. 175). Chapman (1986) also includes the idea of search in defining optimal spiritual health. Spiritual health includes " . . . our ability to discover and articulate our own basic purpose in life, learn how to experience love, joy, peace and fulfillment . . . ." (p. 41)

Spiritual Well-Being

Spiritual well-being is a condition marked by an affirmation of life, peace, harmony, and a sense of interconnectedness with God, self, community, and environment that nurtures and celebrates wholeness (Moberg, 1979). In the hierarchy of human needs, spiritual well-being appears to connote fulfillment of needs beyond the self-actualization level. For example, Hunglemann and coworkers' (1985) study of older adults also found that harmony and interconnectedness were the two major determinants of spiritual well-being with healthy as well as with terminally ill clients. All the subjects expressed a belief in a Supreme Being, had some means of communication with that entity through prayer and worship, and had an extensive social support system of meaningful personal relationships.

Normal Spiritual Pattern

Part of a person's spiritual functional pattern relates to his or her values, beliefs, and faith. Beliefs may range from **atheism** (the denial of the existence of God) to **agnosticism** (the belief that the reality of God is unknown and unknowable) or to **theism** (the belief that the reality of God is personal, without a body, perfect in all things, and creator and sustainer of the universe).

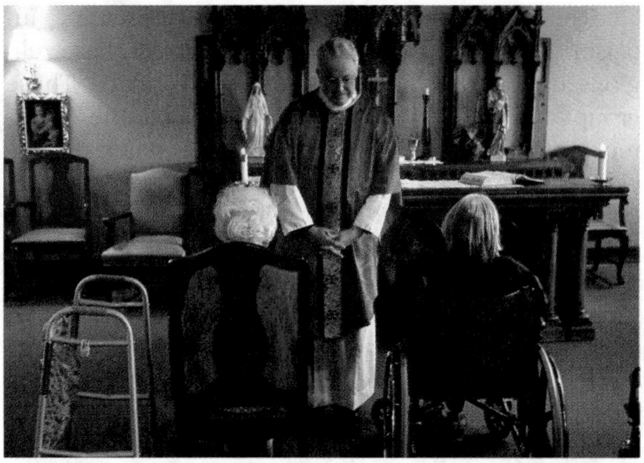

Figure 53-2 • *One's spiritual dimension is lived out in one's belief, faith, and values.*

For example, Christians, Jews, and Muslims are all theists, although each group further delineates distinctive beliefs about God's nature and activity. **Faith**, however, is more than belief; it is the way that beliefs are acted out in one's life. It involves "one's dynamic way of making meaning" (Fowler, 1981). It is the personal expression of living out one's spiritual dimension (Fig. 53-2). Thus, beliefs, faith, and values are interconnected, because what one sets one's heart on, believes in, or lives out is also what one values. Faith is central to the way the person makes meaning.

The expression of spirituality, often through a specific religious group, usually follows an established order of practices. These practices may range from simple meditation and relaxation to more formal worship, such as church services or rituals at shrines. Many observances take place within the home, in privacy or with the family. Some traditions involve special foods or ceremonies as part of the celebration of special holy days. These celebrations hold symbolic meaning and a sense of deep mystery or miracle to those who follow the religion.

Some people may practice their form of spirituality daily, whereas others may formally observe only one or two holy days; still others may answer a "call" to full-time service in a specific religious group. Whatever the spiritual or religious beliefs the person holds and practices, these beliefs fulfill the following needs:

- Give meaning to life, illness, other crises, and death
- Contribute a sense of security for present and future
- Guide daily living habits
- Drive acceptance or rejection of other people
- Furnish psychosocial support within a group of like-minded people
- Provide strength in meeting life's crises
- Give healing strength and support

The major world religions include Christianity, Judaism, Hinduism, Buddhism, and Islam. All these religions are found in the United States and Canada. These groups have many branches, which reflect the occurrence of historical events. For example, when the ancient Roman Empire fell, the church was divided, becoming the Eastern Orthodox Church and the Roman Catholic Church. Still later, the Roman Catholic Church was split again, forming the Anglican Church or the Church of England, when King Henry VIII of England decided to rule the church himself in place of the Pope. During the Protestant Reformation, begun by a monk named Martin Luther, more Christian groups were formed, including such denominations as Lutheran, Presbyterian, and Methodist. Today, a fourth Protestant group, the Baptists, is the largest denomination in the United States. Judaism has three main branches: Reformed, Conservative, and Orthodox. Islam also has several branches in the United States. The newest form of Islam, the American Muslim Mission, sometimes called the Black Muslims, developed as a consequence of the West African slave trade.

Most religious groups have a spiritual leader. That person may range from a pastor, priest, or rabbi, educated in spiritual direction or pastoral counseling, to a shaman or spiritual healer, trained in ancient cultural traditions. Shamans and spiritual healers are found among Native Americans and many southeast Asian groups. This leader is often the center of the spiritual or religious community, leading in worship, teaching, and healing.

Factors Affecting Normal Spiritual Expression

A number of factors affect a person's expression of spiritual needs. These include such things as culture, gender, and previous experience. Individual reactions vary, depending on personality style and past coping styles. Other contributing factors to spiritual health include appropriate religious education, a firm spiritual identity, a dynamic and adaptable belief system, maintenance of belief systems in times of adversity or under questioning by others, recognition of spiritual assistance when needed, empathy for others' beliefs and values, and a sense of spiritual fulfillment (Houldin, et al., 1987).

Culture. Attitudes, beliefs, and values arise out of one's sociocultural background. Usually, but not always, people follow the spiritual and religious traditions of the family. The child learns the importance of religious practices, including moral values, from the family's relationships and participation in religious forms. In an interfaith marriage, the child may follow the practices of one parent over the other. Some parents try to instill the strengths of both religions in their offspring.

Often, a person's religious preference is tied to the family's ethnic background. For example, many Italians and Irish are Roman Catholics, many Scandinavians and Germans are Lutherans, and many East Indians are Hindus. No matter what religious tradition or belief system the person follows, the inner spiritual experience is uniquely personal.

Gender. One's spiritual expression also depends on the society's and religious group's beliefs and teachings about gender or expected behaviors in male and female roles. If one's religion has dietary laws, it probably is the woman's responsibility to see that the family follows the laws. A person's organized religion may also determine how each sex dresses, and whether one wears a head covering. In some cases, the spiritual leader is always male. Some mainline religions now encourage women to assume pastoral positions. This change, however, rises from political processes, particularly the equal rights movement.

Previous Experience. Fowler (1981) and others observe that many people direct their lives based on values that have been appropriated more or less uncritically. If something disruptive occurs, the person's "meaning-in-life assumptions" are called into question. This is sometimes called a "test of faith." Thus, it would appear that if one's faith and values are confronted, then the deeper spiritual needs will arise. During a crisis period, past coping styles or learned ways of handling situations are likely to be in evidence. These coping patterns can be healthy and adaptive, or they can be maladaptive. Life experiences in general are an influence. Such experiences may or may not be related to age.

Crisis. A crisis may strengthen a person's spirituality (Toth, 1992). This often happens when people face death, for example, as a soldier on a battlefield or as a terminally ill client. One study (Reed, 1986) has shown that terminally ill clients or those who have life-threatening medical diagnoses demonstrate that spirituality is potentially a very significant variable. When these clients confronted their own mortality, reliance on spiritual assets such as faith and prayer increased compared with nonterminally ill hospitalized clients or healthy, nonhospitalized people. The disorienting experience of being near death enabled members of this group to reorient their lives spiritually, and in one sense there was healing.

Lifespan Considerations

The expression of the spiritual dimension is also influenced by the person's level of growth and development. Fowler (1981), building on the theories of Erik-

Table 53-1 • Stages of Human Development: Optimal Parallels

Eras (years)	*Erikson*	*Piaget*	*Fowler*
Infancy (0–1.5)	Trust (hope) Autonomy (will)	Sensorimotor	Undifferentiated–Primal
Early childhood (2–6)	Initiative (purpose)	Intuitive/Preoperational	Intuitive–Projective
Childhood (7–12)	Industry (competence)	Concrete Operational	Mythic–Literal Faith
Adolescence (13–21)	Identity (fidelity)	Formal Operational	Synthetic–Conventional
Young adulthood (21–35)	Intimacy (love)		Individuative–Reflective Faith
Adulthood (35–60)	Generativity (care)		Conjunctive Faith
Maturity (60–)	Integrity (wisdom)		Universalizing Faith

Adapted from Fowler, J. (1981). ***Stages of faith*** (p. 52). New York: Harper and Row.

son and Piaget, has formulated a theory of faith development as the person's integrating center of valuing. Fowler's theory does not address the content of a person's faith, such as a specific religious belief system, but looks at faith as another way of knowing the world, a spiritual knowing based on the particular phase of psychological and cognitive development. The stages of faith knowing have parallels with the stages of cognitive development of Piaget and psychosocial development of Erikson. Table 53-1 is adapted from *Stages of Faith* (Fowler, 1981). The following discussion integrates faith stage concepts with growth and development, and identifies spiritual needs arising from these stages.

Newborn and Infant

Trust in the caregiver is the basis not only for development of a sense of safety, security of self in the world, and interpersonal relationships, but is the basis for faith development. Human beings' initial knowing of the world is through relationships; if basic trust needs are met by parents who themselves are secure and have a sense of meaning and commitment, infants will sense this kinesthetically and incorporate this feeling into their "innermost being." This sense of trust will later broaden and deepen into trust in the world, the universe, and a "higher power."

Toddler and Preschooler

The first stage of faith development is the Intuitive–Projective, which is characterized by a continuing differentiation of self from others and an awakening of consciousness and memory. The introduction of language and gestures facilitates the ability to participate in some rituals of faith in the parents' religious belief systems. Children will respond to the routine of grace before meals, bedtime stories and prayers, special celebrations, and holy days if these are offered as a consistent, natural part of family life. The child also responds positively to those who treat their questions about the world, life, and death seriously. Although children do not know about such matters in a rational way, they intuitively sense the deeper spiritual questions of existence.

Child and Adolescent

Children notice the difference between themselves as individuals and others in like or in different groups. Belonging and acceptance in one's own group is important for children, although they are still primarily oriented to the parents' authority. They continue to be sensitive to good–bad issues, often trying to "make up" for wrongdoing in a concrete, literal way (Fowler, 1981).

Children at these ages can now think in a historical perspective, and see themselves as a part of their family tree. The use of "story" is a major strategy for bringing meaning to experience. It is a period when the lore, legends, language, and symbols of a particular religious group are best presented. Wishes, needs, facts, and fantasy may appear somewhat confused, but again, the child is attempting to make sense out of the world. This period is the Mythic–Literal period.

The major change in adolescence is the beginning of or the potential for the ability to think abstractly, conceptualize, and synthesize. Adolescents can ask more sophisticated, philosophic questions, testing the truth, evaluating others' behavior, and noting the incongruities. It is a time during which they develop their own personal style, based on their beliefs, attitudes, and values. Although the adolescent is individually involved in this personal synthesis of identity, it is carried out mainly in the peer group, where mutuality and interpersonal relationships have a major impact. This process is therefore both individualistic and conventional, insofar as it conforms to the peer group. Authority has moved away from the parents to the peer group. Thus, the name for this stage is Synthetic–Conventional.

Adult and Older Adult

In the Individuative–Reflective stage, the young adult is moving away from the conforming peer group and clarifying boundaries of selfhood and commitment. This shift away from the group is often precipitated by an encounter with people or groups other than those that supported the person in the previous stage. One's values, beliefs, and attitudes change as a result of interacting in a more pluralistic setting. Some of the situations precipitating this upheaval include such experiences as a new job, international travel, advanced study or education, or a new religious affiliation. In addition, this may be intertwined with achievement of intimate relationships, choosing a career, and starting a family. The faith challenge during this stage is to establish one's own sense of faith and commitment based on personal experience and reflection on personal meaning in life (Fowler, 1981).

The middle years are fulfilled through productive activity—in Erikson's term, generativity. However, it is still a time of growth and renewed questioning, in some ways very similar to adolescence. This time the adult is not dealing with group conformity as much as with a broader world view. The older adult notices the polarities or extremes in life; these include such things as young and old, rich and poor, masculine and feminine, war and peace, constructive and destructive, and self-awareness and self-denial. These tensions, enhanced or precipitated by personal and environmental situations, demand integration and resolution; this is referred to as Conjunctive Faith (Fowler, 1981).

The final stage of faith, Universalizing, is seldom achieved by most people; usually only great leaders, such as Gandhi, Martin Luther King, and Mother Theresa appear to have reached this world view. One's social perspective expands to include everyone as God's children, and there is a more radical living-out of one's vision of the earth community. Terms such as justice, love, and compassion describe the goals of this person.

Nursing Research
Spirituality

Selected Nursing Research Studies

Emblen, J. D., & Halstead, L. (1993). Spiritual needs and interventions: Comparing the view of patients, nurses, and chaplains. *Clinical Nurse Specialist, 7,* 175–182.

Hall, C., & Lanig, H. (1993). Spiritual caring behaviors as reported by Christian nurses. *Western Journal of Nursing Research, 15,* 730–741.

Reed, P. (1991). Preferences for spiritually related nursing interventions among terminally ill and non-terminally ill hospitalized adults and well adults. *Applied Nursing Research, 4*(3), 122–128.

Saudia, T. L., Kinney M. R., & Young-Ward, L. (1991). Health locus of control and helpfulness of prayer. *Heart-Lung, 20,* 60–65.

Possible Topics for Nursing Inquiry

- What are spiritual needs?
- Do there need to be additional spiritual care nursing diagnoses?
- What are modalities for teaching spiritual caregiving?

Altered Spiritual Function

Many factors can effect a change in a person's spiritual health and well-being; however, those life situations to which the person is personally connected are subjective. For example, one person's sense of meaning may be challenged by a job change, whereas another's may be influenced by a broken relationship.

Potential for Altered Spiritual Function

Crisis and Change. Just as crisis may strengthen one's faith, it may also deal it a blow. Many people do not consciously reflect on their personal philosophy of life. They live life as if it were going to continue forever. "Often it is not until the crisis, illness, aging, loss, limitation or suffering occurs that the illusion [or security] is shattered . . . Therefore, illness, suffering, aging, loss, and ultimately death, by their very nature, become spiritual experiences as well as physical and emotional experiences" (Grandstrom, 1985, p. 12).

Crisis may be related to pathophysiologic changes, the treatment required, or situations affecting the person. The diagnosis of a debilitating, disfiguring, or terminal illness can lead to the person's questioning his or her personal belief system. Sudden trauma, miscarriage, or stillbirth may cause the person to doubt the presence of a Higher Being. Various treatments required for trauma and illness can lead to a sense of isolation or uncertainty. Many treatments generate additional problems, such as amputation, surgery, medication administration, dietary restrictions, and other procedures.

Personal changes resulting from death or illness of a loved one, opposition to personal religious beliefs by significant others, or change in personal status can become other sources of spiritual distress. Being hospitalized can interrupt the person's usual religious practices at a time when they are needed the most, thus adding to the client's spiritual distress.

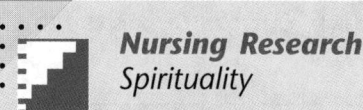

Separation From Spiritual Ties. The experience of being a client in an acute care facility or a resident in a retirement or nursing home can initially be shattering. To some extent one is isolated from personal freedom, personal privileges, and social support systems. The person may be in a private room without familiar surroundings, and may feel insecure. Daily habits may be changed. The person may not be able to attend formal services, have the accoutrements of the faith, or receive the support of the familiar group. This separation from spiritual ties places the person at risk for altered spiritual function.

Moral Issues Regarding Therapy. For most of the major religions, the healer and the healing process are seen as parts of God's way of working in the world. However, certain religious groups object to some modern medical interventions. For example, Jehovah's Witnesses do not accept blood transfusions because of their belief in Old Testament teachings. Some Christians do not condone abortion because of their belief that the soul enters the body at conception. The Amish may refuse expensive treatment because the cost would impose a severe financial hardship on the community. There are many other medical procedures that may be affected by religious teachings, such as right-to-die decisions, organ transplants, circumcision, birth control, sterilization, autopsies, and handling of the deceased. Some groups, such as the Christian Scientists and the Amish, have been legally exempted from immunizations; however, many medical decisions are reviewed on a case-by-case basis, depending on the client's age and the imminence of death. The choice to treat may be difficult to make if the religious beliefs say "no" and the healthcare system says "yes." Many hospitals now have an ethics committee that can clarify and review such situations, so that more adequate and informed decisions can be made.

Inadequate or Inappropriate Care. Peterson (1985) states, "There are some pitfalls . . . to be avoided in providing spiritual care . . . . The first is doing nothing . . . [and the second] is to jump in too quickly" (p. 26). In general, when people become clients they depend on the nurse and the healthcare team. Nurses attempt to overcome this inherent dependency by being a client advocate, and by involving the client as much as possible in mutual goal-setting and care-planning. However, the client is a captive audience. Thus, either of the aforementioned positions may result in inadequate or inappropriate care.

There are several reasons why nurses may avoid spiritual care. These include insecurity in their own spiritual lives, assigning less value and importance to spiritual care, having little or no educational preparation in spiritual care, or believing that it is the clergy's territory. Grandstrom (1985) elaborates on these reasons when she identifies five fairly complex values issues between nurses and clients:

- Pluralism: nurses and clients embrace a wide spectrum of beliefs and creeds
- Fear: related to not being able to handle situations, intruding on client's privacy, or becoming confused in one's own belief and value system
- Awareness of Own Spiritual Quest: what gives meaning, purpose, hope, and sense of love in one's own life
- Confusion: confusion over differences between religious and spiritual concepts
- Basic Attitudes: attitudes relative to illness, aging, and suffering

Mathai (1980) studied spirituality in relation to nurses' own coping strategies when dealing with suffering clients. She concluded that nurses who function in a spiritual vacuum feel frustrated, helpless, and anxious when caring for suffering clients. Because relief of suffering is an essential goal in nursing, there is a clear need to help nurses face and work effectively with this situation. Kreidler (1984) states that, "nurses need reassurance that groping for meaning in suffering . . . [is] . . . a sign of strength . . . . Our spiritual distress when facing suffering must be explored and understood if we are to be able to minister to our clients' needs" (p. 174). And again, Kreidler (1984) states, "Spiritual distress is met through the encouragement and preservation of life coupled with the belief that every human life does have meaning; that no one ever lives, suffers or dies in vain" (p. 175). Thus, nurses need opportunities to reflect on their own philosophy and belief systems. Useful questions (Richardson & Noland, 1984) for this kind of reflection include

What do I believe?
What gives meaning to my life?
How is my belief system working for me?
Is my behavior compatible with my belief system?
How does my belief system relate to my future?
Is there a relationship between my belief system and my healthcare behavior?

Manifestations of Altered Spiritual Function

Various behaviors and expressions should alert the nurse to the fact that clients may be experiencing spiritual concerns. Table 53-2 is a compilation of categorizations regarding adaptive and maladaptive expressions of spiritual needs. The seven areas of spiritual need identified earlier are included. The table may aid the nurse in examining potential spiritual distress manifested in the client or that may appear in the support person or family.

Verbalization of Distress

The person suffering spiritual dysfunction may verbalize that distress or express a need for help. The manifestation may be precise: "I feel guilty because I should have realized earlier he was having a heart attack." A person may state that he or she misses Sunday church services and the beautiful music of the choir, or may

Table 53-2 • Adaptive and Maladaptive Expressions of Spiritual Needs

Needs	Signs of Adaptive Behavior or Patterns	Signs of Maladaptive Behavior or Patterns
Trust	Trust in self and own endurance Accepts that others will be able to meet needs Trust in life even if evidence is against it Acceptance of outcome of life Openness to God	Discomfort with self-awareness Gullibility Inability to be open to others Feels that only certain people and certain places are safe Expects people to be unkind and undependable Wants needs met promptly, cannot wait Lack of openness to God Fears God's intentions
Forgiveness	Accepts self and others as fallible Nonjudgmental Views illness realistically Experiences self-forgiveness Offers to forgive others Accepts God's forgiveness Realistic perspective on the past	Feels illness is a punishment Feels God is judgmental Feels that forgiveness is qualified by behavior Is unable to accept self Either self-blaming or projecting of blame Feels others are judging him or her Self-destructive behavior
Love and relatedness	Expresses feelings of being loved by other/God Able to accept help Self-accepting Seeks the good of others	Fears dependence on others Refuses to cooperate with health regimen Worries about separation from family Self-rejecting or false pride and selfishness Inability to believe that self is lovable by God, lacks love relationship with God Dependent, magical relationship with God Feelings of distance and separation from God Expresses ambivalent feelings about God
Faith	Dependency on divine wisdom/God Motivated for growth Expresses satisfaction with explanation of life after death Expresses need to enter into and/or understand larger drama of human history Expresses need for the symbolic, ritual Expresses need for sense of a shared faith/community	Lack of faith in a transcendent power/God Fear of death/life after death Senses isolation from faith community Bitterness, frustration, and anger with God Unclear values, beliefs and goals Values conflicts Lack of commitment
Creativity and hope	Asks for information about condition Talks about condition realistically Uses time during hospitalization/illness constructively Seeks ways for self-expression Finds comfort in inner self rather than physical self or worldly criteria Expresses hope in the future Open to the possibility of peace	Expresses fear of loss of control Expresses boredom Lacks vision of possible alternatives Fearful of therapy Despairing Cannot help self or accept self Cannot enjoy anything Has put life/major decisions on hold
Meaning and purpose	Expresses contentment with life Lives life in accordance with value system Accepts or uses suffering for self-understanding Expresses meaning in life/death Expresses commitment and goal orientation Clearer sense of what is important	Expresses no reason to live Cannot find any meaning in suffering Questions the meaning of suffering Questions the purpose of illness Cannot form goals or has unattainable goals Abuses drugs/alcohol Jokes about life after death
Grace	Alive in the moment Sense of blessing/abundance Sense of mercy given beyond self from God Sense of harmony/wholeness	Anxious about the past/future Oriented towards achievement/production Focused on regrets/remorse Talks about doing better/trying harder Perfectionistic

say, "I've never missed a service in 20 years." The manifestation may be more subjective, as in the case of the client's rambling speech about life, death, and worth. A client may ask the nurse to pray for him or her or to notify a spiritual leader of his or her illness.

Altered Behavior

A change in behavior may be a manifestation of spiritual dysfunction. A client who is nervous about the outcome of a diagnostic test or who shows anger after hearing the results may be suffering from spiritual distress. Some people will become more introspective; they may reason out the situation and search for facts in available literature. Some will react emotionally and seek out information and support from friends and family. Still others may appear not to "hear," and show no outward signs of recognition of the problem, but it may surface in sleeplessness or lack of concentration. Guilt, fear, depression, and anxiety may indicate altered spiritual function. Table 53-2 gives other specifics.

Impact of Spiritual Dysfunction on Activities of Daily Living

Individual Considerations

In one sense, the activities of daily living may not appear to vary from client to client. All clients need some orientation and understanding of the structure of their day; however, the attitude and mood of clients toward their day influence their acceptance and expectation of care. Clients may go through the motions of daily living, but their involvement in living is changed. Their "spirit" level has changed. For example, if the client is experiencing spiritual distress related to love and relatedness, he or she may refuse to cooperate with the health regimen or not ask for help. If the client questions the pain or the meaning of illness, or expresses no reason to live, he or she may be expressing spiritual distress related to loss of meaning and hope. Thus, it is the process of daily living, rather than the actual tasks, that is influenced by spiritual distress.

Family Considerations

Clients and families may have divergent spiritual beliefs and practices and not really be aware of these differences on a day-to-day basis (Spiritual Care Work Group, 1990). Thus, for example, if family members become involved in home care, there may be unspoken assumptions and expectations regarding the spiritual dimension of life. Depending on the ages and maturity of family members, they may or may not be able to articulate such needs as hope, meaning, or forgiveness. Spiritual distress may be experienced as a subtle, "gnawing" feeling of inadequacy. In the case at the beginning of the chapter, spiritual distress among family members might be evidenced as anger and blame.

Assessment

Stoll (1979) cautions that the timing of the spiritual assessment is important, and that it should come after the psychosocial assessment. Then, if the client has some questions about this portion of the interview, the nurse can explain that one's spiritual beliefs are also an important part of maintaining health.

Subjective Data

Functional Pattern Identification

Several nurses have developed spiritual assessment tools. Stoll's (1979) Guidelines for Spiritual Assessment is probably the most widely recognized tool. Four areas are identified, and questions for each are suggested: 1) concept of God or deity, 2) source of hope and strength, 3) religious practices and rituals, and 4) relationship between spiritual beliefs and state of health. Some of the questions include

- Is religion or God significant to you?
- To whom do you turn when you need help?
- Do you feel your faith (religion) is helpful to you? If yes, tell me how.
- Has being sick (or what has happened to you) made any difference in your feeling about God or the practice of your faith?

Fish and Shelly (1983) also developed an assessment tool; the questions are similar to Stoll's, but the following represent some differences in focus:

- Why are you in the hospital [or healthcare agency]?
- Has being ill affected your outlook in any way?
- Has your illness affected your relationship to the most significant person(s) in your life?
- Has being ill affected the way in which you view yourself?
- What is your greatest need at this time?

Tools have also been modified for various populations. For example, Still (1984) uses different questions to assess children's spiritual needs. Some of the questions include

- How do you feel when you are in trouble?
- To whom do you turn when you are scared (in addition to your parents)?
- What are the favorite things you like to do when you are happy? When you are sad?
- Do you know who God is? What is He like?

Spiritual Assessment

Client Name ______________________________ Date ____________
Days in Treatment ____________ Religious Preference ______________________
Marital Status __________ Children __________ Age __________

Part I. Spiritual Assessment Guide: In the beginning, share with the client that people have several personal aspects, such as physiologic, emotional, and spiritual, and that this is an interview dealing with the spiritual needs. If the client appears to be very uncomfortable, clarify his or her concern and listen.

1. Spiritual Ecology of Childhood
   A. Developmental History: Examples of some questions might be: Describe some early memories of how your family "kept" Sunday (or Saturday) or other Holy Days. How did you feel about yourself? your family? God? Eternity? Who taught you about spiritual things? Can you remember any religious symbols, hymns, stories that had an impact on you? How did these experiences change as your got older?
   B. Current religious practice: Do you participate in a religious organization? Do you pray or meditate, or participate in some spiritual exercise?
2. Awareness of the Spiritual: Client's awareness of some universal power greater than himself or herself and his or her experience of that power. What do you think or feel about God? Is there an image or a song that expresses how you feel?
3. Meaning and Purpose: Client's concept of the direction of his or her life has taken, the present direction, and who is responsible for its direction. What meaning does your life have for you right now? When you're feeling down or discouraged, what gives life meaning?
4. Faith and Trust: Client's ability to accept life's uncertainties and his or her willingness to trust and be trustworthy. How do you view the changes in your life? If you were to get a box labeled "Your Next Major Change," what would you do with it?
5. Forgiveness and Grace: Client's acceptance of others and self that allows him or her to confess and admit mistakes. What does the word "sin" mean to you?
6. Hope and Creativity: Client's desire to make changes in life/lifestyle. When you think of the future, how does it make you feel?
7. Love and Relatedness: Client's quality of relationships with family, friends, work associates, community, self, and God. How would you describe your relationship with people?
8. Crises and Peak Experiences: Client's coping abilities and strengths. Have you ever had a time of crisis or suffering when you felt life had no meaning? What happened to you during these times? Did you feel the same or different after these experiences? Did you try to get help from any idea or person? Was there a spiritual thought or expression that was helpful to you during this time? Have you ever had moments of great joy or breakthrough? How has this affected you? Is there any spiritual image, music, or art that expresses your experience?

Part II. Closing: Because this interview will stimulate a lot of thoughts and feelings, be sure to offer some clarification and summary time. Is there anything we haven't discussed that you would like to add? Do you have any questions?

Adapted from Davis, M. C. (1981). Another look at spiritual assessment: A behavior adaptation model currently in use in a chemical association, *45*, 19–26; and Leean, C. (1985). ***Faith development in the adult life cycle.*** Module 2 (Rev.) Prepared for the Religious Education Association of the United States and Canada.

An example of a spiritual assessment tool is given in the accompanying display.

In addition to the collection of data using assessment tools, other cues can be drawn from sensitive observation and listening. Other cues regarding children's spiritual needs might include the refusal to attend activities, preoccupation with another's situation or illness, reference to Sunday School, statements made in passing by the parents about God's will, and symbolic drawings (Shelly, 1982b).

In one sense, all clients who are suffering from ill health are at risk for spiritual distress. They may be physically separated from sources of spiritual help, such as a faith community where relationships are maintained and rituals of worship are performed. They may be emotionally separated as well, especially if they have not led a self-examined life. Even for those who have spiritual strengths, however, the time of illness and attendant crises bring on increased anxiety. Certainly those clients with critical or terminal illnesses, who are facing death or other profound physical changes, face ultimate, meaning-in-life questions. Westberg (1956) identifies nine situations indicative of a client at spiritual risk:

- One who is lonely and has few, if any visitors
- One who expresses some apprehensions and fears
- One whose illness may have some connection with his or her emotions or religious attitudes
- One who is facing surgery
- One whose surgery or illness forces him or her to change his or her way of living
- One who seems to be doing more than the average amount of thinking about the relationship of his or her religion to his or her health
- One whose pastor is unable to call on him or her, or who has no church affiliation and so would receive no pastoral care
- One whose illness has obvious social implications
- One whose illness is terminal

Dysfunction Identification

The discovery of actual spiritual distress depends on the nurse's observation of the client's verbal and nonverbal responses to the nursing history interview. Clients need to be assisted in understanding that the nursing history is a review of their whole being, and that the questions will be wide-ranging, including not only physical and emotional health, but spiritual health as well. Clients who appear angry, anxious, depressed, or defensive when the spiritual questions are asked may need to hear something like, "I can see from your response that you might not have expected these questions; however, they do let you know that we are interested in how you are experiencing your current situation. Do you have a question or concern in this area?" Some clients may appear relieved to know that the spiritual aspect of their being is worthy of the nurse's concern. Still other clients may indicate that they have a spiritual concern, but that they will deal with it in their own time and way.

Identifying which spiritual need is lacking is related to the nurse's ability to "listen with a third ear." This means that the content or facts of the interview, in combination with the nonverbal behavior, evolve into a theme or a feeling tone such as distrust, judgment, isolation, or bitterness. These themes can then be linked with spiritual needs such as trust, forgiveness, love and relatedness, and faith.

Objective Data

There are objective data that can be helpful in assessing spiritual health; however, because of the qualities of the spiritual dimension, the nurse must verify the objective assessment with subjective information. Sometimes, in a client reluctant to verbalize, the objective data are the only clues to a difficulty.

The nurse can glean much information about the client from general appearance, facial expression, eye contact, body posture and movement, sleeplessness, anxiety, crying, and inappropriate humor or anger. Materials such as religious articles, books, cards, and pictures also indicate the spiritual dimension, as do visitors from the church or clergy.

> ***Safety Alert***
> *Spirituality*
>
> - Be aware of your client's spiritual or religious beliefs.
> - Be aware of any religious beliefs or practices that may be violated by various treatments and therapies.
> - Be mindful of religious beliefs regarding diet or dietary restrictions. Such knowledge may prevent nutritional problems or spiritual distress.
> - Be attentive to the client's religious practices or preferences regarding death, especially if death is imminent.
> - Be aware of significance clothing, jewelry, and other apparel. Some clothing may have religious significance for the client.
> - Care needs to be taken with regard to removal or disposal of clothing.

Nursing Diagnoses

Spiritual Distress and Potential for Enhanced Spiritual Well-Being are North American Nursing Diagnosis Association (NANDA) nursing diagnoses used for acknowledging and identifying the spiritual dimension and needs of clients.

Diagnostic Statement: Spiritual Distress (Distress of the Human Spirit)

Definition

Spiritual Distress is disruption in the life principle that pervades a person's entire being and that integrates and transcends one's biologic and psychosocial nature (NANDA, 1994). The distress may be related to the inability to practice spiritual rituals, a conflict between religious or spiritual beliefs and prescribed health regimens, or a crisis of illness, suffering, and death (Carpenito, 1995).

Defining Characteristics

The major defining characteristic that must be present is that the client experiences a disturbance in belief system (Carpenito, 1995). (This may involve a particular religious belief, or for the nonreligious person it may be a belief in the world, the family, or work—whatever it is that gives them strength, hope, and meaning.) There are nine minor defining characteristics that may be present: if the client questions credibility of belief system; demonstrates discouragement or despair; is unable to practice usual religious rituals; has ambivalent feelings or doubts about beliefs; expresses that there is no reason to live; feels a sense of spiritual emptiness; shows emotional detachment from self and others; expresses concern—anger, resentment, fear—over meaning of life or suffering death; and requests spiritual assistance for a disturbance in belief system.

Related Factors

Certain pathophysiologic, treatment-related, or situational factors may precipitate spiritual distress (Carpenito, 1995). For example, loss of a body part or function, a terminal illness, a debilitating disease, pain, trauma, or a miscarriage or stillbirth may be considered pathologic states that raise questions of meaning and purpose. High-risk treatment-related situations may include abortion, surgery, blood transfusions, dietary restrictions, isolation, amputation, medications, and other medical procedures. The distress in these situations may be a result of beliefs about health, illness, and healing. Situations, either personal or environmental, such as death or illness of a significant other; childbirth; beliefs opposed by family, peers, or healthcare providers; divorce or separation from a loved one; or embarrassment at practicing spiritual rituals may cause spiritual distress. Hospitals (or other healthcare facilities) may also present barriers to practicing spiritual rituals; these include restrictions of intensive care, confinement to bed or room, lack of privacy, or lack of availability of special foods or diet.

Diagnostic Statement: Potential for Enhanced Spiritual Well-Being

Definition

Spiritual Well-Being is the process of an individual's developing/unfolding or mystery through harmonious interconnectedness that springs from inner strengths (NANDA, 1994). A sense of spiritual well-being affirms life and all of its experiences. It also means that we are not alone in life's journey, but that there is a sense of spiritual interconnection with the larger universe.

Defining Characteristics

The major defining characteristics are inner strengths, unfolding mystery, and harmonious interconnectedness. Words used to describe inner strengths include a sense of awareness, self-consciousness, or inner core and a sense of the transcendent, a sacred source, or unifying force. Unfolding mystery connotes the perspective that life experiences of struggles and uncertainty have an ultimate meaning and purpose; however, it may be difficult or impossible to understand it through reason alone. A sense of peace, order, and union with self, others, the environment, and God/Higher Power describes what is meant by harmonious interconnectedness.

Related Factors

Specific related factors have not been established yet by NANDA, but factors related to spiritual well-being in general have been discussed earlier in this chapter.

Related Nursing Diagnoses

Because of the variety of causes, manifestations, and results of spiritual distress, other nursing diagnoses may be evident. Possible diagnoses include the following: Anxiety; Decisional Conflict; Ineffective Denial; Dysfunctional Grieving; Altered Family Processes; Fatigue; Fear; Hopelessness; Noncompliance; Parental Role Conflict; Personal Identity Disturbance; Powerlessness; Altered Role Performance; Self-Esteem Disturbance; Sleep Pattern Disturbance; and Social Isolation.

Outcome Identification and Planning

After nursing diagnoses and related factors are identified, the client and nurse plan outcomes and interventions. Goals for the client with spiritual distress should focus on providing an environment that supports the person's usual religious practices and beliefs. Goals need to be individualized, taking into consideration the client's history, areas of risk, evidence of dysfunction, and related objective data. Examples of goals for the client with spiritual distress include

The client will express satisfaction with spiritual condition.
The client will relate feelings of support in decision regarding health regimen.
The client will describe satisfaction with meaning and purpose of illness, suffering, and death.

Goals for enhancing spiritual well-being can be very similar to those for a client in spiritual distress. The focus should be on supporting the client's strengths. However, there may also be an opportunity for spiritual growth as the client explores creative ways to deal with pain and suffering. Some goals might include

The client will express a sense of wholeness or integrity during the illness and recovery process.
The client will relate feelings of intimacy or closeness with others.

Planning
Examples of Nursing Interventions for Common Problems of Spirituality

- Listen empathetically and sensitively.
- Encourage verbalization about faith and hope.
- Identify the client's personal coping mechanisms.
- Arrange for opportunities for privacy to express spiritual beliefs.
- Refer to appropriate resources for spiritual support.

The client will describe feelings for acceptance and respect when working through questions of meaning, purpose, and mystery.

Among the interventions used in planning are those listed in the accompanying display. They are discussed in the next section.

Implementation

Some of the qualities essential in implementing spiritual care are commitment to the nurse–client relationship, good communication skills, trust, empathy, self-awareness, and an acceptance of a broad definition of spirituality. This is the qualitative aspect of providing spiritual care, and it largely rests with the individual nurse to assess and meet spiritual needs.

Although the qualitative aspects play a large part in performing nursing interventions, implementation also includes continuing data collection, maintaining current documentation, and collaborating with the healthcare team. These steps are important because they ensure consistency and continuity in client care. Spiritual care is not one individual nurse's project.

The process should affirm the individual. If the nurse has been an effective communicator, then either facilitating the client's use of his or her own spiritual resources or finding someone else to help the client will more naturally evolve. The timing will not be forced, but will demonstrate sensitivity and empathy.

Nursing Interventions to Promote Spiritual Health and Function

Spiritual care can be defined as a mutual process that is a potentially healing or integrating experience in which the client's spiritual needs are met. The word "potential" is inserted here, because Penrose and Barret (1982) state: "Ultimately, it is God (or the Supreme Being as one understands it) who fulfills spiritual needs; people are merely His channels to this end" (p. 39).

Use of Self

Spiritual care occurs within the nurse–client relationship. This relationship does not consist only of talking with clients; it is the purposeful use of self to help another person grow in his or her ability to face reality and discover potential solutions to problems. Spiritual care is a relationship that the nurse perceives as a valuable part of therapy and to which a commitment exists.

Qualities such as trust and empathy are partially built on good communication skills and an understanding of the processes and phases of the nurse–client relationship. For example, making oneself and one's time available to the client is necessary to build trust in the initial phase of the relationship. Through active listening, the nurse can gain an understanding of the client's perspective, and thus be more sensitive to a variety of needs, including spiritual needs. Without the establishment of trust and empathy in the first phase of the relationship, the nurse will not be able to discern the deeper concerns, such as meaning and purpose.

In discussing spiritual care of older adults, Peterson (1985) states that "being" with the client is a much more important aspect of spiritual care than "doing" (Fig. 53-3) "Sharing in people's lives is still one of the greatest privileges and responsibilities of nursing" (p. 27). This supports the idea of Burkhardt and Nagai-Jacobson (1985), who state "that the very definition of spiritual issues implies not answers, but the need to struggle with the questions . . . ." (p. 193) Thus, involvement in the meeting of spiritual needs is very personal for both the nurse and the client.

Spiritual Support

Nurses also need to have a broad definition of spirituality so that they can be discerning with a variety of clients. Nurses cannot rely on their own spiritual tradi-

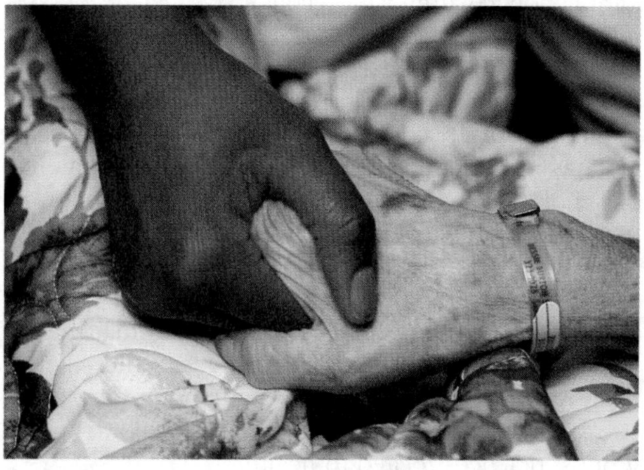

Figure 53-3 • *Being with the client when the client needs someone is an important aspect of spiritual care.*

tions; they must also be knowledgeable about other spiritual expressions and other religious traditions that express these needs. The expression of spiritual needs and the level or depth of spiritual care will vary with the client. Therefore, the nurse needs to be sensitive to this variability and offer appropriate care.

Peck (1981) describes situations in which spiritual faith and belief are beyond the scope of scientific explanation, yet appear to be helpful. She states that the nurse should "do nothing to destroy a constructive faith already present . . . ." The nurse should support and build on the client's faith. If faith is removed, the client will lose hope, and without the will to live, a person frequently is beyond the help of the most potent medical powers. Shelton (1981, p. 58) offers a moderating statement by saying,

> . . . encouraging clients to elaborate on the emotional and spiritual aspects of their faith enhances their growth and personality integration. It is important, however, that these conversations not be judgmental or controversial. If clients feel accepted and affirmed in their religious beliefs, the possibility of their opening up other, perhaps more intimate, areas of concern is increased . . .

Piepgras (1984, p. 2,613) gives the major principle in dealing with the ethical issue of personal witness in the nurse–client relationship:

> Discussion should be confined to the client's ideas, the client's needs, and to whatever level of religious terminology and frame of reference the client wishes to use. Personal witness by the nurse should be used, if at all, only after a common ground and easy dialogue have been established between the client and the nurse.

Support of Spiritual Practices

During the assessment, the nurse should have obtained information regarding the client's spiritual needs and religious preference. To facilitate the meeting of spiritual needs through specific religious practices, the nurse should also become familiar with the various religious groups within the community. Special religious considerations include beliefs about birth, death, sacraments, diet, holy days, and holy objects; a full description of these cannot be covered in this text. For example, dietary practices reflect dietary laws (eg, no pork or beef), as well as celebration of holy days by fasting or feasting. If the food required is so specialized that the dietary department cannot accommodate the client's needs, the family may ask to bring in their own food. Table 53-3 gives a brief overview of the major religious groups' practices related to health.

In general, it is the client's right to be able to practice personal spiritual expressions in private, such as reading holy scriptures, praying, or meditating while in the hospital. The wearing of special amulets or garments on areas exposed to tests, treatments, or surgery may call for a special consultation with the family and spiritual leader, rather than automatically removing them.

If the spiritual leader or healer plans to visit, the client's room and religious articles should be readied appropriately. If the sacraments or other rituals are to be performed, the bedside stand or table may need to be cleared.

Nursing Interventions for Altered Spiritual Function

In considering the implementation of spiritual care, the nurse must prioritize emergent client needs. For example, basic survival needs, such as maintaining an airway, take priority over growth needs that have to do with self-actualization. However, if the client has found no meaning in suffering, is experiencing hopelessness, or is unable to take part in his or her faith community, the spiritual dimension can become a central need. The client may have regained physical strength, but the spirit remains unfulfilled.

Listening and Supporting

The simplest definition of spiritual care is care given that meets spiritual needs. This includes support, comfort, and help. Shelly (1982a, p. 15) summarizes spiritual care as follows:

> Spiritual care is an integrating factor in healthcare. Respecting and encouraging a person's spiritual and religious interest and concerns enhances the healing process. Spiritual support includes communicating love, forgiveness, meaning, purpose, and hope in a time of discouragement and anxiety.

Thus, active listening with empathy and sensitivity becomes one of the most valuable interventions for the nurse. Through purposeful listening, the nurse allows the client to define personal spiritual questions and to direct the type of support that would be most useful at that point in time (Fig. 53-4). The following situation, adapted from Frye and Long (1985), illustrates the intervention of listening and support as an integral part of spiritual caregiving.

> *Robert, the son of a practicing physician and the eldest of four children, was a junior medical student. He is a handsome, popular young man with a keen, satirical sense of humor. Robert was scheduled to be at his first family practice clinic, but he didn't make it.*

Table 53-3 • Practices of Major Religious Groups Related to Health

Religious Faiths	Dietary Rules	Birth Control and Abortion	Organ Transplants	Death and Dying
Observant Jews	Orthodox Jews observe Kosher dietary laws; Reform Jews usually do not observe dietary restrictions.	Orthodox Jews do not encourage birth control; abortion may be performed only to save mother's life.	Organ transplants generally not permitted by Orthodox or Reform Jews without rabbinical consent.	Advocate use of life support without heroic measures. Believe that family or friends should be with the dying patient. There are special procedures for care of the body after death.
Roman Catholics	Observe fasting and abstinence from meat on certain Holy Days. Hospitalized patients are excused from dietary obligations.	Birth control prohibited except for abstinence and natural family planning. Abortion is prohibited.	Organ donation and transplantation are acceptable.	Each Roman Catholic should have the anointing of the sick as well as the Eucharist and penance by a priest before death.
Mainline Protestants (eg, Baptist, Nazarene, Lutheran, Methodist, Presbyterian, Episcopal)	Use of alcohol and tobacco is forbidden by many denominations. Episcopalians may observe fasting and abstinence from meat on some days.	Birth control is generally left as a matter of personal choice. Abortion is generally discouraged, but there may be some exceptions.	Organ donation and transplantation are acceptable.	Notification of clergy, Scripture reading, and prayer are appropriate.
Islam (Muslims)	Pork and alcohol are forbidden.	Contraception is permitted by Islamic law. Abortion is forbidden.	Donation of body parts or organs is generally not allowed. Vigilant attitude is required to avoid misuse.	Believe family should be with the dying patient so they can read the Koran and pray. There are special procedures for care of body after death. Men wash male bodies and women wash female bodies and perform a variety of other rituals.
Other Western Faiths				
Christian Science	Alcohol and tobacco are prohibited.	Personal choice.	Donations of organs unlikely.	A Christian Science practitioner may be called.
	Special Concerns: Normally do not seek medical care.			
Jehovah's Witnesses	Use of alcohol and tobacco discouraged.	Birth control is personal choice. Abortion is opposed.	Organ transplant is a personal decision but must be cleansed with a nonblood product.	No special practices.
	Special Concerns: Blood transfusions are not allowed.			
Church of Jesus Christ of Latter Day Saints (Mormons)	Abstinence from tobacco, alcohol, and caffeine-containing beverages such as coffee, tea, and cola.			Church elder should be notified.
	Special Concerns: A sacred undergarment must be worn at all times.			

(continued)

Table 53-3 (Continued)

Religious Faiths	Dietary Rules	Birth Control and Abortion	Organ Transplants	Death and Dying
Seventh Day Adventists	Alcohol, tobacco, coffee and tea prohibited. Most members are vegetarians.	Personal choice.	Personal choice.	No special practices. Clergy may be notified.
Other Eastern Faiths				
Hinduism represents a 5,000-year tradition. It has many different beliefs and practices depending on the culture and tribal unit. One of the medical traditions is the Ayurveda system. Illness and wellness are viewed as a state of balance. In this world view, the human being is continuous with the environment.	Ranges from complete vegetarian to restrictions on certain foods, such as poultry and milk products. Traditional foods include many legumes, yogurt, and spices. There is also a belief system of "hot" and "cold" food, depending on how the body responds. Balancing tastes is also important (eg, sour, bitter). In some places, to refuse food means that one is angry or hurt.	All of life is sacred, so generally not practiced; however, there is preference for male children, and female infant sacrifices have been known. There may be some concern that amniocentesis could be used to preference male children. Because India has a population problem, both birth control and abortion are permitted but not generally practiced. Abortion has been legal since 1972.	In the Hindu tradition, often ancient myths are reinterpreted to fit current circumstances. At present, there is no information available as to how this procedure is viewed; however, the wealthy may go to other countries for medical care.	There is a belief in reincarnation, so life never ends. Untimely death is regarded with fear and sorrow. The family participates in mourning rituals both before and after mortal death. At death, some place the body on the floor or the earth, to facilitate the soul's journey. Cremation is the common practice; fire purifies the body, and the family gives the ashes to the holy waters.
Buddhism began in the 6th century B.C. in northeast India and expanded along trade routes to the south, southeast Asia, China, and Japan and in the latter 19th century to the west. The medical system that was used is the Ayurveda system. The path of health is right living and thinking. There are many different Buddhist groups who follow different leaders.	Diet is an issue of balance, similar to Hindu beliefs. Alcohol and other drugs are forbidden because they can lead to moral carelessness. The laity may consume fairly heavily, however, and recent attempts at reform have not been taken seriously.	There is ambiguity about when life begins so there is no clear-cut view on abortion. They are against killing or injuring humans and animals. Both birth control and abortion have been known and practiced. The practice may not reflect the faith as much as current social and political policies.	At present there is no stated view about organ transplants. The principles guiding such decisions would include: "all is interdependent (family, donor, healthcare people, society) and suffering." (Personal communication from Ronald Nakasone, Ph.D., Institute of Buddhist Studies, Berkeley, CA)	Life is a temporary state as a combination of body/mental elements, thus death is temporary also; it is necessary for rebirth. Family needs to be present, certain prayers need to be said by the priest. The color white means death, so the use of white by healthcare personnel may cause increased anxiety for some patients/families. Priest visits family home every day for prayers until burial. Prayers are said at certain times and up to 1 year after death, and then every year.

Special Concerns: Most Buddhists have no hesitation about seeking medical advice from non-Buddhist physicians. Thus, some see medical interventions, such as organ transplants, as a technologic issue only.

Derived from Anles, P. (1989). Medicine and living tradition of Islam. In L. E. Sullivan (Ed.), ***Healing and restoring, health and medicine in the world's religious traditions*** (p. 189). New York: Macmillan; Carson, J. B. (1989). ***Spiritual dimensions of nursing practice*** (pp. 76–112). Philadelphia, W. B. Saunders; Desai, P. N. (1989). ***Health and medicine in the Hindu tradition.*** New York, Crossroad Publishing Company; Kitagawa, J. M. (1989). Buddhist medical history. In L. E. Sullivan (Ed.), ***Healing and restoring, health and medicine in the world's religious traditions*** (pp. 9–32). New York: Macmillan.

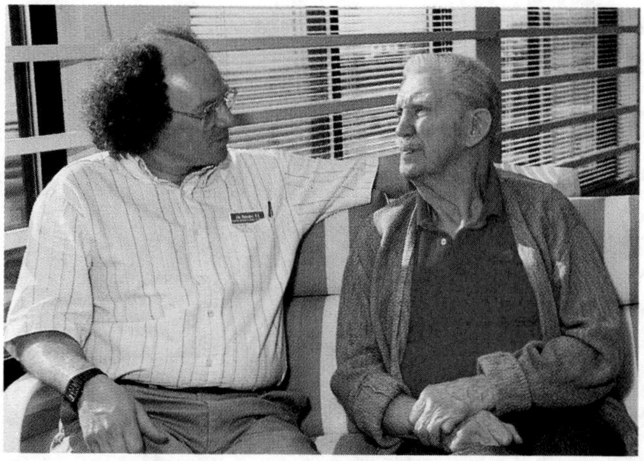

Figure 53-4 • Listening and supporting are important nursing interventions. (Courtesy of Seattle University School of Nursing)

Traffic was heavy on the freeway, and Robert found himself between a truck and a semi-trailer with cars on either side. He tried to swerve into an adjacent lane, rear-ending a large truck. The impact propelled him off and under his motorcycle, resulting in instant unconsciousness. When he arrived at the emergency room, both pupils were fixed and the outlook was grim.

The next 5 months were a battle. Fluctuating intracranial pressures with complications, pervading depression, and thoughts of suicide haunted him. Having deeply religious parents and a strong background in religious education, Robert seemed to have the spiritual strengths to deal with this crisis . . . until one day when the depth of his loneliness and doubt surfaced.

His nurse approached him, suspecting that he needed permission to and acceptance of doubt of previous convictions. As a result, there was an outpouring of questions. Where was God when he needed Him? Why had God let him down?

Many conversations followed with Robert's mother, the nurses, doctor, therapists, and chaplain. Family, friends, and staff supported him in his questions. Robert identified with the story of Job and began to talk of his hope.

As part of this denial of his former convictions, Robert frequently requested pain medication during the day to help him sleep. He stated, "I just don't want to be awake." The nurse confronted him, asking him if he was truly in pain or trying to escape from the realities of his situation. She recommended that they work together on a different approach.

Referral

The nurse should be comfortable in listening to the client's spiritual needs and in hearing religious requests. If the client or family members ask for prayer or scripture reading, and the nurse is comfortable in doing that, the nurse should identify the special focus or topic before he or she begins. When the client and family appear to have no religious tradition, the nurse may ask to assist the client or family in a quiet, reflective moment. The nurse may also respond to a request to see the hospital chaplain, or initiate a referral to see one. For an effective referral, it is helpful if the nurse has a working knowledge of the chaplaincy program and knows the chaplain(s) personally. The chaplain is also a resource for finding representatives for other religious groups as well.

Age-Specific Interventions

Nursing interventions need to be tailored to the stage of faith development of the individual client

Newborn and Infant. Hospitalization and illness potentially disrupt the infant's basic trust in parents. It is the nurse's role to support the spiritual needs of the parents, which in turn will meet the needs of the infant. This can best be done by listening, offering support, and promoting stability in the family support system. To accomplish this, the parents must be encouraged to be present with the infant as much as possible and involved in the caring process (Betz, 1981; Shelly, 1982b).

Toddler and Preschooler. Carrying out established routines and responding to concrete questions are important considerations with the toddler and preschooler. The role of the nurse is to support the family in carrying out the rituals of faith. If the family is not available to do this, then it is helpful if the nurse can carry them out. For example, bedtime, often a difficult transition for children at this age, but especially so in the hospital, is a crucial time of the day to offer support (Betz, 1981; Shelly, 1982b).

Children in early childhood are also very sensitive to good–bad issues. They should not be told that painful or scary treatments are in any way a punishment, even though they might feel that. It should be affirmed that they are still loved by their parents, the nurse, and God or Jesus, or whatever is appropriate given the source of the family's faith (Shelly, 1982b).

Child and Adolescent. The nurse continues to be of major support to the family unit, carrying out the familiar religious rituals in the healthcare setting. It is also important that the nurse clarify fact and fantasy when it comes to all of the medical interventions and procedures (Betz, 1981; Shelly, 1982b). Often, a "story" about

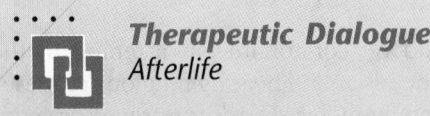

Therapeutic Dialogue
Afterlife

Scenes for Thought

Jeremy Gaston is 17 years old and is in the hospital for his third chemotherapy treatment for leukemia. He is lying in bed and seems very quiet today when you stop in during your morning rounds.

Effective

Nurse: *Hi, Jeremy, how are you this morning? (Checking his central venous catheter and the drip rate of the medication.)*
Client: *I was just thinking about dying.* Looking off into space.
Nurse: *(Stops to look at him in surprise, then continues checking the IV drip.) What were you thinking?*
Client: *What it was like, just in case I don't make it through this cancer.*
Nurse: *What do you think it would be like? (Sitting down next to the bed.)*
Client: *My father almost died from a heart attack and said he could see himself on the emergency room table with everyone working on him. He said it wasn't scary, just weird.*
Nurse: *You've talked about this with your dad?*
Client: *Yeah. A few years ago. But my family isn't religious at all, so I'm not sure about the bright light or angels or heaven or anything like that.* Sounds worried.
Nurse: *You sound a little worried about that.*
Client: *Yeah, I am. I'd hate to think there was nothing.*
Nurse: *So you're worried there might be nothing after death but you're not sure. Is that right?*
Client: *Yeah.*
Nurse: *You know, you and I have talked about pain and the chemo and the leukemia, but I don't think we've talked about this. What kind of help do you need right now?*
Client: Smiles. *Maybe a philosophy course! Could we just talk a little about what you think death is?*
Nurse: *Sure. (They continue . . . .)*

Less Effective

Nurse: *Hi, Jeremy, how are you this morning? (Checking his central venous catheter and the drip rate of the medication.)*
Client: *I was just thinking about dying.* Looking off into space.
Nurse: *(Stops to look at him in surprise, then continues checking the IV drip.) What were you thinking?*
Client: *What it was like, just in case I don't make it through this cancer.*
Nurse: *I thought we talked about how much better you're getting?*
Client: Looks at her, sheepishly. *Yeah, I know, but sometimes it gets to me, all the chemo and how long it's taking and the pain. Sorry.*
Nurse: *You don't have to apologize, Jeremy. I know you get discouraged, but I also know you have Someone (points up) watching over you and caring for you. I feel that very strongly. So don't worry about dying just yet. (Has tears in her eyes that Jeremy doesn't see.)*
Client: *Okay.* Looks off into space again.
Nurse: *I'll let you rest now. Think good thoughts and this treatment will be over in a jiffy. (Leaves the room.)*

Critical Thinking Challenges

• From the conversation of the second nurse, detect who she was reassuring and how the client responded to her reassurance. • Analyze what the first nurse helped the client do. • Construct your own thoughts about an afterlife and how they affect the way you live your life. • Analyze how your thoughts affect the way you care for your clients.

a similar situation will aid in this reality-orienting process. Local libraries usually have a variety of books in which children experience going to the health clinic or the hospital. Again, it is imperative that the child not associate illness and hospitalization with wrongdoing and punishment, becoming in the process more anxious about themselves and fearful of their surroundings. Acceptance and clarification of the experiences are the effective modes in offering meaning to the child.

Development of a personal style and interaction with peers remain priorities even when the adolescent is ill. The nurse can be available to the adolescent's peers, involving them by encouraging them to remain available, either through visits, letters, or telephone. If a long-term illness, accident, or some other severe condition is involved, other networks of support might also be useful, such as the school or the church. For example, the youth group might make a commitment to be a communication link for the adolescent while he or she is in the hospital. It is also possible that the peers might need an opportunity to explore their own responses to illness and accidents to work through their feelings about life. The youth leaders or the hospital chaplain are resources for this kind of experience (Huber & Healy, 1992).

Adolescents are capable of conceptualizing a personal relationship with God (Betz, 1981; Shelly, 1982b). In a time of illness, they may question the meaning of the experience, trying to integrate it into their lives, much as many adults would do under similar circumstances. These issues can often be discerned during a nursing history and assessment. The nurse can either follow up on the data or involve the hospital chaplain or the adolescent's spiritual counselor.

Adult and Older Adult. The young adult is clarifying personal beliefs and commitments based on experience and relationships. The faith challenge is to establish and reflect on personal faith and the meaning of life. Perhaps it is too much to expect that a nurse can perform a mentoring relationship with many clients. However, in some long-term relationships, being available to listen, support, and validate feelings and experiences would facilitate exploration of meaning-in-life or meaning-in-death experiences. At the very least, it is important for the nurse to understand that young adults have this need, and to be open to explore with the client possibilities as to who might fulfill this role. It is also important to continue to be supportive to the client's family and social network, because these relationships also give meaning to the client's life (Shelly, 1982b).

During the middle years, the adult becomes more concerned with a broader world view and more concerned about polarities. The resolution of these polarities lies in being able to see the paradoxes and live with them, not threatened by diversity, but open to it. Such people might be described as "wise-hearted," and in some ways they have much to offer others. For example, a young adult nurse might gain personally by spending time with an adult who was working through a paradox of health and illness. By being available to listen, support, and reflect with the client, the nurse could gain understanding of the client's struggle. By accepting the possibility of mutuality in the relationship, the nurse has the opportunity to give new meaning and hope to the client. Risking mutuality demonstrates true respect and care, which in turn enhances the selves of both client and nurse (Fowler, 1981).

As in other age groups, listening and support are an essential part of the nurse's role as the client deals with the health–illness situation. An additional aspect could be the use of a life review strategy, in which the client is given the opportunity to recollect past experiences and come to an understanding of them. As infirmity increases, the older adult may not be able to participate in his or her faith community as much as previously. At this point, the nurse needs to facilitate connections with people or groups in this community who can either visit regularly or assist with transportation. Connections such as this provide meaning and hope for the older person, for some rituals of faith can be satisfactorily performed only in a group setting.

Often, other family members and friends have died in the last few years, and the older adult not only needs to be able to form new relationships with the younger generations, but may want to come to terms with his or her own mortality. Again, the nurse does not need to have the "answer," but does need to provide an opportunity for the client to discuss death and make his or her own choices about how arrangements should be handled (Shelton, 1981).

Community-Based Care

Assessing and planning for spiritual care is an ongoing process. Probably the place where this can occur most consistently is where the nurse and the client have established a relationship over time. This may be in a clinic, as a case manager, a team leader in a long-term care facility, or as a visiting nurse in a community hospice program. In acute care settings, the nurse most certainly will become aware of spiritual needs and begin to address them. However, the most important part of the care will be the discharge summary and a plan of care that identifies the areas of spiritual distress, so follow-up care can be more holistic. The client may want the nurse to prearrange a visit by a pastor, priest, or members of the religious community after the person arrives at home or at the next healthcare facility. In some areas of the United States, churches have developed a parish nurse program. These nurses can assist clients and families, not only in dealing with appropriate care in the community, but in meeting spiritual needs as well. Clients do not need to be members of the church to have a parish nurse visit; they can be referred by geographic area.

Much healing and spiritual growth can occur in a person without professional assistance, for some clients may have already found ways to meet their spiritual needs. The nurse, therefore, should be sensitive and nonintrusive—the client cannot be forced to deal with spiritual issues or assume religious beliefs, whether in hospital or community settings. "Sometimes [nurses] may set goals for the client and the family which are inflexible and unrealistic; this may inhibit spontaneity and impede the development a sensitive spiritual relationship" (Spiritual Care Work Group, 1990). Spiritual health is one area that cannot be put onto a specific "road map" or trajectory.

Evaluation

Specific outcome criteria are the evaluative tools for measuring the attainment of goals for the client in spiritual distress. Examples of outcome criteria are listed in the following, and use "Robert" (see the section on Listening and Supporting) as the client example. Outcome criteria need to be specifically tailored to the client so that the criteria will uniquely measure the attainment of that client's goals.

Goal

- The client will express acceptance of current life situation.

Possible Outcome Criteria

- Client exhibits feelings of despair, anger, and fear during the first few days.

Nursing Plan of Care
The Client With Spiritual Distress*

Nursing Diagnosis

Spiritual Distress related to crisis of illness as evidenced by loss of meaning in life, suicidal thoughts, and overuse of pain medication.

Client Goal

Client will express increased understanding and acceptance of current life situation.

Client Outcome Criteria

- Client verbalizes feelings of despair, anger, and fear after 3 weeks.
- Client identifies support provided by staff, family, and friends during periods of questioning and despair after 5 weeks.
- Client identifies some alternative coping mechanisms other than requesting pain medications after 10 weeks.

Nursing Intervention	Scientific Rationale
1. Offer client opportunity for one-on-one nurse–client relationship. Actively listen to the client. Allow expression of negative feelings.	1. Initiating a one-on-one relationship establishes a climate of acceptance and builds trust and safety.
2. Plan and coordinate a multidisciplinary team conference, including the chaplain. Facilitate a care-planning conference involving the social support network, including family and friends.	2. Initiating a multidisciplinary social network of conferences facilitates a sense of acceptance, love, and belonging.
3. Explore past coping mechanisms, including use of music, scripture, prayer, and relaxation techniques. Help client identify times when he or she can use a variety of these alternative strategies.	3. Building on past positive coping mechanisms enhances a sense of self-control and self-esteem.
4. Use the "life review" technique focusing on faith/spiritual development. Help client explore ways to use this experience in a unique way, such as sharing in a group or with medical students or other healthcare professional students.	4. By focusing on personal faith/spirit, the client can gain new insights into his or her relationship with God, sensing hope and the potential for creativity or self-actualization.

*Refers to the patient situation of "Robert."

- Client identifies support provided by staff, family, and friends during periods of questioning and despair during the rehabilitation period.

Goal

- The client will participate in spiritual practices that are personally supportive.

Possible Outcome Criteria

- Within the first month, client asks to speak to his or her spiritual advisor.
- Client demonstrates spiritual practices, such as prayer, scripture reading, and the sacraments within the second month.
- Client expresses satisfaction with being able to maintain relationships with his or her faith community within second month.

Key Concepts

- The role of philosophy is not to answer questions but to help people ask the right questions and develop a view of life. Spirituality does the same thing, in part.

- The spiritual dimension is the essence of a person. It is expressed in the need to seek meaning in experiences and to make a spiritual journey through life.
- Spiritual well-being is the condition in which a person is at peace with God, self, community, and environment.
- Fowler's stages of faith have parallels to Piaget's stages of cognitive development and Erikson's stages of psychosocial development.
- Nurses may provide inadequate or inappropriate care if they have not fully addressed their own spirituality and spiritual well-being, and if they hesitate to encourage the client to speak of personal spirituality.
- Altered spiritual function may be expressed in various verbalizations of distress and a variety of altered behaviors.
- Every client has the right to practice his or her spirituality according to personal preference. The nurse should not be judgmental, but should assist the client in fulfilling those needs.
- Nursing interventions include use of self, spiritual support, support of religious practices, listening and supporting, and referral.

Critical Thinking Challenges

Spiritual health and its relationship to the functioning person are now a part of your knowledge base of nursing. Using other information concerning holism, you should be able to think critically about the client in the drug rehabilitation program.Turn back to the situation at the beginning of the chapter, and consider the following:

1. *As you reflect on this situation, describe what might be some of the underlying spiritual issues.*
2. *Consider the potential spiritual issues from the client's point of view, the family's and the injured brother.*
3. *Reflect on your own spiritual perspective.*
4. *Construct ideas for how you would respond to this client.*

References

Assagioli, R. (1971). *Psychosynthesis.* New York: Penguin Books.

Betz, C. L. (1981). Faith development in children. *Pediatric Nursing, 7,* 22–25.

Brallier, L. W. (1978). The nurse as holistic health practitioner. *Nurs Clin North Am, 13,* 643–655.

Burkhardt, M., & Nagai-Jacobson, M. G. (1985). Dealing with spiritual concerns of clients in the community. *J Community Health, 2,* 191–198.

Carson, V. B. (1989). *Spiritual dimensions of nursing practice* (pp. 76–112). Philadelphia: W. B. Saunders.

Carpenito, L. J. (1995). *Nursing diagnosis: Application to clinical practice* (6th ed.). Philadelphia: J. B. Lippincott.

Chapman, L. S. (1986). Spiritual health: A component missing from health promotion. *American Journal of Health Promotion, 1* (1), 38–41.

Fish, S., & Shelly, J. A. (1983). *Spiritual care: The nurse's role* (2nd ed.). Downer's Grove, IL: InterVarsity Press.

Fowler, J. W. (1981). *Stages of faith.* San Francisco: Harper & Row.

Fromm, E. (1968). *The revolution of hope.* New York: Harper & Row.

Frye, B., & Long, L. (1985). Spiritual counseling approaches following brain-injury. *Rehabilitation Nursing, 10,* 14–16.

Grandstrom, S. L. (1985). Spiritual care of oncology clients. *Topics in Clinical Nursing, 7* (1), 39–45.

Houldin, A., Saltstein, W. A., & Ganley, K. M. (1987). *Nursing diagnoses for wellness.* Philadelphia: J. B. Lippincott.

Huber, L., & Healy, M. (1992). Grow days: Nurturing spiritually healthy teens. *Journal of Christian Nursing, 9* (3), 18–21.

Hunglemann, J., Kenke-Rossi, E., Klassen, L., et al. (1985). Spiritual well-being in older adults: Harmonious interconnectedness. *Journal of Religion and Health, 24,* 147–153.

Kreidler, M. (1984). Meaning in suffering . . . philosophy for nurses. *Int Nurs Rev, 31,* 174–176.

Mathai, M. K. (1980). *Spirituality in relation to nurses' perception of their own coping strategies when clients are perceived to be suffering.* Ann Arbor, MI: University of Michigan.

Moberg, D. O. (Ed.). (1979). *Spiritual well-being: Sociological perspectives.* Washington, D. C.: University Press of America.

Murray, R. B., & Zentner, J. P. (1985). *Nursing concepts for health promotion* (3rd ed.). Englewood Cliffs, NJ: Prentice-Hall.

North American Nursing Diagnosis Association (NANDA). (1994). *Nursing diagnoses: Definitions and classification 1995–1996.* Philadelphia: Author.

Ozmon, H. A., & Craver, S. M. (1994). *Philosophical foundations of education* (5th ed.). Columbus, OH: Charles E. Merrill.

Peck, M. L. (1981). The therapeutic effect of faith. *Nurs Forum, 20,* 153–166.

Penrose, V., & Barret, S. (1982). Spiritual needs: "In sickness I lack myself." *Nursing Mirror, 10,* 38–39.

Peterson, E. A. (1985). The physical . . . the spiritual . . . can you meet all of your client's needs? *Journal of Gerontological Nursing, 11,* 23–27.

Piepgras, R. (1984). The other dimension: Spiritual help. *Am J Nurs, 68,* 2610–2613.

Reed, P. (1986). Spirituality and well-being in terminally ill hospitalized adults. *Res Nurs Health, 10,* 335–344.

Richardson, G. R., & Noland, W. P. (1984). Treating the spiritual dimension through educational imagery: Health education. *Health Values, 8,* 25–30.

Ruffing-Rahal, M. A. (1984). The spiritual dimension of well-being: Implications for the elderly. *Home Health Nurse, 2,* 12–16.

Shelly, J. A. (1982a). Spiritual care . . . planting seeds of hope. *Critical Care Update, 9,* 7–17.

Shelly, J. A. (1982b). *The spiritual needs of children: A guide for nurses, parents and teachers.* Downer's Grove, IL: InterVarsity Press.

Shelton, R. L. (1981). The client's need of faith at death. *Topics in Clinical Nursing, 3,* 55–59.

Spiritual Care Work Group. (1990). Assumptions and principles of spiritual care. *Death Studies, 14,* 75–81.

Still, J. V. H. (1984). How to assess spiritual needs of children. *Journal of Christian Nursing, 1,* 4–6.

Stoll, R. I. (1979). Guidelines for spiritual assessment. *Am J Nurs, 79,* 1574–1577.

Tillich, P. (1969). *What is religion?* New York: Harper & Row.

Toth, J.C. (1992) Faith in recovery: Spiritual support after an acute MI. *Journal of Christian Nursing,* 9 (4), 28–31.

Westberg, G. (1956). *Nurse, pastor and client: A hospital chaplain talks with nurses.* Rock Island, IL: Augustina Press.

Bibliography

Burkhardt, M. A. (1994). Becoming and connecting: Elements of spirituality for women. *Holistic Nursing Practice, 8* (4), 12–21.

Burkhardt, M. A., & Nagai-Jacobson, M. G. (1994). Reawakening spirit in clinical practice. *Journal of Holistic Nursing, 12* (1), 9–21.

Corcoran, E. (1993). Spirituality: An important aspect of emergency nursing. *Journal of Emergency Nursing, 19,* 183–184.

Kaye, J., & Robinson, K. M. (1994). Spirituality among caregivers. *Image, 26,* 218–221.

Mansen, T. G. (1993). The spiritual dimension of individuals: Conceptual development. *Nursing Diagnosis, 4* (4), 140–147.

Young, C. (1993). Spirituality and chronically ill Christian elderly. *Geriatric Nursing, 14,* 298–303.

Zerwekh, J. (1993). Transcending life: The practice wisdom of nursing hospice experts. *American Journal of Hospice and Palliative Care, 10* (5), 26–31.

Appendices

APPENDIX A

Equivalents

Outline of the Metric System

Prefix	*Meaning*	*Example(s)*
Kilo	1000	1 kilogram 1000 grams (g)
Hecto	100	1 hectogram 100 grams (g)
Deca	10	1 decaliter 10 liters (L)
	1	1 gram 1 liter 1 meter
Deci	0.1	1 deciliter 0.1 liter (L)
Centi	0.01	1 centimeter 0.01 meter (m)
Milli	0.001	1 milligram 0.001 gram (g)
Micro	0.000001 (10^{6})	1 microgram 0.000001 gram (g) 1 micrometer 0.000001 meter (m)
Nano	0.000000001 (10^{9})	1 nanogram 0.000000001 gram (g)
Pico	0.000000000001 (10^{12})	1 picogram 0.000000000001 gram (g)

Approximate Weight Equivalents

Metric	*Apothecaries*	*Metric*	*Apothecaries*
0.0001 gram —0.1	mg—1/640 grain (1/600 grain)	0.02 gram —20	mg—1/3 grain
0.0002 gram —0.2	mg—1/320 grain (1/300 grain)	0.025 gram —25	mg—3/8 grain
0.0003 gram —0.3	mg—1/210 grain (1/200 grain)	0.03 gram —30	mg—2/5 grain (1/2 grain)
0.0004 gram —0.4	mg—1/150 grain	0.04 gram —40	mg—3/5 grain (2/3 grain)
0.0005 gram —0.5	mg—1/120 grain	0.05 gram —50	mg—3/4 grain
0.0006 gram —0.6	mg—1/100 grain	0.06 gram —60	mg—9/10 grain (1 grain)
0.0007 gram —0.7	mg—1/90 grain	0.7 gram —70	mg—1 1/20 grains
0.0008 gram —0.8	mg—1/80 grain	0.08 gram —80	mg—1 1/5 grains
0.0009 gram —0.9	mg—1/75 grain	0.09 gram —90	mg—1 1/3 grains
0.001 gram —1	mg—1/64 grain (1/60 grain)	0.2 gram —200	mg—3 grains
0.0011 gram —1.1	mg—1/60 grain	0.3 gram —300	mg—4 1/2 grains
0.0016 gram —1.6	mg—1/40 grain (1.5 mg)	0.4 gram —400	mg—6 grains
0.0020 gram —2	mg—1/32 grain (1/30 grain)	0.5 gram —500	mg—7 1/2 grains
0.0022 gram —2.2	mg—1/30 grain	0.6 gram —600	mg—9 grains
0.003 gram —3	mg—1/20 grain	0.80 gram —800	mg—12 grains (0.75 gram)
0.004 gram —4	mg—1/16 grain (1/15 grain)	1.0 gram —1000	mg—15 grains
0.005 gram —5	mg—1/12 grain	1.50 grams—1500	mg—22 grains
0.006 gram —6	mg—1/10 grain	2 grams—2000	mg—30 grains (1/2 dram)
0.008 gram —8	mg—1/8 grain	4 grams	—1 dram (60 grains)
0.01 gram —10	mg—1/6 grain	5 grams	—75 grains
0.016 gram —16	mg—1/4 grain (15 mg)	30 grams	—1 ounce

Approximate Volume Equivalents: Liquid Measures

Metric		Apothecaries
0.06 cubic centimeter	—1	minim
0.25 cubic centimeter	—4	minims
0.3 cubic centimeter	—5	minims
0.5 cubic centimeter	—8	minims
0.6 cubic centimeter	—10	minims
0.75 cubic centimeter	—12	minims
1 cubic centimeter	—15	minims
2 cubic centimeters	—30	minims
3 cubic centimeters	—45	minims
4 cubic centimeters	—1	fluid dram
8 cubic centimeters	—2	fluid drams
10 cubic centimeters	—2½	fluid drams
15 cubic centimeters	—4	fluid drams
20 cubic centimeters	—5½	fluid drams
25 cubic centimeters	—⅚	fluid ounce
30 cubic centimeters	—1	fluid ounce
60 cubic centimeters	—2	fluid ounces
100 cubic centimeters	—3½	fluid ounces
120 cubic centimeters	—4	fluid ounces
200 cubic centimeters	—7	fluid ounces
250 cubic centimeters	—8	fluid ounces
500 cubic centimeters	—1	pint
1000 cubic centimeters	—1	quart

Note: A cubic centimeter (cc) and a milliliter (mL) are approximate equivalents. The terms are used interchangeably.

APPENDIX B

Laboratory Values*

Laboratory values may vary according to the techniques used in different laboratories.

Abbreviations

Conventional Units

kg = kilogram
gm = gram
mg = milligram
μg = microgram
μμg = micromicrogram
ng = nanogram
pg = picogram
dL = 100 milliliters
mL = milliliter
cu mm = cubic millimeter
fL = femtoliter
mM = millimole
nM = nanomole
mOsm = milliosmole
mm = millimeter
μ = micron or micrometer
mm Hg = millimeters of mercury
U = unit
mU = milliunit
μU = microunit
mEq = milliequivalent
IU = International Unit
mIU = milliInternational Unit

SI Units

g = gram
L = liter
d = day
h = hour
mol = mole
mmol = millimole
μmol = micromole
nmol = nanomole
pmol = picomole

Reference Ranges—Hematology

Determination	Reference Range: Conventional units	Reference Range: SI units	Clinical Significance
A_2 hemoglobin	1.5%–3.5% of total hemoglobin	Mass fraction: 0.015–0.035 of total hemoglobin	Increased in certain types of thalassemia
Bleeding time	1–9 min	2–8 min	Prolonged in thrombocytopenia, defective platelet function, and aspirin therapy
Factor V assay (proaccelerin factor)	60%–140%		
Factor VIII assay (antihemophiliac factor)	50%–200%		Deficient in classic hemophilia
Factor IX assay (plasma thromboplastin component)	75%–125%		Deficient in Christmas disease (pseudohemophilia)
Factor X (Stuart factor)	60%–140%		Deficient in Stuart clotting defect

(continued)

Determination	Reference Range: Conventional units	Reference Range: SI units	Clinical Significance
Fibrinogen	200–400 mg/dL	2–4 g/dL	Increased in pregnancy, infections accompanied by leukocytosis, nephrosis Decreased in severe liver disease, abruptio placentae
Fibrin split products	Less than 10 mg/L	Less than 10 mg/L	Increased in disseminated intravascular coagulation
Fibrinolysins (whole blood clot lysis time)	No lysis in 24 h		Increased activity associated with massive hemorrhage, extensive surgery, transfusion reactions
Partial thromboplastin time (activated)	20–45 sec		Prolonged in deficiency of fibrinogen, factors II, V, VIII, IX, X, XI, and XII, and in heparin therapy
Prothrombin consumption	Over 20 sec		Impaired in deficiency of factors VIII, IX, and X
Prothrombin time	9.5–12 sec		Prolonged by deficiency of factors, I, II, V, VII, and X, fat malabsorption, severe liver disease, coumarin-anticoagulant therapy
Erythrocyte count	Males: 4,600,000–6,200,000/ cu mm	$4.6–6.2 \times 10^{12}$/L	Increased in severe diarrhea and dehydration, polycythemia, acute poisoning, pulmonary fibrosis
	Females: 4,200,000–5,400,000/ cu mm	$4.2–5.4 \times 10^{12}$/L	Decreased in all anemias, in leukemia, and after hemorrhage, when blood volume has been restored
Erythrocyte indices			
Mean corpuscular volume (MCV)	80–94 (cu μ)	80–94 fL	Increased in macrocytic anemias: decreased in microcytic anemia
Mean corpuscular hemoglobin (MCH)	27–32 $\mu\mu$g/cell	27–32 pg	Increased in macrocytic anemias; decreased in microcytic anemia
Mean corpuscular hemoglobin concentration (MCHC)	33%–38%	Concentration fraction: 0.33–0.38	Decreased in severe hypochromic anemia
Reticulocytes	0.5%–1.5% of red cells	Number fraction: 0.005–0.015	Increased with any condition stimulating increase in bone marrow activity (ie, infection, blood loss [acute and chronic]); after iron therapy in iron deficiency anemia, polycythemia rubra vera Decreased with any condition depressing bone marrow activity, acute leukemia, late stage of severe anemias
Erythrocyte sedimentation rate (ESR)—Westergren method	Males under 50 yr; <5 mm/h	<15 mm/h	Increased in tissue destruction, whether inflammatory or degenerative; during menstruation and pregnancy; and in acute febrile diseases
	Males over 50 yr; <20 mm/h	<20 mm/h	
	Females under 50 yr; <20 mm/h	<20 mm/h	
	Females over 50 yr; <30 mm/h	<30 mm/h	
Erythrocyte sedimentation ratio–Zeta centrifuge	41%–54% in both sexes	Fraction: 0.41–0.54	Significance similar to ESR
Hematocrit	Males: 42%–50%	Volume fraction: 0.42–0.5	Decreased in severe anemias, anemia of pregnancy, acute massive blood loss

Determination	Reference Range: Conventional units	Reference Range: SI units	Clinical Significance
	Females: 40%–48%	Volume fraction: 0.4–0.48	Increased in erythrocytosis of any cause, and in dehydration or hemoconcentration associated with shock
Hemoglobin	Males: 13–18 gm/dL Females: 12–16 gm/dL	2.02–2.79 mmol/L 1.86–2.48 mmol/L	Decreased in various anemias, pregnancy, severe or prolonged hemorrhage, and with excessive fluid intake Increased in polycythemia, chronic obstructive pulmonary diseases, failure of oxygenation because of congestive heart failure, and normally in people living at high altitudes
Hemoglobin F	Less than 2% of total hemoglobin	Mass fraction: <0.02	Increased in infants and children, and in thalassemia and many anemias
Leukocyte alkaline phosphatase	Score of 40–100		Increased in polycythemia vera, myelofibrosis, and infections Decreased in chronic granulocytic leukemia, paroxysmal nocturnal hemoglobinuria, hypoplastic marrow, and viral infections, particularly infectious mononucleosis
Leukocyte count	Total: 5000–10,000/cu mm	$5–10 \times 10^9/L$	Elevated in acute infectious diseases, predominantly in the neutrophilic fraction with bacterial diseases, and in the lymphocytic and monocytic fractions in viral diseases Elevated in acute leukemia, after menstruation, and after surgery or trauma Depressed in aplastic anemia, agranulocytosis, and by toxic agents such as chemotherapeutic agents used in treating malignancy Eosinophils elevated in collagen disease, allergy, intestinal parasitosis
Neutrophils	60%–70%	Number fraction: 0.6–0.7	
Eosinophils	1%–4%	Number fraction: 0.01–0.04	
Basophils	0%–0.5%	Number fraction: 0.00–0.05	
Lymphocytes	20%–30%	Number fraction: 0.2–0.3	
Monocytes	2%–6%	Number fraction: 0.02–0.06	
Osmotic fragility of red cells	Increased in hemolysis occurs in over 0.5% NaCl Decreased if hemolysis is incomplete in 0.4% NaCl		Increased in congenital spherocytosis, idiopathic acquired hemolytic anemia, isoimmune hemolytic disease, ABO hemolytic disease of newborn Decreased in sickle cell anemia, thalassemia
Platelet count	100,000–400,000/cu mm	$0.1–0.4 \times 10^{12}/L$	Increased in malignancy, myeloproliferative disease, rheumatoid arthritis, and postoperatively, about 50% of clients with unexpected increase of platelet count will be found to have a malignancy Decreased in thrombocytopenic purpura, acute leukemia, aplastic anemia, and during cancer chemotherapy, infections, and drug reactions

Reference Ranges—Serum, Plasma, and Whole Blood Chemistries

Determination	Normal Adult Reference Range: Conventional Units	Normal Adult Reference Range: SI Units	Clinical Significance: Increased	Clinical Significance: Decreased
Acetoacetate	0.2–1.0 mg/dL	19.6–98 μmol/L	Diabetic acidosis Fasting	
Acetone	0.3–2.0 mg/dL	51.6–344.0 μmol/L	Toxemia of pregnancy Carbohydrate-free diet High-fat diet	
Adrenocorticotropic hormone (ACTH) (plasma)—RIA*	Less than 50 pg/mL	Less than 50 mg/L	Pituitary-dependent Cushing's syndrome Ectopic ACTH syndrome Primary adrenal atrophy	Adrenocortical tumor Adrenal insufficiency secondary to hypopituitarism
Aldolase	3–8 Sibley-Lehninger U/dL at 37°C	22–59 mU/L at 37°C	Hepatic necrosis Granulocytic leukemia Myocardial infarction Skeletal muscle disease	
Aldosterone (plasma)—RIA	Supine: 3–10 ng/dL Upright: 5–30 ng/dL Adrenal vein: 200–800 ng/dL	0.80–0.30 nmol/L 0.14–0.90 nmol/L 5.54–22.16 nmol/L	Primary aldosteronism (Conn's syndrome) Secondary aldosteronism	Addison's disease
Alpha-1-antitrypsin	200–400 mg/dL	2–4 g/L		Certain forms of chronic lung and liver disease in young adults
Alpha-1-fetoprotein	None detected		Hepatocarcinoma Metastatic carcinoma of liver Germinal cell carcinoma of the testis or ovary Fetal neural tube defects—elevation in maternal serum	
Alpha-hydroxybutyric dehydrogenase	Up to 140 U/mL	Up to 140 U/mL	Myocardial infarction Granulocytic leukemia Hemolytic anemias Muscular dystrophy	
Ammonia (plasma)	40–80 μg/dL (enzymatic method); varies considerably with method	22.2–44.3 μmol/L	Severe liver disease Hepatic decompensation	
Amylase	60–160 Somogyi UdL	111–296 U/L	Acute pancreatitis Mumps Duodenal ulcer Carcinoma of head of pancreas Prolonged elevation with pseudocyst of pancreas Increased by drugs that constrict pancreatic duct sphincters: morphine, codeine, cholinergics	Chronic pancreatitis Pancreatic fibrosis and atrophy Cirrhosis of liver Pregnancy (2nd and 3rd trimesters)
Arsenic	6–20 μg/dL; if 50 μg/dL, suspect toxicity	0.78–2.6 μmol/L	Accidental or intentional poisoning Excessive occupational exposure	
Ascorbic acid (vitamin C)	0.4–1.5 mg/dL	23–85 μmol/L	Large doses of ascorbic acid as a prophylactic against the common cold	
Bilirubin	Total: 0.1–1.2 mg/dL Direct: 0.1–0.2 mg/dL	1.7–20.5 μmol/L 1.7–3.4 μmol/L	Hemolytic anemia (indirect) Biliary obstruction and disease	

Reference Ranges—Serum, Plasma, and Whole Blood Chemistries (continued)

Determination	Normal Adult Reference Range: Conventional Units	Normal Adult Reference Range: SI Units	Clinical Significance: Increased	Clinical Significance: Decreased
	Indirect: 0.1–1 mg/dL	1.7–17.1 μmol/L	Hepatocellular damage (hepatitis) Pernicious anemia Hemolytic disease of newborn	
Blood gases				
Oxygen, arterial (whole blood)				
Partial pressure (PaO_2)	95–100 mm Hg	12.64–13.30 kPa	Polycythemia	Anemia
Saturation (SaO_2)	94%–100%	Volume fraction: 0.94–1	Anhydremia	Cardiac decompensation Chronic obstructive pulmonary disease
Carbon dioxide, arterial (whole blood): partial pressure ($PaCO_2$)	35–45 mm Hg	4.66–5.99 kPa	Respiratory acidosis Metabolic alkalosis	Respiratory alkalosis Metabolic acidosis
pH (whole blood, arterial)	7.35–7.45	7.35–7.45	Vomiting Hyperpnea Fever Intestinal obstruction	Uremia Diabetic acidosis Hemorrhage Nephritis
Calcitonin	Basal: nondetectable 400 pg/mL	400 ng/L	Medullary carcinoma of the thyroid Some nonthyroid tumors Zollinger-Ellison syndrome	
Calcium	8.5–10.5 mg/dL	2.125–2.625 mmol/L	Tumor or hyperplasia of parathyroid Hypervitaminosis D Multiple myeloma Nephritis with uremia Malignant tumors Sarcoidosis Hyperthyroidism Skeletal immobilization Excess calcium intake: milk-alkali syndrome	Hypoparathyroidism Diarrhea Celiac disease Vitamin D deficiency Acute pancreatitis Nephrosis After parathyroidectomy
CO_2, venous	Adults: 24–32 mEq/L Infants: 18–24 mEq/L	24–32 mmol/L 18–24 mmol/L	Tetany Respiratory disease Intestinal obstruction Vomiting	Acidosis Nephritis Eclampsia Diarrhea Anesthesia
Carcinoembryonic antigen (CEA)—RIA	0–2.5 ng/mL (nonsmoker) 0–5 ng/mL (smoker)	0–2.5 μg/L (nonsmoker) 0–5 μg/L (smoker)	The repeatedly high incidence of this antigen in cancers of the colon, rectum, pancreas, and stomach suggests that CEA levels may be useful in the therapeutic monitoring of these conditions.	
Catecholamines (plasma)—RIA	Epinephrine random: up to pg/mL Norepinephrine, random 100–550 pg/mL Dopamine, random up to 130 pg/mL	Up to 490 pmol/L 590–3240 pmol/L Up to 850 pmol/L	Pheochromocytoma	

(continued)

Reference Ranges—Serum, Plasma, and Whole Blood Chemistries (continued)

	Normal Adult Reference Range		Clinical Significance	
Determination	Conventional Units	SI Units	Increased	Decreased
Cerruloplasmin	30–80 mg/dL	300–800 mg/L		Wilson's disease (hepatolenticular degeneration)
Chloride	95–105 mEq/L	95–105 mmol/L	Nephrosis Nephritis Urinary obstruction Cardiac decompensation Anemia	Diabetes Diarrhea Vomiting Pneumonia Heavy metal poisoning Cushing's syndrome Burns Intestinal obstruction Febrile conditions
Cholesterol	150–200 mg/dL	3.9–5.2 mmol/L	Lipemia Obstructive jaundice Diabetes Hypothyroidism	Pernicious anemia Hemolytic anemia Hyperthyroidism Severe infection Terminal states of debilitating disease
Cholesterol esters	60%–70% of total	Fraction of total cholesterol 0.6–0.7		The esterified fraction decreases in liver diseases
Cholinesterase	Serum: 0.6–1.6 delta pH Red cells: 0.6–1 delta pH	0.6–1.6 U 0.6–1 U	Nephrosis Exercise	Nerve gas intoxication (greater effect on red cell activity) Insecticides, organic phosphates (greater effect on plasma activity)
Chorionic gonadotropin, beta subunit—RIA	0–5 IU/L	0–5 IU/L	Pregnancy Hydatidiform mole Choriocarcinoma	
Complement, human C_3	70–150 mg/dL	880–2520 mg/L	Some inflammatory diseases, acute myocardial infarction, cancer	Acute glomerulonephritis Disseminated lupus erythematosus with renal involvement
Complement C_4	16–45 mg/dL	140–510 mg/L	Some inflammatory diseases, acute myocardial infarction, cancer	Often decreased in immunologic disease, especially with active systemic lupus erythematosus Hereditary angioneurotic edema
Complement, total (hemolytic)	90%–94% complement	25–70 U/mL	Some inflammatory diseases	Acute glomerulonephritis Epidemic meningitis Subacute bacterial endocarditis
Copper	70–165 μg/dL	11–25.9 μmol/L	Cirrhosis of liver Pregnancy	Wilson's disease

Reference Ranges—Serum, Plasma, and Whole Blood Chemistries *(continued)*

Determination	Normal Adult Reference Range: Conventional Units	Normal Adult Reference Range: SI Units	Clinical Significance: Increased	Clinical Significance: Decreased
Cortisol—RIA	8 A.M. 7–25 μg/dL 4 P.M. 2–9 μg/dL	193–690 nmol/L 55–248 nmol/L	Stress: infectious disease, surgery, burns, etc. Pregnancy Cushing's syndrome Pancreatitis Eclampsia	Addison's disease Anterior pituitary hypofunction
C-peptide reactivity	1.5–10 ng/mL	1.5–10 μg/L	Insulinoma	Diabetes
Creatine	0.2–0.8 mg/mL	15.3–61 μmol/L	Pregnancy Skeletal muscle necrosis or atrophy Starvation Hyperthroidism	
Creatine phosphokinase (CPK)	Males: 50–325 mU/mL Females: 50–250 mU/mL	50–325 U/L 50–250 U/L	Myocardial infarction Skeletal muscle diseases Intramuscular injections Crush syndrome Hypothyroidism Alcohol withdrawal delirium Alcoholic myopathy Cerebrovascular disease	
Creatine phosphokinase isoenzymes	MM band present (skeletal muscle); MB band absent (heart muscle)		MB band increase in myocardial infarction, ischemia	
Creatinine	0.7–1.4 mg/dL	62–124 μmol/L	Nephritis Chronic renal disease	Kidney diseases
Creatinine clearance	100–150 mL of blood cleared for creatinine per min	1.67–2.5 mL/s		
Cryoglobulins, qualitative	Negative		Multiple myeloma Chronic lymphocytic leukemia Lymphosarcoma Systemic lupus erythematosus Rheumatoid arthritis Infective subacute endocarditis Some malignancies Scleroderma	
11-Deoxycortisol	1 μg/dL	<0.029 μmol/L	Hypertensive form of virilizing adrenal hyperplasia due to an 11-β-hydroxylase defect	
Dibucaine number	Normal: 70%–85% inhibition Heterozygote: 50%–65% inhibition Homozygote: 16%–25% inhibition			Important in detecting carriers of abnormal cholinesterase activity who are susceptible to succinyldicholine anesthetic shock
Dihydrotestosterone	Males: 50–210 ng/dL Females: none detectable	1.72–7.22 nmol/L		Testicular feminization syndrome
Estradiol—RIA	Females: Follicular: 10–90 pg/mL Midcycle: 100–500 pg/mL	 37–370 pmol/L 367–1835 pmol/L	Pregnancy	Depressed or failure to peak—ovarian failure

(continued)

Reference Ranges—Serum, Plasma, and Whole Blood Chemistries *(continued)*

Determination	Normal Adult Reference Range: Conventional Units	Normal Adult Reference Range: SI Units	Clinical Significance: Increased	Clinical Significance: Decreased
	Luteal: 50–240 pg/mL Follicular phase: 2–20 ng/dL Midcycle: 12–40 ng/dL Luteal phase: 10–30 ng/dL Postmenopausal: 1–5 ng/dL Males: 0.5–5 ng/dL	184–881 pmol/L		
Estriol—RIA	Nonpregnant females: < 0.5 ng/mL Pregnant females: 1st trimester: up to 1 ng/mL 2nd trimester: 0.8–7 ng/mL 3rd trimester: 5–25 ng/mL	< 1.75 nmol/L Up to 3.5 nmol/L 2.8–24.3 nmol/L 17.4–86.8 nmol/L	Pregnancy	Depressed or failure to peak—ovarian failure
Estrogens, total—RIA	Females: cycle days: Day 1–10: 61–394 pg/mL Day 11–20: 122–437 pg/mL Day 21–30; 156–350 pg/mL Males: 40–115 pg/mL	61–394 ng/L 122–437 ng/L 156–350 ng/L 40–115 ng/L	Pregnancy Measured on a daily basis, can be used to evaluate response of hypogonadotropic, hypoestrogenic women to human menopausal or pituitary gonadotropin	Fetal distress Ovarian failure
Estrone—RIA	Females: Day 1–10: 4.3–18 ng/dL Day 11–20: 7.5–19.6 ng/dL Day 21–30: 13–20 ng/dL Males: 2.5–7.5 ng/dL	15.9–66.6 pmol/L 27.8–72.5 pmol/L 48.1–74 pmol/L 9.3–27.8 pmol/L	Pregnancy	Depressed or failure to peak—ovarian failure
Ferritin–RIA	Males: 29–438 ng/mL Females: 9–219 ng/mL	29–438 μg/L 9–219 μg/L	Nephritis Hemochromatosis Certain neoplastic diseases Acute myelogenous leukemia Multiple myeloma	Iron deficiency
Folic acid—RIA	2.5–20 ng/mL	6–46 nmol/L		Megaloblastic anemias of infancy and pregnancy Inadequate diet Liver disease Malabsorption syndrome Severe hemolytic anemia
Follicle stimulating hormone (FSH)—RIA	Males: 2–10 mIU/mL Females: Follicular phase: 5–20 mIU/mL Peak of middle cycle: 12–30 MIU/mL	5–20 IU/L 12–30 IU/L	Menopause and primary ovarian failure	Pituitary failure

Reference Ranges—Serum, Plasma, and Whole Blood Chemistries *(continued)*

Determination	Normal Adult Reference Range: Conventional Units	Normal Adult Reference Range: SI Units	Clinical Significance: Increased	Clinical Significance: Decreased
	Luteinic phase: 5–15 mIU/mL Menopausal females: 40–200 mIU/mL	5–15 IU/L 40–200 IU/L		
Galactose	<5 mg/dL	<0.28 mmol/L		Galactosemia
Gamma glutamyl transpeptidase	Males: <45 IU/L Females: <30 IU/L	45 U/L 30 U/L	Hepatobiliary disease Anicteric alcoholics Drug therapy damage Myocardial infarction Renal infarction	
Gastrin—RIA	Fasting 50–155 pg/mL Postprandial: 80–170 pg/mL Zollinger-Ellison syndrome: 200–over 2000 pg/mL Pernicious anemia; 130–2260 pg/mL (mean 912)	50–155 ng/L 80–170 ng/L 200–over 2000 ng/L 130–2260 ng/L (mean 912)	Zollinger-Ellison syndrome Peptic ulceration of the duodenum Pernicious anemia	
Glucose:	Fasting: 60–110 mg/dL Postprandial (2 h): 65–140 mg/dL	3.3–6.05 mmol/L 3.58–7.7 mmol/L	Diabetes Nephritis Hyperthyroidism Early hyperpituitarism Cerebral lesions Infections Pregnancy Uremia	Hyperinsulinism Hypothroidism Late hyperpituitarism Pernicious vomiting Addison's disease Extensive hepatic damage
Glucose tolerance (oral)	Features of a normal response: 1. Normal fasting between 60–110 mg/dL 2. No sugar in urine 3. Upper limits of normal: Fasting = 125 1 hour = 190 2 hours = 140 3 hours = 125	 3.3–6.05 mmol/L 6.88 mmol/L 10.45 mmol/L 7.70 mmol/L 6.88 mmol/L	(Flat or inverted curve) Hyperinsulinism Adrenal cortical insufficiency (Addison's disease) Anterior pituitary hypofunction Hypothyroidism Sprue and celiac diseases	(High or prolonged curve) Diabetes Hyperthyroidism Primary adrenal cortical tumor or hyperplasia Severe anemia Certain central nervous system disorders
Glucose-6-phosphate dehydrogenase (red cells)	Screening: Decolorization in 20–100 min Quantitative: 1.86–2.5 IU/mL RBC	 1860–2500 U/L		Drug-induced hemolytic anemia Hemolytic disease of newborn
Glycoprotein (alpha-1-acid)	40–110 mg/dL	400–1100 mg/L	Neoplasm Tuberculosis Diabetes complicated by degenerative vascular disease Pregnancy Rheumatoid arthritis Rheumatic fever Infectious liver disease Lupus erythematosus	
Growth hormone—RIA	<10 ng/mL	<10 mg/L	Acromegaly	Failure to stimulate with arginine or insulin—hypopituitarism

(continued)

Reference Ranges—Serum, Plasma, and Whole Blood Chemistries *(continued)*

	Normal Adult Reference Range		Clinical Significance	
Determination	*Conventional Units*	*SI Units*	*Increased*	*Decreased*
Haptoglobin	50–250 mg/dL	0.5–2.5 g/L	Pregnancy Estrogen therapy Chronic infections Various inflammatory conditions	Hemolytic anemia Hemolytic blood transfusion reaction
Hemoglobin (plasma)	0.5–5 mg/dL	5–50 mg/L	Transfusion reactions Paroxysmal nocturnal hemoglobinuria Intravascular hemolysis	
Hemoglobin A1 (Glycohemoglobin)	Nondiabetics & diabetics whose control of glucose is: Good: 4.4%–8.2% Fair: 8.3%–9.2% Poor: >9.2%			
Hexosaminidase, total	Controls: 333–375 mM/mL/h Heterozygotes: 288–644 nM/mL/h Tay-Sachs disease: 284–1232 nM/mL/h Diabetics: 567–3560 mM/mL/h	 333–375 μmol/L/h 288–644 μmol/L/h 284–1232 μmol/L/h 567–3560 μmol/L/h	Diabetes Tay-Sachs disease	
Hexosaminidase A	Controls 49%–68% of total Heterozygotes: 26%–45% of total Tay-Sachs disease 0%–4% of total Diabetics: 39%–59% of total	Fraction of total: 0.49–0.68 0.26–0.45 0–0.4 0.39–0.59		Tay-Sachs disease and heterozygotes
High-density lipoprotein cholesterol (HDL cholesterol)				HDL cholesterol is lower in patients with increased risk for coronary heart disease

Age (yr)	Males (mg/dL)	Females (mg/dL)	Males (mmol/L)	Females (mmol/L)
0–19	30–65	30–70	0.78–1.68	0.78–1.81
20–29	35–70	35–75	0.91–1.81	0.91–1.94
30–39	30–65	35–80	0.78–1.68	0.91–2.07
40–49	30–65	40–85	0.78–1.68	1.04–2.2
50–59	30–65	35–85	0.78–1.68	0.21–2.2
60–69	30–65	35–85	0.78–1.68	0.91–2.2

17-Hydroxyprogesterone—RIA	Males: 0.4–4 ng/mL Females: 0.1–3.3 ng/mL Children: 0.1–0.5 ng/mL	1.2–12 nmol/L 0.3–10 nmol/L 0.3–1.5 nmol/L	Congenital adrenal hyperplasia Pregnancy Some cases of adrenal or ovarian adenomas	
Immunoglobulin A	Adults: 50–300 mg/dL (in children the normals are lower and vary with age)	0.5–3 g/L	Gamma A myeloma Wiskott-Aldrich syndrome Autoimmune disease Hepatic cirrhosis	Ataxia telangiectasis Agammaglobulinemia Hypogammaglobulinemia, transient Dysgammaglobulinemia Protein-losing enteropathies

Reference Ranges—Serum, Plasma, and Whole Blood Chemistries *(continued)*

Determination	Normal Adult Reference Range: Conventional Units	Normal Adult Reference Range: SI Units	Clinical Significance: Increased	Clinical Significance: Decreased
Immunoglobulin D	0–30 mg/dL	0–300 mg/L	IgD multiple myeloma Some patients with chronic infectious diseases	
Immunoglobulin E	20–740 ng/mL	20–740 μg/L	Allergic patients and those with parasitic infestations	
Immunoglobulin G	Adults: 565–1765 mg/dL	6.35–14 g/L	IgG myeloma After hyperimmunization Autoimmune disease states Chronic infections	Congenital and acquired hypogammaglobulinemia IgA myelomas, Waldenstrom's (IgM) macroglobulinemia Some malabsorption syndromes Extensive protein loss
Immunoglobulin M	Adults: 55–375 mg/dL	0.4–2.8 g/L	Waldenstrom's macroglobulinemia Parasitic infections Hepatitis	Agammaglobulinemias Some IgG and IgA myelomas Chronic lymphatic leukemia
Insulin—RIA	5–25 μU/mL	0.2–1 μg/L	Insulinoma Acromegaly	Diabetes mellitus
Iron	50–160 μg/dL	9–29 μmol/L	Pernicious anemia Aplastic anemia Hemolytic anemias Hepatitis Hemochromatosis	Iron deficiency anemia
Iron-binding capacity	IBC: 150–235 μg/dL TIBC: 230–410 μg/dL % Saturation: 20–50	26.9–42.1 μmol/L 41–73 μmol/L Fraction of total iron-binding capacity: 0.2–0.5	Iron deficiency anemia Acute and chronic blood loss Hepatitis	Chronic infectious diseases Cirrhosis
Isocitric dehydrogenase	50–180 U	0.83–3 U/L	Hepatitis: cirrhosis Obstructive jaundice Metastatic carcinoma of the liver Megaloblastic anemia	
Lactic acid (whole blood)	Venous: 5–20 mg/dL Arterial: 3–7 mg/dL	0.6–2.2 mmol/L 0.3–0.8 mmol/L	Increased muscular activity Congestive heart failure Hemorrhage Shock Some varieties of metabolic acidosis Some febrile infections May be increased in severe liver disease	
Lactic dehydrogenase (LDH)	100–225 mU/mL	100–225 U/L	Untreated pernicious anemia Myocardial infarction Pulmonary infarction Liver disease	
Lactic dehydrogenase isoenzymes				
Total lactic dehydrogenase	100–225 mU/mL	100–255 U/L Fraction of total LDH:	LDH-1 and LDH-2 are increased in myocardial infarction, megaloblastic anemia, and hemolytic anemia	
LDH-1	20%–35%	0.2–0.35		

(continued)

Reference Ranges—Serum, Plasma, and Whole Blood Chemistries (continued)

Determination	Normal Adult Reference Range: Conventional Units	SI Units	Clinical Significance: Increased	Decreased
LDH-2	25%–40%	0.25–0.4	LDH-4 and LDH-5 are increased in pulmonary infarction, congestive heart failure, and liver disease	
LDH-3	20%–30%	0.2–0.3		
LDH-4	0–20%	0–0.2		
LDH-5	0%–25%	0–0.25		
Lead (whole blood)	Up to 40 μg/dL	Up to 2 μmol/L	Lead poisoning	
Leucine aminopeptidase	80–200 U/mL	19.2–48 U/L	Liver or biliary tract diseases Pancreatic disease Metastatic carcinoma of liver and pancreas Biliary obstruction	
Lipase	0.2–1.5 U/mL	55–417 U/L	Acute and chronic pancreatitis Biliary obstruction Cirrhosis Hepatitis Peptic ulcer	
Lipids, total	400–1000 mg/dL	4–10 g/L	Hypothyroidism Diabetes Nephrosis Glomerulonephritis Hyperlipoproteinemias	Hyperthyroidism

Lipoprotein Phenotype: Summary of Findings in the Primary Hyperlipoproteinemias

Type	Frequency	Appearance	Triglyceride	Cholesterol	Lipoprotein Staining: Beta	Pre-Beta	Alpha	Chylomicrons	Secondary Causes
Normal		Clear	Normal	Normal	Moderate	Zero to moderate	Moderate	Weak	
I	Very rare	Creamy	Markedly increased	Normal to moderately increased	Weak	Weak	Weak	Markedly increased	Dysglobulinemia
II	Common	Clear	Normal to slightly increased	Slightly to markedly increased	Strong	Zero to strong	Moderate	Weak	Hypothyroidism, myeloma, hepatic syndrome, macroglobulinemia, and high dietary cholesterol
III	Uncommon	Clear, cloudy, or milky	Increased	Increased	Broad intense band	Extends into beta	Moderate	Weak	
IV	Very common	Clear, cloudy, or milky	Slightly to markedly increased	Normal to slightly increased	Weak to moderate	Moderate to strong	Weak to moderate	Weak	Hypothyroidism, diabetes mellitus, pancreatitis, glycogen storage diseases, nephrotic syndrome, myeloma, pregnancy, and oral contraceptives
V	Rare	Cloudy to creamy	Markedly increased	Increased	Weak	Moderate	Weak	Strong	Diabetes mellitus, pancreatitis, and alcoholism

Types I and II are fat induced; types III and IV are carbohydrate induced; type V is fat and carbohydrate induced.

Determination	Conventional Units		SI Units	Increased	Decreased
Lithium	Usual maintenance level; 0.5–1 mEq/L		0.5–1 mmol/L		
Low-density lipoprotein cholesterol (LDL cholesterol)	Age (yr)	mg/dL	mmol/L	LDL cholesterol is higher in patients with increased risk for coronary heart disease	
	0–19	50–170	1.30–4.40		
	20–29	60–170	1.55–4.40		
	30–39	70–190	1.80–4.92		

Reference Ranges—Serum, Plasma, and Whole Blood Chemistries (continued)

Determination	Normal Adult Reference Range: Conventional Units	Normal Adult Reference Range: SI Units	Clinical Significance: Increased	Clinical Significance: Decreased
	40–49 80–190 50–59 80–210	2.07–4.92 2.07–5.44		
Luteinizing hormone—RIA	Males: 4.9–15 mIU/mL Females Follicular phase: 2–3 mIU/mL Ovulatory peak: 40–200 mIU/mL Luteal phase: 0–20 mIU/mL Postmenopausal: 35–120 mIU/mL	4.9–15 mg/L 0.5–6.9 mg/L 0.2–46 mg/L 0–5 mg/L 8–27.5 mg/L	Pituitary tumor Ovarian failure	Depressed or failure to peak—pituitary failure
Lysozyme (muramidase)	2.8–8 μg/mL	2.8–8 mg	Certain types of leukemia (acute monocytic leukemia) Inflammatory states and infections	Acute lymphocytic leukemia
Magnesium	1.3–2.4 mEq/L	0.7–1.2 mmol/L	Excess ingestion of magnesium-containing antacids	Chronic alcoholism Severe renal disease Diarrhea Defective growth
Manganese	0.04–1.4 μg/dL	72.9–255 nmol/L		
Mercury	Up to 10 μg/dL	Up to 0.5 μmol/L	Mercury poisoning	
Myoglobin—RIA	Up to 85 ng/mL	Up to 85 μg/mL	Myocardial infarction Muscle necrosis	
5′ Nucleotidase	3.2–11.6 IU/mL	3.2–11.6 U/L	Hepatobiliary disease	
Osmolality	280–300 mOsm/kg	280–300 mmol/L	Useful in the study of electrolyte and water balance	Inappropriate secretion of antidiuretic hormone
Parathyroid hormone	160–350 pg/mL	160–350 ng/L	Hyperparathyroidism	
Phenylalanine	1.2–3.5 mg/dL 1st week 0.7–3.5 mg/dL thereafter	0.07–0.21 mmol/L 0.04–0.21 mmol/L	Phenylketonuria	
Phosphatase, acid, total	0–11 U/L	0–11 U/L	Carcinoma of prostate Advanced Paget's disease Hyperparathyroidism Gaucher's disease	
Phosphatase, acid, prostatic—RIA	0–10 ng/mL Borderline: 2.5–3.3 IU/L	0–10 μg/L	Carcinoma of prostate	
Phosphatase, alkaline	Adults: 30–115 mU/mL	30–115 μ/L	Conditions reflecting increased osteoblastic activity of bone Rickets Hyperparathyroidism Liver disease	
Phosphatase, alkaline, thermostable fraction	Thermostable fraction >35%; hepatic disease and combined disease with predominant hepatic component Thermostable fraction between 25% and 35%;		Hepatic disease	

(continued)

Reference Ranges—Serum, Plasma, and Whole Blood Chemistries *(continued)*

	Normal Adult Reference Range		Clinical Significance	
Determination	Conventional Units	SI Units	Increased	Decreased
	combined hepatic and skeletal disease Thermostable fraction <25%; skeletal disease with increased osteoblastic activity			
Phosphohexose isomerase	20–90 IU/L	20–90 U/L	Malignancy Disease of heart, liver, and skeletal muscles	
Phospholipids	125–300 mg/dL	1.25–3 g/L	Diabetes Nephritis	
Phosphorus, inorganic	2.5–4.5 mg/dL	0.8–1.45 mmol/L	Chronic nephritis Hypoparathyroidism	Hyperparathyroidism Vitamin D deficiency
Potassium	3.8–5 mEq/L	3.8–5 mmol/L	Addison's disease Oliguria Anuria Tissue breakdown or hemolysis	Diabetic acidosis Diarrhea Vomiting
Progesterone—RIA	Follicular phase: up to 0.8 ng/mL Luteal phase: 10–20 ng/mL End of cycle: <1 ng/L Pregnant: up to 50 ng/mL in 20th	2.5 nmol/L 31.8–63.6 nmol/L <3 nmol/L Up to 160 nmol/L	Useful in evaluation of menstrual disorders and infertility and in the evaluation of placental function during pregnancies complicated by toxemia, diabetes mellitus, or threatened miscarriage	
Prolactin—RIA	6–24 ng/mL	6–24 μg/L	Pregnancy Functional or structural disorders of the hypothalamus Pituitary stalk section Pituitary tumors	
Prostate-specific antigen (PSA)	<4 ng/mL		Prostatic cancer, benign prostatic hyperplasia, prostatitis	
Protein, total	6–8 gm/dL	60–80 g/L	Hemoconcentration	Malnutrition
Albumin	3.5– gm/dL	35–50 g/L	Shock	Hemorrhage
Globulin	1.5–3 gm/dL	15–30 g/L	Multiple myeloma (globulin fraction) Chronic infections (globulin fraction) Liver disease (globulin)	Loss of plasma from burns Proteinuria
Electrophoresis (cellulose acetate)				
Albumin	3.5–5 gm/dL	35–50 g/L		
Alpha-1 globulin	0.2–0.4 gm/dL	2–4 g/L		
Alpha-2 globulin	0.6–1 gm/dL	6–10 g/L		
Beta globulin	0.6–1.2 gm/dL	6–12 g/L		
Gamma globulin	0.7–1.5 gm/dL	7–15 g/L		
Protoporphyrin erythrocyte (whole blood)	15–100 μg/dL	0.27–1.80 μmol/L	Lead toxicity Erythropoietic porphyria	
Pyridoxine	3.6–18 ng/mL			A wide spectrum of clinical conditions such as mental depression, peripheral neuropathy,

Reference Ranges—Serum, Plasma, and Whole Blood Chemistries *(continued)*

	Normal Adult Reference Range		Clinical Significance	
Determination	Conventional Units	SI Units	Increased	Decreased
				anemia, neonatal seizures, and reactions to certain drug therapies
Pyruvic acid (whole blood)	0.3–0.7 mg/dL	34–80 μmol/L	Diabetes Severe thiamine deficiency Acute phase of some infections, possibly secondary to increased glycogenolysis and glycolysis	
Renin (plasma)—RIA	Normal diet: Supine 0.3–1.9 ng/mL/h Upright: 0.6–3.6 ng/mL/h Low salt diet: Supine: 0.9–4.5 ng/mL/h Upright: 4.1–1.9 ng/mL/h	0.08–0.52 ng/L/sec 0.16–1.00 μg/L/sec 0.25–1.25 μg/L/sec 1.13–2.53 μg/L/sec	Renovascular hypertension Malignant hypertension Untreated Addison's disease Primary salt-losing nephropathy Low-salt diet Diuretic therapy Hemorrhage	Frank primary aldosteronism Increased salt intake Salt-retaining steroid therapy Antidiuretic hormone therapy Blood transfusion
Sodium	135–145 mEq/L	135–145 mmol/L	Hemoconcentration Nephritis Pyloric obstruction	Alkali deficit Addison's disease Myxedema
Sulfate (inorganic)	0.5–1.5 mg/dL	0.05–0.15 nmol/L	Nephritis Nitrogen retention	
Testosterone—RIA	Females: 25–100 ng/dL Males: 300–800 ng/dL	0.9–3.5 nmol/L 10.5–28 nmol/L	Females: Polycystic ovary Virilizing tumors	Males: Orchidectomy for neoplastic disease of the prostate or breast Estrogen therapy Klinefelter's syndrome Hypopituitarism Hypogonadism Hepatic cirrhosis
T_3 (triiodothyronine) uptake	25%–35%	Relative uptake fraction: 0.25–0.35	Hyperthyroidism TBG deficiency Androgens and anabolic steroids	Hypothyroidism Pregnancy TBG excess Estrogens and antiovulatory drugs
T_3, total circulating—RIA	75–200 ng/dL	1.15–3.1 nmol/L	Pregnancy Hyperthyroidism	Hypothyroidism
T_4 (thyroxine)—RIA	4.5–11.5 μg/dL	58.5–150 nmol/L	Hyperthyroidism Thyroiditis Elevated thyroxine; binding proteins caused by oral contraceptives Pregnancy	Primary and pituitary hypothyroidism Idiopathic involvement Cases of diminished thyroxine-binding proteins caused by androgenic and anabolic steroids Hypoproteinemia Nephrotic syndrome

(continued)

Reference Ranges—Serum, Plasma, and Whole Blood Chemistries (continued)

	Normal Adult Reference Range		Clinical Significance	
Determination	Conventional Units	SI Units	Increased	Decreased
T_4, free	1–2.2 ng/dL	13–30 pmol/L	Euthyroid patients with normal free thyroxine levels may have abnormal T_3 and T_4 levels caused by drug preparations	
Thyroid-stimulating hormone (TSH)—RIA		0.3–5 m/IU/L	Hypothyroidism	Hyperthyroidism
Thyroid-binding globulin	10–26 μg/dL	100–260 μg/L	Hypothyroidism Pregnancy Estrogen therapy Oral contraceptives Genetic and idiopathic	Androgens and anabolic steroids Nephrotic syndrome Marked hypoproteinemia Hepatic disease
Transaminase, serum glutamic-oxalo-acetate (SGOT) aspartate amino-transferase)	7–40 U/mL	4–20 U/L	Myocardial infarction Skeletal muscle disease Liver disease	
Transaminase, serum glutamic-oxaloacetate (SGPT, alanine aminotransferase)	10–40 U/mL	5–20 U/L	Same conditions as SGOT, but increase is more marked in liver disease than SGOT	
Transferrin	230–320 mg/dL	2.3–3.2 g/L	Pregnancy Iron-deficiency anemia due to hemorrhaging Acute hepatitis Polycythemia Oral contraceptives	Pernicious anemia in relapse Thalassemic and sickle cell anemia Chromatosis Neoplastic and hepatic diseases
Triglycerides	10–150 mg/dL	0.10–1.65 mmol/L	See *Lipoprotein Phenotype*	
Tryptophan	1.4–3 mg/dL	68.6–147 nmol/L		Tryptophan-specific malabsorption syndrome
Tyrosine	0.5–4 mg/dL	27.6–220.8 mmol/L	Tyrosinosis	
Urea nitrogen (BUN)	10–20 mg/dL	3.6–7.2 mmol/L	Acute glomerulonephritis Obstructive uropathy Mercury poisoning Nephrotic syndrome	Severe hepatic failure Pregnancy
Uric acid	2.5–8 mg/dL	0.15–0.5 mmol/L	Gouty arthritis Acute leukemia Lymphomas treated by chemotherapy Toxemia of pregnancy	Xanthinuria Defective tubular reabsorption
Viscosity	1.4–1.8 relative to water at 37°C (98.6°F)		Patients with marked increases of the gamma globulins	
Vitamin A	50–220 μg/dL	1.75–7.7 μmol/L	Hypervitaminosis A	Vitamin A deficiency Celiac disease Obstructive jaundice Giardiasis Parenchymal hepatic disease

Reference Ranges—Serum, Plasma, and Whole Blood Chemistries *(continued)*

Determination	Normal Adult Reference Range		Clinical Significance	
	Conventional Units	SI Units	Increased	Decreased
Vitamin B_1 (thiamine)	1.6–4 μg/dL	47.4–135.7 nmol/L		Anorexia Beriberi Polyneuropathy Cardiomyopathies
Vitamin B_6 (pyridoxal phosphate)	3.6–18 ng/mL	14.6–72.8 nmol/L		Chronic alcoholism Malnutrition Uremia Neonatal seizures Malabsorption, such as celiac syndrome
Vitamin B_{12}—RIA	130–785 pg/mL	100–580 pmol/L	Hepatic cell damage and in association with the myeloproliferative disorders (the highest levels are encountered in myeloid leukemia)	Strict vegetarianism Alcoholism Pernicious anemia Total or partial gastrectomy Ileal resection Sprue and celiac disease Fish tapeworm infestation
Vitamin E	0.5–2 mg/dL	11.6–46.4 μmol/L		Vitamin E deficiency
Xylose absorption test	2 hr, 30–50 mg/dL	2–3.35 mmol/L		Malabsorption syndrome
Zinc	55–150 μg/dL	7.65–22.95 μmol/L	Zinc is essential for the growth and propagation of cell cultures and the functioning of several enzymes	

*By radioimmunoassay.

Reference Ranges—Immunodiagnostic Tests

Determination	Normal Value	Clinical Significance
Acetylcholine receptor binding antibody	Negative or <0.03 nmol/L	Considered to be diagnostic for myasthenia gravis in clients with symptoms
Anti-ds-DNA antibody	<70 units by ELISA <1:20 by indirect fluorescence	Valuable in supporting diagnosis or monitoring disease activity and prognosis of systemic lupus erythematosus (SLE)
Anti-glomerular basement membrane antibody	Negative or less than 10 units	Primarily used in the differential diagnosis of glomerular nephritis induced by antiglomerular basement membrane antibodies from other types of glomerular nephritis
Anti-insulin antibody	<3% binding of labeled beef and pork insulin by patient's serum; or <9 MIU/L	Helpful in determining the best therapeutic agent in diabetics and the cause of allergic manifestations. Also used to identify insulin resistance
Anti-mitochondrial antibody and anti-smooth muscle antibody	<1:5 and <1:20 respectively	Increased in cirrhosis, autoimmune disease, thyroiditis. pernicious anemia

(continued)

Reference Ranges—Immunodiagnostic Tests *(continued)*

Determination	Normal Value	Clinical Significance
Anti-nuclear antibody	Negative, <1:20	Increased in SLE, chronic hepatits, scleroderma, leukemia, and mononucleosis
Anti-parietal cell antibody	Negative, <1:20	Helpful in diagnosing chronic gastric disease and differentiating autoimmune pernicious anemia from other megaloblastic anemias
Anti-ribonucleoprotein antibody	Negative	Helpful in differential diagnosis of systemic rheumatic disease
Anti-scleroderma antibody	Negative	Highly diagnostic for scleroderma
Anti-Smith antibody	Negative	Highly diagnostic of SLE
Anti-SS-A anti-SS-B antibody	Negative	SS-A antibodies are found in Sjogren's syndrome alone or associated with lupus. SS-B antibodies are associated with primary Sjogren's syndrome
Antithyroglobulin and antimicrosomal antibodies	<1:100 titer by gelatin or hemagglutination	Presence and concentration are important in evaluation and treatment of various thyroid disorders such as Hashimoto's thyroiditis and Grave's disease. May also be indicative of previous autoimmune disorders
Ca 15-3 tumor marker	<22 IU/mL	Increased in metastatic breast cancer
Ca 19-9 tumor marker	<37 IU/mL	Increased in pancreatic, hepato-biliary, gastric, and colorectal cancer; gallstones; cirrhosis
Ca 125	0–35 IU/mL	Increased in colon, upper GI, ovarian, and other gynecologic cancers; pregnancy, peritonitis
Cold agglutinins	<1:16	Increased in mycoplasma pneumonia, viral illness, mononucleosis, multiple myeloma, scleroderma
C-reactive protein	<0.8 mg/dL	Increase indicates presence of active inflammation
Hepatitis A virus antibodies, IgM (HAV-Ab/IgM)	Negative	Positive in acute stage hepatitis A; develops early in disease
Hepatitis A virus antibodies, IgG (HAV-Ab/IgG)	Negative	Positive if previous exposure and immunity to hepatitis A
Hepatitis B surface antigen (HBsAg)	Negative	Positive in acute stage hepatitis B
Hepatitis B surface antibody (HBsAb)	Negative	Positive if previous exposure and immunity to hepatitis B
Infectious mononucleosis tests (monospot, mono-test, heterophile antigen test, EBV antiviral capsid antigen IgM and IgG)	Negative, <1:80	Positive monospot and monotest are presumptive; positive Epstein-Barr virus (EBV) IgM and IgG indicate acute and recent or past infection, respectively
Lyme disease titer	Negative, <1:256 by indirect fluorescent antibody method <0.8 by ELISA	Positive results help diagnose Lyme disease. False-positives may occur with high rheumatoid factor titers or syphilis. Positive ELISA confirmed by Western blot test
Pyroglobulin test	Negative	These abnormal proteins may be associated with myeloma, lymphoma, polycythemia vera, and SLE

Reference Ranges—Immunodiagnostic Tests *(continued)*

Determination	Normal Value	Clinical Significance
Rheumatoid factor	Negative or less than 60 IU/mL	Elevated in rheumatoid arthritis, lupus, endocarditis, tuberculosis, syphilis, sarcoidosis, cancer
T- and B-cell lymphocyte surface markers T-helper/T-suppressor ratio	T- and B-surface markers: Percent T cells (CD2) 60%–88% Percent helper cells (CD4) 34%–67% Percent suppressor cells (CD8) 10%–42% Percent B cells (CD19) 3%–21% Absolute counts: Lymphocytes 0.66–4.60 thou/mL T cells 644–2201 cells/mL Helper cells 493–1191 cells/mL Suppressor T cells 182–785 cells/mL B cells 92–392 cells/mL Lymphocyte ratio: T/T ratio > 1	Done to evaluate immune system by identifying the specific cells involved in the immune response. Valuable in diagnosis of lymphocytic leukemia, lymphoma, and immunodeficiency diseases including AIDS, and in the assessment of client response to chemotherapy and radiation

Reference Ranges—Urine Chemistry

Determination	Normal Adult Reference Range		Clinical Significance	
	Conventional Units	SI Units	Increased	Decreased
Acetone and acetoacetate	Zero		Uncontrolled diabetes Starvation	
Acid mucopolysaccharides	Negative		Hurler's syndrome Marfan's syndrome Morquio-Ulrich disease	
Aldosterone	Normal salt: Normal: 4–20 μg/24 h Renovascular: 10–40 μg/24 h Tumor: 20–100 μg/24 h	 11.1–55.5 nmol/24 h 27.7–111 nmol/24 h 55.4–277 nmol/24 h	Primary aldosteronism (adrenocortical tumor) Secondary aldosteronism Salt depletion Potassium loading ACTH in large doses Cardiac failure Cirrhosis with ascites formation Nephrosis Pregnancy	
Alpha amino nitrogen	50–200 mg/24 h	3.6–14.3 mmol/24 h	Leukemia Diabetes Phenylketonuria Other metabolic diseases	
Amylase	35–260 units excreted per h	6.5–48.1 U/h	Acute pancreatitis	
Arylsulfatase A	>2.4 U/mL			Metachromatic leukodystrophy
Bence-Jones protein	None detected		Myeloma	
Calcium	<150 mg/24 h	<3.75 mmol/24 h	Hyperparathyroidism Vitamin D intoxication Fanconi syndrome	Hypoparathyroidism Vitamin D deficiency
Catecholamines	Total: 0–275 μg/24 h Epinephrine: 10%–40%	0–275 μg/24 h Fraction total: 0.10–8.4	Pheochromocytoma Neuroblastoma	

(continued)

Reference Ranges—Urine Chemistry (continued)

Determination	Normal Adult Reference Range: Conventional Units	SI Units	Clinical Significance: Increased	Decreased
	Norepinephrine: 60%–90%	Fraction total: 0.60–0.90		
Chorionic gonadotropin qualitative (pregnancy test)	Negative		Pregnancy Chorionepithelioma Hydatidiform mole	
Copper	20–70 μg/24 h	0.32–1.12 μmol/24 h	Wilson's disease Cirrhosis Nephrosis	
Coproporphyrin	50–300 μg/24 h	0.075–0.45 μmol/24 h	Poliomyelitis Lead poisoning Porphyria hepatica Porphyria erythropoietica Porphyria cutanea tarda	
Cortisol, free	20–90 μg/24 h	55.2–248.4 nmol/d	Cushing's syndrome	
Creatine	0–200 mg/24 h	0–1.52 mmol/24 h	Muscular dystrophy Fever Carcinoma of liver Pregnancy Hyperthyroidism Myositis	
Creatinine	0.8–2 gm/24 h	7–17.6 mmol/24 h	Typhoid fever Salmonella infections Tetanus	Muscular atrophy Anemia Advanced degeneration of kidneys Leukemia
Creatinine clearance	100–150 mL of blood cleared of creatinine per min	1.67–2.5 mL/s		Measures glomerular filtration rate Renal diseases
Cystine and cysteine	10–100 mg/24 h	0.08–0.83 mmol/24 h	Cystinuria	
Delta aminolevulinic acid	0–0.54 mg/dL	0–40 μmol/L	Lead poisoning Porphyria hepatica Hepatitis Hepatic carcinoma	
11-Desoxycortisol	20–100 μg/24 h	0.6–2.9 μmol/d	Hypertensive form of virilizing adrenal hyperplasia due to an 11-beta hydroxylase defect	
Estriol (placental)	(see table below)			Decreased values occur with fetal distress of many conditions, including preeclampsia, placental insufficiency, and poorly controlled diabetes mellitus
Estrogens, total (fluorometric)	Females: Onset of menstruation: 4–25 μg/24 h Ovulation peak: 24 μg/24 h Luteal peak:	 4–25 μg/24 h 28 μg/24 h	Hyperestrogenism due to gonadal or adrenal neoplasm	Primary or secondary amenorrhea

Estriol (placental):

Weeks of pregnancy	μm/24 h	nmol/24 h
12	<1	<3.5
16	2–7	7–24.5
20	4–9	14–32
24	6–13	21–45.5
28	8–22	28–77
32	12–43	42–150
36	14–45	49–158
40	19–46	66.5–160

Reference Ranges—Urine Chemistry *(continued)*

Determination	Normal Adult Reference Range: Conventional Units	Normal Adult Reference Range: SI Units	Clinical Significance: Increased	Clinical Significance: Decreased
	22–105 μg/24 h	22–105 μg/24 h		
	Menopausal: 1.4–19.6 μg/24 h	1.4–19.6 μg/24 h		
	Males: 5–28 μg/24 h	5–18 μg/24 h		
Etiocholanolone	Males: 1.9–6 mg/24 h Females: 0.5–4 mg/24 h	6.5–20.6 μmol/24 h 1.7–13.8 μmol/24 h	Adrenogenital syndrome Idiopathic hirsutism	
Follicle stimulating hormone—RIA	Females: Follicular: 5–20 IU/24 h Luteal: 5–15 IU/24 h Midcycle: 15–60 IU/24 h Menopausal: 50–100 IU/24 h Males: 5–25 IU/24 h	 5–20 IU/d 5–15 IU/d 15–60 IU/d 5–25 IU/d 5–25 IU/d	Menopause and primary ovarian failure	Pituitary failure
Glucose	Negative		Diabetes mellitus Pituitary disorders Intracranial pressure Lesion in floor of 4th ventricle	
Hemoglobin and myoglobin	Negative		Extensive burns Transfusion of incompatible blood Myoglobin increased in severe crushing injuries to muscles	
Homogentisic acid, qualitative	Negative		Alkaptonuria Ochronosis	
Homovanillic acid	Up to 15 mg/24 h	Up to 82 μmol/d	Neuroblastoma	
17-hydroxycorticosteroids	2–10 mg/24 h	5.5–27.5 μmol/d	Cushing's disease	Addison's disease Anterior pituitary hypofunction
5-Hydroxyindoleacetic acid, qualitative	Negative		Malignant carcinoid tumors	
Hydroxyproline	15–43 mg/24 h	0.11–0.33 μmol/d	Paget's disease Fibrous dysplasia Osteomalacia Neoplastic bone disease Hyperparathyroidism	
17-ketosteroids, total	Males: 10–22 mg/24 h Females: 6–16 mg/24 h	35–76 μmol/d 21–55 μmol/d	Interstitial cell tumor of testes Simple hirsutism, occasionally Adrenal hyperplasia Cushing's syndrome Adrenal cancer, virilism Arrhenoblastoma	Thyrotoxicosis Female hypogonadism Diabetes mellitus Hypertension Debilitating disease of mild to moderate severity Eunuchoidism Addison's disease

(continued)

Reference Ranges—Urine Chemistry *(continued)*

Determination	Normal Adult Reference Range		Clinical Significance	
	Conventional Units	SI Units	Increased	Decreased
				Panhypopituitarism Myxedema Nephrosis
Lead	Up to 150 μg/24 h	Up to 60 μmol/24 h	Lead poisoning	
Luteinizing hormone	Males: 5–18 IU/24 h Females Follicular phase: 2–25 IU/24 h Ovulatory peak: 30–95 IU/24 h Luteal phase: 2–20 IU/24 h Postmenopausal: 40–110 IU/24 h	 2–25 IU/d 30–95 IU/d 2–20 IU/d 40–110 IU/d	Pituitary tumor Ovarian failure	Depressed or failure to peak—pituitary failure
Metanephrines, total	Less than 1.3 mg/24 h	Less than 6.5 μmol/d	Pheochromocytoma; a few clients with pheochromocytoma may have elevated urinary metanephrines but normal catecholamines and VMA	
Osmolality	Males: 390–1090 mM/kg Females: 300–1090 mM/kg	 390–1090 mmol/kg 300–1090 mmol/kg	Useful in the study of electrolyte and water balance	
Oxalate	Up to 40 mg/24 h	Up to 456 μmol/d	Primary hyperoxaluria	
Phenylpyruvic acid qualitative	Negative		Phenylketonuria	
Phosphorus, inorganic	0.8–1.3 gm/24 h	26–42 mmol/24 h	Hyperparathyroidism Vitamin D intoxication Paget's disease Metastatic neoplasm to bone	Hypoparathyroidism Vitamin D deficiency
Porphobilinogen, qualitative	Negative		Chronic lead poisoning Acute porphyria Liver disease	
Porphobilinogen, quantitative	0–1 mg/24 h	0–4.4 μmol/24 h	Acute porphyria Liver disease	
Porphyrins, qualitative	Negative		See *porphyrins, quantitative*	
Porphyrins, quantitative (coproporphyrin and uroporphyrin)	Coproporphyrin: 50–160 μg/24 h Uroporphyrin: up to 50 μg/24 h	 0.075–0.24 μmol/24 h Up to 0.06 μmol/24 h	Porphyria hepatica Porphyria erythropoietica Porphyria cutanea tarda Lead poisoning (only coproporphyrin increased)	
Potassium	40–65 mEq/24 h	40–65 mmol/24 h	Hemolysis	
Pregnanediol	Females: Proliferative phase: 0.5–1.5 mg/24 h Luteal phase: 2–7 mg/24 h Menopause 0.2–1 mg/24 h	 1.6–4.8 μmol/24 h 6–22 μmol/24 h 0.6–3.1 μmol/24 h	Corpus luteum cysts When placental tissue remains in the uterus after parturition Some cases of adrenocortical tumors	Placental dysfunction Threatened abortion Intrauterine death

Reference Ranges—Urine Chemistry *(continued)*

Determination	Normal Adult Reference Range: Conventional Units	Normal Adult Reference Range: SI Units	Clinical Significance: Increased	Clinical Significance: Decreased
	Pregnancy:			

Weeks of gestation	mg/24 h	μmol/24 h
10–12	5–15	15.6–47
12–18	5–25	15.6–78.0
18–24	15–33	47.0–103.0
24–28	20–42	62.4–131.0
28–32	27–47	84.2–146.6

Determination	Conventional Units	SI Units	Increased	Decreased
	Males: 01.–2 mg/24 h0.	3–6.2 μmol/24 h		
Pregnanetriol	0.4–2.4 mg/24 h	1.2–7.1 μmol/24 h	Congenital adrenal androgenic hyperplasia	
Protein	Up to 100 mg/24 h	Up to 100 mg/24 h	Nephritis Cardiac failure Mercury poisoning Bence-Jones protein in multiple myeloma Febrile states Hematuria	
Sodium	130–200 mEq/24 h	130–200 mmol/24 h	Useful in detecting gross changes in water and salt balance	
Titratable acidity	20–40 mEq/24 h	20–40 mmol/24 h	Metabolic acidosis	Metabolic alkalosis
Urea nitrogen	9–16 gm/24 h	0.32–0.57 mol/L	Excessive protein catabolism	Impaired kidney function
Uric acid	250–750 mg/24 h	1.48–4.43 mmol/24 h	Gout	Nephritis
Urobilinogen	Random urine: <0.25 mg/dL 24-hour urine: up to 4 mg/24 h	<0.42 mol/24 h Up to 6.76 μmol/24 h	Liver and biliary tract disease Hemolytic anemias	Complete or nearly complete biliary obstruction Diarrhea Renal insufficiency
Uroporphyrins	Up to 50 μg/24 h	Up to 0.06 μmol/24 h	Porphyria	
Vanillylmandelic acid (VMA)	0.7–6.8 mg/24 h	3.5–34.3 μmol/24 h	Pheochromocytoma Neuroblastoma Coffee, tea, aspirin, bananas, and several different drugs	
Xylose absorption test (5 hour)	16%–33% of ingested xylose	Fraction absorbed: 0.16–0.33		Malabsorption syndromes
Zinc	0.15–1.2 mg/24 h	2.3–18.4 mmol/24 h	Zinc is an essential nutritional element	

Reference Ranges—Cerebrospinal Fluid (CSF) *(continued)*

Determination	Normal Adult Reference Range: Conventional Units	SI Units	Clinical Significance: Increased	Decreased
Albumin	15–30 mg/dL	150–300 mg/L	Certain neurologic disorders Lesion in the choroid plexus or blockage of the flow of CSF Damage to the blood–CNS barrier	
Cell count	0–5 mononuclear cells per cu mm	$0–5 \times 10^6$/L	Bacterial meningitis Neurosyphilis Anterior poliomyelitis Encephalitis lethargica	
Chloride	100–130 mEq/L	100–300 mmol/L	Uremia	Acute generalized meningitis Tuberculous meningitis
Glucose	50–75 mg/dL	2.75–4.13 mmol/L	Diabetes mellitus Diabetic coma Epidemic encephalitis Uremia	Acute meningitides Tuberculous meningitis Insulin shock
Glutamine	6–15 mg/dL	0.41–1 mmol/L	Hepatic encephalopathies, including Reye's syndrome Hepatic coma Cirrhosis	
IgG	0–6.6 mg/dL	0–66 mg/L	Damage to the blood–CNS barrier Multiple sclerosis Neurosyphilis Subacute sclerosing panencephalitis Chronic phases of CNS infections	
Lactic acid	<24 mg/dL	<2.7 mmol/L	Bacterial meningitis Hypocapnia Hydrocephalus Brain abscesses Cerebral ischemia	
Lactic dehydrogenase	1/10 that of serum	Activity fraction: 0.1 of serum	CNS disease	
Protein			Acute meningitides Tubercular meningitis Neurosyphilis Poliomyelitis Guillain-Barré syndrome	
Lumbar	15–45 mg/dL	150–450 mg/L		
Cisternal	15–25 mg/dL	150–250 mg/L		
Ventricular	5–15 mg/dL	50–150 mg/L		
Protein electrophoresis (cellulose acetate)	% of total:	Fraction:	An increase in the level of albumin alone can be the result of a lesion in the choroid plexus or a blockage of the flow of CSF. An elevated gamma globulin value with a normal albumin level has been reported in multiple sclerosis, neurosyphilis, subacute sclerosing panencephalitis, and the chronic phase of CNS infections. If the blood–CNS barrier has been damaged severely during the course of these diseases, the CSF albumin level may also be elevated.	
Prealbumin	3–7	0.03–0.07		
Albumin	56–74	0.56–0.74		
$Alpha_1$ globulin	2–6.5	0.02–0.065		
$Alpha_2$ globulin	3–12	0.03–0.12		
Beta globulin	8–18.5	0.08–0.185		
Gamma globulin	4–14	0.04–0.14		

Gastric Analysis

Determination	Normal Adult Reference Range		Clinical Significance	
	Conventional Units	SI Units	Increased	Decreased
pH	2	2		Pernicious anemia
Basal acid output	0–6 mEq/h	0–6 mmol/h	Peptic ulcer	Gastric carcinoma
Maximum acid	5–40 mEq/h	5–40 mmol/h	Zollinger-Ellison syndrome	Chronic atrophic gastritis Decreased normally with age

Miscellaneous Value

Determination	Normal Value	Clinical Significance	
		Conventional Units	SI Units
Acetaminophen	Zero	Therapeutic level 10–20 mg/mL	10–20 mg/L
Aminophylline (theophylline)	Zero	Therapeutic level 10–20 mg/mL	10–20 mg/L
Bromide	Zero	Therapeutic level 5–50 mg/dL	50–500 mg/L
Carbamazepine	Zero	Therapeutic level 8–12 μg/mL	34–51 μmol/L
Carbon monoxide	0%–2%	Symptoms with 20% saturation	
Chlordiazepoxide	Zero	Therapeutic level 1–3 mg/mL	1–3 mg/L
Diazepam	Zero	Therapeutic level 0.5–2.5 mg/dL	5–25 mg/L
Digitoxin	Zero	Therapeutic level 5–30 ng/mL	5–30 mg/L
Digoxin	Zero	Therapeutic level 0.5–2 ng/mL	0.5–2 mg/L
Ethanol	0%–0.01%	Legal intoxication level 0.10% or above 0.3%–0.4% marked intoxication 0.4%–0.5% alcoholic stupor	
Gentamicin	Zero	Therapeutic level 4–10 mg/mL	4–10 mg/L
Lithium	Zero	Therapeutic level 0.6–1.2 mEq/L	0.6–1.2 nmol/L
Methanol	Zero	May be fatal in concentration as low as 10 mg/dL	100 mg/L
Phenobarbital	Zero	Therapeutic level 15–40 mg/mL	10–20 mg/L
Phenytoin	Zero	Therapeutic level 10–20 mg/mL	10–20 mg/L
Primidone	Zero	Therapeutic level 5–12 mg/mL	5–12 mg/L
Quinidine	Zero	Therapeutic level 0.2–0.5 mg/dL	2–5 mg/L
Salicylate	Zero	Therapeutic level 2–25 mg/dL	20–250 mg/L
		Toxic level 30 mg/dL	300 mg/L
Sulfonamide	Zero	Therapeutic levels:	
		Sulfadiazine 8–15 mg/dL	80–150 mg/L
		Sulfaguanidine 3–5 mg/dL	30–50 mg/L
		Sulfamerazine 10–15 mg/dL	100–150 mg/L
		Sulfanilamide 10–15 mg/dL	100–150 mg/L

*Reprinted with permission: *The Lippincott manual of nursing practice* (6th ed.). Philadelphia: J.B. Lippincott. Prepared by Goodman, D. B. P., MD, PhD, Professor and Department Chief, Department of Pathology and Laboratory Medicine, Hospital of the University of Pennsylvania, Philadelphia, PA.

APPENDIX C

Medical Terminology: Prefixes, Roots, and Suffixes

Medical terms are made up of components that are derived mostly from Latin or Greek. The root is the main part of the word. Prefixes precede the root and suffixes follow the root to modify its meaning. The roots are presented here with combining vowels that are used to ease pronunciation when a suffix is added.

Prefixes

Prefix	*Meaning*	*Example*	*Definition of Example*
a-, an-	without, not	aseptic	Sterile; free of infection
		anoxia	Lack of oxygen
ab-	away from	abduct	To move away from the midline
acro-	extremity	acromegaly	Disease marked by enlargement of the extremities
ad-	to, toward	adduct	To move toward the midline
ambi-	both	ambidextrous	Able to use either hand
ante-	before	antenatal	Occurring before birth; prenatal
anti-	against	antidote	Substance that neutralizes a poison
auto-	self	autoimmunity	An immune response to one's own body tissues
bi-	two, double	binocular	Pertaining to both eyes
brady-	slow	bradycardia	Slow heart rate
circum-	around	circumduction	Circular movement of a limb at a ball-and-socket joint
co-	together	coherent	Sticking together; logical
contra-	against	contraindication	A condition that makes it inadvisable to use a certain for of treatment
de-	without, removal	dehydration	Removal of water
di-	two, twice	diatomic	Having two atoms
dia-	through	dialysis	Separation of substances by passage through a semipermeable membrane
diplo-	double, two	diplopia	Double vision
dis-	removal, separation	disinfect	Remove infectious organisms from
dys-	abnormal, difficult, painful	dysmenorrhea	Painful menstruation
ecto-	outside	ectopic	Outside the normal position
endo-	within	endoscope	Instrument for viewing the inside of a body space
epi-	above	epigastric	Above the stomach
eryth/r/o-	red	erythema	Redness of the skin
		erythrocyte	Red blood cell
eu-	normal, good, true	eupnea	Normal breathing
ex/o-	out, out of	excise	To remove surgically
extra-	outside, in addition to	extracellular	Outside the cell

Prefixes (continued)

Prefix	Meaning	Example	Definition of Example
hemi-	half	hemiplegia	Paralysis of one half of the body
hetero-	other, different	heterosexual	Pertaining to the opposite sex
homo-, homeo-	same	homograft	Transplant of tissue from same species
		homeostasis	State of internal constancy
hyper-	high, excessive	hypertension	High blood pressure
hypo-	under, decreased	hypoglycemia	Low blood sugar
in, im-	in, within	inhale	To breathe in
		impacted	Held firmly
in-, im-	not	indigestion	Incomplete digestion
		impermeable	Unable to be penetrated
infra-	below	infrared	Pertaining to heat waves beyond the red spectrum
inter-	between	interstitial	Between cells
intra-	within	intracranial	Within the skull
iso-	equal, same	isotonic	Having the same concentration as cellular fluids
juxta-	near	juxtaglomerular	Neat the glomerulus of the kidney
leuk/o-	white, colorless	leukemia	Malignant overgrowth of white blood cells (leukocytes)
macro-	large	macromolecule	Large molecule composed of subunits
mal-	bad, poor	malnutrition	Poor nutrition
melan/o-	black, dark	melanin	Dark pigment found in skin, hair, the brain, and the eye
mega/lo-	large, enlarged	megalocyte	Large red blood cell
mes/o-	middle	mesoderm	Middle germ layer of the embryo
meta-	beyond, over, change	metamorphosis	Change in form or structure; passage from one stage to another
micr/o-	small, one millionth	microscope	Instrument for viewing extremely small objects
mon/o-	one	monocyte	White blood cell with a single large nucleus
multi-	many	multipara	Woman who has borne more than one viable fetus
neo-	new	neoplasm	A new, abnormal growth of tissue; a growth or tumor
noct/i-	night	nocturnal	Occurring at night
non-	not	nontoxic	Not poisonous
olig/o-	little, deficiency	oliguria	Decreased amount of urine formation
ortho-	straight, correct	orthopedics	Medical specialty that deals with prevention and correction of deformities
pan-	all	pandemic	Presence of a disease in most of a large population
para-	beside, near	paramedic	Trained medical assistant
per-	by, through	percutaneous	Through the skin
peri-	around	perioral	Around the mouth
poly-	many	polydactyly	Having more than the normal number of fingers or toes
post-	after, behind	postpartum	Occurring after birth
pre-	before	pre-existing	Present or occurring before a given time
prim/i-	first	primigravida	Woman during her first pregnancy
pro-	before	prognosis	Prediction of the outcome of a disease
pseud/o-	false	pseudostratified	Appearing to be in layers
quad/r/i-	four	quadriplegia	Paralysis of all four limbs
re-	back, again	reflux	Backward flow

(continued)

Prefixes (continued)

Prefix	Meaning	Example	Definition of Example
retro-	backward, behind	retroperitoneal	Behind the peritoneum
scler/o-	hard, hardening	scleroderma	Disease characterized by hardening of the skin
semi-	half	semilunar	Shaped like a half moon
sub-	below, under	subcutaneous	Under the skin
super-	above, excessive	superinfection	Second infection after an initial infection and caused by a different organism
supra-	above	suprapubic	Above the pubis
syn-, sym-	together	synthesis	Union of elements or molecules; a joining of parts
		symmetry	Correspondence in position of parts
tachy-	fast	tachypnea	Rapid respiration rate
trans-	through, across	transfusion	Injection of a substance into the bloodstream
tri-	three	tricuspid	Having three points or cusps
ultra-	beyond	ultrasound	Sound waves beyond the audible range
un-	not	unconscious	Lacking in awareness; insensible
uni-	one	unicellular	Having one cell

Roots

Root	Meaning	Example	Definition of Example
aden/o	gland	adenoma	A neoplasm of glandular epithelium
angi/o	vessel	angioplasty	Surgical repair of a blood vessel
arteri/o	artery	endarteritis	Inflammation of the lining of an artery
arthr/o	joint	arthroscope	Instrument for examining the interior of a joint
audio/o	hearing	audiologist	Specialist in the study and treatment of hearing disorders
bio	life	biopsy	Removal and examination of living tissue
blast/o	immature form, growing form	osteoblast	A growing cell that produces bone tissue
brachi/o	arm	antebrachium	Forearm
bronch/o, bronchi/o	bronchus	bronchogenic	Originating in a bronchus
		bronchiectasis	Chronic dilation of the bronchi
carcin/o	cancer	carcinogen	Agent that causes cancer
cardi/o	heart	cardiomyopathy	Any disease affecting the heart muscle
cerebr/o	brain	cerebrospinal	Pertaining to the brain and spinal cord
cephal/o	head	hydrocephalus	Accumulation of excess cerebrospinal fluid in the brain
cervic/o	neck, cervix	cervical	Pertaining to the neck or cervix
chol/e	bile	cholelithiasis	Presence or formation of gallstones
cholecyst/o	gallbladder	cholecystectomy	Surgical removal of the gallbladder
chondr/o	cartilage	endochondral	Located or occurring within cartilage
cleid/o	clavicle	cleidomastoid	Pertaining to the clavicle and mastoid process
col/o	colon	colostomy	Surgical formation of an opening between the colon and the surface of the body

Roots *(continued)*

Root	Meaning	Example	Definition of Example
colp/o	vagina	colpocele	Hernia into the vagina
cost/o	rib	intercostal	Between the ribs
crani/o	skull	craniotomy	Surgery on the cranium
cyst/o	sac, bladder	cystitis	Inflammation of the urinary bladder
cyt/o	cell	cytology	Study of cells
derm, dermat/o	skin	hypodermic	Beneath the skin
		dermatosis	Any skin disease
encephal/o	brain	encephalitis	Inflammation of the brain
enter/o	intestine	enterotoxin	Toxin that acts on the cells lining the intestine
gastr/o	stomach	epigastric	Above the stomach
genesis	origin	spermatogenesis	Formation of sperm cells
glomerul/o	glomerulus	glomerulonephritis	Inflammation of the glomeruli of the kidney
gloss/o	tongue	hypoglossal	Under the tongue
hem/o, hemat/o	blood	hemoglobin	The pigment that carries oxygen in red blood cells
		hematoma	Localized collection of clotted blood
hepat/o	liver	hepatomegaly	Enlargement of the liver
hist/o	tissue	histologist	One who studies tissue
hydro/o	water, fluid	hydrophilic	Readily absorbing water
hyster/o	uterus	hysterectomy	Surgical removal of the uterus
ile/o	ileum	ileocecal	Pertaining the ileum and cecum
ili/o	ilium	iliac	Pertaining to the ilium
kerat/o	cornea, horny layer of the skin	keratoplasty	Plastic surgery of the cornea; corneal grafting
		keratosis	Any horny growth, such as a wart or callus
labi/o	lip, labium	labiodental	Pertaining to the lips and teeth
lact/o	milk	lactogenic	Promoting formation of milk
laryng/o	larynx	laryngospasm	Spasmodic closing of the larynx
lith/o	stone	sialolith	Stone in a salivary gland or duct
lymph/o	lymph	lymphadenopathy	Any disease of a lymph node
mast/o	breast	mastectomy	Surgical removal of a breast
medull/o	central part, medulla oblongata	medullary	Pertaining to the central region of a structure or to the medulla oblongata
men/o	menses	menarche	Beginning of menstrual cycles
mening/o	meninges	meningocele	Hernia of the meninges
metr/o	uterus	endometrium	Lining of the uterus
my/o	muscle	myofiber	Muscle cell
myc/o	fungus	dermatomycosis	Any fungal infection of the skin
myel/o	marrow, spinal cord	myelogenous	Originating in bone marrow
		myelodysplasia	Defective formation of the spinal cord
myring/o	tympanic membrane	myringotomy	Incision of the tympanic membrane
nas/o	nose	paranasal	Near the nose
necr/o	death	necrosis	Death of tissue
nephr/o	kidney	hydronephrosis	Accumulation of fluid in the renal pelvis due to obstruction
neur/o	nerve	neuralgia	Pain along the path of a nerve
ocul/o	eye	oculomotor	Pertaining to eye movements
odont/o	tooth	orthodontics	Branch of dentistry that deals with prevention and correction of irregularities in the teeth
onc/o	tumor, swelling	oncolytic	Destructive of tumor cells
onych/o	nail	paronychia	Infection of the area around a nail
oo	egg, ovum	oocyte	Developing ovum
oophor/o	ovary	oophorectomy	Removal of an ovary
opthalm/o	eye	exophthalmia	Protrusion of the eyeball

(continued)

Roots (continued)

Root	Meaning	Example	Definition of Example
orchi/o, orchid/o	testis	orchiopexy	Surgical fixation of an undescended testis in the scrotum
		orchidoptosis	Dropping of the testis
os, oste/o	bone	ossification	Formation of bone
		periosteum	Membrane that covers bone
ot/o	ear	otosclerosis	Formation of bone tissue in the inner ear leading to hearing loss
ovari/o	ovary	ovariorrhexis	Rupture of an ovary
path/o	disease	pathophysiology	Study of the physiology of disease
ped/o	child, foot	pediatrics	Branch of medicine that deals with care of children
		pedometer	Instrument for recording numbers of steps
phag/o	eating	phagocyte	Cell that takes in and destroys waste or foreign particles
phak/o, phac/o	lens of the eye	phacolysis	Destruction of the lens
phleb/o	vein	phlebotomist	One who draws blood from a vein
pneum/o, pneumon/o	lung, air, breathing	pneumothorax	Accumulation of air in the pleural space
		pneumonia	Inflammation of the lung
proct/o	rectum	proctoscopy	Endoscopic examination of the rectum
psych/o	mind	psychogenic	Of mental or emotional origin
ptosis	dropping	blepharoptosis	Drooping of the eyelid
py/o	pus	empyema	Accumulation of pus in a body cavity
pyel/o	pelvis, renal pelvis	pyelography	X-ray study of the renal pelvis and ureter
pylor/o	pylorus	pylorospasm	Spasm of the pylorus
rachi/o	spine	rachiocentesis	Lumbar tap
ren/o	kidney	suprarenal	Above the kidney
rhin/o	nose	rhinorrhea	Discharge of thin mucus from the nose
salping/o	tube, oviduct	salpingectomy	Surgical removal of the oviduct
scler/o	hardening	arteriosclerosis	Hardening of the arteries
splen/o	spleen	splenectomy	Removal of the spleen
thorac/o	chest, thorax	thoracotomy	Surgical incision of the chest wall
thromb/o	blood clot	thrombosis	Formation or presence of a blood clot, usually causing obstruction of a vessel
tox/o, toxic/o	poison	toxoid	Modified bacterial toxin used to produce immunity
		toxicology	The study of poisons
trache/o	trachea	tracheostomy	Surgical creation of an opening into the trachea
trich/o	hair	trichology	Study of hair
ureter/o	ureter	ureterectasis	Dilation of the ureter
urethr/o	urethra	urethrostenosis	Narrowing of the urethra
ur/o	urine	anuria	Lack of urine formation
vas/o	vessel, duct	vasomotor	Pertaining to changes in the diameter of a vessel
vesic/o	urinary bladder	vesical	Pertaining to the urinary bladder

Suffixes

Suffix	Meaning	Example	Definition of Example
-algia	pain	gastralgia	Pain in the stomach
-cele	tumor, hernia, swelling	cystocele	Hernia of the bladder
-centesis	puncture, tap	paracentesis	Surgical puncture of a cavity for removal of fluid
-cide	killing	bactericide	Agent that kills bacteria
-ectasis	dilation, stretching	atelectasis	Incomplete expansion of the lungs
-ectomy	excision	tonsillectomy	Surgical removal of the tonsils
-emia	blood	ischemia	Insufficient blood supply to an area
-esthesia	pertaining to sensation	anesthesia	Loss of sensation
-form	shaped like	cruciform	Shaped like a cross
-gen, -genic	formation, origin, producing	fibrinogen	Substance in the blood that is converted to fibrin during blood clotting
		cardiogenic	Originating in the heart
-gram	record	echocardiogram	Record produced by echocardiography
-graph	recording instrument	pneumograph	Instrument for recording the rate and depth of respiration
-graphy	recording of data	radiography	The taking of x-ray pictures
-iasis	condition	helminthiasis	Infestation with worms
-ism	condition	embolism	Blockage of a blood vessel, usually by a blood clot
-itis	inflammation	pericarditis	Inflammation of the pericardium
-logy	study	etiology	Study of the origin of disease
-lysis	separation, disintegration	hemolysis	Rupture of red blood cells
-malacia	softening	osteomalacia	Softening of the bones
-megaly	enlargement	splenomegaly	Enlargement of the spleen
-meter	measuring instrument	calorimeter	Instruction for measuring heat production
-metry	measurement	pelvimetry	Measurement of the pelvis
-odynia	pain	cephalodynia	Pain in the head; headache
-oid	like, resembling	rheumatoid	Similar to rheumatism
-oma	tumor	sarcoma	Tumor of connective tissue
-osis	condition	narcosis	Unconsciousness due to narcotics
-pathy	disease	myopathy	Any disease of muscle
-penia	lack of	leukopenia	Abnormal decrease in the number of white blood cells
-pexy	surgical fixation	hysteropexy	Surgical fixation of the uterus
-phagia	eating	dysphagia	Difficulty in swallowing
-phil, -philic	attracting	basophil	White blood cell that stains with basic stain
-plasia	formation, molding	hyperplasia	Excessive growth of cells
-plasty	plastic repair	rhinoplasty	Plastic surgery of the nose
-plegia	paralysis	paraplegia	Paralysis of both legs and the lower part of the body
-pnea	breathing	apnea	Absence of breathing
-poiesis	formation, production	erythropoiesis	Formation of red blood cells
-ptosis	dropping	nephroptosis	Dropping of the kidney
-rhage, -rhagia	bursting forth	hemorrhage	Bursting forth of blood
		menorrhagia	Excessive menstrual bleeding
-rhaphy	surgical repair	herniorrhaphy	Surgical repair of a hernia
-rhea	discharge	pyorrhea	Discharge of pus
-rhexis	rupture	amniorrhexis	Rupture of the amnion
-scope	instrument for examining	cystoscope	Instrument for examining the bladder
-scopy	visual examination	bronchoscopy	Examination of the bronchi
-stasis	stoppage of flow	hemostasis	Prevention of blood loss
-stomy	surgical formation of an opening	colostomy	Surgical formation of an opening in the colon
-tomy	incision into	tracheotomy	Incision into the trachea
-trophy	nourishing	atrophy	Wasting or decrease in size of an organ or tissue
-tropic	acting on	gonadotropic	Acting on the gonads
-tripsy	crushing	lithotripsy	Crushing of a stone
-uresis	urination	diuresis	Elimination of large amounts of urine
-uria	urine	hematuria	Presence of blood in the urine

Word Roots According to Body System

Circulatory System
angi/o
arteri/o
cardi/o
hem/o, hemat/o
lymph/o
myel/o
phleb/o
thromb/o
vas/o

Digestive System
chol/e
cholecyst/o
col/o
enter/o
gastr/o
gloss/o
hepat/o
ile/o
lith/o
odont/o
proct/o

Integumentary System
derm, dermat/o
onych/o
trich/o

Musculoskeletal System
arthr/o
brachi/o
cervic/o
chondr/o
cleid/o
cost/o
crani/o
ili/o
my/o
myel/o
os, oste/o
ped/o
rachi/o
sarc/o

Nervous System
audi/o
cerebr/o
encephal/o
kerat/o
medull/o
mening/o
myring/o
neur/o
ocul/o
opthalm/o
ot/o
phac/o, phak/o
psych/o

Reproductive System
cervic/o
colp/o
hyster/o
labi/o
lact/o
mast/o
men/o
metr/o
oo
oophor/o
orchi/o, orchid/o
ovari/o
salping/o

Respiratory System
bronch/o
laryng/o
nas/o
pneum/o, pneumon/o
rhin/o
thora, thorac/o
trache/o

Urinary System
cyst/o
glomerul/o
nephr/o
pyel/o
ren/o
ureter/o
urethr/o
ur/o
vesic/o

Prepared by Barbara Janson Cohen, MS, Delaware County Community College, Media PA and Thomas Jefferson University, Philadelphia PA.

APPENDIX D

Recommended Dietary Allowances, USA

Summary Table: Estimated Safe and Adequate Daily Dietary Intakes of Selected Vitamins and Minerals*

Category	Age (yr)	Vitamins: Biotin (μg)	Vitamins: Pantothenic Acid (mg)
Infants	0–0.5	10	2
	0.5–1	15	3
Children and adolescents	1–3	20	3
	4–6	25	3–4
	7–10	30	4–5
	11+	30–100	4–7
Adults		30–100	4–7

Category	Age (yr)	Trace Elements†: Copper (mg)	Man-ganese (mg)	Fluoride (mg)	Chromium (μg)	Molybdenum (μg)
Infants	0–0.5	0.4–0.6	0.3–0.6	0.1–0.5	10–40	15–30
	0.5–1	0.6–0.7	0.6–1.0	0.2–1.0	20–60	20–40
Children and adolescents	1–3	0.7–1.0	1.0–1.5	0.5–1.5	20–80	25–50
	4–6	1.0–1.5	1.5–2.0	1.0–2.5	30–120	30–75
	7–10	1.0–2.0	2.0–3.0	1.5–2.5	50–200	50–150
	111	1.5–2.5	2.0–5.0	1.5–2.5	50–200	75–250
Adults		1.5–3.0	2.0–5.0	1.5–4.0	50–200	75–250

*Because there is less information on which to base allowances, these figures are not given in the main table of RDA and are provided here in the form of ranges of recommended intakes.

†Because the toxic levels for many trace elements may be only several times usual intakes, the upper levels for the trace elements given in this table should not be habitually exceeded.

Food and Nutrition Board, National Academy of Sciences—National Research Council Recommended Dietary Allowances, Revised 1989*

Designed for the maintenance of good nutrition of practically all healthy people in the United States

Category	Age (yr) or Condition	Weight† (kg)	Weight† (lb)	Height† (cm)	Height† (in)	Protein (g)	Fat-Soluble Vitamins: Vitamin A (μg RE)‡	Vitamin D (μg)§	Vitamin E (mg α-TE)‖	Vitamin K (μg)
Infants	0.0–0.5	6	13	60	24	13	375	7.5	3	5
	0.5–1.0	9	20	71	28	14	375	10	4	10
Children	1–3	13	29	90	35	16	400	10	6	15
	4–6	20	44	112	44	24	500	10	7	20
	7–10	28	62	132	52	28	700	10	7	30
Males	11–14	45	99	157	62	45	1000	10	10	45
	15–18	66	145	176	69	59	1000	10	10	65
	19–24	72	160	177	70	58	1000	10	10	70
	25–50	79	174	176	70	63	1000	5	10	80
	51+	77	170	173	68	63	1000	5	10	80
Females	11–14	46	101	157	62	46	800	10	8	45
	15–18	55	120	163	64	44	800	10	8	55
	19–24	58	128	164	65	56	800	10	8	60
	25–50	63	138	163	64	50	800	5	8	65
	51+	65	143	160	63	50	800	5	8	65
Pregnant						60	800	10	10	65
Lactating	1st 6 months					65	1300	10	12	65
	2nd 6 months					62	1200	10	11	65

*The allowances, expressed as average daily intakes over time, are intended to provide for individual variations among most normal persons as they live in the United States under usual environmental stresses. Diets should be based on a variety of common foods to provide other nutrients for which human requirements have been less well defined. See test for detailed discussion of allowances and of nutrients not tabulated.

†Weights and heights of Reference Adults are actual medians for the U.S. population of the designated age, as reported by NHANES II. The median weights and heights of those under 19 years of age were taken from Hamill et al. (1979) (see pages 16–17). The use of these figures does not imply that the height-to-weight ratios are ideal.

‡Retinol equivalents. 1 retinol equivalent = 1 μg retinol or 6 μg β-carotene. See text for calculation of vitamin A activity of diets as retinol equivalents.

§As cholecalciferol. 10 μg cholecalciferol = 400 IU of vitamin D.

‖α-Tocopherol equivalents. 1 mg-d-α tocopherol = 1 α-TE. See text for variation in allowances and calculation of vitamin E activity of the diet as α-tocopherol equivalents.

¶ 1 NE (niacin equivalent) is equal to 1 mg of niacin or 60 mg of dietary tryptophan.

Water-Soluble Vitamins							*Minerals*						
Vitamin C (mg)	*Thiamin (mg)*	*Riboflavin (mg)*	*Niacin (mg NE)¶*	*Vitamin B_6 (mg)*	*Folate (μg)*	*Vitamin B_{12} (μg)*	*Calcium (mg)*	*Phosphorus (mg)*	*Magnesium (mg)*	*Iron (mg)*	*Zinc (mg)*	*Iodine (μg)*	*Selenium (μg)*
30	0.3	0.4	5	0.3	25	0.3	400	300	40	6	5	40	10
35	0.4	0.5	6	0.6	35	0.5	600	500	60	10	5	50	15
40	0.7	0.8	9	1.0	50	0.7	800	800	80	10	10	70	20
45	0.9	1.1	12	1.1	75	1.0	800	800	120	10	10	90	20
45	1.0	1.2	13	1.4	100	1.4	800	800	170	10	10	120	30
50	1.3	1.5	17	1.7	150	2.0	1200	1200	270	12	15	150	40
60	1.5	1.8	20	2.0	200	2.0	1200	1200	400	12	15	150	50
60	1.5	1.7	19	2.0	200	2.0	1200	1200	350	10	15	150	70
60	1.5	1.7	19	2.0	200	2.0	800	800	350	10	15	150	70
60	1.2	1.4	15	2.0	200	2.0	800	800	350	10	15	150	70
50	1.1	1.3	15	1.4	150	2.0	1200	1200	280	15	12	150	45
60	1.1	1.3	15	1.5	180	2.0	1200	1200	300	15	12	150	50
60	1.1	1.3	15	1.6	180	2.0	1200	1200	280	15	12	150	55
60	1.1	1.3	15	1.6	180	2.0	800	800	280	15	12	150	55
60	1.0	1.2	13	1.6	180	2.0	800	800	280	10	12	150	55
70	1.5	1.6	17	2.2	400	2.2	1200	1200	300	30	15	175	65
95	1.6	1.8	20	2.1	280	2.6	1200	1200	355	15	19	200	75
90	1.6	1.7	20	2.1	260	2.6	1200	1200	340	15	16	200	75

APPENDIX E

Nutrition Recommendations for Canadians

Recommended Nutrient Intake Based on Age and Body Weight Expressed as Daily Rates

Age	*Sex*	*Weight (kg)*	*Protein (g)*	*Vit. A (RE*)*	*Vit. D (μg)*	*Vit. E (mg)*	*Vit. C (mg)*	*Folate (μg)*	*Vit. B_{12} (μg)*	*Calcium (mg)*	*Phosphorus (mg)*	*Magnesium (mg)*	*Iron (μg)*	*Iodine (mg)*	*Zinc (mg)*
Months															
0–4	Both	6.0	12†	400	10	3	20	25	0.3	250‡	150	20	0.3§	30	2§
5–12	Both	9.0	12	400	10	3	20	40	0.4	400	200	32	7	40	3
Years															
1	Both	11	13	400	10	3	20	40	0.5	500	300	40	6	55	4
2–3	Both	14	16	400	5	4	20	50	0.6	550	350	50	6	65	4
4–6	Both	18	19	500	5	5	25	70	0.8	600	400	65	8	85	5
7–9	M	25	26	700	2.5	7	25	90	1.0	700	500	100	8	110	7
	F	25	26	700	2.5	6	25	90	1.0	700	500	100	8	95	7
10–12	M	34	34	800	2.5	8	25	120	1.0	900	700	130	8	125	9
	F	36	36	800	2.5	7	25	130	1.0	1100	800	135	8	110	9
13–15	M	50	49	900	2.5	9	30‖	175	1.0	1100	900	185	10	160	12
	F	48	46	800	2.5	7	30‖	170	1.0	1000	850	180	13	160	9
16–18	M	62	58	1000	2.5	10	40‖	220	1.0	900	1000	230	10	160	12
	F	53	47	800	2.5	7	30‖	190	1.0	700	850	200	12	160	9
19–24	M	71	61	1000	2.5	10	40‖	220	1.0	800	1000	240	9	160	12
	F	58	50	800	2.5	7	30‖	180	1.0	700	850	200	13	160	9
25–49	M	74	64	1000	2.5	9	40‖	230	1.0	800	1000	250	9	160	12
	F	59	51	800	2.5	6	30‖	185	1.0	700	850	200	13	160	9
50–74	M	73	63	1000	5	7	40‖	230	1.0	800	1000	250	9	160	12
	F	63	54	800	5	6	30‖	195	1.0	800	850	210	8	160	9
75+	M	69	59	1000	5	6	40‖	215	1.0	800	1000	230	9	160	12
	F	64	55	800	5	5	30‖	200	1.0	800	850	210	8	160	9
Pregnancy (additional)															
1st Trimester			5	0	2.5	2	0	200	0.2	500	200	15	0	25	6
2nd Trimester			15	0	2.5	2	10	200	0.2	500	200	45	5	25	6
3rd Trimester			24	0	2.5	2	10	200	0.2	500	200	45	10	25	6
Lactation (additional)			20	400	2.5	3	25	100	0.2	500	200	65	0	50	6

*Retinol equivalents.
†Protein is assumed to be from breast milk and must be adjusted for infant formula.
‡Infant formula with high phosphorus should contain 375 mg calcium.
§Breast milk is assumed to be the source of the mineral.
‖Smokers should increase vitamin C by 50%.
Nutrition Recommendations: The Report of the Scientific Review Committee 1990, p. 204. Published by the authority of the Minister of National Health and Welfare.

APPENDIX F

Selected Resources for Community-Based Care

ACTION
806 Connecticut Avenue, NW
Washington, DC 20525

Administration on Aging
Department of Health and Human Services
330 Independence Avenue, SW
Washington, DC 20201

Al-Anon Family Group Headquarters
P.O. Box 182
Madison Square Station
New York, NY 10159

Alcoholics Anonymous
468 Park Avenue South
New York, NY 19916

American Anorexia/Bulimia Association Inc.
133 Cedar Lane
Teaneck, NJ 07666

American Association of Retired Persons (AARP)
601 E. Street, NW
Washington, DC 20049

American Burn Association
Shriner's Burn Institute
University of Cincinnati
202 Goodman Street
Cincinnati, OH 45219

American Cancer Society
1599 Clifton Road NE
Atlanta, GA 30329

American Diabetes Association
149 Madison Avenue
New York, NY 10016

American Dietetic Association
216 West Jackson Boulevard
Suite 800
Chicago, IL 60606

American Foundation for the Blind
15 West 16th Street
New York, NY 10016
212-620-2000

American Lung Association
1740 Broadway
New York, NY 10019

American Nurses Association
600 Maryland Avenue, SW
Suite 100 West
Washington, DC 20024

American Psychiatric Nurses' Association
6900 Grove Road
Thorofare, NJ 08086

American Public Health Association (APHA)
1015-15th Street, NW
Washington, DC 20005

American Red Cross
431 18th Street, NW
Washington, DC 20005

American Speech-Language-Hearing Association
10801 Rockville Pike
Dept AP
Rockville, MD 20852
301-897-5700

American Spinal Injury Association
2020 Peachtree Road NW
Atlanta, GA 30309

Arthritis Foundation
1314 Spring Street, NW
Atlanta, GA 30309

Asociacion Nacional por Personas Mayores (for Hispanic Seniors)
3325 Wilshire Boulevard, Suite 800
Los Angeles, CA 90010

Association for Death Education and Counseling
638 Prospect Avenue
Hartford, CT 60105-4298

Asthma and Allergy Foundation of America
1717 Massachusetts Avenue, NW, No. 305
Washington, DC 20036

Canadian Federation of Mental Health Nurses
331 Montgomery Avenue
Winnipeg, Manitoba R3L 1T6

Candlelighters Foundation
7910 Woodmont Avenue
Suite 460
Bethesda, MD 20814

Centers for Disease Control and Prevention
Department of Health and Human Services
U.S. Public Health Service
1600 Clifton Road, NE
Atlanta, GA 30333

Community Health Nurses Association of Canada
1049 Flintlock Court
London, Ontario M6H 4M3

The Compassionate Friends, Inc. (A nationwide support group for bereaved parents and siblings)
P.O. Box 3696
Oak Brook, IL 60522-3696

Concern for Dying
250 W. 57th Street
New York, NY 10107

Cystic Fibrosis Foundation
6931 Arlington Road
Bethesda, MD 20814

Digestive Diseases Clearinghouse
1555 Wilson Blvd.,
Suite 600
Rosslyn, VA 22209-2461

Elderhostel International
75 Federal Street
Boston, MA 02110

Hospice Action
PO Box 32331
Washington, DC 20007

Juvenile Diabetes Foundation International
432 Park Avenue
New York, NY 10016

Leukemia Society of America
600 Third Avenue
New York, NY 10016

Lions International
300 22nd Street
Oak Brook, IL 60521-8842
708-571-5466

March of Dimes Birth Defects Foundation
1275 Marmaroneck Avenue
White Plains, NY 10605

Muscular Dystrophy Association
3561 E. Sunrise Ave
Tucson, AZ 85718

National Association to Control Epilepsy
22 East 67th Street
New York, NY 10012

National Association for Home Care (NAHC)
510 C Street NE
Stanton Park
Washington, DC 20002

National Association for Retarded Citizens
2501 Ave J
Arlington, TX 76011

National Association for Sickle Cell Disease
4221 Wilshire Boulevard, Suite 360
Los Angeles, CA 90010

National Cancer Institute
Office of Cancer Communications
Building 31, Room 10A24
National Institutes of Health
Bethesda, MD 20892

National Clearinghouse for Drug Abuse Information
P.O. Box 2345
11400 Rockville Pike
Rockville, MD 20852

National Council on Alcoholism
12 West 21st Street
New York, NY 10010

National Easter Seal Society
2023 W Ogden Ave
Chicago, IL 60612

National Head Injury Foundation
333 Turnpike Road
Southborough, MA 01722

National Hemophilia Foundation
110 Greene Street, Suite 406
New York, NY 10012

National Hospice Organization
765 Prospect Street
New Haven, CT 06511

National Hydrocephalus Foundation
22427 South River Road
Joilet, IL 60436

National Indian Council on Aging
PO Box 2088
Albuquerque, NM 87103

National Institute on Alcohol Abuse and Alcoholism
National Institute on Drug Abuse (NIDA)
5600 Fishers Lane
Rockville, MD 20857

National Institute of Allergy and Infectious Diseases
Building 10, National Institutes of Health
Bethesda, MD 20892

National Institute of Arthritis and Musculoskeletal and Skin Diseases
National Institutes of Health
Bethesda, MD 20892

National Kidney Foundation
30 East 33rd Street, Suite 1100
New York, NY 10016
212-889-2210

National League for Nursing
350 Hudson Street
New York, NY 10014

National Mental Health Association
1021 Prince Street
Alexandria, VA 22314-2971

National Pacific/Asian Resource Association
2033 6th Avenue, Suite 410
Seattle, WA 98121

National Psoriasis Foundation
6443 SW Beaverton Hwy, Suite 210
Portland, OR 97221

National Safety Council
1121 Spring Lake Drive
Itasca, IL 60143

National Scoliosis Foundation
93 Concord Avenue, PO Box 547
Belmont, MA 02187

National Spinal Cord Injury Association
600 West Cumming Park, #3200
Woburn, MA 01801

National Society to Prevent Blindness
500 East Remington Road
Schaumburg, IL 60173
312-843-2020

Office for Handicapped Individuals
Department of Education
Room 3106, Switzer Bldg
400 Maryland Ave SW
Washington, DC 20202

Osteoporosis Foundation
612 North Michigan Avenue, Suite 510
Chicago, IL 60611

Parkinson's Disease Foundation
Medical Center
William Black Medical Research Bldg.
640 West 168th Street
New York, NY 10032

Retinitis Pigmentosa Foundation
1401 Mount Royal Avenue
4th Floor
Baltimore, MD 21217-4245

Scoliosis Association
PO Box 51353
Raleigh, NC 27609

Spina Bifida Association of America
1700 Rockville Pike, Suite 250
Rockville, MD 20852

Sudden Infant Death Syndrome Clearinghouse
8201 Greensboro Drive
Suite 600
McLean, VA 22102

United Cerebral Palsy Association
1522 K St NW
Washington, DC 20005

United Ostomy Association
36 Executive Park, Suite 120
Irvine, CA 92714

Visiting Nurse Association of America (VNAA)
3801 E. Florida Avenue
Suite 900
Denver, CO 80210

Glossary of Terms

Abduction Movement of a body part away from the midline of the body.

Abrasion Wound in which skin or mucous membranes are rubbed or scraped away.

Abscess Collection of debris from local tissues, dead and dying white blood cells, and bacteria without a blood supply to the center.

Absorption Process by which a medication enters the body.

Abstract thinking Level of thought that involves an idea apart from any material object.

Acid Any substance capable of releasing hydrogen ions in solution.

Acidosis Excessive acidity of body fluids; pH below 7.38.

Acne vulgaris Inflammatory disorder of the sebaceous glands; usually occurs in adolescence.

Acronym A type of mnemonic in which a word is formed from the initial letters of each of the successive parts or major parts of a compound term.

Action The performance of a specific function, step, or procedure.

Active range of motion Exercise or movement of joints done independently.

Active transport Movement of substances across a cell membrane against an electrochemical gradient.

Activities of daily living (ADLs) Activities frequently performed on a daily basis, such as bathing, grooming, eating, and toileting.

Activity tolerance Physical ability to withstand activity.

Actual nursing diagnosis An existing human response to a health problem identified by the nurse that is amenable to nursing intervention.

Acute Having a short and relatively severe course.

Acute pain Pain that lasts less than 6 months; usually associated with physical findings.

Adaptation Process by which a person changes to conform to the environment.

Addiction A psychological dependence with behavioral pattern of compulsive drug use or physical dependence to maintain self without signs and symptoms of withdrawal.

Adduction Movement of a body part toward the midline of the body.

Adenosine triphosphate (ATP) Nucleotide involved in energy metabolism, required for DNA synthesis, and used to store energy.

Administration Top-level management of an organization.

Adult day care An interdisciplinary service provided in congregate settings during specific daytime hours to disabled or impaired adults who need stimulation, supervision, socialization, or recreational therapy.

Adventitious breath sounds Abnormal lung sounds heard on auscultation.

Adverse effect Secondary effect of a drug (e.g., sensitivity, allergy, or idiosyncratic reactions).

Advocacy Communicating and acting on behalf of the welfare of another, especially a patient in the healthcare system; keeping the patient informed about treatment and nursing care.

Aerobic Exercise requiring oxygen for energy; involves elevation of heart rate for an extended period.

Aerosol Fine mist or spray of water, saline, or medication inhaled for therapeutic effects.

Affective Refers to emotional reactions (feeling as opposed to knowing).

Agonist Drug that has affinity for a receptor and is capable of eliciting a pharmacologic response.

Air embolus Air bubble in the vascular space that may obstruct circulation.

Airway resistance Increased work of breathing caused by narrowing of airway diameter.

Albuminuria Presence of albumin, a protein, in urine.

Aldosterone Adrenal cortex hormone that regulates sodium reabsorption.

Alkalosis Excessive alkalinity of body fluids; pH above 7.42.

Allodynia Enhanced sensation of pain produced by an innocuous stimulus, such as a light touch.

Alternative healthcare Nontraditional treatments.

Alveoli Spherical, saclike epithelial structures in the lungs through which gas exchange occurs.

Ambulatory care Healthcare services (community, personal or combined) provided to a person who is not an in-patient in a healthcare institution.

American Nurses Association Professional nursing organization concerned with all aspects of professional nursing; provides standards and leadership for the profession. ANA is comprised of individual state nursing associations and also has nursing specialty bodies representing all nursing practice areas.

Amino acids Building blocks from which proteins are constructed; end-products of protein digestion.

Ampule Small, sealed glass container.

Anabolism Building phase of metabolism in which the body converts simple substances into more complex substances (e.g., tissue repair, growth).

Anaerobic exercise Exercise in which muscles cannot extract enough oxygen, and anaerobic pathways are used to provide additional energy for a short time; useful in endurance training.

Analgesia Blockage of pain.

Analgesic Something that relieves pain.

Anaphylaxis Exaggerated allergic reaction to a foreign substance (drug or food); requires immediate medical intervention.

Andragogy Adult learning theory.

Anemia Insufficient number of red cells in the blood.

Anergy Inability to mount an immune response; seen in severe nutritional deficits.

Anesthesia Loss of sensation due to injury, disease, or a drug.

Anesthesiologist Physician who specializes in anesthesia administration.

Aneurysm Dilation or weakness of a blood vessel; occasionally seen as a localized ballooning.

Angina Pain and discomfort about the heart, characteristic of myocardial ischemia; severe pain felt in the anterior chest, shoulder, left arm, neck, and jaw.

Angiogram X-ray of blood vessels injected with radiopaque dye.

Anion Negatively charged ion.

Anonymity Protection of a research participant in such a way that the participant cannot be linked to the information provided.

Anorexia Loss of appetite.

Anorexia nervosa Eating disorder in which a person refuses to eat because of a fear of becoming overweight, even in the presence of normal or less than ideal body weight.

Antagonist A pharmacologic agent that binds with a receptor but does not produce a physiologic response or block the effect of an agonist. (e.g., naloxone).

Anthropometric measurements Comparative body measurements (eg, height and weight, skinfold measurements, limb circumference measurements).

Antibiotic Medication that can prevent the growth of or destroy bacterial organisms.

Antibody Protective substance produced by the body to protect it from an antigen.

Anticipatory grief Pattern of psychological and physiologic responses a person makes to the impending loss (real or imagined) of a significant person, object, belief, or relationship.

Anticipatory guidance Information given to a client about a situation before the situation occurs so that the client can develop problem-solving and coping strategies.

Anticoagulation Prevention of clot formation.

Antidiuretic hormone (ADH) Hypothalamic hormone stored in the posterior pituitary that promotes reabsorption of water by the kidney; also called vasopressin.

Antiemetic Drug given to prevent or relieve vomiting.

Antigen Substance that provokes irritation or damage to the body tissues and induces the formation of antibodies.

Antipyretic Medication used to reduce body temperature.

Antiseptic Agent that stops or slows the growth of microorganisms on living tissue. Most commonly used for handwashing, skin preparation before invasive procedures, and to pack or irrigate wounds.

Anuria Formation and excretion of less than 100 cc of urine in 24 hours.

Aorta Largest artery in the body; carries blood from the left ventricle to the body.

Aphasia Communication disorder that may affect speech, reading, and writing.

Apnea Absence of respiration.

Apneustic respirations Pattern of breathing characterized by a long inspiratory period that is gasping in nature and a short expiratory period.

Aquathermia pad Heating pad through which water circulates; used to apply local heat.

Arrhythmia Abnormal heart rate, rhythm, or pattern.

Arterial blood gases Set of blood tests used to assess acid–base balance and/or respiratory status.

Arteriosclerosis Disease characterized by thickening of arterioles with loss of elasticity and contractility due to fatty deposits and lesions.

Arthroscopy Direct visualization of a joint by insertion of a scope.

Articulation Enunciation of words and sentences.

Ascites Abnormal accumulation of fluid in the abdominal cavity.

Asepsis Absence of disease-producing microorganisms.

Asphyxiation Lack of oxygen, leading to cell death.

Aspiration Act of inhaling fluid or particulate matter into the bronchi.

Assault Threat of touching a person without his or her consent.

Assessment First phase of the nursing process. Data are gathered to identify actual or potential health problems.

Assisted range of motion Exercises that the client can perform with help from another person.

Ataxia Abnormal lack of muscle coordination.

Atelectasis Collapse of alveoli.

Atrophy Wasting away of an organ, muscle, or body tissue.

Attention span deficit Inability to concentrate; client is highly distractible and cannot screen out competing stimuli.

Audit Review of records.

Auricle Portion of the ear outside the head; the flap of the ear.

Auscultation Technique of listening to body sounds with a stethoscope.

Auscultatory gap Absence of audible sounds during blood pressure measurement that may cause inaccurate readings.

Autism State in which the client is withdrawn and preoccupied with inner thoughts, daydreams, fantasies, delusions, and hallucinations.

Autonomy Degree of discretion and independence a practitioner has.

Axillae Armpits.

Bacteremia Presence of bacteria in the blood.

Bactericidal Able to kill bacteria.

Bacteriostatic Able to inhibit the growth of bacteria.

Bacteriuria Presence of bacteria in the urine that can cause infection of the urinary tract.

Bandage Piece of gauze or other material used to cover an injured body part.

Barium Contrast medium used in x-rays of the gastrointestinal system.

Barrel chest Increased diameter of the chest caused by air trapping; common in COPD.

Basal body temperature Temperature of the body taken early in the morning before getting out of bed. This temperature rises during ovulation.

Basal metabolic rate Amount of energy used by the body during absolute rest in an awake state.

Base Any substance that can combine with and decrease hydrogen ions in solution; alkali.

Battery Unlawful touching a person's body without his or her consent.

Bedrest Restriction of activity to resting in bed.

Behaviors Observable actions.

Beliefs Ideas that a person accepts as true.

Belongingness and love needs Developing relationships with others and seeking friendship, love, and intimacy.

Bereavement Response to the death of a significant other.

Binder Large bandage used to support a body part or hold a dressing in place.

Biofeedback A technique in which the client learns voluntary control over autonomic functions.

Biopsy Specimen of tissue or cells, or the procedure used to obtain the sample.

Biot's respiration Cyclic pattern of breathing characterized by periods of shallow breathing alternating with periods of apnea.

Biotransformation Chemical change of a drug, usually to a less active state.

Blended family Two parents with unrelated children who are being raised together.

Blood gases Studies performed on arterial blood to evaluate the client's oxygenation, ventilation, and metabolic (acid–base) status.

Blood pressure Force exerted by the blood against the walls of the blood vessels.

Blood transfusion Administration of blood or blood components into the circulatory system.

Body image Feelings about one's body.

Body mechanics Positioning or movement of the body to prevent or correct problems related to activity or immobilization.

Body substance isolation Protocol that recommends wearing gloves for contact with moist body membranes, nonintact skin, and moist body substances from all clients at all times. Gowns, masks, and goggles should be worn when splashing or soiling of the caregiver's face or clothing with the client's body fluids is likely.

Bolus Small volume of medication given intravenously in a controlled fashion in a relatively short period of time (IV push).

Borborygmus Loud rumbling sound produced by the normal movement of gas through the intestines referred to as "stomach growling" (plural: borborygmi).

Bradycardia Abnormally slow heart rate (usually less than 60 beats per minute in adults).

Bradypnea Abnormally slow respiratory rate (usually less than 10 breaths per minute in adults).

Bronchioles Narrow airways that conduct air into alveolar ducts and alveoli.

Bronchospasm Narrowing of the bronchioles caused by tightening of smooth muscles in the airways.

Bronchovesicular breath sounds Muffled, blowing sounds of medium pitch normally heard over the mainstem bronchi.

Bruit Abnormal swishing or blowing sound heard on auscultation of veins or arteries; caused by increased turbulence of blood.

Buccal Pertaining to the inside cheek.

Buffer Compound that helps stabilize the pH of a solution by neutralizing added acid or base.

Bulla Serous skin elevation greater than 1 cm in size or diameter.

Burn Injury caused by exposure to thermal, chemical, electrical, or radioactive energy.

Burnout Depletion of energy and low morale.

Butterfly bandage Butterfly-shaped adhesive strip used to hold wound edges together.

Calorie (kilocalorie) Unit of heat; commonly used to describe the energy value of food.

Capillary Smallest peripheral blood vessel.

Carbohydrates Food group containing simple sugars and complex sugars composed of carbon, hydrogen, and oxygen.

Cardiopulmonary response Pulse, blood pressure, and respiratory rate.

Care plan conference Meeting held to discuss plan of care revisions and coordination of care.

Caregiver Person, usually a family member, responsible for providing day-to-day care, especially hygiene, nutrition, supervision and nurturance, for someone who has a functional or instrumental ADL impairment.

Carrier Person from whom a microorganism can be cultured but who shows no sign of disease.

Case finding Activities undertaken to identify people who need health or social services.

Case management Professional approach to providing care in which a client's services are coordinated by one provider.

Catabolism Breaking-down process of metabolism in which energy is released by converting complex substances to simpler substances.

Catheter Tube placed into a body cavity or vessel for evacuating or injecting fluid.

Cation Positively charged ion.

Cellulitis Reddened area resulting from the inflammatory response with small vessel dilation, leakage of fluid from the endothelium, and WBC infiltration; usually a sign of infection.

Cerebrospinal fluid Fluid that circulates in the subarachnoid space and protects the brain and spinal cord from injury.

Certification Achievement of competence in a specialty area evidenced by successful completion of a variety of testing measures specified by the organization granting certification.

Change theory A variety of theories that state that subtle, continuous changes happen daily; they involve modification or alterations and may be planned or unplanned.

Change-of-shift report Information passed between nurses at change of shift about client status and plan of care.

Charge nurse Nurse responsible for the functioning of a nursing unit for a particular work shift.

Charting by exception Charting in which the nurse documents only those findings that fall outside the standard of care and norms that have been developed by the institution.

Chemical drug name Name that gives a drug's molecular structure.

Chemoreceptors Nerve receptors that respond to chemical changes.

Chemotaxis Chemical attraction of the neutrophil toward the bacterial cell to be phagocytized.

Chemotherapeutic agents Chemicals used for therapeutic purposes in the body, such as antiviral medications and antibiotics; also used to refer to drugs used in cancer therapy.

Chest physiotherapy Treatment designed to facilitate removal of mucus from lungs; usually involves postural drainage.

Cheyne–Stokes respiration Respiratory pattern characterized by periods of respirations of increased rate and depth alternating with periods of apnea.

Chief complaint Client's specific reason for seeking medical attention.

Cholesterol Type of animal fat; needed for specific body functions, but an excess is harmful to the arteries.

Chronic Persisting over a long period of time.

Chronic bronchitis Disease characterized by cough, greatly increased mucus production, and chronic inflammation and infection of larger airways.

Chronic obstructive pulmonary disease (COPD) Usually a combination of chronic bronchitis and emphysema.

Chronic pain Pain that lasts more than 6 months.

Chyme Partially digested food and digestive secretions of the stomach and small intestine.

Circadian rhythm Regular occurrence of certain phenomena in cycles of about 24 hours.

Circadian thermal rhythm Fluctuations in normal body temperature occurring over a 24-hour period.

Circle of confidentiality Professionals with whom client information can be shared.

Circumcision Surgical removal of the foreskin from the head of the penis.

Clean-catch urine sample Small amount of voided urine that has been obtained after the urinary meatus has been cleansed with soap or disinfectant.

Client Person requiring the services of a healthcare provider.

Climacteric Menopause.

Clinical judgment Process of evaluating a client cues to make an accurate nursing diagnosis.

Clinical nurse specialist Registered nurse who holds a master's degree in a nursing specialty and has advanced clinical experience.

Clitoris Small erectile organ located just above the urinary meatus in females; plays a key role in female orgasm.

Clustering Combining client data into meaningful patterns.

Coagulation Blood clotting.

Cognition Thinking and awareness; system by which sensory input, past experiences, and emotions are integrated and made meaningful.

Cognitive Refers to rational thought (knowing as opposed to feeling).

Cognitive function Ability to think, understand, and communicate with the environment.

Cognitive level Degree of ability to know, think, and remember.

Coitus interruptus Withdrawal of the penis from the vagina just before ejaculation; an ineffective means of contraception.

Collaboration Actions taken in coordination with other professionals.

Collaborative health problem Problems based on medical diagnoses, medically ordered treatments, or other related problems that require interdependent standards and activity to be addressed.

Colloid Fluids that contain proteins or starch molecules.

Colonization State in which a microorganism is present but no immune reaction or tissue destruction occurs.

Colostomy Opening of a part of the colon onto the abdominal skin surface.

Coma Abnormally deep stupor occurring in illness or as a result of injury. The client cannot be aroused by external stimuli.

Communal family Related and unrelated people with common goals and beliefs sharing a household.

Communicable disease Disease transmissible between hosts.

Communication Interchange of information.

Communication channel Medium through which a message is sent (eg, television, writing, speaking).

Community Social group whose members may or may not share common geographic boundaries but interact because of common interests or shared values to meet their needs within a larger society.

Community-acquired infections Infections that are present and symptomatic on admission to the hospital or within 24 hours after admission.

Community-based healthcare Healthcare directed toward a specific group within the community.

Complete protein Protein that contains sufficient amounts of essential amino acids to maintain body tissues and to promote body growth.

Compliance 1. Adherence to recommended plan. 2. Measure of the "stretchiness" of the lung.

Comprehension Capacity for understanding and reasoning.

Conceptual framework Formal explanation that links concepts and emphasizes relationships among them.

Concrete thinking Objects or groups of things that can be perceived by the senses; objective reality.

Condom catheter (external, Texas) Noninvasive urinary collection device for incontinent male clients; consists of a thin flexible sheath placed over the penis and attached to tubing and a collection bag.

Confidentiality Practice of keeping client information private.

Confusion Impaired cognition; ranges from mild memory or orientation deficits to profoundly disorganized thinking.

Consultation Conferring with another professional to obtain his or her assessment of a situation or client.

Consumer Person who engages the services of another while retaining rights and responsibilities related to the service provided.

Consumerism Public's expectation that they will have a voice in determining the type, quality, and cost of care being provided.

Contact Person who has been near an infected person and may have been exposed to an infectious disease.

Contamination State in which microorganisms are present on an inanimate object or on the body surface without tissue invasion.

Continuing education Education beyond basic preparation; purpose is to remain current in knowledge and practice.

Continuity of care Provision of uninterrupted service as a client moves between settings.

Contraception Any method of preventing pregnancy.

Contract Negotiated agreement between nurse and client in which roles and responsibilities of each are delineated.

Contractility Force of contraction.

Contracture Shortening of a muscle and loss of joint mobility from fibrotic changes in the tissues surrounding the joint.

Contralateral stimulation Stimulation of the opposite side from the pain. Pressure, massage, cold, heat, and other methods may be used.

Contrast medium Material that appears solid in x-rays; used to outline cavities and blood vessels to show abnormalities.

Controlling Management function that involves checking that plans are being carried out effectively and evaluating the outcomes of the actions.

Coordination Act of assembling and directing activities of others so that services are provided harmoniously.

Coping Problem-solving process a person uses to manage stresses or events.

Coping mechanism Effort used to manage stress.

Core temperature Internal temperature of the body.

Crackles Abnormal breath sounds; rales.

Credentialing Method of ensuring quality healthcare services (eg, licensure, certification, degrees).

Crepitus Crunching or grating sounds that occur when bones rub against one another during movement or when air deposits in subcutaneous tissue.

Critical pathway Standard plan of care used to establish and monitor the extent and timing of care; includes key elements such as diagnostic tests, consultations, treatments, activities, procedures, and discharge planning and teaching. Also called clinical paths, collaborative care plans, CareMap (TM), multidisciplinary care plan, and case management plan.

Critical thinking Purposeful process that is disciplined, active, multidimensional, reasonable, rational, and reflective to arrive at insight and draw conclusions.

Crystalloid Fluids that are clear.

Cue Piece of data, subjective or objective, about a client.

Cultural relativity Principle that meaning is created by one's culture and truth is culture specific; the same experience may carry different meanings to people of different cultures.

Cultural sensitivity Acceptance of a culture other than one's own.

Culture 1. Behavior and institutions of a given society. 2. Growth of microorganisms in a specialized medium under precise conditions.

Culture shock Failure to comprehend the culture in which one is living.

Data Pieces of information.

Debridement Removal of foreign material or dying tissue from a wound.

Decision-making process Method of analyzing a problem, determining alternatives, and selecting the appropriate action.

Decoding Process of understanding a message.

Decompression Removal of pressure caused by an accumulation of gas and fluids.

Decontamination Removal of potential pathogens.

Decubitus ulcer Breakdown of the surface of body tissue; caused by prolonged pressure on a body part (pressure sore).

Deductive theory Process by which specific predictions are developed from general principles.

Defecation Elimination of solid waste from the bowels.

Defecation reflex Involuntary response of intestinal contraction and anal sphincter relaxation to rectal distention.

Defendant Person being sued or accused.

Deglutition Swallowing.

Dehiscence Accidental separation of wound edges, especially a surgical wound.

Dehydration Condition resulting from excessive loss of body water or saline.

Delirium Reversible disorder of cognition; confusion.

Delusion Belief that is not based in reality and that reflects an unconscious need or fear.

Demands of daily living (DDLs) Responsibilities generated by job, house, car, pets, environment, and so on.

Dementia Cognitive impairment as the result of irreversible organic changes in brain cell function.

Deontology Theory of philosophy that examines our duty to moral law or moral principles.

Dependent variable Variable (or item of interest that varies) that is the outcome; hypothesized to depend on or be caused by another variable.

Depressive pseudodementia Dementialike syndrome due to depression rather than cerebral degeneration.

Dermatitis Various skin conditions involving inflammation.

Dermis Layer of skin beneath the epidermis; composed of dense connective fibers, blood vessels, nerves, hair follicles, and glands.

Detrusor Smooth muscle of the urinary bladder.

Development Process of ongoing change throughout a person's life.

Developmental stages Points in life when old responsibilities are discarded and new ones are taken on.

Developmental tasks Psychomotor, psychosocial, or cognitive skills attained at certain stages of life that are prerequisites for successive skill development.

Diagnosis-related groups (DRGs) Categories or classifications of illnesses, disorders, procedures, or other conditions necessitating hospitalization from which cost of care is predetermined.

Diagnostic process Skills used to make nursing diagnoses.

Diaphragmatic breathing Breathing exercise using the diaphragm to obtain a deep breath.

Diastole Period of rest in the cardiac cycle, when the ventricles are not contracting and the coronary arteries are filling with blood.

Diastolic blood pressure Pressure in the blood vessels during cardiac ventricular relaxation.

Diffusion Movement of molecules from an area of higher concentration to one of lower concentration.

Digestion Mechanical and chemical processes necessary to convert food to an absorbable state.

Direct care Care that requires the professional to interact directly with the client.

Directing Management function of supervision and ongoing decision-making to get people to carry out plans.

Directive leadership Leadership style in which the leader makes all the decisions and tells subordinates what to do.

Disability Degree of physical or mental impairment.

Discharge planner Health professional who coordinates services for clients making the transition from one healthcare setting to another setting.

Discharge planning Process of coordinating, planning, and arranging for the transition from one healthcare setting to another setting.

Disinfectant Chemical used to kill microorganisms on lifeless objects.

Disinfection Reduction in the number of microorganisms by physical or chemical means.

Disorganized thinking Disorder manifested by inappropriate interactions and conversations with others, talking or gesturing to oneself, performing inappropriate activities, or other confused or bizarre behavior.

Disorientation Lack of awareness of identity or environment (person, place, time).

Distention Condition of being stretched or inflated.

Distress Too much or too little arousal of a person's mind and body, resulting in harm to the mind or body.

Distressor Demand on the mind or body leading to distress.

Distribution Process by which a drug passes from the circulation of blood and lymphatic systems across cell membranes to a specified tissue.

Disuse osteoporosis Decrease in bone density due to lack of activity or stress on bones.

Diuresis Formation and excretion of large amounts of urine.

Diuretics Drugs that cause the kidney to form and excrete more urine.

Doppler Hand-held transducer that directs high-frequency sound waves to the organ or vessel being scanned during ultrasonography.

Dorsiflexion Bending at the ankle joint so as to point toes upward.

Drain Device used to remove excess fluid from a wound or body area.

Drug Substance that alters physiologic function with the potential for affecting health.

Dualism Theory that divides concepts into two mutually irreducible elements.

Duodenocolic reflex Involuntary response of intestinal contraction and motility to duodenal distention.

Dysarthria Disorders affecting either single or combined motor control of the muscles of speech.

Dysfunction Action that does not meet expected norms.

Dysfunctional grief Grief that falls outside normal parameters; may be manifested as absence of grief, delayed grief, exaggerated grief, or prolonged grief.

Dyspareunia Painful sexual intercourse.

Dyspnea Breathing that requires marked effort.

Dysuria Painful voiding.

Eczema Inflammatory skin condition characterized by erythema, papules, vesicles, scales, and crusts.

Edema Accumulation of fluid in the interstitial tissues.

Effective communication Transfer of meaning between two or more people.

Elective surgery Surgical procedure performed at the desire of the client but not needed to preserve life or function.

Electrocardiogram (EKG, ECG) Record of heart action showing specific patterns of electrical activity in the heart muscle.

Electroencephalogram (EEG) Record of electrical activity in the brain.

Electrolyte Chemical compound that dissociates into ions when in solution; usually refers to extracellular sodium, potassium, and chloride.

Embolus Foreign substance, usually a blood clot, circulating in the blood and lodging in small arterial vessels.

Embryo Stage of development from the second week after conception to about 8 weeks, during which time major structures and organs are formed.

Emergent surgery Situation in which surgery must be performed immediately to preserve the function of a body part or the life of the client.

Empathy Ability to understand how another person sees a situation, while maintaining objectivity.

Emphysema Disease characterized by loss of bronchiolar smooth muscle tone, destruction of alveoli, and air trapping.

Encoding Process of translating the purpose of a communication into a message that can be sent.

Endemic Infectious disease restricted to a particular nation, region, or group; found in a community all the time but does not spread.

Endocardium Innermost layer of the heart muscle; covers all internal surfaces of the heart and is lined by endothelium continuous with that of the blood vessels.

Endogenous (autogenous) From a source inside the client.

Endorphins Endogenous opiates that alter pain perception.

Endoscopy Procedure allowing visual inspection of the hollow body organs using a fiberoptic instrument.

Endothelium Single layer of cells lining the blood vessels and the heart.

Endurance Ability to withstand physical or other stressors over time.

Enema Insertion of fluid into the rectum and colon.

Enteral nutrition Delivery of nutrition into the gastrointestinal system, usually in the form of tube feedings.

Enuresis Involuntary voiding with underlying pathophysiologic origin after the age that bladder control is usually achieved. Nocturnal enuresis is bedwetting.

Environment Context in which a person lives; includes social and inanimate characteristics.

Epicardium Serous, external layer of the heart.

Epidemic Disease that breaks out in a large proportion of the population.

Epidemiology Study of the causative agents of disease, occurrence of disease, and distribution of health and disease in population; also concerned with defining risks for contracting diseases.

Epidermis Thin, avascular, outermost layer of skin.

Erythema Redness of the skin.

Eschar Black, leathery crust of dead tissue covering a wound.

Esophagus Muscular tube connecting the pharynx and the stomach.

Esteem needs Two types: esteem derived from others and self-esteem (feelings of self-worth marked by the perception of confidence, competence, achievement, and productivity).

Ethics Professional standards of behavior related to right and wrong.

Ethnicity or ethnic identity Shared cultural characteristics that symbolize a common group origin.

Ethnocentrism Use of one's own culture to judge the beliefs, behaviors, attitudes, and values of people of another culture.

Etiology Cause or origin.

Evaluation Judgment of the effectiveness of nursing care in achieving client goals.

Eversion Turning the feet outward so toes are pointed away from the midline.

Evisceration Protrusion of internal organs through an open wound.

Exanthem Sink rash or eruption occurring in certain infectious diseases.

Excitement phase First phase in the human sexual response cycle, according to Master and Johnson, in which there is initial response to physiologic or psychological stimuli.

Excoriation Loss of superficial skin layers.

Excretion Process by which a drug or urine is eliminated from the body.

Exogenous From a source other than the client.

Extension Straightening a joint.

External rotation Lateral rotation of the anterior surface of a limb.

Extracellular fluid (ECF) compartment Body fluid outside the cells; mainly interstitial fluid and plasma.

Extracellular fluid volume The intravascular fluid, which consists of the fluid inside the blood and lymphatic vessels, and interstitial fluid which is the fluid between the cells.

Exudate Fluid that has penetrated from blood vessels into surrounding tissues as the result of inflammation.

Facilitation A method used to eliminate problems or barriers or to make something easier.

Faith Belief held; a relational phenomenon.

Family Basic human social unit; membership is based on mutual commitment, heredity, or legal arrangements.

Family development tasks Activities that usually occur at pre-expansion, expansion, dispersion, and replacement stages of family life. The failure to accomplish these tasks may identify families at risk for dysfunction.

Fasting Doing without food for a period of time.

Fatigue A subjective state of weariness, lack of energy.

Fats Lipid organic substances composed of carbon, hydrogen, and oxygen.

Febrile With an elevated temperature.

Fecal impaction Hard stool lodged in the rectum.

Feces Solid waste products of digestion; stool.

Feedback loop Output is rerouted back to the system as input.

Fetus Stage of development from 8 weeks after conception to birth.

Fever State in which the body's core temperature rises above the normal level for that person during rest.

Fiber Component of food that adds bulk to the diet and is not broken down by digestion.

Fight-or-flight response Sympathetic physiologic response that prepares a person to fight or to flee from a stressor.

Filtration Passage of a solution through a semipermeable membrane from a region of higher pressure to a region of lower pressure.

Filtration pressure Hydrostatic pressure minus osmotic pressure; determines the direction of flow across a membrane or vessel wall.

Fistula Abnormal tubelike passage between organs or between an organ and the body surface, often as the result of poor wound healing.

Flaccid Without muscle tone or resistance.

Flatus Gas in the gastrointestinal tract.

Flexibility Ability to bend without excessive resistance.

Flexion Bending or being bent so as to decrease the angle between two bones at a joint.

Flora Microorganisms.

Flowsheet Form for charting routine nursing procedures.

Fluid overload Condition of excessive extracellular fluid that can be due to the rapid administration of IV fluids.

Fluid volume deficit Abnormal reduction in isotonic extracellular fluid; also called hypovolemia, saline deficit, or isotonic dehydration.

Fluid volume excess Abnormal increase in isotonic extracellular fluid.

Fluoroscopy X-ray visualization of organs or movement within organs.

Food Guide Pyramid Recommendation for healthy eating by the U. S. Department of Agriculture. Guidelines suggest appropriate number of servings a day for the five major food groups: bread, cereal, rice, and pasta; vegetable; fruit; meat, poultry, dry beans, eggs, and nuts; milk, yogurt, and cheese.

Foot drop Temporary or permanent plantar flexion due to weakness or paralysis.

Foreskin Loose skin at the head of the penis, removed during circumcision; prepuce.

Fowler's position Semisitting position in bed.

Frequency 1. Measurement of vibrations. 2. Voiding more often than usual.

Functional health patterns A framework for collecting and organizing nursing assessment data to ascertain the strengths of the client as well as any dysfunction or potentially dysfunctional patterns that exist.

Gait Character of one's walk.

General adaptation syndrome Responses to stress composed of three stages: alarm reaction, stage of resistance, and stage of exhaustion.

General anesthetic Agent used to induce complete loss of sensation and consciousness.

General Systems Theory A systems framework that assumes all systems must be goal directed; a system is more than the sum of its parts; a system is ever changing and any change in one part affects the whole; and boundaries are implicit and in human systems are open and dynamic.

Generic drug name Product or medication not protected by trademark; nonproprietary name assigned to a drug.

Genetics Characteristics determined by the DNA code inherited from biologic mother and father.

Germicide Agent that destroys microorganisms, particularly pathogens; used on both living tissue and inanimate objects.

Glomerular filtrate Plasma fluid that is filtered out by the glomerular capillaries of the nephron and passes in the nephron tubule.

Glucosuria Presence of an abnormal amount of sugar, specifically glucose, in urine.

Glycogenesis Anabolic process of glycogen storage; formation of glycogen from glucose.

Glycogenolysis Catabolic process that converts stored glycogen into glucose so it can be used as an energy source.

Glyconeogenesis Catabolic process occurring in the liver that forms glycogen from noncarbohydrate sources such as amino acids or fatty acids.

Goal Aim or expected end to which the nurse and client work together.

Gram stain Process to identify microorganisms in which a slide of a specimen is stained with identifying chemicals.

Granulation tissue Soft, pink, highly vascularized connective tissue formed during wound repair.

Granuloctyes Polymorphonuclear white blood cells: neutrophils, eosinophils, and basophils.

Grief Psychological and physiologic response after the loss of a significant person, object, belief, or relationship.

Ground To connect electricity between an electrical conductor and the ground or earth.

Growth Progressive increase in physical size or psychosocial development.

Guaiac Test to reveal the presence of blood in feces.

Half-life Time required for a drug or substance to lose 50% of its activity through metabolism or elimination.

Hallucination False sensory perception; seeing, hearing, smelling, feeling, or tasting objects that are not there.

Head nurse Department head or manger responsible for all operations of a client-care unit; provides a vital communication link between the client, the direct-care providers, and the administration.

Health 1. State of well-being and optimal functioning. 2. Interactive process between the person and the internal and external environment. The person responds to changes in the environment to maintain integrity and harmony.

Healthcare delivery system People, institutions, and associated businesses responsible for providing healthcare to the public.

Healthcare reform Reform directed at cost control, providing health insurance for the poor, and pooling the health insurance risks of the nonpoor while reforming the insurance industry.

Health insurance Protection against the cost of medical care and hospitalization.

Health maintenance Positive health behaviors to preserve a current state of health.

Health maintenance organization (HMO) Organization that provides comprehensive health services to members for a set monthly fee.

Health promotion Health behaviors that enhance a person's level of health.

Health status Level of health.

Hematocrit Percent of red blood cells in a given volume of whole blood.

Hematology Study of blood components.

Hematoma Localized accumulation of blood in a body tissue, organ, or space as a result of broken blood vessel.

Hematuria Presence of blood in urine.

Hemoglobin Oxygen-carrying component of the red blood cell.

Heterosexual Person who relates sexually to a member of the opposite sex.

High-level wellness Way of living in which a person strives toward the highest potential in physical, mental, emotional, and spiritual health.

Holism Seeing the universe—and the client—as a system of connected parts rather than a sum of isolated parts.

Home health aide Person hired to provide basic hygiene for homebound clients.

Home health care Healthcare services provided at home.

Home management Ability to maintain oneself in a safe, nurturing home environment.

Homebound Unable to leave home because of poor health.

Homeless Lacking a permanent residence or having no shelter.

Homeostasis State of balance in the body, including the balance of body fluids and their chemical constituents.

Homosexual Person who relates sexually to a member of the same sex.

Hormonal dyssynchrony Situation in which the circadian rhythms of different hormones adjust to changes in sleeping time at different rates.

Hospice Family-focused health service that provides care for terminally ill clients.

Hospital Information System (HIS) Computer system developed for the needs of hospitals.

Host Person or animal who harbors and nourishes a microorganism.

Human need Physiologic or psychological factor necessary for a healthy existence.

Human sexual response cycle Pattern of physiologic responses to sexual stimulation proceeding from arousal to orgasm.

Humidification Addition of water vapor to inspired air to prevent drying of the respiratory mucosa.

Hydrostatic pressure Pressure exerted by a fluid against the wall of its container (eg, against vessel walls).

Hyperalgesia Enhanced sensation of pain produced by a noxious stimulus.

Hypercalcemia High concentration of calcium in the blood.

Hyperextension Extension of a joint beyond its normal (or intended) range of motion.

Hyperglycemia High concentrations of glucose in the blood.

Hyperkalemia High concentration of potassium in the blood.

Hyperlipoproteinemia Excessive fat-protein molecules in the blood; includes fat-protein combinations such as high-density lipoproteins (HDL), low-density lipoproteins (LDL), and triglycerides.

Hypermagnesemia High concentration of magnesium in the blood.

Hypernatremia High concentration of sodium in the blood; also called water deficit.

Hyperosmolar One compartment contains a greater concentration of a dissolved substance (hyperosmolar) than the other compartment (hypoosmolar).

Hyperpyrexia Fever that becomes life-threatening.

Hyperresonant Increased propagation of sound on percussion.

Hypertension Abnormally high blood pressure.

Hyperthermia Above-normal core temperature.

Hypertonic Of greater concentration than in body fluids.

Hyperventilation Breathing in excess of metabolic demands, resulting in removal of too much carbon dioxide from the blood; indicated by decreased $PaCO_2$.

Hypnotic Medication that induces or maintains sleep.

Hypocalcemia Low concentration of calcium in the blood.

Hypokalemia Low concentration of potassium in the blood.

Hypomagnesemia Low concentration of magnesium in the blood.

Hyponatremia Low concentration of sodium in the blood; also called water excess.

Hypoosmolar One compartment contains a lesser concentration of a dissolved substance (hypoosmolar) than the other compartment (hyperosmolar).

Hypotension Abnormally low blood pressure.

Hypothermia Below-normal core temperature.

Hypothesis Statement that predicts the relationships between the variables under study.

Hypotonic Of lower concentration than in body fluids.

Hypoventilation Breathing insufficient to meet metabolic demands and adequately remove carbon dioxide from the blood; indicated by elevated $PaCO_2$.

Hypovolemia Abnormally decreased volume of circulating plasma.

Hypoxemia Below-normal amount of oxygen in the blood.

Hypoxia Decreased amount of oxygen available to the tissues.

Hypoxic drive Stimulus to breathe based on decreased PaO_2; found in some COPD clients.

Iatrogenic disease Caused as the result of receiving healthcare treatment.

ICU psychosis State of delirium and agitation that can occur after several days in an ICU; caused by obtrusive stimuli, sleep deprivation, and acute illness. Usually reverses a few days after leaving the ICU.

Ideal body weight Body weight optimal for functioning and health.

Identity Awareness of self, as separate and distinct from others.

Ileostomy Opening of the ileum onto the abdominal skin surface via a stoma.

Illiteracy Inability to read or write, found among all races and socioeconomic levels.

Illness Subjective symptoms of disease, such as malaise, nausea, and vomiting.

Illness prevention Positive behaviors to prevent illness or disease; also known as health promotion.

Imagery Focusing the mind on a series of images for self-awareness, relaxation, and healing.

Immobility State in which the client cannot or does not move.

Immunity Resistance to a specific infection; may be naturally or artificially acquired.

Immunosuppression Unresponsiveness of the body's immune system to the presence of a foreign substance.

Impetigo Highly contagious skin infection characterized by bullae and pustules.

Implementation Action phase of the nursing process, in which nursing care is provided.

Impotence Inability to attain or maintain an erection long enough to have satisfactory sexual intercourse.

Incentive spirometer Breathing exercise device that uses sustained maximal inspiration to prevent or reverse atelectasis.

Incidence Rate or range of occurrence of a disease.

Incident Unusual happening to a client or visitor at a healthcare facility.

Incision Cut or wound made by a sharp instrument, usually during a surgical procedure.

Incomplete protein Protein that does not contain enough amino acid to independently maintain life, build tissue, or promote growth.

Incontinence Inability to control excretion from the bowel or bladder.

Independence Ability to carry out activities of daily living autonomously.

Independent variable Variable that causes or affects the dependent variable.

Indirect care Care provided in which the professional does not interact with the client; rather, the care is given by people under the professional's direction.

Inductive theory Process by which specific observations lead to more general rules.

Indwelling catheter Tube left in the bladder to drain urine.

Infarction Dead tissue resulting from ischemia due to lack of circulation.

Infection Organ or tissue dysfunction caused by microorganisms.

Infectious disease Process resulting from infection that produces manifestations such as fever, leukocytosis, inflammation, or tissue damage.

Infectivity Ability of a microorganism to invade and multiply within the host.

Infiltration Abnormal or accidental seepage or deposition of a substance into the tissues; accidental administration of IV fluids into subcutaneous tissues that occurs when the needle or catheter becomes dislodged from the vein.

Influence Power to bring about a change in others.

Information processing theory Method of organizing information so that cues can be used to make accurate diagnoses.

Informed consent Legal document giving permission for surgical or diagnostic procedure signed by client or legal guardian; before signing the physician has explained all aspects of the surgery, including the risks.

Inpatient Client who occupies a hospital bed.

Insensible evaporation Body water that is continuously being lost through evaporation from the skin and lungs.

In-service education Education provided at a healthcare facility to orient and update employees.

Insomnia Difficulty sleeping; may be characterized by trouble falling asleep or staying asleep, or waking too early.

Inspection Systematic visual examination of the client.

Integument Skin.

Intellectual function Memory, comprehension, and concentration.

Intelligence Measurable product of intellectual functioning.

Intensity Loudness of sound.

Interaction Response or action between a drug and the body cells.

Interdisciplinary Involving members of different fields or specialties, who interact to maximize the effectiveness of healthcare.

Interferon Protein that retards viral replication. It is produced by body cells on exposure to viruses, and it triggers a reaction that neutralizes the virus.

Intermittent positive pressure breathing (IPPB) Treatment that provides deep breaths under pressure to improve air distribution in the lungs.

Internal rotation Rotation toward the midline of the anterior surface of a limb.

International Council of Nurses Nursing organization concerned with health and nursing care throughout the world.

Interview Goal-directed conversation in which the nurse questions the client.

Intracellular fluid (ICF) compartment Portion of body fluid contained within the cells.

Intradermal Involving administration of a medication into the dermis located just beneath the skin surface.

Intraoperative period Time that starts when the client is transferred to the operating room bed and ends with transfer to the postanesthesic area.

Intraspinal Involving administration of a medication within the area of the spinal column; also called intrathecal.

Intravenous (IV) Involving administration of fluid or medication within a vein.

Intravenous therapy Infusion of a fluid into a vein to treat or prevent fluid and electrolyte or nutritional imbalances; may be used to deliver medications or blood products.

Intuition Use of insight, instincts, and clinical experience to make judgments.

Invasiveness Ability of microorganisms to enter tissues.

Inversion Turning the feet inward so toes are pointing toward the midline.

Ion Charged particle formed by the dissociation of electrolytes in solution.

Irrigation 1. The cleansing of a wound or body cavity by flushing with fluid. 2. The cleansing of a tube with solution to clear a blockage.

Ischemia Insufficient blood supply to a body part due to obstruction of circulation.

Isolation Techniques used to prevent or limit the spread of infection.

Isolation systems Procedures used to prevent the spread of infection. Systems developed through the years include Universal Precautions, category-specific isolation, disease-specific isolation, and body-substance isolation. The CDC in 1995 developed a new two-tiered system to combine the former systems. The new system includes Standard Precautions and Transmission-Based Precautions.

Isometric exercise Exercise involving muscle contraction without a change in muscle length (often occurs against resistance).

Isotonic Osmotic concentration equal to that of body fluids.

Isotonic exercise Dynamic form of exercise in which there is constant muscle tension, muscle contraction, and active movement.

IV time strip Strip of tape placed on an IV solution container marked to indicate the amount of fluid expected to infuse each hour.

Judgment Process of reasoning; ability to process incoming stimuli and determine meanings that encompass many aspects of a situation.

Kardex Trade name of a care plan documentation system.

Kegel exercises Exercises to strengthen the muscles of the pelvic floor.

Key informant Person who knows and will discuss certain aspects of his or her culture with someone outside that culture.

Kinship Relationship between people based on common blood ties.

Korotkoff sounds Sounds heard during auscultation that indicate the systolic and diastolic blood pressure.

Kussmaul respirations Pattern of breathing characterized by respirations of increased rate and depth.

Kyphosis Exaggerated curvature of the thoracic spine; hunchback.

Labia Fleshy border of the female external genitalia; divided into labia majora and labia minora.

Laceration Wound caused by tearing of body tissue.

Language A prescribed way of using words; a means of expressing thoughts and feelings.

Lacrimal fluid Tears.

Laryngectomy Excision of the larynx.

Laws Standards of human conduct established and enforced by the authority of an organized society through its government.

Laxative Medication that causes bowel elimination.

Leadership Ability to influence others to strive for a goal or to change.

Leadership style Manner in which the leader interacts with subordinates.

Learning Process of acquiring knowledge; a multidimensional process that depends on symbols, language, classifications, concepts, and other concrete operations along with abstract functions.

Learning nursing care plan Educational tool to help students learn the nursing process.

Lesbian Female homosexual.

Lesion Injured or diseased area of the skin or other body tissue.

Leukocytosis Increase in production of white blood cells.

Leukopenia Insufficiency of white blood cells in the blood.

Level of care The intensity and permanence of care required to maintain, restore, or promote health.

Liability Responsibility for one's actions; an obligation one is bound to perform.

Licensed practical nurse Person licensed by a state after completing a state-approved nursing program to provide technical nursing care under the direct supervision of a registered nurse.

Licensure Process for ensuring safe practice in nursing. States grant permission via licensure for qualified professionals to practice professional nursing. Qualification is determined by successful completion of the licensure examination developed by each state's board of nursing.

Lipid emulsion Isotonic mixture of fats for hyperalimentation infusion.

Literature review Process of selecting published materials about the concepts to be examined in a research project.

Local adaptation syndrome Localized expression of the three stages of the general adaptation syndrome.

Long-term care Healthcare services provided over a period of time to clients who need ongoing care; generally provided in institutions such as nursing homes.

Lordosis Exaggerated curvature of the lumbar spine; swayback.

Lumbar puncture Puncture, usually between the third and fourth lumbar vertebrae, to obtain cerebrospinal fluid.

Maceration Softening of tissue due to excessive moisture.

Macrodrip IV tubing that delivers 10, 15, or 20 drops per milliliter, depending on the manufacturer.

Macula Spotted, nonelevated discoloration of the skin.

Malignant hyperthermia Severe body temperature elevation after administration of certain anesthetics.

Malignant pain Pain with recurrent acute episodes, or persistent chronic pain, or both acute and persistent pain associated with a progressive malignant-type process.

Malpractice Professional misconduct; causing harm or injury to a person from lack of experience, skill, knowledge, or judgment.

Mammogram Radiograph of the breast; used to detect breast tumors or cysts.

Managed care Model of client care delivery in which the care of an individual from the time of contact with the healthcare system to discharge is carefully planned and monitored to ensure that standards are followed and cost is minimized.

Management Getting the job done or accomplishing a goal through the functions of planning, organizing, directing, and controlling.

Mastication Chewing.

Masturbation Autostimulation of the genitals.

Maturation Process of development.

Meconium First feces of a newborn.

Medicaid Government-funded health insurance plan that provides financial assistance to the disabled or financially needy.

Medical diagnosis Identified disease or pathologic process; treatment focuses on correcting or preventing specific pathology of specific organs or body systems.

Medicare Federally funded program that provides medical and hospital insurance to people age 65 or older or those who are disabled.

Medication Drug given for its therapeutic effects. All medications are drugs.

Meditation Purposeful quieting of the mind to experience inner peace.

Melanin Pigment found normally in the skin that gives it a brown color and protects it from ultraviolet light.

Menarche First menstrual period.

Menopause Permanent cessation of menstruation.

Mental health Mental or emotional well-being in terms of interpersonal relationships, role fulfillment, and achievement in work, family, and community.

Metabolism 1. Chemical reactions in the cells that produce heat as a byproduct. 2. Breakdown of a drug (usually in the liver) to an inactive form.

Metacognition Thinking about thinking.

Metacommunication Meanings beyond the literal level of communication, such as the roles of the communicators and the context in which the communication is taking place.

Method Procedure a researcher follows to gather and analyze data.

Microdrip IV tubing that delivers 60 drops per milliliter.

Micturition Urination.

Milliequivalent (mEq) Unit used to give the concentration of an electrolyte in solution; commonly expressed as mEq/L.

Minority Smaller segment of a society.

Mnemonic A memory tool.

Mode of transmission Way in which a microorganism moves from the source to the host.

Monosaccharides Simple sugars.

Montgomery straps (or ties) Adhesive strips with ties used to hold dressings in place; they allow frequent changes without the need for tape removal.

Moral Involving correct behavior.

Motivation Something that provides drive or incentive.

Mourning Behavior after the death of a significant other. Mourning behaviors vary from culture to culture.

Mucociliary escalator Mucus blanket that lies on top of ciliated cells in airways. It traps bacteria and dust and moves them upward toward the mouth for expectoration.

Mucosa Mucous membrane lining many tubular body structures; capable of secreting mucus.

Multidisciplinary Involving people of different specialties who work together.

Multi-infarct dementia Dementia that results from multiple small infarcts in cerebral vessels.

Myelogram Radiographic procedure to evaluate the subarachnoid space around the spinal cord.

Myocaridum Layer of cardiac muscle that forms the walls of the heart.

Myoclonus Uncontrolled muscle movements.

Narcolepsy Sleep disorder characterized by sudden uncontrollable episodes of sleep.

National League of Nursing Organization that serves as the accrediting body for nursing education programs.

Nebulizer Device that breaks liquids into tiny droplets for aerosol therapy.

Necrosis Localized areas of dead tissue, dying leukocytes, bacteria, and cellular debris.

Negative nitrogen balance State in which nitrogen excretion is greater than intake; can occur due to impaired protein synthesis or excessive breakdown (eg, with intense physical stress).

Negligence Not doing something that a reasonably prudent person would do, or doing something that a reasonably prudent person would not do.

Neonate Infant from birth to about 1 month.

Nephron Functional unit of the kidney; contains the glomerulus and the tubule.

Neuropathic pain Pain caused by nerve damage.

Neutropenia Decrease in the neutrophils in the blood, the white blood cells, responsible for quick response to invasion by infectious organisms.

Nightmare Frightening dream occurring during REM sleep.

Night terrors Repeated episodes of sudden wakening accompanied by screaming and acute anxiety, occurring during slow wave sleep.

Nitrogen balance State of equilibrium in which the amount of nitrogen taken in is equal to the amount of nitrogen excreted.

Nits Eggs of lice.

Nociceptors Free nerve endings that sense and respond to potentially noxious thermal, electrical, mechanical, or chemical stimuli.

Nocturnal Occurring at night.

Noncompliance Failure to adhere to a recommended plan.

Noninvasive Not entering a body cavity or breaking the skin.

Nonproprietary name Not protected by trademark; synonymous with generic name.

Non-REM sleep Non-rapid-eye-movement sleep, the four stages of quiet sleep in which brain waves slow but muscle tone is maintained.

Nonverbal communication Messages sent without words (eg, via gestures, facial expressions, body postures, silence).

Normal flora Microorganisms commonly found in a body location that ordinarily cause no harm to the person.

Nosocomial infection Infection acquired during receipt of healthcare.

NPO Nothing by mouth; oral food or liquids are forbidden.

Nuclear scan Radiographic procedure in which organs are visualized through the use of radioactive dye.

Nurse administrator Nurse who supervises the organization of nursing care to ensure overall safety and quality; requires at least a baccalaureate degree in nursing.

Nurse anesthetist (CRNA) Nurse who specializes and is certified in the administration of anesthesia.

Nurse educator Nurse responsible for nursing and healthcare education in a variety of settings; requires a master's or doctoral degree.

Nurse executive Top administrative nursing position in an organization.

Nurse midwife Nurse with advanced education and certification in the care of women during pregnancy and childbirth.

Nurse practice acts State guidelines that govern the practice of professional nursing.
Nurse practitioner Nurse with advanced education and certification. May practice independently in a variety of healthcare areas.
Nurse researcher Nurse responsible for continued development of nursing knowledge and improvement of practice through research; usually requires a doctoral degree.
Nursing Profession that involves diagnosis and treatment of human responses to actual or potential health problems.
Nursing centers Free-standing centers that provide nursing services on an independent basis.
Nursing diagnosis Actual, potential, or possible health problem identified by the nurse that is amenable to nursing intervention.
Nursing history Process in which the nurse interviews the client to elicit a description of his or her current and past health status.
Nursing monitor Review by a nurse of a client's care or records to determine the extent to which the care or records meet established standards.
Nursing orders Prescribed interventions in the nursing plan of care.
Nursing process Systematic approach to providing nursing care using assessment, planning, outcome identification, intervention, and evaluation.
Nursing research Research that focuses on establishing a scientific base for the practice of nursing.
Nursing theory Explanation or description of nursing issues that defines and predicts nursing practice.
Nutrients Food containing elements for normal body functioning.

Obesity Weight more than 20% over ideal body weight.
Objective data Observable, measurable information that can be validated or verified.
Observation Art of noticing client cues.
Obstructive disease Lung disorder characterized by narrowed airways, such as asthma, emphysema, or bronchitis.
Occult Hidden; not visible to the naked eye.
Official drug name Name of medication as listed in official publications.
Oliguria Formation and excretion of less than 500 mL or urine in 24 hours.
One-day surgery center Medical facility where admission, surgery, and discharge occur on the same day; also known as surgicenter.
Open family People who recognize a commitment to each other but are not necessarily related by blood.
Ophthalmoscope Instrument for examining the interior of the eye.
Opportunistic organisms Organisms that invade the tissues when body defenses are suppressed.
Opsonization Preparation of the bacterial cell wall to facilitate engulfment by phagocytes.
Oral administration Given by mouth.
Organizing Arranging the work to be done in small units so it can be accomplished.
Orgasm Climax phase of the human sexual response cycle; the man experiences expulsive contractions of the entire length of the urethra, and the woman experiences contractions in the outer third of the vagina and labia minora, as well as uterine contractions.
Orientation Awareness to time, place, situation, and self.
Orthopnea Ability to breathe easily only when in an upright position.
Orthostatic hypotension Fall in blood pressure associated with a change in position (from lying to sitting to standing).
Osmolality Concentration of solutes in a solution; expressed as milliosmosis per kilogram.
Osmolarity Concentration of solutes in a solution; expressed as milliosmols per liter.
Osmosis Movement of a fluid through a semipermeable membrane from a region of lower to higher solute concentration.
Osmotic pressure Pressure exerted by nondiffusible particles in a solution across a semipermeable membrane; tends to hold fluid within its container and is opposed by hydrostatic pressure.
Osteoporosis Reduction in bone mass due to loss of calcium.
Otoscope Instrument for examining the ear.
Outcome criteria Specific, measurable, realistic statement of goal attainment.
Outcome identification The formulation of goals and measurable outcomes which provides the basis for evaluation.
Outpatient Person who is having diagnostic or laboratory tests, receiving therapy, or attending a clinic, but does not occupy a bed.
Ovaries Almond-shaped bodies that contain the female gonads; they lie on either side of the pelvic cavity.
Over-the-counter (OTC) medication Medication that can be bought without a prescription.
Oxygenation Provision of oxygen to the blood or tissues.

$PaCO_2$ Partial pressure of carbon dioxide in arterial blood.
PaO_2 Partial pressure of oxygen in arterial blood.
Pain Body's response to events that threaten body tissue.
Pain threshold Lowest intensity at which a certain person perceives a stimulus to be painful.
Pain tolerance Highest intensity of pain that the person is willing to tolerate.
Palpation Use of the sense of touch to ascertain the size, shape, and configuration of underlying body structures.
Pandemic Worldwide epidemic.
Papule Small, solid skin elevation.
Paracentesis Puncture of the abdomen to remove excess fluid.
Paradoxical blood pressure Significant decrease in systolic blood pressure with inspiration.
Paraplegia Paralysis of both legs and the lower part of the body.
Parasomnias Group of disorders, such as somnambulism (sleepwalking) and enuresis (bedwetting) involving autonomic and motor activity associated with partial arousal from sleep.
Parenteral administration Medication given by injection, usually intravenously or intramuscularly.
Parenteral nutrition Nutritional elements supplied through an intravenous route, usually into a central vein.
Parenting Process of nurturing children to enhance development.
Participative leadership Style of a leader who involves subordinates in setting goals, solving problems, and making decisions.
Passive range of motion Exercises in which body parts are moved by another person.

Pathogen Microorganism that can harm humans.

Pathogenicity Ability to induce a disease.

Pedagogy Teaching as applied to children or adolescent learners.

Pediculosis Infestation with lice.

Peer review Evaluation and judgment of performance by other nurses.

Penis Male organ of copulation; urine and semen flow from the body through it.

Perceiving Process of recognizing and interpreting sensory stimuli; basis for understanding, knowing, or learning.

Perceptions How we view ourselves and the world; influenced by culture, religion, family, past experiences, expectations, and knowledge.

Percussion Examination by tapping the body surface with the fingertips and evaluating the sounds obtained.

Perfusion Passing of blood through an area.

Perineal care Cleansing of the perineum.

Perineum Area of the body containing the external pelvic structures: in a girl or woman, the area between the vulva and the anus; in a boy or man, the area between the penis and anus.

Perioperative period Period that begins with the decision to have surgery and ends with recovery.

Peripheral parenteral nutrition Infusion of isotonic solutions into the peripheral vessels to meet nutritive requirements.

Peristalsis Motility and movement of the intestines.

Peritonitis Inflammation of the membranous lining of the abdominal cavity.

pH Measure of the degree of acidity or alkalinity of a solution; as the pH increases, the acidity decreases.

Phagocytosis Process of engulfing microorganisms and other antigens.

Pharmacokinetics Study of how a medication changes as it passes through the body and undergoes absorption, distribution, metabolism, and excretion.

Phlebitis Inflammation or infection of a vein, manifested by redness, swelling, and tenderness along the course of the vein.

Phonation Process by which humans create vocal sounds.

Physical examination Use of one's senses through the techniques of inspection, palpation, percussion, and auscultation to obtain information about the structure and function of body parts.

Physical fitness State of health in which a person can perform normal and strenuous daily activities.

Physiologic needs Needs for air, food, water, elimination, sleep and rest, temperature maintenance, and sex.

Piggyback Diluted intravenous medication given over an intermediate length of time (ie, 30 minutes).

Placebo Inactive substance given to client for its psychological benefit.

Plaintiff Person who sues another.

Plan Written nursing diagnoses, outcome criteria, and interventions necessary to provide nursing care.

Planning Management function of deciding what to do, when, where, how, by whom, and with what resources.

Plantar flexion Bending at the ankle so as to point toes downward.

Plateau phase Phase of the human sexual response cycle that follows the excitement phase and precedes the orgasmic phase.

Pleximeter In percussion, the finger placed between the area to be percussed and the finger creating the vibrations.

Plexor Finger creating the vibrations during percussion.

Pneumonia Inflammation of the tissues in the lungs caused by bacteria, viruses, chemicals, fluids, or other irritants.

Pneumothorax Collection of air in the pleural space, usually as a result of perforation of the chest wall or the pleura covering the lung.

Poison Substance or gas that can injure or kill.

Pollution Substances in air, water, or land that are potentially harmful to health.

Polygraph recordings Graphic recordings of electrophysiologic changes in brain waves, eye movements, and muscles.

Polymicrobial infections Infections caused by a variety of organisms growing synergistically, often of mixed anaerobic and aerobic species.

Polysaccharides Complex sugars.

Polyuria Formation and excretion of large amounts of urine in the absence of a concurrent increase in fluid intake.

Portal of entrance Site of deposition of a microorganism.

Portal of exit Means of escape of a microorganism, such as body fluids.

Positive nitrogen balance State in which intake of nitrogen is greater than the amount excreted; occurs in growth, athletic training, or pregnancy.

Positive regard Warmth, caring, interest, and respect for another person; a nonjudgmental attitude toward others.

Possible nursing diagnosis Health problem amenable to nursing intervention that requires additional data collection and validation before it can be confirmed or deleted as a nursing diagnosis.

Postoperative period Phase that begins with transfer to the surgical recovery area and ends with recovery.

Precordium Part of the chest that overlies the heart and lower thorax.

Preferred Provider Organization (PPO) Group of physicians and possibly one or more hospitals which offers a prepaid healthcare plan to employers.

Premature ejaculation Condition in which the man cannot delay ejaculation long enough for the woman to reach orgasm, or for satisfactory sexual intercourse to occur.

Preoperative checklist Form summarizing a client's preoperative preparation; ensures that all necessary information is in the chart.

Preoperative period Phase that begins with the decision to have surgery and ends with transfer to the operating room bed.

Prepuce Loose skin at the head of the penis; foreskin.

Prescription Directive written by a physician.

Pressure sore Sore or ulcer caused by prolonged pressure and decreased blood flow to skin and underlying tissue; also known as decubitus ulcer or bedsore.

Prevalence Extent to which a condition exists within a population.

Preventable infection Infection that could have been prevented if some event related to the infection had been altered.

Primary intention Healing process that occurs in wounds with little tissue loss and well-approximated edges; results in minimal granulation tissue and scar formation.

Primary nursing Model of nursing care in which a professional nurse develops a 24-hour nursing plan of care and integrates that plan with the therapy plan of other healthcare professionals.

Priority Nursing problem that takes on a position of prominence.

Problem-oriented medical record Charting system in which everyone caring for the client uses the client problem list as a guide.

Problem-solving Systematic process that involves identifying and analyzing the problem, determining and weighing the possible solutions, choosing and implementing a solution, and evaluating the results.

Pronation 1. Rotation of the forearm, turning the palm to face downward. 2. Assuming a face-down position.

Prone Lying face down.

Proprietary name Name protected by trademark; synonymous with brand name or trade name.

Proprioceptors Nerve receptors that respond to position or movement.

Proprioception Awareness of the position and movements of body parts in space, sensed by sensory nerve terminals in muscles, tendons, and the labyrinth of the ear.

Prospective payment Method of reimbursing a fixed dollar amount for client care based on diagnosis-related groups (DRGs).

Protein Organic compound composed of polymers of amino acids connected by peptide bonds.

Protein-sparing action Body's use of carbohydrates rather than protein as an energy source.

Proteinuria Presence of protein in urine.

Pruritus Severe itching.

Psoriasis Skin disease involving overproduction of epidermal cells.

Psychomotor Relating to muscle movements resulting from a mental process.

Psychosomatic Involving the integration of mind and body.

Puberty Period of life in which the sex organs mature, secondary sex characteristics appear, and reproduction becomes possible.

Pulmonary system System designed for ventilation and gas exchange; includes the lungs, their vasculature, and the structures required for their proper function.

Pulse deficit Mathematical difference between apical and radial pulse.

Pulse pressure Mathematical difference between systolic and diastolic blood pressure.

Purpose statement Clear, concise statement that defines the limits of a study.

Pursed-lip breathing Exhalation of air against resistance that clients with obstructive diseases use to reduce trapping of air; done by forming a small "O" with lips and exhaling slowly.

Purulent Producing or containing pus.

Pus Thick liquid product of inflammation that contains dead white blood cells, dead liqufied tissue, and living or dead bacteria.

Pustule Small, pus-filled skin elevation.

Pyuria Presence of pus in urine.

Quadriplegia Paralysis of arms and legs.

Quality assurance Systematic evaluation of healthcare designed to ensure excellence.

Quality assurance monitors Mechanisms that ensure that acceptable client care is provided and standards are upheld.

Race Group defined by biologic characteristics (eg, Asian, black, or caucasian).

Racism Oppression and exploitation of people of a different skin color or ethnic origin.

Radioisotope Radioactive chemical used in diagnostic tests.

Radiopaque Impenetrable to x-ray.

Rales Crackling breath sounds heard on inhalation that indicate fluid in alveoli or alveoli that are partially collapsed between breaths.

Range of motion Extent to which joints and muscles can be moved.

Range-of-motion exercises Systematic movement of joints to maintain flexibility and prevent muscle contractures.

Rationale Reason for a nursing intervention, supported by clinical research.

Reality orientation Nursing technique to help restore the client's awareness of reality.

Rebound phenomenon In relation to sleep, the tendency for stage 4 and REM sleep to be recovered at the expense of the other stages.

Recall and recognition Abilities used to retrieve information in long- and short-term memory.

Recommended Dietary Allowances (RDAs) Nutritive requirements for kilocalories, proteins, and selected vitamins and minerals determined by research to support health.

Record Permanent document of client information and care.

Referral Request of another professional to provide a service outside the scope of the professional making the referral.

Regional anesthetic Agent used to induce loss of sensation in a selected body area.

Registered nurse Person licensed by a state to practice professional nursing. Steps toward licensure include completing a state-approved nursing program and passing the state licensure examination.

Rehabilitation Actions taken to restore, to the extent possible, a person to a former state of functioning.

Relativism Theory that knowledge is relative to individuals, groups, and conditions and that there are a variety of effective approaches to any situation.

Reliability Degree to which an instrument or test consistently or dependably measures the attribute it is intended to measure.

REM sleep Sleep characterized by rapid eye movements and very low muscle activity.

Reminiscence therapy Use of recall of the client's past to help clarify meaning in the present or reconcile conflict.

Reporting Sharing of client information by two or more healthcare professionals.

Research design Overall plan for collecting and analyzing data.

Reservoir Place where microorganisms collect, reproduce, and grow.

Residential care Health and social services provided to clients who live in a group-housing setting.

Residual urine Amount of urine remaining in the bladder after voiding.

Resistance In microbiology, lack of response by a microorganism to a drug that is intended to slow its growth or destroy it.

Resolution phase Final phase of the human sexual response cycle; immediately follows orgasm and is marked by rapid loss of vasocongestion.

Resonance Echoing of sound through passages.

Respiration Exchange of carbon dioxide for oxygen in lungs and in the tissues.

Respiratory failure Inability of the pulmonary system to meet the metabolic demands of carbon dioxide elimination and tissue oxygenation.

Respite care Healthcare services provided to a client to give the regular caregiver a temporary relief from responsibility.

Respondeat superior "Let the master answer"; doctrine in which a hospital is held liable for an employee's negligence.

Rest Physical and emotional state of decreased muscle and cognitive activity.

Restraint Device that prevents a client from moving or from gaining normal access to a body part.

Restrictive disease Lung disorder characterized by decreased ability to stretch the lungs, such as pneumonia or fibrosis.

Reticular activating system (RAS) Part of the brain responsible for bringing together information from the cerebellum and other parts of the brain and from the sense organs.

Rh factor Group of antigens on the erythrocytes of most people; a person is designated Rh + or Rh − based on the absence or presence of this factor.

Rhonchi Rumbling breath sounds caused by air passing through secretions in the airways.

Risk nursing diagnosis State of being at risk for the development of a health problem amenable to nursing intervention; formerly called a potential nursing diagnosis or a high-risk nursing diagnosis.

Roentgenogram X-ray.

Role Expected function and behavior of a person.

Role play Therapeutic enactment of a problematic situation.

Rotation Movement of a bone or body part about an axis.

Safety needs Freedom from fear, anxiety, and danger.

Sanguineous Pertaining to or containing blood.

Sanitizing Cleaning an item, generally by use of chemical agents.

Satiety Satisfaction; often used to describe gratification of hunger or thirst.

Scabies Highly contagious, inflammatory skin disease caused by mites.

Scoliosis Abnormal lateral curvature of the spine.

Scrotum Loose, pouchlike sac in the male external genitalia that contains the testes.

Seamless care System in which all levels of care are available in an integrated form.

Sebaceous glands Oil-secreting glands of the dermis.

Secondary intention Wound healing by filling in with granulation tissue.

Self-actualization Process of developing one's maximum potential and managing one' life confidently.

Self-awareness Knowing and caring for oneself; recognizing one's strengths and limitations.

Self-concept Mental image of oneself.

Self-efficacy An individual's belief that he or she is capable of doing something.

Self-esteem Evaluation and judgment of one's worth.

Self-evaluation Conscious assessment of the self.

Self-expectation The self a person wants to be.

Self-knowledge Basic understanding of oneself.

Self-perception A person's awareness or identification of self; the filtering process of evaluating events and entering them into the subconscious.

Semipermeable membrane Membrane that permits passage of some molecules in a solution while excluding others.

Sensation information Telling a client what he or she will see, hear, smell, taste, or feel in a particular situation.

Sensitivity Identification of the antibiotic that will destroy specific cultured microorganisms.

Sensoristasis State of optimal sensory input; differs for each person.

Sensory deprivation Lack of meaningful sensory stimuli; monotonous input, or interference with the processing of information; leads to behavioral changes ranging from boredom to psychosis.

Sensory overload State of arousal in which a person cannot manage the intensity or quantity of incoming sensory stimuli.

Sepsis Poisoning of body tissues; usually refers to blood-borne organisms or their toxic products.

Septicemia Bacterial infection in the bloodstream, leading to fever, chills, malaise, and collapse; may proceed to septic shock.

Serosanguineous Containing serum and blood.

Serous Thin, water, serumlike.

Sexuality Persons' characteristics and perceptions concerning sexual expression.

Shearing force Force applied when tissues move against each other, causing stretching of vasculature in the subcutaneous tissues. Occurs when a client slides up or down in bed.

Shock Severe circulatory insufficiency.

Shock (electrical) Interruption of body functions due to electrical current.

Sims' position Side-lying with the upper leg flexed.

Single-parent family Family consisting of a parent and child or children.

Skilled nursing facility Inpatient facility that provides long-term nursing care.

Sleep Readily reversible state of altered consciousness in which awareness and responsiveness to the environment is decreased.

Sleep apnea Condition in which, at least five times an hour, the client stops breathing for 10 seconds or more during sleep.

Sleep deprivation State of having less sleep than needed.

Sleep latency Time it takes to get to sleep after going to bed.

Sleep pattern disturbance Disruption in quantity or quality of sleep, causing discomfort or interfering with life.

Sleep–wake cycle Alternating periods of sleep and wakefulness in 24-hour period.

SOAP note Method of organizing charting entries so that subjective, objective, assessment, and planning information is included in each entry.

Social isolation State in which a person's desire for interpersonal relationships is perceived as unattainable; negative feelings of being alone.

Social self One's behavior and interaction with others in social situations.

Social worker Professional trained to assess and assist people regarding public assistance, social or family crisis, and access to social service programs.

Socialization Process in which a person is familiarized with the ways of a specific culture or group.

Somnambulism Sleepwalking.

Somnolence Sleepiness.

Source Place from which the infectious agent passes to the host.

Source recording Type of medical record system in which each healthcare specialty records in a separate area of the chart.

Spasticity Sudden involuntary increase in muscle tone or contractions due to central nervous system lesions.

Specific gravity Measure of the weight of a substance in comparison to an equal volume of water; indicates relative concentration of a fluid.

Sphincter Circular muscle that surrounds and constricts an opening.

Spiritual distress Condition in which a person's value system, from which he or she draws strength and hope, is disturbed.

Spiritual well-being Condition marked by an affirmation of life and a sense of unity with God, self, community, and environment.

Spirituality Personal striving toward unity and God in an attempt to find meaning in life.

Sputum Expectorated respiratory secretions, including mucus and saliva.

Standard Precautions The latest CDC isolation system which combines the major features of Universal Precautions (blood-borne transmissions) and Body Substance Isolation (moist body substances transmission), thus protecting against blood and body-fluid transmission of potential infective agents.

Standards Statements of the required quality of nursing care that serve as the model for others to follow.

Standing order Order to be implemented until canceled by a physician or by agency policy.

Stasis Stagnation or slowing of body fluid.

Stat order Directive to be carried out immediately.

Stenosis Narrowing of an opening.

Stereotype Preconceived belief about a person or people.

Sterilization 1. Destruction of all bacteria, spores, fungi, and viruses on an item; accomplished by heat, chemicals, or gas. 2. Rendered unable to reproduce biologically.

Steristrip Small adhesive strip used to hold wound edges in approximation.

Stethoscope Instrument used to amplify sounds produced in the body.

Stimulus Something that rouses the mind or spirit.

Stoma Artificially created opening of bowel on the abdominal skin surface.

Stool Solid waste products of digestion; feces.

Straight catheter Tube placed through the urethra into the bladder to drain urine temporarily.

Strategic planning Planning major long-range goals, objectives, and directions for an organization.

Stress State of arousal of mind and body in response to demands made on the person.

Stressor Stimulus or event that requires coping and adaptation.

Stria Thin streak or line; often associated with stretch marks from pregnancy or obesity (plural: striae).

Stridor Harsh crowing sound heard on inspiration, caused by upper airway obstruction; common in croup.

Stroke Cerebrovascular accident (CVA); involves a sudden onset of hemorrhage, blood clots, or other vascular lesions causing damage to the brain.

Stroke volume Amount of blood ejected from each cardiac ventricle with each contraction of the heart.

Subclinical infection Infection that produces an immune response without overt disease.

Subculture Beliefs held by a portion of the larger population (eg, an occupational or ethnic group).

Subcutaneous Pertaining to the layer of tissue under the dermis.

Sublingual Under the tongue.

Substantia gelatinosa Area in the dorsal horn of the spinal cord that is thought to be the "gate" for pain transmission.

Substrate Substance on which an enzyme works to produce changes.

Suffering An emotional response to increased pain; associated with events that threaten the intactness of a person, as differentiated from pain, which threatens body tissue.

Suffocation Oxygen deprivation.

Sundown syndrome Nocturnal delirium; state of disorientation and agitation that occurs at night in institutionalized clients who are oriented during the day.

Superinfection State in which susceptible microbes are suppressed by an antibiotic, allowing overgrowth of strains that are resistant to the antibiotic.

Supination Rotation of the forearm, turning the palm upward.

Suppository Medication inserted into the rectum or vagina.

Suppuration Production or discharge of pus.

Surgery Treatment of disease and injury by invasive manual and operative techniques.

Surgical holding area Area outside the operating room where final preparations are made before surgery.

Suture Material used to stitch together the edges of traumatic or surgical wounds.

Symbiotic Living in harmony, with no harm to host or organism.

Symmetry Correspondence in size, shape movement, and other qualities on opposite sides of the body.

System Set of interacting parts that make up a whole.

Systems theory Way of viewing the world or an organization in which the parts are seen in relation to the whole.

Systole Period of contraction of the ventricles.

Systolic blood pressure Pressure in the blood vessels during cardiac ventricular contraction.

Tachycardia Abnormally rapid heart rate, usually above 100 beats per minute in an adult.

Tachypnea Abnormally rapid respiratory rate, usually more than 20 breaths per minute in an adult.

Tangential lighting Light shining from the side to create shadows over the area being examined; accentuates subtle differences in contour and movement.

Taxonomy Classification system to organize information.

Teaching To communicate and impart knowledge by instruction, lesson, or demonstration.

Team conference Gathering of healthcare providers to discuss a specific client.

Team nursing Model of nursing care in which a team of nurses, licensed practical nurses, and nursing assistants are assigned specific functions or procedures to do for a group of clients.

Teleology Theory of philosophy in which the consequences of actions are considered in judging right and wrong.

Terminal ends Values regarded as good in themselves; they transcend immediate needs and shape long-term goals.

Testes Male gonads.

Testosterone Male hormone.

Theory Explanation of the relationships among phenomena.

Therapeutic communication Interactions that help a person express feelings and work out problems.

Thermoreceptors Nerve receptors that respond to temperature changes.

Thinking Mental activity in which one forms thoughts or intentions, determines by reflection, or attains clear ideas.

Third spacing Loss of intravascular fluid into an area of the body (a "third space") where it cannot be reabsorbed (eg, into the abdominal cavity).

Thoracentesis Puncture of the thoracic cavity to remove fluid.

Thought processes Cognitive functions under cerebral cortical control, including short- and long-term memory, use of language, attention span, judgment, and the ability to solve problems.

Thrombocytopenia Deficiency of platelets in the blood.

Thrombocytosis Excessive number of platelets in the blood.

Thrombosis Presence of a blood clot that completely or partially obstructs a blood vessel.

Thrombus Blood clot in a blood vessel.

Tidal volume Amount of air moving in and out of the lungs with each breath.

Tissue turgor Ability of the skin to return to normal position after begin pinched; reflects skin elasticity and/or hydration status.

Titration A method of medication administration in which the dosage is adjusted based on the client's response to the medication.

Tolerance Decreased physiologic response to repeated administration of a drug; an increase in dosage is needed to maintain a given therapeutic effect.

Topical administration Application directly to a body site.

Tort Wrong committed against a person or property; is subject to action in a civil court.

Total parenteral nutrition (TPN) Administration of hypertonic solutions containing dextrose, proteins, vitamins, and minerals to provide for nutritional deficits; also known as hyperalimentation.

Toxicity Harmful effect of a drug.

Tracheostomy Permanent or temporary opening into the trachea through the neck.

Tracheotomy Incision through the neck to create a temporary opening in the trachea; usually performed in an emergency.

Trade name Synonymous with brand name; name designated by drug manufacturer.

Transcribe To write orders and treatments on the nursing Kardex, medication administration records, or treatment records.

Transcutaneous electrical nerve stimulation (TENS) A mild electrical impulse to an area or over the pain zone and controlled by the client.

Transdermal medication Topical medication that is released through the epidermis and dermis to the blood.

Transfusion reaction Adverse physiologic response occurring as a result of blood transfusions.

Transient ischemic attack (TIA) Temporary cerebral ischemia due to transient interruption in blood supply.

Transient flora Microorganisms not normally found on the surface of the tissue that have not become attached to the tissue and are not growing or replicating.

Transmission-Based Precautions The latest CDC isolation system which protects against the transmission of highly transmissible or epidemiologically significant pathogens in clients with documented or suspected infections.

Transsexual Person who psychologically sees himself or herself as a member of the opposite sex.

Tremor Involuntary trembling or convulsive movement due to alternating contractions of opposing muscle groups.

Tympany Hollow, drumlike sound heard on percussion over an organ containing air or fluid.

Ultrasonography Diagnostic technique in which the reflection of sound waves is used to view organs and blood flow.

Unit dose Individual medication dose that is packaged and labeled in its own container.

Universal Precautions Practice in which blood and cerain body fluids, particularly those containing visible blood, of all clients are considered potentially infectious for blood-borne pathogens.

Urgency Inability to voluntarily delay voiding.

Urgent care centers Newer form of healthcare offered in shopping areas and malls and operating during regular business hours.

Urgent surgery Surgery performed for a health problem that is not immediately life-threatening.

Urticaria Hypersensitivity to food, drugs, or emotional factors manifested by pruritus and elevated patches (wheals); hives.

Uterus Muscular pear-shaped organ in which the fetus develops; womb.

Vagina Tube extending from the uterus to the vulva; its walls stretch to accommodate the penis in sexual intercourse and the baby at birth.

Vaginismus Involuntary contraction of the muscles around the vaginal orifice; makes sexual intercourse painful or impossible.

Validation Re-examining information to check its accuracy.

Validity Degree to which something measures what it is intended to measure.

Valsalva maneuver Forceful exhalation against a closed glottis, nose, and mouth, as during defecation.

Values Personal standards for decision-making.

Values conflict Different views on a decision or course of action.

Values system Enduring set of personal principles and rules.

Valve Structure that temporarily closes an opening; flaps or cusps that allow fluid to move in only one direction.

Vasoconstriction Decrease in diameter of a vessel due to the contraction of smooth muscle cells.

Vasodilation Increase in diameter of a vessel due to the relaxation of smooth muscle cells.

Venipuncture Insertion of a needle or catheter into a vein.

Ventilation Movement of air in and out of the lungs; breathing.

Ventilator Breathing machine used in clients with respiratory failure.

Verbal ability Use of language to store, process, and communicate thought content.

Vesicle Serous skin elevation less than 1 cm in diameter.

Vial Small plastic or glass bottle for medication.

Virulence Ability of a microorganism to cause disease; depends on the quality of the environment and the vigor of the organism.

Vitamins Organic compounds that do not supply energy but are necessary to the body in small amounts for growth, development, maintenance, and reproduction.

Vulva Collective term for the external female genitalia.

Water Balance Two aspects of body fluid monitored and controlled by the body: 1. the volume of fluid in the extracellular space, and 2. the water concentration (osmolarity) of body fluid.

Wheeze Musical breath sound indicating narrowed airways; commonly heard in asthma and COPD.

Working nursing care plan Concise, practical working tool for the practicing nurse that focuses on client needs.

Wound Break in tissue continuity secondary to trauma or injury.

Wound approximation Bringing wound edges into close proximity.

Wound healing Process of restoring tissue to normal structure and function.

Index

Note: Page numbers followed by f indicate figures; those followed by t indicate tables.

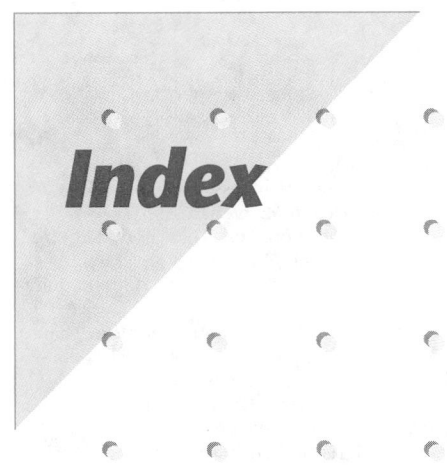

D

E

I

J

K

L

M

P

Q

S

U

W

X

Y

Z

Photo Credits

Custom Medical Stock Photo, Inc.

Section One
Figure 1-1 (2 parts)
Unit II
Unit IV
Unit V
Figure 23-1
Figure 23-5
Section Two
Unit XIII

United States Department of Agriculture

Figures 37-2*B*, 37-3, 49-9, 50-4

Isadore Faven

Figures 18-2, 19-2, 19-4, 19-6, 29-2, 29-3, 29-9, 31-3*A*, 47-4, 49-2

Debra Broadwell Jackson

Figure 49-5

Rebecca Saunders

Figures 37-2*A*, 49-6

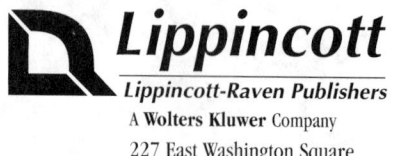

Fundamentals of Nursing: Human Health and Function

Self-Study Computer Program Instructions

This electronic self-study program has been designed for use with an IBM or IBM-compatible computer, and requires DOS version 3.0 or higher, 512KB RAM, a 3.5 inch disk drive, and a CGA graphics card or better.

To start the program, insert the diskette in your drive and type "a:" (or the appropiate letter for your disk drive—usually a or b), and press the <Enter> key. At the prompt (A:\> or B:\>), type "go" and press the <Enter> key to start the program.

This self-study program enables you to answer approximately 350 questions in a manner similar to the way you will take the NCLEX examination. As in the NCLEX, all questions in this program are multiple choice. To answer the questions, you will need to use only the up and down arrow keys and the <Enter> key. Use the arrow keys to highlight the answer you wish to select, and press <Enter> to make the selection. Instructions are provided at the bottom of the screen.

The Main Menu of the program looks like this:

1. Instructions
2. Choose a Test
3. Review Results
4. Quit

Highlight your choice using the arrow keys, and press <Enter> to select it. Selecting the **Instructions** option will display an instructions screen.

Selecting the **Choose a Test** option will provide you with a list of 17 tests, each corresponding to a unit in the text. To begin taking a test, use the arrow keys to highlight the name of the test you wish to take, and press the <Enter> key.

After you have selected a topic, you will be asked if you wish to take the test in *Study Mode* or *Test Mode*. To select a mode, press the <Alt> key at the same time as the underlined letter in your choice (<Alt>S for *Study Mode*, <Alt>T for *Test Mode*).

Study Mode lets you know immediately if the answer you selected was correct and provides you with the feedback for correct and incorrect choices. If you select an incorrect answer, try again until you find the correct answer.

If you select *Test Mode*, you will be given the option of having the test timed (press <Alt>I), having the screen display the time remaining (press <Alt>R), and having the screen display the number of questions remaining in the test (press <Alt>Q). While in *Test Mode*, you will not recieve immediate feedback on your answers. When you have answered all the questions, or when time has expired, you will be shown how many questions you have answered correctly.

After seeing your test results in *Test Mode*, you will have the option of printing the results of the test (press <Alt>P), reviewing the questions again in *Study Mode* (press <Alt>S), or returning to the main menu (press <Alt>M).

If you choose to review the question in *Study Mode*, you will see all the questions in that particular test again. The questions you answered correctly will be indicated with a check mark in front of the question number. All questions without a check mark were either answered incorrectly or not answered. In this mode, you will receive instant feedback on the answers you select.

The results for each test taken in a single session are temporarily stored in memory. Choosing the **Review Results** option from the Main Menu will show you the results for any test you have taken during this session.

Selecting the **Quit** option from the Main Menu will end the session and return you to DOS.